a LANGE medical book

CURRENT
Surgical
Diagnosis & Treatment

11th Edition

Edited by

Lawrence W. Way, MD
Professor & Vice Chair
Department of Surgery
University of California, San Francisco
San Francisco, California

Gerard M. Doherty, MD
N.W. Thompson Professor of Endocrine Surgery
Chief, Division of Endocrine Surgery
Section Head, General Surgery
Department of Surgery
University of Michigan Medical School
Ann Arbor, Michigan

Lange Medical Books/McGraw-Hill
Medical Publishing Division

New York   Chicago   San Francisco   Lisbon   London   Madrid   Mexico City
Milan   New Delhi   San Juan   Seoul   Singapore   Sydney   Toronto

Current Surgical Diagnosis & Treatment, Eleventh Edition

1 2 3 4 5 6 7 8 9 0 DOC/DOC 0 9 8 7 6 5 4 3 2

ISBN: 0-8385-1456-1
ISSN: 0894-2277

Notice

Medicine is an ever-changing science. As new research and clinical experience broaden our knowledge, changes in treatment and drug therapy are required. The authors and the publisher of this work have checked with sources believed to be reliable in their efforts to provide information that is complete and generally in accord with the standards accepted at the time of publication. However, in view of the possibility of human error or changes in medical sciences, neither the authors nor the publisher nor any other party who has been involved in the preparation or publication of this work warrants that the information contained herein is in every respect accurate or complete, and they disclaim all responsibility for any errors or omissions or for the results obtained from use of the information contained in this work. Readers are encouraged to confirm the information contained herein with other sources. For example and in particular, readers are advised to check the product information sheet included in the package of each drug they plan to administer to be certain that the information contained in this work is accurate and that changes have not been made in the recommended dose or in the contraindications for administration. This recommendation is of particular importance in connection with new or infrequently used drugs.

This book was set in Garamond by Pine Tree Composition.
The editors were Shelley Reinhardt, Jim Ransom, and John Williams.
The production supervisor was Phil Galea.
The illustration manager was Charissa Baker.
The text designer was Eve Siegel.
The cover designer was Mary McKeon.
RR Donnelley was printer and binder.

This book is printed on acid-free paper.

ISBN: 0-07-112444-6 (International Edition)

Contents

Authors vii

Preface xvii

1. Approach to the Surgical Patient 1
   J. Englebert Dunphy, MD, & Lawrence W. Way, MD

2. Preoperative Care 6
   Gerard M. Doherty, MD, & Robert H. Demling, MD

3. Postoperative Care 14
   Gerard M. Doherty, MD, Sean J. Mulvihill, MD, & Carlos A. Pellegrini, MD

4. Postoperative Complications 23
   Gerard M. Doherty, MD, Sean J. Mulvihill, MD, & Carlos A. Pellegrini, MD

5. Special Medical Problems in Surgical Patients 38
   Endocrine Disease & the Surgical Patient 38   Hematologic Disease & the Surgical Patient 52
     Gerard M. Doherty, MD   *Julie Hambleton, MD, & Pearl T.C.Y. Toy, MD*
   Heart Disease & the Surgical Patient 41   Pregnancy & the Surgical Patient 62
     Barry M. Massie, MD   *Aaron B. Caughey, MD, MPP, MPH, & Edward C. Hill, MD*
   Respiratory Disease & the Surgical Patient 46   Management of the Older Surgical Patient 67
     Robert F. Hickey, MD   *Gerard M. Doherty, MD, & Edmund T. Lonergan, MD*
   Renal Disease & the Surgical Patient 48
     Daniel C. Brennan, MD

6. Legal Medicine for the Surgeon 72
   Suzanne C. Will, JD, & Jack Nagan, JD

7. Wound Healing 86
   David D. Zabel, MD, Thomas K. Hunt, MD, Reid V. Mueller, MD, & William H. Goodson III, MD

8. The Metabolic & Neuroendocrine Responses to Trauma & Operations 100
   Arthur E. Baue, MD

9. Inflammation, Infection, & Antibiotics 112
   J. Perren Cobb, MD, Robert Schmieg, MD, Thomas K. Hunt, MD, & Linda M. Mundy, MD

10. Fluid & Electrolyte Management 142
    Michael H. Humphreys, MD

11. Surgical Metabolism & Nutrition 156
    Julie A. Margenthaler, MD, Virginia M. Herrmann, MD, & Michael S. Hickey, MD

12. Anesthesia 191
    Ronald D. Miller, MD

13. Shock & Acute Pulmonary Failure in Surgical Patients 203
    James W. Holcroft, MD, & David H. Wisner, MD

14. **Management of the Injured Patient** 230
James R. Macho, MD, William C. Krupski, MD, & Frank R. Lewis, Jr., MD

15. **Burns & Other Thermal Injuries** 267
Robert H. Demling, MD

16. **Head & Neck Tumors** 282
Samuel W. Beenken, MD, & Marshall M. Urist, MD

17. **Thyroid & Parathyroid** 298
Orlo H. Clark, MD

18. **Breast** 319
Armando E. Giuliano, MD

19. **Thoracic Wall, Pleura, Mediastinum, & Lung** 344
David Jablons, MD, Robert B. Cameron, MD & Kevin Turley, MD

20. **The Heart**
   I. Acquired Diseases 408
Scot H. Merrick, MD
   II. Congenital Heart Disease. 439
Ronald K. Woods, MD, & Edward Verrier, MD

21. **Esophagus & Diaphragm** 472
Gerard M. Doherty, MD, Carlos A. Pellegrini, MD, & Lawrence W. Way, MD

22. **The Acute Abdomen** 503
Gerard M. Doherty, MD, & John H. Boey, MD

23. **Peritoneal Cavity** 517
Gerard M. Doherty, MD, & John H. Boey, MD

24. **Stomach & Duodenum** 533
Gerard M. Doherty, MD, & Lawrence W. Way, MD

25. **Liver & Portal Venous System** 565
Gerard M. Doherty, MD, & Lawrence W. Way, MD

26. **Biliary Tract** 595
Gerard M. Doherty, MD, & Lawrence W. Way, MD

27. **Pancreas** 625
Gerard M. Doherty, MD, & Lawrence W. Way, MD

28. **Spleen** 652
Gerard M. Doherty, MD, Douglas L. Fraker, MD, & David C. Hohn, MD

29. **Appendix** 668
Lawrence W. Way, MD

30. **Small Intestine** 674
Andrew A. Shelton, MD, Theodore R. Schrock, MD, & Mark Lane Welton, MD

31. Large Intestine 705
George J. Chang, MD, Andrew Shelton, MD, Theodore R. Schrock, MD, & Mark Lane Welton, MD

32. Anorectum 756
Mark Lane Welton, MD

33. Hernias & Other Lesions of the Abdominal Wall 783
Karen E. Deveney, MD

34. Adrenals 797
Quan-Yang Duh, MD, Chienying Liu, MD, J. Blake Tyrrell, MD,& Edward G. Biglieri, MD

35. Arteries 813
William C. Krupski, MD

36. Amputation 859
William C. Krupski, MD,& Mark R. Nehler, MD

37. Veins & Lymphatics 871
Laura K. Pak, MD, Louis M. Messina, MD, & Thomas W. Wakefield, MD

38. Neurosurgery & Surgery of the Pituitary 888
Mitchel S. Berger, MD

Diagnosis & Management of Depressed States
  of Consciousness 888
  Cornelia S. von Koch, MD, PhD, & Julian T. Hoff, MD
Neurodiagnostic Procedures 892
  William P. Dillon, MD
Intraoperative Neurophysiologic Monitoring 897
  Charles D. Yingling, PhD
Craniocerebral Trauma 900
  Martin C. Holland, MD
Spinal Cord Injury 908
  *Geoffrey T. Manley, MD, PhD, Alexander M.
  Papanastasio, MD, & Russ P. Nockels, MD*
Traumatic Peripheral Nerve Lesions 913
  Nicholas M. Barbaro, MD
Brain Tumors 915
  *Michael W. McDermott, MD, Sandeep Kunwar, MD,
  & Mitchel S. Berger, MD*
Tumors of the Spinal Cord 927
  Philip R. Weinstein, MD, & Harold Rosegay, PhD, MD

Tumors of Peripheral Nerves 929
  *Nicholas M. Barbaro, MD, & Charles B. Wilson, MD, DSc,
  MSHA*
Pituitary Tumors 930
  Charles B. Wilson, MD, DSc, MSHA
Pediatric Neurosurgery 931
  Nalin Gupta, MD, PhD, & Warwick J. Peacock, MD
Intracranial Aneurysms 937
  Philip V. Theodosopolous, MD, & Michael T. Lawton, MD
Arteriovenous Malformations 943
  G. Edward Vates, MD, PhD, & Michael T. Lawton, MD
Movement Disorders Responsive to Surgery 947
  Philip Starr, MD
Pain 950
  Nicholas M. Barbaro, MD
Intervertebral Disk Disease 952
  Philip R. Weinstein, MD, & Julian T. Hoff, MD
Surgical Infections of the Central Nervous System 958
  Cornelia S. von Koch, MD, PhD, & Mark L. Rosenblum, MD

39. Otolaryngology—Head & Neck Surgery 962
Lee D. Rowe, MD

40. The Eye & Ocular Adnexa 999
Stephen A. Kamenetzky, MD, Linda M. Tsai, MD, & Khalid F. Tabbara, MD

41. Urology 1013
Richard D. Williams, MD, Christopher S. Cooper, MD, & James F. Donovan, Jr., MD

42. Gynecology 1085
Edward C. Hill, MD, & Elena A. Gates, MD

Congenital Anomalies of the Female Reproductive
  System 1085
  Edward C. Hill, MD, & Elena A. Gates, MD

Correction of Infertility Due to Tubal Abnormalities 1086
  Marcelle Cedars, MD

Abnormal Uterine Bleeding 1087
  Abner Korn, MD
Chronic Pelvic Pain 1089
  Lee Learman, MD, PhD
Contraception 1090
  Philip D. Darney, MD
Pelvic Organ Prolapse & Urinary Incontinence 1092
  Sharon Knight, MD, & Elaine Waetjen, MD
Fistulas 1093
  Robert Domush, MD
Benign Tumors of the Vulva & Vagina 1095
  Elena A. Gates, MD

Endometriosis 1095
  Marcelle Cedars, MD
Adenomyosis 1098
  Lee Learman, MD, PhD
Leiomyomas of the Uterus 1099
  Alison Jacoby, MD
Adnexal Masses 1100
  Lisa Everson, MD
Ectopic Pregnancy 1102
  Mindy Goldman, MD
Gynecologic Malignancies 1104
  Lee-May Chen, MD, & Bethan Powell, MD

43. Orthopedics 1116
Bobby K-B Tay, MD, William W. Colman, MD, Sigurd Berven, MD, Roger Fontes, Jr., MD, Stephen B. Gunther, MD, William Holmes, MD, Hubert T. Kim, MD, PhD, Lisa Lattanza, MD, Edward Diao, MD, Serena S. Hu, MD, & David S. Bradford, MD

44. Plastic & Reconstructive Surgery 1230
Luis O. Vasconez, MD, & Henry C. Vasconez, MD

45. Hand Surgery 1270
David M. Young, MD, Mahesh Mankani, MD, John T. Alexander, MD, Eugene S. Kilgore, MD, William P. Graham III, MD, & Robert E. Markison, MD

46. Pediatric Surgery 1293
Craig T. Albanese, MD, Roman M. Sydorak, MD, & Michael R. Harrison, MD

47. Oncology 1352
Steven Hunt, MD, & Gerard M. Doherty, MD

48. Organ Transplantation 1372
John P. Roberts, MD, Nancy L. Ascher, MD, Nicholas J. Feduska, MD, Fraser M. Keith, MD, Juliet Melzer, MD, & Oscar Salvatierra, Jr., MD

Index 1387

Authors

Craig T. Albanese, MD
Associate Professor of Surgery, Pediatrics, & Obstetrics, Gynecology, & Reproductive Sciences; Co-Director, Fetal Treatment Center, Department of Surgery, University of California, San Francisco
albanese@surgery.ucsf.edu
Pediatric Surgery

John T. Alexander, MD
Consulting Staff, Department of Plastic Surgery, Scripps Memorial Hospital La Jolla, La Jolla, California
jta2@alexandersurgery.com
Hand Surgery

Nancy L. Ascher, MD
Professor and Chair, Department of Surgery, University of California, San Francisco
aschern@surgery.ucsf.edu
Organ Transplantation

Nicholas M. Barbaro, MD
Associate Professor of Neurological Surgery, University of California, San Francisco; Co-Director, Functional Neurosurgery Program; Director, CNS Infections & AIDS Program; Principal Investigator, Center for Neurological Injury & Repair; Co-Director, Program for Research on Epilepsy & Parkinsonism
barbaron@neurosurgery.ucsf.edu
Neurosurgery & Surgery of the Pituitary: Traumatic Peripheral Nerve Lesions; Neurosurgery & Surgery of the Pituitary: Tumors of Peripheral Nerves; Neurosurgery & Surgery of the Pituitary: Pain

Arthur E. Baue, MD
Professor, Division of Cardiothoracic Surgery, Department of Surgery, Saint Louis University School of Medicine, St. Louis, Missouri
The Metabolic & Neuroendocrine Responses to Trauma & Operations

Samuel W. Beenken, MD
Professor of Surgery, University of Alabama at Birmingham; Head, Section of Head & Neck Surgery, Veterans Affairs Medical Center, Birmingham, Alabama
samuel.beenken@ccc.uab.edu
Head & Neck Tumors

Mitchel S. Berger, MD
Professor & Chairman, Department of Neurological Surgery, University of California, San Francisco; Director, Brain Tumor Surgery Program; Director, Neurosurgical Research Centers; Brain Tumor Research Center; and Center for Neurological Injury & Repair
bergerm@neurosurg.ucsf.edu
Neurosurgery & Surgery of the Pituitary; Neurosurgery & Surgery of the Pituitary: Brain Tumors

Sigurd Berven, MD
Assistant Professor, Department of Orthopedic Surgery, University of California, San Francisco
bervens@orthosurg.ucsf.edu
Orthopedics

Edward G. Biglieri, MD
Professor Emeritus, Department of Medicine, University of California, San Francisco
Adrenals

John H. Boey, MD
Former Reader in Surgery, University of Hong Kong, Hong Kong
jboey@netvigator.com
The Acute Abdomen; Peritoneal Cavity

David S. Bradford, MD
Chair & Professor, Department of Orthopedic Surgery, University of California, San Francisco
Bradford@orthosurg.ucsf.edu
Orthopedics

Daniel C. Brennan, MD
Associate Professor, Division of Renal Diseases, Department of Medicine, Washington University School of Medicine, St. Louis; Director, Transplant Nephrology; Medical Director, Pharmacoeconomic Transplant Research
Brennand@msnotes.wustl.edu
Special Medical Problems in Surgical Patients: Renal Disease & the Surgical Patient

Robert B. Cameron, MD
Associate Professor, Divisions of Cardiothoracic
Surgery and Surgical Oncology, Department of
Surgery, David Geffen School of Medicine, University
of California, Los Angeles; Chief, General
Thoracic Surgery and Thoracic Oncology, University
of California, Los Angeles Medical Center and West
Los Angeles Veterans Affairs Medical Center
rcameron@mednet.ucla.edu
Thoracic Wall, Pleura, Mediastinum, & Lung

Aaron B. Caughey, MD, MPP, MPH
Clinical Instructor, Maternal-Fetal Medicine, Department of Obstetrics, Gynecology, & Reproductive Sciences, University of California, San Francisco
abcmd@uclink.berkeley.edu
*Special Medical Problems in Surgical Patients: Pregnancy
& the Surgical Patient*

Marcelle Cedars, MD
Director, Division of Reproductive Endocrinology,
Department of Obsetrics, Gynecology, &
Reproductive Sciences, University of California,
San Francisco
cedarsm@obgyn.ucsf.edu
*Gynecology: Correction of Infertility Due to Tubal
Abnormalities; Gynecology: Endometriosis*

George J. Chang, MD
Resident in Surgery, Department of Surgery,
University of California, San Francisco
gc1473@itsa.ucsf.edu
Large Intestine

Lee-May Chen, MD
Assistant Clinical Professor in Gynecologic Oncology,
Department of Obstetrics, Gynecology, &
Reproductive Sciences, Comprehensive Cancer Center,
University of California, San Francisco
Lee-may.chen@ucsfmedctr.org
Gynecology: Gynecologic Malignancies

Orlo H. Clark, MD
Professor & Vice Chair, Department of Surgery,
University of California, San Francisco; Chief of
Surgery, University of California, San Francisco/Mt.
Zion Medical Center
clarko@surgery.ucsf.edu
Thyroid & Parathyroid

J. Perren Cobb, MD
Associate Professor, Department of Surgery; Director,
Cellular Injury & Adaptation Laboratory,
Washington University School of Medicine, St. Louis,
Missouri
cobb@msnotes.wustl.edu
Inflammation, Infection, & Antibiotics

William W. Colman, MD
Assistant Professor, Department of Orthopedic
Surgery, University of California, San Francisco
colmanw@orthosurg.ucsf.edu
Orthopedics

Christopher S. Cooper, MD
Assistant Professor of Pediatric Urology, Department
of Urology, University of Iowa College of Medicine
and Children's Hospital of Iowa, Iowa City
Christopher-cooper@uiowa.edu
Urology

Philip D. Darney, MD
Professor, Department of Obstetrics, Gynecology, &
Reproductive Sciences, University of California, San
Francisco; Division Director & Chief, Department of
Obstetrics, Gynecology, & Reproductive
Sciences, San Francisco General Hospital
darney@ob.ucsf.edu
Gynecology: Contraception

Robert H. Demling, MD
Professor of Surgery, Harvard Medical School, Boston;
Director, Burn Center, Department of Surgery,
Brigham & Women's Hospital, Boston,
Massachusetts
rhdemling@partners.org
Preoperative Care; Burns & Other Thermal Injuries

Karen E. Deveney, MD
Professor of Surgery, Oregon Health Sciences
University, School of Medicine, Portland, Oregon
deveneyk@ohsu.edu
Hernias & Other Lesions of the Abdominal Wall

Edward Diao, MD
Associate Professor, Department of Orthopedic
Surgery, University of California, San Francisco; Chief
of Service, Hand, Upper Extremity, & Microvascular
Surgery Service; Medical Director, University of
California, San Francisco/Mt. Zion Ambulatory
Orthopedics
diaoe@orthosurg.ucsf.edu
Orthopedics

William P. Dillon, Jr., MD
Professor, Department of Radiology, University of California, San Francisco
Bill.Dillon@radiology.ucsf.edu
Neurosurgery & Surgery of the Pituitary: Neurodiagnostic Procedures

Gerard M. Doherty, MD
N.W. Thompson Professor of Endocrine Surgery; Chief, Division of Endocrine Surgery; Section Head, General Surgery, Department of Surgery, University of Michigan Medical School, Ann Arbor, Michigan
gerardd@umich.edu
Preoperative Care; Postoperative Care; Postoperative Complications; Special Medical Problems in Surgical Patients: Endocrine Disease & the Surgical Patient; Special Medical Problems in Surgical Patients: Management of the Older Surgical Patient; Esophagus & Diaphragm; The Acute Abdomen; Peritoneal Cavity; Stomach & Duodenum; Liver & Portal Venous System; Biliary Tract; Pancreas; Spleen; Oncology

Robert Domush, MD
Associate Professor, Department of Ostetrics, Gynecology, & Reproductive Sciences, University of California, San Francisco
Gynecology: Fistulas

James F. Donovan, Jr., MD
Associate Professor of Urology, University of Iowa College of Medicine, Iowa City
Urology

Quan-Yang Duh, MD
Professor, Department of Surgery, University of California, San Francisco; Attending Surgeon, University of California, San Francisco Veterans Affairs Medical Center
quan-yang.duh@med.va.gov
Adrenals

J. Englebert Dunphy, MD (Deceased)
Formerly Professor of Surgery Emeritus, University of California, San Francisco
Approach to the Surgical Patient

Lisa Everson, MD
Assistant Clinical Professor, Department of Obstetrics, Gynecology, & Reproductive Sciences, University of California San Francisco
eversonl@obgyn.ucsf.edu
Gynecology: Adnexal Masses

Nicholas J. Feduska, MD
General Surgery, Sunrise Hospital & Medical Center, Las Vegas, Nevada
Organ Transplantation

Roger Fontes, Jr., MD
Assistant Professor, Department of Orthopedic Surgery, University of California, San Francisco
Orthopedics

Douglas L. Fraker, MD
Jonathan E. Rhoads Associate Professor of Surgery & Chief, Division of Surgical Oncology, University of Pennsylvania School of Medicine, Philadelphia
fraker@mail.med.upenn.edu
Spleen

Elena A. Gates, MD
Professor of Obstetrics, Gynecology, & Reproductive Sciences, Vice Chair, and Division Director, General Gynecology, University of California, San Francsico
gatese@obgyn.ucsf.edu
Gynecology; Gynecology: Congenital Anomalies of the Female Reproductive System; Gynecology: Benign Tumors of the Vulva & Vagina

Armando E. Giuliano, MD
Director, Joyce Eisenberg Keefer Breast Center; Clinical Professor of Surgery, University of California, Los Angeles; Chief of Surgical Oncology, John Wayne Cancer Institute, Santa Monica, California
giulianoa@jwci.org
Breast

Mindy Goldman, MD
Assistant Clinical Professor, Division of Obstetrics, Gynecology, & Reproductive Sciences, University of California, San Francisco
goldmanm@obgyn.ucsf.edu
Gynecology: Ectopic Pregnancy

William H. Goodson III, MD
Senior Clinical Research Scientist (Surgery), California Pacific Medical Research Institute, San Francisco, California
whg3@cooper.cpmc.org
Wound Healing

William P. Graham III, MD
Section of Plastic & Reconstructive Surgery, Department of Surgery, Pennsylvania State University College of Medicine, Hershey, Pennsylvania
wgraham@psghs.edu
Hand Surgery

Stephen B. Gunther, MD
Assistant Clinical Professor, Department of Orthopedic Surgery, University of California, San Francisco; Chief, University of California, San Francisco Shoulder & Elbow Service; Co-Director, Sports Medicine Fellowship
guntherS@orthosurg.ucsf.edu
Orthopedics

Nalin Gupta, MD, PhD
Assistant Professor, Dennis Bruce Dettmer Endowed Chair, Principal Investigator, Brain Tumor Research Center, Department of Neurological Surgery, University of California, San Francisco
guptan@neurosurg.ucsf.edu
Neurosurgery & Surgery of the Pituitary: Pediatric Neurosurgery

Julie Hambleton, MD
Associate Professor of Medicine, University of California, San Francisco
jsh@medicine.ucsf.edu
Special Medical Problems in Surgical Patients: Hematologic Disease & the Surgical Patient

Michael R. Harrison, MD
Professor of Surgery, Pediatrics, & Obstetrics, Gynecology, & Reproductive Sciences; Director, Fetal Treatment Center; Chief, Division of Pediatric Surgery, University of California, San Francisco
harrisonm@surgery.ucsf.edu
Pediatric Surgery

Virginia M. Herrmann, MD
Professor of Surgery, Washington University School of Medicine, St. Louis, Missouri
herrmannv@msnotes.wustl.edu
Surgical Metabolism & Nutrition

Michael S. Hickey, MD, FACS
Trauma Surgery Service, Harris Methodist Forth Worth Hospital, Fort Worth, Texas
Surgical Metabolism & Nutrition

Robert F. Hickey, MD
Professor and Vice-Chairman, Department of Anesthesia, University of California, San Francisco
hickeyr@anesthesia.ucsf.edu
Special Medical Problems in Surgical Patients: Respiratory Disease & the Surgical Patient

Edward C. Hill, MD
Professor Emeritus, Department of Obstetrics, Gynecology, & Reproductive Sciences, University of California, San Francisco
Special Medical Problems in Surgical Patients: Pregnancy & the Surgical Patient; Gynecology; Gynecology: Congenital Anomalies of the Female Reproductive System

Julian T. Hoff, MD
Professor & Chair, Department of Neurosurgery, University of Michigan, School of Medicine, Ann Arbor
jthoff@umich.edu
Neurosurgery & Surgery of the Pituitary: Diagnosis & Management of Depressed States of Consciousness; Neurosurgery & Surgery of the Pituitary: Intervertebral Disk Disease

David C. Hohn, MD
President & CEO, Roswell Park Cancer Institute, Buffalo, New York
david.hohn@roswellpark.org
Spleen

James W. Holcroft, MD
Professor of Surgery, University of California, Davis, School of Medicine, Sacramento
jwholcroft@ucdavis.edu
Shock & Acute Pulmonary Failure in Surgical Patients

Martin C. Holland, MD
Assistant Professor of Neurological Surgery; Director, Neurosurgical Central Nervous System Injury Program; Acting Chief of Neurosurgery, San Francisco General Hospital; Principal Investigator, Center for Neurological Injury & Repair, Neurotrauma Program, University of California, San Francisco
hollandm@neurosurg.ucsf.edu
Neurosurgery & Surgery of the Pituitary: Craniocerebral Trauma

William Holmes, MD
Assistant Professor, Department of Orthopedic Surgery, University of California, San Francisco
holmesw@orthosurg.ucsf.edu
Orthopedics

Serena S. Hu, MD
Associate Professor, Department of Orthopedic Surgery, University of California, San Francisco
hus@orthosurg.ucsf.edu
Orthopedics

Michael H. Humphreys, MD
Professor of Medicine, University of California, San Francisco; Chief, Division of Nephrology, San Francisco General Hospital
mhhsfgh@itsa.ucsf.edu
Fluid & Electrolyte Management

Steven Hunt, MD
House Officer, Department of Surgery, Washington University School of Medicine, St. Louis, Missouri
hunts@msnotes.wustle.edu
Oncology

Thomas K. Hunt, MD
Professor of Surgery & Vice Chair for Research Affairs, Department of Surgery, University of California, San Francisco
wound@itsa.ucsf.edu
Wound Healing; Inflammation, Infection, & Antibiotics

David Jablons, MD
Associate Professor of Surgery; Chief, General Thoracic Surgery; Ada Endowed Chair & Program Leader, Thoracic Oncology, Comprehensive Cancer Center, University of California, San Francisco
jablonsd@surgery.ucsf.edu
Thoracic Wall, Pleura, Mediastinum, & Lung

Alison Jacoby, MD
Assistant Clinical Professor, Department of Obstetrics, Gynecology, & Reproductive Sciences, University of California, San Francisco
jacobya@obgyn.ucsf.edu
Gynecology: Leiomyomas of the Uterus

Steven A. Kamenetzky, MD
Associate Professor of Clinical Ophthalmology & Visual Sciences, Department of Ophthalmology, Washington University School of Medicine, St. Louis, Missouri
kamenet@mindspring.com
The Eye & Ocular Adnexa

Fraser M. Keith, MD
Director, Division of Cardiothoracic Surgery, LifeLink Transplant Institute, Tampa, Florida
keith@lifelinkfound.org
Organ Transplantation

Eugene S. Kilgore, MD
Clinical Professor of Surgery, University of California, San Francisco
Hand Surgery

Hubert T. Kim, MD, PhD
Assistant Professor, Department of Orthopedic Surgery, University of California, San Francisco
kim.hubert_t@sanfrancisco.va.gov
Orthopedics

Sharon Knight, MD
Clinical Instructor, Department of Obstetrics, Gynecology, & Reproductive Sciences, University of California, San Francisco
knights@obgyn.ucsf.edu
Gynecology: Pelvic Organ Prolapse & Urinary Incontinence

Abner Korn, MD
Professor, Department of Obstetrics, Gynecology, & Reproductive Sciences, University of California, San Francisco
korna@obgyn.ucsf.edu
Gynecology: Abnormal Uterine Bleeding

William C. Krupski, MD
Professor of Surgery & Chief, Division of Vascular Surgery, University of Colorado, School of Medicine, Denver
william.krupski@uchsc.edu
Management of the Injured Patient; Arteries; Amputation

Sandeep Kunwar, MD
Assistant Professor of Neurological Surgery; Principal Investigator, Brain Tumor Research Center, University of California, San Francisco
kunwars@neurosurg.ucsf.edu
Neurosurgery & Surgery of the Pituitary: Brain Tumors

Lisa Lattanza, MD
Assistant Clinical Professor, Department of Orthopedic Surgery, University of California, San Francisco
lattanza@orthosurg.ucsf.edu
Orthopedics

Michael T. Lawton, MD
Assistant Professor of Neurological Surgery; Tong Po Kan Endowed Chair; Director, Cerebrovascular Disorders Program; Principal Investigator, Center for Neurological Injury & Repair, University of California, San Francisco
lawtonm@neurosurg.ucsf.edu
Neurosurgery & Surgery of the Pituitary: Intracranial Aneurysms; Neurosurgery & Surgery of the Pituitary: Arteriovenous Malformations

Lee Learman, MD, PhD
Associate Professor, Department of Obstetrics, Gynecology, & Reproductive Sciences, University of California, San Francisco
Learmanl@obgyn.ucsf.edu
Gynecology: Chronic Pelvic Pain; Gynecology: Adenomyosis

Frank R. Lewis, Jr., MD
Executive Director, American Board of Surgery, Philadelphia, Pennsylvania
flewis@absurgery.org
Management of the Injured Patient

Chienying Liu, MD
Fellow in Endocrinology & Metabolism, University of California, San Francisco
cliu@itsa.uscf.edu
Adrenals

Edmund T. Lonergan, MD
Professor of Clinical Medicine, University of California, San Francisco; Chief, Geriatrics Section, San Francisco Veterans Affairs Medical Center
Special Medical Problems in Surgical Patients: Management of the Older Surgical Patient

James R. Macho, MD
Emeritus Professor of Surgery, University of California, San Francisco; Director of Bothin Burn Center and Attending Surgeon, Saint Francis Memorial Hospital, San Francisco, California
jmacho@webmd.com
Management of the Injured Patient

Mahesh Mankani, MD
Assistant Professor, Department of Surgery, University of California, San Francisco
mmankani@sfghsurg.ucsf.edu
Hand Surgery

Geoffrey T. Manley, MD, PhD
Assistant Professor of Neurological Surgery; Director, Central Nervous System Injury Research Program, San Francisco General Hospital; Principal Investigator, Center for Neurological Injury & Repair, University of California, San Francisco
manleyg@neurosurg.ucsf.edu
Neurosurgery & Surgery of the Pituitary: Spinal Cord Injury

Julie A. Margenthaler, MD
Resident in Surgery, Washington University School of Medicine, St. Louis, Missouri
margenthaler@msnotes.wustl.edu
Surgical Metabolism & Nutrition

Robert E. Markison, MD
Associate Clinical Professor of Surgery, University of California, San Franicsco
Hand Surgery

Barry M. Massie, MD
Professor of Medicine, University of California, San Francisco; Chief, Cardiology Division, San Francisco Veterans Affairs Medical Center
barry.massie@med.va.gov
Special Medical Problems in Surgical Patients: Heart Disease & the Surgical Patient

Michael W. McDermott, MD
Associate Professor of Neurological Surgery, Halperin Endowed Chair; Neurosurgical Director, Gamma-Knife Radiosurgery Program; Principal Investigator, Brain Tumor Research Center, University of California, San Francisco
mcdermottm@neurosurg.ucsf.edu
Neurosurgery & Surgery of the Pituitary: Brain Tumors

Juliet Melzer, MD
Formerly, Associate Professor of Surgery, University of California, San Francisco, and Director, Pancreas Transplant Program. Graduate student, School of Public Health, University of California, Berkeley
Organ Transplantation

Scot H. Merrick, MD
Professor of Clinical Surgery, University of California, San Francisco
merricks@surgery.ucsf.edu
The Heart: I. Acquired Diseases

Louis M. Messina, MD
Professor and Chief, Division of Vascular Surgery;
Edwin J. Wylie Chair in Surgery, University of
California, San Francisco
messina@surgery.ucsf.edu
Veins & Lymphatics

Ronald D. Miller, MD
Professor & Chairman, Department of Anesthesia &
Perioperative Care, & Professor of Cellular & Molecular Pharmacology, University of California, San Francisco
millerr@anesthesia.ucsf.edu
Anesthesia

Reid V. Mueller, MD
Assistant Professor of Surgery, Division of Plastic &
Reconstructive Surgery, Oregon Health Sciences Uni-
versity, School of Medicine, Portland
Reid@reidmueller.com
Wound Healing

Sean J. Mulvihill, MD
Professor & Chair, Department of Surgery, University
of Utah School of Medicine, Salt Lake City
sean.mulvihill@hsc.utah.edu
Postoperative Care; Postoperative Complications

Linda M. Mundy, MD
Assistant Professor of Medicine, Department of Medi-
cine, Washington University School of Medicine, St.
Louis, Missouri
lmundy@im.wustl.edu
Inflammation, Infection, & Antibiotics

Jack Nagan, JD
Chief Executive Officer, Northern California Institute
for Research & Education, San Francisco, California
Legal Medicine for the Surgeon

Mark R. Nehler, MD
Assistant Professor of Surgery, University of Colorado
School of Medicine, Denver
mark.nehler@uchsc.edu
Amputation

Russ P. Nockels, MD
Associate Professor & Vice Chair, Department of Neu-
rological Surgery; Chief, Division of Neurological
Spinal Disorders; Director, Spinal Cord Injury & Re-
pair Laboratory, Loyola University, Stritch School of
Medicine, Maywood, Illinois
*Neurosurgery & Surgery of the Pituitary: Spinal Cord
Injury*

Laura K. Pak, MD
Clinical Instructor, Division of Vascular Surgery,
University of California, San Francisco
pakl@surgery.ucsf.edu
Veins & Lymphatics

Alexander M. Papanastasio, MD
Department of Neurological Surgery, University of
California, San Francisco
*Neurosurgery & Surgery of the Pituitary: Spinal Cord
Injury*

Warwick J. Peacock, MD
Professor Emeritus of Pediatric Neurological Surgery,
University of California, San Francisco
*Neurosurgery & Surgery of the Pituitary: Pediatric
Neurosurgery*

Carlos A. Pellegrini, MD
Professor & Chairman, Department of Surgery,
University of Washington, Seattle
*Postoperative Care; Postoperative Complications; Esopha-
gus & Diaphragm*

Bethan Powell, MD
Associate Professor in Gynecologic Oncology, Compre-
hensive Cancer Center, University of California, San
Francisco
Bethan.powell@ucsfmedctr.org
Gynecology: Gynecologic Malignancies

John P. Roberts, MD
Professor of Surgery & Chief, Transplant Service,
University of California, San Francisco
robertsj@surgery.ucsf.edu
Organ Transplantation

Harold Rosegay, PhD, MD
Professor Emeritus, Department of Neurological
Surgery, University of California, San Francisco
*Neurosurgery & Surgery of the Pituitary: Tumors of the
Spinal Cord*

Mark L. Rosenblum, MD
Chair, Department of Neurological Surgery, Henry
Ford Hospital, Detroit, Michigan
*Neurosurgery & Surgery of the Pituitary: Surgical
Infections of the Central Nervous System*

Lee D. Rowe, MD
Private Practice, General Otolaryngology, Philadelphia,
Pennsylvania
Otolaryngology—Head & Neck Surgery

Oscar Salvatierra, Jr., MD
Department of Surgery, University of California, San
Francisco
Organ Transplantation

Robert Schmieg, MD
Assistant Professor, Department of Surgery, Washington University School of Medicine, St. Louis,
Missouri
schmiegr@msnotes.wustl.edu
Inflammation, Infection, & Antibiotics

Theodore R. Schrock, MD
J. Englebert Dunphy Professor of Surgery; Associate
Dean for Clinical Services; Chief Medical Officer,
University of California, San Francisco
ted.schrock@ucsfmedctr.org
Small Intestine; Large Intestine

Andrew A. Shelton, MD
Assistant Professor of Surgery (General Surgery),
Stanford University, School of Medicine, Stanford,
California
shelton@stanford.edu
Small Intestine; Large Intestine

Philip Starr, MD
Assistant Professor of Neurological Surgery, University
of California, San Francisco; Co-Director, Functional
Neurosurgery Program for Epilepsy, Movement Disorders, Pain, & Nerve Disorders; Chief, Neurological
Surgery, San Francisco Veterans Affairs Medical Center; Principal Investigator, Center for Neurological Injury & Repair Research on Movement Disorders
*Neurosurgery & Surgery of the Pituitary: Movement
Disorders Responsive to Surgery*

Roman M. Sydorak, MD
Postgraduate Research Fellow, Fetal Treatment Center,
Department of Surgery, University of California, San
Francisco
Pediatric Surgery

Khalid F. Tabbara, MD, FCOphth
Professor & Chairman, Department of Ophthalmology, College of Medicine, King Saud University,
Riyadh, Saudi Arabia
The Eye & Ocular Adnexa

Bobby K-B Tay, MD
Assistant Professor, Department of Orthopedic
Surgery, University of California, San Francisco
tayb@orthosurg.ucsf.edu
Orthopedics

Philip V. Theodosopolous, MD
Resident, Department of Neurological Surgery,
University of California, San Francisco
*Neurosurgery & Surgery of the Pituitary: Intracranial
Aneurysms*

Pearl T.C.Y. Toy, MD
Professor, Department of Laboratory Medicine; Chief,
Blood Bank & Donor Center, University of
California, San Francisco
Pearl.toy@clinlab.ucsfmedctr.org
Special Medical Problems in Surgical Patients: Hematologic Disease & the Surgical Patient

Linda M. Tsai, MD
Instructor in Clinical Ophthalmology & Visual Sciences, Department of Ophthalmology, Washington
University School of Medicine, St. Louis, Missouri
The Eye & Ocular Adnexa

Kevin Turley, MD
Formerly, Chief, Pediatric Cardiovascular Surgery,
California Pacific Medical Center, San Francisco
Thoracic Wall, Pleura, Mediastinum, & Lung

J. Blake Tyrrell, MD
Clinical Professor of Medicine; Chief, Clinical
Endocrinology & Metabolism, Division of Endocrinology & Metabolism & Metabolic Research Unit,
University of California, San Francisco
blaket@medicine.ucsf.edu
Adrenals

Marshall M. Urist, MD
Professor & Vice-Chairman, Department of Surgery;
Chief, Section of Surgical Oncology, University of Alabama at Birmingham
mmurist@ccc.uab.edu
Head & Neck Tumors

Henry C. Vasconez, MD
Professor & Chief, Division of Plastic & Reconstructive Surgery; Program Director, Plastic Surgery, University of Kentucky, College of Medicine, Lexington
hcvasc@uky.edu
Plastic & Reconstructive Surgery

Luis O. Vasconez, MD
Professor & Director, Division of Plastic Surgery, University of Alabama School of Medicine, Birmingham
Plastic & Reconstructive Surgery

G. Edward Vates, MD, PhD
Resident, Department of Neurological Surgery, University of California, San Francisco
Neurosurgery & Surgery of the Pituitary: Arteriovenous Malformations

Edward Verrier, MD
Vice Chairman, Department of Surgery; William K. Edmark Professor of Cardiovascular Surgery; Chief, Division of Cardiothoracic Surgery, University of Washington Medical Center, Seattle
edver@u.washington.edu
The Heart: II. Congenital Heart Disease

Cornelia S. von Koch, MD, PhD
Resident, Department of Neurological Surgery, University of California, San Francisco
Neurosurgery & Surgery of the Pituitary: Diagnosis & Management of Depressed States of Consciousness; Neurosurgery & Surgery of the Pituitary: Surgical Infections of the Central Nervous System

Elaine Waetjen, MD
Department of Obstetrics, Gynecology, & Reproductive Sciences, University of California, San Francisco
Gynecology: Pelvic Organ Prolapse & Urinary Incontinence

Thomas W. Wakefield, MD
S. Martin Lindenauer Collegiate Professor in Vascular Surgery, Section of Vascular Surgery, Department of Surgery, University of Michigan Medical Center and Ann Arbor Veterans Administration Medical Center, Ann Arbor
thomasww@umich.edu
Veins & Lymphatics

Lawrence W. Way, MD
Professor & Vice-Chair, Department of Surgery, University of California, San Francisco
lwway@aol.com
Approach to the Surgical Patient; Esophagus & Diaphragm; Stomach & Duodenum; Liver & Portal Venous System; Biliary Tract; Pancreas; Appendix

Philip R. Weinstein, MD
Professor of Neurological Surgery; Co-Director, Neurospinal Disorders Program; Principal Investigator, Center for Neurological Injury & Repair Research on Ischemia & Neurologic Repair, University of California, San Francisco
weinsteinp@neurosurg.ucsf.edu
Neurosurgery & Surgery of the Pituitary: Tumors of the Spinal Cord; Neurosurgery & Surgery of the Pituitary: Intervertebral Disk Disease

Mark Lane Welton, MD
Associate Professor & Chief, Section of Colon & Rectal Surgery, Department of Surgery, Stanford University School of Medicine, Stanford, California
mwelton@stanford.edu
Small Intestine; Large Intestine; Anorectum

Suzanne C. Will, JD
Member, California Bar Association, San Francisco, California
Legal Medicine for the Surgeon

Richard D. Williams, MD
Rubin H. Flocks Chair & Professor, Department of Urology, University of Iowa College of Medicine, Iowa City, Iowa
richard-williams@uiowa.edu
Urology

Charles B. Wilson, MD, DSc, MSHA
Professor Emeritus, Department of Neurological Surgery, University of California, San Francisco
wilsonc@neurosurg.ucsf.edu
Neurosurgery & Surgery of the Pituitary: Tumors of Peripheral Nerves; Neurosurgery & Surgery of the Pituitary: Pituitary Tumors

David H. Wisner, MD
Professor of Surgery & Chief of Trauma Surgery, University of California, Davis, School of Medicine, Sacramento, California
Shock & Acute Pulmonary Failure in Surgical Patients

Ronald K. Woods, MD
Specialist Registrar, Pediatric Cardiothoracic Surgery, Great Ormond Street Hospital for Children, London, England
woodsronaldk@hotmail.com
The Heart: II. Congenital Heart Disease

Charles D. Yingling, PhD
Professor of Neurological Surgery; Principal Investigator, Neurosurgical Research Centers, University of California, San Francisco
Neurosurgery & Surgery of the Pituitary: Intraoperative Neurophysiologic Monitoring

David M. Young, MD
Assistant Professor, Department of Surgery, University of California, San Francisco and San Francisco General Hospital
dyoung@sfghsurg.ucsf.edu
Hand Surgery

David D. Zabel, MD
Advanced Plastic Surgery Center, Newark, Delaware
Wound Healing

Preface

Current Surgical Diagnosis & Treatment is intended to serve as a ready source of information about diseases managed by surgeons. Like other books in this Lange series, it emphasizes quick recall of major diagnostic features and brief descriptions of disease processes, followed by procedures for definitive diagnosis and treatment. Epidemiology, pathophysiology, and pathology are discussed to the extent that they contribute to the book's ultimate purpose, which is patient care.

Not quite a third of the book is given over to general medical and surgical topics important in the management of all patients.

References to the current journal literature are provided for the reader who wishes to explore specific matters in greater detail than would be appropriate in a concise text of this sort.

OUTSTANDING FEATURES

- After some delays, the text will again be revised and updated frequently. With each revision, particular subjects are completely, substantially, partially, or minimally rewritten as called for by the progress in each field. This edition in particular has been extensively updated because of the longer period since last publication.
- Illustrations have been judiciously chosen to clarify anatomic and surgical concepts.
- Over 1000 diseases and disorders are covered.
- Thorough coverage is provided of the role of the many new minimally invasive surgical procedures in treatment.

INTENDED AUDIENCE

- **Students** will find this book to be an authoritative introduction to surgery as it is taught and practiced at major teaching institutions.
- **House officers** will find many occasions to refer to the concise discussions of the diseases they must deal with every day as well as less common ones calling for quick study on the spot.
- **Medical practitioners** who must occasionally deal with surgical problems or counsel patients needing surgical referrals will have many uses for this book; practicing surgeons will find it useful as a guide to the most current management strategies.

ORGANIZATION

This book is organized chiefly by organ system. Lists of subjects taken up in the longer chapters are presented in the table of contents, but for some users the more convenient portal of entry to the text will be the index.

Early chapters provide general information about the relationship between surgeons and their patients (Chapter 1), preparation for surgery (Chapter 2), postoperative care (Chapter 3), and surgical complications (Chapter 4). Chapter 5 deals with the problems of medically ill patients who require surgery. Chapter 6 summarizes the main features of the surgeon's legal obligations and tort law. Then follow chapters on wound healing (Chapter 7), a new chapter on the metabolic and neuroendocrine responses to surgery (Chapter 8), inflammation, infection, and antibiotics (Chapter 9), fluid and electrolyte management (Chapter 10), surgical metabolism and nutrition (Chapter 11), anesthesia (Chapter 12), and shock and acute pulmonary failure (Chapter 13). Chapter 14 discusses management of trauma and Chapter 15, management of burns. The main series of body system topics begins with Chapter 16 (head and neck tumors) and ends with Chapter 45 (hand surgery). Pediatric surgery (Chapter 46), oncology and cancer chemotherapy (Chapter 47), and organ transplantation (Chapter 48) round out the main text.

NEW TO THIS EDITION

Along with the customary revision of all sections as called for by changing concepts in each field covered in this book, the following can be mentioned specifically:

- This has been a particularly complete revision with extensive changes to every chapter to update the material.
- Chapter 5 has several sections regarding Special Medical Problems in Surgical Patients, which have each been extensively rewritten to provide optimal guidance to the practitioner or trainee.
- Chapter 8, Metabolic & Neuroendocrine Systems in Surgery, is a new chapter covering material not previously included in the text.
- Chapter 9, Inflammation, Infections, & Antibiotics, has been completely rewritten, reflecting current concepts and practice in the management of surgical infections and antimicrobial therapy.
- Chapter 11, Surgical Metabolism & Nutrition, has been completely rewritten to simplify the approach to nutritional support of the surgical patient.
- Head & Neck Tumors (Chapter 16) has been extensively revised, including up-to-date combined modality therapy information.
- Oncology (Chapter 47) is entirely new, with added coverage of lymphomas, melanoma, sarcoma, and systemic cancer therapy.

ACKNOWLEDGMENTS

The editors and the contributors continue to acknowledge their gratitude to J. Englebert Dunphy, MD, for his inspiration and lifetime of service to the practice and teaching of surgery. We are also particularly grateful for the important contributions that Jim Ransom, who has served as copy editor for over 25 years, has made to the quality of this text, and especially to this extensive revision. We are grateful also to our colleagues and readers who have offered comments and criticisms for our guidance in preparing future editions. We hope that anyone with an idea, suggestion, or criticism regarding this book will contact us. Finally, we welcome the new association of the Lange series with McGraw-Hill, and appreciate the constant support and encouragement of the Editor-in-Chief, Shelley Reinhardt, without whom this project might not have been completed.

Gerard M. Doherty, MD
Lawrence W. Way, MD

Ann Arbor, Michigan and San Francisco, California
August, 2002

Approach to the Surgical Patient

1

J. Englebert Dunphy, MD, & Lawrence W. Way, MD

The management of surgical disorders requires not only the application of technical skills and training in the basic sciences to the problems of diagnosis and treatment but also a genuine sympathy and indeed love for the patient. The surgeon must be a doctor in the old-fashioned sense, an applied scientist, an engineer, an artist, and a minister to his or her fellow human beings. Because life or death often depends upon the validity of surgical decisions, the surgeon's judgment must be matched by courage in action and by a high degree of technical proficiency.

■ THE HISTORY

At their first contact, the surgeon must gain the patient's confidence and convey the assurance that help is available and will be provided. The surgeon must demonstrate concern for the patient as a person who needs help and not just as a "case" to be processed through the surgical ward. This is not always easy to do, and there are no rules of conduct except to be gentle and considerate. Most patients are eager to like and trust their doctors and respond gratefully to a sympathetic and understanding person. Some surgeons are able to establish a confident relationship with the first few words of greeting; others can only do so by means of a stylized and carefully acquired bedside manner. It does not matter how it is done, so long as an atmosphere of sympathy, personal interest, and understanding is created. Even under emergency circumstances, this subtle message of sympathetic concern must be conveyed.

Eventually, all histories must be formally structured, but much can be learned by letting the patient ramble a little. Discrepancies and omissions in the history are often due as much to overstructuring and leading questions as to the unreliability of the patient. The enthusiastic novice asks leading questions; the cooperative patient gives the answer that seems to be wanted; and the interview concludes on a note of mutual satisfaction with the wrong answer thus developed.

BUILDING THE HISTORY

History taking is detective work. Preconceived ideas, snap judgments, and hasty conclusions have no place in this process. The diagnosis must be established by inductive reasoning. The interviewer must first determine the facts and then search for essential clues, realizing that the patient may conceal the most important symptom—eg, the passage of blood by rectum—in the hope (born of fear) that if it is not specifically inquired about or if nothing is found to account for it in the physical examination, it cannot be very serious.

Common symptoms of surgical conditions that require special emphasis in the history taking are discussed in the following paragraphs.

Pain

A careful analysis of the nature of pain is one of the most important features of a surgical history. The examiner must first ascertain how the pain began. Was it explosive in onset, rapid, or gradual? What is the precise character of the pain? Is it so severe that it cannot be relieved by medication? Is it constant or intermittent? Are there classic associations, such as the rhythmic pattern of small bowel obstruction or the onset of pain preceding the limp of intermittent claudication?

One of the most important aspects of pain is the patient's reaction to it. The overreactor's description of pain is often obviously inappropriate, and so is a description of "excruciating" pain offered in a casual or jovial manner. A patient who shrieks and thrashes about is either grossly overreacting or suffering from renal or biliary colic. Very severe pain—due to infection, inflammation, or vascular disease—usually forces the patient to restrict all movement as much as possible.

Moderate pain is made agonizing by fear and anxiety. Reassurance of a sort calculated to restore the patient's confidence in the care being given is often a more effective analgesic than an injection of morphine.

Vomiting

What did the patient vomit? How much? How often? What did the vomitus look like? Was vomiting projec-

I

tile? It is especially helpful for the examiner to see the vomitus.

Change in Bowel Habits

A change in bowel habits is a common complaint that is often of no significance. However, when a person who has always had regular evacuations notices a distinct change, particularly toward intermittent alternations of constipation and diarrhea, colon cancer must be suspected. Too much emphasis is placed upon the size and shape of the stool—eg, many patients who normally have well-formed stools may complain of irregular small stools when their routine is disturbed by travel or a change in diet.

Hematemesis or Hematochezia

Bleeding from any orifice demands the most critical analysis and can never be dismissed as due to some immediately obvious cause. The most common error is to assume that bleeding from the rectum is attributable to hemorrhoids. The character of the blood can be of great significance. Does it clot? Is it bright or dark red? Is it changed in any way, as in the coffee-ground vomitus of slow gastric bleeding or the dark, tarry stool of upper gastrointestinal bleeding? The full details and variations cannot be included here but will be emphasized under separate headings elsewhere.

Trauma

Trauma occurs so commonly that it is often difficult to establish a relationship between the chief complaint and an episode of trauma. Children in particular are subject to all kinds of minor trauma, and the family may attribute the onset of an illness to a specific recent injury. On the other hand, children may be subjected to severe trauma though their parents are unaware of it. The possibility of trauma having been inflicted by a parent must not be overlooked.

When there is a history of trauma, the details must be established as precisely as possible. What was the patient's position when the accident occurred? Was consciousness lost? Retrograde amnesia (inability to remember events just preceding the accident) always indicates some degree of cerebral damage. If a patient can remember every detail of an accident, has not lost consciousness, and has no evidence of external injury to the head, brain damage can be excluded.

In the case of gunshot wounds and stab wounds, knowing the nature of the weapon, its size and shape, the probable trajectory, and the position of the patient when hit may be very helpful in evaluating the nature of the resultant injury.

The possibility that an accident might have been caused by preexisting disease such as epilepsy, diabetes, coronary artery disease, or hypoglycemia must be explored.

When all of the facts and essential clues have been gathered, the examiner is in a position to complete the study of the present illness. By this time, it may be possible to rule out (by inductive reasoning) all but a few possible diagnoses. A novice diagnostician asked to evaluate the causes of shoulder pain in a given patient might include ruptured ectopic pregnancy in the list of possibilities. The experienced physician will automatically exclude that possibility on the basis of sex or age.

Family History

The family history is of great significance in a number of surgical conditions. Polyposis of the colon is a classic example, but diabetes, Peutz-Jeghers syndrome, chronic pancreatitis, multiglandular syndromes, other endocrine abnormalities, and cancer are often better understood and better evaluated in the light of a careful family history.

Past History

The details of the past history may illuminate obscure areas of the present illness. It has been said that people who are well are almost never sick, and people who are sick are almost never well. It is true that a patient with a long and complicated history of diseases and injuries is likely to be a much poorer risk than even a very old patient experiencing a major surgical illness for the first time.

In order to make certain that important details of the past history will not be overlooked, the system review must be formalized and thorough. By always reviewing the past history in the same way, the experienced examiner never omits significant details. Many skilled examiners find it easy to review the past history by inquiring about each system as they perform the physical examination on that part of the body.

In reviewing the past history, it is important to consider the nutritional background of the patient. There is an increasing awareness throughout the world that the underprivileged malnourished patient responds poorly to disease, injury, and operation. Indeed, there is some evidence that various lesions such as carcinoma may be more fulminating in malnourished patients. Malnourishment may not be obvious on physical examination and must be elicited by questioning.

Acute nutritional deficiencies, particularly fluid and electrolyte losses, can be understood only in the light of the total (including nutritional) history. For example, a low serum sodium may be due to the use of diuretics or a sodium-restricted diet rather than to acute loss. In this connection, the use of any medications must be carefully recorded and interpreted.

A detailed history of acute losses by vomiting and diarrhea—and the nature of the losses—is helpful in estimating the probable trends in serum electrolytes. Thus, the patient who has been vomiting persistently with no evidence of bile in the vomitus is likely to have acute pyloric stenosis associated with benign ulcer, and hypochloremic alkalosis must be anticipated. Chronic vomiting without bile—and particularly with evidence of changed and previously digested food—is suggestive of chronic obstruction, and the possibility of carcinoma should be considered.

It is essential for the surgeon to think in terms of nutritional balance. It is often possible to begin therapy before the results of laboratory tests have been obtained, because the specific nature and probable extent of fluid and electrolyte losses can often be estimated on the basis of the history and the physician's clinical experience. Laboratory data should be obtained as soon as possible, but a knowledge of the probable level of the obstruction and of the concentration of the electrolytes in the gastrointestinal fluids will provide sufficient grounds for the institution of appropriate immediate therapy.

The Patient's Emotional Background

Psychiatric consultation is seldom required in the management of surgical patients, but there are times when it is of great help. Emotionally and mentally disturbed patients require surgical operations as often as others, and full cooperation between psychiatrist and surgeon is essential. Furthermore, either before or after an operation, a patient may develop a major psychotic disturbance that is beyond the ability of the surgeon to appraise or manage. Prognosis, drug therapy, and overall management require the participation of a psychiatrist.

On the other hand, there are many situations in which the surgeon can and should deal with the emotional aspects of the patient's illness rather than resorting to psychiatric assistance. Most psychiatrists prefer not to be brought in to deal with minor anxiety states. As long as the surgeon accepts the responsibility for the care of the whole patient, such services are superfluous.

This is particularly true in the care of patients with malignant disease or those who must undergo mutilating operations such as amputation of an extremity, ileostomy, or colostomy. In these situations, the patient can be supported far more effectively by the surgeon and the surgical team than by a consulting psychiatrist.

Surgeons are becoming increasingly more aware of the importance of psychosocial factors in surgical convalescence. Recovery from a major operation is greatly enhanced if the patient is not worn down with worry about emotional, social, and economic problems that have nothing to do with the illness itself. Incorporation of these factors into the record contributes to better total care of the surgical patient.

■ THE PHYSICAL EXAMINATION

The complete examination of the surgical patient includes the physical examination, certain special procedures such as gastroscopy and esophagoscopy, laboratory tests, x-ray examination, and follow-up examination. In some cases, all of these may be necessary; in others, special examinations and laboratory tests can be kept to a minimum. It is just as poor practice to insist on unnecessary thoroughness as it is to overlook procedures that may contribute to the diagnosis. Painful, inconvenient, and costly procedures should not be ordered unless there is a reasonable chance that the information gained will be useful in making clinical decisions.

THE ELECTIVE PHYSICAL EXAMINATION

The elective physical examination should be done in an orderly and detailed fashion. One should acquire the habit of performing a complete examination in exactly the same sequence, so that no step is omitted. When the routine must be modified, as in an emergency, the examiner recalls without conscious effort what must be done to complete the examination later. The regular performance of complete examinations has the added advantage of familiarizing the beginner with what is normal so that what is abnormal can be more readily recognized.

All patients are sensitive and somewhat embarrassed at being examined. It is both courteous and clinically useful to put the patient at ease. The examining room and table should be comfortable, and drapes should be used if the patient is required to strip for the examination. Most patients will relax if they are allowed to talk a bit during the examination, which is another reason for taking the past history while the examination is being done.

A useful rule is to first observe the patient's general physique and habitus and then to carefully inspect the hands. Many systemic diseases show themselves in the hands (cirrhosis of the liver, hyperthyroidism, Raynaud's disease, pulmonary insufficiency, heart disease, and nutritional disorders).

Details of the examination cannot be included here. The beginner is urged to consult special texts.

Inspection, palpation, and auscultation are the time-honored essential steps in appraising both the normal and the abnormal. Comparison of the two sides of the body often suggests a specific abnormality. The slight droop of one eyelid characteristic of Horner's syndrome can only be recognized by comparison with the opposite side. Inspection of the female breasts, particularly as the patient raises and lowers her arms, will often reveal slight dimpling indicative of an infiltrating carcinoma barely detectable on palpation.

Successful palpation requires skill and gentleness. Spasm, tension, and anxiety caused by painful examination procedures may make an adequate examination almost impossible, particularly in children.

Another important feature of palpation is the laying on of hands that has been called part of the ministry of medicine. A disappointed and critical patient often will say of a doctor, "He hardly touched me." Careful, precise, and gentle palpation not only gives the physician the information being sought but also inspires confidence and trust.

When examining for areas of tenderness, it may be necessary to use only one finger in order to precisely localize the extent of the tenderness. This is of particular importance in examination of the acute abdomen.

Auscultation, once thought to be the exclusive province of the physician, is now more important in surgery than it is in medicine. Radiologic examinations, including cardiac catheterization, have relegated auscultation of the heart and lungs to the status of preliminary scanning procedures in medicine. In surgery, however, auscultation of the abdomen and peripheral vessels has become absolutely essential. The nature of ileus and the presence of a variety of vascular lesions are revealed by auscultation. Bizarre abdominal pain in a young woman can easily be ascribed to hysteria or anxiety on the basis of a negative physical examination and x-rays of the gastrointestinal tract. Auscultation of the epigastrium, however, may reveal a murmur due to obstruction of the celiac artery.

Examination of the Body Orifices

Complete examination of the ears, mouth, rectum, and pelvis is accepted as part of a complete examination. Palpation of the mouth and tongue is as essential as inspection. Inspection of the rectum with a sigmoidoscope is now regarded as part of a complete physical examination. Every surgeon should acquire familiarity with the use of the ophthalmoscope and sigmoidoscope and should use them regularly in doing complete physical examinations.

THE EMERGENCY PHYSICAL EXAMINATION

In an emergency, the routine of the physical examination must be altered to fit the circumstances. The history may be limited to a single sentence, or there may be no history if the patient is unconscious and there are no other informants. Although the details of an accident or injury may be very useful in the total appraisal of the patient, they must be left for later consideration. The primary considerations are the following: Is the patient breathing? Is the airway open? Is there a palpable pulse? Is the heart beating? Is massive bleeding occurring?

If the patient is not breathing, airway obstruction must be ruled out by thrusting the fingers into the mouth and pulling the tongue forward. If the patient is unconscious, the respiratory tract should be intubated and mouth-to-mouth respiration started. If there is no pulse or heartbeat, start cardiac resuscitation.

Serious external loss of blood from an extremity can be controlled by elevation and pressure. Tourniquets are rarely required.

Every victim of major blunt trauma should be suspected of having a vertebral injury capable of causing damage to the spinal cord unless rough handling is avoided.

Some injuries are so life-threatening that action must be taken before even a limited physical examination is done. Penetrating wounds of the heart, large open sucking wounds of the chest, massive crush injuries with flail chest, and massive external bleeding all require emergency treatment before any further examination can be done.

In most emergencies, however, after it has been established that the airway is open, the heart is beating, and there is no massive external hemorrhage—and after antishock measures have been instituted, if necessary—a rapid survey examination must be done. Failure to perform such an examination can lead to serious mistakes in the care of the patient. It takes no more than 2 or 3 minutes to carefully examine the head, thorax, abdomen, extremities, genitalia (particularly in females), and back. If cervical cord damage has been ruled out, it is essential to turn the injured patient and carefully inspect the back, buttocks, and perineum.

Tension pneumothorax and cardiac tamponade may easily be overlooked if there are multiple injuries.

Upon completion of the survey examination, control of pain, splinting of fractured limbs, suturing of lacerations, and other types of emergency treatment can be started.

■ LABORATORY & OTHER EXAMINATIONS

Laboratory Examination

Laboratory examinations in surgical patients have the following objectives: (1) screening for asymptomatic disease that may affect the surgical result (eg, unsuspected anemia or diabetes); (2) appraisal of diseases that may contraindicate elective surgery or require treatment before surgery (eg, diabetes, heart failure); (3) diagnosis of disorders that require surgery (eg, hyperparathyroidism, pheochromocytoma); and (4) evaluation of the nature and extent of metabolic or septic complications.

Patients undergoing major surgery, even though they seem to be in excellent health except for their surgical disease, should have a complete blood and urine examination. A history of renal, hepatic, or heart disease requires detailed studies. Latent, asymptomatic renal insufficiency may be missed, since many patients with chronic renal disease have varying degrees of nitrogen retention without proteinuria. A fixed urine specific gravity is easily overlooked, and preoperative determination of the blood urea nitrogen and serum creatinine is frequently required. Patients who have had hepatitis may have no jaundice but may have severe hepatic insufficiency that can be precipitated into acute failure by blood loss or shock.

Medical consultation is frequently required in the total preoperative appraisal of the surgical patient, and there is no more rewarding experience than the thorough evaluation of a patient with heart disease or gastrointestinal disease by a physician and a surgeon working together. It is essential, however, that the surgeon not become totally dependent upon a medical consultant for the preoperative evaluation and management of the patient. The total management must be the surgeon's responsibility and is not to be delegated. Moreover, the surgeon is the only one with the experience and background to interpret the meaning of laboratory tests in the light of other features of the case—particularly the history and physical findings.

Imaging Studies

Modern patient care calls for a variety of critical radiologic examinations. The closest cooperation between the radiologist and the surgeon is essential if serious mistakes are to be avoided. This means that the surgeon must not refer the patient to the radiologist, requesting a particular examination, without providing an adequate account of the history and physical findings. Particularly in emergency situations, review of the films and consultation are needed.

When the radiologic diagnosis is not definitive, the examinations must be repeated in the light of the history and physical examination. Despite the great accuracy of x-ray diagnosis, a negative gastrointestinal study still does not exclude either ulcer or a neoplasm; particularly in the right colon, small lesions are easily overlooked. At times, the history and physical findings are so clearly diagnostic that operation is justifiable despite negative imaging studies.

Special Examinations

Special examinations such as cystoscopy, gastroscopy, esophagoscopy, colonoscopy, angiography, and bronchoscopy are often required in the diagnostic appraisal of surgical disorders. The surgeon must be familiar with the indications and limitations of these procedures and be prepared to consult with colleagues in medicine and the surgical specialties as required.

Preoperative Care

Gerard M. Doherty, MD, & Robert H. Demling, MD

The care of the patient with a major surgical problem commonly involves distinct phases of management that occur in the following sequence:

(1) Preoperative care
Diagnostic workup
Preoperative evaluation
Preoperative preparation
(2) Anesthesia and operation
(3) Postoperative care
Postanesthetic observation
Intensive care
Intermediate care
Convalescent care

DEFINITIONS & OBJECTIVES
Preoperative Care

The **diagnostic workup** is concerned primarily with determining the cause and extent of the present illness. **Preoperative evaluation** consists of an overall assessment of the patient's general health in order to identify significant abnormalities that might increase operative risk or adversely influence recovery. **Preoperative preparation** includes interventions dictated by the findings on diagnostic workup and preoperative evaluation and by the nature of the expected operation.

Postoperative Care

The **postanesthetic observation** phase of management is the few hours immediately after operation during which the acute reaction to operation and the residual effects of anesthesia subside. A recovery room with special staff and equipment is usually provided for this purpose. Patients who need continued cardiopulmonary support or continued invasive monitoring to avoid major morbidity and death should be transferred to the intensive care unit. For most postoperative patients, the duration of stay in the ICU is 1–2 days. However, a stay in excess of 2 weeks can result if organ failure develops.

Intermediate care is usually provided on an inpatient nursing unit until the patient's recovery can continue at home during the convalescent phase.

The Continuum of Surgical Care

The continuum of surgical care has been represented above as progressing through a series of pre- and postoperative phases. In practice, these phases merge, overlap, and vary in relative importance from patient to patient. Complications, death, and the therapeutic end result in the surgical patient depend upon the competence with which each succeeding phase is managed. The rapid progression and severe episodic stress of major surgical illness leave small margin for errors in management. The care immediately preceding and following operation, which includes preoperative evaluation and preparation and postanesthetic observation and intensive care, is especially critical. The increased complexity of surgical critical care has resulted in a team approach to the ICU patient, with management directed by the primary surgeon and the critical care specialists in the ICU, whose role it is to maintain optimum care.

PREOPERATIVE EVALUATION
General Health Assessment

The initial diagnostic workup of the surgical patient is concerned chiefly with determining the cause of the presenting complaints. Except in strictly minor surgical illness, this initial workup should be supplemented by a complete assessment of the patient's general health. Such an evaluation, which should be completed prior to all major operations, seeks to identify abnormalities that may influence operative risk or may have a bearing on the patient's future well-being. Preoperative evaluation includes at least a complete history and physical examination. Patients over 40 should also have complete blood counts and serum electrolyte measurements. Patients over 50 should have chest x-rays and electrocardiograms as well. Open wounds and infections usually require culture and determination of antibiotic sensitivity. Surface cultures of open wounds are usually of little help, particularly when closure of the wound with a skin graft is contemplated or primary closure will be allowed to occur. Quantitative cultures of punch biopsies from the wound are much more precise indicators. Greater than 10^5 organisms per gram of tissue correspond to a greater than 50% graft failure, whereas values below 10^5 organisms per gram correspond to a greater than 80% graft take. To minimize cost, this workup should be done before admission.

All significant complaints, physical findings, and test abnormalities should be adequately evaluated by appropriate further tests, examinations, and consultations. The adequacy of circulating blood volume needs to be evaluated and can be determined by the adequacy of peripheral perfusion, the fullness of neck veins in the supine and partially erect positions, and tests for orthostatic changes in blood pressure and pulse. Severe cardiovascular disease will make these parameters much more difficult to interpret. Patients (other than those with acute blood loss) who are prone to a hypovolemic state include those with significant weight loss as a result of cancer, gastrointestinal disease, or drugs such as diuretics. A hemoglobin of 8 g/dL is generally physiologically safe for tissue oxygen delivery. However, this may be inadequate in the patient with reduced cardiac output. The adequacy of liver and kidney function should be tested if impairment is suspected, as each organ plays a major role in the response to and clearance of various anesthetic agents both preoperatively and intraoperatively. Selection of the ideal agent depends on recognition of liver or renal impairment in the preoperative period. Bleeding tendencies, medications currently being taken, and allergies and reactions to antibiotics and other agents should be noted and prominently displayed on the chart. Psychiatric consultation should be considered in patients with a past history of significant mental disorder that may be exacerbated by operation and in patients whose complaints may have a psychoneurotic basis.

The physical examination should be thorough and must include neurologic examination and check of peripheral arterial pulses (carotid, radial, femoral, popliteal, posterior tibial, and dorsalis pedis). Peripheral vascular disease should be suspected if there is a history of transient ischemic attacks, claudication, or diabetes. If a carotid bruit is found, other studies may be indicated to specifically assess stenosis. A rectal examination should always be done, and a pelvic examination should be performed unless contraindicated by age, virginity, or other valid reason. An annual Papanicolaou smear of the cervix should be obtained in women over 30 years of age. Sigmoidoscopy is required for completeness of evaluation when there are rectal or colonic complaints.

If a procedure is planned that will or may require blood replacement, the preoperative preparation should include planning for that procedure. Appropriate strategies may include storing the patient's blood in the weeks prior to operation to allow autologous transfusion, directed-donor blood storage for transfusion, or phlebotomy and hemodilution immediately preoperatively with subsequent reinfusion.

In summary, the preoperative evaluation should be comprehensive in order to assess the patient's overall state of health, to determine the risk of the impending surgical treatment, and to guide the preoperative preparation.

Fischer SP: Cost-effective preoperative evaluation and testing. Chest 1999;115:96S.

Specific Factors Affecting Operative Risk

A. THE COMPROMISED OR ALTERED HOST

Patients may be considered compromised or altered hosts if significant impairment of systems and tissues does not permit a normal response to operative trauma or infection. Preoperative recognition of an abnormal nutritional or immune state is of obvious importance.

1. Nutritional Assessment—It has long been documented that malnutrition leads to a significant increase in the operative death rate. Weight loss of more than 20% caused by illness such as cancer or intestinal disease not only results in a higher death rate but also a greater than threefold increase in the postoperative infection rate. Although there is still no uniformity of opinion about the best way to determine nutritional status, it is clear that dietary history is of major importance in the assessment, as is a working knowledge of the basic nutritional deficiencies associated with certain disease states, particularly vitamin deficiencies. Standard biochemical parameters that indicate impairment in the visceral protein mass include a serum albumin of less than 3 g/dL or a serum transferrin of less than 150 mg/dL.

Even when malnutrition is diagnosed, there is no uniformity of opinion about when short-term (7–10 days) preoperative hyperalimentation is indicated. It is known that nutrition can improve wound healing and immune function. Current indications for supportive measures before elective surgery include a history of weight loss in excess of 10% of body weight or an anticipated prolonged postoperative recovery period during which the patient will not be fed orally.

2. Assessment of immune competence—Increased knowledge and appreciation of immune defenses has led to a greater awareness of the increased postoperative rates of complications and death due to infection in patients with immune deficiency disorders. Many immune deficiency states are linked to malnutrition. Total lymphocyte count and cell-mediated immunity measurement are the two most commonly performed tests. Anergy or impaired immunity is diagnosed if no response is noted to any of the skin tests, whereas a positive response (5 mm or more of induration at the test site) to one or more skin tests indicates normal lymphocyte activity. Anergy is associated with an increased susceptibility to infectious complications. Other more specific tests include neutrophil chemotaxis and measurements of specific lymphocyte populations. Patients at high risk for immune deficiency in whom this information is helpful include elderly patients and those with malnutrition, severe trauma or burns, or cancer. Other than for a course of preoperative hyperalimentation, no stimulants of the immune system are consistently being used in the preoperative period, though research activity in this area is extensive. The AIDS patient may also be severely immunocompromised and presents a risk to health care workers. Since preoperative AIDS testing is not required even for high-risk patient groups, universal precautions are practiced, especially when dealing with blood and body secretions.

3. Other factors leading to increased infection— Certain drugs may reduce the patient's resistance to infection by interfering with host defense mechanisms. Corticosteroids, immunosuppressive agents, cytotoxic drugs, and prolonged antibiotic therapy are associated with an increased incidence of invasion by fungi and other organisms not commonly encountered in infections. A combination of irradiation and corticosteroid therapy is found experimentally to predispose to lethal fungal infections. It is possible that the synergistic combination of irradiation, corticosteroids, and serious underlying disease may set the stage for clinical fungal infection. A high rate of wound, pulmonary, and other infections is observed in renal failure, presumably as a result of decreased host resistance. Granulocytopenia and diseases that may produce immunologic deficiency—eg, lymphomas, leukemias, and hypogammaglobulinemia—are frequently associated with septic complications. The uncontrolled diabetic patient is also observed clinically to be more susceptible to infection (see Chapter 5).

B. PULMONARY DYSFUNCTION

The patient with compromised pulmonary function preoperatively is susceptible to postoperative pulmonary complications, including hypoxia, atelectasis, and pneumonia. Preoperative evaluation of the degree of respiratory impairment is necessary in patients at high risk for postoperative complications. These include a history of heavy smoking and cough, obesity, advanced age, major intrathoracic or upper abdominal surgery, and known pulmonary disease. Pertinent factors in the history include the presence and character of cough and excessive sputum production, history of wheezing, and exercise tolerance. Pertinent physical findings include the presence of wheezing or prolonged expiration. A chest x-ray, ECG, blood gases, and some basic pulmonary function tests are indicated. Although an evaluation of arterial

oxygen tension is very helpful, the major reason for obtaining preoperative blood gases is to determine whether CO_2 retention is present. This indicates severe pulmonary dysfunction, and the need for an elective operative procedure must be reevaluated. If surgery is necessary, oxygen must be used carefully in the postoperative period, as overuse may accentuate CO_2 retention and aggravate concomitant respiratory acidosis. The most helpful screening pulmonary function tests are forced vital capacity (FVC) and forced expiratory volume in 1 second (FEV_1). Values less than 50% of predicted outcome based on age and body size indicate significant airway disease with a high risk for complications.

Preoperative pulmonary preparation for a period as short as 48 hours has been shown to significantly decrease postoperative complications. Even a few days of abstinence from smoking will decrease sputum production. Oral or inhaled bronchodilators along with twice-daily chest physical therapy and postural drainage will help clear inspissated secretions from the airway. Before surgery, patients should be instructed in techniques of coughing, deep breathing, and use of one of the incentive spirometry devices that increase inspiratory effort. The use of intermittent positive-pressure breathing (IPPB) has been found to be no more effective than the much less expensive incentive spirometers when used properly.

C. DELAYED WOUND HEALING

This problem can be anticipated in certain categories of patients whose tissue repair process may be compromised. Many factors have been alleged to influence wound healing. Important factors include protein depletion, ascorbic acid deficiency, marked dehydration or edema, severe anemia, diabetes mellitus, and smoking. It has been shown experimentally that hypovolemia, vasoconstriction, increased blood viscosity, and increased intravascular aggregation and erythrostasis resulting from remote trauma will interfere with wound healing by reducing tissue oxygen tension. The most important component is maintenance of adequate blood volume and perfusion. Decreased perfusion results in a marked decrease in tissue oxygen tension, which in turn impairs collagen deposition. Often the decrease is not clinically evident, but it can be expected to occur in patients receiving chronic diuretic therapy or those with underlying myocardial dysfunction. Large doses of corticosteroids have been shown to depress wound healing in humans. It is therefore reasonable to assume that wounds in patients who have received appreciable doses of corticosteroids preoperatively should be closed with special care to prevent disruption and managed postoperatively as though healing will be delayed.

Operation may be required on a patient receiving cancer chemotherapy with cytotoxic drugs. These drugs usually interfere with cell proliferation and (theoretically at least) tend to decrease the tensile strength of the surgical wound. Although experimental evidence to support this assumption is equivocal, it is wise to manage wounds in patients receiving cytotoxic drugs as though healing will be slower than normal.

Decreased vascularity and other local changes occur after a few weeks or months in tissues that have been heavily irradiated. These are potential deterrents to wound healing, a point that should be kept in mind in planning surgical incisions in patients who have been irradiated. Radiation therapy at levels of 3000 cGy or more are injurious to skin and to connective and vascular tissues. Chronic changes include scarring, damage to fibroblasts and collagen, and degenerative changes with subsequent hyalinization in the walls of blood vessels. Angiogenesis, seen as the capillary budding in granulation tissue and collagen formation, is inhibited when these changes are well established, so that surgical wounds in heavily irradiated tissues will heal slowly or may break down in the presence of infection. When radiation is given prior to operation, it is generally agreed that there is an optimal delay period (2–12 weeks) after completion of the radiation therapy before operation is performed in order to minimize wound complications. Technical problems in correctly timed operations for cancer are not usually increased by low-dosage (2000–4000 cGy) adjunctive radiotherapy. With radiation dosage in the therapeutic range (5000–6000 cGy), an increased incidence of wound complications can be expected, though this can be minimized by careful surgical technique and proper timing.

D. Drug Effects

Drug allergies, sensitivities, and incompatibilities and adverse drug effects that may be precipitated by operation must be foreseen and, if possible, prevented. A history of skin or other untoward reactions or sickness after injection, oral administration, or other use of any of the following substances should be noted so they can be avoided:

Penicillin or other antibiotic
Morphine, codeine, meperidine, or other opioid
Procaine or other anesthetic
Aspirin or other analgesic
Barbiturates
Sulfonamides
Tetanus antitoxin or other serum
Iodine, thimerosal (Merthiolate), or other germicide
Any other medication
Any foods such as eggs, milk, or chocolate
Adhesive tape

A personal or strong family history of asthma, hay fever, or other allergic disorder should alert the surgeon to possible hypersensitivity to drugs.

Drugs currently or recently taken by the patient may require continuation, dosage adjustment, or discontinuation. Medications such as digitalis, insulin, and corticosteroids must usually be maintained and their dosage carefully regulated during the operative and postoperative periods. Prolonged use of corticosteroids (even though discontinued 1 month or more preoperatively) may be associated with hypofunction of the adrenal cortex, which impairs the physiologic responses to the stress of anesthesia and operation. The standard stress dose of hydrocortisone (100 mg three times daily) is more than is required during surgical stress; however, such a patient should receive corticosteroids immediately before, during, and after operation. Anticoagulants should be discontinued for most patients and most operations. If the interval of anticoagulant discontinuation must be minimized, heparin can be used in the perioperative period.

The anesthesiologist is concerned with the long-term preoperative use of central nervous system depressants (eg, barbiturates, opioids, and alcohol), which may be associated with increased tolerance for anesthetic drugs; tranquilizers (eg, phenothiazine derivatives such as chlorpromazine); and antihypertensive agents, which may be associated with hypotension in response to anesthesia.

E. Risks of Thromboembolism

Increased risk factors for deep vein thrombophlebitis and pulmonary embolus include cancer, obesity, myocardial dysfunction, age over 45 years, and a prior history of thrombosis. Prophylaxis and treatment of venous thrombotic disease are discussed in Chapter 37.

F. The Pediatric Patient

See Chapter 46.

G. The Elderly Patient

(See also discussion in Chapter 5.) Operative risk should be judged on the basis of physiologic rather than chronologic age, and an elderly patient should not be denied a needed operation because of age alone. The hazard of the average major operation for the patient over age 60 years is increased only slightly provided there is no cardiovascular, renal, or other serious systemic disease. Assume that every patient over 60—even in the absence of symptoms and physical signs—has some generalized arteriosclerosis and potential limitation of myocardial and renal reserve. Accordingly, the preoperative evaluation should be comprehensive. Occult cancer is not infrequent in this age group; therefore, even minor gastrointestinal and other complaints should be thoroughly investigated by the physician.

Administer intravenous fluids with care so as not to overload the circulation. Monitoring of intake, output, body weight, serum electrolytes, and central venous pressure is important in evaluating cardiorenal response and tolerance in this age group.

Aged patients generally require smaller doses of strong narcotics and are frequently depressed by routine doses. Codeine is usually well tolerated. Sedative and hypnotic drugs often cause restlessness, mental confusion, and uncooperative behavior in the elderly and should be used cautiously. Preanesthetic medications should be limited to atropine or scopolamine in the debilitated elderly patient, and anesthetic agents should be administered in minimal amounts.

H. The Obese Patient

Obese patients have an increased frequency of concomitant disease and a high incidence of postoperative wound complications. A controlled preoperative weight loss program is often beneficial before elective procedures.

Kearon C, Hirsh I: Management of anticoagulation before and after elective surgery. N Engl J Med 1997;336:1506.

Consultations

The opinion of a qualified consultant should be obtained when it may be of benefit to the patient, when requested by the patient or family members, or when it may be of medicolegal importance. The physician should take the initiative in arranging consultation when the treatment proposed is controversial or exceptionally risky, when dangerous complications occur, or when the physician senses that the patient or family members are unduly apprehensive regarding the plan of management or the course of events. Consultation with cardiac or other medical or surgical specialists preoperatively is important if the patient has abnormal findings in their fields of competence. It is also beneficial for the specialist consultant to become acquainted with the patient and the condition preoperatively when the possibility exists that the consultant will be called upon for advice later in connection with a postoperative complication or development. Second-opinion programs for elective surgery have recently become more popular, with many programs being initiated by insurance companies. The purpose is to assist patients in making an informed decision when elective surgery has been recommended. The second opinion can be requested either by the patient or by the physician and is of particular assistance in difficult cases.

Anesthesia consultation is always requested prior to major surgery if an anesthesiologist is available. In poor-risk patients, this consultation should be requested several days in advance of operation if possible. The patient's prospects for a smooth and uncomplicated anesthetic experience are greatly improved by the anesthesiologist's preoperative evaluation and advice. The assessment classifies the patient as follows:

Class 1: Healthy

Class 2: Mild systemic disease

Class 3: Severe but not incapacitating disease

Class 4: Severe disease, constant threat to life

Class 5: Moribund patient not expected to survive for 24 hours

Preoperative Note

When the diagnostic workup and preoperative evaluation have been completed, all details should be reviewed and a preoperative note written in the chart. The note summarizes the pertinent findings and decisions, gives the indications for the operation proposed, and attests that there has been a discussion of the complications and risks of the operation between surgeon and patient (ie, informed consent has been obtained). This constitutes a final check on the adequacy of the analysis of the patient's problem, the need for treatment, and the patient's understanding of these facts.

PREOPERATIVE PREPARATION

Major operations create surgical wounds and cause severe stress, subjecting the patient to the hazard of infection and metabolic and other derangements. Appropriate preoperative preparation facilitates wound healing and systemic recovery by making certain that the patient's condition is optimal. Operation also results in psychic trauma to the patient and to family members and has significant medicolegal implications, all of which deserve special consideration preoperatively to avoid postoperative repercussions. In emergency conditions, time for preparation is limited but is usually sufficient to permit the principles of good surgical preparation to be followed. In elective operation, meticulous preoperative preparation is both possible and mandatory and includes the following steps.

Informing the Patient

Surgery is a frightening prospect for both patient and family. Their psychologic preparation and reassurance should begin at the initial contact with the surgeon. Appropriate explanation of the nature and purpose of preoperative studies and treatments establishes confidence. When all pertinent information has been gathered, it is the surgeon's responsibility to describe the planned surgical procedure and its risks and possible consequences in understandable terms to the patient and usually also to the next of kin. The potential need for blood transfusion must be addressed. Preferably, the patient has already donated his or her own blood before scheduled surgery. This discussion must be documented in the chart. It is also very helpful to explain to the patient what will happen in the operating room before induction of anesthesia and in the recovery room. The patient should be told that an endotracheal tube may be in place and that speech may not be possible for that reason. Similarly, prompt postoperative interpretation of pertinent findings and prospects to patient and family contributes to rapport and to cooperation during the recovery period.

Operative Permit

The patient or the patient's legal guardian must sign (in advance) a permit authorizing a major or minor operation or a procedure such as thoracentesis, lumbar puncture, or sigmoidoscopy. The nature, risk, and probable result of the operation or procedure must be made clear to the patient or a legally responsible relative or guardian so that the signed permit will constitute informed consent. A separate anesthesia consent is required. A signed consent is not valid except for the specific operation or procedure for which it was obtained.

Therapeutic abortions and operations that adversely affect the sexual or childbearing functions should usually be undertaken with the concurrence in writing of the marital partner.

Emergency lifesaving operations or procedures may have to be done without a permit. In such cases, every effort should be made to obtain adequate consultation. The situation should be carefully documented in the chart.

Legal and institutional requirements regarding permits vary. It is essential that the physician know and follow local regulations.

Asepsis & Antisepsis in the Prevention of Wound Infection

Protection of the surgical patient from infection is a primary consideration throughout the preoperative, operative, and postoperative phases of care. The factor of host resistance that influences the individual patient's susceptibility to infection has been discussed above. The incidence and severity of infection, particularly wound sepsis, are related also to the bacteriologic status of the hospital environment and to the care with which basic principles of asepsis, antisepsis, and surgical technique are implemented. The entire hospital environment must be protected from undue bacterial contami-

nation in order to avoid colonization and cross-infection of surgical patients with virulent strains of bacteria that will invade surgical wounds in the operating room in spite of aseptic precautions taken during operation. Prevention of wound infection therefore involves both application of general concepts and techniques of antisepsis and asepsis in the hospital at large and the use of specific procedures in preparation for operation.

A. STERILIZATION

The only completely reliable methods of sterilization in wide current use for surgical instruments and supplies are (1) steam under pressure (autoclaving), (2) dry heat, and (3) ethylene oxide gas.

1. Autoclaving—Saturated steam at a pressure of 750 mm Hg (14.5 psi above atmospheric pressure) at a temperature of 120 °C destroys all vegetative bacteria and most resistant dry spores in 13 minutes. Sterilization time is markedly shortened by the high-vacuum or high-pressure autoclaves now widely used.

2. Dry heat—Exposure to continuous dry heat at 170 °C for 1 hour will sterilize articles that would be spoiled by moist heat or are more conveniently kept dry. If grease or oil is present on instruments, safe sterilization calls for 4 hours' exposure at 160 °C.

3. Gas sterilization—Liquid and gaseous ethylene oxide as a sterilizing agent will destroy bacteria, viruses, molds, pathogenic fungi, and spores. It is also flammable and toxic, and it will cause severe burns if it comes in contact with the skin. Gas sterilization with ethylene oxide is an excellent method for sterilization of most heat-sensitive materials, including telescopic instruments, plastic and rubber goods, sharp and delicate instruments, and miscellaneous items such as electric cords and sealed ampules. It has largely replaced soaking in antiseptics as a means of sterilizing materials that cannot withstand autoclaving. Gas sterilization is normally carried out in a pressure vessel (gas autoclave) at slightly elevated pressure and temperature. It requires 1¾ hours for sterilization in a gas autoclave utilizing a mixture of 12% ethylene oxide and 88% dichlorodifluoromethane (Freon 12) at a temperature of 55 °C and a pressure of 410 mm Hg (8 psi above atmospheric pressure). Following sterilization, a variable period of time is required for dissipation of the gas from the materials sterilized. Solid metal or glass items such as knives, drills, and thermometers may be used immediately following sterilization. Lensed instruments and packs including cloth, paper, rubber, and other porous items must usually be kept on the shelf exposed to air for 24–48 hours before use. Certain types of materials or complex instruments, such as a cardiac pacemaker, may require 7 days of exposure to air before use.

B. SKIN ANTISEPTICS

The most important applications of skin antisepsis are the hand scrub of the operating team and the preparation of the operative field.

1. Hand scrub routine—Although the duration of the hand scrub is not universally defined, a 5-minute scrub before the first case—provided a brush is used—appears to be sufficient. Greatest attention should be paid to the fingertips and nails, since these areas harbor the greatest numbers of bacteria. A 2-minute scrub is adequate between cases. Solutions containing chlorhexidine or one of the iodophors appear to be most effective.

2. Preparation of the operative field—Initial preparation of the skin is usually done the afternoon or evening before operation. The area should be washed with soap and water, making sure that it is grossly quite clean. A shower is satisfactory. The type of soap used makes little difference. Soap is a weak antiseptic and is useful because of its nonirritating detergent action, especially when washing is combined with mechanical friction.

For elective operations involving areas with high levels of resident bacteria (eg, hands, feet) or likely to be irritated by strong antiseptics (eg, face, genitalia), preoperative degerming of the skin can be improved by repeated use of chlorhexidine gluconate (Hibiclens). Instruct the patient to wash the area several times daily with one of these preparations (and with nothing else) for 3–5 days before the scheduled day of operation. It has been established that shaving the surgical area the night before or within several hours before surgery increases the skin bacterial flora. Therefore, it is recommended that shaving be performed immediately before the operation, preferably in an adjacent preparation area. Shaving may be eliminated if only fine hairs are present, as their presence has not been found to increase the incidence of infection.

3. In the operating room—A 1-minute skin preparation using either 70% alcohol or 2% iodine in 90% alcohol—followed by a polyester adherent wound drape—has been shown to be as effective in controlling wound infections as the more traditional 5- to 10-minute wound scrub with povidone-iodine.

Iodine is one of the most efficient skin antiseptics available. It rarely causes skin reactions in this concentration. Avoid streaming of iodine outside of the operative field. Do not use iodine on the perineum, genitalia, or face; on irritated or delicate skin (eg, small children); or when the patient has a history of iodine sensitivity. For iodine-sensitive patients, one can use 80% isopropyl or 70% ethyl alcohol. Apply to the skin with a gauze swab for 3 minutes and allow to dry before draping. Alternatively, tinted tincture of benzalkonium (1:750) may be used.

For sensitive areas (perineum, around the eyes, etc), apply iodophor, chlorhexidine, or 1:1000 aqueous benzalkonium solution.

Disease transmission to patients and health care workers—especially with the hepatitis virus and the AIDS virus—is a major problem in the operating room environment. Both can be transmitted to the patient and care providers by blood. Transmission to the surgeon or nurse via a needle or cut is of major concern because of the frequent occurrence of accidental punctures. Since the infected patient cannot readily be detected in the absence of a mandatory preoperative testing program, universal precautions are required, including the following:

a. All health care workers should routinely use appropriate barrier precautions—gloves, masks, goggles, etc—to prevent skin and mucous membrane exposure when contact with blood or body fluids is anticipated.

b. Immediate hand and other skin surface washing is necessary if contamination occurs.

c. Special precautions must be taken to avoid accidental injuries, eg, needle punctures and cuts.

d. Workers who have any open wounds should avoid direct patient contact.

e. If a glove is torn, it should be removed and changed as promptly as patient safety permits and the needle or instrument removed from the sterile field.

C. CONTROL OF HOSPITAL ENVIRONMENT

Hospital cross-infection with hemolytic, coagulase-positive *Staphylococcus aureus* and other organisms is always a potential problem. Strains endemic in hospitals are often resistant to many antimicrobial drugs as a consequence of the widespread use of these agents. Relaxation of aseptic precautions in the operating room and an unwarranted reliance on "prophylactic" antibiotics contribute to the development of resistant strains. The result may be a significant increase in the incidence of hospital-acquired wound infection, pneumonitis, and septicemia, the latter two complications especially affecting infants, the aged, and the debilitated.

Although pyogenic cocci are major offenders, enteric gram-negative bacteria (particularly the coliform and proteus groups and *Pseudomonas aeruginosa*) are increasingly prominent in hospital-acquired infections.

1. Hospital administration

a. The surgical infection control program should be coordinated closely with that of other services through a hospital infection committee set up to promulgate and enforce regulations.

b. All significant infections must be reported immediately. A clean wound infection rate of more than 1% indicates a need for more effective control measures. The wound infection rate should be continuously monitored on the surgical services.

2. Cultures—Obtain culture and antibiotic sensitivity studies on all significant infections.

3. Isolation—Isolate every patient with a significant source of communicable bacteria; every case of suspected communicable infection until the diagnosis has been ruled out; and every patient in whom cross-infection will be serious.

4. Aseptic technique

a. **Operating room**—The operating room should be considered an isolation zone that may be entered only by persons wearing clean operating attire (which may not be worn elsewhere).

b. **Patient unit procedures**—All open wounds should be aseptically dressed to protect them from cross-infection and to prevent heavy contamination of the environment. Eliminate dressing carts containing supplies and equipment for multiple bedside dressings.

c. **Hand washing**—Hand washing before and after each contact with a patient is a simple but important routine measure in control of infection.

5. Antibiotics—Prophylactic antibiotics are indicated for clean contaminated or contaminated cases. Even for clean cases, prophylactic antibiotics appear to decrease the rate of infection. When possible, antibiotic therapy should be based on sensitivity studies. Antibiotics should be given in adequate doses and discontinued as soon as it is appropriate to do so.

6. Epidemiology

a. Personnel with active staphylococcal infections should be excluded from patient contact until they have recovered. Personnel carrying staphylococci in their nasal passages or gastrointestinal tracts must observe personal hygiene but need not be removed from duty unless they prove to be a focus of infection. The advisability of treatment of the carrier is uncertain, since the carrier state is frequently transient or recurrent in spite of treatment.

b. Every significant infection acquired in the hospital should be investigated to determine its origin and spread, possible contacts and carriers, and whether improper techniques may have been responsible.

Postoperative Care

3

Gerard M. Doherty, MD, Sean J. Mulvihill, MD, & Carlos A. Pellegrini, MD

The recovery from major surgery can be divided into three phases: (1) an immediate, or postanesthetic phase; (2) an intermediate phase, encompassing the hospitalization period; and (3) a convalescent phase. During the first two phases, care is principally directed at maintenance of homeostasis, treatment of pain, and prevention and early detection of complications. The convalescent phase is a transition period from the time of hospital discharge to full recovery. The trend toward earlier postoperative discharge after major surgery has added new importance to this period.

THE IMMEDIATE POSTOPERATIVE PERIOD

The major causes of early complications and death following major surgery are acute pulmonary, cardiovascular, and fluid derangements. The postanesthetic recovery room is staffed by specially trained personnel and provided with equipment for early detection and treatment of these problems. All patients undergoing major procedures should be initially monitored in this specialized unit. While en route from the operating room to the recovery room, the patient should be accompanied by a physician and other qualified attendants. In the recovery room, the anesthesiologist generally exercises primary responsibility for the patient's cardiopulmonary function. The surgeon is responsible for the operative site and all other aspects of the patient's care not directly related to the effects of anesthesia. The patient can be discharged from the recovery room when cardiovascular, pulmonary, and neurologic function have returned to baseline, which usually occurs 1–3 hours following operation. Patients who require continuing ventilatory or circulatory support or who have other conditions that require frequent monitoring are transferred to the intensive care unit. In this setting, nursing personnel specially trained in the management of respiratory and cardiovascular emergencies are available, and the staff:patient ratio is higher than it is on the wards. Monitoring equipment is available to ensure early detection of cardiorespiratory derangements.

Postoperative Orders

Detailed treatment orders should be written upon arrival in the recovery room. Unusual or particularly important orders should also be communicated to the nursing team orally. The nursing team must also be advised of the nature of the operation and the patient's condition. Postoperative orders should cover the following:

A. MONITORING

1. Vital signs—Blood pressure, pulse, and respiration should be recorded every 15–30 minutes until stable and then hourly until the patient is discharged from the recovery room. The frequency of vital sign measurements thereafter depends upon the nature of the operation and the patient's course in the recovery room. When an arterial catheter is in place, blood pressure and pulse should be monitored continuously. Continuous electrocardiographic monitoring is indicated for most patients in the recovery room. Any major changes in vital signs should be communicated to the anesthesiologist and surgeon immediately.

2. Central venous pressure—Central venous pressure should be recorded periodically in the early postoperative period if the operation has entailed large blood losses or fluid shifts. A Swan-Ganz catheter for measurement of pulmonary artery wedge pressure is indicated under these conditions if the patient has borderline cardiac or respiratory function.

3. Fluid balance—A record is maintained by the anesthesiologist of all fluid administered and all blood loss and urine output during the operation. This record should be continued in the postoperative period and should also include fluid losses from drains and stomas. This information aids in assessing hydration and guides intravenous fluid replacement. In operations where fluid shifts are great or when renal function is marginal, a bladder catheter should be placed for frequent measurement of urine output. In the absence of a bladder catheter, the surgeon should be notified if the patient is unable to void within 6–8 hours after operation.

4. Other types of monitoring—Depending on the nature of the operation and the patient's preexisting conditions, other types of monitoring may be necessary. Examples include measurement of intracranial pressure and level of consciousness following cranial surgery and monitoring of distal pulses following vascular surgery or in patients with casts.

B. Respiratory Care

In the early postoperative period, the patient may remain mechanically ventilated or treated with supplemental oxygen by mask or nasal prongs. These orders should be specified. In intubated patients, tracheal suctioning or other forms of respiratory therapy should be ordered as required. Patients who are not intubated should be encouraged to take deep breaths frequently to prevent atelectasis.

C. Position in Bed and Mobilization

The postoperative orders should describe any required special positioning of the patient. Unless doing so is contraindicated, the patient should be turned from side to side every 30 minutes until conscious and then hourly for the first 8–12 hours to minimize atelectasis. Early ambulation is encouraged to reduce venous stasis. Venous stasis may also be minimized by intermittent compression of the calf by a pneumatic device (see Chapter 37).

D. Diet

Patients undergoing thoracic or abdominal surgery and critically ill patients should have nothing by mouth until normal gastrointestinal function has returned (usually within 4 days). Other patients usually can tolerate liquids by mouth shortly after full return to consciousness.

E. Administration of Fluid and Electrolytes

Orders for postoperative intravenous fluids should be based on maintenance needs and the replacement of gastrointestinal losses from drains, fistulas, or stomas (see Chapter 10).

F. Drainage Tubes

The care required for drains should be included in the postoperative orders. Details such as type and pressure of suction, irrigation fluid and frequency, and skin exit site care should be specified. The surgeon should examine drains frequently, since the character or quantity of drain output may herald the development of postoperative complications such as bleeding or fistulas.

G. Medications

Orders should be written for antibiotics, analgesics, and sedatives. If appropriate, preoperative medications should be reinstituted. Careful attention should be paid to replacement of corticosteroids in patients at risk, since postoperative adrenal insufficiency may be life-threatening. Gastric stress ulcer prophylaxis with antacids or histamine H_2 receptor antagonists should be considered for patients in the intensive care unit. The incidence of stress ulcer formation is too low to justify the use of these agents routinely after all elective operations. Other medications such as antipyretics, laxatives, and stool softeners should not be ordered routinely but should be used selectively as indicated.

H. Laboratory Examinations and Imaging

The use of postoperative laboratory and radiographic examinations should be aimed at the detection of specific abnormalities in high-risk groups. Routine use of daily chest radiographs, blood counts, electrolytes, and renal or liver function panels is not indicated.

THE INTERMEDIATE POSTOPERATIVE PERIOD

The intermediate phase starts with complete recovery from anesthesia and lasts for the rest of the hospital stay. During this time, the patient recovers most basic functions and becomes self-sufficient and able to continue convalescence at home.

Care of the Wound

Within hours after a wound is closed, the wound space fills with an inflammatory exudate. Epidermal cells at the edges of the wound begin to divide and migrate across the wound surface. By 48 hours after closure, deeper structures are completely sealed off from the external environment. Sterile dressings applied in the operating room provide protection during this period. Dressings over closed wounds should be removed on the third or fourth postoperative day. If the wound is dry, dressings need not be reapplied; this simplifies periodic inspection. Dressings should be removed earlier if they are wet, because soaked dressings increase bacterial contamination of the wound. Dressings should also be removed if the patient has manifestations of infection (eg, fever, unusual wound pain). The wound should then be inspected and the adjacent area gently compressed. Any drainage from the wound should be examined by culture and Gram-stained smear. Removal of the dressing and handling of the wound during the first 24 hours should be done with aseptic technique. Medical personnel should wash their hands before and after caring for any surgical wound. Gloves should always be used when there is contact with open wounds or fresh wounds.

Generally, skin sutures or skin staples may be removed by the fifth or sixth postoperative day and replaced by tapes. Sutures should be left in longer (eg, for 2 weeks) with incisions across creases (eg, groin, popliteal area); with incisions closed under tension; with some incisions in the extremities (eg, the hand); and with incisions of any kind in debilitated patients. Sutures should be removed if suture tracts show signs of infection. If the incision is healing normally, the patient may be allowed to take a shower or bath by the seventh postoperative day.

Fibroblasts proliferate in the wound space quickly, and by the end of the first postoperative week, new collagen is abundant in the wound. On palpation of the wound, connective tissue can be felt as a prominence (the healing ridge) and is evidence that healing is normal. Tensile strength is minimal for the first 5 days. It increases rapidly between the fifth and twentieth postoperative days and more slowly thereafter. Wounds continue to gain tensile strength slowly for about 2 years. In otherwise healthy patients, the wound should be subjected to only minor stress for 6–8 weeks. When wound healing is expected to be slower than normal (eg, in elderly or debilitated patients or those taking corticosteroids), activity should be delayed even further.

Adequate tissue perfusion is important for wound healing. In a patient with venous stasis, for example, tissue perfusion will increase, and a wound of the lower extremity will heal faster if the extremity is elevated and edema is eliminated. Oxygen tension has a profound effect on healing tissue. Indolent healing in an amputation stump may be substantially improved by arterial surgery that increases blood supply to the extremity.

When a wound has been contaminated with bacteria during surgery, it is often best to leave the skin and subcutaneous tissues open and either to perform delayed primary closure or allow secondary closure to occur. The wound is loosely packed with fine-mesh gauze in the operating room and is left undisturbed for 4–5 days; the packing is then removed. If at this time the wound contains only serous fluid or a small amount of exudate, the skin edges can be approximated with tapes. If drainage is considerable or infection is present, the wound should be allowed to close by secondary intention. In this case, the wound should be packed with moist-to-dry dressings, which are changed once or twice daily. The patient can usually learn how to care for the wound and should be discharged as soon as his or her general condition permits. Most patients do not require visiting nurses to assist with wound care at home.

Wound healing is faster if the state of nutrition is normal and there are no specific nutritional deficits. For example, vitamin C deficiency interferes with collagen synthesis and vitamin A deficiency decreases the rate of epithelialization. Deficiencies of copper, magnesium, and other trace metals decrease the rate of scar formation. Supplemental vitamins and minerals should be given postoperatively when deficiencies are suspected, but wound healing cannot be accelerated beyond the normal rate by nutritional supplements.

Wound problems should be anticipated in patients taking corticosteroids, which inhibit the inflammatory response, fibroblast proliferation, and protein synthesis

in the wound. Maturation of the scar and gain of tensile strength occur more slowly. Extra precautions include using nonabsorbable suture materials for fascial closure, delaying removal of skin stitches, and avoiding stress in the wound for 3–6 months.

Management of Drains

Drains are used either to prevent or to treat an unwanted accumulation of fluid such as pus, blood, or serum. Drains are also used to evacuate air from the pleural cavity so that the lungs can reexpand. When used prophylactically, drains are usually placed in a sterile location. Strict precautions must be taken to prevent bacteria from entering the body through the drainage tract in these situations. The external portion of the drain must be handled with aseptic technique, and the drain must be removed as soon as it is no longer useful. When drains have been placed in an infected area, there is a smaller risk of retrograde infection of the peritoneal cavity, since the infected area is usually walled off. Drains should usually be brought out through a separate incision, because drains through the operative wound increase the risk of wound infection.

Soft latex drains are held in place by skin stitches and are prevented from slipping into the abdominal cavity by a safety pin placed through the external part of the drain or a suture between the drain and the skin. If the amount of drainage is expected to be more than about 50 mL every 8 hours, a bag should be placed over the drain site. The quantity and quality of drainage may be noted, and contamination is minimized. If drainage is scant, drains may be covered with a dressing, which should be changed often enough to prevent it from becoming soaked through or at least once every 24 hours. When drains are no longer needed, they may be withdrawn entirely at one time if there has been little or no drainage or may be progressively withdrawn over a period of a few days. Penrose drains should not be left in place longer than about 14 days, since at this point the drain tract will begin to firm up and a soft pliable drain will act as a plug. If drains are needed for more than 2 weeks, soft drains should be replaced with rubber catheters, which can be irrigated periodically.

Closed drainage is possible with a firm catheter that passes through a small, snug hole in the skin. Closed drainage minimizes retrograde movement of bacteria from the external environment into the area being drained. Flow through the tube may be aided with suction, but unless a sump tube is used, the drain often becomes plugged if drainage is thicker than a thin serous fluid. Closed drainage is ideal when drainage is serous and in a location especially vulnerable to infection (eg, the subcutaneous space after mastectomy). Rigid tubes in the abdomen may erode into adjacent intestine after approximately 4 weeks and should therefore be positioned carefully during surgery.

Sump drains have an airflow system that keeps the lumen of the drain open when fluid is not passing through it, and they must be attached to a suction device. Sump drains are especially useful when the amount of drainage is large or when drainage is likely to plug other kinds of drains. Some sump drains have an extra lumen through which saline solution can be infused to aid in keeping the tube clear. After infection has been controlled and the discharge is no longer purulent, the large-bore catheter is progressively replaced with smaller catheters, and the cavity eventually closes.

Postoperative Pulmonary Care

The changes in pulmonary function observed following anesthesia and surgery are principally the result of decreased vital capacity, functional residual capacity (FRC), and pulmonary edema. Vital capacity decreases to about 40% of the preoperative level within 1–4 hours after major intra-abdominal surgery. It remains at this level for 12–14 hours, slowly increases to 60–70% of the preoperative value by 7 days, and returns to the baseline level during the ensuing week. FRC is affected to a lesser extent. Immediately after surgery, FRC is near the preoperative level, but by 24 hours postoperatively it has decreased to about 70% of the preoperative level. It remains depressed for several days and then gradually returns to its preoperative value by the tenth day. These changes are accentuated in patients who are obese, who smoke heavily, or who have preexisting lung disease. Elderly patients are particularly vulnerable because they have decreased compliance, increased closing volume, increased residual volume, and increased dead space, all of which enhance the risk of postoperative atelectasis. In addition, reduced FEV_1 impairs the aged patient's ability to clear secretions and increases the chance of infection postoperatively.

The postoperative decrease in FRC is caused by a breathing pattern consisting of shallow tidal breaths without periodic maximal inflation. Normal human respiration includes inspiration to total lung capacity several times each hour. If these maximal inflations are eliminated, alveolar collapse begins to occur within a few hours and atelectasis with transpulmonary shunting is evident shortly thereafter. Pain is thought to be one of the main causes of shallow breathing postoperatively. Complete abolition of pain, however, does not completely restore pulmonary function. Neural reflexes, abdominal distention, obesity, and other factors that limit diaphragmatic excursion appear to be as important.

The principal means of minimizing atelectasis is deep inspiration. Periodic hyperinflation can be facilitated by using an incentive spirometer. This is particu-

larly useful in patients with a higher risk of pulmonary complications (eg, elderly, debilitated, or markedly obese patients). Intermittent positive-pressure breathing (IPPB) has lost popularity because it is expensive and no more effective than simpler measures. Early mobilization, encouragement to take deep breaths (especially when standing), and good coaching by the nursing staff suffice for most patients.

Postoperative pulmonary edema is caused by high hydrostatic pressures (due to left ventricular failure, fluid overload, decreased oncotic pressure, etc), increased capillary permeability, or both. Edema of the lung parenchyma narrows small bronchi and increases resistance in the pulmonary vasculature. In addition, pulmonary edema may increase the risk of pulmonary infection. Adequate management of fluids postoperatively and early treatment of cardiac failure are important preventive measures.

Systemic sepsis increases capillary permeability and leads to pulmonary edema. In the absence of deranged cardiac function or fluid overload, the development of pulmonary edema postoperatively should be regarded as evidence of sepsis.

RESPIRATORY FAILURE

Most patients tolerate the postoperative changes in pulmonary function described above and recover from them without difficulty. Patients who have marginal preoperative pulmonary function may be unable to maintain adequate ventilation in the immediate postoperative period and may develop respiratory failure. In these patients, the operative trauma and the effects of anesthesia reduce respiratory reserve below levels that can provide adequate gas exchange. In contrast to acute respiratory distress syndrome (see Chapter 13), early postoperative respiratory failure (which develops within 48 hours after the operation) is usually only a mechanical problem, ie, there are minimal alterations of the lung parenchyma. However, this problem is life-threatening and requires immediate attention.

Early respiratory failure develops most commonly in association with major operations (especially on the chest or upper abdomen), severe trauma, and preexisting lung disease. In most of these patients, respiratory failure develops over a short period (minutes to 1–2 hours) without evidence of a precipitating cause. By contrast, late postoperative respiratory failure (which develops beyond 48 hours after the operation) is usually triggered by an intercurrent event such as pulmonary embolism, abdominal distention, or opioid overdose.

Respiratory failure is manifested by tachypnea above 25–30 breaths per minute with a low tidal volume of less than 4 mL/kg. Laboratory indications are acute elevation of PCO_2 above 45 mm Hg, depression of PO_2

below 60 mm Hg, or evidence of low cardiac output. Treatment consists of immediate endotracheal intubation and ventilatory support with a volume ventilator to ensure adequate alveolar ventilation. As soon as the patient is intubated, it is important to determine whether there are any associated pulmonary problems such as atelectasis, pneumonia, or pneumothorax that require immediate treatment.

Prevention of respiratory failure requires careful postoperative pulmonary care. Atelectasis must be minimized using the techniques described above. Patients with preexisting pulmonary disease must be carefully hydrated to avoid hypovolemia. These patients must hyperventilate in order to compensate for the inefficiency of the lungs. This extra work causes greater evaporation of water and dehydration. Hypovolemia leads to dry secretions and thick sputum, which are difficult to clear from the airway. High FIO_2 in these patients removes the stabilizing gas N_2 from the alveoli, predisposing to alveolar collapse. In addition, it may impair the function of the respiratory center, which is driven by the relative hypoxemia, and thus further decrease ventilation. The use of epidural blocks or other methods of local analgesia in patients with COPD may prevent respiratory failure by relieving pain and permitting effective respiratory muscle function.

Postoperative Fluid & Electrolyte Management

Postoperative fluid replacement should be based on the following considerations: (1) maintenance requirements, (2) extra needs resulting from systemic factors (eg, fever, burns), (3) losses from drains, and (4) requirements resulting from tissue edema and ileus (third space losses). Daily maintenance requirements for sensible and insensible loss in the adult are about 1500–2500 mL depending on the patient's age, sex, weight, and body surface area. A rough estimate can be obtained by multiplying the patient's weight in kilograms

times 30 (eg, 1800 mL/24 h in a 60-kg patient). Maintenance requirements are increased by fever, hyperventilation, and conditions that increase the catabolic rate.

For patients requiring intravenous fluid replacement for a short period (most postoperative patients), it is not necessary to measure serum electrolytes at any time during the postoperative period, but measurement is indicated in complicated cases (patients with extra fluid losses, sepsis, preexisting electrolyte abnormalities, or other factors). Assessment of the status of fluid balance requires accurate records of fluid intake and output and is aided by weighing the patient daily.

As a rule, 2000–2500 mL of 5% dextrose in normal saline or in lactated Ringer's solution is given daily. Potassium should usually not be added during the first 24 hours after surgery, because increased amounts of potassium enter the circulation during this time as a result of operative trauma and increased aldosterone activity.

In most patients, fluid loss through a nasogastric tube is less than 500 mL/d and can be replaced by increasing the infusion used for maintenance by a similar amount. About 20 meq of potassium should be added to every liter of fluid used to replace these losses. One must remember, however, that with the exception of urine, body fluids are isosmolar and that if large volumes of gastric or intestinal juice are replaced with normal saline solution, electrolyte imbalance will eventually result. Whenever external losses from any site amount to 1500 mL/d or more, electrolyte concentrations in the fluid should be measured periodically, and the amount of replacement fluids should be adjusted to equal the amount lost. Table 3–1 lists the compositions of the most frequently used solutions.

Losses that result from fluid sequestration at the operative site are usually adequately replaced during operation, but in a patient with a large retroperitoneal dissection, severe pancreatitis, etc, third space losses may be substantial and should be considered when postoperative fluids are given.

Table 3–1. Composition of frequently used intravenous solutions.

Solution	Glucose (g/dL)	Na$^+$ (meq/L)	Cl$^-$ (meq/L)	HCO$_3^-$ (meq/L)	K$^+$ (meq/L)
Dextrose 5% in water	50	...	...	...	...
Dextrose 5% and sodium chloride 0.45%	50	77	77	...	...
Sodium chloride 0.9%	...	154	154	...	...
Sodium chloride 0.45%	...	77	77	...	...
Lactated Ringer's solution	...	130	109	28	4
Sodium chloride 3%	...	513	513	...	...

Fluid requirements must be evaluated frequently. Intravenous orders should be rewritten every 24 hours or more often if indicated by special circumstances. Following an extensive operation, fluid needs on the first day should be reevaluated every 4–6 hours. Other aspects of fluid and electrolyte therapy are discussed in Chapter 10. Postoperative nutrition is discussed in Chapter 11.

Postoperative Care of the Gastrointestinal Tract

Following laparotomy, gastrointestinal peristalsis temporarily decreases. Peristalsis returns in the small intestine within 24 hours, but gastric peristalsis returns more slowly. Function returns in the right colon by 48 hours and in the left colon by 72 hours. After operations on the stomach and upper intestine, propulsive activity of the upper gut remains disorganized for 3–4 days. In the immediate postoperative period, the stomach may be decompressed with a nasogastric tube. Nasogastric intubation was once used in almost all patients undergoing laparotomy to avoid gastric distention and vomiting, but it is now recognized that routine nasogastric intubation is unnecessary and may cause postoperative atelectasis and pneumonia. For example, following cholecystectomy, pelvic operations, and colonic resections, nasogastric intubation is not needed in the average patient, and it is probably of marginal benefit following operations on the small bowel. On the other hand, nasogastric intubation is probably useful after esophageal and gastric resections and should always be used in patients with marked ileus or a very low level of consciousness (to avoid aspiration) and in patients who manifest acute gastric distention or vomiting postoperatively.

The nasogastric tube should be connected to low intermittent suction and irrigated frequently to ensure patency. The tube should be left in place for 2–3 days or until there is evidence that normal peristalsis has returned (eg, return of appetite, audible peristalsis, or passage of flatus). The nasogastric tube enhances gastroesophageal reflux, and if it is clamped overnight for assessment of residual volume, there is a slight risk of aspiration.

Once the nasogastric tube has been withdrawn, fasting is usually continued for another 24 hours, and the patient is then started on a liquid diet. Opioids may interfere with gastric motility and should be stopped in patients who have evidence of gastroparesis beyond the first postoperative week.

Gastrostomy and jejunostomy tubes should be connected to low intermittent suction or dependent drainage for the first 24 hours after surgery. Absorption of nutrients and fluids by the small intestine is not affected by laparotomy, and enteral nutrition through a jejunostomy feeding tube may therefore be started on the second postoperative day even if motility is not entirely normal. Gastrostomy or jejunostomy tubes should not be removed before the third postoperative week, because firm adhesions should be allowed to develop between the viscera and the parietal peritoneum.

After most operations in areas other than the peritoneal cavity, the patient may be allowed to resume a regular diet as soon as the effects of anesthesia have completely worn off.

Postoperative Pain

Severe pain is a common sequela of intrathoracic, intra-abdominal, and major bone or joint procedures. About 60% of such patients perceive their pain to be severe, 25% moderate, and 15% mild. In contrast, following superficial operations on the head and neck, limbs, or abdominal wall, less than 15% of patients characterize their pain as severe. The factors responsible for these differences include duration of surgery, degree of operative trauma, type of incision, and magnitude of intraoperative retraction. Gentle handling of tissues, expedient operations, and good muscle relaxation help lessen the severity of postoperative pain.

While factors related to the nature of the operation influence postoperative pain, it is also true that the same operation produces different amounts of pain in different patients. This varies according to individual physical, emotional, and cultural characteristics. Much of the emotional aspect of pain can be traced to anxiety. Feelings such as helplessness, fear, and uncertainty contribute to anxiety and may heighten the patient's perception of pain.

It was once thought that anesthesia and analgesia in neonates and infants was too risky and that these young patients did not perceive pain. It is now known that reduction of pain with appropriate techniques actually decreases morbidity from major surgery in this age group.

The physiology of postoperative pain involves transmission of pain impulses via splanchnic (not vagal) afferent fibers to the central nervous system, where they initiate spinal, brain stem, and cortical reflexes. Spinal responses result from stimulation of neurons in the anterior horn, resulting in skeletal muscle spasm, vasospasm, and gastrointestinal ileus. Brain stem responses to pain include alterations in ventilation, blood pressure, and endocrine function. Cortical responses include voluntary movements and psychologic changes, such as fear and apprehension. These emotional responses facilitate nociceptive spinal transmission, lower the threshold for pain perception, and perpetuate the pain experience.

Postoperative pain serves no useful purpose and may cause alterations in pulmonary, circulatory, gastrointestinal, and skeletal muscle function that set the stage for postoperative complications. Pain following thoracic and upper abdominal operations, for example, causes voluntary and involuntary splinting of thoracic and abdominal muscles and the diaphragm. The patient may be reluctant to breathe deeply, promoting atelectasis. The limitation in motion due to pain sets the stage for venous stasis, thrombosis, and embolism. Release of catecholamines and other stress hormones by postoperative pain causes vasospasm and hypertension, which may in turn lead to complications such as stroke, myocardial infarction, and bleeding. Prevention of postoperative pain is thus important for reasons other than the pain itself. Effective pain control may improve the outcome of major operations.

A. PHYSICIAN-PATIENT COMMUNICATION

Close attention to the patient's needs, frequent reassurance, and genuine concern help minimize postoperative pain. Spending a few minutes with the patient every day in frank discussions of progress and any complications does more to relieve pain than many physicians realize.

B. PARENTERAL OPIOIDS

Opioids administered intramuscularly are the mainstay of therapy for postoperative pain. Their analgesic effect is via two mechanisms: (1) a direct effect on opioid receptors and (2) stimulation of a descending brain stem system that contributes to pain inhibition. Although substantial relief of pain may be achieved with opioids, they do not modify reflex phenomena associated with pain, such as muscle spasm. Opioids administered intramuscularly, while convenient, result in wide variations in plasma concentrations. This, as well as the wide variations in dosage required for analgesia among patients, reduces analgesic efficacy. Physician and nurse attitudes reflect a persistent misunderstanding of the pharmacology and psychology of pain control. Frequently, the dose of opioid prescribed or administered is too small and too infrequent. When opioid usage is limited to temporary treatment of postoperative pain, drug addiction is extremely rare.

Morphine is the most widely used opioid for treatment of postoperative pain. Adequate pain relief with minimal side effects is achieved in about two-thirds of patients with severe pain following an intramuscular dose of 10 mg. The remaining one-third of patients require higher doses. Peak analgesic effect is achieved in 1–2 hours after intramuscular injection. The recommended dosing interval is every 3–4 hours.

Morphine may also be administered intravenously, either intermittently or continuously. Except as discussed below in the section on patient-controlled analgesia, these last methods require close supervision and are impractical except in the recovery room or intensive care unit. Side effects of morphine include respiratory depression, nausea and vomiting, and clouded sensorium. In the setting of severe postoperative pain, however, respiratory depression is rare, because pain itself is a powerful respiratory stimulant.

Meperidine is an opioid with about one-eighth the potency of morphine. It provides a similar quality of pain control with similar side effects. The usual dosage of meperidine in the treatment of severe pain is 75–100 mg intramuscularly. The duration of pain relief is somewhat shorter than with morphine. The dosing interval should be no longer than every 3 hours. Like morphine, meperidine may be given intravenously, but the same requirements for monitoring apply.

Other opioids useful for postoperative analgesia include hydromorphone and methadone. Hydromorphone is usually administered in a dose of 1–2 mg intramuscularly every 2–3 hours. Methadone is given intramuscularly or orally in an average dose of 10 mg every 4–6 hours. The main advantage of methadone is its long half-life (6–10 hours) and its ability to prevent withdrawal symptoms in patients with morphine dependence.

C. NONOPIOID PARENTERAL ANALGESICS

Ketorolac tromethamine is a nonsteroidal anti-inflammatory drug (NSAID) with potent analgesic and moderate anti-inflammatory activities. It is available in injectable form suitable for postoperative use. In controlled trials, ketorolac (30 mg) has demonstrated analgesic efficacy roughly equivalent to that of morphine (10 mg). A potential advantage over morphine is its lack of respiratory depression. Gastrointestinal ulceration, impaired coagulation, and reduced renal function—all potential complications of NSAID use—have not yet been reported with short-term perioperative use of ketorolac.

D. OTHER AGENTS

Hydroxyzine is an anxiolytic and ataractic occasionally useful as an adjunct to potent opioids for postoperative pain. Hydroxyzine potentiates the analgesic (and respiratory depressant) properties of morphine. It produces a calming effect and has antiemetic properties.

E. ORAL ANALGESICS

Within several days following most abdominal surgical procedures, the severity of pain decreases to a point where oral analgesics suffice. Aspirin should be avoided as an analgesic postoperatively, since it interferes with platelet function, prolongs bleeding time, and interferes with the effects of anticoagulants. For most patients, a combination of acetaminophen with codeine (eg, Tylenol No. 3) or propoxyphene (Darvocet-N 50 or -N 100) suffices. Hydrocodone with acetaminophen (Vicodin) is a synthetic opioid with properties similar to those of codeine. For more severe pain, oxycodone is available in combination with aspirin (Percodan) or acetaminophen (Percocet, Tylox). Oxycodone is an opioid with slightly less potency than morphine. As with all opioids, tolerance develops with long-term use.

F. Patient-Controlled Analgesia

Prospective surveys of postoperative patients indicate that up to 40% have inadequate analgesia with conventional techniques such as intermittent subcutaneous opioid injections. This prompted the development of patient-controlled analgesia (PCA), which puts the frequency of analgesic administration under the patient's control but within safe limits. A device containing a timing unit, a pump, and the analgesic medication is connected to an intravenous line. By pressing a button, the patient delivers a predetermined dose of analgesic (usually morphine, 1–3 mg). The timing unit prevents overdosage by interposing an inactivation period (usually 6 minutes) between patient-initiated doses. The possibility of overdosage is also limited by the fact that the patient must be awake in order to search for and push the button that delivers the morphine. The dose and timing can be changed by medical personnel to accommodate the needs of the patient. This method appears to improve pain control and even reduces the total dose of opioid given in a 24-hour period. The addition of a background continuous infusion to the patient-directed administration of analgesic appears to offer no advantage over PCA alone.

G. Continuous Epidural Analgesia

Opioids are also effective when administered directly into the epidural space. Topical morphine does not depress proprioceptive pathways in the dorsal horn, but it does affect nociceptive pathways by interacting with opioid receptors. Therefore, epidural opioids produce intense, prolonged segmental analgesia with relatively less respiratory depression or sympathetic, motor, or other sensory disturbances. In comparison with parenteral administration, epidural administration requires similar dosage for control of pain, has a slightly delayed onset of action, provides substantially longer pain relief, and is associated with better preservation of pulmonary function. Epidural morphine is usually administered as a continuous infusion at a rate of 0.2–0.8 mg/h with or without the addition of 0.25% bupivacaine. Analgesia produced by this technique is superior to that of intravenous or intramuscular opioids. Patients managed in this way are more alert and have better gastrointestinal function. Side effects of continuous epidural adminis-

tration of morphine include pruritus, nausea, and urinary retention. Respiratory depression may occur. Because the patient is unable to urinate, bladder catheterization is almost always required.

H. Intercostal Block

Intercostal block may be used to decrease pain following thoracic and abdominal operations. Since the block does not include the visceral afferents, it does not relieve pain completely, but it does eliminate muscle spasm induced by cutaneous pain and helps to restore respiratory function. It does not carry the risk of hypotension—as does continuous epidural analgesia—and it produces analgesia for periods of 3–12 hours. The main disadvantage of intercostal blocks is the risk of pneumothorax and the need for repeated injections. These problems can be minimized by placing a catheter in the intercostal space or in the pleura through which a continuous infusion of bupivacaine 0.5% is delivered at a rate of 3–8 mL/h.

REFERENCES

Wound Healing

Clark MA, Plank LD, Hill GL: Wound healing associated with severe surgical illness. World J Surg 2000;24:648.

Hunt TK, Hopf HW: Wound healing and wound infection. What surgeons and anesthesiologists can do. Surg Clin North Am 1997;77:587.

Singer AJ, Clark RA: Cutaneous wound healing. N Engl J Med 1999;341:738.

Wilmore DW: Metabolic response to severe surgical illness: overview. World J Surg 2000;24:705.

Witte MB, Barbul A: General principles of wound healing. Surg Clin North Am 1997;77:509.

Fluid Therapy

Kim PK, Deutschman CS: Inflammatory responses and mediators. Surg Clin North Am 2000;80:885.

Plank LD, Hill GL: Sequential metabolic changes following induction of systemic inflammatory response in patients with severe sepsis or major blunt trauma. World J Surg 2000;24:630.

Rooke GA: Autonomic and cardiovascular function in the geriatric patient. Anesthesiol Clin North Am 2000;18:31.

Pain

Austrup ML, Korean G: Analgesic agents for the postoperative period. Opioids. Surg Clin North Am 1999;79:253.

Buggy DJ, Smith G: Epidural anaesthesia and analgesia: better outcome after major surgery? Growing evidence suggests so. BMJ 1999;319:530.

Etches RC: Patient-controlled analgesia. Surg Clin North Am 1999;79:297.

Grass JA: The role of epidural anesthesia and analgesia in postoperative outcome. Anesthesiol Clin North Am 2000;18:407.

Krauss B, Green SM: Sedation and analgesia for procedures in children. N Engl J Med 2000;342:938.

Power I, Barratt S: Analgesic agents for the postoperative period. Nonopioids. Surg Clin North Am 1999;79:275.

Rawal N: Epidural and spinal agents for postoperative analgesia. Surg Clin North Am 1999;79:313.

Sorkin LS, Wallace MS: Acute pain mechanisms. Surg Clin North Am 1999;79:213.

Wiklund RA, Rosenbaum SH: Anesthesiology. First of two parts. N Engl J Med 1997;337:1132.

Wiklund RA, Rosenbaum SH: Anesthesiology. Second of two parts. N Engl J Med 1997;337:1215.

Postoperative Complications*

4

Gerard M. Doherty, MD, Sean J. Mulvihill, MD, & Carlos A. Pellegrini, MD

Postoperative complications may result from the primary disease, the operation, or unrelated factors. Occasionally, one complication will result from another previous one (eg, myocardial infarction following massive postoperative bleeding). The usual clinical signs of disease are often blurred in the postoperative period. Early detection of postoperative complications requires repeated evaluation of the patient by the operating surgeon and other team members.

Prevention of complications starts in the preoperative period with evaluation of the patient's disease and risk factors. Efforts should be made to improve the health of the patient before surgery. For example, cessation of smoking for 6 weeks before surgery decreases the incidence of postoperative pulmonary complications from 50% to 10%. Correction of gross obesity decreases intra-abdominal pressure and the risk of wound and respiratory complications and improves ventilation postoperatively.

The surgeon should explain the operation and the expected postoperative course to the patient at this time. The preoperative hospital stay, if one is necessary, should be as short as possible both to reduce costs and to minimize exposure to antibiotic-resistant microorganisms. Adequate training in respiratory exercises should be provided, as this substantially decreases the incidence of postoperative pulmonary complications. At operation, good technique practiced by a disciplined team is critical to the prevention of complications.

Early mobilization, proper respiratory care, and careful attention to fluid and electrolyte needs are important postoperatively. On the evening after surgery the patient should be encouraged to sit up, cough, breathe deeply, and walk. The upright position permits expansion of basilar lung segments, and walking increases the circulation of the lower extremities and lessens the danger of venous thromboembolism. In severely ill patients, complications may be avoided by continuous monitoring of systemic blood pressure and cardiac performance. Other aspects of prevention of complications are discussed in Chapters 3 and 5.

---

* Coagulation disorders and postoperative renal failure are discussed in Chapter 5, postoperative wound infection and other aspects of wound sepsis in Chapter 9, acute respiratory distress syndrome in Chapter 13, and pulmonary embolism in Chapter 37.

WOUND COMPLICATIONS

Hematoma

Wound hematoma, a collection of blood and clot in the wound, is one of the most common wound complications and is almost always caused by imperfect hemostasis. Patients receiving aspirin or minidose heparin have a slightly higher risk of developing this complication. The risk is much higher in patients who have been given anticoagulants and those with preexisting coagulopathies. Vigorous coughing or marked arterial hypertension immediately after surgery may contribute to the formation of a wound hematoma.

Hematomas produce elevation and discoloration of the wound edges, discomfort, and swelling. Blood sometimes leaks through skin sutures. Neck hematomas following operations on the thyroid, parathyroid, carotid artery, etc, are particularly dangerous, because they may expand rapidly and deviate the trachea. Hematomas in this area must be evacuated early, before ventilation is compromised. Small hematomas may resorb, but they increase the incidence of wound infection. Treatment in most cases consists of evacuation of the clot under sterile conditions, ligation of bleeding vessels, and reclosure of the wound.

Seroma

A seroma is a fluid collection in the wound other than pus or blood. Seromas often follow operations that involve elevation of skin flaps and transection of numerous lymphatic channels (eg, mastectomy, operations in the groin). Seromas delay healing and increase the risk of wound infection. Those located under skin flaps can usually be evacuated by needle aspiration. Compression dressings should then be applied to seal lymphatic leaks and prevent reaccumulation. Small seromas that recur may be treated by evacuation and injection of tetracycline (1 g in 150 mL saline) as a sclerosant solution. Seromas of the groin, which are common after vascular operations, are best left alone, since the risks of introducing a needle (infection, disruption of vascular structures, etc) are greater than the risk associated with the seroma itself. If seromas persist—or if they start leaking through the wound after several days—the wound should be explored in the operating room and the lymphatics ligated.

3

Wound Dehiscence

Wound dehiscence is partial or total disruption of any or all layers of the operative wound. Rupture of all layers of the abdominal wall and extrusion of abdominal viscera is called evisceration. Wound dehiscence occurs in 1–3% of abdominal surgical procedures. Systemic and local factors contribute to the development of this complication.

A. SYSTEMIC RISK FACTORS

Dehiscence is rare in patients under age 30 but affects about 5% of patients over age 60 having laparotomy. It is more common in patients with diabetes mellitus, uremia, immunosuppression, jaundice, sepsis, hypoalbuminemia, and cancer; in obese patients; and in those receiving corticosteroids.

B. LOCAL RISK FACTORS

The three most important local factors predisposing to wound dehiscence are inadequate closure, increased intra-abdominal pressure, and deficient wound healing. Dehiscences often result from a combination of these factors rather than from a single one. The kind of incision (transverse, longitudinal, etc) does not influence the incidence of dehiscence.

1. Adequacy of closure—This is the single most important factor. The fascial layers give strength to a closure, and when fascia disrupts, the wound separates. Accurate approximation of anatomic layers is essential for adequate wound closure. Most wounds undergo dehiscence because the sutures cut through the fascia. Prevention of this problem includes performing a neat incision, avoiding devitalization of the fascial edges by careful handling of tissues during the operation, placing and tying sutures correctly, and selecting the proper suture material. Sutures must be placed 2–3 cm from the wound edge and about 1 cm apart. *Dehiscence is often the result of using too few stitches and placing them too close to the edge of the fascia.* It is unusual for dehiscence to recur following reclosure, implying that adequate closure was technically possible at the initial procedure. In patients with risk factors for dehiscence, the surgeon should "do the second closure at the first operation," ie, take extra care to prevent dehiscence. Modern synthetic suture materials (polyglycolic acid, polypropylene, and others) are clearly superior to catgut for fascial closure. In infected wounds, polypropylene sutures are more resistant to degradation than polyglycolic acid sutures and have lower rates of wound disruption. Wound complications are decreased by obliteration of dead space. Ostomies and drains should be brought out through separate stab incisions to reduce the rate of wound infection and disruption.

2. Intra-abdominal pressure—After any intra-abdominal operation, some degree of ileus is inevitable. High abdominal pressures may occur in patients with chronic obstructive pulmonary disease who use their abdominal muscles as accessory muscles of respiration. In addition, coughing produces sudden increases in intra-abdominal pressure. Other factors contributing to increased abdominal pressure are postoperative bowel obstruction, obesity, and cirrhosis with ascites formation. Extra precautions are necessary to avoid dehiscence in such patients.

3. Deficient wound healing—Infection is an associated factor in more than half of wounds that rupture. The presence of drains, seromas, and wound hematomas also delays healing. Normally, a "healing ridge" (a palpable thickening extending about 0.5 cm on each side of the incision) appears near the end of the first week after surgery. The presence of this ridge is clinical proof that healing is adequate, and it is invariably absent from wounds that rupture.

C. DIAGNOSIS AND MANAGEMENT

Although wound dehiscence may occur at any time following wound closure, it is most commonly observed between the fifth and eighth postoperative days, when the strength of the wound is at a minimum. Wound dehiscence may occasionally be the first manifestation of an intra-abdominal abscess. The first sign of dehiscence is discharge of serosanguineous fluid from the wound or, in some cases, sudden evisceration. The patient often describes a popping sensation associated with severe coughing or retching. Thoracic wounds, with the exception of sternal wounds, are much less prone to dehiscence than are abdominal wounds. When a thoracotomy closure ruptures, it is heralded by leakage of pleural fluid or air and paradoxic motion of the chest wall. Sternal dehiscences, which are almost always associated with infection, produce an unstable chest and require early treatment. If infection is not overwhelming and there is minimal osteomyelitis of the adjacent sternum, the patient may be returned to the operating room for reclosure. Continuous mediastinal irrigation through small tubes left at the time of closure appears to reduce the failure rate. In cases of overwhelming infection, the wound is best treated by debridement and closure with a pectoralis major flap, which increases vascular supply to the area.

Patients with dehiscence of a laparotomy wound and evisceration should be returned to bed and the wound covered with moist towels. With the patient under general anesthesia, any exposed bowel or omentum should be rinsed with lactated Ringer's solution containing antibiotics and then returned to the abdomen. After mechanical cleansing and copious irrigation of the wound, the previous sutures should be removed and the wound reclosed using additional measures to prevent recurrent dehiscence, such as full-thickness retention sutures of No. 22 wire or heavy nylon. Evisceration carries a 10% mortality rate due both to contributing factors (eg, sepsis and cancer) and to resulting local infections.

Wound dehiscence without evisceration is best managed by prompt elective reclosure of the incision. If a partial disruption (ie, the skin is intact) is stable and the patient is a poor operative risk, treatment may be delayed and the resulting incisional hernia accepted. It is important in these patients that skin stitches not be removed before the end of the second postoperative week and that the abdomen be wrapped with a binder or corset to prevent further enlargement of the fascial defect or sudden disruption of the covering skin. When partial dehiscence is discovered during treatment of a wound infection, repair should be delayed if possible until the infection has been controlled, the wound has healed, and 6–7 months have elapsed. In these cases, antibiotics specific for the organisms isolated from the previous wound infection must be given at the time of hernia repair.

Recurrence of evisceration after reclosure of disrupted wounds is rare, though incisional hernias are later found in about 20% of such patients—usually those with wound infection in addition to dehiscence.

Miscellaneous Problems of the Operative Wound

Every new operative wound is painful, but those subject to continuous motion (eg, incisions that cross the costal margin) may be more painful than others. In general, the pain of an operative wound decreases substantially during the first 4–6 postoperative days. Chronic pain localized to one portion of an apparently healed wound may indicate the presence of a stitch abscess, a granuloma, or an occult incisional hernia. Abnormalities on examination of the wound usually allow for easy diagnosis; when this is difficult, ultrasound scanning may help detect a fascial defect or a collection of fluid associated with granulomas or abscesses. Rarely, a neuroma in the wound is responsible for focal pain and tenderness late in the postoperative course. Persistent localized pain is best treated by exploring the area, usually under local anesthesia, and removing a stitch, draining an abscess, or closing a hernia defect. Small sinus tracts usually result from stitch abscesses. The infected stitch can usually be removed with a clamp or crochet hook passed down the tract. If drainage continues, it is occasionally necessary to reopen the skin for better exposure and to remove a series of infected stitches.

Patients with ascites are at risk of fluid leak through the wound. Left untreated, **ascitic leaks** increase the incidence of wound infection and, through retrograde contamination, may result in peritonitis. Prevention in susceptible patients involves closing at least one layer of the wound with a continuous suture and taking measures to avoid the accumulation of ascites postoperatively. If an ascitic leak develops, the wound should be explored and the fascial defect closed. The rest of the wound, including the skin, should also be closed.

RESPIRATORY COMPLICATIONS

Respiratory complications are the most common single cause of morbidity after major surgical procedures and the second most common cause of postoperative deaths in patients older than 60 years. Patients undergoing chest and upper abdominal operations are particularly prone to pulmonary complications. The incidence is lower after pelvic surgery and even lower after extremity or head and neck procedures. Pulmonary complications are more common after emergency operations. Special hazards are posed by preexisting chronic obstructive pulmonary disease (chronic bronchitis, emphysema, asthma, pulmonary fibrosis). Elderly patients are at much higher risk because they have decreased compliance, increased closing and residual volumes, and increased dead space, all of which predispose to atelectasis.

Atelectasis

Atelectasis, the most common pulmonary complication, affects 25% of patients who have abdominal surgery. It is more common in patients who are elderly or overweight and in those who smoke or have symptoms of respiratory disease. It appears most frequently in the first 48 hours after operation and is responsible for over 90% of febrile episodes during that period. In most cases, the course is self-limited and recovery uneventful.

The pathogenesis of atelectasis involves obstructive and nonobstructive factors. Obstruction may be caused by secretions resulting from chronic obstructive pulmonary disease, intubation, or anesthetic agents. Occasional cases may be due to blood clots or malposition of the endotracheal tube. In most instances, however, the cause is not obstruction but closure of the bronchioles. Small bronchioles (≤ 1 mm) are prone to close when lung volume reaches a critical point ("closing volume"). Portions of the lung that are dependent or compressed are the first to experience bronchiole closure since their regional volume is less than that of nondependent portions. Shallow breathing and failure to periodically hyperinflate the lung result in small alveolar size and decreased volume. The closing volume is higher in older patients and in smokers owing to the loss of elastic recoil of the lung. Other nonobstructive factors contributing to atelectasis include decreased functional residual capacity and loss of pulmonary surfactant.

The air in the atelectatic portion of the lung is absorbed, and since there is minimal change in perfusion, a ventilation/perfusion mismatch results. The immediate effect of atelectasis is decreased oxygenation of blood; its clinical significance depends on the respiratory and cardiac reserve of the patient. A later effect is the propensity of the atelectatic segment to become infected. In general, if a pulmonary segment remains atelectatic for over 72 hours, pneumonia is almost certain to occur.

Atelectasis is usually manifested by fever (pathogenesis unknown), tachypnea, and tachycardia. Physical examination may show elevation of the diaphragm, scattered rales, and decreased breath sounds, but it is often normal. Postoperative atelectasis can be largely prevented by early mobilization, frequent changes in position, encouragement to cough, and use of an incentive spirometer. Preoperative teaching of respiratory exercises and postoperative execution of these exercises prevents atelectasis in patients without preexisting lung disease. Intermittent positive pressure breathing is expensive and less effective than these simpler exercises.

Treatment consists of clearing the airway by chest percussion, coughing, or nasotracheal suction. Bronchodilators and mucolytic agents given by nebulizer may help in patients with severe chronic obstructive pulmonary disease. Atelectasis from obstruction of a major airway may require intrabronchial suction through an endoscope, a procedure that can usually be performed at the bedside with moderate sedation.

Pulmonary Aspiration

Aspiration of oropharyngeal and gastric contents is normally prevented by the gastroesophageal and pharyngoesophageal sphincters. Insertion of nasogastric and endotracheal tubes and depression of the central nervous system by drugs interferes with these defenses and predisposes to aspiration. Other factors, such as gastroesophageal reflux, food in the stomach, or position of the patient, may play a role. Trauma victims are particularly likely to aspirate regurgitated gastric contents when consciousness is depressed. Patients with intestinal obstruction and pregnant women—who have increased intra-abdominal pressure and decreased gastric motility—are also at high risk of aspiration. Two-thirds of cases of aspiration follow thoracic or abdominal surgery, and of these, one-half result in pneumonia. The death rate for grossly evident aspiration and subsequent pneumonia is about 50%.

Minor amounts of aspiration are frequent during surgery and are apparently well tolerated. Methylene blue placed in the stomach of patients undergoing ab-

dominal operations can be found in the trachea at completion of the procedure in 15% of cases. Radionuclide techniques have shown aspiration of gastric contents in 45% of normal volunteers during sleep.

The magnitude of pulmonary injury produced by aspiration of fluid, usually from gastric contents, is determined by the volume aspirated, its pH, and the frequency of the event. If the aspirate has a pH of 2.5 or less, it causes immediate chemical pneumonitis, which results in local edema and inflammation, changes that increase the risk of secondary infection. Aspiration of solid matter produces airway obstruction. Obstruction of distal bronchi, though well tolerated initially, may lead to atelectasis and pulmonary abscess formation. The basal segments are affected most often. Tachypnea, rales, and hypoxia are usually present within hours; less frequently, cyanosis, wheezing, and apnea may appear. In patients with massive aspiration, hypovolemia caused by excessive fluid and colloid loss into the injured lung may lead to hypotension and shock.

Aspiration has been found in 80% of patients with tracheostomies and may account for the predisposition to pulmonary infection in this group. Patients who must remain intubated for long periods should have a low-pressure, high-volume type of cuff on their tube, as this prevents aspiration and avoids pressure necrosis of the trachea.

Aspiration can be prevented by preoperative fasting, proper positioning of the patient, and careful intubation. A single dose of cimetidine before induction of anesthesia may be of value in situations where the risk of aspiration is high. Treatment of aspiration involves reestablishing patency of the airway and preventing further damage to the lung. Endotracheal suction should be performed immediately, as this procedure confirms the diagnosis and stimulates coughing, which helps to clear the airway. Bronchoscopy may be required to remove solid matter. Fluid resuscitation should be undertaken concomitantly. Hydrocortisone, 30 mg/kg/d intravenously, may be useful for the first 3 days. Antibiotics are used initially when the aspirate is heavily contaminated; they are used later to treat pneumonia.

Postoperative Pneumonia

Pneumonia is the most common pulmonary complication among patients who die after surgery. It is directly responsible for death—or is a contributory factor—in more than half of these patients. Patients with peritoneal infection and those requiring prolonged ventilatory support are at highest risk for developing postoperative pneumonia. Atelectasis, aspiration, and copious secretions are important predisposing factors.

Host defenses against pneumonitis include the cough reflex, the mucociliary system, and the activity of alveolar macrophages. After surgery, cough is usually weak and may not effectively clear the bronchial tree. The mucociliary transport mechanism is damaged by endotracheal intubation, and the functional ability of the alveolar macrophage is compromised by a number of factors that may be present during and after surgery (oxygen, pulmonary edema, aspiration, corticosteroid therapy, etc). In addition, squamous metaplasia and loss of ciliary coordination further hamper antibacterial defenses. More than half of the pulmonary infections that follow surgery are caused by gram-negative bacilli. They are frequently polymicrobial and usually acquired by aspiration of oropharyngeal secretions. Although colonization of the oropharynx with gram-negative bacteria occurs in only 20% of normal individuals, it is frequent after major surgery as a result of impaired oropharyngeal clearing mechanisms. Aggravating factors are azotemia, prolonged endotracheal intubation, and severe associated infection.

Occasionally, infecting bacteria reach the lung by inhalation—eg, from respirators. *Pseudomonas aeruginosa* and klebsiella can survive in the moist reservoirs of these machines, and these pathogens have been the source of epidemic infections in intensive care units. Rarely, contamination of the lung may result from direct hematogenous spread from distant septic foci.

The clinical manifestations of postoperative pneumonia are fever, tachypnea, increased secretions, and physical changes suggestive of pulmonary consolidation. A chest x-ray usually shows localized parenchymal consolidation. Overall mortality rates for postoperative pneumonia vary from 20% to 40%. Rates are higher when pneumonia develops in patients who had emergency operations; are on respirators; or develop remote organ failure, positive blood cultures, or infection of the second lung.

Maintaining the airway clear of secretions is of paramount concern in the prevention of postoperative pneumonia. Respiratory exercises, deep breathing, and coughing help prevent atelectasis, which is a precursor of pneumonia. Although postoperative pain is thought to contribute to shallow breathing, neither intercostal blocks nor epidural narcotics prevent atelectasis and pneumonia when compared with traditional methods of postoperative pain control. The prophylactic use of antibiotics does not decrease the incidence of gram-negative colonization of the oropharynx or that of pneumonia. Treatment consists of measures to aid the clearing of secretions and administration of antibiotics. Sputum obtained directly from the trachea, usually by endotracheal suctioning, is required for specific identification of the infecting organism.

Postoperative Pleural Effusion & Pneumothorax

Formation of a very small pleural effusion is fairly common immediately after upper abdominal operations and is of no clinical significance. Patients with free peritoneal fluid at the time of surgery and those with postoperative atelectasis are more prone to develop effusions. In the absence of cardiac failure or a pulmonary lesion, appearance of a pleural effusion late in the postoperative course suggests the presence of subdiaphragmatic inflammation (subphrenic abscess, acute pancreatitis, etc). Effusions that do not compromise respiratory function should be left undisturbed. If there is a suspicion of infection, the effusion should be tapped. When an effusion produces respiratory compromise, it should be drained with a thoracostomy tube.

Postoperative pneumothorax may follow insertion of a subclavian catheter or positive-pressure ventilation, but it sometimes appears after an operation during which the pleura has been injured (eg, nephrectomy or adrenalectomy). Pneumothorax should be treated with a thoracostomy tube.

FAT EMBOLISM

Fat embolism is relatively common but only rarely causes symptoms. Fat particles can be found in the pulmonary vascular bed in 90% of patients who have had fractures of long bones or joint replacements. Fat embolism can also be caused by exogenous sources of fat, such as blood transfusions, intravenous fat emulsion, or bone marrow transplantation. **Fat embolism syndrome** consists of neurologic dysfunction, respiratory insufficiency, and petechiae of the axillae, chest, and proximal arms. It was originally described in trauma victims—especially those with long bone fractures—and was thought to be a result of bone marrow embolization. However, the principal clinical manifestations of fat embolism are seen in other conditions. The existence of fat embolism as an entity distinct from posttraumatic pulmonary insufficiency has been questioned.

Fat embolism syndrome characteristically begins 12–72 hours after injury but may be delayed for several days. The diagnosis is clinical. The finding of fat droplets in sputum and urine is common after trauma and is not specific. Decreased hematocrit, thrombocytopenia, and other changes in coagulation parameters are usually seen.

Once symptoms develop, supportive treatment should be provided until respiratory insufficiency and central nervous system manifestations subside. Respiratory insufficiency is treated with positive end-expiratory pressure ventilation and diuretics. The prognosis is related to the severity of the pulmonary insufficiency.

CARDIAC COMPLICATIONS

Cardiac complications following surgery may be life-threatening. Their incidence is reduced by appropriate preoperative preparation.

Dysrhythmias, unstable angina, heart failure, or severe hypertension should be corrected before surgery whenever possible. Valvular disease—especially aortic stenosis—limits the ability of the heart to respond to increased demand during operation or in the immediate postoperative period. When aortic stenosis is recognized preoperatively—and assuming that the patient is monitored adequately (Swan-Ganz catheterization, central venous pressure, etc)—the incidence of major perioperative complications is small. Thus, patients with preexisting heart disease should be evaluated by a cardiologist preoperatively. Determination of cardiac function, including indirect evaluation of the left ventricular ejection fraction, identifies patients at higher risk for cardiac complications. Continuous electrocardiographic monitoring during the first 3–4 postoperative days detects episodes of ischemia or dysrhythmia in about a third of these patients. Oral anticoagulant drugs should be stopped 3–5 days before surgery, and the prothrombin time should be allowed to return to normal. Patients at high risk of thromboembolic disease should receive heparin until approximately 6 hours before the operation, when heparin should be stopped. If needed, heparin can be restarted 36–48 hours after surgery along with oral anticoagulation.

General anesthesia depresses the myocardium, and some anesthetic agents predispose to dysrhythmias by sensitizing the myocardium to catecholamines. Monitoring of cardiac activity and blood pressure during the operation detects dysrhythmias and hypotension early. In patients with a high cardiac risk, regional anesthesia may be safer than general anesthesia for procedures below the umbilicus.

The duration and urgency of the operation and uncontrolled bleeding with hypotension have been individually shown to correlate positively with the development of serious postoperative cardiac problems. In patients with pacemakers, the electrocautery current may be sensed by the intracardiac electrode, causing inappropriate pacemaker function.

Noncardiac complications may affect the development of cardiac complications by increasing cardiac demands in patients with a limited reserve. Postoperative sepsis and hypoxemia are foremost. Fluid overload can produce acute left ventricular failure. Patients with coronary artery disease, dysrhythmias, or low cardiac output should be monitored postoperatively in the intensive care unit.

Dysrhythmias

Most dysrhythmias appear during the operation or within the first 3 postoperative days. They are especially likely to occur after thoracic procedures.

A. Intraoperative Dysrhythmias

The overall incidence of intraoperative cardiac dysrhythmias is 20%; most are self-limited. The incidence is higher in patients with preexisting dysrhythmias and in those with known heart disease (35%). About one-third of dysrhythmias occur during induction of anesthesia. These dysrhythmias are usually related to anesthetic agents (eg, halothane, cyclopropane), sympathomimetic drugs, digitalis toxicity, and hypercapnia.

B. Postoperative Dysrhythmias

These dysrhythmias are generally related to reversible factors such as hypokalemia, hypoxemia, alkalosis, digitalis toxicity, and stress during emergence from anesthesia. Occasionally, postoperative dysrhythmias may be the first sign of myocardial infarction. Most postoperative dysrhythmias are asymptomatic, but occasionally the patient complains of chest pain, palpitations, or dyspnea.

Supraventricular dysrhythmias usually have few serious consequences but may decrease cardiac output and coronary blood flow. Patients with atrial flutter or fibrillation with a rapid ventricular response who are in shock require cardioversion. If they are hemodynamically stable, they should have the heart rate controlled with digitalis, beta-blockers, or calcium channel blockers. Associated hypokalemia should be treated promptly.

Ventricular premature beats are often precipitated by hypercapnia, hypoxemia, pain, or fluid overload. They should be treated with oxygen, sedation, analgesia, and correction of fluid losses or electrolyte abnormalities. Ventricular dysrhythmias have a more profound effect on cardiac function than supraventricular dysrhythmias and may lead to fatal ventricular fibrillation. Immediate treatment is with lidocaine, 1 mg/kg intravenously as a bolus, repeated as necessary to a total dose of 250 mg, followed by a slow intravenous infusion at a rate of 1–2 mg/min. Higher doses of lidocaine may cause seizures.

Postoperative complete heart block is usually due to serious cardiac disease and calls for the immediate insertion of a pacemaker. First- or second-degree heart block is usually well tolerated.

Postoperative Myocardial Infarction

Approximately 0.4% of all patients undergoing an operation in the USA develop postoperative myocardial infarction. The incidence increases to 5–12% in patients undergoing operations for other manifestations of atherosclerosis (eg, carotid endarterectomy, aortoiliac graft). Other important risk factors include preoperative congestive heart failure, ischemia identified on dipyridamole-thallium scan or treadmill exercise test, and age over 70 years. In selected patients with angina, consideration should be given to coronary revascularization before proceeding with a major elective operation on another organ.

Postoperative myocardial infarction may be precipitated by factors such as hypotension or hypoxemia. Clinical manifestations include chest pain, hypotension, and cardiac dysrhythmias. Over half of postoperative myocardial infarctions, however, are asymptomatic. The absence of symptoms is thought to be due to the residual effects of anesthesia and to analgesics administered postoperatively.

Diagnosis is substantiated by electrocardiographic changes, elevated serum creatine kinase levels—especially the MB isoenzyme—and serum troponin I levels. The mortality rate of postoperative myocardial infarction is as high as 67% in high-risk groups. The prognosis is better if it is the first infarction and worse if there have been previous infarctions. Prevention of this complication includes postponing elective operations for 3 months or preferably 6 months after myocardial infarction, treating congestive heart failure preoperatively, and controlling hypertension perioperatively.

Patients with postoperative myocardial infarction should be monitored in the intensive care unit and provided with adequate oxygenation and precise fluid and electrolyte replacement. Anticoagulation, though not always feasible after major surgery, prevents the development of mural thrombosis and arterial embolism after myocardial infarction. Congestive heart failure should be treated with digitalis, diuretics, and vasodilators as needed.

Postoperative Cardiac Failure

Left ventricular failure and pulmonary edema appear in 4% of patients over age 40 undergoing general surgical procedures with general anesthesia. Fluid overload in patients with limited myocardial reserve is the most common cause. Postoperative myocardial infarction and dysrhythmias producing a high ventricular rate are other causes. Clinical manifestations are progressive dyspnea, hypoxemia with normal CO_2 tension, and diffuse congestion on chest x-ray.

Clinically inapparent ventricular failure is frequent, especially when other factors predisposing to pulmonary edema are present (massive trauma, multiple transfusions, sepsis, etc). The diagnosis may be sus-

pected from a decreased PaO_2, abnormal chest x-ray, or elevated pulmonary artery wedge pressure. The treatment of left ventricular failure depends on the hemodynamic state of the patient. Those who are in shock require transfer to the intensive care unit, placement of a pulmonary artery line, monitoring of filling pressures, and immediate pre- and afterload reduction. Preload reduction is achieved by diuretics (and nitroglycerin if needed); afterload reduction, by administration of sodium nitroprusside. Dopamine is the best drug for inotropic support. Patients who are not in shock may, instead, be digitalized. Rapid digitalization (eg, divided intravenous doses of digoxin to a total of 1–1.5 mg over 24 hours, with careful monitoring of the serum potassium level), fluid restriction, and diuretics may be enough in these cases. Fluids should be restricted, and diuretics may be given. Respiratory insufficiency calls for ventilatory support with endotracheal intubation and a mechanical respirator. Although pulmonary function may improve with the use of positive end-expiratory pressure, hemodynamic derangements and decreased myocardial reserve preclude it in most cases.

PERITONEAL COMPLICATIONS

Hemoperitoneum

Bleeding is the most common cause of shock in the first 24 hours after abdominal surgery. Postoperative hemoperitoneum—a rapidly evolving, life-threatening complication—is usually the result of a technical problem with hemostasis, but coagulation disorders may play a role. For example, most of these patients have experienced substantial intraoperative blood loss, and several transfusions have already been given. As a consequence, changes usually observed after transfusion, such as thrombocytopenia, may be present. Other causes of coagulopathy such as mismatched transfusion, administration of heparin, etc, should also be considered. In these cases, bleeding tends to be more generalized, occurring in the wound, venipuncture sites, etc.

Hemoperitoneum usually becomes apparent within 24 hours after the operation. Its manifestations are those of hypovolemia: tachycardia, decreased blood pressure, decreased urine output, and peripheral vasoconstriction. If bleeding continues, abdominal girth may increase. Changes in the hematocrit are usually not obvious for 4–6 hours and are of limited diagnostic help in patients who sustain rapid blood loss.

The manifestations may be so subtle that the diagnosis is overlooked. Only a high index of suspicion, frequent examination of patients at risk, and a systematic investigation of patients with postoperative hypotension will result in early recognition of the problem. Preexisting disease and drugs taken before surgery as well as those administered during the operation may cause hypotension. The differential diagnosis of immediate postoperative circulatory collapse also includes pulmonary embolism, cardiac dysrhythmias, pneumothorax, myocardial infarction, and severe allergic reactions. Infusions to expand the intravascular volume should be started as soon as other diseases have been ruled out. If hypotension or other signs of hypovolemia persist, one must reoperate promptly. At operation, bleeding should be stopped, clots evacuated, and the peritoneal cavity rinsed with saline solution.

Complications of Drains

Postoperative drainage of the peritoneal cavity is indicated to prevent fluid accumulation such as bile or pancreatic juice or to treat established abscesses. Drains may be left to evacuate small amounts of blood, but this process cannot be used to provide a reliable estimate of the rate of bleeding. The trend recently has been away from the use of drains in uncomplicated operations such as splenectomy and cholecystectomy. The use of drains in these settings increases the rate of postoperative intraabdominal and wound infection. These problems can be minimized with the use of closed suction drains brought out of the abdomen through separate stab incisions. Latex Penrose drains, which were once popular, should be avoided because of the risk of introducing infection. Large rigid drains may erode into adjacent viscera or vessels and cause fistula formation or bleeding. This risk is lessened with the use of softer Silastic drains, which are removed as early as possible. Drains should not be left in contact with intestinal anastomoses, as they promote anastomotic leakage and fistula formation.

POSTOPERATIVE PAROTITIS

Postoperative parotitis—-a rare but serious staphylococcal infection of the parotid gland—is limited almost entirely to elderly, debilitated, malnourished patients with poor oral hygiene. It appears in the second postoperative week and is associated with prolonged nasogastric intubation. The triggering factors are dehydration and poor oral hygiene, and the pathogenesis consists of a decrease in the secretory activity of the gland with inspissation of parotid secretions that become infected by staphylococci or gram-negative bacteria from the oral cavity. This results in inflammation, accumulation of cells that obstruct large and medium-sized ducts, and, eventually, formation of multiple small abscesses. These lobular abscesses, separated by fibrous bands, may dissect through the capsule and spread to the periglandular tissues to involve the auditory canal, the superficial skin, and the neck. If the disease is not treated at this stage, it may produce acute respiratory failure from tracheal obstruction.

Clinically, parotitis first appears as pain or tenderness at the angle of the jaw. With progression, high fever and leukocytosis develop, and there is swelling and redness in the parotid area. The parotid usually feels firm, and even after abscesses have formed, fluctuance is uncommon.

Prophylaxis includes adequate fluid intake, avoiding the use of anticholinergics, minimizing trauma during intubation, and, most importantly, good oral hygiene (frequent gargles, mouth irrigation, and other mouth cleansing and moistening measures). Stimulation of salivary flow with chewing gum, hard candy, etc, may also be useful. Routine observance of these simple preventive measures has virtually eliminated parotitis, which was once a common postoperative complication.

When signs of acute parotitis appear, fluid obtained from Stensen's duct by gentle compression of the gland should be cultured. Vancomycin should be started while the results of cultures are awaited. Warm moist packs and mouth irrigations may be helpful. In most instances, the disease responds promptly to these measures. If the disease progresses, the parotid must be surgically drained. The procedure consists of elevating a skin flap over the gland and making multiple small incisions parallel to the branches of the facial nerve. The wound is then packed open.

COMPLICATIONS CAUSED BY POSTOPERATIVE ALTERATIONS OF GASTROINTESTINAL MOTILITY

The presence, strength, and direction of normal peristalsis are governed by the enteric nervous system. Anesthesia and surgical manipulation result in a decrease of the normal propulsive activity of the gut, or **postoperative ileus.** Several factors worsen ileus or prolong its course. These include medications—especially opioids—electrolyte abnormalities, inflammatory conditions such as pancreatitis or peritonitis, and pain. The degree of ileus is related to the extent of operative manipulation.

Gastrointestinal peristalsis returns within 24 hours after most operations that do not involve the abdominal cavity. After laparotomy, gastric peristalsis returns in about 48 hours. Colonic activity returns after 48 hours, starting at the cecum and progressing caudally. The motility of the small intestine is affected to a lesser degree, except in patients who have had small bowel resection or who were operated on to relieve bowel obstruction. Normal postoperative ileus leads to slight abdominal distention and absent bowel sounds. Return of peristalsis is often noted by the patient as mild cramps, passage of flatus, and return of appetite. Feedings should be withheld until there is evidence of return of normal gastrointestinal motility. There is no specific therapy for postoperative ileus.

Gastric Dilation

Gastric dilation, a rare life-threatening complication, consists of massive distention of the stomach by gas and fluid. Predisposing factors include asthma, recent surgery, gastric outlet obstruction, and absence of the spleen. Infants and children in whom oxygen masks are used in the immediate postoperative period and adults subjected to forceful assisted respiration during resuscitation are also at risk. Occasionally, gastric dilation develops in patients with anorexia nervosa or during serious illnesses without a specific intercurrent event.

As the air-filled stomach grows larger, it hangs down across the duodenum, producing a mechanical gastric outlet obstruction that contributes further to the problem. The increased intragastric pressure produces venous obstruction of the mucosa, causing mucosal engorgement and bleeding and, if allowed to continue, ischemic necrosis and perforation. The distended stomach pushes the diaphragm upward, which causes collapse of the lower lobe of the left lung, rotation of the heart, and obstruction of the inferior vena cava. The acutely dilated stomach is also prone to undergo volvulus.

The patient appears ill, with abdominal distention and hiccup. Hypochloremia, hypokalemia, and alkalosis may result from fluid and electrolyte losses. When the problem is recognized early, treatment consists of gastric decompression with a nasogastric tube. In the late stage, gastric necrosis may require gastrectomy.

Bowel Obstruction

Failure of postoperative return of bowel function may be the result of paralytic ileus or mechanical obstruction. Mechanical obstruction is most often caused by postoperative adhesions or an internal (mesenteric) hernia. Most of these patients experience a short period of apparently normal intestinal function before manifestations of obstruction supervene. About half of cases of early postoperative small bowel obstruction follow colorectal surgery, probably owing to the more extensive peritoneal stripping involved.

Diagnosis may be difficult because the symptoms are difficult to differentiate from those of paralytic ileus. If plain films of the abdomen show air-fluid levels in loops of small bowel, mechanical obstruction is a more likely diagnosis than ileus. Enteroclysis or an ordinary small bowel series with barium sulfate may aid diagnosis.

Strangulation is uncommon because the adhesive bands are broader and less rigid than in the average case of late small bowel obstruction. The death rate is high

(about 15%), however, probably because of delay in diagnosis and the postoperative state. Treatment consists of nasogastric suction for several days and, if the obstruction does not resolve spontaneously, laparotomy.

Small bowel intussusception is an uncommon cause of early postoperative obstruction in adults but accounts for 10% of cases in the pediatric age group. Ninety percent of postoperative intussusceptions occur during the first 2 postoperative weeks, and more than half in the first week. Unlike idiopathic ileocolic intussusception, most postoperative intussusceptions are ileoileal or jejunojejunal. They most often follow retroperitoneal and pelvic operations. The cause is unknown. The symptom complex is not typical, and x-ray studies are of limited help. The physician should be aware that intussusception is a possible explanation for vomiting, distention, and abdominal pain after laparotomy in children and that early reoperation will avoid the complications of perforation and peritonitis. Surgery is the only treatment, and provided the bowel is viable, reduction of the intussusception is all that is needed.

Postoperative Fecal Impaction

Fecal impaction after operative procedures is the result of colonic ileus and impaired perception of rectal fullness. It is principally a disease of the elderly but may occur in younger patients who have predisposing conditions such as megacolon or paraplegia. Postoperative ileus and the use of opioid analgesics and anticholinergic drugs are aggravating factors. Early manifestations are anorexia and obstipation or diarrhea. In advanced cases, marked distention may cause colonic perforation. The diagnosis of postoperative fecal impaction is made by rectal examination. The impaction should be manually removed, enemas given, and digital examination then repeated.

Barium remaining in the colon from an examination done before surgery may harden and produce **barium impaction.** This usually occurs in the right colon, where most of the water is absorbed, and is a more difficult management problem than fecal impaction. The clinical manifestations are those of bowel obstruction. Treatment includes enemas and purgation with polyethylene glycol-electrolyte solution (eg, CoLyte, GoLYTELY). Diatrizoate sodium (Hypaque), a hyperosmolar solution that stimulates peristalsis and increases intraluminal fluid, may be effective by enema if other solutions fail. Surgery is rarely needed.

POSTOPERATIVE PANCREATITIS

Postoperative pancreatitis accounts for 10% of all cases of acute pancreatitis. It occurs in 1–3% of patients who have operations in the vicinity of the pancreas, and with higher frequency after operations on the biliary tract.

For example, pancreatitis occurs in about 1% of patients undergoing cholecystectomy and in 8% of patients undergoing common bile duct exploration. In the latter cases, it does not appear to be related to the performance of intraoperative cholangiograms or choledochoscopy. Postoperative pancreatitis after biliary surgery is worse in patients who have had biliary pancreatitis preoperatively. Pancreatitis is occasionally observed following cardiopulmonary bypass, parathyroid surgery, and renal transplantation. Postoperative pancreatitis is frequently of the necrotizing type. Infected pancreatic necrosis and other complications of pancreatitis develop with a frequency three to four times greater than in biliary and alcoholic pancreatitis. The reason postoperative pancreatitis is so severe is unknown, but the mortality rate is 30–40%.

The pathogenesis in most cases appears to be mechanical trauma to the pancreas or its blood supply. Nevertheless, manipulation, biopsy, and partial resection of the pancreas are usually well tolerated, so why some patients develop pancreatitis is unclear. Prevention of this complication includes careful handling of the pancreas and avoidance of forceful dilation of the choledochal sphincter or obstruction of the pancreatic duct. The 2% incidence of pancreatitis following renal transplantation is probably related to special risk factors such as use of corticosteroids or azathioprine, secondary hyperparathyroidism, or viral infection. Acute changes in serum calcium are thought to be responsible for pancreatitis following parathyroid surgery. Hyperamylasemia develops in about half of patients undergoing heart surgery with extracorporeal bypass, but clinical evidence of pancreatitis is present in only 5% of these patients.

The diagnosis of postoperative pancreatitis may be difficult in patients who have recently had an abdominal operation. Hyperamylasemia may or may not be present. One must be alert to renal and respiratory complications and the consequences of necrotizing or hemorrhagic pancreatitis. Because of the high frequency with which complications develop, frequent monitoring of the pancreas and retroperitoneum with CT scans is useful.

See Chapter 27 for diagnosis and treatment of acute pancreatitis.

POSTOPERATIVE HEPATIC DYSFUNCTION

Hepatic dysfunction, ranging from mild jaundice to life-threatening hepatic failure, follows 1% of surgical procedures performed under general anesthesia. The incidence is greater following pancreatectomy, biliary bypass operations, and portacaval shunt. Postoperative hyperbilirubinemia may be categorized as prehepatic jaundice, hepatocellular insufficiency, and posthepatic obstruction (Table 4–1).

Table 4–1. Causes of postoperative jaundice.

Prehepatic jaundice (bilirubin overload)
  Hemolysis (drugs, transfusions, sickle cell crisis)
  Reabsorption of hematomas
Hepatocellular insufficiency
  Viral hepatitis
  Drug-induced (anesthesia, others)
  Ischemia (shock, hypoxia, low-output states)
  Sepsis
  Liver resection (loss of parenchyma)
  Others (total parenteral nutrition, malnutrition)
Posthepatic obstruction (to bile flow)
  Retained stones
  Injury to ducts
  Tumor (unrecognized or untreated)
  Cholecystitis
  Pancreatitis

Prehepatic Jaundice

Prehepatic jaundice is caused by bilirubin overload, most often from hemolysis or reabsorption of hematomas. Fasting, malnutrition, hepatotoxic drugs, and anesthesia are among the factors that impair the ability of the liver to excrete increased loads of bilirubin in the postoperative period.

Increased hemolysis may result from transfusion of incompatible blood but more often reflects destruction of fragile transfused red blood cells. Other causes include extracorporeal circulation, congenital hemolytic disease (eg, sickle cell disease), and effects of drugs.

Hepatocellular Insufficiency

Hepatocellular insufficiency, the most common cause of postoperative jaundice, occurs as a consequence of hepatic cell necrosis, inflammation, or massive hepatic resection. Drugs, hypotension, hypoxia, and sepsis are among the injurious factors. Although posttransfusion hepatitis is usually observed much later, this complication may occur as early as the third postoperative week.

Benign postoperative intrahepatic cholestasis is a vague term used to denote jaundice following operations that often involve hypotension and multiple transfusions. Serum bilirubin ranges from 2–20 mg/dL and serum alkaline phosphatase is usually high, but the patient is afebrile and postoperative convalescence is otherwise smooth. The diagnosis is one of exclusion. Jaundice clears by the third postoperative week.

Hepatocellular damage is occasionally seen after intestinal bypass procedures for morbid obesity. Cholestatic jaundice may develop in patients receiving total parenteral nutrition.

Posthepatic Obstruction

Posthepatic obstruction can be caused by direct surgical injury to the bile ducts, retained common duct stones, tumor obstruction of the bile duct, or pancreatitis. Acute postoperative cholecystitis is associated with jaundice in one-third of cases, though mechanical obstruction of the common duct is usually not apparent.

One must determine if a patient with postoperative jaundice has a correctable cause that requires treatment. This is particularly true for sepsis (where decreased liver function may sometimes be an early sign), lesions that obstruct the bile duct, and postoperative cholecystitis. Liver function tests are not helpful in determining the cause and do not usually reflect the severity of disease. Liver biopsy, ultrasound and CT scans, and transhepatic or endoscopic retrograde cholangiograms are the tests most likely to sort out the diagnostic possibilities. Renal function must be monitored closely, since renal failure may develop in these patients. Treatment is otherwise expectant.

POSTOPERATIVE CHOLECYSTITIS

Acute postoperative cholecystitis may follow any kind of operation but is more common after gastrointestinal procedures. Acute cholecystitis develops shortly after endoscopic sphincterotomy in 3–5% of patients. Chemical cholecystitis has been observed in patients undergoing hepatic arterial chemotherapy with mitomycin and floxuridine with such frequency that cholecystectomy should always be performed before infusion of these agents is begun. Fulminant cholecystitis with gallbladder infarction may follow percutaneous embolization of the hepatic artery for malignant tumors of the liver or for arteriovenous malformation involving this artery.

Postoperative cholecystitis differs in several respects from the common form of acute cholecystitis: It is frequently acalculous (70–80%), more common in males (75%), progresses rapidly to gallbladder necrosis, and is not likely to respond to conservative therapy. The cause is clear in cases of chemical or ischemic cholecystitis but not in other forms. Factors thought to play a role include biliary stasis (with formation of sludge), biliary infection, and ischemia. Diagnosis and treatment are discussed in Chapter 26.

CLOSTRIDIUM DIFFICILE COLITIS

Postoperative diarrhea due to *Clostridium difficile* is a common nosocomial infection in surgical patients. The spectrum of illness ranges from asymptomatic colonization to—rarely—severe toxic colitis. Transmission from hospital personnel probably occurs. The main risk factor is perioperative antibiotic use. The diagnosis is established by identification of a specific cytopathic toxin in the stool or culture of the organism from stool samples or rectal swabs. In severely affected patients, colonoscopy reveals pseudomembranes. Prevention is accomplished by strict handwashing, enteric precautions, and minimizing antibiotic use. Treatment of established infection is with intravenous metronidazole or, for infections with resistant pathogens, oral vancomycin.

URINARY COMPLICATIONS

Postoperative Urinary Retention

Inability to void postoperatively is common, especially after pelvic and perineal operations or operations conducted under spinal anesthesia. Factors responsible for postoperative urinary retention are interference with the neural mechanisms responsible for normal emptying of the bladder and overdistention of the urinary bladder. When its normal capacity of approximately 500 mL is exceeded, bladder contraction is inhibited. Prophylactic bladder catheterization should be performed whenever an operation is likely to last 3 hours or longer or when large volumes of intravenous fluids are anticipated. The catheter can be removed at the end of the operation if the patient is expected to be able to ambulate within a few hours. When bladder catheterization is not performed, the patient should be encouraged to void immediately before coming to the operating room and as soon as possible after the operation. During abdominoperineal resection, operative trauma to the sacral plexus alters bladder function enough so that an indwelling catheter should be left in place for 4–5 days. Patients with inguinal hernia who strain to void as a manifestation of prostatic hypertrophy should have the prostate treated before the hernia.

The treatment of acute urinary retention is catheterization of the bladder. In the absence of factors that suggest the need for prolonged decompression, such as the presence of 1000 mL of urine or more, the catheter may be removed.

Urinary Tract Infection

Infection of the lower urinary tract is the most frequently acquired nosocomial infection. Preexisting contamination of the urinary tract, urinary retention, and instrumentation are the principal contributing factors. Bacteriuria is present in about 5% of patients who undergo short-term (< 48 hours) bladder catheterization, though clinical signs of urinary tract infection occur in only 1%. Cystitis is manifested by dysuria and mild fever and pyelonephritis by high fever, flank tenderness, and, occasionally, ileus. Diagnosis is made by examination of the urine and confirmed by cultures. Prevention involves treating urinary tract contamination before surgery, prevention or prompt treatment of urinary retention, and careful instrumentation when needed. Treatment includes adequate hydration, proper drainage of the bladder, and specific antibiotics.

CENTRAL NERVOUS SYSTEM COMPLICATIONS

Postoperative Cerebrovascular Accidents

Postoperative cerebrovascular accidents are almost always the result of ischemic neural damage due to poor perfusion. They often occur in elderly patients with severe atherosclerosis who become hypotensive during or after surgery (from sepsis, bleeding, cardiac arrest, etc). Normal regulatory mechanisms of the cerebral vasculature can maintain blood flow over a wide range of blood pressures down to a mean pressure of about 55 mm Hg. Abrupt hypotension, however, is less well tolerated than a more gradual pressure change. Irreversible brain damage occurs after about 4 minutes of total ischemia.

Strokes occur in 1–3% of patients after carotid endarterectomy and other reconstructive operations of the extracranial portion of the carotid system. Embolization from atherosclerotic plaques, ischemia during carotid clamping, and postoperative thrombosis at the site of the arteriotomy or of an intimal flap are usually responsible. Aspirin, which inhibits platelet aggregation, may prevent immediate postoperative thrombosis.

Open heart surgery using extracorporeal circulation or deep cooling is also occasionally followed by stroke. The pathogenesis of stroke is thought to be related to hypoxemia, emboli, or poor perfusion. The presence of a carotid bruit preoperatively increases the risk of postoperative stroke after coronary bypass by a factor of 4. Previous stroke or transient ischemic attacks and postoperative atrial fibrillation also increase the risk. For patients undergoing noncardiac, noncarotid surgery, the risk of stroke has been estimated at 0.2%. Predictors of risk in these patients are the presence of cerebrovascular, cardiac, or peripheral vascular disease and arterial hypertension.

Convulsions

Epilepsy, metabolic derangements, and medications may lead to convulsions in the postoperative period. For unknown reasons, patients with ulcerative colitis and Crohn's disease are peculiarly susceptible to convulsions with loss of consciousness after surgery. Convulsions should be treated as soon as possible to minimize their harmful effects.

PSYCHIATRIC COMPLICATIONS

Anxiety and fear are normal in patients undergoing surgery. The degree to which these emotions are experienced depends upon diverse cultural and psychologic variables. Underlying depression or a history of chronic pain may serve to exaggerate the patient's response to surgery. The boundary between the normal manifestations of stress and **postoperative psychosis** is difficult to establish, since the latter is not really a distinct clinical entity.

Postoperative psychosis (so-called) develops in about 0.5% of patients having abdominal operations. It is more common after thoracic surgery, in the elderly, and in those with chronic disease. About half of these patients suffer from mood disturbances (usually severe depression). Twenty percent have delirium. Drugs given in the postoperative period may play a role in the development of psychosis; meperidine, cimetidine, and corticosteroids are most commonly implicated. Patients who develop postoperative psychosis have higher plasma levels of β-endorphin and cortisol than those who do not. These patients also lose, temporarily, the normal circadian rhythms of β-endorphin and cortisol. Specific psychiatric syndromes may follow specific procedures, such as visual hallucinations and the "black patch syndrome" after ophthalmic surgery. Preexisting psychiatric disorders not apparent before the operation sometimes contribute to the motivation for surgery (eg, circumcision or cosmetic operations in schizophrenics).

Clinical manifestations are rare on the first postoperative day. During this period, patients appear emotionless and unconcerned about changes in the environment or in themselves. Most overt psychiatric derangements are observed after the third postoperative day. The symptoms are variable but often include confusion, fear, and disorientation as to time and place. Delirium presents as altered consciousness with cognitive impairment. These symptoms may not be readily apparent to the surgeon, as this problem is usually seen in sick patients whose other problems may mask the manifestations of psychosis. Early psychiatric consultation should be obtained when psychosis is suspected so that adequate and prompt assessment of consciousness and cognitive function can be done and treatment instituted. The earlier the psychosis is recognized, the easier it is to correct. Metabolic derangements or early sepsis (especially in burn patients) must be ruled out as the cause. Severe postoperative emotional disturbances may be avoided by appropriate preoperative counseling of the patient by the surgeon. This includes a thorough discussion of the operation and the expected outcome, acquainting the patient with the intensive care unit, etc. Postoperatively, the surgeon must attend to the patient's emotional needs, offering frequent reassurance, explaining the postoperative course, and discussing the prognosis and the outcome of the operation.

Special Psychiatric Problems

A. THE ICU SYNDROME

The continuous internal vigilance that results from pain and fear and the sleep deprivation from bright lights, monitoring equipment, and continuous noise causes a psychologic disorganization known as ICU psychosis. The patient whose level of consciousness is already decreased by illness and drugs is more susceptible than a normal individual, and the result is decreased ability to think, perceive, and remember. When the cognitive processes are thoroughly disorganized, delirium occurs. The manifestations include distorted visual, auditory, and tactile perception; confusion and restlessness; and inability to differentiate reality from fantasy. Prevention includes isolation from the environment, decreased noise levels, adequate sleep, and removal from the intensive care unit as soon as possible.

B. POSTCARDIOTOMY DELIRIUM

Mental changes that occasionally follow open heart surgery include impairment of memory, attention, cognition, and perception and occasionally hysteria, depressive reaction, and anxiety crisis. The symptoms most often appear after the third postoperative day. The type of operation, the presence of organic brain disease, prolonged medical illness, and the length of time on extracorporeal circulation are related to the development of postcardiotomy psychosis. Mild sedation and measures to prevent the ICU syndrome may prevent this complication. In more severe cases, haloperidol (Haldol) in doses of 1–5 mg given orally, intramuscularly, or intravenously may be required. Haloperidol is preferred over phenothiazines in these patients because it is associated with a lower incidence of cardiovascular side effects.

C. DELIRIUM TREMENS

Delirium tremens occurs in alcoholics who stop drinking suddenly. Hyperventilation and metabolic alkalosis contribute to the development of the full-blown syndrome. Hypomagnesemia and hypokalemia secondary to alkalosis or nutritional deficits may precipitate seizures. Readaptation to ethanol-free metabolism requires about 2 weeks, and it is during this period that alcoholics are at greatest risk of developing delirium tremens.

The prodrome includes personality changes, anxiety, and tremor. The complete syndrome is characterized by agitation, hallucinations, restlessness, confusion, overactivity, and, occasionally, seizures and hyperthermia. The syndrome also causes a hyperdynamic cardiorespiratory and metabolic state. For example, cardiac index, oxygen delivery, and oxygen consumption double during delirium tremens and return to normal 24–48 hours after resolution. The wild behavior may precipitate dehiscence of a fresh laparotomy incision. Diaphoresis and dehydration are common, and exhaustion may herald death.

Withdrawal symptoms may be prevented by giving small amounts of alcohol, but benzodiazepines are the treatment of choice. Vitamin B_1 (thiamine) and magnesium sulfate should also be given.

The aims of treatment are to reduce agitation and anxiety as soon as possible and to prevent the development of other complications (eg, seizures, aspiration pneumonia). General measures should include frequent assessment of vital signs, restoration of nutrition, administration of vitamin B, correction of electrolyte imbalance or other metabolic derangements, and adequate hydration. Physical restraint, though necessary for seriously violent behavior, should be as limited as possible. With proper care, most patients improve within 72 hours.

D. SEXUAL DYSFUNCTION

Sexual problems commonly occur after certain kinds of operations, such as prostatectomy, heart surgery, and aortic reconstruction. The pathogenesis is unclear. In abdominoperineal resection, severance of the peripheral branches of the sacral plexus may cause impotence. It is important to discuss this possibility with the patient before any operation with a risk of impotence is performed. When sexual dysfunction is psychogenic, reassurance is usually all that is needed. If psychogenic impotence persists beyond 4–6 weeks, psychiatric consultation is indicated.

COMPLICATIONS OF INTRAVENOUS THERAPY & HEMODYNAMIC MONITORING

Air Embolism

Air embolism may occur during or after insertion of a venous catheter or as a result of accidental introduction of air into the line. Embolized air lodges in the right atrium, preventing adequate filling of the right heart. This is manifested by hypotension, jugular venous distention, and tachycardia. This complication can be avoided by placing the patient in the Trendelenburg position when a central venous line is inserted. Emergency treatment consists of aspiration of the air with a syringe. If this is unsuccessful, the patient should be positioned right side up and head down, which will help dislodge the air from the right atrium and return circulatory dynamics to normal.

Phlebitis

A needle or a catheter inserted into a vein and left in place will in time cause inflammation at the entry site. When this process involves the vein, it is called phlebitis. Factors determining the degree of inflammation are the nature of the cannula, the solution infused, bacterial infection, and venous thrombosis. Phlebitis is one of the most common causes of fever after the third postoperative day. The symptomatic triad of induration, edema, and tenderness is characteristic. Visible signs may be minimal. Prevention of phlebitis is best accomplished by observance of aseptic techniques during insertion of venous catheters, frequent change of tubing (ie, every 48–72 hours), and rotation of insertion sites (ie, every 4 days). Silastic catheters, which are the least reactive, should be used when the line must be left in for a long time. Hypertonic solutions should be infused only into veins with substantial flow, such as the subclavian, jugular, or vena cava. Venous catheters should be removed at the first sign of redness, induration, or edema. Because phlebitis is most frequent with cannulation of veins in the lower extremities, this route should be used only when upper extremity veins are unavailable. Removal of the catheter is adequate treatment.

Suppurative phlebitis may result from the presence of an infected thrombus around the indwelling catheter. Staphylococci are the most common causative organisms. Local signs of inflammation are present, and pus may be expressed from the venipuncture site. High fever and positive blood cultures are common. Treatment consists of excising the affected vein, extending the incision proximally to the first open collateral, and leaving the wound open.

Cardiopulmonary Complications

Perforation of the right atrium with cardiac tamponade has been associated with the use of central venous lines. This complication can be avoided by checking the position of the tip of the line, which should be in the superior vena cava, not the right atrium. Complications associated with the use of the flow-directed balloon-tipped (Swan-Ganz) catheter include cardiac perforation (usually of the right atrium), intracardiac knotting of the catheter, and cardiac dysrhythmias. Pulmonary hemorrhage may result from disruption of a branch of the pulmonary artery during balloon inflation and may be fatal in patients with pulmonary hypertension. Steps in prevention include careful placement, advancement under continuous pressure monitoring, and checking the position of the tip before inflating the balloon.

Ischemic Necrosis of the Finger

Continuous monitoring of arterial blood pressure during the operation and in the intensive care unit requires insertion of a radial or femoral arterial line. The hand receives its blood supply from the radial and ulnar arteries, and because of the anatomy of the palmar arches, patency of one of these vessels is usually enough to provide adequate blood flow through the hand. Occasionally, ischemic necrosis of the finger has followed use of an indwelling catheter in the radial artery. This serious complication can usually be avoided by evaluating the patency of the ulnar artery (Allen's test) before establishing the radial line and by changing arterial line sites every 3–4 days. After an arterial catheter is withdrawn, a pressure dressing should be applied to avoid formation of an arterial pseudoaneurysm.

POSTOPERATIVE FEVER

Fever occurs in about 40% of patients after major surgery. In most patients the temperature elevation resolves without specific treatment. However, postoperative fever may herald a serious infection, and it is therefore important to evaluate the patient clinically. Features often associated with an infectious origin of the fever include preoperative trauma, ASA class above 2, fever onset after the second postoperative day, an initial temperature elevation above 38.6 °C, a postoperative white blood cell count greater than 10,000/μL, and a postoperative serum urea nitrogen of 15 mg/dL or greater. If three or more of the above are present, the likelihood of associated bacterial infection is nearly 100%.

Fever within 48 hours after surgery is usually caused by atelectasis. Reexpansion of the lung causes body temperature to return to normal. Because laboratory and radiologic investigations are usually unrevealing, an extensive evaluation of early postoperative fever is rarely appropriate if the patient's convalescence is otherwise smooth.

When fever appears after the second postoperative day, atelectasis is a less likely explanation. The differential diagnosis of fever at this time includes catheter-related phlebitis, pneumonia, and urinary tract infection. A directed history and physical examination complemented by focused laboratory and radiologic studies usually determine the cause.

Patients without infection are rarely febrile after the fifth postoperative day. Fever this late suggests wound infection or, less often, anastomotic breakdown and intra-abdominal abscesses. A diagnostic workup directed to the detection of intra-abdominal sepsis is indicated in patients who have high temperatures (> 39 °C) and wounds without evidence of infection 5 or more days postoperatively. CT scan of the abdomen and pelvis is the test of choice and should be performed early, before overt organ failure occurs.

Fever is rare after the first week in patients who had a normal convalescence. Allergy to drugs, transfusion-related fever, septic pelvic vein thrombosis, and intra-abdominal abscesses should be considered.

REFERENCES

Deysine M: Pathophysiology, prevention, and management of prosthetic infections in hernia surgery. Surg Clin North Am 1998;78:1105.

Emparan C et al: Infective complications after abdominal surgery in patients infected with human immunodeficiency virus: role of CD4+ lymphocytes in prognosis. World J Surg 1998; 22:778.

Carlson MA: Acute wound failure. Surg Clin North Am 1997; 77:607.

Eagle KA et al: Guidelines for perioperative cardiovascular evaluation for noncardiac surgery: an abridged version of the report of the American College of Cardiology/American Heart Association Task Force on Practice Guidelines. Mayo Clin Proc 1997;72:524.

Shibata Y et al: Patterns of intestinal motility recovery during the early stage following abdominal surgery: clinical and manometric study. World J Surg1997;21:806.

McGuire BE et al: Intensive care unit syndrome: a dangerous misnomer. Arch Intern Med 2000;160:906.

Rabinowitz RP, Caplan ES: Management of infections in the trauma patient. Surg Clin North Am 1999;79:1373.

Sitges-Serra A, Girvent M: Catheter-related bloodstream infections. World J Surg 1999;23:589.

Special Medical Problems in Surgical Patients

5

■ ENDOCRINE DISEASE & THE SURGICAL PATIENT

Gerard M. Doherty, MD

DIABETES MELLITUS

Diabetic patients undergo more surgical procedures than do nondiabetics, and management of the diabetic patient before, during, and after surgery is an important responsibility of the surgeon. Fortunately, because close control of fluids, electrolytes, glucose, and insulin is now possible in the operating room, control of blood glucose levels during the perioperative period is usually relatively simple. Marked hyperglycemia should be avoided during surgery; the greater danger, however, is from severe unrecognized hypoglycemia.

Preoperative Workup

Blood glucose concentrations may be elevated in diabetic patients during the preoperative period. Physical trauma, if present, combined with the emotional and physiologic stress of the illness may cause epinephrine and cortisol levels to rise, in each case resulting in increased blood glucose levels. If exogenous cortisol is being administered (eg, to a renal or pancreatic transplant recipient), marked insulin resistance and elevations of blood glucose levels regularly result. Infections may also increase blood glucose concentrations, occasionally to dangerous levels. Inactivity in bedridden patients can increase blood glucose levels by causing insulin resistance. Hypokalemia—frequently the result of diuretic therapy but also of epinephrine release induced by trauma—may prevent B cells from secreting adequate amounts of insulin and may thereby raise blood glucose levels in patients with type 2 diabetes.

The preoperative workup of patients with diabetes mellitus should include a thorough physical examination, with special care to discover occult infections; an ECG to rule out myocardial infarction; and a chest x-ray to identify hidden pneumonia or pulmonary edema. A complete urinalysis should be done to rule out urinary tract infection and proteinuria, the earliest signs of diabetic renal disease. Serum potassium levels should be measured to check for hypokalemia or hyperkalemia, the latter usually resulting from hyporeninemic hypoaldosteronism, a relatively common syndrome in diabetics. Serum creatinine levels should be measured to assess renal function. The serum glucose concentration should ideally be between 100 and 200 mg/dL, but operation can be safely performed in patients whose serum glucose is as high as 350–400 mg/dL preoperatively.

Preoperative & Intraoperative Management of Diabetic Patients

A. TYPE 2 (NON-INSULIN-DEPENDENT) DIABETES MELLITUS

Approximately 85% of diabetics over age 50 years have only a moderately decreased ability to produce and secrete insulin, and when at home they can usually be controlled by diet or by sulfonylureas. If the serum glucose level is below 250 mg/dL on the morning of surgery, sulfonylureas should be withheld; long-acting sulfonylurea drugs—glipizide, glyburide, and chlorpropamide—should be discontinued on the day before surgery; and 5% glucose solution should be administered intravenously at a rate of about 100 mL/h. This means that over a 10-hour period, only 50 g of glucose would be given; by contrast, during an average day, a diabetic on a normal diet would consume four to five times as much carbohydrate (ie, 200–250 g). During any but the most extensive surgery, the pancreas should be able to produce enough insulin to handle this modest glucose load and at the same time prevent undue gluconeogenesis.

If the fasting glucose level is above 250–300 mg/dL or if the patient is taking small doses of insulin but does not actually require insulin to prevent ketoacidosis, an alternative approach would be to add 5 units of insulin directly to each liter of 5% glucose solution being given at 100 mL/h. If the operation is lengthy, blood glucose levels should be measured every 3–4 hours during surgery to ensure adequate glucose control. The goal is to maintain glucose levels between 100 and 200 mg/dL, but there is little harm in allowing levels to go as high as 250 mg/dL.

B. TYPE 1 (INSULIN-DEPENDENT) DIABETES MELLITUS

Type 1 patients require insulin during surgery. It can be administered by any of the following methods: (1) subcutaneous administration of long-acting insulin; (2) constant infusion of a mixture of glucose and insulin; or (3) separate infusions of glucose and insulin. Intravenous boluses of regular insulin are rarely, if ever, indicated. The effect of single boluses of insulin given intravenously typically lasts only minutes, leading to the danger of acute hypoglycemia followed shortly thereafter by recurrent hyperglycemia. With either technique, blood glucose levels should be monitored at least every 2 hours during the procedure to avoid hypoglycemia below 60 mg/dL and hyperglycemia above 250 mg/dL. Blood glucose levels can be measured rapidly during surgery with a portable electronic glucose analyzer.

1. Conventional procedure for insulin administration—The first and still most widely used method of controlling blood glucose levels during surgery is to administer subcutaneously, on the morning of the operation, one-third to one-half the patient's usual dose of long-acting insulin plus one-third to one-half the usual dose of short-acting insulin. This is followed by intravenous infusion of 5% or even 10% glucose at a rate of 100 mL/h preoperatively and intraoperatively. If the operation is prolonged, potassium chloride should be added at a rate of 20 meq/h.

There are a number of disadvantages to this procedure, which results in giving the full day's insulin requirement preoperatively. First, after subcutaneous administration, the absorption of NPH and regular insulin varies greatly in individual patients, especially when they are inactive. Second, although surgeons are aware that operations on diabetics should be scheduled early in the day, all too often the procedure must be delayed until afternoon. The relatively small amounts of glucose being administered are then inadequate to compensate for the 18–20 hours the patient has been without food, with the result that the insulin causes severe afternoon hypoglycemia. In the average diabetic, the peak action of regular insulin occurs about 6 hours after its administration—not 1–2 hours afterward, as stated in older textbooks. Therefore, if regular insulin is given subcutaneously at 7 AM, its peak action in an average patient will occur at about 1 PM. As a result, following subcutaneous administration of regular insulin in the early morning, the patient's glucose concentration may be inadequately controlled early in the morning; and if surgery is delayed, the peak action of regular insulin in the early afternoon and of NPH insulin in the later afternoon may result in severe hypoglycemia. If surgery must be delayed, it is imperative that blood glucose levels be carefully monitored for hypoglycemia and additional glucose given as necessary.

2. Intravenous infusion of insulin in glucose solution—There is an increasing tendency to treat type 1 diabetics undergoing surgery by giving an infusion of 5% or 10% glucose solution containing 5, 10, or even 15 units of insulin per liter, depending on the patient's initial blood glucose concentration. At an infusion rate of 100 mL/h, insulin is thereby administered at a rate of 0.5, 1, or 1.5 units/h, respectively. In patients receiving corticosteroids, as much as 20 units per liter of insulin may be required.

There are a number of advantages to this regimen. First, the problem of absorption of insulin is avoided, since it is given intravenously. As a result, instead of an average 6-hour lag for maximal response to regular insulin, the effect starts within 10–15 minutes and is relatively constant. Second, unlike the fixed insulin dose with subcutaneous administration, the insulin infusion can be changed at any time in response to changes in blood glucose levels. Third, the dangers of hypo- and hyperglycemia are minimized, because if the intravenous solution is stopped (if the needle is inadvertently removed or the tubing clamped), both the glucose and the insulin are discontinued simultaneously. Since only 10% of insulin adsorbs to glass or plastic, the resulting reduction in dosage is of little therapeutic importance. A similar continuous intravenous infusion of insulin has also become a common way to treat diabetic ketoacidosis.

3. Use of insulin "piggy-backed" into the glucose infusion—Instead of mixing insulin in the same bottle as the glucose, an insulin solution is infused ("piggy-backed") into the tubing delivering the 5% or 10% glucose. Generally, 50 units of regular insulin are mixed with 500 mL of normal saline—a solution containing 1 unit of insulin per 10 mL of solution. The glucose solution is given at a rate of 100 mL/h, and the insulin infusion is adjusted (usually by IVAC pump) to deliver a total of 5 mL (0.5 units), 10 mL (1 unit), 30 mL (30 units) per hour, etc, depending on the results of blood glucose determinations obtained approximately hourly during the surgical procedure. Of the three techniques, this one is the most flexible, allows the closest control of blood glucose levels, and is therefore increasingly being recommended as the method of choice. It requires careful monitoring of the pump delivery rate, because too rapid infusion of insulin will cause hypoglycemia. A number of simple algorithms have been recommended for adjusting the rate of insulin infusion according to the previous plasma glucose levels. This approach is especially useful during prolonged operations. The simplest and most practical procedure is to give no insulin if plasma glucose is less than 90 mg/dL. Above values of 90 mg/dL, the dosage of regular insulin in units per hour should equal 1% of the previous hour's plasma glucose (mg/dL)—eg, at a glucose level of 200 mg/dL, give 2 units/h; at 300 mg/dL, give 3 units/h, etc.

Postoperative Care

With either of the intravenous infusion techniques, it is best to continue the glucose-insulin infusion until the patient is eating. Hypoglycemia, the most common postoperative complication, most often follows the use of long-acting insulin given subcutaneously before surgery. Although hypoglycemia may also occur if the intravenous insulin infusion is excessive in relation to that of the glucose, an infusion of 1.5 units or less of insulin per hour, when given with 5% glucose, rarely results in hypoglycemia. Blood glucose levels should be measured every 2–4 hours and the patient monitored for signs and symptoms of hypoglycemia (eg, anxiety, tremulousness, profuse sweating without fever). When hypoglycemia is detected, the amount of glucose infused should be promptly increased and the insulin decreased. It is rarely advisable to stop the insulin infusion completely for mild hypoglycemia, since a smoother transition to euglycemia results if the insulin is continued but at a lower dose.

A marked increase in glucose and insulin requirements postoperatively suggests the presence of occult infection (eg, wound infection, cellulitis at the intravenous site, urinary tract infection, or unrecognized aspiration pneumonia).

The use of a "sliding scale" based on urine glucose values to judge insulin requirements is no longer justified for postoperative diabetic management. Problems of urine retention, failure to obtain a double-voided specimen, and variations in the renal threshold for glucose excretion confuse the interpretation of urine glucose values; this makes it extremely dangerous to base insulin requirements on these measurements. Adjustments in the rate of glucose or insulin administration must be based on *blood* glucose levels.

Hyperosmolar Coma

Hyperosmolar coma, the result of severe dehydration, may occur in undiagnosed diabetics who have been given large amounts of glucose during surgery. The resulting osmotic diuresis leads to disproportionate water loss, dehydration, and hyperosmolarity. Hyperosmolar coma rarely occurs until the serum glucose level exceeds 800 mg/dL and the osmolarity exceeds 340 meq/L. Hyperosmolar coma may be best avoided by monitoring fluid input and output, measuring blood glucose levels, and instituting treatment promptly if the value exceeds 400 mg/dL.

Golden SH et al: Perioperative glycemic control and the risk of infectious complications in a cohort of adults with diabetes. Diabetes Care 1999; 22:1408.

Hirsch IB et al: Diabetes management in special situations. Endocrinol Metab Clin North Am 1997;26:631.

Kaufman FR et al: Perioperative management with prolonged intravenous insulin infusion versus subcutaneous insulin in children with type I diabetes mellitus. J Diabetes Complications 1996;10:6.

Vanhaeverbeek M: Peri-operative care: management of the diabetic patient. A novel controversy about tight glycemic control. Acta Clin Belg 1997;52:313.

THYROID DISEASE

Both hyper- and hypothyroidism represent serious problems for patients undergoing surgery. It may be difficult to establish an adequate airway in patients with large goiters. The hyperthyroid patient undergoing surgery is apt to develop hypertension, severe cardiac dysrhythmias, congestive heart failure, and hyperthermia.

Life-threatening thyrotoxicosis (thyroid storm) may be precipitated by any operation but especially by thyroidectomy, which accentuates thyroxine release. It is therefore preferable to bring hyperthyroid patients into a euthyroid state before surgery. This takes 1–6 weeks and is best accomplished by treatment with propylthiouracil, 800–1000 mg/d for about 1 week, followed by a maintenance dose of 200–400 mg/d. If emergency surgery is required, adequate sedation and potassium iodide plus a β-adrenergic blocking agent such as propranolol should be given in addition to propylthiouracil.

Hypothyroid patients are subject to acute hypotension, shock, and hypothermia during surgery; if the patient is allowed to breathe spontaneously, severe CO_2 retention may result from hypoventilation. **Myxedema coma** should be suspected in patients who fail to awaken promptly from anesthesia and who manifest CO_2 retention, even to the point of CO_2 narcosis, accompanied by hypothermia. Increased tissue friability, poor wound healing, and even wound dehiscence may also occur. It is highly advisable to treat myxedematous patients with levothyroxine before elective surgery. In an emergency (eg, severe myxedema requiring immediate surgery), treatment should consist of levothyroxine sodium, 500 μg (0.5 mg) intravenously, by nasogastric tube, or orally. If there is no emergency, the euthyroid state may be gradually restored with levothyroxine, 25 μg/d, with the dose increased over several weeks to a maintenance dose of 150–200 μg/d. It is also always advisable to obtain a baseline cortisol level before treatment of myxedema to rule out coexistent Addison's disease (Schmidt's syndrome), since levothyroxine therapy can precipitate addisonian crisis in this setting.

Attia J et al: Diagnosis of thyroid disease in hospitalized patients: a systematic review. Arch Intern Med 1999;159:658.

Cooper DS: Antithyroid drugs for the treatment of hyperthyroidism caused by Graves' disease. Emerg Med Clin North Am 1998;27:225.

Ladenson PW et al: Complications of surgery in hypothyroid patients. Am J Med 1984;77:261.

Kahaly GJ et al: Cardiac risks of hyperthyroidism in the elderly. Thyroid 1998;8:1165.

Koutras DA: Subclinical hyperthyroidism. Thyroid 1999;9:311.

ADRENAL INSUFFICIENCY

Patients with adrenal insufficiency undergoing the stress of operation are at risk of addisonian crisis, manifested by salt wastage, decreased blood volume, hypotension, shock, and death. For at least 2–3 days preoperatively, they should receive fluid and sodium chloride replacement intravenously (usually 1–3 L of normal saline per day) and cortisol therapy (20 mg each morning and 10 mg each afternoon). On the day of surgery, 100 mg of cortisol is administered intramuscularly or intravenously just before the operation, followed by 50–100 mg every 6 hours during surgery—a regimen that mimics the normal endogenous cortisol response to stress (up to 300 mg/d). Saline is continued postoperatively at a rate of at least 2–3 L/d, with careful monitoring of blood pressure, serum electrolyte concentrations, and urine output. In the absence of complications, the cortisol dosage can be decreased by half each day until the usual maintenance dose of about 30 mg/d is reached.

Patients receiving chronic corticosteroid therapy may present with severe hypokalemia and at times serious hypertension, both of which should be corrected before surgery. Stress doses of cortisol (approximately 300 mg/d) must be administered during surgery according to the protocol described for addisonian patients. If the patient is diabetic, large doses of insulin (eg, 3 units/h) may be required to control blood glucose levels during surgery. Postoperatively, slow wound healing and a predisposition to infection should be anticipated. Infections in these patients may occur without fever.

PITUITARY INSUFFICIENCY

Patients with **panhypopituitarism** must be treated for thyroid and adrenocorticosteroid insufficiency with the doses of levothyroxine and cortisol set forth in the preceding sections.

■ HEART DISEASE & THE SURGICAL PATIENT

Barry M. Massie, MD

Anesthesia and surgery present a finite risk to any patient, but this risk is increased in the patient with preexisting heart disease, whether clinically apparent or undiagnosed. Indeed, complications related to heart disease are the major cause of nonsurgical perioperative deaths.

Cardiac disease may be exacerbated by many of the physiologic changes accompanying surgery, including fluctuations in heart rate, blood pressure, blood volume, oxygenation, pH, and coagulability. These may lead to myocardial ischemia due to increased myocardial O_2 demand or reduced coronary blood flow, impaired myocardial contractility, and altered cardiac performance due to changes in preload or afterload. Increased circulating catecholamines or sympathetic nervous system activity may precipitate arrhythmias as well as increase heart rate and blood pressure. Anesthesia and medications such as vagolytics and muscle relaxants have direct effects on myocardial contractility, automaticity, and conduction.

While it is often felt that the operative period itself is the most stressful, intraoperative cardiac complications have become in fact relatively uncommon as a result of careful monitoring and improved understanding of the risk of the accompanying hemodynamic alterations. The greatest risk occurs in the first 72 hours after operation, when fluid volume shifts, fluctuations in heart rate and blood pressure, and medication changes are greatest and the ability to control them is compromised. The best approach to minimizing cardiac complications is to maintain one's awareness of the presence and severity of preexisting heart disease and of the risk of asymptomatic and unrecognized disease.

Given this information, the medical consultant, anesthesiologist, and surgeon can weigh the following key questions: (1) Is the operation urgent, essential but with elective timing, or optional? (2) Does the patient have heart disease, manifest or silent? (3) What additional risk does heart disease impose? (4) Can this risk be reduced by additional treatment or by delaying surgery? The answers to these questions will determine the appropriate management strategy. Urgent surgery must proceed, so the problem for the consultant and anesthesiologist is to minimize risk. Elective surgery may need to be delayed or canceled depending on the risk:benefit ratio.

Cardiac Conditions Masquerading as Surgical Illnesses

It is important to recognize that cardiovascular diseases may occasionally produce symptoms that mimic surgical conditions, and this possibility must be considered before operation. Such presentations include the following:

(1) Myocardial infarction or angina pectoris presenting with epigastric pain, suggesting peptic ulcer, gallbladder disease, or other surgical abdominal disease.

(2) Right heart failure presenting as right upper quadrant pain due to hepatic congestion, suggesting gallbladder disease.

(3) Nonspecific gastrointestinal symptoms such as anorexia, nausea, early satiety, and weight loss due to severe heart failure, suggesting cancer or other abdominal surgical disease.

(4) Ascites due to heart failure or pericardial disease.

(5) Dysphagia due to left atrial enlargement or diseases of the aorta.

(6) Back and abdominal pain due to aortic dissection.

(7) Abdominal pain due to splenic, renal, or mesenteric emboli from infective endocarditis, emboli of cardiac origin, or atrial myxoma.

(8) Upper abdominal pain and even jaundice due to pulmonary infarction.

Most of these conditions will be readily recognized if they are considered. More typical associated symptoms are usually present. The ECG should reveal evolving or recent infarction, and the physical examination and chest x-ray should demonstrate heart failure or signs of pericardial disease. Echocardiography will confirm the presence of left or right ventricular failure, valvular disease, and pericardial disease and may reveal a source of emboli.

Preoperative Evaluation of the Surgical Patient for Cardiovascular Disease

All patients should be evaluated for possible cardiovascular disease preoperatively. The extent of this evaluation will depend on the statistical likelihood of previously unrecognized disease if the patient is asymptomatic and the nature of the heart condition if the diagnosis is known. A careful history is the primary screening procedure. Key areas of inquiry include the presence of

dyspnea, exercise tolerance (and what limits it), chest discomfort and other ischemic equivalents (epigastric, throat, shoulder, or arm discomfort), edema, syncope or presyncope, or a history of heart murmur, hypertension, or failing an employment or insurance physical examination. Patients with a family history of premature coronary disease or with associated peripheral vascular disease should be assumed to be at high risk for ischemic heart disease, as should patients with a long history of diabetes. Patients with hyperlipidemia or hypertension are also at increased risk.

The physical examination will occasionally demonstrate a previously unrecognized heart murmur, mitral valve prolapse, irregular heart rhythm, or hypertension. In patients with heart disease, it will reveal the severity and degree of compensation of heart failure and provide a guide to the severity of valvular disease.

Most patients should have a preoperative ECG, though the yield is low in young patients with negative histories and examinations. Important findings include abnormal rhythms and conduction, left ventricular hypertrophy, myocardial infarction, and "nonspecific" ST segment and T wave abnormalities. A routine preoperative chest x-ray has a low yield in healthy subjects but may be useful in patients with symptoms or an abnormal physical examination. Additional noninvasive tests or procedures that may be indicated to diagnose and define the severity of cardiac abnormalities include echocardiography, exercise testing, stress (exercise or dipyridamole) thallium scintigraphy, radionuclide ejection fraction measurements, and ambulatory monitoring. In some patients, cardiac catheterization and coronary arteriography are indicated to determine the severity of heart disease and the need for additional medical or other intervention before surgery.

The evaluation and management of specific cardiac diseases and abnormalities are discussed below.

Relative Contraindications to Surgery

There are no absolute contraindications to surgery, but a number of cardiac conditions substantially increase the risks and become relative contraindications. These include recent myocardial infarction, an unstable or progressive pattern of angina pectoris, decompensated heart failure, severe aortic or mitral stenosis, and severe hypertension. Most heart diseases do not themselves prohibitively increase the surgical risk, but when they are progressive, unstable, or decompensated, the level of risk rises abruptly.

Several approaches have been proposed for quantifying operative risk. The most widely used of these is the Goldman Index, which provides a point score for findings associated with additional risk:

Finding	Points
S_2 gallop or elevated venous pressure	11
Myocardial infarction in previous 6 months	10
More than five VPCs/min on any ECG	7
Nonsinus rhythm or APCs on last ECG	7
Age > 70 years	5
Emergency operation	4
Intrathoracic, intraperitoneal, or aortic surgery	3
Significant aortic stenosis	3
Poor general medical condition	3

The risk of cardiac death and life-threatening cardiac complications rises progressively with the total point score—from less than 1% when the score is 0–5 points, to 7% for 6–12 points, 13% (2% mortality rate) with 13–25 points, to 78% (including a 56% mortality rate) in patients with scores over 26 points.

Detsky has modified this multifactorial index to take into account the nature of the operation. However, it should be recognized that these indices serve two functions: to identify factors of risk and to provide probabilities for populations. In assessing the individual patient, the physician must make a judgment based upon the specific cardiac disease, its severity, and its stability.

Specific Cardiac Conditions

A. CORONARY ARTERY DISEASE

Coronary artery disease is the most common cardiac disease and the major cause of morbidity and mortality in patients undergoing surgery. Several categories of patients must be considered: those with prior myocardial infarction, those with angina pectoris, and those with possible asymptomatic coronary disease. Virtually all patients who have had a myocardial infarction have coronary artery disease and are at risk for further ischemia or reinfarction. This risk is highest in patients in whom the infarction is most recent, declining from approximately 20–30% (or higher in earlier studies) in the first 3 months, to 10–15% after 4–6 months, and to 5% thereafter. With advances in medical therapy, better diagnostic testing, and improved perioperative management, these numbers are falling, but it is still preferable to delay elective surgery for 3–6 months after myocardial infarction. The propensity for ischemia and reinfarction are higher following nontransmural infarctions, in which the volume of residual ischemic myocardium is greater. If the infarction is recent, such patients should undergo stress testing with exercise or dipyridamole thallium scintigraphy to identify individuals with large areas of ischemia before major surgery; these patients should undergo coronary angiography

and revascularization if indicated. It may be helpful to assess left ventricular function noninvasively in patients with anterior transmural infarctions, since they may have significantly decreased ejection fractions in the absence of symptomatic heart failure.

Angina pectoris also reflects underlying coronary artery disease and is just as important an indicator of risk as is prior infarction. When the pattern is progressive or unstable or the activity threshold is very low, operation should be postponed at least until the angina can be stabilized by medical therapy. If major noncardiac surgery is planned, coronary arteriography is usually indicated in patients with unstable or severely limiting angina to detect critical lesions.

Patients with *stable* mild to moderate angina pectoris, old myocardial infarctions, or multiple risk factors without overt coronary artery disease represent a group with intermediate perioperative risk. When major surgery (especially vascular procedures) is planned or if additional risk factors such as age over 70 years, diabetes mellitus, or heart failure are present, further evaluation may be warranted. Since exercise testing is often not feasible, pharmacologic stress with dipyridamole or adenosine in association with perfusion scintigraphy or echocardiography are usually employed. Individuals with demonstrable ischemia, especially when it involves multiple or large areas, are at increased risk; coronary arteriography or additional medical therapy may be indicated.

However, before additional noninvasive diagnostic procedures are performed, there are several things to consider. First, in *stable* patients with mild or even moderate symptoms, the risk of a major cardiac event (cardiac death, nonfatal infarction) as a complication of surgery averages just 2%, rising to only 5% with the most stressful (eg, vascular) operations. Consequently, myocardial revascularization by coronary artery bypass surgery or percutaneous transluminal angioplasty is rarely justified in such patients preoperatively. Although noninvasive imaging procedures could theoretically identify high-risk subgroups, experience has not been consistently good (Table 5–1). Therefore, routine stress testing for risk stratification is not warranted, and imaging tests should generally be reserved for instances where the results are likely to alter management, such as to postpone surgery or change the planned procedure. Decisions concerning evaluation for coronary revascularization should be based upon the patient's symptoms or other accepted indications, such as multivessel disease in a patient with underlying left ventricular dysfunction, rather than specifically for decreasing perioperative risk. Therefore, all patients with cardiac risk factors who are undergoing major operations must be managed carefully during and after surgery whether or not noninvasive studies are normal. And there is no convincing evidence that preliminary

Table 5–1. Significance of a reversible dipyridamole ^{201}T1 defect.

Reference		N	Sensitivity (%)	Specificity (%)	PPV (%)	NPV (%)	RR
Boucher	N Engl J Med 1985;312:389	48	100	80	50	100	16.0
Cutler	J Vasc Surg 1987;5:91	101	100	69	23	100	14.3
Leppo	J Am Coll Cardiol 1987;9:269	89	93	62	33	98	15.7
Eagle	JAMA 1987;257:2185	200	83	66	30	96	7.2
Mangano	Circulation 1991;84:493	60	46	66	27	82	1.5
Marwick[1]	Clin Cardiol 1990;13:14	86	30	75	14	89	1.2
Fleischer	Anesthesiology 1990;73(3A):A75	19	0	46	0	38	0.0
Bertrand[2]	Anesthesiology 1990;73(3A):A85	71	43	77	55	63a	1.3

[1]Fixed or reversible defect considered positive.
[2]Compared with coronary arteriography.

PPV = Predictive value of a positive test for subsequent outcome event.
NPV = Predictive value of negative test for absence of an outcome event.
RR = Relative risk for an outcome event of patients with a positive test compared with those with a negative test.

coronary revascularization improves the outcome even in high-risk patients.

Patients with coronary artery disease or a high probability of coronary artery disease need to be managed carefully. Preoperative medications—including beta-blockers in particular but also nitrates and calcium channel blockers—should be continued throughout the perioperative period. Aspirin should be continued unless concerns about hemostasis are overriding; addition of aspirin postoperatively may be useful, since many infarcts may be caused by a postoperative hypercoagulable state. Excessive tachycardia, hypertension, and hypotension should be avoided. Complications are most common in the second to fifth postoperative days, so vigilance must be maintained.

B. CONGESTIVE HEART FAILURE

Severe or decompensated congestive heart failure is an important risk factor for perioperative cardiac death. Surgery should be postponed until congestive heart failure is stable, pulmonary edema is absent, and excessive fluid is eliminated. A stable regimen of diuretics, angiotensin-converting enzyme inhibitors, and digoxin when indicated should be instituted. Underlying reversible causes (such as valvular lesions, ischemia, or uncontrolled hypertension) should be identified and treated. For major surgery, hemodynamic monitoring intraoperatively and postoperatively is essential. Decompensation is most common during and after the second postoperative day, when extravascular fluid begins to be mobilized. Weights, fluid balance, and oxygenation must be followed closely and diuretic therapy reinstituted early unless hypotension is present.

C. VALVULAR HEART DISEASE

Valvular heart disease in the absence of congestive heart failure is usually well tolerated during surgery. The exceptions are critical aortic stenosis and mitral stenosis. The former can be associated with hypotension and heart failure, while the latter often causes pulmonary edema when the heart rate increases, atrial fibrillation occurs, or excessive fluid volume is administered. Nonetheless, patients with moderate obstructions (eg, aortic valve area > 0.8 cm^2; mitral area > 1.2 cm^2) usually do well, and those with even more severe stenoses can be managed successfully with careful monitoring if the need for surgery is urgent. Mitral valve prolapse is an indication for antibiotic prophylaxis in nonsterile procedures but does not increase the risk of surgery.

D. DYSRHYTHMIAS AND CONDUCTION ABNORMALITIES

Supraventricular arrhythmias can usually be managed with agents such as verapamil and esmolol as well as with digoxin. Frequent ventricular ectopy does indicate increased risk, but this usually reflects associated myocardial disease, which should be sought and evaluated. It is not necessary to suppress asymptomatic nonsustained ventricular arrhythmias preoperatively. Ventricular ectopy and ventricular tachycardia occurring during or after surgery often reflect arrhythmias that were present preoperatively. Treatment is required only when they result in symptoms or hemodynamic compromise. Electrolyte imbalance, hypoxia, and electrocardiographic evidence of bigeminy or infarction should be sought and treated. Prophylactic antiarrhythmic activity has not been shown to be beneficial.

Left bundle branch block or bifascicular block also indicates higher risk, since these findings often indicate myocardial disease. However, progression to advanced atrioventricular block during surgery is rare. Prolonged PR intervals, Mobitz I (Wenckebach) atrioventricular block, or sinus bradycardia (heart rate less than 45–50/ min) often reflects excessive medication effect from digoxin, β-adrenergic blocking agents, and calcium channel-blocking agents. These dosages should be adjusted downward if possible. Higher degrees of atrioventricular blockade should usually be managed with temporary or permanent pacing.

E. CONGENITAL HEART DISEASE

Space does not permit discussion of the impact of various congenital lesions on perioperative risk. In general, if these lesions are associated with heart failure, severe pulmonary hypertension (systolic pulmonary pressure above 80 mm Hg), or hypoxemia, the risk of surgery is high.

F. HYPERTENSION

Patients with uncomplicated and controlled hypertension usually tolerate surgery well. The presence of left ventricular hypertrophy with repolarization changes indicates mildly increased risk, perhaps because of a higher incidence of associated coronary artery disease. Indeed, untreated and suboptimally treated hypertension do not appear to significantly increase risk when the pressure is below 160/105 mm Hg, since it is relatively easy to reduce it with anesthesia and parenteral agents. When the pressure exceeds 180/110 mm Hg, the incidence of severe perioperative hypertension increases along with the need for prolonged parenteral treatment and observation as well as the risk of complications.

Antihypertensive medications should be continued to avoid withdrawal syndromes, especially when the patient is receiving central sympatholytics or beta-blockers. This can usually be accomplished with oral medication, but transdermal clonidine, sublingual nifedipine, and intravenous calcium channel blockers (verapamil and diltiazem) and parenteral beta-blockers and converting enzyme inhibitors are available.

Special Issues Related to Monitoring & Anesthesia

A. MEDICATIONS

As noted above, it is feasible and desirable to continue most medications in the perioperative period. This is especially true with medications for coronary artery disease, congestive heart failure, and hypertension. If additional medications are needed, parenteral therapy is should be provided.

B. HEMODYNAMIC MONITORING

Hemodynamic monitoring of high-risk patients during major surgical procedures has become routine. This is essential in patients with congestive heart failure, impaired left ventricular function (ejection fraction below 40%), critical valve disease, and recent myocardial infarction when the surgery is major. It probably is not necessary in patients at risk for ischemia with preserved left ventricular function except in the case of major vascular procedures. Perhaps the most valuable period for hemodynamic monitoring in high-risk patients is the immediate postoperative period, when appropriate parameters for fluid administration and blood pressure can be difficult to define.

C. TRANSESOPHAGEAL ECHOCARDIOGRAPHY

This technique is being increasingly used in the operating room. It permits excellent visualization of the left ventricle and can provide continuous monitoring of cavity size, contractile function, and segmental wall motion. In experienced hands, transesophageal echocardiography allows early detection of heart failure and myocardial ischemia, but its additional value beyond hemodynamic monitoring in noncardiac surgery has not been proved, and for that reason its routine use even in high-risk patients is not indicated.

D. CHOICE OF ANESTHETICS

There is no conclusive evidence that the choice of anesthetics affects outcomes in patients with heart disease, and the selection of the route of anesthesia and the choice of agent are best left to the anesthesiologist. Epidural anesthesia may be preferable when a low spinal level is adequate for the procedure, but hypotension is a problem with higher levels. Narcotics have little myocardial depressant action and may be preferable to the volatile gases in patients with diminished contractility.

E. ANTIBIOTIC PROPHYLAXIS

Patients with valvular heart disease and prosthetic heart valves require antibiotic prophylaxis for potentially bacteremic events, including genitourinary, gastrointestinal, oropharyngeal, and gallbladder surgery. The usual regimen is ampicillin, 2 g intravenously, plus gentamicin, 1.5 mg/kg intravenously 30 minutes before operation. This may be repeated after 8 hours. Vancomycin, 1 g intravenously over 60 minutes, may be substituted in patients allergic to penicillin.

F. ANTICOAGULATION

Patients with prosthetic valves and other heart conditions may be receiving chronic anticoagulation. In the former case, interruption of anticoagulation should be as brief as possible. Such patients should have their warfarin withdrawn 5 days prior to surgery and be maintained on intravenous heparin from the time their prothrombin time falls below 1½ times control until 6 hours before operation. Heparin can usually be resumed 12 hours postoperatively. Anticoagulation for other indications can usually be withdrawn safely for the perioperative period.

Abraham S et al: Coronary risk of noncardiac surgery. Prog Cardiovasc Dis 1991;34:205.

Ashton CM et al: Incidence of perioperative myocardial infarction in men undergoing noncardiac surgical procedures. Ann Intern Med 1993;118:504.

Baron J-F et al: Dipyridamole-thallium scintigraphy and gated radionuclide angiography to assess cardiac risk before abdominal aortic surgery. N Engl J Med 1994;330:663.

Massie BM et al: Assessment of perioperative risk: have we put the cart before the horse? J Am Coll Cardiol 1993;21:1353.

Wong T et al: Perioperative cardiac risk assessment for patients having peripheral vascular surgery. Ann Intern Med 1992; 116:745.

■ RESPIRATORY DISEASE & THE SURGICAL PATIENT

Robert F. Hickey, MD

Risk Factors

The most common perioperative complications involve the pulmonary system. The relatively high incidence of pulmonary complications is associated with anesthesia and surgery, and the two primary determinants are the operative site and the presence of lung disease. The correlation between the site of surgical incision and the incidence of pulmonary complications—from high to low—is thoracotomy, upper abdomen, lower abdomen, and periphery. The introduction of laparoscopic surgery has altered this basic paradigm, introducing a possible technique for reducing postoperative respiratory complications in high-risk patients. However, in these same patients, the complexity of intraoperative management may be increased. The implications of laparoscopic surgery for patients at high risk of postoperative respiratory complications is discussed below. Pulmonary complications occur least frequently in patients with normal lung function who are undergoing peripheral surgery.

Secondary determinants of perioperative pulmonary complications include a history of smoking, age, obesity, and cooperativeness of the patient in postoperative care. These factors probably facilitate the development of lung disease, decrease the ability of the patient to co-

operate in common maneuvers used to prevent or treat pulmonary complications, and compromise laryngeal integrity. (See also Chapter 4.)

Laparoscopic Surgery

The advantage of laparoscopic surgery is that the use of smaller incisions and reduction in surgical trauma results in less postoperative pain and earlier recovery of bowel function. Thus, the impact of laparoscopic surgery on postoperative respiratory function may be intermediate between that of peripheral surgery and a lower abdominal incision and thus reduce postoperative respiratory complications. The disadvantage of this technique is its impact on both circulation and ventilation intraoperatively. Laparoscopic surgery requires the introduction of a pneumoperitoneum, distending the abdomen (usually with carbon dioxide) to intra-abdominal pressures of 11–15 mm Hg. Measurements in relatively healthy patients have shown that this maneuver results in a reduction of lung volume, systemic hypercapnia, reduction in cardiac index, and an increase in cardiac filling pressures and systemic vascular resistance. In these healthy patients, it is recommended that ventilation be increased to normalize $PaCO_2$. In patients with serious lung disease, the impact of introduction of a pneumoperitoneum is unknown. Additionally, attempts to normalize $PaCO_2$ have the potential to introduce air trapping with resultant circulatory collapse. At present, we would recommend that in patients with severe lung disease laparoscopic surgery may require extensive intraoperative monitoring with the possibility of converting to an open procedure if so indicated.

Specific Diseases & Problems

A. ACUTE UPPER RESPIRATORY TRACT INFECTIONS

Both anesthesia and surgery provide opportunities for the spread of infection because respiratory defense mechanisms are compromised and instrumentation of the airway may be required. Therefore, the presence of a cold, pharyngitis, or tonsillitis is a relative contraindication to elective surgery, since viral infections decrease defense mechanisms against bacterial infections. If surgery is necessary, the appropriate antibiotic should be administered and manipulation of the infected area avoided when possible. No studies document the rate of complications or the preferred anesthetic techniques applicable to this situation.

B. ACUTE LOWER RESPIRATORY TRACT INFECTIONS (TRACHEITIS, BRONCHITIS, PNEUMONIA)

These infections are absolute contraindications to elective surgery. For emergency surgery, therapy includes humidification of inhaled gases, removal of lung secretions, and continued administration of bronchodilators and antibiotics. If surgery is not absolutely necessary, the course of action is uncertain because no information is available concerning the incidence and severity of pulmonary complications.

C. Chronic Obstructive Pulmonary Disease (COPD) (Bronchitis, Emphysema, Bronchiectasis)

In patients with chronic obstructive pulmonary disease, the well-documented increase in the incidence and severity of postoperative pulmonary complications is related to the degree of lung disease. Two studies have investigated the influence of preoperative treatment of lung disease on the incidence of postoperative pulmonary complications. In both studies, patients underwent upper abdominal or thoracic surgery, and lung disease was defined by pulmonary function testing. In one study, therapy lasted 1 week and consisted of cessation of smoking, administration of antibiotics for purulent sputum, administration of bronchodilators, and physical therapy. In the second study, therapy lasted for 2 days and consisted of administration of antibiotics and bronchodilators and physical therapy. Both studies reported marked reduction in the incidence and severity of complications. The 1-week study reported decreased length of hospitalization for its patients.

Two other studies demonstrated the interaction between lung disease and the surgical site. They suggest that in peripheral surgery, lung disease is not a factor in the production of pulmonary complications unless disease is very severe (eg, severe enough to result in elevated PaCO$_2$). However, both of these studies were performed on a limited number of patients.

The results of these four studies indicate that patients with lung disease who are scheduled for elective upper abdominal or thoracic surgery should have preoperative treatment. Treatment should decrease the incidence and severity of postoperative pulmonary complications and shorten the hospital stay. A minimum of 1 week of therapy should include cessation of smoking; administration of antibiotics for purulent sputum and bronchodilators when indicated, and physical therapy to help remove excess sputum. Therapy can be performed on an outpatient basis. While any patient with lung disease should be treated regardless of plans for surgery, the focus here is on the prevention of death and illness from pulmonary complications in the surgical patient along with reduction of hospital time required to recover from surgical procedures.

D. Bronchial Asthma

Retrospective studies indicate that patients with bronchial asthma who are undergoing surgery are at increased risk of pulmonary complications. Preoperative management includes adjustment of bronchodilator medication, cessation of smoking, and treatment of infection. Intraoperative bronchoconstriction from mechanical stimulation of the airway must be prevented so that appropriate anesthetics can be given in adequate concentrations. Since intraoperative use of bronchodilators may be necessary, adverse interactions between anesthetic agents and bronchodilators must be avoided. Many patients with bronchial asthma have been treated with corticosteroids and require corticosteroid therapy in the perioperative period.

E. Restrictive Lung Disease (Caused by Pulmonary Fibrosis or Obesity)

Little information exists on perioperative pulmonary complications secondary to restrictive lung disease. Restrictive lung disease reduces lung volumes and decreases arterial oxygen tension; the decrease in arterial oxygen tension is particularly noticeable with exercise. Preoperative preparation is similar to that for any other lung disease and consists of treatment of infection, removal of sputum, and discontinuance of smoking. When controlled ventilation is required for patients with pulmonary fibrosis, it may be necessary to use smaller tidal volumes and more rapid respiratory rates than normal.

When the administration of the antitumor chemotherapeutic agent bleomycin causes pulmonary fibrosis, patients may be susceptible to oxygen toxicity; therefore, inspired oxygen concentrations should be carefully controlled.

The effects of obesity on the development of perioperative pulmonary complications are most easily demonstrated in the massively obese patient. Obesity exists when the body weight is 1.2 times the normal weight; in morbid obesity, the weight is at least twice the normal weight. Pulmonary compromise is mostly due to reduction in lung volumes, leading to hypoxemia, airway obstruction from encroaching soft tissues in the airway, and perhaps an increase in gastric contents and acidity. If the problems are recognized and evaluated preoperatively, complications can be minimized. The massively obese patient should be mobilized as soon as possible postoperatively.

Preoperative Evaluation of Pulmonary Function

The purpose of preoperative pulmonary evaluation is to assess the risk of perioperative lung complications. This information not only guides perioperative pulmonary care but also selects patients for specific preoperative treatment that will decrease the risk of pulmonary complications and the length of the hospital stay. Such evaluations should be made before hospital admission to allow time for treatment if indicated.

Ideally, pulmonary evaluation is performed by the referring physician or surgeon (or both) at the time surgery is proposed. The site of surgery is a major consideration in the decision to perform pulmonary function tests and institute treatment (see Risk Factors, above). Other indications for pulmonary function testing arise primarily from the patient's history and physical examination and include factors present in lung disease, such as exertional dyspnea, exercise tolerance, cough, production of sputum, history of smoking, previous pulmonary complications, asthma, age, and body weight. Patients with mild pulmonary compromise who are to undergo peripheral surgery (not abdominal or thoracic surgery) probably do not require pulmonary function testing. When testing is necessary, simple spirometry with measurement of forced expiratory airflow is usually all that is required. If airflow on forced expiration is reduced significantly, the response to bronchodilators should be measured and arterial blood gases determined. More extensive tests such as diffusing capacity, radioisotopic ventilation-perfusion scans, and pulmonary artery catheterization are usually necessary only in patients with pulmonary hypertension or life-threatening lung disease or in those who require thoracic surgery.

Many studies have been done to try to determine which pulmonary function tests are the most reliable indicators of surgical and anesthetic risk and which reveal the greatest risk. Specific tests are usually correlated with perioperative complications, but for the most part these studies are not definitive, and as yet there are no absolute criteria for "operability." Tests can provide guidelines but are not reliable predictors for the following reasons:

(1) Patients with normal pulmonary function may develop perioperative pulmonary complications, though the incidence is low.

(2) Criteria developed for one surgical procedure (eg, thoracotomy) may not be accurate for another procedure.

(3) Pulmonary function tests cannot take into account intangibles such as patient cooperativeness. Tests do not measure the amount of sputum produced or predict the likelihood of pulmonary aspiration.

In general, simple spirometry with some measurement of impairment of airflow provides the best and least expensive screening test. Patients undergoing thoracic surgery without lung resection are at increased risk if FEV_1 or maximum breathing capacity is less than 50% of normal. For peripheral surgery, these values are lower (about 30% of predicted normal values). $PaCO_2$ greater than 45 mm Hg in patients not receiving ventilatory depressant drugs who are undergoing abdominal surgery or thoracotomy without lung tissue rejection indicates potential life-threatening pulmonary complications.

Surgery on these patients should proceed only after adequate consultation. In peripheral surgery as well, elevated $PaCO_2$ indicates a greater likelihood of pulmonary complications and the possible need for postoperative mechanical ventilation and special monitoring.

Bartlett RH: Pulmonary pathophysiology in surgical patients. Surg Clin North Am 1980;60:1323.

Celi BR et al: A controlled trial of intermittent positive pressure breathing, incentive spirometry, and deep breathing exercises in preventing pulmonary complications after abdominal surgery. Am Rev Respir Dis 1984;130:12.

Craig DB: Postoperative recovery of pulmonary function. Anesth Analg 1981;60:46.

Cunningham AJ et al: Laparoscopic cholecystectomy: anesthetic implications. Anesth Analg 1993;76:1120.

Ford GT et al: Toward prevention of postoperative pulmonary complications. (Editorial.) Am Rev Resp Dis 1984;130:4.

Joris JL et al: Hemodynamic changes during laparoscopic cholecystectomy. Anesth Analg 1993;76:1067.

Keagy BA et al: Correlation of preoperative pulmonary function testing with clinical course in patients after pneumonectomy. Ann Thorac Surg 1983;36:253.

Kimball WR et al: Dynamic hyperinflation and ventilator dependence in chronic obstructive pulmonary disease. Am Rev Respir Dis 1982;126:991.

Miller JI et al: Pulmonary function test criteria for operability and pulmonary resection. Surg Gynecol Obstet 1981;153:893.

Odeberg S et al: Haemodynamic effects of pneumoperitoneum and the influence of posture during anesthesia for laparoscopic surgery. Acta Anaesth Scand 1994;38:276.

Okeson GC: Pulmonary dysfunction and surgical risk: how to assess and minimize the hazards. Postgrad Med 1983;74:75.

Poe RH et al: Small airway testing and smoking in predicting risk in surgical patients. Am J Med Sci 1982;283:57.

Shah DM et al: Prevention of pulmonary complications in high risk patients. Surg Clin North Am 1980;60:1359.

Tisi GM: Preoperative evaluation of pulmonary function: Validity, indications, and benefits. Am Rev Respir Dis 1979;119:293.

RENAL DISEASE & THE SURGICAL PATIENT

Daniel C. Brennan, MD

The discussion of renal disease and the surgical patient is primarily concerned with two clinical situations: management of the surgical patient with preexisting renal disease and management of the surgical patient who develops renal complications perioperatively. To understand the management of patients with renal disease, it is first necessary to have a fundamental knowledge of the normal function of the kidney and the implications of various degrees of renal insufficiency.

NORMAL RENAL FUNCTION & ASSESSMENT OF RENAL DISEASE

The principal task of the kidney is to maintain physiologic homeostasis through regulation of body fluids, osmolarity, electrolyte concentration, and acidity. The kidney accomplishes this through filtration of blood, formation of a plasma ultrafiltrate, and processing of the ultrafiltrate via secretion, reabsorption, and excretion. The kidney controls regulation of salt, water, and body pH as well as the excretion of water-soluble metabolic end products, toxins, and drugs. It is responsible also for the production of several hormones, including renin, erythropoietin, and 1,25-dihydroxyvitamin D_3. Renin is produced by the juxtaglomerular apparatus and catalyzes the formation of angiotensin, a potent vasoconstrictor peptide involved in salt balance and blood pressure regulation. Erythropoietin is produced by renal cortical interstitial cells and stimulates maturation of erythrocytes in the bone marrow, thus preventing anemia. 1,25-dihydroxyvitamin D_3 is formed by the proximal tubular cells and is involved in the regulation of calcium and phosphorus.

Renal disease manifests as a perturbation of these normal functions. It should be suspected if there is evidence of hypertension, volume dysregulation (edema or volume contraction), electrolyte disturbances, proteinuria, hypoalbuminemia, hematuria, pyuria, anemia, or an elevated serum urea nitrogen or creatinine. Initial evaluation of renal disease should include a comprehensive history and physical examination, urinalysis, and determination of serum electrolytes, including calcium, phosphorus, and magnesium, as well as uric acid, urea nitrogen, creatinine, and albumin and an assessment of renal function or glomerular filtration rate (GFR).

Urinalysis of a freshly voided urine specimen includes (1) dipstick assessment of pH, specific gravity, glycosuria, proteinuria, hematuria, and pyuria; and (2) microscopic examination for cells, casts, or crystals. The physiologic urine pH ranges from 4.5–8.0. An alkaline pH should make one suspect the presence of a urinary tract infection with a nitrate-splitting bacterium such as proteus. The specific gravity may range from 1.001–1.035 and corresponds to osmolalities of 50–1000 mosm/kg. These represent roughly the minimum and maximum concentrating abilities of the kidney. A specific gravity of 1.010 denotes isosthenuria—ie, the urine osmolality matches the plasma osmolality. In the absence of proteinuria, glucosuria, or iodinated contrast administration, a specific gravity > 1.018 implies preserved concentrating ability. Measurement of the urine specific gravity is useful in differentiating between prerenal azotemia (high specific gravity) and acute tubular necrosis (ATN), which is associated with isosthenuria. The specific gravity also aids in the interpretation of proteinuria as detected on a dipstick. The normal protein excretion rate is less than 150 mg/d. It is important to realize that the dipstick detects the concentration of protein. Thus, detection of protein in a concentrated urine specimen may not represent overt proteinuria. Glucose, cells, casts, and crystals are not normally observed on urinalysis. Glucosuria generally indicates uncontrolled diabetes or tubular dysfunction. White blood cells indicate infection or interstitial nephritis. Red blood cells may be of glomerular or nonglomerular origin and may indicate tumor, infection, trauma, stones, prostatitis, or primary renal disease. White cell casts indicate pyelonephritis; red cell casts indicate glomerulonephritis; and coarse-granular or "muddy-brown" casts indicate ATN.

The normal GFR is 80–120 mL/min. Thus, dividing 100 by the serum creatinine can give a very rough estimation of renal function. This is usually all that is necessary to estimate drug dosages or anticipate fluid and electrolyte problems in the perioperative period. For example, a serum creatinine of 1 mg/dL correlates with a GFR of 100 mL/min. Similarly, a serum creatinine of 2 mg/dL would correlate with a GFR of 50 mL/min. A more accurate estimation of renal function, however, can be made by using the Cockroft-Gault equation for creatinine clearance, which is an estimate of GFR:

$$\text{Creatinine clearance (mL/min)} = \frac{(140 - \text{Age}) \times (\text{Weight in kg})}{72 \times \text{Serum creatinine in mg/dL}}$$

As can be seen from this formula, a 70-year-old man would be expected to have a GFR of 50 based on age alone.

An even more accurate method is to perform a timed (usually 24 hours) calculation:

$$\text{Creatinine clearance (mL/min)} = \frac{\text{Urine Cr (mg/dL)} \times \text{dL)} \times \text{Volume (mL)}}{\text{Plasma Cr (mg/dL)} \times \text{Time (minutes)}}$$

This is rarely necessary and often unreliable in the acute situation.

Disturbances of electrolytes, difficulties with fluid regulation, and anemia are unusual until the GFR decreases to 20–40 mL/min. Thus, surgical management of patients with this level of renal insufficiency is similar to that of patients with normal renal function. Patients with GFRs below 20 mL/min require careful preoperative hydration and blood transfusion to raise the hemoglobin concentration above 11 mg/dL. Most patients with GFRs below 10 mL/min have end-stage renal disease (ESRD) and are on dialysis. Preoperative hydration should be avoided in these patients, and blood transfusions should be administered during hemodialysis to avoid volume overload. All renal transplant recipients or potential renal transplant recipients should receive blood transfusions that have been leukopoor-filtered to reduce exposure to white cells that may sensitize patients to HLA (transplant) antigens or transmit viral diseases such as cytomegalovirus. Erythropoietin (epoetin alfa) is not effective for the rapid correction of anemia in chronic renal failure and ESRD.

Renal ultrasonography is noninvasive and commonly used to assess kidney size and rule out obstruction, vascular stenosis, or thrombosis. The normal kidney size is 10–13 cm in length. Small kidneys reflect chronic disease. Large kidneys are seen with diabetes, amyloidosis, multiple myeloma, lymphoma, polycystic kidney disease, and renal vein thrombosis.

IMPACT OF SPECIFIC RENAL DISEASES

Certain renal diseases present unique hazards. Patients with diabetes are more susceptible to infection and cardiovascular complications such as stroke and acute myocardial infarction and have poorer wound healing. Intravenous contrast administration is more likely to produce acute renal failure (ARF) in patients with diabetes. Contrast nephropathy is manifested as a rise in serum creatinine within 24 hours that peaks by 5 days after administration of the contrast medium. Other risk factors for contrast nephropathy include a history of congestive heart failure, age greater than 65 years, nephrotic syndrome, a serum creatinine above 2 mg/dL, and a contrast load that exceeds 125 mL. Digital subtraction angiography, carbon dioxide angiography, or MRI or angiography should be considered for imaging in patients with two or more of these risk factors.

The abrupt onset of ARF following intra-arterial invasive procedures (eg, cardiac catheterization, aortography) may also result from atheromatous emboli. Atheromatous emboli are associated with circulating eosinophilia, eosinophiluria, elevated amylase, and peripheral embolization resulting in "blue toe syndrome." Renal failure from atheromatous embolization is associated with a stuttering, gradual, and often irreversible increase in serum creatinine.

Patients with nephrotic range proteinuria (> 3 g/d) are hypercoagulable and at increased risk for venous thrombosis because of the loss of antithrombotic clotting factors, including antithrombin III, protein C and S, and hyperhomocysteinemia. In addition to use of pneumatic compression stockings and anticoagulation, serum vitamin B_{12} and folate levels should be evaluated because a deficiency of these vitamins may lead to hyperhomocysteinemia.

ACUTE RENAL FAILURE: DEFINITION, DIAGNOSIS, PREVENTION, & MANAGEMENT

Acute renal failure represents a recent rise in serum creatinine greater than 0.5 mg/dL when the baseline serum creatinine is less than 3 mg/dL or at least a 1 mg/dL rise when the serum creatinine is greater than 3 mg/dL. Chronic renal failure occurs when ARF persists. Acute renal failure may be oliguric (< 500 mL/d) or nonoliguric. The high mortality and morbidity rates due to ARF in surgical patients can be significantly reduced in three ways: (1) by identification of patients who are at high risk for acute renal failure and careful planning and treatment to prevent it; (2) by early diagnosis of intrinsic renal failure; and (3) by early institution of fluid restriction and dialysis. The approach to patients with ARF is simplified by classifying it as prerenal, intrarenal, or postrenal (usually obstructive). The most common prerenal causes include volume depletion, hypotension, severe heart failure, and liver disease. Intrarenal causes can be considered anatomically and include vasculitis and direct vascular injury, stenosis, or thrombosis; tubular injury from ATN or tubular blockade from uric acid or myeloma proteins; rapidly progressive glomerulonephritis; and interstitial nephritis from drugs, infection, or cholesterol embolization. Postrenal obstruction is most commonly associated with ureteral obstruction, which may be extrinsic, from tumor, retroperitoneal fibrosis, or hemorrhage; or intrinsic, from thrombus, stone, or papillary necrosis. Bladder outlet obstruction related to neurogenic bladder, prostatic hyperplasia, tumor, stone, thrombus, or stricture also causes postrenal ARF.

The evaluation of ARF follows the approach to renal disease, as set forth above. The initial management of ARF is prevention. The best means to prevent ARF is to guarantee that the patient is volume-repleted. This should be accomplished with adequate preoperative hydration of at least 1 L of normal saline and transfusion. Nonsteroidal anti-inflammatory drugs (NSAIDs) should be avoided, particularly if volume depletion is present or the patient is receiving a concomitant angiotensin-converting enzyme inhibitor or angiotensin receptor blocker. Aminoglycosides and amphotericin B are particularly nephrotoxic and should be avoided if possible.

Once ARF occurs—in addition to the studies above—simultaneous serum and urine for sodium and creatinine should be obtained to calculate a fractional excretion of sodium (FE_{Na^+}) to help determine the volume status:

$$FE_{Na^+} = \frac{\text{Urine Na}^+ \times \text{Plasma Cr}}{\text{Urine Cr} \times \text{Plasma Na}^+} \times 100\%$$

A FE_{Na^+} less than 1% may be normal or indicative of prerenal azotemia. A FE_{Na^+} greater than 1% is indicative of ATN. A urine sodium less than 20 meq/L or a ratio of urine creatinine to plasma creatinine greater than 40:1 is also indicative of prerenal azotemia. If clinical and supporting studies indicate that a prerenal state exists, a fluid challenge with normal saline may reverse the ARF. Alternatively, 5% dextrose with three ampules of sodium bicarbonate per liter is also isotonic and avoids the acid load of saline. In ARF and renal insufficiency, these solutions are preferable to lactated Ringer's solution, which contains potassium. Hemodynamic monitoring may be necessary to demonstrate that the central venous pressure is 15–20 cm of water and indicative of volume repletion. Although controversial, low-dose dopamine (> 3–5 μ/kg/min) preferentially dilates the renal vasculature and may be tried to treat or prevent ARF. Oliguric renal failure may be converted to nonoliguric renal failure with chlorthalidone (500 mg intravenously twice daily) or metolazone (5 mg orally twice daily) followed by furosemide (80–200 mg intravenously twice daily) to make management easier.

Conservative treatment of renal failure begins with dietary restrictions. Fluid intake is restricted to urine output plus insensible losses, usually 1.5–2 L/d. Protein is restricted to 0.7–1.2 g/kg/d—as dictated by the surgical catabolic state—to decrease the rise in BUN. Sodium chloride is restricted to 2 g/d (sodium, 35 meq/d), potassium chloride to 2 g/d (potassium, 25 meq/d), and phosphorus, magnesium, and aluminum are avoided as much as possible. Control of serum phosphorus can be accomplished through use of calcium carbonate (500–2500 mg orally within 30 minutes of meals and at bedtime or four times daily if the patient is NPO). Sodium bicarbonate (650 mg orally twice to four times daily) is used to control acidosis when the serum bicarbonate is less than 20 mg/dL and also helps to prevent protein breakdown. Diuretics may be used as above.

When conservative management is insufficient, dialysis may be initiated. In general, the indications for dialysis can be recalled by the mnemonic AEIOU-PP: *A*cidosis. Dialysis should be considered when the serum bicarbonate is less than 10 mg/dL and administration of further alkalis is contraindicated.

*E*lectrolyte disturbance with serum potassium greater than 6 meq/dL, when sodium polystyrene sulfonate (Kayexalate) is contraindicated, is the most common electrolyte indication for dialysis. Sodium, calcium, and magnesium levels may also be corrected dialytically.

*I*ntoxicants commonly dialyzed include lithium, ethanol, methanol, ethylene glycol, salicylates, and theophylline.

*O*verload with fluid—unresponsive to diuretics—is another indication for dialysis.

*U*remia is an indication for dialysis and constitutes a syndrome of vomiting, anorexia, nausea, itching, listlessness, and asterixis associated with renal failure. Symptoms do not correlate directly with the degree of azotemia.

*P*ericarditis and *p*olyneuropathy from uremia are absolute indications for dialysis.

Dialysis may be initiated earlier and performed routinely three to five times per week if the protein requirements are such that dialysis is needed to control the BUN. Most studies have failed to show a clear survival advantage to early dialysis with ARF.

DRUGS & THE KIDNEY

Water-soluble drugs and non-protein-bound drugs require dose adjustments with renal insufficiency. Cefazolin and imipenem are two commonly used antibiotics that accumulate in renal insufficiency and may cause seizures. Although protein-bound, digitalis and phenytoin require special adjustment with renal insufficiency and ESRD. Reference books should be consulted. Many drugs are particularly toxic to the kidney. Aminoglycosides, amphotericin B, and NSAIDs are among the most toxic. Halogenated anesthetics such as methoxyflurane (which is no longer used) may be toxic. Pain management is best accomplished with hydromorphone. Meperidine metabolites accumulate with renal insufficiency and cause seizures. Fentanyl and morphine are particularly sedating in renal insufficiency. Traditional nonspecific NSAIDs inhibit the enzymes COX-1 and COX-2 and commonly cause ARF and should be avoided. The COX-2 specific inhibitor celecoxib has less gastrointestinal toxicity and may be less nephrotoxic.

Aronoff G et al: *Drug Prescribing in Renal Failure: Dosing Guidelines for Adults,* 4th ed. American College of Physicians, 1999.

Aronson S et al: Perioperative renal dysfunction and cardiovascular anesthesia: concerns and controversies. J Cardiothorac Vasc Anesth 1998;12:567.

Ayus JC et al: Abnormalities of water metabolism in the elderly. Semin Nephrol 1996;16:277.

Conger JD: Interventions in clinical acute renal failure: what are the data? Am J Kidney Dis 1995;26:565.

Dennis V et al: Homocysteinemia and vascular disease in end-stage renal disease. Kidney Int Suppl 1996;57:S11.

Klahr S et al: Acute renal failure. N Engl J Med 1998;338:671.

Slapak M: Acute renal failure in general surgery. J R Soc Med 1996;89(Suppl 29):13.

Vane JR et al: Anti-inflammatory drugs and their mechanism of action. Inflamm Res 1998;47(Suppl 2):S78.

■ HEMATOLOGIC DISEASE & THE SURGICAL PATIENT

Julie Hambleton, MD, & Pearl T.C.Y. Toy, MD

PREOPERATIVE HEMOSTATIC EVALUATION

The preoperative evaluation of a surgical patient should always include a review of the patient's personal and family history for abnormal bleeding tendencies. Questions that may uncover an undiagnosed bleeding disorder include the following: Does the patient think he or she bleeds or bruises too easily? Has the patient ever been told by a health care professional that he or she bleeds too easily? Has the patient bled abnormally after a previous surgical procedure? Has the patient ever required a blood transfusion because of abnormal bleeding?

Many bleeding disorders manifest with abnormal hemostasis after oral trauma or surgery. Therefore, all patients should be asked if they have ever experienced prolonged bleeding after dental extractions or tonsillectomy. A history of abnormal bleeding with other surgeries or after minor cuts, development of spontaneous ecchymoses, or development of massive lip or tongue swelling after a biting injury should be elicited. Patients should also be asked if there are any "bleeders" in the family.

An initial screen for patients with positive bleeding histories includes a platelet count, prothrombin time (PT), activated partial thromboplastin time (aPTT), and hematology consultation. The bleeding time does not predict surgical bleeding, nor is it sensitive for mild disorders that are often associated with a prolonged bleeding time. Therefore, this test is not routinely recommended in the preoperative evaluation of a patient. While many bleeding disorders will manifest with an abnormal screening test, this is not a universal finding. Therefore, patients with suggestive histories and normal screening tests may require further workup before once can proceed with a recommended surgical procedure.

For surgery in anatomic areas where bleeding would be life-threatening, routine preoperative hemostasis tests have been advocated. The cause of an abnormal platelet count, PT, or aPTT must be identified before proceeding with surgery in order to determine appropriate therapy.

Klopfenstein CE: Preoperative clinical assessment of hemostatic function in patients scheduled for a cardiac operation. Ann Thorac Surg 1996;62:1918.

SURGERY IN PATIENTS WITH ANEMIA

In general, moderate anemia (hematocrit < 30%) does not increase the hazards associated with surgery. If time permits, deficiencies of iron, folic acid, and vitamin B_{12} should be repleted before surgery. In the case of megaloblastic anemias (pernicious anemia and folic acid deficiency), surgery should be deferred if possible until specific therapy (vitamin B_{12} or folic acid) has repleted the generalized tissue defect, because in these two conditions all the cells of the body are affected by the vitamin deficiency, and transfusions alone do not make surgery safe. It probably takes 1–2 weeks to reach adequate tissue levels.

In patients with sickle cell disease, red cell sickling may be precipitated by anoxia and acidosis. Although this occurs infrequently during surgery with careful anesthetic management, partial exchange with normal packed red cells decreases the concentration of sickle hemoglobin—ideally to less than 30%—and may be considered before general anesthesia in patients with sickle cell disease.

The decision to transfuse a specific patient is largely a matter for the consulting hematologist's, surgeon's, and anesthesiologist's clinical judgment. Pertinent considerations include the duration of anemia, the patient's intravascular volume, the extent of the operation, the probability of massive blood loss, and the presence of coexisting conditions such as impaired pulmonary function, inadequate cardiac output, myocardial ischemia, or cerebrovascular or peripheral circulatory disease.

There are no rigid rules or guidelines about which patients with anemia should definitely undergo perioperative transfusion. Much of the decision depends on the specific clinical scenario and the judgment of the attending physicians. However, current experience suggests that otherwise healthy patients with hemoglobin values of 10 g/dL or greater rarely require perioperative transfusion, whereas those with acute anemia with resulting hemoglobin values of less than 7 g/dL frequently do require red blood cell transfusions. The decision to transfuse red blood cells will depend on clinical assessment aided by laboratory data such as arterial oxygenation, mixed venous oxygen tension, cardiac output, the oxygen extraction ratio, and blood volume, when indicated.

Practice Guidelines for blood component therapy: a report by the American Society of Anesthesiologists Task Force on Blood Component Therapy. Anesthesiology 1996;84:732.

Vichinsky EP et al: A comparison of conservative and aggressive transfusion regimens in the perioperative management of sickle cell disease. The Preoperative Transfusion in Sickle Cell Disease Study Group. N Engl J Med 1995;333:206.

Weiskopf RB: Practice guidelines for blood component therapy summarized. West J Med 1997;166:204.

HEMATOLOGIC DISORDERS THAT MAY SIMULATE ACUTE ABDOMINAL SURGICAL CONDITIONS

Sickle Cell Anemia

Painful abdominal crises in sickle cell anemia may suggest appendicitis, cholecystitis, a ruptured viscus, or other acute abdominal conditions. In a patient with this kind of pain, helpful diagnostic points are the following: (1) In patients with sickle cell anemia, the abdomen may be rigid and tender but peristalsis is typically normal. (2) The leukocytosis in sickle cell anemia is associated with a relatively normal differential count—eg, with a white count of 20,000/μL, only 65% granulocytes. (3) Leukocyte counts above 20,000/μL are seen in many patients with sickle cell anemia who are not acutely ill. (4) An elevated leukocyte alkaline phosphatase level suggests infection rather than painful crisis.

Henoch-Schönlein Purpura & Nonthrombocytopenic Purpura

These conditions are usually associated with obvious skin lesions or perhaps hematuria but may on occasion present with acute abdominal pain. The symptoms are apparently due to bleeding into the bowel wall. Intussusception may occur and may require operation. No reliably effective treatment is available to prevent or treat abnormal bleeding, though prednisone may be tried.

Lead Poisoning

Lead poisoning may cause acute abdominal pain. A history of possible exposure to lead may be of great importance. Laboratory clues are moderate anemia with basophilic stippling of the red blood cells and a marked elevation of urinary coproporphyrin. The diagnosis is established by finding elevated lead levels in blood and urine.

Porphyria

The porphyrias are a group of inherited diseases that arise from errors in heme biosynthesis and are caused by a specific enzymatic defect leading to overproduction of a porphyrin species. Acquired forms of porphyria disorders may be caused by drugs, chemicals, or heavy metals such as lead.

While most of the porphyrias manifest with cutaneous light sensitivity, patients with either of two forms may present with abdominal colic or an acute abdomen syndrome. Acute intermittent porphyria typically manifests in young adulthood with episodic abdominal colic, polyneuropathy, psychiatric disturbances, electrolyte abnormalities, and hypertension. Patients with variegate porphyria may also present with intermittent episodes of abdominal colic and psychiatric disturbances. Both disorders may be precipitated by ingestion of alcohol or certain drugs, such as barbiturates, anticonvulsants, and sulfonamide derivatives.

Abdominal Wall Hemorrhage

Hemorrhage into the abdominal wall may simulate acute appendicitis in patients with thrombocytopenia, hemophilia, or other severe coagulation disorders or in patients receiving anticoagulation therapy.

SURGERY IN PATIENTS WITH HEMATOLOGIC MALIGNANT DISORDERS

It is occasionally necessary to operate on patients who have leukemia, lymphoma, myeloma, or related disorders. Such patients can always undergo surgery without increased risk if they are in hematologic remission, and surgery may be relatively safe in patients who are in partial remission. In acute leukemia, the risk of surgery is low if the white count is not excessive and the neutrophil count is greater than 1000/μL, the hemoglobin is over 10 g/dL, and the platelet count is near 100,000/μL. Other coagulation factors are not typically disturbed in acute leukemia. An exception is the promyelocytic subtype of acute myelogenous leukemia, which may be complicated by disseminated intravascular coagulation.

Bleeding may be a complication in patients with chronic myelogenous leukemia whose platelet counts are above 1 million/μL or whose white counts are above 100,000/μL. In patients with chronic lymphocytic leukemia and a normal platelet count, excessive white cell counts greater than 100,000/μL are not a contraindication to surgery as long as the patient is not neutropenic.

Very high platelet counts may be encountered in polycythemia vera and essential thrombocytosis. Most patients with these myeloproliferative disorders will suffer from thrombotic complications, including arterial thromboses and venous thromboses in unusual locations. A minority of patients, however, will experience abnormal bleeding secondary to an acquired qualitative platelet defect. If surgery is urgently necessary, plateletpheresis to achieve a platelet count below 1 million/μL may be considered before surgery. If surgery can be deferred for a week, therapy with hydroxyurea, 30 mg/kg/d orally, may be used.

Interestingly, patients with polycythemia vera may have very high packed cell volumes (over 60%). This may result in a falsely prolonged prothrombin time and activated partial thromboplastin time unless allowance is made for the relatively small plasma volume by reducing the amount of citrate in the test tube. Similarly, fibrinogen may be too low for the volume of whole blood. When blood counts normalize with therapy (phlebotomy or chemotherapy), surgery is safer, but the incidence of complications, especially thrombotic, is still increased.

Patients with multiple myeloma or macroglobulinemia may bleed excessively in surgery because of their elevated paraprotein, which may interfere with coagulation. Plasmapheresis before surgery should be considered if the procedure cannot be delayed to allow institution of adequate chemotherapy.

Patients with the hematologic diseases described above generally have normal wound healing, and an increased incidence of postoperative infections is not expected as long as the total granulocyte count is at least 1500/µL. An exception is the patient with chronic lymphocytic leukemia and secondary hypogammaglobulinemia. These patients are at increased risk for developing recurrent infections with encapsulated organisms, which may impact on their postoperative course. The common anticancer chemotherapeutic agents, such as mercaptopurine, busulfan, melphalan, methotrexate, and cyclophosphamide, do not interfere with wound healing unless they have rendered the patient neutropenic.

SURGERY IN PATIENTS RECEIVING ANTICOAGULANTS

Heparin

Oftentimes, a patient receiving full-dose anticoagulant therapy will need to go to emergent or semi-emergent surgery. Unfractionated heparin, given as a continuous intravenous infusion, has a relatively short half-life of approximately 1 hour. Therefore, one option is to discontinue the infusion 4–6 hours prior to planned surgery. If, however, a large dose of unfractionated heparin has been administered or the patient suddenly becomes a candidate for emergency surgery, it may be necessary to neutralize the effect of unfractionated heparin with protamine sulfate.

Immediately after an intravenous dose of heparin, the amount of protamine sulfate required (in milligrams) is equal to one-hundredth of the last dose of heparin (in units). Because of the relatively short half-life of unfractionated heparin, the dose of protamine is reduced if some time has elapsed since the last dose of heparin. For example, in 30 minutes, only about half the amount of protamine is required; in 4–6 hours, there is seldom a need for neutralization. Protamine

should always be given by slow intravenous injection. Rapid injection may result in an anaphylactic type of reaction or thrombocytopenia. If given in excessive amounts, protamine may act as a weak anticoagulant.

During open heart surgery and extracorporeal circulation, large doses of unfractionated heparin are required to prevent coagulation in the pump oxygenator and the patient's circulatory system. At the end of the procedure, this large dose of heparin must be neutralized. The dose of protamine should be based on the amount of heparin used. Heparin neutralization is not required in some vascular operations if the heparin dosage is calculated and timed so as to lose its effect by the end of the operation.

Low-Molecular-Weight Heparins

Unfractionated heparin is a heterogeneous mixture of long- and short-chained heparin molecules. The main anticoagulant activity of unfractionated heparin is via an antithrombin III-dependent inactivation of activated factors X and II (thrombin). The low-molecular-weight heparins (LMWH) such as enoxaparin, dalteparin, and tinzaparin contain predominantly the shorter chains of heparin molecules. Therefore, the inactivation of thrombin is less complete because a trimolecular complex cannot be formed. Subsequently, LMWH drugs have primarily anti-Xa activity and do not result in a prolonged aPTT. They are, however, very effective anticoagulants that bind nonspecific plasma and cell surface proteins less well, resulting in a longer half-life and more predictable pharmacokinetics. Monitoring of the anticoagulant effect of these drugs is generally not necessary unless the patient is obese or has renal insufficiency or failure, as the drugs will accumulate in the setting of renal disease. Low-molecular-weight heparins have been found to be safe and efficacious in the setting of postsurgical deep vein thrombosis prophylaxis, acute coronary syndrome, and acute venous thrombosis. However, because their anticoagulant activity cannot be entirely neutralized by protamine sulfate, because they have a longer half-life, and because they are relatively expensive, their use should be limited in critically ill or hospitalized patients or in patients who may need emergent procedures or surgery.

Heparin-Induced Thrombocytopenia With Thrombosis Syndrome (HIT/TS)

One of the greatest challenges in caring for the surgical patient is the development of thrombocytopenia while the patient is receiving heparin therapy. Surgical patients typically have several reasons for developing thrombocytopenia, such as sepsis, drugs, postoperative state, hypersplenism, and platelet consumption due to disseminated intravascular coagulation. Approximately 9% of patients will develop heparin-associated thrombocytopenia within the first few days of exposure to the drug. This drop in platelet count is transient and benign. The troublesome syndrome of heparin-induced thrombocytopenia (HIT) is defined by a fall in the platelet count of 50% or to less than 150×10^9/L after 5 days of heparin exposure. The heparin may be in the form of unfractionated or low-molecular-weight heparin given as a continuous intravenous infusion, by subcutaneous injection, or as a flush for a venous catheter. Approximately 2–3% of patients exposed to heparin will develop HIT associated with the development of antibodies directed against the heparin-platelet factor 4 complex. This antibody-antigen complex then binds the Fc receptor on adjacent platelets, forming platelet aggregates that circulate and become activated. Venous or arterial thrombotic complications ensue, causing deep venous thromboses, pulmonary emboli, myocardial infarctions, mesenteric infarctions, etc. Lepirudin, a direct thrombin inhibitor, is the drug of choice for acute anticoagulation in this setting.

Coumarin Anticoagulants

Patients being maintained on oral anticoagulant therapy with coumarin derivatives should be instructed to discontinue their therapy approximately 4–6 days prior to a planned surgical procedure. Surgery may then proceed relatively safely if the prothrombin time is prolonged by less than 50% (eg, INR < 1.5). In patients with higher values, prophylactic measures are in order if surgery is necessary. Vitamin K$_1$, 5 mg orally or parenterally, will return the prothrombin time to safe levels (40% or better) in approximately 4 hours and to normal levels in 24–48 hours. However, its administration may render the patient refractory to all coumarin therapy for a week or more. For immediate restoration of normal prothrombin values, one should infuse 500–1000 mL of plasma (generally 10 mL/kg body weight). However, treatment with plasma alone will result in only a transient correction of the prothrombin time due to the short half-life of factor VII. Administration of vitamin K is required as an adjunct to plasma therapy if complete reversal is desired, and the prothrombin time should be monitored every 6–8 hours until correction is maintained. Factors II, VII, IX, and X—the vitamin K-dependent factors lowered by coumarin therapy—are quite stable in banked plasma. Blood products that can be transfused for warfarin reversal include fresh frozen plasma and liquid plasma.

Hirsh J et al: Oral anticoagulants: mechanism of action, clinical effectiveness, and optimal therapeutic range. Chest 1998; 114:445S.

Kearon C et al: Management of anticoagulation before and after elective surgery. N Engl J Med 1997;336:1506.
Warkentin TE: Heparin-induced thrombocytopenia: pathogenesis, frequency, avoidance and management. Pharmacoepidemiology 1997;17:325.
Weitz JI: Low-molecular-weight heparins. N Engl J Med 1997; 337:688.

SURGERY IN PATIENTS WITH DISORDERS OF HEMOSTASIS

Platelet Disorders

A. THROMBOCYTOPENIA

Depending on the cause of the thrombocytopenia, surgery can be performed safely in patients with platelet counts as low as 50,000/μL, especially if they have shown no clinical signs of bleeding (eg, purpura, ecchymoses) before the operation. Hematologic consultation should be requested to assist in determining the cause of thrombocytopenia and whether surgery could be safely performed. Surgery in patients with certain types of drug-induced thrombocytopenia (but not heparin-induced) and immune-mediated thrombocytopenia may be safely undertaken. Microangiopathic causes of thrombocytopenia such as disseminated intravascular coagulation and thrombotic thrombocytopenic purpura (TTP) are relative contraindications to surgery unless the disease process in under control.

For rapid restoration of the platelet count in a patient with profound thrombocytopenia of immune etiology, infusion of intravenous immune globulin or high-dose steroids is indicated. Preoperative platelet transfusions are futile in this disease until the splenic pedicle has been clamped, at which time the transfusion is unnecessary. The indications for splenectomy in various hematologic diseases are discussed in Chapter 28.

B. QUALITATIVE PLATELET DEFECTS

Aspirin and NSAIDs may cause slight prolongation of the bleeding time, which is clinically significant in a minority of normal persons. Renal failure is frequently associated with severe platelet dysfunction, and patients with bleeding require dialysis to improve platelet function. Desmopressin, 0.3 μg/kg, may reverse the defect. Administration of conjugated estrogens, 0.6 mg/kg intravenously daily for 5 days, is also useful, but the hemostatic response is somewhat delayed.

Von Willebrand's disease is the most common inherited bleeding disorder, affecting approximately 1% of the population. Patients with this disorder have a bleeding diathesis similar to that seen in patients with platelet defects, with mucosal bleeding being the norm. Surgery in these patients can be performed safely, and the perioperative and postoperative pharmacologic management of these patients depends on the severity of their disease and the procedure to be done. For example, patients with mild type I disease may only require pre- and postoperative desmopressin infusions, while more severely affected patients will need an intermediate-pure, plasma-derived factor VIII product that contains von Willebrand factor. Surgery in patients with congenital disorders of platelet function requires preoperative platelet transfusions. Unfortunately, these patients have often been transfused with platelets on numerous occasions in the past because of their bleeding diathesis or surgery. Subsequently, they have become alloimmunized and thus refractory to future platelet transfusions.

Thrombocytopenia with or without abnormal platelet function may develop in patients who have undergone cardiac bypass surgery. Desmopressin, 0.3 μg/kg intravenously post bypass, increases von Willebrand factor levels and reduces blood loss in patients undergoing complex cardiac operations. Prophylactic platelet concentrates are not indicated, but if diffuse microvascular oozing occurs at raw wounds, mucosa, and puncture sites, platelet concentrates may be given.

Patients with uremia are often anemic and have platelet dysfunction with or without mild thrombocytopenia. Consultation is recommended with hematologists or transfusion medicine experts knowledgeable about the use of erythropoietin (epoetin alfa), estrogens, and platelet transfusion in these situations. For major elective surgery with large anticipated blood loss, anemia can be corrected with the preoperative administration of recombinant erythropoietin. In addition, platelet dysfunction should be treated preoperatively with dialysis. Conjugated estrogens, 0.6 mg/kg intravenously daily for 5 days, also improve platelet dysfunction for about 14 days; the mechanism of action is unclear. Intraoperatively, desmopressin acetate, 0.3 μg/kg administered intravenously, may release von Willebrand factor from the blood vessel wall. The effect occurs within 30 minutes and lasts several hours. One or two doses can be repeated every 12–24 hours, with close monitoring for the development of resultant hyponatremia. Postoperatively, dialysis is the treatment of choice for uremic platelet dysfunction, when estrogens and desmopressin have been used before and during the procedure.

Mild thrombocytopenia may also occur in patients with uremia, and the platelet count should probably be maintained at 70,000–100,000/μL. However, infused platelets will be affected by the patient's uremic state unless the patient is being actively dialyzed.

Mannucci PM: Hemostatic drugs. N Engl J Med 1998;339:245.

Norfolk DR et al: Consensus Conference on Platelet Transfusion; Royal College of Physicians of Edinburgh, 27–28 November 1997. Synopsis of background papers. Br J Haematol 1998; 101:609.

Weiskopf RB: Practice guidelines for blood component therapy summarized. West J Med 1997;166:204.

Coagulation Factors

Patients with congenital bleeding disorders, such as hemophilia A (factor VIII deficiency), B (factor IX deficiency), and C (factor XI deficiency), can be safely operated on in a hospital setting where adequate hematologic consultation and pharmacologic support can be provided.

Patients with hemophilia A may have surgery if enough factor VIII concentrate is given to bring the preoperative factor VIII level to about 100%, depending on the procedure to be done. Each unit of factor VIII administered to a patient raises the level approximately 2%. Therefore, the amount of factor VIII concentrate given either as a plasma-derived or recombinant product is typically 50 units per kilogram of body weight, assuming a normal hemoglobin and a starting baseline factor level of less than 1%. Smaller doses are needed for patients with mild or moderate disease, those whose baseline levels are greater than 1%, or prior to minor surgical procedures in which the target factor VIII level is only 50–75%. Because of their greater plasma volumes, larger doses are required for patients who are significantly anemic. After a loading dose of factor VIII with documentation of the peak level, 50% of the dose is repeated every 12 hours for 7–10 days, depending on the procedure and the need for ongoing physical rehabilitation.

Factor IX-deficient patients are treated in a similar manner with plasma-derived or recombinant products, except that twice the dose of factor is required but at longer intervals because of its longer half-life. Patients with factor XI deficiency must be treated with plasma, since purified factor XI products are not readily available in the United States.

The perioperative and postoperative management of patients with hemophilia is complicated and specialized. Therefore, these patients should always be managed by a hematologist knowledgeable in the management of this disease.

SPECIAL PROBLEMS IN PATIENTS WITH LIVER DISEASE

Patients with liver disease from any cause may develop abnormal bleeding on the basis of several conditions. Factors II, V, VII, VIII, IX, X, XI, XIII, and fibrinogen are all synthesized in the liver. Moderately severe liver disease can lead to a deficiency of any combination of these factors and produce a bleeding diathesis. Liver disease can also increase a patient's risk for bleeding by causing thrombocytopenia (due to congestive spleno-megaly), increased baseline fibrinolysis (due to deficiencies of other liver-derived factors that inhibit fibrinolysis such as the α_2 plasminogen inhibitor), and acquired dysfibrinogenemias. Factor VIII is generally not lowered by liver disease.

Bleeding from the gastrointestinal tract in patients with cirrhosis of the liver is most commonly due not to abnormal coagulation but to an underlying structural defect such as esophageal varices, gastritis, or hemorrhoids.

Platelets may be severely reduced in number—below 30,000/μL—in acute alcoholism, which may be responsible for bleeding problems, but the count rises spontaneously to normal levels in a few days of abstinence from alcohol. Moderate thrombocytopenia (50,000–100,000/μL) that does not remit spontaneously may be a sign of hypersplenism secondary to cirrhosis and accompanying portal hypertension. This modest decrease in platelet count generally does not result in a bleeding diathesis. More profound thrombocytopenia suggests additional abnormalities, such as concomitant nutritional deficiencies or a primary bone marrow defect. Acquired qualitative defects of platelet function have also been described in patients with liver disease, but they are probably uncommon and difficult to diagnose in this population.

Patients with end-stage liver disease often suffer from easy bruising and mucosal bleeding. Acquired deficiencies of one or multiple clotting proteins, as mentioned above, is one cause. Factor VII has the shortest half-life; therefore, early liver disease accompanied by coagulopathy presents with an isolated prolongation of the prothrombin time (PT). As the patient's liver disease and synthetic function continue to deteriorate, other clotting proteins become lacking, the prothrombin time will be further prolonged, and the activated partial thromboplastin time (aPTT) will be prolonged as well.

A more troublesome complication of liver disease is acute generalized oozing. There are three main causes for this: **Disseminated intravascular coagulation (DIC),** characterized by prolonged PT and thrombin time, prolonged aPTT (depending on the degree of factor consumption and decreased factor synthesis), low plasma fibrinogen, a low platelet count, and the presence of fibrin degradation products—specifically the D-dimer. A second cause is **primary fibrinolysis,** in which the necrotic liver fails to clear plasminogen activators. Elevated levels of fibrin degradation products are not diagnostic of primary fibrinolysis; their clearance may be impaired by severe liver disease without bleeding. In general, platelets and factors V and VIII are less strikingly reduced in primary fibrinolysis than in DIC. However, distinguishing end-stage liver disease

from DIC or primary fibrinolysis can be a troublesome challenge for the treating physician.

Acute hemodilution, in which blood loss is replaced by packed red blood cells and saline, is another cause of generalized oozing in liver disease. Because these patients already have decreased levels of coagulation factors, hemodilution can result in significant further reduction in coagulation factors. Acquired dysfibrinogenemia may also occur as a result of abnormal posttranslational processing of the fibrinogen molecule in liver disease. Patients may present with generalized oozing from mucous membranes that is out of proportion to the degree of coagulopathy and thrombocytopenia. A prolonged thrombin time or reptilase time would confirm this abnormality.

Treatment of the bleeding complications associated with liver disease is generally reserved for clinically significant episodes of bleeding and not epistaxis or easy bruising per se. However, if a patient is to undergo an invasive procedure or surgery, prophylactic therapy must be instituted. Clotting factor deficiency resulting from liver damage does not respond to vitamin K even when it is given parenterally in large doses. If fresh frozen plasma is used, 10 mL/kg or approximately four units of plasma must be infused to fully impact on the patient's coagulopathy. The peak effect on coagulation times with infused plasma is within 2 hours posttransfusion. The PT and aPTT should be measured before and within 2 hours after transfusion of fresh frozen plasma. Given the short half-life of factor VII, the hemostatic effect of a plasma infusion will wane after 4–6 hours, necessitating repeated transfusions if clinically indicated. Desmopressin acetate, 0.3 μg/kg, shortens the bleeding time in cirrhotics and may improve the bleeding diathesis. These patients, however, must be closely monitored for the development of hyponatremia. Infusion of cryoprecipitate may be necessary for patients with liver disease complicated by an acquired hypo- or dysfibrinogenemia and bleeding. For patients who undergo a liver transplant procedure, administration of conjugated estrogens (100 mg intravenously) may ameliorate the coagulopathy and decrease blood product transfusion requirements.

Frenette L et al: Conjugated estrogen reduces transfusion and coagulation factor requirements in orthotopic liver transplantation. Anesth Analg 1998;86:1183.

DISSEMINATED INTRAVASCULAR COAGULATION (DEFIBRINATION SYNDROME; DIC)

The coagulation mechanism in disseminated intravascular coagulation differs from normal clotting in three principal ways: (1) It is diffuse instead of localized;

(2) it damages the site of clotting instead of protecting it; and (3) it consumes enough of some clotting factors that plasma concentrations fall, resulting in diffuse bleeding. DIC is a syndrome characterized by escape of the clotting process from its normal inhibitory controls, resulting in the dysregulation of the clotting and fibrinolytic pathways. The manifestations include complications from either bleeding or thrombosis, depending on the degree of imbalance. Bleeding is characteristic of DIC associated with sepsis, whereas thrombotic complications are typical of cancer-associated DIC. The paradoxical situation of bleeding from excessive intravascular coagulation is a result of many factors.

Disseminated intravascular coagulation occurs following acute hemolytic transfusion reactions, some types of surgery (particularly involving the lung, brain, or prostate), and certain obstetric catastrophes. It sometimes occurs in patients with malignant tumors (especially adenocarcinomas of the prostate and pancreas) and in patients with septicemia. Many patients with severe liver disease have some degree of disseminated intravascular coagulation, though it is very difficult to truly distinguish DIC from end-stage liver disease (see above).

The most common clinical manifestation is diffuse bleeding from many sites at surgery and from needle punctures. Uncontrollable postpartum hemorrhage may be a manifestation. In the laboratory, the combination of reduced platelets on the blood smear and a prolonged prothrombin time is very suggestive of DIC. The aPTT may be prolonged and fibrinogen levels fall to severely decreased levels, usually well below 75 mg/dL. The thrombin time is prolonged, and fibrin monomer and fibrin degradation fragments are present.

In the differential diagnosis, a prolonged prothrombin time with or without a prolonged aPTT may be due to vitamin K deficiency, so a trial of vitamin K may be indicated. On rare occasions, circulating anticoagulants and accidental excessive heparin administration may simulate disseminated intravascular coagulation.

Treatment of DIC focuses on treatment of the underlying cause, such as sepsis, cancer, or an obstetric emergency. When the fibrinogen deficiency is severe and the patient is bleeding, cryoprecipitate must be given. A unit of cryoprecipitate contains about 250 mg of fibrinogen; one unit per 10 kg of body weight is usually necessary to correct the defect. Occasionally, platelet transfusions are also necessary, and it may be necessary to use low-dose heparin to stop the pathologic clotting. Typically, no loading dose of heparin is used, and the patient is started on a low infusion rate at about 200–500 units/h. However, the acute treatment of DIC is controversial and not well established. Hematology consultation should be obtained for these complicated cases.

Bick RL: Disseminated intravascular coagulation: pathophysiological mechanisms and manifestations. Semin Thromb Hemost 1998;24:3.

Carey MJ et al: Disseminated intravascular coagulation: clinical and laboratory aspects. Am J Hematol 1998;59:65.

TRANSFUSION OF BLOOD, BLOOD COMPONENTS, & PLASMA SUBSTITUTES

Transfusion of blood, blood components, and plasma substitutes for surgical patients may be required for one or more of the following reasons: (1) to restore and maintain normal blood volume, (2) to correct severe anemia, or (3) to correct bleeding and coagulation disorders.

Decisions about the need for transfusion and selection of the proper type and amount of transfusion material must be based upon careful evaluation of the individual patient. Urgency of need and the availability of diagnostic and therapeutic resources are obviously the determining factors. Attention must be given to the total clinical picture.

Goodnough LT et al: Transfusion medicine. First of two parts—blood transfusion. N Engl J Med 1999;340:438.

Serologic Considerations (Blood Typing)

A. EMERGENCY TRANSFUSIONS

In an emergency, type-specific packed red cells or whole blood is the product of choice. The patient's ABO and Rh types can be determined in 5 minutes, and type-specific blood can be issued in 10 minutes. Although O-negative packed red cells can be transfused to any patient, only 6% of the population is O-negative, and this rare universal donor blood should therefore be reserved for critically bleeding patients from whom a blood sample cannot be obtained.

B. ELECTIVE TRANSFUSIONS

When red cell transfusion can be postponed for an hour, maximal compatibility of donor red cells is ensured by performing an antibody screen and cross-match. In the antibody screen, the patient's serum is tested for red cell antibodies other than those in the ABO system. The antibody screen takes about 45 minutes. If the antibody screen is negative, donor red cells are cross-matched with patient serum in 5 minutes, and cross-matched compatible blood can be issued in 10 minutes. In elective surgical patients in whom a type and screen has been performed within the last 48 hours, if the antibody screen is negative, cross-matched blood can be available in 10 minutes.

Amount of Blood for Transfusion

A. ADULTS

One unit of packed red cells will raise the hemoglobin by 1 g/dL and the hematocrit by 3% in the average adult (70 kg).

B. CHILDREN

The amount of whole blood to be given is as follows: Children over 25 kg, 50 mL/kg; children under 25 kg, 20 mL/kg; and premature infants, 10 mL/kg.

Rate of Transfusion

Blood is normally given at a rate of 500 mL in 1½–2 hours. In patients with heart disease, one should allow 2–3 hours for the transfusion. For rapid transfusions in emergencies, it is best to use a 15-gauge plastic cannula and allow the blood to run freely. The use of added pressure to increase flow is dangerous unless it can be applied by gentle compression of collapsible plastic blood containers. Central venous pressure monitoring is a safeguard against over-transfusion; it is a measure of the heart's ability to handle venous return.

Massive Transfusions

Bleeding from one site is usually due to a structural defect and should be corrected by sutures and cautery. Bleeding from multiple sites suggests a hemostatic disorder, which is usually manifested by diffuse microvascular oozing from raw wounds, mucosa, and puncture sites. Development of abnormal bleeding correlates strongly with the duration of hypotension. Primary treatment of coagulopathy due to hypoperfusion is by restoring blood volume.

Whole blood is the product of choice for massive transfusion (ie, giving more than one blood volume in rapid succession). Since whole blood is devoid of platelets, thrombocytopenia can occur from dilution. Loss of two clotting factors in stored whole blood is usually less important. For factor V, only 5–10% of normal levels are adequate for hemostasis; reductions to this level rarely result from multiple transfusions if whole blood is used. For factor VIII, the level usually rises with the stress of surgery. Thus, when primarily whole blood is used in massive transfusion, any coagulopathy is usually due to thrombocytopenia rather than deficient coagulation factors.

Platelet concentrates are indicated in patients with diffuse microvascular bleeding and thrombocytopenia. Prophylactic administration of platelet concentrates in the absence of abnormal bleeding is not recommended. Platelet counts rarely fall below 50,000/µL on the basis of hemodilution alone unless more than 15–20 units

have been given or the patient was thrombocytopenic before the massive transfusion.

If whole blood is administered in massive transfusion, prophylactic use of fresh frozen plasma is not necessary. However, if only packed red blood cells or cell-saver red cells (or both) have been transfused, dilution of platelets and coagulation factors can be expected with massive transfusion, and fresh frozen plasma is often needed when more than one blood volume has been transfused.

Fibrinogen levels may decrease due to dilution if only red blood cells or cell-saver red cells are given in massive transfusion. In addition, consumption may occur associated with shock. If diffuse microvascular bleeding occurs and the fibrinogen level is less than 100 mg/dL, cryoprecipitate can be given. If the PT is more than 1½ times normal, fresh frozen plasma can be administered.

Leslie SD et al: Laboratory hemostatic abnormalities in massively transfused patients given red blood cells and crystalloid. Am J Clin Pathol 1991;96:770.

Complications of Blood Transfusion

Acute hemolysis due to transfusion of the wrong unit of blood to the wrong patient is the most common cause of immediate deaths due to transfusion. Hepatitis is the most common cause of late deaths.

A. HEMOLYTIC REACTIONS

Hemolytic reactions are a serious complication of blood transfusion. The most severe immediate reactions are due to ABO incompatibility, but serious hemolytic delayed reactions (1 week after transfusion) may also be due to antibodies resulting from isoimmunization following previous transfusion or pregnancy. Symptoms may include apprehension, headache, fever, chills, pain at the injection site or pain in the back, chest, and abdomen, and shock; but in the anesthetized patient, spontaneous bleeding from different areas and changes in vital signs may be the only clinical evidence of transfusion reactions. Posttransfusion blood counts fail to show the anticipated rise in hemoglobin. Free hemoglobin can be detected in the plasma within a few minutes. Hemoglobinuria and oliguria may occur. Exact identification of the offending antibody should be made, and this is usually possible when the Coombs test is positive.

Some studies suggest that osmotic diuretics such as mannitol can prevent renal failure following a hemolytic transfusion reaction. After an apparent reaction and in oliguric patients, a test dose of 12.5 g of mannitol (supplied as 25% solution in 50-mL ampules) is administered intravenously over a period of 3–5 minutes;

this dose may be repeated if no signs of circulatory overload develop. A satisfactory urinary output following the use of mannitol is 60 mL/h or more. Mannitol can be safely administered as a continuous intravenous infusion; each liter of 5–10% mannitol should be alternated with 1 L of normal saline to which 40 meq of KCl has been added to prevent serious salt depletion. If oliguria develops despite these efforts, treat as for acute renal failure.

B. FEVER

Fever is the most common immediate transfusion reaction and is due chiefly to recipient reaction against white cells in the donor blood. Treatment is with antipyretics. If fever occurs after transfusion of three different units despite pretreatment with antipyretics, leukocyte-poor blood products should be used.

C. ALLERGIC REACTIONS

Allergic reactions occur in about 1% of transfusions. They are usually mild and associated with itching, urticaria, and bronchospasm, but they may be severe or even fatal. (The cause is an antigen-antibody reaction between a protein in the donor plasma and a corresponding antibody in the patient. Some of these reactions are caused by an antibody to IgA.) If reactions are mild, the transfusion may be cautiously continued. Antihistamines, epinephrine, and corticosteroids may be required.

D. CIRCULATORY PROBLEMS

Too rapid transfusions of large quantities of blood may result in circulatory complications (eg, cardiac or respiratory failure). This is particularly true of elderly or debilitated patients. Careful monitoring should help prevent this complication.

E. VIRAL HEPATITIS

Viral hepatitis can be acquired from blood transfusion. Hepatitis A does not have a chronic carrier state, and transmission from donor to transfusion recipient is rare. After implementation in 1999 of nucleic acid testing of donors, the risk is estimated to be 1:63,000 per unit for hepatitis B and from 1:1,000,000 to 1:500,000 for hepatitis C. Among patients who develop hepatitis and who survive their primary illness, it is estimated that half develop chronic liver disease. About 10% of those with chronic liver disease develop cirrhosis.

F. INFECTIONS

Testing of blood donors for HIV antibody began in 1985 in the United States. Improved donor questioning, improved antibody tests, and additional antigen and nucleic acid tests have reduced the risk to about 1:1,000,000–1:500,000 per unit in 1999. The risk of

human T cell lymphotropic virus (HTLV I and II) is estimated to be 1:641,000 with antibody testing of blood donors.

Bacterial contamination of blood may occur through improper collection, storage, and administration. Reactions—noted early in the course of transfusions—are serious and may be fatal. Treat as for septic shock. Patients develop fever, chills, and hypotension after the contaminated transfusion.

Schreiber GB et al: The risk of transfusion-transmitted viral infections. N Engl J Med 1996;334:1685.

Whole Blood

When banked blood is transfused, cells damaged from storage are removed within 24 hours, and the remainder survive normally. Whole blood can be stored for up to 35 days and is the product of choice for massive transfusions. The increased content of citrate and potassium in stored blood is usually clinically insignificant.

Most coagulation factors are stable in stored blood, but platelets and factors V and VIII deteriorate. Bank blood that has been stored in the refrigerator for more than 2 days is essentially devoid of viable platelets.

Packed Red Blood Cells

Packed red cells have a storage (shelf) life of 42 days. They are the component of choice for the treatment of anemia without hypovolemia. Most blood transfusions can be given as packed red cells, even to patients with moderate degrees of blood loss, if adequate crystalloid is given concomitantly. A hematocrit of 30% or a hemoglobin concentration of 10 g/dL is considered acceptable in surgical patients. However, lower levels may be acceptable as well.

In assessing the need for perioperative red blood cell transfusion, the patient's age and cardiopulmonary status, the hemoglobin concentration, and the amount of anticipated further perioperative blood loss should be considered. In selected patients without cardiovascular disease and with little or no further bleeding, a hemoglobin level of 7 g/dL may be adequate. In the Canadian randomized study of patients in critical care, a transfusion trigger of 7 g/dL was at least as effective as and possibly superior to a transfusion trigger of 9 g/dL in patients under 55 years of age without acute myocardial infarction or unstable angina.

Anemia does not adversely affect wound healing, provided that peripheral perfusion is maintained by adequate volume replacement. Human and animal studies show that collagen deposition did not correlate with postoperative hematocrit but correlated with oxygen tension in wounds.

Hebert PC et al: A multicenter, randomized, controlled clinical trial of transfusion requirements in critical care. N Engl J Med 1999;340:409.

Spence RK for the Blood Management Practice Guidelines Conference: surgical red blood cell transfusion practice policies. Am J Surg 1995;170(Suppl):3S.

Prehospital Donation for Autologous Transfusion

Patients can donate blood for themselves before surgery that requires transfusion. Patients with hematocrits above 34% who will require transfusion for an elective procedure can predeposit if they have arm veins that can accommodate a 16-gauge needle. Patients should not donate if the need for transfusion is unlikely. Healthy patients can donate one unit a week starting 5 weeks before surgery if given ferrous sulfate, 325 mg orally three times daily between meals. The earlier the donation, the greater the amount of red blood cell mass regenerated before surgery. If time or iron is limited, the patient will be anemic before surgery and will need more red cell transfusions—autologous and possibly allogeneic. Recombinant erythropoietin (epoetin alfa) may be effective but is expensive.

Forgie MA et al: Preoperative autologous donation decreases allogeneic transfusion but increases exposure to all red blood cell transfusion: results of a meta-analysis. International Study of Perioperative Transfusion (ISPOT) investigators. Arch Intern Med 1998;158:610.

Jafar-Fesharaki M et al: Effect and cost of subcutaneous recombinant human erythropoietin in preoperative patients. Orthopedics 1997;20:1159.

Intraoperative Autotransfusion

Intraoperative autotransfusion may be a valuable adjunct in the management of vascular surgery and major trauma. Several commercially available devices can be used to implement this procedure. Intracavitary blood is incoagulable; it has virtually no fibrinogen; systemic anticoagulation is unnecessary; and emboli should be entirely preventable when the available devices are used properly. Intraoperative salvage should not be used in cases where little blood is salvaged. Washed cell-saver red blood cells contain virtually no platelets or coagulation factors, and the platelet count, PT, and PTT should be monitored.

Valbonesi M et al: Intraoperative blood salvage in cardiac and vascular surgery. Int J Artific Organs 1995;18:130.

Goodnough LT et al: Transfusion medicine. Second of two parts—blood conservation. N Engl J Med 1999;340:525.

Platelet Transfusion

The goal of platelet transfusion is to achieve a hemostatic level of platelets in the circulation. Generally, a platelet count of 50,000/μL is adequate for surgical hemostasis. The platelet count should be maintained higher—above 100,000/μL—during the perioperative period of patients undergoing surgery in a critical area (eg, brain, eye, upper airway). Platelet transfusions should be given, when necessary, 4 hours or less before the surgical procedure, and a 10-minute to 1-hour posttransfusion platelet count should be done to document efficacy of the platelet transfusion. The usual adult dose is six units, which should raise the patient's platelet count by approximately 40,000/μL. Absence of a rise in platelet count after platelet transfusion is a serious finding and may be due to alloantibody, autoantibody, posttransfusion purpura, DIC, or other causes of platelet consumption. To determine the reason for refractoriness to platelet transfusion, hematology consultation is recommended.

American Society of Anesthesiologists Task Force on Blood Component Therapy. Practice guidelines for blood component therapy. Anesthesiology 1996;84:732.

Coagulation Factor Concentrates

Solvent-detergent or heat-treated plasma-derived factor VIII concentrates and recombinant factor VIII are the products of choice for patients with severe hemophilia A. Treatment of factor VIII in this manner inactivates HIV and the hepatitis viruses. Treated and filtered plasma-derived factor IX products and recombinant factor IX are also available for patients with hemophilia B.

Cryoprecipitate, a concentrate prepared by freeze-thawing the plasma from a single donor, contains 80–120 units of factor VIII, 250 mg of fibrinogen, and an unknown amount of von Willebrand factor per bag (15–25 mL). It is effective in the treatment of classic hemophilia and von Willebrand's disease and the rare case of fibrinogen deficiency in need of therapy. One unit of the cryoprecipitate for each 6 kg body weight raises the AHF level to 50%—enough for most surgical procedures. For difficult cases, it may have to be followed by half that amount every 12 hours given as long as necessary. An adequate dose for hypofibrinogenemia is 5 g, or 20 bags.

Fibrin glue is a blood product that has high concentrations of fibrinogen which when mixed with thrombin forms a fibrin clot at the site of bleeding. Fibrin glue is usually made by freeze-thawing of plasma and can be made from the patient's own (autologous) blood donated at least 3 days before surgery. Fibrin glue is a useful operative sealant in a variety of procedures, including cardiovascular surgery (mediastinal spray application, sealing of vascular anastomoses and prostheses), thoracic surgery (treatment of bronchopleural fistula), trauma management (repair of liver or splenic injury), transplantation procedures (transplant of partial hepatectomy specimen), plastic repair (skin grafts), central nervous system repair (repair of dural or peripheral nerve injury, pituitary tumor removal), and orthopedic operations (repair of osteochondral fracture or of the Achilles tendon). Fibrin glue has achieved hemostasis in a few patients with coagulation disorders. In patients with coagulopathy due to multiple coagulation deficiency, fibrin glue was effective in controlling liver hemorrhage and bleeding from splenorrhaphy. Unless fibrin glue is made from the patient's own blood, it carries the same risks of viral transmission as are associated with administration of other blood products.

Felfernig M et al: Coagulation support: fresh frozen plasma versus clotting factor concentrate. Anesthesia 1998;53(Suppl 2):54.

Plasma

The proper use of plasma is confined to the management of certain coagulation problems. There is no justification for the use of fresh frozen plasma as a volume expander or as a nutritional source, because safer and cheaper alternatives exist. For volume expansion, crystalloid solutions are preferable to fresh frozen plasma.

Indications for use of fresh frozen plasma include the following:

(1) For patients in whom the effects of warfarin must be reversed rapidly. Immediate hemostasis can be achieved in patients receiving anticoagulant therapy who are actively bleeding or who require emergency surgery.

(2) As an adjunct to massive blood transfusions when only packed red cells are available. Bleeding in patients whose entire blood volume has been replaced over a few hours can be due to thrombocytopenia or depletion of coagulation factors, and when a factor deficiency occurs as demonstrated by prolonged PT or PTT, fresh frozen plasma can be used for correction.

(3) In surgical patients with liver disease who still have abnormal prothrombin times after administration of vitamin K, fresh frozen plasma may be given, though it often fails to correct the abnormality.

(4) In patients requiring replacement of specific factors such as antithrombin III, factor XI, or factor XIII and in the management of thrombotic thrombocytopenic purpura, fresh frozen plasma may be used.

Graftstein E et al: Guidelines for red blood cell and plasma transfusion for adults and children: an emergency physician's overview of the 1997 Canadian Blood Transfusion Guidelines. Part 2: Plasma transfusion and infectious risk. J Emerg Med 1998;16:239.

BLOOD SUBSTITUTES
Artificial Colloids

Artificial colloids (dextran, gelatin, hetastarch [hydroxyethyl starch]) are inexpensive, effective plasma expanders without infectious risks. They have been used extensively in Europe. Their infrequent use in the USA has been due to the anaphylactoid or anaphylactic reactions of all these colloids, the antithrombotic effect of the dextrans, and the unknown long-term effects of hetastarch, which remains in the reticuloendothelial system. Hetastarch was found to be a cheaper alternative to albumin. The safety and efficacy of albumin has been questioned, and randomized trials are needed to resolve the issue.

Offringa M: Excess mortality after human albumin administration in critically ill patients. Clinical and pathophysiological evidence suggests albumin harmful. BMJ 1998;317:223.

Electrolyte Solutions

Experimental and clinical studies have shown that substantial blood losses can be effectively replaced with balanced salt solutions. With careful monitoring of central venous pressure, vital signs, urinary output, and serum electrolyte determinations, specific fluid and electrolyte abnormalities may be corrected and normal blood volume maintained. The volume of normal salt replacement solutions used must be two to three times the volume lost.

Future Blood Substitutes

Red cell substitutes are not yet available, but research is being performed on hemoglobin solutions and perfluorocarbons. Platelet substitutes are being developed also. However, because of difficulty in demonstrating efficacy, it is unlikely that synthetic products will replace the use of donor red cells or platelets in the foreseeable future.

Cohn SM: The current status of haemoglobin-based blood substitutes. Ann Intern Med 1997;29:371.

■ PREGNANCY & THE SURGICAL PATIENT

Aaron B. Caughey, MD, MPP, MPH, & Edward C. Hill, MD

The incidence of surgical illness in pregnant and nonpregnant women of the same age group is similar and equals about 1:500 gestations. Pregnancy may alter or mask the signs and symptoms of the particular presentation or course of disease, so that diagnosis is made more difficult. Furthermore, the fetus and changes in maternal physiology and anatomy must be considered in the use of diagnostic tests, medical therapy, and the planning of surgical procedures. Any major operation represents a risk not only to the mother but to the fetus as well. One study based upon the Swedish Health Registry suggested an increase in both preterm delivery and growth restriction in infants that resulted from pregnancies which involved a surgical procedure.

Although there is no evidence that congenital anomalies are induced in the developing fetus by anesthesia, semielective procedures should be deferred until the second trimester of pregnancy, exercising the greatest precautions to prevent hypoxia and hypotension. Emergent surgical procedures should proceed as necessary; however, changes in maternal physiology—particularly in cardiac output and maternal blood volume—as well as of the size of the gravid uterus must be considered.

Radiologic Investigation

If possible, one should avoid diagnostic radiologic examinations of the lower abdomen and pelvis, especially during the first 6 weeks when the fetus is particularly susceptible to irradiation. Radioactive isotopes pose a particular hazard to the fetus. Radioactive iodine or pertechnetate for thyroid scanning and bone scanning with radioactive strontium or calcium are contraindicated because these agents cross the placenta and are taken up by fetal tissues. Alternative modalities such as sonography and MRI are useful in many circumstances.

Laparoscopic Surgery

Laparoscopy for a variety of surgical problems, including diagnostic exploration, cholecystectomy, appendectomy, and ovarian cystectomy, has been used increasingly in the past 2 decades. Most of the evidence regarding safety of laparoscopy comes from case series, but common sense suggests guidelines about the use of laparoscopic surgery during pregnancy. The primary issues to consider when using laparoscopy in pregnancy are (1) placement of the initial trocar or Veress needle so as to avoid the uterus; (2) having adequate visualization to operate; (3) keeping CO_2 pressures as low as possible to preserve blood flow to and from the uterus; and (4) avoiding manipulation of the gravid uterus, which may induce preterm labor or cause uterine injury and kinking off the blood supply to the uterus. Placement of the initial trocar can be best managed by the open technique after the first rimester. Avoiding trocar injuries and preserving laparoscopic viewing angles is easiest prior to 18–20 weeks.

Medical Management

There are a variety of medications that are contraindicated in pregnancy and many whose use during pregnancy has not been studied. Furthermore, because of increases in the maternal blood volume, creatinine clearance, and hepatic metabolism, dosing regimens may need to be modified. Other than in the emergent setting, one should seek obstetric consultation before starting medical therapy of a pregnant patient with a surgical illness. Specialists in perinatology and maternal-fetal medicine are available for this purpose.

Doll DC et al: Management of cancer during pregnancy. Arch Intern Med 1988;148:2058.

Fatum M et al: Laparoscopic surgery during pregnancy. Obstet Gynecol Surv 2001;56:50.

Mazze RI et al: Reproductive outcome after anesthesia and operation during pregnancy: a registry study of 5,405 cases. Am J Obstet Gynecol 1989;161:1178.

Reedy MB et al: Laparoscopy during pregnancy: a study of laparoendoscopic surgeons. J Reprod Med 1997;42:33.

Reedy MB et al: Laparoscopy during pregnancy: a study of five fetal outcome parameters with use of the Swedish Health Registry. Am J Obstet Gynecol 1997;177:673.

SPECIFIC SURGICAL ISSUES IN PREGNANCY

1. Appendicitis

Acute appendicitis occurs about once in every 2000 pregnancies. The signs and symptoms are similar to those that occur in nonpregnant women, but they may be modified. First, the symptoms of early appendicitis may be disregarded because of the nausea, vomiting, and lower abdominal discomfort often present in the first and second trimesters of normal pregnancy. Moderate leukocytosis and sedimentation rate elevation are common during pregnancy. Moreover, the enlarging uterus often carries the appendix higher in the abdomen, so that McBurney's point can no longer be used. This can lead to misdiagnosis of appendicitis as cholecystitis, chorioamnionitis, or gastroenteritis. The differential diagnosis also includes ectopic pregnancy, ruptured corpus luteum cyst, adnexal torsion, round ligament syndrome, degenerating myoma, and pyelonephritis.

Peritoneal signs should only be seen with a ruptured cyst, ectopic pregnancy, or appendicitis. However, there may be relatively little rigidity associated with inflammation of the appendix, and rebound tenderness may be hard to define. Thus, the sensitivity of peritoneal signs for appendicitis is decreased, though specificity is still high. Adler's sign may be helpful. The pain is located while the patient is in the supine position. If the pain shifts to the left when she turns on her left side, the cause may be uterine or adnexal. If the pain remains in the same location, appendicitis should be suspected. A positive Bryan sign, indicative of acute appendicitis, is exacerbation of pain when the uterus is shifted to the right side. Ultrasonographic imaging of the appendix may be useful in confirming the diagnosis. If ultrasound is of no use and acute appendicitis is suspected, the risks of radiation exposure to the fetus in the second and third trimester of a spiral CT may be outweighed by the benefits of its diagnostic accuracy. However, early in pregnancy, if the physical signs are significant, then it is preferable to perform diagnostic laparoscopy.

The course of the disease may vary as well. In particular, the gravid uterus may effectively displace the omentum and loops of small intestine. Thus, rupture of the appendix is more often associated with widespread dissemination of infection, generalized peritonitis, and a higher mortality rate in gravid than in nongravid patients. If an abscess does form following perforation, the gravid uterus forms the medial wall of the abscess. The intense inflammatory process can initiate uterine contractions, resulting in loss of the fetus or preterm delivery.

The management of acute appendicitis during pregnancy is appendectomy. Because of the seriousness of perforation, aggressive management of suspected appendicitis is preferable. Perforation of the appendix occurs most commonly in the third trimester and is often associated with a delay in performing laparotomy. If generalized peritonitis exists, depending on the gestational age, delivery by cesarean section may be considered since the incidence of premature labor is high and fetal death in utero due to bacterial sepsis is not uncommon. Beyond 34 weeks of gestation, there is little to be gained by expectant management of the pregnancy; however, before 32–34 weeks, continuous fetal monitoring throughout the period of surgical management and postoperatively until the patient has defervesced will ensure continuation of the pregnancy.

Throughout the first trimester until about 18–20 weeks of gestation, a laparoscopic approach to appendectomy is reasonable. There are more than 20 laparoscopic appendectomies reported in the literature. The most common complication is spontaneous abortion, though it is difficult to estimate what percentage can actually be attributed to the operation itself as opposed to the infectious disease process. If an open approach is used, regional anesthesia is preferred, and the transverse or oblique muscle-splitting incision should be placed somewhat higher than would be the case in a nonpregnant patient.

Blaakaer J et al: Abruptio placentae as complication to acute appendicitis. Int J Gynaecol Obstet 1989;29:179.

Curet MJ et al: Laparoscopy during pregnancy. Arch Surg 1996;31:546.

Dornhoffer JL et al: Appendicitis complicating pregnancy. Kans Med 1988;89:139.

Masse RI et al: Appendectomy during pregnancy: a Swedish Registry study of 778 cases. Obstet Gynecol 1991;77:835.

2. Cholecystitis & Cholelithiasis

Acute cholecystitis in pregnancy occurs with a prevalence of about one in 3500–6500 pregnancies. However, the incidence of biliary colic is higher in pregnant than in nonpregnant patients (at least 1:1000 pregnancies). It is associated with gallstones in 50% of cases.

Sonographic studies show that the volume of the gallbladder is twice the normal size beyond 14 weeks of gestation, and both the rate of emptying and the percentage emptied are lower during pregnancy.

The symptoms are the same as in the nonpregnant patient, with an abrupt onset of right upper quadrant abdominal pain radiating to the right scapula, low-grade fever, and nausea and vomiting. Cholecystitis may be difficult to distinguish from acute appendicitis, with the high position of the appendix associated with the third trimester of pregnancy. Ultrasound may be helpful in diagnosis.

Unlike appendicitis, however, acute cholecystitis in the first trimester of pregnancy is best managed conservatively, with hospitalization, parenteral fluids, nasogastric suction, antispasmodics, analgesics, and broad-spectrum antibiotics. In three out of four patients treated conservatively, there will be improvement within 2 days, and a definitive surgical procedure can be deferred until the second trimester or the postpartum period. Surgery should be done whenever there is doubt regarding the differentiation from acute appendicitis or if there is no response to conservative therapy as manifested by an enlarging mass (empyema), jaundice (common duct obstruction), evidence of rupture, or associated pancreatitis. Gallstone-induced pancreatitis increases both fetal and maternal death rates. Cholecystectomy is the procedure of choice, but cholecystostomy may be performed if technical difficulties warrant it, gallbladder excision being delayed until the puerperium.

As with appendectomy, the laparoscopic approach is now commonly used in pregnant patients. One advantage over laparoscopic appendectomy is that the operative field is less likely to be obstructed by the gravid uterus before 20 weeks, so that manipulation of the uterus is less common. Conversely, surgeons are more likely to attempt laparoscopic cholecystectomy at later gestations because of the seemingly better exposure then achieved than with laparoscopic surgery in the lower abdomen and pelvis. A number of laparoscopic procedures in the third trimester have been reported, with the most common complications being preterm contractions and preterm labor. Rarely, uterine injury with Veress needle and trocar placement has been reported. In the third trimester, further consideration should be given to expectant management of cholecystitis with antibiotic therapy, and if surgical intervention is indicated an open procedure may be preferable to laparoscopy in most cases.

Baillie J et al: Endoscopic management of choledocholithiasis during pregnancy. Surg Gynecol Obstet 1990;171:1

Elderling SC: Laparoscopic cholecystectomy in pregnancy. Am J Surg 1993;165:625.

Gouldman JW et al: Laparoscopic cholecystectomy in pregnancy. Am Surg 1998;64:93.

Morrell DG et al: Laparoscopic cholecystectomy during pregnancy in symptomatic patients. Surgery 1992;112:856.

Steinbrook RA et al: Laparoscopic cholecystectomy during pregnancy. Surg Endosc 1996;10:511.

3. Intestinal Obstruction

Intestinal obstruction occurs infrequently during pregnancy. Adhesive bands are the most common cause of intestinal obstruction, and displacement of the intestine is most likely to occur when uterine growth carries the pregnancy into the abdomen around the fourth or fifth month of gestation; near term, when the fetus moves into the pelvis; or postpartum, with sudden reduction in the size of the uterus. Other causes during pregnancy are volvulus, intussusception, and large bowel cancer.

The symptoms and signs of intestinal obstruction are the same as those that occur in the nonpregnant woman, though the clinical picture may be obscured by the nausea and vomiting of early pregnancy, round ligament pain, and the abdominal distention already produced by the pregnancy. Radiologic investigation of the abdomen may be diagnostic and must be obtained. The gestational age and the benefit to the particular clinical situation of the diagnostic studies should be weighed.

Management of bowel obstruction is similar to that of the nonpregnant patient. If the patient has no signs of perforation or bowel necrosis, bowel rest (nothing by mouth) with or without nasogastric decompression can be used as first line management, and many patients will recover with this conservative management. However, if this fails and exploratory surgery is indicated, it should be performed without delay. Consideration of gestational age can inform the surgical plan. Near term, a cesarean section may be required to obtain necessary exposure. If the fetus is undelivered, continuous fetal monitoring is indicated postoperatively until the patient has recovered.

Coleman MT et al: Nonobstetric emergencies in pregnancy: trauma and surgical conditions. Am J Obstet Gynecol 1997; 177:497.

Lopez Carral JM et al: Volvulus of the right colon in pregnancy. Int J Clin Pract 1998;52:270.

Lord SA et al: Sigmoid volvulus in pregnancy. Am Surg 1996; 62:380.

4. Hernias

Hiatal hernia is common during pregnancy; perhaps 15–20% of pregnant women develop this condition as a result of pressure against the stomach by the enlarging uterus. The principal symptom is reflux esophagitis, with severe heartburn aggravated by recumbency or ingestion of a large meal and relieved by an upright position or antacids. Very rarely, hematemesis may result from ulceration of the esophageal mucosa.

Elevation of the upper half of the body while reclining, frequent small meals, and antacids given liberally are usually effective treatment. The gastroesophageal reflux caused by the hiatal hernia may also be treated with H_2 blockers or proton pump antagonists. Most hiatal hernias disappear following the pregnancy. Surgical correction is required only for those that persist postpartum and remain symptomatic.

Umbilical, inguinal, and ventral hernias usually are accompanied by symptomatic exacerbations during pregnancy. The increase in abdominal pressure during pregnancy may make them more obvious to the patient or clinician, leading to their diagnosis. Repair can be done electively after delivery. Surgery during pregnancy is indicated only in the rare event of an incarcerated or strangulated hernia.

Firstenberg MS et al: Gastrointestinal surgery during pregnancy. Gastroenterol Clin North Am 1998;27:73.

Katz PO et al: Gastroesophageal reflux disease during pregnancy. Gastroenterol Clin North Am 1998;27:153.

Mayer IE et al: Abdominal pain during pregnancy. Gastroenterol Clin North Am 1998;27:1.

5. Cancer of the Breast

The rate of breast cancer during pregnancy has increased as a result of the increased average age of pregnant women. The rate was estimated to be 1:3000 pregnancies in the mid 1980s and has recently been estimated as high as 1:2000–1:1500. The breast changes that occur during gestation make detection of early breast carcinoma much more difficult. Since there may be considerable delay in diagnosis, many cases are advanced by the time the diagnosis is made. In one study, the rate of node-positive disease was 61% in pregnant or lactating patients versus 38% in nonpregnant patients.

Breast cancer in pregnancy is found on self-examination in the majority of cases. Diagnostic management is similar to that in nonpregnant patients, though the efficacy of mammography is reduced in pregnancy because of the increased radiographic density. Ultrasound is useful. Biopsy and appropriate surgical treatment should be undertaken as soon as cancer is suspected.

The overall cure rate for breast cancer developing during pregnancy or lactation is significantly lower than that of nonpregnant women of comparable age. This is most likely because delay in diagnosis results in more advanced disease. Cure rates of 90% have been achieved in pregnant patients with stage I disease. While the breast cancer itself does not seem to affect pregnancy outcome, management of the disease needs to consider the pregnancy.

Therapeutic abortion is not indicated in the patient with localized disease of a favorable microscopic type. Interruption of an early pregnancy as part of estrogen ablation may be of some palliative benefit to the woman with advanced disease, but there is no specific evidence to support this. Thus, the decision about pregnancy termination in the setting of breast cancer management needs to be made via a series of counseling sessions involving a team including a perinatologist and an oncologist.

The surgical management of breast cancer is not likely to affect the pregnancy other than exposure to anesthesia; thus, the resection (mastectomy or breast conservation) should proceed as indicated at any stage of gestation. However, chemotherapy and particularly radiation therapy may affect the fetus.

Finley JL et al: Fine-needle aspiration cytology of breast masses in pregnant and lactating women. Diagn Cytopathol 1989; 5:255.

Gallenberg MM et al: Breast cancer and pregnancy. Semin Oncol 1989;16:369.

Higgins S et al: Pregnancy and lactation after breast-conserving therapy for early-stage breast cancer. Cancer 1994;73:2175.

Michels KB et al: Prospective assessment of breastfeeding and breast cancer incidence among 89,877 women. Lancet 1996; 347:431.

Parente JT et al: Breast cancer associated with pregnancy. Obstet Gynecol 1988;71(Part 1):861.

Tretli S et al: Survival of breast cancer patients diagnosed during pregnancy or lactation. Br J Cancer 1988;58:382.

Zemlickis D et al: Maternal and fetal outcomes after breast cancer in pregnancy. Am J Obstet Gynecol 1992;166:781.

6. Ovarian Tumors & Ovarian Torsion

A cystic corpus luteum is the most frequent cause of ovarian enlargement during pregnancy. This structure rarely exceeds 6 cm in diameter and gradually diminishes in size as the pregnancy progresses. The corpus luteum is responsible for secreting the hormones that maintain the pregnancy until about 10 weeks of gestation. It is usually asymptomatic, and careful observation is required to distinguish it from a proliferative type of cystic enlargement. Adnexal masses that are not corpus luteum cysts are encountered in approximately 1:1000 pregnancies. Only 2–5% of these are actually ovarian cancer, making that incidence between 1:50,000 and 1:20,000 pregnancies.

Adnexal masses are often asymptomatic unless there is hemorrhage into the tumor, rupture of the cyst, or torsion of the pedicle—complications that are definitely increased during pregnancy (see Chapter 42). Thus, adnexal masses in pregnancy are most commonly identified either on initial examination or upon routine ultrasound. However, some are not found until the immediate postpartum period, when the uterine size no longer masks their presence and the abdominal wall is flaccid. When a pelvic mass separate from the uterus is identified in pregnancy, the next step in diagnosis is ultrasound. Whether seen on routine ultrasound or identified on physical examination, determining whether an ovarian lesion is malignant or benign is of the utmost importance.

Most ovarian neoplasms are cystic; solid tumors are quite rare. The cystic neoplasms most often seen during pregnancy are benign cystic teratomas (about 40% are of this variety), serous and mucinous cystadenomas, and endometrial cysts. Ovarian cancer is quite uncommon in pregnancy (< 1:20,000 pregnancies), but of the three major subtypes—epithelial, stromal, and germ cell—during pregnancy, germ cell tumors seem to be more common. Dysgerminoma is the most frequently encountered solid tumor. Serous and mucinous cystadenocarcinomas and endometrioid carcinomas are the most common histologic types.

Management of the asymptomatic adnexal mass in pregnancy is controversial. If there is no ultrasonographic evidence of malignancy, the mass can be followed expectantly during through the first trimester. Serial ultrasound examination is used to follow the growth or resolution of the adnexal mass. At any point, surgical management of the adnexal mass needs to be weighed against increased risk of complications of the pregnancy. In general, because of the increased risk of adnexal torsion, ovarian cysts and tumors larger than 6 cm are removed via cystectomy in the mid second trimester. Depending on the size of the mass, either laparotomy or laparoscopy can be used. It is important to evaluate the mass via ultrasound immediately before operation to reassess both the indication and the surgical approach.

If a true ovarian neoplasm is suspected, consultation with a gynecologic oncologist should be obtained, and a staging and diagnostic procedure can usually be performed in the second trimester. A conservative staging procedure has been described consisting of removal of the ovary containing the mass, peritoneal washings, and extensive pelvic and abdominal examination. Depending on the stage of disease, termination of the pregnancy should be considered.

An ovarian mass may be diagnosed when a patient presents with abdominal pain. Operation may be indicated if there is an acute abdominal emergency caused by ovarian torsion or rupture or hemorrhage of an ovarian cyst. Again, a laparoscopic approach is reasonable. If the pregnancy is early (less than 10 weeks gestation) and termination is not wanted, it is optimal to avoid cystectomy because of the contribution of the corpus luteum to the pregnancy. In the setting of ovarian torsion, untwisting the adnexa results in a viable ovary in most cases.

Bider D et al: Outcome of pregnancy after unwinding of ischemic hemorrhagic adnexum. Br J Obstet Gynaecol 1989;96:426.

Buller RE et al: Conservative surgical management of dysgerminoma concomitant with pregnancy. Obstet Gynecol 1992; 79:887.

Busine A et al: Conservative laparoscopic treatment of adnexal torsion during pregnancy. J Obstet Biol Reprod 1994;23:918.

El Yahia AR et al: Ovarian tumors in pregnancy. Aust N Z J Obstet Gynecol 1991;31:327.

Farahmand SH et al: Case report: ovarian endodermal sinus tumor associated with pregnancy: review of the literature. Gynecol Oncol 1991;41:156.

Fleischer AC et al: Sonographic evaluation of maternal disorders during pregnancy. Radiol Clin North Am 1990;28:51.

Hess L et al: Adnexal mass occurring with intrauterine pregnancy: report of fifty-four patients requiring laparotomy for definitive management. Am J Obstet Gynecol 1996;174:1499.

Horbelt D et al: Mixed germ cell malignancy of the ovary concurrent with pregnancy. Obstet Gynecol 1994;84:662.

Malfetano JH et al: Cisplatinum combination chemotherapy during pregnancy for advanced epithelial ovarian carcinoma. Obstet Gynecol 1990;75:545.

Platek DN et al: The management of a persistent adnexal mass in pregnancy. Am J Obstet Gynecol 1995;173:123.

Soriano D et al: Laparoscopy versus laparotomy in the management of adnexal masses during pregnancy. Fertil Steril 1999;71:955.

■ MANAGEMENT OF THE OLDER SURGICAL PATIENT

Gerard M. Doherty, MD,
& Edmund T. Lonergan, MD

Advances in perioperative management have made surgery available for an increasing number of persons 65 years of age and older, and recent figures for the USA show more than 600,000 operations on geriatric patients each year. Despite a 50% improvement in surgical mortality for this population since the 1960s, older patients account for about 70% of postoperative deaths and complications. Diminished physiologic reserves associated with aging may contribute to complications, but most of the increased risk is due to chronic illness.

Older patients should undergo the same preoperative and postoperative evaluations as younger adults, but a number of other factors should receive attention as well: (1) age-related changes in organ function, (2) functional status, and (3) special problems of the aged.

Age-Related Changes in Organ Function

The most important of these are summarized in Table 5–2. As a rule, organ function decreases with aging, though it usually remains adequate to meet the stress of surgery, and age as such is rarely a contraindication to operative management.

A. PULMONARY FUNCTION

Decreased pulmonary function due to aging should pose no risk to surgical candidates who are otherwise free of pulmonary disease. However, diminished pulmonary reserve may exaggerate conditions that would be better tolerated by younger patients, with attendant risk of postoperative hypoxia, atelectasis, and pneumonia. Pain, oversedation, infection, and intrathoracic or upper abdominal surgical procedures may increase this risk.

B. CARDIOVASCULAR FUNCTION

In healthy older persons, cardiac output rises in response to exercise well into the ninth decade. Since the maximal heart rate is diminished in the aged (220 – Age) and increased cardiac output depends upon stroke volume, cardiac performance is vulnerable to volume depletion (hemorrhage, dehydration, excessive diuresis).

Diminished sinus node activity and loss of cardiac conducting tissue increase the likelihood of arrhythmias. Decreased responsiveness to catecholamines, heightened vascular resistance, and reduced left ventricular compliance may limit the ability of the aging cardiovascular system to cope with stress. Blunted baroreceptor reflexes increase the risk of postural hypotension, especially during ambulation shortly after surgery.

A history of myocardial infarction or angina is a major risk factor. The prevalence of arteriosclerotic heart disease (often asymptomatic) in men aged 60 or older is about 20%, rising to 40% after age 80. Arrhythmias, heart failure, myocardial ischemia (often asymptomatic) and infarction, and thromboembolism

Table 5–2. Age-related changes in selected organ systems.

Organ System	Change With Age	Potential Clinical Consequences
Pulmonary	Decreased compliance of thorax Increase in dead space, residual volume, closing volume (> age 45) FEV_1 decreases by 10 mL/yr > age 30	Increased alveolar-arterial Po_2 gradient; increased vulnerability to hypoxia Decreased clearance of secretions
Cardiovascular	Decreased sinus node P cells; decreased cells in AV node, bundle of His, Purkinje network Decreased response to catecholamines; blunted baroreceptor activity (especially > age 75) Increased rigidity of arterial tree; decreased LV compliance	Increased risk of arrhythmias Increased vulnerability to volume loss, postural hypotension Diminished response to volume overload
Renal	≥ 30% decrease in GFR (note exceptions) Decreased ability to concentrate or dilute urine Decreased formation of NH_4^+ Decreased renin response to volume loss	Increased risk of renal failure Decreased excretion of some drugs Increased vulnerability to dehydration and to overhydration Decreased defense against acidosis Increased vulnerability to volume depletion
Central nervous system	Decreased cerebral blood flow autoregulation over age 65 Decreased acetylcholine stores (especially Alzheimer's disease)	Increased vulnerability to cerebral ischemia with hypotension Increased risk of confusion with anticholinergic drugs

are the most serious cardiovascular problems in older patients.

In addition to the classic findings, cardiac problems in the aged may be manifested as acute confusion, weakness and hypotension, severe fatigue, dyspnea, neurologic changes, arrhythmias, and pulmonary edema. Any of these states should be investigated (eg, by CK, serial ECGs, isotope studies) as possible signs of myocardial ischemia. The hours immediately after surgery are especially dangerous for patients with ischemic heart disease, and during this time the patient should be monitored with great care for pain, hypoxia, hypotension, and other conditions that may increase cardiac work.

The risk of postoperative cardiac failure is increased in the presence of an S_3 gallop or distended external jugular veins, a heart rate of less than 100/min after 2 minutes of stationary bicycle exercise in the supine position, or the presence of ischemic changes (which may occur in the absence of symptoms) on the ECG in the immediate postoperative period.

Patients at increased risk for postural hypotension often have elevated systolic blood pressures and may be identified by a drop of 20 mm Hg or more in systolic pressure after 2–3 minutes in the upright position following a 5-minute period in the supine position. If postural hypotension is detected, ambulation should be al-

lowed with caution. Volume status and hypotensive drugs must be attended to in the immediate postoperative period.

Control of hypertension, arrhythmias, angina, and cardiac failure will reduce perioperative mortality and morbidity in older patients. Unless contraindicated, cardiac medications should be continued until the morning of surgery. Monitoring of cardiovascular status following surgery (eg, blood gases, Swan-Ganz line, ECGs) is often necessary and should be instituted earlier for suspected cardiac embarrassment in patients aged 65 and above.

Good management of pain decreases catecholamine release and arrhythmias, but it is equally important to guard against oversedation and hypoxia.

Early ambulation of older patients protects them against deconditioning, and together with low-dose heparin prophylaxis (5000 units every 8–12 hours) reduces the frequency of thromboembolism.

C. RENAL FUNCTION

Most persons experience a decline in glomerular filtration rate (GFR) of at least 30% by the eighth decade, though one-third of older persons who are free of renal and cardiovascular disease have a well-preserved GFR as attested by serial creatinine clearance measurements. A reduction in GFR and renal blood flow may predispose geriatric patients to postoperative renal failure and toxicity from drugs cleared by the kidney. Impaired thirst perception, decreased urine concentration, and reduced renin response to volume contraction weaken the older patient's defense against hypotension when challenged by hemorrhage, nasogastric drainage, third-space sequestration of fluid, or dehydration.

Decreased dilutional capacity may lead to overhydration and hyponatremia after vigorous fluid administration, with serious cardiovascular (pulmonary edema) or central nervous system (cerebral edema) complications. Reduced NH_4^+ secretion impairs the aged patient's ability to correct acidosis.

A history of renal disease is present in a minority of patients who develop postoperative renal failure; detection of subclinical renal insufficiency in older surgical candidates is an important priority to protect them against this potentially catastrophic event.

Because muscle mass and creatinine production are much less in many older patients, serum creatinine levels may be normal despite a 60% or more decline in GFR. Nomograms and formulas that estimate creatinine clearance without the need for urine collections have proved unreliable. Therefore, if incipient renal failure is suspected, a 12- to 24-hour creatinine clearance determination should be obtained before nonemergent surgery.

A 50% or more reduction in GFR (< 50–60 mL/min) reflects in increased risk of postoperative renal failure. Operations lasting more than 3 hours or involving clamping of the aorta above the renal arteries are additional risk factors.

Avoiding volume depletion or overhydration, limiting the use of nephrotoxic drugs or drugs cleared by the kidney, monitoring acid-base status and urine output, and maintaining urine volume at 1 mL/min all help minimize renal complications postoperatively.

D. CENTRAL NERVOUS SYSTEM FUNCTION

The aged brain (Table 5–2) has a diminished ability to maintain cerebral blood flow during hypotension and a decreased acetylcholine content in many areas of the cerebrum and associated structures.

Because autoregulatory control of cerebral blood flow is impaired in older patients, signs of cerebral ischemia may appear when mean arterial pressure (MAP) falls below 80 mm Hg.

MAP =
0.33 × [Systolic blood pressure – Diastolic blood pressure]
   + Diastolic blood pressure

Geriatric surgical patients whose systolic blood pressure is 105 mm Hg or less should be closely monitored for

Table 5–3. Activities of daily living.

Bathing	Being continent of stool and urine
Feeding oneself	Transferring from bed to chair
Dressing	Going to the toilet
Grooming	

cognitive impairment or confusion, and corrective action should be taken as appropriate (eg, decrease vasodilator therapy, improve volume status).

The risk of bladder obstruction in older men with enlarged prostates who receive anticholinergic drugs (eg, diphenhydramine, some antidepressants, opioids) is well known, but these drugs may also lead to acute confusion in the elderly (especially those with Alzheimer's disease) as a consequence of age-related depletion of acetylcholine in the cerebrum and elsewhere in the central nervous system. Postoperatively, older patients receiving anticholinergics should be examined for acute confusion, and these drugs should be used only when absolutely required.

Functional Status of Older Patients

About 23% of older persons are unable to perform one or more activities of daily living (ADLs) (Table 5–3). This is true for only 7% of those under age 74, but the percentage rises to 50% or more after age 85.

Pre- and postoperative evaluation of persons age 65 and older should include attention to ADLs; rehabilitation therapy and appropriate support (eg, home care, visiting nurse) should be provided when patients are deficient in one or more activities of self-care. For example, an older patient who is unable to move from bed to chair after successful surgery may have to be rehospitalized or admitted to a nursing home if the disability is not corrected or no provision is made to assist the family or the patient's aged spouse with the necessary care.

SPECIAL PROBLEMS OF OLDER PATIENTS

See also Table 5–4.

Altered Drug Disposition

Changes in body composition, renal function, hepatic function, and nutritional status may lead to increased risks when older surgical patients receive drugs.

A. CHANGES IN BODY COMPOSITION

Increased fat and decreased muscle mass in old age result in diminished total body water and a contracted

Table 5–4. Special problems of older patients.

Decreased drug metabolism and elimination
Delirium
Falls
Pressure sores
Infection

volume of distribution for water-soluble drugs such as nitrates, aminoglycosides, and some antihypertensive agents. To avoid overdosing with water-soluble drugs, therapy should begin at the low end of the dosage scale, with regular monitoring of drug levels in older subjects.

B. DIMINISHED RENAL FUNCTION

Diminished renal function is common in old age, and unless this is borne in mind patients may receive excessive doses of nephrotoxic agents (eg, nonsteroidal anti-inflammatory agents, aminoglycosides) or drugs cleared by the kidney (eg, digoxin, some calcium channel blockers) that accumulate and cause side effects.

C. DECREASED LIVER FUNCTION

Hepatic mass and function decline by about 30% by the eighth decade. This poses little danger unless it is exacerbated by decreased blood flow (hypotension, volume contraction) or by drugs that inhibit hepatic enzymes (eg, cimetidine) or that reduce liver blood flow (eg, cimetidine, propranolol). In such cases, there is a risk of toxicity from drugs (eg, nitrates, propranolol, morphine) cleared by rapid hepatic inactivation.

D. MALNUTRITION

Malnutrition is present in 20% of hospitalized older patients, and decreased serum albumin levels associated with malnutrition (or with acute phase reactions to infection) may lead to an increase in the free serum levels of drugs that are highly protein-bound (eg, quinidine, warfarin, rifampin, propranolol), with attendant risks of toxicity. Patients with hypoalbuminemia who receive such drugs should be monitored closely for toxic side effects.

Delirium

Postoperative confusion and delirium are common in the aged and occur more often among patients with diminished cognition. Delirium carries a poor prognosis in older patients. Although it is often self-limited, all patients with delirium should be examined for reversible causes (oversedation, hypoxia, infection, pain, decreased cardiac output, anticholinergic drugs). Low-dose haloperidol (0.5 mg every 8–12 hours) may be useful for severe agitation, but on occasion it will increase confusion in cognitively impaired patients.

Falls

One-third of the geriatric population experience a fall at least once a year, with a resulting one million fractures. Weakness, hypotension, deconditioning, and pain on movement may increase the risk of falling among older postoperative patients. Surgical candidates should be questioned closely for a history of falls (a predictor of subsequent falls); the blood pressure should be taken while standing in all subjects aged 75 or older (to detect positional hypotension); and patients should be observed for postural defects, awkwardness on arising from a chair, and ataxic gait.

Pressure Sores

Immobilization, urinary and fecal incontinence, and malnutrition expose aged patients to the development of pressure sores. Patients with predisposing factors should have daily inspection of pressure points for evidence of early skin ischemia (blanching erythema), stage I pressure sores (nonblanching erythema; shallow ulcers), or more extensive dermal defects. Patients at high risk should be protected by being kept dry, by frequent turning to relieve skin pressure, and by the use of air or foam mattresses. Treatment of skin ulcers involves wet-to-dry dressings to remove dead tissue, protective coverings, and surgical debridement and skin grafting for advanced lesions.

Infection

Patients of advanced age who are infected in the perioperative period may have atypical or nonspecific manifestations, including failure to develop elevated core temperatures. Often, the presenting picture is one of slowness to recover function after surgery, cognitive impairment, or persistent weakness. If infection is suspected, the triad of fever, leukocytosis, and elevated band count strongly support the diagnosis of bacterial invasion, and the absence of these indicators is good evidence against infection.

Fried LP et al: Disability in older adults: evidence regarding significance, etiology, and risk. J Am Geriatr Soc 1997;45:92.

Gerson MC et al: Prediction of cardiac and pulmonary complications related to elective abdominal and noncardiac thoracic surgery in geriatric patients. Am J Med 1990;88:101.

Gustafson Y et al: A geriatric-anesthesiologic program to reduce acute confusional states in elderly patients treated for femoral neck fracture. J Am Geriatr Soc 1991;39:655.

Lonergan ET (editor): *Extending Life, Enhancing Life. A National Research Agenda on Aging.* National Academy Press, 1991.

Mandavia D et al: Geriatric trauma. Emerg Med Clin North Am 1998;16:257.

Odenheimer GL: Geriatric neurology. Neurol Clin 1998;16:561.

Rorbackmadsen M et al: General surgery in patients 80 years and older. Br J Surg 1992;79:1216.

Small GW et al: Diagnosis and treatment of Alzheimer disease and related disorders. Consensus statement of the American Association for Geriatric Psychiatry, the Alzheimer's Association, and the American Geriatrics Society. JAMA 1997; 278:1363.

Suter-Gut D et al: Post-discharge care planning and rehabilitation of the elderly surgical patient. Clin Geriatr Med 1990;6:669.

Vellas B et al: The Mini Nutritional Assessment (MNA) and its use in grading the nutritional state of elderly patients. Nutrition 1999;15:116.

Vestal RE: Aging and pharmacology. Cancer 1997;80:1302.

Legal Medicine for the Surgeon

6

Suzanne C. Will, JD, & Jack Nagan, JD

Surgery entails risks. The surgeon recognizes that a good outcome is never certain, even in the most skilled hands, but this is not always appreciated by patients. Bad results, whether real or perceived, generate malpractice litigation against 40% of all physicians in the USA at some point during their careers. Many others serve as expert witnesses or peer reviewers. Consequently, most physicians eventually become involved in legal proceedings developed to determine medical liability. To reduce the chances of being sued, to increase the chances of successfully defending a lawsuit, and to maximize the effectiveness of one's efforts, all physicians should understand the legal principles of medical practice. This chapter is intended to sharpen awareness of those principles. Because the law varies from state to state and changes over time, the physician is strongly advised to retain legal counsel for the defense of any legal action, when contemplating bringing a legal action against another party, and for advice when dealing with issues affecting licensing, privileging, statutory reporting, and other legal matters affecting professional practice.

OVERVIEW: CIVIL & CRIMINAL LAW

There are two kinds of law: civil and criminal. Medical malpractice belongs in the former category. When lay people discuss medical negligence, however, the two areas are often confused. For example, one is not *guilty* of negligence but *liable for* negligence; guilt is a criminal finding, and negligence is a civil wrong. Other essential distinctions between civil and criminal law should also be kept in mind. For example, the party who brings the complaint is always the *plaintiff*, but the civil complainant is a person or entity seeking redress for a personal injury whereas in criminal law the people bring the action against the defendant. That is why criminal cases bear titles such as *People versus Smith* and civil cases *Jones versus Smith*. The victim in a criminal case is said to be the state—ie, even though a particular individual may have been murdered or raped, the crime is, in theory, one against society.

The purpose of the criminal suit is punishment and deterrence of crime; the object of civil litigation is generally to remedy a wrong so as to place the plaintiff in the same position he or she would have occupied if the wrong had not occurred. The idea is to make the plaintiff whole. Thus, civil redress is usually seen in terms of compensation, although there are certain narrowly restricted situations in which punishment is allowed in the form of exemplary damages (discussed below).

The scale used to judge the plaintiff's allegations differs in criminal and civil law. In both criminal and civil law, of course, the plaintiff bears the burden of proving each element of the case. Every cause of action, whether it be a complaint for murder, robbery, negligence, or breach of contract, is composed of certain required elements which, taken as a whole, are known as the prima facie case for that cause of action. Both the civil and the criminal plaintiff bear the burden of establishing their prima facie case, but the standard by which the plaintiff's case is judged is different in civil and criminal proceedings. In a criminal case, the defendant is assumed to be innocent until and unless the state can prove each element of its prima facie case beyond a reasonable doubt. In a civil action, the defendant remains blameless and free of liability until and unless the plaintiff can establish each element of the prima facie case by a preponderance of the evidence. Obviously, there is a significant difference between the two standards, although an exact definition of reasonable doubt remains elusive. It is quite clear that "beyond a reasonable doubt" is meant to be very close to certainty, as opposed to a "preponderance of the evidence," which requires only that a fact be established as more likely to be true than not to be true.

The sanctions imposed for criminal guilt and civil liability are also different. Criminal guilt may be punished by death, imprisonment, or fine, whereas civil liability in most cases is imposed in the form of a judgment for money damages.

It is possible that the same act may involve both a criminal and a civil wrong, as, for instance, in the case of rape. That act may be prosecuted in a criminal court as rape and may also be the subject of a civil action for the intentional tort of battery. Where an act results in the possibility of both criminal and civil actions, the two cases must be tried separately and, given the difference in the required levels of proof, might well result in a judgment for damages but a verdict of not guilty on the criminal charge.

LITIGATION

The legal process in the USA is characterized by the adversary system. The adversary system does not guarantee justice, just as the physician practicing medicine does not guarantee a cure. Both the legal and medical systems employ sets of procedures that have been tested and found by experience to be sound. All of these procedures are constantly under review and are continually being refined in an attempt to improve the result. In the adversary system, the assumption is that a contest between two equally knowledgeable and equally well prepared adversaries, judged by an impartial third party, affords a thorough airing of each issue of fact and law, which in most cases leads to a finding or reconstruction of what actually happened. It is this process that is the immediate goal of the legal system, with "justice" generally appearing as the ultimate product. It is well to remember that in law the result depends on what is *proved* rather than what *is*.

The roles of the participants in a civil trial are easily explained. Each client's attorney presents evidence of facts most favorable to that side, minimizing by deletion or explanation any unfavorable evidence and rebutting damaging evidence produced by opposing counsel. Testimonial evidence is presented by witnesses to fact (called percipient witnesses), who relate their first-hand experience of relevant subjects within lay comprehension. As to matters outside lay understanding, testimony is limited to expert witnesses (eg, physicians), who alone can offer opinions as evidence. Where there is a judge and a jury, the judge sits as the trier of law only; it is not the judge's task to decide which evidence presented, whether testimonial or physical, is true and which is not true. That decision is reserved for the jury, which sits as the trier of fact. After all of the evidence has been presented, the jury decides which are the facts based on the evidence. It disbelieves some evidence, believes other evidence, and weighs every piece of evidence according to each juror's knowledge, experience, and understanding.

The judge, as trier of law, controls the conduct of the trial and, most importantly, determines the admissibility of evidence sought to be presented to the jury by counsel for each side. If, at the completion of the plaintiff's presentation of the case, the judge finds that the plaintiff has not met the burden of proof in establishing a prima facie case, a nonsuit against the plaintiff may be directed, which terminates the action in favor of the defendant. The judge may also find that, although the plaintiff's presentation has met the burden of proof, the defendant's presentation substantially rebutted the plaintiff's evidence, and the judge may thus direct a verdict in favor of the defendant. The defendant may fail so completely to rebut the plaintiff's case that a directed verdict is entered by the judge in favor of the plaintiff. The judge also has the option of allowing the jury to reach its own verdict, but even then, if the judge believes that there is no rational basis for the jury's decision, a judgment may be directed "notwithstanding the verdict" in favor of either party.

When the plaintiff and defendant have concluded their presentations and the judge has decided to let the case go to the jury, it is the judge's duty to instruct the jury on matters of law relevant to the case. These instructions are generally framed to indicate that certain findings of fact by the jury require certain conclusions of law. The judge even has the power to reduce the amount of the jury's money verdict (remittitur) or to increase it (additur). Although there must be agreement by the plaintiff to remittitur and agreement by the defendant to additur, the judge can "jaw-bone" the agreement of either party by indicating that unless agreement is reached, a motion for a new trial will be granted and the judgment of the jury set aside. There are, of course, numerous other decisions of law that must be made by the judge, such as matters of jurisdiction, venue, and appropriateness of parties to the action, which can greatly affect the initiation, location, and outcome of the litigation.

In cases where there is no jury, the judge acts as finder of fact as well as trier of law.

The physician's defense counsel in a medical negligence action may prefer to present the case to a judge sitting as trier of fact as well as of law. A trial to the judge alone is conducted with a great deal more flexibility than a trial before a judge and jury, because the judge is not concerned so much about evidence that may be prejudicial. That is, a jury of lay people may be biased in favor of or against a party by emotionally charged evidence or confused by technical or complex evidence. The evidence may be so technical, as in many medical malpractice cases, that it is hopelessly beyond lay understanding (perhaps even with the assistance of expert witnesses). The judge is probably better informed than the average juror and may be familiar with medical terminology from other cases. The judge is much less likely to be influenced by emotional testimony or evidence that might be prejudicial to one of the parties. As a result, questions of admissibility before a judge alone are more likely to be resolved in favor of admission, whereas a judge might hesitate to admit the same evidence in a jury trial because of the possibility of an effect on the jury out of proportion to the real weight of the evidence.

The matter of appeal is sometimes misunderstood by those unfamiliar with the legal process. When a case is appealed, the facts are no longer in dispute. The trier of fact has already heard all of the evidence and made its decision, and the facts are as found. Unless it can be said that there was no rational basis for the finding of fact, which is an exceedingly difficult standard to meet, the findings as to facts will stand on appeal. The issues being contested by an appeal are questions of law decided by the trial judge. Any of the trial judge's decisions referred to above may become the basis for an appeal to a higher court. It then becomes a question of the opinion of an appellate judge, or panel of appellate judges, against that of the trial judge. Trial judges do not like to be overruled on appeal, so they try to make their decisions and instructions on law conform to acceptable, frequently used standards.

Although criminal law in the USA is almost exclusively governed by the state penal codes, civil law is still largely based on the common law system, which began with decisions of English courts and acts of Parliament and was adopted by the American states at the time of the Revolution. This inherited body of common law has since been augmented by decisions of appellate courts at both the state and federal levels. The key to understanding the common law system is the doctrine of stare decisis, which is the rule of legal precedent requiring lower courts to adopt decisions consistent with those of higher courts. When the issue is "on all fours" with an earlier appellate court decision in the same jurisdiction, the earlier decision will control the present case.

CONTRACT BASIS OF THE PHYSICIAN-PATIENT RELATIONSHIP

Civil law obligations are of three types: contract, quasi-contract, and tort. A basic understanding of these areas is useful to physicians because the doctor-patient relationship is a complex one that may involve all of them. The essence of a contractual relationship is voluntary agreement between the parties, expressed orally or in writing, or implied by conduct. A quasi-contractual relationship is the result of a voluntary commitment of only one of the parties and the imposition of an agreement on the other party to avoid unjust enrichment. The ordinary purchase of goods or services is the simplest example of a contractual relationship, where one party agrees to furnish the goods or services and the other party agrees to pay for them. An example of a quasi-contractual situation is providing essential medical care for a patient who is incapable of contractual assent, such as an unconscious person, a minor, or an incompetent. The law will impose a quasi-contractual obligation on the patient or his or her legal representative (eg, parent or guardian) to pay for the medical care (*Greenspan v Slate*, 97 A2d 390 [NJ 1957]; *Schroeder v Perkel*, 432 A2d 834 [NJ 1981]).

If the doctor and patient enter into a written contract for treatment, or if a verbal exchange takes place in which the patient promises to pay and the physician promises to treat, or if there is conduct in place of a promise (patient comes to doctor's office, doctor treats), the doctor-patient relationship is contractual. Subsequent failure of the patient to pay would amount to a breach of contract. Once having undertaken the obligation to treat the patient, a physician who fails to do so commits a particular type of breach known as abandonment. This is true no matter how the physician-patient relationship was created. The fact of that relationship imposes the obligation.

The relationship that is formed is one of fiduciary trust, based on the unavoidable reliance of the lay person on the professional. This means that, unlike the usual "arm's length" sales transaction, there is a special obligation on the part of the physician: a duty of affirmative disclosure. Physicians deal with patients at all times in the context of this special trust. The relationship continues in the ordinary course of events until the treatment is completed. However, there may be situations where the patient wishes to terminate earlier. The patient can terminate at any time without notice or may decide at any time for any reason not to see that doctor any more, and that is the end of it.

There is, however, the possibility that a patient who demonstrates an intent to terminate unilaterally might later claim abandonment by the physician when, for example, an incision is slow in healing or the doctor's bill is higher than expected. To guard against this situation, the physician should confirm the patient's intent to terminate by written notification to the patient with a return receipt to document the change in relationship for the office file.

The physician can also terminate the relationship unilaterally, but special conditions apply. Notice must first be given to the patient and information on past treatment provided to the new physician. In one case, a patient was brought to an emergency room with a gunshot wound in the neck. The patient was examined, admitted, and sent to the ward by the surgeon, who then went home. The surgeon was called shortly thereafter and told that the patient was having difficulty breathing and needed a tracheostomy. The admitting physician failed to return, and by the time another surgeon got the patient to the operating room it was too late. The patient died 4 hours after admission. Even though only a few hours had passed and there had been no formed intent on the part of the admitting doctor to permanently discontinue treatment, the court nevertheless ruled that the doctor had abandoned the patient (*Johnson v Vaughn*, 370 SW2d 591 [Ky 1963]; see also 57 ALR 432, supp sec). So the definition of abandonment is highly flexible. For instance, if a fracture has been set by an orthopedic surgeon, treatment might include checking the patient every few months until healing and rehabilitation are complete. Even though there is no contact between doctor and patient for months, the relationship remains intact. Thus, for a doctor to be protected in terminating the physician-patient relationship, notice must first be given to the patient. How much notice is required varies with the case. In general, the courts have held that 30 days is sufficient.

Of course, there are difficult situations, like the doctor who is working in a small community where there is literally no other doctor available, in which case termination may be impossible. The period of reasonable notice is based in large part on the availability of adequate medical coverage; it is the responsibility of the terminating physician not only to give the patient enough notice to find another physician but also to furnish information to the successor fast enough so that there is no delay in treatment. What constitutes unreasonable delay may also vary with the details of the illness. In the average case, a routine mailing of the records to the new physician and being available for telephone consultation would be sufficient.

It is important to understand the legal distinction between referral and consultation. A referral usually transfers responsibility for care of the patient to a new physician. The referring doctor (legally) drops out of the picture (after documenting that the new physician has accepted responsibility for care). A consultation does not shift responsibility from one physician to another. Instead, it adds another doctor to the treating team until the consultation is complete. Thereafter, there is no continuing relationship between consultant and patient—only the original physician-patient relationship remains.

Occasionally, a physician who does not intend to terminate care waits too long to start the necessary treatment, with resultant injury to the patient. In this case, the legal issue concerns a possible breach of the standard of care. There are situations where abandonment may result in both contractual liability and tort liability, and damages may be recovered for either.

Once the doctor-patient relationship is formed, the obligation of the physician is defined as the possession and application of care, skill, and knowledge common to other physicians of good standing. However, a physician may increase the level of this obligation by expressly promising or "warranting" a particular result or a cure, in which event the failure to achieve the promised result will render the physician liable in contract for breach of warranty. The prima facie case for breach of contract is simple, since it only requires proof of the contract and that the physician made a particular promise and then substantially failed to perform. Thus, there is a considerable legal difference between the ob-

stetrician who promises to perform a tubal ligation and one who promises to sterilize the patient. However successful the surgeon's experience with a given procedure, the discussion of treatment objectives with the patient should be limited to the results expected and hoped for, the statistical probabilities, and the sincere promise to spare no effort to achieve a satisfactory outcome.

Money judgments for breach of contract in most states are limited to the value of the patient's "loss of the bargain" (which assumes that the promised treatment was obtained elsewhere at a greater cost) or "out of pocket" cost to the patient for securing the treatment elsewhere. A minority of jurisdictions do, however, allow recovery of money damages for pain and suffering where it was foreseeable at the time of the breach that failure of the doctor to perform, or delay in performance, would result in such pain and suffering for the patient. Actions for breach of contract against physicians are rare. They may be brought by patients who wish to "punish" a physician for a bad result although they know the physician was not negligent, or may be the only recourse in instances where a negligence action is barred by the shorter statute of limitations for tort.

INTENTIONAL TORTS

The third—and by far the most important—area of civil law for the physician is tort law. There are two kinds of tort: intentional and negligent. Although some categories of torts involve invasions of property rights, our concern here will be solely with invasions of personal rights, ie, those of the patient.

The category of intentional torts includes assault, battery, false imprisonment, defamation, invasion of privacy, infliction of emotional distress, and intentional misrepresentation. The prima facie case for the intentional torts is established by proving that the defendant's conduct was deliberate. If the conduct results in actual injury to the plaintiff, it is compensable in money damages. If conduct is established but injury is not, the damages will be limited to a nominal sum. But if the act (or omission) was particularly outrageous, punitive damages may be awarded in addition to compensatory or nominal damages. It should be emphasized that the only intent required for the commission of an intentional tort is the intent to commit the act, not an intent to bring about the ultimate injury. Another way of saying this is that the intention to bring about the ultimate injury is presumed from the commission of the act.

The act required to establish an **assault** is that which places another in immediate apprehension of harm. Traditionally, words alone without supporting gestures do not establish a cause of action for assault. A **battery** is simply an unauthorized touching of another. Of course, the authorization or consent for contact may not always be expressed. For instance, the fact that a patient has visited a physician for treatment implies consent to reasonable physical contact necessary for the examination. However, when the physician's treatment entails more than such customary contact, as in surgery, invasive diagnostic procedures, and drug treatment involving the risk of special harm, the consent of the patient to the specific procedures must first be obtained. In the absence of such consent, treatment by the physician would be battery, as would also be the case where consent was obtained to operate on a specific site and the consent was exceeded by operating on a different site, either instead of or in addition to the area of original consent. In situations where the issue is not whether any consent was obtained from the patient but rather whether the physician disclosed *enough* information for a reasonable patient to make an intelligent choice, the trend of the courts is to view the lack of so-called informed consent as a form of negligence in the disclosure of information by the physician. The matter of informed consent has been the subject of so much attention that it will be discussed below under its own heading.

The intentional tort of **false imprisonment** consists of an invasion of the personal interest in freedom from restraint of movement. Thus, a physician who orders a patient placed in restraints or drugged to the point of immobility by mistake or without a good medical reason may be liable for damages for false imprisonment. The physician most often involved in false imprisonment actions is the psychiatrist who orders involuntary commitment.

The intentional tort of **defamation** consists of injury to reputation by means of slanderous (oral) or libelous (written) statements to another person that diminish the respect in which the plaintiff is held by others and lessen his or her standing in the community. The extent of the injury caused by verbal defamation must be proved by the plaintiff except in the case of slander involving an accusation of criminal conduct, loathsome disease (eg, syphilis, leprosy), acts incompatible with one's business, trade, or profession, or unchastity of a woman. These are the four categories of slander per se from which general damages are presumed to result without need of proof.

Special (actual) damages need not be proved in the case of libel inherent on the face of a publication, but where reference to extrinsic information is needed to create the libelous meaning (known as libel per quod), general damages will be presumed only in the same four areas as above. Otherwise, special injury must be proved to establish the prima facie case of libel. The defendant may avoid liability for defamation by establishing a privilege of immunity that covers the statement or by establishing that the statement was true. It should be noted that one who repeats or "republishes" defamatory statements faces the same liability as the original purveyor.

Invasion of privacy is a new and still developing area of tort law dating in broad acceptance from the 1930s. The types of invasion recognized in this category are public use for profit of personal information about another or some type of intrusion on one's physical solitude. The most common defenses to an action for invasion of privacy are the privileges that exist for publication of information of public interest or concerning public figures. Specific state statutes define exceptions to the restrictions of defamation and invasion of privacy law. Such laws, known as **reporting statutes,** commonly include specific communicable diseases, gunshot and stab wounds, seizure disorders, and child abuse. (*Examples:* California Penal Codes 11160, 11161; California Health and Safety Codes 103900, 120250.) Giving out details of medical treatment concerning patients (eg, celebrities), even if the information is truly newsworthy, can exceed the privilege. Without a signed release from the patient or a court order, caution is the rule: "If in doubt, don't give it out." The same caution extends to identifying a patient if a description of the case is published. Also, no outsiders are allowed in the operating room without the patient's advance consent. (Standard consent forms usually allow observers to view surgery for educational purposes.)

Infliction of mental distress as a cause of action independent of contemporaneous physical injury has only recently achieved judicial recognition. The conduct or language must be outrageous and extreme and the emotional upset apparent (most successful suits have involved resulting physical illness). The law requires an individual to be somewhat tough-skinned, and annoyance or insult alone is not actionable. Nevertheless, the special closeness and reliance that characterized the fiduciary relationship between doctor and patient add weight to possible liability for ill-considered conduct by physicians, who have a duty to protect and comfort their patients.

Intentional torts are not covered by professional insurance and are not included in the protection afforded by governmental immunity statutes. Where liability for an intentional tort is established, the judgment comes out of the doctor's own pocket.

NEGLIGENT TORTS

Although few physicians will ever have to face a suit for intentional tort, fewer still will complete a career without some involvement in a medical negligence action, whether as defendant, percipient witness, expert witness, or forensic consultant. A basic understanding of negligence law lessens the physician's chances of becoming a defendant and increases the prospects for making an effective, rational response if a legal proceeding does become necessary.

The prima facie case for negligence consists of four elements: duty, breach, causation, and damages. Each of these elements must be proved by the plaintiff by a preponderance of the evidence, and failure to do so will be fatal to the plaintiff's cause of action. In the case of a medical negligence action, the duty owed is coextensive with the doctor-patient relationship. It consists of the obligation on the doctor's part to acquire and maintain the same level of skill, care, and knowledge possessed by other members of the profession in good standing and to exercise that skill, care, and knowledge in the treatment of patients. There is no duty to accept a patient for treatment, and the physician may refuse to accept any person as a patient for any reason or for no reason at all.

There is one situation in which a physician may undertake treatment of an individual without creating a doctor-patient relationship and thus without incurring the obligation to treat, ie, by rendering emergency treatment outside the normal scope of practice. Public policy in favor of physicians stopping to aid accident victims is so strong that the states have enacted special statutes, known generally as Good Samaritan Acts, which provide immunity from liability arising out of ordinary negligence in treatment of such victims and often even for injury due to gross negligence. In addition, some states have enacted special statutes that provide for immunity of medical specialists who are called in emergencies as consultants to "bail out" another physician whose patient has deteriorated despite (or as a result of) earlier treatment. The following statutes enacted in California are typical examples: Section 2395 of the Business and Professions Code, entitled "Emergency Care at Scene of Accident," contains the following wording: "No licensee, who in good faith renders emergency care at the scene of an emergency, shall be liable for any civil damages as result of any acts or omissions by such person in rendering the emergency care." Note that "scene of an emergency" encompasses not only location but also normal scope of employment. Therefore, if a doctor treats a patient while performing normal duties in the emergency room or as part of the responding "crash cart" team in a hospital, the Good Samaritan statute would not apply (*Colby v Schwartz*, 144 *California Reporter* 624 [1978]; *McKenna v Cedars of Lebanon Hospital*, 155 *California Reporter* 631 [1979]).

Section 2396 of the Business and Professions Code, entitled "Emergency Care for Complication Arising From Prior Care by Another," reads as follows: "No li-censee, who in good faith upon the request of another person so licensed, renders emergency medical care to a person for medical complication arising from prior care by another person so licensed, shall be liable for any civil damages as a result of any acts or omissions by such licensed person in rendering such emergency medical care." Scene of an emergency is defined as above.

One problem under the general heading of the physician's duty is the *unintentional* formation of a physician-patient relationship. This situation usually arises where a doctor is consulted very briefly and usually very casually by an individual seeking a quick (and free) "curbstone opinion." Where such an opinion is rendered by a physician in surroundings that quite clearly indicate that no professional relationship was intended, such as a social gathering, the courts have not found the existence of a doctor-patient relationship. The findings may be otherwise, however, where the doctor is consulted in the hospital and—for example—instead of telling the questioner to come to the office for a regular appointment or referring to another doctor for medical advice, or even saying nothing at all, gives an opinion on which the "patient" relies. Even late-at-night advice by telephone to call another doctor in the morning may be held to constitute treatment, since it assumes that the patient can afford to wait until morning before seeking care. The best course to follow when confronted with such a request, unless the doctor does intend to treat the patient, is to offer no advice at all other than an immediate referral to another source of medical treatment (eg, a hospital emergency room).

The physician's duty to the patient is performed within the "standard of care," and it is the failure of a physician to meet the standard of care in a given case that constitutes the "breach" element of the prima facie case for negligence. In the great majority of medical negligence cases, determining what the specific standard of care should be is beyond the comprehension of the lay persons on the jury. In these cases, the law requires that the standard be established by expert medical testimony. This method of setting the standard requires a physician to take the witness stand and testify about the treatment required in the particular case. Although technically any physician may testify as an expert on any medical specialty, in practice, the medical expert will be of the particular specialty appropriate to the facts of the case.

At one time the standard of care was established by comparison with good medical practice in the same community in which the defendant was practicing. This so-called **locality rule** has undergone extensive change, until today most jurisdictions have broadened the standard to include treatment by physicians in good standing **under similar circumstances**—one of those circumstances being similarity of locale in terms of proximity to major medical centers and accessibility of medical information generally. Some states have gone so far as to abolish the locality rule entirely, holding that dissemination of medical advances, especially in the newer specialties, is so effective today that there is, in effect, a national standard of care for those fields of medicine. The well-established trend is away from the narrow confines of the locality rule and toward a national standard (and perhaps, eventually, an international standard of care, beginning with English-speaking countries). Obviously, it is the efficacy of the treatment that is important in setting the standard of care and not the country or city where the treatment occurred. The courts have increasingly recognized that geographic isolation should not offer protection for the use of modes of treatment that have been discredited and discarded by physicians in general.

Even in situations where one mode of therapy is preferred by the majority of specialists in the field, the law does not require that this particular form of treatment be adopted as the standard of care by which all physicians in that field shall be judged. It is sufficient that the treatment actually rendered be approved by a respected school of medical thought in order for it to come within the standard of care.

The requirement of expert medical testimony to establish the standard of care has one well-established exception, ie, where the alleged negligence is within the lay understanding of the jury. In such cases, which include the "foreign object" cases, the judge must decide as a matter of law whether a medical expert will be required to establish the prima facie case in any particular respect. The judge may let the jury decide whether leaving a sponge, needle, clamp, or other object inside the patient is negligent (ie, a breach of the standard of care) but may require medical expert testimony on the element of causation.

The standard of care based on the modes of treatment employed by members of the medical specialty group in good standing is a **minimum standard.** There are two situations in which that minimum standard can be raised to require a higher level of treatment by a medical defendant. The first is that a physician who has made representations to the patient of greater skill or experience than is the case will be bound by them. In other words, a generalist who claims to possess the skill and experience of a specialist (or, if a specialist, that of a subspecialist) will be bound as a matter of law by the higher standard of care. The second situation arises in rare cases when the court itself determines that the standard of treatment in current use is simply not high enough to protect society. The likelihood of such a finding by a court is increased in cases where the added burden on the physician in meeting the higher standard proposed is very slight and the benefit to patients is

very great. Where the existing standard of care is not adequate to protect the patient, the court may impose a stricter standard. This type of reasoning was demonstrated in the informed consent case of *Cobbs v Grant,* 502 P2d 1, 8 (Cal 1972).

It is plain from the decisions on standard of care that the law requires every physician to know his or her own limitations. The physician who attempts too much in a nonemergency case is risking liability for failure to consult or refer.

The element of causation has been the source of considerable confusion in the law. The plaintiff's case must include two types of causation: causation in fact and proximate cause. The test used most often in determining the presence of factual causation is simply that the defendant's conduct must be a substantial factor in bringing about the injury complained of. A minority of jurisdictions approach factual causation somewhat differently and require that the defendant's conduct be an indispensable antecedent to the plaintiff's injury, but in most cases the result is the same whichever test is used. Under either of these tests, the substance of the factual causation element is the same: proof of a sequence of events that connects breach of duty to conform to the standard of care with injury to the plaintiff.

The importance of the factual causation element is demonstrated by cases in which the treatment rendered is palliative and does not affect the course of the underlying disease process. In such cases where the patient dies as a result of the disease, a breach of the standard of care by the physician in administering the palliative treatment does not as a matter of law lead to liability for the death because the treatment was not a cause in fact of the patient's death.

For the purposes of this discussion, it is best to think of the second type of causation, known as either proximate cause or legal cause, as a set of limitations on causation in fact. Having established causation in fact, the court may nevertheless fail to find liability if the injury is too far removed from the physician's conduct or where some abnormal force intervenes to break the chain of events connecting the conduct with the result. The effect of the proximate cause requirement is that, in addition to proving the chain of events connecting the conduct and the result, the plaintiff must also establish a close and direct relationship between the conduct and the result.

RES IPSA LOQUITUR

The three elements of duty, breach, and causation are commonly referred to collectively as the liability aspect of a negligence case. With two basic exceptions, the plaintiff must establish the defendant's liability by a preponderance of the evidence in order to recover. The first of these exceptions is the doctrine of **res ipsa loquitur** ("the thing speaks for itself"). Considering the reams of print and judicial contention that have been generated by this doctrine, its origin was rather prosaic. The term was first applied by Baron Pollack in the 1863 case of *Byrne v Boadle* (2 H & C 772, 159 *English Reports* 299 [1863]), tried on appeal before the English Court of Exchequer. In the words of Pollack: "There are certain cases of which it may be said res ipsa loquitur, and this seems one of them." In some cases the courts have held that the mere fact of the accident having occurred is evidence of negligence: ". . . The present case upon the evidence comes to this, a man is passing in front of the premises of a dealer in flour, and there falls down upon him a barrel of flour. I think it apparent that the barrel was in the custody of the defendant who occupied the premises, and who is responsible for the acts of his servants who had the control of it; and in my opinion the fact of its falling is prima facie evidence of negligence."

The doctrine evolved steadily from that case down to the landmark decision of the California Supreme Court in *Ybarra v Spangard* (154 P2d 687 [Cal 1944]), a case which applied the doctrine of res ipsa loquitur to medical negligence. The holding of the court in *Ybarra* was that "where a plaintiff receives unusual injuries while unconscious and in the course of medical treatment, all those defendants who had any control over his body or the instrumentalities which might have caused the injuries may properly be called upon to meet the inference of negligence by giving an explanation of their conduct."

The doctrine itself serves as a substitute for the elements of breach and causation, although the plaintiff must still establish the existence of the duty element and must show damages. In order to gain the benefit of this substitution, the plaintiff must establish, first, that the accident is of a kind that ordinarily does not occur in the absence of someone's negligence; second, that it must be caused by an instrumentality within the exclusive control of the defendant; and third, that it must not have been due to any voluntary action on the plaintiff's part. If the court finds as a matter of law that these requirements have been met by the plaintiff, the court will instruct the jury that it may infer breach and causation by the defendant unless the inference is successfully rebutted by defendant's proof. As an inference of negligence, the doctrine of res ipsa loquitur operates as a substitute for evidence that would be especially difficult for the plaintiff to produce. The threshold issue— whether the injury is of a type that ordinarily does not occur in the absence of negligence—may itself call for expert testimony. If such testimony establishes that the injury occurs as an inherent risk in a documented percentage of cases not involving negligence, the doctrine will not be applied.

VICARIOUS LIABILITY

The other method of bypassing the prima facie case for negligence against a particular defendant is by imputed negligence. This method relies on the rule of law known as **respondeat superior,** which holds the principal responsible for the acts of his or her agents. This doctrine is manifested in the operating room in the form of the so-called captain of the ship doctrine. As the captain of the ship, the surgeon is held responsible for negligent injury to the patient while the surgeon is directing the operation. It is the exercise of control over others by the surgeon that is the key to the application of the doctrine. For this reason, the actions of the anesthesiologist are generally not imputed to the surgeon. Of course, to the extent that the surgeon issues specific orders to the anesthesiologist, a secondary liability is assumed if the anesthesiologist is negligent in carrying out the orders. In addition, in a medical partnership, the negligence of one partner is imputed to the other partners, and all partners become equally liable for damages that ensue. These instances of vicarious liability are exceptions to the general rule requiring that the elements of the prima facie case be established against the particular defendant only in the sense that once they are established as to one defendant, they may fix liability on another defendant as well, based on the legal relationship of the parties.

DAMAGES

Of course, even when the plaintiff has established the elements of duty, breach, and causation by a preponderance of the evidence as to each, there is still the requirement of proving the last element of the prima facie case: damages. Considering that the average cost today of bringing a medical malpractice case through trial is over $75,000, it is plainly impractical for a plaintiff's attorney to bring a case to trial unless the alleged injury to the plaintiff has been substantial and offers a potential money judgment well in excess of expenses incurred.

The two categories of compensatory damages in personal injury cases are general damages, which include such intangible elements as pain and suffering; and special damages, which include documented economic loss from costs of medical care and diminished income. Because there are no mathematical formulas or other objective criteria for placing a dollar value on pain and suffering, this type of damage award is a frequent target for tort reform. In fact, since 1975, more than half of the states have enacted statutory limits or "caps" on medical malpractice damage awards for pain and suffering. For instance, the ceiling for awards for pain and suffering in California is $250,000 (California Civil

Code 3333.2) and under Hawaii law it is $375,000 (Hawaii Revised Statute 663-8.7). In a wrongful death action, the general damages do not include pain and suffering but do include the family's loss of "comfort and society"; and the special damages include loss of economic support along with funeral expenses. In both personal injury and wrongful death actions, proof of gross negligence or especially outrageous conduct may result in exemplary (punitive) damages, which are fixed in relation to the wealth of the defendant.

According to Department of Treasury statistics for fiscal year 2000, the United States Government paid settlements and judgments in the sum of over $185 million dollars to claimants in medical malpractice cases. The two largest federal health care providers, the Department of Defense and the Department of Veterans Affairs, paid $101 million and $68 million dollars, respectively. Although the total amount of damages paid to individuals who received nonfederal governmental and private health care services has not been calculated, when compared with the comparatively small percentage of health care services received in federal hospitals, the amount must be of staggering proportions.

DEFENSES

Common defenses to medical negligence actions are the statutes of limitations and contributory or comparative negligence. The purpose of **statutes of limitations** is to avoid litigation over stale claims by requiring a plaintiff to initiate suit within a fixed number of years after the negligent act or omission. Although the number of years varies from state to state, the effect of the running of the statutory period is the same everywhere—the plaintiff is forever barred from instituting suit based on that particular act or omission. The period begins to run on the date of the occurrence of the alleged negligence unless the negligence results in an injury that the plaintiff would typically be unaware of, such as the foreign body type of case. To cover this situation, most states and all federal jurisdictions apply the "discovery rule," under which the statutory period does not begin to run until the plaintiff knows, or in the exercise of reasonable diligence should have known, that the injury suffered was the result of treatment. Also, in many states the statutory period is tolled (suspended) by a legal disability on the part of the plaintiff such as minority or incompetency, by misrepresentation of the facts surrounding the treatment by the defendant physician, or by the "continuing care rule," which tolls the statute until the physician-patient relationship is terminated. The importance of a detailed medical record to the maintenance of a statute of limitations defense cannot be overemphasized. The absence of an ap-

propriate medical record favors the patient, the theory being that months or years later, the patient's memory of events that uniquely affect personal health and safety is generally superior to the memory of the physician, who treats a multitude of patients.

The defense of **contributory negligence** operates in a minority of jurisdictions as a complete bar to the maintenance of the plaintiff's action when it is established that the injury was in any way the result of the plaintiff's negligence. Thus, even if it were found that the surgeon was 75% responsible for the injury and the plaintiff only 25% responsible, a verdict for the defendant must result. A bare majority of states now employ the **comparative negligence** approach, which apportions the total amount of damages according to the relative negligence of the plaintiff and the defendant. Thus, in comparative negligence jurisdictions, if it is found that the plaintiff has been injured to the extent of $100,000 in damages but was 25% negligent, the defendant would be assessed $75,000 in damages.

INFORMED CONSENT

Much attention has been paid to the topic of informed consent in recent years, but, for all the reams of analysis, the new case law on consent does not actually affect the basic process of securing consent for medical treatment. The big question has always been, "How much should the patient be told?"

The new cases on consent, founded on *Canterbury v Spence* (464 F2d 772 [DC Cir 1972]) and *Cobbs v Grant* (supra), do not change the priority of the question; neither do they answer it. Common sense is still the best guideline. The exchange between physician and patient in securing consent need be no different for any given treatment now than it was 15 years ago. The requirements are a description of the procedure, its chances of success, the risks, and the alternatives. The physician has always compared risks and benefits in deciding what mode of treatment to recommend. Explaining them to the patient in plain language is all that was ever required and is as sound in law today as it has always been good medical practice.

Traditionally, courts in the USA have used the "customary practice" standard to determine whether enough information was presented to the patient to support a rational decision. The new line of cases, which now constitutes a growing minority trend, holds that reliance on the custom of doctors in good standing is an illusory standard. These courts have substituted a standard of materiality to the patient. Under this minority approach, the test becomes whether a reasonable person would have refused the treatment if the risk of the complication that occurred had been clearly explained.

The effect of this materiality test is that the more important the procedure is to the patient's health, the less credible the claim that the procedure would have been refused. Conversely, the less important the procedure, the more credible will be a later complaint that it would have been refused had the risks been fully identified.

Put in its simplest form, a fully detailed informed consent is less crucial where the procedure may save life or limb and more important where the treatment objective is cosmetic. The principle finds its ultimate expression in the long-established rule that consent is implied in a medical emergency. There is one caveat to the rule of implied consent: the physician cannot assume that consent is implied if a competent adult refuses treatment.

The above discussion of the consent process is rooted in two basic premises. The first is that the physician determines which forms of treatment are appropriate for the patient's condition. The second is that once these therapeutic options have been explained to the patient, the patient will decide which of the options (including the option of no treatment at all) will be elected. The legal right of a competent adult to accept or decline proposed medical treatment has its foundation in the common-law and constitutionally guaranteed right of personal privacy. The patient's right to refuse treatment is not affected by the gravity of the consequences of refusal. Even if pain, disability, or death will be a probable consequence of a refusal of consent, a competent adult has the legal right to make that decision.

The first court decisions on cessation of life support generally involved patients in a persistent vegetative state being maintained on respirators. These cases, beginning with *Matter of Quinlan*, 355 A2d 647 (1976), sided with the patient's (or legal representative's) right to refuse such treatment. Later cases have involved patients who were seriously ill but not curable (or whose prognoses could not be improved) and refused less intrusive life support such as nasogastric tube feeding or intravenous hydration, further refining the patient's right to refuse treatment. From these cases has evolved what is now known as the **doctrine of proportionality,** which states that artificial life support should be initiated and maintained so long as it constitutes "proportionate treatment," ie, treatment which, in the patient's view, has at least a reasonable chance of providing benefits to the patient that outweigh the burdens attendant upon treatment. Thus, even if a proposed course of treatment might be extremely painful or intrusive, it would still be proportionate treatment if the prognosis was for complete cure or significant improvement in the patient's condition. On the other hand, a treatment course that is only minimally painful or intrusive may nonetheless be considered disproportionate to the potential benefits if the prognosis is virtually hopeless for any significant improvement in condition. (*Barber v Superior Court,* 147 Cal App 3d 1006, 1019 [1983]).

The words of the patient himself in one of these cases impressed the court and are instructive here: "While I have no wish to die, I find intolerable the living conditions forced upon me by my deteriorating lungs, heart and blood vessel systems, and I find intolerable my being continuously connected to this ventilator, which sustains my every breath and my life for the past six and one-half . . . weeks. Therefore, I wish this court to order that the sustaining of my respiration by this mechanical device violates my constitutional right, is contrary to my every wish, and constitutes a battery upon my person. I fully understand that my request to have the ventilator removed and discontinued, which I have frequently made to my wife and my doctors, will very likely cause respiratory failure and ultimately lead to my death. I am willing to accept that risk rather than to continue the burden of this artificial existence which I find unendurable, degrading and dehumanizing." (*Bartling v Superior Court,* 163 Cal App 3d 186, 191 [1984]).

In October 1990, the United States Supreme Court decided its first "right-to-die" case, *Cruzan v Director, Missouri Department of Health,* 110 S.Ct. 2841 (1990), confirming the right of a competent adult to accept or refuse medical care but leaving to the states the power to set the standard of proof for evidence that a patient has made such a decision. The best way to prove that treatment has been refused is by means of a written, signed, and witnessed instruction by the patient, executed while competent. Instructions such as this are termed **advance directives** and include durable powers of attorney for health care, living wills, and natural death directives, depending on state law. There is now a new federal law, the Patient Self-Determination Act, effective December 1, 1991 (42 U.S. Code 1395cc et seq), that requires Medicare or Medicaid providers to give their adult patients information on advance directives at the time of initial care or admission under applicable state law. The law does not change the rights of the patient. It does make the health care provider responsible for informing the patient of those rights.

In cases involving patients whose condition is irreversibly and imminently terminal, there may be no treatment the physician can offer. Where there is a consensus among the treatment team, next-of-kin, and the known wishes of the patient, a "do-not-resuscitate" or "no code" order may be appropriate. If such an order is given by the attending physician, it should be a written order in the patient's chart. The order should be supported with a progress note that includes diagnosis and prognosis, wishes (if known) of the patient and family, consensus of the treatment team, and confirmation of the patient's competence.

If a person in need of medical treatment is incapable of giving informed consent, substituted consent must be obtained from the next of kin. In most states, the order of intestate succession controls the identity of next of kin. The order is generally spouse, adult child, parent, sibling. For a person who has been adjudicated incompetent, consent of the court-appointed guardian must be obtained. If a minor is in need of care, consent of one parent is required. The courts have recognized, however, that refusal by parents to consent to emergency care for a child is subject to judicial review.

The signed consent form is merely evidence that the consent process occurred. It should always be backed up by the physician's own brief entry in the progress notes, with date and time. If the need to alter an entry arises, there is only one safe method: Line out the error (without obliterating it), initial and date the deletion, and enter the correct information.

MEDICAL INSURANCE

Discussions of the present status of availability of medical malpractice insurance are usually phrased in terms of crisis. Physicians and other health care practitioners employed by government entities are generally covered by laws that protect them from personal liability. For instance, the Federal Tort Claims Act, 28 USC 1346(b), 2671 through 2680, provides a legal defense and pays any settlement or judgment for federally employed physicians provided they were working within the scope of their employment at the time the negligent act or omission occurred. For the physician approaching private practice, sufficient understanding of the basics of professional insurance is imperative so that at least the right questions can be asked.

The insurance crisis was generated by the loss of profitability of medical liability insurance. This resulted from reduction of surpluses owing to investment losses by the insurance companies, large increases in the cost to the primary insurer of reinsurance (beginning in 1970), and the combination of unpredictability of occurrence claims and the small physician base from which to generate the premium pool. Of the many proposals to remedy the problem, several have found nationwide application. First, there has been a direct shift in the type of policy written from "occurrence" to "claims made."

Briefly, an occurrence policy provides coverage for events that become the basis for claims in the year that the event occurs, while the claims made policy provides coverage only for the year in which a claim is presented to the insurer, regardless of when the underlying event took place. The practical effect of the change from occurrence to claims made policies is that the physician is only secure so long as coverage continues to be purchased every year without lapse. For claims made policies, therefore, it is imperative that the insurance contract include provision for purchase by the doctor of the "tail" of coverage. In other words, there must be liability coverage for the years following the doctor's retirement or change in practice from patient care to nonpatient care. Care should also be taken that "presentation" of a claim under a claims made policy be defined, since some contracts allow presentation only by a third party (plaintiff or attorney) and not by the physician. Attention must also be given to exclusions from coverage, which may place certain high-risk operations outside the scope of the policy.

The purposes of medical liability insurance are protection against costs of defending a suit (commonly as high as $75,000 to $100,000) and payment of adverse judgments. Any physician considering "going bare" (practicing without liability coverage) must weigh the potential impact of these costs. As difficult to achieve as it is, attaining "judgment-proof" status (eg, irrevocable transfer of assets to another person prior to threat of suit) only protects against payment of a judgment. The only way to avoid litigation costs as well would be to submit to default judgment. The hazards of going bare thus make the cost of insurance more palatable.

Following the medical liability insurance "crisis" of the mid 1970s, the number of malpractice claims filed actually leveled off between the years 1976 to 1978. Unfortunately, claims-filed activity rose again in 1979 and has continued to rise steadily. We are faced now with a new crisis in medical insurance. Largely because of the growth of doctor-owned insurance companies, there is no availability problem. There is, however, a serious affordability problem, which is getting worse. With increasing claims activity and the uncertainty of long "tail" coverage, the cost of liability insurance may actually prevent newly licensed physicians from practicing in high-risk surgical specialties. One possible solution that has worked well in some areas is state-sponsored reinsurance pools for coverage of awards over a certain amount (eg, $250,000). Another solution may be found in state-run physician-supported patient compensation funds set up to cover amounts over a statutory limit on what can be awarded.

HOSPITAL STAFF PRIVILEGES

The nature of the physician-hospital relationship has changed drastically since the turn of the century as the hospital's status has graduated from that of essentially a quarantine facility for the isolation of the ill to the modern health care center. With this development, the importance of access to the hospital facility (ie, staff privileges) by the individual physician has become a professional and economic necessity. Until the Illinois Supreme Court decision in *Darling v Charleston Community Memorial Hospital,* 211 NE2d 253 (1965), *cert denied* 383 US 946 (1966), it was generally accepted by the courts that the private physician with staff privileges was an independent contractor with the hospital and that the hospital would not be vicariously liable for contractors' malpractice under the doctrine of respondeat superior. This left no cause of action at all against the hospital. *Darling* and its progeny now represent the majority position in the USA, creating a cause of action for direct hospital liability for failure to adequately supervise the quality of care in the hospital, including evaluation of the abilities of the physicians granted staff privileges. Since the *Darling* decision, the Joint Committee on Accreditation of Health Organizations (JCAHO) has increased pressure on hospitals to tailor staff privileges to the ability of the individual physician in order the raise the quality of care. There has also been increased emphasis by medical malpractice insurance carriers on the limitation of privileges in the hope of reducing exposure from high-risk specialties. These factors will undoubtedly result in closer scrutiny by hospitals of applications for new privileges and for renewal of privileges. Those applications that are granted will be more narrowly drawn than in the past to match the applicants' education, training, and experience. We can also expect to see a proliferation of "closed shop" specialty units in hospitals, such as hemodialysis and cardiac intensive care units.

The physician whose application for staff privileges has been denied or restricted is entitled to a fair hearing before a reasonably impartial tribunal of the hospital with adequate notice of the reasons for denial or restriction; a right to examine documentary evidence in the case; and a right to cross-examine adverse witnesses. Such a hearing provides the minimum procedural due process without which the denial or restriction of privileges would constitute an improper infringement of the physician's liberty or property interests under the 14th Amendment of the United States Constitution. The standard the hospital must meet when restricting or denying staff privileges is that there must be a rational basis for the action which is reasonably related to the hospital's operation. Hospital action that is unreasonable, arbitrary, or capricious is likely to be reversed on judicial review.

Physicians with staff privileges should be aware that hospitals must now comply with new rules that require reporting of negligent acts or omissions. In 1996, in an effort to establish a medical error analysis system, the Joint Committee on Accreditation of Health Organizations implemented its Sentinel Event Policy. See "JCAHO, Facts about the Sentinel Event Policy" (revised April 11, 2000) at http://www.jcaho.org. A sentinel event is defined as "an unexpected occurrence involving death or severe physical or psychological injury, or the risk thereof." The JCAHO Sentinel Event Policy expects a hospital to report all sentinel events by completing a form and delivering it to JCAHO.

FEES FOR MEDICAL WITNESSES

The single most common source of dispute between physicians and attorneys is the medical witness fee. This is due to the lack of understanding by doctors of the rights and duties of such witnesses and the willingness of the trial bar to take advantage of that ignorance. A treating physician is a percipient witness in any suit in which the patient's condition is at issue, and in that role the physician has the same duty to testify as if, for example, an automobile accident were witnessed by the physician. If subpoenaed, the physician must testify. That is the obligation of every citizen, and the standard witness fee (presently $40 per day and 25 cents per mile in federal courts) is all the physician is entitled to.

On the other hand, if a physician is hired by either side as a medical expert to analyze and render an opinion on treatment rendered to the patient by others, reasonable compensation is justified. A physician who is approached by an attorney seeking the services of a medical expert to testify or a medical consultant to evaluate the case and report to the attorney should reach agreement with the attorney *in advance and in writing* on hourly charges for medicolegal services. The hourly fee paid by the federal government for medical expert and consultant services in 2000 is between $400 and $500 per hour for consultation and between $2500 and $5000 per trial day for testimony. Remember that the AMA Code of Medical Ethics does not allow a physician to charge a fee contingent on the outcome of the trial.

Today, most local medical societies have panels of physicians available to the trial bar for the impartial review of medicolegal cases. If these panels find substandard care, they will furnish medical experts to testify in the case. The establishment of such panels should be supported by all physicians because the panels benefit patients deserving compensation, the public image of the medical profession, and the private conscience of the expert medical witness.

CORONER'S INVESTIGATION

The coroner or medical examiner is a county government officer acting under statutory authority to investigate certain classes of deaths. These classes generally include violent deaths such as homicide, suicide, and accidents. Also included are deaths for which no physician can certify the cause, either because no physician was in attendance, the physician was in attendance for less than 24 hours before death, or the physician is *unable* to state the cause of death. (*Note:* This means truly unable, not merely unwilling.) Often the coroner is charged with investigation of deaths in operating rooms, deaths where a patient has not fully recovered from an anesthetic, and deaths in which the patient is comatose throughout the period of the physician's attendance. When a death falls within one of these statutory classes, it must be reported promptly to the coroner. The coroner makes a brief inquiry, perhaps by telephone, and decides whether to take jurisdiction over the case. Thus, simply reporting the case to the coroner does not make it a "coroner's case." The coroner may decide not to take the case and may instruct the reporting physician to sign the death certificate. When a physician is instructed by the coroner to sign the certificate, the contact, the instruction, and the identity of the coroner's official must be immediately entered in the physician's or hospital's patient chart.

MALPRACTICE

The Institute of Medicine, a component of the National Academy of Sciences, published a report in November of 1999 in which it was concluded that between 44,000 and 98,000 deaths each year in the United States are directly attributable to medical errors. The report (Institute of Medicine: *To Err is Human: Building a Safer Health Care System,* edited by Linda T. Kohn et al, 1999) also estimates that one in every 30 patients admitted to United States hospitals is injured by medical errors. About 10% of these incidents are fatal. Most are caused by preventable systemic faults rather than carelessness. The report cites as the most common problems illegible prescription writing, the existence of drugs with similar names, poor communication during shared care, and the routine stocking of full-strength drugs in hospital pharmacies. Referring to the report, President Clinton ordered federal health agencies to reduce the number of medical errors by 50% in 5 years. Private insurers and other major purchasers of health care are also getting involved. Executives of the largest companies have organized the "Leapfrog Group," a program whereby health care entities will be urged to make the reduction of medical errors a top priority. Several states (New York, California, Colorado, Massachusetts, and Florida) have mandated hospital disclosure of serious mistakes and have worked with health care providers to identify and analyze the reasons for those errors.

An earlier study yet published on medical malpractice in the USA is the Report of the Secretary's Commission on Medical Malpractice (DHEW Publication No. [OS] 73-88, 1973). The commission found that the primary factor generating medical malpractice claims was injurious or adverse results of treatment. Factors such as poor physician-patient rapport, patient frustration with the handling of specific complaints concerning treatment and complications, unrealistic expectations about what can be achieved with treatment, and increased patient suit-consciousness are of only secondary importance. A rational prescription for curing the medical malpractice problem would be to reduce patient injury by instituting aggressive risk management programs (especially in the hospital setting), improving personal communication between health care providers and their patients, and adoption of arbitration provisions at the outset of the physician-patient relationship.

When the physician recognizes that the patient has been injured as a result of iatrogenic error, the best course is to tell the patient right away and in plain language exactly what happened. The explanation should stick to the facts and avoid opinions and conclusions of law (such as admissions of negligence). It is essential to document in writing that this discussion has occurred, because the statute of limitations in most jurisdictions is much shorter when the patient has knowledge of the treatment error than when the patient is left to discover that a mistake has been made.

NATIONAL PRACTITIONER DATA BANK REPORTING

The National Practitioner Data Bank (NPDB) was created by Congress in 1986 (42 USC 11131 et seq). The information collected by the NPDB was intended solely to improve the quality of health care. There are three different ways a physician is reportable to the NPDB. First, a health care facility (including an insurance company) that makes payment in settlement or partial settlement of a medical malpractice claim or in satisfaction of a judgment in a medical malpractice action must report the name of the physician for whose benefit the payment was made. The name of the hospital with which the physician is affiliated and a description of the negligent acts or omissions must also be described in the report. Second, each Board of Medical Examiners that revokes or suspends a physician's license or censures, reprimands, or places on probation a physician must report the name of the physician and a description of the acts or omissions resulting in the Board's actions. The reason for Board action is only reportable if it is related to the physician's professional competence or professional conduct. Finally, health care facilities are required to report any professional review action that adversely affects the clinical privileges of a physician for a period longer than 30 days. If a physician voluntarily surrenders privileges while under investigation by the health care facility for possible incompetence or improper professional conduct, the physician nevertheless must be reported. Additionally, the physician is not allowed to escape reporting by agreeing to surrender privileges in exchange for an agreement by the health care entity not to conduct an investigation. There are serious penalties for failure to report.

The health care facility must report the physician not only to the NPDB but also to the physician's state licensing board in the state where the claim arose as well as the state where the health care facility is located (if they are different).

It is the responsibility of a hospital to request information from the NPDB regarding the physician at the time of initial application for clinical privileges as well as once every 2 years during the time the physician continues as a member of the medical staff. Information may also be supplied to health care entities that have or may be entering into an employment or affiliation relationship with the physician. With these exceptions, the information is considered confidential and cannot be otherwise disclosed. Sanctions will be imposed for wrongful disclosure of the information.

REFERENCES

AMA/Medical Professional Liability Insurance; the Informed Physician's Guide to Coverage Decisions. American Medical Association, 1998.

FMS/Judgment Fund Group: All MedMal Cases for Fiscal Year 2000. Financial Management Service, United States Department of Treasury, 2000.

Horn C: Law for Physicians; an Overview of Medical Legal Issues. American Medical Association, 2000.

JCAHO, Facts about the Sentinel Event Policy. http://www.jcaho. org. (Revised April 11, 2000.)

Kessler DP, McClellan MB: How Liability Affects Medical Productivity. NBER Working Paper W7533, 2000.

Kohn LT et al: To Err Is Human: Building a Safer Health Care System. Institute of Medicine, 1999.

Lewis CJ: Medical Negligence: A Practical Guide. Lexis Law Publications, 1998.

Patterson RM: Harney's Medical Malpractice. Lexis Law Publications, 1999.

Pozgar GD: Legal Aspects of Health Care Administration. Aspen Publishers, 1999.

Rothenberg MA: Emergency Medicine Malpractice. Aspen Publishers, 1999.

Rubsamen DS: Diagnostic Errors in Primary Care: 84 Case Illustrations. Professional Liability Newsletter, 1999.

Scott RW: Health Care Malpractice: A Primer on Legal Issues for Professionals. McGraw-Hill, 1999.

Showalter JS: Southwick's the Law of Healthcare Administration. Health Administration Press, 1999.

Smith JT: Medical Malpractice: Psychiatric Care. Aspen Publishers, 2000.

Uribe CG: The Health Care Provider's Guide to Facing Malpractice Deposition. CRC Press, 2000.

Wound Healing

7

David D. Zabel, MD, Thomas K. Hunt, MD, Reid V. Mueller, MD, & William H. Goodson III, MD

Only a century ago, complicated and incomplete healing after injury was the rule rather than the exception. Surgeons had little choice but to accept draining wounds and invasive infections. The evolution of wound care and antisepsis in the 18th and 19th centuries changed surgery as dramatically as the discovery of anesthesia. Even so, poor healing, infection, and excessive scarring continue to be leading causes of disability and death.

Knowledge of the basic mechanisms of healing has grown rapidly. A detailed knowledge of these mechanisms allows surgeons to influence healing and anticipate and prevent problems of infection and incomplete or excessive repair.

FORMS OF HEALING

Surgeons customarily divide types of wound healing into first and second "intention." **First intention (primary) healing** occurs when tissue is cleanly incised and reapproximated and repair occurs without complication. **Second intention (secondary) healing** occurs in open wounds through formation of granulation tissue* and eventual coverage of the defect by spontaneous migration of epithelial cells. Most infected wounds and burns heal in this manner. Primary healing is simpler and requires less time and material than secondary healing. It sometimes happens that primary healing is possible but there is insufficient vascular or nutritional reserve to support secondary healing. For example, an ischemic limb may heal primarily, but if the wound opens and becomes secondarily infected, it may not heal. These two forms may be combined in **delayed primary closure,** when a wound is allowed to heal open for about 5 days and is then closed as if primarily. Such wounds are less likely to become infected than if closed immediately.

THE NATURE OF REPAIR

The major components of repair are shown in Figure 7–1. The lines in the diagram indicate signaling processes that include growth factors, complement, classic

---

*Granulation tissue is the red, granular, moist tissue that appears during healing of open wounds. Microscopically, it contains new collagen, new blood vessels, fibroblasts, and inflammatory cells, especially macrophages.

inflammatory mediators, and metabolic signals such as hypoxia and accumulated lactate. Often several signals are capable of controlling any given step, showing that many wound healing mechanisms are redundant. The following describes the complex process of wound healing as a stepwise process proceeding from coagulation and inflammation through fibroplasia, matrix deposition, angiogenesis, epithelialization, collagen maturation, and finally wound contraction.

THE INITIAL RESPONSE: COAGULATION & INFLAMMATION

Immediately after injury, the coagulation products fibrin, fibrinopeptides, fibrin split products, and complement components begin to attract inflammatory cells—particularly macrophages—into the wound. Platelets activated by thrombin release IGF-1, TGFα, TGFβ, and PDGF, which then attract leukocytes and fibroblasts into the wound. Damaged endothelial cells respond to a signal cascade involving complement product C5a, TNFα, IL-1, and IL-8 and express receptors for integrin molecules on the cell membranes of leukocytes. This allows circulating leukocytes to adhere to the endothelium and then migrate into the wounded tissue. Their interleukins and other inflammatory components, such as histamine, serotonin, and bradykinin, cause vessels first to constrict in aid of hemostasis, and later dilate, becoming so porous that blood plasma and leukocytes can move freely into the area.

The newly arrived inflammatory cells increase metabolic demand. Since the local microvasculature has been damaged, a local energy sink results, and PaO_2 falls while CO_2 and lactate accumulate. Lactate in particular plays a critical role. These conditions persist throughout repair, and—together with other stimulants such as fibrin, foreign bodies, bacteria, etc—they direct leukocytes, particularly macrophages, to release a variety of cytokines, chemoattractants, and growth factors. New information leads to a picture of wound healing as a reaction to severe metabolic stress.

These events trigger reparative processes and ensure their continuation, because macrophages, which secrete most of the growth-promoting products, assume the control of repair as the flood of coagulation-mediated growth substances begins to ebb. Furthermore,

6

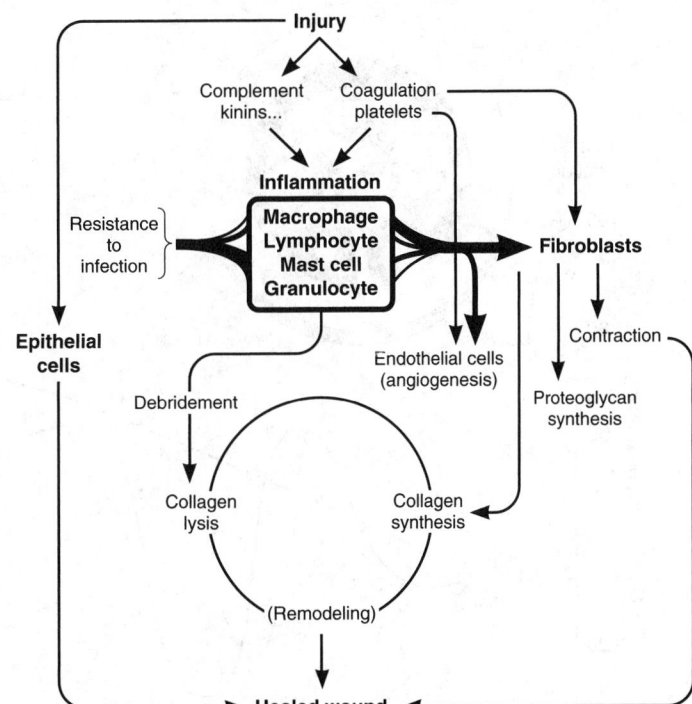

Figure 7–1. Schematic diagram of the sequence of events in wound healing. (Modified and reproduced, with permission, from Hunt TK, van Winkle W Jr: *Fundamentals of Wound Management.* Vol 1. Chirurgecom Press, 1976.)

macrophages, stimulated by fibrin, release large quantities of lactate. Though hypoxia may contribute, this process continues even in the presence of oxygen, thereby maintaining the environment of injury. The environment causes them to release growth promoters and more lactate, a surrogate of hypoxia, which in turn by itself stimulates angiogenesis and collagen deposition.

By the third or fourth day after injury, the reparative cells become loosely arranged in a characteristic spatial relationship as shown in Figure 7–2, a diagram of a wound made in a rabbit's ear and enclosed in a thin, optically clear chamber and allowed to heal for a week. In this constricting apparatus, wound cells must proceed in orderly single file—leaders first, followers next. Unless the wound has become infected, its granulocyte population, which dominated on the first day, has diminished. Macrophages now cover the cut surface. Immature fibroblasts, the product of growth signals, lie just beneath, mixed with buds of new vessels. More mature fibroblasts are scattered behind. The spatial relations of cells with respect to oxygen and lactate concentrations define zones of reparative activities.

These spatial relationships show how macrophages condition an acidic, hypoxic, high-lactate growth-promoting environment to construct a growth center. Farther back are mature fibroblasts synthesizing and depositing new collagen in an area still rich in lactate but better oxygenated as required for maximal collagen synthesis and deposition.

FIBROPLASIA & MATRIX DEPOSITION

Fibroplasia

During the course of healing, fibroplasia (replication of fibroblasts) is stimulated by multiple mechanisms, starting with PDGF, IGF-1, and TGFβ released by platelets and later by the continual release of numerous peptide growth factors from macrophages and fibroblasts within the wound. FGF, IGF-1, VEGF, IL-1, IL-2, IL-8, PDGF, TGFα, TGFβ, and TNFα all seem to be potential contributors from other sources.

Dividing fibroblasts are seen mainly near the wound edge, where they are exposed to the growth environment and to an oxygen tension of approximately 40 mm Hg in normally healing wounds. In cell culture, this PaO_2 is optimal for fibroblast replication.

Fibroblasts originate locally by replication. However, if there is such a thing as a fibrocyte, it is not recognized. Smooth muscle cells are likely progenitors because fibroblasts seem to stream from the adventitia and media of vessels. Lipocytes, pericytes, and others are also candidates. Perhaps all contribute.

Figure 7–2. Diagram of oxygen tension and lactate concentration in a cross-section of a rabbit ear chamber wound. Macrophages lead into the dead space. Fibroblasts and new blood vessels follow. In hypovolemia (as shown by the dashed line) the distal capillaries shut down and the fragile leading edge of the wound literally becomes anoxic.

Matrix Deposition

The newly replicated fibroblasts secrete the collagen and proteoglycans of the connective tissue matrix that weld wound edges together. Both assume high-molecular-weight polymeric forms and become the physical basis of wound strength. Collagen synthesis is not a constitutive property of fibroblasts but must be stimulated. The mechanisms that regulate the stimulation and synthesis of collagen are not clear, but they are probably multifactorial and include both growth factors and metabolic inputs. The collagen gene promoter has binding sites to corticoids, TGFβ, and retinoids, which presumably by this mechanism control collage gene expression, whereas other growth factors regulate glycosaminoglycan, tissue inhibitors of metalloproteinase (TIMP), and fibronectin synthesis. A more basic observation, however, is that mere accumulation of lactate in the extracellular environment directly stimulates transcription of collagen genes as well as posttranslational processing of collagen peptide. This mechanism, which is not pH-dependent, rests on the size of the intracellular pool of adenosine diphosphoribose (ADPR), a key regulatory substance which normally inhibits collagen mRNA synthesis and other vital steps that facilitate collagen export from fibroblasts.

ADPR results when the nicotinamide moiety is removed from NAD^+. Accumulation of lactate converts NAD^+ to NADH. As a consequence, less NAD^+ is available to be converted to ADPR. When ADPR in the nucleus is depleted for any reason—as it is when the NAD^+ pool is diminished—this inhibitory control is released, and more collagen mRNA is formed. The cause of decreased NAD^+ can be hypoxia, accumulation of lactate, excessive conversion of NAD^+ to ADPR, and probably others.

Evidence indicates that the increase in collagen mRNA leads to an increased procollagen peptide. This, however, is not sufficient to increase collagen deposition because procollagen peptide cannot be transported from the cell to the extracellular space until, in a posttranslational step, some of its prolines are hydroxylated. In this reaction, performed by the dioxygenase prolyl hydroxylase, an oxygen atom derived from dissolved O_2 is inserted into selected collagen prolines in the presence of ascorbic acid, iron, and α-ketoglutarate. The activity of this enzyme is normally suppressed by cytoplasmic ADPR. Thus, accumulation of lactate—or any other process that decreases the NAD^+ pool—leads to production of collagen mRNAs, increased collagen peptide synthesis, and (provided enough ascorbate and oxygen is present) increased posttranslational modification and secretion of collagen monomers into the extracellular space.

Another dioxygenase, lysyl hydroxylase, hydroxylates a number of the procollagen lysines and sets the stage for later lysyl to lysyl cross-binding between collagen molecules and fibers, thereby endowing them with considerable strength. It too requires adequate amounts of ascorbate and oxygen. These oxygenase reactions proceed only as fast as the local concentration of oxygen (PaO_2) will allow. The rates are half-maximal at about 20 mm Hg and maximal at about 200 mm Hg. They can be forced to supernormal rates by tissue hyperoxia. Clinically, elevating wound PaO_2 accelerates collagen deposition.

ANGIOGENESIS

Angiogenesis is a necessary feature of repair. It becomes visible about 4 days after injury but begins 2 or 3 days earlier when new capillaries sprout out of preexisting venules and grow toward the injury in response to chemoattractants released by platelets and macrophages. In primarily closed wounds, sprouting vessels soon meet counterparts migrating from the other side of the wound, and blood flow across the wound is established. In unclosed wounds or those not well closed, the new capillaries fuse only with neighbors migrating in the same direction, and granulation tissue is formed instead (Figure 7–3).

Wound angiogenesis is inducible in unwounded tissue by the addition of chemoattractants to endothelial cells. Examples found in wounds include PDGF (homodimer BB), FGF, TNFα, TGFβ, and VEGF.

Wound angiogenesis appears to be a response to local energy depletion, and its mechanism is remarkably similar in outline to the regulation of collagen deposition. In reducing conditions (hypoxia or increased lactate), macrophages secrete at least one peptide chemoattractant to endothelial cells that causes angiogenesis in a corneal assay. Maintenance of the NAD^+ pool severely inhibits the process. Thus, unmet metabolic needs lead through a growth factor mechanism, probably VEGF, to an anatomic response probably of general biologic significance.

Numerous growth factors and cytokines are said to stimulate angiogenesis, but animal experiments indicate that the dominant angiogenic stimulants in wounds are derived first from platelets in response to coagulation and then from macrophages in response to hypoxia or high lactate, fibrin, etc.

Figure 7–3. Photomicrograph of granulation tissue grown into a dead space surrounded by wire mesh. All the tissue is newly made. Note the rich vascular network, especially at the edge of the tissue in the upper left corner, where several open capillaries are leaking red cells into the wound.

EPITHELIALIZATION

Epithelial cells respond to many of the same stimuli as do fibroblasts and endothelial cells. A variety of growth factors regulate replication. TGFβ, for instance, tends to keep epithelial cells from differentiating and thus may potentiate and perpetuate mitogenesis, though it is not itself a mitogen for these cells. TGFα and keratinocyte growth factor (KGF) are epithelial cell mitogens.

In healing, mitoses appear in epithelium a few cells away from the wound edge. The new cells migrate over the cells at the edge and into the unhealed area, perhaps attracted by a growth factor or cytokine, and anchor on the first unepithelialized place, forming a new wound edge. The PaO_2 on the underside of the cell at the anchor point is likely to be low. Low PaO_2 stimulates squamous epithelial cells to produce TGFβ, presumably hindering terminal differentiation and favoring mitosis. This process repeats itself until the wound is closed.

Squamous epithelialization and differentiation proceed maximally when the local PaO_2 approaches about 700 mm Hg and when surface wounds are kept moist.

Contrary to classic thought, even short periods of drying can impair the process. Wounds should be kept moist. The exudate from acute, uninfected superficial wounds also contains growth factors and lactate and therefore recapitulates the growth environment found internally.

COLLAGEN FIBER MATURATION, LYSIS, & CONTRACTION

Replacement of an extracellular matrix is a complex process. First, fibroblasts replace the provisional fibrin extracellular matrix with collagen monomers. Extracellular enzymes, some of which are PaO_2-dependent, quickly polymerize these monomers but in a pattern that is much more random than normal, thus leaving young wounds weak and brittle. This brittleness is overcome when the hastily placed matrix is replaced with a more mature one consisting of larger, better organized, stronger, and more durable fibers (Figure 7–4).

Turnover and reorganization of new matrix is an important feature of healing, and fibroblasts and leukocytes secrete collagenases that ensure the lytic component. Turnover occurs rapidly at first and then more slowly. Even in simple wounds, increased turnover can be detected chemically for as long as 18 months. Healing is successful when a net excess of matrix is deposited despite concomitant lysis. Lysis, being destructive, is less dependent upon energy and nutrition. If synthesis is impaired, lysis weakens wounds. In some tissues (eg, colon), lysis unnecessarily weakens tissue structure, and inhibition of lysis with orally administrable agents leads

Figure 7–4. Schematic representation of collagen synthesis, deposition, and polymerization. The molecules polymerize with a "three-fourths stagger" overlap, which accounts for the cross banding visible on electron microscopy.

to quicker gain of tensile strength. This is one of many features of healing that has not yet been clinically exploited.

During rapid turnover, wounds gain strength and durability but also are vulnerable to contraction and stretching. Fibroblasts provide the motive force for contraction. Fibroblasts attach to collagen and each other and pull the collagen network together when the cell membranes shorten as the fibroblasts migrate. The fibers are then fixed in the packed positions by a variety of cross-linking mechanisms. Both open and closed wounds tend to contract if not subjected to a superior distorting force. The phenomenon is best seen in surface wounds, which in areas of loose skin may close 90% or more by contraction alone. For instance, the result of a large open wound on the back of the neck may be a very small area of epithelialization. On the back, the buttock, or the neck, this is often a beneficial process, whereas in the face and about joints, the results may be disabling or disfiguring. This undesirable result is usually termed a contracture or a stricture. Skin grafts, especially thick ones, impede but do not totally stop the process. Dynamic splints, passive or active stretching, or insertion of flaps containing dermis and subdermis may be needed to counteract contraction. The force can be quite strong, though even severely contracted joints can usually be straightened with countertraction. Prevention of a stricture in a ureteric repair, for example, depends on ensuring that the opposing tissue edges are well perfused so that healing can proceed quickly to completion and contraction can stop.

Healing wounds may also stretch during active turnover when tension overcomes contraction. This may account for the laxity of scars in ligaments of injured but unsplinted joints and the tendency for hernia formation in abdominal wounds of obese patients. If wounds are traumatized when passively stretched, contraction or weakness may continue for long periods and may become troublesome.

COMPLETION OF HEALING

Healing and growth of malignancies are strikingly similar processes. As opposed to their role in oncogenesis, however, growth factors in wound healing generally obey basic controls, and healing stops at an appropriate point. Normally, the final stimuli to release of growth factors and cytokines seem to be local hypoxia and lactic acidosis. When these stimuli disappear as the new microcirculation matures, healing should stop. However, the reason for cessation of healing is debated.

Keloids, local overgrowths of connective tissue, and hypertrophic scars, which occur particularly in pigmented skin, probably represent a loss of normal control over the healing process, but few facts are known. Hypertrophic scars are generally self-limited and may regress after a year or so. The last areas of a burn to heal are the ones most often hypertrophic, but traction and reinjury due to tension, and it may be that immune mechanisms also play a role. Prolonged inflammatory reactions are the mechanism that they all have in common.

ROLE OF TISSUE HYPOXIA

Healing is not a unique process. The injury environment recruits normal cellular mechanisms, which become self-reinforcing. Partly because of its redundancy, healing is almost foolproof. The few vulnerable spots are related to perfusion and oxygenation, nutrition, and aberrations of inflammation. However, the rate of repair is easily influenced, being most rapid in well-perfused tissues and almost static in ischemic tissue.

Impaired perfusion and oxygenation are the most frequent causes of healing failure. Oxygen is required for successful inflammation, angiogenesis, epithelialization, and matrix deposition. The critical oxygenases involved have Km values for oxygen of about 20 mm Hg and maximums of about 200 mm Hg, which means that their reaction rates are governed by PaO_2 and blood perfusion throughout the entire physiologic range. The

PaO_2 of wound fluid in human wounds is about 30–40 mm Hg, implying that these enzymes normally function just beyond half capacity. Furthermore, wound PaO_2 is depressed by blood volume deficiency, catecholamine infusion, or cold. On the other hand, under ideal conditions, wound fluid PaO_2 can be raised above 100 mm Hg by improved perfusion and breathing of oxygen. Collagen deposition in human wounds is proportionate to wound PaO_2. Human healing is profoundly influenced by local blood supply, vasoconstriction, and all other factors that govern perfusion and blood oxygenation.

Cardiopulmonary diseases affect wound healing, but vasoconstriction due to sympathetic nervous system activity is the principal source of clinical problems. Prevention or resolution of problems can be achieved by turning off sympathetic activity by correcting blood volume deficits, alleviating pain, and avoiding hypothermia. Wounds in highly vascularized tissues (eg, head, anus) heal rapidly and are remarkably resistant to infection.

IMPAIRED HEALING IN DISORDERS OF INFLAMMATION

The growth signals and lytic enzymes released by inflammatory cells are necessary for repair. Excessive and inadequate inflammatory responses can pose problems. Failure to heal is common in patients taking anti-inflammatory corticosteroids, immune suppressants, or cancer chemotherapeutic agents and whose inflammatory responses are blunted. Open wounds suffer more than primarily healing ones. The administration of these agents after inflammation has been established is less detrimental. Healing impaired by inadequate inflammation, especially that due to corticosteroids, can be accelerated by vitamin A systemically or locally. Experimentally, this appears to pertain to diabetics as well. In experiments, some of the growth factors have also had this effect. Both growth factors and vitamin A increase the number of inflammatory cells in the wound.

Inflammation may also be excessive. A mild excess may produce a hypertrophic scar. Prolonged inflammation due to infection or foreign bodies is a common cause of excess scarring. A major excess (eg, in response to endotoxin) can excite inflammatory cells to produce cytolytic amounts of cytokines and large amounts of proteinases with the consequence of lysis of newly formed tissue. In gram-negative wound infections or septic shock, granulation tissue may not develop or it may be lysed.

Massive injuries give rise to large inflammatory reactions, and cytokines from large but otherwise uncomplicated wounds can produce systemic symptoms. Extensive wounds can produce large amounts of lactate that must be reconverted to glucose in the liver—a process that contributes to the hypermetabolism of trauma.

Debridement of damaged tissue and early immobilization of fractures minimize the above effects. Stimulation of the reticuloendothelial system, major amounts of injured tissue, and failure to debride can produce the systemic inflammatory response syndrome (SIRS) even in the absence of infection.

EFFECT OF MALNUTRITION

Malnutrition impairs healing, since healing depends on cell replication, specific organ function (liver, heart, lungs), and matrix synthesis. Weight loss and protein depletion have been shown experimentally to be risk factors for poor healing. Still, healing may be normal in patients who have lost weight over a long period. Deficient healing is seen mainly in patients with acute malnutrition (ie, in the weeks just before or after an injury or operation). Even a few days of starvation measurably impairs healing, and an equally short period of repletion can reverse the deficit. Wound complications increase in severe malnutrition. A period of preoperative total parenteral nutrition is generally recommended for patients who have recently lost 10% or more of their body weight. This subject is covered in detail in Chapter 11.

HEALING OF SPECIALIZED TISSUES

Nerves

The brain heals largely through connective tissue scar formation in which glial and perivascular cells seem to differentiate into fibroblasts. When a peripheral nerve is severed, the distal nerve degenerates, leaving the axon sheaths to heal together by inosculation. The axon then regenerates from the nerve cell through the rejoined sheaths, advancing as much as 1 mm/d. Unfortunately, because individual neural sheaths have no means of seeking out their original distal ends, the axon sheaths reconnect randomly, and motor nerve axons may regenerate in vain into a sensory distal sheath and end organ. The functional result of neural regeneration, therefore, is more satisfactory in the purer peripheral nerves and in nerves rejoined by microscopic surgical techniques. Recent advances in growth factor technology and the ischemic, hypoxic nature of wounds suggests that means may be devised to improve nerve regeneration. This is currently one of the forefronts of surgical research.

Intestine

The rate of repair varies from one part of the intestine to the other in proportion to vascularity. Anastomoses of the colon and esophagus are precarious and likely to leak, whereas leakage of stomach or small intestine anastomoses is rare. Intestinal anastomoses usually regain strength rapidly. By 1 week they resist bursting more strongly than the more normal surrounding tissue. However, the surrounding intestine participates in the reaction to injury, loses a large portion of its collagen by lysis, and consequently loses strength. For this reason, leakage is about as likely to occur a few millimeters from the anastomosis as it is in the anastomosis itself, especially at the site of excessively tight sutures or staples. Drugs such as fluorouracil limit lysis and in experimental conditions appear to prevent the early loss of strength in colonic wounds.

Any event that delays collagen synthesis or exaggerates collagen lysis is likely to increase the risk of perforation and leakage (Figure 7–5). The danger of leakage is greatest from the fourth to seventh days, when tensile strength normally would rise rapidly but is prevented from doing so by increased lysis or compromised collagen deposition. Local infection, which often occurs near esophageal and colonic anastomoses, promotes lysis and delays synthesis, thus increasing the likelihood of perforation.

Though the surgeon aims for primary healing in anastomoses, much of the healing actually occurs by second intention in both sutured and stapled anastomoses. Fine surgical technique is more likely to promote primary repair.

Adhesions are assumed to be an almost inevitable consequence of abdominal surgery. While they are common, they are not inevitable. The most powerful stimuli are ischemic tissues (which attract a new blood supply that takes the form of vascularized adhesions), abscesses, and foreign bodies. All attract nests of macrophages which are activated to generate a fibrotic process.

Simple peritoneal defects are insufficient to cause adhesions, but when trauma, large defects, infection, is-

Figure 7–5. Tensile strength is the resultant between the strength of old collagen as affected by lysis and new collagen as affected by synthesis and lysis.

chemia, or foreign bodies are added, the process becomes more intense. Trauma and inflammation excite plasma leaks and deposition of fibrin. If allowed to remain, the fibrin increases the volume of ischemic tissue. Peritoneum normally produces plasminogen activator, which quickly leads to fibrin lysis. Exogenous plasminogen activator has decreased the occurrence of adhesions in experimental circumstances, but side effects discourage its clinical use.

Attempts to prevent adhesions by suturing peritoneal defects usually worsen the problem by causing local ischemia and suture granulomas. Starch powder used in most surgical gloves as a lubricant was a great improvement over talc, but severe peritoneal (as well as pericardial, pleural, and meningeal) inflammatory reactions due to starch and leading to adhesions have been well documented. Evidence indicates that lymphocytes participate in healing more so in intestinal wounds than in wounds of other tissues. Immunologic contribution is proportionately greater.

Bone

Bone healing is controlled by many of the same mechanisms that control soft tissue healing. It too occurs in three morphologic stages: an inflammatory stage, a reparative stage, and a remodeling stage. The duration of each stage varies depending on the location and nature of the fracture.

Injury (fracture) leads to hematoma formation from the damaged blood vessels of the periosteum, endosteum, and surrounding tissues. Within hours, an inflammatory infiltrate of neutrophils and macrophages is recruited into the hematoma as in soft tissue injuries. Monocytes and granulocytes debride and digest necrotic tissue and debris, including bone, on the fracture surface. This process continues for days to weeks depending on the amount of necrotic tissue.

During the reparative stage, the hematoma is gradually replaced by specialized granulation tissue that has the power to form bone. This tissue, known as **callus,** develops from both sides of the fracture and is composed of fibroblasts, endothelial cells, and bone-forming cells (chondroblasts, osteoblasts). The extent to which callus forms from the medulla, the periosteum, or cortical bone depends upon the site of fracture, the degree of immobilization, and the type of bone injured. As macrophages phagocytose the hematoma and injured tissue, fibroblasts deposit a collagenous matrix, and chondroblasts deposit proteoglycans in a process called enchondral bone formation. This step, prominent in some bones, is then converted to bone as osteoblasts condense hydroxyapatite crystals on specific points on the collagen fibers, and endothelial cells form a vasculature characteristic of bone with an end result

analogous to reinforced concrete. Eventually the fibrovascular callus is completely replaced by new bone. Unlike healing of soft tissue, bone healing has features of regeneration, and bone often heals without leaving a scar.

Bone healing also depends on blood supply. The ends of fractured bone are avascular. Osteocyte and vessel lacunae become vacant for several millimeters from the fracture. New blood vessels must sprout from preexisting ones and migrate into the area of injury. When new blood vessels cross the bone ends, they are preceded by osteoclasts just as macrophages precede them in soft tissue repair. In bone, this unit is called the cutting cone because it literally bores its way through bone in the process of connecting with other vessels. Excessive movement of the bone ends during this revascularization stage will break the delicate new vessels and delay healing. Osteomyelitis originates most often in ischemic bone fragments. Hyperoxygenation hastens fracture healing and aids in the cure (and potentially the prevention) of osteomyelitis. Acute or chronic hypoxia slows bone repair.

Once the fracture has been bridged, the new bone remodels in response to the mechanical stresses upon it, with restoration to normal or near-normal strength. During this process, as in soft tissue, bone and its vascular network are simultaneously removed and replaced. Increased bone turnover may be detected as long as 6–9 years after injury. Although remodeling is efficient, it cannot correct deformities of angulation or rotation in misaligned fractures. Careful fracture reduction is still necessary.

Fibroblasts, chondroblasts, and osteoblasts in healing fractures are derived from surrounding primitive mesenchyme. The origin of the mesenchyme is less clear. It seems to arise from muscle, fascia, periosteum, endothelium, marrow, even from circulating cells, as well as directly from fibrous tissue. The differentiation of these mesenchymal cells into bone-forming cells appears to be governed by specific growth factors such as bone morphogenetic protein (BMP), TGFβ, IGF-1, GM-CSF, and PDGF, all of which stimulate proliferation and induce the differentiation of osteoblasts in cell culture. BMP (which belongs to the TGFβ supergene family) appears to be the most specific for bone and is found in large quantity in bone matrix. BMP induces ectopic bone formation in the absence of preexisting bone and induces cartilage formation in vivo.

Bone repair may occur through primary or secondary intention. Primary repair can occur only when the fracture is stable and aligned and its surfaces closely apposed. This situation is rarely present in normal bone healing but is the goal of rigid plate fixation. When these conditions are met, capillaries can grow across the fracture and rapidly reestablish a vascular supply. Little or no callus forms. Secondary repair with abundant callus is more common.

Bone repair can be manipulated. Electrical stimulation, growth factors, and distraction osteogenesis are three promising new tools for this purpose. Electrical currents applied directly (through implanted electrodes) or induced by external alternating electromagnetic fields accelerate repair by inducing new bone formation in much the same way as small piezoelectric currents produced by mechanical deformation of intact bone controls remodeling along lines of stress. The technique of electrical stimulation has been used successfully to treat nonunion of bone (where new bone formation between bone ends fails, often requiring long periods of bed rest). BMP-impregnated implants have accelerated bone healing in animals and have been used with encouraging results to treat large bony defects and nonunions.

The **Ilizarov technique** of linear distraction osteogenesis can lengthen bones, stimulate bone growth across a defect, or correct defects of angulation. The Ilizarov device is an external fixator attached to the bones through metal pins or wires. A surgical break is created and then slowly pulled apart (1 mm/d) or reangulated. The vascular supply and subsequent new bone formation migrate along with the moving segment of bone.

SUTURES

The ideal suture material would be flexible, strong, easily tied, and securely knotted. It would excite little tissue reaction and would not serve as a nidus for infection.

Stainless steel wire is inert and maintains strength for a long time. It is difficult to tie and may have to be removed late postoperatively because of pain. It does not harbor bacteria, and it can be left in granulating wounds, when necessary, and will be covered by granulation tissue without causing abscesses.

Silk is an animal protein but is relatively inert in human tissue. It is commonly used because of its favorable handling characteristics. It loses strength over long periods and is unsuitable for suturing arteries to plastic grafts or for insertion of prosthetic cardiac valves. Silk sutures are multifilament and provide a potential haven for bacteria. Occasionally, silk sutures form a focus for small abscesses that migrate and "spit" through the skin, forming small sinuses that will not heal until the suture is removed.

Catgut (made from the submucosa of bovine intestine) will eventually resorb, but the resorption time is highly variable. It excites considerable inflammatory reaction and tends to potentiate infections. Catgut also loses strength rapidly and unpredictably in the intestine and in infected wounds as a consequence of acid and enzyme hydrolysis. There is little need for catgut suture in modern surgery, though a considerable amount is still used.

Synthetic nonabsorbable sutures are generally inert and retain strength (do not fracture) longer than wire. However, their handling characteristics are not as good as those of silk, and they must usually be knotted at least four times, resulting in large amounts of retained foreign body. Multifilament plastic sutures are just as apt to become infected and migrate to the surface as silk sutures. Monofilament plastic, like wire, will not harbor bacteria. Nylon monofilament is extremely nonreactive, but it is difficult to tie. Monofilament polypropylene is intermediate in these properties. Plastic sutures are required for cardiovascular work because they are not absorbed. Vascular anastomoses to prosthetic vascular grafts rely indefinitely on the strength of sutures; therefore, use of absorbable sutures may lead to aneurysm formation. Even monofilament sutures will "spit." However, this disadvantage is generally confined to sizes of 00 and larger.

Synthetic absorbable sutures are strong, have predictable rates of loss of tensile strength, incite a minimal inflammatory reaction, and may have special usefulness in gastrointestinal, urologic, and gynecologic surgery. Compared with catgut, polyglycolic acid and polyglactin retain tensile strength longer in gastrointestinal anastomoses. Polydioxanone sulfate, polyglycolate, and poliglecaprone 25 sutures are monofilament and lose about half their strength in 50 days, thus solving the problem of premature breakage in fascial closures. Poliglecaprone 25 is a newer monofilament synthetic suture with faster reabsorption, retaining 50% tensile strength at 7 days, and 0% at 21 days. This suture is suitable for soft tissue approximation but is not intended for fascial closure.

Tapes are the skin closure of choice for clean or contaminated wounds. They minimize the probability of infection by not introducing a foreign body in the form of a skin suture that connects the skin surface to the wound dead space. They cannot be used on actively bleeding wounds or wounds with complex surfaces, such as those in the perineum.

Staples, whether for internal use or skin closure, are mainly steel-tantalum alloys that incite a minimal tissue reaction. The technique of staple placement is different from sutures, but the same basic rules pertain. There are no real differences in the healing that follows suture or stapled closures. Stapling devices tend to minimize errors in technique, but at the same time they do not offer a feel for tissue and have limited ability to accommodate to exceptional circumstances.

Staples are preferable to sutures for skin closure, since they do not provide a conduit for contaminating organisms. Staples are not preferable to skin tapes.

IMPLANTABLE MATERIALS

Although prosthetic materials are constantly being improved, none are ideal in regard to tissue compatibility, permanent fixation, and resistance to infection. Two principles are paramount: biocompatibility and a fabric that is incorporated into tissue. Biocompatibility is the foremost consideration. Both specific and nonspecific immune mechanisms are involved in the inflammatory reaction to foreign materials. Highly incompatible materials, such as wood splinters, are rejected immediately with an acute inflammatory process that includes massive local release of proteolytic enzymes. Consequently, the foreign body is never incorporated and lies loosely in a fibrous pocket. Mechanical irritation may induce a similar reaction, which accounts for the occasional spontaneous rejection of large (usually larger than 00), stiff suture materials from soft tissue sites. In less severe incompatibility, rejection is not so vigorous and proteolysis not so prominent. Mononuclear cells and lymphocytes—the major components of wound inflammatory tissue—direct a response that creates a fibrous capsule which may be acceptable in a joint replacement but which may distort a breast reconstruction severely.

Most implants must become anchored to adjacent normal tissues by allowing ingrowth of fibrous tissue or bone. This requires biocompatibility and interstices large enough to incite ingrowth just as in a wound and to allow pedicles of vascularized tissue to enter and join similar units.

In bone this imparts stability. In vascular grafts, the invading tissue supports neointima formation, which retards mural thrombosis and distal embolization. Soft tissue will grow into pores larger than about 50 μm in diameter and even faster into larger ones. Of the vascular prostheses, woven Dacron is best for tissue incorporation. In bone, sintered, porous metallic surfaces are best. Large-screen polypropylene mesh can be used to support the abdominal wall or chest even in the presence of infection and is usually well incorporated into the granulation tissue that penetrates the mesh. Microporous polytetrafluoroethylene (Teflon) sheets are often not well incorporated and are not suitable for use in infected tissues.

Unfortunately, when the mechanical properties of the implant do not match those of the host tissue, shear forces may overcome delicate biologic unions, with loosening of anchoring sites, especially with orthopedic prostheses.

The implantation space remains vulnerable to infection for years and is a particular problem in implants that cross the body surface. Mesh cuffs around vascular access devices that incite incorporation have successfully forestalled infection for months, but infections that arise from bacteria entering the body along "permanently" implanted foreign bodies which traverse the skin surface remain an unsolved problem.

Plastic implants are often chosen for texture and flexibility. Silastic materials are highly compatible, but fixation and material fatigue are problems. Cosmetic implants—particularly silicone breast implants—have a low but troublesome incidence of deforming fibrotic capsule formation. In addition to idiosyncratic healing responses, there is also the problem of toxic responses to trace components such as plasticizers and hardeners. Potential complications include cancers if materials such as asbestos are present even in small amounts. The case for systemic complications from Silastic implants has not been proved.

DECUBITUS & OTHER CHRONIC ULCERS

Decubitus Ulcers

Decubitus ulcers are disastrous complications of immobilization. They result from prolonged pressure that robs tissue of its blood supply. Irritative or contaminated injections and prolonged contact with moisture, urine, and feces also play a prominent role. Most patients who develop decubitus ulcers are also poorly nourished. Pressure ulcers are common in paraplegics, immobile elderly patients, and drug addicts who take overdoses and lie immobile for hours. The ulcers vary in depth and often extend from skin to a bony pressure point such as the greater trochanter or the sacrum.

Most decubitus ulcers are preventable. Hospital-acquired ulcers are nearly always the result of inadequate nursing care or inappropriate positioning on operating tables.

Treatment is difficult and usually prolonged. The first important step is to incise and drain any infected spaces or necrotic tissue. Dead tissue is then debrided until the exposed surfaces are viable and granulating. Many will then heal spontaneously. However, deep ulcers may require surgical closure, sometimes with removal of underlying bone. The defect may require closure by judicious movement of thick, well-vascularized tissue into the affected area. Musculocutaneous flaps are the treatment of choice when chronic infection and significant tissue loss are combined. However, recurrence is common because the flaps are usually insensate.

Chronic Wounds

Chronically unhealed wounds, especially on the lower extremity, are common in the setting of vascular, immunologic, and neurologic disease. Venous ulcers, largely of the medial lower leg, reflect poor perfusion and perivascular leakage of plasma into tissue. This is the result of venous hypertension produced by incompetent venous valves. Most venous ulcers will heal if the venous congestion and edema are relieved by bed rest, compression stockings, or surgical procedures that eliminate incompetent feeding vessels.

Arterial or ischemic ulcers, which tend to occur on the lateral ankle or foot, are best treated by revascularization. Hyperbaric oxygen, which provides a temporary source of oxygen and enhances angiogenesis, is an effective though expensive alternative when revascularization is not possible. Useful information can be obtained by transcutaneous oximetry. Tissues with a low PaO_2 will not heal spontaneously. However, if oxygen tension can be raised into a relatively normal range by oxygen administration even intermittently, the lesion will probably respond to oxygen therapy. Sensory loss, especially of the feet, leads to ulceration and bony deformities due to fractures, the so-called Charcot deformity. Ulcers in patients with diabetes mellitus may have two causes. Patients with neuropathic ulcers usually have good circulation, and their lesions will heal if protected from weight trauma by bed rest, special shoes, or splints. Recurrences are common, however. Diabetics with ischemic disease, whether they have neuropathy or not, are at risk for gangrene, and they frequently require amputation if revascularization is not possible. Insulin dressings have been advocated. More recently, intermittent warming has been helpful.

In pyoderma gangrenosum, granulomatous inflammation with or without arteritis kills skin and subcutaneous skin, possibly by a mechanism involving excess cytokine release. These ulcers are associated with inflammatory bowel disease and certain types of arthritis and chondritis. Corticosteroids or other anti-inflammatory drugs are helpful. Anti-inflammatory corticosteroids can also contribute to poor healing by inhibiting cytokine release. Topical or systemic vitamin A restores the inflammatory mechanism and may induce healing of the lesions. Distinguishing between these possibilities in patients with inflammatory bowel disease may be difficult.

Infection may contribute to the lack of healing of chronic ulcers or may be a complication. Antibiotics should be part of initial therapy in most cases. They are not effective as continuous therapy in chronic wounds, however.

The first principle in managing chronic wounds is to diagnose and treat any underlying circulatory disease. The second principle is never to allow open wounds to dry (ie, use moist dressings). Moist dressings may also relieve pain. A third principle is to control any infection with systemic antibiotics. Topical barriers to infection are useful but not always necessary. A fourth principle is to recognize that chronically scarred tissue is usually poorly perfused. Debridement of unhealthy tissue, often followed by skin grafting, may be required

for healing. A fifth principle is to disarm autonomic vasoconstriction by means of warmth, moisture, pain relief, vasodilating or air flow-promoting medications.

A number of growth factors have been shown to accelerate healing of acute wounds in animals. They include FGFs, TGFβ, IGF-1, PDGF, and EGF, and the list is growing. However, in the setting of chronic human wounds, with the perfusion problems noted above, "proof" of efficacy has been difficult to develop, and no clear-cut advantage to any formulation has yet been convincingly demonstrated. The one exception is the recent randomized, prospective, double-blind, placebo-controlled, multicenter trial by the Diabetic Ulcer Study Group, which demonstrated that daily topical application of recombinant human PDGF-BB homodimer moderately accelerates healing and resulted in more wounds that healed completely.

SURGICAL TECHNIQUE

The most important means of achieving optimal healing after operation is good surgical technique. Many cases of healing failure are due to technical errors. Tissue should be protected from drying and internal or external contamination. The surgeon should use fine instruments; should perform clean, sharp dissection; and should make minimal, skillful use of electrocautery, ligatures, and sutures. All these precautions contribute to the most important goal of surgical technique—gentle handling of tissue. Even the best ligature or suture is a foreign body that may strangulate tissue if tied tightly. The skillful operator who uses sutures minimally and gently will be rewarded with the best results. Good hemostasis is a laudable objective, but excessive sponging, electrocautery, and tying of small vessels are traumatic and invite infection.

Wound Closure

As with many surgical techniques, the exact method of wound closure may be less important than how well it is performed. The tearing strength of sutures from fascia is no greater than 3–4 kg. There is little reason for use of sutures of greater strength than this. Excessively tight closure strangulates tissue and leads to hernia formation and infection.

If surgeons could foresee the future, dehiscence (undesired spontaneous separation of wound edges) would not occur, since techniques to prevent it are well known. The surgeon can choose the techniques to meet the needs and risks of the individual wound (Figures 7–6 and 7–7). The most common technical causes of dehiscence are infection and excessively tight sutures.

The ideal closure for small wounds in healthy patients is with fine interrupted sutures placed loosely and

Figure 7–7. Skin closure with interrupted subdermal sutures and Steri-Strips.

Figure 7–6. Closure of peritoneum with continuous sutures. Fascia closure with figure-of-eight sutures (top) and simple interrupted sutures (bottom) is illustrated. "Running" closures are also useful, and the suture "bites" should be similar to those illustrated, 1 and 1.5 cm apart and 1–1.5 cm apart.

conveniently close to the wound edge. In abdominal wounds, the peritoneum need not be sutured, but posterior and anterior fasciae are sutured with nonabsorbable or slowly absorbable sutures.

Unfortunately, surgeons often must operate on patients who have impaired wound healing. In these cases, closures must be stronger. A more secure closure begins with a running or mattress absorbable suture in the posterior sheath, joint capsule, or submucosa. The closure is continued with simple buried retention sutures through the fascia in which the farthest point of penetration is at least 1 cm from the wound edge. When the tension is placed this far back, the fascial fibers that become weakened by postinjury collagen lysis are not expected to provide critical support. The lytic effect extends for about 5 mm to each side of the wound edge. The skin is preferably closed with adhesive strips unless bleeding from the wound or an uneven surface makes adherence of the strips precarious, in which case staples are the next choice. With this fascial closure, the skin can easily be left open for delayed

primary or secondary closure. Subcutaneous tissues rarely need to be sutured closed.

In all closures, sutures should be placed as far apart as possible consistent with approximation of tissue. Sutures placed too tightly and too close together obstruct blood supply to the wound. In most cases of dehiscence, suture material cuts through tissue and is not broken or untied.

It is useful to assess wound risk in advance, so that the proper choice of closure can be made easily (Table 7–1).

Delayed primary closure is a technique by which the subcutaneous portion of the wound is left open for 4–5 days and then closed with skin tapes. The environs of the wound are inspected daily to be sure that invasive infection is absent. It is left in place until the fourth or fifth day, when, under sterile conditions, the wound is closed, usually with skin tapes. During the delay period, angiogenesis and healing start, and bacteria are cleared from the wound. The success of this method depends on the ability of the surgeon to detect minor signs of infection. Merely leaving the wound open for 4 days does not guarantee that it will not become infected, and some wounds (eg, fibrin-covered or inflamed wounds) should not be closed but should be left open for secondary closure.

POSTOPERATIVE CARE

The appearance of delayed wound infection—weeks to years after operation—emphasizes that all wounds are contaminated and that the line between apparent infec-

Table 7–1. Controllable factors affecting healing.

Factors that decrease collagen synthesis
  Smoking
  Starvation (protein depletion)
  Corticosteroids
  Infection[1]
  Hypoxemia and hypovolemia
  Radiation injury
  Trauma, including the operation itself
  Uremia
  Diabetes mellitus
  Drugs: dactinomycin, fluorouracil, methotrexate, others
  Advanced age
Operative factors
  Tissue injury
  Poor blood supply
  Poor apposition of surrounding tissues (pelvic anastomosis, unreduced fracture, unclosed dead space)
Factors that increase collagen synthesis
  Starvation
  Severe trauma
  Inflammation
  Infection
  Steroids

---

[1]Some infections may in time cause excess collagen deposition.

tion and apparent normal repair is a fine one. A minor setback such as a period of cardiac failure or of malnutrition will often allow infection to become established. Most frequently, however, poor tissue perfusion and oxygenation of the wound during the postoperative period weaken host resistance. Regulation of perfusion is due—more than anything—to sympathetic nervous activity. The instigators are cold, pain, hypovolemia, fear, and cigarette smoking. Recent tests show that special efforts to remove or limit these factors reduce the wound infection rate by more than half. Maintenance of normothermia and blood volume is particularly important. Appropriate assurance that peripheral perfusion is adequate is best obtained from peripheral tissues rather than urine output, central venous pressure, or wedge pressure—none of which correlate with wound tissue oxygenation. What does correlate with tissue oxygenation is capillary refill time on the forehead or patella, which should be less than 2 seconds and 5 seconds, respectively; or true thirst and eye globe turgor (which should match the observer's). Collagen deposition is increased also by the addition of oxygen breathing (nasal prongs or light mask) but only in well-perfused patients. Unfortunately, there are as yet no convenient clinical means of measuring wound PaO_2.

Postoperative care of the wound also involves cleanliness, protection from trauma, and maximal support of the patient. Even closed wounds can be infected by surface contamination of bacteria, particularly within the first 2–3 days. Bacteria gain entrance most easily through suture tracts. If a wound is likely to be traumatized or contaminated, it should be protected during this time. Such protection may require special dressings such as occlusive sprays or repeated cleansings as well as dressings.

Some mechanical stress enhances healing. Even fracture callus formation is greater if slight motion is allowed. Patients should move and stress their wounds a little. Early ambulation and return to normal activity are, in general, good for repair.

The ideal care of the wound begins in the preoperative period and ends only months later. The patient must be prepared so that optimal conditions exist when the wound is made. Surgical technique must be clean, gentle, skillful, and ingenious. Postoperatively, wound care includes maintenance of nutrition, blood volume, and oxygenation. Although wound healing is in many ways a local phenomenon, ideal care of the wound is essentially ideal care of the patient.

REFERENCES

Allen DB et al: Wound hypoxia and acidosis limit neutrophil bacterial killing mechanisms. Arch Surg 1997;132:991.

Cho M et al: Hydrogen peroxide stimulates macrophage vascular endothelial growth factor release. Am J Physiol Heart Circ Physiol 2001;280:H2357.

Constant JS et al: Lactate elicits vascular endothelial growth factor from macrophages: a possible alternative to hypoxia. Wound Repair Regen 2000;8:353.

Demling RH et al: Micronutrients in critical illness. Crit Care Clin 1995;11:651.

Feng JJ et al: Angiogenesis in wound healing. J Surg Pathol 1998;3:1.

Gailit J et al: TGF-beta 1 stimulates expression of keratinocyte integrins during re-epithelialization of cutaneous wounds. J Invest Dermatol 1994;103:221.

Gibson JJ et al: Increased oxygen tension and wound fluid vascular endothelial growth factor levels. Surg Forum 1998;89:607.

Greif R et al: Supplemental perioperative oxygen to reduce the incidence of surgical wound infection. N Engl J Med 2000; 342:161.

Hammarlund C et al: Hyperbaric oxygen reduced size of chronic leg ulcers: a randomized double-blind study. Plast Reconstr Surg 1994;93:829.

Hartmann M et al: Effect of tissue perfusion and oxygenation on accumulation of collagen in healing wounds. Randomized study in patients after major abdominal operations. Eur J Surg 1992;158:521.

Hopf H et al: Subcutaneous perfusion and oxygen during acute severe isovolemic hemodilution in healthy volunteers. Arch Surg 2000;135:1443.

Hopf HW et al: Wound tissue oxygen tension predicts the risk of wound infection in surgical patients. Arch Surg 1997;132: 997.

Hunt TK et al: Postoperative adhesive disease. Perspect Colon Rectal Surg 1998;11:83.

Hunt TK et al: Wound healing and wound infection: what surgeons and anesthesiologists can do. Surg Clin North Am 1997;77:587.

Israelsson LA et al: Closure of midline laparotomy incisions with polydioxanone and nylon: the importance of suture technique. Br J Surg 1994;81:1606.

Schaffer M et al: Neuropeptides. Mediators of inflammation and tissue repair? Arch Surg 1998;133:1107.

Sheikh AY et al: Effect of hyperoxia on vascular endothelial growth factor in a wound model. Arch Surg 2000;135:1293.

Steed DL: Clinical evaluation of recombinant human platelet-derived growth factor for the treatment of lower extremity diabetic ulcers. Diabetic Ulcer Study Group. J Vasc Surg 1995; 21:71.

Unemori EN et al: Relaxin induces vascular endothelial growth factor expression and angiogenesis selectively at wound sites. Wound Repair Regen 2000;8:361.

Wicke C et al: Effects of steroids and retinoids on wound healing. Arch Surg 2000;135:1256.

The Metabolic & Neuroendocrine Responses to Trauma & Operations

8

Arthur E. Baue, MD

The metabolic and neuroendocrine responses to injury are important parts of the stress reaction in that they improve the individual organism's chances of surviving under adverse circumstances or when injured. Over two centuries ago, John Hunter described the reactions to injury as inducing "both the disposition and the means of cure." He suggested that injury initiates a sequence of responses that is both the result of the injury and the means by which the organism survives and heals. He continues: "Inflammation in itself is not to be considered as a disease . . . and in disease where it can alter the diseased mode of action it likewise leads to a cure; but where it cannot accomplish that salutary purpose, . . . it does mischief." The results of this complex but coordinated sequence of responses to injury are maintenance of blood flow, oxygen delivery, and organ perfusion, with mobilization and use of substrates for healing and recovery. By understanding these events and their clinical manifestations and by observing how the patient responds, surgeons are better equipped to care for their patients.

An injury and a major operation represent similar pathophysiologic threats to the victim or patient. Thus, the term "injury" as used here will be considered synonymous with a traumatic event such as a motor vehicle accident or a planned elective therapeutic but still traumatic event in the operating room. The extent of injuries, the number of organs involved, the suddenness of the event, whether or not a body cavity has been entered or damaged, and the unplanned experience of trauma will differ in each case, but the biologic responses to injury or surgery are similar. The magnitude of the response will vary according to the severity of the injury. A clean elective operation produces a level of stress beyond that associated with the fasting, resting state. Stress produced by a multisystem injury, however, is much more severe. The nervous, endocrine, and immune systems interact to adapt to tissue injury, infection, and inflammation. The metabolic response to injury is dynamic.

The mammalian acute phase response (acute phase reactants) to inflammation (infection or physical trauma) is characterized by fever and by changes in vascular permeability along with changes also in the biosynthetic, metabolic, and catabolic profiles of many organs. Thus, there seems to be an organized, sequential, describable, and understandable system of biologic responses to moderate injury—such as nonfatal trauma or a major operation followed by healing. However, patients may now survive injuries or operations that formerly would have been fatal, or they may survive for days to weeks only to die of multiple organ failure and infection. With severe or overwhelming injury, there is a biologic disintegration with excessive mediators of inflammation and remote organ damage (dyshomeostasis). The system then seems disorderly or out of control (Table 8–1).

Baue AE: Injury, inflammation, sepsis—is there a natural organized and sequential progression of neuroendocrine, metabolic and cytokine mediator events leading to organ system failure? In: *Sepsis and Organ Dysfunction.* Baue AE et al (editors). Springer, 1999.

Reichlin S: Neuroendocrine-immune interactions. N Engl J Med 1993;329:1246.

■ THE PHASES OF INJURY

Four phases in the response to injury were described originally by Francis Moore (Table 8–2). The first phase begins at the time of injury or, for an elective operation, during preparation, when the patient stops oral intake, becomes anxious about the experience, and receives preoperative medication. The injury phase normally lasts 2–5 days depending on the magnitude or "dose" of injury and the presence or absence of complications. In normal convalescence, the second phase—the "turning point"—is a transient period marked physiologically by a turning off of the neuroendocrine response and clinically by the appearance of getting well. The third phase is marked by gain in muscular strength, or positive nitrogen balance; and the fourth phase by gain in weight and body fat, or positive caloric balance. These patterns seem to be specific to trauma and are not observed in medical patients with sepsis.

Table 8–1. Metabolic responses to injury.

Extent of Injury	Neuroendocrine, Metabolic, Cytokine, and Immune Responses
Minimal surgery: Laparoscopy, thoracoscopy, inguinal hernia repair, no large incision into body cavity	Minimal and appropriate. Minor changes in the homeostatic thermostat.
Major surgery and non-life-threatening injury: Large incision into a body cavity or multisystem injury	Major changes that seem to be interrelated and coordinated. Homeostasis as we understand it seems evident.
Life-threatening injuries, operations, or illnesses	Biologic chaos—dyshomeostasis. The individual is overwhelmed by the multiplicity of changes that should be protective but become self-destructive.

INJURY PHASE (PHASE 1): THE STIMULI RESULTING FROM INJURY

A number of stimuli trigger the biologic response to injury, tending to reset the homeostatic thermostat at a higher metabolic and circulatory rate and a higher level of functioning (Table 8–3). Anxiety, fear, and pain initiate the response, and starvation, immobilization, and anesthetic agents add to it. Injury or operation damages tissue, causes blood and body fluid loss, and reduces extracellular fluid volume and vascular volume. Pain, fear, fatigue, anesthesia, drugs, immobilization, and transient starvation produce only minor or short-term changes similar to what occurs with an inguinal hernia repair. A patient who undergoes inguinal hernia repair

Table 8–2. Phases of the response to moderate injury.

1. Injury phase. Lasts 2–5 days or longer. Duration is related to the magnitude or "dose" of injury and the presence or absence of complications.
2. Turning point. The neuroendocrine response turns off. A transient period. May occur overnight or develop over 1 or 2 days.
3. Anabolic phase. Gain in muscular strength. Phase of positive nitrogen balance. Lasts 3–12 weeks or longer.
4. Late anabolism. Gain in weight and body fat. Phase of positive caloric balance. Lasts months to years.

Table 8–3. Stimuli resulting from injury.

1. An injury and a major operation are similar in that they produce the same stimuli. Factors that trigger a biologic response and reset the homostatic thermostat are as follows:
   Anxiety, fear, pain
   Starvation
   Immobilization
   Anesthetic agents
   Tissue injury
   Blood and body fluid (extracellular fluid) loss
   Drugs
   Infection
2. Factors that produce only minor transient changes (an inguinal hernia, laparoscopic cholecystectomy, open cholecystectomy, modified radical mastectomy):
   Pain, fear, fatigue
   Anesthesia and drugs
   Immobilization
   Transient starvation
3. Factors that produce major, extensive efforts:
   Multisystem injury
      Long bone and pelvic fractures
      Organ injury—spleen, liver, lung, bowel, heart
   The wound
      Tissue injury
      Tissue necrosis
      Major burns
   Invasive sepsis
   Shock
   Prolonged starvation

with local anesthesia and is discharged to home care shortly after the procedure will barely have the biologic thermostat changed. The reason is that the hernia operation is a minor procedure performed on the surface of the body under local anesthesia—ie, body cavities are not entered. This better result is now with procedures performed in the body cavities (peritoneal or thoracic) via thoracoscopic or laparoscopic approaches. Small incisions for invasive procedures that do not disturb the peritoneal or thoracic cavities produce a minimal response to injury. Thus, such patients, if they have no complications the day after these procedures and feel and look well, can be discharged from the hospital. An uneventful convalescence would be expected. Laparoscopic cholecystectomy, a minimal operation, causes a lesser response to injury as evidenced by less interleukin-6 (IL-6) production and unimpaired immune functions—as compared with a standard or open cholecystectomy. However, tissue injury with necrosis, invasive sepsis, shock, and other aspects of injury with ischemia have major effects such as occurs in an

Figure 8–1. Afferent stimuli after an operation or an injury that induce the neuroendocrine response to injury.

automobile accident with multiple fractures, rupture of the spleen, and head injury. One of the most severe threats to survival which produces a maximum response to injury is a major body burn. The severity or "dose" of the injury determines the magnitude of response. The surgical objective of minimal tissue necrosis, a clean wound, and support for normal organ function is intended to blunt the extent of injury and its response.

The Afferent Pathways

The stimuli of injury provide neural and mediator signals to the central nervous system primarily by way of nociceptors, baroreceptors, chemoreceptors, and from the wound (Figure 8–1). These stimuli initiate the response to injury. The nociceptor (pain) input plays a role in escaping, avoiding further injury, and initiating the generalized sympathetic nervous or stress response. Stimuli to the spinothalamic tracts are transmitted to the thalamus and thence to the cortex for pain perception and to the hypothalamus and medullary sympathetic centers for neuroendocrine stimulation. Epidural or spinal anesthesia for lower abdominal operations inhibits some of the neuroendocrine responses such as hypercortisolemia and the extent of negative nitrogen balance but does not alter acute-phase protein responses. Thus, spinal cord blockade decreases the endocrine response to injury but not the response to tissue injury, which is mediated by local factors from the wound.

Both high-pressure and low-pressure baroreceptors in the central circulation signal the cardiovascular control areas. Arterial receptors found primarily in the aortic arch at bifurcations and in the carotid sinuses respond to both pulsatile and mean arterial pressures. Venous receptors in the left and right atria, the interatrial septum, and the portal system provide information on both the rate and extent of atrial filling. Atrial natriuretic factor, or atriopeptin, is involved in this process. The surgical wound or the area of injury also has an afferent arc of stimulation of central responses. Tissue injury and an operation, infection, or an attack by foreign antigens or foreign bodies causes an acute inflammatory response. Wound healing requires an inflammatory response. The categories of agents involved in this process are listed in Table 8–4.

The Wound as an Organ; The Wound Hormones

The area of injury, incision, or operated organs—called collectively the wound—may usefully be considered an organ. The wound functions as a somewhat independent organ calling on the rest of the body for support. It establishes a high biologic priority for itself and initiates many of the changes in metabolism and responses

Table 8–4. Mediators of injury, inflammation, and infection.

Cytokines
Platelet-activating factor (PAF)
Complement
Kinins and kallikreins
Endorphins
Neutrophils, superoxides, proteases
Immune complexes
Histamine
Nitric oxide (NO_2), endothelium-derived relaxing factor (EDRF)
Myocardial depressant factor (MDF)
Adhesion molecules
Coagulation cascades
Serotonin

to injury. Thus, it provides afferent stimuli to the central nervous system. It also provides efferent stimuli to the liver, the temperature control center, and elsewhere. These signals come from a variety of mediators produced by cells in the wound or in organs, including macrophages, monocytes, neutrophils (PMNs), endothelial cells, and others. The mediators constitute the factors in inflammation (Tables 8–5 and 8–6). They have an autocrine function along with paracrine activity. When produced in larger amounts, there is also a remote endocrine function. Many of these wound mediators—particularly the cytokines—stimulate the hypothalamus-pituitary-adrenal (HPA) axis. A tissue injury (wound) initiates and requires an inflammatory process to heal. Should infection develop later, it exaggerates the inflammatory response.

Endocrine & Mediator Correlates; The Efferent Pathways

The injury phase begins with the stress response and normal neuroendocrine alterations and activities in the hypothalamic-pituitary-adrenal axis. Hormonal changes resulting from injury are listed in Table 8–5, and Table 8–6 sets forth a summary of the most important changes. The complex reactions occurring in the hypothalamic-pituitary-adrenal axis are shown in Figure 8–2. The components of the catabolic response are listed in Table 8–7.

Hypothalamic activation leads to arginine vasopressin (AVP) or antidiuretic hormone (ADH) release from the neurohypophysis, epinephrine secretion from the adrenal medulla, and norepinephrine release from sympathetic nerve endings. Corticotropin-releasing hormone (CRH) travels to the adenohypophysis, stimulating adrenocorticotropic hormone (ACTH) production.

Table 8–5. Hormonal mediator changes with injury.

Hypothalamus (neural control)
  Corticotropin-releasing factor (CRF): stimulates
    release of adrenocorticotropin
  Thyroid-releasing hormone (TRH): no recog-
    nized role
  Luteinizing hormone-releasing hormone
    (LHRH): no recognized role
  Somatostatin (growth hormone [somatotropin]-
    releasing inhibitory factor; SRIF): uncertain role
  Arginine vasopressin, antidiuretic hormone (ADH):
    increased production in hypothalamus and release
    from posterior pituitary gland
  Epinephrine: secretion from adrenal medulla increased
  Norepinephrine: secretion from sympathetic nerve
    endings increased
**Endorphins (enkephalins) and Pituitary (neural
and hormonal control)**
  Corticotropin: increased
  Growth hormone (somatotropin): increased
  Prolactin: increased; function obscure
  Follicle-stimulating hormone-luteinizing hormone
    (FSH-LH): decreased
  Alpha-melanocyte-stimulating hormone: unknown
    function
  Beta-lipotropin hormone: unknown
  Thyroid-stimulating hormone (TSH): no change or
    decrease
  Arginine vasopressin: increased
Adrenal Gland
 Cortex (hormonal control)
  Cortisol: increased
  Aldosterone: increased
  Adrenal estrogens and androgens: no change or
    decreased
 Medulla (autonomic control)
  Catecholamines: increased
Thyroid Gland (hormonal gland)
  Thyroxine: no change
  Triiodothyronine: decreased
  Reverse triiodothyronine: increased

Pancreas (autonomic, hormonal, and substrate control)
  Glucagon: increased
  Insulin: less increase than hyperglycemia would produce
Kidney (autonomic and local control)
  Erythropoietin produced
  Renin-angiotensin activation
Wound (endogenous mediators, enzymes)
  Prostaglandins (prostacyclins, thromboxane)
  Leukotrienes
  Histamine
  Serotonin
  Kallikreins (bradykinin)
  Monokines (cytokines)
  Pro- and anti-inflammatory mediators: IL-1, IL-15
  Interleukin-1 from monocytes
  Hepatocyte-stimulating factor
  IL-6
  Cachectin (tumor necrosis factor) from macrophages
  Chemokines
  Lymphotoxin (a tumorilytic protein derived from
    leukocytes)
  Interferons (alpha [leukocyte], beta [fibroblast], gamma
    [T lym-phocyte])
  Granulocyte-macrophage colony-stimulating factor
  Neopterin
  Others

Although the normal or primary stimulus to ACTH secretion is CRH, with injury ADH and angiotensin II from the kidneys also stimulate ACTH. ACTH acts on the adrenal cortex, producing cortisol release. Among the many profound effects of cortisol are included restoration of blood volume after hemorrhage, inhibition of extrahepatic protein synthesis, potentiation of glucose production, and inhibition of various immune responses. Angiotensin II and aldosterone also serve as direct stimulants for cortisol secretion with injury. The immunosuppressive and anti-inflammatory properties of the glucocorticoids are well known. It has been sug-gested that they prevent the normal responses to trauma from proceeding to a stage of producing tissue damage and threatening homeostasis.

Circulating levels of endorphin (opioid peptides) rise after operation for as long as 72 hours. They produce some analgesia and a calming effect, along with other receptor interactions. The endogenous opioid system modulates noxious stimuli and the sympathetic response. Beta-endorphins from the central nervous system may contribute to hyperglycemia and glucose intolerance after injury. Alkaloid compounds similar to morphine and codeine are also produced in the central

Table 8–6. Hormonal changes and systemic effects of injury.

Major changes
  Stress hormones increased
    Cortisol
    Catecholamines
    Glucagon
  Volume control hormones increased
    Renin-angiotensin, aldosterone
    Arginine vasopressin (ADH)
  Sex hormones decreased
  Thyroid T_3 decreased
  Thyroid rT_3 increased
  Wound mediators increased
Results
  Hypermetabolism
  Proteolysis
  Wound healing begins in spite of negative nitrogen
    balance
  Lipolysis
  Extracellular water gain
  High glucose production for anaerobic cells of wound
    healing

Table 8–7. Components of the catabolic or acute phase response.

Skeletal muscle proteolysis through the ubiquitin-
  proteasome pathway
Decreased muscle protein synthesis
Initial increased gut mucosal synthesis and export
Hepatic protein synthesis (acute phase reactants)
Hepatic gluconeogenesis
Lung response (glutamine)
Kidney response

nervous system. These neurotransmitters help integrate the response to injury. Other pituitary hormones seem to have no major role after injury. Growth hormone concentration is decreased after severe injury and during hyperglycemic, hypermetabolic states. Some investigators have found increased growth hormone with less severe injury. Hormones related to reproduction are suppressed, an effect consistent with the observed depression of reproductive function and menses and libido after injury.

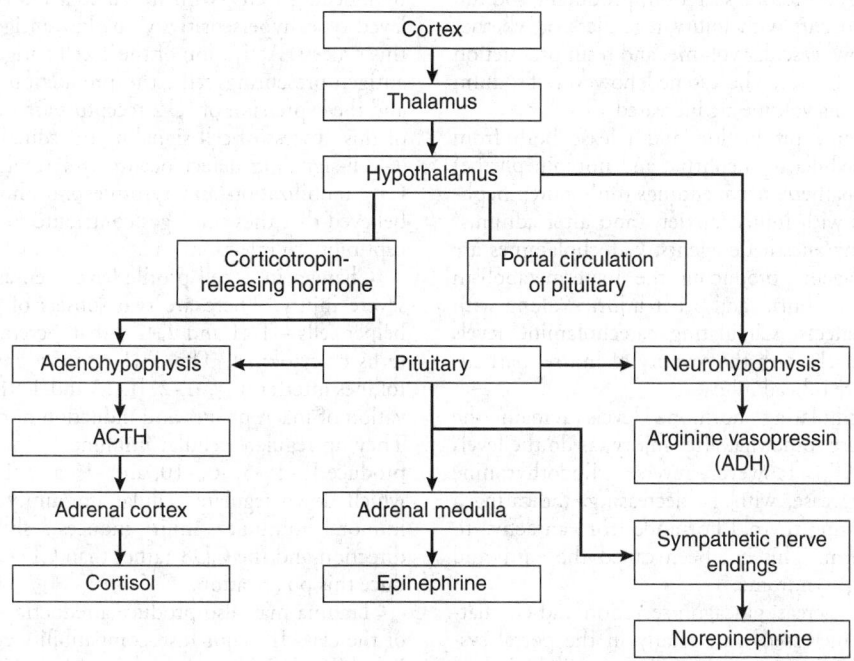

Figure 8–2. The complex series of reactions occurring in the hypothalamic-pituitary-adrenal axis (efferent stimuli) after injury or operation.

During homeostasis, the primary stimulus for ADH secretion is increased plasma osmolality, which is sensed in the osmoreceptors of the hypothalamus. With injury, other factors become more important in ADH release. Fear, pain, hemorrhage; decreased atrial, arterial, and portal pressures; and certain drugs, including morphine, barbiturates, and anesthetic agents, stimulate ADH through the hypothalamus, leading to water conservation. The primary stimulant after injury is decreased effective blood volume. Angiotensin II may also effect ADH release. Aldosterone secretion increases greatly with injury. In homeostasis, the renin-angiotensin system controls its production. Sympathetic system or local stimulation of the myoepithelial cells of the juxtaglomerular apparatus results in renin production. Renin circulates and cleaves an α_1-globulin produced in the liver to form angiotensin I. Angiotensin-converting enzyme converts angiotensin I to the active form, angiotensin II, in the lungs, kidneys, or blood. Angiotensin II, which has a very short half-life, is a potent general vasoconstrictor that has direct chronotropic and inotropic effects on the heart. This agent also seems to have an endocrine effect, increasing vasopressin secretion and sympathetic and adrenal medullary activity. Angiotensin II is the major stimulus for aldosterone secretion from the zona glomerulosa of the adrenal cortex. ACTH, which has a minor role in stimulating aldosterone secretion in normal individuals, is more important after injury or operation. Aldosterone secretion, producing sodium conservation, occurs with injury regardless of whether renal blood flow, vascular volume, and resin production are altered. Secretion can be lessened, however, if sodium intake and plasma volume are increased.

Catecholamine production and release both from the adrenal medulla (epinephrine and norepinephrine) and from sympathetic nerve endings (only norepinephrine) increases with injury, anxiety, and after administration of many anesthetic agents. Catecholamines are the primary agents producing the hypermetabolism that accompanies burns and other injuries, along with many other effects. Circulating catecholamine levels correlate positively with the severity of injury, particularly when there is head injury.

Thyroid-stimulating hormone levels remain the same or decrease somewhat after injury, as do the levels of thyroxine (T_4). However, reverse triiodothyronine (rT_3) levels increase, with T_3 decreasing, indicating a shift of circulating thyroid hormone from an active to an inactive form. This has been called the euthyroid sick (or low T_3) syndrome.

From the pancreas, glucagon secretion and circulating levels are increased, particularly in the portal system. Insulin levels remain normal or increase slightly but do not respond proportionately to the hyperglycemia that occurs with injury. Thus, a period of

insulin resistance resembling diabetes mellitus is a consequence of injury. Cortisol, glucagon, and the catecholamines have been called the counterregulatory or catabolic hormones.

The Psychoneuroimmunologic System

The relationships of psychologic and pathologic stress on the neuroendocrine and immune systems are well established. Many of the hormones and mediators just described produce immune modulation. The sympathetic nervous system and the hypothalamic-pituitary-adrenal system affect immunoreactivity.

Specific immunity was once attributed to the activities of thymus-derived (T) cells and monocyte-macrophages (cellular immunity) and bursa-equivalent (B) cells, which are part of the humoral system producing antibodies. It is now recognized that there are complex interactions and relationships of these systems.

The specific or cell-mediated immune system is suppressed after injury. Glucocorticoids may adversely affect cell nuclear events, leading to inhibition of interleukin-2 (IL-2) production and T cell proliferation. Within 30 minutes after injury, prostaglandin E_2 (PGE_2) is increased. This suppresses IL-2 and lymphocyte stimulation. Increased PGE_2, decreasing IL-2 mRNA and IL-2 production in T cells, has been demonstrated in trauma and burn patients. This process can be reversed by blocking PGE_2 with indomethacin. The loss of delayed-type hypersensitivity to skin antigens is part of this process. Activation of the T cell antigen receptor by antigen-presenting cells, the production of mediators, and the expression of IL-2 receptors are important parts of this process of cell-signaling transduction. The basic T cell-signaling defect occurs as a result of decreased Ca^{2+} mobilization and tyrosine phosphorylation. It is believed that these changes contribute to increased susceptibility to infection.

Changes in T cell profile have been associated with severe injury. There are two subsets of committed T helper cells—TH1 and TH2—that secrete different patterns of cytokines. The TH1 response involves the cytokines interferon-γ, IL-2, IL-12 and TNF-α, with activation of macrophages and induction of cytotoxic cells. They up-regulate cellular immune responses. TH2 cells produce IL-4, -5, -6, -10, and -13 as well as antibodies which down-regulate cellular immunity but augment humoral immunity. Injury induces a shift in the TH2 direction and the CD8 rather than CD4 cells that produce this polarization.

Trauma may also produce a reduction in expression of the class II major histocompatibility complex molecule HLA-DR in monocytes and reduction also in expression of soluble HLA-DR molecules. They are up-regulated by TH1 cytokines. In addition, B cells become differentiated into plasma cells that produce antibodies to specific antigens.

The nonspecific immune system is activated after injury. Polymorphonuclear leukocytes (PMNs) increase and are activated. There is early evidence of circulating self-destructive or toxic mediators such as PMN elastase and oxygen radicals along with nitric oxide (NO_2). PMN priming and activation may play a major role in remote organ damage after ischemia and reperfusion and severe injury.

Magnitude of the Response

The magnitude of the neuroendocrine response is proportionate to the severity of injury or operation, to body fluid and blood loss, sequestration of fluid into the wound (so-called third-spacing), and other factors. If infection (sepsis) develops, the injury phase is prolonged or exaggerated. A severe infection such as peritonitis can induce an inflammatory response which is similar to the response to injury and will exaggerate an injury response.

Physiologic Correlates

The physiologic correlates of the neuroendocrine response during the injury phase are (1) blood pressure and cardiac output maintenance by cardiovascular compensation and capillary refilling; (2) salt and water retention to maintain vascular and extracellular fluid volume; (3) increased metabolic rate (hypermetabolism); (4) altered metabolism, with insulin resistance, hyperglycemia, gluconeogenesis, excess catabolism, and negative nitrogen balance, with release of intracellular components; (5) mobilization of fats; (6) beginning of wound healing; and (7) immunomodulation.

A. Cardiovascular Compensation

The initial emergency response of the sympathoadrenal system and the circulation is to maintain blood pressure by increasing peripheral vascular resistance and heart rate. Inotropy for the ventricles maintains cardiac output and capillary refilling, and venoconstriction shifts blood volume from the splanchnic bed to the central circulation. The splanchnic bed (gut) is a major reservoir of available blood. An otherwise normal individual can tolerate blood loss of roughly 1000 mL if kept quiet. With more severe blood loss, cardiovascular compensation cannot maintain an adequate circulation and shock will develop. An individual will not survive without treatment after blood loss of 1500 mL or more.

B. Salt and Water Retention

ADH and aldosterone secretion attempt to maintain the internal environment, particularly the extracellular fluid and vascular volume. Extracellular fluid volume is maintained, however, at the expense of tonicity. Maximum sodium retention occurs if the injury has been significant. Urine sodium losses are then very low (10 meq/L). Urinary potassium loss is greater but water is retained, with relative oliguria. Bicarbonate is conserved, so the urine tends to be acid. During this time the patient is unable to handle a free water load, tending toward hypotonicity and metabolic alkalosis. Administration of excess free water (as 5% dextrose and water) can produce water intoxication, manifested by convulsions, brain damage, and death. Despite maximal salt retention, hyponatremia tends to develop because the patient produces free water through metabolism and lipolysis. Furthermore, some sodium may enter cells at the injury site or with muscle breakdown from catabolism. Likewise, hyperkalemia tends to occur despite significant potassium losses in the urine because of red cell breakdown, transfused blood, and muscle catabolism, which releases potassium.

C. Hypermetabolism

Increased catecholamine secretion mediates in good part the increased metabolic rate, which can be significant with severe injury. Heat production, body temperature, oxygen consumption ($\dot{V}O_2$), and circulatory demand increase. Temperature elevation of 0.5–1 °C accounts for 10–20% of the increased $\dot{V}O_2$. Synthesis of glucose and protein in the liver accounts for most of the increased $\dot{V}O_2$. The respiratory quotient is usually 0.7–0.76, indicating primarily fat oxidation. In burn patients, catecholamines are the major factor elevating thermogenesis and metabolism, with cortisol playing a less prominent role. Some believe that impairment or loss of the cutaneous evaporative cooling barrier also affects thermoregulation. Initially after injury, resting energy expenditure may be low or low-normal. It quickly increases, but— with an elective uncomplicated operation—elevations are only 10% or so of preoperative values for 5–7 days. With injuries such as multiple fractures, measured metabolic rate elevations are 10–25% for 10–14 days. With major infections such as peritonitis, the elevation is 15–50% for as long as the infection continues; with major burns, expenditure is 40–100% above normal until the burn is covered. This hypermetabolism requires increased cardiac output (cardiac index) and increased blood flow, a hyperdynamic circulation. If the patient cannot meet this circulatory requirement because of limitations in cardiovascular reserve function, the circulation becomes inadequate and complications of decreased organ blood flow (ischemia) occur.

D. Altered Metabolism

Insulin resistance, glucagon secretion, excessive catabolism, negative nitrogen balance, and breakdown and release of intracellular components of lean body mass (primarily skeletal muscle) are the major metabolic alterations with injury. These alterations go far beyond what starvation and bed rest alone would predict. Immediately after injury, glucose production and circulating levels of glucose increase—with relative hyperglycemia—probably because epinephrine stimulates glycogen breakdown in the liver. Glycogen stores are used up quickly. This is followed by increased gluconeogenesis. During the injury phase, rapid breakdown of body protein from skeletal muscle occurs if the injury is severe. Infusions of hydrocortisone, glucagon, and epinephrine in normal human volunteers produce many of the metabolic alterations seen in critically ill patients. These include hypermetabolism, increased nitrogen loss, glucose intolerance, and insulin resistance—but not net muscle breakdown. The total picture of muscle breakdown of protein, decreased muscle amino acid uptake, increased uptake of amino acids in the liver, and acute phase protein synthesis is caused by a combination of glucocorticoids, glucagon, and cytokines from macrophages and white cells, particularly tumor necrosis factor (TNF-α), IL-1, and IL-6. The IL-6 superfamily is the major factor in producing acute-phase proteins or reactants by the liver. These reactants include C-reactive protein, serum amyloid A, metal-binding proteins, proteinase inhibitors, and coagulation proteins. Intracellular protection from stress is provided by a family of heat shock proteins that can be induced by stimulation of the hypothalamic-pituitary-adrenal axis.

With modest injury, the body burns a balanced fuel, including both protein and fat. With severe injury, the catabolism of muscle protein becomes more pronounced, leading to a decrease in lean body cell mass or muscle. This contributes to the feeling of weakness that an injured and operated patient experiences. The injured patient does not adjust to starvation in the same way as a normal individual. With starvation alone, there is an adjustment to conserve body protein and burn fat for fuel, thereby producing ketone bodies which are used by the brain and other tissues. Injured patients do not adapt, as does the starving patient, with high fat utilization, ketosis, and protein conservation. They are in a catabolic state because of this greatly increased rate of whole body protein catabolism, compensated for in part by a modest increase in protein synthesis. Nutritional support in such patients minimizes the rate of protein loss, but loss continues nevertheless. Muscle protein goes to the liver for gluconeogenesis. There is a great need for glucose, primarily for the wound, where all of the tissues (the cells of repair—macrophages, fibroblasts, capillary buds) must work in an anaerobic environment. Anaerobic glycolysis utilizing glucose is an important part of wound healing and repair of injury. The wound is thus a glucose sump. The mechanisms producing catabolism are not completely understood. As lean body mass decreases, weakness may become profound, with difficulty in ambulation and decreased ventilatory reserve. Wound healing begins and progresses despite the negative nitrogen balance. Catabolism also produces endogenous water that is sodium-free. There is also some fat mobilization. Free fatty acids increase and are used by muscle for fuel. Glycerol is extracted by the liver for glucose production.

The entire specific immune system is suppressed after injury. The reasons for this are not well understood. A major factor in this immunosuppression along with cortisol is increased production of PGE_2, which suppresses IL-2 expression, which then cannot stimulate T cell proliferation. Catabolism produces protein-calorie malnutrition with altered immunoglobulins and altered T and B cell function. Anesthetic agents may also contribute to immunosuppression. Shock alters PMN function and lung and liver macrophage function.

Clinical Correlates

The clinical correlates of the neuroendocrine and physiologic responses to injury are important. Observing the patient during this time can indicate whether the response is normal or complications are developing. During the injury phase, patients are quiet, lethargic, and look ill. They are not interested in their surroundings or appearance. They do not turn on television and are not interested in newspapers. Women will not consider applying makeup during this time. Men will not comb their hair or shave. ("Let me alone. I hurt. I don't feel good. I want to curl up and get over this.") This is most likely due to pain, beta-endorphins, the enkephalins, and IL-1 production. People who witness an injury (an accident) are often excited and running about, but the victim is lying quietly waiting for help. People who have pets may have observed that an injured animal wants to lie quietly and be left alone, allowing the metabolic and neuroendocrine response to preserve its internal environment. The neuroendocrine response to injury functions to enhance the possibility of survival without treatment.

During the injury phase the patient's pulse increases modestly; temperature increases, with low grade fever of 37.7–38.3 °C, oliguria tends to develop, appetite decreases, the gastrointestinal tract and peristalsis are quiet, and pain is present. A temperature elevation greater than 38.3 °C suggests other problems such as atelectasis.

When a patient looks ill and is going through the injury phase, it is important just to observe him before vital signs and other laboratory data are reviewed. Much can be learned by talking to and observing the patient in the intensive care unit or on rounds. Look first for illness and then for wellness. If the injury phase continues, weight loss, fatigue, and weakness progress. The patient may have difficulty ambulating without help and eventually could be bedridden with an altered sensorium, impaired ventilatory reserve, and impaired ability to cough. Initially, body weight increases each day for 1–3 days as extracellular fluid and blood normally are sequestered in the injury site. After that time, daily body weight loss is equal to catabolism unless nutrition is provided. The fluids sequestered as initial third-space accumulation gradually come back into the circulation, with diuresis on the second to fourth days. The patient could then have circulatory overload if the previous loss was great.

It is critical to maintain adequate blood and extracellular fluid volumes by intraoperative and postoperative administration of sodium-containing solutions for the third-space requirements of the wound. Attempts to block third-space fluxes and excess catabolism have been ineffective and counterproductive.

The normal response may become abnormal if the injury phase is prolonged because of tissue necrosis, infection, continuing tissue injury, other complications, or ill-advised therapy. Problems in the injury phase include fluid overload, hypotonicity or water intoxication, acute and chronic desalting water loss, dehydration, metabolic alkalosis, and volume deficits.

The problems of infection after injury are a major contribution to multiple organ failure. Susceptibility to infection increases because of tissue injury, necrosis, contamination, and altered host resistance. If the injury phase is prolonged, nutritional support should be provided by the enteral route if the gut is working.

Baumann H et al: The acute phase response. Immunol Today 1994;15:74.

Decker D et al: Surgical stress induces a shift in the type 1/type 2 T-helper cell balance, suggesting down-regulation of cell-mediated and up-regulation of antibody-mediated immunity commensurate to the trauma. Surgery 1996;119:316.

Voerman HJ et al: Time course and variability of the endocrine and metabolic response to severe sepsis. Surgery 1993;114:951.

Woolf PD: The catecholamine response to multisystem trauma. Arch Surg 1992;127:899.

Turning Point (Phase 2)

If the patient stabilizes after injury, homeostasis is adequate, the wound is controlled, and complications such as sepsis are not developing, the turning point is reached. Survival is likely, and at this time the neuroendocrine stimulation shuts off. This has also been called the corticoid withdrawal phase or the endorphin withdrawal phase. In addition, the beginning of wound healing decreases the inflammatory response. Local mediators produced by the wound are decreased and no longer have any systemic effects.

This transitional phase may occur suddenly and dramatically overnight or may last 1–2 more days or longer. After a clean elective operation, the turning point is often clearly evident. One morning, the patient suddenly looks better. This may be obscured, however, with massive injury or with an overwhelmingly severe or extensive burn. Neuroendocrine withdrawal can be observed more clearly after an operation such as an open cholecystectomy or colectomy rather than after generalized peritonitis. The plasma concentrations of epinephrine, norepinephrine, cortisol, growth hormone, somatomedin, and vasopressin return to normal. Insulin levels begin to rise and then peak 1 week or so after injury. The physiologic correlates of the endocrine withdrawal phase include water diuresis, increased sodium in the urine, normal retention of potassium, decreased nitrogen excretion, and, depending upon nitrogen intake, a return toward zero or positive nitrogen balance.

Many clinical correlates characterize this phase. The patient looks as if he or she is recovering, regains appetite, and becomes interested in the surroundings. The patient becomes interested in personal grooming and wants to get up and move about. Pulse and temperature return to normal, and the patient has a sense of well-being. If a patient does not experience such a turning point by 2–3 days after an elective, otherwise uncomplicated operation, the surgeon should investigate the possible presence of complications. Burn patients are the exception, because epinephrine levels return to normal after hypovolemia is corrected but norepinephrine levels remain high until the burn is covered. There may be a prolonged increased in cortisol levels and persistent insulin resistance in elderly patients.

If the patient does not stabilize; if circulation and homeostasis are not adequate; if the injury or wounding continues, as with fractures that are not immobilized, with tissue necrosis or an open necrotic wound; or if complications develop—in these circumstances, the turning point will be delayed, and the injury phase will continue. Obviously, the integrity of fracture fixation, nutritional support, oral intake, the possibility of sepsis, and other factors influence the timing and magnitude of the response. With major burns, some aspects of the injury phase continue until the eschar is removed, the burn area is grafted, and the wounds are healed. The injury phase will continue as long as there is a wound that is not clean or closed or is not immobilized.

Can a patient go through the turning point, appear to be getting well, and then have a life-threatening complication? This is unlikely. A late pulmonary embolus, a delayed wound dehiscence, or other problems could arise but not commonly. There is no better sign of an uneventful recovery than the observation that the patient reached the turning point and is beginning to look and feel well.

Anabolic Phase (Phase 3)

Anabolism begins immediately after the turning point, particularly if the patient can take nourishment or is provided with parenteral nutrition. The patient at this time may begin to ambulate but feels weak and tired. Weakness is in good part due to the previous hypermetabolic catabolic response, loss of lean body mass, and duration of bed rest. It is not unlike a febrile illness such as the flu, with loss of appetite, decreased oral intake, and inactivity with bed rest. This has been called the period of ambition without fulfillment. Patients may feel great, feel like they are convalescing, and believe they should be able to get out of bed and go home. Recovery of strength, positive nitrogen balance, and restoration of muscle protein are slow procedures. Initially, little weight is gained because muscle water is lost as muscle is rebuilt. Furthermore, the rate of weight gain is three to eight times slower than the rate of loss. Positive nitrogen balance may average 3–4 g of nitrogen per day, 19–25 g of protein, or 90–120 g of lean body mass. If enteral or parenteral caloric intake during this period exceeds expenditure, some fat may be deposited as well. Describing this early anabolic phase to patients is helpful for them because they may become discouraged by their inability to return to normal as fast as they hoped.

Late Anabolism (Phase 4)

Distinguishing between phases 3 and 4 is not always easy. The final phase after injury is one of positive caloric and carbon balance. Fat stores are replaced. Although the fat gain may continue for months or years, some fat is restored earlier, along with protein. After nitrogen balance has been achieved, it becomes zero. Weight gain accelerates, but the extent of injury or operation may dictate the amount of weight restored. For example, in a patient with an upper gastrointestinal operation, weight may not return to the preoperative level but rather reset itself at 6.8–9 kg less than before because of altered nutrition, a smaller gastric reservoir, or diminished interest in food.

Treatment & Methods to Decrease the Response to Injury

Prompt operative care is the first step toward recovery. Correcting blood loss, repairing injured organs, supporting damaged organs, closing wounds, and cleaning body cavities should stop the wounding and shorten the injury phase.

Careful surgical technique will lighten the load of necrotic tissue and minimize the risk of postinjury or postoperative infection, either in the wound or elsewhere. Debridement, irrigation, and cleaning and stopping continued pleural, peritoneal, bone, or muscle contamination are critical.

Minimal surgical procedures will decrease the response to stress and injury. In general, laparoscopic surgery reduces the stress response to injury compared with comparable procedures performed via an open approach. Measured improvements include reduced inflammatory response (C-reactive protein, IL-6) and immunomodulatory response, improved pulmonary function with less hypoxemia, and a lesser risk of infectious complications.

The immune response with minimal procedures has been evaluated extensively. Again, in general, the immunosuppressive response that is common after open operations is largely absent after laparoscopic procedures.

Epidural or spinal anesthesia and agents such as fentanyl and morphine decrease the response to injury by decreasing the cortisol, cAMP, and glucose responses. Epidural analgesia also prevents the sensitization of the spinal cord by pain. This effect may be enough to decrease morbidity. In one study, a combination of prednisolone, epidural analgesia, and indomethacin decreased the stress response in patients having colon operations. In that experience there was decreased pain, decreased hyperthermia, and better pulmonary function; fatigue was less pronounced, and there was less PGE$_2$, IL-6, and C-reactive protein production. Thus, a combined neural and hormonal blockade inhibited the global stress response to operation. Epidural anesthesia appears to attenuate the hormonal response to stress by blocking afferent pain stimuli that may still elicit a subconscious sympathetic response even in a patient under general anesthesia.

It has also been established that even mild hypothermia during an operation is deleterious. Normothermia should be maintained during major surgery because it reduces the incidence of morbid cardiac events, reduces the incidence of surgical wound infection, and shortens hospitalization. Trauma patients should be rewarmed rapidly, because doing so improves survival.

Pain relief, intravenous fluids to compensate for third-space requirements, and mobilization are important. Nutritional support will decrease total protein loss. Early postinjury enteral feeding should be provided whenever possible, particularly if the patient will not be able to resume normal nutrition after 3–4 days or is severely hypermetabolic. Evidence is accumulating that additives such as glutamine, arginine, omega-3 fatty acids, branched-chain amino acids, and antioxidants (vitamins C, A, and E and glutathione) may decrease the incidence of infection and provide immune enhancement. However, total parenteral or enteral nutrition cannot abolish the hypermetabolic, hyperglycemic response to the catabolic hormones. Hormonal manipulations with the anabolic hormones such as exogenous insulin, growth hormone, and insulin-like growth hormone have been shown to have some positive effects in reducing protein loss, preserving body composition, increasing strength, and decreasing complications such as infection. These agents are not recommended as yet for general use in injured and operated patients.

Frank SM et al: Perioperative maintenance of normothermia reduces the incidence of morbid cardiac events. A randomized clinical trial. JAMA 1997;277:1127.

Hill GL et al: Metabolic basis for the management of patients undergoing major surgery. World J Surg 1993;17:146.

Iwanaka T et al: Evaluation of operative stress and peritoneal macrophage function in minimally invasive operations. J Am Coll Surg 1997;184:357.

Kehlet H et al: Impact of laparoscopic surgery on stress responses, immunofunction, and risk of infectious complications. New Horiz 1998;6(2 Suppl):S80.

Kurz A et al: Perioperative normothermia to reduce the incidence of surgical-wound infection and shorten hospitalization. Study of Wound Infection and Temperature Group. N Engl J Med 1996;334:1209.

Variations in the Response to Injury

Patients with chronic diseases before injury or before a major operation are at increased risk for prolonged recovery, complications, or death. Their response to injury may be exaggerated. An injured patient with heart disease may not tolerate the salt and water retention and venous congestion that occurs. A patient with liver disease having an operation or sustaining an injury will require a much higher cardiac output than normal. Liver disease is associated with decreased peripheral resistance, hyperaldosteronism, and increased cardiac output. Oliguria may be a significant problem because the hyperaldosteronism of liver disease is added to that of injury. Such a patient may not increase urine output after a saline challenge. A fluid challenge may produce ascites. Diuretics may be required. A patient with chronic obstructive pulmonary disease and respiratory insufficiency who was operated upon or injured has a tendency toward hypoxemia in addition to the inability to maintain normal ventilation that accompanies injury. An injured patient with renal insufficiency has the additional problem of a rapid rise in the products of cell breakdown such as urea and potassium. Further renal injury from inadequate resuscitation can occur. In patients with prolonged starvation, failure of body cell mass may be added to the usual response of protein-calorie malnutrition. Elderly patients may have insufficient recovery of strength after injury, which could put them at risk of respiratory and cardiovascular complications.

Inappropriate activity of the neuroendocrine system may also jeopardize the individual, such as inappropriate ADH secretion, or failure of ADH production, as in acute diabetes insipidus. The massive neuroendocrine, metabolic, and mediator response that occurs with an overwhelming injury or a major operation with complications has raised the possibility that the biologic responses which should protect us can have destructive consequences. Many of the mediators of inflammation such as IL-1 and TNF, when infused into normal human volunteers, produce a flu-like syndrome. Activation of other mediator systems can also decrease microcirculatory blood flow and cause tissue damage and other problems. Severe multisystem injury, infection, or inflammation can produce remote organ failure or dysfunction. This was originally called multiple organ failure and may be the result of excessive mediator activation of cytokines, complement, histamine, prostanoids, leukotrienes, bradykinin, and others. Thus, an overwhelming inflammatory response can be a destructive phenomenon. This has raised the possibility of trying to block some of these mediators, which are necessary for survival but become toxic in excess. Various "magic bullets" have been suggested such as monoclonal antibodies to endotoxin, a monoclonal antibody to TNF, the use of an IL-1 receptor antagonist, or soluble receptors to TNF and other cytokines. So far, when these agents have been subjected to prospective randomized clinical trials, they have not improved survival. Natural antagonists or anti-inflammatory agents are currently being studied. These include IL-4, IL-10, IL-13, and bactericidal permeability-increasing protein, which is a naturally occurring endotoxin-binding agent. Much more will be learned about this in the near future. Originally, the term infection was limited to invasion by an organism that attacked the patient. If this infection was systemic, it was called sepsis. Severely ill or inflamed patients may have all the characteristics of sepsis without bacterial infection. This was then called the sepsis syndrome. Some years ago it became evident that patients who developed complications after injury and operation were developing a multiple organ failure problem. The ability to support individual organ function in an ICU (ventilators, dialysis, circulatory support, etc) led to patients dying of multiple organ problems rather than of the initial failure. It is now proposed to use the terms systemic inflammatory response syndrome (SIRS) and multiple organ dysfunction syndrome (MODS). There is some evidence that the care of such patients is now improving.

Baue AE et al: Systemic inflammatory response syndrome (SIRS), multiple organ dysfunction syndrome (MODS), multiple organ failure (MOF): are we winning the battle? Shock 1998;10:79.

Demling RH et al: Physiologic support of the septic patient. Surg Clin North Am 1994;74:637.

Weigent DA et al: Associations between the neuroendocrine and immune systems. J Leukoc Biol 1995;58:137.

Inflammation, Infection, & Antibiotics

9

J. Perren Cobb, MD, Robert Schmieg, MD, Thomas K. Hunt, MD, & Linda M. Mundy, MD

■ INFLAMMATION & INFECTION

SURGICAL INFECTIONS

A surgical infection is an infection that (1) is unlikely to respond to nonsurgical treatment (it usually must be excised or drained) and occupies an unvascularized space in tissue or (2) occurs in an operated site. Common examples of the first group are appendicitis, empyema, gas gangrene, and most abscesses.

Surgeons are regrettably familiar with the vicious circle of operation or injury, infection, malnutrition, immunosuppression, organ failure, reoperation, further malnutrition, and further infection. One of the fine arts of surgery is to know when to intervene with excision, drainage, physiologic support, antibiotic therapy, and nutritional therapy. For infections arising in a space or in dead tissue, by far the most important aspect of treatment is to establish surgical drainage.

Pathogenesis

Three elements are common to surgical infections: (1) an infectious agent, (2) a susceptible host, and (3) a closed, unperfused space.

A. THE INFECTIOUS AGENT

Although a few pathogens cause most surgical infections, many organisms are capable of doing so. Among the aerobic organisms, streptococci may invade even minor breaks in the skin and spread through connective tissue planes and lymphatics. *Staphylococcus aureus* is the most common pathogen in wound infections and around foreign bodies. Klebsiella often invades the inner ear and enteric tissues as well as the lung. Enteric organisms, especially the Enterobacteriaceae and enterococci, are often found together with anaerobes. Among the anaerobes, bacteroides species and peptostreptococci are often present in surgical infections, and clostridium species are major pathogens in ischemic tissue.

Pseudomonas and serratia are usually nonpathogenic surface contaminants but may be opportunistic and even lethal invaders in critically ill or immunosuppressed patients. Some fungi (histoplasma, coccidioides) and yeasts (candida), along with nocardia and actinomyces, cause abscesses and sinus tracts, and even animal parasites (amebas and echinococcus) may cause abscesses, especially in the liver. Destructive granulomas, such as tuberculosis, once required excision, but antibiotic therapy has now superseded operation for this purpose in most cases. Other rare diseases such as cat-scratch fever, psittacosis, and tularemia may cause suppurative lymphadenitis and require drainage or excision.

Identification of the pathogen by smear and culture remains a cardinal step in therapy. The surgeon must inform the microbiologist of peculiar circumstances associated with any given specimen, so that appropriate smears and cultures can be done; serious errors may otherwise result.

B. THE SUSCEPTIBLE HOST

Surgical infections such as appendicitis and furuncles occur in patients whose only defect in immunity is a closed space in tissue. However, patients with suppressed immune systems are being seen with increasing frequency, and their problems have become a major surgical challenge. **Immunosuppression** seems a simple concept but in fact usually represents a combination of defects of the multifaceted immune mechanism.

1. Specific immunity—The immune process that depends upon prior exposure to an antigen involves detection and processing of antigen by macrophages, mobilization of T and B lymphocytes, synthesis of specific antibody, and other functions. Its importance is illustrated in AIDS, transplant immunosuppression, and agammaglobulinemia, each of which is associated with only a slight increase in the frequency and severity of some surgical infections. Specific abnormalities of cell-mediated and humoral immunity have been reported in almost every imaginable form of surgical infection. For instance, severe injury in animals and patients is associated with a subsequent decrease in T cell-dependent immune cell function and thus depressed adaptive immunity. Unfortunately, the clinical significance of this and other isolated defects of specific immunity is obscure, and their clinical importance in the complex immune system is difficult to determine (see Systemic Inflammatory Response System, below). In general, isolated defects contribute little to the severity of ordinary surgical infections. Major defects contribute substantially, but only to long-term morbidity and to deaths due to more widespread infections such as pneumonia, meningitis, and viral diseases, for which specific immune mechanisms constitute the principal mode of defense.

2. Nonspecific immunity—Also known as innate immunity, nonspecific immunity serves to limit damage during the first few hours after infection. Despite the emphasis in the literature on specific immune mechanisms, nonspecific immunity, which depends on phagocytic leukocytes seeking out, ingesting, and killing microorganisms, is the principal means by which the host defends against abscess-forming and necrotizing infections. Only recently has nonspecific immunity generated considerable interest, in part because it is an ancient, evolutionary defense system with many features common to both insects and humans.

a. Chemoattraction and phagocytosis—Invading microbes display molecular patterns that are shared among groups of pathogens. Examples include lipopolysaccharides (LPS) of gram-negative bacteria, lipoteichoic acid of gram-positive bacteria, mannans of yeast, and double-stranded RNA of certain viruses. To control infection, the host uses an array of pattern recognition receptors (complement, collectins, bactericidal permeability-increasing protein [BPI], LPS-binding protein [LBP]) that bind to these molecular patterns, acting together with effector cells to eliminate them. Typically, granulocytes internalize these pattern-receptor complexes by engulfment into a phagocytic vacuole. The subsequent release of chemoattractants causes the movement (diapedesis) of leukocytes from the bloodstream to the tissue, increasing leukocyte numbers locally and the likelihood that the invading microbe will be destroyed. These steps require little or no oxygen, but chemotaxis is vulnerable to a number of disorders, particularly anti-inflammatory steroid hormones and malnutrition, which reduce the number of granulocytes that arrive at a contaminated site in a given time.

b. Killing mechanisms—Once the phagosome is formed, other cytoplasmic granules (lysosomes) fuse with it and release into it preformed and increasingly

acidic proteolytic solutions that kill most bacteria and fungi.

A second process, termed "oxidative killing," is particularly important to the killing of organisms such as staphylococci which are commonly responsible for surgical infections. This mechanism consumes and requires molecular oxygen, which it converts to superoxide anion. In this process, a membrane-bound NADPH oxidase is activated, and a burst of respiration (oxygen consumption) follows. Part of the consumed oxygen is converted to a series of oxygen radicals (including superoxide, hydroxyl radical, and hypochlorite), which are released into phagosomes and assist in bacterial killing. This process is progressively inhibited when extracellular oxygen tension falls below about 30 mm Hg. When oxygen tension is 0 mm Hg, the antibacterial capacity of normal granulocytes for *S aureus* and *E coli*, for instance, falls by half—to the same capacity observed in granulocytes taken from victims of chronic granulomatous disease, which results from the genetic absence of membrane-bound oxidase and which without aggressive antibiotic therapy is lethal in early childhood.

Whether a given inoculum will establish an infection and become invasive depends to a great extent on how well tissue perfusion—and therefore oxygenation—can meet the increased metabolic demands of the granulocytes. Inflammatory signals from complement factors and histamine, for instance, dilate vessels and help direct blood flow to infected areas, but if blood volume or regional vascular supply is so poor that tissue perfusion cannot increase, invasive infection soon follows. Tissue oxygen supplies can often be raised by increasing blood volume and arterial PO_2 and are lowered by hypovolemia and pulmonary insufficiency. Tests in animals show that correcting arterial hypoxia aborts bacterial infections as effectively as does use of specific antibiotics and that antibiotics are far more effective when phagocytes have an adequate oxygen supply.

Patients with pulmonary disease, severe trauma, congestive heart failure, hypovolemia, or excessive levels of vasopressin, angiotensin, or catecholamines have hypoxic peripheral tissues and are unusually susceptible to infection. They are truly immunosuppressed. Support of the circulation is just as important to immune defense as is nutrition or antibiotic therapy.

3. Anergy—Anergy is defined as the lack of inflammatory response to skin test antigens. It characterizes a population of immunosuppressed patients who tend to develop infections and die from them. The skin tests used to diagnose anergy are those often used to test recall antigens and delayed hypersensitivity—but in fact they test much of the spectrum of antibacterial immunologic events, including antigen detection and processing by macrophages, release of lymphokines, antibody synthesis, and the inflammatory response, including leukocyte chemotaxis. One event they do not detect is, conspicuously, the final crucial step of actually killing bacteria. Anergy has many causes, including defective T and B lymphocytes, the presence of excess anti-inflammatory corticosteroids, defective antigen processing, and increased numbers of suppressor T cells. Among surgical patients, severe malnutrition, trauma, shock and sepsis suppress skin test responses, which become active again after resolution of the acute process.

4. Immunity in diabetes mellitus—Diabetes mellitus impairs immunity. Well-controlled diabetics resist infection normally except in tissues made ischemic by arterial disease, while uncontrolled diabetics do not. The mechanism is unknown, except that leukocytes from poorly controlled diabetics adhere, migrate, and kill bacteria poorly. They improve their performance when control is regained. Leukocytes also function poorly without insulin, and insulin is consumed in wounds and other poorly perfused spaces, resulting in low ambient insulin levels.

C. THE CLOSED SPACE

Most surgical infections start in a susceptible, usually poorly vascularized place in tissue such as a wound or a natural space. The common denominators are poor perfusion, local hypoxia, hypercapnia, and acidosis. Some natural spaces with narrow outlets, such as those of the appendix, gallbladder, ureters, and intestines, are especially prone to becoming obstructed and then infected.

The peritoneal and pleural cavities are potential spaces, and their surfaces slide over one another, thereby dispersing contaminating bacteria. However, foreign bodies, dead tissue, and injuries interfere with this mechanism and predispose to infection. Fibrin inhibits the clearing of bacteria. It polymerizes around bacteria, trapping them; this encourages abscess formation but at the same time prevents dangerous spread of infection.

Foreign bodies may have spaces in which bacteria can reside. Infarcted tissue is markedly susceptible to infection. Thrombosed veins, for example, rarely become infected unless intravenous catheters enter them and act as entry points for bacteria.

Spread of Surgical Infections

Surgical infections usually originate as a single focus and become dangerous by spreading and releasing toxins. Spreading occurs by several mechanisms.

A. NECROTIZING INFECTIONS

Necrotizing infections tend to spread along anatomically defined paths. Necrotizing fasciitis spreads along poorly perfused fascial and subcutaneous planes, its toxins causing thrombosis even of large vessels ahead of the necrotic area, thus creating more ischemic and vulnerable tissue.

B. ABSCESSES

If not promptly drained, abscesses enlarge, killing more tissue in the process. Leukocytes contribute to necrosis by releasing lysosomal enzymes during phagocytosis. Natural boundaries can be breached; eg, intestinal cutaneous fistulas may form, or blood vessel walls may be penetrated.

C. PHLEGMONS AND SUPERFICIAL INFECTIONS

Phlegmons contain little pus but much edema. They spread along fat planes and by contiguous necrosis, combining features of both of the above kinds of spread. Retroperitoneal peripancreatic inflammation or infection is typical. Superficial infections may spread along skin not only by contiguous necrosis but also by metastasis.

D. SPREAD OF INFECTION VIA THE LYMPHATIC SYSTEM

Lymphangitis produces red streaks in the skin and travels proximally along major lymph vessels. However, it may also occur in hidden places such as the retroperitoneum in puerperal sepsis.

E. SPREAD OF INFECTION VIA THE BLOODSTREAM

Empyema and endocarditis caused by intravenously injected contaminated drugs are now common. Brain abscesses resulting from infections elsewhere in the body (especially the face) occur in infants and diabetics. Liver abscesses may complicate appendicitis and inflammatory bowel disease, sometimes as a result of suppurative phlebitis of the portal vein (pylephlebitis).

Complications

A. FISTULAS AND SINUS TRACTS

Fistulas and sinus tracts often result when abdominal abscesses contiguous to bowel open to the skin. When tissue necrosis compounds the development of sinus tracts and erodes major blood vessels, severe bleeding may occur. This is most troublesome in irradiated tissue of nonhealing neck wounds and in infected groin wounds after vascular surgery.

Some intestinal fistulas originate in poorly fashioned or necrotic suture lines, and some result from contiguous abscesses that eventually penetrate both bowel and skin, often helped along by the surgeon who must drain the abscess.

B. SUPPRESSED WOUND HEALING

Suppressed wound healing is a consequence of infection. The mechanism is probably stimulation by bacteria of cytokines, which in turn stimulates proteolysis, especially collagenase production.

C. IMMUNOSUPPRESSION AND SUPERINFECTION

Immunosuppression is a common consequence of injury, which includes surgery, trauma, shock, or infection or sepsis. Superinfection occurs when immunosuppression provides an opportunity for invasion by opportunistic, often antibiotic-resistant organisms.

D. BACTEREMIA

The term bacteremia denotes the presence of bacteria in blood. The significance of bacteremia is variable. That which follows dental work is usually rapidly cleared and harmless, except in patients with damaged heart valves, cardiac, vascular, or orthopedic prostheses, or impaired immunity. It occurs predictably during instrumentation of the gastrointestinal tract or infected urinary tract. Patients in these groups are at increased risk and should receive an appropriate prophylactic antibiotic regimen.

E. ORGAN DYSFUNCTION, SEPSIS, AND THE SYSTEMIC INFLAMMATORY RESPONSE SYNDROME

Infection and tissue damage initiate the inflammatory response, a very tightly controlled, adaptive response to eliminate dead or infected tissue. At the site of injury, endothelial cells and leukocytes coordinate the local release of mediators of the inflammatory response, including cytokines (tumor necrosis factor-α), interleukins, interferons, leukotrienes, prostaglandins, nitric oxide, reactive oxygen species, and products of the classic inflammatory pathway (complement, histamine, and bradykinin) (Table 9–1). When localized to diseased tissue, these mediators are highly effective at recruiting and arming cells of the innate and adaptive immune systems to destroy invading organisms and elicit reparative mechanisms in wounded tissue. However, if the degree of the infectious or traumatic insult exceeds the ability of the host to contain it, the inflammatory response becomes systemic. The result is whole body activation of the inflammatory response, with resultant disruption of normal cellular metabolism and microcirculatory perfusion. This leads to clinical deterioration, manifested as dysfunction of the brain (delirium), lungs (hypoxia), heart and blood vessels (shock and edema), kidneys (oliguria), intestines (ileus), liver (hyperbilirubinemia), and the hematologic (coagulopathy, anemia)

and immunologic systems (immunosuppression). This syndrome is referred to as **multiple organ dysfunction syndrome (MODS).** The risks of organ failure in general are directly proportionate to the duration and severity of shock and inversely proportionate to the age and underlying health of the patient. It is frequently difficult or impossible to determine whether the cause of organ dysfunction in critically ill patients is severe infection or inflammation. Consensus definitions were therefore established in 1992. The term **sepsis** is used when the systemic response results from infection. In contrast, when the systemic response occurs in the absence of infection, as it does in severe burns, trauma, and pancreatitis, it is called **systemic inflammatory response syndrome (SIRS).** The interrelationships between infection, bacteremia, sepsis, and SIRS are depicted in Figure 9–1.

Diagnosis

The aim of management is to detect and treat sepsis before it evolves into more advanced stages.

A. PHYSICAL EXAMINATION

Physical examination is the easiest way to localize a surgical infection. When infection is suspected but cannot be found initially, repeated examination will often reveal subtle warmth, erythema, induration, tenderness, or splinting due to a developing abscess. Failure to repeat the physical examination is the most common reason for delayed diagnosis and therapy.

B. LABORATORY FINDINGS

1. General findings—Laboratory data are of limited value. Leukocytosis may give way to leukopenia when the infection is severe. Acidosis is helpful in diagnosis, and signs of disseminated intravascular coagulation are useful as well. Otherwise unexplained respiratory, hepatic, renal, and gastric (ie, stress ulcers) failure is strong evidence for sepsis.

2. Cultures—Positive cultures help to differentiate SIRS from sepsis even though 50% of cases of sepsis are culture-negative. If infection is suspected, cultures of blood, sputum, and urine are collected routinely initially, especially in hospitalized patients given the high frequency of nosocomial pneumonia and urinary tract infections (see below). Other fluids such as cerebrospinal fluid, pleural and joint effusions, and ascites can be aspirated and cultured based upon signs or symptoms that specifically indicate these sites as potential sources of infection. In general, pus from abscesses should be cultured unless the causative organism is known. In rapidly advancing cases, two separate blood cultures should be taken within 15 minutes. In less

Table 9–1. Cytokines and growth factors.

Peptide	Site of Synthesis	Regulation	Target Cells	Effects
G-CSF	Fibroblasts, monocytes	Induced by IL-1, LPS, IFN-α	Committed neutrophil progenitors (CFU-G, Gran)	Supports the proliferation of neutrophil-forming colonies. Stimulates respiratory burst.
GM-CSF (IL-3 has almost identical effects)	Endothelial cells, fibroblasts, macrophages, T lymphocytes, bone marrow	Induced by IL-1, TNF	Granulocyte-erythro-cyte-monocyte-megakaryocyte progenitor cells (CFU-GEMM, CFU-MEG, CFU-Eo, CFU-GM)	Supports the proliferation of macrophage-, eosinophil-, neutrophil-, and monocyte-containing colonies
IFNα, -β, -γ	Epithelial cells, fibroblasts, lymphocytes, macrophages, neutrophils	Induced by viruses (foreign nucleic acids), microbes, microbial foreign antigens, cancer cells	Lymphocytes, macrophages, infected cells, cancer cells	Inhibits viral multiplication. Activates defective phagocytes, direct inhibition of cancer cell multiplication, activation of killer leukocytes, inhibition of collagen synthesis.
IL-1	Endothelial cells, keratinocytes, lymphocytes, macrophages	Induced by TNF-α, IL-1, IL-2, C5a. Suppressed by IL-4, TGF-β	Monocytes, macrophages, T cells, B cells, NK cells, LAK cells	Stimulates T cells, B cells, NK cells, LAK cells. Induces tumoricidal activity and production to other cytokines, endogenous pyrogen (via PGE_2 release). Induces steroidogenesis, acute phase proteins, hypotension; chemotactic neutrophils. Stimulates respiratory burst.
IL-1ra	Monocytes	Induced by GM-CSF, LPS, IgG	Blocks type 1 IL-1 receptors on T cells, fibroblasts, chondrocytes, endothelial cells	Blocks type 1 IL-1 receptors on T cells, chondrocytes, endothelial cells. Ameliorates animal models of arthritis, septic shock, and inflammatory bowel disease.
IL-2	Lymphocytes	Induced by IL-1, IL-6	T cells, NK cells, B cells, activated monocytes	Stimulates growth of T cells, NK cells, and B cells
IL-4	T cells, NK cells, mast cells	Induced by cell activation, IL-1	All hematopoietic cells and many others express receptors	Stimulates B cell and T cell growth. Induces HLA class II molecules.
IL-6	Endothelial cells, fibroblasts, lymphocytes, some tumors	Induced by IL-1, TNF-α	T cells, B cells, plasma cells, keratinocytes, hepatocytes, stem cells	B cell differentiation. Induction of acute phase proteins, growth of keratinocytes. Stimulates growth of T cells and hematopoietic stem cells.
IL-8	Endothelial cells, fibroblasts, lymphocytes, monocytes	Induced by TNF, IL-1, LPS, cell adherence (monocytes)	Basophils, neutrophils, T cells	Induces expression of endothelial cell LECAM-1 receptors, β_2 integrins, and neutrophil transmigration. Stimulates respiratory burst.
M-CSF	Endothelial cells, fibroblasts, monocytes	Induced by IL-1, LPS, IFN-α	Committed monocyte progenitors (CFU-M, Mono)	Supports the proliferation of monocyte-forming colonies. Activates macrophages.
MCP-1, MCAF	Monocytes. Some tumors secrete a similar peptide.	Induced by IL-1, LPS, PHA	Unstimulated monocytes	Chemoattractant specific for monocytes

(continued)

Table 9–1. Cytokines and growth factors. (continued)

Peptide	Site of Synthesis	Regulation	Target Cells	Effects
TNF-α (LT has almost identical effects)	Macrophages, NK cells, T cells, transformed cell lines, B cells (LT)	Suppressed by PGE₂, TGF-β, IL-4. Induced by LPS.	Endothelial cells, monocytes, neutrophils	Stimulates T cell growth. Direct cytotoxin to some tumor cells. Profound proinflammatory effect via induction of IL-1 and PGE₂. Systemic administration produces many symptoms of sepsis. Stimulates respiratory burst and phagocytosis.

Key:
CFU   = Colony-forming unit
G-CSF   = Granulocyte colony-stimulating factor
GM-CSF = Granulocyte-macrophage colony-stimulating factor
IFN   = Interferon
IL   = Interleukin
IL1ra   = Interleukin-1 receptor antagonist
LPS   = Lipopolysaccharide
LT   = Lymphotoxin

MCAF   = Monocyte chemotactic and activating factor
M-CSF   = Macrophage colony-stimulating factor
MCPO-1 = Monocyte chemotactic peptide-1
NK   = Natural killer (cell)
PHA   = Phytohemagglutinin
TGF-β   = Transforming growth factor beta
TNF-α   = Tumor necrosis factor alpha

urgent situations, cultures should be taken over a 24-hour period, and up to six should be taken if the patient has a cardiac or joint prosthesis or vascular shunt. False-negative blood culture results occur in about 20% of cases. False-positive results are difficult to define, since skin commensals (even some diphtheroids and *Staphylococcus epidermidis*), regarded as contaminants in the past, have proved occasionally to be true pathogens. Arterial blood cultures may be necessary to detect fungal endocarditis.

C. Imaging Studies

Radiologic examination is frequently helpful, particularly for the diagnosis of pulmonary infections. Whenever infection is close to bone, radiologic examination is indicated to detect early signs of osteomyelitis, which might require more aggressive surgical or antibiotic therapy. CT scanning is useful for detecting abscesses in solid organs. CT scanning and ultrasonography are particularly useful in localizing occult infection. Numerous radionuclide scans have been tested, all with fair results. The best radionuclides for labeling leukocytes are gallium (⁶⁷Ga) and indium (¹¹¹In).

D. Source of Infection

An early diagnosis of sepsis is usually based on a combination of suspicion and inconclusive evidence, since the results of blood cultures are often unavailable during this stage. An important initial step is to identify the source. Surgical or traumatic wounds, surgical infections in the abdomen or thorax, and clostridial infections are all common, but so are urinary tract infections, pneumonia, and even sinus infections. Once identified, any septic focus amenable to surgical therapy should be excised or drained.

Treatment

A. Incision and Drainage

Abscesses must be opened and bacteria, necrotic tissue, and toxins drained to the outside. The pressure and the number of bacteria in the infected space are lowered; this decreases the spread of toxins and bacteria. An abscess with systemic manifestations is a surgical emergency.

Fluctuation is a reliable but late sign of a subcutaneous abscess. Abscesses in the parotid or perianal area may never become fluctuant, and if the surgeon waits for this sign, serious sepsis may result. Drainage creates an open wound, but the tissue will heal by second intention with remarkably little scarring. Deep abscesses

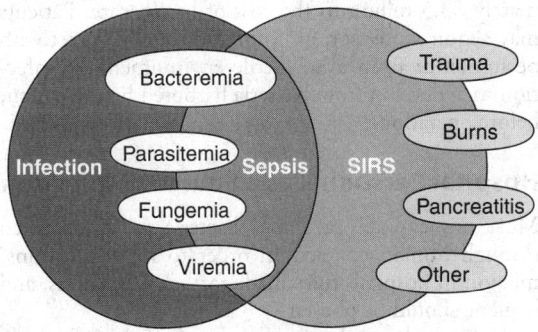

Figure 9–1. Interrelationships among systemic inflammatory response syndrome (SIRS), sepsis, and infection. (Modified, with permission, from Crit Care Med 1992;20:864.)

difficult to drain surgically may be drained by a catheter placed percutaneously under guidance by CT scanning or ultrasonography.

It may appear that a patient with sepsis cannot withstand operation. In fact, operation to drain an abscess may be the most important of all therapeutic measures. One can hardly imagine delaying removal of infarcted bowel because the patient is in shock. There is no substitute for obliteration of the focus of infection when it is surgically accessible.

B. EXCISION

Some surgical infections may be excised (eg, an infected appendix or gallbladder). In these cases, drainage may not be necessary, and the patient is cured on the operating table. Clostridial myositis may require amputation of the infected limb. The success of such operations is greatly facilitated by intensive specific antimicrobial therapy.

C. CIRCULATORY ENHANCEMENT

Just as infections due to vascular ischemia are cured by restoring arterial patency, chronic infections in poorly vascularized areas, as in osteoradionecrosis, may be cured by transplanting a functioning vascular bed (eg, a musculocutaneous flap or omental transposition) into the affected area.

D. ANTIBIOTICS

Antibiotics are not necessary for simple surgical infections that respond to incision and drainage alone—furuncles and uncomplicated wound infections. Infections likely to spread or persist require antibiotic therapy, best chosen on the basis of sensitivity tests. In "toxic" infections, including septic shock, antibiotics must be started promptly and empirically and the regimen modified later from the results of blood cultures. The choice of drugs must take into account the organisms most often cultured from similar infections in previous patients, the results of gram-stained smears, and specific characteristics of the patient. (See Antibiotics, below.)

E. NUTRITIONAL SUPPORT

In malnourished, septic, or severely traumatized patients, the ability to ward off or recover from infection is often enhanced by aggressive nutritional therapy. Specific measurable effects include improved immunocompetency and blunting or reversal of catabolism. Protection or restoration of visceral and skeletal muscle allows the patient to cough better and be more mobile.

Prognosis

The mortality rate ranges from 10% in septic patients with manifestations limited to fever, chills, and toxicity, to almost 100% in those who manifest shock and multiple organ failure. Factors that have independent influences on outcome include the causative microorganism, blood pressure, body temperature (inverse relationship), primary site of infection, age, predisposing factors, and place of acquisition of infection (hospital or home). Of patients with low-grade fever and an elevated leukocyte count after antibiotics have been discontinued, 60% will have a relapse. Nevertheless, continuation of antibiotics in questionable cases is often contraindicated because it only delays recognition of infection and may enhance its morbidity, as well as increasing antibiotic resistance.

American College of Chest Physicians/Society of Critical Care Medicine Consensus Conference: Definitions for sepsis and organ failure and guidelines for the use of innovative therapies in sepsis. Crit Care Med 1992;20:864.

Bone RC. Sir Isaac Newton, sepsis, SIRS, and CARS. Crit Care Med 1996;24:1125.

Bone RC et al: Definitions for sepsis and organ failure and guidelines for the use of innovative therapies in sepsis. The ACCP/SCCM Consensus Conference Committee. American College of Chest Physicians/Society of Critical Care Medicine. Chest 1992;101:1644.

Hoffman JA et al: Phylogenetic perspectives in innate immunity. Science 1999;284:1313.

Lederer JA et al: The effects of injury on the adaptive immune response. Shock 1999;11:153.

O'Grady NP et al: Practice parameters for evaluating new fever in critically ill adult patients. Task Force of the American College of Critical Care Medicine of the Society of Critical Care Medicine in collaboration with the Infectious Disease Society of America. Crit Care Med 1998;26:392.

NOSOCOMIAL INFECTIONS & INFECTION CONTROL

Nosocomial infections affect approximately 2 million patients annually in the United States and add approximately $3.5 billion to the cost of health care. Patients may acquire infection in hospital through contact with personnel or from a nonsterile environment, or infection may develop from bacteria harbored by the patient before operation.

Hospital Personnel as a Source of Infection

Most nosocomially acquired bacteria are transmitted through human contact. In order to minimize transmission in hospital, rules made for behavior, dress, and hygiene should be obeyed.

Unwashed hands are by far the most frequent sources of nosocomial infections such as pneumonia, intravenous catheter-related sepsis, burn wound infections, and even pseudomembranous colitis. Therefore, hand washing is the single most important procedure for preventing nosocomial infections. Routine hand washing should be a matter of reflex conditioning. In today's atmosphere, failure to wash one's hands between patient contacts in a hospital is essentially an unethical act.

The Operating Room as a Source of Infection

Any break in operative technique noted by any member of the operating team should be corrected immediately. Members of the team should not operate if they have cutaneous infections or upper respiratory or viral infections that may cause sneezing or coughing.

Scrub suits should be worn only in the operating room and not in other areas of the hospital. If they must be worn outside the operating room, they should be changed before reentering. Physicians and nurses should always wash their hands between patients. Careful hand washing should follow all contact with infected patients. For preoperative preparation, hands and forearms up to the elbows should be scrubbed for 2–5 minutes with any approved agent if the surgeon has not scrubbed within the past week. Shorter scrubs are allowable between operations. Traffic and talking in the operating room should be minimized.

Though many parts of the operating environment are sterile, the operative field is not—it is merely as sterile as it can be made. Attempts to achieve a level of sterility beyond normal standards have not led to further reductions in wound infection rates. This reflects the fact that bacteria are also present in the patient, and immune variables are also important determinants of infection not affected by more aggressive attempts to achieve sterility.

Many special and expensive techniques have been devised to minimize bacterial contamination in the operating room. Ultraviolet light, laminar flow ventilation, and elaborate architectural and ventilation schemes have been advocated, but none have proved more effective than common sense and surgical discipline.

The only completely reliable methods for sterilization of surgical instruments and supplies are steam under pressure (autoclaving), dry heat, and ethylene oxide gas. Saturated steam at 2 atm pressure and a temperature of 120 °C destroys all vegetative bacteria and most resistant dry spores in 13 minutes, but exposure of surgical instrument packs should usually be extended to 30 minutes to allow heat and moisture to penetrate to the center of the package. Shorter times are allowable for unwrapped instruments with the vacuum-cycle or high-pressure autoclaves now widely used. Continuous dry heat at 170 °C for 1 hour sterilizes articles that cannot tolerate moist heat. If grease or oil is present on in-struments, safe dry-heat sterilization requires 4 hours at 160 °C.

Gaseous ethylene oxide destroys bacteria, viruses, fungi, and various spores. It is used for heat-sensitive materials, including telescopic instruments, plastic and rubber goods, sharp and delicate instruments, electrical cords, and sealed ampules. It damages certain plastics and pharmaceuticals. The technique requires a special pressurized-gas autoclave, with 12% ethylene oxide and 88% Freon-12 at 55 °C, 8 psi pressure above atmospheric pressure. Most items must be aerated in sterile packages on the shelf for 24–48 hours before use in order to rid them of the dissolved gas. Implanted plastics should be stored for 7 days before use. Ethylene oxide is toxic and represents a safety hazard unless it is used according to strict regulations.

Miscellaneous sterilization procedures include soaking in antiseptics such as 2% glutaraldehyde to remove viruses from instruments with lenses. Total sterilization by this method requires 10 hours. Chemical antiseptics are often used to clean operating room surfaces and instruments that need not be totally sterile. Other disinfectant solutions include synthetic phenolics, polybrominated salicylanilides, iodophors, alcohols, other glutaraldehyde preparations, and 6% stabilized hydrogen peroxide. These agents maintain high potency in the presence of organic matter and usually leave effective residual antibacterial activity on surfaces. They are also used to clean anesthetic equipment that cannot be sterilized. Prepackaged instruments and supplies can be sterilized with gamma radiation by manufacturers. Synthetic fabrics have now proved to be superior barriers to bacteria and less costly than the traditional cotton. They can be used in gowns and drapes.

The Patient as a Source of Infection

When possible, preexisting infections should be treated before operation. Secretions from patients with a history of respiratory tract infections should be cultured and appropriate treatment given. The urinary tract should be cultured and specific antibiotics administered before instruments are introduced; this precaution has eliminated septic shock as a complication of urologic surgery. The colon should be prepared as discussed in Chapter 32.

Commensal bacteria on the patient's skin are a common cause of infection. Preoperative showers or baths with antiseptic soap reduce the infection rate in clean wounds by 50%. Shaving of the operative field hours prior to incision is associated with a 50% increase in wound infection rates and should not be done. If the patient has a heavy growth of hair, an area just large enough to accommodate the wound and its closure should be clipped rather than shaved immediately before operation. Razor shaving more than a few minutes before operation clearly raises the wound infection rate.

The skin to be included in the operative field should be cleansed with antiseptic. Nonirritating agents such as benzalkonium salts should be used in or around the nose or eyes. For other skin areas, the iodophors (eg, povidone-iodine) and chlorhexidine are used most commonly.

Isolation Procedures: Universal Precautions

Traditionally, patients with infection were individually isolated. In 1985—partly in response to the HIV epidemic—a more general kind of isolation called "universal precautions" has been substituted. In this system, *any* procedure involving close contact with *any* patient—and especially those involving contact with blood—is performed by hospital personnel wearing gloves and other protective devices. As blood is the single most important source of HIV and other blood-borne pathogens (eg, hepatitis B virus), the concept of universal precautions emphasizes (1) prevention of needlestick injuries, (2) the use of traditional barriers such as gloves and gowns, (3) the use of masks and eye coverings to prevent mucous membrane exposure during procedures, and (4) the use of individual ventilation devices when the need for resuscitation is predictable. The Centers for Disease Control and Prevention (CDC) recommends that universal precautions apply to blood, semen, and vaginal secretions; to amniotic, cerebrospinal, pericardial, peritoneal, pleural, and synovial fluids; and to other body fluids contaminated with blood. Universal precautions are not recommended for feces, nasal secretions, sputum, sweat, tears, urine, or vomitus unless they contain visible blood. The need for hand washing is not diminished by this system.

http://www.cdc.gov/ncidod/hip/isolat/isolat.htm

Antibiotic Prophylaxis Against Surgical Infections

Prophylactic use of antibiotics can decrease the incidence of infections, especially surgical site infections, but at the risk of toxic and allergic reactions to the drug, drug interactions, bacterial resistance, and superinfection. The principles of antibiotic prophylaxis are simple: (1) Choose antibiotics effective against the expected type of contamination. (2) Use antibiotics only if the risk of infection justifies doing so. (3) Give antibiotics in appropriate doses and at appropriate times. (4) Stop dosing before the risk of side effects outweighs benefits.

Antibiotics for preventive use must not be highly toxic and should not be "first-line" antibiotics for treatment of established infection. Because resistance to antibiotics may develop quickly, agents that have been used frequently for prophylaxis are likely to lose their effectiveness for later treatment. Prophylactic agents should be chosen for cost-effectiveness and safety as well as for efficacy.

Prophylactic antibiotics should be selected to combat the organisms most likely to be encountered in the anticipated operative procedure. A first-generation cephalosporin (eg, cefazolin) is preferred for most procedures since it is effective against common gram-positive and gram-negative bacteria and has a moderately long serum half-life. The routine use of vancomycin for prophylaxis is discouraged in light of the emergence of vancomycin-resistant organisms—especially enterococcus and staphylococcus. Agents with better gram-negative and anaerobic bacterial activity (eg, cefoxitin, cefotetan) are preferred for colorectal and gynecologic procedures. A single dose of antibiotic given 30 minutes prior to making the skin incision should provide adequate tissue concentrations for most procedures. Additional doses are advisable for longer procedures (over 4 hours) or those that require large volumes of resuscitative fluids (larger volume of distribution). Postoperative doses of prophylactic antibiotics are usually not necessary. The American Heart Association recommends that patients with valvular heart disease or prosthetic heart valves receive antibiotics prior to procedures that result in bacteremia in order to prevent endocarditis. A similar argument has been made for patients with indwelling prosthetic joints.

Antibiotic prophylaxis cannot and is not intended to eliminate bacteria. Use of multiple antibiotics increases the risk of drug reactions, diminishes effectiveness in the long run by promoting the emergence of resistant strains, and increases costs. Antibiotics should be given only when a significant rate of infection is encountered without them or when the consequences of infection would be disastrous, as with placement of vascular, cardiac, or joint prostheses.

The surgeon may be tempted to give every patient antibiotics in order to have an infection-free record, but there are several reasons why this strategy is not appropriate: (1) Clean wounds may become infected with organisms for which prophylactic antibiotics are ineffective. (2) Resistant organisms will eventually develop, creating a higher risk of infection within the hospital. (3) The expense and risks associated with antibiotics (eg, kidney failure, hearing loss, anaphylaxis, skin rashes, fungal infections, enterocolitis) overshadow the minimal beneficial effects of using antibiotics in clean cases. The number of antibiotic-resistant strains has been correlated with the number of kilograms of antibiotics used in any given hospital.

In the usual case, prophylactic antibiotics should be stopped a few hours after operation. If contamination will be possible for an extended period—as when intravascular lines remain in patients with cardiac prostheses—prophylaxis may be continued. However, the longer the period of contamination, the less effective will be the antibiotics.

Control of Infection Within the Hospital

Considering the cost of infection in both lives and money, infection control is a very sound investment. Data indicate that infection control programs can prevent approximately one-third of nosocomial infections. Consequently, the Joint Commission on Accreditation of Hospitals in the USA requires each hospital to have an infection control committee. This committee is expected to establish infection control procedures, with rules for isolation of infected patients and for protection of hospital personnel exposed to infection. In addition, the committee establishes procedures for disposal of materials contaminated by bacteria as well as guidelines for limiting the spread of infection. Infection control personnel usually record and analyze patterns of infection. Isolates of bacteria cultured from patients are routinely analyzed for potential significance to the hospital environment. Attempts are made to determine the source of "epidemics." These efforts are coordinated at the national level by the CDC's National Nosocomial Infections Surveillance (NNIS) system, established in 1970 to monitor and report nosocomial infection trends. These data are then used to generate recommendations and guidelines to improve outcomes.

Antimicrobial prophylaxis in surgery. Med Lett Drugs Ther 1999;41:75.

CDC Guidelines on Prevention of Nosocomial Infections, Hospital Infections Program, Centers for Disease Control and Prevention: http://www.cdc.gov/ncidod/hip/

■ SPECIFIC TYPES OF INFECTIONS

SURGICAL SITE INFECTIONS

Surgical site infections, previously called postoperative wound infections, result from bacterial contamination during or after a surgical procedure. The most recent data from the NNIS of the CDC indicate that surgical site infections are the third most frequently reported nosocomial infection, accounting for 14–16% of all nosocomial infections in acutely hospitalized patients. Among surgical patients, surgical site infections are the most frequent cause of such infections, accounting for 38% of the total.

Infection usually is confined to the subcutaneous tissues. Despite every effort to maintain asepsis, most surgical wounds are contaminated to some extent. However, infection rarely develops if contamination is minimal, if the wound has been made without undue injury, if the subcutaneous tissue is well perfused and well oxygenated, and if there is no dead space. The criteria used to define surgical site infections have been standardized and describe three different anatomic levels of infection (see Table 9–2).

The degree of intraoperative contamination can be divided into four categories: (1) clean (no gross contamination from exogenous or endogenous sources); (2) lightly contaminated (clean-contaminated); (3) heavily contaminated; and (4) infected (in which obvious infection has been encountered during operation). The infection rate is about 1.5% in clean cases. Clean-contaminated wounds (eg, with gastric or biliary surgery) are infected about 2–5% of the time. Heavily contaminated wounds, as in operations on the unprepared colon or emergency operations for intestinal bleeding or perforation, may have an infection risk of 5–30%. Wise use of isolation techniques, preoperative antibiotics, and delayed primary closure will keep rates of surgical site infections within acceptable limits. Since even a minor surgical site infection significantly prolongs hospitalization and increases economic loss, all reasonable efforts must be made to keep the infection rate as low as possible.

The risk of wound infection is influenced but not entirely determined by the degree of contamination. Multiple patient risk factors and perioperative characteristics can increase the likelihood of surgical site infections (Table 9–3)

The susceptibility of the host is usually but not always local. Susceptibility is also proportionate to the oxygen tension in the operative wound. Wound tissue P_{O_2} in turn is proportionate to arterial P_{O_2} and the per-

Table 9–2. Types of surgical site infections (SSIs).

Incisional SSIs
Superficial incisional (skin and subcutaneous tissues)
Deep incisional (deeper soft tissues of the incision)
Organ/space SSIs
Any part of the anatomy other than body wall layers that was manipulated during the procedure

Table 9–3. Surgical site infection risk factors.

Patient characteristics
   Diabetes mellitus
   Nicotine (cigarette smoking)
   Steroids
   Malnutrition
   Nares colonization with *S aureus*
   Poor skin hygiene
Perioperative characteristics
   Operative site shaving the night before surgery
   Breaks in operative sterile technique
   Infected or colonized surgical personnel (skin or surgical
      attire)
   Poor operating room air quality (contaminated ventilation)
   Colonized operating room instruments or environment
   Poor wound care postoperatively

---

fusion rate. The perfusion rate is generally determined by the cardiac output and by the tone of the sympathetic nervous system. Sympathetic tone, ie, the degree of peripheral vasoconstriction, is determined by the patient's surface temperature, the degree of pain, the blood volume, and the degree of fear. Therefore, susceptibility to infection can be reduced by such simple methods as rapid infusion of additional fluids, warming, better pain control, and oxygen administration (but only after perfusion has been ensured). Contrary to popular opinion, urinary output correlates poorly with the incidence of wound infection. When the infection risk is high, wound tissue PO_2 can be measured, monitored, and supported. Appropriate technology is available.

Clinical Findings

Wound infections usually appear between the fifth and tenth days after surgery, but they may appear as early as the first postoperative day or even years later. The first sign is usually fever, and postoperative fever requires inspection of the wound. The patient may complain of wound pain. The wound rarely appears severely inflamed, but edema may be obvious because the skin sutures appear tight.

Palpation of the wound may disclose an abscess. A good method is to pour surgical soap on the wound and, using it as a lubricant, palpate gently with the gloved hand. Firm or fluctuant areas, crepitus, or tenderness can be detected with minimal pain and contamination. The rare infection deep to the fascia may be difficult to recognize. In doubtful cases, one can carefully open the wound in the suspicious area using meticulous sterile technique. If no pus is present, the wound can be closed immediately with skin tapes. Cul-

tures even of clean wounds that are successfully reclosed are often positive.

Differential Diagnosis

Differential diagnosis includes all other causes of postoperative fever, wound dehiscence, and wound herniation (see Chapter 4).

Prevention

Detailed recommendations for the prevention of surgical site infections (and the relevant supporting data) have been published by the CDC. In general, there are three main aspects to prevention of infection: (1) careful, gentle, clean surgery; (2) reduction of contamination; and (3) support of the patient's defenses, including use of prophylactic antibiotics. The surgeon who traumatizes tissue, leaves foreign bodies or hematomas in wounds, uses too many ligatures, and exposes the wound to drying or pressure from retractors is exposing patients to needless risks of infection.

The purpose of sutures is to approximate tissues and hold them securely, and the right number to use is as few as will accomplish this aim. Since sutures strangulate tissue, they should be tied as loosely as the requirements of approximation permit. Subcutaneous sutures should be used rarely. Using skin tapes instead of skin sutures or staples lowers infection rates, especially in contaminated wounds.

Severely contaminated wounds in which subcutaneous infection is likely to develop are best left open initially and managed by delayed primary closure. This means that the deep layers are closed while skin and subcutaneous tissues are left open, dressed with sterile gauze, inspected on the fourth or fifth day, and then closed (preferably with skin tapes) if no sign of infection is seen. A clean granulating open wound is preferable to a wound infection. Scarring from secondary healing is usually minimal.

Prophylactic antibiotics are indicated whenever wound contamination during the operation can be predicted to be high (eg, operations on the colon). Excessively liberal use of antibiotics is not reasonable. The incidence of postoperative infections in clean operations is not diminished by administration of antimicrobials, and the prophylactic use of these drugs must be reserved for selected cases at high risk for infection.

Treatment

The basic treatment of established wound infection is to open the wound and allow it to drain. Antibiotics are not necessary unless the infection is invasive, manifested by a surrounding zone of soft tissue inflammation (erythema and edema). Culture should be performed to help locate the source and prevent further infection in other patients; to gain a preview of bacterial flora in case other infections develop deep to the wound or in case the existing infection becomes invasive; and to select preoperative antibiotics in case the wound must be entered again.

Prognosis

Most wound infections make illness more severe. Wound infection correlates positively with death rates but is not often the cause of death. It may tip the scales against successful operation.

Bergamini TM et al: The importance of tissue antibiotic activity in the prevention of operative wound infection. J Antimicrob Chemother 1989;23:303.

Culver DH et al: Surgical wound infection rates by wound class, operative procedure, and patient risk index. National Nosocomial Infections Surveillance System. Am J Med 1991; 91:152S.

CELLULITIS

Cellulitis is a common invasive nonsuppurative infection of connective tissue. The term is loosely used and often misapplied. The microscopic picture is one of severe inflammation of the dermal and subcutaneous tissues. Although PMNs predominate, there is no gross suppuration except perhaps at the portal of entry.

Clinical Findings

Cellulitis usually appears on an extremity as a brawny red or reddish-brown area of edematous skin. It advances rapidly from its starting point, and the advancing edge may be vague or sharply defined (eg, in erysipelas). A surgical wound, puncture, skin ulcer, or patch of dermatitis is usually identifiable as a portal of entry. The disease often occurs in susceptible patients, eg, alcoholics with postphlebitic leg ulcers. Most cases are caused by streptococci or staphylococci, but other bacteria have been involved. A moderate or high fever is almost always present.

Lymphangitis arising from cellulitis produces red, warm, tender streaks 3–4 mm wide leading from the infection along lymphatic vessels to the regional lymph nodes. There is no suppuration. Bacteria are difficult to obtain for culture, but blood culture is sometimes positive.

Differential Diagnosis

Since the visible features of cellulitis are all due to inflammation, the words inflammation and cellulitis have sometimes been used imprecisely as synonyms. Some forms of inflammation are associated with suppuration

requiring incision and drainage, whereas cellulitis as such is not.

Thrombophlebitis is often difficult to differentiate from cellulitis, but phlebitic swelling is usually greater, and tenderness may localize over a vein. Homans' sign does not always make the differentiation—nor does lymphadenopathy. Fever is usually greater with cellulitis, and pulmonary embolization does not occur in cellulitis.

Contact allergy, such as poison oak, may mimic cellulitis in its early phase, but dense nonhemorrhagic vesiculation soon discloses the allergic cause.

Chemical inflammation due to drug injection may also mimic streptococcal cellulitis.

The appearance of hemorrhagic bullae and skin necrosis suggests necrotizing fasciitis.

Treatment

Therapy should consist of rest, elevation, warm packs, and an oral or intravenous antibiotic. Warm packs elevate subcutaneous tissue temperature, and if regional blood supply is normal they can raise local oxygen tension, which should support clearing of infection. Semisynthetic penicillins or first-generation cephalosporins are usually effective. If a clear response has not occurred in 12–24 hours, one should suspect an abscess or consider the possibility that the causative agent is a gram-negative rod or resistant organism. The patient must be examined once daily or more often to detect a hidden abscess masquerading within or under an area of cellulitis.

DIFFUSE NECROTIZING INFECTIONS

These infections are particularly dangerous because they frequently are difficult to diagnose, extremely toxic, and spread rapidly, often leading to limb amputation. It is for these reasons that the popular press recently characterized the causative bacteria as "flesh-eating" or "meat-eating." Although several classification systems for diffuse necrotizing infections have been published, most are not practical since they are based upon historical descriptions and eponyms. The American College of Surgeons recently published a classification system based on clinical presentation, anatomic site of primary tissue involvement, and the microbiology of the causative organisms (Table 9–4). The four known pathogenic factors are the presence of an anaerobic wound, bacterial exotoxins, bacterial synergy, and thrombosis of nutrient bridging vessels.

Classification & Clinical Findings

A. CLOSTRIDIAL INFECTIONS

Clostridia are saprophytes. Vegetative and spore forms are widespread in soil, sand, clothing, and feces. They

Table 9–4. Classification of diffuse necrotizing infections.

Clostridial
Necrotizing cellulitis
Myositis
Nonclostridial
Necrotizing fasciitis
Streptococcal gangrene

are generally fastidious anaerobes requiring a low redox potential to grow and to initiate conversion of the spores into vegetative, toxin-producing pathogens. Tissue redox potentials in vivo are diminished by impaired blood supply, muscle injury, pressure from casts, severe local edema, foreign bodies, or oxygen-consuming organisms. On Gram stain they appear as relatively large, gram-positive, rod-shaped bacteria. Clostridial infections frequently occur in the presence of other bacteria, especially gram-negative bacilli. A broad spectrum of disease is caused by clostridia, ranging from negligible surface contamination through invasive cellulitis of connective tissue to invasive anaerobic infection of muscle with massive tissue necrosis and profound shock. Six species cause infection in humans; *Clostridium perfringens* (80% of cases), *C novyi,* and *C septicum* are the species most frequently isolated.

Clostridia proliferate and produce toxins that diffuse into the surrounding tissue. *C tetani* and *C botulinum* produce extremely potent biologic toxins. As the pathogens responsible for tetanus and food-borne botulism, respectively, they owe their virulence to their toxigenicity (see below). Other clostridia, however, are highly invasive. For example, *C perfringens* produces a large number of exotoxins that destroy the local microcirculation. This allows further invasion, which can advance at an astonishing rate. The alpha toxin, a necrotizing lecithinase, is thought to be particularly important in this sequence, but other toxins, including collagenase, hyaluronidase, leukocidin, protease, lipase, and hemolysin, also contribute. When the disease has advanced sufficiently, toxins enter the systemic circulation, causing the features of SIRS and, if untreated, ultimately septic shock, multiple organ dysfunction syndrome (MODS), and death. The severity and progress of the local lesion can be judged by the general state of the patient as well as by the local signs of infection. Immunosuppressed patients are particularly susceptible.

Many open wounds are superficially infected or contaminated with clostridia without developing significant infections. The condition is not invasive because the surrounding tissue is basically healthy and the clostridia are confined to necrotic surface tissue. De-

bridement of dead surface tissue is usually the only treatment necessary. A crepitant abscess or cellulitis has a characteristic brown seropurulent exudate and mousy odor. Invasion is usually superficial to the deep fascia and may spread very quickly, producing discoloration of the skin. Delayed or inadequate debridement of injured tissue after devascularizing injury is the most common setting. Severe pain suggests extension into muscle compartments (myositis). The disease characteristically progresses rapidly, with loss of blood supply to the infected muscle. Profound shock can appear early, rapidly leading to organ dysfunction (MODS). Air bubbles—often visible on plain radiographs (gas gangrene)—and crepitus may be present. However, gas in the tissues is not a good differentiating point, since some clostridial species do not produce gas (eg, *C novyi*); since nonclostridial organisms often produce gas (eg, *E coli*); and since air can enter tissues through a penetrating wound.

B. NONCLOSTRIDIAL INFECTIONS

Necrotizing fasciitis is caused by multiple nonclostridial bacterial pathogens. Infection usually involves a mixed microbial flora, often including microaerophilic streptococci, staphylococci, aerobic gram-negative bacteria, and anaerobes, especially peptostreptococci and bacteroides. Fasciitis usually begins in a localized area such as a puncture wound, leg ulcer, or surgical wound. The infection spreads along the relatively ischemic fascial planes, leading to thrombosis of penetrating vessels. Overlying subcutaneous tissue and skin are thus devascularized. Externally, hemorrhagic bullae are usually the first sign of skin death. The skin is usually anesthetic, and crepitus is occasionally present. The fascial necrosis is usually wider than the skin appearance indicates. The patient often seems alert and unconcerned but appears toxic. At operation, the finding of edematous, dull-gray, and necrotic fascia and subcutaneous tissue confirms the diagnosis. Thrombi in penetrating vessels are often visible.

Group A streptococcus *(S pyogenes)* is a bacterium frequently found on the skin and in the throat. Severe invasive infections with group A streptococci associated with shock and organ failure (streptococcal gangrene) are uncommon but have been reported with increasing frequency since the 1980s. This type of infection is also referred to as streptococcal toxic shock syndrome. The incidence of these infections was one to ten cases per 100,000 population in the United States in 1998. Those with chronic immunosuppressive illnesses such as cancer, diabetes, and end-stage renal disease and those taking corticosteroids are at increased risk.

Streptococcal organisms release at least five different types of exotoxins. The sudden onset of severe pain is the most common presenting symptom, usually in an extremity associated with a wound. Fever and other signs of systemic infection are frequently present at the time of presentation. Shock and renal dysfunction are usually present within the first 24 hours after admission. Invasion of deeper layers, especially muscle, is uncommon.

Treatment

The major emphasis in treatment is inevitably surgical. Suspicion should be directed toward any wound incurred out of doors and contaminated with a foreign body, soil, or feces and any wound in which tissue (particularly muscle) has been extensively injured. This type of wound should be carefully examined, with the patient under sufficient anesthesia to permit full inspection and debridement of devitalized tissue, including muscle.

It is often difficult to distinguish necrotic from edematous tissue. Careful daily inspections of the wound will determine whether repeated debridement will be necessary. Daily debridement under anesthesia may be required, since these lesions are extensive and the degree of tissue viability is often difficult to assess in the operating room. Tight fascial compartments must be decompressed. Wide-open drainage is essential and may require extensive denudation. A functional extremity can usually be salvaged in fasciitis; if not, amputation can be safely performed later.

It is important to avoid confusing fasciitis with deep gangrene. It is a tragic error to amputate an extremity when removal of dead skin and fascia will suffice. Immediate amputation is necessary when there is diffuse myositis with complete loss of blood supply or when adequate debridement would clearly leave a useless limb. When viability of the remaining tissue is assured and the infection has been controlled, soft tissue deficits can be covered with skin grafts.

Antibiotics are often essential but are ineffective without surgical control of the disease. Given the polymicrobial nature of many necrotizing infections and the difficulty of distinguishing them clinically, broad-spectrum antibiotic therapy is indicated. Two useful regimens are (1) intravenous penicillin and an aminoglycoside plus clindamycin; and (2) intravenous imipenem-cilastatin. Some authorities recommend also giving immune globulin (400 mg/kg/d intravenously for 5 days) for documented streptococcal toxic shock syndrome. Gram stain and culture of the infected tissue will help to narrow the antibiotic spectrum once bacterial sensitivities are available.

In severe cases of infection, the importance of resuscitative therapy cannot be overemphasized. Debridement often leaves a large raw surface that may bleed extensively and contribute to massive insensible water losses. Intravascular volume must be maintained by infusions of crystalloid; plasma and blood are transfused as needed to correct coagulopathy or anemia. Diabetes mellitus, if present, must be treated aggressively.

Hyperbaric oxygenation has been reported anecdotally to be beneficial in treating clostridial infections, but it cannot replace surgical therapy since no amount of increased arterial PO_2 can force oxygen into dead tissue. Hyperbaric oxygen inhibits bacterial invasion but does not eliminate the focus of infection.

Prognosis

Diffuse necrotizing infections are potentially lethal diseases. With adequate treatment, deaths should occur only when treatment is delayed or when patients are already severely ill with other comorbidities (eg, diabetes mellitus) or have advanced bacterial invasion of vital structures. About 20% of patients with necrotizing fasciitis and more than half of patients with streptococcal toxic shock syndrome die. The prognosis for salvage of functioning limbs is not favorable. Limbs affected with myonecrosis often become useless and must be amputated to save life.

Stevens DL: Streptococcal toxic-shock syndrome: spectrum of disease, pathogenesis, and new concepts in treatment. Emerg Infect Dis 1995;1:69.

FURUNCLE, CARBUNCLE, & HIDRADENITIS

Furuncles and carbuncles are cutaneous abscesses (primary pyodermas) that begin in skin glands and hair follicles. Hair follicles normally contain bacteria. Furuncles (boils) usually start in infected hair follicles, though some are caused by retained foreign bodies and other injuries. If the pilosebaceous apparatus becomes obstructed at the skin level, the development of a furuncle can be anticipated. Because the base of the hair follicle may lie in subcutaneous tissue, the infection can spread as cellulitis or it can form a subcutaneous abscess. If a furuncle results from confluent infection of hair follicles, a central core of skin may become necrotic and will slough when the abscess is drained. Furuncles may take a phlegmonous form, ie, extend into the subcutaneous tissue, forming a long, flat abscess. A carbuncle is a deep-seated mass of fistulous tracts between infected hair follicles. Furuncles are the most common surgical infections, but carbuncles are rare.

Furuncles can be multiple and recurrent (furunculosis). Furunculosis usually occurs in young adults and is associated with hormonal changes resulting in impaired skin function. The commonest organisms are staphylococci and anaerobic diphtheroids.

Hidradenitis suppurativa is a serious skin infection of the axillae or groin consisting of multiple abscesses of the apocrine sweat glands. The condition often becomes chronic and disabling. The cause is unknown but may involve a defect of terminal follicular epithelium.

Clinical Findings

Furuncles itch and cause pain. The skin first becomes red and then turns white and necrotic over the top of the abscess. There is usually some surrounding erythema and induration. Regional nodes may become enlarged. Systemic symptoms are rare.

Carbuncles usually start as furuncles, but the infection dissects through the dermis and subcutaneous tissue in a myriad of connecting tunnels. Many of these small extensions open to the surface, giving the appearance of large furuncles with many pustular openings. As carbuncles enlarge, the blood supply to the skin is destroyed and the central tissue becomes necrotic. Carbuncles on the back of the neck are seen almost exclusively in diabetic patients or other relatively immunocompromised patients. The patient is usually febrile and mildly toxic. This is a serious problem that demands immediate surgical attention. Diabetes or some other immunosuppressive condition (eg, HIV disease) must be suspected and treated when a carbuncle is found.

Differential Diagnosis

On occasion, the surgeon may be confronted with a localized area of erythema and induration without obvious suppuration. Many such lesions will go on to central suppuration and become obvious furuncles. On the other hand, when these lesions are located near joints or over the tibia or when they are widely distributed, one must consider such differential diagnoses as rheumatoid nodules, gout, bursitis, synovitis, erythema nodosum, fungal infections, some benign or malignant skin tumors, and inflamed (but not usually infected) sebaceous or epithelial inclusion cysts.

Hidradenitis is differentiated from furunculosis by skin biopsy, which shows typical involvement of the apocrine sweat glands. One suspects hidradenitis when abscesses are concentrated in the apocrine gland areas, ie, the axillae, groin, and perineum. Carbuncles are rarely confused with any other condition.

Complications

Any of these infections may cause suppurative phlebitis when located near major veins. This is particularly important when the infection is located near the nose or eyes. Central venous thrombosis in the brain is a serious complication, and abscesses on the face usually must be treated with antibiotics as well as by prompt incision and drainage.

Hidradenitis may disable the patient but rarely has systemic manifestations. Carbuncles on the back of the neck may in rare cases lead to epidural abscess and meningitis.

Treatment

The classic therapy for furuncle is drainage, not antibiotics. Invasive carbuncles, however, must be treated by excision and antibiotics. Between these two extremes, the use of antibiotics depends on the location of the abscess and the extent of infection.

Patients with recurrent furunculosis may be diabetic or immunodeficient. Approximately 50% of patients in a recent study had impaired neutrophil function; treatment with vitamin C appeared to improve neutrophil function and the clinical response. Frequent washing with soaps containing hexachlorophene or other disinfectants is advisable. It may also be necessary to advise extensive laundering of all personal clothing and disinfection of the patient's living quarters in order to reduce the reservoirs of bacteria.

When an abscess fails to resolve after a superficial incision, the surgeon must look for a small opening to a deeper and larger subcutaneous abscess, ie, a **collar-button abscess.**

Carbuncles are often more extensive than the external appearance indicates. Incision alone is almost always inadequate, and excision with electrocautery is required. Excision is continued until the many sinus tracts are removed—usually far beyond the cutaneous evidence of suppuration. It is sometimes necessary to produce a large open wound. This may appear to be drastic treatment, but it achieves rapid cure and prevents further spread. The large wound usually contracts to a small scar and does not usually require skin grafting, because carbuncles tend to occur in loose skin on the back of the neck and on the buttocks, where contraction is the predominant form of repair.

Hidradenitis is usually treated by drainage of the individual abscess followed by careful hygiene. The patient must avoid astringent antiperspirants and deodorants. Painting with mild disinfectants is sometimes helpful. Fungal infections should be searched for if healing after drainage does not occur promptly. If none of these measures is successful, the apocrine sweat-bearing skin must be excised; if the deficit is large, closure with a skin graft may be indicated. The choice of antibiotic must reflect the frequent polymicrobial origin of these infections, including mixed aerobic and anaerobic bacteria. Topical clindamycin was beneficial in a randomized controlled trial. In a separate trial, systemic therapy with tetracycline yielded similar results when compared with topical clindamycin. Isotretinoin may be useful in some cases.

Brook I et al: Aerobic and anaerobic microbiology of axillary hidradenitis suppurativa. J Med Microbiol 1999;48:103.

Brown TJ et al: Hidradenitis suppurativa. South Med J 1998; 91:1107.

Jemec GB et al: Topical clindamycin versus systemic tetracycline in the treatment of hidradenitis suppurativa. J Am Acad Dermatol 1998;39:971.

Levy R et al: Vitamin C for the treatment of recurrent furunculosis in patients with impaired neutrophil functions. J Infect Dis 1996;173:1502.

ANTIBIOTIC-ASSOCIATED COLITIS

The incidence of colonic dysfunction secondary to antibiotic use is increasing. Aminopenicillins, cephalosporins, and clindamycin are most often implicated. Illness results from antibiotic-induced decreases in normal colonic flora, with resultant overgrowth of the responsible organism, usually *C difficile.* These bacteria, normally present in the feces of 5% of healthy persons, can release two types of toxins (cytotoxin A and cytotoxin B) that induce inflammation and mucosal damage. The spectrum of disease ranges from diarrhea to severe, potentially life-threatening colitis associated with mucosal ulceration, bacteremia, and septic shock. The pathognomonic finding on colonoscopy is an elevated, yellow pseudomembrane of necrotic mucosa ("pseudomembranous colitis"). The clinical presentation is characterized by fever, abdominal distention, and usually copious diarrhea in postoperative patients who are being given or have been given antibiotics. Stool smear shows many leukocytes and may show gram-positive bacilli. The stool shows a rising titer of *C difficile* toxin. Other organisms that rarely cause colitis include salmonella species, *Clostridium perfringens, Candida albicans,* and *Staphylococcus aureus.*

Treatment includes intravenous fluid resuscitation, correction of electrolyte disorders, and withdrawal of antibiotics. Severe cases are treated with metronidazole, 250 mg orally four times per day, until either toxin titers or culture results are available. Ten days of oral therapy completes a full course of treatment. Oral vancomycin is also effective but should be reserved for those who are critically ill or who have not responded to metronidazole—or in whom this agent is contraindicated because of allergy. Recurrence of symptoms, which occurs in up to 20% of cases, requires repeated antibiotic treatment; many experts also recommend adjunctive attempts to normalize colonic flora.

Spread is nosocomial, and poor hand washing has been implicated in several outbreaks.

Cleary RK: *Clostridium difficile*-associated diarrhea and colitis: clinical manifestations, diagnosis, and treatment. Dis Colon Rectum 1998;41:1435.

Cunha BA: Nosocomial diarrhea. Crit Care Clin 1998;14:329.

Frost F et al: Increasing hospitalization and death possibly due to *Clostridium difficile* diarrheal disease. Emerg Infect Dis 1998; 4:619.

Surawicz CM et al: Pseudomembranous colitis: causes and cures. Digestion 1999;60:91.

TETANUS

Tetanus is a specific anaerobic infection mediated by a neurotoxin that causes nervous irritability and tetanic muscular contractions. The causative organism, *Clostridium tetani,* enters and flourishes in hypoxic wounds contaminated with soil or feces (eg, deep puncture from stepping on a nail). The tetanus-prone wound is usually a puncture wound or one containing devitalized tissue or a foreign body. The occurrence of tetanus in the United States has dropped over the last 5 decades; the lowest annual average ever was reported recently (41 cases, 1995–1997). This improvement is attributed to the increasingly widespread use of tetanus toxoid and improved wound management (see below), including the use of prophylaxis against tetanus in emergency rooms. Tetanus continues to be a severe disease primarily of older adults who are unvaccinated or inadequately vaccinated; during 1995–1997, a disproportionately high number of cases (35%) were reported in persons aged 60 or older.

Tetanus is a clinical diagnosis, as confirmatory laboratory tests are not routinely available. Wound isolation of the organism is neither sensitive nor specific. Symptoms of tetanus may occur as soon as 1 day following exposure or as long as several months later; the median incubation period is 7 days. The first symptoms are usually pain or tingling in the area of injury, limitation of movements of the jaw ("lockjaw"), and spasms of the facial muscles (risus sardonicus). These are followed typically by stiffness of the neck, dysphagia, and laryngospasm. In more severe cases, spasms of the muscles of the back produce opisthotonos. As chest and diaphragm spasms occur, longer and longer periods of apnea follow. The temperature is normal or slightly elevated. The severity of cases varies widely; some are very mild and barely recognizable.

The Centers for Disease Control and Prevention regularly revises its recommendations for the prevention and treatment of tetanus (www.cdc.gov/nip). Importantly, serosurveys indicate that at least 40% of adults over the age of 60 may lack protective levels of circulating tetanus antitoxin. Because people of all ages are exposed to tetanus, each person should be actively immunized with tetanus toxoid, beginning with routine childhood immunization and continuing with booster injections every 10 years. It is thus imperative that all patients with traumatic wounds be queried regarding previous tetanus prophylaxis. Tetanus prophylaxis in injured patients depends on the history of immunization and the type of wound. A tetanus-diphtheria (Td) booster (active immunization for clean wounds), tetanus immune globulin (TIG; passive immunization for contaminated wounds), or both may be indicated.

If established tetanus is suspected, intensive treatment should be started immediately. Mainstays of therapy include neutralization of the toxin with TIG, excision and debridement of the suspected wound, intravenous high-dose penicillin, ventilatory support if indicated, and protection from sudden stimuli. The death rate is approximately 18% in established tetanus. An attack of tetanus does not confer lasting immunity, and patients who have recovered from the disease require active immunization according to the usual recommended schedules.

[CDC National Immunization Program—Epidemiology and Prevention of Vaccine-Preventable Diseases]

http://www.cdc.gov/nip/publications/pink/tetanus.pdf

Diphtheria, tetanus, and pertussis: recommendations for vaccine use and other preventive measures: recommendations of the Immunization Practices Advisory Committee (ACIP), Centers for Disease Control. MMWR Morb Mortal Wkly Rep 1991;40(RR-10):1.

Tetanus surveillance: United States, 1991–1994. MMWR Morb Mortal Wkly Rep 1997;46(SS-2):15.

Tetanus surveillance: United States, 1995–1997. MMWR Morb Mortal Wkly Rep 1998;47(SS-2):1.

RABIES

Rabies is a preventable viral encephalitis of mammals transmitted through the saliva of an infected animal. Humans are usually inoculated by the bite of a rabid bat, raccoon, skunk, fox, or other wild animal; however, about 30% of victims have no memory or evidence of a bite. Other reported modes of transmission include mucous membranes (eyes, nose, mouth), aerosolization, and corneal transplantation. In 1997, there were 8513 reported cases of rabies (93% in wild animals), but only four were in humans. The number of human deaths due to rabies in the United States decreased dramatically during the 20th century, down to one to four deaths per year in the late 1990s.

Since the established disease is almost invariably fatal, early preventive measures are essential. The wound should be washed thoroughly with soap and water. Information useful in determining the risk of potential rabies infection includes the geographic location of the incident, the type of animal involved, how the exposure occurred, the vaccination status of the animal, and whether it can be safely captured and tested for rabies. Rabies prophylaxis has proved nearly 100% successful, as most human deaths now occur in people who fail to seek medical assistance. Each year, approximately 18,000 people receive rabies vaccine prophylaxis before exposure, and an additional 40,000 receive prophylaxis (vaccine plus immune globin) after exposure. The latest information regarding both pre- and postexposure prophylaxis is available at the CDC's Rabies Section website (http://www.cdc.gov/ncidod/dvrd/rabies).

The rabies virus has a distinctive bullet shape and a nonsegmented, negative-stranded RNA genome. After local (primary) infection, the virus enters peripheral nerves and is transported to the central nervous system, making it difficult to detect (eclipse phase). The subsequent incubation period varies in humans from several days to typically 1–3 months. Clinical symptoms begin with pain and numbness around the site of the wound, followed by nonspecific flu-like symptoms of fever, irritability, malaise, and progressive cerebral dysfunction. Delirium, hallucinations, insomnia, paralysis, and convulsions occur terminally.

The direct fluorescent antibody (dFA) test on brain tissue is used most frequently to diagnose rabies in animals. A complement of tests are used routinely in humans, because no single test can rule out rabies absolutely: serum and cerebrospinal fluid are tested for antibodies, skin biopsy is examined by dFA, and saliva can be tested by nested reverse transcription polymerase chain reaction (RT-PCR).

Rabies Section, Viral and Rickettsial Zoonoses Branch, Division of Viral and Rickettsial Diseases, National Center for Infectious Diseases, Centers for Disease Control and Prevention, Atlanta, Georgia. http://www.cdc.gov/ncidod/dvrd/rabies

ECHINOCOCCOSIS

Echinococcosis (hydatid disease) is caused by the microscopic cestode parasites *Echinococcus granulosus* and *E multilocularis* (1–4 mm tapeworms), which form larval cysts in mammalian tissue. Foxes, coyotes, dogs, and cats are the definitive hosts that harbor the adult tapeworms in their intestines; these animals are not harmed by the worms and have no symptoms. Ova are passed in the feces and are ingested by intermediate hosts such as cattle, humans, rodents, and particularly sheep. The ova penetrate the intestine and pass via the portal vein to the liver (75%) and then to the lung (15%) or other tissues. In the liver, the ovum typically develops into a cyst filled with clear fluid. Brood capsules containing scoleces bud into the cyst lumen. Such "endocysts" may cause secondary intraperitoneal cyst formation if spilled into the peritoneal cavity. Because the cysts grow slowly, patients may be asymptomatic for several years. Pain or discomfort in the upper abdominal region and weight loss may occur as a result of the cyst enlarging. Eosinophilia is present in about 40% of patients. Serologic diagnosis may be substantiated by immunoassays. Ultrasonography and CT scanning readily demonstrate cysts. In some patients, the parasite dies, the cyst wall calcifies, and therapy is not required. However, surgery is most often required, though removal of the cyst is not usually 100% effective. Excision of the cyst intact, if practical, is preferred. Because of the dangers of anaphylaxis or implantation, care must be taken to avoid rupturing the cyst and spilling its contents into the peritoneal cavity. In some cases, the cyst fluid can be aspirated and replaced by a scolicidal agent (hypertonic sodium chloride solution or sodium hypochlorite solution). After surgery, medication (albendazole) may be necessary to keep the cyst from growing back. The overall death rate is about 15%, but it is only 4% in surgically treated cases.

Ammann RW et al: Cestodes. Echinococcus. Gastroenterol Clin North Am 1996;25:655.

Clarkson MJ. Hydatid disease. J Med Microbiol 1997;46:24.

Taylor BR et al: Current surgical management of hepatic cyst disease. Adv Surg 1997;31:127.

ACTINOMYCOSIS & NOCARDIOSIS

Actinomycosis and nocardiosis are chronic, slowly progressive infections that may involve many tissues, resulting in the formation of granulomas and abscesses that drain through sinuses and fistulas. Although the causative organisms are true bacteria, the lesions resemble those produced by mycobacteria, fungi, and cancer, making accurate diagnosis difficult.

Actinomyces israelii is a gram-positive, non-acid-fast, filamentous organism that usually shows branching and may break up into short bacterial forms. It is a strict anaerobe and part of the normal flora of the human oropharynx and upper intestinal tract. Inflammatory nodular masses, abscesses, and draining sinuses occur most commonly in the head and neck. One-fifth of patients with actinomycosis have primary lesions in the chest and an equal proportion in the abdomen, most commonly involving the appendix and cecum. Multiple sinuses are commonly formed, and the pus may contain "sulfur granules," yellow granules of tangled filaments. The inflammatory lesions are often hard and relatively painless and nontender. Systemic symptoms, including fever, are variably present. The discharging sinus tracts or fistulas usually become secondarily infected with other bacteria. Abdominal actinomycosis may produce an abdominal mass mimicking a malignant process or may give rise to appendicitis. If the appendix perforates, multiple lesions and sinuses of the abdominal wall form. Thoracic actinomycosis may give rise to cough, pleural pain, fever, and weight loss, simulating mycobacterial or mycotic infection. Later in the course of the disease, the sinuses perforate the pleural cavity and the chest wall, often involving ribs or vertebrae. CT scanning and needle aspiration may be helpful diagnostically. All forms of actinomycosis are treated with penicillin G for many weeks. Although long-term antibiotic therapy appears to be very successful and can avoid the need for operation, preoperative exclusion of other diagnoses is difficult. Surgical extirpation or drainage of lesions therefore is frequently performed.

Nocardiae are gram-positive, branching, filamentous organisms that may be acid-fast; *Nocardia asteroides* is the most common isolate. The filaments often fragment into bacillary forms. They are aerobes rarely found in the normal flora of the respiratory tract. Nocardiosis may present in two forms. One is localized, chronic granuloma with suppuration, abscess, and sinus tract formation resembling actinomycosis. A specialized disorder occurs in the extremities as Madura foot (mycetoma), with extensive bone destruction but little systemic illness. The second form is a systemic infection, usually beginning as pneumonitis with suppuration and progressing via the bloodstream to involvement of other organs, eg, meninges or brain. Systemic nocardiosis produces fever, cough, and weight loss and resembles mycobacterial or mycotic infections. The mortality rate of nocardial bacteremia is as high as 50%. It is particularly apt to occur as a complication of immunodeficiency in patients with chronic obstructive pulmonary disease, cancer, HIV-associated disease, or corticosteroid-induced immunosuppression. Nocardiosis is best treated with sulfonamides (eg, trimethoprim-sulfamethoxazole) or, when severe, with imipenem and amikacin, for many weeks. Surgical drainage of abscesses, excision of fistulas, and repair of defects are essential features of management.

Cintron JR et al: Abdominal actinomycosis. Dis Colon Rectum 1996;39:105.

Conant EF et al: Actinomycosis and nocardiosis of the lung. J Thorac Imaging 1992;7:75.

Kontoyiannis DP et al: *Nocardia* bacteremia. Report of 4 cases and review of the literature. Medicine 1998;77:255.

Lerner PI: Nocardiosis. Clin Infect Dis 1996;22:891.

Menendez R et al: Pulmonary infection with *Nocardia* species: a report of 10 cases and review. Eur Respir J 1997;10:1542.

Smego R Jr et al: Actinomycosis. Clin Infect Dis 1998;26:1255.

Tarabichi M, Schloss M: Actinomycosis otomastoiditis. Arch Otolaryngol 1993;119:561.

Threlkeld SC et al: Update on management of patients with *Nocardia* infection. Curr Clin Top Infect Dis 1997;17:1.

Warren NG: Actinomycosis, nocardiosis, and actinomycetoma. Dermatol Clin 1996;14:85.

■ VENOMOUS BITE INJURIES

SNAKEBITE

About 8000 people a year in the United States are bitten by venomous snakes. About one-third of these snakebites do not result in envenomation, as the snake may bite but not inject venom, or may eject it onto the skin in a superficial fashion. Death from serious envenomation occurs in only 9–15 victims per year in the United States. In comparison, there are about 120 United States deaths a year from wasp and bee stings and about 150 deaths per year from lightning.

Identification of Snake

The vast majority of snakebites in the United States are from nonvenomous snakes. Distinguishing whether the patient has been bitten and envenomed by a venomous snake, bitten but not envenomed, or bitten by a nonvenomous snake is critical prior to starting treatments that may not only cause discomfort but may also produce serious side effects. These distinctions require identification of the attacking snake through knowledge of snake taxonomy, anatomy, and geographic distribution. Coloration patterns and fang or tooth marks are deceptive and unreliable identification criteria.

There are about 120 species of snakes in the United States, of which 26 are venomous. The indigenous venomous snakes of North America can be placed in four groups. Three groups are pit vipers of the subfamily Crotalidae: rattlesnakes, with multiple species within the two genera (*Crotalus* and *Sistrurus*); the cottonmouth or water moccasin *(Agkistrodon piscivorus);* and the copperhead *(Agkistrodon contortrix).* Pit vipers can be distinguished from nonvenomous snakes by a round mouth and a pit between the eyes and the nares on each side. They have retractable canaliculated fangs that can rapidly spring into biting position and deliver venom. The large venom glands also give the head a triangular or diamond appearance. North American pit vipers have vertically oriented elliptiform irises. The vast majority of North American pit vipers have a primarily hemotoxic venom, but some, particularly the Mojave rattlesnake, have primarily neurotoxic venom.

The coral snake is the fourth group of indigenous North American venomous snake. It is a member of the family Elapidae, which also includes the much more dangerous cobras and kraits. Two different genera of coral snakes (the Western coral snake, *Micruroides euryxanthus,* and the Eastern coral snake, *Micrurus fulvius)*are found chiefly in the western and southern states, respectively, with distinct nonoverlapping geographic distributions. Coral snakes have small mouths, short teeth, and deliver secreted venom into prey through created lacerations. A coral snake bite lacks the characteristic fang marks of bites by pit vipers, sometimes making the bite hard to detect. The degree of envenomation depends upon the size of the snake and the duration of contact; rapid removal of the snake from the victim reduces the risk of significant poisoning. Coral snake venom is primarily neurotoxic and unrelated to that of the pit vipers. Victims may experience respiratory paralysis, one of the hazards of neurotoxic venom.

Some nonpoisonous snakes such as the red milk snake and the scarlet king snake mimic the bright red, yellow, and black coloration of the coral snake. True coral snakes will have red bands immediately adjacent to yellow bands; the nonvenomous mimics will have black bands immediately adjacent to the red bands, thus giving rise to the colloquial mnemonic: "Red on black, venom lack; red on yellow, kill a fellow." This rhyming maxim applies only to North American coral snakes.

The family Elapidae includes the cobras, kraits, and mambas, common in Asia and Africa. Their fangs are at the front of the mouth and are small to moderate in size. Cobra venoms are quite toxic and internationally are a major cause of human snakebite morbidity and mortality.

Sea snakes of the family Hydrophiidae are closely related to the cobras. They are native to the Indian and Pacific oceans, live primarily in an aquatic—usually marine—environment, and have short fixed fangs and flattened tails. Their venom is quite toxic, and envenomation is a significant risk for fishermen in areas where these snakes are indigenous.

The family Atractaspidae consists of the side-fanged vipers, including the mole vipers and stiletto snakes. They are confined to Africa and the Middle East. Their venom contains sarafotoxins, which are endothelin-like compounds causing potent smooth muscle contraction and vasoconstriction.

Snake Venom

The poison glands of snakes are modified salivary glands that secrete a complex mixture of specialized proteins and enzymes. Snake venom has several functions, including rapid immobilization of prey, predigestion of prey, and defense against predators. Snake venom effects are often broadly and superficially classified as primarily hemotoxic or neurotoxic. Caution should be used, as a combination of multiple effects may present either concurrently or consecutively.

Hemotoxic effects are mediated by proteolytic enzymes, peptides, and metalloproteins that can cause local tissue destruction directly and by intimal injury to blood vessels, followed by thrombosis and necrosis. Activation of the coagulation cascade can occur at multiple points, resulting in net anticoagulation. Direct lysis of red blood cells can cause acute hemolytic anemia and produce acute tubular necrosis. Bites on extremities may cause subcutaneous tissue destruction and loss of digits. Myotoxins can cause compromise of muscle compartments from direct myonecrosis as well as from local pressure effects. Secondary edema can develop rapidly in tissues from both cytokine release and from hemorrhage into local tissues. Systemic effects can include pulmonary edema. Intravascular injection can cause a more severe systemic reaction, with diffuse bleeding from thrombocytopenia and hypofibrinogenemia.

Snake venom neurotoxins often act upon the acetylcholine receptor system, with different components causing postsynaptic antagonism and acetylcholinesterase activity. Other components may cause direct presynaptic nerve cell destruction.

Clinical Findings

Bites by nonvenomous snakes are much more common than bites by venomous snakes. These should be treated as simple puncture wounds, employing an appropriate antitetanus agent.

The excitement and hysteria associated with any snakebite may give rise to symptoms of disorientation, faintness, dizziness, hyperventilation, a rapid pulse, and even primary shock even with nonvenomous snakebites.

A bite by a venomous snake results in envenomation in only 50–70% of cases. Envenomation may be classified as mild (scratch followed by minimal swelling and not much pain), moderate (fang marks, local swelling, and definite pain), or severe (fang marks, severe and progressive swelling and pain).

Most rattlesnakes, copperheads, water moccasins and coral snakes tend to bite superficially, but a few bites penetrate muscle. The severity of the poisoning will depend upon the species and size of the snake; the age and size of the victim; the location, depth, nature, and number of bites; the amount of venom injected; the victim's sensitivity to the venom; the microbes present in the snake's mouth; and the availability of appropriate first-aid treatment and subsequent medical care.

Local signs of envenomation include puncture marks, local ecchymosis and discoloration, vesicles and bullae, and rapid appearance of swelling and edema at the injured area, with further progression to adjacent areas. The pain of the bite can be quite severe. Additional signs of hypotension, diaphoresis, nausea, weakness, and faintness are common. Perioral or peripheral paresthesias, taste changes, and fasciculations can be seen. Signs suggestive of neurotoxic envenomation include dysphagia, dysphonia, diplopia, headache, weakness, and respiratory distress. Laboratory findings may include hemoconcentration initially due to fluid shifts, with later decreases in red blood cells and platelets. Urinalysis may show hematuria, glycosuria, and proteinuria. Prothrombin and partial thromboplastin times are often abnormal.

Treatment

The presence and degree of envenomation dictate treatment measures; other factors, such as time elapsed since being bitten, prehospital care, and the age and size of the victim, are also critical.

Wash the bite with soap and water or an antiseptic if available. Apply a broad, firm compressing bandage over the bite which does not restrict arterial and venous blood flow, and immobilize the bitten area at a level below the heart. Remove rings and constrictive devices, and keep the victim at rest and warm. Popular conceptions of first aid measures including tourniquets, wound incision and suction, application of ice, cryotherapy, electrical shock, and ingestion of alcohol are of no proved value and may be hazardous to both the patient and the caregiver, particularly in the field setting. Transporting the patient to a medical facility is an important field management objective. Identification of the snake is helpful but of lower priority.

Standard evaluation and support of respiratory and cardiovascular function are initial priorities. Laboratory evaluation should include blood typing and crossmatching, coagulation studies, a complete blood count, and urinalysis. Local wound management includes cleansing and disinfection. Systemic measures include administration of antitetanus agent for tetanus prophylaxis and broad-spectrum antibiotic therapy. Fasciotomy should be reserved only for the uncommon compartment syndrome with compartment pressures documented above 30–40 mm Hg. Local bite area excision is not useful and should not be done.

The decision to use antivenin is based upon identification of the offending snake as venomous, discernment of the degree and manifestations of envenomation, time elapsed since the bite, and laboratory abnormalities. Several grading systems have been proposed but are inadequate at present, and the decision to use antivenin must be individualized to each patient and his or her specific reaction to the snakebite.

Effective specific antivenins are available for the bites of both pit vipers and Eastern coral snakes. Crotalidae polyvalent antivenin is effective against all North American pit vipers; North American coral snake antivenin is effective only for the Eastern coral snake. Because these equine antivenins have serious potential side-effects, including both allergic reactions and serum sickness, their administration should be reserved for patients with significant bites or after early signs of envenomation have appeared.

Antivenin should ideally be administered early and as a diluted continuous intravenous infusion; local injection in or around the bite is contraindicated. Crotalidae polyvalent antivenin is most effective if given within 4 hours after a bite, of less value after 8 hours, and of questionable value after 30 hours. Severe envenomations may require over 30 vials; antivenin may be appropriate for moderate envenomation, but the risks outweigh the benefits if envenomation is minimal. Coral snake antivenin may be started prior to any neurologic symptoms if the offending snake is suspected or confirmed to be a coral snake.

Chippaux JP et al: Venoms, antivenoms and immunotherapy. Toxicon 1998;36:823.

Consroe P, et al: Comparison of a new ovine antigen binding fragment (Fab) antivenin for United States Crotalidae with the commercial antivenin for protection against venom-induced lethality in mice. Am J Trop Med Hyg 1995;53:507.

Gold BS et al: Snake venom poisoning in the United States: a review of therapeutic practice. South Med J 1994;87:579.

Goldstein EJ: Bite wounds and infection. Clin Infect Dis 1992; 14:633.

Holstege CP et al: Crotalid snake envenomation. Crit Care Clin 1997;13:889.

Thwin MM et al: Snake envenomation and protective natural endogenous proteins: a mini review of the recent developments (1991–1997). Toxicon 1998;36:1471.

Walter FG et al: Envenomations. Crit Care Clin 1999;15:353.

Weisman RS et al: Snake and spider antivenin: risks and benefits of therapy. J Fla Med Assoc 1996;83:192.

Whitley RE: Conservative treatment of copperhead snakebites without antivenin. J Trauma 1996;41:219.

ARTHROPOD BITES

Stings and bites of arthropods are most often merely a nuisance. Some arthropods, however, can produce death by direct toxicity or by hypersensitivity reactions. Because of their prevalence and numbers, bees and wasps kill more people than any other venomous animal, including snakes.

Bees & Wasps

When a bee stings, it becomes anchored by the two barbed lancets, so that withdrawal is impossible. In the struggle, a bee will usually avulse its stinging apparatus and die. After being stung by a bee, one should scrape the exuded poison sac with a sharp knife. Any attempt to pull the poison apparatus out will simply cause more venom to be squeezed into the tissue. The stinger, once embedded, remains present. If this has occurred in an eyelid, it may irritate the globe of the eye months after the sting.

The stinging lancets of the wasp are not barbed and can easily be withdrawn by the insect to allow it to reinsert or to escape. It is unusual, therefore, to find a stinger left in place after a wasp sting. The females of the variety called yellow jackets are very aggressive. These insects sometimes bite before stinging.

The venom of bees and wasps contains histamine, basic protein components of high molecular weight, free amino acids, hyaluronidase, and acetylcholine. Antigenic proteins are species-specific and may lead to cross-reactivity between insects. Symptoms of arthropod stings may vary from minimal erythema to a marked local reaction of severe systemic toxicity (especially from multiple stings). Infection may occur. A generalized allergic reaction has been described that resembles serum sickness.

Early application of ice packs to reduce swelling is indicated. Elevation of the extremity is also useful. Oral antihistamines may be of some use in reducing urticaria. Parenteral corticosteroids may reduce delayed inflammation. If infection occurs, treatment consists of local debridement and antibiotics. Moderately severe reactions will present as generalized syncope or urticarial reactions. If an anaphylactic reaction or severe reaction is present, aqueous epinephrine, 0.5–1 mL of 1:1000 solution, should be given intramuscularly. A repeat dose may be given in 5–10 minutes, followed by 5–20 mg of diphenhydramine slowly intravenously. Administration of corticosteroids and general supportive measures such as oxygen administration, plasma expanders, and pressor agents may be required in case of shock. Previously sensitized patients should carry identifying tags and a kit for emergency intramuscular injection of epinephrine.

It is possible to immunize persons against bee and wasp stings, but cost-benefit analyses indicate that this is rarely if ever indicated.

Spiders

While all spiders have poison glands and use venom for killing prey, only a few spider venoms are harmful to humans. As with all toxic exposures, the very young, the elderly, and patients with comorbid medical conditions are at greatest risk for adverse outcomes.

A. LACTRODECTISM

The bite of the lactrodectus species of spiders (widow and red-back spiders), including the black widow (*La-*

trodectus mactans) and the red-backed spider *(L hasseltii),* has primarily systemic neurotoxic effects. The female black widow spider can be identified by its characteristic black body with a red hourglass-like pattern on the abdomen; the male of the species does not bite, and is smaller. The potent venom of this genus acts by destabilization of cell membranes and degranulation at nerve terminals with release of neurotransmitters. Neuromuscular toxic effects of black widow venom occur by presynaptic motor end plate neurotransmitter release, with release of norepinephrine and acetylcholine causing excessive stimulation and eventual fatigue of the motor end plate and muscle.

Symptoms of envenomation begin with pain at the bite location, followed by later development of abdominal wall muscle rigidity, abdominal pain and cramping, respiratory difficulty with potential paralysis, and lower extremity weakness. Massive hemolysis, severe hypotension, and cardiovascular collapse can be seen. Local skin changes are often minimal and can make identification of the bite difficult.

Intravenous administration of calcium gluconate may relieve muscle pain and spasm, but similar relief can be obtained from intravenous opioids and benzodiazepines. Ice packs may improve localized pain from the bite. Most symptoms are self-limited and, with appropriate supportive therapy, resolve within 48 hours, though full recovery may take over a week. A horse antivenin is available but may cause allergic reactions. Antivenin may be indicated in severely symptomatic patients to speed recovery and perhaps to prevent development of long-term symptoms related to neurologic dysfunction.

B. Loxoscelism

The brown recluse spider *(Loxosceles reclusa)* is dark tan and has a violin-shaped mark on the back of the main body. Envenomation can have significant and prolonged local dermonecrotic effects, with development of deep necrotic wounds at the bite site that are very slow to heal. Systemic loxoscelism with intravascular coagulation and renal failure has been seen but is uncommon. The venom appears to cause local tissue necrosis by dissociating normal neutrophil responses of adhesion and degranulation from transmigration and shape changes. Phospholipase D and sphingomyelinase D also contribute to the local necrosis, as well as venom-induced platelet aggregation. Alterations in complement activation and binding of venom to erythrocyte membranes contribute to hemolysis.

The bite may have local signs of erythema and edema but usually minimal associated pain. With serious envenomation, hemorrhagic bullae surrounded by localized ischemia develop over the next 24–48 hours. The local lesion usually progresses to a very slowly healing ulcer. Systemic effects of fever, urticaria, lymphangitis, nausea, and emesis can develop. Hemolysis and disseminated intravascular coagulation are rare.

Loxoscelism is managed by supportive measures. Cleansing of the bite, rest, elevation of the affected area, and prophylactic antibiotics (eg, erythromycin) are appropriate. While tissue loss is common, early excision of lesions is also associated with poor wound healing. Conflicting data exist regarding systemic treatment with either corticosteroids or dapsone (50–100 mg/d), which may be indicated if ulcers develop or if there is rapid progression of the local reaction.

Anderson PC: Spider bites in the United States. Dermatol Clin 1997;15:307.

Bond GR: Snake, spider, and scorpion envenomation in North America. Pediatr Rev 1999;20:147.

Clark RF et al: Clinical presentation and treatment of black widow spider envenomation: a review of 163 cases. Ann Emerg Med 1992;21:782.

Gendron B: *Loxosceles reclusa* envenomation. Am J Emerg Med 1990;8:51.

Gomez HF et al: Loxosceles spider venom induces the production of alpha and beta chemokines: implications for the pathogenesis of dermonecrotic arachnidism. Inflammation 1999; 23:207.

Hobbs GD et al: Comparison of hyperbaric oxygen and dapsone therapy for loxosceles envenomation. Acad Emerg Med 1996; 3:758.

Phillips S et al: Therapy of brown spider envenomation: a controlled trial of hyperbaric oxygen, dapsone, and cyproheptadine. Ann Emerg Med 1995;25:363.

Wilson DC et al: Spiders and spider bites. Dermatol Clin 1990; 8:277.

Wright SW et al: Clinical presentation and outcome of brown recluse spider bite. Ann Emerg Med 1997;30:28.

■ ANTIMICROBIAL CHEMOTHERAPY

PRINCIPLES OF SELECTION OF ANTIMICROBIAL DRUGS

Initial & Subsequent Selection of Antimicrobial Agents

For optimal treatment of an infectious process, a suitable antimicrobial agent must be administered as early as possible. This involves a series of decisions: (1) The judgment, on the basis of clinical impression, that a microbial infection probably exists. (2) Formulation of a differential diagnosis and possible microbial pathogens. (3) Procurement of specimens likely to provide a microbiologic diagnosis. (4) Selection of the drug most

Table 9–5. Tetanus immunization and prophylaxis.

Indication	Immunization or Prophylaxis[1]
Routine adult immunization	Td 0.5 mL every 10 years (or a single booster at age 50)[2]
Clean minor wounds Prior immunization unknown or < 3 doses	Td 0.5 mL
Prior immunization > 3 doses	Td 0.5 mL if last dose > 10 years age
Other wounds Prior immunization unknown or < 3 doses	Td 0.5 mL and TIG
Prior immunization > 3 doses	Td 0.5 mL (unless last dose < 5 years ago)

[1]Td = adult tetanus-diphtheria booster; TIG = tetanus immune globulin 250 units IM. If given concurrently with Td, give at separate site.
[2]Patients who have never received an initial vaccination series should receive the complete series.

likely to be effective against the suspected organisms ("empiric therapy"). (5) Observation of the clinical response to the prescribed antimicrobial and laboratory identification of a putative microbial pathogen. (6) Continuation of the empiric regimen or a switch to pathogen-directed therapy.

Although laboratory data need not always overrule a decision based on clinical and empiric grounds, judicious targeted use of antimicrobial therapy reduces the risk of multidrug-resistant infections during future care.

A separate but often related issue is the decision regarding tetanus immunization and prophylaxis. Guidelines are presented in Table 9–5.

Selection of an Antimicrobial Drug by Laboratory Tests

When an etiologic pathogen has been isolated from a specimen, it is often possible to select the drug of choice on the basis of current clinical experience. Such a listing of drug choices is given in Table 9–6. Given the rising rates of multidrug-resistant bacteria and geographic differences in antibiogram data (tables setting forth the antibiotic sensitivities of pathogens), laboratory tests for antimicrobial drug susceptibility are necessary, particularly if the isolated organism is of a type

that often exhibits drug resistance, eg, enteric gram-negative rods.

Antimicrobial drug susceptibility tests may be done on solid media as disk tests, in broth in tubes, or in wells of microdilution plates. The latter method yields results expressed as the MIC (minimal inhibitory concentration), and the technique can be modified to also permit determination of the MBC (minimal bactericidal concentration). When performed in a well-controlled setting, disk tests indicate whether a microbial culture is susceptible or resistant to drug concentrations achievable in vivo with conventional dosage regimens. This can provide valuable guidance in selecting therapy. At times, however, there is a marked discrepancy between the results of the test and the clinical response of the patient given the chosen drug. Some possible explanations for such discrepancies are listed below.

(1) The organism isolated from the specimen may not be the one responsible for the infectious process. The usual cause is failure to culture tissue instead of pus.

(2) There may have been failure to drain a collection of pus, debride necrotic tissue, or remove a foreign body. Antimicrobials can never take the place of surgical drainage and removal.

(3) Superinfection may occur in the course of prolonged chemotherapy. New microorganisms may have replaced the original infectious agent. This is particularly common with open wounds or sinus tracts.

(4) The drug may not reach the site of active infection in adequate concentration. The pharmacologic properties of antimicrobials determine their absorption and distribution. Certain drugs penetrate phagocytic cells poorly and thus may not reach intracellular organisms. Some drugs may diffuse poorly into the eye, central nervous system, or pleural space unless injected directly into the area.

(5) At times, two or more microorganisms participate in an infectious process but only one may have been isolated from the specimen. The antimicrobial being used may be effective only against the less virulent organism.

(6) In the course of drug administration, resistant microorganisms may have been selected from a mixed population, and these drug-resistant organisms continue to grow in the presence of the drug.

Assessment of Drug & Dosage

An adequate therapeutic response is an important but not always sufficient indication that the right drug is being given in the right dosage. Proof of drug activity in serum against the original infecting organisms may provide important support for a selected drug regimen

Table 9–6. Drugs of choice for suspected and empiric regimens. Pathogen-directed therapy should utilize antibiogram data from clinical microbiology laboratory.*

Suspected or Proved Etiologic Agent	Drugs of First Choice	Alternative Drugs
Gram-negative cocci		
Moraxella catarrhalis	Amoxicillin-clavulanic acid or TMP-SMZ[1]	Cephalosporins,[2] erythromycin,[3] tetracycline[4]
Gonococcus	Ceftriaxone	Cefixime, ciprofloxacin, spectinomycin
Meningococcus	Penicillin[5]	Cephalosporins,[2] ampicillin, chloramphenicol
Gram-positive cocci		
Streptococcus pneumoniae (penicillin-susceptible)	Penicillin,[5] ceftriaxone ± vancomycin (combination therapy may be indicated)	Erythromycin,[3] cephalosporin,[6] vancomycin
S pneumoniae (penicillin-resistant)		
Streptococcus, hemolytic, groups A, B, C, G	Penicillin[5]	Erythromycin,[3] cephalosporin,[6] vancomycin
Viridans streptococci	Penicillin[5] ± aminoglycosides[7]	Cephalosporin,[6] vancomycin
Staphylococcus, methicillin-resistant	Vancomycin + gentamicin or rifampin (or both)	TMP-SMZ, ciprofloxacin
Staphylococcus, non-penicillinase-producing	Penicillin	Cephalosporin, vancomycin
Staphylococcus, penicillinase-producing	Penicillinase-resistant penicillin[8]	Vancomycin, cephalosporin[6]
Enterococci	Ampicillin ± gentamicin	Vancomycin + gentamicin
Gram-negative rods		
Acinetobacter	Aminoglycoside[7] + imipenem	Minocycline, TMP-SMZ[1]
Bacteroides, oropharyngeal strains	Penicillin,[5] clindamycin	Metronidazole, cephalosporin[2,6]
Bacteroides, gastrointestinal strains	Metronidazole	Cefoxitin, chloramphenicol, clindamycin, TMP-SMZ[1]
Brucella	Tetracycline[4] + streptomycin	Tetracycline,[4] ciprofloxacin
Campylobacter	Erythromycin[3]	Imipenem, newer cephalosporins[2]
Enterobacter	TMP-SMZ,[1] aminoglycoside[7]	Ampicillin, TMP-SMZ[1]
Escherichia coli (sepsis)	Aminoglycoside,[7] newer cephalosporins[2]	Ampicillin, cephalosporin[6]
E coli (first urinary infection)	Sulfonamide,[9] TMP-SMZ[1]	Ampicillin and chloramphenicol[1]
Haemophilus (meningitis, respiratory infections)	Cephalosporins[2]	TMP-SMZ,[1] aminoglycoside[7]
Klebsiella	Cephalosporins[2]	TMP-SMZ
Legionella (pneumonia)	Macrolide + rifampin	Chloramphenicol
Pasteurella (Yersinia) (plague, tularemia)	Streptomycin, tetracycline[4]	Cephalosporins,[2] aminoglycoside[7]
Proteus mirabilis	Ampicillin	Aminoglycoside[7]
Proteus vulgaris and other species	Newer cephalosporins[2]	Ceftazidime or cefoperazone + aminoglycoside; imipenem + aminoglycoside; aztreonam
Pseudomonas aeruginosa	Aminoglycoside[7] + antipseudomonal penicillin[10]	Chloramphenicol, tetracycline,[4] TMP-SMZ
Burkholderia pseudomallei (melioidosis)	Ceftazidime	Chloramphenicol + streptomycin
Burkholderia mallei (glanders)	Streptomycin + tetracycline[4]	TMP-SMZ,[1] ciprofloxacin, ampicillin, chloramphenicol
Salmonella	Ceftriaxone	TMP-SMZ[1]
Serratia, Providencia	Cephalosporins,[2] aminoglycoside[7]	Ampicillin, tetracycline,[4] ciprofloxacin, chloramphenicol
Shigella	TMP-SMZ[1]	
Stenotrophomonas maltophilia	TMP-SMZ[11]	
Vibrio (cholera, sepsis)	Tetracycline[4]	TMP-SMZ[1]

(continued)

Table 9–6. Drugs of choice for suspected and empiric regimens. Pathogen-directed therapy should utilize antibiogram data from clinical microbiology laboratory.* (continued)

Suspected or Proved Etiologic Agent	Drugs of First Choice	Alternative Drugs
Gram-positive rods		
Actinomyces	Penicillin[5]	Tetracycline[4]
Bacillus (eg, Anthrax)	Penicillin[5]	Erythromycin[3]
Clostridium (eg, gas gangrene, tetanus)	Penicillin[5]	Metronidazole, chloramphenicol, clindamycin
Corynebacterium diphtheriae	Erythromycin[3]	Penicillin[5]
Corynebacterium jeikeium	Vancomycin	Ciprofloxacin
Listeria	Ampicillin + aminoglycoside[7]	TMP-SMZ[1]
Acid-fast rods		
Mycobacterium tuberculosis	INH + rifampin + pyrazinamide + ethambutol	Other antituberculosis drugs
Mycobacterium leprae	Dapsone + rifampin, clofazimine	Ethionamide
Mycobacterium kansasii	INH + rifampin + ethambutol	Other antituberculosis drugs
Mycobacterium avium-intracellulare	Ethambutol + rifampin + clarithromycin	Other antituberculosis drugs
Mycobacterium fortuitum-chelonei	Amikacin + doxycycline	Cefoxitin, erythromycin, sulfonamide
Nocardia	Sulfonamide,[9] TMP-SMZ[1]	Minocycline
Spirochetes		
Borrelia (Lyme disease, relapsing fever)	Tetracycline,[4] ceftriaxone	Penicillin,[5] erythromycin[3]
Leptospira	Penicillin[5]	Tetracycline[4]
Treponema (syphilis, yaws, etc)	Penicillin[5]	Erythromycin,[3] tetracycline[4]
Mycoplasmas	Macrolide or tetracycline[4]	
Chlamydiae		
C psittaci	Tetracycline[4]	Chloramphenicol
C trachomatis (urethritis or pelvic inflammatory disease)	Doxycycline or erythromycin[3]	Ofloxacin or azithromycin
C pneumoniae	Tetracycline[4]	Erythromycin[3]
Rickettsiae	Tetracycline[4]	Chloramphenicol

*N Eng J Med 1997;336:708.

[1]TMP-SMZ is a mixture of 1 part trimethoprim and 5 parts sulfamethoxazole.

[2]Cephalosporins include cefotaxime, cefuroxime, ceftriaxone, ceftazidime, ceftizoxime, and others.

[3]Erythromycin estolate is best absorbed orally but carries the highest risk of hepatitis; erythromycin stearate and erythromycin ethylsuccinate are also available.

[4]All tetracyclines have similar activity against microorganisms. Dosage is determined by rates of absorption and excretion of various preparations.

[5]Penicillin G is preferred for parenteral injection; penicillin V for oral administration—to be used only in treating infections due to highly sensitive organisms.

[6]Older cephalosporins are cephalothin, cefazolin, cephapirin, and cefoxitin for parenteral injection; cephalexin and cephradine can be given orally.

[7]Aminoglycosides—gentamicin, tobramycin, amikacin, netilmicin—should be chosen on the basis of local patterns of susceptibility.

[8]Parenteral nafcillin or oxacillin; oral dicloxacillin, cloxacillin, or oxacillin.

[9]Oral sulfisoxazole and trisulfapyrimidines are highly soluble in urine; parenteral sodium sulfadiazine can be injected intravenously in treating severely ill patients.

[10]Antipseudomonal penicillins: ticarcillin, carbenicillin, mezlocillin, azlocillin, piperacillin.

[11]First choice for previously untreated urinary tract infection is a highly soluble sulfonamide or TMP-SMZ.

even if fever or other signs of infection are continuing. In sepsis, extended-interval administration of aminoglycosides has efficacy and toxicity similar to what is associated with traditional dosing regimens, but costs are less and convenience is increased. This dosing regimen is not recommended for patients with endocarditis, pregnancy, cystic fibrosis, burns covering more than 20% of body surface area, mycobacterial infections, and anasarca. The initial dose is gentamicin or tobramycin, 5 mg/kg intravenously, or amikacin, 15 mg/kg intravenously. A follow up random serum drug level 6–14 hours later is compared with a nomogram to determine follow-up dosing intervals.

Determining Duration of Therapy

The duration of drug therapy depends on the nature of the infection and the severity of the clinical presentation. Treatment of acute uncomplicated infections should be continued until the patient has been afebrile and clinically well for at least 72 hours. Infections at certain sites (eg, endocarditis, septic arthritis, osteomyelitis) require more prolonged therapy. In evaluating the patient's clinical response, the possibility of adverse reactions to drugs must be considered. Such reactions may mimic continuing activity of the infectious process by causing fever, skin rashes, central nervous system disturbances, and changes in blood and urine. In the case of many drugs, it is desirable to assess hepatic and renal function at intervals. Adverse events may require dose reduction or drug discontinuation.

Oliguria & Renal Failure

Oliguria and renal failure have an important influence on antimicrobial drug dosage, since most of these drugs are excreted—to a greater or lesser extent—by the kidneys. Some drugs require minor adjustments in dosage or frequency of administration. Others, such as aminoglycosides (eg, tobramycin), tetracyclines, and vancomycin, must be drastically reduced in dosage or frequency of administration if toxicity is to be avoided in the presence of nitrogen retention. General guidelines for the administration of such drugs to patients with renal failure are set forth in Table 9–7. The administration of particularly nephrotoxic antimicrobials such as aminoglycosides to patients in renal failure may have to be guided by frequent direct assays of serum drug concentrations.

In the newborn or premature infant, excretory mechanisms for some antimicrobials are poorly developed, and for this reason special dosage schedules must be used in order to avoid accumulation of drugs.

Prevention & Control of Spread of Vancomycin-Resistant Genes

In an attempt to limit the emergence of vancomycin-resistant genes, six judicious uses of vancomycin have been identified. Vancomycin should not be used routinely in the following circumstances: (1) for routine surgical prophylaxis in a patient without a severe beta-lactam allergy; (2) for empiric therapy of a febrile neutropenic patient unless initial evidence suggests an infection with gram-positive bacteria; (3) for treatment of a single positive blood culture with a coagulase-negative staphylococcus; (4) for continued empiric administration against presumed infection when cultures do not confirm a beta-lactam-resistant gram positive organism; (5) as prophylaxis against infection of a central or peripheral intravascular catheter; (6) for routine treatment of *Clostridium difficile* colitis; and (7) for topical application or irrigation.

ANTIMICROBIAL DRUGS USED IN COMBINATION

Indications

Possible reasons for employing two or more antimicrobials simultaneously instead of a single drug are as follows:

(1) The necessity for prompt treatment in a severely ill patient suspected of having a serious microbial infection. A good guess about the most probable two or three pathogens is made, and drugs are empirically targeted to those organisms. Before such treatment is started, it is essential that adequate specimens be obtained for identifying the etiologic agent in the laboratory.

(2) The need to delay the emergence of antimicrobial resistance to one drug in chronic infections by the use of a second or third non-cross-reacting drug. Treatment of active tuberculosis is a good example.

(3) The presence of mixed infections, particularly those following massive trauma. Each drug is aimed at an important pathogenic microorganism likely to cause bacteremia.

(4) To achieve bactericidal synergism (see below). In a few infections, eg, enterococcal sepsis, a combination of drugs is more likely to eradicate the infection than either drug used alone. Unfortunately, such synergism is unpredictable, and a given drug pair may be synergistic for only a single microbial strain.

Disadvantages

The following disadvantages of using antimicrobial drugs in combinations must always be considered:

Table 9–7. Use of antibiotics in patients with renal failure and hepatic failure.

	Principal Mode of Excretion or Detoxification	Approximate Half-Life in Serum		Proposed Dosage Regimen in Renal Failure		Removal of Drugs by Hemodialysis	Dose After Hemodialysis	Dosage in Hepatic Failure[3]
		Normal	Renal Failure[1]	Initial Dose[2]	Maintenance Dose			
Acyclovir	Renal	2.5–3.5 hours	20 hours	2.5 mg/kg	2.5 mg/kg q24h	Yes	2.5 mg/kg	NC
Ampicillin	Tubular secretion	0.5–1 hour	8–12 hours	1 g	1 g q8–12h	Yes	1 g	NC
Azlo-, mezlo-, piperacillin	Renal 50–70%; biliary 20–30%	1 hour	3–6 hours	3 g	2 g q6–8h	Yes	1 g	1–2 g q8h
Aztreonam	Renal	1.7 hours	6 hours	1–2 g	0.5–1 g q6–8h	Yes	0.5–1 g	NC
Carbenicillin	Tubular secretion	1 hour	16 hours	4 g	2 g q12h	Yes	2 g	NC
Chloramphenicol	Mainly liver	3 hours	4 hours	0.5 g	0.5 g q6h	Yes	0.5 g	0.25–0.5 g q12h
Ciprofloxacin	Renal and liver	4 hours	8.5 hours	0.5 g	0.25–0.75 g q24h	No	None	NC
Clindamycin	Liver	2–4 hours	2.4 hours	0.6 g IV	0.6 g q8h	No	None	0.3–0.6 q8h
Erythromycin	Mainly liver	1.5 hours	1.5 hours	0.5–1 g	0.5–1 g q6h	No	None	0.25–0.5 g q6h
Fluconazole	Renal	30 hours	98 hours	0.2 g	0.1 g q24h	Yes	Give q24h dose	NC
Ganciclovir	Renal	3 hours	11–28 hours	1.25 mg/kg	1.25 mg/kg q24h	Yes	Give q24h dose	NC
Imipenem	Glomerular filtration	1 hour	3 hours	0.5 g	0.25–0.5 g q12h	Yes	0.25–0.5 g	NC
Metronidazole	Liver	6–10 hours	6–10 hours	0.5 g IV	0.5 g q8h	Yes	0.25 g	0.25 g q12h

Drug	Elimination	Half-life (normal)	Half-life (renal failure)[1]	Normal dose	Dose in renal failure[1]	Dialysis	Supplemental dose[2]	Change
Nafcillin	Liver 80%, Kidney 20%	0.75 hour	1.5 hours	1.5 g	1.5 g q5h	No	None	2–3 g q12h
Penicillin G	Tubular secretion	0.5 hour	7–10 hours	1–2 million units	1 million units q8h	Yes	500,000 units	NC
Ticarcillin	Tubular secretion	1.1 hour	15–20 hours	3 g	2 g q6–8 h	Yes	1 g	NC
Trimethoprim-sulfamethoxazole	Some liver	TMP 10–12 hours; SMZ 8–10 hours	TMP 24–48 hours; SMZ 18–24 hours	320 mg TMP + 1600 mg SMZ	80 mg TMP + 400 mg SMZ q12h	Yes	80 mg TMP + 400 mg SMZ	NC
Vancomycin	Glomerular filtration	6 hours	6–10 days	1 g	1 g q6–10 days based on serum levels	None	None	NC
Cefazolin	Renal	90 min		0.5 g	0.5 g qd	Yes	0.5 g	NC
Cefuroxime	Renal	80 min		1–2 g	1–2 g qd	Yes	0.5 g	NC
Cefotetan	Renal	150 min		0.5–1 g	0.5–1 g qd	Yes	0.5 g	NC
Cefoxitin	Renal	60 min		1–2 g	1–2 g qd	Yes	0.5 g	NC
Ceftriaxone	Renal and liver	480 min		1–2 g	1–2 g qd	No	None	NC
Ceftazidime	Renal	120 min		0.5–1 g	0.5–1 g qd	Yes	0.5 g	NC

[1]Considered here to be marked by creatinine clearance of 10 mL/min or less.
[2]For a 70-kg adult with a serious systemic infection.
[3]NC = No change.

(1) The more drugs administered, the greater the chance for drug reactions to occur or for the patient to become sensitized to drugs.

(2) Combined drug regimens may be unnecessarily expensive.

(3) Antimicrobial combinations often accomplish no more than an effective single drug.

(4) Empiric, broad-spectrum antimicrobial coverage may compromise the effort to establish a specific etiologic diagnosis.

(5) On rare occasions, one drug may antagonize a second drug given simultaneously. Antagonism resulting in increased rates of illness and death has been observed mainly in bacterial meningitis when a bacteriostatic drug (eg, tetracycline or chloramphenicol) was given with (or prior to) a bactericidal drug (eg, penicillin or ampicillin). However, antagonism can usually be overcome by giving a larger dose of one of the drugs in the pair and is therefore an infrequent problem in clinical therapy.

Synergism

Antimicrobial synergism occurs in the situations listed below. Synergistic drug combinations must be selected by specialized laboratory procedures.

(1) One drug inhibits a microbial enzyme that might destroy a second drug. For example, clavulanic acid inhibits bacterial β-lactamase and protects simultaneously administered amoxicillin from destruction.

(2) Sequential block of a metabolic pathway. Sulfonamides inhibit utilization of extracellular p-aminobenzoic acid by susceptible bacteria. Trimethoprim inhibits the reduction of folates, the next metabolic step. Simultaneous use of sulfamethoxazole and trimethoprim can be strikingly more effective in some bacterial infections than use of either drug alone. Similarly, sulfamethoxazole plus pyrimethamine has greatly enhanced activity in pneumocystis and toxoplasma infections.

(3) One drug enhances greatly the uptake of a second drug. Cell-wall inhibitor (β-lactam) drugs enhance the penetration of various bacteria by aminoglycosides and thus increase the overall bactericidal effect. Eradication of infections by enterococci are enhanced by combinations of a cell wall-active agent and an aminoglycoside. Similarly, the control of sepsis by pseudomonas and other gram-negative rods may be enhanced by combination of a cephalosporin and an aminoglycoside.

Antifungal Therapy

The selection of an antifungal drug is usually based on the result of a culture obtained for clinical indications or persistent systemic symptoms in a host already receiving broad-spectrum antibacterial therapy. Given the extensive and prolonged use of antibacterial agents, the rising number of immunocompromised hosts, and the availability of antifungal therapeutic options, there has been an increasing need for the judicious use of antifungal therapeutic agents. Since in vitro testing of fungi is not well standardized, recommendations for treatment will depend upon the characterization of the yeast in the mycology laboratory. Assessment of drug, dosage, duration of therapy, and evaluation of adverse events is often best done in consultation with an infectious disease specialist. Drug options include the following.

A. Amphotericin B

Amphotericin B is a polyene antimicrobial agent that disrupts the fungal cell by binding to ergosterol in the plasma membrane. This is the drug of choice for most systemic mycoses except *Pseudallescheria boydii* and some fusarium species. Amphotericin B is poorly absorbed and must be administered intravenously except for topical therapy in AIDS patients with oral candidiasis. The intravenous infusion dose is often determined by the severity of the infection. An initial infusion dose is often determined by the severity of the infection. An initial dose of 0.5–1 mg/kg is usually given over 2–4 hours. In most instances, daily prehydration with 500 mL of normal saline solution will reduce the risk of nephrotoxicity. Recognized adverse events (fever, chills, headache, myalgias, nausea and vomiting) may be reduced by premedicating the patient with acetaminophen, 600 mg orally, and diphenhydramine, 50 mg orally, plus hydrocortisone, 25–100 mg intravenously. Nephrotoxicity may occur over time in the form of distal renal tubular acidosis, hyperkalemia, hypermagnesemia, or impairment of glomerular filtration.

B. Lipid Preparations of Amphotericin B

These formulations include amphotericin B lipid complex, amphotericin B colloidal dispersion, and liposomal amphotericin B. These formulations alter the pharmacokinetics and distribution of the drug and are often substituted for treatment of infections in patients intolerant of or not responding to regular amphotericin B.

C. Flucytosine

Flucytosine, 25–37.5 mg/kg orally every 6 hours, is an effective agent against some isolates of candida species and *Cryptococcus neoformans*. This drug, when used in combination with amphotericin B, will enhance fungicidal activity. Flucytosine is not recommended as monotherapy and is excreted in the kidney, thus requiring alteration of dosage with renal insufficiency. The primary adverse effect is bone marrow suppression, which is dose-related and occurs with peak serum levels greater than 100 µg/mL.

D. AZOLES

There are three fungistatic azoles: ketoconazole, fluconazole, and itraconazole. Ketoconazole is the oldest of these drugs, has the highest frequency of drug interactions, and is markedly hepatotoxic.

Fluconazole is widely distributed in the body and penetrates readily into the cerebrospinal fluid. It has been effective in the treatment of fungal urinary tract infections, oropharyngeal and esophageal candidiasis, and fungal peritonitis. For most indications, one gives 200 mg orally or intravenously as a loading dose followed by a maintenance dose of 100 mg intravenously or orally daily. Adverse events include headache, gastrointestinal side effects, elevated serum aminotransferases, and rashes.

Itraconazole is a triazole with a broad antifungal spectrum. This drug is approved by the Food and Drug Administration (FDA) for the treatment of histoplasmosis and blastomycosis both in immunocompetent and in immunocompromised hosts. Formulations exist both as tablets and as an elixir and are best taken on an empty stomach, with absorption improved by increased gastric acidity. Adverse events include nausea, vomiting, rash, and early hepatitis.

Antiviral Agents

Eleven drugs have been approved by the FDA for the treatment of viral infections (other than those known for the human immunodeficiency virus type 1). Antiviral drugs can be used for prophylaxis, suppression, preemptive therapy, or treatment of overt disease. The goals of treating acute viral infections in immunocompromised patients are to reduce the severity of illness and potential complications as well as reduction of viral transmission. The goal of antiviral therapy in patients with chronic viral infections is to prevent damage to visceral organs, especially the liver, lungs, gastrointestinal tract, and the central nervous system. The currently most commonly used drugs are acyclovir, valacyclovir, and famciclovir.

A. ACYCLOVIR

Acyclovir is active against herpes simplex virus (HSV) and varicella zoster virus (VZV). This drug is used for the treatment of primary and recurrent genital herpes, severe herpes dermatitis, and herpes simplex encephalitis in normal hosts as well as disseminated VZV and herpes zoster ophthalmicus. For severe systemic infections, the dose is 5 mg/kg intravenously every 8 hours for HSV infections to 10 mg/kg intravenously every 8 hours for HSV encephalitis or VZV infections. The

oral dose is 400 mg three times daily for HSV infection and 800 mg five times daily for localized herpes zoster infections. Dosage must be adjusted in renal failure. Side effects are uncommon.

B. VALACYCLOVIR

Valacyclovir is an orally administered prodrug of acyclovir approved for treatment of a first herpes zoster infection or for recurring episodes of genital HSV.

C. FAMCICLOVIR

Famciclovir is an oral drug that has activity against VZV, HSV, and Epstein-Barr virus (EBV). It is approved for acute herpes zoster and treatment of recurring episodes of genital HSV at a dosage of 500 mg orally every 8 hours for 7 days or, in recurring HSV episodes, 100 mg orally every 12 hours for 5 days. Headache, nausea, and diarrhea have been reported as adverse events.

Antimycobacterial Therapy

Depending on the location of the surgical practice, antituberculous empiric or pathogen-directed therapy may be a common necessity. Effective treatment of *Mycobacterium tuberculosis* infections requires combination chemotherapy, and initial four-drug regimens are recommended in geographic areas where the prevalence of multidrug-resistant tuberculosis is greater than 4%. Primary treatment regimens include isoniazid, rifampin, ethambutol, and pyrazinamide—with or without streptomycin. Surgical patients suspected of having tuberculosis need to be placed in negative pressure rooms for the protection of health care workers and other patients. Given the public health ramifications, it is often best for the surgical team to include an infectious disease specialist in the initiation and follow-up of patients receiving antituberculous therapy.

Bailey TC et al: A meta-analysis of extended-interval dosing versus multiple daily dosing of aminoglycosides. Clin Infect Dis 1997;24:786.

Balfour HH: Antiviral drugs. N Engl J Med 1999;340:1255.

Bass JB Jr et al: Treatment of tuberculosis and tuberculosis infection in adults and children. Am J Respir Crit Care Med 1994;149:1359.

Quagliarello VJ et al: Drug therapy: treatment of bacterial meningitis. N Engl J Med 1997;336:708.

Recommendations for preventing the spread of vancomycin resistance. Hospital Infection Control Practices Advisory Committee (HICPAC). MMWR Morb Mortal Wkly Rep 1995; 44(RR-12):1.

Sun KO et al: Management of tetanus: a review of 18 cases. J R Soc Med 1994;87:135.

Fluid & Electrolyte Management 10

Michael H. Humphreys, MD

The surgical patient is liable to develop numerous disorders of body fluid volume and composition, some of which may be iatrogenic. Understanding the physiologic mechanisms that regulate the composition and volume of the body fluids and the principles of fluid and electrolyte therapy is therefore essential for patient management.

BODY WATER & ITS DISTRIBUTION

Total body water comprises 45–60% of body weight; the percentage in any individual is influenced by age and the lean body mass, but in health it remains remarkably constant from day to day. Table 10–1 lists the average values of total body water as a percentage of body weight for men and women of different ages. Total body water is divided into intracellular (ICF) and extracellular (ECF) compartments. Intracellular water represents about two-thirds of total body water, or 40% of body weight. The remaining one-third of body water is extracellular. ECF is divided into two compartments: (1) plasma water, comprising approximately 25% of ECF, or 5% of body weight; and (2) interstitial fluid, comprising 75% of ECF, or 15% of body weight.

The solute composition of the intracellular and extracellular fluid compartments differs markedly (Figure 10–1). ECF contains principally sodium, chloride, and bicarbonate, with other ions in much lower concentrations. ICF contains mainly potassium, organic phosphate, sulfate, and various other ions in lower concentrations.

Even though plasma water and interstitial fluid have similar electrolyte compositions, plasma water contains more protein than interstitial fluid. This results in slight differences in electrolyte concentrations, as governed by the Gibbs-Donnan equilibrium. The plasma proteins, chiefly albumin, account for the high colloid osmotic pressure of plasma, which is an important determinant of the distribution of fluid between vascular and interstitial compartments, as defined by the Starling relationships.

The kidneys maintain constant volume and composition of body fluids by two distinct but related mechanisms: (1) filtration and reabsorption of sodium, which adjusts urinary sodium excretion to match changes in dietary intake; and (2) regulation of water excretion in response to changes in secretion of antidiuretic hormone. These two mechanisms allow the kidneys to keep the volume and osmolality of body fluid constant within a few percentage points despite wide variations in intake of salt and water. A corollary is that analysis of the composition and volume of the urine usually provides valuable clues in the diagnosis of disorders of body fluid volume and composition.

Although the movement of certain ions and proteins between the various body fluid compartments is restricted, water is freely diffusible. Consequently, the osmolality (total solute concentration) of all the body compartments is identical—normally, about 290 mosm/kg H_2O. The solutes dissolved in body fluids contribute to total osmolality in proportion to their molar concentration: In ECF, sodium and its salts account for most of the osmolality, whereas in ICF salts of potassium are chiefly responsible. Control of osmolality occurs through regulation of water intake (thirst) and water excretion (urine volume, insensible loss, and stool water), with the kidneys being the chief regulator. If water intake is low, the kidneys can reduce urine volume and raise urine solute concentration fourfold above plasma (ie, to 1200–1400 mosm/kg H_2O). If water intake is high, the kidneys can excrete a large volume of dilute (50 mosm/kg H_2O) urine.

Concentrations of electrolytes are usually expressed as equivalent weights: A 1-molar (M) solution contains 1 gram molecular weight of a compound dissolved in 1 liter (L) of fluid; 1 equivalent (eq) of an ion is equal to 1 mole (mol) multiplied by the valence of the ion. For example, in the case of the monovalent sodium ion, 1 eq is equal to 1 mol. In the case of calcium, which is divalent, 1 eq is equal to 0.5 mol. In the relatively dilute conditions of body fluids, the sum of the molar concentrations of ions is approximately equal to total fluid osmolality. However, because the chemical activities of these solutes differ, it is usually more accurate to estimate osmolality by multiplying the serum sodium concentration by 2.

The sensitive regulation of salt and water excretion by the kidney produces an intimate relationship between body fluid osmolality and volume. Edelman and his coworkers showed that the osmolality of plasma or

Table 10–1. Total body water (as percentage of body weight) in relation to age and sex.

Age	Male	Female
10–18	59	57
18–40	61	51
40–60	55	47
Over 60	52	46

any other body fluid can be closely approximated by the sum of exchangeable sodium (Na_e^+) and its anions (A^-) plus exchangeable potassium (K_e^+) and its anions divided by total body water (TBW):

$$\text{Osmolality} = \frac{(Na_e^+ + A^-) + (K_e^+ + A^-)}{\text{TBW}} \quad (1)$$

The plasma sodium concentration (P_{Na}) can be determined by the expression shown in equation 2:

$$P_{Na} = \frac{(Na_e^+ + (K_e^+)}{\text{TBW}} \quad (2)$$

Although it is neither practical nor necessary to measure exchangeable sodium, exchangeable potassium, or total body water routinely, equation 2 illustrates the major factors that affect the serum sodium concentration and helps one to understand the cause and therapy of many fluid and electrolyte disturbances.

In a steady state, the volume and composition of the urine depend upon the intake of water and dietary solutes. An average North American diet generates about 600 mosm of solute daily that must be excreted by the kidneys. Most people ingest more than 5 g of sodium chloride per day, equivalent to about 85 meq of Na^+ (1 g NaCl = 17 meq Na^+). Potassium excretion averages 40–60 meq/d. Water intake is more variable but usually amounts to about 2 L/d; an additional 400 mL of water per day is generated from cellular metabolism. Extrarenal (insensible) water loss amounts to 10 mL/kg body weight/24 h equally divided among losses from the lungs, from the skin, and in the stool. Losses from the lungs and skin may vary under physiologic conditions, but stool water rarely exceeds 200 mL/d in health. Thus, a typical 24-hour urine volume is 1500 mL and has the approximate solute concentrations shown in Table 10–2.

Figure 10–1. Electrolyte composition of human body fluids. Note that the values are in meq/L of water, not of body fluid. (Reproduced, with permission, from Leaf A, Newburgh LH: *Significance of the Body Fluids in Clinical Medicine*, 2nd ed. Thomas, 1955.)

Table 10–2. Typical daily solute balances in normal subjects.

	Concentration	Total Amount	
Intake			
Water			
Ingested	...	2	L
Cell metabolism	...	0.4	L
Total solute	...	600	mosm
Sodium	...	100	meq
Potassium	...	60	meq
Urinary excretion			
Water		1.5	L
Total solute	400 mosm/kgH$_2$O	600	mosm
Sodium	60 meq/L	90	meq[1]
Potassium	36 meq/L	54	meq[1]

[1]Small amounts of sodium and potassium are lost extrarenally (stool, sweat).

■ VOLUME DISORDERS

RECOGNITION & TREATMENT OF VOLUME DEPLETION

Since volume depletion is common in surgical patients, a general approach to the diagnosis and treatment of volume depletion should be developed and applied to each patient systematically. The clinical manifestations of volume depletion are low blood pressure, narrow pulse pressure, tachycardia, poor skin turgor, and dry mucous membranes. The history may suggest the reason for volume depletion. Records of intake and output, changes in body weight, urine specific gravity, and analysis of the chemical composition of the urine should confirm the clinical impression and be useful when a treatment plan is being devised. Therapy must aim to correct the volume deficit and associated aberrations in electrolyte concentrations.

VOLUME DEPLETION

The simplest form of volume depletion is water deficit without accompanying solute deficit. However, in surgical patients, water and solute deficits more often occur together. Pure water deficits occur in patients who are unable to regulate intake. They may be debilitated or comatose or may have increased insensible water loss from fever. Patients given tube feedings without adequate water supplementation and those with diabetes insipidus may also develop this syndrome. Pure water deficit is reflected biochemically by hyperna-

tremia; the magnitude of the deficit can be estimated from the P$_{Na}$ (equations 2, 3).

Associated findings are an increase in the plasma osmolality, concentrated urine, and a low urine sodium concentration (< 15 meq/L) despite hypernatremia. The clinical manifestations are chiefly caused by hypernatremia, which can depress the central nervous system, resulting in lethargy or coma. Muscle rigidity, tremors, spasticity, and seizures may occur. Since many patients suffering from water deficit have primary neurologic disease, it is often difficult to tell if the symptoms were caused by hypernatremia or by the underlying disease.

Treatment involves replacement of enough water to restore the plasma sodium (P$_{Na}$) concentration to normal. The excess sodium for which water must be provided can be estimated from equation 3:

$$\Delta Na = (140 - P_{Na}) \times TBW \qquad (3)$$

The ΔNa represents the total milliequivalents of sodium in excess of water. Divide ΔNa by 140 to obtain the amount of water required to return the serum sodium concentration to 140 meq/L. Because of the dehydration, an estimate of total body water (TBW) should be used that is somewhat lower than the normal values listed in Table 10–1. In addition to correction of the existing water deficit, ongoing obligatory water losses (due to diabetes insipidus, fever, etc) must be satisfied. Treat the patient with 5% dextrose in water unless hypotension has developed, in which case hypotonic saline should be used. Rarely, isotonic saline may be indicated to treat shock due to dehydration even though the patient is hypernatremic.

VOLUME & ELECTROLYTE DEPLETION

Combined water and electrolyte depletion may occur from gastrointestinal losses due to nasogastric suction, enteric fistulas, enterostomies, or diarrhea. Other causes are excessive diuretic therapy, adrenal insufficiency, profuse sweating, burns, and body fluid sequestration following trauma or surgery. Diagnosis of combined volume and electrolyte deficiency can be made from the history, physical signs, and records of intake and output. The clinical findings are similar to those of pure volume depletion. However, the urine Na$^+$ concentration is often less than 10 meq/L, a manifestation of renal sodium conservation resulting from the action of aldosterone on the renal tubule. The urine is usually hypertonic (sp gr > 1.020), with an osmolality greater than 450–500 mosm/kg. The decreased blood volume diminishes renal perfusion and often produces prerenal azotemia, reflected by elevated blood urea nitrogen (BUN) and serum creatinine. Prerenal azotemia is characterized by a disproportionate rise of BUN compared to creatinine; the normal BUN/creatinine ratio of 10:1 is exceeded and may go as high as 20–25:1. This relationship helps differentiate prerenal azotemia from acute tubular necrosis, in which the BUN/creatinine ratio remains close to normal as the serum levels of both substances rise.

Combined water-electrolyte deficits are corrected by restoring volume and the deficient electrolytes. The magnitude of the volume deficit can be estimated by serial measurements of body weight, since acute changes in body weight primarily reflect changes in body fluid. Central venous or pulmonary artery pressure may be low in blood volume deficits and may be useful for monitoring replacement therapy.

The composition of the replacement fluid should take into account the plasma sodium concentration: If the P_{Na} is normal, fluid and electrolyte losses are probably isotonic, and the replacement fluid should be isotonic saline or its equivalent. Hyponatremia may result from salt loss exceeding water loss (ie, the decrease in Na_e^+ will be greater than the decrease in TBW; equation 2) or from previous administration of hypotonic solutions. In this situation, the magnitude of the salt deficit can be calculated from equation 3.

Replacement therapy should be planned in two steps: (1) the sodium deficit should be calculated, and (2) the volume deficit should be estimated from clinical signs and changes in body weight. From these calculations, a hypothetical replacement solution can be devised in which the sodium deficit is administered as NaCl and the volume deficit as isotonic NaCl solution. Then administer isotonic NaCl solutions and monitor the patient's response (ie, urine volume and composition, serum electrolytes, and clinical signs). With restoration of ECF volume, renal perfusion improves, and excretion of water will occur while Na^+ continues to be reabsorbed. When replacement is adequate, renal function and serum Na^+ and Cl^- concentrations will return to normal.

VOLUME OVERLOAD

Hormonal and circulatory responses to surgery result in postoperative conservation of sodium and water by the kidneys that is independent of the status of the ECF volume. Antidiuretic hormone, released during anesthesia and surgical stress, promotes water conservation by the kidneys. Renal vasoconstriction and increased aldosterone activity reduce sodium excretion. Consequently, if fluid intake is excessive in the immediate postoperative period, circulatory overload may occur. The tendency for water retention may be exaggerated if heart failure, liver disease, renal disease, or hypoalbuminemia is present. Clinical manifestations of volume overload include edema of the sacrum and extremities, jugular venous distention, tachypnea (if pulmonary edema develops), increased body weight, and elevated pulmonary artery and central venous pressure. A gallop rhythm would indicate cardiac failure.

Volume overload may precipitate prerenal azotemia and oliguria. Examination of the urine usually shows low sodium and high potassium concentrations consistent with enhanced tubular reabsorption of Na^+ and water.

Management of volume overload depends upon its severity. For mild overload, sodium restriction will usually be adequate. If hyponatremia is present, water restriction will also be necessary. Diuretics must be used for severe volume overload. If cardiac failure is present, other measures must be employed, and a cardiology consultation may be necessary.

Inappropriate secretion of antidiuretic hormone (which may occur with head injury, some cancers, and burns) will produce a syndrome characterized by hyponatremia, concentrated urine, elevated urine sodium concentration, and a normal or mildly expanded ECF volume. The serum Na^+ values may drop below 110 meq/L and produce confusion and lethargy. In most cases, restriction of water intake alone will be sufficient to correct the abnormality. Occasionally, a potent diuretic (eg, furosemide) should be given and intravenous isotonic saline infused at a rate equal to the urine output; this will rapidly correct the hyponatremia. Patients with intracranial disease may also develop the syndrome of cerebral salt wasting and present with hyponatremia. However, these patients are volume-depleted, and correct treatment is sodium and volume replacement rather than water restriction.

■ SPECIFIC ELECTROLYTE DISORDERS

SODIUM

Regulation of the sodium concentration in plasma or urine is intimately associated with regulation of total body water (equation 2) and clinically reflects the balance between total body solute and TBW.

Hypernatremia represents chiefly loss of water; this condition has been discussed above. Current neurosurgical management of traumatic brain injury utilizes controlled hypernatremia by infusion of hypertonic saline to maintain serum Na^+ between 155 and 160 meq/L.

In addition to dilutional hyponatremia and isotonic dehydration, apparent hyponatremia developed in patients with marked hyperlipidemia or hyperproteinemia due to earlier measurement techniques since fat and protein contribute to plasma bulk even though they are not dissolved in plasma water. The sodium concentration of plasma water in this situation is usually normal. Current laboratory techniques use ion-specific electrode measurements of the serum electrolytes, so apparent hyponatremia is no longer a clinical concern.

Hyponatremia in severe hyperglycemia results from the osmotic effects of the elevated glucose concentration, which draws water from the intracellular space to dilute ECF sodium. In hyperglycemia, the magnitude of this effect can be estimated by multiplying the blood glucose concentration in mg/dL by 0.016 and adding the result to the existing serum sodium concentration. The sum represents the predicted serum sodium concentration if the hyperglycemia were corrected. A recent study has suggested that this correction factor may be even higher, particularly at very high (> 400 mg/dL) glucose concentrations.

Acute, severe hyponatremia occasionally develops in patients undergoing elective surgery. In these patients, the hyponatremia results from excessive intravenous sodium-free fluid administration coupled with the postsurgical stimulation of antidiuretic hormone release and causes severe permanent brain damage. Premenopausal women are at greater risk for developing this complication. This outcome underscores the need to limit postoperative free water administration and monitor serum electrolytes.

In most cases, hyponatremia can be successfully treated by administering the calculated sodium needs in isotonic solutions. Infusion of hypertonic saline solutions is rarely indicated and could precipitate circulatory overload. Only when severe hyponatremia (usually with P_{Na} < 120 meq/L) produces mental obtundation and seizures should the patient be treated with hypertonic sodium solutions. The rate of correction of hyponatremia is a major factor in determining outcome. Rapid correction of severe hyponatremia may cause permanent brain damage due to the osmotic demyelination syndrome. For this reason, serum Na^+ should be increased at a rate not to exceed 10–12 meq/L/h. Hyponatremia with volume overload usually indicates impaired renal ability to excrete sodium.

POTASSIUM

The potassium in extracellular fluids constitutes only 2% of total body potassium (Figure 10–1); the remaining 98% is within body cells.

The serum potassium concentration ($[K^+]$) is thought to be determined primarily by the pH of ECF and the size of the intracellular K^+ pool (Figure 10–2). With extracellular acidosis from administration of inorganic (strong) acids, it has been shown that a large pro-

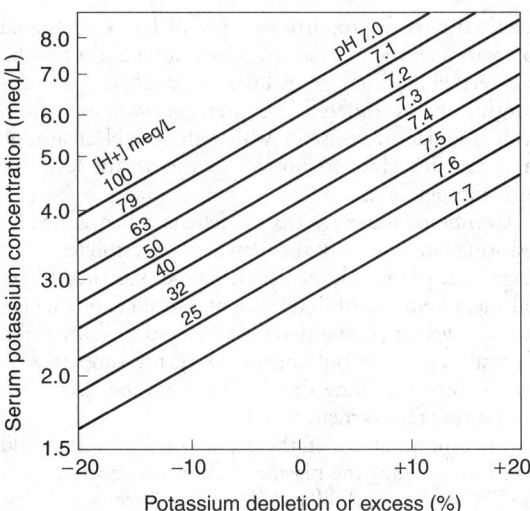

Figure 10–2. Relationship of serum potassium to total body potassium stores at different blood pH levels. (Reprinted, with permission, from *University of Washington Teaching Syllabus for the Course on Fluid and Electrolyte Balance*. Edited by Belding Scribner, MD.)

portion of the excess hydrogen is buffered intracellularly by an exchange of intracellular K^+ for extracellular H^+; this movement of K^+ may produce dangerous hyperkalemia. However, states of clinical metabolic acidosis result from derangements in intracellular metabolism to produce organic acidosis, which may not exert the same effects on the serum K^+. Likewise, simple alkalosis does not regularly result in hypokalemia from movement of K^+ into cells.

In the absence of an acid-base disturbance, serum K^+ reflects the total body pool of potassium (Figure 10–2). With excessive external losses of potassium (eg, from the gastrointestinal tract) (Table 10–3), the serum $[K^+]$ falls: A loss of 10% of total body K^+ drops the serum $[K^+]$ from 4 to 3 meq/L at a normal pH.

Although pH and body composition influence potassium metabolism, measurements of potassium intake and urinary potassium excretion allow the clinician to control potassium balance. Renal excretion of potassium is regulated by mineralocorticoid (aldosterone) levels. Renal failure—particularly acute oliguric renal failure—results in potassium retention and hyperkalemia. Adrenal insufficiency may produce hyperkalemia through impaired renal excretion. Hypokalemia from excessive renal excretion may follow administration of diuretics, adrenal steroid excess, and certain renal tubular disorders associated with potassium wasting. Rarely, potassium deficiency can arise from defi-

Table 10–3. Volume and electrolyte content of gastrointestinal fluid losses.[1]

	Na$^+$ (meq/L)	K$^+$ (meq/L)	Cl$^-$ (meq/L)	NCO$_3^-$ (meq/L)	Volume (mL)
Gastric juice, high in acid	20 (20–30)	10 (5–40)	120 (80–150)	0	1000–9000
Gastric juice, low in acid	80 (70–140)	15 (5–40)	90 (40–120)	5–25	1000–2500
Pancreatic juice	140 (115–180)	5 (3–8)	75 (55–95)	80 (60–110)	500–1000
Bile	148 (130–160)	5 (3–12)	100 (90–120)	35 (30–40)	300–1000
Small bowel drainage	110 (80–150)	5 (2–8)	105 (60–125)	30 (20–40)	1000–3000
Distal ileum and cecum drainage	80 (40–135)	8 (5–30)	45 (20–90)	30 (20–40)	1000–3000
Diarrheal stools	120 (20–160)	25 (10–40)	90 (30–120)	45 (30–50)	500–17,000

[1]Average values/24 h with range in parentheses.

cient dietary potassium intake, as in alcoholic patients or in those receiving total parenteral nutrition with inadequate potassium replacement.

1. HYPERKALEMIA

Hyperkalemia is a treatable problem that may prove fatal if undiagnosed. Blood potassium levels must be closely monitored in susceptible patients such as those with severe trauma, burns, crush injuries, renal insufficiency, or marked catabolism from other causes. Hyperkalemia may also be due to Addison's disease. Clinical evidence of significant hyperkalemia is usually not present. Nausea and vomiting, colicky abdominal pain, and diarrhea may occur. The electrocardiographic changes are the most helpful indicators of the severity of the disorder: Early changes include peaking of the T waves, widening of the QRS complex, and depression of the ST segment. With further elevation of the blood potassium level, the QRS widens to such a degree that the tracing resembles a sine wave, a finding that portends imminent cardiac standstill.

A number of factors must be rapidly considered in assessing the hyperkalemic patient. First, one should determine whether the serum potassium level is a true metabolic abnormality or has been elevated by hemolysis, marked leukocytosis, or thrombocytosis. Platelet counts greater than 1 million/μL may elevate the serum potassium, since the ion is liberated from platelets as they are consumed during clotting. Second, the acid-

base status should be assessed to ascertain its influence (Figure 10–2). Finally, the rapidity with which the elevated serum potassium should be corrected must be determined.

There are five approaches to the emergency treatment of hyperkalemia. Initially, an intravenous infusion of 100 mL of 50% dextrose solution containing 20 units of regular insulin will lower extracellular K$^+$ by promoting its intracellular transport in association with glucose. Intravenous NaHCO$_3$ solutions may lower serum K$^+$ as acidosis is corrected, though this point remains controversial. Calcium antagonizes the tissue effects of potassium; an infusion of calcium gluconate will transiently reverse cardiac depression from hyperkalemia without changing the serum potassium concentration. A slower method of controlling hyperkalemia is to administer the cation exchange resin sodium polystyrene sulfonate (Kayexalate) orally or by enema at a rate of 40–80 g/d. This drug binds potassium in the intestine in exchange for sodium. It is often given with sorbitol to induce osmotic diarrhea and enhance the rate of potassium removal. Finally, when hyperkalemia is a manifestation of renal failure, hemodialysis is often necessary; beta-adrenergic stimulation with inhaled albuterol is also helpful in these patients.

2. HYPOKALEMIA

Hypokalemia usually results from renal wasting of potassium; potassium deficiency and hypokalemia from inadequate dietary intake occur only after weeks of a deficient diet. Alcoholics and elderly people with restricted diets are at risk for potassium depletion due to insufficient dietary intake. The clinical manifestations of hypokalemia relate to neuromuscular function: Decreased muscle contractility and muscle cell potential develop, and in extreme cases death may result from paralysis of the muscles of respiration.

When the clinician assesses hypokalemia, the initial goal is to identify the cause. If alkalosis is present, the K^+ needs can be estimated from the nomogram in Figure 10–2. If there is no acid-base imbalance, or if hypokalemia persists after alkalosis is corrected, renal losses are probably excessive. Urine potassium excretion of more than 30 meq/24 h associated with a serum $[K^+]$ under 3.5 meq/L indicates renal potassium wasting. The primary problem in this situation is usually diuretic therapy, alkalosis, or increased aldosterone activity. If renal potassium excretion is less than 30 meq/24 h, the kidneys are conserving potassium appropriately, and hypokalemia reflects a total body deficit.

Treatment consists of correcting the cause of hypokalemia and administering potassium. If the patient is able to eat, potassium should be given orally; otherwise, it should be given intravenously. Usually, potassium concentrations in intravenous solutions should not exceed 40 meq/L. In moderate to severe hypokalemia ($[K^+] < 3$ meq/L), potassium may be administered at a rate of 20–30 meq/h. With mild hypokalemia ($[K^+]$ 3–3.5 meq/L), potassium should be replaced slowly to avoid hyperkalemia. Potassium should usually be administered intravenously as the chloride salt; in metabolic alkalosis, potassium chloride is specific, since it helps to correct the acid-base abnormality as well as the hypokalemia. Occasional patients may have persistent hypokalemia refractory to replacement therapy because of coexistent magnesium deficiency. Therefore, serum magnesium concentration should be measured in hypokalemic patients, particularly since many of the causes of potassium deficiency will also result in magnesium depletion (see below).

CALCIUM

Calcium is an important mediator of neuromuscular function and cellular enzyme processes even though most of the body calcium is contained in the skeleton. The usual dietary intake of calcium is 1–3 g/d, most of which is excreted unabsorbed in the feces.

The normal serum calcium concentration (8.5–10.3 mg/dL, 4.2–5.2 meq/L) is maintained by humoral factors, mainly vitamin D, parathyroid hormone, and calcitonin. Acidemia increases and alkalemia decreases the serum ionized calcium concentration. Approximately half of the total serum calcium is bound to plasma proteins, chiefly albumin; a small amount is complexed to plasma anions, such as citrate; and the remainder (approximately 40%) of the total serum calcium is free, or ionized, calcium, which is the fraction responsible for the biologic effects. The ionized calcium usually remains constant when the total serum calcium concentration changes with different serum albumin concentrations. Unless the ionized calcium is measured, the serum calcium can only be reliably assessed if accompanied by measurement of the serum albumin concentration.

Severe disturbances of calcium concentration are uncommon in surgical patients, although transient asymptomatic hypocalcemia is common. After operations on the thyroid or parathyroids, the serum calcium concentration should be measured at regular intervals to detect hypocalcemia early if it appears.

1. HYPOCALCEMIA

Hypocalcemia occurs in hypoparathyroidism, hypomagnesemia, severe pancreatitis, chronic or acute renal failure, severe trauma, crush injuries, and necrotizing fasciitis. The clinical manifestations are neuromuscular: hyperactive deep tendon reflexes, a positive Chvostek sign, muscle and abdominal cramps, carpopedal spasm, and, rarely, convulsions. Hypocalcemia is reflected in the ECG by a prolonged QT interval.

The initial step is to check the whole blood pH; if alkalosis is present, it should be treated. Intravenous calcium, as calcium gluconate or calcium chloride, may be needed for the acute problem (eg, after parathyroidectomy). Chronic hypoparathyroidism requires vitamin D, oral calcium supplements, and often aluminum hydroxide gels to bind dietary phosphate in the intestine.

2. HYPERCALCEMIA

Hypercalcemia most frequently is caused by hyperparathyroidism, cancer with bony metastases, ectopic production of parathyroid hormone, vitamin D intoxication, hyperthyroidism, sarcoidosis, milk-alkali syndrome, or prolonged immobilization (especially in young patients or those with Paget's disease). It is also a rare complication of thiazide diuretics.

The symptoms of hypercalcemia are fatigability, muscle weakness, depression, anorexia, nausea, and constipation. Long-standing hypercalcemia may impair renal concentrating mechanisms, resulting in polyuria and polydipsia and in metastatic deposition of calcium. Severe hypercalcemia can cause coma and death. *A serum calcium concentration above 12 mg/dL should be regarded as a medical emergency!*

With severe hypercalcemia (Ca^{2+} > 14.5 mg/dL), intravenous isotonic saline should be given to expand ECF, increase urine flow, enhance calcium excretion, and reduce the serum level.

Furosemide and intravenous sodium sulfate are other methods of increasing renal calcium excretion. Plicamycin is particularly useful for hypercalcemia associated with metastatic cancer. Adrenal corticosteroids are useful for hypercalcemia associated with sarcoidosis, vitamin D intoxication, and Addison's disease. Calcitonin is indicated in patients with impaired renal and cardiovascular function. When renal failure is present, hemodialysis may be required.

MAGNESIUM

Magnesium is largely present in bone and cells, where it serves an important role in cellular energy metabolism. The normal plasma magnesium concentration is 1.5–2.5 meq/L. Magnesium is excreted primarily by the kidneys. The serum magnesium concentration reflects total body magnesium. Serum magnesium levels may be elevated in hypovolemic shock as magnesium is liberated from cells.

1. HYPOMAGNESEMIA

Hypomagnesemia occurs with poor dietary intake, intestinal malabsorption of ingested magnesium, or excessive losses from the gut (eg, severe diarrhea, enteric fistulas, use of purgatives, or nasogastric suction). It may also be caused by excessive urinary losses (eg, from diuretics), chronic alcohol abuse, hyperaldosteronism, and hypercalcemia. Hypomagnesemia occasionally develops in acute pancreatitis, in diabetic acidosis, in burned patients, or after prolonged total parenteral nutrition with insufficient magnesium supplementation. The clinical manifestations resemble those of hypocalcemia: hyperactive tendon reflexes, a positive Chvostek sign, and tremors that may progress to delirium and convulsions.

The diagnosis of hypomagnesemia depends on clinical suspicion with confirmation by measurement of the serum magnesium. Treatment consists of administering magnesium, usually as the sulfate or chloride. In moderate magnesium deficiency, oral replacement is adequate. In more severe deficits, parenteral magnesium must be administered intravenously (40–80 meq of $MgSO_4$ per liter of intravenous fluid). When large doses are infused intravenously, there is a risk of producing hypermagnesemia, with tachycardia and hypotension. The ECG should be inspected for prolongation of the QT interval. Magnesium should be administered cautiously to oliguric patients or those with renal failure and only after magnesium deficiency has been unequivocally documented. Magnesium deficiency may also be accompanied by refractory hypokalemia.

2. HYPERMAGNESEMIA

Hypermagnesemia usually occurs in patients with renal disease; it is rare in surgical patients. In patients with renal insufficiency, serum magnesium levels should be monitored closely. Strict attention must be paid to excess magnesium intake, which can occur from a variety of commonly administered antacids and laxatives and which may produce severe and even fatal hypermagnesemia in renal insufficiency.

The initial signs and symptoms of hypermagnesemia are lethargy and weakness. Electrocardiographic changes resemble those in hyperkalemia (widened QRS complex, ST segment depression, and peaked T waves). When the serum level reaches 6 meq/L, deep tendon reflexes are lost; with levels above 10 meq/L, somnolence, coma, and death may ensue.

Treatment of hypermagnesemia consists of giving intravenous isotonic saline to increase the rate of renal magnesium excretion. This may be accompanied by slow intravenous infusion of calcium, since calcium antagonizes some of the neuromuscular actions of magnesium. Patients with hypermagnesemia and severe renal failure may need dialysis.

PHOSPHORUS

Phosphorus is primarily a constituent of bone, but it is also an important intracellular ion with a role in energy metabolism. The serum phosphorus level is only an approximate indicator of total body phosphorus and can be influenced by a number of factors, including the serum calcium concentration and the pH of blood. In urine, phosphorus is an important buffer that facilitates the excretion of acids formed by intermediary metabolism. Urine phosphate buffer is reflected by the excretion of titratable acid.

1. HYPOPHOSPHATEMIA

Clinically important hypophosphatemia may follow poor dietary intake (especially in alcoholics), hyperparathyroidism, and antacid administration (antacids bind phosphate in the intestine). Hypophosphatemia was at one time a frequent complication of total parenteral nutrition until phosphate supplementation became routine. Clinical manifestations appear when the serum phosphorus level falls to 1 mg/dL or less. Neuromuscular manifestations include lassitude, fatigue, weakness, convulsions, and death. Red blood cells hemolyze, oxygen delivery is impaired, and white cell phagocytosis is depressed. Cardiac contractility may be impaired, and rhabdomyolysis can occur. Chronic phosphate depletion has been implicated in the development of osteomalacia.

2. HYPERPHOSPHATEMIA

Hyperphosphatemia most often develops in severe renal disease, after trauma, or with marked tissue catabolism. It is rarely caused by excessive dietary intake. Hyperphosphatemia is usually asymptomatic. Because it raises the calcium-phosphorus product, the serum calcium concentration is depressed. A high calcium-phosphate product predisposes to metastatic calcification of soft tissues. Treatment of hyperphosphatemia is by diuresis to increase the rate of urinary phosphorus excretion. Administration of phosphate-binding antacids, such as aluminum hydroxide gels, will diminish the gastrointestinal absorption of phosphorus and lower the serum phosphorus concentration. In patients with renal disease, dialysis may be required.

■ ACID-BASE BALANCE

NORMAL PHYSIOLOGY

During the course of daily metabolism of protein and carbohydrate, approximately 70 meq (or 1 meq/kg of body weight) of hydrogen ion is generated and delivered into the body fluids. In addition, a large amount of carbon dioxide is formed that combines with water to form carbonic acid (H_2CO_3). If efficient mechanisms for buffering and eliminating these acids were not available, the pH of body fluids would fall rapidly. Although mammals have a highly developed system for handling daily acid production, disturbances of acid-base balance are common in disease.

Hydrogen ions generated from metabolism are buffered through two major systems. The first involves intracellular protein, eg, the hemoglobin in red blood cells. More important is the bicarbonate/carbonic acid system, which can be understood from the Henderson-Hasselbalch equation:

$$pH = pK + \log \frac{[HCO_3^-]}{0.03 \times P_{CO_2}} \qquad (4)$$

where pK for the $\dfrac{HCO_3^-}{H_2CO_3}$ system is 6.1.

Hydrogen ion concentration is related to pH in an inverse logarithmic manner. The following transforma-

tion of equation 4 is easier to use, because it eliminates the logarithms:

$$[H^+] = \frac{24 \times P_{CO_2}}{[HCO_e^-]} \qquad (5)$$

There is an approximately linear inverse relationship between pH and hydrogen ion concentration over the pH range of 7.9–7.50: For each 0.01 decrease in pH, the hydrogen ion concentration increases 1 nmol. Remembering that a normal blood pH of 7.40 is equal to a hydrogen ion concentration of 40 nmol/L, one can calculate the approximate hydrogen ion concentration for any pH between 7.10 and 7.50. For example, a pH of 7.30 is equal to a hydrogen ion concentration of 50 nmol/L. This estimation introduces an error of approximately 10% at the extremes of this pH range. (See also Figure 10–2.)

A consideration of the right-hand side of equation 5 demonstrates that hydrogen ion concentration is determined by the ratio of the P_{aCO_2} to the plasma bicarbonate concentration. In body fluids, CO_2 is dissolved and combines with water to form carbonic acid, the acid part of the acid-base pair. If any two of these three variables are known, the third can be calculated using this expression.

Equation 5 also illustrates how the body excretes acid produced from metabolism. Blood P_{CO_2} is normally controlled within narrow limits by pulmonary ventilation. The plasma bicarbonate concentration is regulated in the renal tubules by three major processes: (1) Filtered bicarbonate is reabsorbed, mostly in the proximal tubule, to prevent excessive bicarbonate loss in the urine; (2) hydrogen ions are secreted as titratable acid to regenerate the bicarbonate that was buffered when these hydrogen ions were initially produced and to provide a vehicle for excretion of about one-third of the daily acid production; and (3) the kidneys also excrete hydrogen ion in the form of ammonium ion by a process that regenerates bicarbonate initially consumed in the production of these hydrogen ions. Volume depletion, increased P_{aCO_2}, and hypokalemia all favor enhanced tubular reabsorption of HCO_3^-.

ACID-BASE ABNORMALITIES

The management of clinical acid-base disturbances is facilitated by the use of a nomogram (Figure 10–3) that relates the three variables in equation 5.

Primary respiratory disturbances cause changes in the blood P_{aCO_2} (the numerator in equation 5) and produce corresponding effects on the blood hydrogen ion concentration. Metabolic disturbances primarily affect the plasma bicarbonate concentration (the denomi-

Figure 10–3. Acid-base nomogram for use in evaluation of clinical acid-base disorders. Hydrogen ion concentration (top) or blood pH (bottom) is plotted against plasma HCO_3^- concentration; curved lines are isopleths of CO_2 tension (Pa_{CO_2}, mm Hg). Knowing any two of these variables permits estimation of the third. The circle in the center represents the range of normal values; the shaded bands represent the 95% confidence limits of four common acid-base disturbances: I, acute respiratory acidosis; II, acute respiratory alkalosis; III, chronic respiratory acidosis; IV, sustained metabolic acidosis. Points lying outside these shaded areas are mixed disturbances and indicate two primary acid-base disorders. (Courtesy of Anthony Sebastian, MD, University of California Medical Center, San Francisco.

nator in equation 5). Whether the disturbance is primarily respiratory or metabolic, some degree of compensatory change occurs in the reciprocal factor in equation 5 to limit or nullify the magnitude of perturbation of acid-base balance. Thus, changes in blood P_{CO_2} from respiratory disturbances are compensated for by changes in the renal handling of bicarbonate. Conversely, changes in plasma bicarbonate concentration are blunted by appropriate respiratory changes.

Because acute respiratory changes allow insufficient time for compensatory renal mechanisms to respond, the resulting pH disturbances are often great and the abnormalities may be present in pure form. By contrast, chronic respiratory disturbances allow the full range of compensatory mechanisms by the kidneys to come into play, so that blood pH may remain near normal despite wide variations in the blood P_{CO_2}. On the other hand, respiratory compensation for metabolic disturbances occurs almost instantaneously, so that there is little difference in the acid-base variables between acute and chronic disorders.

1. RESPIRATORY ACIDOSIS

Acute respiratory acidosis occurs when respiration suddenly becomes inadequate. CO_2 accumulates in the blood (the numerator in equation 5 increases), and hydrogen ion concentration increases. This occurs most often in acute airway obstruction, aspiration, respiratory arrest, certain pulmonary infections, and pulmonary edema with impaired gas exchange. There is acidemia and an elevated blood P_{CO_2} but little change in the plasma bicarbonate concentration. Over 80% of the carbonic acid resulting from the increased Pa_{CO_2} is buffered by intracellular mechanisms—about 50% by intracellular protein and another 30% by hemoglobin. Because relatively little is buffered by bicarbonate ion, the plasma bicarbonate concentration may be normal. An acute increase in the Pa_{CO_2} from 40 to 80 mm Hg will increase the plasma bicarbonate by only 3 meq/L. This is why the 95% confidence band for acute respiratory acidosis (I in Figure 10–3) is nearly horizontal; ie, increases in Pa_{CO_2} directly increase hydrogen ion concentration and decrease pH with little change in plasma bicarbonate concentration. Treatment involves restoration of adequate ventilation. If necessary, tracheal intubation and assisted ventilation or controlled ventilation with sedation should be employed.

Chronic respiratory acidosis arises from chronic respiratory failure in which impaired ventilation gives a sustained elevation of blood P_{CO_2}. Renal compensation raises plasma bicarbonate to the extent illustrated by the 95% confidence limits in Figure 10–3 (the area marked by III). Rather marked elevations of Pa_{CO_2} produce small changes in blood pH, because of the increase in plasma bicarbonate concentration. This is achieved primarily by increased renal excretion of ammonium ion, which enhances acid excretion and regenerates bicarbonate, which is returned to the blood. Chronic respiratory acidosis is generally well tolerated until severe pulmonary insufficiency leads to hypoxia. At this point, the long-term prognosis is very poor. Paradoxically, the patient with chronic respiratory acidosis appears better able to tolerate additional acute increases in blood P_{CO_2}.

Treatment of chronic respiratory acidosis depends largely on attention to pulmonary toilet and ventilatory status. Rapid correction of chronic respiratory acidosis, as may occur if the patient is placed on controlled ventilation, can be dangerous, since the Pa_{CO_2} is lowered rapidly and the compensated respiratory acidosis may be converted to a severe metabolic alkalosis (posthypercapnic metabolic acidosis).

2. RESPIRATORY ALKALOSIS

Acute hyperventilation lowers the $PaCO_2$ without concomitant changes in the plasma bicarbonate concentration and thereby lowers the hydrogen ion concentration (II in Figure 10–3). The clinical manifestations are paresthesias in the extremities, carpopedal spasm, and a positive Chvostek sign. Acute hyperventilation with respiratory alkalosis may be an early sign of bacterial sepsis.

Chronic respiratory alkalosis occurs in pulmonary and liver disease. The renal response to chronic hypocapnia is to decrease the tubular reabsorption of filtered bicarbonate, increasing bicarbonate excretion, with a consequent lowering of plasma bicarbonate concentration. As the bicarbonate concentration falls, the chloride concentration rises. This is the same pattern seen in hyperchloremic acidosis, and the two can only be distinguished by blood gas and pH measurements. Generally, chronic respiratory alkalosis does not require treatment; if the $PaCO_2$ is allowed to return to normal rapidly, posthypocapnic metabolic acidosis with hyperchloremia may occur.

3. METABOLIC ACIDOSIS

Metabolic acidosis is caused by increased production of hydrogen ion from metabolic or other causes or from excessive bicarbonate losses. In either case, the plasma bicarbonate concentration is decreased, producing an increase in hydrogen ion concentration (see equation 5). With excessive bicarbonate loss (eg, severe diarrhea, diuretic treatment with acetazolamide or other carbonic anhydrase inhibitors, certain forms of renal tubular disease, and in patients with ureterosigmoidostomies), the decrease in plasma bicarbonate concentration is matched by an increase in the serum chloride, so that the anion gap (the sum of chloride and bicarbonate concentrations subtracted from the serum sodium concentration) remains at the normal level, below 15 meq/L. On the other hand, metabolic acidosis from increased acid production is associated with an anion gap exceeding 15 meq/L. Conditions in which this occurs are renal failure, diabetic ketoacidosis, lactic acidosis, methanol ingestion, salicylate intoxication, and ethylene glycol ingestion. The lungs compensate by hyperventilation, which returns the hydrogen ion concentration toward normal by lowering the blood PCO_2. In long-standing metabolic acidosis, minute ventilation may increase sufficiently to drop the $PaCO_2$ to as low as 10–15 mm Hg. The shaded area marked IV on the nomogram (Figure 10–3) represents the confidence limits for sustained metabolic acidosis.

Treatment of metabolic acidosis depends on identifying the underlying cause and correcting it. Often, this is sufficient. In some conditions, particularly when there is an increased anion gap, alkali administration is required. The amount of sodium bicarbonate required to restore the plasma bicarbonate concentration to normal can be estimated by subtracting the existing plasma bicarbonate concentration from the normal value of 24 meq/L and multiplying the resulting number by half the estimated total body water. This is a useful empiric formula. In practice, it is not usually wise to administer enough bicarbonate to return the plasma bicarbonate completely to normal. It is better to raise the plasma bicarbonate concentration by 5 meq/L initially and then reassess the clinical situation. The administration of sodium bicarbonate may cause fluid overload from the large quantity of sodium and may overcorrect the acidosis. The long-term management of patients with metabolic acidosis entails providing adequate alkali, either as supplemental sodium bicarbonate tablets or by dietary manipulation. In all cases, attempts should be made to minimize the magnitude of bicarbonate loss in patients with chronic metabolic acidosis.

4. METABOLIC ALKALOSIS

Metabolic alkalosis is probably the most common acid-base disturbance in surgical patients. In this condition, the blood hydrogen ion concentration is decreased as a result of accumulation of bicarbonate in plasma. The pathogenesis is complex but involves at least three separate factors: (1) loss of hydrogen ion, usually as a result of loss of gastric secretions rich in hydrochloric acid; (2) volume depletion, which is often severe; and (3) potassium depletion, which almost always is present.

HCl secretion by the gastric mucosa returns bicarbonate ion to the blood. Gastric acid, after mixing with ingested food, is subsequently reabsorbed in the small intestine, so that there is no net gain or loss of hydrogen ion in this process. If secreted hydrogen ion is lost through vomiting or drainage, the result is a net delivery of bicarbonate into the circulation. Normally, the kidneys are easily able to excrete the excess bicarbonate load. However, if volume depletion accompanies the loss of hydrogen ion, the kidneys work to preserve volume by increasing tubular reabsorption of sodium and whatever anions are also filtered. Consequently, because of the increased sodium reabsorption, the excess bicarbonate cannot be completely excreted. This perpetuates the metabolic alkalosis. At first, some of the filtered bicarbonate escapes reabsorption in the proximal tubule and reaches the distal tubule. Here it promotes potassium secretion and enhanced potassium loss in the urine. The urine pH will be either neutral or alkaline, because of the presence of bicarbonate. Later, as volume depletion becomes more severe, the reabsorption of filtered bicarbonate in the proximal tubule becomes virtually complete. Now, only small amounts of sodium, with little bicarbonate, reach the distal tubule. If potassium depletion is severe, sodium is reabsorbed in exchange for hydrogen ion. This results in the paradoxically acid urine sometimes observed in patients with advanced metabolic alkalosis.

Assessment should involve examination of the urine electrolytes and urine pH. In the early stages, bicarbonate excretion will obligate excretion of sodium as well as potassium, so the urine sodium concentration will be relatively high for a volume-depleted patient and the urine pH will be alkaline. In this circumstance, the urine chloride will reveal the extent of the volume depletion: A urine chloride of less than 10 meq/L is diagnostic of volume depletion and chloride deficiency. Later, when bicarbonate reabsorption becomes virtually complete, the urine pH will be acid, and urine sodium, potassium, and chloride concentrations will all be low. The ventilatory compensation in metabolic alkalosis is variable, but the maximal extent of compensation can only raise the blood P_{CO_2} to about 55 mm Hg. A Pa_{CO_2} greater than 60 mm Hg in metabolic alkalosis suggests a mixed disturbance also involving respiratory acidosis.

To treat metabolic alkalosis, fluid must be given, usually as saline solution. With adequate volume repletion, the stimulus to tubular sodium reabsorption is diminished, and the kidneys can then excrete the excess bicarbonate. Most of these patients are also substantially potassium-depleted and will require potassium supplementation. This should be administered as KCl, since chloride depletion is another hallmark of this condition and potassium given as citrate or lactate will not correct the potassium deficit.

5. MIXED ACID-BASE DISORDERS

In many situations, mixed disorders of acid-base balance develop. The most common example in surgical patients is metabolic acidosis superimposed on respiratory alkalosis. This problem can arise in patients with septic shock or hepatorenal syndrome. Since the two acid-base disorders tend to cancel each other, the disturbance in hydrogen ion concentration is usually small. The reverse situation, ie, respiratory acidosis combined with metabolic alkalosis, is less common. Combined metabolic and respiratory acidosis occurs in cardiorespiratory arrest and obviously constitutes a medical emergency. Circumstances involving both metabolic and respiratory alkalosis are rare. The clue to the presence of a mixed acid-base disorder can come from plotting the patient's acid-base data on the nomogram in Figure 10–3. If the set of data falls outside one of the confidence bands, then by definition the patient has a mixed disorder. On the other hand, if the acid-base data fall within one of the confidence bands, it suggests (but does not prove) that the acid-base disturbance is pure or uncomplicated.

■ PRINCIPLES OF FLUID & ELECTROLYTE THERAPY

The development of a rational plan of fluid and electrolyte therapy requires an understanding of the principles developed earlier in this chapter. First, maintenance fluid requirements must be determined. Second, existing deficits of volume or composition should be calculated. This involves the analysis of four aspects of the patient's fluid and electrolyte status based on weight changes, serum electrolyte concentrations, and blood pH and P_{CO_2}: (1) the magnitude of the volume deficit present, (2) the pathogenesis and treatment of abnormal sodium concentration, (3) assessment of any potassium requirement, and (4) management of any coexistent acid-base disturbance. Finally, therapy must also recognize the presence of ongoing obligatory fluid losses and include these losses in the daily plan of treatment.

Normal maintenance requirements can be determined using the guidelines in Table 10–2. Fever or elevated ambient temperature will increase insensible losses and thereby increase these requirements. The normal response to the stress of surgery is to conserve water and electrolytes, so maintenance requirements are decreased in the immediate postoperative period. In addition, increased catabolism will deliver more potassium to the circulation, so that this ion can be omitted from maintenance solutions for several days postoperatively.

Correction of preexisting deficits must be based on the four factors listed above. Volume deficit is best estimated on the basis of acute changes in weight or from clinical estimates; the clinician should remember that deficits less than 5% of body water will not be detectable and that loss of 15% of body water will be associated with severe circulatory compromise. The relationship of net sodium to net fluid deficit is given by the serum sodium concentration according to equation 3. If the serum sodium concentration is normal, fluid losses have been isotonic; if hyponatremia is present, more sodium than water has been lost. In either case, initial replacement should be with isotonic saline solutions. Any potassium excess or deficit must be assessed in the light of the blood pH according to Figure 10–2. If hypokalemia exists at normal pH, the magnitude of the total body potassium deficit can also be estimated using Figure 10–2. For example, a serum potassium concentration of 2.5 meq/L at pH 7.40 suggests a 20%

depletion of total body potassium. A normal human has a potassium capacity of 45 meq/kg body weight; a moderately wasted patient, 35 meq/kg. For a normal 70-kg man, total potassium capacity is 45 × 70, or 3150 meq; the deficit is 20% of this, or 630 meq, and this amount must be considered in therapy calculations. Principles of acid-base therapy have already been outlined.

Two rules of thumb should be applied in prescribing parenteral therapy for fluid and electrolyte deficits. The first is that for most problems, half of the calculated deficits should be replaced in a 24-hour period, with subsequent reassessment of the clinical situation. The second is that a fluid or electrolyte abnormality should take as long to correct as it took to develop. By adherence to these guidelines, overly vigorous replacement will be avoided and, along with it, the production of a different (iatrogenic) electrolyte abnormality.

Ongoing losses must be considered also in the daily fluid therapy plan, with regard to both volume and composition. Characteristic measurements for fluids removed from different segments of the gastrointestinal tract are shown in Table 10–3.

ILLUSTRATIVE EXAMPLE

A 40-year-old man whose normal weight is 70 kg is admitted to the hospital after 5 days' protracted vomiting, during which time he has been able to ingest nothing but an occasional glass of water. Physical examination shows evidence of dehydration, and diagnostic studies confirm the admitting impression of a duodenal ulcer with pyloric obstruction. Weight on admission is 65 kg. Initial laboratory studies include the following:

Serum Na^+ 122 meq/L, K^+ 2 meq/L, Cl^- 80 meq/L, HCO_3^- 35 meq/L, urea nitrogen 42 mg/dL, creatinine 1.7 mg/dL.

Arterial blood pH 7.50, PCO_2 44 mm Hg.

Urine Na^+ 27 meq/L, Cl^- 8 meq/L, K^+ 64 meq/L, pH 7.0.

Discussion

Volume depletion is suggested by weight loss of 5 kg, evidence of volume depletion, elevation of BUN and creatinine, and urine Cl^- less than 10 meq/L. The underlying abnormality is metabolic alkalosis and chloride depletion from loss of gastric juice. Hyponatremia results from loss of sodium (gastric juice and urine) with ingestion only of water. Urine pH is neutral because of bicarbonate excretion, obligating sodium excretion, and the high urine potassium is reflective of the potassium wasting occurring in metabolic alkalosis despite hypokalemia.

Parenteral fluid therapy for the first 24 hours should consider the following:

Maintenance requirements will be unchanged from normal in the absence of fever. Based on weight, the volume deficit is about 5 L. The sodium deficit, calculated from equation 3, is 585 meq; this amount is required to restore the serum sodium concentration to 140 meq/L. To this must be added the amount of sodium in 5 L of isotonic replacement fluid, or 700 meq, for a total sodium deficit of 1285 meq. The serum potassium, when corrected to normal pH, would be about 2.4 meq/L, consistent with a 20% deficit, or about 630 meq. The alkalosis in this setting will be responsive merely to volume replacement and requires no special therapy; sodium and potassium replacements, however, must be with chloride as the anion. If gastric losses via nasogastric suction continue in the hospital, they should be included in the plan (Table 10–3). These considerations result in the following:

	Volume (L)	Na^+ (meq/L)	K^+ (meq/L)
Maintenance	2	100	60
Correction of deficit	5	1285	630
Ongoing losses (estimated)	2	40	20

Using the rule of thumb that half of deficits should be replaced in 24 hours, the physician should issue initial orders for intravenous therapy of about 6.5 L of fluid, 780 meq of sodium, and 260 meq of potassium; this last figure is not sufficient to replace half of the potassium deficit but limits the potassium concentration in intravenous fluid to 40 meq/L, the highest concentration routinely advisable. This combination can be approximated with 4 L of 5% dextrose in isotonic sodium chloride and 2.5 L of 5% dextrose in 0.5 N saline, with potassium added to each bottle to achieve a concentration of 40 meq/L. These fluids should then be administered at a rate of 250 mL/h and the situation then reassessed after 24 hours.

REFERENCES

General

Seldin DW, Giebisch G (editors): *The Kidney: Physiology and Pathophysiology,* 3rd ed. Lippincott Williams & Wilkins, 2000.

Fluid Volume & Sodium Concentration

Adrogue HJ et al: Hypernatremia. N Engl J Med 2000;342:1493.
Adrogue HJ et al: Hyponatremia. N Engl J Med 2000;342:1581.

Anderson RJ: Hospital-associated hyponatremia. Kidney Int 1986; 29:1237.

Arieff AI: Hyponatremia, convulsions, respiratory arrest, and permanent brain damage after elective surgery in healthy women. N Engl J Med 1986;314:1529.

Ayus JC et al: Postoperative hyponatremic encephalopathy in menstruant women. Ann Intern Med 1992;117:891.

Ayus JC et al: Chronic hyponatremic encephalopathy in postmenopausal women. Association of therapies with morbidity and mortality. JAMA 1999;281:2342.

Brater DC: Use of diuretics in cirrhosis and nephrotic syndrome. Semin Nephrol 1999;19:575.

Doyle JA et al: The use of hypertonic saline in the treatment of traumatic brain injury. J Trauma 2001;50:367.

Ellison DH: Diuretic resistance: physiology and therapeutics. Semin Nephrol 1999;19:581.

Fried LF et al: Hyponatremia and hypernatremia. Med Clin North Am 1997;81:585.

Harrigan MR: Cerebral salt wasting syndrome: a review. Neurosurgery 1996;38:152.

Hilliard TA et al: Hyponatremia: evaluating the correction factor for hyperglycemia. Am J Med 1999;106:399.

Hirshberg B et al: The syndrome of inappropriate antidiuretic hormone secretion on the elderly. Am J Med 1997;103:270.

Katz MA: Hyperglycemia-induced hyponatremia—calculation of expected serum sodium depression. N Engl J Med 1973;289: 843.

Knochel JP: Hypoxia is the cause of brain damage in hyponatremia. JAMA 1999;281:2342.

Kumar S et al: Sodium. Lancet 1998;352:220.

Palevsky PM: Hypernatremia. Semin Nephrol 1998;18:20.

Palevsky PM et al: Hypernatremia in hospitalized patients. Ann Intern Med 1996;124:197.

Singer I et al: The management of diabetes insipidus in adults. Arch Intern Med 1997;157:1293 .

Steele A et al: Postoperative hyponatremia despite near-isotonic saline infusion: a phenomenon of desalination. Ann Intern Med 1997;126:20.

Wilcox CS: Metabolic and adverse effects of diuretics. Semin Nephrol 1999;19:557.

Acid-Base Disturbances & Potassium

Adrogue HJ et al: Management of life-threatening acid-base disorders. (Two parts.) N Engl J Med 1998;338:26, 107.

Greenberg A: Hyperkalemia: treatment options. Semin Nephrol 1998;18:46.

Ishihara K et al: Anion gap acidosis. Semin Nephrol 1998;18:83.

Krapf R et al: Plasma potassium response to acute respiratory alkalosis. Kidney Int 1995;47:217.

Krapf R et al: Chronic respiratory alkalosis. The effect of sustained hyperventilation on renal regulation of acid-base equilibrium. N Engl J Med 1991;324:1394.

Kruse JA et al: Rapid correction of hypokalemia using concentrated intravenous potassium chloride infusions. Arch Intern Med 1990;150:613 .

Potkin RT et al: Resuscitation from severe acute hypercapnia: determinants of tolerance and survival. Chest 1992;102:1742.

Luft FC: Lactic acidosis update for critical care clinicians. J Am Soc Nephrol 2001;12: S 15.

Whang R et al: Refractory potassium repletion: a consequence of magnesium deficiency. Arch Intern Med 1992;152:40.

Calcium, Magnesium, & Phosphorus

Aguilera IM et al: Calcium and the anaesthetist. Anaesthesia 2000;55:779.

Barri YM et al: Hypercalcemia and electrolyte disturbances in malignancy. Hematol Oncol Clin North Am 1996;10:775.

Bilezikian JP: Management of acute hypercalcemia. N Engl J Med 1992;326:1196.

Body JJ: Current and future directions in medical therapy: hypercalcemia. Cancer 2000;88(12 Suppl):3054.

Brooks MJ et al: The refeeding syndrome: an approach to understanding its complications and preventing its occurrence. Pharmacotherapy 1995;15:713 .

Brown DL et al: Developments in the therapeutic applications of bisphosphonates. J Clin Pharmacol 1999;39:651.

Bugg NC et al: Hypophosphataemia. Pathophysiology, effects and management on the intensive care unit. Anaesthesia 1998; 53:895.

Kelepouris E et al: Hypomagnesemia: renal magnesium handling. Semin Nephrol 1998;18:58.

Miller DW et al: Hypophosphatemia in the emergency department therapeutics. Am J Emerg Med 2000;18:457.

Subramanian R et al: Severe hypophosphatemia. Pathophysiologic implications, clinical presentations, and treatment. Medicine 2000;79:1

Whang R: Clinical disorders of magnesium metabolism. Compr Ther 1997;23:168.

Ziegler R: Hypercalcemic crisis. J Am Soc Nephrol 2001;12(Suppl 17):S3.

Surgical Metabolism & Nutrition 11

Julie A. Margenthaler, MD, Virginia M. Herrmann, MD, & Michael S. Hickey, MD

The effect of disease on body composition and immune status is well recognized. Protein-calorie malnutrition in surgical patients is associated with decreased lean muscle mass, altered respiratory mechanics, impaired immune function, and intestinal atrophy. Surgical patients who have acutely lost more than 10% of their customary body weight will have delayed wound healing and an increased incidence of postoperative complications. More dramatic weight loss (> 20% of usual body weight) is associated with an increase in both morbidity and mortality.

NUTRITIONAL ASSESSMENT

Nutrition screening is the process of identifying patients who are either malnourished or at risk for developing malnutrition. Patients with recent operations or traumas may be at risk from changes in intake and absorption of nutrients. The scope of this problem has been well documented in studies demonstrating a 30–55% incidence of malnutrition in hospitalized patients.

Following screening, a comprehensive nutrition assessment is essential to determine the patient's nutritional status and develop a plan of nutritional support (Table 11–1).

History & Physical Examination

The nutritional assessment is based on information from the history and physical examination. A complete medical history is essential to identify factors that predispose the patient to an altered nutritional status. Chronic illnesses such as alcoholism are associated with general protein-calorie malnutrition as well as vitamin and mineral deficiencies. Previous operative procedures such as gastrectomy or ileal resection may predispose to malabsorption and isolated vitamin or mineral deficiencies. In most cases, the possibility of malnutrition is suggested by the underlying disease or by a history of recent weight loss. Liver and kidney diseases are often associated with deficiencies of protein, vitamins, and trace metals. Patients with renal failure who require hemodialysis also lose amino acids, vitamins, trace metals, and carnitine in the dialysate. Patients with inflammatory bowel disease—especially those with ileal involvement—often suffer from deficiencies of protein (due to

a combination of poor intake, chronic diarrhea, and treatment with corticosteroids), fat, vitamins, calcium, magnesium, and trace elements. About 30% of patients with cancer have protein, calorie, and vitamin deficiencies due either to the underlying disease or to antimetabolite chemotherapy (eg, methotrexate). Patients infected with HIV are frequently malnourished and have protein, trace metal (selenium and zinc), mineral, and vitamin deficiencies.

A complete history of current medications is essential to alert caregivers to potential underlying deficiencies as well as drug-nutrient interactions. Information about socioeconomic factors and a dietary history may uncover other risk factors.

A careful physical examination begins with an overall assessment of the patient's appearance. Patients with severe malnutrition may appear emaciated, but more subtle signs of malnutrition include temporal muscle wasting, skin pallor, edema, and generalized loss of body fat. Protein status is evaluated from the bulk and strength of the extremity muscles and visible evidence of temporal muscle wasting. Vitamin malnutrition may be manifested by changes in the texture of the skin, the presence of follicular plugging or a skin rash, corneal vascularization, cracks at the corners of the mouth (cheilosis), hyperemia of the oral mucosa (glossitis), cardiac enlargement and murmurs, altered sensation in the hands and feet, absence of vibration and position sense (dorsal and lateral column deficits), and abnormal quality and texture of the hair. Trace metal deficiencies produce cutaneous and neurologic abnormalities similar to those associated with vitamin deficiency plus changes in mental status.

Anthropometric Measurements

Anthropometry is the science of assessing body size, weight, and proportions. Anthropometric measurements assess body cell mass or body composition with the intent of providing specific information on lean body mass and fat stores. Body composition studies may be used to determine total body water, nitrogen, and potassium. Typically, anthropometric measurements include assessment of body weight, body height, and body mass index, and these values will allow the clinician to assess the patient's visceral and somatic protein mass and fat reserve.

Table 11–1. Nutritional assessment.

History

$$\text{Present illness} = \frac{\text{Actual weight} \times 100}{\text{Ideal weight}}$$

$$\text{Percentage usual body weight} = \frac{\text{Actual weight} \times 100}{\text{Usual weight}}$$

Past illness predisposing to malnutrition

Physical Examination

Skin: Quality, texture, rash, follicles, hyperkeratosis, nail deformities

Hair: Quality, texture, recent loss

Eyes: Keratoconjunctivitis, night blindness

Mouth: Cheilosis, glossitis, mucosal atrophy, dentition

Heart: Chamber enlargement, murmurs

Abdomen: Hepatomegaly, abdominal mass, ostomy, fistulas

Rectum: Stool color, perineal fistula

Neurologic: Peripheral neuropathy, dorsolateral column deficit

Extremities: Muscle size and strength, pedal edema

Laboratory Tests

CBC: Hemoglobin, hematocrit, red cell indices, white count and differential, total lymphocyte count,[1] platelet count

Electrolytes: Sodium, potassium, chloride, calcium, phosphate, magnesium

Liver function tests: AST (SGOT), ALT (SGPT), alkaline phosphatase, bilirubin, albumin,[2] prealbumin,[3] retinol-binding protein,[4] prothrombin

Miscellaneous: BUN, creatinine, triglycerides, cholesterol, free fatty acids, ketones, uric acid, calcium, copper, zinc, magnesium, transferrin[5]

---

[1]Total lymphocyte count (normal = 1500–4000 cells/μL)
  Mild malnutrition: 1200–2000 cells/μL
  Moderate malnutrition: 800–1200 cells/μL
  Severe malnutrition: < 800 cells/μL
[2]Albumin (normal = > 3.5 g/dL)
  Mild malnutrition: 2.8–3.2 g/dL
  Moderate malnutrition: 2.1–2.7 g/dL
  Severe malnutrition: < 2.1 g/dL
[3]Prealbumin (normal = 17–42 mg/dL): Values < 17 mg/dL represent malnutrition
[4]Retinol-binding protein (normal = 4.1–6.1 mg/dL): Values < 4.1 mg/dL represent malnutrition
[5]Transferrin (normal = > 250 mg/dL)
  Mild malnutrition: 200–250 mg/dL
  Moderate malnutrition: 100–200 mg/dL
  Severe malnutrition: < 100 mg/dL

A. BODY WEIGHT AND HEIGHT

Accurate measurement of height, either directly or by alternative means (arm span, body part summation, or knee-height measurement) is essential for nutrition assessment. Accurate weight is similarly important, as is current weight expressed as a percentage of usual body weight. Actual weight should be compared with ideal body weight, available from standardized life insurance tables.

The BMI is used to measure protein-calorie malnutrition as well as overnutrition (obesity), and is calculated by the following equation:

$$\text{BMI} = \frac{\text{Weight (kg)}}{\text{Height (m)}^2}$$

Dual-energy x-ray absorptiometry (DEXA) is increasingly available in hospitals and can be used to assess various body compartments (mineral, fat, lean muscle mass).

Somatic (skeletal) protein reserve—most protein resides in skeletal muscle—is estimated by measuring the mid arm circumference. This measurement is corrected to account for subcutaneous tissue, which gives the mid arm muscle circumference (MAMC). The result is compared with normal values for the patient's age and sex to determine the extent of protein depletion or reserve.

Fat reserve is estimated from the thickness of the triceps skin fold (TSF).

Laboratory Data

The visceral protein reserve is estimated from the serum total protein, albumin, and transferrin levels; total lymphocyte count; and antigen skin testing (Table 11–2). The serum albumin level provides a rough estimate of the patient's nutritional status but is a better prognostic indicator than a tool for nutrition assessment. Decreased serum albumin correlates with increased morbidity and mortality and increased length of stay. Because albumin has such a long half-life (20 days), other serum proteins such as transferrin, prealbumin, retinol-binding protein, and ceruloplasmin, which have half-lives of a few hours, are more sensitive indices of acute changes in nutritional status. Transferrin has a shorter half-life (8–10 days) and is a more sensitive indicator of nutrition status than albumin. Prealbumin has a half-life of 2–3 days, and retinol-binding protein has a half-life of 12 hours. Unfortunately, their serum levels are

also influenced by other factors, so they have limited utility.

A. TWENTY-FOUR-HOUR NITROGEN BALANCE DETERMINATION

Protein synthesis or breakdown can be determined by measuring the nitrogen balance (nitrogen intake minus nitrogen excretion) (Table 11–3; Figure 11–1). Nitrogen intake is the sum of nitrogen delivered from enteral and parenteral feedings. Nitrogen output is the sum of nitrogen excreted in urine, fistula drainage, diarrhea, etc. The usual approach is to measure the urea nitrogen concentration of an aliquot of a 24-hour urine collection and then calculate nitrogen content from the urine volume. A correction factor is added to account for nitrogen losses in the stool and from skin exfoliation. The difference—nitrogen intake minus output—estimates the 24-hour nitrogen balance. The result is not very precise, however, because it represents a small difference between two large numbers. Accuracy can be improved if the calculations are extended to cover a period of several weeks. When losses of nitrogen are large (eg, diarrhea, hematochezia, protein-losing enteropathy, fistula, or burn exudate), measurements of nitrogen balance lose accuracy because of the difficulty in collecting

Table 11–2. Clinical staging of malnutrition.

Clinical and Laboratory Parameters	Extent of Malnutrition		
	Mild	Moderate[1]	Severe[1]
Albumin (g/dL)[2]	2.8–3.2	2.1–2.7	< 2.1
Transferrin (mg/dL)[2]	200–250	100–200	< 100
Total lymphocyte count (cells/μL)[2]	1200–2000	800–1200	< 800
Creatinine/height index (%)[3]	60–80	30–60	< 40
Ideal body weight (%)	80–90	70–80	< 70
Usual body weight (%)	85–95	75–85	< 75
Weight loss/unit time	< 5%/month < 7.5%/3 months < 10%/6 months	< 2%/week > 5%/month > 7.5%/3 months > 10%/6 months	> 2%/week
Skin tests (No. reactive ÷ No. placed)	4/4 (normal)	1–2/4 (weak)	0/0 (anergic)
Normal anthropometric measurements	Male	Female	
Triceps skin fold (mm)[4]	12.5	16.5	
Midarm circumference (cm)	29.3	28.5	

[1]Nutritional therapy indicated.
[2]Visceral protein reserve.
[3]Somatic protein reserve (see Table 11–3).
[4]Fat reserve.

Table 11–3. Special tests for nutritional assessment.

1. Anthropometrics:

Body Mass Index (BMI) $= \dfrac{\text{Wt (Kg)}}{\text{Ht}^2 (\text{m}^2)}$

Triceps skin fold (TSF)
Midhumeral circumference (MHC)

Arm muscle circumference $= \dfrac{\text{MHC} - (\pi)(\text{TSF})}{10}$

Creatinine - height index $= \dfrac{24 \text{ - hour urine creatinine excretion}}{\text{Ideal creatinine excretion for height}}$

2. Energy:

Total energy expenditure (Table 10–4)

Weir formula (REE): kcal / min $= 3.9 (\dot{V}_{O_2})^1 + 1.1\,(V_{CO_2}) - 2.2$ (urine N)[1]

Nonprotein RQ: $\dfrac{\dot{V}_{CO_2}\ \dot{V}_{CO_2} - 4.8\,(\text{urine N})}{\dot{V}_{O_2} - 5.9\,(\text{urine N})}$

3. Protein:

Nitrogen balance = Nitrogen intake − Nitrogen output (refer to text for equation)
3-Methylhistidine urinary excretion
Isotopic determination of protein turnover (^{15}N glycine, ^{15}N lysine, and ^{4}C leucine infusion)

4. Body Composition:

Total body water (TBW): ^{3}H or ^{2}H H_2O isotope dilution
Extracullular water (ECW): ^{22}Na isotope dilution

Lean body mass (LBM): $\dfrac{\text{TBW}}{0.73}$

Body cell mass (BCM): $(K_e)(0.083)$ or $(TBN)(6.25)(4)$
Total body potassium: ^{42}K isotope dilution; ^{40}K whole body counting; K_e (exchangeable potassium)
Total body nitrogen (TBN): Neutron activation

5. Immunologic testing:

Skin tests	Immunoglobulin levels
Lymphocyte blastogenesis	Complement levels
Mixed lymphocyte response	Lymphokine production

6. Miscellaneous laboratory tests:

Prealbumin[2]
Retinol-binding protein[3]
Transferrin[4]

---

[1]$\dot{V}_{O_2}$ and $\dot{V}_{CO_2}$ are oxygen consumption and CO_2 production in mL/min; urine nitrogen is in g/min.
[2]Prealbumin (normal = 17–42 mg/dL): Values < 4.1 mg/dL represent malnutrition.
[3]Retinol-binding protein (normal = 4.1–6.1 mg/dL): Values < 4.1 mg/dL represent malnutrition.
[4]Transferrin (normal = > 250 mg/dL):
  Mild malnutrition: 200–250 mg/dL
  Moderate malnutrition: 100–200 mg/dL
  Severe malnutrition: < 100 mg/dL

$$\text{Nitrogen balance} = \text{Nitrogen}^{(\text{intake})} - \text{Nitrogen}^{(\text{output})}$$

$$\text{Nitrogen}^{(\text{intake})} = \frac{\text{g protein}}{6.25 \text{ g protein/g nitrogen}}$$

$$\text{Nitrogen}^{(\text{output})} = \text{UUN}^1 \times \frac{1000 \text{ mL}}{\text{L}} \times 24\text{-hour urine volume (L)} \times \frac{\text{g nitrogen}}{1000 \text{ mg nitrogen}} + 3$$

$$^1\text{UUN} = \frac{\text{mg nitrogen}}{100 \text{ mL urine}}$$

Figure 11–1. Twenty-four-hour nitrogen balance determination.

all of the secretions. Despite these shortcomings, a 24-hour urine collection for nitrogen balance determination is the best practical means of measuring net protein synthesis and breakdown.

A nitrogen balance determination is helpful in assessing efficacy of nutritional therapy and is particularly helpful in critically ill patients.

B. Creatinine-Height Index (CHI)

CHI may be used to determine the degree of malnutrition. A 24-hour urinary creatinine excretion is measured and compared with normal standards. CHI is calculated by the following equation:

$$\text{CHI} = \frac{\text{Actual 24-hour creatinine excretion}}{\text{Expected creatine excretion}}$$

$$> 80\% = \text{Zero to mild depletion}$$
$$60–80\% = \text{Moderate depletion}$$
$$< 60\% = \text{Severe depletion}$$

CHI is less valid in patients with renal disease or who are severely catabolic.

The urinary excretion of 3-methylhistidine is a more precise measurement of protein status. The amino acid histidine is irreversibly methylated in muscle. During tissue breakdown, histidine (ie, within 3-methylhistidine) is not reincorporated into protein, so the urinary excretion of 3-methylhistidine correlates well with muscle protein breakdown. Unfortunately, measuring 3-methylhistidine is too expensive to use as a clinical test.

C. Immune Function

Immune function may be assessed by hypersensitivity skin testing as well as total lymphocytic count, which reflects T and B cell status. A low total lymphocyte count (TLC) correlates directly with the degree of malnutrition, though the count may be altered by infection, chemotherapy, and other factors, thus limiting its usefulness.

$$\text{TLC} = \frac{\% \text{ Lymphocytes} \times \text{White blood cells (WBC)}}{100}$$

$$1500–1800/\mu\text{L} = \text{Mild depletion}$$
$$900–1500/\mu\text{L} = \text{Moderate depletion}$$
$$< 900/\mu\text{L} = \text{Severe depletion}$$

D. Subjective Global Assessment (SGA)

SGA is based on five features of the medical history (weight loss in past 6 months, dietary intake, gastrointestinal symptoms, functional status or energy level, and metabolic demands) along with four features of the physical examination (loss of subcutaneous fat, muscle wasting, edema, and ascites). SGA very accurately predicts clinical outcome.

E. Prognostic Nutrition Indicator (PNI)

The PNI correlates nutrition status with operative mortality and morbidity. PNI > 40% is associated with a significant increase in complications and mortality.

$$\text{PNI\%} = 158 - 16.6 \text{ (albumin g/dL)}$$
$$- 0.78 \text{ (triceps skinfold mm)}$$
$$- 0.20 \text{ (transferrin mg/dL)}$$
$$- 5.8 \text{ (delayed hypersensitivity)}$$

Determining Energy Requirements

The adult daily caloric requirement is calculated by using the total energy expenditure (TEE) equation, which is a modified version of the Harris-Benedict equation (Table 11–4). It includes three variables—height (cm), weight (kg), and age (yr)—and makes allowances for specific activity, injury factors, and gender.

Indirect calorimetry is the most accurate method for determining an adult's daily caloric requirements. It calculates the production of O_2 ($\dot{V}O_2$) and CO_2 ($\dot{V}CO_2$)

Table 11–4. Total energy expenditure equation for adults.

Estimated:
Calories (total kcal) (male or female)
  25–30/kg (weight loss)
  30–35/kg (weight maintenance)
  35–40/kg (weight gain)
Protein (g) (male or female)
  0.8–2.0/kg

Calculated:
Calories (total kcal) for weight maintenance
  Male = [66.5 + (13.7 × wt kg) + (5 × ht cm)
    − (6.7 × age yr)] × AF[1] × IF[2]
  Female = [665.1 + (9.6 × wt kg) + (1.8 × ht cm)
    − (4.7 × age yr)] × AF[1] × IF[2]

  Note: Add 500 kcal to the above equations for weight gain.

Protein (g)

$$\text{Male or female} = \text{Total kcal} \times \frac{\text{g nitrogen}}{150 \text{ kcal}} \times \frac{6.25 \text{ g protein}}{\text{g nitrogen}}$$

[1]Activity factor		[2]Injury factor	
Confined to bed	1.2	Surgery	1.1–1.2
Ambulatory	1.3	Infection	1.2–1.6
Fever factor (>37°C)	1.3	Trauma	1.1–1.8
		Sepsis	1.4–1.8

from the timed volumetric collection of expired O_2, CO_2, and urinary nitrogen. The resting energy expenditure (REE) in kilocalories (kcal) per minute is derived from the Weir formula:

$$\text{kcal/min} = 3.9(\dot{V}_{O_2}) + 1.1(\dot{V}_{CO_2}) - 2.2(\text{urine N})$$

$$\text{Nonprotein RQ} = \frac{\dot{V}_{CO_2} - 4.8(\text{urine N})}{\dot{V}_{CO_2} - 5.9(\text{urine N})}$$

where $\dot{V}_{O_2}$ and $\dot{V}_{CO_2}$ are oxygen consumption and carbon monoxide production in milliliters per minute and urine nitrogen is in grams per minute.

The nonprotein respiratory quotient (RQ) is the percentage of carbohydrate and fat used for energy production. When the RQ is 1, pure carbohydrate is being oxidized. When the RQ is 0.7, only fat is being oxidized. The nonprotein RQ is used to gauge the patient's metabolic response to nutritional therapy. Theoretically, the administration of large amounts of glucose to patients with sepsis and chronic obstructive pulmonary disease (COPD) could result in CO_2 retention due to the increased $\dot{V}_{CO_2}$.

NUTRIENT REQUIREMENTS & SUBSTRATES

Calories

The body requires an energy source to remain in a steady state. About 50% of the basal metabolic rate (BMR) reflects the work of ion pumping; 30% represents protein turnover; and the remainder represents recycling of amino acids, glucose, lactate, and pyruvate. Total energy expenditure is the sum of energy consumed in basal metabolic processes, physical activity, the specific dynamic action of protein, and extra requirements resulting from injury, sepsis, or burns. Energy consumed in physical activity constitutes 10–50% of the total in normal subjects but drops to 10–20% for hospitalized patients. The increment above basal needs resulting from injury or trauma is about 10% for elective operations, 10–30% for trauma, 50–80% for sepsis, and 100–200% for burns (depending on the extent of the wound).

Calories can come from glucose or fat. The metabolism of 1 g glucose yields 3.4 kcal. The metabolism of 1 g fat yields 9.2 kcal. Glucose, the primary source of calories, stimulates insulin secretion, which in turn influences protein synthesis. Fat can be used to provide as much as 60% of daily caloric requirements, but more than that could impair polymorphonuclear, macrophage, and reticuloendothelial cell function.

Protein

Protein balance reflects the sum of protein synthesis and protein breakdown. By changing the levels of metabolic substrates, hormones, or cytokines, the body adjusts protein stores in response to changes in the basal state, level of activity, operations, trauma, sepsis, or burns. Because protein turnover is in constant flux, the published requirements for protein, amino acids, and nitrogen are only approximations.

The quality of a protein is related to its amino acid composition. The 20 amino acids are divided into essential amino acids (EAAs) and nonessential amino acids (NEAAs) depending on whether they can be synthesized de novo in the body. They are further divided into aromatic (AAAs), branched chain (BCAAs), and sulfur-containing amino acids. Amino acids contain highly reactive thiol, imidazole, aromatic, and dicarboxylic acid groups, which catalyze chemical reactions and help determine the tertiary structures of protein molecules via polar, hydrophobic, nonionic, disulfide, and hydrogen bonds. Certain amino acids have unique metabolic functions. For example, alanine and glutamine participate in a cycle with glucose that preserves carbon during starvation; leucine stimulates protein synthesis and inhibits catabolism; and BCAAs are the fuels preferred by cardiac and skeletal muscle during starvation.

Glutamine

Although classified as a nonessential amino acid, glutamine plays an important role in the metabolically stressed patient. Glutamine is the crucial respiratory fuel for the gastrointestinal cell or enterocyte. Glutamine is metabolized in the small intestine to ammonia, citrulline, alanine, and proline, and the carbon skeleton serves as an energy precursor for the enterocyte.

Following injury, operation, sepsis, and other catabolic events, intracellular glutamine stores may decrease by over 50% and plasma levels by 25%. The decline exceeds that of any other amino acid and persists during recovery after the concentrations of other amino acid have returned to normal. Glutamine-supplemented nutrition formulas help prevent the stress-induced decrease in muscle and plasma glutamine. Supplementation with glutamine maintains intestinal cell integrity, villous height, and mucosal DNA activity and helps minimize reduction in numbers of T and B cells during stress.

Glutamine is avidly consumed by replicating cells, such as fibroblasts, lymphocytes, tumor cells, and intestinal epithelial cells. Catabolic states, such as trauma, sepsis, major burns, and uncontrolled diabetes mellitus, are characterized by accelerated skeletal muscle proteolysis and translocation of amino acids from the periphery to the visceral organs. Glutamine accounts for a major portion of the amino acids released by muscle in these states.

Glutamine supplementation may improve neutrophil and macrophage function in burn patients and other critically ill traumatized patients. Individuals with short gut syndrome may also benefit from glutamine with epidermal growth factor, which improves nitrogen retention, intestinal cell integrity, and DNA and protein content of mucosal cells. Investigation of glutamine supplementation in cancer patients is ongoing.

Arginine

Arginine is a substrate for the urea cycle and nitric oxide production and a secretagogue for growth hormone, prolactin, and insulin. Arginine supplementation formulas have been shown to improve nitrogen balance and wound healing, to stimulate T cell response, and to reduce the incidence of infectious complications. T cell proliferation and T cell function in humans are stimulated in response to arginine supplementation, and albumin synthesis has also been shown to improve with additional amounts of this amino acid. The effects of arginine on T cells may be very important in maintaining the gut barrier. Arginine has been

identified as the sole precursor of nitric oxide. Nitric oxide from arginine serves as an effector molecule in tumor cell cytotoxicity, and nitrogen oxide production from tumors may influence tumor growth, differentiation, and metastases and may enhance tumor responsiveness to chemotherapy and radiation therapy.

Arginine supplementation has also been shown to increase interleukin-2 (IL-2) production and up-regulate the interleukin-2 receptor (IL-2R). T cell function is measured in part by its ability to secrete IL-2 and upregulate IL-2R, and IL-2 in turn stimulates T cell proliferation. Cytotoxic T cell lymphocytes express the CD8 molecule and are important in helping effector cells recognize and reject tumor cells. Arginine supplementation has, however, been demonstrated to stimulate tumor growth. Some tumor lines produce nitric oxide (NO), and NO may regulate tumor growth, cell differentiation, metastatic capability, and sensitivity to chemotherapy. Therefore, tumor stimulation with arginine may be therapeutically beneficial and improve our ability to deliver cell-cycle-specific chemotherapy or radiation therapy.

Nucleotides

Nucleotides are precursors of DNA and RNA and participate in a number of metabolic reactions fundamental to cellular activity.

Nucleic acids have generally not been considered essential for human growth and development. However, the need for dietary nucleotides increases in severe stress and critical illness. Nucleotides are formed from purines and pyrimidines and play a crucial role in many biochemical reactions. Immunosuppression has been reported in renal transplant patients being maintained on nucleotide free diets. Dietary nucleotides are necessary for helper-inducer T lymphocyte activity. Diets supplemented with RNA or uracil (precursors to nucleotide production) have been shown to restore delayed hypersensitivity and augment both lymphoproliferative response and IL-2 receptor expression. Nucleotides may facilitate recovery from infection, as shown in animal studies where increased resistance to *Candida albicans* and *Staphylococcus aureus* infections occurred in groups receiving diets enriched with uracil or RNA. These substrates are incorporated into enteral formulas as potential immunomodulators. It should be noted that in the solid organ transplant population, immune enhancement may not be a desirable goal, and nucleotides should be avoided.

Fatty Acids

Dietary fats are the sole precursors to eicosanoid production and as such are potent immunomodulators.

Fats or fatty acids are hydrocarbon chains ranging from two carbons to twenty-four carbons in length. Fatty acids are classified as short-chain, medium-chain, or long-chain. The body is able to synthesize fats from other dietary substrates, but two of the long-chain fatty acids (linoleic and α-linolenic) are essential. Deficient intake of these essential fats will lead to fatty acid deficiency and can be prevented by supplying 2–4% of the total caloric intake as essential fatty acids.

The essential polyunsaturated fatty acids (PUFAs) are grouped into two families: ω-6 and ω-3 fatty acids. Linoleic acid is an example of the ω-6 PUFAs; α-linolenic acid of the ω-3 PUFAs. Vegetable oils such as corn, safflower, sunflower, and soybean oils are good sources of linoleic acid (ω-6 PUFA). Linseed, canola, walnut, and soybean oils are good sources of α-linolenic acid (ω-3 PUFA). Cold water fish are a rich source of ω-3 fatty acids, specifically eicosapentaenoic acid (EPA) and docosahexaenoic acid (DHA). Linoleic acid (ω-6 PUFA) is desaturated by δ-6 desaturase and elongated to form arachidonic acid. Arachidonic acid is a precursor to the synthesis of eicosanoids—specifically, the series-2 prostaglandins and series-4 leukotrienes. Eicosanoids are potent biochemical mediators of cell-to-cell communication and are involved in inflammation, infection, tissue injury, and immune system modulation.

Delta-6 desaturase also regulates the conversion of α-linolenic acid (ω-3 PUFA) to EPA, a precursor of less potent eicosanoids, the series-3 prostaglandins, and series-5 leukotrienes. These mediators compete with or inhibit the effects of the eicosanoids produced by the ω-6 PUFA.

Efficient functioning of the immune system depends upon a balance of eicosanoid production between the ω-6 and ω-3 PUFA. Eicosanoids modulate numerous events involving cell-mediated and humoral immunity and can be synthesized in varying amounts by all immune cells, especially macrophages and monocytes. Diets high in ω-6 fatty acids suppress immune function by inhibiting mitogenesis due to increased prostaglandin E_2 synthesis, which inhibits T cell proliferation. The administration of additional ω-3 PUFAs negates this effect.

Platelet function and inflammatory response are not aggravated by ω-3 fatty acids, and ω-3 fatty acids are associated with a significant decrease in IL-1 and TNF. ω-3 fatty acids decrease fibrinogen levels, blood pressure, and cell proliferation and improve arterial compliance and endothelial function by modulating NO metabolism.

Medium-chain fatty acids are generally not components of most ordinary diets but are widely used in enteral tube feedings. They are easily digested, absorbed, and oxidized and are not precursors to the inflammatory or immunosuppressive eicosanoids.

Vitamins

Vitamins are involved in metabolism, wound healing, and immune function. They are essential parts of the diet because they cannot be synthesized de novo. The normal requirements for vitamins (Table 11–5) may increase in disease. For example, increased amounts of vitamins are excreted in the urine of patients with trauma, burns, and sepsis.

A. FAT-SOLUBLE VITAMINS

Vitamins A, D, E, and K are absorbed in the proximal small bowel in association with bile salt micelles and fatty acids. After absorption, they are delivered to the tissues in chylomicrons and stored in large quantities in the liver (vitamins A and K) or subcutaneous tissue and skin (vitamins D and E). Fat-soluble vitamins participate in immune function and wound healing.

B. WATER-SOLUBLE VITAMINS

Vitamins B_1, B_2, B_6, and B_{12}, vitamin C, and niacin, folate, biotin, and pantothenic acid are absorbed in the duodenum and proximal small bowel, transported in portal vein blood, and utilized in the liver and peripherally. Only vitamin B_{12} is stored to any extent. Water-soluble vitamins serve as cofactors that facilitate reactions involved in the generation and transfer of energy and in amino acid and nucleic acid metabolism. Because of their limited storage, water-soluble vitamin deficiencies are common.

Trace Elements

The daily requirements for the trace elements (Table 11–5) vary geographically owing to differences in soil composition. Trace elements have important functions in metabolism, immunology, and wound healing. Subclinical trace element deficiencies occur in many common diseases.

Iron, which is essential for hemoglobin synthesis, serves as the core of the heme prosthetic group in hemoglobin and the respiratory chain cytochromes. Impaired cerebral, muscular, and immunologic function can occur in patients with iron deficiency before anemia becomes evident.

Zinc is a cofactor for a number of metalloenzymes involved in carbohydrate, fat, amino acid, and nucleic acid metabolism. Deficiency may develop in patients with large fecal losses (eg, those with AIDS) or after prolonged total parenteral nutrition (TPN) in the absence of zinc supplements. Clinically, zinc deficiency is characterized by a diffuse maculopapular rash (similar to that of acrodermatitis enteropathica), poor wound healing, cutaneous anergy, hair loss, and taste and smell disturbances.

Copper is a component of a number of metalloenzymes, including cytochrome oxidase (the terminal en-

Table 11-5. Daily electrolyte, trace element, vitamin, and mineral requirements for adults.

	Enteral	Parenteral
Electrolytes		
Sodium	90–150 meq	90–150 meq
Potassium	60–90 meq	60–90 meq
Trace elements		
Chromium[1,2]	5–200 µg	10–15 µg
Copper[1,2]	2–3 mg	0.15–0.5mg
Manganese[1,2]	2.5–5.0 mg	0.15–0.8 mg
Zinc[1]	15 mg	2.5–4.0 mg
Iron	10 mg	2.5 mg
Iodine	150 µg	...
Fluoride[2]	1.5–4.0 mg	...
Selenium[2]	0.05–0.20 mg	20–40 µg
Molybdenum[2]	0.15–0.50 mg	20–120 µg
Tin[3]	...	...
Vanadium[3]	...	...
Nickel[3]	...	...
Arsenic[3]	...	...
Silicon[3]	...	...
Vitamins		
Ascorbic acid (C)[4]	60 mg	100 mg
Retinol (A)[4]	1000 µg	3300 IU
Vitamin D[4]	5.0 µg	200 IU
Thiamin (B_1)[4]	1.4 mg	3.0 mg
Riboflavin (B_2)[4]	1.7 mg	3.6 mg
Pyridoxine (B_6)[4]	2.2 mg	4.0 mg
Niacin[4]	19 mg	40 mg
Pantothenic acid[4]	4–7 mg	15 mg
Vitamin E[4]	10.0 mg	10 IU
Biotin[2,4]	100–200 µg	60 µg
Folic acid[2]	400 µg	400 µg
Cyanobalamin (B_{12})[4]	2.0 µg	5.9 µg
Vitamin K[5]	70–149 µg	10 mg
Minerals		
Calcium	800 mg	0.20–0.30 meq/kg
Phosphorus	800 mg	300–400 mg/kg
Magnesium	350 mg	0.34–0.45 meq/kg
Sulfur	2–3 g	...

[1]Multitrace 5 mL provides the normal daily requirement.
[2]Estimated safe and adequate dose.
[3]No data available regarding human requirements.
[4]M.V.I.-12 10 mL parenterally provides the normal daily requirement.
[5]Weekly requirement.

zyme of the electron transport chain), dopamine hydroxylase (a key enzyme in catecholamine metabolism), and lysyl oxidase (which is involved in collagen cross-linkage). Copper deficiency is manifested by anemia (unresponsive to iron) or pancytopenia.

Chromium forms a complex with a small peptide containing nicotinic acid to produce glucose tolerance factor (GTF). GTF facilitates the binding of insulin to membrane receptors. Chromium may improve glucose tolerance in patients with adult-onset diabetes mellitus. Chromium deficiency presents as sudden glucose intolerance during prolonged unsupplemented TPN without evidence of sepsis, in which case chromium therapy returns glucose tolerance to normal.

Selenium is part of the enzyme glutathione peroxidase. A decrease in the activity of this enzyme leads to peroxidation of membrane lipids, resulting in elevated concentrations of pentane in expired air. Selenium deficiency, which can occur in patients receiving TPN for a prolonged period, is manifested by proximal neuromuscular weakness or cardiac failure with electrocardiographic changes.

Manganese is the cofactor for the metalloenzymes pyruvate carboxylase and manganese-superoxide dismutase, being involved in the initial step in gluconeogenesis and in cellular antioxidant capability. Manganese deficiency is associated with weight loss, altered hair pigmentation, nausea, and low plasma levels of phospholipids and triglycerides.

Molybdenum is involved in uric acid, purine, and amino acid metabolism as a cofactor for the metalloenzymes xanthine oxidase and aldehyde oxidase. Deficiency results in elevated plasma methionine levels and depressed uric acid concentrations, producing a syndrome consisting of nausea, vomiting, tachycardia, and central nervous system disturbances.

Iodine is a key component of thyroid hormone. Deficiency is rare in the USA because of the widespread use of iodized salt. Chronically malnourished patients can become iodine-deficient, and since thyroxine participates in the neuroendocrine response to trauma and sepsis, iodine should be included in TPN solutions.

NUTRITIONAL PATHOPHYSIOLOGY

Physiologic processes, immunocompetence, wound healing, and recovery from critical illness depend upon adequate nutrient intake. A working knowledge of nutritional pathophysiology is essential in planning nutritional regimens.

Starvation

After an overnight fast, liver glycogen is rapidly depleted because of a fall in insulin and a rise in glucagon levels in plasma (Figure 11–2). Concomitantly, there is an increase in hepatic gluconeogenesis from amino acids derived from the breakdown of muscle protein. Hepatic glucose production must satisfy the energy demands of the hematopoietic system and the central nervous system, particularly the brain, which is dependent on glucose oxidation during acute starvation. The release of amino acids from muscle is regulated by insulin, which stimulates amino acid uptake, polyribosome formation, and protein synthesis. The periodic rise and fall of insulin associated with ingestion of nutrients stimulates muscle protein synthesis and breakdown. During starvation, chronically low insulin levels result in a net loss of amino acids from muscle (ie, protein synthesis drops while protein catabolism remains

unchanged). Hepatic gluconeogenesis requires energy, which is supplied by the oxidation of FFA. The fall in insulin along with a rise in plasma glucagon levels results in an increase in the concentration of cAMP in adipose tissue, which stimulates a hormone-sensitive lipase to hydrolyze triglycerides and release FFA. Gluconeogenesis and FFA mobilization require the presence of ambient cortisol and thyroid hormone (a permissive effect).

During starvation, the body attempts to conserve substrate by recycling metabolic intermediates. The hematopoietic system utilizes glucose anaerobically and increases lactate production. Lactate is recycled back to glucose in the liver via the glucogenic (not gluconeogenic) Cori cycle (Figure 11–3). The glycerol re-

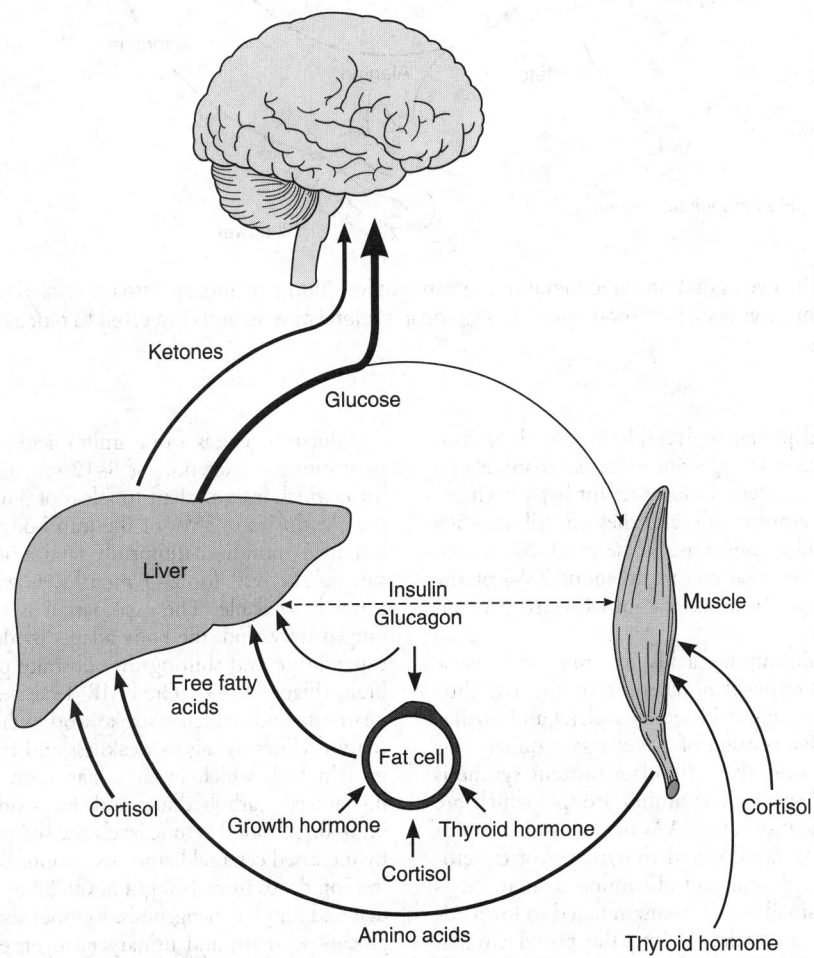

Figure 11–2. The plasma substrate concentrations and hormone levels following an overnight fast. The brain is dependent on glucose, which is supplied by gluconeogenesis from amino acids. These amino acids are derived from the breakdown of skeletal muscle protein.

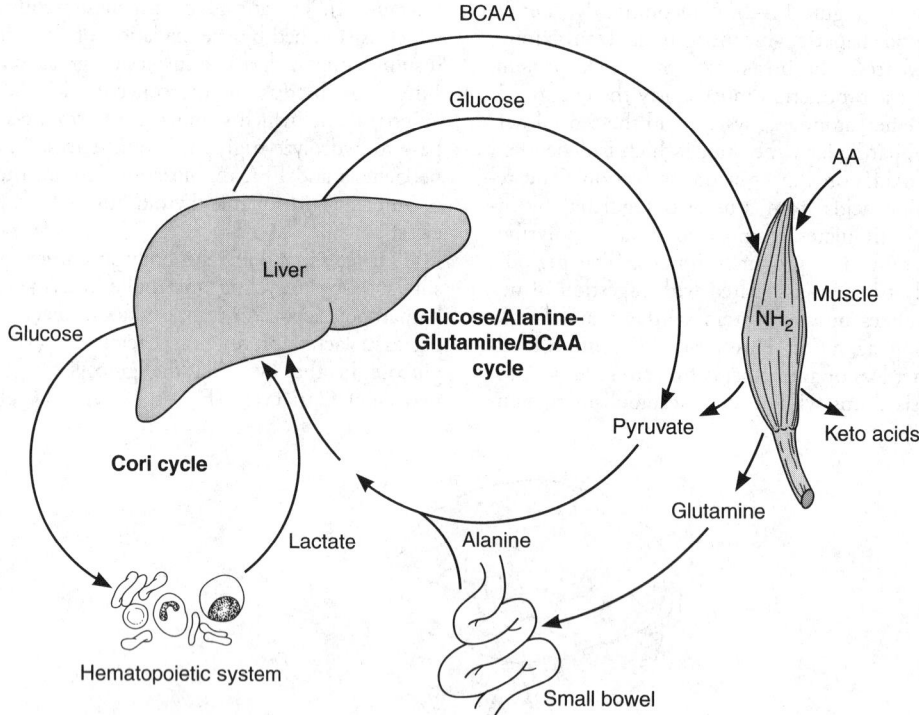

Figure 11–3. The cycles that preserve metabolic intermediates during fasting. Lactate is recycled to glucose via the Cori cycle, while pyruvate is transaminated to alanine in skeletal muscle and converted to glucose by hepatic gluconeogenesis.

leased during peripheral triglyceride hydrolysis is converted into glucose via gluconeogenesis. Alanine and glutamine are the preferred substrates for hepatic gluconeogenesis from amino acids, and they contribute 75% of the amino acid carbon for glucose production. Alanine and glutamine also constitute about 75% of the amino acids released from skeletal muscle during starvation.

Branched-chain amino acids are unique because they are secreted rather than taken up by the liver during starvation; they are oxidized by skeletal and cardiac muscle to supply a portion of the energy requirements of these tissues; and they stimulate protein synthesis and inhibit catabolism. The amino groups, which are derived from oxidation of BCAAs or transamination of other amino acids, are donated to pyruvate or α-ketoglutarate to form alanine and glutamine. Glutamine is taken up by the small bowel, transaminated to form additional alanine, and released into the portal circulation. These amino acids plus glucose participate in the glucose-alanine/glutamine-BCAA cycle, which shuttles amino groups and carbon from muscle to liver for conversion into glucose.

Gluconeogenesis from amino acids results in a urinary nitrogen excretion of 8–12 g/d, predominantly as urea, which is equivalent to a loss of 340 g/d of lean tissue. At this rate, 35% of the lean body mass would be lost in 1 month, a uniformly fatal amount. Starvation can be survived for 2–3 months, however, as long as water is available. The explanation is that during prolonged starvation, the body adapts by decreasing energy expenditure and shifting the substrate preference of the brain (Figure 11–4). The BMR decreases by slowing the heart rate and reducing stroke work, while voluntary activity declines owing to weakness and fatigue. The nonprotein RQ, which in early starvation is 0.85 (reflecting mixed carbohydrate and fat oxidation), falls to 0.70–0.73. Blood ketone levels rise sharply, accompanied by increased cerebral ketone oxidation. Brain glucose utilization drops from 140 g/d to 60–80 g/d, decreasing the demand for gluconeogenesis. Ketones also inhibit hepatic gluconeogenesis, and urinary nitrogen excretion falls to 2–3 g/d. The main component of urine nitrogen is now ammonia (rather than urea), derived from renal transamination and gluconeogenesis from glutamine, and it buffers the acid urine that results from ketonuria.

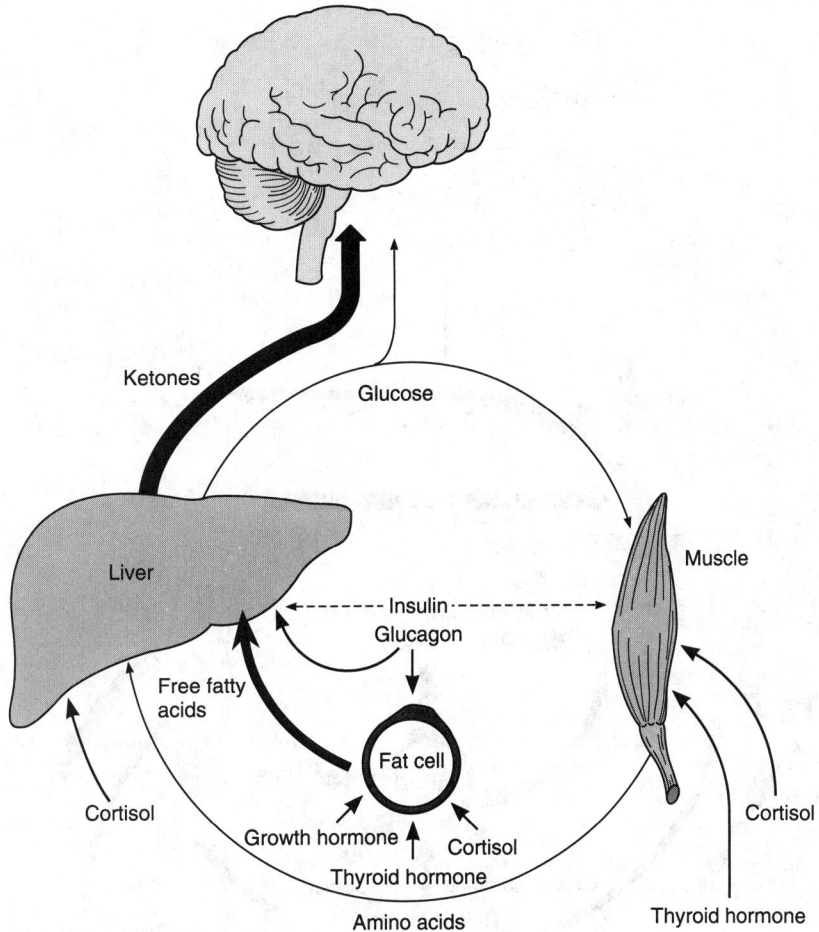

Figure 11–4. The metabolic adaptation to chronic starvation whereby the brain shifts its substrate preference to ketones produced by the liver. Hepatic gluconeogenesis falls and protein breakdown is diminished, which conserves lean tissue.

Acute or chronic starvation is characterized by hormone and fuel alterations orchestrated by changing blood substrate levels and can be thought of as "substrate-driven" processes. In summary, the adaptive changes in uncomplicated starvation are a decrease in energy expenditure, a change in type of fuel consumed (which maximizes the caloric potential), and preservation of protein.

Elective Operation or Trauma

The effects of elective operations and trauma (Figure 11–5) differ from those of simple starvation due to activation of neural and endocrine systems, which accelerates the loss of lean tissue and inhibits adaptation.

Following injury, neural impulses carried via spinothalamic pathways activate the brain stem, thalamic centers, and cortical centers, which in turn stimulate the hypothalamus. The control center for the sympathetic nervous system and the trophic nuclei of the pituitary is in the hypothalamus. Consequently, hypothalamic stimulation triggers a combined neural and endocrine discharge. Norepinephrine is released from sympathetic nerve endings, epinephrine from the adrenal medulla, aldosterone from the adrenal cortex, ADH from the posterior pituitary, insulin and glucagon from the pancreas, and ACTH, TSH, and growth hormone from the anterior pituitary. This causes secondary elevations of cortisol, thyroid hormone, and somatomedins. This heightened neuroendocrine secretion produces (1) pe-

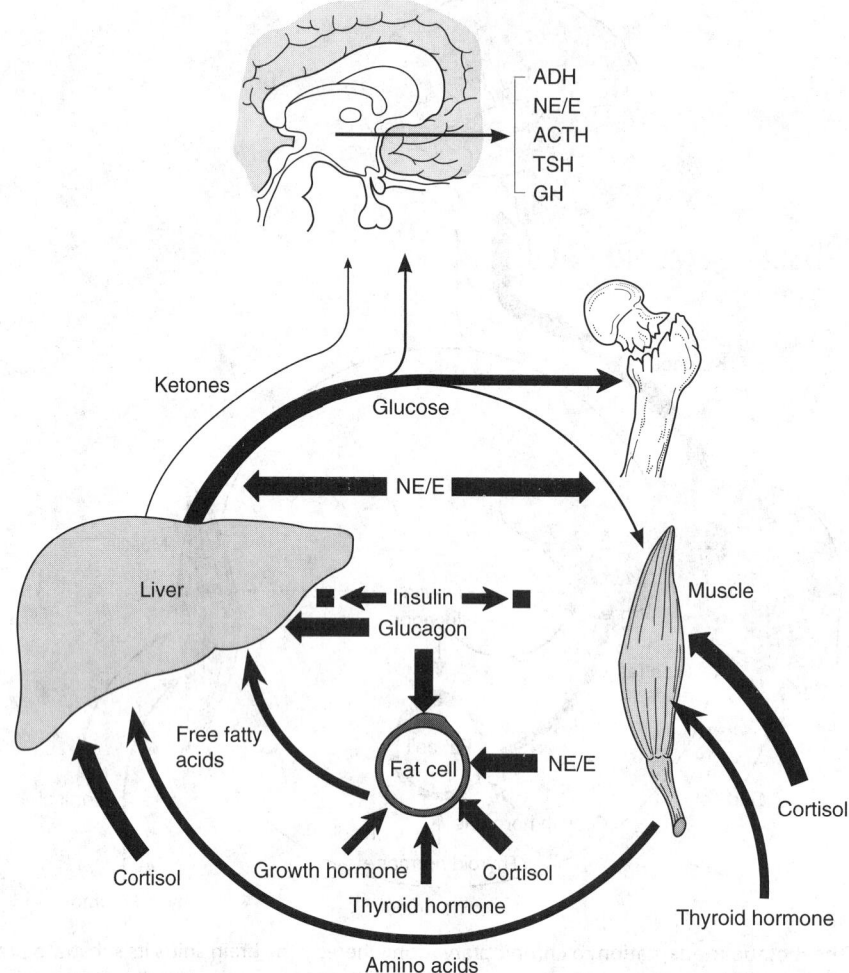

ADH
NE/E
ACTH
TSH
GH

Ketones

Glucose

NE/E

Liver

Insulin

Glucagon

Muscle

Free fatty
acids

Fat cell

NE/E

Cortisol

Cortisol

Growth hormone

Cortisol

Thyroid hormone

Thyroid hormone

Amino acids

Figure 11–5. The metabolic response to trauma is a result of neuroendocrine stimulation, which accelerates protein breakdown, stimulates gluconeogenesis, and produces glucose intolerance.

ripheral lipolysis, by the synergistic activation of hormone-sensitive lipase by glucagon, epinephrine, cortisol, and thyroid hormone; (2) accelerated catabolism, consisting of a rise in proteolysis, stimulated by cortisol; and (3) decreased peripheral glucose uptake due to insulin antagonism by growth hormone and epinephrine. These peripheral effects result in a marked rise in plasma concentrations of FFA, glycerol, glucose, lactate, and amino acids. The liver responds by an increase in substrate uptake and glucose production, owing to glucagon-stimulated glycogenolysis and to enhanced gluconeogenesis induced by cortisol and glucagon.

This accelerated glucose production, along with inhibited peripheral uptake, produces the glucose intolerance of trauma. The kidney avidly retains water and

sodium because of the effects of ADH and aldosterone. Urinary nitrogen excretion increases to 15–20 g/d in severe trauma, equivalent to a lean tissue loss of 750 g/d. Without exogenous nutrients, the median survival under these circumstances is about 15 days.

The difference in the metabolic response to accidental trauma and to elective operation is related to the intensity of the neuroendocrine stimulus. The REE rises only 10% in postoperative patients, compared with 25–30% after severe accidental trauma. The liberal use of analgesia and immobilization of injured extremities decreases the intensity of neuroendocrine stimuli, helping to spare the loss of lean body tissue.

The neuroendocrine response to trauma results in an exaggerated mobilization of metabolic substrates and a loss of the adaptive decrease in REE and nitrogen excretion seen in starvation. In contrast to the substrate dependency of uncomplicated starvation, operation and trauma are "neuroendocrine-driven" processes.

Sepsis

The metabolic changes during sepsis are somewhat different (Figure 11–6). The REE rises 50–80% above control values, and urinary nitrogen excretion reaches 20–30 g/d, equivalent to a median survival of 10 days without nutritional input. The plasma glucose, amino acid, and FFA levels increase more than in trauma, while there is an enormous increase in muscle protein

catabolism along with a profound depression of protein synthesis. Hepatic protein synthesis is stimulated, with both enhanced secretion of export protein and accumulation of structural protein. The nonprotein RQ falls to 0.69–0.71, indicative of intense FFA oxidation. This enhanced FFA oxidation is unresponsive to exogenous nutrients. During nutritional therapy, septic patients fail to demonstrate a rise in RQ to 1 or greater, indicating FFA synthesis from glucose. This unresponsiveness of the RQ can result in large increases in $\dot{V}CO_2$ and can even precipitate respiratory failure when these patients are supported with a glucose-based TPN system. Septic patients also have an abnormal plasma amino acid pattern (ie, increased levels of AAAs and decreased levels of

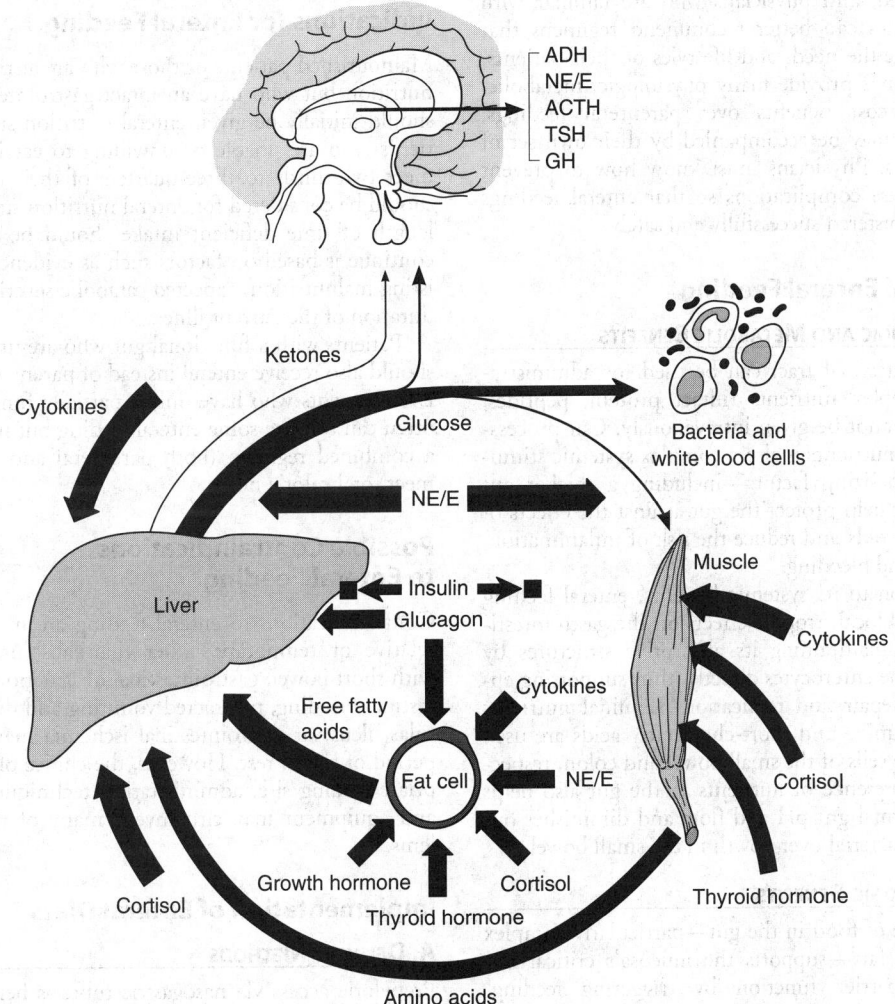

Figure 11–6. During sepsis, cytokines (IL-1, IL-2, TNF) released by lymphocytes and macrophages contribute to catabolism of muscle protein and adipose tissue and amplify the neuroendocrine response to antecedent trauma.

BCAAs) similar to that of patients with liver failure. Terminal sepsis results in a further increase in plasma amino acids and a fall in glucose concentration, as hepatic amino acid clearance declines and gluconeogenesis stops.

NUTRITIONAL SUPPORT

Enteral Nutrition

Use of an intact gastrointestinal tract for nutritional support should be the initial step in alimentation. The appropriate enteral dietary regimen depends upon the patient's diagnosis, nutritional status, nutrient and fluid requirements, and alimentary tract function. There are various ways that enteral feedings can be administered and scheduled, and physicians who are familiar with these schedules can better recommend regimens that accommodate the needs and lifestyles of their patients. Enteral feedings provide many physiologic, metabolic, safety, and cost benefits over parenteral feedings, though they may be accompanied by their own set of complications. Physicians must know how to prevent and treat these complications so that enteral feedings can be administered successfully and safely.

Benefits of Enteral Feeding

A. PHYSIOLOGIC AND METABOLIC BENEFITS

The gastrointestinal tract can be used for administration of complex nutrients (intact protein, peptides, fiber) that cannot be given intravenously. Gut processing of intact nutrients is also a complex systemic stimulus for synthesizing factors—including a thicker gut barrier—that help protect the gut against the effects of stress and steroids and reduce the risk of inflammation, ulceration, and bleeding.

In addition to its systemic benefits, enteral feeding has beneficial local, trophic effects on the gastrointestinal mucosa, maintaining its absorptive structures by nourishing the enterocytes directly, thus supporting epithelial cell repair and replication. Luminal nutrients such as glutamine and short-chain fatty acids are used as fuel by the cells of the small bowel and colon, respectively. The presence of nutrients in the gut also helps maintain normal gut pH and flora and diminishes opportunistic bacterial overgrowth in the small bowel.

B. IMMUNOLOGIC BENEFITS

The presence of food in the gut—particularly complex proteins and fats—supports the mucosa's critical immunologic barrier function by triggering feeding-dependent neuroendocrine activity. Subsequently, this appears to stimulate the manufacture of immunoglobulins in the gut—particularly secretory immunoglobulin A, which is important for preventing bacterial adherence and translocation.

C. SAFETY BENEFITS

Enteral feeding is generally considered safer than parenteral feeding when it is administered cautiously. However, enteral feeding has its own potential complications.

D. COST BENEFITS

Enteral nutrition generally costs less than parenteral feeding, including costs for formula, equipment, and administration both in the hospital and in other settings.

Indications for Enteral Feeding

Malnourished patients or those who are at risk for malnutrition but who have an intact gastrointestinal tract should initially be given enteral nutrition support. Patients who are unable or unwilling to eat in order to meet two-thirds to three-quarters of their daily needs should be considered for enteral nutrition support. The length of time deficient intake should be allowed to continue is based on factors such as evidence of preexisting malnutrition, expected catabolic severity, and the duration of the current illness.

Patients with a functional gut who are unable to eat should also receive enteral instead of parenteral feeding. Even patients who have only a partially functional gut often can tolerate some enteral feeding but may require a combined regimen (both parenteral and enteral) to meet total caloric needs.

Possible Contraindications to Enteral Feeding

Contraindications to enteral feeding are in most cases relative or temporary rather than absolute. Patients with short bowel, gastrointestinal obstruction, gastrointestinal bleeding, protracted vomiting and diarrhea, fistulas, ileus, or gastrointestinal ischemia may require a period of bowel rest. However, the choice of an appropriate feeding site, administration technique, formula, and equipment may circumvent many of these problems.

Implementation of Enteral Diets

A. DELIVERY METHODS

Prepyloric access via nasogastric tubes is beneficial because it is less expensive, easier to secure and maintain, and less labor-intensive than small bowel access. Contraindications to gastric feeding are delayed gastric emptying, gastrointestinal reflux, gastric outlet obstruction, and a history of repeated aspiration of tube feedings due to reflux. Patients with nasal obstruction or severe facial fractures should not have these tubes inserted nasally but can have the tube inserted orally.

Postpyloric access via nasoenteric tubes (duodenal or jejunal) is preferred when gastric feedings are not tolerated, when patients are at risk for reflux or aspiration, and when early enteral nutrition is desired. In general, a jejunal tube is preferable since the shorter duodenal tubes have an increased incidence of reflux of feedings or reflux of the tube itself into the stomach. Contraindications to enteral feeding are small or large bowel obstruction, peritonitis, and hemodynamic instability. In times of physiologic stress, the body shunts blood away from the gut. Feeding a patient who is hemodynamically unstable or taking vasopressors may stress the bowel so much that it may become ischemic.

When long-term gastric or enteral feeding is needed, permanent gastrostomy or jejunostomy tubes may be inserted. Often they are inserted at the time of laparotomy for a separate indication when the patient is expected to have a prolonged ileus or a complicated postoperative course.

Although a number of bedside methods (eg, auscultation, feeding tube aspirate pH measurements, observation for patient coughing) have been described to check tube placement, these are often unreliable. Therefore, before infusing an enteral diet, it is recommended that tube position is confirmed radiographically.

Formulas

Currently available dietary formulations for enteral feedings may be divided into polymeric commercial formulas (blenderized and nutritionally complete), chemically defined formulas (elemental diets), and modular formulas (Table 11–6).

Blenderized tube feedings may be composed of any food that can be blenderized. Caloric distribution of these formulas should parallel a normal diet.

Nutritionally complete commercial formulas (standard enteral diets) vary in protein, carbohydrate, and fat composition. Several formulas use sucrose or glucose as carbohydrate sources and are suitable for lactose-deficient patients. Commercial formulas are convenient, sterile, and low in cost. They are recommended for patients experiencing minimal metabolic stress who have normal gut function.

Chemically defined formulas are commonly called elemental diets. The nutrients are provided in a predigested and readily absorbed form. They contain protein in the form of low-molecular-weight free amino acids

or polypeptides. Amino acid (elemental) and polypeptide diets are efficiently absorbed in the presence of compromised gut function. However, they are more expensive than nutritionally complete commercial formulas and are hyperosmolar, which may cause cramping and diarrhea.

Modular formulations include special formulas used for specific clinical situations (eg, pulmonary, renal, or hepatic failure or immune dysfunction).

The available preparations (Table 11–6) vary in (1) caloric and protein content; (2) protein, carbohydrate, and fat composition; (3) nonprotein carbohydrate calorie-to-gram nitrogen ratio; (4) osmolality; (5) content of minor trace metals (selenium, chromium, and molybdenum); (6) glutamine or glutamic acid (glutamate) content; and (7) branched-chain amino acid content.

Initiating Feedings

In the past, elaborate protocols for initiating tube feedings were used. It is currently recommended that feedings be started with full-strength formula begun at a slow rate and steadily advanced. This approach reduces the risk of microbial contamination and achieves full nutrient intake earlier. Formulas are generally introduced at full strength at 10–40 mL/h initially and advanced to the goal rate in increments of 10–20 mL every 8–12 hours as tolerated. This approach can also be used with high-osmolality or elemental products. Conservative initiation and advancement rates are recommended for patients who are critically ill, those who have not been fed for some time, and those who are receiving high-osmolality or calorie-dense formula.

Monitoring Feedings

Assessment of gastrointestinal tolerance includes monitoring for symptoms or signs of abdominal discomfort, nausea and vomiting, abdominal distention, and abnormal bowel sounds or stool patterns. Gastric residuals are used to evaluate gastric emptying of enteral feedings. High residuals raise concerns about intolerance to gastric feedings and the potential risk for regurgitation and aspiration. When a residual value reaches > 200 mL with a nasogastric tube or > 100 mL with a gastrostomy tube with associated signs or symptoms of intolerance, feedings should be interrupted. Further workup with radiographs may be indicated. If the abdominal examination is unremarkable, feedings should be postponed for at least an hour and the residual volume should be rechecked. If high residuals persist without associated clinical signs and symptoms, a promotility agent (eg, erythromycin, metoclopramide) may be added.

Table 11–6. Enteral formulas.

Product and Description	kcal/mL	mosm/kg H₂O	Protein g (% kcal)	CHO g (% kcal)	Fat g (% kcal)	H₂O (mL)	Na⁺ (meq)	K⁺ (meq)	Ca²⁺ (mg)	PO₄⁻ (mg)	Vit K (mg)	U.S. RDAs (mL)
						Per 1000 mL						
Standard												
Ensure (lactose-free, low-residue, flavored)	1.06	470	37.2 (14)	145 (54.5)	37.2 (31.5)	845	36.8	40.0	530.0	530.0	43.0	1887
Osmolite (isotonic, lactose-free, low-residue)	1.06	300	37.2 (14)	145 (54.6)	38.5 (31.4)	841	27.6	25.9	530.0	530.0	43.0	1887
Jevity (isotonic, lactose-free, high dietary fiber [14.4 g/L], high nitrogen content)	1.06	310	44.4 (16.7)	151.7 (53.3)	36.8 (30)	833	40.4	40.0	909.0	756.0	61.0	1321
Glucerna (lactose-free, low-CHO, high-fiber [14.4 g/L], (vanilla flavor)	1.0	375	41.8 (16.7)	93.7 (33.3)	55.7 (50)	873	40.3	40.0	703.0	703.0	57.0	1422
Volume-restricted												
Ensure Plus (lactose-free, low-residue, flavored)	1.5	690	54.9 (14.7)	200 (53.3)	53.3 (32)	769	45.9	49.7	704.0	704.0	57.0	1420
Magnacal (lactose-free, low-residue, vanilla flavor)	2.0	590	70 (14)	250 (50)	80 (34)	690	43.5	32.0	1000.0	1000.0	300.0	1000
Volume-restricted, high-nitrogen												
Ensure Plus HN (lactose-free, low-residue, flavored)	1.5	650	62.6 (16.7)	199.9 (53.3)	50 (30)	769	51.5	46.5	1056.0	1056.0	85.0	947
Perative[1] (lactose-free, low-residue, unflavored)	1.3	425	66.6 (20.5)	177 (54.5)	37.3 (25)	789	45.2	44.3	867.0	867.0	70.0	1155

Very high nitrogen												
Replete with Fiber (lactose-free, high-fiber [14 g/L], unflavored)	1.0	300	62.5 (25)	113 (45)	34 (30)	840	21.7	40.0	1000.0	1000.0	80.0	1000
Sustacal (lactose-free, low-residue, flavored)	1.01	650	61 (24)	140 (55)	23 (21)	840	40.0	54.0	1010.0	930.0	240.0	1060
Elemental												
Vivonex TEN (elemental, low-fat, low-residue)	1.0	630	38.2 (15.3)	205.6 (82.2)	2.77 (2.5)	845	20.0	20.0	500.0	500.0	22.3	2000
Pudding (per 5 oz serving)												
Ensure Pudding (contains lactose)	250.0	...	6.8	34.0	9.7	...	10.4	8.5	200.0	200.0	12.0	...
Modulars (analysis per tablespoon)												
Polycose Liquid (glucose polymer)	30.0	...	...	7.5	...	...	...	1.0	...	...	...	...
Promod (protein supplement)	17.0	...	3.0	0.4	0.4	...	0	1.0	15.6	15.6	...	...
Microlipid (fat supplement)	67.5	...	...	...	7.5	...	...	...	...	...	...	...
MCT Oil (MCT supplement)	115.5	...	...	...	14.0	...	...	...	...	...	...	...

RDA = recommended daily allowance; MCT = medium-chain triglyceride

[1] Perative may be contraindicated in transplant patients.

PROTOCOL FOR NASOGASTRIC FEEDING

1. Insert a nasointestinal feeding tube.
2. Obtain a stat portable KUB postinsertion to confirm the position of the nasointestinal feeding tube in the small bowel. Notify the physician when a plain film of the abdomen is obtained.
3. Begin_____(enteral diet) at _____ (strength) at a rate of _____mL/h continuously per volumetric pump via the nasointestinal feeding tube when notified by the physician that the feeding tube is positioned in the small bowel.
4. Elevate the head of the bed 30 degrees or more while administering the enteral diet.
5. Only liquid medications or powdered solids suspended in liquid by a pharmacist should be administered via the feeding tube.
6. Flush the feeding tube every 4 hours with 20 mL of sterile water.
7. Check on the amount of residual fluid by aspirating the feeding tube every 4 hours. If the residual is > 150 mL, discontinue the infusion for 2 hours. After 2 hours, recheck again for residual. If the residual is < 150 mL, restart the enteral diet infusion. If the residual remains > 150 mL, do not restart the infusion until the physician is notified.
8. Inform the physician about persistent residuals > 150 mL, increasing abdominal distention, nausea, vomiting, diarrhea, or an oral temperature > 38°C.
9. Record intake and output (I/O) with strict accuracy. Total the I/O every 24 hours.
10. Record the patient's weight weekly on the vital signs sheet.
11. Check the urine for sugar and acetone daily and record the results on the vital signs sheet. If the urine sugar is 4+, obtain a stat serum glucose determination. If the serum glucose is > 160 mg/dL, contact the physician for treatment orders.
12. Begin (per the nasointestinal feeding tube):
    a. Neutra-Phos (phosphate supplement): 1 or 2 capsules (250 mg/capsule) dissolved in 75-150 mL of the enteral diet 4 times daily.
    b. Zinc sulfate (zinc supplement): 200 mg added to the enteral diet twice daily.
    c. Titralac (calcium supplement): 2 tsp added to the enteral diet twice daily.
13. Routine enteral diet laboratory tests should be drawn weekly and as indicated by the patient's clinical condition.

Complications of Enteral Feeding

Technical complications occur in about 5% of enterally fed patients and include clogging of the tube; esophageal, tracheal, bronchial, or duodenal perforation; and tracheobronchial intubation with tube feeding aspiration. Patients with decreased consciousness, impaired gag reflexes, or those who have undergone endotracheal intubation are at increased risk. The tip of the feeding tube must be positioned and verified radiographically—any other method is unreliable.

Functional complications include nausea, vomiting, abdominal distention, constipation, and diarrhea. These occur in up to 25% of tube-fed patients and are the main reason for intolerance to enteral diets. Nausea, vomiting, and abdominal distention can be minimized by infusing the duodenum rather than the stomach and giving the diet continuously rather than as a bolus.

Diarrhea is usually the result of polypharmacy (eg, multiple antibiotics), mechanical gut dysfunction (eg, partial small bowel obstruction), intestinal bacterial overgrowth (eg, *Clostridium difficile*), protein content or osmolality of the diet, intrinsic bowel disease (eg, inflammatory bowel disease), or systemic disease (eg, HIV infection, amyloidosis). Treatment consists of stopping any medications at fault, correcting gut dysfunction, giving appropriate antibiotics, modifying the protein content (intact protein versus amino acid or polypeptide formula) or osmolality of the diet, adding pectin or fiber to the diet, or administering antidiarrheal agents.

In the case of the surgical patient, *C difficile* is a frequent cause of diarrhea due to the common use of perioperative antibiotics. Laboratory confirmation is by *C difficile* toxin assay. Treatment options include either metronidazole (oral or intravenous) or oral vancomycin.

Electrolyte abnormalities (principally hypernatremia and hyponatremia, hyperkalemia and hypokalemia, hypophosphatemia, and hypomagnesemia) occur in about half of patients. Hyperglycemia severe enough to cause hyperosmolar nonketotic acidosis may also occur.

Alverdy J: Effect of nutrition on gastrointestinal barrier function. Semin Respir Infect 1994;9:248.

Coghlin Dickson TM et al: Effect of oral glutamine supplementation during bone marrow transplantation. JPEN J Parenter Enteral Nutr 2000;24:61.

Cresci GA: The use of probiotics with the treatment of diarrhea. Nutr Clin Pract 2001;16:30.

Cui XL et al: Arginine-supplemented diet decreases expression of inflammatory cytokines and improves survival in burned rats. JPEN J Parenter Enteral Nutr 2000;24:89.

DeLegge MH: Enteral access—the foundation of feeding. J Parenter Enteral Nutr 2001;25:58.

Fuhrman MP: Diarrhea and tube feeding. Nutr Clin Pract 1999; 14:83.

Gianotti L et al: A prospective, randomized clinical trial on perioperative feeding with an arginine-, omega-3 fatty acid-, and RNA-enriched enteral diet: effect on host response and nutritional status. JPEN J Parenter Enteral Nutr 2001;23:314.

Granato D et al: Effects of parenteral lipid emulsions with different fatty acid composition on immune cell functions in vitro. JPEN J Parenter Enteral Nutr 2000;24113.

Ibanez J et al: Incidence of gastroesophageal reflux and aspiration in mechanically ventilated patients using small-bore nasogastric tubes. JPEN J Parenter Enteral Nutr 2000;24:103.

Johnson CC et al: Postoperative feeding: a clinical review. Obstet Gynecol Surv 2000;55:571.

McClave SA et al: Enteral tube feeding in the intensive care unit: factors impeding adequate delivery. Crit Care Med 1999; 27:1252.

McClave SA et al: Use of residual volume as a marker for enteral feeding intolerance: prospective blinded comparison with physical examination and radiographic findings. JPEN J Parenter Enteral Nutr 1992;16:99.

McClave SA: The effects of immune-enhancing diets (IEDs) on mortality, hospital length of stay, duration of mechanical ventilation, and other parameters. JPEN J Parenter Enteral Nutr 2001;25:544.

Metheny NA et al: Bedside methods for detecting aspiration in tube-fed patients. Chest 1997;111:724.

Ochoa JB et al: Effect of L-arginine on the proliferation of T lymphocyte subpopulations. JPEN J Parenter Enteral Nutr 2001; 25:23.

Orlando R: Gastrointestinal motility and tube feeding. Crit Care Med 1998;26:1472.

Sax HC: Effect of immune enhancing formulas (IEF) in general surgery patients. JPEN J Parenter Enteral Nutr 2001;25:519.

Schloerb PR: Immune-enhancing diets: products, components, and their rationales. JPEN J Parenter Enteral Nutr 2001;25:53.

Williams MS et al: Diarrhea management in enterally fed patients. Nutr Clin Pract 1998;13:225.

PARENTERAL NUTRITION THERAPY

When the gastrointestinal tract cannot be used, nutrients must be given parenterally. Since parenteral nutrition is more expensive, is associated with more technical, metabolic, and septic complications, and requires more expertise than enteral nutrition, it should only be used when the gut cannot be used. Parental formulas deliver 75–150 nonprotein carbohydrate calories per gram of nitrogen infused—a ratio that maximizes carbohydrate and protein assimilation and minimizes metabolic complications (aminoaciduria, hyperglyce-mia, and hepatic glycogenesis). There are two methods: peripheral parenteral nutrition (PPN) and total parenteral nutrition (TPN). (See Table 11–7.) In addition to route of administration, the two differ in (1) the dextrose and amino acid (protein) content of the parenteral solution, (2) the primary caloric source (glucose versus fat), (3) the frequency of fat administration, (4) the infusion schedule, and (5) the potential complications.

1. PERIPHERAL PARENTERAL NUTRITION (PPN)

Indications

PPN therapy is safe, easy, and indicated for patients with compromised gut function who require short-term (< 10–14 days) nutrition because they are unable to ingest adequate nutrients.

PPN Solution Formulation

One liter of standard PPN solution contains $D_{20}W$, 500 mL, and 10% amino acids, 500 mL, plus electrolytes, vitamins, minerals, and trace metals. $D_{20}W$ contains 20 g glucose per 100 mL (100 g per 500 mL). Since the metabolism of 1 g glucose yields 3.4 kcal, the metabolism of 500 mL of $D_{20}W$ yields 340 kcal. Therefore, 1 L of standard PPN solution ($D_{20}W$ 500 mL plus 10% amino acids 500 mL) provides 340 kcal.

A carbohydrate source less commonly used in peripheral parenteral nutrition is glycerol, which provides 4.3 kcal/g and a 10% amino acid solution containing 10 g protein per 100 mL or 50 g protein per 500 mL. Since 1 g of nitrogen is equivalent to 6.25 g of protein, 50 g of protein is equivalent to 8 g of nitrogen. Therefore, 1 L of standard PPN solution ($D_{20}W$ 500 mL plus 10% amino acids 500 mL) provides approximately 8 g of nitrogen.

The ratio of nonprotein carbohydrate calories to grams of nitrogen in 1 L of standard PPN solution is approximately 43:1 (340 kcal per 8 g nitrogen supplies 43 kcal/g nitrogen).

Since 1 L of standard PPN solution contains adequate nitrogen but inadequate calories, the daily PPN regimen should also include 500 mL of 20% fat emulsion (2 kcal/mL). Table 11–8 lists the various PPN additives and gives the basic formulation of a standard liter of PPN solution. By giving PPN solution at 125 mL/h and supplementing it with 500 mL of 20% fat emulsion daily, PPN provides about 2200 kcal and 150 g protein (24 g nitrogen) daily.

Fat is an excellent source of calories, but—as mentioned earlier—fat generally should provide 20–40% of the total caloric requirement and should not be used to provide more than 60% of the patient's estimated daily caloric requirement.

Table 11–7. Partial (PPN) versus total (TPN) therapy: Indications, contraindications, and characteristic features.

	Standard PPN Therapy	Standard TPN Therapy
Clinical indications	Short-term (< 10 days) supplemental or total nutritional therapy.	Long-term (> 10 days) supplemental or total nutritional therapy.
Clinical contraindications	(1) Patients who are able to consume their daily caloric, protein, and other required nutrients per oral or enteral feedings. (2) Patients who require long-term (> 10 days) total nutritional therapy because of gut dysfunction.	(1) Patients who are able to consume their daily caloric, protein, and other required nutrients per oral or enteral feedings. (2) Patients who require short-term (< 10 days) total nutritional therapy because of gut dysfunction.
Primary source of calories	Fat metabolism.	Dextrose metabolism.
Dextrose content	$D_{20}W$	$D_{50}W$
Protein content	10% amino acids (essential and nonessential).	8.5% amino acids (essential and non-essential).
Fat therapy	Fat emulsion 20% 500 mL daily.[1]	Fat emulsion 20% 500 mL every Monday, Wednesday, and Friday.[2]
Route of administration	Peripheral 18-gauge intravenous cannula or a central intravenous infusion catheter with the distal tip positioned in the superior or inferior vena cava.	Central intravenous infusion catheter with the distal tip positioned in the superior or inferior vena cava.
Infusion schedule (mL/h via pump)	Day 1: 100–125[3]	Day 1: 40–100
Therapeutic monitoring	CBC, blood chemistries, and 24-hour nitrogen balance determination.	CBC, blood chemistries, and 24-hour nitrogen balance determination.
Complications	Technical, infectious, and metabolic (Tables 11–10 and 11–11).[4]	Technical, infectious, and metabolic (Tables 11–10 and 11–11).[4]
Rebound hypoglycemia	No risk.[5]	Risk.[6]

[1]Fat emulsion therapy provides the major source of calories.
[2]Fat emulsion 20% 500 mL is administered intravenously via at least an 18-gauge peripheral intravenously or central venous catheter positioned in the superior vena cava per pump over 4–6 hours. Fat therapy should provide at least 4–6% of the daily caloric requirement to prevent the development of a fatty acid deficiency. The frequency and quantity of fat administered weekly may be increased depending on the patient's estimated daily caloric requirement.
[3]The final infusion rate is dependent upon the patient's calculated daily caloric and protein requirements, age, and overall cardiovascular status.
[4]Phlebitis is the most common complication.
[5]PPN therapy can be discontinued at any time without the risk of rebound hypoglycemia.
[6]The discontinuance of central TPN therapy may result in rebound hypoglycemia if the patient is either NPO or has inadequate enteral caloric intake. To avoid rebound hypoglycemia in these patients, the central TPN solution must be tapered or replaced with a $D_{10}W$ infusion at the previous infusion rate.

Table 11–8. PPN solution formulation.

Components in 1 L of PPN:

Routine additives

$D_{20}W^1$	500 mL
10% amino acid[1]	500 mL
Sodium chloride[2]	0–140 meq
Sodium phosphate[3]	0–20 mmol
Potassium chloride[4]	0–40 meq
Magnesium sulfate[5]	0–12 meq
Calcium gluconate[5,6]	4.5 or 9.0 meq
M.V.I.-12[7]	10 mL
Multitrace[7]	5 mL

Optional additives

Sodium acetate[2]	0–140 meq
Potassium acetate[4]	0–40 meq
H_2 antagonist[8]	Variable[8]
Regular insulin[9]	0–40 units

Administration schedule for standard PPN:

Day of Therapy	Rate (mL/h)
1	40
2	80
3	100–125[10]

Fat emulsion schedule:

Infuse a 20% fat emulsion 500 mL intravenously via pump over 6–8 hours at least daily via either an 18-gauge peripheral intravenous cannula or piggyback per the central infusion catheter.

---

[1]The solution is formulated to deliver 43 nonprotein carbohydrate calories per gram of nitrogen infused.
[2]Add sodium chloride if the serum CO_2 > 25 meq/L. Add sodium acetate if the serum $CO_2 \le$ 25 meq/L.
[3]The total phosphate dosage should not exceed 20 mmol/L or 60 mmol daily.
[4]Add KCl if the serum CO_2 > 25 meq/L. Add potassium acetate if the serum $CO_2 \le$ 25 meq/L. The potassium dosage should not exceed 40 meq/L.
[5]Added to each liter.
[6]Add calcium gluconate 9 meq to each liter if the serum calcium < 8.5 meq/L. Add 4.5 meq if the serum calcium $\ge$ 8.5 meq/L.
[7]Administered in only 1 L per day.
[8]Dosage depends upon the H_2 antagonist selected. Divide the daily dosage equally in all liters of PPN administered.
[9]Total dosage should not exceed 40 units/L.
[10]The final infusion rate is dependent upon the patient's calculated daily caloric and protein requirements and overall cardiovascular status.

Administration

PPN is infused via an 18-gauge intravenous cannula in a peripheral vein. A 16-gauge single-lumen central venous catheter (SLCVC) positioned in the superior vena cava via the subclavian or internal jugular vein may also be used. A peripheral PPN catheter site is dressed like any other peripheral intravenous site. A central PPN catheter site is dressed like a TPN catheter site (discussed below). Standard PPN therapy orders (Figure 11–7) should include the administration schedule for the PPN solution and fat supplement as well as explicit catheter care orders and monitoring guidelines.

Special PPN Solutions

Since the final dextrose concentration of a PPN solution cannot exceed 12.5%, it is impossible to formulate a concentrated PPN solution for patients on restricted

1. PPN components:

ROUTINE ADDITIVES	Recommended Dosage Ranges per Liter PPN	BAG #___	BAG #___	BAG #___
$D_{20}W$	500 mL	500 mL	500 mL	500 mL
AA 10%	500 mL	500 mL	500 mL	500 mL
NaCl	0–140 meq	meq	meq	meq
NaPO₄	0–20 mmol	mmol	mmol	mmol
K⁺Cl	0–40 meq	meq	meq	meq
MgSO₄	0–12 meq	meq	meq	meq
Ca gluconate	4.5 or 9 meq	meq	meq	meq
MVI-12®	10 mL/d	10 mL		
Multitrace®	5 mL/d	5mL		
OPTIONAL ADDITIVES				
Na acetate	0–140 meq	meq	meq	meq
K⁺ acetate	0–40 meq	meq	meq	meq
Regular insulin	0–40 units	units	units	units
H_2 antagonist**				
NURSE'S SIGNATURE				

* TOTAL POTASSIUM CONTENT PER LITER OF PPN SHOULD NOT EXCEEED 40 meq.
**DIVIDE THE DAILY DOSAGE EQUALLY INTO EACH LITER OF PPN.

RATE:___100–125___ mL/h via pump.
Final dextrose concentration___10___%   Final AA concentration___10___%

2. Pharmacy to add vitamin K 10 mg to 1 L of PPN solution every Mon. and Thurs.
3. Insert at least an 18-gauge peripheral IV and begin the PPN infusion at 100–125 mL/h per pump.
4. Infuse 500 mL 20% fat emulsion daily IVPB over 6–8 hours via at least an 18-gauge peripheral IV.
5. Strict I/O every shift. Total the I/O every 24 hours.
6. Record the daily weight in kilograms on the vital signs sheet.
7. Check the urine for sugar and acetone every shift and record on the vital signs sheet. If the urine sugar is 4+, request a STAT serum glucose measurement to be drawn by the physician. If the serum glucose is > 160 mg/dL, contact the physician for treatment orders.
8. Notify the physician if the oral temperature is >38°C (>100.4°F).
9. Routine PPN laboratory tests are to be drawn weekly on the days and times specified below:
   Sun. AM: CBC, SMAC-20
   Tues. AM: Electrolytes, BUN, creatinine, and glucose
   Thurs. AM: CBC, SMAC-20, copper, zinc, magnesium, transferrin, and triglycerides
10. Begin a 24-hour urine collection for urinary urea nitrogen (UUN) at 6:00 AM every Mon. for nitrogen balance determination.
11. PPN catheter dressing and tubing changes per the hospital IV protocol.
12. Contact the physician for all problems related to PPN.
13. All changes in PPN therapy must be approved by the physician.

Figure 11–7. PPN therapy orders.

fluid intake (eg, cardiac disease, renal failure). Consequently, PPN is contraindicated in the treatment of fluid-restricted patients.

A. NONOLIGURIC RENAL FAILURE

Patients in nonoliguric renal failure (serum creatinine > 2 mg/dL) who can tolerate the PPN regimen of 3500 mL daily and who cannot be dialyzed should receive a special renal failure PPN solution and daily fat supplements. One liter of this solution should contain a combination of $D_{20}W$ 500 mL and renal failure amino acids (essential amino acids only) 500 mL plus limited amounts of sodium, potassium, magnesium, and phosphate.

B. HEPATIC FAILURE

Patients with hepatic encephalopathy who can tolerate the daily 3500 mL infusion should receive a special hepatic failure PPN solution that contains $D_{20}W$ 500 mL and hepatic failure amino acids (primarily branched-chain amino acids) 500 mL plus additives, with the exception that sodium content is limited to 40 meq/L.

2. TOTAL PARENTERAL NUTRITION (TPN)

Indications

TPN is indicated for patients who cannot be nourished enterally and require more than 10 days of nutritional support.

Solution Formulation

TPN may be provided in individual liter units, with fat given separately, or (more commonly) as a 3:1 admixture. Various concentrations of dextrose are illustrated in the accompanying table.

Characteristics of TPN Solutions

Dextrose	kcal/L	Osmolality (mosm/L)
5	170	250
10	340	500
20	680	1000
50	1700	2500
70	2380	3500

One liter of standard TPN solution contains $D_{50}W$ 500 mL and 8.5% amino acids 500 mL plus electrolytes, vitamins, minerals, and trace metals.

$D_{50}W$ contains 50 g of glucose per 100 mL or 250 g per 500 mL (and thus 850 kcal). An 8.5% amino acid solution contains 8.5 g of protein per 100 mL or 42.5 of protein (or 6.8 g of nitrogen) per 500 mL. Therefore, 1 L of standard TPN solution ($D_{50}W$ 500 mL

plus 8.5% amino acids 500 mL) provides approximately 1000 kcal and 6.8 g of nitrogen; and the ratio of nonprotein carbohydrate calories to grams of nitrogen is approximately 125:1. General guidelines for recommended additives to TPN are as depicted in the accompanying table.

Total Parenteral Nutrition

Daily Requirements	
Amino acids	60–80 g
Dextrose	250 g
Na^+	60–80 meq
K^+	30–60 meq
Cl^-	80–100 meq
Acetate	Variable
Ca^{2+}	4.6–9.2 meq
Mg^{2+}	8.1–20 meq
PO_4^-	12–24 mmol

Patients receiving TPN should also receive 3–5% of their daily caloric requirement as fat in order to prevent a fatty acid deficiency. This is accomplished by giving 500 mL of 20% fat emulsion (2 kcal/mL) intravenously over 6–8 hours at least three times per week. More commonly, fat is given in an admixture (3:1) with the dextrose and amino acid solution, where fat will provide 20–30% of the daily caloric requirement. TPN therapy also includes additives as listed in Table 11–9.

Administration

In patients over age 10, TPN solutions are routinely administered via a single-lumen central venous catheter with a Luer-Lok connection. The distal port of a triple-lumen central venous catheter may be used, but this results in a higher incidence of catheter infection.

The TPN catheter is inserted either into the superior vena cava via the internal jugular or subclavian vein or into the inferior vena cava via the femoral vein. Because of the discomfort and increased risk of infection associated with neck and groin insertions, they are not recommended. The TPN catheter site is dressed with a sterile gauze or transparent occlusive polyurethane dressing.

The solution is initially infused at a rate of 40 mL/h via a constant infusion pump. The rate should be 40 mL/h on the first day, 80 mL/h on the second day, and 100–125 mL/h on the third day. The final rate, achieved within 72 hours, depends on the patient's daily caloric and protein requirements, age, and cardiovascular status. Standard TPN therapy orders (Figure 11–8) should include the administration schedule for the TPN solution and fat supplement as well as explicit catheter care orders and monitoring guidelines.

Table 11–9.   TPN solution formulation.

Components in 1 L of standard TPN:

Routine additives

$D_{50}W^1$	500 mL
8.5% amino acid[1]	500 mL
Sodium chloride[2]	0–140 meq
Sodium phosphate[3]	0–20 mmol
Potassium chloride[4]	0–40 meq
Magnesium sulfate[5]	0–12 meq
Calcium gluconate[5,6]	4.5 or 9.0 meq
M.V.I.-12[7]	10 mL
Multitrace[7]	5 mL

Optional additives

Sodium acetate[2]	0–140 meq
Potassium acetate[4]	0–40 meq
H_2 antagonist[8]	Variable[8]
Regular insulin[9]	0–40 units

Administration schedule for standard TPN:

Day of Therapy	Rate (mL/h)
1	40
2	80
3	100–125[10]

Fat emulsion schedule:

Infuse a 20% fat emulsion 500 mL intravenously via pump over 6–8 hours at least 3 times per week via either an 18-gage peripheral intravenous cannula or piggyback per the central infusion catheter.

[1]The solution is formulated to deliver 125 nonprotein carbohydrate calories per gram of nitrogen infused.

[2]Add sodium chloride if the serum CO_2 > 25 meq/L. Add sodium acetate if the serum $CO_2 \leq 25$ meq/L.

[3]The total phosphate dosage should not exceed 20 mmol/L or 60 mmol daily.

[4]Add KCl if the serum CO_2 > 25 meq/L. Add potassium acetate if the serum $CO_2 \leq 25$ meq/L. The potassium dosage should not exceed 40 meq/L.

[5]Added to each liter.

[6]Add calcium gluconate 9 meq to each liter if the serum calcium < 8.5 meq/L. Add 4.5 meq if the serum calcium $\geq$ 8.5 meq/L.

[7]Administered in only 1 L per day.

[8]Dosage depends upon the H_2 antagonist selected. Divide the daily dosage equally in all liters of TPN administered.

[9]Total dosage should not exceed 40 units/L.

[10]The final infusion rate is dependent upon the patient's calculated daily caloric and protein requirements and overall cardiovascular status.

Special TPN Solutions

The TPN solution must be more concentrated for patients who require fluid restriction (eg, those with pulmonary and cardiac failure). One liter of concentrated TPN solution usually contains a combination of $D_{60}W$ or $D_{70}W$ 500 mL and 10% or 15% amino acids 500 mL plus additives.

---

1. TPN components:

ROUTINE ADDITIVES	Recommended Dosage Ranges per Liter TPN	BAG #___	BAG #___	BAG #___
$D_{50}W$	500 mL	500 mL	500 mL	500 mL
AA 8.5%	500 mL	500 mL	500 mL	500 mL
NaCl	0–140 meq	meq	meq	meq
$NaPO_4$	0–20 mmol	mmol	mmol	mmol
K⁺Cl	0–40 meq	meq	meq	meq
$MgSO_4$	0–12 meq	meq	meq	meq
Ca gluconate	4.5 or 9 meq	meq	meq	meq
MVI-12®	10 mL/d	10 mL		
Multitrace®	5 mL/d	5mL		
OPTIONAL ADDITIVES				
Na acetate	0–140 meq	meq	meq	meq
K⁺ acetate	0–40 meq	meq	meq	meq
Regular insulin	0–40 units	units	units	units
H_2 antagonist**				
25% albumin***	25 g	g	g	g
NURSE'S SIGNATURE				

* TOTAL POTASSIUM CONTENT PER LITER OF TPN SHOULD NOT EXCEEED 40 meq.
** DIVIDE THE DAILY DOSAGE EQUALLY INTO EACH LITER OF TPN.
*** ONLY IF THE SERUM ALBUMIN < 2.5g/dL AND ENTERAL DIET THERAPY IS ANTICIPATED.

RATE: ___40___ mL/h via pump.
Final dextrose concentration __25__%   Final AA concentration __4.25__%

2. Pharmacy to add vitamin K 10 mg to 1 L of TPN solution every Mon. and Thurs.
3. Fat emulsion 20% 500 mL every Mon., Wed., and Fri. IVPB per pump over 6–8 hours via at least an 18-gauge peripheral IV or via the subclavian catheter.
4. STAT upright and expirational portable chest x-ray to check the position of the subclavian catheter and to rule out a pneumothorax. Notify the physician when the chest x-ray is completed.
5. Heparin lock the TPN catheter with 2 mL of heparin (100 units/mL) until notified by the physician to start the first liter of TPN solution.
6. Strict I/O every shift. Total the I/O every 24 hours.
7. Record the daily weight in kilograms on the vital signs sheet.
8. Check the urine for sugar and acetone every shift and record on the vital signs sheet. If the urine sugar is 4+, request a STAT serum glucose measurement to be drawn by the physician. If the serum glucose is > 160 mg/dL, contact the physician for treatment orders.
9. Notify the physician if the oral temperature is >38°C (>100.4°F).
10. Routine TPN laboratory tests are to be drawn weekly on the days and times specified below:
   Sun. AM: CBC, SMAC-20
   Tues. AM: Electrolytes, BUN, creatinine, and glucose
   Thurs. AM: CBC, SMAC-20, copper, zinc, magnesium, transferrin, and triglycerides
11. Begin a 24-hour urine collection for urinary urea nitrogen (UUN) at 6:00 AM every Mon. and Thurs. for nitrogen balance determination.
12. TPN catheter dressing and tubing changes per the hospital TPN protocol.
13. Contact the physician for all problems related to TPN.
14. All changes in TPN therapy must be approved by the physician.

Figure 11–8.   TPN therapy orders.

A. RENAL FAILURE

Patients in renal failure (serum creatinine 2 mg/dL) who cannot be dialyzed and who require fluid restriction should receive a special renal failure TPN solution. Each liter of solution contains a combination of $D_{60}W$ or $D_{70}W$ 500 mL and renal failure amino acids (essential amino acids only) 500 mL plus limited amounts of sodium, potassium, magnesium, and phosphate.

Table 11–10. Nutritional therapy complications.

Enteral Nutrition	Total Parenteral Nutrition
Technical	**Technical**
Abscess of nasal septum	Air embolus
Acute sinusitis	Arterial laceration
Aspiration pneumonia	Arteriovenous fistula
Bacterial contamination of formula	Brachial plexus injury
Esophagitis-ulceration-stenosis	Cardiac perforation
Gastrointestinal perforation	Catheter embolism
Gastrostomy/jejunostomy dislodgment	Catheter malposition
Hemorrhage	Pneumothorax
Hoarseness	Subclavian vein thrombosis
Inadvertent tracheobronchial intubation	Thoracic duct laceration
Intestinal obstruction	Venous laceration
Intracranial passage of tube	
Knotting of tube	
Laryngeal ulceration	
Nasal erosions	
Necrotizing enterocolitis	
Otitis media	
Pneumatosis intestinalis	
Rupture of varices	
Skin excoriation	
Tracheoesophageal fistula	
Functional	**Infectious**
Nausea	Catheter fever
Vomiting	Catheter tip infection
Abdominal distention	Catheter exit site infection
Constipation	Catheter tip infection with bac-
Diarrhea	teremia infection
Metabolic	**Metabolic**
Dehydration	Azotemia
EFA deficiency	EFA deficiency
Hyperglycemia	Fluid overload
Hyperkalemia	Hyperchloremic metabolic acidosis
Hypernatremia	Hypercalcemia
Hyperosmolar nonketotic coma	Hyperkalemia
Hyperphosphatemia	Hypermagnesemia
Hypokalemia	Hypernatremia
Hypocupremia	Hyperosmolar nonketotic coma
Hypoglycemia	Hyperphosphatemia
Hypomagnesemia	Hypervitaminosis A
Hyponatremia	Hypevitaminosis D
Hypophosphatemia	Hypocalcemia
Hypozincemia	Hypokalemia
Liver function test elevation	Hypomagnesemia
Overhydration	Hyponatremia
Vitamin K deficiency	Hypophosphatemia
	Liver function test elevation
	Metabolic bone disease
	Trace element deficiency
	Ventilatory failure

Patients in renal failure who can undergo dialysis should receive a TPN solution that contains $D_{60}W$ or $D_{70}W$ and 8.5% standard amino acids (a combination of essential and nonessential) 500 mL plus additives, with limited amounts of sodium, potassium, magnesium, and phosphate.

B. HEPATIC FAILURE

Patients with hepatic encephalopathy should receive a hepatic failure TPN solution that contains a combination of $D_{30}W$ or $D_{40}W$ 500 mL and a special hepatic failure amino acid solution (branched-chain amino acids) 500 mL plus additives, with the exception of limited amounts of sodium (< 40 meq/L).

COMPLICATIONS OF PARENTERAL NUTRITION

PPN Therapy

Technical complications of PPN are few (see Table 11–10). The most common problem is maintenance of venous access. Because it causes phlebitis, the PPN infusion catheter must often be moved to another site. Since most patients have few usable peripheral veins, prolonged PPN (> 10 days) is rarely possible. The addition of fat, heparin, or corticosteroids to PPN solutions has not decreased the incidence of phlebitis.

Infectious complications such as catheter site skin infections and septic phlebitis develop in 5% of patients.

TPN Therapy

Technical, infectious, and metabolic complications each occur in 5% of patients, and the overall mortality rate directly attributable to TPN is 0.2%.

The most common technical complications are inability to cannulate the subclavian vein, malposition of the catheter, pneumothorax, bleeding, and air embolism (Table 11–11).

Air embolism—a rare but often lethal complication of subclavian vein catheterization—is characterized by sudden, severe respiratory distress (tachypnea), hypotension, and a cogwheel murmur. To prevent air embolism, the subclavian line should be inserted only with the patient tilted into a head-down position. It is also critical that the line not be disconnected when the patient is upright. This is easier to ensure if Luer-Lok connections are used.

Treatment of air embolism involves placing the patient with left side down, head down, and feet (Durant position) elevated and aspirating blood and air through the subclavian catheter (Figure 11–9).

Catheter site infection is characterized by mild fever (37.5–38 °C), pus around the catheter tract, and erythema and tenderness of the surrounding skin. Late changes include induration of the skin and systemic sepsis.

Primary line (catheter) infection is more difficult to diagnose than is local catheter site infection. Because catheter infections are twice as common (10% versus 5%) with triple-lumen than with single-lumen catheters, the latter are much preferred. The principal findings are (1) unexplained hyperglycemia (serum glucose 160 mg/dL), (2) a plateau pattern of fever (38–38.5 °C) for 12–24 hours, (3) leukocytosis (10,000/μL), and (4) positive blood cultures from a remote vein as well as from the suspect catheter. Skin changes are rare.

Patients with a suspected catheter infection who have negative blood cultures and no cardiovascular compromise should have the catheter exchanged over a guidewire and the tip sent for bacterial and fungal cultures. If the fever resolves and subsequent cultures are negative (colony count 15), no further therapy is necessary. If the patient remains febrile after the catheter exchange or continues to have positive blood or catheter cultures, a new central catheter should be inserted at another site. The most common metabolic complications (Tables 11–10 and 11–11) are hyperglycemia (serum glucose 160 mg/dL), electrolyte and mineral abnormalities, and acidosis.

Patients with severe malnutrition and weight loss (> 30% of their usual weight) may develop sudden cardiopulmonary failure during TPN, a complication known as the refeeding syndrome. In starvation, energy is derived principally from fat metabolism. TPN results in a shift from fat to glucose as the predominant fuel, which increases the production of phosphorylated intermediates of glycolysis and inhibits fat metabolism, thereby trapping phosphate and resulting in hypophosphatemia. Hypophosphatemia decreases ventricular stroke work and mean arterial pressure and produces severe congestive cardiomyopathy as a consequence of deficient ATP production and subsequent cell and tissue damage.

Because of these risks, the rate of TPN for a severely malnourished patient (< 70% of usual weight) should be slowly increased over several days. Instead of trying to meet the patient's nutritional requirements within 72 hours, the infusion should be raised by increments of 5–10 mL daily and only if the patient's heart rate is less than 100 beats/min.

Severely malnourished patients should also receive intravenous fat supplements and sodium phosphate—the latter to prevent hypophosphatemic cardiomyopathy. The daily phosphate dosage should not exceed 60 mmol. When oral nutrient intake is low, discontinuation of TPN may cause rebound hypoglycemia unless the infusion is decreased gradually.

Table 11–11. Complications of TPN.

Complication	Treatment

Catheter sepsis
Incidence
  Single-lumen catheter: 3–5%
  Triple-lumen catheter: 10%
Diagnosis:
  • Unexplained hyperglycemia (> 160 mg/dL)
  • "Plateau" temperature elevation (> 38°C) for several hours or days. (**Note:** *An isolated spike or "picket fence" temperature pattern is usually not indicative of an infected catheter.*)
  • Leukocytosis (> 10,000/μL)
  • Exclusion of other potential sources of infection,
 	
  or
 	
  • A positive blood culture (> 15 colony count) aspirated via the TPN catheter or obtained peripherally,
 	
  or
 	
  • Catheter site induration, erythema, or purulent drainage.
	Algorithms:
	Negative blood cultures and no cardiovascular signs of sepsis:
	(1) Aspirate a blood specimen via the TPN catheter and peripherally for bacterial and fungal culture and then sterilely exchange the preexisting TPN catheter for a new catheter over a guidewire; submit the previous catheter tip for bacterial and fungal culture and colony count; and continue the TPN infusion.
	
	then
	
	(2) Monitor the patient's temperature closely. If the patient defervesces, no further therapy is necessary. If the fever continues or recurs, remove the catheter and insert a new one on the contralateral side and continue the TPN infusion.
	
	Positive blood culture or cardiovascular signs of sepsis:
	(1) Aspirate a blood specimen via the TPN catheter and peripherally for bacterial and fungal culture. Then remove the catheter immediately, and submit the catheter tip for bacterial and fungal culture and colony count.
	
	then
	
	(2) Insert a new TPN infusion catheter on the contralateral side and continue the TPN infusion.
	
	then
	
	(3) Initiate appropriate antibiotic therapy.

Hyperglycemia (> 160 mg/dL)	**Algorithms:** (1) Maintain the current TPN infusion rate and begin adding regular insulin to the TPN solution in 10-unit increments until the serum glucose is maintained at ≤ 160 mg/dL. (**Note:** *The maximum allowable insulin dosage per liter of TPN is 40 units.*) Until the hyperglycemia is controlled by adding insulin to the TPN solution, simultaneously administer intravenous regular insulin. (**Note:** *One unit of regular insulin results in an approximately 10 mg/dL increase in the serum glucose. The maximum intravenous dose of regular insulin should not exceed 15 units.*) If the serum glucose remains > 160 mg/dL despite the addition of a total of 40 units of regular insulin per liter of TPN and intravenous regular insulin therapy. *then* (2) Maintain the current TPN infusion rate but begin gradually decreasing the final dextrose concentration of the TPN solution. (**Note:** *The lower limit for the final dextrose concentration is 15%.*) In addition, begin adding regular insulin to the TPN solution in 10-unit increments until the serum glucose is maintained at ≤ 160 mg/dL or the maximum allowable insulin dosage (40 units) is reached. Regular insulin should also be simultaneously administered intravenously as in (1) above until the hyperglycemia is controlled by adding insulin to the TPN solution. If the serum glucose remains > 160 mg/dL despite the addition of 40 units of regular insulin per liter of TPN solution, decreasing the final TPN dextrose concentration to 15%, and intravenous regular insulin therapy. *then*

Table 11–11. Complications of TPN. (continued)

Complication	Treatment
	(3) Restart the original TPN solution as in (1) above but begin decreasing the TPN infusion rate. Also begin insulin therapy as discussed in (2) above while simultaneously increasing the frequency of fat emulsion therapy from every Monday, Wednesday and Friday to daily to provide adequate caloric intake.
Hypoglycemia (< 65 mg/dL)	May occur with the sudden discontinuance of TPN infusion. If the TPN infusion administered to either an NPO patient or a patient consuming inadequate oral calories is suddenly discontinued, immediately begin an infusion of D_{10} NS at the previous TPN infusion rate via either the TPN catheter or a peripheral IV to prevent rebound hypoglycemia.
Hypernatremia (> 145 meq/L)	Determine the cause. Hypernatremia secondary to dehydration is treated by administering additional "free water" and providing only the daily maintenance sodium requirements (90–150 meq/L) via the TPN infusion. Hypernatremia secondary to increased sodium intake is treated by reducing or deleting sodium from the TPN solution until the serum sodium ≤ 145 meq/L.
Hyponatremia (< 135 meq/L)	Determine the cause. Hyponatremia secondary to dilution is treated by fluid restriction and by providing only the daily maintenance sodium requirements (90–150 meq/L). Hyponatremia secondary to inadequate sodium intake is treated by increasing the sodium content of the TPN solution until the serum sodium ≥ 135 meq/L. (**Note:** *The maximum sodium content per liter of TPN should not exceed 154 meq.*)
Hyperkalemia (> 5 meq/L)	Immediately discontinue the current TPN infusion containing potassium and begin an infusion of D_{10}NS at the previous TPN infusion rate. Then reorder a new TPN solution without potassium and continue to delete potassium from the TPN solution until the serum potassium ≤ 5 meq/L.
Hypokalemia (< 3.5 meq/L)	A TPN solution should not be utilized for the primary treatment of hypokalemia. The potassium content per liter of TPN solution should not exceed 40 meq. If additional potassium is necessary, it should be administered via another route, eg, IV interrupts.
Hyperphosphatemia (> 4.5 mg/dL)	Immediately discontinue the present phosphate-containing TPN infusion and begin an infusion of D_{10}NS at the previous infusion rate. Then reorder a new TPN solution without phosphate and continue to delete phosphate from the TPN solution until the serum phosphate ≤ 4.5 mg/dL.
Hypophosphatemia (< 2.5 mg/dL)	Increase the phosphate content of the TPN solution to a maximum of 20 mmol/L. (**Note:** *The total daily phosphate dosage should not exceed 60 mmol.*) If severe hypophosphatemia exists, carbohydrate infusion or delivery should be restricted.
Hypermagnesemia (> 3 mg/dL)	Immediately discontinue the present magnesium-containing TPN infusion and begin an infusion of D_{10}NS at the previous infusion rate.
Hypomagnesemia (<1.6 mg/dL)	Increase the magnesium content of the TPN solution to a maximum of 12 meq/L. (**Note:** *The total daily dosage of magnesium should not exceed 36 meq.*)
Hypercalcemia (> 10.5 mg/dL)	Immediately discontinue the present calcium-containing TPN infusion and begin an infusion of D_{10}NS at the previous TPN infusion rate. Then reorder a new TPN solution without calcium and continue to delete calcium from the TPN dilution until the serum calcium ≤ 10.5 mg/dL.
Hypocalcemia (< 8.5 mg/dL)	Increase the calcium content of the TPN solution to a maximum of 9 meq/L. (**Note:** *The total daily calcium dosage should not exceed 27 meq.*)
High serum zinc (> 150 µg/L)	Discontinue the trace metal supplement (Multitrace 5 mL) in the TPN solution until the serum zinc ≤ 150 µg/L.
Low serum zinc (< 55 µg/dL)	Add elemental zinc 2–5 mg daily to 1 L of TPN solution only until the serum zinc ≥ 55 µg/dL. (**Note:** *The elemental zinc is added in addition to the daily supplement.*)

(continued)

Table 11–11. Complications of TPN. (continued)

Complication	Treatment
High serum copper (> 140 µg/dL)	Discontinue the trace metal supplement in the TPN solution until the serum copper ≤ 140 µg/dL.
Low serum copper (< 70 µg/dL)	Add elemental copper 2–5 mg daily to 1 L of TPN solution only until the serum copper ≥ 70 µg/dL. (***Note:*** *The elemental copper is added in addition to the daily Multitrace 5 mL.*)
Hyperchloremic metabolic acidosis (CO_2 < 22 mmol/L and Cl^- > 110 meq/L)	Reduce the chloride intake by administering the Na^+ and K^+ in the acetate form as either sodium or potassium acetate (or both) until the acidosis resolves (serum CO_2 ≥ 22 mmol/L) and the serum chloride level returns to normal (< 110 meq/L).

The recommended tapering schedule for a patient with no oral nutrient intake (NPO) who is receiving TPN at an infusion rate of 125 mL/h is as follows: Start an infusion of $D_{10}NS$ at 40 mL/h via pump into a peripheral vein. Then proceed as follows: (1) Decrease the TPN infusion rate to 80 mL/h and continue the $D_{10}NS$ at 40 mL/h for 2 hours; (2) then decrease the TPN infusion rate to 40 mL/h and increase the $D_{10}NS$ infusion rate to 80 mL/h for 2 hours; and (3) discontinue the TPN infusion and increase the $D_{10}NS$ infusion rate to 125 mL/h. Once the TPN infusion is discontinued, the central catheter can be used to infuse the $D_{10}NS$ (peripheral intravenous catheter is removed or preserved with a heparin lock).

The TPN infusion rate does not need to be tapered if the patient has adequate oral nutrient intake.

Harris WS et al: Cardioprotective effects of omega-3 fatty acids. Nutr Clin Pract 2001;16:6.

Maxfield D et al: Effect or oral glutamine supplementation during bone marrow transplantation. JPEN J Parenter Enteral Nutr 2000;24:61.

Nagel M: Nutrition screening: identifying patients at risk for malnutrition. Nutr Clin Pract 1998;8:171.

Nakamura K et al: Influence of preoperative nutritional state on inflammatory response after surgery. Nutrition 1999;15:834.

Seidner DL et al: Parenteral nutrition-associated metabolic bone disease: pathophysiology, evaluation and treatment. Nutr Clin Pract 2000;15:163.

Van Acker BA et al: Response of glutamine metabolism to glutamine-supplemented parenteral nutrition. Am J Clin Nutr 2000;72:79.

The Veterans Affairs Total Parenteral Nutrition Cooperative Study Group: Perioperative total parenteral nutrition in surgical patients. N Engl J Med 1991;325:527.

Wanten GJ et al: Phagocytosis and killing of *Candida albicans* by human neutrophils after exposure to structurally different lipid emulsions. JPEN J Parenter Enteral Nutr 2001;25:9.

Weinsier RI et al: Hospital malnutrition: a prospective evaluation of general medical patients during the course of hospitalization. Am J Clin Nutr 1979;32:418.

DIETS

Optimal Diet

An optimal diet should have the following distribution of energy sources: carbohydrate 55–60%, fat 30%, protein 10–15%. Refined sugar should constitute no more than 15% of dietary energy and saturated fats no more

Trendelenburg position
Left lateral decubitus
Syringe aspiration

Figure 11–9. Durant position for treatment of air embolism than 10%, the latter balanced by 10% monounsaturated and 10% polyunsaturated fats. Cholesterol intake should be limited to about 300 mg/d (one egg yolk contains 250 mg of cholesterol). The amount of salt in the average American diet, 10–18 g, far exceeds the recommended 3 g. For Western societies to meet the criteria for an optimal diet, consumption of fat would have to decrease (from 40%) and carbohydrate (principally complex carbohydrates such as potatoes and whole grain bread) would have to increase. As a source of protein, meat is presently overemphasized at the expense of grain, legumes, and nuts. Diets that chronically include substantial fish intake have been associated with a decrease in numbers of deaths from cardiovascular disease. The active ingredient is ω-3 fatty acids, principally eicosapentaenoic and docosahexaenoic acids.

Many adults, particularly those who drink no milk, consume inadequate amounts of calcium. In women this may result in calcium deficiency and skeletal calcium depletion, which in later years predispose to osteoporosis and possibly fractures (eg, of the hip or vertebrae).

The amount of fiber in Western diets averages 25 g/d, but some persons ingest as little as 10 g/d. Fiber is a chemically complex group of indigestible carbohydrate polymers, which includes cellulose, hemicellulose, lignins, pectins, gums, and mucilages. It is thought that people who consume low-fiber diets are more prone to the development of chronic constipation, appendicitis, diverticular disease, diabetes mellitus, colonic neoplasms, and irritable bowel syndrome. Thus, increased fiber intake would probably be beneficial, though the evidence for this is not conclusive. Fiber can be obtained in the form of bran in cereals and bread. It can also be obtained from fruit, potatoes, rice, and leafy vegetables.

Many therapeutic diets are archaic and based on currently unaccepted concepts of illness. For example, low-residue diets are no longer considered to be useful for diverticulitis. The "progressive diet," designed for postoperative feeding and consisting of a clear liquid (high in sodium), then a full liquid (high in sucrose), then a regular diet, is based on outmoded concepts. When peristalsis returns after operation, as evidenced by bowel sounds and ability to tolerate water, most patients are able to ingest a regular diet. The following paragraphs describe briefly the therapeutic diets most commonly prescribed in clinical practice.

Regular Diets

Regular diets have an unrestricted spectrum of foods and are most attractive to the patient. An average regular hospital diet for 1 day contains 230–275 g of carbohydrate, 70–75 g of fat, and 95–110 g of protein, with a total caloric content of 2000–2500 kcal. This composition reflects the nutritional needs of healthy persons of average height and weight and will not meet the increased demands imposed by malnutrition or disease.

Lactose Intolerance & Lactose-Free Diets

A lactose-free diet is indicated for patients who have symptoms such as diarrhea, bloating, or flatulence after the ingestion of milk or milk products. Lactose intolerance is genetically determined and in adults is found in 5–10% of European Caucasians, 60% of Ashkenazic Jews, and 70% of blacks. A previously subclinical lactose intolerance commonly becomes unmasked by an unrelated disease or operation on the gastrointestinal tract. For example, following gastrectomy, symptomatic relief from nonspecific complaints may be obtained by interdicting lactose-containing foods. Similar advice is often useful in managing patients with Crohn's disease, ulcerative colitis, and AIDS. The frequency of lactose intolerance is high enough in the general population that it should be considered as a possible cause of flatulence and diarrhea in many clinical circumstances. The efficiency of lactose digestion and absorption can be measured by giving 100 g of lactose orally and measuring the blood lactose concentration at 30-minute intervals for 2 hours. Patients with lactose intolerance exhibit a rise in blood glucose of 20 mg/dL or less. However, unpredictable variations in gastric emptying interfere with the reliability of this test, so in most cases it is better to observe the results of eliminating lactose from the diet than to perform a lactose tolerance test. A lactose-free diet may be deficient in Ca^{2+}, vitamin D, and riboflavin.

DISEASE-SPECIFIC NUTRITION SUPPORT

Burns

Thermal injury has a tremendous impact on metabolism because of prolonged, intense neuroendocrine stimulation. Extensive burns raise the REE 100–200% above baseline and urinary nitrogen excretion to 30–40 g/d, equivalent to a loss of 1500 g/d of lean tissue and a median survival of 7–10 days without nutritional support. The increase in metabolic demands following thermal injury is proportionate to the extent of ungrafted body surface. The principal mediator of burn hypermetabolism is elevated levels of catecholamines, which return to baseline only when skin coverage is complete. Decreasing the intensity of neuroendocrine stimulation by providing analgesia and thermoneutral environments lowers the accelerated metabolic rate in many of these patients and helps to decrease catabolic protein loss until the burned surface can be grafted.

Burned patients are also prone to infection, and cytokines activated by sepsis augment catabolism. The keratinized layer of skin contains large amounts of interleukin-1, which are released during thermal injury, and cytokine activity may be an important stimulus of burn catabolism.

Because infection so often complicates TPN therapy in burn patients, enteral nutrition is preferred whenever tolerated. Aggressive enteral feeding should be started within the first 6–12 hours postburn to reduce the hypermetabolic response and improve postburn survival. Gastric ileus is not a problem if the tip of the nasointestinal feeding tube is passed into the duodenum.

Burn patients have increased caloric requirements (Table 11–12). In addition to maintenance needs (females, 22 kcal/kg/d; males, 25 kcal/kg/d), they require an additional 40 kcal per percent of total body surface area burned, and these patients often require 40–60 kcal per kg body weight. During the hypermetabolic phase of burn injury (0–14 days), the ability to metabolize fat is restricted, so a diet that derives calories primarily from carbohydrate is preferable. Following the hypermetabolic phase, the metabolism of fat becomes normal. The burn patient should also be given supplemental arginine, nucleotides, and ω-3 polyunsaturated fat to maintain and stimulate immunocompetence.

Table 11–12. Daily caloric and protein requirements for burn patients.

Estimated:
  Calories (total kcal) (male or female)
    Maintenance + 40 kcal per % TBSA[1] burned
  Protein (g) (male or female)
    1.5–2.5/kg
Calculated:
  Calories (total kcal) for weight maintenance
    Male = (25 kcal × preburn wt kg × BMR[2] age factor) + (40 kcal × % TBSA[1])
    Female = (22 kcal × preburn wt kg × BMR[2] age factor) + (40 kcal × % TBSA[1])
    Note: Add 500 kcal to the above equations for weight gain.
  Protein (g)
    Male or female = (1 g protein × preburn wt kg) + (3 × % TBSA[1] burn)

---

[1]TBSA = Total body surface area.
[2]BMR = Basal metabolic rate:
  20–40 yr = 1.00
  40–50 yr = 0.95
  50–75 yr = 0.90
  > 75 yr = 0.80

Cancer

Annually in every country, cancer will account for one of the leading diagnoses and causes of death in adult patients. Over two-thirds of patients with cancer will develop nutritional depletion and weight loss at some time during the course of the illness, and protein-calorie malnutrition in patients presenting with cancer has been estimated to be as high as 48%. Malnutrition and its sequelae are directly related to the cause of death in 20–40% of these patients. The effects of cancer and its treatment comprise a significant portion of the budget of any nation—not only in direct medical costs but also in loss of productivity, treatment of morbidity, and support of terminally ill patients. Length of stay is nearly two to three times as long for patients with cancer who are admitted with dehydration and malnutrition. Weight loss alone predicts a poor prognosis in many malignancies.

Nutrition support has become an essential adjunct in caring for the cancer patient. Many studies have evaluated the effectiveness of nutrition support in patients with cancer, with varying results. Klein reported a meta-analysis of 28 prospective, randomized, controlled clinical trials evaluating TPN in patients with cancer. Only one of ten surgical trials showed a significant decrease in mortality in the patients receiving TPN, and no other significant benefit was seen in survival, tolerance to treatment, toxicity, or tumor response in patients receiving chemotherapy or radiation therapy. Increasing efforts have been directed to using enteral nutrition because it is simpler, presumably safer, and less costly. Seven prospective controlled randomized trials of enteral nutrition in patients with cancer undergoing surgery showed little if any difference in mortality or morbidity in patients who received enteral feedings.

Patients with cancer may have decreased energy expenditure and abnormalities of protein and carbohydrate metabolism. REE increases by 20–30% in certain malignant tumors yet in the absence of other disease neuroendocrine activity is normal. The increase in REE can occur even in patients with extreme cachexia in whom a similar degree of uncomplicated starvation would produce a profound decrease in REE. Whether or not the increase in REE is proportionate to the extent of disease and the volume of tumor is unsettled.

Patients with cancer avidly retain nitrogen despite losses in most lean tissue. Animal carcass analysis has shown that the retained nitrogen resides in the tumor, which behaves as a nitrogen trap. Synthesis, catabolism, and turnover of body protein are all increased, but the change in catabolism is greatest.

The changes in carbohydrate metabolism consist of impaired glucose tolerance, elevated glucose turnover rates, enhanced Cori cycle activity, and gluconeogenesis from alanine. Owing to the high rate of anaerobic glucose metabolism in neoplastic tissue, patients with extensive tumors are susceptible to lactic acidosis when given large glucose loads during TPN.

More recently, efforts have been directed to identification of the biochemical mechanism of cancer cachexia and to examination of the effects of immune modulation in patients with cancer and route of feeding as a possible immunomodulating tool. While TPN became the mainstay of nutritional therapy in the last decade, eventual awareness of the morbidity associated with mechanical and septic complications—as well as of the immune dysfunction associated with TPN—led to its falling into disfavor. However, many studies of TPN use in patients with cancer were poorly designed and evaluated a heterogeneous population, with marked variations in the degree of malnutrition and the treatments used. A number of studies support the use of enteral nutrition to maintain gastrointestinal mucosal integrity, enhance IgA production, maintain systemic immunity, and reduce the cost of therapy.

Glutamine metabolism in the cancer model has been extensively studied. Just as glutamine is the primary fuel for the intestinal cell, it is also a primary fuel for many tumors. Progressive tumor growth is associated with significant changes in glutamine metabolism. As the cancer progresses, total body glutamine is depleted. Glutamine transport from muscle is increased, but intestinal utilization of glutamine decreases. The tumor continually competes with the host for glutamine. As the tumor grows, the muscle responds to glutamine depletion by increasing glutamine synthetase activity and increasing glutamine transport. As glutamine uptake by the intestine decreases, this may have deleterious effects on the gut mucosal barrier and gastrointestinal immune function.

Investigators have attempted to use tumor dependence on glutamine to develop glutamine analogs that will function as antineoplastic agents. Unfortunately, the toxicity of these agents has prevented their clinical application clinical. Some investigators have demonstrated protection from intestinal damage and toxicity from whole body radiation therapy with the use of enteral formula supplemented with glutamine. Others have shown protective effects and improved response to chemotherapy with glutamine-supplemented nutrition. Some of the most impressive work demonstrating the protective effects of glutamine has been with bone marrow transplant recipients, in whom glutamine-supplemented TPN is associated with improved nitrogen balance, decreased length of hospital stay, and reduced cost of hospitalization.

Caution should be used, however, in recommending glutamine supplementation for all cancer patients. Glutamine promotes intestinal mucosa turnover, integrity, and growth and therefore may not be an ideal substrate in patients with intestinal or colonic tumors. One study demonstrated increased colon cancer cell proliferation, decreased cell differentiation, and decreased cellular adhesion with glutamine supplementation. Further work needs to be done in various oncology populations before final recommendations can be made.

Many studies have used diets with combinations of various substrates (glutamine, arginine, ω-3 fatty acids, RNA) to alter outcome with varying results. Despite the conflicting information, many studies suggest that supplemented diets alter the immune response and may reduce morbidity and length of stay in some patients with cancer. Further studies examining the effects of particular substrates need to be done before the routine use of supplemented formulas should be recommended for all patients with cancer.

Renal Failure

Whether nutritional support improves the outcome of acute renal failure is difficult to determine because the metabolism of renal failure is so complex.

Patients with acute renal failure can have a normal or increased metabolic rate. Renal failure precipitated by x-ray contrast agents, antibiotics, aortic or cardiac surgery, or moderate periods of hypotension is associated with a normal or slightly elevated REE and a moderately negative nitrogen balance (4–8 g/d). When renal failure follows severe trauma, rhabdomyolysis, or sepsis, the REE may be markedly increased and the nitrogen balance sharply negative (15–25 g/d). When dialysis is frequent, losses into the dialysate of amino acids, vitamins, glucose, trace metals, and lipotrophic factors can be substantial.

The method of measuring nitrogen balance in renal failure is presented in Table 11–13. Nitrogen output is calculated from the urea nitrogen appearance (UNA) and the application of a correction factor for nitrogen

Table 11–13. Calculation of nitrogen balance in renal failure.

Nitrogen balance (g/d) = Nitrogen intake – Nitrogen output
Nitrogen output (g/d) = (0.97) (UNA) + 1.93
UNA (g/d) = Urine urea nitrogen + Dialysate urea nitrogen[1] + Change in body urea nitrogen
Change in body urea nitrogen = $(BUN_f - BUN_i) (BW_i)^2 (0.6)^3 + (BW_f - BW_i) (BUN_i)^4$

[1]UNA (urea nitrogen appearance) is determined between dialysis runs, so this term can be dropped in final calculations.
[2]BW = body weight.
[3]0.6 = the volume of distribution of urea.
[4]f= final; i = initial.

loss in stool, skin, and feces. The UNA is the difference in BUN levels between dialysis intervals multiplied by a factor for the volume of distribution of urea in total body water plus the change in weight (assuming weight change is due entirely to water).

Patients in renal failure (serum creatinine > 2 mg/dL) with a normal metabolic rate (UNA 4–8 g/d) who cannot undergo dialysis should receive a concentrated (maximum calories and protein per milliliter of diet) enteral or parenteral diet containing just the essential amino acids (EAAs), dextrose, and limited amounts of sodium, potassium, magnesium, and phosphate.

In contrast, patients with a normal metabolic rate who can undergo dialysis should receive a concentrated enteral or parenteral diet that contains a combination of EAAs and nonessential amino acids (NEAAs), dextrose, and limited amounts of sodium, potassium, phosphate, and magnesium.

Hepatic Failure

Most patients with hepatic failure present with acute decompensation superimposed on chronic hepatic insufficiency. Liver disease or poor diet has usually contributed to depletion of protein, vitamins, and trace elements. Total body protein is often diminished because of poor dietary habits (eg, in alcoholics) or iatrogenic protein restriction intended to control encephalopathy. Water-soluble vitamins, including folate, ascorbic acid, niacin, thiamin, and riboflavin, are especially likely to be deficient. Fat-soluble vitamin deficiency may be a result of malabsorption due to bile acid insufficiency (vitamins A, D, K, and E), deficient storage (vitamin A), inefficient utilization (vitamin K), or failure of conversion to active metabolites (vitamin D). Hepatic iron stores may be depleted either from poor intake or as a result of gastrointestinal blood loss. Total body zinc is decreased owing to the above factors plus increased urinary excretion.

The contribution of amino acid abnormalities to hepatic encephalopathy is discussed in Chapter 25.

The use of BCAA-enriched amino acid formulations for TPN in patients with liver disease is controversial because the results of controlled trials are inconclusive. Patients without clinical signs of encephalopathy should receive a concentrated enteral or parenteral diet that has a reduced carbohydrate content, a combination of EEAs and NEAAs, and limited amounts of sodium and potassium. In contrast, patients with clinical signs of encephalopathy should receive a concentrated enteral or parenteral diet that has a reduced carbohydrate content, only branched-chain amino acids, and limited amounts of sodium and potassium.

Hepatorenal Failure

Hepatorenal failure patients who cannot undergo dialysis and have clinical signs of encephalopathy should receive a concentrated enteral or parenteral diet that has a reduced carbohydrate content, only BCAAs, and limited amounts of sodium, potassium, magnesium, and phosphate.

Cardiac Disease

Myocardial dysfunction may complicate malnutrition, especially in the late stages, and fatal cardiac failure can develop in extreme cachexia.

Cardiac muscle uses FFAs and BCAAs as preferred metabolic fuels instead of glucose. During starvation, the heart rate slows, cardiac size decreases, and the stroke volume and cardiac output fall. As starvation progresses, cardiac failure ensues, along with chamber enlargement and anasarca.

The profound nutritional depletion that may accompany chronic heart failure—particularly in valvular disease—is the result of anorexia from chronic disease and passive congestion of the liver; malabsorption due to venous engorgement of the small bowel mucosa; and enhanced peripheral proteolysis due to chronic neuroendocrine secretion.

Attempts at aggressive nutritional repletion in patients with cardiac cachexia—before or after operation—have produced inconclusive results. Concentrated dextrose (eg, 35% rather than 25%) and 7.5% amino acid preparations should be used to avoid fluid overload. Nitrogen balance should be measured to ensure adequate nitrogen intake. Lipid emulsions should be administered cautiously because they can produce myocardial ischemia and negative inotropy.

Gastrointestinal Disease

Gastrointestinal disease (eg, inflammatory bowel disease, fistula, pancreatitis) often presents nutritional problems due to intestinal obstruction, malabsorption, or anorexia. In each situation, the patient would benefit from nutritional therapy.

Chronic involvement of the ileum in inflammatory bowel disease leads to malabsorption of fat-soluble and water-soluble vitamins, calcium and magnesium, anions (phosphate), and the trace elements iron, zinc, chromium, and selenium. Protein-losing enteropathy, accentuated by transmural destruction of lymphatics, can add to protein depletion. The REE is increased by 25–30%, which prevents the adaptive hypometabolism of chronic starvation and causes a negative caloric balance. Treatment with sulfasalazine can produce folate deficiency, and glucocorticoid administration may accelerate breakdown of lean tissue and enhance glucose intolerance owing to stimulation of gluconeogenesis. Patients with inflammatory bowel disease who require elective surgery should be evaluated, and those with a recent loss of 10% of body weight should be given nutritional therapy preoperatively.

Parenteral nutrition therapy for 4–6 weeks combined with bowel rest, metronidazole, and sulfasalazine is the treatment of choice for patients with acute exacerbations of inflammatory bowel disease without bowel obstruction or perforation. Patients who fail to respond to medical therapy or develop intestinal obstruction or perforation require operation and postoperative parenteral diet therapy.

Patients with gastrointestinal fistulas can develop electrolyte, protein, fat, vitamin, and trace metal deficiencies; dehydration; and acid-base imbalance. They require fluid replacement and aggressive nutritional therapy.

Antidiarrheal agents usually fail to reduce fluid losses from enterocutaneous fistulas, but octreotide acetate, a synthetic octapeptide analog of somatostatin, is more effective. Octreotide suppresses the secretion of serotonin, vasoactive intestinal polypeptide, gastrin, insulin, glucagon, growth hormone, secretin, and pancreatic polypeptides and exerts widespread effects on gastrointestinal function. It prolongs intestinal transit, regulates intestinal water and electrolyte transport, and decreases splanchnic blood flow. In a dose of 50–300 μg every 6 hours (intravenously or subcutaneously), it is quite useful in the management of high-output fistulas.

Patients with fistulas also require nutritional therapy, which differs depending on the level of bowel involved. Patients with a proximal enterocutaneous fistula (ie, from the stomach to the mid ileum) should receive TPN with no oral intake. Patients with a low enterocutaneous fistula (ie, distal ileum or colon) should receive TPN initially, but after infection is brought under control they can often be switched to an enteral formula or even a low-residue diet. The management of enterocutaneous fistulas is discussed further in Chapter 30.

Short Bowel Syndrome

Short bowel syndrome is defined as malabsorption resulting from extensive small intestinal resection. Excessive water loss, electrolyte losses, and malnutrition result. There is a large reserve capacity in the small intestine such that resection of up to half of the small bowel is reasonably well tolerated. Typically, short bowel syndrome is defined as less than 200 cm of anatomic small bowel remnant. However, short bowel syndrome may also result from functional abnormality of the small bowel resulting from severe inflammation or motility disorder.

The optimal nutritional therapy for a patient with short bowel syndrome must be tailored individually and depends upon the underlying disease process and the remaining anatomy. Short bowel syndrome patients can be divided into three groups according to their particular needs: (1) those who require nutritional supplements to remain in good health; (2) those who need parenteral supplements of fluid and electrolytes but can maintain satisfactory nutritional status with ordinary food; and (3) those who require parenteral fluid, electrolytes, and nutrition.

The goals of therapy, in the short term include stabilization of fluids, electrolytes, vitamins (thiamin), and minerals (magnesium). The long-term aim of nutritional management in patients with short bowel syndrome is to provide a good quality of life with the minimum medical interventions necessary to prevent thirst and malnutrition. The nutrition support necessary for a patient with short bowel syndrome is a dynamic process, and changes in requirements can be expected in the early phases.

Pancreatic Disease

Patients with acute pancreatitis who present with fewer than three Ranson criteria (see Chapter 27) should be treated with fluid replacement, nasogastric suction, and bowel rest for at least a week before considering parenteral nutrition. Most of these patients can resume an oral diet and do not benefit from TPN. Patients with more than three Ranson criteria should receive TPN. Enteral diets, including elemental and polypeptide formulas, are not recommended because they stimulate the pancreas and may aggravate the disease.

AIDS

Patients with AIDS develop protein-calorie malnutrition and lose weight. Many factors contribute to deficiencies of electrolytes (sodium and potassium), trace metals (copper, zinc, and selenium), and vitamins (A, C, E, pyridoxine, and folate). Dehydration occurs as a consequence of refractory diarrhea.

Enteropathy may impair fluid and nutrient absorption and produce a voluminous life-threatening diarrhea. Standard antidiarrheal agents do not control the diarrhea in AIDS patients, but octreotide often helps.

Malnourished AIDS patients require 35–40 kcal and 2–2.5 g protein/kg/d. In addition to the required electrolytes, vitamins, and minerals, they should receive glutamine, arginine, nucleotides, ω-3 polyunsaturated fats, branched-chain amino acids, and trace metal supplements. Those with normal gut function should be given a high-protein, high-calorie, low-fat, lactose-free oral diet. Patients with compromised gut function require an enteral (amino acid or polypeptide) diet or TPN.

Obesity

Massively obese patients—those who weigh more than twice the calculated ideal weight—are handicapped physically, emotionally, socially, and economically. This degree of excessive weight has been termed morbid obesity to emphasize the life-threatening seriousness of the condition. Complications such as arthritis, hypertension, diabetes mellitus, hyperlipidemia, and Pickwickian syndrome may develop. The death rate is greater for morbidly obese people than for people of average weight.

Obesity is quantified according to the body mass index (BMI), which is calculated as follows:

$$BMI = \frac{\text{Weight (kg)}}{\text{Height (m)}^2}$$

The average BMI in our society is 25; 28 is considered the threshold for obesity.

The standard approach to therapy for obesity begins with reducing diets and medical counseling. Unfortunately, these measures are almost uniformly unsuccessful in patients with severe obesity. Weight loss is usually disappointing, and in the 5–10% of cases where a large amount of weight is lost on a rigid dieting program, it is almost always regained quickly. Surgical therapy is acceptable for patients whose BMI exceeds 40 if they strongly desire surgery in order to improve the quality of their lives. Surgery may be appropriate also for patients with a BMI between 30 and 40 in order to improve serious comorbid conditions such as severe sleep apnea or obesity-related cardiomyopathy.

The first operation for obesity that gained widespread acceptance was jejunoileal bypass, in which the jejunum was transected 14 inches from the ligament of Treitz and anastomosed to the terminal ileum 4 inches from the ileocecal valve. Weight loss resulted from malabsorption due to the shortened bowel and from decreased food intake. However, late follow-up demonstrated an unacceptable rate of serious metabolic complications. Protein deficiency occurred in about 25% of patients, sometimes causing liver disease that occasionally progressed to hepatic cirrhosis. Renal stones were very common. Consequently, jejunoileal bypass is now rarely used. Patients suffering from late complications of a jejunoileal bypass should have the bypassed intestine put back into continuity. A concomitant gastric bypass is necessary if weight loss from the earlier procedure is to be maintained.

Alverdy J: Effect of nutrition on gastrointestinal barrier function. Semin Respir Infect 1994;9:248.

Bozzetti F et al: Perioperative total parenteral nutrition in malnourished gastrointestinal cancer patients: a randomized, clinical trial. JPEN J Parenter Enteral Nutr 2000;24:7.

Byrne TA et al: Beyond the prescription: optimizing the diet of patients with short bowel syndrome. Nutr Clin Pract 2000; 15:306.

Clark RH et al: Nutritional treatment for acquired immunodeficiency virus-associated wasting using beta-hydroxy beta-methylbutyrate, glutamine, and arginine: a randomized, double-blind, placebo-controlled study. JPEN J Parenter Enteral Nutr 2000;24:133.

Curreri PW et al: Dietary requirements of patients with major burns. Nutr Clin Pract 2001;16:169.

Fischer JE: Branched-chain-enriched amino acid solutions in patients with -liver failure. JPEN J Parenter Enteral Nutr 1990; 14(Suppl):226.

Klein S et al: Nutrition support in patients with cancer: what do the data really show? Nutr Clin Pract 1994;9:91.

Martindale RG et al: Use of immune-enhancing diets in burns. JPEN J Parenter Enteral Nutr 2001;25:524.

Moore FA: Effects of immune-enhancing diets on infectious morbidity and multiple organ failure. JPEN J Parenter Enteral Nutr 2001;25:536.

Anesthesia

Ronald D. Miller, MD

Anesthesiology is concerned not only with the administration of anesthesia for surgery but also with many other areas of patient care, including critical care medicine, management of chronic pain, and respiratory therapy. In this chapter, the discussion will be limited to anesthesia during surgery and the overall perioperative period.

The development of anesthesia represents one of the most interesting aspects of United States medical history. In 1842, Crawford Long was the first physician to administer diethyl ether by inhalation to produce surgical anesthesia, but his work went largely unrecognized. In 1846, a dentist, William Morton, administered diethyl ether for the removal of a submandibular tumor by surgeon John Warren. This event took place at the Massachusetts General Hospital before an audience of surgeons, medical students, and a newspaper reporter and was therefore well publicized. Another dentist, Horace Wells, allowed nitrous oxide to be administered to him by Gardner Colton, a showman, while a fellow dentist performed a painless tooth extraction. Unfortunately, Wells failed to appreciate the marginal potency of nitrous oxide and was unable to reproduce surgical anesthesia during a demonstration at the Massachusetts General Hospital. Between 1844 and 1886, nitrous oxide continued to be used by showmen who staged public displays of the exhilarating effects of the gas. Diethyl ether was often used for similar purposes. Since then, many techniques for general anesthesia have been developed and improved upon.

In the late 19th century, within a year after Karl Koller, a Viennese surgeon, discovered the topical anesthetic properties of cocaine, William Halsted, of Johns Hopkins University, gave the drug by injection for the production of peripheral nerve block. In 1898, after a trial on himself that led to the first-described lumbar puncture headache, August Bier, in Germany, administered the first spinal anesthetic. In the years that followed, the development of local anesthetics with different durations of action led to the widespread use of regional anesthesia.

Kitz RJ, Vandam LD: A history and the scope of anesthetic practice. In: *Anesthesia*, 5th ed. Miller RD (editor). Churchill Livingstone, 1990.

OVERALL ANESTHETIC RISK

Anecdotal reports of anesthetic mishaps are difficult to evaluate, partly because morbidity and mortality resulting from problems related to the anesthesia itself are difficult to distinguish from those due to the surgical procedure. Yet, in an age of increasing assessment and accountability, data bases are being analyzed to determine the benefit and hazards of surgery in general and anesthesia specifically. Anesthetic-related deaths have decreased dramatically in the past 2 decades and are now rare. The Institute of Medicine's analysis of medical errors recently complimented anesthesia for its marked decrease in morbidity and mortality.

Nevertheless, anesthesiologists worry about issues regarding difficult airway management, neurologic deficits, patients with coronary artery disease, giving anesthesia in remote locations (eg, offices and radiology laboratories), and inadequate times for preoperative evaluation.

Despite these problems, with proper care, the overall anesthetic risk is extremely low, leading one writer to state that "perhaps the most insidious hazard of anesthesia is its relative safety."

Stoelting R: Results of APSF survey regarding anesthesia patient safety issues. Anesthesic Patient Safety Foundation Newsletter 1999;13:6.

Voelker R: Anesthesia-related risks have plummeted. JAMA 1995; 275:445.

PREOPERATIVE PROCEDURES ASSOCIATED WITH ANESTHESIA

Preoperative Evaluation for Anesthetic Risk

Anesthetic risk is difficult to ascertain precisely in most cases. Perioperative complications and deaths are frequently caused by a combination of factors, including concurrent disease, complexity of the operation, and adverse effects of anesthesia. A few complications are due entirely to anesthesia, such as aspiration pneumonitis and hypoxemia due to failure to maintain a patent airway. While many classifications exist, the patient's physical status according to the criteria given in Table 12–1 is the most widely known. This classification system was not specifically designed to estimate anesthetic risk but does provide a "common language" of evaluation for use by different institutions.

A. Method and Site of Evaluations

Historically, patients were evaluated the night before surgery in the hospital. That approach has mostly been abandoned because most patients (even for complicated surgery) enter the hospital the morning of surgery. Low-risk patients are interviewed by telephone, while higher-risk patients may be evaluated in a preoperative evaluation clinic one or more days preoperatively. The end result is that the anesthesiologist who will be delivering the anesthetic will actually meet the patient in person for the first time 1 hour or less before surgery. This places tremendous emphasis on the adequacy of the telephone and clinic visits to make certain that patients are adequately prepared for anesthesia and surgery.

B. History and Physical Examination

The history should include a review of the patient's previous experiences with anesthesia, and data should be elicited regarding any allergic reactions, delayed awakening, prolonged paralysis from neuromuscular blocking agents, and jaundice. The presence and severity of any concurrent diseases (eg, hepatitis), coagulopathies,

Table 12–1. Physical status classification of the American Society of Anesthesiologists.

Class	Physical Status
1	Patient has no organic, physiologic, biochemical, or psychiatric disturbance.
2	Patient has mild to moderate systemic disturbances that may or may not be related to the disorder requiring surgery (eg, essential hypertension, diabetes mellitus).
3	Patient has severe systemic disturbances that may or may not be related to the disorder requiring surgery (eg, heart disease that limits activity, poorly controlled essential hypertension).
4	Patient has severe systemic disturbance that is life-threatening with or without surgery (eg, congestive heart failure, persistent angina pectoris).
5	Patient is moribund and has little chance for survival, but surgery is to be performed as a last resort (resuscitative effort) (eg, uncontrolled hemorrhage, as from a ruptured abdominal aneurysm).
E	Patient requires emergency operation.

endocrine abnormalities (eg, diabetes mellitus), or cardiorespiratory dysfunction should be noted.

The physical examination should focus on the cardiovascular system, lungs, and upper airway. It should include measurements of heart rate and of arterial blood pressure obtained in both the supine and standing positions and auscultation for cardiac murmurs, carotid artery bruits, or abnormal breathing. If abnormalities are found, additional tests (electrocardiography, pulmonary function tests, etc) may be indicated. The airway, head, and neck should be examined for factors that could make endotracheal intubation difficult, eg, fat or short neck, limited temporomandibular mobility. Since over 50% of all anesthetic-induced morbidity and mortality is related to inability to maintain the airway, examination of the airway demands special emphasis. The most common scoring of the airway as a prediction of difficult endotracheal intubation is the "Mallampati classification." When the patient's uvula is visible with the mouth open, the score is grade I (easy intubation); in contrast, grade IV exists when the hard palate is visible but not the soft palate. Grade IV suggests a technically difficult endotracheal intubation.

Peripheral venous sites, including the external jugular vein, should also be checked. If regional anesthesia is planned, the proposed site of injection should be examined for abnormalities and signs of infection, and a limited neurologic examination should be performed.

C. Evaluation of Concurrent Drug Therapy

Concurrent drug therapy must be reviewed, since many drugs can interact with anesthetic drugs (Table 12–2). For example, acute cocaine intoxication can increase anesthetic requirements; long-term use of an antihypertensive drug can reduce anesthetic requirements; and ethanol use can either increase (long-term use) or decrease (acute intoxication) the requirements. Smoking and alcohol are well-known factors influencing anesthetic requirement and the postoperative outcome. Antiarrhythmics, local anesthetics, and especially antibi-

Table 12–2. Mechanisms by which drugs may influence effects of anesthesia.

Anesthetic requirements may be increased or decreased.
Neuromuscular blockade from muscle relaxants may be enhanced.
Cardiovascular response to sympathomimetics and anesthetics may be exaggerated.
Peripheral sympathetic nervous system activity may be reduced, and cardiovascular depressant reactions to anesthetics may be augmented.
Metabolism may be enhanced or impaired.

otics may enhance the neuromuscular blockade from neuromuscular blocking drugs. Tricyclic antidepressants exaggerate the sympathomimetic response of many vasopressors, but antihypertensive and antiarrhythmic drugs can decrease peripheral sympathetic activity and augment the depressant effect of anesthetics. Patients whose hypertension is being treated with angiotensin receptor antagonists seem to have more trouble with hypotension intraoperatively. Current practice is to continue most pharmacologic therapy until the evening before surgery and to anticipate the need for less anesthetic agent, including monoamine oxidase inhibitors. Barbiturates can enhance the metabolism of anesthetic drugs and thereby increase the possibility of a toxic reaction. Echothiophate may prolong the response to certain neuromuscular blocking drugs. Obviously, the safety of continuing drug therapy depends on awareness of potential drug interactions.

D. LABORATORY TESTS

In the past, hospital rules mandated that a large battery of screening laboratory tests be given prior to anesthesia; however, many of these tests have been found to be unnecessary, and the advisability of others has been questioned. For example, one common rule is that elective surgery should not be performed if the hemoglobin concentration is less than 10 g/dL. There is no evidence, however, that correction of normovolemic anemia decreases perioperative morbidity and mortality rates. More important is the need to determine why the patient is anemic. Administering blood preoperatively in an effort to increase the hemoglobin concentration above 10 g/dL is of questionable medical benefit and exposes the patient to the risks of allogeneic blood.

The history and physical examination are the most valuable guides for determining which laboratory tests are necessary (eg, a long history of smoking dictates a thorough examination of pulmonary status by means of pulmonary function tests). Men aged 40 years or younger with no history of problems with anesthesia and normal findings on physical examination usually require no laboratory tests; women of this age and health status usually require only hemoglobin measurements.

Questionnaires are a useful means of identifying patients likely to have complications who would therefore benefit from preoperative laboratory testing. This is especially important with increasing emphasis on same-day surgery. Blue Cross/Blue Shield estimates that several billion dollars a year are wasted in the USA on unnecessary preoperative tests and subsequent evaluation of trivial abnormal results. Excessive testing can even be hazardous, because borderline abnormalities may lead to additional—sometimes invasive—tests or therapy. An example is potassium treatment for borderline low potassium levels.

E. SUMMARY

The three major goals of preoperative evaluation can be briefly stated as follows: (1) to make certain that the patient is in optimal condition for anesthesia (eg, antibiotic therapy for respiratory infection in a patient with emphysema); second,(2) to understand the patient's concurrent diseases and drug therapy; and (3) to ensure that all of the patient's questions and concerns are adequately dealt with.

Brabant SM et al: Refractory hypotension after induction of anesthesia in a patient chronically treated with angiotensin receptor antagonists. Anesth Analg 1999;89:887.

Smetana GW: Preoperative pulmonary evaluation. N Engl J Med 1999;340:937.

Wyatt WJ, Reed DN Jr, Apelgren KN: Pitfalls in the role of standardized pre-admission laboratory screening for ambulatory surgery. Am Surg 1989;55:343.

Informed Consent

Informed consent involves advising the patient of what to expect from administration of anesthesia and of possible adverse effects and risks. The general scenario of the perioperative period should be described, and the patient should be allowed to ask questions. Table 12–3 lists concerns that the anesthesiologist should routinely address. A signed consent form should be obtained, and the physician should make notes and file them in the patient's medical record (see Chapter 6). Many hospitals use a common consent form for both surgery and anesthesia. Although that procedure is acceptable, a separate consent form for anesthesia is increasingly being recommended.

Table 12–3. Issues that should be discussed with patients preoperatively.

Risks of anesthesia (dental, heart, vomiting)
Preoperative insomnia and its treatment
Preoperative medication (time, route of administration, and effect)
Anticipated time of transport to the operating room
Sequence of events prior to induction of anesthesia
Anticipated duration of surgery
Description of where awakening from anesthesia will occur
Presence of catheters (eg, epidural, tracheal, bladder, arterial) on awakening
Expected time of return to hospital ward room
Likelihood of postoperative nausea and vomiting
Magnitude of postoperative pain and methods for treatment
Whether they will receive blood transfusions, with associated risks

"Informed consent" is a term that is becoming increasingly difficult to define for both surgery and anesthesia. While one might argue that a patient should be informed of every possible complication, in actuality this is not practical and may even be harmful by causing undue worry. In anesthesia, patient autonomy must be balanced with medical needs in deciding what constitutes informed consent. This balance should be based on the anesthesiologist's best judgment. The anesthesiologist's conversation with the patient should be recorded as a separate note in the chart.

IMMEDIATE PREOPERATIVE MANAGEMENT

Selection of Preoperative Medication

The principal goals of preoperative medication are (1) to relieve anxiety and provide sedation; (2) to induce amnesia; (3) to decrease secretion of saliva and gastric juices; (4) to increase the gastric pH; and (5) to prevent allergic reactions to anesthetic drugs. Medication is usually given 0.5–2 hours before the induction of anesthesia. It is not necessary to give medication specifically to facilitate the induction of anesthesia. The selection of drugs is largely subjective. Sedation can be achieved by benzodiazepines or opioids (or both). To avoid an intramuscular injection, diazepam, 0.12 mg/kg, is especially effective for sedation when given orally 1–2 hours preoperatively. Midazolam is a benzodiazepine with powerful amnestic properties, but it cannot be given orally and so must be administered intramuscularly or intravenously. Gastric secretion can be decreased by H_2 receptor antagonists such as cimetidine. Anticholinergics such as atropine or scopolamine are rarely indicated. The traditional practice of prolonged fasting (eg, NPO after midnight or for 8 hours before induction of anesthesia) in patients without risk factors (eg, obesity, bowel obstruction, severe pain) is being reevaluated. The volume and pH of gastric contents are not affected by fluids ingested more than 2 hours previously. Although it is reasonable to allow clear fluids orally up to 2 hours before induction of anesthesia, this does not apply to patients with known risks for aspiration or those who have ingested solid food.

The anesthesiologist's explanation to the patient of what will occur can substantially alleviate fears about anesthesia and surgery. In fact, it has been shown that a thorough explanation has a calming effect comparable to that of medications given to relieve anxiety.

For some other conditions associated with surgery, it is better to give medication as the need arises. Cardiac vagal activity is best controlled with glycopyrrolate given just before anticipated vagal stimulation. Postoperative analgesia is better achieved by giving opioids intravenously just before they are needed, and antiemetics should be given just before postoperative nausea and vomiting are expected to occur.

Selection of Anesthesia

Many factors influence the choice of anesthesia for a given patient, and it is common practice to discuss the question with the patient preoperatively. The site of surgery and positioning of the patient on the operating table are obviously important factors. A regional nerve block may be contraindicated in a patient with neuropathy due to diabetes mellitus. Spinal anesthesia is inappropriate for thyroidectomy. Different types of anesthesia may be given for elective or emergency surgery, particularly if the patient requiring emergency surgery has a full stomach. Coexisting diseases (eg, hypertension, cardiac disease) must be considered. The age and preferences of the patient must also be taken into account.

The need for pain management and the incidence of nausea and vomiting postoperatively may influence the choice of anesthesia (eg, epidural opioids for pain or propofol for nausea and vomiting).

Preparation for Administration of Anesthesia

Anesthesia usually begins by starting an intravenous infusion and engaging standard monitors, which include noninvasively measured arterial blood pressure, electrocardiography, pulse oximetry, and in some cases peripheral nerve stimulation and body temperature.

The machine for administering anesthesia must be checked for proper functioning, and drugs and other necessary supplies must be at hand (eg, the apparatus needed to suction the pharynx and ventilate the lungs with oxygen via a cuffed endotracheal tube).

National standards are evolving for patient monitoring during anesthesia. In general, minimum monitoring dictates measurement of arterial blood pressure and heart rate every 5 minutes, and the ECG should be displayed continuously.

In addition, standard practice during anesthesia is the use of pulse oximetry, capnography, an oxygen analyzer in the anesthetic circuit, a disconnect alarm, and measurement of body temperature. Other monitors, such as transcutaneous PaO_2, intra-arterial blood pressure, central venous pressure, transesophageal echocardiography, and bispectral index are optimal depending on the anticipated extent of surgery and the anticipated duration and depth of anesthesia. In early development is the use of automated anesthetic records, in which all vital sign and other data are downloaded to a common record that can be connected to all activities in the perioperative period (eg, the postanesthetic care unit).

Positioning of the Patient on the Operating Table

It is important that the patient be positioned properly on the operating table to avoid physical or physiologic complications. Immediate complications (eg, decreased cardiac output) or long-term complications (eg, peripheral neuropathy) can result from improper positioning. Nerve damage can be caused by placing the patient in a position that stretches or applies pressure to a nerve. Pressure on a vulnerable area may lead to skin necrosis and ulceration, which in rare cases requires skin grafting. Damage to the toes or fingers may occur when positioning of equipment (eg, Mayo stand) is adjusted. Because anesthesia blunts the normal compensatory mechanisms, a sudden change in the patient's position can cause cardiovascular changes (eg, a shift from the supine to a sitting position may result in hypotension and cerebral hypoperfusion).

A. COMMON NERVE INJURIES DUE TO IMPROPER POSITIONING

Some peripheral nerves are at risk of trauma during anesthesia. Ulnar nerve injury is the most common postoperative peripheral neuropathy. If the elbow is allowed to hang over the edge of the operating table, the ulnar nerve, which runs superficially along the medial aspect of the elbow, may be compressed between the medial epicondyle and the operating table. Injury to the brachial plexus nerves usually results from extension of the arm more than 90 degrees while the patient is supine. The radial nerve may be injured if the patient's arm slips off the operating table or if pressure is applied to the nerve at the point where it traverses the spiral groove of the humerus.

The sciatic nerve may be damaged if the patient is in the lithotomy position with thighs and legs extended outward and rotated or if the knees are extended. The common peroneal nerve is typically damaged by compression between the fibula and the metal brace used in the lithotomy position.

B. INJURIES DUE TO IMPROPER PLACEMENT OF ANESTHETIC EQUIPMENT

Complications can also occur from improper application of the anesthetic mask, mask strap, or tracheal tube connector. Necrosis of the bridge of the nose due to excessive pressure by the mask is the most common injury. This can be minimized if the mask is removed every 5 minutes and the bridge of the nose gently massaged. The outer third of the eyebrow may be lost, often permanently, owing to pressure from the mask strap; this can be avoided by putting a pad under the strap. Excessive pressure on the buccal branch of the fa-

cial nerve can cause loss of function of the orbicularis oris muscle or necrosis of the ear.

Cheney FW et al: Nerve injury associated with anesthesia. Anesthesiology 1999;90:1062.

Particular requirements for anesthesia workstations and their components. American Society for Testing and Materials, 1998.

Warner MA et al: Practice guidelines for preoperative fasting and the use of pharmacologic agents to reduce the risk of pulmonary aspiration: application to healthy patients undergoing elective procedures. Anesthesiology 1999;90:896.

MANAGEMENT OF GENERAL ANESTHESIA DURING OPERATION

Induction of General Anesthesia

General anesthesia can be induced by giving drugs intravenously, by inhalation, or by a combination of both methods.

A. RAPID-SEQUENCE INDUCTION

Anesthesia is most commonly induced by the method of rapid-sequence induction, in which rapid administration of an ultra-short-acting barbiturate (eg, thiopental) is followed by a depolarizing muscle relaxant (eg, succinylcholine). While other drugs (eg, ketamine, propofol, etomidate) can be used for rapid-sequence induction of anesthesia, the combination of thiopental and succinylcholine is the standard against which others must be compared. This approach allows anesthesia to be induced within 30 seconds and the trachea to be intubated within 60–90 seconds. Oxygen is usually given by mask beforehand to allow maximum time for intubation while the patient is apneic. A nondepolarizing neuromuscular blocking drug (eg, rocuronium) can be substituted for succinylcholine, but the onset of paralysis is delayed by about 60 seconds.

Rapid-sequence induction of anesthesia minimizes the time during which the trachea is unprotected. Consequently, this method is often used in emergency surgery in patients who have eaten recently. The disadvantage of giving depressant drugs rapidly is that hypotension may occur in patients with questionable cardiovascular status or marginal circulatory volume.

B. INHALATION INDUCTION

Inhalation of nitrous oxide plus a potent volatile anesthetic (eg, halothane, sevoflurane, desflurane, or isoflurane) can produce anesthesia within 3–5 minutes. After induction, a depolarizing or nondepolarizing neuromuscular blocking drug can be given intravenously to facilitate tracheal intubation. If there is some question about the difficulty of intubation, it can be attempted while the patient is breathing spontaneously, without giving a muscle relaxant. Although conditions for intubation may not be as good with this method, the patient will still be breathing if difficulties with intubation prolong the time before complete airway control is achieved.

The advantage of inhalation induction is that anesthetic drugs can be titrated according to the patient's needs. This allows for administration of more precise doses and minimizes the risk of an accidental overdose with resultant cardiovascular depression. The disadvantages are a slower induction time and lack of protection for the airway for a longer period of time.

C. COMBINED INTRAVENOUS-INHALATION INDUCTION

Short-acting anesthetic drugs such as thiopental, propofol, or midazolam are often administered intravenously before inhalation of a volatile anesthetic. This is done to minimize the discomfort of wearing the anesthetic mask and to facilitate inhalation of the anesthetic agent, which many people consider to have an offensive odor. This technique combines the advantages of both the intravenous and inhalation approaches. Anesthesia is induced rapidly, and anesthetic drug dosages can be titrated according to the patient's requirements.

Maintaining the Airway

Historically, administering general anesthesia without endotracheal intubation was uncommon. While this approach avoids the complications of intubation, it has many disadvantages. If the patient vomits even a small amount, the airway is unprotected and aspiration will occur. Furthermore, the anesthesiologist must hold the mask with one hand during the entire procedure, and this hinders performance of the many other tasks required (eg, administration of other drugs or blood, record keeping, and monitoring).

A. APPROACH TO AIRWAY MANAGEMENT OTHER THAN TRADITIONAL ENDOTRACHEAL INTUBATION

In the last 10 years, many other options have become available for managing the airway in both the awake and the anesthetized patient. The two most important are the laryngeal mask airway (LMA) and the fiberoptic laryngoscope. The LMA is an alternative to endotracheal intubation when less invasive approaches are desired or when endotracheal intubation is difficult or impossible; it provides an excellent airway but does not protect against pulmonary aspiration of gastric contents. The fiberoptic laryngoscope represents a major advance in the management of difficult airways in both awake and anesthetized patients. Other valuable but less often used devices include the lighted stylet (lightwand), the Bullard intubatory laryngoscope, and many types of endotracheal tests.

B. INDICATIONS FOR ENDOTRACHEAL INTUBATION

Endotracheal intubation is now almost routinely performed during general anesthesia (Table 12–4). Clearly, any patient who has recently eaten or has intestinal obstruction should be managed by rapid intubation. Tracheal intubation is usually mandatory also for patients requiring positive pressure ventilation (eg, during thoracotomy or when neuromuscular blocking drugs are given). When the patient must be placed in a position other than supine, intubation is often required.

C. COMPLICATIONS OF ENDOTRACHEAL INTUBATION

The most important complication is failure to intubate the trachea, the most common cause of serious anesthesia-induced morbidity. The difficulty of tracheal intubation is related to body weight, head and neck movement, jaw movement, receding mandible, and buck teeth. A variety of techniques are available, including fiberoptic laryngoscopy, to facilitate intubation. Complications occurring during direct laryngoscopy and passage of the tube most often involve injuries to the teeth. The laryngoscope blade should not be used as a lever on the teeth. If a tooth is dislodged, it must be removed. If the tooth cannot be located, radiographs of the chest and abdomen should be obtained to ascertain that the tooth has not passed through the glottic opening.

Hypertension and tachycardia may be associated with endotracheal intubation, but they are usually transient and of no clinical significance. They can be minimized by ensuring that the depth of anesthesia is adequate and by giving lidocaine, 100 mg/70 kg intravenously, to susceptible patients. Administration of small doses of a potent opioid (eg, 150 μg/70 kg of fentanyl) during induction of anesthesia will attenuate the cardiovascular responses to tracheal intubation.

The endotracheal tube can be obstructed or accidentally removed. If it has been incorrectly placed (eg, into

Table 12–4. Indications for endotracheal intubation.

To provide a patent airway
To prevent aspiration of gastric contents
To provide tracheal or bronchial suctioning
To facilitate positive-pressure ventilation
To provide adequate ventilation—
    when the position of the patient is other than supine
    when ventilation provided by mask or laryngeal mask
       airway is not sufficient
    when disease of the upper airway is present

the bronchus or esophagus), hypoxemia will result. Auscultation of the lungs and stomach will determine whether the tube is in the esophagus. If too much pressure is applied by the balloon cuff to the tracheal wall, the tracheal mucosa may become ischemic. Previously, endotracheal tubes had "high-pressure cuffs" that required 80–250 mm Hg of pressure before they expanded enough to seal the tracheal lumen. The currently available "low-pressure cuffs" adapt to irregularities in the tracheal circumference and produce a seal at pressures of 15–30 mm Hg. With these cuffs, the incidence of tracheal ischemia is minimal. However, there is no way to entirely avoid laryngotracheal damage. For example, ciliary denudation can occur over the tracheal rings with only 2 hours of intubation and tracheal pressures of less than 25 mm Hg.

The most common complications following extubation are laryngospasm, aspiration of gastric contents, pharyngitis (sore throat), laryngitis, and laryngeal or subglottic edema. Later complications include laryngeal ulceration with or without granuloma formation, tracheitis, tracheal stenosis, vocal cord paralysis, and arytenoid cartilage dislocation.

The incidence of many of these complications can be reduced by using low-pressure endotracheal tube cuffs to minimize tissue damage and by performing prompt extubation when clinically possible.

Maintaining General Anesthesia

The main objectives of general anesthesia are analgesia, unconsciousness, skeletal muscle relaxation, and control of sympathetic nervous system responses to noxious stimulation. Inhaled and intravenous anesthetics, opioids, and muscle relaxants should be selected with specific pharmacologic goals in mind.

A. NITROUS OXIDE, VOLATILE ANESTHETICS, AND NARCOTICS

Since nitrous oxide does not provide total anesthesia, it is frequently given in combination with a volatile anes-

thetic or opioid. The main disadvantage of most volatile anesthetics is dose-dependent decrease in arterial blood pressure; when they are used in combination with nitrous oxide, which is relatively free of cardiovascular effects, their total dose can be decreased. Delivery of potent volatile anesthetics is controlled by a machine that allows the anesthesiologist to titrate the dose to the needs of the patient.

Narcotics, which generally do not depress the cardiovascular system, are often combined with nitrous oxide. However, in patients with normal ventricular function, the lack of opioid-induced cardiovascular depression in the face of unblocked sympathetic nervous system responses may produce hypertension. If this happens, the addition of low concentrations of a volatile anesthetic will usually control the blood pressure. With a combined opioid-nitrous oxide anesthetic, muscle relaxants are more frequently needed to facilitate skeletal muscle relaxation.

B. MONITORING THE DEPTH OF ANESTHESIA

Signs for assessing the depth of anesthesia are listed in Table 12–5. Although paralysis by muscle relaxants simplifies exposure of the operative site and decreases the need for volatile anesthetics, many signs of anesthesia are absent in the paralyzed patient. It is essential that the anesthesiologist continuously assess the depth of anesthesia. Failure to do so may result in the patient being awake but paralyzed during the procedure.

The bispectral index is a monitor that can be used in many cases to assess anesthetic depth. It is measured from superficial scalp electrodes and is a processed electroencephalogram. It is possible that this monitor will be increasingly used to assess anesthetic depth.

C. NEUROMUSCULAR BLOCKADE

One of the greatest challenges for the anesthesiologist is to administer the proper dosage of muscle relaxant—ie, a dosage high enough to facilitate the surgical procedures but not so high as to cover up inadequate doses of anesthetic drugs and thereby expose the patient to the risk of

Table 12–5. Signs indicating depth of anesthesia.[1]

	Blood Pressure	Heart Rate	Respiration	Sweating	Muscle Relaxation	Pupil Size	Pupil Movement
Desflurane	++	0	+	0	++	+	±
Sevoflurane	++	++	+	0	++	+	±
Isoflurane	++	+	0	++	+	±	±
N$_2$O–narcotic	+	+	+	+	0	0	0
N$_2$O–ketamine	0	0	+	0	0	0	+

[1]Usefulness of signs of graded as follows: ++, very useful; +, moderately useful; ±, questionably useful; 0, not useful.

prolonged postoperative paralysis. A peripheral nerve stimulator is of help in gauging the extent of neuromuscular blockade intraoperatively. Usually, the ulnar nerve is stimulated, and adduction of the thumb is observed. If anesthesia is sufficient, obliteration of 90% of the response will in general result in adequate relaxation. The increasing need for profound muscular relaxation has increased the incidence of weakness causing inadequate ventilation in the recovery room. This can be partly ascribed to difficulties in reversing profound neuromuscular blockade. As a result, the surgical team should also take all other measures to aid in exposure (eg, correct positioning and adequate depth of anesthesia), so that the amount of muscle relaxant can be kept to a minimum. This decreases the incidence of prolonged paralysis and dependence on mechanical ventilation postoperatively.

Benumof JL: Laryngeal mask airway and the ASA difficult airway algorithm. Anesthesiology 1996;84:686.

Crosby ET et al: The unanticipated difficult airway with recommendations for management. Can J Anaesth 1998;45:757.

Ericksson LI: The effects of residual neuromuscular blockade and volatile anesthetics on the control of ventilation. Anesth Analg 1999;89:243.

Hunter JM: New neuromuscular blocking drugs. N Engl J Med 1995;332:1691.

REGIONAL ANESTHESIA DURING OPERATION

A regional anesthetic is used when it is desirable that the patient remain conscious during the operation. Skeletal muscle relaxation is usually excellent, especially with spinal and epidural anesthesia. Thus, muscle relaxants (eg, vecuronium) are unnecessary. Patients often have misconceptions about regional anesthesia that require detailed explanation of the safety of this technique. One disadvantage of regional anesthesia is the occasional failure to produce adequate anesthesia; another is hypotension due to sympathetic blockade. Regional anesthesia is used most often for surgery of the lower abdomen or lower extremities, since the effect of sympathetic blockade of these areas is minimal.

Despite its limitations, regional anesthesia does have many attractive features. Anesthetizing only the part of the body upon which surgery is being performed (eg, spinal anesthesia for lower abdominal surgery or brachial plexus nerve block for arm surgery) may decrease postoperative morbidity. Some examples are as follows:

(1) Blood loss from total hip arthroplasty or prostatectomy is decreased by spinal or epidural anesthesia.

(2) Thromboembolic complications after hip and prostate operations are less.

(3) Lung function may be less affected.

(4) Decreased hospital stay for colon surgery.

(5) Postoperative impairment of immune function is avoided.

(6) Convalescence may be shorter.

Spinal & Epidural Blocks

Spinal anesthesia is achieved by injecting a local anesthetic into the lumbar intrathecal space. This blocks the spinal nerve roots and dorsal root ganglia and probably also blocks the periphery of the spinal cord. Epidural anesthesia is accomplished by injecting a local anesthetic into the extradural (epidural) space. The epidural space is usually identified via the lumbar approach. The gastrointestinal tract is usually contracted with spinal and epidural anesthesia, facilitating exposure of the surgical site. A limitation not only of spinal and epidural anesthesia but of regional anesthesia generally is the need to provide some sedation. Proper selection will eliminate those patients who need excessive sedation. When enough sedatives are given, the result is a comfortable-appearing, sleep-like state in which there is no spontaneous verbalization. Excess sedation can produce respiratory insufficiency leading to cardiac arrest. Monitoring with a pulse oximeter should allow detection of more subtle degrees of respiratory insufficiency.

There are several complications of spinal anesthesia. Headache is the most common and is seen most frequently in young patients. The incidence is only 1% when a 25-gauge needle is used. For severe headache, a "blood-patch" epidural injection should be performed. This involves injecting 5–10 mL of the patient's blood into the epidural space at the site of the previous lumbar puncture. Pain relief is usually prompt, and headache usually does not recur. This technique is thought to plug the leak of cerebrospinal fluid, restoring pressure in the subarachnoid space to normal.

Because spinal anesthesia blocks innervation of the bladder, administration of large amounts of intravenous fluids may cause bladder distention, and a urethral catheter may be required. This usually occurs with minor operations such as inguinal hernia repairs and can be avoided by keeping fluids to a minimum. Nausea and vomiting may occur when a spinal anesthetic is begun, especially if hypotension is present. If nausea and vomiting persist despite successful treatment of hypotension, diazepam or droperidol may be effective. Peripheral nerve damage is rare, occurring in one out of 10,000 cases.

In the past few years, epidurals have increasingly been used not so much for their intraoperative advantages but for their ability to provide excellent postoperative analgesia via opioids administered epidurally. For example, patients frequently can ambulate more rapidly following epidural anesthesia versus general anesthesia and still have pain relief. One of the problems with epidurals is the increasing use of low-molecular-weight heparin (eg, enoxaparin) to prevent deep vein thrombosis, especially in hip surgery. If used, the incidence of epidural hematomas may increase.

Recently, the technique of combined spinal-epidural anesthesia has been used. It provides the intense block from spinal anesthesia intraoperatively but also allows the advantages of epidural analgesia to occur postoperatively.

Complications from epidural anesthesia are the same as those for spinal anesthesia, with the exception of headache.

Nerve Blocks

Nerve blocks are most appropriate for surgery of the upper extremities. Intercostal nerve blocks are useful for postoperative pain relief. Overall, nerve blocks play a minor role in anesthesia because of the discomfort they cause the patient and the time they require. However, in a well-organized anesthesia department, nerve blocks can be performed with a minimum of turnaround time between cases, and patient comfort can be assured with adequate premedication.

MONITORED ANESTHETIC CARE DURING OPERATION (STANDBY ANESTHESIA)

Monitored (standby) anesthesia is the use of local anesthesia by the surgeon along with administration of sedative-hypnotics (eg, diazepam, midazolam) and opioids (eg, morphine) by the anesthesiologist. In elderly or fragile patients—especially those with unprotected airways—these cases can become quite challenging. When unexpectedly large amounts of sedative-hypnotics are required, the decision to interrupt surgery and convert to a general anesthetic with endotracheal intubation is often difficult but obviously crucial.

Carpenter RL et al: Incidence and risk factors for side effects of spinal anesthesia. Anesthesiology 1992;76:906.

Chan WBS et al: Comparison of ropivacaine and lidocaine for intravenous regional anesthesia in volunteers. Anesthesiology 1999;90:1602.

Mulroy MF, Norris MC, Lui SS: Safety steps for epidural injection or local anesthesics. Anesth Analg 1997;85:1346.

POSTOPERATIVE PROCEDURES ASSOCIATED WITH ANESTHESIA

Postanesthetic Care Unit (PACU)

The PACU is designed for the monitoring and care of patients during the period immediately following anesthesia and surgery. The PACU must be near the operating room, so that the physician is available for consultation and assistance. The size of the PACU depends on the number and kind of operations performed, with approximately one and one-half beds for each operating room.

Equipment and drugs must be available to provide routine care and advanced organ support. An electrical defibrillator, appropriate airway equipment, and drugs must be available to provide cardiopulmonary resuscitation. In a way, the PACU functions like an intensive care unit with special emphasis on the immediate postoperative period. Of course, appropriate personnel (eg, nurses and an anesthesiologist) must be available to provide care. Standards for PACU care have been formulated by many professional organizations, including the American Society of Anesthesiologists and the American Society of Post Anesthesia Nurses.

Recovery from anesthesia begins in the operating room with the discontinuation of anesthetic drugs and extubation of the trachea. Volatile anesthetics are eliminated by the lungs and intravenous anesthetics by metabolism or renal excretion. Residual activity of muscle relaxants should be assessed with a peripheral nerve stimulator, and any residual blockade should be treated with antagonists. Patients frequently enter the PACU in a state of hypothermia. Rewarming is important to minimize the adverse effects of shivering on oxygen consumption. Surgeons could help keep their patients from becoming hypothermic by allowing operating room temperatures to be warmer. Postoperative shivering can be treated with body surface warming with devices such as the Bair Huggar system or with meperidine, 10–25 mg/70 kg intravenously.

The most common immediate postoperative complications are upper airway obstruction, arterial hypoxemia, alveolar hypoventilation, hypotension, hypertension, cardiac dysrhythmias, and agitation (delirium tremens).

The physician must make sure that the patient is breathing adequately before initiating the transfer from the PACU to the ward, where monitoring is much less intense. While discharge from the PACU requires clinical judgment, a commonly used scoring system is the Aldrete Score, which quantitates the ability of the patient to move the extremities, the adequacy of breathing and circulation, consciousness, and oxygen saturation as measured by pulse oximetry.

Nausea & Vomiting

Nausea and vomiting is a common problem in the immediate postoperative period. Most pharmacologic therapy (eg, small doses of droperidol) are reactive instead of preventive. This problem can be ameliorated by preoperative administration of antiemetics (eg, droperidol, ondansetron) to high-risk patients (eye surgery, gynecologic surgery). Also, the intraoperative use of opioids augments the incidence of nausea and vomiting. Ketorolac tromethamine, a nonsteroidal, nonopioid anti-inflammatory drug, can produce postoperative analgesia (ie, equivalent to morphine) without respiratory depression and minimal nausea and vomiting. A variety of drugs can be used in the PACU for treatment of nausea and vomiting, including ondansetron, tropisetron, granisetron, and droperidol, the last of which could induce sedation that might delay discharge from the PACU.

Pain Relief

The adequacy of pain management has received national attention, including that of the Joint Commission on the Accreditation of Healthcare Organizations. Most certainly, postoperative pain relief will receive prime attention. Historically, morphine has been the foundation of postoperative analgesia. Opioids are first given intravenously and later intramuscularly. Regional anesthesia can also be used for postoperative pain relief. For example, after a cholecystectomy, intercostal nerve blocks with 0.5% bupivacaine will often provide 12–18 hours of pain relief.

Epidural or occasionally intrathecal administration of opioids is an important advance in pain relief. Complete analgesia can be obtained for 12–24 hours with no interference with autonomic or motor function. If the epidural catheter remains in place postoperatively, the analgesia can be sustained for several days. Several complications can occur from epidural opioids. Pruritus is common but seldom bothersome. Although not caused by histamine release, antihistamines often provide symptomatic relief. Naloxone is reliably effective in doses that do not reverse the analgesia (eg, 0.05 mg/70 kg), but it may have to be repeated frequently or infused. These small doses of naloxone may reverse urinary retention, though some patients may require bladder catheterization. Nausea and vomiting can be relieved by antiemetics or transdermal scopolamine. Inadequate analgesia can be treated by administration of fentanyl, 50 μg, into the epidural catheter. Lastly, respiratory depression is always to be feared and can be detected by standard nursing care, with specific monitoring orders, on the ward. Even smaller community hospitals that do not have continuous physician coverage are now using this technique. However, epidural catheters should be used cautiously in patients receiving prophylactic small doses or low-molecular-weight heparin against venous thromboembolism.

The addition of clonidine, an α_2-adrenergic agonist, to epidural opioids markedly reduces the required dose of opioid. The ultimate role of clonidine has yet to be determined. Also, a small dose of local anesthetic may be infused that will reduce the dose of opioid and improve the quality of analgesia. The analgesics can be given by intermittent injections or, more commonly, by a continuous infusion.

Patient-controlled analgesia is another technique used to control postoperative pain. With this technique, the patient can regulate his or her analgesic dose within limits that prevent excessive administration of opioids. Devices are now available that allow the patient to self-administer small bolus doses of opiates. The dose is preset by the physician or nurse and is delivered when the patient presses a button at the bedside. After the dose is given, a preselected "lockout" interval must elapse before another dose can be administered. Another technique is intrapleural injection (ie, through a catheter) of local anesthetics.

To achieve such profound analgesia postoperatively, the complexity of pain management has markedly increased. This has led to the development of acute pain management teams, usually but not always led by anesthesiologists. As a result, standards for postoperative analgesia have been established, including standard order and evaluation forms.

Aldrete JA: The post anaesthesia recovery score revisited. J Clin Anesth 1995;7:89.

Desilva PHDP et al: The efficacy of prophylactic ondansetron, droperidol, perphenazine, and metoclopramide after major gynecologic surgery. Anesth Analg 1995;81:139.

Dexter F et al: Computer simulation to determine how rapid anesthetic recovery protocols to decrease the time for emergence or increase the phase I postanesthetic care unit bypass rate affect staffing of an ambulatory surgery center. Anesth Analg 1999;88:1053.

Scuderi PE et al: Multimodal antiemetic management prevents early postoperative vomiting after outpatient laparoscopy. Anesth Analg 2000;91:1408.

Sinclair DR, Chung F, Mezei G: Can post-operative nausea and vomiting be predicted? Anesthesiology 1999;91:109.

OUTPATIENT SURGERY: HOSPITAL, SURGICENTER, OR OFFICE-BASED

To decrease the cost of hospitalization, outpatient surgery is conducted in a variety of settings, including within a hospital or satellite (surgicenter) unit that is either part of the hospital or free-standing. Physician's offices have increasingly been used for surgery and even general anesthesia. If surgery is performed in an office, the same high standards should be observed as are required in a hospital operating room or surgicenter-based outpatient facility. When this option is used, access to a hospital is needed for the rare unexpected hospitalization that may be required.

Patients who report to the hospital on the day of surgery must be given detailed instructions well in advance (Table 12–6). Local or general anesthesia is usually used in ambulatory surgical procedures. Peripheral nerve blocks are often ideal (especially intravenous Bier block) for superficial surgery of the extremities. Although epidural anesthesia can be used, spinal anesthesia may be followed by postanesthesia headache.

Recovery from anesthesia is accompanied by return of vital signs to normal, normal level of consciousness, and ability to walk without assistance. After regional anesthesia, it is important to document complete return of sensory and motor function. Nausea, vomiting, and vertigo should be absent, and the patient should not have excessive pain. The patient should be able to drink fluids. Hoarseness or stridor in a patient who was intubated must be watched carefully. Significant laryngeal edema, if present, typically becomes evident within the first hour following extubation of the trachea. Most patients with stridor improve and can be discharged without hospitalization.

The patient should be reminded that mental clarity and dexterity may remain impaired for 24–48 hours, despite an overall feeling of well-being. Driving motor vehicles or operating complex equipment should not be attempted during this period. The use of alcohol or depressant drugs should be avoided, since additive interactions with residual amounts of anesthetic are possible. Oral analgesics should be provided when appropriate. Lastly, the patient should be given the physician's telephone number and instructed to report any new symptoms or other concerns.

Table 12–6. Written instructions given to patients receiving anesthesia on an outpatient basis.

Complete all laboratory tests requested prior to surgery.
Notify the surgeon if your medical condition changes before surgery.
Do not eat solids for 6 hours or more before surgery.
Clear fluids can be taken up to 2 hours before induction of anesthesia if approved by the anesthesiologist.
Do not wear cosmetics or jewelry.
Report for surgery _____ [where and when] _____ .
The estimated time of discharge will be ____ [when] ____ .
You must be accompanied by an adult when you leave the hospital or clinic after surgery.
Following surgery, eat when hungry, starting with fluids and progressing to solid food.
Do not drive or make important decisions during the 24–48 hours following surgery.
Contact the physician in case of complications: [phone number]

Dexter F, Traub RD: The lack of systematic month-to-month variation over one-year periods in ambulatory surgery caseload. Anesth Analg 2000;91:1426.

Marshall SI, Chung F: Discharge criteria and complications after ambulatory surgery. Anesth Analg 1999;88:508.

Pavlin DJ et al: Factors affecting discharge times in outpatients. Anesth Analg 1998;816.

White PE: Criteria for fast-tracking outpatients after ambulatory surgery. J Clin Anesth 1999;11:78.

COMPLICATIONS

Aspiration Pneumonitis

A significant percentage of anesthesia-related deaths are the result of aspiration of food particles, foreign bodies, blood, gastric acid, oropharyngeal secretions, or bile during induction of anesthesia.

Aspiration pneumonitis usually takes one of two forms. Undigested food may be aspirated, producing airway obstruction and respiratory distress. Depending on the amount of material aspirated, respiratory distress can be severe, with cyanosis and cardiac arrest. Other cases may follow a milder, chronic course, leading to lobar pneumonia and lung abscess formation. Treatment involves removal of the particles by suction and bronchoscopy, followed by intensive care support. The second (more common) form of aspiration pneumonitis is caused by aspiration of gastric secretions with a pH less than 2.50, producing sudden bronchospasm, tachypnea, labored respiration, diffuse rales, cyanosis, and hypotension. Cardiac arrest may occur in severe cases.

Prevention is obviously most desirable. Generally, any patient who has eaten solid food within 8 hours should be considered to have a full stomach and therefore at risk of vomiting during induction. However, it should be recognized that 8 hours of fasting does not guarantee a low gastric volume. In traumatized or pregnant patients, gastric emptying may be delayed, and the interval between eating and elective surgery should be lengthened to 12 hours. Premedication with H_2 receptor blockers such as cimetidine and other drugs such as metoclopramide is frequently recommended. Drinking sodium citrate will increase the gastric pH in most patients, but this must be done 45–75 minutes before induction. If time does not permit such a wait, either endotracheal intubation with the patient awake or rapid-sequence induction must be performed.

Warner MA et al: Practice guidelines for preoperative fasting and the use of pharmacologic agents to reduce the risk of pulmonary aspirations. Anesthesiology 1999;90:896.

Malignant Hyperthermia

Malignant hyperthermia associated with anesthesia is an inherited disease manifested by a rapid increase in body temperature, which is often lethal if not promptly treated. The caffeine-halothane contracture test, which measures the concentration of caffeine required to trigger contracture in freshly biopsied skeletal muscle, is the standard test used to establish susceptibility to malignant hyperthermia. A linkage has been established between the human gene for malignant hyperthermia and the ryanodine receptor gene. This receptor is a protein that comprises the calcium release channel of skeletal muscle sarcoplasmic reticulum. Genetic studies suggest that the caffeine-halothane contracture test may yield many false-positive results. In any event, the incidence during anesthesia is approximately 1:15,000 for pediatric patients and 1:50,000 for adult patients. This disease is due to a defect in excitation-contraction coupling in skeletal muscles and high calcium concentrations in the myoplasm. Exposure to a triggering drug such as a volatile anesthetic, succinylcholine, or an amide local anesthetic causes unusually high and sustained levels of calcium in the myoplasm and persistent skeletal muscle contraction. This results in hypermetabolism, including tachycardia, arterial hypoxemia, metabolic and respiratory acidosis, and profound hyperthermia. Dantrolene, up to 10 mg/kg intravenously, is the treatment of choice.

Patients who will require anesthesia and are susceptible to malignant hyperthermia should be pretreated with dantrolene, 5 mg/kg/d orally in four divided doses for 1–3 days; drugs known to trigger the syndrome should be avoided during anesthesia. No anesthetic approach is completely safe in these patients, though the drugs usually used are opioids, barbiturates, nitrous oxide, and local anesthetics.

Fulminant malignant hyperthermia is increasingly rare because of sophisticated monitoring in the operating room and systematic education by groups such as the North American and European Malignant Hyperthermia Group of anesthesiologists and nurse anesthetists. The mortality rate has decreased from about 38% to almost zero with proper management.

Larach MG et al: A clinical grading scale to predict malignant hyperthermia susceptibility. Anesthesiology 1994;80:771.

Ørding HD et al: Between-center variability of results of the in vitro contracture test for malignant hyperthermia susceptibility. Anesth Analg 2000;91:452.

Pessah IN, Lynch C, Gronert GA: Complex pharmacology of malignant hyperthermia. Anesthesiology 1996;84:1275.

Shock & Acute Pulmonary Failure in Surgical Patients

13

James W. Holcroft, MD, & David H. Wisner, MD

■ I. SHOCK

Severe cardiovascular failure, or shock, can be caused by (1) depletion of the vascular volume, (2) compression of the heart or great veins, (3) intrinsic failure of the heart itself, (4) loss of autonomic control of the vasculature, (5) severe untreated sepsis, and (6) severe but partially compensated sepsis. Depending on the type and severity of cardiovascular failure and on the success of initial management, shock can go on to compromise other organ systems. For discussion of gastrointestinal failure, see Chapter 3; for hepatic failure and psychiatric problems, see Chapter 4; for kidney failure, see Chapter 5; for problems of catabolism and the resulting musculoskeletal debility, see Chapter 11; and for infection in seriously ill surgical patients, see Chapter 9.

This chapter discusses the cardiovascular and pulmonary disorders associated with shock.

DIAGNOSIS & TREATMENT OF THE CARDIOVASCULAR CONSEQUENCES OF SHOCK

HYPOVOLEMIC SHOCK

Pathophysiology

Hypovolemic shock (shock caused by inadequate circulating blood volume) can arise from bleeding, protracted vomiting or diarrhea, sequestration of fluid in the gut lumen (eg, bowel obstruction), or loss of plasma into injured tissues (eg, burns or trauma). Depletion of vascular volume, which results in collapse of systemic venules and small veins, decreases the driving pressure for return of blood to the heart, decreases end-diastolic ventricular volumes, and decreases stroke volumes and cardiac output.

In mild to moderate shock, the body compensates through discharge of the cardiovascular adrenergic nerves and release of vasopressin and angiotensin, which constrict venules and small veins throughout the body and selectively constrict arterioles to the skin, fat, connective tissue, bone, skeletal muscle, gut, pancreas, spleen, and liver (but not the brain or heart). Venular constriction displaces blood to the heart and thus helps reestablish end-diastolic volumes, stroke volumes, and cardiac output; the selective arteriolar constriction diverts blood away from organs that withstand ischemia relatively well to those that withstand it poorly. In addition, aldosterone is released. It and vasopressin stimulate tubular reabsorption of water and sodium and thus minimize urinary losses of plasma constituents.

Diagnosis

Although compensatory responses to arrested **mild shock** (a deficit of less than 20% of the blood volume) are almost always adequate to ensure survival even without treatment, recognition of an untreated cause early in mild shock can prevent fatal progression. The signs of early hypovolemic shock are postural hypotension, cutaneous vasoconstriction, sweat gland stimulation, collapse of the neck veins, concentration of the urine, oliguria, and a decreasing hematocrit with administration of fluids (Table 13–1). These are manifestations either of the shock itself (such as postural hypotension, neck vein collapse, and serial falling hematocrits) or represent compensatory responses to shock (cutaneous vasoconstriction and sweat production and urine concentration and oliguria).

The blood pressure in a supine mildly hypovolemic patient is usually normal but will fall by at least 10 mm Hg when the patient sits up, and the lower level typically persists for several minutes. (The blood pressure in a euvolemic patient may fall transiently when the patient sits up rapidly but will return to normal levels within 1 minute.) Postural hypotension is a sensitive sign of hypovolemia and can be elicited by nonphysician personnel. It cannot be used in patients with multiple injuries, however, and its use is limited mostly to patients who are suspected of being hypovolemic from either dehydration or occult internal blood loss (eg, in a patient who might have gastrointestinal bleeding).

Table 13–1. Clinical classification
of hypovolemia.

Mild hypovolemia (deficit < 20% of blood volume)
Pathophysiology: Decreased perfusion of organs that withstand ischemia well (skin, fat, skeletal muscle, bone).
Manifestations: Patient complains of feeling cold. Postural changes in blood pressure and pulse. Pale, cool, clammy skin. Flat neck veins. Concentrated urine.
Moderate hypovolemia (deficit = 20–40% of blood volume)
Pathophysiology: Decreased perfusion of organs that withstand ischemia poorly (pancreas, spleen, kidneys).
Manifestations: Patient complains of being thirsty. Occasionally, low blood pressure and rapid pulse in supine position. Oliguria.
Severe hypovolemia (deficit > 40% blood volume)
Pathophysiology: Decreased perfusion of brain and heart.
Manifestations: Patient is restless, agitated, confused, obtunded, or "drunk." Low blood pressure and sometimes rapid, weak, irregular pulse. Deep breaths at rapid rate. Cardiac arrest.

The skin manifestations of adrenergic discharge are sensitive and can be noted in any patient, including one with multiple injuries. They are easiest to detect in the feet. The subcutaneous veins collapse, which causes difficulty in inserting venous cannulas as an early finding in shock, and the skin becomes cold, clammy, and pale, with delayed microvascular filling. Coldness and clamminess are usually obvious. Pallor is best detected on the plantar surfaces of the toes or in the nail beds, where color changes can be seen in all patients, including those with dark skin. Compressing the toe to produce blanching and then releasing the compression and watching for color return can usually resolve any uncertainty. In a normovolemic patient without peripheral vascular disease, the color should return within 2 seconds; refill takes longer than 2 seconds in hypovolemic patients. The test should be done with the foot of the bed at the level of the heart.

Although examination of the skin can help in diagnosis of hypovolemia, it can sometimes be misleading. Fright, exposure to a cold environment, and difficulty in deciding if the skin really is pale are potentially confusing factors.

Looking for collapsed neck veins—an index of low central venous pressure—is best done with the patient's head, neck, and torso elevated 30 degrees. Whether or not pulsations are present in the internal jugular vein gives a clue to filling pressures of the right heart, as there are no valves between the internal jugular vein and the right atrium. A normal right atrial pressure will distend the neck veins to about 4 cm above the manubrium.

A urine specimen should be promptly obtained in any patient suspected of being hypovolemic, and a Foley catheter should be inserted. Even in mild hypovolemia, the urine will be concentrated and the patient oliguric. Oliguria is defined as urine output less than 0.5 mL/kg/h in adults; less than 1 mL/kg/h in children; or less than 2 mL/kg/h in infants. It is an early and specific sign of hypovolemia.

The initial hematocrit is of no value in diagnosing hypovolemia except in chronic bleeding, when vascular equilibration has had time to dilute the hematocrit. Acute hemorrhage does not immediately reduce the hematocrit, so repeated measurements are required.

The hematocrit will always fall as asanguineous fluids are administered. A fall of 3–4% indicates that the blood volume has been depleted by about 10%; a fall of 6–8% indicates a deficit of about 20% (or 1 L in an average adult). These calculations assume that the patient has been given enough fluid to correct the hypovolemia.

Additional manifestations in **moderate hypovolemia** (a deficit of 20–40% of the blood volume) include thirst and sometimes moderate hypotension with the patient supine (Table 13–1). **Severe hypovolemia** (a deficit of more than 40% of blood volume) can produce signs of inadequate cerebral and cardiac perfusion. The former includes changes in mental status, eg, restlessness, agitation, confusion, lethargy, or the appearance of inebriation; the latter includes an irregular heartbeat or electrocardiographic evidence of myocardial ischemia, such as ST–T segment depression or the appearance of Q waves. Patients in severe hypovolemic shock will almost always be hypotensive, even when supine (Table 13–1).

Although the heart rate in some species increases proportionately in response to graded hemorrhage, there is little correlation between severity of hypovolemia and heart rate in humans. For example, hypovolemic patients often have normal heart rates, and severe hypovolemia can even produce bradycardia as a preterminal event. Thus, tachycardia can be taken as weak confirmation of the presence of shock, but a normal rate is not evidence against hypovolemia.

If the patient is inebriated, hypovolemia may be difficult to diagnose (Table 13–2). High blood ethanol levels produce warm, flushed, and dry skin and promote diuresis of dilute urine—ie, alcohol ablates two of the principal signs. Postural hypotension—if it can be elicited—will remain, however, and supine hypotension occurs with less severe hypovolemia in inebriation.

Like hypovolemia, insulin shock also stimulates adrenergic discharge and release of vasoactive hormones (Table 13–2). The cold, clammy, oliguric, and hypotensive type 1 diabetic who has just been in an automobile accident could be hypovolemic, hypoglycemic,

Table 13–2. Manifestations of cardiovascular disorders in critically ill patients.

Condition	Skin	Neck Veins
Hypovolemia	Cold, clammy	Flat
Cardiac compression	Cold, clammy	Distended[1]
Cardiogenic	Cold, clammy	Distended
Neurogenic	Warm[2]	Flat
High-output sepsis	Warm	Flat to normal
Low-output sepsis	Cold, clammy	Flat
Hypoglycemia	Cold, clammy	Flat to normal
Inebriation[3]	Warm	Normal

[1]May be flat if patient is also hypovolemic.
[2]In denervated areas.
[3]Listed only to emphasize that alcohol can mask signs of other conditions.

or both. Blood glucose levels should be measured in such patients, and an intravenous bolus of 50 mL of 50% glucose should be administered while the patient is being evaluated for hypovolemia.

Treatment

Resuscitation of patients in hemorrhagic shock should begin with establishment of an airway, which can usually be accomplished by hyperextending the neck and supporting the jaw. Many hypovolemic patients can breathe adequately, and they may even hyperventilate. Supplemental nasal oxygen is usually all that is needed. Some patients, however, require tracheal intubation and mechanical ventilation. Trauma victims may require insertion of chest tubes. External hemorrhage, if present, should be controlled, and preparations should be made to operate on patients bleeding internally.

Percutaneously placed venous catheters should be used for mild hypovolemia; large-bore intravenous catheters placed by cut-down, for severe hypovolemia. The saphenous veins at the ankles provide an accessible site unless the extremity is badly traumatized. Catheters in the saphenous vein should be removed within 24 hours to avoid phlebitis.

Percutaneously placed central venous catheters should not be used for initial resuscitation, because a central line is not required to administer fluids and because technical problems during placement could produce complications. Central venous catheters may be inserted later, when they can be used to measure right atrial pressures. Large-bore (14-gauge or larger) catheters should be used. The commonly used 16-gauge subclavian lines are too long and narrow to permit rapid infusion of fluids.

Crystalloid solution with a sodium concentration approximating that of plasma (eg, lactated Ringer's so-

lution or normal saline) should be used for initial resuscitation. The lactate buffers the metabolic acidemia of shock by absorbing hydrogen ion to form lactic acid. The lactic acid is then oxidized to carbon dioxide and water in the Krebs cycle. Although, in theory, shock-induced hepatic hypoperfusion might impair metabolism of lactic acid, metabolism is in fact rapid, probably because liver blood flow is quickly reestablished with the initial resuscitation. However, patients with cirrhosis should be given normal saline instead of lactated Ringer's solution. Glucose should not be used in initial resuscitation (except to treat hypoglycemia) because it may induce osmotic diuresis.

The severity of shock should determine the rate and amount of fluid given. Two liters of crystalloid should be given as fast as possible in patients in severe shock, followed by a third liter infused over 10 minutes. Three liters of fluid will resuscitate most patients in whom hemorrhage has been arrested. Incomplete resuscitation indicates continued bleeding and probably the need for operative control of hemorrhage. Less severe shock requires proportionately less fluid.

Resuscitation should begin with a crystalloid solution even if blood is available—indeed, even if the patient is bleeding. By restoring peripheral perfusion, the initial fluid bolus flushes into the circulation products of anaerobic and catabolic metabolism, which can temporarily depress the myocardium. Cold, acidotic, hyperkalemic banked blood at this point would compromise the myocardium even further.

In general, blood should be withheld until bleeding has been controlled, to minimize loss of transfused red blood cells. Young patients without heart disease tolerate hemodilution well as long as the plasma volume is fully expanded. Hematocrits as low as 15% are safe for the 20 minutes or so required to control major hemorrhage.

Blood transfusion should be started, however, in patients who remain unstable after the initial crystalloid infusion—even if bleeding has not yet been contained. In young patients with normal coronary arteries, the hematocrit should be brought into the mid 20s. If bleeding is liable to continue, the objective should be a hematocrit in the low 30s. If the patient has coronary artery disease or shows signs of myocardial ischemia on electrocardiography, the hematocrit should be increased to the mid 30s. The heart is the first organ to show the ill effects of a hematocrit that is too low.

The freshest possible blood should be used, especially if more than a few units will be necessary. Fresh blood minimizes coagulation abnormalities. If blood must be given before it can be cross-matched, type-specific non-cross-matched blood, which can usually be obtained within 10 minutes, should be used. The risk of a transfusion reaction is negligible compared with the risks of inadequate oxygen delivery to the tissues. If type-specific blood is not available, Rh-negative type O red blood cells reconstituted in normal saline may be used. Whole blood, if available, should be given to resuscitate severely bleeding patients because of the time required to administer packed cells.

Albumin-containing solutions (other than blood) should not be used in the initial resuscitation since, during shock, they have little effect on plasma oncotic pressure and do not retain fluids within the vascular space, as was once thought. Instead, the protein extravasates into the interstitial space. Dextran, starch solutions, fluorocarbons, and stroma-free hemoglobin solutions have not been adequately evaluated, and their role in resuscitation is undefined.

In some cases, the total amount of fluid required for resuscitation is 20–30 L, especially in the presence of massive injuries. Much of this fluid ends up in the interstitium because of trauma-induced microvascular endothelial disruption. To minimize the increase in endothelial permeability, every effort should be made to rapidly control bleeding, immobilize fractures, and debride necrotic tissue. The combination of shock and tissue trauma stimulates coagulation and inflammation, which is manifested by generalized edema.

Elevation of the lower extremities above the level of the heart (Trendelenburg's position) may shift some blood to the right heart, but there is little lasting benefit, and the left ventricle must work harder to pump blood back to the elevated extremities. This time-honored procedure is best abandoned for treatment of hypovolemia. Neither is the pneumatic antishock garment—an inflatable overall enclosing the lower extremities and abdomen—useful in reversing the cardiovascular changes in shock, because it hinders blood return by compressing the inferior vena cava and perhaps the renal and hepatic veins, and it makes left ventricular emptying more difficult by compressing the arterioles in the lower body. Although in normovolemic subjects the garment displaces blood from subdiaphragmatic to supradiaphragmatic organs, this shift will already have been accomplished by adrenergic mechanisms in hypovolemic patients, and some residual blood flow to splanchnic viscera may be essential to prevent late organ failure. The garment precludes use of the saphenous vein as a site for venous access, and it may push the diaphragm into the thorax and interfere with ventilation. It may be effective, however, in splinting fractures and in tamponading bleeding in the parts of the body that it encloses, and its use should therefore be restricted to these indications.

Treatment of nonhemorrhagic hypovolemic shock is similar to that of hemorrhagic shock. Blood is unnecessary, and in some cases, such as severe burns, one goal of therapy is to decrease the hematocrit. Asanguineous fluids should be given to eliminate postural hypotension, restore peripheral perfusion, and reestablish urine output. For hypovolemia caused by protracted vomiting or loss of fluid into the gut, volume replenishment should also take into account the need to correct electrolyte abnormalities. (See Chapter 10.)

CARDIAC COMPRESSIVE SHOCK

Pathophysiology

Shock can arise from any condition that compresses the heart or great veins, including pericardial tamponade; positive-pressure ventilation; tension pneumothorax; distention of the abdomen with compression of the inferior vena cava and elevation of the diaphragm into the chest; and rupture of the diaphragm with displacement of abdominal viscera into the chest. Compression of the inferior or superior vena cava or the pulmonary veins retards blood return to the heart; compression of the heart itself, especially the thin-walled atria and right ventricle, prevents adequate chamber filling.

Diagnosis

The signs of shock are present—ie, postural hypotension, poor cutaneous perfusion, oliguria, hypotension, mental status changes, or electrocardiographic signs of myocardial ischemia—combined with distended neck veins (Table 13–2). The only other condition that can produce this pattern is cardiogenic shock, which rarely poses a problem in differential diagnosis because cardiac compression usually follows trauma or occurs in a setting where mechanical compromise of the heart or great veins is a known risk, such as mechanical ventilation or massive ascites. Cardiogenic shock usually develops against a background of evident disease that predisposes to primary myocardial dysfunction (see Cardiogenic Shock, below).

Confirmation of cardiac compression can be made by observing the neck veins and measuring the systolic blood pressure while the patient takes a deep breath. Inspiration in a normovolemic patient without cardiac compression decreases right atrial pressure, which can be detected by observing the neck veins. The decrease in pressure arises from the balance of three different influences: First, as the lungs pull away from the extrapericardial great veins, blood tends to surge into the right atrium and increase the pressure within the chamber. Second, the pressure inside the atrium tends to increase with a deep breath because a fully expanded lung compresses the interalveolar pulmonary vasculature and makes it difficult for the right ventricle to contract; blood tends to back up in the right heart and increase right atrial pressure. Third, the lungs pull away from the pericardium and from the enclosed thin-walled right heart chambers, which tends to decrease right atrial pressure. Under normal conditions, this last effect predominates.

In the presence of cardiac compression, however, the effect of the lungs pulling away from the heart is lost. An engorged pericardium acts as a barrier so that decreased pressure on the outside of the pericardium is no longer reflected by pressure changes on the heart. The effects of inspiration on the extrapericardial great veins and pulmonary vasculature, however, are not influenced by the tamponade. The overall result is increased right atrial pressure and further distention of the neck veins. This **Kussmaul sign** is pathognomonic of pericardial tamponade.

The so-called **paradoxic pulse** can also be helpful in diagnosis. A spontaneous breath in a normovolemic patient without cardiac compression produces little effect on systemic blood pressure. A fall in systolic pressure of more than 10 mm Hg ("pulsus paradoxus") supports the diagnosis of pericardial tamponade. As the lungs expand, the walls of the extra-alveolar pulmonary capacitance vessels are pulled apart, and blood pools within the vasculature. This transient pulmonary sequestration of blood decreases left atrial filling, reduces stretching of the atrial myocardium and the effectiveness of atrial contraction, and reduces the amount of blood delivered into the left ventricle. Left ventricular end-diastolic volume and stroke volume decrease. On the other hand, a spontaneous inspiration tends to increase stretching of the atrial myocardial fibers as the lungs pull away from the heart, which tends to increase left heart filling and left ventricular stroke volume.

These two opposing effects usually cancel each other out, and the stroke volumes associated with inspiration and expiration—and the corresponding blood pressures—are about the same. In the presence of pericardial tamponade, however, blood pressure can fall considerably because tamponade leaves unopposed the inspiration-induced pooling of blood in the pulmonary vasculature.

The diagnosis of cardiac compression is facilitated if the patient can be monitored in an intensive care unit with a Swan-Ganz catheter (see Swan-Ganz Catheter, below), where a low cardiac output in the face of high filling pressures can be documented by direct measurement. In addition, the catheter can be used to compare pressures in the left and right atria. Under normal circumstances, the pressure in the left atrium is about 5 mm Hg higher than in the right. In tamponade, the pressures are identical, because cardiac compression dominates all other influences. This finding is sensitive but not specific, especially if the patient is being mechanically ventilated.

Positive-pressure ventilation has three potential adverse effects on cardiac output: (1) Inflation of the lungs compresses the superior and inferior vena cava and impedes filling of the right heart (in contrast, a spontaneous inspiration augments filling); (2) lung inflation compresses the thin-walled atria and right ventricle, decreases end-diastolic myocardial stretch, and decreases stroke volumes (again in contrast to a spontaneous inspiration); and (3) expansion of the lung compresses the interalveolar vessels and hinders right ventricular emptying. In extreme cases, these three effects can decrease cardiac output to the point that it can no longer meet metabolic needs, especially if the patient is hypovolemic.

Tension pneumothorax produces shock by kinking the great veins and by compressing the atria and right ventricle. Ascites, intra-abdominal bleeding, or distention of the gut compresses the inferior vena cava and pushes the diaphragm directly against the heart. Rupture of the diaphragm with displacement of abdominal viscera into the chest also directly compresses the heart. The clinical diagnosis of these conditions is discussed in Chapter 14; the hemodynamic changes that help make the diagnosis are shock in the presence of distended neck veins, sometimes with a Kussmaul sign or a paradoxic pulse.

Treatment

Infusion of fluid can transiently overcome some of the ill effects of cardiac compression, but the cause of shock in these patients is mechanical, and definitive treatment must correct the mechanical abnormality. Pericardial tamponade, tension pneumothorax, and ruptured diaphragm are discussed in Chapter 14; bowel obstruction in Chapter 30. Treatment of compressive shock caused by large-volume mechanical ventilation is discussed later in this chapter in the section on mechanical ventilation.

CARDIOGENIC SHOCK

Pathophysiology

Cardiogenic shock can arise from an arrhythmia, ischemia-induced myocardial failure, valvular or septal defects, systemic or pulmonary hypertension, myocarditis, or myocardiopathies. The diagnosis is usually made on the basis of a known history of cardiovascular disease in conjunction with an abnormal ECG in a patient in shock with distended neck veins (Table 13–2).

A slow heart rate (< 50 beats/min in an adult) can cause inadequate cardiac output because cardiac output is the product of stroke volume and heart rate. A rapid heart rate—one that exceeds the maximum aerobic limit of 0.8 multiplied by 230 minus the patient's age in years—can cause inadequate output because the ventricles have inadequate time to fill and the coronary arteries receive too little blood during diastole. Myocardial ischemia can cause shock because the myocardium lacks adequate oxygen; anatomic defects, because of wasted pumping; hypertension, because of an excessive load on the ventricles and because of superimposed abnormalities that develop in the myocardium with hypertrophy or dilation; and myocardial disease, because of intrinsic failure of the heart muscle.

Diagnosis

The diagnosis of cardiogenic shock usually depends on recognition of the underlying medical condition. Shock, distended neck veins, peripheral edema, an enlarged and tender liver, a third heart sound, rales, electrocardiographic signs of ischemia, and an enlarged heart on x-ray can all be helpful. The diagnosis is usually easy, but two common situations may pose a problem.

The first is a ruptured abdominal aortic aneurysm in a patient with coronary artery disease. The patient might have abdominal pain consistent with a myocardial infarction and electrocardiographic signs of ischemia—the ischemia caused by hypovolemia and severe shock. The key is to observe the neck veins.

The second is to ascribe shock to myocardial contusion in a patient who has just suffered a major chest injury. Although blunt chest trauma can damage the heart, damage of this kind is usually fatal at the scene of the injury. A contusion that produces failure but not death is rare. Shock after blunt trauma in a patient who survives to reach the hospital is almost never caused by contusion—it is far more likely to be caused by hypovolemia or cardiac compression.

Treatment

A. OPIOIDS

Opioids relieve pain, provide sedation, block adrenergic discharge, decrease right ventricular filling, and lessen stress on the heart. They can be especially effective in treating cardiac failure after myocardial infarction.

B. DIURETICS

By decreasing vascular volume, diuretics decrease right and left atrial pressures and alleviate peripheral and pulmonary edema. Pulmonary vascular pressures and volumes decrease; effectiveness of right ventricular contraction may increase. Coronary blood flow increases as coronary sinus pressure drops. Diuretics are ideal therapy in congestive heart failure with expanded vascular volumes; they are obviously contraindicated in cardiovascular disorders caused by hypovolemia, trauma, cardiac compression, sepsis, or loss of microvascular tone,

even though these forms of shock are frequently associated with oliguria.

C. CHRONOTROPIC AGENTS

Patients in cardiac failure with bradycardia may on rare occasion temporarily benefit from administration of a chronotropic agent such as atropine or isoproterenol. Isoproterenol increases heart rate, augments myocardial contractility, and dilates the systemic arterioles. Chronotropic agents should be used to increase the heart rate only to levels that can be tolerated comfortably. A 60-year-old patient with normal coronary arteries should be able to tolerate a heart rate of 120/min; the limit is about 90/min in the presence of coronary artery disease.

Chronotropic agents increase myocardial work and shorten the time during diastole for coronary blood flow and ventricular filling and usually should not be used except as a temporary expedient. If they are used for more than 30 minutes, a Swan-Ganz catheter should be inserted. The goal of therapy is a normal or supranormal cardiac index. Cardiac indices should be determined at different heart rates produced by different doses of drug and the results compared with timing of chest pain and electrocardiographic signs of myocardial ischemia.

D. INOTROPIC AGENTS

Many patients in cardiac failure benefit from administration of an inotropic agent such as dobutamine or milrinone. The principal use of these drugs is to increase flow in the cardiovascular system.

Dobutamine and milrinone must be used with caution, and the patient should be monitored in an intensive care unit.

If it is necessary to use inotropic agents for more than 1 hour, a Swan-Ganz catheter should be inserted. Filling pressures and cardiac indices should be determined at different infusion rates. If any question remains about the adequacy of volume resuscitation, filling pressures and cardiac indices should be measured before and after a fluid bolus is given.

Digitalis compounds should not be used in acute cardiac failure except to control dysrhythmias. Toxicity may develop, especially when pH and electrolyte changes are unpredictable. The inotropic actions of digitalis are no different from those of dopamine and milrinone.

E. VASODILATORS

The most useful vasodilating agents in surgical patients with cardiac failure are morphine, nitroprusside, and nitroglycerin, all of which are either easily reversible or short-acting. These drugs should be used as primary vasodilators only if systemic vascular resistance is known to be elevated (ie, only if a Swan-Ganz catheter is in place). They are usually used in patients with high mean systemic arterial pressures but can occasionally be used (with caution) in patients with normal arterial pressures as long as the blood pressure is adequate for perfusion of the brain and heart.

Vasodilators decrease systemic vascular resistance, allowing the left heart to pump more efficiently. These agents may also reduce pulmonary vascular resistance and increase pulmonary vascular compliance, improving right heart performance. Nitroglycerin and, to a lesser extent, nitroprusside dilate the systemic venules and small veins and decrease right heart filling.

All of these effects decrease myocardial work and oxygen demands. In some patients, however, excessive venous dilation can decrease cardiac filling enough that cardiac output falls. Cardiac filling pressures and cardiac output should be measured before and after starting treatment. Excessive arteriolar dilation may lead to inadequate perfusion pressures for the coronary arteries and myocardial ischemia. The patient should be monitored for chest pain and electrocardiographic evidence of myocardial ischemia while the drugs are being given.

F. Beta-Blocking Agents

Many patients in cardiac failure with ischemia and a rapid heart rate will benefit from a beta-adrenergic blocking agent (eg, esmolol or propranolol), which may reduce myocardial oxygen consumption and salvage marginal myocardium.

G. Vasoconstrictors

Vasoconstrictors are occasionally useful to increase perfusion pressures for atherosclerotic coronary arteries, though endogenous adrenergic mechanisms usually bring forth a maximum response. Because vasoconstrictors can decrease the efficiency of left ventricular pumping and produce ischemic necrosis of digits or extremities, they should be used only when absolutely necessary and not for more than 60 minutes unless a pulmonary arterial catheter is in place.

H. Transaortic Balloon Pump

The transaortic balloon pump is effective in resuscitating selected patients with severe reversible left ventricular dysfunction (eg, after cardiopulmonary bypass or acute myocardial infarction). It should only be used if a Swan-Ganz catheter is in place.

NEUROGENIC SHOCK

Shock caused by failure of the autonomic nervous system can arise from regional anesthetics, injuries to the spinal cord, or administration of autonomic blocking agents. The cardiac output decreases because the

venules and small veins lose tone. Blood pools in the periphery, ventricular end-diastolic volumes decrease, and stroke volumes fall. The adrenergic nervous system above the level of denervation is activated, increasing heart rate and contractility to compensate for peripheral pooling of blood if the lesion is below the midthoracic sympathetic outflow. If the sympathetic nerves to the heart are also blocked, the patient may develop an absolute or relative bradycardia. Loss of perivenular support by paralyzed skeletal muscle tone can aggravate venous pooling. The blood pressure in neurogenic shock can plummet to very low levels because arteriolar as well as venular tone will also be lost.

The diagnosis rests on knowledge of the circumstances preceding the onset of shock and on the physical examination. The patient will always be hypotensive, and the skin will be warm and flushed in the denervated areas (Table 13–2). The cause is usually obvious.

Head injury—as opposed to spinal cord injury—does not produce neurogenic shock or any other kind of shock. In fact, increased intracranial pressure typically increases blood pressure and slows the heart rate (Cushing reflex). Hypotension and tachycardia should never be attributed to head injury—even severe head injury with cerebral dysfunction—until concomitant hypovolemia has been ruled out.

Neurogenic shock is the only type in which vasoconstrictors are usually useful. The goal is to restore tone in the venules and small veins and to increase blood pressure to the point that coronary perfusion is sustained, as judged by normal ST–T segments on electrocardiography and absence of chest pain. Either norepinephrine or phenylephrine can be used. If vasoconstrictors are expected to be needed for more than 1 hour, the patient should be placed in an intensive care unit with Swan-Ganz monitoring. Trendelenburg's position can also be temporarily useful.

HIGH-OUTPUT SEPTIC SHOCK

Bowel perforation, necrotic intestine, abscesses, gangrene, and soft tissue infections can produce high-output septic shock. Early or adequately treated sepsis presents with fever and compensatory cutaneous vasodilation. Systemic vascular resistance and arterial blood pressure fall, but cardiac output increases because the left ventricle has little resistance to pump against. Although adrenergic activity increases somewhat, the need to decrease core temperature predominates, and flow to the skin remains high. Cardiac output remains elevated as long as the blood volume is maintained. This high-output septic state is frequently associated with deranged metabolism, so that the tissue's metabolic needs are not met even though the circulation is hyperdynamic.

Early sepsis is manifested by fever and hypotension in a patient who appears pink and well perfused (Table 13–2). If vascular volume is maintained, the cutaneous veins will be full, urine output adequate, and the pulse rate high. The patient is often anxious and confused. Intermittent chills and fever are common.

Treatment consists of administration of intravenous fluids and antibiotics, correction of gastrointestinal leaks, debridement of dead tissue, and drainage of pus. If the vascular volume can be maintained, the patient will remain well perfused; if treatment is delayed or if the infection cannot be controlled, late sepsis will develop. Treatment consists of transfer to an intensive care unit, insertion of systemic and pulmonary arterial catheters, administration of fluid, and, if necessary, use of inotropes. Vasoconstrictors should be used only if hypotension is threatening the brain, the heart, or an organ with an obstructed arterial supply, such as the small intestine in a patient with known atherosclotic occlusive disease of the superior mesenteric artery or one with a thoracoabdominal aneurysm with occlusion of the arteries that supply the spinal cord.

LOW-OUTPUT SEPTIC SHOCK

Untreated or late systemic sepsis, from either Gram-positive or Gram-negative bacteria, can disrupt the microvascular endothelium, prompt the loss of plasma into the interstitium, and produce shock similar to that associated with hypovolemia (Table 13–2). Pulmonary vascular resistance increases and hinders right ventricular emptying. In addition, in some patients, circulating plasma factors might depress myocardial contractility. (It is unlikely that myocardial depression plays any role in hypovolemic, cardiac compressive, or neurogenic shock.) The cardiovascular findings of low-output sepsis are identical to those of hypovolemic shock. The diagnosis is usually clear from the clinical circumstances. The initial cardiovascular resuscitation for low-output septic and hypovolemic shock is the same. The goal is to perfuse the infected tissues with adequate power so that the product of the cardiac output and the mean arterial pressure is normal. The blood pressure can be low as long as the cardiac output is high.

NEUROHUMORAL & CELLULAR RESPONSES TO SHOCK

The neurohumoral responses to shock include discharge of the cardiovascular nerves and release of vasoactive, metabolically active, and volume-conserving hormones. The responses can be life-saving before therapy begins and serve to maintain homeostasis once

therapy has started. The responses, however, can also contribute to postshock organ failure.

CARDIOVASCULAR ADRENERGIC DISCHARGE

Adrenergic discharge constricts the venules and small veins, constricts arterioles in all parts of the body except the brain and heart, and increases cardiac contractility. The result is increased cardiac output and blood pressure and diversion of flow to the brain and heart.

RELEASE OF VASOACTIVE HORMONES

The vasoactive hormones, angiotensin II and vasopressin, act in concert with discharge of the cardiovascular adrenergic nerves. Activation of angiotensin II begins with release of renin from the kidneys. Renin stimulates the liver to synthesize and release angiotensinogen, which is converted to angiotensin I; enzymes in the pulmonary endothelium convert angiotensin I to angiotensin II. Angiotensin II constricts the vasculature in the skin, kidneys, and splanchnic organs and diverts blood flow to the heart and brain.

Systemic hypotension and hyperosmolality (see below) stimulate the posterior pituitary to release vasopressin. Vasopressin, like adrenergic discharge and angiotensin II, constricts the vascular sphincters in the skin and splanchnic organs (it does not constrict the renal vasculature) and diverts blood flow to the heart and brain.

RELEASE OF METABOLICALLY ACTIVE HORMONES

Hypovolemia, hypotension, pain, and other stresses of critical illness stimulate the release of three metabolically active hormones—cortisol, glucagon, and epinephrine—all of which increase extracellular glucose concentrations. The glucose provides fuel for nervous system function, metabolism of blood cells, and wound healing; the increased extracellular osmolality helps to replenish vascular volume (see below).

Cortisol, glucagon, and epinephrine increase the extracellular glucose concentration by several mechanisms. All three hormones induce breakdown of hepatic glycogen into glucose, which is released into the hepatic veins and made available to the rest of the body. Cortisol and epinephrine induce breakdown of muscle glycogen into glucose, which is metabolized to lactate. Lactate is then carried to the liver, where it is converted into glucose (via the Cori cycle). Cortisol and epinephrine also induce breakdown of skeletal muscle protein into its constituent amino acids; the amino acids then lose their amino groups and form keto acids and alanine, which are carried to the liver, where they are converted into glucose by gluconeogenesis. To a certain extent, depending on perfusion of the adipose tissue, cortisol and epinephrine induce the breakdown of triglycerides in fat into glycerol and free fatty acids. Glycerol is carried to the liver, where it is converted into glucose, and the free fatty acids serve as an energy source for muscle and viscera.

The result is to increase blood glucose levels at the expense of liver glycogen, muscle glycogen, and muscle protein. If the illness persists, the patient will become debilitated. If the illness does not become too severe and if resuscitation proceeds well, metabolic priorities will be restored to normal. Oxygen consumption and energy expenditure will increase, and the augmented glucose levels will support wound healing and fight infection.

Other hormones with potential metabolic actions, including insulin and growth hormone, are also released during critical illnesses. They have little effect, however, compared with cortisol, glucagon, and epinephrine. Indeed, infusion of cortisol, glucagon, and epinephrine in normal subjects can produce most of the metabolic changes of critical illness.

RELEASE OF VOLUME-CONSERVING HORMONES

Vasopressin, besides being a selective vasopressor, potentiates reabsorption of water by the kidneys. Aldosterone, which is released in response to angiotensin II and corticotropin, stimulates tubular reabsorption of sodium and bicarbonate. These two hormones compensate for hypovolemia in critically ill patients by conserving (but not replenishing) vascular volume.

REPLENISHMENT OF VASCULAR VOLUME

Vascular volume is replenished in hypovolemic patients by the influx of fluid from the cells and interstitium. These fluid shifts are mediated by two mechanisms. The first—and probably the more effective—is initiated by the increased extracellular glucose concentrations of shock. Extracellular hyperosmolality draws water out of the cells, increases interstitial hydrostatic pressure, and drives interstitial protein into the lymphatics and from there into the vascular space. Interstitial oncotic pressure falls, and plasma oncotic pressure rises. The augmented oncotic gradient between the vascular and interstitial spaces draws water, sodium, and chloride into the vascular space. Vascular volume is replenished. This replenishment will continue as long as interstitial hydrostatic pressures are maintained and as

long as interstitial protein stores, which constitute more than half of the total extracellular protein content, can be recruited.

A second—probably less important—mechanism for replenishment of vascular volume arises from arteriolar constriction and the low-flow state of many types of shock. Capillary hydrostatic pressure falls, and water, sodium, and chloride are drawn into the vascular space. The amount of fluid recovered by this mechanism is limited, however. The shift of protein-free fluid from the interstitium to the plasma increases interstitial oncotic pressure and decreases plasma oncotic pressure. The resultant unfavorable oncotic gradient opposes further recovery of fluid.

DILATION OF SYSTEMIC ARTERIOLES

In severely ill patients, three responses—dilation of systemic arterioles, failure of cell membrane function, and disruption of the vascular endothelium—serve to worsen the patient's condition. In decompensated shock, the systemic arterioles lose their ability to constrict, while the postcapillary sphincters remain constricted. Capillary hydrostatic pressure rises. Water, sodium, and chloride are driven out of the vascular space and into the interstitium. The process is limited, however, because the oncotic gradient, which increases as fluid is lost from plasma, prevents further fluid losses.

FAILURE OF CELL MEMBRANE FUNCTION

Cell membrane potentials deteriorate in severely ill patients, and water, sodium, and chloride shift from the extracellular space into the cells even in the face of high extracellular glucose concentrations. This membrane failure accounts for the loss of perhaps 2 L of interstitial fluid, which can be critical because it decreases interstitial hydrostatic pressure, the driving pressure that normally would force interstitial protein back into the vascular space. Membrane failure can thus eliminate the most effective mechanism for replenishment of vascular volume.

DISRUPTION OF VASCULAR ENDOTHELIUM

Trauma and sepsis activate coagulation and inflammation, which can disrupt endothelial integrity in severely ill patients. Platelet and white cell microaggregates that form in injured or infected tissues embolize to the lungs or liver, where they lodge in the capillaries. The microaggregates, endothelium, and plasma in the regions of embolization release kinins, fibrin degradation products, thromboxanes, prostacyclin, prostaglandins, complement, leukotrienes, lysosomal enzymes, oxygen radicals, and other toxic factors, which damage the endothelium and dilate the vasculature in the region of the emboli and distally. Protein, water, sodium, and chloride extravasate into the interstitium. The amount of extravasation is unlimited: As long as the endothelium is damaged, protein will extravasate, and water and electrolytes will follow. The edema that results can be massive and can involve any tissue in the body.

■ II. ACUTE PULMONARY FAILURE

CAUSES OF PULMONARY FAILURE IN SURGICAL PATIENTS

There are nine causes of severe pulmonary failure in the surgical patient: the acute respiratory distress syndrome, inability to effectively expand the lungs because of mechanical abnormalities, atelectasis, aspiration, pulmonary contusion, pneumonia, pulmonary embolus, cardiogenic pulmonary edema, and, rarely, neurogenic pulmonary edema.

ACUTE RESPIRATORY DISTRESS SYNDROME

Acute respiratory distress syndrome (ARDS) typically follows shock and either trauma or sepsis, which activate coagulation and inflammation in the injured or infected tissues and release coagulative and inflammatory mediators into the circulation. The lungs bear the brunt of the insult from any process that involves the nonsplanchnic portions of the body because they receive all the venous blood that returns to the heart and because they contain the first microvasculature encountered by the mediators. (The liver bears the initial brunt of mediators released into the portal venous system.) The mediators disrupt the microvascular endothelium, and plasma extravasates into the interstitium and alveoli. The resultant pulmonary edema impairs both ventilation and oxygenation; the embolization to the lungs impairs perfusion. Arterial oxygen saturation decreases and carbon dioxide content increases—assuming that no compensatory mechanisms come into play.

A number of different mediators of coagulation and inflammation have been implicated as causes of the increased permeability. Platelet and white cell aggregates formed in response to injury or infection are trapped in the lungs, where they engender an inflammatory response. Proteases, kinins, complement, oxygen radicals, prostaglandins, thromboxanes, leukotrienes, lysosomal enzymes, and other mediators are released from the aggregates or from the endothelium or plasma as a consequence of the interaction between the aggregates and the vessel wall. Some of these substances are chemoattractants of more platelets and white blood cells, and a vicious cycle of inflammation develops that worsens the disruption of the vascular endothelium. Infection, disease, injury, and ischemia in nonpulmonary tissues thus lead to damage and dysfunction in previously healthy lungs.

The diagnosis is made by the development of hypoxemia approximately 24 hours after resuscitation from shock and either trauma or sepsis in the absence of other common causes of hypoxemia under these conditions—mechanical failure, atelectasis, aspiration, and pulmonary contusion. The chest x-ray usually shows a diffuse infiltrate. The lungs develop a nonspecific inflammatory reaction. Interstitial edema appears within a few hours after injury or sepsis, and alveolar flooding is florid within 1 day. Monocytes and neutrophils invade the interstitium, and scar tissue begins to form within a week. If the process is unchecked, the lungs become sodden and resemble liver tissue on gross inspection; they eventually may become fibrotic. If treatment is effective, the lungs can return to normal, both grossly and microscopically. The process of diagnosis and the pathologic features of ARDS are identical to those of the so-called **fat embolism syndrome,** which is, for practical purposes, merely a special case of ARDS in which the release of marrow fat into the blood contributes to the development of pulmonary microvascular damage. Nothing is gained by making a distinction between the two entities.

MECHANICAL FAILURE

Mechanical failure can arise from chest wall trauma, pain and weakness after surgery and anesthesia, debility caused by the catabolic metabolism of long-term illness, or bronchopleural fistula. Massive trauma to the chest with multiple fractures of multiple ribs or bilateral disruption of the costochondral junctions can result in a free-floating segment of chest wall known as a **flail chest:** Expansion and relaxation of the rest of the chest wall with spontaneous breathing results in paradoxic motion of the free segment in response to changes in intrathoracic pressure; ventilation becomes compromised; and the arterial PCO_2 increases. Lesser degrees of chest wall injury can lead to hypoventilation because of pain associated with breathing. Prolonged mechanical ventilation with loss of muscle mass and power in the diaphragm and the accessory muscles of respiration can require ventilatory support until muscle function returns to normal. A bronchopleural fistula—a communication from the airway to the pleural cavity to the atmosphere, either through a chest tube or through a hole in the chest wall—can develop after pulmonary surgery, trauma, or infection. Large air leaks can compromise ventilation to the uninvolved lung as well as to the diseased side because insufflated air preferentially goes to the side with the fistula.

ATELECTASIS

Atelectasis—localized collapse of alveoli—can develop with prolonged immobilization, as during anesthesia or in association with bed rest. The problem is usually full-blown within a few hours after the initiating event. Only mechanical failure (to which it is related), aspiration, cardiogenic pulmonary edema, and pulmonary embolism can produce equivalent levels of hypoxemia so soon. The diagnosis is supported by auscultation of bronchial breath sounds at dependent portions of the lung and occasionally, if severe enough, by x-ray confirmation of plate-like collapse of pulmonary parenchyma. The most reliable confirmation of the diagnosis, however, comes with response to therapy, which can include encouragement of deep breathing and coughing, ambulation, bronchoscopy, and intubation and mechanical ventilation. Atelectasis should respond within a few hours. No other form of pulmonary insufficiency responds as quickly.

ASPIRATION

Aspiration of gastric contents or blood can occur in any patient who cannot protect the airway, eg, one who has just been injured or anesthetized or who is debilitated or obtunded for any reason. Gastric acid or particulate matter in the airways leads to disruption of the alveolar and microvascular membranes, causing interstitial and alveolar edema. The resultant hypoxemia is usually evident within a few hours and is associated with a localized infiltrate on x-ray. Recovery of gastric contents by suctioning from the endotracheal tree confirms the diagnosis.

PULMONARY CONTUSION

Pulmonary contusion arises from direct trauma to the chest wall and the underlying lung parenchyma. Hypoxemia associated with a localized infiltrate on x-ray develops over 24 hours as the injured lung becomes edematous.

PNEUMONIA

Pneumonia can arise primarily or can be superimposed on aspiration, pulmonary contusion, or ARDS. The diagnosis is made by recovery of bacteria and purulent material from the endotracheal tree, hypoxemia, signs of systemic sepsis, and a localized infiltrate on x-ray.

PULMONARY EMBOLISM

(See also Chapter 37.)

Sudden deterioration of pulmonary function 5 days or more after an event—such as an operation, injury, or the beginning of immobilization—that can stimulate deposition of clot in a large systemic vein should suggest the possibility of pulmonary embolism. Patients with cancer are at particularly high risk, and in any patient the greater the magnitude of operation or injury, the greater the chance of venous thrombosis and embolization. The chest film is usually nonspecific. Definitive diagnosis can on rare occasions be made by a radionuclide perfusion scan, but this approach can only be successful in the face of a completely normal chest x-ray—an unusual occurrence after a major procedure. High-definition computed tomograms of the chest can sometimes make the diagnosis but carry the risks associated with transfer to the radiology suite and the use of large amounts of radiographic contrast material. Pulmonary arteriography carries the same risks—transfer to the radiology suite and use of contrast—but has the enormous advantage of giving a definitive diagnosis with one diagnostic test. Treatment can sometimes be initiated as well during arteriography by infusing lytic agents into the clot and placing a filter into the inferior vena cava as the pulmonary arterial catheter is withdrawn. Pulmonary angiography is necessary for diagnosis in most hospitalized surgical patients.

Clot emboli must be organized to be clinically significant; embolism to the lung of fresh soft clot rarely causes any difficulty. The pulmonary endothelium contains potent fibrinolysins that can break up any poorly organized embolus. Sudden deterioration in pulmonary function sooner than 5 days after an event that stimulates clot formation is only rarely caused by an embolus; the deterioration is more likely to be caused by mechanical failure, atelectasis, aspiration, or pneumonia.

CARDIOGENIC PULMONARY EDEMA

Cardiogenic pulmonary edema arises from high left atrial and pulmonary microvascular hydrostatic pressures. Patients who have suffered an acute myocardial infarction can present this way, as can patients with underlying myocardial or coronary artery disease when faced with fluid shifts and surgical stress. Occasionally, the rapid administration of intravenous fluid—especially in elderly patients with poor myocardial performance—will outstrip the heart's ability to pump, and pulmonary edema will result. Acute valvular disease, though quite rare after injury or cardiac surgery, is another possible cause of inability of the left heart to pump effectively. The diagnosis is made on the basis of hypoxemia, rales, a third heart sound, perihilar infiltrates, Kerley's lines, and cephalization of blood flow on x-ray along with elevated pulmonary arterial wedge pressures on Swan-Ganz catheterization.

NEUROGENIC PULMONARY EDEMA

Neurogenic pulmonary edema is associated both experimentally and clinically with head injury and increased intracranial pressure. The exact mechanism by which this occurs is unknown, but it is probably related to sympathetic discharge with postmicrovascular vasoconstriction in the lungs and a resultant increase in pulmonary microvascular hydrostatic pressure. This form of pulmonary edema and oxygenation defect is rare, and other causes should be considered also in patients with head injury.

USE OF THE MECHANICAL VENTILATOR

INDICATIONS

Intubation of the airway and mechanical ventilation are indicated for treatment of established pulmonary failure, prophylaxis against potential failure, airway protection, and pulmonary toilet. Pulmonary insufficiency will usually require mechanical ventilation if on room air the patient has a $PaCO_2$ of 45 mm Hg or more or a PaO_2 of 60 mm Hg or less, but these guidelines should be related to the clinical status of the patient. A $PaCO_2$ of 40 mm Hg in a patient breathing 40 times per minute is as alarming as a $PaCO_2$ of 60 mm Hg in a patient with a respiratory rate of 10/min. A PaO_2 of 60 mm Hg on room air in an elderly patient with chronic lung disease may be acceptable; the same value in a young patient who is tensing the sternocleidomastoid and intercostal muscles with each breath and who seems to be struggling to draw in enough air, making excessive or dyscoordinated use of the abdominal musculature, would mandate immediate intubation. A postoperative patient after debridement of necrotizing fasciitis should remain ventilated until it is clear that the overall clinical status is improving even if the patient is capable of independent oxygenation and ventilation in the immediate postoperative period. A patient with stridor or with maxillofacial trauma or pharyngeal edema may need intubation to maintain the airway. A patient with a severe head injury and depressed mental status may require intubation to protect the airway

from aspiration. Intubation may also be indicated for repeated suctioning of the tracheobronchial tree in a patient with a weak gag reflex or inability to cough and clear secretions.

The indications for intubation should be more liberal for a surgical patient than for a medical patient. The medical patient with an exacerbation of chronic obstructive lung disease can be poorly served by placement of a foreign body in his trachea. Airway resistance increases, coughing effectiveness decreases, and opportunistic organisms obtain a foothold on and near the tube. Benefit from intubation may be minimal in that the patient may respond to treatment without mechanical ventilation.

Circumstances for the seriously ill surgical patient are usually different. The patient who has multiple injuries, for example, can temporarily tolerate the increased airway resistance, loss of cough, and increased likelihood of tracheobronchial infection. What cannot be tolerated is respiratory arrest during trauma resuscitation. Furthermore, in all likelihood, such patients will eventually require mechanical ventilation anyway. ARDS strikes the lungs 2 days after the injury, not initially. It is safest to secure the airway early; the tube can be removed later if the patient's condition improves faster than expected.

TYPES OF INTUBATION

The trachea can be intubated via the mouth, the nose, the cricothyroid membrane (cricothyroidostomy), or directly (tracheostomy). Orotracheal and nasotracheal intubation involve passage of a tube through the oropharynx and nasopharynx, respectively; cricothyroidostomy and tracheostomy are surgical procedures requiring a neck incision.

The orotracheal route allows for passage of a larger tube than the nasotracheal route. Nasotracheal intubation requires the presence of spontaneous ventilation in order to guide tube placement and therefore cannot be accomplished in many situations. Conversely, nasotracheal intubation is more comfortable for the awake patient and avoids any need for paralysis and heavy sedation. Nasotracheal tubes can lead to sinusitis by interfering with normal sinus drainage, a complication not seen with orotracheal intubation. Nasotracheal tubes can lead to pressure necrosis of the skin of the nares. Pressure necrosis can also occur in the corner of the mouth with orotracheal tubes but is less common than with nasotracheal intubation, because moving the tube from one side of the mouth to the other is possible. Nasotracheal intubation requires no neck extension and may be preferable to orotracheal intubation in patients with suspected cervical spine fractures. Under no circumstances, however, should concern about the cervical spine lead to prolonged unsuccessful attempts at nasotracheal intubation in critically injured patients. The risk of respiratory arrest outweighs the risk of exacerbating cervical spine injury in such situations. The limited neck extension required for orotracheal intubation is safe even in most cases of unstable cervical spine fracture. Flexion and rotation of the neck, on the other hand, put the unstable cervical spine at risk for increased neurologic damage. Axial traction should be maintained during intubation to guard against flexion and rotation.

Cricothyroidostomy is indicated when an urgent surgical airway is needed. Tracheostomy is more difficult than cricothyroidostomy and should not be done in such situations. Patients with extensive maxillofacial trauma can be impossible to intubate by the orotracheal or nasotracheal route. Intubation can also be difficult because of poor patient cooperation, altered anatomy, or airway or laryngeal swelling—or because of inexperience on the part of the person trying to do the intubating. When the patient is in extremis and respiratory collapse is imminent, prolonged attempts at orotracheal or nasotracheal intubation should be avoided. If orotracheal intubation is not successful after one or two attempts, cricothyroidostomy should be done. The cricothyroid membrane in the midline is bounded superiorly by the lower border of the thyroid cartilage. It is located by palpation and is incised by a stab incision. After the hole has been enlarged with the knife handle, a No. 4 or No. 6 tracheostomy tube should be inserted into the trachea. The patient can then be supported with mechanical ventilation and supplemental oxygen as necessary. Cricothyroidostomies maintained for longer than 2 or 3 days may produce glottic and subglottic stenosis; therefore, cricothyroidostomies should be converted to tracheostomies as soon as is safe and practical when intubation beyond 2–3 days is necessary.

Tracheostomies have several advantages over translaryngeal (orotracheal or nasotracheal) intubation: Airway resistance is lower; nursing care is simpler; accidental extubation is less serious—a well-established tracheostomy tract can usually be easily reintubated, and the patient can usually breathe through the stoma while the tube is being replaced; suctioning is more direct; and the tubes do not damage the vocal cords or larynx.

Tracheostomy is also of benefit when weaning from mechanical ventilation is very slow and the patient has been on and off the ventilator a number of times. The presence of a tracheostomy allows for prolonged periods off the ventilator without the requirement for extubation. If the patient develops respiratory distress off the ventilator and a tracheostomy is present, the ventilator can simply be reconnected to the tracheostomy tube.

Translaryngeal intubation, however, has three major advantages over tracheostomies: First, because the tube can be repositioned, the balloon on the end of the tube does not always compress the same area of tracheal mucosa; the tube moves up and down with tracheal motion, minimizing axial friction by the balloon. The result is a much lower incidence of late tracheal stenosis and tracheo-innominate artery and tracheoesophageal fistulas. Second, because the opening of the tube is well away from the neck and chest, intravenous catheters in these areas can be kept sterile. Third, in patients with poor pulmonary compliance and high inspiratory pressures, the need for maintenance of intrapulmonary volume and avoidance of volume leak around the tube cuff is minimized with translaryngeal intubation.

The timing of conversion from a translaryngeal intubation to a tracheostomy is controversial. Recommendations as short as 3 days have been made, but large numbers of patients have been intubated for months by the orotracheal or nasotracheal route without serious sequelae. Patients should be converted when airway protection, pulmonary toilet, or any of the other indications outlined above are present. If, in addition, the need for more than 2–3 weeks of intubation is obvious, the threshold for performing tracheostomy should be lowered. Conversion to tracheostomy should be done only as an elective procedure under controlled conditions. A transverse incision overlying the upper trachea is developed by separating the strap muscles of the neck in the midline. After exposure of the anterior surface of the trachea, a tracheostomy tube is placed through the second or third tracheal ring. Often the thyroid isthmus must be either retracted upward or divided to allow for adequate exposure of the trachea in the proper location.

Endotracheal tubes of all types come with either of two different types of cuffs. High-pressure, low-volume cuffs are useful for short-term intubation and ventilation. Because of the high cuff pressure, however, they interfere with tracheal blood supply and can lead to tracheomalacia, erosion into the innominate artery (tracheo-innominate fistula), erosion into the esophagus (tracheoesophageal fistula), or airway stenosis. They should not be used for long-term intubation; low-pressure, high-volume cuffs are preferable in this circumstance.

VOLUME VENTILATORS

Ventilators can be constructed either to deliver a preset volume (volume ventilators) or to deliver flow continuously until a preset pressure is reached (pressure ventilators). In the past, volume ventilators were commonly used. Today they are used less frequently. They are still quite useful, however, in situations in which the ventilation needs to be kept simple, as in the acutely injured or ill patient. The four main parameters that need to be set on volume ventilators are the rate of ventilation, the tidal volume of each ventilation, the inspired oxygen concentration (FIO_2), and the level of positive end-expiratory pressure (PEEP). Although an oversimplification, ventilator management can be easily understood by dividing these parameters into those concerned primarily with ventilation (rate and tidal volume) and those concerned primarily with oxygenation (FIO_2 and PEEP).

Setting the ventilatory rate tells the ventilator how many times it should cycle per minute. Doubling the rate doubles the minute volume, or the amount of volume delivered by the ventilator each minute. It can be turned up or down depending on the patient's needs. In patients who do not breathe spontaneously, the ventilator rate will equal the total respiratory rate; in patients with spontaneous breaths, the ventilator rate will ensure a certain number of machine-delivered breaths per minute, but the respiratory rate will be greater than the machine rate because of spontaneous breaths. The ventilator rate should be set between 12 and 15 breaths per minute in most patients beginning mechanical ventilation. The rate can be increased or decreased as necessary based on analysis of arterial blood gases. The PCO_2 should be kept close to 40 mm Hg unless hyperventilation is desired, as may be indicated in some in patients with increased intracranial pressure.

Setting the tidal volume dictates how much volume will be delivered with each machine ventilation. The normal tidal volume during resting spontaneous ventilation is 7 mL/kg; the tidal volume in a ventilated patient should be set at the same value. Larger tidal volumes associated with higher airway pressures can damage the epithelium lining the small airways and alveoli. If more ventilation is needed, it is preferable to increase the other determinant of ventilation, the ventilatory rate. If ventilation remains less than normal, as manifested by a persistently elevated $PaCO_2$, it is usually better to accept the hypercapnia as long as the arterial pH exceeds 7.20. Increasing the tidal volume solely for the purpose of creating a normal $PaCO_2$ is ill-advised as long as the pH is acceptable. Hyperexpansion of the alveoli is more damaging to the lungs than hypercapnia is to the body. Occasionally, very high tidal volumes are necessary when a bronchopleural fistula is present. To compensate for the volume lost through the fistula, tidal volume as well as ventilatory rate must be increased.

Inspired oxygen concentration is set by adjusting the oxygen percentage of inspired gas. Oxygen leads to chronic pulmonary fibrosis when administered in concentrations above 50% for prolonged periods, and the FIO_2 should be kept as low as possible consistent with adequate oxygenation. All of the nonoxygen volume of ventilator gas is made up of nitrogen, which, unlike oxygen, is not absorbed from alveoli. When nitrogen is replaced by increasing concentrations of oxygen, increased atelectasis caused by oxygen absorption can occur. For this reason, ventilation with 80–100% oxygen for periods of greater than 1–2 hours should be avoided.

Positive end-expiratory pressure is the other primary determinant of arterial oxygenation. A valve placed in the expiratory circuit of the ventilator ensures that the airway pressure remains above a preset level even at the end of expiration. This keeps the airway pressure above the closing pressure of small airways and minimizes alveolar collapse at end-expiration.

Positive end-expiratory pressure, however, can decrease cardiac output, as described in the section on cardiac compressive shock, and can rupture the lungs. The remedy for decreased cardiac output is usually fluid infusion; the remedy for lung rupture is more of a problem. The ruptures are associated more with peak inspiratory airway pressures than with mean pressures. The patient may develop tension pneumothorax or mediastinal or subcutaneous emphysema, caused by rupture of a bronchus with decompression into the mediastinum. Occasionally, PEEP can even decrease the peak inspiratory pressure by expanding atelectatic areas of the lungs. In most cases, however, the PEEP increases the peak airway pressure by an amount equivalent to the level of the PEEP. This increase in the peak pressure is usually proportionately small, and, fortunately, rupture of the lung caused by PEEP is uncommon in surgical patients, who are likely to have the consolidated lungs of ARDS and not likely to have many pulmonary blebs. Medical patients with emphysema are at much greater risk.

Placement of an endotracheal tube bypasses the normal physiologic PEEP present during spontaneous ventilation from closure of the glottis at the end of expiration. Low levels of "physiologic" PEEP (5 cm H_2O) should probably be used in most intubated patients with severe pulmonary dysfunction to maintain arterial oxygen saturation and to keep the inspired oxygen concentration below 50%. Balancing the complications of high inspired oxygen concentration and high PEEP can be difficult in patients with major defects in oxygenation, but if possible the inspired oxygen concentration should be kept below 50% and the level of PEEP below 20 cm H_2O.

The oxygen saturation of arterial blood should be kept above 90% in most cases. Patients with chronic obstructive pulmonary disease and long-standing CO_2 retention are an exception. Such patients have lost the ability to increase their respiratory drive in response to increases in PCO_2 and rely instead on their response to hypoxemia. Increasing the arterial oxygen saturation by adding exogenous oxygen takes away this hypoxic ventilatory stimulus and makes weaning from ventilatory support more difficult.

The two basic modes available on most volume ventilators are assist or control mode ventilation (assist-control ventilation) and intermittent mandatory ventilation (IMV). Assist-control ventilation is designed to assist any ventilatory efforts made by the patient by delivering a machine breath. Whenever the patient begins to inspire, the ventilator is triggered and the preset machine tidal volume is given. A machine backup rate is also set to ensure a minimal number of machine breaths in the absence of spontaneous ventilatory efforts. Assist-control mode ventilation requires minimal ventilatory effort from the patient and minimizes the work of breathing. It is useful in patients recovering from anesthesia and in patients with flail chest. Assist-control mode ventilation, by assisting all of the patient's ventilatory efforts, minimizes pain and paradoxic motion of the flail segment. A disadvantage of assist-control ventilation is that hyperventilation can occur if the patient's respiratory rate increases. It is also difficult to wean a patient from ventilatory support when assist-control ventilation is being used because the ventilator continually compensates for weak or absent spontaneous ventilatory efforts.

Intermittent mandatory ventilation was designed to overcome the limitations of the assist-control mode. Intermittent machine breaths are delivered at a predetermined rate and—unlike assist-control—are given to the patient regardless of the spontaneous respiratory rate. Between the intermittent mandatory ventilations, however, the patient's spontaneous respiratory efforts are not assisted, and the patient thus generates his or her own tidal volume. Synchronized intermittent mandatory ventilation (SIMV) is a modification of IMV designed to deliver the preset number of machine breaths in synchrony with some of the patient's own ventilatory efforts, but the principle of spontaneously generated tidal volumes between machine breaths is the same as with IMV. Intermittent mandatory ventilation requires increased work of breathing by the patient as compared with assist-control, and the rate of machine breaths can be varied to increase or decrease the patient's contribution to ventilation. At very high IMV rates, all ventilation is done by the ventilator, and the patient's contribution is minimal. As the rate is gradually decreased, the patient must increasingly ventilate himself to maintain minute volume. Incrementally decreasing the IMV rate can be used as a means of weaning from the ventilator. Clinical status, respiratory rate, and the arterial PCO_2 are used to guide the weaning process.

The four basic parameters to be set on a volume ventilator—ventilatory rate, tidal volume, FIO_2, and PEEP—and the two basic modes of ventilation—assist-control and IMV—thus need to be adjusted in relation to each other and in response to the patient's blood gases and clinical condition. As an example, the typical patient who requires mechanical ventilation after a major injury should be started on assist-control with a backup rate of 15 breaths/min and a tidal volume of 7 mL/kg. The FIO_2 should initially be set at 1.00, and no PEEP should be used. As blood gas measurements become available, the tidal volume should be kept at 7 mL/kg; the respiratory rate should be adjusted to keep the $PaCO_2$ around 40 mm Hg. The FIO_2 can be lowered to bring an excessively high PaO_2 down, but the value should be kept between 90 and 120 mm Hg until the patient is hemodynamically stable. Once stability is achieved and once the patient is in an ICU, the FIO_2 should be lowered to bring the PaO_2 into the range of 65–90 mm Hg. PEEP should be added as full monitoring becomes available and increased to levels as high as 20 cm H_2O, if necessary, to bring the FIO_2 to less than 0.50. When the patient becomes a candidate for weaning, he or she can be switched to IMV.

PRESSURE VENTILATORS

Pressure ventilators are now commonly used in patients who require long-term ventilation—in whom it becomes critical to avoid high airway pressures and large tidal volumes. Pressure support ventilation and pressure control with inverse ratio ventilation (IRV) are two of the new modes used with these ventilators. Pressure support can be used with IMV and provides the patient with a constant predetermined level of airway pressure during spontaneous inspiration. Machine IMV breaths are unaffected. It can also be used as the sole means of ventilatory support in patients who require long-term mechanical ventilation as long as the patient can initiate spontaneous breaths. The pressure support is typically supplied for approximately 90% of the time during which the patient inspires. The interval is determined by analog circuits within the ventilator and usually cannot be adjusted by the physician. Providing pressure support by assisting the patient during spontaneous breathing increases spontaneous tidal volumes and decreases the work of breathing. It also helps overcome resistance to inspiratory flow in the endotracheal tube and the ventilatory apparatus. Although its role is still being defined, pressure support seems to be useful in managing patients who have been difficult to wean from the ventilator. Arbitrary levels of pressure support between 5 and 25 cm H_2O can be provided, or the amount of pressure support necessary can be set by determining a desired level of spontaneous tidal volume and then gradually adjusting the pressure support until that tidal volume is reached.

Pressure control ventilation is similar conceptually to pressure support ventilation but provides a constant inspiratory pressure during machine breaths and for the entirety of the breath. It is generally used in conjunction with inverse ratio ventilation (IRV). In addition to ventilatory rate and tidal volume, the relative amounts of time in the ventilatory cycle spent in inspiration and expiration (I:E) must be set. In standard modes of ventilation, this ratio is set at 1:2 to approximate spontaneous ventilation. Inverse ratio ventilation increases the proportion of the ventilatory cycle spent in inspiration and changes this relationship to anywhere between 1:1 and 4:1. Pressure control ventilation is used with IRV in order to maintain a constant inspiratory airway pressure and safely allow initiation of a new inspiration before expiratory flow from the previous ventilatory cycle has reached zero. The resultant air trapping with each ventilatory cycle is thought to minimize alveolar collapse and improve the distribution of inspired volume. Pressure control and IRV are primarily useful in patients with profound oxygenation defects and poor compliance. Paralysis is usually required to tolerate IRV, and care must be taken to ensure that uncontrolled air trapping does not lead to barotrauma.

WEANING FROM MECHANICAL VENTILATION

Weaning from mechanical ventilation depends on the type of ventilatory support being provided. When the patient is on IMV, weaning is accomplished by gradually decreasing the IMV rate. Decreasing the rate with the object of removing the patient from the ventilator is generally not appropriate until oxygen requirements are at or below an FIO_2 of 40% and a PEEP of 5 cm H_2O. When these requirements have been met, the weaning process can begin and the IMV rate can be reduced. As outlined above, this requires the patient to contribute increasingly to the maintenance of adequate minute ventilation. The patient's overall clinical status, respiratory rate, and arterial PCO_2 should be used as guidelines to determine the rate of weaning. When an IMV of 4/min or less is well tolerated for long periods, a trial of spontaneous ventilation without any machine support should be conducted. This is done by putting the patient on a T-piece trial in which the endotracheal tube forms the long arm of the T and is connected to a blow-by oxygen source. All ventilation must be done by the patient, and if the trial is well tolerated for 30 minutes that is usually an indication that the patient is extubatable. The patient should not be stressed excessively during trials of spontaneous ventilation. The ventilatory rate should not exceed 25/min, and breathing should not be allowed to become labored. T-piece trials should be limited to no more than 30 minutes. If the patient

can be extubated at the end of the trial, the tube should be removed. If the patient cannot be extubated, mechanical ventilation should be reinstituted.

"Wind sprints" are another method for weaning patients who have required extended periods of mechanical ventilation. The patient is managed with intermittent periods on a T-piece alternating with periods of assist-control ventilation or IMV. The length and frequency of the T-piece periods are gradually increased as the patient's ability to ventilate spontaneously improves. When 30-minute periods on a T-piece with continuous positive airway pressure (CPAP) are well tolerated, the patient can be extubated.

Pressure support in conjunction with IMV is useful in weaning patients who have required mechanical ventilation for a long time. After it has been instituted, pressure support should be maintained while the IMV rate is gradually decreased. When the IMV rate has been reduced to 4/min or less, gradual decreases in the level of pressure support can be started. The patient can be tried on a T-piece when the pressure support is minimal or has been completely discontinued. As with weaning from IMV without pressure support, the patient's clinical status, respiratory rate, degree of dyspnea, and PCO_2 are the guidelines used during the weaning process.

If the patient is on pure pressure support ventilation, the weaning process becomes quite straightforward. The amount of pressure support is gradually reduced, and the patient's ability to tolerate extubation (see below) is assessed daily. When the amount of pressure needed to sustain adequate ventilation over a 24-hour period is less than 10 cm H_2O and when the patient meets the criteria for extubation as listed below, the patient is extubated.

Patients who seem to be doing well and who have required mechanical ventilation for less than 24 hours can frequently be extubated quickly after going straight to a single T-piece trial. Patients on IRV are not candidates for weaning from the ventilator until they improve enough to allow for their return to one of the standard modes of ventilation.

EXTUBATION

Both objective and subjective criteria are used to determine if a patient is ready for extubation. Objective measures of pulmonary function include the respiratory rate, the arterial PCO_2, and the patient's ability to oxygenate. The respiratory rate on a T-piece should be less than 25/min if extubation is being considered and in ideal circumstances should be below 20/min. In most instances, the PCO_2 should be 42 mm Hg or less with an acceptably low respiratory rate. In patients with chronic CO_2 retention or metabolic alkalosis with respiratory compensation, higher P_{CO_2} levels are acceptable as long as the arterial pH is 7.34 or greater. A pH lower than this indicates that the elevation in P_{CO_2} is acute and poorly tolerated. The patient should have an arterial oxygen saturation of greater than 90% on an F_{IO_2} of 40% or less and a PEEP of 5 cm H_2O or less.

Subjective criteria for extubation are also important. The patient's underlying disease process will often dictate whether extubation is appropriate. A critically ill patient requiring further operative procedures and with a guarded prognosis may require continued intubation and mechanical ventilatory support in spite of current fairly good pulmonary function. Inability to protect the airway is another indication for continued intubation even when the patient's ability to oxygenate and ventilate are adequate. Finally, there is a gestalt determination of a patient's ability to tolerate extubation and spontaneous ventilation. A patient who can lift his head off the pillow, has a sparkle in his eye, and obviously wants the endotracheal tube removed is a good candidate for extubation; a lethargic, diaphoretic patient is not.

ADJUVANT TREATMENT OF PULMONARY INSUFFICIENCY

Mechanical ventilation is the mainstay of therapy for treatment of severe pulmonary insufficiency in the surgical patient. Mechanical ventilation, however, introduces problems, such as bacterial colonization of the tracheobronchial tree, that may require adjuvant treatment. The underlying disease process may also require adjuvant treatment.

ANTIBIOTICS

Bacteria can be recovered from tracheal secretions of any patient who has been intubated and on mechanical ventilation for several days. The question is when to treat with antibiotics. Indications include purulent sputum associated with abundant white cells on Gram-stained smears; pathogenic organisms recovered from suctioning; signs of systemic sepsis with increasing fluid requirements and increasing blood glucose concentrations; worsening pulmonary function, as judged by the need to increase inspired oxygen concentrations or end-expiratory pressure; and worsening signs on chest x-ray. If all of these are present, antibiotics should be started. If only one or two are present, antibiotics are probably best withheld to avoid overgrowth of resistant organisms that could later cause fatal pneumonia.

Older patients may have only one chance to survive a critical period of illness and should probably be given antibiotics sooner than younger patients, who are better able to recover after prolonged illness. Thus, an 80-year-old patient with flail chest should probably be given antibiotics early; a 20-year-old patient who was hospitalized for a gunshot wound involving the colon and who develops questionable pneumonia 2 weeks later should probably be given antibiotics only when infection is definitely confirmed and the causative organisms are identified.

CLOTTING FACTORS

After severe trauma or major sepsis, many patients will demonstrate signs of intravascular coagulation, with prolonged clotting times, low platelet counts, decreased fibrinogen levels, and production of fibrin degradation products or fibrin monomers. Nevertheless, if the patient is not bleeding, fresh-frozen plasma and platelets should not be given; they will only add fuel to the fire of systemic inflammation and coagulation. They should, however, be given to patients who are bleeding and to those with severe head injuries who could develop a sudden irretrievable and devastating hemorrhage.

MUSCLE RELAXANTS

Muscle relaxants sometimes greatly simplify ventilatory management in patients with severe pulmonary insufficiency, particularly those with recent injuries or sepsis. Because struggling against the ventilator can compromise ventilatory and cardiovascular function, it may be necessary to paralyze the patient when mechanical ventilation is being instituted. Muscle relaxants are dangerous, however, and should only be used when absolutely necessary and for the shortest possible time. Undetected malfunction of a ventilator may mean death for the paralyzed patient.

CHEST X-RAYS

Chest x-rays should be obtained daily in patients being treated with mechanical ventilation. Films are unreliable in differentiating cardiogenic from noncardiogenic edema, however, and visible changes lag behind clinical changes. Films are helpful in diagnosing contusion, aspiration, and pneumonia and may demonstrate a small pneumothorax or mediastinal emphysema. They show positioning of endotracheal tubes, nasogastric tubes, feeding tubes, central venous catheters, and pulmonary arterial catheters. They may show dilation of the trachea at the site of the balloon on the end of the endotracheal tube.

■ III. EVALUATION OF SHOCK & PULMONARY FAILURE IN THE ICU

Serious pulmonary failure in the surgical patient can be associated with concomitant cardiac dysfunction and is almost always associated with hypoxemia, hypercapnia, or acidemia. The Swan-Ganz catheter can be very useful in evaluating cardiac function; an understanding of hypoxemia, hypercapnia, and acidemia rests on an understanding of (1) the relationship between the Po_2, the oxygen saturation of hemoglobin, and the oxygen content of blood; (2) the relationship between the Pco_2 in systemic arterial blood and the concept of alveolar ventilation; (3) the causes of hypoxemia; and (4) the relationship between hydrogen ion concentration ($[H^+]$), Pco_2, and bicarbonate concentration ($[HCO_3^-]$).

SWAN-GANZ CATHETER

The balloon- and thermistor-tipped pulmonary arterial catheter permits measurement of the cardiac output; right atrial, pulmonary arterial, and pulmonary arterial wedge pressures; and mixed venous oxygen contents. Knowledge of the cardiac index (cardiac output divided by body surface area) and filling pressures can be used to assess ventricular function as fluid is administered or withheld. The mixed venous oxygen saturation reflects the adequacy of oxygen delivery to the periphery; a value less than 60% indicates inadequate peripheral oxygenation and can be used to evaluate adequacy of the cardiac index and of systemic arterial oxygen content. It can also be used to determine oxygen consumption, which is calculated as the cardiac index multiplied by the difference of the oxygen contents of blood in the systemic and pulmonary arteries. Oxygen consumption can fall in severely ill patients, and measurements of consumption can help assess the patient's response to resuscitation (Table 13–3).

The catheter is particularly useful when treatment of one organ system might harm another. For example, fluid administration might be needed to treat septic shock, but excess fluid might contribute to pulmonary failure; a diuretic might be indicated in an oliguric patient in congestive heart failure, but excessive diuresis might decrease the cardiac output to the point that the kidneys fail; and fluid might be needed for cardiovascular resuscitation in a patient with multiple injuries, but too much fluid might exacerbate cerebral edema. The pulmonary arterial catheter can be extremely helpful in these situations.

Data obtained from the Swan-Ganz catheter can be misleading, however, if mistakes are made in performing the measurements. The cardiac output, as measured by thermodilution, is obtained by injecting a known volume of a solution cooler than blood into the right atrium and measuring the temperature drop in the blood as it flows past a thermistor on the end of the pulmonary arterial catheter. The greater the area under the temperature curve, the less the amount of flow through the right heart. Injections should be made at the same time in the ventilatory cycle, because flow through the right heart varies with the phase of ventilation. Calculations of the cardiac output are made by computer.

When one is obtaining pulmonary arterial or mixed venous blood, the balloon on the end of the catheter should be deflated, and the blood should be withdrawn slowly. If the blood is withdrawn too quickly, the walls of the pulmonary artery will collapse around the end of the catheter, and the specimen will be contaminated by blood that is pulled back, in a retrograde manner, past ventilated and nonperfused alveoli.

All pressures measured with the pulmonary arterial catheter should be recorded from tracings displayed on an oscilloscope. The number recorded should be the pressure at end-expiration regardless of the patient's ventilatory mode.

Of the five pressures obtained from the catheter, only two—the right atrial and the mean pulmonary arterial pressures—can be taken at face value; the other three—the pulmonary arterial systolic, diastolic, and wedge pressures—are subject to errors of measurement and interpretation. The pulmonary arterial wedge pressure usually is the same as the left atrial pressure. The wedge pressure will not reflect left atrial pressure, however, if the catheter is in a portion of the vasculature occluded by inflated alveoli. If the wedge pressure varies by more than 10 mm Hg with cycles of mechanical ventilation one should assume that the tip of the catheter is facing the pressure in the alveoli rather than the pressure in the left atrium.

OXYHEMOGLOBIN DISSOCIATION

The concentration of oxygen in the blood, or oxygen content (Co_2), is expressed as milliliters of O_2/dL of blood, or vol%. This quantity is the most important of the three different measures of oxygenation of the blood. The Co_2 can be measured directly, but the measurement is time-consuming, and the content is usually calculated on the basis of the other two measures of blood oxygenation, the oxygen saturation (So_2) and the Po_2. The Co_2 is related to these other quantities by the following formula:

$$Co_2 = 1.34 \times [Hb] \times So_2 + 0.0031 \times Po_2$$

Table 13–3. Normal values obtained from commonly used monitors.[1]

Variable	Abbreviation or Deviation	Normal Value	Units
Partial pressure of oxygen in systemic arterial blood	Pao_2	Varies (eg, 95 for young adult, 80 for elderly)	mm Hg
Partial pressure of carbon dioxide in arterial blood	$Paco_2$	40; does not vary with age	mm Hg
Oxygen saturation in arterial blood	Sao_2	97%	Dimensionless
Oxygen content in arterial blood	Cao_2[2] $^4/_3 \times$ [Hb] $\times Sao_2$	20	mL O_2/dL blood, or vol%
Partial pressure of oxygen in mixed venous blood	$Pmvo_2$	40	mm Hg
Partial pressure of carbon dioxide in mixed venous blood	$Pmvco_2$	46	mm Hg
Oxygen saturation in mixed venous blood	$Smvo_2$	75%	Dimensionless
Oxygen content in mixed venous blood	$Cmvo_2$[2] $^4/_3 \times$ [Hb] $\times Smvo_2$	15	mL O_2/dL blood, or vol %
pH (arterial blood)		7.4	Dimensionless
Hydrogen ion concentration	See Table 13–5	40	nmol/L
Bicarbonate ion concentration	$(24 \times Pco_2) \div [H^+]$	24	mmol/L
Cardiac index	CI	3	$L \cdot min^{-1} \cdot min^{-2}$
Mean systemic arterial pressure	Pa	93	mm Hg
Mean right atrial pressure	P_{RA}	3[3]	mm Hg
Mean pulmonary arterial pressure	P_{PA}	15[3]	mm Hg
Mean wedge pressure	P_{wedge}	8[3]	mm Hg
Systemic vascular resistance	$(Pa-P_{RA}) \div CI$	30	$mm Hg \cdot L \cdot min^{-1} \cdot m^{-2}$
Oxygen transport	$CI \times Cao_2$	600	$mL O_2 \cdot min^{-1} \cdot m^{-2}$
Oxygen return	$CI \times Cmvo_2$	450	$mL O_2 \cdot min^{-1} \cdot m^{-2}$
Oxygen consumption	$CI \times (Cao_2-Cmvo_2)$	150	$mL O_2 \cdot min^{-1} \cdot m^{-2}$

[1]Reproduced, with permission, from Abrams JH, Cerra F, Holcroft JW: Cardiopulmonary monitoring, in: *Care of the Surgical Patient.* Vol 1. Critical Care, Section II. Care in the ICU. Wilmore DW et al (editors). Scientific American, 1989.
[2]Oxygen contents calculated on the assumption that [Hb] equals 15 g % and that O_2 consumption and cardiac index are normal.
[3]Values given are for when the patient is breathing spontaneously. Pressures, on average, will be 5 mm Hg higher if the patient is being mechanically ventilated.

where [Hb] is expressed as g/dL and the P_{O_2} as mm Hg. Thus, for example, the C_{O_2} of a blood specimen with a [Hb] of 12 g/dL, an S_{O_2} of 90%, and a P_{O_2} of 60 mm Hg is 14.7 vol%.

The first term in the equation represents the O_2 carried by the hemoglobin molecule; the second, the O_2 dissolved in the blood water. This second term is small compared with the first as long as the [Hb] is greater than (say) 7 g/dL and the P_{O_2} is less than (say) 100 mm Hg. Omitting the second term then simplifies the formula to read as follows:

$$C_{O_2} = 1.34 \times [Hb] \times S_{O_2}$$

For the previous set of blood gases, this would give a C_{O_2} of 14.5 vol%.

The formula can be made even simpler by substituting the fraction ⁴⁄₃ for the decimal 1.34:

$$C_{O_2} = {}^4\!/_3 \times [Hb] \times S_{O_2} \qquad \textbf{(1)}$$

Because [Hb] and the S_{O_2} can usually be approximated by integers with little loss of accuracy, the calculation frequently allows cancellation of the three and can be done mentally. For the previous example, the C_{O_2} would be 14.4 vol%.

Calculation of the C_{O_2} requires knowledge of the S_{O_2}. Many pulmonary arterial catheters are now equipped with sensors mounted on their tips that directly measure the saturation of the blood in the pulmonary artery. Alternatively, blood can be withdrawn from the tip of the catheter and sent to the laboratory, where the S_{O_2} can be easily measured by an instrument known as a co-oximeter. Most laboratories will make this measurement by specific request, but some will calculate the S_{O_2} from the P_{O_2}. This calculation is frequently inaccurate for mixed venous specimens but is usually accurate for arterial blood. The calculation is made from equations that are based on the oxyhemoglobin dissociation curve (Figure 13–1), an empirically derived relationship between the S_{O_2} of human blood and its P_{O_2}. The saturation for a given P_{O_2} depends on blood temperature, [H⁺], and P_{CO_2} and on the red cell concentration of 2,3-diphosphoglycerate (2,3-DPG). The laboratory should be told the temperature, and it will measure the [H⁺] and P_{CO_2}. It will then calculate the S_{O_2} from the P_{O_2} with the assumption that the 2,3-DPG concentration is normal.

It is helpful, however, to have some guidelines for converting back and forth between S_{O_2} and P_{O_2}. Five approximations for points on the dissociation curve for a patient with normal temperature, [H⁺], P_{CO_2}, and 2,3-

Figure 13–1. Oxyhemoglobin dissociation curve for human blood at 37 °C with a P_{CO_2} of 40 mm Hg, a pH of 7.40, and a normal 2,3-DPG red cell concentration. Approximate values from Table 13–4 fall close to the idealized curve.

DPG level are given in Table 13–4. The P_{50} of human hemoglobin—the P_{O_2} at which the molecule is half-saturated—is 27 mm Hg (approximated as 25 mm Hg in the table). The P_{O_2} and S_{O_2} for mixed venous blood in a person with a [Hb] of 15 g/dL and a normal O_2 consumption and cardiac output are 40 mm Hg and 75%, respectively. A P_{O_2} of 60 mm Hg—a value that should be exceeded by most patients in an ICU—corresponds to an S_{O_2} of 90%. A P_{O_2} of 80 mm Hg corresponds to an S_{O_2} of 96%. Remembering the values in the table allows construction of a dissociation curve and facilitates conversion from one measure of oxygenation to the other. For example, in a patient with a normal temperature, [H⁺], P_{CO_2}, and 2,3-DPG and a [Hb] of 10 g/dL, a P_{O_2} of 60

Table 13-4. Approximate correlations for partial pressures of oxygen and oxygen saturation in blood at 37 °C with a pH of 7.4, a P_{CO_2} of 40 mm Hg, and a normal 2,3-DPG red cell concentration.

P_{O_2}	S_{O_2}
0 mm Hg	0%
25 mm Hg	50%
40 mm Hg	75%
60 mm Hg	90%
80 mm Hg	95%

mm Hg in the systemic arterial blood would create a CO_2 of 12 vol% (from Equation 1), a value that would be adequate if the patient had normal coronary arteries and a good heart. Such a value would be inadequate, however, in the face of underlying heart disease.

CAUSES OF AN ELEVATED Paco₂

The arterial P_{CO_2} is proportionate to CO_2 production divided by alveolar ventilation—defined as the volume of air exchanged per unit time in functioning alveoli. Since CO_2 production is usually fairly constant in adequately perfused patients, the P_{CO_2} comes to be inversely proportionate to alveolar ventilation. An elevated P_{CO_2} in the presence of normal CO_2 production means inadequate alveolar ventilation. Ventilation should be assessed with respect to how much work is required to generate the P_{CO_2}. In the case of spontaneous ventilation, this assessment involves the frequency and depth of breathing; in the case of mechanical ventilation, the frequency of the machine-generated breaths and the tidal volume of those breaths.

The P_{CO_2} also gives an indication of dead space ventilation—the ventilation of nonperfused airways. Since minute or total ventilation is dead space ventilation plus alveolar ventilation, a normal P_{CO_2} combined with a normal minute ventilation implies a normal dead space ventilation. A normal P_{CO_2} that must be generated by a supranormal minute ventilation implies increased dead space ventilation. Normal dead space ventilation is one-third of total ventilation, but many critically ill surgical patients will have a dead space ventilation that is up to two-thirds of total ventilation. Increased dead space ventilation can be caused by hypovolemia with poor perfusion of nondependent alveoli, ARDS, pulmonary emboli, pulmonary vasoconstriction, and mechanical ventilation-induced compression of the pulmonary vasculature. Hypovolemia should be treated by expansion of the vascular volume. Emboli should be treated by anticoagulation or by elimination of their source. Dead space generated by mechanical ventilation should be minimized by adjustment of the ventilator, usually by decreasing tidal volumes or end-expiratory pressures, while at the same time maintaining enough mechanical support to generate a normal P_{CO_2} and alveolar ventilation.

CAUSES OF A LOW Pao₂

There are five causes of arterial hypoxemia: low inspired O_2 concentration, diffusion block between alveolar gas and capillary blood, subnormal alveolar ventilation, shunting of blood through completely nonventilated portions of the lung or bypassing of blood past the lung, and perfusion of parts of the lung that have low ventilation/perfusion ratios. In addition, any process that decreases the mixed venous CO_2 in the presence of any of the above can lower the arterial P_{O_2} even further. Low mixed venous CO_2 can be caused by a low arterial CO_2, low cardiac output, or high O_2 consumption.

Arterial hypoxemia in the surgical patient is usually caused by shunting, low ventilation/perfusion ratios, low mixed venous CO_2, or a combination of these factors. Low inspired O_2 concentrations at sea level are impossible so long as the ventilator is functioning properly. (This must be checked, however, as the first step in diagnosing and correcting the cause of a low P_{O_2}.) Diffusion block is exceedingly rare in surgical patients. Subnormal alveolar ventilation can be ruled out with a normal arterial P_{CO_2} assuming CO_2 production is not depressed. Thus, shunting and areas of low ventilation/perfusion ratios, along with low mixed venous CO_2, remain as causes for almost all cases of hypoxemia in the surgical patient. Shunting and low ventilation/perfusion ratios do not need to be distinguished from each other very often, but the distinction can be made by increasing the inspired O_2 concentration to 100%: Hypoxemia caused by areas of low ventilation/perfusion ratios will be at least partially corrected by 100% O_2; hypoxemia caused by shunting will not. The mixed venous CO_2 can be measured with the Swan-Ganz catheter. The causes of a low value can be evaluated by measuring the blood hemoglobin concentration, the cardiac output, and the O_2 consumption.

ACID-BASE BALANCE

Hypercapnia represents inadequate alveolar ventilation assuming a normal CO_2 production and, as such, should be a cause for concern, but the elevated P_{CO_2} by itself actually does no harm. It is the acidemia that usually accompanies the hypercapnia which disrupts vital metabolic processes. Thus, it is important to normalize not only the P_{CO_2} and P_{O_2} in the critically ill patient but also the $[H^+]$.

The $[H^+]$, P_{CO_2}, and $[HCO_3^-]$ equilibrate with one another in the plasma water, and if two of the quantities are known, the third can be calculated. In practice, the P_{CO_2} and $[H^+]$ are measured directly, and the $[HCO_3^-]$ is calculated by the Henderson-Hasselbalch equation, which can be written in the following form (see Chapter 10):

$$[HCO_3^-] = \frac{24 \times P_{CO_2}}{[H^+]}$$

(2)

where $[HCO_3^-]$ is expressed as mmol/L, P_{CO_2} as mm Hg, and $[H^+]$ as nmol/L. This form of the equation requires conversion of pH, the more common expression of [H⁺], into nmol/L, the more logical expression, but the conversion is not difficult (Table 13–5). The values in the table are easy to remember if one notes that each value in the column under $[H^+]$ is 80% of the value immediately above, with the exception of 80 and 63, which is off by 1. Thus, by Equation 2, if the P_{CO_2} is 60 mm Hg and the pH is 7.30, the $[HCO_3^-]$ is 29 mmol/L.

The $[HCO_3^-]$ calculated by this equation is the actual amount of bicarbonate ion dissolved in the plasma water and can be obtained only from a specimen of blood that is obtained and processed without exposure to the atmosphere. The "CO_2 combining power" that is typically measured along with electrolyte concentrations in blood that is not processed anaerobically includes not only the $[HCO_3^-]$ but any CO_2 gas and carbonic acid that is dissolved in the plasma as well. The CO_2 combining power is usually about 2 mmol/L greater than the calculated (and actual) $[HCO_3^-]$.

The base deficit or excess is determined by comparing the calculated $[HCO_3^-]$ with the $[HCO_3^-]$ that might be expected in a patient with a given P_{CO_2} and $[H^+]$. These expected values have been determined by analyzing blood obtained from patients with a wide variety of pulmonary disorders. For example, the kidneys in a patient with chronic respiratory acidemia can usually compensate to the extent that a chronic elevation in P_{CO_2} of 10 mm Hg will generate an increase in $[HCO_3^-]$ of 3 mmol/L. A patient with chronic obstructive lung disease and a chronically elevated P_{CO_2} of 60 mm Hg would be expected to have a $[HCO_3^-]$ of 30 mmol/L—6 mmol/L more than a normal value of 24. If such a patient had a pH of 7.30, the actual $[HCO_3^-]$ would be 29 mmol/L (from Equation 2; see the example in the preceding paragraph). That is, the observed value would be 1 mmol/L less than predicted, and the patient would be said to have a base deficit of 1 mmol/L.

The difficulty with the concept of base deficit and excess is that it rests on historically determined values, which may not be applicable to the patient at hand. For example, if a surgical patient with previously normal lungs lost his or her airway after an operation and began to hypoventilate, one would expect the $[HCO_3^-]$ to be normal—24 mmol/L—because the kidneys would not have had time to compensate for the hypercapnia. If the P_{CO_2} were 60 mm Hg and the pH 7.30, the physician should be concerned because the $[HCO_3^-]$ is 29 mmol/L (these values are the same as in the preceding paragraphs). A value of 29 mmol/L should alert the physician to the fact that the $[HCO_3^-]$ is too high, perhaps because $NaHCO_3$ had been given unnecessarily. The base deficit, however, would be 1 mmol/L, suggesting that the patient's $[HCO_3^-]$ was appropriate. The base deficit would be misleading.

The use of base deficit and excess should probably be abandoned in surgical patients. Errors in patient evaluation are more likely to be minimized if the physician concentrates on the $[HCO_3^-]$ and interprets that value in the light of a particular patient's situation. If a chronically ill patient in the ICU has severe ARDS and a P_{CO_2} of 60 mm Hg with a pH of 7.30, no attempt should be made to change the accompanying $[HCO_3^-]$ of 29 mmol/L—that value represents the expected renal compensation for such a chronic hypercapnia (though the impaired alveolar ventilation should be of concern). On the other hand, if the patient's P_{CO_2} is 60 mm Hg and the pH is 7.45, the patient has an inappropriately high $[HCO_3^-]$ of approximately 40 mmol/L (calculated from Equation 2), perhaps because of unreplaced losses of hydrogen ion from the stomach, chronic use of a loop diuretic, or administration of excessive amounts of acetate in the patient's parenteral nutrition. In this situation, the $[HCO_3^-]$ should be brought down into the low 30s. The excessively high $[HCO_3^-]$ and its resultant alkalemia may be blunting the patient's ventilatory drive.

RISK ASSESSMENT

Predicting the likelihood of survival in critically ill surgical patients is best accomplished by evaluating clinical and laboratory findings. Computation of a severity of illness score is usually unnecessary. Nonetheless, several scoring systems have been developed with the intention of increasing the precision of the estimate. All such systems assign a mathematical probability for survival in groups of patients, and many are useful for research purposes because they allow comparisons of patients between different institutions. None of them are accurate enough to predict survival for an individual patient, however, though some are still clinically useful for assessing the effects of therapy.

Table 13–5. Conversion of pH to hydrogen ion concentration.

pH	Hydrogen Ion Concentration (nmol/L)	
7.0		100
7.1	$100 \times 0.8 =$	80
7.2	$80 \times 0.8 =$	63
7.3	$63 \times 0.8 =$	50
7.4	$50 \times 0.8 =$	40
7.5	$40 \times 0.8 =$	32
7.6	$32 \times 0.8 =$	25

Note: Values not indicated in the table can be derived by interpolation. For example, a pH of 7.35 corresponds to a hydrogen ion concentration of approximately 45.

The APACHE II score, in which clinical data and 14 measured variables are entered into a formula to assess the probability of survival, takes about 30 minutes to calculate by hand—less by computer. The score can predict survival in critically ill medical patients; it has not been found to be of value in the usual surgical patient, and in any case it is too cumbersome unless one has a particular interest in this kind of methodology.

Methods for predicting survival in trauma patients are well established, though most trauma systems are designed to evaluate all trauma patients and not the specific subset of critically ill trauma patients. The Injury Severity Score, the Revised Trauma Score, and the ASCOT score have proved to be most reliable. The Glasgow Coma Score is quite accurate for predicting survival in patients with head injuries. Combining the Glasgow Coma Score with a simple measurement of fluid requirement has also proved to be accurate in critically injured trauma patients.

■ IV. CASE EXAMPLES

Case No. 1: Acute Trauma

A 20-year-old man is involved in a motor vehicle accident. He was the unrestrained driver of a car that hit a tree. On arrival in the emergency room, he has evidence of maxillofacial trauma and is agitated and cyanotic.

Question: *Does this patient need intubation? What intubation route should be used?*

Agitation and cyanosis indicate the need for an airway. Nasotracheal intubation is difficult in an uncooperative patient with poor respiratory effort and is contraindicated in the presence of maxillofacial trauma because of concern that the nasotracheal tube might be unintentionally passed backward into the cranial vault. Depending on the severity of facial trauma, one or two attempts at orotracheal intubation might be justified. Severe maxillofacial trauma or difficulties in passing an orotracheal tube should prompt the rapid placement of a surgical airway. Cricothyroidostomy is the procedure of choice because of its simplicity and the rapidity with which it can be done.

A cricothyroidostomy is done, and the patient's agitation and cyanosis improve. He will not follow commands but does respond to pain, and his abdomen is distended. The blood pressure is 90/60 mm Hg, and both femurs are broken.

Question: *Should the patient be mechanically ventilated? What type of ventilator and what settings should be used?*

The patient is hypotensive and has evidence of head, abdominal, and orthopedic injuries. He requires mechanical ventilation with a volume ventilator. An FIO_2 of 100% should be used to ensure maximal oxygen delivery in the face of shock and a head injury. The benefits of maximal oxygenation outweigh the risks of short-term administration of 100% oxygen. Because it may increase intracranial pressure by increasing central venous back pressure, PEEP should not be used. A tidal volume of 7 mL/kg should be used initially. The small tidal volume can be increased later, when the patient is hemodynamically stable.) Assist-control ventilation can be used with a backup rate of 25/min.

The patient is placed on mechanical ventilation using the settings described above. Shortly thereafter, his systolic blood pressure drops to 60 mm Hg. There are no breath sounds over the left chest.

Question: *What is the problem, and how should it be dealt with?*

The patient has a tension pneumothorax on the left. The initiation of positive-pressure mechanical ventilation has rapidly increased the size of the pneumothorax and resulted in high intrathoracic pressure. This in turn interferes with venous return and leads to worsening of shock. The pneumothorax should be relieved with needle decompression of the left chest followed by a chest tube.

The patient is taken to the operating room for exploratory celiotomy and removal of a ruptured spleen. His leg fractures are treated with open reduction and internal fixation. No abnormalities are seen on CT scan of the head. His mental status clears rapidly, and no intracranial pressure monitoring is necessary. He is taken to the intensive care unit.

Question: *What ventilator settings should now be used? When and how should he be weaned from the ventilator?*

All of the injuries have been repaired, and rapid recovery is expected. The patient's mental status has cleared. He is initiating his own breaths, and there is minimal evidence of head injury. The patient can be placed on pure pressure support, with the pressure adjusted so that his tidal volumes will be approximately 7 mL/kg. Hyperventilation and a high FIO_2 are no longer necessary, and both the pressure support and the FIO_2 should be reduced gradually. Arterial PO_2 and PCO_2 as well as the patient's clinical status should be used to guide the rapidity with which weaning is carried out. When the pressure support is less than 10 cm H_2O and the patient is receiving an FIO_2 of 40% or less, a T-piece trial should be done for 30 minutes. If the patient tolerates the T-piece trial well, the prognosis for recovery remains good; and if the mental status is completely normal, the patient is ready for extubation. Weaning parameters can be obtained if desired to document the appropriateness of extubation.

Case No. 2: Intra-abdominal Sepsis

A 50-year-old man develops gallstone pancreatitis. He receives supportive care, but his condition worsens during his first 24 hours of hospitalization. He becomes increasingly tachypneic, and his respiratory rate reaches 35/min. His breathing is shallow, and he is using his accessory muscles of respiration. Because of concern about his respiratory status, an arterial blood gas measurement is obtained. His Po_2 on 70% oxygen by mask is 40 mm Hg (75% saturated). The Pco_2 is 40 mm Hg and the pH is 7.34.

> **Question:** *Does this patient require intubation and ventilatory support? What mode of ventilation should be used, and what should his ventilator settings be? When and how should he be weaned from the ventilator?*

The patient requires intubation and mechanical ventilation for several reasons. The Po_2 of only 40 mm Hg on 70% oxygen by mask indicates a large pulmonary shunt. A Pco_2 of 40 mm Hg, though it would be normal if the respiratory rate were normal, is a sign of impending respiratory arrest at a respiratory rate of 35/min. The rate of 35/min cannot be maintained indefinitely and is itself a sign of impending collapse. Furthermore, the patient's disease process and the prognosis are unclear, and the subjective impression that he is clearly getting worse argues for intubation. Pressure support ventilation is appropriate, and the pressure should be adjusted to give tidal volumes of approximately 7 mL/kg. The patient will set his own respiratory rate to maintain a satisfactory pH. (If he develops severe respiratory acidemia, he can be converted to pressure control ventilation with an IRV.) The Fio_2 should initially be set between 70% and 100%, and PEEP should be instituted at 5 cm H_2O. Using the Po_2 as a guide, the inspired oxygen concentration should then be decreased to as low a level as possible compatible with an oxygen saturation above 90%. If necessary, PEEP should be increased in an attempt to reduce the inspired oxygen concentration to at least 50%.

The patient is intubated and mechanical ventilation begun with tidal volumes of approximately 7 mL/kg. His respiratory rates vary between 18/min and 25/min. His Fio_2 is 90%, and his PEEP is 5 cm H_2O. He is more comfortable, and over the next several hours it is possible to decrease the inspired oxygen concentration to 50%. The PEEP is increased to 10 cm H_2O. A diagnosis of necrotizing pancreatitis is made, which requires operative debridement. On the first postoperative day, the Fio_2 is decreased to 40% and the oxygen saturation is 95%. His pressure support is unchanged.

> **Question:** *Is the patient ready for weaning and extubation?*

The prognosis for this patient is still guarded, and he may well require further operative debridement. Although the decrease in inspired oxygen concentration is encouraging, he remains on a PEEP of 10 cm H_2O. Prior to weaning, an attempt should be made to reduce the level of PEEP. Weaning should await further improvements in the patient's overall status.

Attempts to decrease the level of PEEP over the next several days are unsuccessful. Bilateral pulmonary infiltrates develop within 12 hours after his operation. Multiple further operative debridements of the pancreas and drainage procedures for intra-abdominal abscess are required, and the patient continues to require ventilatory support for the next 3 weeks. He receives several courses of antibiotics and is treated for pneumonia on two occasions. His intra-abdominal sepsis is ultimately controlled, and no further operations are planned. He is off of antibiotics. He is awake and is writing notes. The Fio_2 is 40%, and the PEEP is 5 cm H_2O. His pressure support is unchanged, but now his respiratory rates are between 15/min and 20/min.

> **Question:** *Is the patient now ready for weaning? If so, how should it be done?*

Weaning is now appropriate. The patient is awake and alert, and his prognosis for recovery is good. He is on acceptably low levels of inspired oxygen and PEEP. Pressure support should be gradually decreased, and his clinical status and Pco_2 should be monitored. If the patient tolerates decreases in pressure support to less than 10 cm H_2O, a T-piece trial should be initiated. If this is well tolerated, the patient should be extubated.

The pressure support is decreased to 15 cm H_2O but cannot be decreased further. CO_2 retention develops and the patient becomes agitated, with labored breathing.

> **Question:** *What are the alternatives for further weaning?*

Simply supporting the patient on an adequate amount of pressure support would be one option. A second option would be a regimen of T-piece wind sprints of gradually increasing duration. Regardless of the weaning method chosen, a tracheostomy should be considered if it is anticipated that the patient will remain intubated for 2–3 more weeks.

A tracheostomy is done and a wind sprint regimen begun. The length of the wind sprints is gradually increased over the next 2 weeks until the patient can easily tolerate T-piece with CPAP for a 30-minute period.

He is then successfully removed from the ventilator. The tracheostomy is removed 5 days later.

Case No. 3: Hypovolemic or Cardiogenic Shock

A 60-year-old man with a history of coronary artery disease and peptic ulcer disease presents to the emergency department with a 24-hour history of abdominal pain. The pain was sudden in onset and has become progressively more severe. He has had nothing by mouth for the past 24 hours. There is free air under the diaphragm on admission x-ray, and a presumptive diagnosis of perforated duodenal ulcer is made. On admission the patient is cool, and capillary refill in the toes is 3 seconds. The blood pressure is 80/40 mm Hg. The pulse is thready and 130/min in the supine position. The neck veins are flat, and mentation is poor. A urinary catheter is placed, and only 5 mL of urine are initially drained from the bladder.

Question: *Is the patient in shock? What is the most likely cause of the shock and how should it be treated?*

There are several indications of shock in this patient. Peripheral perfusion is poor. He is hypotensive, tachycardiac, and his neck veins are flat. His mental status is depressed, and there is minimal urine output. Treatment at this point should be directed toward repletion of the intravascular volume with a balanced salt solution such as lactated Ringer's solution or normal saline to replace fluid lost into the peritoneal cavity in response to peritonitis. Although the patient will require surgery, it is important to restore intravascular volume before induction of anesthesia.

The admission hematocrit comes back from the laboratory and is 50%. Two large intravenous catheters are placed, and the patient is given 4 L of lactated Ringer's solution over the next 2 hours. The blood pressure increases to 120/80 mm Hg, and the pulse decreases to 100/min. The toes are somewhat warmer to the touch, and capillary refill time decreases to 2 seconds. The patient undergoes exploratory laparotomy, and a duodenal ulcer is oversewn. Postoperatively, he is taken to the intensive care unit and is extubated the following day.

Question: *Why was the admission hematocrit 50%? How should the patient's volume status be followed in the postoperative period?*

The blood is hemoconcentrated because of the loss of plasma into the peritoneal cavity. In the postoperative period, as in the initial evaluation, blood pressure, pulse, capillary refill, temperature, and neck vein examination can be used to follow the patient. One of the best measures of perfusion, assuming there is no underlying renal disease, is the urinary output.

Initially, the patient does quite well. On the second postoperative day, however, he complains of substernal chest pain and shortness of breath. The blood pressure falls to 90/60 mm Hg, and the pulse increases to 120/min. The neck veins are distended. The arterial PO_2 is 50 mm Hg with the patient on 40% oxygen by face mask.

Question: *What is the most likely cause for this patient's deterioration? How should it be treated?*

The presence of chest pain associated with hypotension and respiratory distress suggests cardiogenic shock, as do the distended neck veins. The patient should initially be treated with increased oxygen and limitation of intravenous fluids. The diagnosis should be confirmed with placement of a Swan-Ganz catheter and determination of the pulmonary arterial wedge pressure and cardiac index. A high wedge pressure and low cardiac index should be treated with diuresis, and inotropic support as needed. The diagnosis should be further confirmed with serial ECGs and cardiac enzymes, looking for signs of myocardial infarction as a cause of cardiogenic shock.

The oxygen concentration is increased to 100% by mask, and a Swan-Ganz catheter is placed. The pulmonary arterial wedge pressure is 40 mm Hg, and the cardiac index is 1.8 L/min/m². The patient is given diuretics to a wedge pressure of 15 mm Hg and dobutamine at a dose of 6 μg/kg/min. The blood pressure increases to 120/80 mm Hg, and the pulse decreases to 80/min. The cardiac index increases to 3.2 L/min/m². Myocardial infarction is confirmed by ECG and cardiac enzymes. The patient continues to improve, recovers completely except for occasional continued angina pectoris, and is discharged home on the 18th postoperative day. Three months later, he undergoes coronary angiography and coronary artery bypass grafting.

Case No. 4: Trauma & Sepsis

A 25-year-old man is shot once in the abdomen. On arrival in the emergency department, he is unresponsive, and his respirations are rapid and shallow. His blood pressure is 80/40 mm Hg, and his abdomen is distended. He is pale and cool to the touch, and there is minimal capillary refill. The neck veins are flat.

Question: *Is the patient in shock? What is the most likely cause, and how should it be treated?*

Hypotension, pallor, coolness, poor capillary refill, and decreased mental status indicate shock. The gunshot wound, abdominal distention, and flat neck veins point to hemorrhage as the likely cause. The patient requires immediate surgery for control of hemorrhage as the best means for correcting his shock.

The patient is intubated and ventilated. Several large intravenous catheters are placed, lactated Ringer's injection is infused as rapidly as possible, and an exploratory laparotomy is done. Two liters of blood are found on entry to the abdomen, and there is an injury to the infrarenal abdominal aorta. There are also several large holes in the transverse colon, with gross fecal contamination of the abdomen. The aorta is repaired and the right and transverse colon are resected, with creation of a diverting ileostomy. The peritoneal cavity is irrigated, and the abdomen is closed. Ten units of blood are transfused intraoperatively, and at the conclusion of the operation the hematocrit is 30%.

> **Question:** *What should be done about the hematocrit of 30%?*

Nothing should be done about the hematocrit. A level of 30% is adequate for a young, otherwise healthy patient such as this one and may even improve perfusion because of decreased blood viscosity.

On the eighth postoperative day, the patient develops ileus, and large volumes of intravenous fluid are needed to maintain urine output and blood pressure. Whenever fluid rates are decreased, hypotension and decreased urine output recur. There is increasing respiratory distress and hypoxemia that requires intubation and mechanical ventilation on an inspired oxygen concentration of 60%. There are diffuse bilateral infiltrates on chest x-ray. The digits are warm, and capillary refill is normal. There are signs of glucose intolerance.

> **Question:** *What kind of shock is this patient suffering from, and how should it be treated?*

This is a case of septic shock. Vigorous fluid administration to compensate for hypotension and decreased urine output has prevented low-output septic shock and resulted in high-output septic shock instead. Aggressive monitoring is indicated, and both an arterial catheter and a pulmonary arterial catheter should be placed. The pulmonary arterial catheter is helpful both in confirming the diagnosis and in monitoring subsequent therapy. In addition, a source of sepsis should be sought.

The pulmonary arterial wedge pressure is 10 mm Hg, and the cardiac index is 3.5 L/min/m^2. Intravenous fluid administration is continued, and the wedge pressure increases to 15 mm Hg. The cardiac index increases to 4.5 L/min/m^2. Positive end-expiratory pressure of 10 cm H_2O is added, and the inspired oxygen concentration is decreased to 50%. CT scan of the abdomen reveals a large subhepatic abscess, and the patient is taken to the operating room for drainage. He does well afterward, and his pulmonary function improves. Fluid requirements remain high for 2 days postoperatively, but spontaneous diuresis begins on postop-

erative day 3. The patient recovers completely and is discharged home 2 weeks later.

REFERENCES

Amato MBP et al: Effect of a protective-ventilation strategy on mortality in the acute respiratory distress syndrome. N Engl J Med 1998;338:347.

Angle N et al: Hypertonic saline resuscitation diminishes lung injury by suppressing neutrophil activation after hemorrhagic shock. Shock 1998;9:164.

Angus DC et al: E5 murine monoclonal antiendotoxin antibody in gram-negative sepsis. A randomized controlled trial. JAMA 2000;283:1723.

Bernard GR et al: Efficacy and safety of recombinant human activated protein C for severe sepsis. N Engl J Med 2001; 344:699.

Bulger EM et al: Current clinical options for the treatment and management of acute respiratory distress syndrome. J Trauma 2000;48:562.

Chang MC et al: Effects of abdominal decompression on cardiopulmonary function and visceral perfusion in patients with intra-abdominal hypertension. J Trauma 1998;44:440.

Chang MC et al: Maintaining survivors' values of left ventricular power output during shock resuscitation: a prospective pilot study. J Trauma 2000;49:26.

Chang MC et al: Redefining cardiovascular performance during resuscitation: ventricular stroke work, power, and the pressure-volume diagram. J Trauma 1998;45:470.

Ciesla DJ et al: Hypertonic saline attenuation of polymorphonuclear neutrophil cytotoxicity: timing is everything. J Trauma 2000;48:388.

Cohn SM. Surgical research review. Blood substitutes in surgery. Surgery 2000;127:599.

Demetriades D et al: Relative bradycardia in patients with traumatic hypotension. J Trauma 1998;45:534.

Diebel LN, Tyburski JG, Dulchavsky SA. Effect of acute hemodilution on intestinal perfusion and intramucosal pH after shock. J Trauma 2000;49:800.

Esteban A et al: A comparison of four methods of weaning patients from mechanical ventilation. N Engl J Med 1995;332:345.

Gausche M et al: Effect of out-of-hospital pediatric endotracheal intubation on survival and neurological outcome. A controlled clinical trial. JAMA 2000;283:783.

Gore DC et al: Influence of glucose kinetics on plasma lactate concentration and energy expenditure in severely burned patients. J Trauma 2000;49:673.

Griffiths RD, Jones C, Palmer TEA. Six-month outcome of critically ill patients given glutamine-supplemented parenteral nutrition. Nutrition 1997;13:295.

Hébert PC et al: A multicenter, randomized, controlled clinical trial of transfusion requirements in critical care. N Engl J Med 1999;340:409.

Ho HS et al: Hypertonic perfusion inhibits intracellular Na and Ca accumulation in hypoxic myocardium. Am J Physiol Cell Physiol 2000;278:C953.

Houdijk APJ et al: Randomised trial of glutamine-enriched enteral nutrition on infectious morbidity in patients with multiple trauma. Lancet 1998;352:772.

Human albumin administration in critically ill patients: systematic review of randomised controlled trials. Cochrane Injuries Group Albumin Reviewers. BMJ 1998;317:235.

Ketoconazole for early treatment of acute lung injury and acute respiratory distress syndrome. A randomized controlled trial. The ARDS Network. JAMA 2000;283:1995.

Kress JP et al: Daily interruption of sedative infusions in critically ill patients undergoing mechanical ventilation. N Eng J Med 2000;342:1471.

Miller PR, Meredith JW, Chang MC. Randomized, prospective comparison of increased preload versus inotropes in the resuscitation of trauma patients: effects on cardiopulmonary function and visceral perfusion. J Trauma 1998;44:107.

Perdue PW et al: "Renal dose" dopamine in surgical patients. Dogma or science? Ann Surg 1998;227:470.

Ranieri VM et al: Effect of mechanical ventilation on inflammatory mediators in patients with acute respiratory distress syndrome. A randomized controlled trial. JAMA 1999;282:54.

Rotstein OD. Novel strategies for immunomodulation after trauma: revisiting hypertonic saline as a resuscitation strategy for hemorrhagic shock. J Trauma 2000;49:580.

Sloan EP et al: Diaspirin cross-linked hemoglobin (DCLHb) in the treatment of severe traumatic hemorrhagic shock. A randomized controlled efficacy trial. JAMA 1999;282:1857.

Tobin MJ. Weaning from mechanical ventilation: what have we learned? Respir Care 2000;45:417.

Vassar MJ et al: A multicenter trial for resuscitation of injured patients with 7.5% sodium chloride. Arch Surg 1993;128:1003.

Vassar MJ et al: Prediction of outcome in intensive care unit trauma patients: a multicenter study of acute physiology and chronic health evaluation (APACHE), trauma and injury severity score (TRISS), and a 24-hour intensive care unit (ICU) point system. J Trauma 1999;47:324.

Velmahos GC et al: Endpoints of resuscitation of critically injured patients: normal or supranormal? A prospective randomized trial. Ann Surg 2000;232:409.

Ventilation with lower tidal volumes as compared with traditional tidal volumes for acute lung injury and the acute respiratory distress syndrome. Acute Respiratory Distress Syndrome Network. N Engl J Med 2000;342:1301.

Wade CE et al: Individual patient cohort analysis of the efficacy of hypertonic saline/dextran in patients with traumatic brain injury and hypotension. J Trauma 1997;42:S61.

Wilmore DW. Metabolic response to severe surgical illness: overview. World J Surg 2000;24:705.

Management of the Injured Patient 14

James R. Macho, MD, William C. Krupski, MD, & Frank R. Lewis, Jr., MD

EPIDEMIOLOGY OF TRAUMA

Injury can be defined as damage to the body caused by acute exposure to energy. Trauma is the medical term used to denote injury and usually refers to life-threatening or serious injuries that require specialized surgical care if the patient is to survive without disability. As a "disease," trauma represents a major public health problem. It is the principal cause of death during the first half of the normal human life span and the fifth leading cause of death for all age groups. In persons under age 30, trauma is responsible for more deaths than all other diseases put together. In the USA, about 146,000 lives are lost per year because of injuries, and an additional 300,000 injured persons suffer some form of permanent disability. Because trauma affects mainly a young population, it results in the loss of more working years than all other causes. The financial costs of injury exceed $224 billion annually, an increase of 42% in the last decade. What is most tragic is that as many as 40% of all trauma deaths could be avoided by preventive measures and by the establishment of regional trauma systems that would expedite the evaluation and treatment of seriously injured people.

Trauma deaths have been classically described as having a trimodal distribution, with peaks that correspond to the types of intervention that would be most effective in reducing mortality. The first peak, the **immediate deaths,** represents patients who die of their injuries before reaching the hospital. The injuries accounting for these deaths include major brain or spinal cord trauma and those resulting in rapid exsanguination. Few of these patients would have any chance of survival even with access to immediate care since almost 60% of these deaths occur at the same time as the injury. Prevention remains the major strategy to reduce these deaths.

The second peak, the **early deaths,** are those that occur within the first few hours after injury. They are mainly caused by internal hemorrhage, and almost all are treatable. However, in most cases, salvage requires prompt and definitive operative care of the sort available at a trauma center, ie, a specialized institution that can provide immediate resuscitation and access to a ready operating room 24 hours a day.

The third peak, the **late deaths,** consists of patients who die days or weeks after injury. Sixty-one percent are caused by sepsis and multiple organ failure. The critical care phase of trauma management is important in reducing these deaths. Evidence suggests that at present, as many as 30% of the late deaths could be prevented by improved critical care management. It is essential that surgeons caring for trauma patients have genuine expertise in surgical critical care.

PREVENTION OF TRAUMA

Prevention of injury has received much less scientific attention than has the treatment of diseases of far less consequence. Unfortunately, prevention programs depending for their success on altering human behavior have been largely unsuccessful because the programs often do not reach the populations most at risk and because they often raise controversial social questions, including the right of individuals to engage in high-risk behavior. Programs mandated by law or official policies have met with greater success. It is estimated that drivers under the influence of alcohol or other drugs cause 50–60% of all fatal motor vehicle accidents. Evidence suggests that stringent measures such as mandatory jail terms and revocation or suspension of a driver's license after a drunk driving conviction decrease the rate of drunk driving (and drunk driving injuries).

Current laws requiring the use of seat belts have demonstrated a clear survival benefit. Seat belts are the most effective safety devices in vehicles today, estimated to save 9500 lives each year. Yet only about 70% of United States motor vehicle occupants are buckled. In 1996, more than 60% of the occupants killed in fatal crashes were unrestrained. In data from the National Pediatric trauma registry, restrained children in vehicle crashes had half the death rate, needed surgery less often, and were hospitalized for fewer days than those who were unrestrained. In some states, deaths from automobile occupants decreased by 25%, after seat belt use was required by law.

Initial experience has shown that the use of air bags as a form of passive restraint has resulted in a decrease in the number of deaths from certain kinds of accidents, such as head-on collisions. Drivers protected by air bags experienced a reduced fatality risk of 31% in purely frontal crashes and 11% in all crashes. Starting in model year 1998, all new passenger cars are required to have dual air bags (driver side and passenger side). Based on the 11% effectiveness in all crashes, it is estimated that more than 6200 people are alive today because of air bags. Unfortunately, air bag designs and deployment systems have also contributed to death and injury in children and smaller adults. In most of these relatively rare cases, the injured persons were determined to have been unrestrained or improperly restrained at the time of the crashes.

Laws mandating the use of motorcycle helmets have generated controversy, but data clearly indicate that they reduce injury severity by decreasing the incidence of head injury. Helmets also decrease the likelihood of death and the overall cost of care. Just like safety belts in cars, helmets will not provide total protection against head injury or death but they do reduce the incidence of both. The National Highway Traffic Safety Administration (NHTSA) estimates that helmets reduce the risk of death in a motorcycle crash by 29% and the risk of fatal head injury by 40%. Helmets are even more effective in preventing nonfatal brain injuries, which often require extensive treatment and may result in lifelong disability. After federal highway safety standards required the use of helmets by motorcycle riders, deaths from this activity decreased by 50%. Where such laws have been repealed or weakened, the mortality rate has increased by a similar percentage. Helmets provide even greater protection for bicycle riders, since nearly all fatal bicycle injuries are due to head injuries.

Total firearms deaths in the United States now number approximately 38,000 each year. Of this total, at least 4% are unintentional deaths, with children comprising many of the deaths in this category. An additional 100,000–200,000 firearm injuries each year are serious but nonfatal. Firearm injuries cost over $20 billion a year in both direct costs for medical care and in indirect costs for long-term disability. At least 80% of these costs are borne by public agencies. These totals are staggering when compared with other industrialized nations with more restrictive gun laws and availability. It is estimated that in the United States, one in three homes has a gun and that one in five are kept loaded and unlocked. Attempts to introduce gun control legislation or even mandatory safety measures such as trigger locks have been met with strong opposition from national gun organizations on the basis that such laws would restrict individual freedoms. Although controversial, gun control legislation to restrict civilian access to weapons designed primarily for interpersonal violence and enforcement of mandatory jail sentences for crimes committed with firearms would probably decrease this source of trauma.

The possibility of preventing injury by modifying the environment has been largely ignored. The record suggests that the nation's health might benefit more by increased emphasis on environmental factors. The few efforts at environmental modification have produced significant results. Motor vehicle crashes are the leading cause of death for people ages 1–24. The effect of highway design is shown by the fact that death rates per vehicle mile on interstate highways are one-third those on other roads. Higher travel speeds also mean more deaths. In states where the speed limits were raised to 65 mph in 1987, the higher limits are causing about 15–20% more deaths on rural interstate highways each year than otherwise would be expected. Speeding reduces the time drivers have to avoid crashes and lengthens stopping distances, increasing both the likelihood of crashing and the severity of the crashes that do occur. In a high-speed crash, a passenger vehicle is subjected to forces so severe that the vehicle structure cannot withstand the force of the crash and thus cannot sufficiently protect occupants from serious injury. Likewise, the performance of restraint systems such as air bags and safety belts are compromised in high-speed crashes. This also is true of roadside safety features such as barriers, crash cushions, and bridge rails, which are designed to reduce crash severity by absorbing crash energy. Future efforts at injury prevention are more likely to be effective if they include consideration of these factors.

TRAUMA SYSTEMS

The purpose of a trauma system is to provide timely, organized care in order to minimize preventable morbidity and mortality following injury. The system includes prehospital care designed to identify, triage, treat and transport victims with serious injuries. Criteria for staging patients with major trauma consist of standardized scoring systems based on readily discernible anatomic and physiologic variables. The criteria are designed to identify not only the more severe and complex single injuries but also combinations of injuries that require tertiary care. Patients are transported to a trauma center organized to provide the highest possible level of care to patients with major injuries. When a patient arrives in the trauma center, additional triage occurs. The most severely injured patients are identified and receive more intensive care. By the most optimistic estimates, only 25% of the United States population is served by regional trauma systems even though there is no disagreement that such systems decrease death and disability. The issue is highlighted by a study in which it was found that the percentage of preventable deaths in a California county dropped from 11% to 1% after establishment of a regionalized trauma care facility. Similar data are available for other areas of the country.

The American College of Surgeons (ACS) has defined three levels of institutional trauma care. **Level I** is the highest designation a trauma center can receive. It indicates that the hospital has committed itself to the care of trauma patients and offers the highest level of skill available in trauma care. A level I trauma center is directed by a board-certified surgeon specializing in trauma care and is staffed by a team of board-certified trauma care specialists available 24 hours a day—including emergency room physicians, trauma surgeons, neurosurgeons and neurologists, orthopedic surgeons, plastic surgeons, anesthesiologists, and radiologists. The level I center maintains a quality improvement program including a trauma registry and has an active commitment to research and teaching. **Level II** trauma centers provide 24-hour care by in-hospital and on-call physicians. They are able to deliver the same quality of care as a level I center but without the same teaching and research obligations. Immediate operating room capability must be maintained 24 hours a day in level II centers. The **level III** trauma center provides prompt assessment, resuscitation, and stabilization followed by surgical treatment or interhospital transfer as appropriate. Although they may not be able to provide definitive care in all circumstances, level III centers serve a valuable function in less populated areas where resuscitation and stabilization before transport may be lifesaving.

Only 20% of the hospitals in the United States have sought certification and received a trauma center level I, II, or III designation since the ACS began the program in 1987.

PREHOSPITAL CARE & TRIAGE

The effectiveness of paramedics in the treatment of trauma victims remains controversial owing to a lack of data regarding the success of specific prehospital treatments. Evidence of improved survival of cardiac arrest victims treated by well-trained paramedical teams has been inappropriately extrapolated to trauma victims. In the urban setting, where transportation from the scene of an accident to the hospital is typically 5–10 minutes, it is questionable whether any treatment by paramedics other than airway management, simple first aid, and splinting is beneficial. The principal causes of immediate death from trauma are head injury (35%), exsanguination (50%), and airway or pulmonary problems (15%). Only the last of these can be treated in the field. Patients with head injury or airway and pulmonary problems benefit from endotracheal intubation to maintain effective ventilation and prevent aspiration and hypercapnia. Most life-threatening injuries require hospital facilities and a well-organized team that can provide immediate treatment, including surgery, and any delay in the field usually worsens the outcome. One study showed that trauma victims with cardiac wounds who were treated by paramedics had longer delays in

transportation and lower survival rates compared with victims treated by emergency medical technicians (EMTs) or nonmedical persons. However, recent information shows that well-trained paramedics can prepare patients for transport quickly and then perform life-support procedures en route with a high rate of patient survival. Further studies are required to identify the procedures other than intubation that would improve the survival of these patients.

IMMEDIATE MEASURES AT THE SCENE OF AN ACCIDENT

When first seen, the victim of an accident may not appear to be badly injured. There may be little external evidence of injury, so when the mechanism of trauma is sufficient to produce severe injury, the victim must be handled as if a severe injury has occurred.

The injured person must be protected from further trauma. First aid at the scene of an accident should be administered by trained personnel whenever possible. The simple act of moving a victim from one position to another, if done improperly, may compress or lacerate the spinal cord, puncture a lung, sever a major blood vessel, or compound a fracture, thereby converting a simple injury into a major one.

Whether the patient is first seen on the battlefield, beside a road, in the emergency ward, or in the hospital, the basic principles of initial management are the same:

(1) Is the victim breathing? If not, provide an airway and establish mouth-to-mouth ventilation.

(2) Is there a pulse or heartbeat? If not, begin closed-chest compression.

(3) Is there gross external bleeding? If so, elevate the part if possible and apply enough external pressure to stop the bleeding. A tourniquet is rarely needed.

(4) Is there any question of injury to the spine? If so, protect the neck and spine before moving the patient.

(5) Splint obvious fractures.

As soon as these steps have been taken, the patient can be safely transported.

Specific details of prehospital management are considered in the following paragraphs.

1. Airway Management

The most important therapy that can be provided before the patient gets to the hospital is airway management. Simple measures such as clearing the airway, positioning the mandible, and the use of oral airways may be all that is necessary to ensure adequate ventilation. This can often be done by simple manipulation of the mandible or traction on the tongue, particularly in unconscious or semiconscious patients. After the mouth is

Figure 14–1. Relief of airway obstruction.

Figure 14–2. Needle in trachea to establish temporary airway.

forced open, the tongue can be grasped between the thumb and forefinger covered with a handkerchief or gauze bandage. The tip of the tongue should be pulled forward beyond the front teeth. The mandible should be manipulated either by pulling forward the angles of the lower jaw or by inserting the thumb between the upper and lower rows of teeth, grasping the mandible in the midline, and drawing it forward until the lower teeth are leading (Figure 14–1).

Suctioning the mouth and pharynx may clear them of blood, mucus, or vomitus so as to permit normal respiration. Repeated suctioning may be required to maintain an adequate airway at the scene of the accident and during transit to a medical facility. Aspiration of vomitus, a frequent cause of sudden death, must be prevented at all costs. A lateral and slightly head-down position is best for patients who are liable to vomit. In respiratory arrest, a clear airway must be provided and mouth-to-mouth breathing instituted if other means of ventilation are not available. In extreme situations, where the upper airway is occluded and the foreign body cannot be removed, it can be lifesaving to insert one or two large-bore needles (14 gauge) through the cricothyroid membrane (Figure 14–2). Emergency tracheotomy should never be attempted at the scene of the accident or in the ambulance. Whenever possible, pa-

tients who are unconscious or in profound shock should have the airway controlled with an endotracheal tube (Figure 14–3). Although endotracheal intubation is the only prehospital treatment proved to benefit trauma victims with potentially lethal injuries, few

Figure 14–3. *Top:* Nasotracheal intubation. *Bottom:* Orotracheal intubation.

paramedics are trained or proficient in this skill. Extensive evaluation of the field use of endotracheal intubation by paramedics in emergency care systems has shown that relatively limited training is needed, that intubation is successful in 85–95% of cases, and that paramedics retain their skill in this technique even when the frequency of field use is only moderate. For these reasons, endotracheal intubation should be taught to all paramedics.

2. Intravenous Lines

Intravenous lines are critical for intravenous volume resuscitation. However, starting intravenous lines in the field is probably counterproductive because the amount of fluid given during a brief trip to the hospital rarely compensates for the loss of blood that occurs during the time it takes to place the line. When long delays to definitive treatment are inevitable because of difficulty in transportation, intravenous infusions are more apt to be of benefit. The infusion should be started after the patient is en route whenever possible. The administration of hypertonic saline may be preferable to conventional isotonic solutions when transport time is long. However, no benefit of hypertonic saline has been demonstrated with short transport times or for in-hospital resuscitations.

3. Prehospital Cardiac Arrest

Cardiac arrest following trauma, when encountered at the scene of an accident, is usually fatal unless a correctable cause such as airway obstruction can be immediately identified. If blunt trauma is the cause of prehospital arrest, the salvage rate almost is nil. If the cause is penetrating trauma—particularly stab wounds—the salvage rate is highest if the patient can be rapidly delivered to a trauma center. In such cases, ventilation by mouth-to-mouth resuscitation or a manual device should be initiated during transport, and closed-chest cardiac compression should be performed.

4. Neck, Spine, & Fracture Immobilization

All patients with major blunt trauma should be suspected of having spinal injury, and precautions should be taken to immobilize the spine and prevent further injury. Recognition and splinting of major fractures and immobilization of all injured parts before transportation are essential features of early management. Improper handling of the injured patient may worsen or prolong shock and aggravate existing trauma beyond the possibility of definitive repair. "Splint' .em where they lie!" is a time-honored rule of emergency care of fractures that has only a few exceptions—when it is necessary to remove an injured patient from imminent danger of fire, explosion, escaping gas, etc. Immobilization should be achieved rapidly and should not delay transfer to the hospital.

5. Triage

Triage at the accident scene seeks to identify the patients who are most at risk of dying from their injuries and thus would benefit most from a trauma center. The ACS has published guidelines for the triage of trauma victims (Figure 14–4). Whenever in doubt, the patient should be transported to a trauma center.

6. Prehospital Transport

Transportation by ground or air ambulance is preferable when feasible. The choice of helicopter or ambulance depends upon time and distance and the level of care that must be provided en route. Ideally, transport should not exceed 15 minutes and the total prehospital time should not exceed 30 minutes. Resuscitation of the seriously injured patient should be continued during transportation, and a constant effort must be made to avoid airway obstruction and aspiration if the patient is vomiting.

If no ambulance is available, a station wagon or truck is preferable to a passenger car. The manipulation necessary to load a seriously injured person into a passenger car may be more harmful than the time lost in waiting for proper transportation. Except in unusual circumstances, injured patients should be transported in the supine position.

■ EVALUATION OF THE TRAUMA PATIENT

In most cases the history is obtained from prehospital personnel via radio communication or when the patient arrives at the hospital. In the case of motor vehicle accidents, for example, it is important to determine the circumstances of the injury, including the speed of impact, the condition of the vehicle, the position of the patient at the scene, evidence of blood loss, and the condition of other passengers. Record the time the injury occurred and the treatment rendered while en route. Every person who may have information about the circumstances of the injury should be questioned. Knowing the mechanism of the injury often gives a clue to concealed trauma. Information regarding serious un-

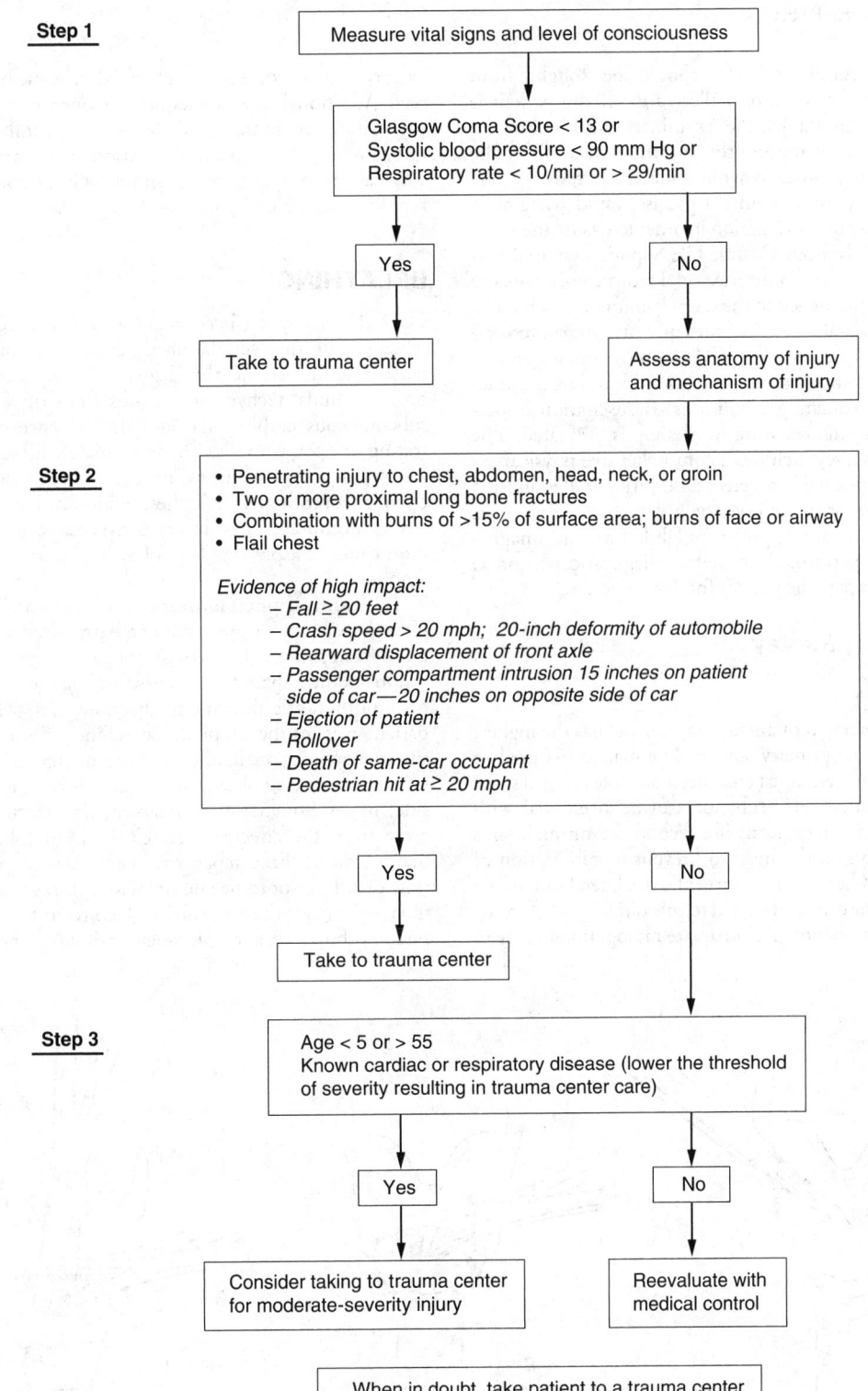

Figure 14–4. Triage scheme for trauma victims as published by the American College of Surgeons Committee on Trauma.

derlying medical problems should be sought from Medic Alert bracelets or wallet cards. If the patient is conscious and stable, the examiner should obtain a complete history and use this information to direct the examination in order to avoid unnecessary tests.

Trauma victims require a precise, rapid, systematic approach to initial evaluation in order to ensure their survival. The Advanced Trauma Life Support system developed by the ACS Committee on Trauma represents the best current approach to the severely injured patient. The sequence of evaluation includes primary survey, resuscitation, secondary survey, and definitive management. The primary survey attempts to identify and treat immediate life-threatening conditions. Resuscitation is performed, and the response to therapy is evaluated. The secondary survey includes a comprehensive physical examination designed to detect all injuries and establish a treatment priority for potentially life-threatening ones. During this phase, appropriate laboratory and imaging studies are performed as well as diagnostic peritoneal lavage to prepare the patient for definitive care.

1. Primary Survey

AIRWAY

The establishment of an adequate airway has the highest priority in the primary survey. The maneuvers used in the trauma patient must consider a possible cervical spine injury. Orotracheal intubation can be attempted with cervical spine precautions if a second person maintains axial traction on the head to prevent destabilization of the spine. When circumstances allow, a lateral film of the cervical spine can be obtained to rule out injury before attempting intubation. An adequate radiographic study to

exclude injury requires that all seven vertebrae be clearly seen. Additional views are required frequently. If ventilatory failure occurs and an adequate airway cannot be obtained readily by orotracheal or nasotracheal intubation, surgical cricothyroidotomy should be performed as rapidly as possible (Figure 14–5).

BREATHING

Once the airway has been established, it is necessary to make certain that ventilation is adequate. Examine the patient to determine the degree of chest expansion, breath sounds, tachypnea, crepitus from rib fractures, subcutaneous emphysema, and the presence of penetrating or open wounds. The immediately life-threatening pulmonary conditions are tension pneumothorax, open pneumothorax, flail chest, and occasionally massive hemothorax. Chest injury is the second most common cause of asphyxia. The following are the chief examples:

(1) **Tension pneumothorax** occurs from air in the pleural space under pressure. The harmful effects result more from shift of the mediastinum and impairment of venous return than from ventilatory failure. Tension pneumothorax is difficult to diagnose even when the patient reaches the hospital. The clinical findings consist of hypotension in the presence of distended neck veins, decreased or absent breath sounds on the affected side, hyperresonance to percussion, and tracheal shift away from the affected side. Cyanosis may be a late manifestation. Emergency treatment consists of insertion of a large-bore needle or plastic intravenous cannula to relieve the pressure and convert the tension pneumothorax to a simple pneumothorax. The needle

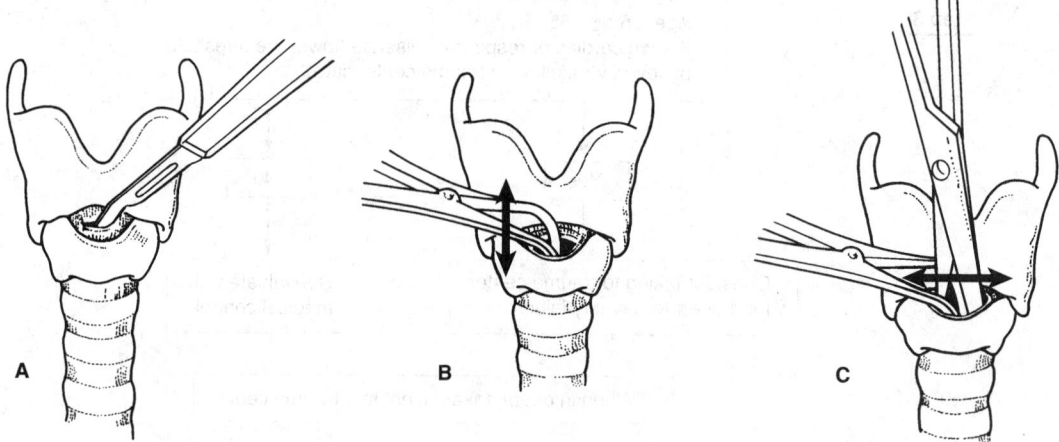

Figure 14–5. Surgical cricothyroidotomy.

or cannula may be left in place while a chest tube is inserted for definitive management (Figure 14–6).

(2) **Open pneumothorax** results from an open wound of the chest wall with free communication between the pleural space and the atmosphere. The resulting impairment of the thoracic bellows results in ineffectual ventilation. With ventilatory efforts, air moves in and out of the chest wall opening instead of through the trachea, producing hypoventilation that can be rapidly fatal. Emergency treatment consists of sealing the wound with a sterile dressing if possible—or with any material if nothing sterile is available. Definitive treatment requires placement of a chest tube to reexpand the lung and surgical closure of the defect.

(3) **Flail chest:** Multiple rib fractures resulting in a free-floating segment may produce instability of the chest wall so that paradoxic motion occurs with ventilatory efforts (Figure 14–7). However, this does not fully

Figure 14–7. Flail chest.

explain the pathophysiology. Associated pulmonary contusion is common and is the major cause of ventilatory failure. The injury is identified by careful inspection and palpation. Patients with large flail segments will almost always require prompt endotracheal intubation and mechanical ventilation, both to stabilize the flail segment and to optimize gas exchange. Smaller flail segments may be well tolerated if supplemental oxygen and adequate analgesia are provided. The work of breathing is increased considerably, and many patients who initially appear to be compensating well may suddenly deteriorate a few hours later. Therefore, most patients with flail chest require monitoring in an intensive care unit.

CIRCULATION

Hemorrhage

Gross hemorrhage from accessible surface wounds is usually obvious and can be controlled in most cases by local pressure and elevation of the part. Firm pressure on the major artery in the axilla, antecubital space, wrist, groin, popliteal space, or at the ankle may suffice for temporary control of arterial hemorrhage distal to these points. When other measures have failed, a tourniquet may rarely be necessary to control major hemorrhage from extensive wounds or major vessels in an extremity. Failure to release it periodically may cause irreparable vascular or neurologic damage. For this reason, the tourniquet must be kept exposed and loosened at least every 20 minutes for 1 or 2 minutes while the patient is in transit and permanently as soon as definitive care is given. It is wise to write the letters "TK" on

Figure 14–6. Relief of pneumothorax. Tension pneumothorax must be immediately decompressed by a needle introduced through the second anterior intercostal space. A chest tube is usually inserted in the midaxillary line at the level of the nipple and is directed posteriorly and superiorly toward the apex of the thorax. The tube is attached to a "three-bottle" suction device, and the rate of escape of air is indicated by the appearance of bubbles in the second of the three bottles. Cessation of bubbling suggests that the air leak has become sealed.

the patient's forehead with a skin-marking pen or on adhesive tape.

Vascular Access

All patients with significant trauma should have a large-caliber intravenous catheter inserted immediately for administration of drugs and fluids as needed. If any degree of shock is present, at least two intravenous lines should be inserted, one of which should be a large-bore catheter placed in a femoral vein using a Seldinger guidewire technique. If severe shock, hypovolemic cardiac arrest, or major vascular lesions are present, three intravenous lines are necessary, and one of the venous lines should be placed so that central venous pressure can be monitored as fluids are administered. Alternatively, lines can be placed percutaneously with 14–16 gauge angiocatheters, usually in the antecubital fossa or by venous cutdown, preferably in the saphenous vein at the ankle, with an 8–10F feeding tube or intravenous extension tube with the tip cut off.

As soon as the first intravenous line is inserted, rapid crystalloid infusion should begin. Adult patients should be given 2 L of normal saline or Ringer's lactate. An additional 2 L of crystalloid may be administered if there is no change in blood pressure or only a transient response. Beyond this amount, whole blood must also be given in combination with crystalloid solutions to avoid excessive hemodilution. Protein-containing solutions are unnecessary in shock or resuscitation and should generally be avoided. For children, the initial administered volume should be 20 mL/kg. Group O, Rh-negative packed red blood cells should be immediately available for any patient with impending cardiac arrest or massive hemorrhage. Type-specific blood should be available within 15 minutes.

NEUROLOGIC DISABILITY

Various stages of coma due to a variety of causes may accompany injury and require treatment during resuscitation. The most common causes are alcoholic intoxication, cerebrovascular accidents, diabetic acidosis, barbiturate poisoning, narcotic overdosage, and hypovolemic shock. Less common causes are epilepsy, eclampsia, and electrolyte imbalances associated with metabolic and systemic diseases. Other causes include anaphylaxis, heavy metal poisoning, electric shock, tumors, severe systemic infections, hypercalcemia, asphyxia, heat stroke, severe heart failure, and hysteria.

The differential diagnosis depends upon (1) a careful history from available informants; (2) a careful and complete physical examination, with particular attention to the neurologic examination; and (3) laboratory tests such as urinalysis, blood counts, blood cultures, blood glucose, BUN, ammonia, electrolytes, and alcohol, and cerebrospinal fluid examination; and (4) urgent head CT scan.

Laboratory studies may be helpful in ruling out the following: blood alcohol levels in acute alcoholism; blood and urine glucose levels in diabetic coma and hypoglycemic shock; and serum potassium, blood urea nitrogen, and creatinine in uremia.

EXPOSURE

All clothing should be removed at once (cut off, usually) from the seriously injured patient, with great care being taken to avoid unnecessary movement. The removal of helmets or other protective clothing may require additional personnel to stabilize the patient and prevent further injury. All surfaces should be examined to identify injuries that may not be readily apparent, such as posterior penetrating trauma or open fractures.

EMERGENCY ROOM THORACOTOMY

Certain injuries are so critical that operative treatment must be undertaken as soon as the diagnosis is made. In these cases, resuscitation is continued as the patient is being operated on. For cardiopulmonary arrest that occurs in the emergency room as a direct result of trauma, external cardiac compression is rarely successful in maintaining effective perfusion of vital organs. An emergency left anterolateral thoracotomy should be performed in the fourth or fifth intercostal space, and the pericardium should be opened anterior to the phrenic nerve (Figure 14–8). Open cardiac massage, cross-clamping of the descending thoracic aorta, repair of cardiac injuries, and in-

Figure 14–8. Emergency thoracotomy and open cardiac massage.

ternal defibrillation can be performed as appropriate. Wounds of the lung producing severe hemorrhage or systemic air embolus may require hilar cross-clamping.

Emergency room thoracotomy is most useful for cardiac arrest due to penetrating thoracic trauma, particularly in patients with pericardial tamponade. This extreme procedure is ineffective for most patients with arrest due to blunt trauma and for all patients who have no detectable vital signs in the field. If vital signs are present in the emergency room but arrest appears imminent, the patient should be transferred rapidly to the operating room, since the conditions there are optimal for operation.

RESUSCITATION PHASE

Shock

Some degree of shock accompanies most severe injuries and is manifested initially by pallor, cold sweat, weakness, lightheadedness, hypotension, tachycardia, thirst, air hunger, and, eventually, loss of consciousness. Patients with any of these signs should be presumed to be in shock and evaluated thoroughly. All patients determined to be in any degree of shock should be reexamined at regular intervals.

A. HYPOVOLEMIC SHOCK

Hypovolemic shock is due to loss of whole blood or plasma. Blood pressure may be maintained initially by vasoconstriction. Tissue hypoxia increases when hypotension ensues, and shock may become irreversible if irreparable damage occurs to the vital organs. Massive or prolonged hemorrhage, severe crushing injuries, major fractures, and extensive burns are the most common causes. The presence of any of these conditions is an indication for prompt intravenous fluid infusions.

The patient must be kept recumbent and given reassurance and analgesics as necessary. If opioids are necessary for pain, they are best administered intravenously in small doses. Subcutaneous injections are poorly absorbed in these circumstances.

The most reliable clinical guide in assessing hypovolemic shock is skin perfusion, In mild or class 1 shock (< 20% blood volume loss), compensatory mechanisms may preserve adequate perfusion and no skin or physiologic changes may be apparent. In moderate or class 2 shock (20–40% blood loss), the skin on the extremities becomes pale, cool, and moist as a result of vasoconstriction and release of epinephrine. Systolic blood pressure is often maintained at near-normal levels, but urine output will usually decrease. With severe or class 3 shock (approximately > 40% blood volume loss), these changes—particularly diaphoresis—become more marked, and urine output decreases significantly. Hy-

potension ensues. In addition, changes in cerebral function become evident, consisting chiefly of agitation, disorientation, and memory loss. A common error is to attribute uncooperative behavior to intoxication or drug use when in fact it may be due to cerebral ischemia from blood loss. With class 4 shock (> 40% blood volume loss), profound hypotension is typically accompanied by loss of consciousness and anuria. In this situation, rapid resuscitation with crystalloid and blood products is necessary to prevent imminent death.

With any degree of shock, balanced salt solution (eg, lactated Ringer's solution) should be given rapidly intravenously until the signs of shock abate and urine output returns to normal. When large volumes of resuscitation fluid are necessary, central venous pressure should be monitored to avoid fluid overload. Two to 4 liters of crystalloid solution can be given rapidly if needed to resuscitate the patient in severe shock. Successful resuscitation is indicated by warm, dry, well-perfused skin, a urine output of 30–60 mL/h, and an alert sensorium.

As a general principle, measurements of blood pressure and pulse are less reliable than changes in urine output in assessing the severity of shock. Young patients and athletic older ones have compensatory mechanisms that often maintain adequate blood pressure even with moderate volume loss. Older patients and those taking cardiac or blood pressure medications often do not exhibit tachycardia even with extreme volume loss. Therefore, a urinary catheter should be inserted for monitoring urine output in any patient with major injuries or shock. Oliguria is the most reliable sign of moderate shock, and successful resuscitation is indicated by a return of urine output to 0.5–1 mL/kg/h. Absence of oliguria is an unreliable index of the absence of shock if the patient has an osmotic diuresis due to alcohol, glucose, mannitol, or intravenous contrast material.

A patient who is receiving intravenous fluids at a high rate may not exhibit signs of shock even in the setting of ongoing hemorrhage. If a patient continues to require high volumes of fluid after initial resuscitation in order to maintain urine output, mental status, and blood pressure, further investigation must be performed to rule out occult hemorrhage.

B. NEUROGENIC SHOCK

Neurogenic shock is due to the pooling of blood in autonomically denervated venules and small veins and is usually due to spinal cord injury. Neurogenic shock is not caused by an isolated head injury, and in those patients other causes of shock should be sought. A patient thought to be in neurogenic shock should be placed in Trendelenburg's position and given a 2 L crystalloid fluid bolus—followed by an additional bolus if the response is suboptimal. If shock persists, phenylephrine or another vasopressor should be given as a drip with the dosage adjusted until the blood pressure is maintained at a satisfactory level. If the patient does not improve quickly, other kinds of shock must be considered. Patients with neurogenic shock will generally require central venous pressure or pulmonary artery monitoring to ensure an optimal volume status.

C. CARDIAC COMPRESSIVE SHOCK

Cardiac compressive shock is caused by compression of the thin-walled chambers of the heart—the atria and the right ventricle—or by compression or distortion of the great veins entering the heart. The usual causes of this type of shock in the trauma patient are pericardial tamponade, tension pneumothorax, massive hemothorax, diaphragmatic rupture with herniation of abdominal contents into the chest, and an elevated diaphragm from massive abdominal hemorrhage. Treatment consists of urgent decompression depending on the specific cause. In severe cases, emergency thoracotomy may be necessary to restore adequate cardiac function.

D. CARDIOGENIC SHOCK

Cardiogenic shock is caused by decreased myocardial contractility and is most commonly caused by myocardial infarction or arrhythmia. Older trauma patients may develop a myocardial infarction as a complication of their injuries. Rarely, a severe myocardial contusion may lead to cardiogenic shock. Treatment is supportive, with volume replacement guided by hemodynamic monitoring and administration of inotropic agents to augment cardiac output as necessary to maintain adequate organ perfusion.

Laboratory Studies

Immediately after intravenous catheters are placed, blood should be drawn for hematocrit, white blood count, creatinine, blood urea nitrogen, and whole blood typing and cross-matching. If the patient has a history of renal or cardiac disease or is taking diuretics, serum electrolytes should be measured. If there is any indication of liver disease, a liver panel is indicated. If the patient has a thoracic injury, any sign of respiratory compromise or distress, or any degree of shock, arterial blood gases should be measured (pH, PaO_2, $PaCO_2$). Urinalysis should be obtained, checking especially for hematuria. Even mild hematuria indicates the need for intravenous urography or abdominal CT scan and, in selected cases, a cystogram and urethrogram.

Imaging Studies

Films of the chest and abdomen are required in all major injuries. Cervical spine films should be obtained in patients at risk for this type of injury who have not been cleared during the primary survey.

CT scanning of the head or abdomen may be considered in patients with altered mental status and hemodynamic stability. An intravenous urogram is critical in abdominal injuries and pelvic fractures.

X-rays of the skull and long bones can usually be deferred until the more critical injuries of the thorax and abdomen have been cared for.

2. Secondary Survey & Treatment Priorities

A rapid and complete history and physical examination (with a written record of the findings) are essential for patients with serious or multiple injuries. Progressive changes in clinical findings are often the key to correct diagnosis, and negative findings that change to positive may be of great importance in revising an initial clinical evaluation. This is particularly true in the case of intra-abdominal, intrathoracic, and head injuries, which frequently do not become manifest until hours after the trauma.

Certain kinds of trauma are apt to cause more than one injury. Fractures of the calcaneus resulting from a fall from a great height are often associated with central dislocation of the hip and fractures of the spine and of the base of the skull. A crushed pelvis is often combined with rupture of the posterior urethra or bladder. Crush injuries of the chest are often associated with lacerations or rupture of the spleen, liver, or diaphragm. Penetrating wounds of the chest may involve not only the thoracic contents but also the abdominal viscera. These combinations occur frequently and should always be suspected.

TREATMENT PRIORITIES

In all cases of multiple injury, there must be a "captain of the team" who directs the resuscitation, decides which x-rays or special diagnostic tests should be obtained, and establishes priority for care by continuous consultation with other surgical specialists and anesthesiologists. A trauma surgeon or a general surgeon experienced in the care of injured patients usually has this role.

If the injuries are extensive and there are signs of hypovolemic shock, coma is apt to be the result of cerebral ischemia. Resuscitation and blood volume replacement have first priority. If there are no signs of shock, coma is probably due to head injury (see Chapter 38).

Deepening stupor in patients under observation should arouse suspicion of an expanding intracranial lesion requiring repeated and thorough neurologic examinations. Too often, obvious signs of acute alcoholism have been assumed to be the cause of unconsciousness, and intracranial hemorrhage has been overlooked.

Cerebral injuries take precedence in care only when there is rapidly deepening coma. Extradural bleeding is a critical emergency, requiring operation for control and cerebral decompression. Subdural bleeding may produce a similar emergency. If the patient's condition permits, CT scanning should be performed for localization of the bleeding. In many cases of combined cerebral and abdominal injury with massive bleeding, laparotomy and craniotomy should be performed simultaneously.

In most cases, fractures of the skull have a low priority and can be dealt with after more critical abdominal or thoracic injuries have been treated.

Most urologic injuries are managed at the same time as associated intra-abdominal injuries. Pelvic fractures present special problems discussed in Chapters 41 and 43.

Unless there is associated vascular injury with threatened ischemia of the limb, fractures of the long bones can be splinted and treated on an urgent basis. Open contaminated fractures should be cleansed and debrided as soon as possible.

Injuries of the hand run the risk of infection that may result in a lifelong handicap without early effective treatment. Early treatment of the hand at the same time as treatment of any life-threatening injuries avoids infection and preserves the means of livelihood.

Tetanus prophylaxis should be given in all instances of open contaminated wounds, puncture wounds, and burns.

Details of definitive management of injuries are discussed in the sections on trauma that follow and in the various organ system chapters of this book.

■ NECK INJURIES

All injuries to the neck are potentially life-threatening because of the many vital structures in this area. Injuries to the neck are classified as blunt or penetrating, and the treatment is different for each.

Penetrating injuries of the neck are divided into three anatomic zones (Figure 14–9). Zone I injuries occur at the thoracic outlet, which extends from the level of the cricoid cartilage to the clavicles. Included in this area are the proximal carotid arteries, the subclavian vessels, and the major vessels in the chest. Proximal control of injuries to vascular structures in this zone requires thoracotomy. Zone II injuries occur in the area between the cricoid and the angle of the mandible. Injuries here are the easiest to expose and evaluate. Zone

Figure 14–9. Zones of the neck.

III injuries are between the angle of the mandible and the base of the skull. Exposure is much more difficult in this zone and in some cases may require disarticulation of the mandible. High injuries can be inaccessible, and control of hemorrhage may require ligation of major proximal vessels. Penetrating trauma to the posterior neck may injure the vertebral column, the cervical spinal cord, the interosseous portion of the vertebral artery, and the neck musculature. Penetrating trauma to the anterior and lateral neck may injure the larynx, trachea, esophagus, thyroid, carotid arteries, subclavian arteries, jugular veins, and subclavian veins.

Blunt cervical trauma may cause fracture or dislocation of the cervical vertebrae (with the risk of spinal cord injury), traumatic occlusion of the carotid arteries, cerebrospinal fluid cysts, or laryngeal and tracheal injuries complicated by hemorrhage and airway obstruction.

The patient must be examined closely for associated head and chest injuries. The initial level of consciousness is of paramount importance; progressive depression of the sensorium signifies intracranial bleeding and requires craniotomy. Trauma to the base of the neck may lacerate major blood vessels. Hemorrhage into the pleural cavity may occur suddenly as contained hematomas rupture.

Clinical Findings

Injuries to the larynx and trachea may be asymptomatic or may cause hoarseness, laryngeal stridor, or dyspnea secondary to airway compression or aspiration of blood. Subcutaneous emphysema may appear if the wall of the larynx or trachea has been disrupted.

Esophageal injuries are rarely isolated and by themselves may not cause immediate symptoms. Severe chest pain and dysphagia are characteristic of esophageal perforation. Hours later, as mediastinitis develops, progressive sepsis may become manifest. Mediastinitis results because the deep cervical space is in direct continuity with the mediastinum. Esophageal injuries can be recognized promptly if the physician is alert to the possibility. Exploration of the neck or radiographic examination of the esophagus with contrast medium confirms the diagnosis.

Cervical spine and cord injuries should always be suspected in deceleration injuries or following direct trauma to the neck. If the patient complains of cervical pain or tenderness or if the level of consciousness is depressed, the head and neck should be immobilized (eg, with sandbags) until cervical x-rays can be taken to rule out cervical fracture.

Injury to the great vessels (subclavian, common carotid, internal carotid, and external carotid arteries; subclavian, internal jugular, and external jugular veins) may follow penetrating trauma. Fractures of the clavicle or first rib may lacerate the subclavian artery and vein. With vascular injuries, the patient typically presents with visible external blood loss and hematoma formation and in varying degrees of shock. Occasionally, bleeding may be contained and the injury may go undetected for a short time. Auscultation may reveal bruits that suggest arterial injury.

Diagnosis

With any penetrating cervical trauma, the likelihood of significant injury is high because there are so many vital structures in such a small space. Any patient with shock, expanding hematoma, or uncontrolled hemorrhage should be taken to the operating room for emergency exploration. The location of the injury suggests which structures may be involved. Vascular injuries at the base of the neck require thoracotomy to obtain proximal control of injured blood vessels before the site of probable injury is exposed. If the patient is stable after resuscitation, additional diagnostic testing may be considered. Arteriography is usually recommended for patients with injuries in zones I and III because precise identification of the location and extent of injury may alter the operative approach. If possible, arteriography should be performed before exploration of any injury in which blood vessels may be damaged below the level of the cricoid cartilage or above a line connecting the mastoid process with the angle of the jaw. Arterial injuries above this line are practically inaccessible. If injury to the carotid artery at the base of the skull is confirmed by arteriography, repair may not be possible and ligation may be required to control bleeding. In addition,

injured carotid arteries that have produced a neurologic deficit should be ligated. Since exposure of injuries in zone II is relatively easy to obtain, a policy of mandatory exploration has been proposed for all injuries penetrating the platysma in this area. Although this approach is safe, reliable, and time-tested, recent studies have demonstrated that a selective approach is safe as well provided that diagnostic testing does not detect a major injury. In the absence of an obvious vascular injury on clinical examination, ultrasound with color flow Doppler has been demonstrated to reliably rule out carotid injuries. Arteriography can also be used in this setting and may offer the advantage of identifying an unsuspected vertebral artery injury. Rigid endoscopy can be used to evaluate the trachea and esophagus. A contrast study of the upper esophagus should be performed to identify esophageal injuries that might not be readily apparent on endoscopy. These injuries can be difficult to detect and are occasionally missed on surgical exploration. In either case, repeated, careful examinations should be performed.

Vertebral artery injuries should also be suspected when bleeding from a posterior or lateral neck wound cannot be controlled by pressure on the carotid artery or when there is bleeding from a posterolateral wound associated with fracture of a cervical transverse process.

X-rays of the soft tissues and cervical spine should be taken routinely. Fractures of the cervical spine can be confirmed by x-ray. X-rays of the soft tissues can locate opaque foreign bodies if present and help determine the route of the missile.

The most important injuries resulting from blunt cervical trauma are (1) cervical fracture, (2) cervical spinal cord injury, (3) vascular injury, and (4) laryngeal and tracheal injury. X-rays of the cervical spine and soft tissues are essential. Careful neurologic examination can differentiate between injuries to the cord, brachial plexus, and brain.

Complications

The complications of untreated neck injuries are related to the individual structures injured. Injuries to the larynx and trachea can result in acute airway obstruction, late tracheal stenosis, and sepsis. Cervicomediastinal sepsis can result from esophageal injuries. Carotid artery injuries can produce death from hemorrhage, brain damage, and arteriovenous fistula with cardiac decompensation. Major venous injury can result in exsanguination, air embolism, and arteriovenous fistula formation if there is concomitant arterial injury. Cervical fracture can result in paraplegia, quadriplegia, or death.

Prevention of these complications depends upon immediate resuscitation by intubation of the airway, prompt control of external hemorrhage and blood replacement, protection of the head and neck when cervical fracture is possible, accurate and rapid diagnosis, and prompt operative treatment when indicated.

Treatment

Any wound of the neck that penetrates the platysma requires prompt surgical exploration or angiography to rule out major vascular injury. In patients with zone II injuries, color flow Doppler imaging may provide a reliable way to assess for vascular injury and may be a safe alternative to routine contrast angiography. If the patient presents with a neurologic deficit that is clearly not due to head injury, primary repair of the artery and reestablishment of blood flow to the brain will make the neurologic deficit worse, since an ischemic area of infarction in the brain is thus converted into a more lethal hemorrhagic infarction; in such cases, the carotid artery should be ligated. Arteries damaged by high-velocity missiles require debridement. End-to-end anastomosis of the mobilized vessels is preferred, but if a significant segment is lost, an autogenous vein graft can be used. Vertebral artery injury presents formidable technical problems because of the interosseous course of the artery shortly after it arises from the subclavian artery. Although unilateral vertebral artery ligation has been followed by fatal midbrain or cerebellar necrosis, because of inadequate communication to the basilar artery, only 3% of patients with left vertebral ligation and 2% of patients with right vertebral ligation develop these complications. Therefore, in the face of massive hemorrhage from a partially severed vertebral artery, the risks of immediate ligation must be accepted.

Subclavian artery injuries are best approached through a combined cervicothoracic incision. Proper exposure is the key to success in the management of these difficult and too often fatal injuries. Ligation of the subclavian artery is relatively safe, but primary repair is preferable.

Venous injuries are best managed by ligation. The possibility of air embolism must be kept constantly in mind. A simple means of preventing this complication is to lower the patient's head until bleeding is controlled.

Esophageal injuries should be sutured and drained. Drainage is the mainstay of treatment. Extensive injury to the esophagus is often immediately fatal, because of associated injuries to the spinal cord. Systemic antibiotics should be administered routinely to patients with esophageal injuries.

Minor laryngeal and tracheal injuries do not require treatment, but immediate tracheotomy should be performed when airway obstruction exists. If there has been significant injury to the thyroid cartilage, a temporary laryngeal stent (Silastic) should be employed to provide support. Mucosal lacerations should be approximated before insertion of the stent. Conveniently located small perforations of the trachea can be utilized for tracheotomy. Otherwise, the wounds can be closed after they are debrided and a distal tracheotomy performed. Extensive circumferential tracheal injuries may require resection and anastomosis or reconstruction using synthetic materials.

Primary neurorrhaphy should be attempted for nerve injury. Bilateral vagal nerve injury results in hoarseness and dysphagia. Cervical spinal cord injury should be managed in such a way as to prevent further damage. When there is cervical cord compression from hematoma formation, vertebral fractures, or foreign bodies, decompression laminectomy is necessary.

Blunt trauma to the neck rarely requires direct surgical treatment. More commonly, the soft tissues are contused, but hematomas may develop and cause tracheal compression and respiratory insufficiency. Tracheotomy is indicated in this instance. Cervical fractures are managed with skull tongs and traction. Surgical stabilization of cervical fractures is rarely indicated before 3 weeks after injury unless there is progressive paraplegia. Vascular injuries may occur in cases of severe or localized blunt neck trauma. The common or internal carotid arteries can be torn or can undergo disruption of the intima and require vascular reconstruction. Carotid arteriograms are essential to the diagnosis and should be considered in selected patients.

Prognosis

Severance of the cervical spinal cord results in paralysis. Injuries to the soft tissues of the neck, trachea, and esophagus have a good to excellent prognosis if promptly treated. Major vascular injuries have a good prognosis if promptly treated before the onset of irreversible shock or neurologic deficit. The overall death rate for cervical injuries is about 10%.

Demetriades D et al: Penetrating injuries of the neck in patients in stable condition. Physical examination, angiography, or color flow Doppler imaging. Arch Surg 1995;130:971.

Eddy VA: Zone 1 Penetrating Neck Injury Study Group: is routine arteriography mandatory for penetrating injury to zone 1 of the neck? J Trauma 2000;48:208.

Edwards MJ et al: Routine cervical spine radiography for trauma victims: does everybody need it? J Trauma 2001;50:529.

Ginzburg E: The use of duplex ultrasonography in penetrating neck trauma. Arch Surg 1996;131:691.

Grossman MD et al: National survey of the incidence of cervical spine injury and approach to cervical spine clearance in U.S. trauma centers. J Trauma 1999,47:684.

Irish JC et al: Penetrating and blunt neck trauma: 10-year review of a Canadian experience. Can J Surg 1997;40:33.

Sofianos C et al: Selective surgical management of zone II gunshot injuries of the neck: a prospective study. Surgery 1996;120:785.

■ THORACIC INJURIES

Thoracic trauma accounts directly for or is a contributing factor in 50% of deaths due to trauma. Early deaths are commonly due to (1) airway obstruction, (2) flail chest, (3) open pneumothorax, (4) massive hemothorax, (5) tension pneumothorax, and (6) cardiac tamponade. Later deaths are due to respiratory failure, sepsis, and unrecognized injuries. Eighty percent of blunt thoracic injuries are caused by automobile accidents. Penetrating chest injuries from knives, bullets, etc, are almost as frequent as those from blunt trauma. The death rate in hospitalized patients with isolated chest injury is 4–8%; it is 10–15% when one other organ system is involved and rises to 35% if multiple additional organs are injured.

Combined injuries of multiple intrathoracic structures are usual. There are often other injuries to the abdomen, head, or skeletal system. Eighty-five percent of chest injuries do not require open thoracotomy, but immediate use of lifesaving measures is often necessary and should be within the competence of all surgeons.

When the physician is confronted with a patient who has sustained thoracic injuries, a rapid estimate of cardiorespiratory status and possible associated injuries gives a valuable overview. For example, patients with upper airway obstruction appear cyanotic, ashen, or gray; examination reveals stridor or gurgling sounds, ineffective respiratory excursion, constriction of cervical muscles, and retraction of the suprasternal, supraclavicular, intercostal, or epigastric regions. The character of chest wall excursions and the presence or absence of penetrating wounds can be observed. If respiratory excursions are not visible, ventilation is probably inadequate. Severe paradoxic chest wall movement in flail chest is usually located anteriorly and can be seen immediately. Sucking wounds of the chest wall should be obvious. A large hemothorax can usually be detected by percussion, and subcutaneous emphysema is easily detected. Both massive hemothorax and tension pneumothorax may produce absent or diminished breath sounds and a shift of the trachea to the opposite side, but in massive hemothorax the neck veins are usually collapsed. If the patient has a thready or absent pulse and distended neck veins, the main differential diagnosis is between cardiac tamponade and tension pneumothorax. In moribund patients, diagnosis must be immediate, and treatment may require chest tube placement, pericardiocentesis, or thoracotomy in the emergency room. The first priority of management should be to provide an airway and restore circulation. One can then reassess the patient and outline definitive measures. A cuffed endotracheal tube and assisted ventilation are required for apnea, ineffectual breathing,

severe shock, deep coma, airway obstruction, flail chest, or open sucking chest wounds. Persistent shock or hypoxia may be due to massive hemorrhage, cardiac tamponade, or tension pneumothorax. Shock due to thoracic trauma may be caused by any of the following: massive hemopneumothorax, cardiac tamponade, tension pneumothorax or massive air leak, or air embolism. If hemorrhagic shock is not explained readily by findings on chest x-ray or external losses, it is almost certainly due to intra-abdominal bleeding.

Types of Injuries

A. CHEST WALL

Rib fracture, the most common chest injury, varies across a spectrum from simple fracture to fracture with hemopneumothorax to severe multiple fractures with flail chest, pulmonary contusion, and internal injuries. With simple fractures, pain on inspiration is the principal symptom; treatment consists of providing adequate analgesia. In cases of multiple fractures, intercostal nerve blocks or epidural analgesia may be required to ensure adequate ventilation. Measures such as strapping the chest wall with adhesive tape or the placement of elastic binders will interfere with adequate ventilation and lead to the development of atelectasis—and they have no place in the modern management of rib fractures. Multiple fractures may be associated with voluntarily decreased ventilation and subsequent pneumonitis, particularly in the elderly patient.

Flail chest occurs when a portion of the chest wall becomes isolated by multiple fractures and moves in and out with inspiration and expiration with a potentially severe reduction in ventilatory efficiency. The magnitude of the effect is determined by the size of the flail segment and the amount of pain with breathing. The rib fractures are usually anterior and there are at least two fractures of the same rib. Bilateral costochondral separation and sternal fractures can also cause a flail segment. An associated lung contusion may produce a decrease in lung compliance not fully manifest until 12–48 hours after injury. Increased negative intrapleural pressure is then required for ventilation, and chest wall instability becomes apparent. If ventilation becomes inadequate, atelectasis, hypercapnia, hypoxia, accumulation of secretions, and ineffective cough occur. Arterial PO_2 is often low before clinical findings appear. Serial blood gas determination is the best way to determine if a treatment regimen is adequate. For less severe cases, intercostal nerve block or continuous epidural analgesia may be adequate treatment. However, most cases require ventilatory assistance for variable periods of time with a cuffed endotracheal tube and a mechanical ventilator. External fixation of the chest wall is less reliable than positive-pressure ventilation for the average case but may be useful for severe sternal flail or other extensive injuries associated with chest wall instability.

B. TRACHEA AND BRONCHUS

Blunt tracheobronchial injuries are often due to compression of the airway between the sternum and the vertebral column in decelerating steering wheel accidents. The distal trachea or main stem bronchi are usually involved. Penetrating tracheobronchial injuries may occur at any location. Most patients have pneumothorax, subcutaneous emphysema, pneumomediastinum, and hemoptysis. Cervicofacial emphysema may be dramatic. Tracheobronchial injury should be suspected when there is a massive air leak or when the lung does not readily reexpand after chest tube placement. In penetrating injuries of the trachea or main stem bronchi, there is usually massive hemorrhage and hemoptysis. Systemic air embolism resulting in cardiopulmonary arrest may occur if a bronchovenous fistula is present. If air embolism is suspected, emergency thoracotomy should be performed with cross-clamping of the hilum on the affected side. The diagnosis is confirmed by aspiration of air from the heart. In blunt injuries, the tracheobronchial injury may not be obvious and may be suspected only after major atelectasis develops several days later. Diagnosis may require tracheobronchoscopy.

Immediate primary repair is indicated for tracheobronchial lacerations.

C. PLEURAL SPACE

Hemothorax (blood within the pleural cavity) is classified according to the amount of blood: minimal, 350 mL; moderate, 350–1500 mL; or massive, 1500 mL or more. The rate of bleeding after evacuation of the hemothorax is clinically even more important. If air is also present, the condition is called hemopneumothorax.

Hemothorax should be suspected with penetrating or severe blunt thoracic injury. There may be decreased breath sounds and dullness to percussion, but a chest x-ray (upright or semiupright, if possible) should be promptly obtained (Figure 14–10). Tube thoracostomy should be performed promptly. Needle aspiration of a hemothorax is never adequate. In 85% of cases, tube thoracostomy is the only treatment required. If bleeding is persistent, as noted by continued output from the chest tubes, it is more likely to be from a systemic (eg, intercostal) rather than a pulmonary artery. When the rate of bleeding is 100–200 mL/h or the total hemorrhagic output exceeds 1000 mL, thoracoscopy or thoracotomy should usually be performed. Thoracoscopy has been shown to be effective in controlling chest tube bleeding in 82% of cases. This technique has also been shown to be 90% effective in evacuating retained hemothoraces. In most of these cases, the chest wall is the source of hemorrhage. Thoracotomy is required for management of injuries to the lungs, heart, pericardium, and great vessels.

Pneumothorax occurs in lacerations of the lung or chest wall following penetrating or blunt chest trauma.

Figure 14–10. Hemopneumothorax. Supine (*left*) and upright films (on different patients).

Hyperinflation (eg, blast injuries, diving accidents) can also rupture the lungs. After penetrating injury, 80% of patients with pneumothorax also have blood in the pleural cavity. Most cases of pneumothorax are readily diagnosed on chest x-ray. In some cases, an occult pneumothorax will be identified on an abdominal CT scan that includes sections of the lower chest. Pneumothorax or hemothorax may be identified on the lateral scans which are performed as part of the ultrasound examination of the abdomen for trauma (see section on abdominal trauma). Most cases of traumatic pneumothorax should be treated with immediate tube thoracostomy.

Tension pneumothorax develops when a flap-valve leak allows air to enter the pleural space but prevents its escape; intrapleural pressure rises, causing total collapse of the lung and a shift of the mediastinal viscera to the opposite side, interfering with venous return to the heart. It must be relieved immediately to avoid impairment of cardiac function. Immediate treatment involves placement of a large-bore needle or plastic angiocatheter in the pleural space with care being taken to avoid injury to the intercostal vessels. After this emergency measure has been instituted, tension pneumothorax should be treated definitively by tube thoracostomy.

Sucking chest wounds, which allow air to pass in and out of the pleural cavity, should be promptly treated by an occlusive dressing and tube thoracostomy. The pathologic physiology resembles flail chest except that the extent of associated lung injury is usually less. Definitive management includes surgical closure of the defect in the chest wall.

D. Lung Injury

Pulmonary contusion due to sudden parenchymal concussion occurs after blunt trauma or wounding with a high-velocity missile. Pulmonary contusion occurs in 75% of patients with flail chest but can also occur following blunt trauma without rib fracture. Alveolar rupture with fluid transudation and extravasation of blood are early findings. Fluid and blood from ruptured alveoli enter alveolar spaces and bronchi and produce localized airway obstruction and atelectasis. Increased mucous secretions and overzealous intravenous fluid therapy may combine to produce copious secretions and further atelectasis. The patient's ability to cough and clear secretions effectively is weakened because of chest wall pain or mechanical inefficiency from fractures. Elasticity of the lungs is decreased, resistance to air flow increases, and, as the work of breathing increases, blood oxygenation and pH drop and $PaCO_2$ rises. The cardiac compensatory response may be compromised, because as many as 35% of these patients have an associated myocardial contusion.

Treatment is often delayed because clinical and x-ray findings may not appear until 12–48 hours after injury. The clinical findings are copious thin, blood-tinged secretions, chest pain, restlessness, apprehensiveness, and labored respirations. Eventually, dyspnea, cyanosis, tachypnea, and tachycardia develop. X-ray changes consist of patchy parenchymal opacification or diffuse linear peribronchial densities that may progress to diffuse opacification ("white-out").

Mechanical ventilatory support permits adequate alveolar ventilation and the use of enriched oxygen mixtures and thus reduces the work of breathing. Blood gases should be monitored frequently and arterial saturation adequately maintained. There is some controversy over the best regimen for fluid management, but excessive hydration or blood transfusion should be avoided. Optimal management may require placement of a pulmonary artery catheter, preferably with a thermistor tip for measurement of cardiac output by thermodilution. Serial measurement of central venous pressure, pulmonary arterial pressure, wedge pressures, mixed venous oxygen saturation, and cardiac output help to avoid either under- or overtransfusion. Despite optimal therapy, about 15% of patients with pulmonary contusion die.

Most lung lacerations are caused by penetrating injuries, and hemopneumothorax is usually present. Tube thoracostomy is indicated to evacuate pleural air or blood and to monitor continuing leaks. Since expansion of the lung tamponades the laceration, most lung lacerations do not produce massive hemorrhage or persistent air leaks.

Lung hematomas are the result of local parenchymal destruction and hemorrhage. The x-ray appearance is initially a poorly defined density that becomes more circumscribed a few days to 2 weeks after injury. Cystic cavities occasionally develop if damage is extensive. Most hematomas resolve adequately with expectant treatment.

E. Heart and Pericardium

Blunt injury to the heart occurs most often from compression by the steering wheel in auto accidents. The injury varies from localized contusion to cardiac rupture. Autopsy studies of victims of immediately fatal accidents show that as many as 65% have rupture of one or more cardiac chambers and 45% have pericardial lacerations. The incidence of myocardial contusion in patients who reach the hospital is unknown but is probably higher than generally suspected.

Early clinical findings include friction rubs, chest pain, tachycardia, murmurs, dysrhythmias, or signs of low cardiac output. Electrocardiograms may be normal or may show nonspecific ST and T wave changes. Serial tracings should be obtained, since abnormalities may not appear for 24 hours. Serum enzyme determinations such as AST, LDH, or CK are not valuable, since elevations can be due to associated musculoskeletal injury.

Management of myocardial contusion should be the same as for acute myocardial infarction. Hemopericardium may occur without tamponade and can be treated by pericardiocentesis. Tamponade in blunt cardiac trauma is often due to myocardial rupture or coronary artery laceration. Tamponade produces distended neck veins, shock, and cyanosis. Immediate thoracotomy and control of the injury are indicated. If cardiopulmonary arrest occurs before the patient can be transported to the operating room, emergency room thoracotomy with relief of tamponade should be performed. Treatment of injuries to the valves, papillary muscles, and septum must be individualized; when tolerated, delayed repair is usually recommended.

Pericardial lacerations from stab wounds tend to seal and cause tamponade, whereas gunshot wounds frequently leave a sufficient pericardial opening for drainage. Gunshot wounds produce more extensive myocardial damage, multiple perforations, and massive bleeding into the pleural space. Hemothorax, shock, and exsanguination occur in nearly all cases of cardiac gunshot wounds. The clinical findings are those of tamponade or blood loss.

Treatment of penetrating cardiac injuries requires prompt thoracotomy, pericardial decompression, and control of hemorrhage. Most patients do not require cardiopulmonary bypass. The standard approach has been to repair the laceration using mattress sutures with pledgets while controlling hemorrhage with a finger on the heart. Suture control of cardiac lacerations may be technically difficult when working with a beating heart or in patients with large or multiple lacerations. Several studies have demonstrated that in most cases, emergency temporary control of hemorrhage from cardiac lacerations can be achieved with the use of a skin stapler (Figure 14–11). Following stabilization of the patient, the staples can be removed after definitive suture repair is performed in the operating room. With either approach, care must be taken to avoid injury to the coronary arteries. Pericardiocentesis or creation of a pericardial window is reserved for selected cases when the diagnosis is uncertain or in preparation for thoracotomy. In approximately 75% of cases of stab wounds and 35% of cases of gunshot cardiac wounds, the patient survives the operation. However, it is estimated that 80–90% of patients with gunshot wounds of the heart do not reach the hospital.

F. Esophagus

Anatomically, the esophagus is well protected, and perforation from external penetrating trauma is relatively infrequent. Blunt injuries are very rare. The most common symptom of esophageal perforation is pain; fever develops within hours in most patients. Regurgitation of blood, hoarseness, dysphagia, or respiratory distress may

Robert E. Markison, M.D.

Figure 14–11. Technique of cardiac stapling. Finger pressure (not shown) is used to maintain hemostasis during stapling. (Reproduced, with permission, from Macho JR, Markison RE, Schecter WP: Cardiac stapling in the management of penetrating injuries of the heart: rapid control of hemorrhage and decreased risk of personal contamination. J Trauma 1993;34:711.)

also be present. Physical findings include shock, local tenderness, subcutaneous emphysema, or Hamman's sign (pericardial or mediastinal "crunch" synchronous with cardiac sounds). Leukocytosis occurs soon after injury. X-ray findings on plain chest films include evidence of a foreign body or missile and mediastinal air or widening. Pleural effusion or hydropneumothorax is frequently seen, usually on the left side. Contrast x-rays of the esophagus should be performed but are positive in only about 70% of proven perforations.

A nasogastric tube should be passed to evacuate gastric contents. If recognized within 24–48 hours after injury, the esophageal perforation should be closed and pleural drainage instituted with large-bore catheters. Repair of these perforations requires special techniques that include buttressing of the esophageal closure with pleural or pericardial flaps; pedicles of intercostal, diaphragmatic, or cervical strap muscles; and serosal patches from stomach or jejunum. Illness and death are due to mediastinal and pleural infection.

G. Thoracic Duct

Chylothorax and chylopericardium are rare complications of trauma but are difficult to manage when they occur. Penetrating injuries of the neck, thorax, or upper abdomen can injure the thoracic duct or its major tributaries.

Symptoms are due to mechanical effects of the accumulations, eg, shortness of breath from lung collapse or low cardiac output from tamponade. The diagnosis is established when the fluid is shown to have characteristics of chyle.

The patient should be maintained on a fat-free, high-carbohydrate, high-protein diet and the effusion aspirated. Chest tube drainage should be instituted if the effusion recurs. Total parenteral nutrition with no oral intake may be effective in treating persistent leaks. Three or 4 weeks of conservative treatment usually are curative. If daily chyle loss exceeds 1500 mL for 5 successive days or persists after 2–3 weeks of conservative treatment, the thoracic duct should be ligated via a right thoracotomy. Intraoperative identification of the leak may be facilitated by preoperative administration of fat containing a lipophilic dye.

H. Diaphragm

Penetrating injuries of the diaphragm outnumber blunt diaphragmatic injuries by a ratio of at least 6:1. Diaphragmatic lacerations occur in 10–15% of cases of penetrating wounds to the chest and in as many as 40% of cases of penetrating trauma to the left chest. Injuries to the right diaphragm are more common than previously thought. The injury is rarely obvious. Wounds of the diaphragm must not be overlooked because they rarely heal spontaneously and because herniation of abdominal viscera into the chest can occur with catastrophic complications either immediately or years after the injuries.

Associated injuries are usually present, and as many as 25% of patients are in shock when first seen. There may be abdominal tenderness, dyspnea, shoulder pain, or unilateral breath sounds. The diagnosis is often missed. Although chest radiography is a sensitive diagnostic tool, it may be entirely normal in 40% of cases. The most common finding is ipsilateral hemothorax, which is present in about 50% of patients. Occasionally, a distended, herniated stomach is confused with a pneumothorax. Passage of a nasogastric tube before x-rays will help to identify an intrathoracic stomach. CT scan or contrast x-rays may be necessary to establish the diagnosis in some cases. Laparoscopy may prove to be a useful technique for detecting occult diaphragmatic injuries in patients who have no other indications for formal laparotomy.

Once the diagnosis is made, a transabdominal surgical approach should be used in cases of acute rupture. Laparoscopic suturing for repair of the injury may be possible in selected cases. The diaphragm should be sutured with closely placed, heavy, nonabsorbable sutures. Chronic herniation is associated with adhesions of the affected viscera to the thoracic structures and should be approached via thoracotomy, with the addition of a separate laparotomy when indicated.

Asensio JA et al: Penetrating cardiac injuries: a prospective study of variables predicting outcomes. J Am Coll Surg 1998;186:24.

Arrillaga A et al: Increased efficiency and cost-effectiveness in the evaluation of the blunt abdominal trauma patient with the use of ultrasound. Am Surg 1999;65:31.

Brasel KJ et al: Treatment of occult pneumothoraces from blunt trauma. J Trauma 1999;46:987.

Cohn SM: Pulmonary contusion: review of a clinical entity. J Trauma 1997;42:973.

Dulchavsky SA et al: Thoracic ultrasound diagnosis in pneumothorax. J Trauma 1999;47:970.

Etoch S et al: Tube thoracostomy. Arch Surg 1995;130:521.

Feliciano DV et al: Advances in the diagnosis and treatment of thoracic trauma. Surg Clin North Am 1999;79:1417.

Fujikawa T et al: Endovascular stent grafting for the treatment of blunt thoracic aortic injury. J Trauma 2001;50:223.

Ho AM et al: Systemic air embolism after lung trauma. Anesthesiology 1999;90:564.

Liu DW et al: Video-assisted thoracic surgery in treatment of chest trauma. J Trauma 1997;42:670.

Macho JR et al: Cardiac stapling in the management of penetrating injuries of the heart: rapid control of hemorrhage and decreased risk of personal contamination. J Trauma 1993;34:711.

Mayrose J et al: Comparison of staples versus sutures in the repair of penetrating cardiac wounds. J Trauma 1999;46:441.

Mansour KA: Trauma to the diaphragm. Chest Surg Clin North Am 1997;7:373.

Murray JA et al: Penetrating left thoracoabdominal trauma: the incidence and clinical presentation of diaphragm injuries. J Trauma 1997;43:624.

Nagy K et al: Guidelines for the diagnosis and management of blunt aortic injury: J Trauma 2000;48:1128.

Newman PG et al: Blunt cardiac injury. New Horizons 1999;7:26

Pape HC et al: Appraisal of early evaluation of chest trauma: development of a standardized scoring system for initial clinical decision-making. J Trauma 2000;49:496.

Rozycki GS et al: The role of ultrasound in patients with possible penetrating cardiac wounds: a prospective, multicenter study. J Trauma 1999;46:543.

Villavicencio RT et al: Analysis of thoracoscopy in trauma. Surg Endosc 1999;13:3.

■ ABDOMINAL INJURIES

Twenty percent of all trauma operations are performed for the management of abdominal injury. The distribution of blunt and penetrating injury in a given population is highly dependent upon geographic location. Blunt injuries predominate in rural areas, while penetrating injuries are more common in urban areas. The specific type of injury varies according to whether the trauma is penetrating or blunt. The mechanism of injury in blunt trauma is rapid deceleration, and noncompliant organs such as the liver, spleen, pancreas, and kidneys are at greater risk of injury due to parenchymal fracture. Occasionally, hollow organs may be injured, with the duodenum and urinary bladder being particularly susceptible. The small bowel occupies a large portion of the total abdominal volume and is more likely to be injured by penetrating trauma. Most blunt abdominal injuries are related to motor vehicle accidents. Although the use of restraints has been associated with a decrease in the incidence of head, chest, and solid organ injuries, their use may be associated with pancreatic, mesenteric, and intestinal injuries due to compression against the spinal column. These injuries should be considered in the evaluation of patients who have signs of seat belt-related abrasions or hematomas. Internal injury may be present in as many as 30% of these cases.

As many as 35% of patents with significant hemoperitoneum may not manifest clinical signs of peritoneal irritation. Retroperitoneal injury may be more subtle and difficult to diagnose during the initial evaluation.

Deaths from abdominal trauma result principally from hemorrhage or sepsis. Most deaths from abdominal trauma are preventable. Patients at risk of abdominal injury should undergo prompt and thorough evaluation. In some cases, dramatic physical findings may be due to abdominal wall injury in the absence of intraperitoneal injury. If the results of diagnostic studies are equivocal, diagnostic laparoscopy or exploratory laparotomy should be considered, since they may be lifesaving if serious injuries are identified early.

Types of Injuries

If the abdomen is the probable source of exsanguinating hemorrhage, the patient should be transferred to the operating room for immediate laparotomy. The hemodynamically stable patent can be more thoroughly assessed within the framework of the secondary survey. Evaluation always includes comprehensive physical examination with pelvic and rectal examinations and may require specific laboratory and radiologic tests. Serially performed examinations may be necessary to detect subtle findings.

A. PENETRATING TRAUMA

Penetrating injuries may cause sepsis if they perforate a hollow viscus. When a full bowel is injured, the con-

tents are evacuated into the peritoneal cavity, and clinical signs of injury are obvious. When an empty bowel is injured or when the retroperitoneal portion of the bowel is penetrated, spillage of bowel contents may be negligible initially, and findings may be minimal. Increasing abdominal tenderness demands surgical exploration. White blood cell count elevations and fever appearing several hours following injury are keys to early diagnosis.

Penetrating injuries cause severe and early shock if they involve a major vessel or the liver. Penetrating injuries of the spleen, pancreas, or kidneys usually do not bleed massively unless a major vessel to the organ (eg, the renal artery) is damaged. Bleeding must be controlled promptly. A patient in shock with a penetrating injury of the abdomen who does not respond to 4 L of fluid resuscitation should be operated on immediately following chest x-ray.

The treatment of hemodynamically stable patients with penetrating injuries to the lower chest or abdomen varies. All surgeons agree that patients with signs of peritonitis or hypovolemia should undergo surgical exploration, but treatment is less certain for patients with no signs of sepsis who are hemodynamically stable.

Most stab wounds of the lower chest or abdomen should be explored, since a delay in treatment of a hollow viscus perforation can result in severe sepsis. Some surgeons have recommended a selective policy in the management of these patients. When the depth of injury is in doubt, local wound exploration may rule out peritoneal penetration. Laparoscopy may ultimately have a role in the evaluation of penetrating injuries. All gunshot wounds of the lower chest and abdomen should be explored, because the incidence of injury to major intra-abdominal structures exceeds 90% in such cases.

B. BLUNT TRAUMA

A major addition in management of blunt trauma has been the Focused Assessment with Sonography for Trauma (FAST) examination. Ultrasound has proven to be an ideal modality in the emergency evaluation of the trauma patient because it is rapid and accurate for the detection of intraabdominal fluid or blood and is readily repeatable. It provides valuable information that augments the surgeon's diagnostic capabilities. The use of ultrasonography for the evaluation of trauma patients is not new and it has been used in Europe for the past 2 decades. Since its introduction in North America in 1989, the technique has been adopted rapidly and a recent survey reports that 78% of United States trauma centers routinely use the FAST examination in the evaluation of patients.

The goal of the FAST examination is the identification of abnormal collections of blood or fluid. In this regard, it obviates the need for diagnostic peritoneal lavage. The primary focus is on the peritoneal cavity, but attention is directed also to the pericardium and to the pleural space. Unclotted blood or fluid allows transmission of ultrasound waves without echoes and thus appears black (Figure 14–12). In the standard FAST examination, four areas are scanned: the right upper quadrant, the subxiphoid area, the left upper quadrant, and the pelvis (Figure 14–13). Most surgeons recommend scanning initially in the right upper quadrant because more than half of the positive tests will reveal blood or fluid in this area. Unstable patients with a positive FAST examination should undergo urgent exploratory laparotomy.

The other diagnostic procedures most commonly used in patients without obvious indications for laparo-

Figure 14–13. Transducer positions for FAST. Pericardial area, right and left upper quadrants, and pelvis. (Reproduced, with permission, from Rozycki GS et al: Surgeon-performed ultrasound for the assessment of truncal injuries: lessons learned from 1540 patients. Ann Surg 1998;228:557.)

tomy include peritoneal lavage, CT scanning, and diagnostic laparoscopy.

Diagnostic Peritoneal Lavage

Diagnostic peritoneal lavage is designed to detect the presence of intraperitoneal blood. Although its use has decreased significantly at many centers with the use of the FAST examination, it is still considered to be an important test in certain circumstances because of its high sensitivity and specificity. Additional determinations of leukocytes, particulate matter, or amylase in the lavage fluid may indicate the presence of a bowel injury. Drainage of lavage fluid from a chest tube or urinary catheter may indicate a lacerated diaphragm or bladder. Lavage can be performed easily and rapidly, with minimal cost and morbidity. It is an invasive procedure that will affect the findings on physical examination, and it should be performed by a surgeon.

The procedure is neither qualitative nor quantitative. It cannot identify the source of hemorrhage, and

Figure 14–12. *Top:* Normal ultrasound of the right upper quadrant. *Bottom:* Right upper quadrant ultrasound revealing blood between the liver and the kidney and between the liver and the diaphragm. (Courtesy of San Francisco General Hospital.)

relatively small amounts of intraperitoneal bleeding may result in a positive study. It may not detect small and large injuries to the diaphragm and cannot rule out injury to the bowel or retroperitoneal organs. The indications for diagnostic peritoneal lavage include abdominal pain or tenderness, low abdominal rib fractures, unexplained hypotension, spinal or pelvic fractures, paraplegia or quadriplegia, and assessment hampered by altered mental status due to neurologic injury or intoxication. The only contraindication is a need for emergency laparotomy.

The procedure may be performed with careful technique on patients with prior abdominal surgery and in pregnant patients. It should usually be performed through a small infra-umbilical incision with placement of the catheter under direct vision (Figure 14–14). Closed techniques of catheter placement utilizing trocars or guidewires have been shown to be about as safe as the open technique, but the rate of failure with the closed technique is higher, thus eliminating most of the potential advantage. After placement of the catheter, 1 L of normal saline solution is instilled into the peritoneal cavity and then allowed to drain by gravity. At least 200 mL of lavage fluid should be recovered to allow for accurate interpretation. A portion of the recovered fluid is sent for laboratory analysis of cell counts, the presence of particulate matter, and amylase. Criteria for evaluation of results are summarized in Table 14–1.

Computed Tomography

CT is noninvasive, qualitative, sensitive, and accurate for the diagnosis of intra-abdominal injury. Modern

Table 14–1. Criteria for evaluation of peritoneal lavage fluid.

Positive
  20 mL gross blood on free aspiration (10 mL in children)
  ≥ 100,000 red cells/μL
  ≥ 500 white cells/μL (if obtained 3 hours or more after injury)
  ≥ 175 units amylase/dL
  Bacteria on Gram-stained smear
  Bile (by inspection or chemical determination of bilirubin content)
  Food particles (microscopic analysis of strained or spun specimen)
Intermediate
  Pink fluid on free aspiration
  50,000–100,000 red cells/μL in blunt trauma
  100–500 white cells/μL
  75–175 units amylase/dL
Negative
  Clear aspirate
  ≤ 100 white cells/μL
  ≤ 75 units amylase/dL

spiral scanners have greatly decreased the time required for obtaining high-quality images. However, CT scanning remains expensive and the scans require an experienced radiologist for proper interpretation. CT scanning requires transport from the acute care area and should not be attempted in the unstable patient.

CT scanning has a primary role in defining the location and magnitude of intra-abdominal injuries related to blunt trauma. It has the advantage of detecting most retroperitoneal injuries, but it may not identify some gastrointestinal injuries. The information provided on the magnitude of injury allows for nonoperative management of patients with solid organ injuries. Nonsurgical therapy is now used in more than 80% of blunt liver and spleen injuries.

Diagnostic Laparoscopy

Laparoscopy has an important diagnostic role in stable patients with penetrating abdominal trauma. It can quickly establish whether peritoneal penetration has occurred and thus reduce the number of negative and nontherapeutic trauma laparotomies performed. In selected patients, therapeutic laparoscopy has been used to repair injuries to the bowel and diaphragm. This approach offers all the advantages of minimally invasive surgery. Laparoscopy has also been applied safely and effectively as a screening tool in stable patients with blunt abdominal trauma. However, its use in this context requires further study. Concerns regarding the use

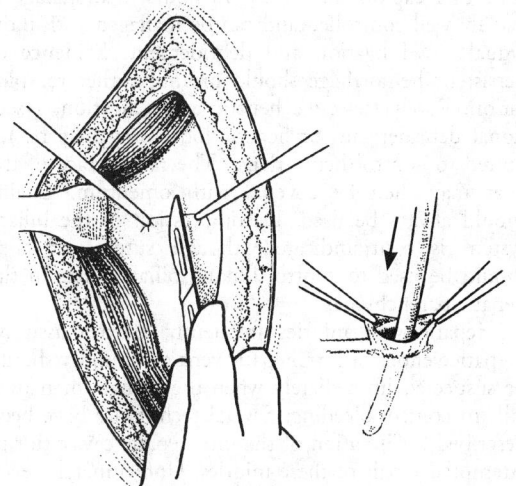

Figure 14–14. Diagnostic pericardial lavage.

of laparoscopy in trauma include the possibility of missed injuries, air embolism, hemodynamic instability related to the pneumoperitoneum, and complications related to trocar placement.

Exploratory Laparotomy

The three main indications for exploration of the abdomen following blunt trauma are peritonitis, unexplained hypovolemia, and the presence of other injuries known to be frequently associated with intra-abdominal injuries. Peritonitis after blunt abdominal trauma is rare but always requires exploration. Signs of peritonitis can arise from rupture of a hollow organ, such as the duodenum, bladder, intestine, or gallbladder; from pancreatic injury; or occasionally from the presence of retroperitoneal blood.

Emergency abdominal exploration should be considered for patients with profound hypovolemic shock and a normal chest x-ray unless extra-abdominal blood loss is sufficient to account for the hypovolemia. In most cases a rapidly performed FAST examination or peritoneal lavage will confirm the diagnosis of intraperitoneal hemorrhage. Patients with blunt trauma and hypovolemia should be examined first for intra-abdominal bleeding even if there is no overt evidence of abdominal trauma. For example, hypovolemia may be due to loss of blood from a large scalp laceration, but it may also be due to unsuspected rupture of the spleen. Hemoperitoneum may present with no signs except hypovolemia. The abdomen may be flat and nontender. Patients whose extra-abdominal bleeding has been controlled should respond to initial fluid resuscitation with an adequate urine output and stabilization of vital signs. If hypovolemia recurs, intra-abdominal bleeding must be considered to be the cause.

Injuries frequently associated with abdominal injuries are rib fractures, pelvic fractures, abdominal wall injuries, and fractures of the thoracolumbar spine (eg, 20% of patients with fractures of the left lower ribs have a ruptured spleen).

Treatment

A. ABDOMINAL WALL INJURIES

Abdominal wall injuries from blunt trauma are most often due to shear forces, such as being run over by the wheels of a tractor or bus. The shearing often devitalizes the subcutaneous tissue and skin, and if debridement is delayed, a serious necrotizing anaerobic infection may develop. The management of penetrating abdominal wall injuries is usually straightforward. Debridement and irrigation are appropriate surgical treatment. Every effort must be made to remove foreign material, shreds of clothing, necrotic muscle, and soft tissue. Abdominal wall defects may require insertion of prosthetic material (eg, polypropylene mesh) or coverage with a myocutaneous flap.

B. LIVER INJURIES

Severe liver injury may result in exsanguinating hemorrhage. At laparotomy, immediate efforts should be directed to control of hemorrhage. In addition to stopping ongoing blood loss, this will allow for stabilization of the patient by restoration of circulating blood volume. The initial techniques for the control of hepatic hemorrhage include manual compression, perihepatic packing, and the Pringle maneuver. Manual compression or perihepatic packing with laparotomy pads will control hemorrhage in most cases. The Pringle maneuver—clamping of the hepatic pedicle—should be performed when life-threatening hemorrhage is encountered and will control all hepatic bleeding except that from the hepatic veins or the intrahepatic vena cava. In most cases, the Pringle maneuver should not be maintained for more than 1 hour in order to prevent ischemic damage to the liver. Hepatic bleeding can be controlled by suture ligation or application of surgical clips directly to the bleeding vessels. Electrocautery or the argon beam coagulator can be used to control bleeding from raw surfaces of the liver. Microfibrillar collagen or hemostatic gelatin foam sponges soaked in thrombin can be applied to bleeding areas with pressure to control diffuse capillary bleeding. Fibrin glue has been used in treating both superficial and deep lacerations and appears to be the most effective topical agent. Reports of fatal anaphylactic reactions have limited its use. When injury has already resulted in massive blood loss, packing of the abdomen with laparotomy pads and planned reexploration should be considered. At the time of reexploration in 24–48 hours, hemorrhage is usually well controlled and can be managed with individual vessel ligation and debridement. Evidence of persistent hemorrhage should prompt earlier reexploration. Rarely, selective hepatic artery ligation, resectional debridement, or hepatic lobectomy may be required to control hemorrhage. The raw surface of the liver may then be covered with omentum. Drains should always be used. Decompression of the biliary system is contraindicated, though sutures or clips should be used to control leaking biliary ducts in the hepatic parenchyma.

Hepatic vein injuries frequently bleed massively. Hepatic venous or intrahepatic vena caval injury should be suspected immediately when the Pringle maneuver fails to control bleeding. Several techniques have been described for isolation of the intrahepatic cava prior to attempted repair of these injuries. Unfortunately, even with the use of these techniques, mortality remains very high.

Approximately 85% of all patients with blunt hepatic trauma are stable following resuscitation. In this group, nonoperative management has been shown to be superior to operation in avoiding complications. The primary requirement for nonoperative therapy is continued hemodynamic stability. Patients are monitored in the intensive care unit with frequent assessment of vital signs and serial hematocrits. If more than two transfusions with packed red blood cells are required, arteriography with possible embolization of bleeding vessels should be considered. Associated injuries are present in 1–4% of patients in whom nonoperative management is attempted. Many of these injuries—particularly those involving bowel—may not be evident on the initial CT scans. Therefore, patients must be monitored carefully for the development of peritoneal irritation and sepsis.

Nonoperative management of blunt hepatic trauma is successful in more than 90% of cases. With more severe injuries, repeat CT scanning may be necessary to evaluate for possible complications such as parenchymal infarction, hematoma, or biloma. Extrahepatic bile collections should generally be drained percutaneously. Intrahepatic collections of blood and bile usually resolve spontaneously over the course of several months.

C. Biliary Tract Injuries

Injury to the gallbladder should be treated in most cases by cholecystectomy, but minor lacerations may be closed with absorbable suture material.

Most injuries to the common bile duct can be treated by suture closure and insertion of a T tube. Avulsion of the common duct due to duodenal or ampullary trauma may require choledochojejunostomy in conjunction with total or partial pancreatectomy, duodenectomy, or other diversion procedures. Segmental loss of the common bile duct is best treated by choledochojejunostomy.

D. Splenic Injuries

The spleen is the most commonly injured organ in cases of blunt abdominal trauma. Splenic injuries in children have been managed traditionally without surgery. Until recently, most splenic injuries in adults were managed with splenorrhaphy or splenectomy. Currently, 50–80% of adults with blunt splenic injuries are treated nonoperatively . Patients must be monitored closely in the intensive care unit, and immediate availability of an operating room is essential. Patients should be evaluated frequently for the possibility of other missed injuries. The severity of splenic trauma evident on CT staging is used to guide nonoperative management. Patients with high-grade injuries are better managed with operation.

Diagnosis and management are covered in detail in Chapter 28.

E. Pancreatic Injuries

Pancreatic injuries may present with few clinical manifestations. Injury should be suspected whenever the upper abdomen has been traumatized, especially when serum amylase levels remain persistently elevated. The best diagnostic study for pancreatic injury (other than exploratory celiotomy) is CT scan of the abdomen. Peritoneal lavage is usually not helpful. Upper gastrointestinal studies with water-soluble contrast material may suggest pancreatic injury by demonstrating widening of the duodenal C-loop. Endoscopic retrograde cholangiopancreatography may be used in selected cases to evaluate for injuries to the major ducts.

The treatment of pancreatic injury depends on its grade and extent. Minor injuries not involving a major duct may be treated nonoperatively. Moderate injuries usually require operative exploration, debridement, and the placement of external drains. More severe injuries, including those with major duct injury or transection of the gland, may require distal resection or external drainage. Traumatic injuries to the head of the pancreas often include associated vascular injuries and carry a high mortality rate. Efforts should be directed at controlling hemorrhage, and drains can be placed in the area of the pancreatic injury. In most cases, pancreaticoduodenectomy should not be attempted in the setting of an unstable patient with multiple injuries.

The late complications of pancreatic injuries include pseudocyst, pancreatic fistula, and pancreatic abscess. Patients treated without resection may require reoperation for resection or Roux-en-Y drainage.

F. Gastrointestinal Tract Injuries

Most injuries of the stomach can be repaired. Large injuries, such as those from shotgun blasts, may require subtotal or total resection.

Duodenal injuries may not be evident from the initial physical examination or x-ray studies. Abdominal films will reveal retroperitoneal gas within 6 hours after injury in most patients. Computed tomography performed with a contrast agent will frequently identify the site of perforation. Most duodenal injuries can be treated with lateral repair, but some may require resection with end-to-end anastomosis. Occasionally, pancreaticoduodenectomy is required to manage a severe injury. A duodenostomy tube is useful in decompressing the duodenum and can be used to control a fistula caused by an injury. Jejunal or omental patches may also aid in preventing a suture line leak.

Duodenal hematomas causing high-grade obstruction usually resolve with nonoperative management. Patients may require total parenteral nutrition. In some cases, a small bore enteral feeding tube can be passed beyond the area of obstruction utilizing interventional radiology techniques. Large hematomas may require operative evacuation, particularly when the obstruction lasts for more than 10–14 days and a persistent hematoma is seen on CT scan.

Most small bowel injuries can be treated with a two-layer sutured closure, though devascularizing injuries to the mesentery or small bowel will require resection. The underlying principle is to preserve as much small bowel as possible.

For injuries to the colon, the standard approach has been to divert the fecal stream or exteriorize the injury. Primary repair of colon injuries can be performed safely in certain circumstances. Wounds that involve less than one-half of the bowel should be considered for primary repair if the blood supply is not compromised. Primary repair should not be attempted in the patient who is in shock with associated hypotension, in the patient requiring multiple transfusions, or if there has been a delay of more than 6 hours between injury and operation—and not in the presence of an extensive retroperitoneal hematoma from pelvic fractures or if there is gross contamination or peritonitis. If the wound is so destructive as to require resection and anastomosis, primary repair is generally contraindicated. Small, clean rectal injuries may be closed primarily if conditions are favorable. The treatment of larger rectal wounds should always include proximal diversion with insertion of presacral drains. In this latter case, direct repair of the rectal injury is not mandatory but should be performed if it can be readily exposed. Irrigation of the distal stump should be performed in most cases unless it would further contaminate the pelvic space.

G. GENITOURINARY TRACT INJURIES

The most commonly injured genitourinary tract organs are the male genitalia, the uterus, the urethra, the bladder, the ureters, and the kidneys. The workup for these injuries consists primarily of radiologic examinations, which may include abdominal CT scan, intravenous urogram, cystogram, and urethrogram. In unstable patients with associated injuries, it may not be possible to obtain these studies prior to emergency laparotomy. In these patients, an intraoperative single-shot intravenous urogram is safe and of high quality in most cases. This study often provides important information that facilitates rapid and accurate decision making. It can confirm function in the noninjured kidney and help in identifying blunt renal injuries that may be safely observed.

1. Injuries to the male genitalia—Injuries to the male genitalia usually result in skin loss only; the penis, penile urethra, and testes are usually spared. Skin loss from the penis should be treated with a primary skin graft. Scrotal skin loss should be treated by delayed re-

construction; an exposed testis can be temporarily protected by placing it subcutaneously in the thigh.

2. Uterine injuries—Injuries of the female reproductive organs are infrequent except in combination with genitourinary or rectal trauma. Injuries to the uterine fundus can usually be repaired with absorbable sutures; drainage is not necessary. In more extensive injuries, hysterectomy may be preferable. The vaginal cuff may be left open for drainage, particularly if there is an associated urinary tract or rectal injury. Injuries involving the uterus in a pregnant woman usually result in death of the fetus. Bleeding may be massive in such patients, particularly in women approaching parturition. Cesarean section plus hysterectomy may be the only alternative.

3. Urethral Injuries—Prostatomembranous urethral disruption is often associated with pelvic fracture or deceleration injuries. Blood at the urethral meatus is the classic sign of injury to the male urethra. The prostate may be elevated superiorly by the pelvic hematoma and will be free-riding and high on rectal examination. If either or both of these signs are present, urethrography should be performed before attempts at catheter placement, which may convert an incomplete injury to a complete disruption. Urethrography will demonstrate free extravasation of blood in the pelvis.

Penetrating injuries are best treated with primary repair. Suprapubic bladder drainage and delayed reconstruction of blunt urethral disruption injuries are safe and effective in the majority of cases. Immediate realignment with cystourethroscopy and placement of a urethral catheter is an attractive minimally invasive alternative. In cases of partial disruption it has been shown to result in stricture-free outcomes.

Major injuries to the bulbous or penile urethra should be managed by suprapubic urinary diversion. A voiding cystourethrogram may later reveal a stricture, but operative correction or dilation is usually not necessary.

4. Bladder injuries—Rupture of the bladder, like urethral disruption, is frequently associated with pelvic fractures. Seventy-five percent of ruptures are extraperitoneal and 25% intraperitoneal. A ruptured bladder should be repaired through a midline abdominal incision. Rupture of the anterior wall of the bladder can be repaired by direct suture; rupture of the posterior wall can be repaired from inside the bladder after an opening has been made in the anterior wall. Care should be taken to avoid entering a pelvic hematoma. Postoperatively, urine should be diverted for at least 7 days via a suprapubic cystostomy.

5. Kidney injuries—Advances in the imaging and staging of renal trauma as well as in treatment strategies have decreased the need for operation and increased renal preservation. More than half of renal injuries can be treated nonoperatively. Management criteria are based on radiographic, laboratory, and clinical findings. Nonoperative treatment of penetrating renal lacerations is appropriate in hemodynamically stable patients without other injuries. Small to moderate injuries can be treated nonoperatively, but severe injuries are associated with a significant risk of delayed bleeding if treated expectantly. Renal exploration should be considered if laparotomy is indicated for associated injuries. A midline transabdominal approach is preferred. The renal artery and vein are secured before Gerota's fascia is opened. The injury should be managed by suture repair, partial nephrectomy, or, rarely, total nephrectomy. Pedicle grafts of omentum or free peritoneal patch grafts can be used to cover defects. Renal vascular injuries require immediate operation to save the kidney. Meticulous attention to reconstructive techniques in renal exploration can ensure an excellent renal salvage rate. Adherence to the principles of early proximal vascular control, debridement of devitalized tissue, hemostasis, closure of the collecting system, and coverage of the defect will maximize the salvage of renal function while minimizing potential complications.

Perirenal hematomas found incidentally at celiotomy should be explored if they are expanding, pulsatile, or not contained by retroperitoneal tissues or if a preexploration urogram shows extensive urinary extravasation.

6. Ureteral injuries—Ureteral injuries are easily missed since urinalysis and imaging studies can be unreliable. Most such injuries can be successfully reconstructed by primary repair, ureteroureterostomy, or ureteral reimplantations

Armenakas NA et al: Indications for nonoperative management of renal stab wounds. J Urol 1999;161: 768.

Asensio JA et al: Approach to the management of complex hepatic injuries. J Trauma 2000;48:66.

Bradley EL et al: Diagnosis and initial management of blunt pancreatic trauma: guidelines for a multiinstitutional review. Ann Surg 1998, 227: 861.

Brandes SB et al: Reconstructive surgery for trauma of the upper urinary tract. Urol Clin North Am 1999;26: 183.

Brasel KJ et al: Trends in the management of hepatic injury. Am J Surg 1997;174:674.

Brown RL et al: Observation of splenic trauma: when is a little too much? J Pediatr Surg 1999;34:1124.

Cathey KL et al: Blunt splenic trauma: characteristics of patients requiring urgent laparotomy. Am Surg 1998;64: 450.

Chen RJ et al: Surgical management of juxtahepatic venous injuries in blunt hepatic trauma. J Trauma 1995;38: 886.

Coburn MC et al: Nonoperative management of splenic and hepatic trauma in the multiply injured pediatric and adolescent patient. Arch Surg 1995;130:332.

Croce MA et al: Nonoperative management of blunt hepatic trauma is the treatment of choice for hemodynamically stable patients. Results of a prospective trial. Ann Surg 1995;221:744.

Fakhry SM et al: Relatively short diagnostic delays produce morbidity and mortality in blunt small bowel injury: an analysis of time to operative intervention in 202 patients in a multicenter experience. J Trauma 1999;47: 207.

Fulcher AS et al: Magnetic resonance cholangiopancreatography in the assessment of pancreatic duct trauma and its sequelae: preliminary findings. J Trauma 2000;48: 1001.

Jacobs IA et al: Nonoperative management of blunt splenic and hepatic trauma in the pediatric population: significant differences between adult and pediatric surgeons? Am Surg 2001; 67:149.

Kielb SJ et al: Evaluation and management of traumatic posterior urethral disruption with flexible cystourethroscopy. J Trauma 2001;50:36.

Malhotra AK et al: Blunt bowel and mesenteric injuries: the role of screening computed tomography. J Trauma 2000;48: 991.

Myers JG et al: Blunt splenic injuries: dedicated trauma surgeons can achieve a high rate of nonoperative success in patients of all ages. J Trauma 2000;48: 801.

Pachter HL et al: The current status of splenic preservation. Adv Surg 2000;34:137.

Patton JH: Pancreatic trauma: a simplified management guideline. J Trauma 1997;43: 234.

Peitzman AB et al: Blunt splenic injury in adults: multi-institutional Study. J Trauma 2000;49: 177.

Richardson JD et al: Evolution in the management of hepatic trauma: a 25-year perspective. Ann Surg 2000;232:324.

Rozycki GS et al: Surgeon-performed ultrasound for the assessment of abdominal injuries. Adv Surg 1999;33:243.

Sartorelli KH et al: Nonoperative management of hepatic, splenic, and renal injuries in adults with multiple injuries. J Trauma 2000;49:56.

Shapiro MB et al: Damage control: collective review. J Trauma 2000;49: 969.

Takishima T et al: Serum amylase level on admission in the diagnosis of blunt injury to the pancreas: its significance and limitations. Ann Surg 1997;226:70.

Uecker J et al: The role of follow-up radiographic studies in nonoperative management of spleen trauma. Am Surg 2001;67:22.

Udobi KF et al: Role of ultrasonography in penetrating abdominal trauma: a prospective clinical study. J Trauma 2001;50:475.

Williams RA et al: Computed tomography-assisted management of splenic trauma. Am J Surg 1997;174:276.

Zantut LF et al: Diagnostic and therapeutic laparoscopy for penetrating abdominal trauma: a multicenter experience. J Trauma 1997;42:825.

ARTERIAL INJURIES

Historical Perspective

Much of our knowledge of blood vessel injuries was developed during the course of military conflicts in the

20th century. Although techniques for the management of vascular injuries were in use prior to World War I, arterial ligation to save a life rather than arterial repair to salvage a limb was generally employed, and amputation frequently resulted after vascular injury. The amputation rate in such cases during World War I was about 20%.

During World War II, only 33% of arterial injuries were repaired. The amputation rate was 49% following arterial ligation and 36% following arterial repair. The lower amputation rate in World War I was due to longer evacuation times and delays before treatment, so that casualties died from exsanguination from vascular injuries and ligation and amputation were not required. In the Korean War, with the advent of antibiotics and advanced vascular surgical techniques, the amputation rate decreased to 13% of cases. The amputation rate associated with arterial injuries during the Vietnam War fell to about 10% due to more rapid evacuation and better resuscitation despite the use of high-velocity weapons. Amputation rates have dropped to less than 10% for arterial injuries in the extremities in many recent civilian series. This is a result of more rapid transport of injured people, improved blood volume replacement, selective use of arteriography, and better operative techniques.

The Epidemiology of Vascular Trauma

The epidemiology of vascular trauma has been studied in three different settings: military conflicts, large urban locations, and, to a lesser extent, rural areas. The types of injuries seen in civilian vascular trauma, once much different from military varieties, are now more similar to military wounds, and the incidence is increasing as a result of the rise in urban violence, motor vehicle crashes, and iatrogenic injuries owing to more frequent use of minimally invasive diagnostic and therapeutic procedures.

Peripheral vascular trauma typically occurs in young men between the ages of 20 and 40 years. In both urban and rural environments, penetrating mechanisms dominate, accounting for 50–90% of vascular injuries. Because many vascular injuries of the head, neck, and torso are immediately fatal, most patients with vascular injuries surviving transport have extremity trauma. This is especially true in the military experience—eg, in Vietnam, extremity vascular injuries accounted for approximately 90% of all arterial trauma. In the urban civilian experience, extremity vascular injuries comprise about 50% of arterial injuries. In rural vascular trauma, blunt injuries occur more frequently than in urban populations.

Mortality and utilization of medical resources is higher among patients with vascular injuries than among patients who do not have blood vessel injuries. Vascular injuries from automobile accidents or falls from heights and crush injuries account for up to half of all noniatrogenic vascular injuries in United States hospitals. The likelihood of vascular injury after blunt trauma correlates with the overall severity of the injury and the presence of specific orthopedic injuries. For example, as many as one-fourth of patients with knee dislocations sustain popliteal artery injury.

The number of iatrogenic vascular injuries has risen dramatically in recent decades. Most involve diagnostic and therapeutic procedures utilizing the femoral (less frequently the brachial or axillary) vessels, which serve as access routes. In order of decreasing frequency, injuries include hemorrhage and hematoma, pseudoaneurysm, arteriovenous fistula formation, vessel thrombosis, and embolization. Rates of injury range from 0.5% for diagnostic procedures to as high as 10% for therapeutic procedures involving large catheters. Increasing age, female gender, use of anticoagulation, and the presence of atherosclerosis increase the risk of these complications. Complications remote from the puncture site include vessel rupture and dissection. Operative procedures (especially hepatic and pancreaticobiliary surgery) are associated with iatrogenic vascular trauma. In addition, anterior and retroperitoneal approaches to the lumbar spine and other orthopedic procedures such as total joint replacement and arthroscopy can produce vascular injuries.

Several strategies to reduce the epidemic incidence of vascular injuries have been proposed. The excessive toll of injuries from gunshot wounds might be decreased by restricting access to firearm ownership to licensed persons, tougher sentences for those convicted of firearm-related crimes, taxing of weapons or ammunition, and legislation to permit lawsuits against gun manufacturers. Seat belt and air bag use has decreased the incidence of ejection during car crashes, which reduces the incidence of some vascular injuries such as disruption of the heart, thoracic aorta, and great vessels. Technologic improvements may result in smaller catheters and delivery systems that will lessen arterial injuries from interventional procedures.

Types of Injuries

A. PENETRATING TRAUMA

The local and regional effects of penetrating wounds are determined by the mechanism of vessel injury. Stab wounds, low-velocity (< 2000 ft/s) bullet wounds, iatrogenic injuries from percutaneous catheterization, and inadvertent intra-arterial injection of drugs produce less soft tissue injury and disrupt collateral circulation less than injuries from sources of greater kinetic energy. The high-velocity missiles responsible for war wounds produce more extensive vascular injuries, which involve massive destruction and contamination of surrounding tissues. The temporary cavitational effect of high-velocity missiles causes additional trauma to the ends of severed arteries and may produce arterial thrombosis due to disrupted intima even when the artery has not been directly hit. This blast effect can also draw material such as clothing, dirt, or pieces of skin along the wound tract, which contributes to the risk of infection. Associated injuries are often major determinants of the eventual outcome.

Shotgun blasts present special problems. Although muzzle velocity is low (about 1200 ft/s), the multiple pellets produce widespread damage, and shotgun wadding entering the wound enhances the likelihood of infection. Similar to high-velocity injuries, the damage is often much greater than might be anticipated from inspection of the entry wound. Moreover, the multiplicity of potential sites of arterial damage often mandates diagnostic arteriography, even in the presence of obvious arterial insufficiency.

B. BLUNT TRAUMA

Motor vehicle accidents continue to increase in frequency and severity and are a major cause of blunt vascular trauma. Multiple injuries include fractures and dislocations; and while direct vascular injury may occur, in most instances the damage is indirect due to fractures. This is especially likely to occur with fractures near joints, where vessels are relatively fixed and vulnerable to shear forces. For example, the popliteal artery and vein are frequently injured in association with posterior dislocation of the knee. Fractures of large heavy bones such as the femur or tibia transmit forces that have cavitation effects similar to those caused by high-velocity bullets. There is extensive damage to soft tissues and neurovascular structures, and edema formation interferes with evaluation of pulses. Delay in diagnosis and the presence of associated injuries decrease the chances of limb salvage. Contusions or crush injuries may result in complete or partial disruption of arteries, producing intimal flaps or intramural hematomas that impede blood flow.

Blunt trauma, chiefly from car crashes, is the principal cause of over 8000 cases of thoracic aortic injuries every year in the United States. About 10–15% of persons who die from automobile accidents sustain an aortic rupture. Most such ruptures occur in patients aged 20–30 years, and males predominate by a ratio of 9:1. Approximately 10–20% of patients with acute thoracic disruptions survive the initial trauma. Of these, about 30% die within 6 hours, 40% within 24 hours, 72% within the first week, and over 90% within 10 weeks if no treatment is instituted. The disruption generally oc-

Table 14–2. Clinical features of traumatic aortic rupture.

History of high-speed deceleration injury
Flail chest
Fractured sternum
Superior vena cava syndrome
Multiple or first or second rib fractures
Upper extremity hypertension or pulse deficits
Hematoma in the carotid sheaths
Interscapular bruits
Hoarseness with normal larynx

curs at the aortic isthmus (between the left subclavian artery and the ligamentum arteriosum) due to a deceleration injury in which the heart, the ascending aorta, and the transverse arch continue to move forward while movement of the isthmus and the descending aorta is limited by their posterior attachments. Clinical findings associated with traumatic rupture of the thoracic aorta are listed in Table 14–2 and radiographic findings in Table 14–3. Blunt traumatic injury to the abdominal aorta is uncommon, but this has been reported from lap seat belt trauma.

Almost any vessel can be injured by blunt trauma, including the extracranial cerebral and visceral arteries. Blunt carotid arterial injuries are associated with mortality rates of 20–30%, with over 50% of survivors having permanent severe neurologic deficits. Whereas in the past vertebral artery injuries were considered innocuous, recent studies have reported devastating complications related to these injuries, including a 70% incidence of coexistent cervical spine injuries. Traumatic injury to the superior mesenteric artery is associated with a 50% mortality rate. The brachial and popliteal arteries, which cross joints and are exposed to direct

Table 14–3. Radiographic features of traumatic aortic rupture.

Widening of mediastinum
Fractured sternum
Multiple or first rib or second rib fractures
Esophageal deviation to the right
Tracheal deviation to the right
Apical cap
Depression of left main stem bronchus
Obliteration of the aortic knob
Obliteration of the descending aorta
Obliteration of the aortopulmonary window
Obliteration of the medial left upper lobe
Widened paravertebral stripe

trauma, are particularly susceptible to injury as a result of fractures and dislocations.

Clinical Findings

A. HEMORRHAGE

When pulsatile external hemorrhage is present, the diagnosis of arterial injury is obvious, but when blood accumulates in deep tissues of the extremity, the thorax, abdomen, or retroperitoneum, the only manifestation may be shock. Peripheral vasoconstriction may make evaluation of peripheral pulses difficult until blood volume is restored. If the artery is completely severed, thrombus may form at the contracted vessel ends and a major vascular injury may not be suspected. The presence of arterial pulses distal to a penetrating wound does not preclude arterial injury; as many as 20% of patients with injuries of major arteries in an extremity have palpable pulses distal to the injury, either because the vessel has not thrombosed or because pulse waves are transmitted through soft clot. Conversely, the absence of a palpable pulse in an adequately resuscitated patient is a sensitive indicator of arterial injury.

B. ISCHEMIA

Acute arterial insufficiency must be diagnosed promptly to prevent tissue loss. Ischemia should be suspected when the patient has one or more of the "five Ps": pain, pallor, paralysis, paresthesia, or pulselessness. The susceptibility of different cells to hypoxia varies (eg, sudden occlusion of the carotid artery results in brain damage within minutes unless collateral circulation can maintain adequate perfusion, but a kidney can survive severe ischemia for up to an hour). Peripheral nerves are quite vulnerable to ischemia because they have a high basal energy requirement to maintain ion gradients over large membrane surfaces and because they have few glycogen stores. Hence, interruption of arterial flow for relatively short periods can result in neural damage due to interrupted substrate delivery. In contrast, skeletal muscle is more tolerant of decreased arterial flow. Muscle can be ischemic for up to 4 hours without developing histologic changes. In general, complete interruption of all arterial inflow (including collateral blood supply) results in neuromuscular ischemic damage after 4–6 hours. Restoration of flow can actually worsen this damage as part of the reperfusion syndrome. With ischemia, the sodium pump fails, cells swell, and the integrity of cellular membranes is lost; intracellular water production increases owing to a shift to anaerobic metabolism; and blood viscosity increases and red blood cells sludge within capillaries. At this stage, restoration of perfusion may increase swelling (reperfusion edema), sometimes causing tissue necrosis. Reperfusion reintroduces oxygen and leads to conversion of accumulated hypoxanthine (the major by-product of ATP metabolism) to xanthine with the generation of large amounts of superoxide anion, a highly reactive oxygen free radical. Superoxide anion injures the microvascular endothelial membrane with loss of endothelial membrane integrity due to lipid peroxidation. In addition, superoxide anion causes accumulation of polymorphonuclear leukocytes in muscle and decreases the production of nitric oxide, leading to vasoconstriction. Inflammatory mediators cause platelet aggregation, increased vascular permeability, and additional neutrophil activation. Activated neutrophils can adhere to the endothelium, resulting in microvascular obstruction. Thus, the events associated with reperfusion after complete ischemia can increase the severity of the original ischemic insult.

Prolonged ischemia can produce muscle necrosis and rhabdomyolysis, which releases potassium and myoglobin into the circulation. Myoglobin is an oxygen-transporting protein similar in structure to hemoglobin; it is innocuous unless it dissociates into hematin, which is nephrotoxic in an acidic milieu. Precipitation of hematin pigment also occurs when urine flow is reduced by hypotension or hypovolemia, obstructing renal tubules and worsening nephrotoxicity. Myoglobinemia can lead to acute tubular necrosis and renal failure, hyperkalemia, and a risk of life-threatening arrhythmias. Thus, in addition to limb loss, acute arterial ischemia can produce organ failure and death.

C. FALSE ANEURYSM

Disruption of an arterial wall as a result of trauma may lead to formation of a false aneurysm. The wall of a false aneurysm is composed primarily of fibrous tissue derived from nearby tissues, not arterial tissue. Because blood continues to flow past the fistulous opening, the extremity is seldom ischemic. False aneurysms may rupture at any time. They continue to expand because they lack elastic fibers. Spontaneous resolution of pseudoaneurysms larger than 3 cm is unlikely, and operative repair becomes increasingly difficult as the aneurysms increase in size and complexity with time. Symptoms gradually appear as a result of compression of adjacent nerves or collateral vessels or from rupture of the aneurysm—or as a result of thrombosis with ischemic symptoms. Iatrogenic false aneurysms after atrial puncture thrombose spontaneously within 4 weeks when they are less than 3 cm in diameter. Simple ultrasound follow-up rather than therapy is indicated. Color flow duplex-guided compression of iatrogenic pseudoaneurysms is successful in 70–90% of attempts, but the procedure is uncomfortable and may take hours of probe pressure. Ultrasound-guided thrombin injection has been effective for thrombosing large false aneurysms in a matter of seconds, but distal arterial thrombosis has also been described using this technique.

D. Arteriovenous Fistula

With simultaneous injury of an adjacent artery and vein, a fistula may form that allows blood from the artery to enter the vein. Because venous pressure is lower than arterial pressure, flow through an arteriovenous fistula is continuous; accentuation of the bruit and thrill can be detected over the fistula during systole. Traumatic arteriovenous fistulas may occur as operative complications (eg, aortocaval fistula following removal of a herniated intervertebral disk). Iatrogenic femoral arteriovenous fistulas after arteriograms and cardiac catheterization are seen with increasing frequency. Long-standing large arteriovenous fistulas may result in cardiac failure. Similar to iatrogenic pseudoaneurysms occurring after arteriography, spontaneous resolution of acute arteriovenous fistulas usually occurs.

Diagnosis

Arterial injury must be considered in any injured patient. Patients who present in shock following penetrating injury or blunt trauma should be assumed to have vascular injury until proved otherwise. Any injury near a major artery should arouse suspicion. A plain film may be helpful in demonstrating a fracture whose fragments could jeopardize an adjacent vessel or a bullet fragment that could have passed near to a major vessel. Before the x-ray is taken, entrance and exit wounds should be marked with radiopaque objects such as safety pins.

Diagnosis is usually established on the basis of physical examination. In addition to checking for obvious hemorrhage and the "five Ps," the physician should listen for a bruit, palpate for a thrill (eg, of an arteriovenous fistula), and look for an expanding hematoma (eg, of a false aneurysm). Secondary hemorrhage from a wound is an ominous sign that may herald massive hemorrhage. The finding of these "hard" signs reliably reflects the presence of a vascular injury; hard signs mandate immediate exploration in most instances. The presence of "soft" signs (history of bleeding, diminished but palpable pulse, injury in proximity to a major artery, neurapraxia) requires further tests or serial observation.

Doppler flow studies have gained importance in the diagnosis of arterial trauma. An ankle brachial index (ABI), determined by dividing the systolic pressure in the injured limb by the systolic pressure in an uninjured arm, is highly reliable for excluding arterial injury after both blunt and penetrating trauma. An ABI < 0.9 has sensitivity of 95%, specificity of 97%, and negative predictive value of 99% for determining the presence of clinically significant arterial injury. Thus, only patients with "soft" signs and an ABI of < 0.9 require arteriography.

Color flow duplex ultrasonography combines real time B mode (brightness modulation) ultrasound imaging with a steerable pulsed Doppler flow detector. This technology can provide images of vessels and velocity spectral analysis. Color flow duplex scanning of an area of injury is noninvasive, painless, portable, and easily repeated for follow-up examinations. When compared with arteriography and performed by experienced examiners, duplex ultrasound identifies nearly all major injuries that require treatment, potentially at considerable cost savings. In addition to screening for arterial trauma, duplex scanning has been used to detect pseudoaneurysms, arteriovenous fistulas, and intimal flaps. However, potential logistical and resource problems exist. The technology is sophisticated and requires skill in operation and interpretation, which is not always immediately available.

Arteriography is the most accurate diagnostic procedure for identifying vascular injuries (Figure 14–15). Arteriography to exclude vascular injury for soft signs results in a negative exploration rate of 20–35% and an arteriography-related complication rate of 2–4%. Proximity as the sole indication for arteriography has an extremely low yield, ranging from nil to 10%. Patients with unequivocal signs of arterial injury on physical examination or plain films should have urgent operation. The false-negative rate of arteriography is low, and a normal arteriogram precludes the need for surgical exploration. Virtually all arteriographic errors are due to false-positives, which occur in 2–8% of patients. Technical considerations in performing arteriography include the following: (1) entrance and exit wounds should be marked with a radiopaque marker; (2) the injection site should not be near the suspected injury; (3) an area 10–15 cm proximal and distal to the suspected injury should be included in the arteriographic field; (4) sequential films should be obtained to detect early

Figure 14–15. Arteriogram showing traumatic pseudoaneurysm of subclavian/axillary artery from penetrating injury.

venous filling; (5) any abnormality should be considered an indication of arterial injury unless it is obviously the result of preexisting disease; and (6) two different projections should be obtained.

Emergency center arteriography not using the Seldinger technique but rather cannulating the artery to be studied with an 18-gauge catheter (antegrade in the lower extremity and prograde in the upper extremity arteries) is quick and surprisingly accurate. The use of fluoroscopy, especially if equipped with subtraction capability, simplifies the timing of contrast injection and x-ray exposure. Fluoroscopy is particularly helpful to visualize distal arteries and minimize the amount of contrast media needed. Arteriography may be particularly useful in differentiating arterial injury from spasm. In general, it is risky to attribute abnormal physical findings in an injured patient to arterial spasm; an arteriogram is indicated in such patients.

Arteriography is also valuable when arterial injuries may have occurred at multiple sites or to localize an injury when a long parallel penetration makes this determination difficult. Complications of arteriography include groin hematomas, iatrogenic pseudoaneurysms, arteriovenous fistulas, embolic occlusions, and delays in diagnosis that may lead to irreversible ischemia in marginally perfused limbs.

Screening isotope angiography has little value in patients with arterial trauma. The technique cannot detect subtle arterial injuries such as intimal fractures and often causes unnecessary delay and confusion in interpretation of results. Digital venous angiography and magnetic resonance angiography lack sufficient resolution to detect significant arterial abnormalities. Placing a critically ill patient in a magnetic resonance scanner is dangerous. Thus, neither technique is practical for accurate diagnosis of arterial trauma. Venography also has little usefulness; if surgical exploration is planned, the vein can be directly inspected. CT scans may reveal intra-abdominal or thoracic hematomas or organ displacement, suggesting the presence of a hematoma. This suggests the need for arteriography or immediate surgery.

Management

A. INITIAL TREATMENT

A rapid but thorough examination should be performed to determine the complete extent of injury. The physician must establish the priority of arterial injury in the overall management of the patient and should remember that delay in arterial repair decreases chances of a favorable outcome. When repair is performed within 12 hours after injury, amputation is rarely necessary; if repair is performed later, the incidence of ampu-

tation is about 50%. Depending on the degree of ischemia, delay in arterial repair will lead to lasting neuromuscular damage after as short a period as 4–6 hours.

Restoration of blood volume and control of hemorrhage are done simultaneously. If exsanguinating hemorrhage precludes resuscitation in the emergency room, the patient should be moved directly to the operating room. External bleeding is best controlled by firm direct pressure or packing. Probes or fingers should not be inserted into the wound because a clot may be dislodged, causing profuse bleeding. Tourniquets occlude venous return, disturb collateral flow, and further compromise circulation and should not be employed. Atraumatic vascular clamps may be applied to accessible vessels, but blind clamping can increase damage and injure adjacent nerves and veins.

After hemorrhage has been controlled and general resuscitation accomplished, further assessment is possible. The extent of associated injuries is determined and a plan of management made. Large-bore intravenous catheters should be placed in extremities with no potential venous injuries. It is prudent to preserve the saphenous or cephalic vein in an uninjured extremity for use as a venous autograft for vascular repair.

B. NONOPERATIVE TREATMENT

Some arterial injuries remain asymptomatic and heal. Data supporting the practice of observation of small or asymptomatic arterial injuries have emerged from experimental animal studies and clinical reports showing resolution, improvement, or stabilization of arterial injuries. In well-defined settings, this strategy has proved safe in follow-up reports covering periods of up to 10 years. Thus, a nonoperative approach may be appropriate for compliant patients willing to return for follow-up who have (1) no active hemorrhage, (2) low-velocity injuries (particularly stab wounds or iatrogenic punctures), (3) minimal arterial wall disruptions (< 5 mm), (4) small (< 5 mm) intimal defects, and (5) intact distal circulation.

Follow-up must include frequent physical examinations and carefully performed noninvasive studies, and patients should be asymptomatic—and the strategy must be reconsidered if symptoms develop. Adjuvant therapy with antiplatelet agents has been shown in animal models to improve patency in experimental intimal flaps.

Endovascular management has assumed a greater role in the treatment of arterial trauma in recent years. Transcatheter embolization with coils or balloons has been successful in managing selected arterial injuries such as pseudoaneurysms, arteriovenous fistulas, and active bleeding from nonessential arteries. Coils are made of stainless steel with wool or polyester tufts. They are extruded at the site of vessel injury through 5F or 7F catheters. After deployment, the coils expand and lodge at the extrusion site and the tufts promote thrombosis. Catheter-based intra-arterial infusion of vasodilators has also been used to treat vasospasm in small distal arteries.

The recent popularity of endovascular grafting in elective vascular surgery (see Chapter 35) has been applied to the treatment of arterial trauma. A fixation device such as a stent is attached to a graft, and the stent-graft is inserted endoluminally from a remote site and deployed at the site of injury to repair false aneurysms or arteriovenous fistulas. Endovascular grafting may improve as technology advances, but the most frequent application is likely to be in stable patients with delayed presentations who have complex false aneurysms or arteriovenous fistulas. Use of stent grafts in the acute setting requires the availability of a wide variety of sizes and lengths of grafts and advanced catheter skills.

C. Operative Treatment

General anesthesia is preferable to spinal or regional anesthesia. When vascular injuries involve the neck or thoracic outlet, endotracheal intubation must be performed carefully to avoid dislodging a clot. Moreover, care is necessary to avoid neurologic damage in patients with associated cervical spine injuries. At least one uninjured extremity should also be prepared for surgery, so that a saphenous or cephalic vein may be obtained if a vein graft is required. Provision should also be made for operative arteriography.

Incisions should be generous and parallel to the injured vessel. Meticulous care in handling incisions is essential to avoid secondary infections; all undamaged tissue should be conserved for use in covering repaired vessels. Preservation of all arterial branches is important in order to maintain collateral circulation. Control of the vessel should be achieved proximal and distal to the injury, so that the injured area may be dissected free of other tissues and inspected without risk of further bleeding. When large hematomas and multiple wounds make exposure and clamping of vessels difficult, it is wise to place an orthopedic tourniquet proximal to the injury that can be inflated temporarily if needed.

The extent of arterial injury must be accurately determined. Arterial spasm generally responds to gentle hydraulic or mechanical dilation. Local application of warm saline or drugs such as papaverine, tolazoline, lidocaine, or nitroglycerin is occasionally effective in relieving spasm. Intra-arterial injection of nitroglycerin is also very effective in alleviating spasm. If spasm persists, however, it is best to assume that it is caused by an intramural injury, and the vessel should be opened for direct inspection. An old adage is that spasm is spelled "c-l-o-t."

All devitalized tissue, including damaged portions of the artery, must be debrided. One should resect only the grossly injured portion of the vessel—margins of healthy vessel do not need to be removed, as was at one time recommended. The method of reconstruction depends on the degree of arterial damage. In some instances, the ends of injured vessels can be approximated and an end-to-end anastomosis created. If the vessels cannot be mobilized well enough to provide a tension-free anastomosis, an interposition graft should be used. Early experience with prosthetic interposition grafts was disappointing since postoperative infection, thrombosis, and anastomotic disruption were common. These problems have decreased considerably with the use of grafts made of expanded polytetrafluoroethylene (PTFE). Nevertheless, most surgeons still prefer to use an autogenous graft (ie, vein or artery) in severely contaminated wounds. Saphenous vein grafts should be obtained from the noninjured leg to avoid impairment of venous return on the side of the injury. Patch angioplasty using saphenous vein is performed when closure of a partially transected vessel would result in narrowing. Suturing should be done with fine monofilament material.

In the unusual circumstance of isolated vascular injury, 5000–10,000 units of intravenous heparin should be given to prevent thrombosis. Otherwise, a small amount of dilute heparin solution (100 units/mL) may be gently injected into the lumen of the injured vessel before clamps are applied. Proximal and distal thrombi are removed with a Fogarty embolectomy catheter. Back-bleeding from the distal artery is not a sure indication that thrombus is absent. A completion operative arteriogram is indicated to determine distal patency and to check on the adequacy of the reconstruction—even when distal pulses are palpable.

It was formerly taught that fractures should be stabilized before vascular injuries were repaired so that manipulation of bones would not jeopardize vascular repair. The disadvantages of this dictum were delay in restoration of flow to ischemic tissue and interference with vascular reconstruction and subsequent arteriographic study of the completed repair by the fixation device. It is currently recommended that vascular repair be performed first, followed by careful application of external traction devices that allow easy access to the wound for observation and dressing changes. Another alternative is to place an intraluminal shunt temporarily across the vascular injury to decrease ischemia while fractures or other injuries are dealt with. There is controversy about the best time to repair injured peripheral nerves; the trend favors concomitant repair except for high-velocity or complicated injuries.

Repaired vessels must be covered with healthy tissue. If left exposed, they invariably desiccate and rupture. Skin alone is inadequate, because subsequent necrosis of the skin would leave the vessels exposed, greatly endangering the reconstruction. Generally, an adjacent muscle (eg, sartorius muscle for coverage of the common femoral artery) can be mobilized and placed over the repair. Musculocutaneous flaps can be constructed by plastic surgeons to cover almost any site. In an extensive or severely contaminated wound, a remote bypass may be routed through clean tissue planes to circumvent difficult soft tissue coverage problems.

D. VENOUS INJURIES

Venous injuries commonly accompany arterial injuries. In order of decreasing frequency, the most common extremity venous injuries are the superficial femoral vein, the popliteal vein, and the common femoral vein. The relative importance and timing of venous repair in an injured extremity is controversial. Advocates of routine venous repair contend that ligation is associated with significant postoperative morbidity, including more frequent failure of arterial repairs due to compromised outflow, venous insufficiency, compartment syndrome, and limb loss. Proponents of venous ligation argue that venous repairs are difficult (requiring interposition, compilation, and spiral grafting), time-consuming (dangerous in the multiply-injured patient), and likely to cause occlusion (patency rates are only about 50%). The presence of postoperative edema after combined arterial and venous injuries is not reliably reduced by attempted venous repair. It seems reasonable to recommend repair of venous injuries when the repair is not too technically difficult and the patient is hemodynamically stable. Thus, the decision to repair the vein depends on the condition of the patient and the condition of the vein. When venous ligation is necessary, postoperative edema can be controlled by elevation of the extremity and use of compression stockings. In patients undergoing venous repair, patency should be monitored using duplex scanning. If thrombosis of the repair is detected and there are no contraindications, anticoagulation should be instituted and maintained for at least 3 months postoperatively.

Fasciotomy is an important adjunctive treatment in many cases of arterial trauma. Indications include the following: (1) combined arterial and venous injury, (2) massive soft tissue damage, (3) delay between injury and repair (4–6 hours), (4) prolonged hypotension, and (5) excessive swelling or high tissue pressure measured by one of several techniques. Whenever compartment pressures (measured with a needle and manometer) approach diastolic pressure, fasciotomy should be performed promptly. Fasciotomies must be performed through adequate skin incisions because when edema is massive the skin envelope itself can compromise neurovascular function.

Fasciotomies are not benign procedures. They create large open wounds, and chronic venous insufficiency is a recognized late complication even in the absence of venous reflux or obstruction. The chronic swelling is thought to be related to loss of integrity of the ensheathing fascia of the calf muscles, reducing the efficiency of the calf muscle pump. Thus, many authorities recommend against routine use of fasciotomies at the initial operation. In the postoperative period, compartmental pressures can be measured using a handheld solid-state transducer as often as clinically indicated. Normal intracompartmental pressure is less than 10 mm Hg. In general, a pressure of 30 mm Hg requires either fasciotomy or continuous monitoring. When the pressure exceeds 45 mm Hg, fasciotomy is mandatory.

E. IMMEDIATE AMPUTATION

High-energy or crush injuries of the extremities are associated with high morbidity and a poor prognosis for useful limb function—there is a high late amputation rate despite initial limb salvage. Vascular injuries are now repaired with a high rate of success, but associated orthopedic, soft tissue, and nerve injuries are the critical factors that determine long-term function. A number of scoring systems or indices have been proposed to help determine when to amputate immediately and thus reduce the number of protracted reconstructive procedures that ultimately fail. Management of the mangled extremity is particularly difficult, and none of the scoring systems are universally accepted. Evaluation and management of these patients should be multidisciplinary.

F. ARTERIAL INJURIES IN ATHLETES

A number of recent reports have addressed the problem of the increased frequency of arterial injuries in athletes due to certain features of soft tissue hypertrophy and overuse. For example, baseball pitchers frequently develop complications related to thoracic outlet syndrome, producing axillary artery aneurysms and occlusions. Popliteal artery entrapment syndrome, producing popliteal artery aneurysms and occlusions, has been reported in soccer players and long-distance runners. Blunt arterial injuries leading to false aneurysms and occlusions occur in athletes participating in martial arts and other contact sports. Finally, repeated leg motion is thought to be responsible for external iliac artery lesions that have been frequently described in avid cyclists.

Abraham P et al: Lower extremity arterial disease in sports. Am J Sports Med 1997;25:581.

Arko FR et al: Vascular complications in high-performance athletes. J Vasc Surg 2001;33:935.

Asensio JA et al: Traumatic injury to the superior mesenteric artery. Am J Surg 1999;178;235.

Asensio JA et al: Operative management and outcome of 302 abdominal vascular injuries. Am J Surg 2000;180:528.

Bastounis E et al: Revascularization of the limbs using vein grafts after vascular injuries. Injury 1998;29:105.

Biffl WL et al: The devastating potential of blunt vertebral arterial injuries. Ann Surg 2000;231:672.

Biffl WL et al: Management of abdominal vascular injuries. Semin Vasc Surg 1998;11:243.

Biffl WL et al: The unrecognized epidemic of blunt carotid arterial injuries: early diagnosis improves neurologic outcome. Ann Surg 1998;228:462.

Brinker MR et al: Tibial shaft fractures with an associated infrapopliteal arterial injury: a survey of vascular surgeons opinions on the need for vascular repair. J Orthop Trauma 2000; 14:194.

Brown KR et al: Determinates of functional disability after complex upper extremity trauma. Ann Vasc Surg 2001;15:43.

Buckman RF Jr et al: Juxtahepatic venous injuries: a critical review of reported management strategies. J Trauma 2000;48:978.

Caps MT: The epidemiology of vascular trauma. Semin Vasc Surg 1998;11:227.

Carlin RE et al: Sural artery pseudoaneurysms after knee arthroscopy: treatment with transcatheter embolization. J Vasc Surg 2001;33:170.

Carrillo EH et al: Common and external iliac artery injuries associated with pelvic fractures. J Orthop Trauma 1999;13:351.

Cox CS Jr et al: Blunt versus penetrating subclavian artery injury: presentation, injury pattern, and outcome. J Trauma 1999; 46:445.

Dennis JW et al: Validation of nonoperative management of occult vascular injuries and accuracy of physical examination alone in penetrating extremity trauma: 5- to 10-year follow-up. J Trauma 1998;44:243.

Demetriades D et al: Penetrating injuries to the subclavian and axillary vessels. J Am Coll Surg 1999;188:290.

Fujikawa T et al: Endovascular stent grafting for the treatment of blunt thoracic aortic injury. J Trauma 2001;50:223.

Gasparri MG et al: Physical examination plus chest radiography in penetrating periclavicular trauma: the appropriate trigger for angiography. J Trauma 2000;49:1029.

Granchi T et al: Prolonged use of intraluminal arterial shunts without systemic anticoagulation. Am J Surg 2000;180:493.

Heges MS et al: Knee dislocation. Complications of nonoperative and operative management. Clin Sports Med 2000;19:519.

Hyre CE et al: Aggressive management of vascular injuries of the thoracic outlet. J Vasc Surg 1998;27:880.

Ishitobi K et al: Extra-anatomic bypass graft for management of axillary artery occlusion in pitchers. J Vasc Surg 2001;33:797.

Kalakuntla V et al: Six-year experience with management of subclavian artery injuries. Am Surg 2000;66:927.

Kang SS et al: Percutaneous ultrasound guided thrombin injections: a new method for treating postcatheterization femoral pseudoaneurysms. J Vasc Surg 1998;27:1032.

Knudsen MM et al: Outcome after major renovascular injuries: a Western trauma association multicenter report. J Trauma 2000;49:1116.

Lyden SP et al: Common iliac artery dissection after blunt trauma: case report of endovascular repair and literature review. J Trauma 2001;50:339.

Makrin V et al: Stab wounds to the gluteal region: a management strategy. J Trauma 2001;50:707.

Martinez D et al: Popliteal artery injury associated with knee dislocations. Am Surg 2001;67:165.

McEwan L et al: Lap belt abdominal aortic trauma. Australas Radiol 1999;43:369.

McIntyre WB, Ballard JL: Cervicothoracic vascular injuries. Semin Vasc Surg 1998;11:232.

McKinley AG et al: Management of proximal axillary and subclavian artery injuries. Br J Surg 2000;87:79.

McQueen MM et al: Acute compartment syndrome. Who is at risk? J Bone Joint Surg Br 2000;82:200.

Mittal VK et al: Carotid artery injuries and their management. J Cardiovasc Surg 2000;41:423.

Modrall JC et al: Diagnosis and management of penetrating vascular trauma and the injured extremity. Emerg Med Clin North Am 1998;16:129.

Naidoo NM et al: Angiographic embolisation in arterial trauma. Eur J Vasc Endovasc Surg 2000;19:77.

Nair R et al: Gunshot injuries of the popliteal artery. Br J Surg 2000;87:602.

Nair R et al: Management of penetrating cervicomediastinal venous trauma. Eur J Vasc Endovasc Surg 2000;19;65.

Nehler MR et al: Iatrogenic vascular injuries from percutaneous vascular suturing devices. J Vasc Surg 2001;33:943.

Nehler MR et al: Iatrogenic vascular trauma. Semin Vasc Surg 1998;11:283.

Ofer A et al: CT angiography of the carotid arteries in trauma to the neck. Eur J Vasc Endovasc Surg 201:401.

Pagan-Marin H et al: Blunt abdominal or pelvic trauma—suspected vascular injury. American College of Radiology. ACR Appropriateness Criteria. Radiology 2000;215(Suppl)41.

Risberg B et al: Management of vascular injuries using endovascular techniques. Eur J Surg 2000;166:196.

Rosengart MR et al: Prognostic factors in patients with inferior vena cava injuries. Am Surg 1999;65:849.

Ruchat P et al: Endovascular treatment of aortic rupture by blunt chest trauma. J Cardiovasc Surg 2001;42:77.

Schneider K et al: An aneurysm involving the axillary artery and its branch vessels in a major league baseball pitcher. A case report and review of the literature. Am J Sports Med 1999; 27:370.

Skudder PA et al: Tibial artery false aneurysm: uncommon result of blunt injury occurring during athletics. Ann Vasc Surg 1999; 13:589.

Sparks SR et al: Arterial injury in uncomplicated upper extremity dislocations. Ann Vasc Surg 2000;14:110.

Tuech JJ et al: Blunt injury to the common iliac artery. Eur J Vasc Endovasc Surg 2000;20:47.

Velmahos GC et al: Angiographic embolization for arrest of bleeding after penetrating trauma to the abdomen. Am J Surg 1999;178:367.

Wahl WL et al: Blunt thoracic aortic injury: delayed or early repair? J Trauma 1999;47:254.

Wascher DC: High-velocity knee dislocation with vascular injury. Treatment principles. Clin Sports Med 2000;19:457.

Yasuhara H et al: Blunt thoracic and abdominal vascular trauma and organ injury caused by road traffic accident. Eur J Vasc Endovasc Surg 2000;20:517.

■ BLAST INJURY

Blast injuries in civilian populations occur as a result of fireworks, household explosions, or industrial accidents. Urban guerrilla warfare or terrorist tactics may take the form of letter bombs, suitcase bombs, car bombs, or truck bombs. Injuries occur from the effects of the blast itself, propelled foreign bodies, or, in large blasts, from falling objects. Military blast injuries may also involve personnel submerged in water. Water increases energy transmission and the possibility of injury to the viscera of the thorax or abdomen. The pathophysiology of blast injuries involves two mechanisms. **Crush injury** results from rapid displacement of the body wall and may result in laceration and contusion of underlying structures. Minor displacements may produce serious injury if the body wall velocity is high. In addition, the motion of the body wall generates waves that propagate within the body and transfer energy to internal sites.

Clinical Findings

A. Symptoms and Signs

The injury is dependent upon proximity to the blast, space confinement, and detonation size. Large explosions cause multiple foreign body impregnations, bruises, abrasions, and lacerations. Gross soilage of wounds from clothing, flying debris, or explosive powder is usual. About 10% of all casualties have deep injuries to the chest or abdomen. Blast-induced circulatory shock may be caused by immediate myocardial depression without a compensatory vasoconstriction. Lung damage usually involves rupture of the alveolus with hemorrhage. Air embolism from bronchovenous fistula may cause sudden death. The mechanisms of lung injury are thought to be due to spalling effects (splintering forces produced when a pressure wave hits a fluid-air interface), implosion effects, and pressure differentials. Hypoxia may result from a ventilation-perfusion mismatch caused by the pulmonary hemorrhage. Patients with pulmonary blast injury may die despite intensive respiratory support.

Blast injury causing pneumatic disruption of the esophagus or bowel has been reported. Tension pneumoperitoneum is a known although rare complication of barotrauma. Letter bombs cause predominantly hand, face, eye, and ear injuries. Energy transmission within the fluid media of the eye can cause globe rupture, dialysis of the iris, hyphema of the anterior chamber, lens capsule tears, retinal rupture, or macular pucker. Ear injuries may consist of drum rupture or cochlear damage. There may be nerve or conduction hearing deficit or deafness. Tinnitus, vertigo, and anosmia are also seen in letter bomb casualties.

B. Imaging Studies

Chest x-ray may initially be normal or may show pneumothorax, pneumomediastinum, or parenchymal infiltrates.

Treatment

Severe injuries with shock from blood loss or hypoxia require resuscitative measures to restore perfusion and oxygenation. The usual criteria for exploring penetrating wounds of the thorax or abdomen are employed. Perforation of hollow organs should be suspected in patients with appropriate histories, particularly those that were submerged at the time of injury. Respiratory insufficiency may result from pulmonary injury or may be secondary to shock, fat embolism, or other causes. Tracheal intubation and prolonged respiratory care with mechanical ventilation may be necessary. In cases of tension pneumoperitoneum, surgical decompression may dramatically improve respiratory and hemodynamic functions. Surgical treatment of extremity injuries requires wide debridement of devitalized muscle, thorough cleansing of wounds, and removal of foreign materials The possibility of gas gangrene in contaminated muscle injuries may warrant open treatment. Eye injuries may require immediate repair. Ear injuries are usually treated expectantly.

Cernak I et al: Recognizing, scoring and predicting blast injuries. World J Surg 1999;23:44.

Coupland RM et al: Mortality associated with the use of weapons in armed conflicts, wartime atrocities, and civilian mass shootings: literature review. BMJ 1999;319:407.

Guy RJ et al: Physiologic responses to primary blast. J Trauma 1998;45:983.

Haywood 1 et al: ABC of major trauma: blast and gunshot injuries. Br Med J 1990;301:1040.

Irwin RJ et al: Cardiopulmonary physiology of primary blast injury. J Trauma 1997;43:650.

Irwin RJ et al: Shock after blast wave injury is caused by a vagally mediated reflex. J Trauma 1999;47:105.

Mallonee S et al: Physical injuries and fatalities resulting from the Oklahoma City bombing. JAMA 1996;276:382.

Oppenheim A et al: Tension pneumoperitoneum after blast injury: dramatic improvement in ventilatory and hemodynamic parameters after surgical decompression. J Trauma 1998;44:915.

■ DROWNING

Drowning is a major cause of accidental death in the United States, particularly in children, and has resulted in 5500 deaths yearly for the last four decades. During summer vacation weekends, the number of deaths may rise to 50 per day. Approximately 25% of drowning victims are teenagers; 20% are less than 10 years of age; and 10% occur in each decade of life from age 20 to age 70. Drowning victims are males in 85% of cases. In the United States, most cases of drowning occur in fresh water, usually lakes, rivers, swimming pools, or spas. Only about one-fourth of drownings occur in seawater. Alcohol ingestion is a factor in as many as 40% of the cases of adult drowning. Inadequate supervision and improperly covered pools or spas are the chief causes of childhood drownings.

The effects of drowning or near-drowning are due principally to hypoxemia and aspiration. The physiologic effects of aspiration differ according to whether the drowning medium is fresh water or salt water, which are hypotonic and hypertonic, respectively, compared with plasma. It is possible for a drowning victim to die of hypoxemia without aspiration, but this occurs rarely. In animal studies, arterial PO_2 falls rapidly after tracheal obstruction, reaching a PO_2 of 10 mm Hg within 3 minutes. In human volunteers who hyperventilated, then held their breath as long as possible, PO_2 declined to 58 mm Hg after 146 seconds of breath holding without exercise but reached 43 mm Hg at 85 seconds if the subject was exercising. Within 3–5 minutes after total immersion in water, this degree of hypoxemia would be enough to cause loss of consciousness in all victims.

If fresh water is aspirated, the fluid is rapidly absorbed from the alveoli, producing intravascular hypervolemia, hypotonicity, dilution of serum electrolytes, and intravascular hemolysis. Animal studies show that the intravascular volume may increase 50% within 3 minutes after fresh water aspiration. In addition, the direct injury to pulmonary surfactant results in increased surface tension and damage to the pulmonary capillary membrane. This can result in a form of noncardiogenic pulmonary edema. Debris and microorganisms are deposited in the alveoli, setting the stage for later infectious complications if the victim survives.

Salt water aspiration produces opposite effects because water is drawn into the alveoli from the vascular space, producing hypovolemia, hemoconcentration, and hypertonicity. Hemolysis is not significant after salt water near-drowning.

Treatment of the near-drowning victim should be directed toward immediate restoration of ventilation, as the degree of hypoxemia and resulting damage increases rapidly. Time should not be wasted in trying to drain the victim's lungs of water, since the actual amount of water aspirated is not large, and in fresh water drowning it is rapidly absorbed from the alveoli in any case.

After restoration of ventilation, the major goals of treatment are to evaluate and correct residual hypoxemia or acidosis and electrolyte abnormalities. If the patient has aspirated significant quantities of fluid, endotracheal intubation and ventilation will usually be necessary. Metabolic acidosis will be self-correcting if the circulation can be restored. In extreme cases, sodium bicarbonate may be given intravenously if the pH is below 7.2. No specific drugs appear to be useful other than those normally used in cardiopulmonary resuscitation. Prophylactic antibiotics and corticosteroids have specifically been shown not to be beneficial.

If immediate resuscitation is successful, the victim is still at high risk of acute respiratory failure if aspiration occurred. This is the major cause of late fatalities. Treatment is identical to that for acute respiratory failure due to any cause—specifically, intubation and the initiation of positive pressure mechanical ventilation with supplemental O_2.

Neurologic damage is the next most common sequela of near-drowning and results from the period of hypoxemia. If the victim never lost consciousness during the drowning episode, the chance of neurologic damage is negligible. In patients who sustain neurologic damage, the neurologic changes and the prognosis are similar to those after cerebral damage from other forms of cardiopulmonary arrest. The kidney may also be affected if significant intravascular hemolysis has occurred. Hemoglobinuria is treated initially by osmotic diuretics and alkalinization of the urine. If acute renal failure occurs, dialysis may be necessary.

Immersion associated with hypothermia may represent a special situation since studies have shown that young, otherwise healthy people can survive accidental deep hypothermia with minimal or no cerebral impairment, even with prolonged circulatory arrest. Rewarming strategies include immersion, body cavity lavage, or, preferably, the use of cardiopulmonary bypass. The latter technique has the advantage of immediately restoring organ perfusion in patients with inadequate circulation.

Biggart NI et al: Effect of hypothermia and cardiac arrest on outcome of near-drowning accidents in children. J Pediatr 1990; 117:179.

Cummings P et al: Trends in unintentional drowning: the role of alcohol and medical care. JAMA 1999;281:2198.

De Nicola LK et al: Submersion injuries in children and adults. Crit Care Clin 1997;13:477.

Gheen KM: Near-drowning and cold water submersion. Semin Pediatr Surg 2001;10:26.

Giesbrecht GG: Cold stress, near drowning and accidental hypothermia: a review. Aviat Space Environ Med 2000;71:733.

Graf WD et al: Outcome of children after near drowning. Pediatrics 1998;101:160.

O'Flaherty JE et al: Prevention of pediatric drowning and near-drowning: a survey of members of the American Academy of Pediatrics. Pediatrics 1997;99:169.

Tipton MJ et al: Human initial responses to immersion in cold water at three temperatures and after hyperventilation. J Appl Physiol 1991;70:317.

Walpoth BH et al: Outcome of survivors of accidental deep hypothermia and circulatory arrest treated with extracorporeal blood warming. N Engl J Med 1997;337:1500.

Weinstein MD et al: Near-drowning: epidemiology, pathophysiology, and initial treatment. J Emerg Med 1996;14:461.

Wyatt JP et al: Resuscitation of drowning victims in south-east Scotland. Resuscitation 1999;41:101.

Burns & Other Thermal Injuries 15

Robert H. Demling, MD

■ BURNS

A severe thermal injury is one of the most devastating physical and psychologic injuries a person can suffer. Over 2 million injuries due to burns require medical attention each year in the USA, with 14,000 deaths resulting. Fires in the home are responsible for only 5% of burn injuries but for 50% of burn deaths—most due to smoke inhalation. About 75,000 patients require hospitalization every year, and 25,000 of those remain hospitalized for over 2 months—evidence of the severity of illness associated with this injury.

ANATOMY & PHYSIOLOGY OF THE SKIN

The skin is the largest organ of the body, ranging in area from 0.25 m² in the newborn to 1.8 m² in the adult. It consists of two layers: the epidermis and the dermis (corium). The outermost cells of the epidermis are dead cornified cells that act as a tough protective barrier against the environment. The second, thicker layer, the corium (0.06–0.12 mm), is composed chiefly of fibrous connective tissue. The corium contains the blood vessels and nerves to the skin and the epithelial appendages of specialized function. Since the nerve endings that mediate pain are found only in the corium, partial-thickness injuries may be extremely painful, whereas full-thickness burns are usually painless.

The corium is a barrier that prevents loss of body fluids by evaporation and loss of excess body heat. Sweat glands help maintain body temperature by controlling the amount of water that evaporates. They also excrete small amounts of sodium chloride and cholesterol and traces of albumin and urea. The corium is interlaced with sensory nerve endings that mediate the sensations of touch, pressure, pain, heat, and cold. This is a protective mechanism which allows an individual to adapt to changes in the physical environment.

The skin produces vitamin D, which is synthesized by the action of sunlight on certain intradermal cholesterol compounds. The skin also acts as a protective barrier against infection by preventing penetration of the subdermal tissue by microorganisms.

DEPTH OF BURNS

The depth of the burn (Figure 15–1) significantly affects all subsequent clinical events. The depth may be difficult to determine and in some cases is not known until after spontaneous healing has occurred or when the eschar is removed and granulation tissue is seen.

Traditionally, burns have been classified as first-, second-, and third-degree, but the current emphasis on burn healing has led to classification as partial-thickness burns, which heal spontaneously, and full-thickness burns, which require skin grafting.

A **first-degree burn** involves only the epidermis and is characterized by erythema and minor microscopic changes; tissue damage is minimal, protective functions of the skin are intact, skin edema is minimal, and systemic effects are rare. Pain, the chief symptom, usually resolves in 48–72 hours, and healing takes place uneventfully. In 5–10 days, the damaged epithelium peels off in small scales, leaving no residual scarring. The most common causes of first-degree burns are overexposure to sunlight and brief scalding.

Second-degree or partial-thickness burns are deeper, involving all of the epidermis and some of the corium. The systemic severity of the burn and the quality of subsequent healing are directly related to the amount of undamaged corium. Superficial burns are often characterized by blister formation, while deeper partial-thickness burns have a reddish appearance or a layer of whitish nonviable dermis firmly adherent to the remaining viable tissue. Blisters, when present, continue to increase in size in the postburn period as the osmotically active particles in the blister fluid attract water. Complications are rare from superficial second-degree burns, which usually heal with minimal scarring in 10–14 days unless they become infected.

Deep dermal burns heal over a period of 25–35 days with a fragile epithelial covering that arises from the residual uninjured epithelium of the deep dermal sweat glands and hair follicles. Severe hypertrophic scarring occurs when such an injury heals; the resulting epithelial covering is prone to blistering and breakdown. Evaporative losses after healing remain high compared with losses in normal skin. Conversion to a full-thickness burn by bacteria is common. Skin grafting of deep dermal burns, when feasible, improves the physiologic quality and appearance of the skin cover.

Figure 15–1. Layers of the skin showing depth of first-degree, second-degree, and third-degree burns.

Full-thickness (third-degree) burns have a characteristic white, waxy appearance and may appear to the untrained eye as unburned skin. Burns caused by prolonged exposure, with involvement of fat and underlying tissue, may be brown, dark red, or black. The diagnostic findings of full-thickness burns are lack of sensation in the burned skin, lack of capillary refill, and a leathery texture that is unlike normal skin. All epithelial elements are destroyed, leaving no potential for reepithelialization.

DETERMINATION OF SEVERITY OF INJURY

Illness and death are related to the size (surface area) and depth of the burn, the age and prior state of health of the victim, the location of the burn wound, and the severity of associated injuries, if any—particularly lung injuries.

The total body surface area involved in the burn is most accurately determined by using the age-related charts designed by Lund and Browder (Figure 15–2). A set of these charts should be filled out for every burn patient on admission and when resuscitation is begun.

A careful calculation of the percentage of total body burn is useful for several reasons. First, there is a general clinical tendency to both underestimate and overestimate the size of the burn and thus its severity. The American Burn Association has adopted a severity index for burn injury (Table 15–1). Second, prognosis is directly related to the extent of injury. Third, the decision about who should be treated in a specialized burn facility or managed as an outpatient is based in part on the estimate of burn size.

Patients under age 2 years and over age 60 years have a significantly higher death rate for any given extent of burn. The higher death rate in infants results from a number of factors. First, the body surface area in children relative to body weight is much greater than in adults. Therefore, a burn of comparable surface area has

a greater physiologic impact on a child. Second, immature kidneys and liver do not allow for removal of a high solute load from injured tissue or the rapid restoration of adequate nutritional support. Third, the incompletely developed immune system increases susceptibility to infection. Associated conditions such as cardiac disease, diabetes, or chronic obstructive pulmonary disease significantly worsen the prognosis in elderly patients.

Burns involving the hands, face, feet, or perineum will result in permanent disability if not properly treated. Patients with such burns should always be admitted to the hospital, preferably to a burn center. Chemical and electrical burns or those involving the respiratory tract are invariably far more extensive than is evident on initial inspection. Therefore, hospital admission is necessary in these cases also.

PATHOLOGY & PATHOPHYSIOLOGY OF THERMAL INJURIES

The microscopic pathologic feature of the burn wound is principally coagulation necrosis. Beneath any obviously charred tissue there are three distinct zones. The first is the zone of "coagulation," with irreversible vessel coagulation and no capillary blood flow. The depth of this most severely damaged zone is determined by the temperature and duration of exposure. Surrounding this is a zone of stasis, characterized by sluggish capillary blood flow. Although damaged, the tissue has not been coagulated. Stasis can occur early or late. Avoiding additional injury from rubbing or dehydration may prevent stasis changes from developing and in that way prevent extension of the depth of the burn. Prevention of venous occlusion is important because it may lead to thrombosis and infarction in this zone. The third zone is that of "hyperemia," which is the usual inflammatory response of healthy tissue to nonlethal injury.

A rapid loss of intravascular fluid and protein occurs through the heat-injured capillaries. The volume loss is greatest in the first 6–8 hours, with capillary integrity returning toward normal by 36–48 hours. In addition, there is an increase in interstitial osmotic pressure that accentuates the edema. A transient increase in vascular permeability also occurs in nonburned tissues, probably as a result of the initial release of vasoactive mediators. However, the edema that develops in nonburned tissues during resuscitation appears to be due in large part to the marked hypoproteinemia caused by protein loss into the burn itself. A generalized decrease in cell energy and membrane potential occurs as a result of the early decrease in tissue perfusion. This leads to a shift of extracellular sodium and water into the intracellular space, which in turn increases fluid requirements. This process is also corrected as hemodynamic stability is restored. Smoke

Relative Percentages of Areas Affected by Growth			
	Age		
Area	**10**	**15**	**Adult**
A = half of head	5 1/2	4 1/2	3 1/2
B = half of one thigh	4 1/4	4 1/2	4 3/4
C = half of one leg	3	3 1/4	3 1/2

Relative Percentages of Areas Affected by Growth			
	Age		
Area	**0**	**1**	**5**
A = half of head	9 1/2	8 1/2	6 1/2
B = half of one thigh	2 3/4	3 1/4	4
C = half of one leg	2 1/2	2 1/2	2 3/4

Figure 15–2. Table for estimating extent of burns. In adults, a reasonable system for calculating the percentage of body surface burned is the "rule of nines": Each arm equals 9%, the head equals 9%, the anterior and posterior trunk each equal 18%, and each leg equals 18%; the sum of these percentages is 99%

Table 15–1. Summary of American Burn Association burn severity categorization.

Major burn injury
 Second-degree burn of > 25% body surface area in adults
 Second-degree burn of > 25% body surface area in children
 Third-degree burn of > 10% body surface area
 Most burns involving hands, face, eyes, ears, feet, or perineum
 Most patients with the following:
  Inhalation injury
  Electrical injury
  Burn injury complicated by other major trauma
 Poor-risk patients with burns
Moderate uncomplicated burn injury
 Second-degree burn of 15–25% body surface area in adults
 Second-degree burn of 10–20% body surface area
 Third-degree burn of < 10% body surface area
Minor burn injury
 Second-degree burn of < 15% body surface area in adults
 Second-degree burn of < 10% body surface area in children
 Third-degree burn of < 2% body surface area

inhalation markedly increases the hemodynamic instability, fluid requirements, and mortality rates.

METABOLIC RESPONSE TO BURNS & METABOLIC SUPPORT

The initial metabolic response appears to be activated by proinflammatory cytokines and in turn oxidants. The secretion of catecholamines, cortisol, glucagon, renin-angiotensin, antidiuretic hormone, and aldosterone is also increased. Early in the response, energy is supplied by the breakdown of stored glycogen and by the process of anaerobic glycolysis.

A profound hypermetabolism occurs in the postburn period, characterized by an increase in metabolic rate that approaches doubling of the basal rate in severe burns. The degree of response is proportionate to the degree of injury, with a plateau occurring when the burn involves about 70% of total body surface. The initiating and perpetuating factors are the mediators of inflammation, especially the cytokines and endotoxin.

Added environmental stresses such as pain, cooling, and sepsis increase the obligatory hypermetabolism.

During the first postburn week, the metabolic rate (or heat production) and oxygen consumption rise progressively from the normal level present during resuscitation and remain elevated until the wound is covered. The specific pathophysiologic mechanism remains undefined, but increased and persistent catecholamine secretion and excessive evaporative heat loss from the burn wound are major factors, as is increased circulating endotoxin from wound or gut.

The evaporative water loss from the wound may reach 300 mL/m^2/h (normal is about 15 mL/m^2/h). This produces a heat loss of about 580 kcal/L of water evaporated. Covering the burn with an impermeable membrane, such as skin substitute, reduces the hypermetabolism. Similarly, placing the burn patient in a warm environment, where convection and radiant loss of heat are minimized, also modestly reduces the metabolic rate. Placing the burn patient in an unwarmed environment (room temperature at or below 27 °C) accentuates heat loss and markedly increases the hypermetabolic state. The persistently elevated circulating levels of catecholamines stimulate an exaggerated degree of gluconeogenesis and protein breakdown. Protein catabolism, glucose intolerance, and marked total body weight loss result.

Aggressive nutritional support along with rapid wound closure and control of pain, stress, and sepsis are the only means available to decrease the hypermetabolic state. The use of selective anti-inflammatory agents may be of some benefit in the future.

IMMUNOLOGIC FACTORS IN BURNS

A number of immunologic abnormalities in burn patients predispose to infection. Serum IgA, IgM, and IgG are frequently depressed, reflecting depressed B cell function. Cell-mediated immunity or T cell function is also impaired, as demonstrated by prolonged survival of homografts and xenografts. A decrease in interleukin-2 production due to circulating mediators may be responsible. An excess of suppressor T cell activity is seen in severely burned patients, and the degree of activity has been found to be a good predictor of sepsis and eventual fatality.

PMN chemotactic activity is suppressed. This has been attributed by some to a circulating inhibitory factor released from the burn wound. A decrease in chemotaxis predates evidence of clinical sepsis by several days. Decreased oxygen consumption and impaired bacterial killing have also been demonstrated in PMNs. Depressed killing is probably due to decreased production of hydrogen peroxide and superoxide; this has been demonstrated by decreased PMN chemiluminescent activity in burn patients.

■ BURN MANAGEMENT

ACUTE RESUSCITATION

The burn patient should be assessed and treated like any patient with major trauma. The first priority is to ensure an adequate airway. If there is a possibility that smoke inhalation has occurred—as suggested by exposure to a fire in an enclosed space or burns of the face, nares, or upper torso—arterial blood gases and arterial oxygen saturation of hemoglobin and carboxyhemoglobin levels should be measured and oxygen should be administered.

Endotracheal intubation is indicated if the patient is semicomatose, has deep burns to the face and neck, or is otherwise critically injured. Intubation should be done early in all doubtful cases, because delayed intubation will be difficult to achieve in cases associated with pharyngeal edema or upper airway injury, and an emergency tracheostomy may become necessary later under difficult circumstances. If the burn exceeds 20% of body surface area, a urinary catheter should be inserted to monitor urine output. A large-bore intravenous catheter should be inserted, preferably into a large peripheral vein. There is a significant complication rate with the use of central lines in burn patients owing to the increased risk of infection.

Severe burns are characterized by large losses of intravascular fluid, which are greatest during the first 8–12 hours. Fluid loss occurs as a result of the altered capillary permeability, severe hypoproteinemia, and the shift of sodium into the cells. Both fluid shifts diminish significantly by 24 hours postburn. The lung appears to be reasonably well protected from the early edema process, and pulmonary edema is uncommon during the resuscitation period unless there is a superimposed inhalation injury.

Initially, an isotonic crystalloid salt solution is infused to counterbalance the loss of plasma volume into the extravascular space and the further loss of extracellular fluid into the intracellular space. Lactated Ringer's solution is commonly used, the rate being dictated by urine output, pulse (character and rate), state of consciousness, and, to a lesser extent, blood pressure. Urine output should be maintained at 0.5 mL/kg/h and the pulse at 120 beats/min or slower.

Swan-Ganz catheters and central venous pressure lines are seldom needed except in the case of severe smoke inhalation injury or unless the patient has sufficient cardiopulmonary disease so that accurate monitoring of volume status would be difficult without measurement of filling pressures or unless a persistent base deficit is present, indicating continued impaired perfusion. It has been estimated that the amount of lactated Ringer's necessary in the first 24 hours for adequate resuscitation is approximately 3–4 mL/kg of body weight per percent of body burn. This is the amount of fluid needed to restore the estimated sodium deficit. At least half of the fluid is given in the first 8 hours because of the greater initial volume loss. It has been demonstrated that patients can be adequately resuscitated with less fluid and, in turn, less edema if a hypertonic salt solution is used instead of lactated Ringer's solution. The main concern with hypertonic salt solutions has been the ease with which an excessive salt load can be administered. Serum sodium must be carefully monitored to avoid exceeding a value of 160 meq/L. Discontinuation of the hypertonic salt solution and a return to Ringer's lactate are required if this occurs. Dextrose-containing solutions are not used initially because of early stress-induced glucose intolerance.

Although the importance of restoring colloid osmotic pressure and plasma proteins is well recognized, the timing of colloid infusion remains somewhat varied. Plasma proteins are ordinarily not infused until after the initial plasma leak in nonburned tissues begins to decrease. This usually occurs about 4–8 hours postburn. The addition of a protein infusion to the treatment regimen after this period will decrease the fluid requirements and—in very young or elderly patients and in patients with massive burns (in excess of 50% of body surface)—will improve hemodynamic stability.

After intravenous fluids are started and vital signs stabilized, the wound should be debrided of all loose skin and dirt. To avoid severe hypothermia, debridement is best done by completing one body area before exposing a second. An alternative is to use an overhead radiant heater, which will decrease heat loss. Cool water is a very good analgesic on a small superficial burn; however, it should not be used for larger burns because of the risk of hypothermia. Pain is best controlled with the use of intravenous rather than intramuscular narcotics. Tetanus toxoid, 0.5 mL, should be administered to patients with any significant burn injury.

POSTRESUSCITATION PERIOD

Intravenous fluid therapy during the second 24 hours should consist of glucose in hypotonic salt solution to replace evaporative losses and of plasma proteins to maintain adequate circulating volume. Evaporative losses are considerable and will continue until the wound is healed or has been grafted. An estimate of these losses in milliliters per hour is arrived at as follows:

$$(25 \times \% \text{ burn}) \times m^2 \text{ body surface}$$

Treatment should aim to decrease excessive catecholamine stimulation and provide enough calories to offset the effects of the hypermetabolism. Hypothermia, pain, and anxiety all need to be aggressively controlled. Hypovolemia should be prevented by giving enough fluid to make up for the body losses.

Nutritional support should begin as early as possible in the postburn period to maximize wound healing and minimize immune deficiency. Patients with moderate body burns may be able to meet nutritional needs by voluntary oral intake. Patients with large burns invariably require calorie and protein supplementation. This can usually be accomplished by administering a formula diet through a small feeding tube. Parenteral nutrition is also occasionally required, but the intestinal route is preferred if needs can be met this way. Early restoration of gut function will also decrease gut bacterial translocation and endotoxin leak. The reader should consult Chapter 11 for detailed information on nutrition.

The use of penicillin prophylactically in burned patient is controversial. It is probably better to treat streptococcal infections in the few patients who acquire them than to cover all patients. Broad-spectrum antibiotics should never be given for prophylaxis.

Vitamins A, E, and C and zinc should be given until the burn wound is closed. Low-dose heparin therapy may have some benefit, as with other immobilized patients with soft tissue injury.

CARE OF THE BURN WOUND

In the management of first- and second-degree burns, one must provide as aseptic an environment as possible to prevent infection. However, superficial burns generally do not require the use of topical antibiotics. Occlusive dressings to minimize exposure to air increase the rate of reepithelialization and decrease pain. If there is no infection, burns will heal spontaneously.

The goals in managing full-thickness (third-degree) burns are to prevent invasive infection (ie, burn wound sepsis), to remove dead tissue, and to cover the wound with skin as soon as possible.

All topical antibiotics retard wound healing to some degree and therefore should be used only on deep second- or third-degree burns or wounds with a high risk of infection.

Topical Antibacterial Agents

Topical agents have definitely advanced the care of burn patients. Although burn wound sepsis is still a major problem, the incidence is lower and the death rate has been reduced, particularly in burns of less than 50% of body surface area. Silver sulfadiazine is now the most widely used preparation. Mafenide, silver nitrate, povidone-iodine, and gentamicin ointments are also used.

Silver sulfadiazine is effective against a wide spectrum of gram-negative organisms and is moderately effective in penetrating the burn eschar. A transient leukopenia secondary to bone marrow suppression often occurs with use of silver sulfadiazine in large burns, but the process is usually self-limiting and the agent does not have to be discontinued.

Mafenide penetrates the burn eschar and is a more potent antibiotic, but there are more complications with its use. Mafenide causes considerable pain upon application in over half of patients. It is also a carbonic anhydrase inhibitor, and metabolic acidosis can result if it is used over a large surface area, particularly in children or the elderly. This agent is used chiefly on burns already infected or when silver sulfadiazine is no longer effective in controlling bacterial growth.

Exposure Versus Closed Management

There are two methods of management of the burn wound with topical agents. In **exposure therapy,** no dressings are applied over the wound after application of the agent to the wound twice or three times daily. The advantages of this method are that bacterial growth is not enhanced, as may be the case under a closed dressing, and the wound remains visible and readily accessible. This approach is typically used on the face and head. Disadvantages are increased pain and heat loss as a result of the exposed wound and an increased risk of cross-contamination.

In the **closed method,** an occlusive dressing is applied over the agent and is usually changed twice daily. The disadvantage of this method is the potential increase in bacterial growth if the dressing is not changed twice daily, particularly when thick eschar is present. The advantages are less pain, less heat loss, and less cross-contamination. The closed method is generally preferred.

Temporary Skin Substitutes

Skin substitutes are another alternative to topical agents for the partial-thickness burn or the clean excised wound. Split-thickness **porcine xenografts** are commercially available and have gained popularity as a biologic dressing that can be applied to clean partial-thickness wounds and to cover primarily excised areas when grafting must be delayed or when autografts are not available. **Homografts (human skin)** work better for this purpose but are difficult to obtain. Other alterna-

tives include a number of synthetic skin substitutes such as Biobrane, a thin plastic membrane that reduces water evaporative loss.

These agents are particularly effective on second-degree burns. After the initial cleansing and removal of blisters, immediate application prevents fluid loss, protects against infection, and stops pain. The patient can walk about in comfort immediately. The resultant healing is associated with minimal scarring.

Hydrotherapy

The use of hydrotherapy for wound management remains controversial. A number of studies have shown that the infection rate is actually increased when patients are immersed in a tub because of the generalized inoculation of burn wounds with bacteria from what was previously a localized infection. Hydrotherapy, however, is a very useful form of physical therapy once the wounds are in the process of being debrided and closed. Showering is also effective for wound cleansing in the more stable patient.

Debridement & Grafting

Burn wound inflammation, even in the absence of infection, can result in organ dysfunction and perpetuation of the hypermetabolic state. Early wound closure would be expected to control this process more effectively. Surgical management of burn wounds has now become much more aggressive, with operative debridement beginning within the first several days postburn rather than after eschar has sloughed. More rapid closure of burn wounds clearly decreases the rate of sepsis and, in full-thickness burn injuries in excess of 60% of body surface, significantly decreases the death rate. The approach to operative debridement varies from an extensive burn excision and grafting within several days of injury to a more moderate approach of limiting debridements to less than 15% of the burned area and no more than four units of blood loss per procedure. Excision can be carried down to fascia or to viable remaining dermis or fat. Excision to fascia has the advantage of allowing for nearly a 100% graft take and also allows the use of wide-meshed grafts if necessary. The procedure can be performed on an extremity, using a tourniquet to decrease blood loss. The mesh can be covered with a biologic dressing to avoid desiccation of the uncovered wound. Excision to viable tissue, referred to as tangential excision, is advantageous because it provides a vascular base for grafting while preserving remaining viable tissue, especially dermis. Blood loss is substantial in view of the vascularity of the dermis.

A number of **permanent skin substitutes** are now being tested that could further facilitate wound closure, particularly in massive burns with insufficient donor sites. Autologous cultures of epithelium have been applied with some success. Permanent skin substitutes composed of both dermis and epidermis have been designed in order to maintain coverage and improve skin function. The efficacy of skin substitutes remains uncertain.

Maintenance of Function

The maintenance of functional motion during evolution of the burn wound is especially desirable to avoid loss of motion at joints. Wound contraction, a normal event during healing, may result in extremity contracture. Immobilization may produce joint stiffness, which at one time was thought to be caused by edema but probably is more due to pain, disuse, or immobilizing dressings. Contracture of the scar, muscles, and tendons across a joint also causes loss of motion and can be diminished by traction, early motion, and pressure distributed directly over the wound to decrease hypertrophic scar formation.

The scar is a metabolically active tissue, continually undergoing reorganization. The extensive scarring that frequently occurs after burns can lead to disfiguring and disabling contractures, but it may be avoided by the use of splints and elevation to maintain a functional position before grafting. Following application of the skin graft, maintenance of proper positioning with splints is indicated. In the convalescent period, application of a pressure dressing and pressure and isoprene splints will result in less hypertrophic scarring and contracture. The pressure should be maintained with elastic garments for at least 6 months and in some cases may be necessary for as long as a year. Early burn contractures can usually be stretched by constant light force.

If reinjury does not occur, the amount of collagen in the scar tends to decrease with time. Stiff collagen becomes softer, and on flat surfaces of the body, where reinjury and inflammation are prevented, remodeling may totally eliminate contracture. However, around joints or the neck, contractures usually persist and plastic surgical reconstruction is often necessary. The sooner granulation tissue can be covered with skin grafts, the less likely is contracture.

MANAGEMENT OF COMPLICATIONS

Infection remains a critical problem in burns, though the incidence has been reduced by modern therapy with topical antibacterial agents. Sequential quantitative cultures of the burn will show when a concentration of 10^5 organisms—the level defining invasive infection—is present. The cultures also show the sensitivity of the bacteria, and when the bacterial concentration passes 10^5 organisms per gram, systemic administration of specific antibiotics should be instituted (Tables 15–2 and 15–3).

Sepsis can be difficult to diagnose, since fever and leukocytosis are often present with a burn alone. Hemodynamic instability is a late sign. The temperature may fall below normal, the appearance of the wound may deteriorate, and the white count may fall, ending finally with septic shock. Aggressive antibiotic therapy must be initiated and an attempt made to identify the source of the infection. Pneumonitis, urinary tract infection, and intravenous catheter sepsis should be considered in the differential diagnosis. If other causes are not found, the wound is usually the septic focus and will have to be debrided. Blood volume, nutrition, and oxygenation must be assessed. Steroids should not be given because they compromise already weakened immune defenses.

Circumferential burns of an extremity or of the trunk pose special problems. Swelling beneath the unyielding eschar may act as a tourniquet to blood and lymph flow, and the distal extremity may become swollen and tense. More extensive swelling may compromise the arterial supply. Escharotomy or excision of the eschar may be required. To avoid permanent damage, escharotomy must be performed before arterial ischemia develops. Constriction involving the chest or abdomen may severely restrict ventilation and may require longitudinal escharotomies. Anesthetics are rarely required, and the procedure can usually be performed in the patient's room.

Acute gastroduodenal (Curling's) ulcers were at one time a frequent complication of severe burns, but the

Table 15–2. Diagnosis of burn wound infection.

Systemic Changes	Colonized or Clean	Wound Infection
Body temperature	Increased	Variable
White blood cell count	Increased Mild left shift	High or low Severe left shift
Wound appearance	Variable—may appear purulent or benign	Purulence may be present, or wound surface may appear dry and pale
Bacterial content Surface	Scant to large amount	Variable
Quantitative Biopsy	Usually < 10^5/g No invasion of normal tissue	Usually > 10^5/g Invasion of normal tissue by organisms

Table 15–3. Most common pathogens in burn infections.

	S aureus	*P aeruginosa*	*C albicans*
Wound appearance	Loss of wound granulation	Surface necrosis; patchy, black	Minimal exudate
Course	Slow onset over 2–5 days	Rapid onset over 12–36 hours	Slow (days)
CNS signs	Disorientation	Modest changes	Often no change
Temperature	Marked increase	High or low	Modest changes
White blood count	Marked increase	High or low	Modest changes
Hypotension	Modest	Often severe	Minimal change
Mortality rate	5%	20–30%	30–50%

incidence is now decreasing, largely as a result of the early and routine institution of antacid and nutritional therapy and the decrease in the rate of sepsis. Management of Curling's ulcers is discussed in Chapter 24.

A complication unique to children is seizures, which may result from electrolyte imbalance, hypoxemia, infection, or drugs; in one-third of cases, the cause is unknown. Hyponatremia, the most frequent cause, is becoming less common with the diminishing use of topical silver nitrate. Drugs that have been implicated include penicillin, phenothiazine antipsychotic agents, diphenhydramine, and aminophylline.

Acute gastric dilation, which occurs in the first week after injury, should be suspected when the patient repeatedly vomits small quantities of food. Fecal impaction resulting from immobilization, dehydration, and narcotic analgesics is a fairly common occurrence. Systemic hypertension occurs in about 10% of cases in the postresuscitation period.

RESPIRATORY TRACT INJURY IN BURNS

Today the major cause of death after burns is respiratory tract injury or complications in the respiratory tract. The problems include inhalation injury, aspiration in unconscious patients, bacterial pneumonia, pulmonary edema, pulmonary embolism, and posttraumatic pulmonary insufficiency.

Direct inhalation injuries, which predispose to other complications, are divided into three categories: carbon monoxide poisoning (Table 15–4), heat injury to the airway, and inhalation of noxious gases (Table 15–5).

Direct inhalation of dry heat is a rare cause of damage below the vocal cords because in most cases the upper airway effectively cools the inspired gases before they reach the trachea and because reflex closure of the cords and laryngeal spasm halt full inhalation of the hot gas. Direct burns to the upper airway are associated with burns of the face, lips, and nasal hairs and necrosis or

swelling of the pharyngeal mucosa. Acute edema of the upper tract may cause airway obstruction and asphyxiation without lung damage. Laryngeal edema must be anticipated in patients with airway burns, and endotracheal intubation should be performed well before manifestations of airway obstruction appear. The endotracheal tube should be large enough to allow removal of thick copious secretions during subsequent care. Tracheostomies performed through burned tissue are associated with a prohibitively high complication rate and should only be done if endotracheal intubation is impossible.

Treatment is primarily supportive, including maintenance of pulmonary toilet, mechanical ventilation (when indicated), and antibiotics.

Carbon monoxide poisoning must be considered in every patient suspected of having inhalation injury on the basis of having been burned in a closed space, physical evidence of inhalation, or dyspnea. Arterial blood gases and carboxyhemoglobin levels must be deter-

Table 15–4. Carbon monoxide poisoning.

Carboxyhemoglobin Level	Severity	Symptoms
< 20%	Mild	Headache, mild dyspnea, visual changes, confusion
20–40%	Moderate	Irritability, diminished judgment, dim vision, nausea, easy fatigability
40–60%	Severe	Hallucinations, confusion, ataxia, collapse, coma
> 60%	Fatal	

Table 15–5. Sources of noxious chemicals in smoke.

Polyethylene, polypropylene	Clean burning combustion to CO_2 and H_2O
Polystyrene	Copious black smoke and soot—CO_2, H_2O, some CO
Wood, cotton	Aldehydes (acrolein)
Polyvinylchloride	Hydrochloric acid
Acrylonitrile, polyurethane, nitrogenous compounds	Hydrogen cyanide
Fire retardants may produce toxic fumes	Halogens (F_2, Cl_2, Br_2), ammonia

mined. Levels of carboxyhemoglobin above 5% in non-smokers and above 10% in smokers indicate carbon monoxide poisoning. Carbon monoxide has an affinity for hemoglobin 200 times that of oxygen, displaces oxygen, and produces a leftward shift in the oxyhemoglobin dissociation curve (P_{50}, the oxygen tension at which half the hemoglobin is saturated with oxygen, is lowered). Measurements of oxyhemoglobin saturation may be misleading because the hemoglobin combined with carbon monoxide is not detected and the percentage saturation of oxyhemoglobin may appear normal.

Mild carbon monoxide poisoning (< 20% carboxyhemoglobin) is manifested by headache, slight dyspnea, mild confusion, and diminished visual acuity. Moderate poisoning (20–40% carboxyhemoglobin) leads to irritability, impairment of judgment, dim vision, nausea, and fatigability. Severe poisoning (40–60% carboxyhemoglobin) produces hallucinations, confusion, ataxia, collapse, and coma. Levels in excess of 60% carboxyhemoglobin are usually fatal.

Various **toxic chemicals** in inspired smoke produce specific respiratory injuries. Inhalation of kerosene smoke, for example, is relatively innocuous. Smoke from a wood fire is extremely irritating because it contains aldehyde gases, particularly acrolein. Direct inhalation of acrolein, even in low concentrations, irritates mucous membranes and produces an outpouring of fluid. A concentration of 10 ppm will cause pulmonary edema. Smoke from some plastic compounds, such as polyurethane, is the most serious kind of toxic irritant. Poisonous gases such as chlorine, sulfuric acid, or cyanides are given off. Cyanide absorption can be lethal. Oxidants are released after all smoke exposures.

Inhalation injury causes severe mucosal edema followed soon by sloughing of the mucosa. The destroyed mucosa in the larger airways is replaced by a mucopurulent membrane. The edema fluid enters the airway and, when mixed with the pus in the lumen, may form casts and plugs in the smaller bronchioles. Terminal bronchioles and alveoli may contain carbonaceous material. Acute bronchiolitis and bronchopneumonia commonly develop within a few days. Sputum smears should be examined daily to detect early bacterial tracheobronchial infection.

When inhalation injury is suspected, early endoscopic examination of the airway with fiberoptic bronchoscopy is helpful in determining the area of injury, ie, whether just the upper airway is involved or the lower airway as well. Unfortunately, the severity of the injury cannot be accurately quantified by bronchoscopy—it can only be shown that an injury is present. Direct laryngoscopy probably gives as much information.

Less common causes of respiratory failure are pulmonary embolus and overload pulmonary edema. Emboli usually occur later in the course of treatment after prolonged bed rest and should be suspected if respiratory function suddenly deteriorates. Heparin anticoagulation is indicated for pulmonary embolism (see Chapter 37). Pulmonary edema from fluid overload during resuscitation usually occurs only in patients with preexisting heart disease. The inhalation-injured lung is very susceptible to edema, which is difficult to manage, since systemic hypoperfusion must be avoided by attempts at diuresis.

Probably the most common cause of respiratory failure is bacterial pneumonia due to either inhalation injury, contamination of the lungs through a tracheostomy or endotracheal tube, airborne infection, or hematogenous spread of bacteria from the burn wound. Alteration of oropharyngeal normal flora with colonization by pathogens and subsequent aspiration of infected secretions is the most common cause of the lung infections.

Pulmonary insufficiency is associated with systemic sepsis. Differentiating acute respiratory distress syndrome (ARDS) from bacterial pneumonia may be difficult. There is damage to the pulmonary capillaries and leakage of fluid and protein into the interstitial spaces of the lung, resulting in loss of compliance and difficulty in oxygenation of the blood. Modern methods of ventilatory support and vigorous pulmonary toilet have significantly reduced the death rate from pulmonary insufficiency.

Treatment

Management of a burn patient should include frequent evaluation of the lungs throughout the hospital course. All patients who initially have evidence of smoke inhalation should receive humidified oxygen in high concentrations. If carbon monoxide poisoning has occurred, 100% oxygen should be given until the carboxyhemoglobin content returns to normal levels and until symptoms of carbon monoxide toxicity resolve. With severe exposures, carbon monoxide may still be bound to the cytochrome enzymes, leading to cell hypoxia even after carboxyhemoglobin levels have returned to near normal. Continued oxygen administration will also reverse this process.

The use of corticosteroids for inhalation injuries is no longer controversial and is clearly contraindicated with the exception of bronchiolitis obliterans.

Bronchodilators by aerosol or aminophylline intravenously may help if wheezing is due to reflex bronchospasm. Chest physical therapy with postural drainage is also required.

When endotracheal intubation is used without mechanical ventilation (eg, for upper airway obstruction), mist and continuous positive pressure ventilatory assistance should be included. The humidity will help loosen the secretions and prevent drying of the airway; the continuous positive pressure will help prevent atelectasis and closure of lung units distal to the swollen airways. Tracheostomy is indicated in the first several days for patients who are expected to require ventilatory support for a few weeks or more. If the neck is burned, excision and grafting followed by tracheostomy is indicated in order to improve pulmonary toilet.

Mechanical ventilation should be instituted early if a significant pulmonary injury is anticipated. A large body burn with chest wall involvement will result in decreased chest wall compliance, increased work of breathing, and subsequent atelectasis. Tracheobronchial injury from inhaled chemicals is accentuated by the presence of a body burn, with a resultant increase in the potential for atelectasis and infection. Controlled ventilation along with sedation will diminish the degree of injury and also conserve energy expenditure. A discussion of ventilatory support is presented in Chapters 3 and 14. Early excision of the deep chest wall burn and wound closure will help remove the constricting component. Wound closure in will decrease the excessive CO_2 production caused by the hypermetabolic state.

REHABILITATION OF THE BURNED PATIENT

Plastic surgical revisions of scars are often necessary after the initial grafting, particularly to release contractures over joints and for cosmetic reasons. The physician must be realistic in defining an acceptable result, and the patient should be told that it may take years to achieve. Burn scars are often unsightly, and—although hope should be extended that improvement can be made—total resolution is not possible in many cases.

Skin expansion techniques utilizing a subdermal Silastic bag that is gradually expanded have greatly improved scar revision management. The ability to enlarge the available skin to be used for replacement of scar improves both cosmetic appearance and function. Advances in microvascular flap surgery have also resulted in substantial improvements in outcome.

The patient must take special care of the skin of the burn scar. Prolonged exposure to sunlight should be avoided, and when the wound involves areas such as the face and hands, which are frequently exposed to the sun, ultraviolet screening agents should be used. Hypertrophic scars and keloids are particularly bothersome and can be diminished with the use of pressure garments, which must be worn until the scar matures—approximately 12 months. Since the skin appendages are often destroyed by full-thickness burns, creams and lotions are required to prevent drying and cracking and to reduce itching. Substances such as lanolin, vitamin A and D ointment, and Eucerin cream are all effective.

Barton R et al: Resuscitation of thermally injured patients with oxygen transport criteria as goals of therapy. J Burn Care Rehabil 1997:18;1.

Boyce S et al: Cultured skin substitutes combined with Integra Artificial Skin to replace native skin autograft and allograft for the closure of excised full thickness burns. J Burn Care Rehabil 1999:20;453.

DeSanti L et al: Development of a burn rehabilitation unit: impact on burn center length of stay and functional outcome. J Burn Care Rehabil 1998:19;414.

Forjuoh SN: The mechanisms, intensity of treatment and outcomes of hospitalized burns: issues for prevention. J Burn Care Rehabil 1998:19;456.

Holm C et al: The relationship between oxygen delivery and oxygen consumption during fluid resuscitation of burn-related shock. J Burn Care Rehabil 2000:21;147.

Kaups KL et al: Base deficit as an indicator of resuscitation needs in patients with burn injuries. J Burn Care Rehabil 1998:19;346.

Kinsky M: The role of interstitial starting focus in the pathogenesis of burn edema. J Burn Care Rehabil 1998:19;1.

Mayes T et al: Clinical nutritional protocols for continuous quality improvements in the outcomes of patients with burns. J Burn Care Rehabil 1997:18;365.

Meyer W et al: Evaluating the psychosocial adjustment of 2 and 3 year old pediatric burn survivors. J Burn Care Rehabil 2000: 21;179.

Nguyen T et al: Current treatment of severely burned patients. Ann Surg 1996:223;14.

Peck MD et al: Surveillance of burn wound infections: a proposal for definitions. J Burn Care Rehabil 1998:19;386.

Schulz JT: A 10-year experience with toxic epidermal necrolysis. J Burn Care Rehabil 2000:21;199.

Smith PD et al: Efficacy of growth factors in the accelerated closure of interstices in explanted meshed human skin grafts. J Burn Care Rehabil 2000:21;5.

Yin HO et al: Comparative evaluation of the antimicrobial activity of ACTICOAT antimicrobial barrier dressing. J Burn Care Rehabil 1999:20;195.

■ ELECTRICAL INJURY

There are three kinds of electrical injuries: electrical current injury, electrothermal burns from arcing current, and flame burns caused by ignition of clothing. Occasionally, all three will be present in the same victim.

Flash or arc burns are thermal injuries to the skin caused by a high-tension electrical current reaching the skin from the conductor. The thermal injury to the skin is intense and deep, because the electrical arc has a temperature of about 2500 °C (high enough to melt bone). Flame burns from ignited clothing are often the most serious part of the injury. Treatment is the same as for any thermal injury.

The damage from electrical current is directly proportionate to its intensity as governed by Ohm's law:

$$\frac{\text{Amperage}}{\text{(intensity of current)}} = \frac{\text{Voltage (tension or potential)}}{\text{Resistance}}$$

Thus, the amperage depends on the voltage and on the resistance provided by various parts of the body. Voltages above 40 V are considered dangerous.

Once current has entered the body, its pathway depends on the resistances it encounters in the various organs. The following are listed in descending order of resistance: bone, fat, tendon, skin, muscle, blood, and nerve. The pathway of the current determines immediate survival; for example, if the current passes through the heart or the brain stem, death may be immediate from ventricular fibrillation or apnea. Current passing through muscles may cause spasms severe enough to produce long-bone fractures or dislocations.

The type of current is also related to the severity of injury. The usual 60-cycle alternating current that causes most injuries in the home is particularly severe. Alternating current causes tetanic contractions, and the patient may become "locked" to the contact. Cardiac arrest is common from contact with house current.

Electrical current injuries are more than just burns. Focal burns occur at the points of entrance and exit through the skin. Once inside the body, the current travels through muscles, causing an injury more like a crush than a thermal burn. Thrombosis frequently occurs in vessels deep in an extremity, causing a greater depth of tissue necrosis than is evident at the initial examination. The greatest muscle injury is usually closest to the bone, where the highest heat of resistance is generated. The treatment of electrical injuries depends on the extent of deep muscle and nerve destruction more than any other factor.

Myoglobinuria may develop with the risk of acute tubular necrosis. The urine output must be kept two to three times normal with intravenous fluids. Alkalinization of the urine and osmotic diuretics may be indicated if myoglobinuria is present.

A rapid drop in hematocrit sometimes follows sudden destruction of red blood cells by the electrical energy. Bleeding into deep tissues may occur as a result of disruption of blood vessels and tissue planes. In some cases, thrombosed vessels disintegrate later and cause massive interstitial hemorrhage.

The skin burn at the entrance and exit sites is usually a depressed gray or yellow area of full-thickness destruction surrounded by a sharply defined zone of hyperemia. Charring may be present if an arc burn coexists. The lesion should be debrided to underlying healthy tissue. Frequently there is deep destruction not initially evident. This dead and devitalized tissue must also be excised. A second debridement is usually indicated 24–48 hours after the injury, because the necrosis is found to be more extensive than originally thought. The strategy of obtaining skin covering for these burns can tax ingenuity, because of the extent and depth of the wounds. Microvascular flaps are now used routinely to replace large tissue losses.

In general, the treatment of electrical injuries is complex at every step, and after initial resuscitation these patients should be referred to specialized centers.

Haberal M: An eleven year survey of electrical burn injuries. J Burn Care Rehabil 1995:16;43.

Shaw J et al: *Electrical Injuries in Total Burn Care.* Herndon D (editor). Saunders, 1997.

■ HEAT STROKE

Heat stroke occurs when core body temperature exceeds 40 °C and produces severe central nervous system dysfunction. Two other related syndromes induced by exposure to heat are heat cramps and heat exhaustion.

Heat cramps—muscle pain after exertion in a hot environment—have usually been attributed to salt deficit. It is probable, however, that many cases are really examples of **exertional rhabdomyolysis.** The latter condition, which may also be a complicating factor in heat stroke, involves acute muscle injury due to severe exertional efforts beyond the limits for which the individual has trained. It often produces myoglobinuria, which rarely affects kidney function except when it occurs in patients also suffering from heat stroke. Complete recovery is the rule after uncomplicated heat cramps.

Heat exhaustion consists of fatigue, muscular weakness, tachycardia, postural syncope, nausea, vomiting, and an urge to defecate caused by dehydration and hypovolemia from heat stress. Although body temperature is normal in heat exhaustion, there is a continuum between this syndrome and heat stroke.

Heat stroke, a result of imbalance between heat production and heat dissipation, kills about 4000 persons yearly in the USA. Exercise-induced heat stroke most often affects young people (eg, athletes, military recruits, laborers) who are exercising strenuously in a hot environment, usually without adequate training. Sedentary heat stroke is a disease of elderly or infirm people whose cardiovascular systems are unable to adapt to the stress of a hot environment. Epidemics of heat stroke in elderly people can be predicted when the ambient temperature surpasses 32.2 °C and the relative humidity reaches 50–76%.

In humans, heat is dissipated from the skin by radiation, conduction, convection, and evaporation. When the ambient temperature rises, heat loss by the first three is impaired; loss by evaporation is hindered by a high relative humidity. Predisposing factors to heat accumulation are dermatitis; use of phenothiazines, beta-blockers, diuretics, or anticholinergics; intercurrent fever from other disease; obesity; alcoholism; and heavy clothing. Cocaine and amphetamines may increase metabolic heat production.

The mechanism of injury is direct damage by heat to the parenchyma and vasculature of the organs. The central nervous system is particularly vulnerable, and cellular necrosis is found in the brains of those who die of heat stroke. Hepatocellular and renal tubular damage are apparent in severe cases. Subendocardial damage and occasionally transmural infarcts are discovered in fatal cases even in young persons without previous cardiac disease. Disseminated intravascular coagulation may develop, aggravating injury in all organ systems and predisposing to bleeding complications.

Clinical Findings

A. Symptoms and Signs

Heat stroke should be suspected in anyone who develops sudden coma in a hot environment. If the patient's temperature is above 40 °C (range: 40–43 °C), the diagnosis of heat stroke is definitive. Measurements of body temperature must be made rectally. A prodrome including dizziness, headache, nausea, chills, and gooseflesh of the chest and arms is seen occasionally but is not common. In most cases, the patient recalls having experienced no warning symptoms except weakness, tiredness, or dizziness. Confusion, belligerent behavior, or stupor may precede coma. Convulsions may occur after admission to the hospital.

The skin is pink or ashen and sometimes, paradoxically, dry and hot; dry skin in the presence of hyperpyrexia is virtually pathognomonic of heat stroke. Profuse sweating is usually present in runners and other athletes who have heat stroke. The heart rate ranges from 140/min to 170/min; central venous or pulmonary wedge pressure is high; and in some cases the blood pressure is low. Hyperventilation may reach 60/min and may give rise to respiratory alkalosis. Pulmonary edema and bloody sputum may develop in severe cases. Jaundice is frequent within the first few days after onset of symptoms.

Dehydration, which may produce the same central nervous system symptoms as heat stroke, is an aggravating factor in about 15% of cases.

B. Laboratory Findings

There is no characteristic pattern to the electrolyte changes: The serum sodium concentration may be normal or high, and the potassium concentration is usually low on admission or at some point during resuscitation. Hypocalcemia is common, and hypophosphatemia may occur. In the first few days, the AST, LDH, and CK may be elevated, especially in exertional heat stroke. Alkalosis may follow hyperventilation; acidosis can result from lactic acidosis or acute renal failure. Proteinuria and granular and red cell casts are seen in urine specimens collected immediately after diagnosis. If the urine is dark red or brown, it probably contains myoglobin. The blood urea nitrogen and serum creatinine rise transiently in most patients and continue to climb if renal failure develops. Hematologic findings may be normal or may be typical of disseminated intravascular coagulation (ie, low fibrinogen, increased fibrin split products, slow prothrombin and partial thromboplastin times, and decreased platelet count).

Prevention

For the most part, heat stroke in military recruits and athletes in training is preventable by adhering to a graduated schedule of increasing performance requirements that allows acclimatization over 2–3 weeks. Heat produced by exercise is dissipated by increased cardiac output, vasodilation in the skin, and increased sweating. With acclimatization there is increased efficiency for muscular work, increased myocardial performance, expanded extracellular fluid volume, greater output of sweat for a given amount of work, a lower salt content of sweat, and a lower central temperature for a given amount of work.

Access to drinking water should be unrestricted during vigorous physical activity in a hot environment. Free water is preferable to electrolyte-containing solutions. Most training regimens should not include the use of supplemental salt tablets, since enough salt (10–15 g/d) will be consumed with food to meet the electrolyte losses in sweat and since hypernatremia can develop if ingested salt tablets are not taken with enough water. Clothing and protective gear should be lightened as heat production and air temperature rise, and heavy exercise should not be scheduled at the hottest times of day, especially at the beginning of a training schedule. Long distance runs with open competition, which attract novice runners, should be held in late summer or fall, when heat acclimatization is more apt to have occurred, and should be started before 8 AM or after 6 PM.

Treatment

The patient should be cooled rapidly. The most efficient method is to induce evaporative heat loss by spraying the patient with water at 15 °C and fanning with warm air. Immersion in an ice water bath or use of ice packs is also effective but causes cutaneous vasoconstriction and shivering and makes patient monitoring more difficult. Monitor the rectal temperature frequently. To avoid overshooting the end point, vigorous cooling should be stopped when the temperature reaches 38.9 °C. Shivering should be controlled with parenteral phenothiazines. Oxygen should be administered, and if the PaO_2 drops below 65 mm Hg, tracheal intubation should be performed to control ventilation. Fluid, electrolyte, and acid-base balance must be controlled by frequent monitoring. Intravenous fluid administration should be based on the central venous or pulmonary artery wedge pressure, blood pressure, and urine output; overhydration must be avoided. On average, about 1400 mL of fluid is required in the first 4 hours of resuscitation. Intravenous mannitol (12.5 g) may be given early if myoglobinuria is present. Renal failure may require hemodialysis. Disseminated intravascular coagulation may require treatment with heparin. Digitalis and occasionally inotropic agents (eg, isoproterenol, dopamine) may be indicated for cardiac insufficiency, which should be suspected if hypotension persists after hypovolemia has been corrected.

Prognosis

Bad prognostic signs are temperature of 42.2 °C or more, coma lasting over 2 hours, shock, hyperkalemia, and an AST greater than 1000 units/L during the first 24 hours. The death rate is about 10% in patients who are correctly diagnosed and treated promptly. Deaths in the first few days are usually due to cerebral damage; later deaths may be from bleeding or may be due to cardiac, renal, or hepatic failure.

Bouchama A, DeVol EB: Acid-base alterations in heatstroke. Intensive Care Med 2001;27:680.

Dematte JE et al: Near-fatal heat stroke during the 1995 heat wave in Chicago. Ann Intern Med 1998;129:173.

Khosla R, Guntupalli KK: Heat-related illnesses. Crit Care Clin 1999;15:251.

■ FROSTBITE

Frostbite involves freezing of tissues. Ice crystals form between the cells and grow at the expense of intracellular water. The resulting cellular dehydration coupled with ischemia due to vasoconstriction and increased blood viscosity are the mechanisms of tissue injury. Skin and muscle are considerably more susceptible to freezing damage than tendons and bones, which explains why the patient may still be able to move severely frostbitten digits.

Frostbite is caused by cold exposure, whose effects can be magnified by moisture or wind. For example, the chilling effects on skin are the same with an air temperature of 6.7 °C) and a 40-mile-per-hour wind as with an air temperature of –40 °C and only a 2-mile-per-hour wind. Contact with metal or gasoline in very cold weather can cause virtually instantaneous freezing; skin will often stick to metal and be lost. The risk of frostbite is increased by generalized hypothermia, which produces peripheral vasoconstriction as part of the mechanism for preservation of core body temperature.

Two related injuries, trench foot and immersion foot, involve prolonged exposure to wet cold above freezing (eg, 10 °C). The resulting tissue damage is produced by ischemia.

Clinical Findings

Frostnip, a minor variant of this syndrome, is a transient blanching and numbness of exposed parts that may progress to frostbite if not immediately detected and treated. It often appears on the tips of fingers, ears, nose, chin, or cheeks and should be managed by rewarming through contact with warm parts of the body or warm air.

Frostbitten parts are numb, painless, and of a white or waxy appearance. With **superficial frostbite,** only the skin and subcutaneous tissues are frozen, so the tissues beneath are still compressible with pressure. **Deep frostbite** involves freezing of underlying tissues, which imparts a wooden consistency to the extremity.

After rewarming, the frostbitten area becomes mottled blue or purple and painful and tender. Blisters appear that may take several weeks to resolve. The part becomes edematous and to a varying degree painful.

Treatment

The frostbitten part should be rewarmed (thawed) in a water bath at 40–42.2 °C for 20–30 minutes. Thawing should not be attempted until the victim can be kept permanently warm and at rest. It is far better to continue walking on frostbitten feet even for many hours than to thaw them in a remote cold area where definitive care cannot be provided. If a thermometer is unavailable, the temperature of the water should be adjusted to be warm but not hot to a normal hand. Never use the frozen part to test the water temperature or expose it to a source of direct heat such as a fire. The risk of seriously compounding the injury is great with any method of thawing other than immersion in warm water.

After thawing has been completed, the patient should be kept recumbent and the injured part left open to the air, protected from direct contact with sheets, clothing, etc. Blisters should be left intact and the skin gently debrided by immersing the part in a whirlpool bath for about 20 minutes twice daily. No scrubbing or massaging of the injured part should be allowed, and topical ointments, antiseptics, etc, are of no value. Vasodilating agents and surgical sympathectomy do not appear to improve healing.

The tissues will heal gradually, and any dead tissue will become demarcated and will usually slough spontaneously. Early in the course, it is nearly impossible, even for someone with considerable experience in the treatment of frostbite, to judge the depth of injury; most early assessments tend to overestimate the extent of permanent damage. Therefore, expectant treatment is the rule, and surgical debridement should be avoided even if evolution of the injury requires many months. Surgery may be indicated to release constricting circumferential eschars, but rarely should the process of spontaneous separation of gangrenous tissue be surgically facilitated. Even in severe injuries, amputation is rarely indicated before 2 months unless invasive infection supervenes. Nuclear scans may be useful to delineate tissue viability.

Concomitant fractures or dislocations create challenging and complex problems. Dislocations should be reduced immediately after thawing. Open fractures require operative reduction, but closed fractures should be managed with a posterior plastic splint. Anterior tibial compartment syndrome, which may develop in patients with associated fractures, may be diagnosed by arteriography and treated by fasciotomy.

After the eschar separates, the skin is noted to be thin, shiny, tender, and sensitive to cold; occasionally it exhibits a tendency to perspire more readily. Gradually it returns toward normal, but pain on exposure to cold may persist indefinitely.

Prognosis

The prognosis for normal function is excellent if appropriate treatment is provided. Individuals who have recovered from frostbite have increased susceptibility to another frostbite injury on exposure to cold.

Affleck DG et al: Assessment of tissue viability in complex extremity injuries: utility of the pyrophosphate nuclear scan. J Trauma 2001;50:263.

Murphy JV et al: Frostbite: pathogenesis and treatment. J Trauma 2000;48:171.

■ ACCIDENTAL HYPOTHERMIA

Accidental hypothermia consists of the uncontrolled lowering of core body temperature below 35 °C by exposure to cold. The syndrome may be seen in elderly people living alone in inadequately heated homes, in alcoholics exposed to the cold during a binge, in those engaged in winter sports, and in others who become lost in cold weather. Alcohol facilitates the induction of hypothermia by producing sedation (inhibiting shivering) and cutaneous dilation. Other sedatives, tranquilizers, and antidepressants are occasionally implicated. Diseases that predispose to hypothermia include myxedema, hypopituitarism, adrenal insufficiency, cerebral vascular insufficiency, mental impairment, and cardiovascular disorders.

The heart is the organ most sensitive to cooling and is subject to ventricular fibrillation or asystole when the temperature drops to 21–24 °C. Hypothermia affects the oxyhemoglobin dissociation curve, so less oxygen is released to the tissues. Cardiac standstill may cause death in less than 1 hour in shipwreck victims immersed in cold water (6.7 °C). Increased capillary permeability, manifested by generalized edema and pulmonary, hepatic, and renal dysfunction, may develop as the patient is rewarmed. Coagulopathies and disseminated intravascular coagulation are seen occasionally. Pancreatitis and acute renal failure are common in patients whose temperature on admission is below 32 °C.

Clinical Findings

A. SYMPTOMS AND SIGNS

The patient is mentally depressed (somnolent, stuporous, or comatose), cold, and pale to cyanotic. The clinical findings are not always striking and may be mistaken for the effects of alcohol. The core temperature ranges from 21 to 35 °C. Shivering is absent when the temperature is below 32 °C. Respirations are slow and shallow. Many patients have bronchopneumonia. The blood pressure is usually normal and the heart rate slow. When the core temperature drops below 32 °C, the patient may appear to be dead. The extremities may be frostbitten or frozen.

B. LABORATORY FINDINGS

Dehydration may increase the concentration of various blood constituents. Severe hypoglycemia is common, and unless detected and treated immediately, it may become dangerously worse as rewarming produces shivering. The serum amylase is elevated in about half of cases, but autopsy studies show that it does not always reflect pancreatitis. Diabetic ketoacidosis becomes a management problem in some patients whose amylase values are elevated on entry. The AST, LDH, and CK enzymes are usually elevated but are of no predictive significance. The ECG shows lengthening of the PR interval, delay in interventricular conduction, and a pathognomonic J wave at the junction of the QRS complex and ST segment.

Treatment

Hypothermic patients should never be considered dead until all measures for resuscitation have failed—prolonged cardiopulmonary arrest in severe hypothermia is compatible with complete recovery.

Mild hypothermia (body temperature 32–35 °C) can be treated in most cases by passive rewarming (heavy clothing and blankets in a warm environment) for a few hours—especially when the patient is shivering. The patient's temperature should be continuously monitored with a rectal or esophageal probe until body temperature reaches normal. Since the volume of intravenous fluids required for resuscitation is often substantial, their temperature can affect the outcome. Consequently, intravenous fluids should be warmed with a heat exchanger during administration.

Active rewarming is indicated for temperature below 32 °C, cardiovascular instability, or failure of passive rewarming. The methods include immersion in a warm water bath, inhalation of heated air, pleural lavage, peritoneal lavage, and blood warming with an extracorporeal bypass machine. Active external rewarming is most often performed by immersion in a warm (40–42 °C) water bath, which will raise body temperature at a rate of 1–2 degrees per hour. A disadvantage of this method is that the core temperature may continue to decline after initiation of the rewarming efforts (known as after-drop), which is associated with worsening cardiovascular function.

Closed pleural irrigation should be performed by flushing the right hemithorax with warm (40–42 °C) saline solution through two large thoracostomy tubes, one anterior and the other posterior. Rewarming by peritoneal lavage involves giving warm (40–45 °C) crystalloid solutions, 6 L/h, which raises core temperature by 2–4 degrees per hour.

Active core rewarming with partial cardiopulmonary bypass, the most efficient technique, is indicated for patients with ventricular fibrillation and severe hypothermia or those with frozen extremities. At a flow rate of 6–7 L/min, core temperature can be raised by 1–2 °C every 3–5 minutes.

In severe cases, endotracheal intubation should be used for better management of ventilation and protection against aspiration, a common lethal complication. Arterial blood gases should be monitored frequently. Bretylium tosylate in an initial dose of 10 mg/kg is the best drug for ventricular fibrillation. Antibiotics are often indicated for coexisting pneumonitis. Serious infections are often unsuspected upon admission, and delay in appropriate therapy may contribute to the severity of the illness. Hypoglycemia calls for intravenous administration of 50% glucose solution. Fluid administration must be gauged by central venous or pulmonary artery wedge pressures, urine output, and other circulatory parameters. Increased capillary permeability following rewarming predisposes to the development of pulmonary edema and compartment syndromes in the extremities. To minimize these complications, the central venous or wedge pressure should be kept below 12–14 cm water. Drugs should not be injected into peripheral tissues, because absorption will not take place while the patient is cold and because drugs may accumulate to produce serious toxicity as rewarming occurs.

As rewarming proceeds, the patient should be continually reassessed for signs of concomitant disease that may have been masked by hypothermia, especially myxedema and hypoglycemia. Any inexplicable failure to respond should suggest adrenal insufficiency.

Prognosis

Survival can be expected in only 50% of patients whose core temperature drops below 32.2 °C. Coexisting diseases (eg, stroke, neoplasm, myocardial infarction) are common and increase the death rate to 75% or more. Survival does not correlate closely with the lowest absolute temperature reached. Death may result from pneumonitis, heart failure, or renal insufficiency.

Farstad M et al: Recovering from accidental hypothermia by extracorporeal circulation: a retrospective study. Eur J Cardiothorac Surg 2001;20:58.

Brunette DD, McVaney K: Hypothermic cardiac arrest: an 11-year review of ED management and outcome. Am J Emerg Med 2000;18:418.

Peng RY, Bongard FS: Hypothermia in trauma patients. J Am Coll Surg 1999;188:685.

Vasallo SU et al: A prospective evaluation of the electrocardiographic manifestations of hypothermia. Acad Emerg Med 2000;18:418.

Head & Neck Tumors

16

Samuel W. Beenken, MD, & Marshall M. Urist, MD

In 2000, an estimated 40,300 people in the United States will develop squamous cell carcinoma of the upper aerodigestive tract. When detected and treated at an early stage, these cancers are curable in 80% of cases, but many patients present with a locally advanced primary cancer or with regional lymph node metastases. Accurate staging is essential to determine the best therapy and to permit comparison of treatment results. Therapy often involves collaboration between many disciplines such as surgery, radiation oncology, medical oncology, maxillofacial prosthetics, and speech therapy. The priorities of treatment are to eradicate the cancer, then to maintain function, and finally to preserve appearance.

BIOLOGY OF HEAD & NECK TUMORS

The great majority of upper aerodigestive tract cancers are squamous cell carcinomas, and they are the emphasis of this chapter. The most important etiologic agents in the development of these tumors are tobacco and alcohol. The combination of tobacco and alcohol use accounts for the development of 75% of all oral cavity, oropharyngeal, and hypopharyngeal cancers. It is estimated that more than 80% of laryngeal cancers are due to cigarette smoking. Premalignant lesions include leukoplakia and erythroplakia, with the most important risk factor being the presence of cellular dysplasia. Because the entire mucosal surface of the upper aerodigestive tract is exposed to the same carcinogens, multiple anatomic sites are at risk for the simultaneous or sequential development of second primary cancers. Second primary cancers develop in 10–15% of cases.

The development of squamous cell carcinoma is a multistep process. Deletions of chromosomes 3p and 18q, amplification of int-2 and bcl-1, mutation of *P53* and overexpression of transforming growth factor-α (TGF-α) and the epidermal growth factor receptor (EGFr) have all been implicated as important components of the carcinogenic process.

16

Beckhardt RN et al: HER-2/neu oncogene characterization in head and neck squamous cell carcinoma. Arch Otolaryngol Head Neck Surg 1995;121:1265.

Koch WM et al: p53 mutation and locoregional treatment failure in head and neck squamous cell carcinoma. J Natl Cancer Inst 1996;88:1580.

Lee DJ et al: Impact of chromosome 14q loss on survival in primary head and neck squamous cell carcinoma. Clin Cancer Res 1997;3:501.

Nawroz H et al: Allelotype of head and neck squamous cell carcinoma. Cancer Res 1994;54:1152.

Shin DM et al: Activation of p53 gene expression in premalignant lesions during head and neck tumorigenesis. Cancer Res 1994;54:321.

Shin DM et al: Dysregulation of epidermal growth factor receptor expression in premalignant lesions during head and neck tumorigenesis. Cancer Res 1994;54:3153.

Xu XC et al: Differential expression of nuclear retinoid receptors in normal, premalignant, and malignant head and neck tissues. Cancer Res 1994;54:3580.

DIAGNOSIS OF HEAD & NECK TUMORS

The evaluation of a patient with an abnormality of the upper aerodigestive tract begins with a complete history and physical examination.

History

Common presenting symptoms are pain, bleeding, obstruction, and a mass. Pain is characterized as to frequency, duration, severity, location, and radiation. The amount and types of analgesics used are determined. Several specific clinical patterns are important. Pain around the eyes can be referred from the nasopharynx. Cancers of the base of the tongue, tonsil, or hypopharynx can cause otalgia. Odynophagia can result from deep penetration by cancers of the base of the tongue or hypopharynx or from extensive cervical lymph node metastases. Hemorrhage is usually mild and intermittent and is most commonly associated with cancers of the nasal cavity, nasopharynx, and oral cavity. Obstruction causing alterations of phonation, breathing, swallowing, or hearing can be a manifestation of either early or advanced cancer. Hoarseness is often an early finding in cancers of the glottis, whereas cancers only a few millimeters away on the false vocal cord can grow and metastasize before causing a change in voice. Trismus usually indicates extension of cancer into the pterygoid muscles. Dysphagia is often a late symptom of cancer growth at the base of the tongue, hypopharynx, or cervical esophagus. Loss of hearing can be the first symptom of cancers arising in or invading the auditory tract from the external auditory canal or nasopharynx.

A history of prior squamous cell carcinoma is common, and accurate documentation of its histologic type, stage, and date of occurrence is necessary. One arising more than 3 years after a previous cancer is considered a new primary cancer. The late appearance of cervical lymph node metastases requires a thorough search for a new primary cancer. The appearance of a lung nodule following treatment of squamous cell carcinoma can signify the development of metastases or a primary lung cancer.

Physical Examination

Examination of the upper aerodigestive tract begins with careful inspection of each anatomic site. Dentures are removed and the lips and tongue retracted to obtain a clear view of the oral cavity. The dimensions of a mass or ulcer can be estimated by placing a tongue blade (2 cm wide) over the area. Bimanual palpation is used to examine the floor of the mouth. Palpation is also used to detect cancers in all areas of the oropharynx, especially the base of the tongue and tonsillar fossas. Parapharyngeal tumors arising from a retromandibular extension of the parotid gland—and from nerves, enlarged lymph nodes, or the carotid body—can present as masses in the tonsillar area. Complete examination of the nasopharynx, larynx, and hypopharynx may require use of a topical anesthetic spray. Although most sites are well seen with a headlight and laryngeal mirror, flexible fiberoptic examination can provide additional information.

A detailed neurologic examination can reveal localizing signs when no other findings are present. Hyposmia (decreased sensitivity to odors) can be caused by primary cancers of the olfactory bulb or cancers of the nasal cavity and paranasal sinuses. Sensory loss in the distribution of the infraorbital nerve can be a manifestation of a maxillary sinus cancer. Dysfunction of cranial nerves III–VII and IX–XII can occur with nasopharyngeal cancer. Horner's syndrome suggests extracapsular invasion of cervical lymph node metastases, extralaryngeal spread of a laryngeal cancer, or involvement of the cervical sympathetic chain by a primary lung cancer.

Jugular chain lymph nodes are best examined by feeling the nodes between the thumb and the index finger while grasping around the sternocleidomastoid muscle. Nevertheless, physical examination of the cervical lymph nodes is not very accurate. Thirty percent of patients with clinically negative cervical lymph nodes have metastases on pathologic staging, and 20% of those with clinically suspicious cervical lymph nodes

will be histologically free of cancer. Cervical lymph node metastases originate from a primary cancer above the clavicles in 85% of cases (Figure 16–1). Squamous cell carcinoma of the skin and melanoma are important causes of enlarged regional nodes and must not be overlooked.

Biopsy

A biopsy for definitive diagnosis can usually be made at the time of the initial examination. Pinch or punch biopsies of mucosal lesions are generally taken from the margin of the lesion, away from areas of necrosis. Fine needle aspiration biopsy (FNA) can also be used, particularly for evaluation of palpable cervical lymphadenopathy. If the FNA is reported as showing malignant cells, treatment based on these results can be started. However, if the FNA is read as benign and the cervical lymphadenopathy is clinically suspicious for cancer, repeat FNA or open biopsy is undertaken.

Additional Studies

Examination under anesthesia is often indicated. In addition to palpation of the oral cavity, oropharynx, and neck, direct laryngoscopy, rigid esophagoscopy, nasopharyngoscopy, and bronchoscopy can also be performed. A search can be made for a second cancer. The

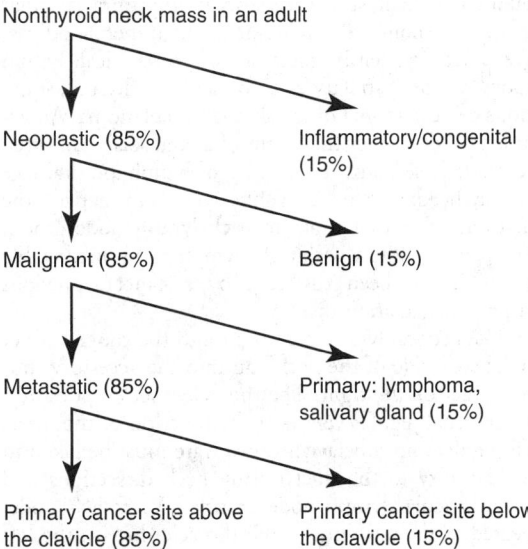

Figure 16–1. Etiology of nonthyroid neck masses in adults.

location and extent of any cancer is described in detail in order to plan appropriate therapy and to assess the results of therapy. A chest x-ray is routine. Barium swallow examination can identify intrinsic or extrinsic compression of the esophagus. Panorex x-rays of the mandible can identify bony invasion from an oral or oropharyngeal cancer. A CT scan of the head and neck is the imaging study of choice for advanced squamous cell carcinoma. Axial and coronal views can demonstrate involvement of the paranasal sinuses, the parapharyngeal and pterygomaxillary spaces, the orbits, and the anterior skull base. MRI is used to determine the extent of cancer involvement at the skull base, in the parapharyngeal space, and in the orbit.

Miller FR et al: Magnetic resonance imaging and the management of parapharyngeal space tumors. Head Neck 1996;18:67.

Weissman JL et al: Current imaging techniques for head and neck tumors. Oncology 1999;13:697.

EXAMINATION OF THE CERVICAL LYMPH NODES

There are three main groups of lymphatic tissue in the head and neck region. The first contains the structures of Waldeyer's ring (palatine tonsils, lingual tonsils, adenoids) and adjacent submucosal lymphatics; the second consists of transitional lymphatics (submental, submandibular, parotid, retroauricular, and occipital nodes); and the third includes the cervical lymph nodes (internal jugular chain, spinal accessory chain, supraclavicular area). Squamous cell carcinoma of the upper aerodigestive tract frequently metastasizes to cervical lymph nodes, as does papillary carcinoma of the thyroid, squamous cell carcinoma of the skin, and melanoma. An accurate prediction of the origin of a metastasis can often be made based on the anatomy of lymphatic drainage in the head and neck. Table 16–1 summarizes the anatomic sites that drain to each lymph node group. The pattern of flow within the lymphatics is predictable unless it has been distorted by a cancer, previous surgery, or radiation therapy.

The cervical lymphatics drain into the thoracic duct on the left side of the neck and into the accessory thoracic duct on the right. The thoracic duct empties into the internal jugular vein near the junction of the internal jugular and subclavian veins. Care must be taken to avoid injury to the duct during neck dissections and supraclavicular lymph node biopsies. Virchow's node, located at the terminus of the thoracic duct in the left supraclavicular region, can sequester metastases from distant primary cancers via the retroperitoneal and posterior mediastinal lymph channels.

WORKUP OF A NECK MASS

The workup of a patient with a neck mass is an orderly progression of examinations and tests aimed at obtaining information about the mass and possible primary sites of cancer should the mass prove to be metastatic from an unknown primary cancer. The site of a cervical lymph node metastasis often suggests the location of the primary cancer because of specific lymphatic flow patterns in the neck (Table 16–1). Following a thorough history and physical examination, including flexible nasopharyngoscopy for visualization of the nasopharynx, hypopharynx, and larynx, FNA of the neck mass is performed for diagnosis. If the diagnosis is squamous carcinoma from an unknown primary cancer, a CT scan of the head and neck is performed. The patient is subsequently examined under anesthesia. Any abnormal areas are biopsied. The most common sites of occult cancers are the nasopharynx, hypopharynx (piriform sinus), and oropharynx (tonsillar fossa and base of tongue). A neck dissection is performed if the cancer is surgically resectable. The neck dissection removes additional ipsilateral cervical lymph nodes that can contain occult metastases. A modified neck dissection may be appropriate, with preservation of the spinal accessory nerve, the stern-

Table 16–1. Cervical lymph node metastases by primary cancer site.

Lymph Node Site	Lymph Node Level	Primary Cancer Sites
Submental, submandibular	Level I	Lip, oral cavity, skin, salivary gland
Upper jugular nodes	Level II	Oral cavity, oropharynx, nasopharynx, hypopharynx, larynx, salivary gland
Mid-jugular nodes	Level III	Oral cavity, oropharynx, hypopharynx, larynx, thyroid
Lower jugular nodes	Level IV	Oropharynx, hypopharynx, larynx, cervical esophagus, thyroid
Accessory nerve nodes	Level V	Nasopharynx, scalp
Supraclavicular nodes	Level V	Breast, lung, gastrointestinal tract
Suboccipital nodes	Level V	Skin
Parotid nodes	Level V	Skin, parotid gland

ocleidomastoid muscle, and the internal jugular vein if these structures are not involved with cancer. If more than two cervical lymph nodes contain metastases, if cervical lymph nodes at two or more levels contain metastases, or if there is extracapsular spread of cervical lymph node metastases, then postoperative radiation therapy is recommended. Prophylactic radiation therapy to all potential primary cancer sites is not recommended.

Only 15% of cervical lymph node metastases in the neck come from primaries below the clavicles (Figure 16–1). Metastases in the lower jugular chain and supraclavicular nodes (levels IV and V) can originate from primary cancers below the clavicle. In this case, the most common primary cancer site is the lung; other sites include the pancreas, esophagus, stomach, breast, ovary, testis, and prostate. CT scans of the chest and abdomen are performed in the search for a primary cancer, but they reveal the primary cancer in only 25% of cases. While many of these cancers cannot be effectively treated, it is important to diagnose lung, breast, prostate, and genital cancers, which often do respond to specific therapy.

Beenken SW et al: Work-up of a patient with a mass in the neck. Adv Surg 1996;28:371.

Colletier PJ et al: Postoperative radiation for squamous cell carcinoma metastatic to cervical lymph nodes from an unknown primary site: outcomes and patterns of failure. Head Neck 1998;20:674.

Califano J et al: Unknown primary head and neck squamous cell carcinoma: molecular identification of the site of origin. J Natl Cancer Inst 1999;91:599.

STAGING OF SQUAMOUS CELL CARCINOMA

Squamous cell carcinoma is staged in order to classify the cancer, to estimate the prognosis, and to plan and assess the results of treatment. This entails an accurate description of the location and size of the primary cancer, the status of the cervical lymph nodes, and the presence or absence of distant metastases. The TNM staging system has done much to standardize the reporting of results of cancer treatment. In the oral cavity, oropharynx, and major salivary glands, T (tumor) stage is defined primarily by cancer size; while in the larynx, hypopharynx, and nasopharynx, T stage depends on the extent of local involvement. The accompanying boxes summarize N (regional lymph nodes) and M (distant metastasis) staging as they apply to squamous cell carcinoma. T stage (primary tumor) is summarized subsequently for the various upper aerodigestive tract anatomic sites. The following definitions are common to all sites: TX: primary tumor cannot be assessed; T0: no evidence of primary tumor; Tis: carcinoma in situ.

N STAGE

NX:	Regional lymph nodes cannot be assessed
N0:	No regional lymph node metastasis
N1:	Metastasis in a single ipsilateral clinically positive node, 3 cm or less in greatest dimension
N2:	Metastasis in–
	N2a: Single ipsilateral lymph node more than 3 cm but not more than 6 cm in greatest dimension
	N2b: multiple ipsilateral lymph nodes, none more than 6 cm in greatest dimension
	N2c: Bilateral or contralateral lymph nodes, none more than 6 cm in greatest dimension
N3:	Metastasis in a lymph node more than 6 cm in greatest dimension

---

M STAGE

MX:	Presence of distant metastasis cannot be assessed
M0:	No distant metastasis
M1:	Distant metastasis

Stage Grouping

Once the TNM classification is established, the cancer stage (Figure 16–2) is defined as follows:

STAGE GROUPING

Stage 0	Tis	N0	M0
Stage I	T1	N0	M0
Stage II	T2	N0	M0
Stage III	T3	N0	M0
	T1	N1	M0
	T2	N1	M0
	T3	N1	M0
Stage IV	T4	N0	M0
	T4	N1	M0
	Any T	N2	M0
	Any T	N3	M0
	Any T	Any N	M1

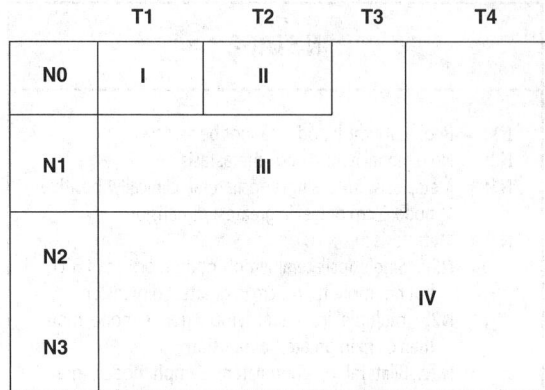

	T1	T2	T3	T4
N0	I	II		
N1		III		
N2				IV
N3				

Figure 16–2. Cancer stage groupings for squamous cell carcinoma of the upper aerodigestive tract.

CANCER OF THE ORAL CAVITY

Anatomy

The vermilion border of the lips is the anterior boundary of the oral cavity, while the anterior tonsillar pillars, the posterior aspect of the hard palate, and the circumvallate papillae of the tongue are the posterior boundary. Subsites are (1) the vermilion surfaces of the lips; (2) the alveolar process of the mandible; (3) the alveolar process of the maxilla; (4) the retromolar trigone, which is the mucosa overlying the ascending ramus of the mandible behind the last lower molar tooth; (5) the hard palate; (6) the buccal mucosa, which lines the cheeks and inner aspects of the lips and includes the upper and lower buccoalveolar gutters; (7) the floor of the mouth; and (8) the anterior two-thirds of the tongue (oral tongue), which is limited posteriorly by the circumvallate papillae and includes the tip, dorsum, lateral borders, and undersurface of the oral tongue. The mucosa of the oral cavity consists of stratified squamous epithelium.

Pathology

Over 95% of cancers of the oral cavity are squamous cell carcinomas. They are predominantly well and moderately well differentiated and can be preceded by premalignant lesions. Leukoplakia ("white patch") is induced by the same factors (tobacco, alcohol) that cause carcinomas. The malignant potential of leukoplakia corresponds to the degree of cellular dysplasia seen on biopsy. Erythroplakia ("red patch") usually shows severe cellular dysplasia and carries a 50% risk of malignant degeneration. Macroscopically, oral cancers can be exophytic growths, flat cancers with central ulceration and indurated edges, or deeply infiltrating ulcers. Verrucous carcinoma is an exophytic lesion that is histolog-

ically well differentiated and has a better prognosis than other oral cancers.

Oral cancers—especially those of the mucosa of the upper and lower alveolar ridges—often invade nearby bone. The mandible is most frequently involved. Minor salivary gland cancers arise in submucosal glands, which are most abundant in the hard palate. Ulceration is a late feature. Melanoma developing in the mucosa of the mouth is rare.

Cancers of the upper lip drain to parotid and submandibular nodes (level I), while those of the lower lip drain to submental and submandibular nodes (level I) and upper and mid jugular nodes (levels II and III). Midline cancers of the lip, the tongue, and the floor of the mouth can drain bilaterally. The incidence of cervical lymph node involvement from cancers of the oral cavity is related to the site and size of the primary cancer. Cancers of the oral tongue and the floor of the mouth have a higher incidence of cervical lymph node involvement than do cancers of the lip, hard palate, or buccal mucosa.

Clinical Findings

Patients with cancer of the oral cavity usually present with ulcerated cancers that have been present for weeks or months. They are typically men aged 50–70 years with a history of heavy tobacco and alcohol use. Dental hygiene is frequently poor, and areas of leukoplakia and erythroplakia can be seen adjacent to the cancer. Submandibular or jugular chain lymph nodes are palpable in 25–35% of patients. Pain is usually not a prominent feature but may become severe with deep infiltration.

T STAGE: ORAL CANCER

- -

T1   Tumor 2 cm or less in greatest dimension

T2   Tumor more than 2 cm but not more than 4 cm in greatest dimension

T3   Tumor more than 4 cm in greatest dimension

T4   Lip: Tumor invaces adjacent structures (eg, through cortical bone, tongue, skin)

T4   Oral cavity: Tumor invades adjacent structures (eg, through cortical bone, into deep [extrinsic] muscle of tongue, maxillary sinus, skin)

Treatment

A. PRIMARY CANCER

Surgical excision is the treatment of choice for most oral cancers. Cancers of the vermilion surface of the lip are best treated with full-thickness excision of the lip.

Lateral margins of 5 mm of uninvolved lip are taken with the cancer. The defect is closed primarily when one-third or less of the lip is excised. When excision of more than one-third of the lip is required, closure is achieved by transposition of a segment of the opposite lip on a vascular pedicle (Abbe flap). When the entire vermilion of the lip has been damaged, vermilionectomy (lip shave) can be performed along with excision of the cancer and a new vermilion surface created by advancing the labial mucosa.

Within the oral cavity, small cancers can usually be excised through the open mouth. Small defects are closed by direct suture or split-thickness skin grafts. Cancers larger than 2 cm in diameter require more extensive excision, aiming for at least 1-cm to 2-cm margins of normal-appearing tissue. The resulting defect requires reconstruction to replace the oral lining and to maintain oral function. For cancers involving bone, marginal or segmental resection of the mandible is performed. A **composite resection** involves resection of an oral cancer, resection of a portion of the mandible, and a neck dissection.

Radiation therapy is an alternative to surgery for oral cancers smaller than 4 cm in diameter (T1 and T2 cancers). The side effects of mucositis, xerostomia, and osteoradionecrosis of the mandible must be balanced against potential advantages. T3 and T4 cancers are usually treated with combined surgery and radiation therapy to improve the rate of local control.

B. Management of Neck Metastases

Cervical lymph node metastases can be treated by radical neck dissection, which involves removal of all the lymphatic tissue of the neck along with the sternocleidomastoid muscle, internal jugular vein, and spinal accessory nerve. To save structures not directly involved by cancer, **modified neck dissection** is performed. A **modified radical neck dissection** always preserves the spinal accessory nerve, while a **functional neck dissection** always preserves the sternocleidomastoid muscle, the internal jugular vein, and the spinal accessory nerve. **Selective neck dissections** involve only certain cervical lymph node levels. For example, levels I, II, and III cervical lymph nodes and cervical lymph nodes in the upper portion of level V are removed with a **supraomohyoid neck dissection** while preserving the sternocleidomastoid muscle, the internal jugular vein, and the spinal accessory nerve (Table 16–2).

When modified neck dissections are performed, adjuvant radiation therapy to the neck is frequently required. It is recommended for use when more than two cervical lymph nodes contain metastases, when more than one level of cervical lymph nodes are involved, or when there is extension of metastases through the capsule of a cervical lymph node. Occult cervical lymph node metastases are present in 20–30% of patients with oral cancers (other than lip, buccal mucosa, or hard palate cancers) who present with a clinically negative neck. **Elective neck dissections** have been advocated for these patients to more accurately stage the cancer and to prevent the need for a later and probably more radical neck dissection when the cervical lymph node metastases becomes clinically apparent. A supraomohyoid neck dissection is the dissection of choice in the elective situation.

Table 16–2. Classification of neck dissections.

Type of Neck Dissection	Node Level of Dissection	Structures Preserved
Radical	I–V	None
Modified radical	I–V	SAN
Functional	II–V (± I)	SCM, IJV, SAN
Anterior	II–IV	SCM, IJV, SAN
Posterior	V	SCM, IJV, SAN
Supraomohyoid	II, III (± I)	SCM, IJV, SAN

SCM = sternocleidomastoid muscle; IJV = internal jugular vein; SAN = spinal accessory nerve.

Prognosis

The five-year survival rates for cancer of the oral cavity with appropriate treatment are as follows: stage I, 72–88%; stage II, 46–80%; stage III, 36–66%; and stage IV, 11–32%. Buccal mucosa cancers have a better prognosis than tongue or hard palate cancers.

Beenken S et al: T1 and T2 squamous cell carcinoma of the oral cavity: prognostic factors and the role of elective lymph node dissection. Head Neck 1999;21:124.

Byers RM et al: Selective neck dissections for squamous carcinoma of the upper aerodigestive tract: patterns of regional failure. Head Neck 1999;21:499.

Byers RM et al: Can we detect or predict the presence of occult nodal metastases in patients with squamous carcinoma of the oral tongue? Head Neck 1998;20:138.

Byers RM, et al: Frequency and therapeutic implications of skip metastases in the neck from squamous carcinoma of the oral tongue. Head Neck 1997;19:14.

Friedlander PL et al: Squamous cell carcinoma of the tongue in young patients: a matched-pair analysis. Head Neck 1998:20:363.

Kraus DH et al: Supraspinal accessory lymph node metastases in supraomohyoid neck dissection. Am J Surg 1996;172:646.

Krontiras H et al: Fatty acid synthetase expression is increased in neoplastic lesions of the oral tongue. Head Neck 1999;21:325.

Parsons JT et al: An analysis of factors influencing the outcome of postoperative irradiation for squamous cell carcinoma of the oral cavity. Int J Radiol Oncol Biol Phys 1997;39:137.

Spiro RH, Morgan GJ: Supraomohyoid neck dissection. Am J Surg 1996;172:650.

CANCER OF THE OROPHARYNX

Anatomy

The oropharynx extends from the hard palate superiorly to the hyoid bone inferiorly. The subsites of the oropharynx are (1) the anterior surface of the soft palate, including the uvula; (2) the posterior pharyngeal wall; (3) the anterior and posterior tonsillar pillars; (4) the tonsils and tonsillar fossas; and (5) the posterior one-third of the tongue, which lies between the circumvallate papillae and the vallecula. The lingual surface of the epiglottis is part of the supraglottic larynx. The mucosa of the oropharynx consists of stratified squamous epithelium.

Pathology

Most oropharyngeal cancers are squamous cell carcinomas, but they tend to be less well differentiated than oral cancers. Deep infiltration is common. Minor salivary gland cancers and lymphomas—particularly non-Hodgkin's lymphoma involving the tonsil and other parts of Waldeyer's ring—also arise in this area. Tumors of the parapharyngeal space may also present as oropharyngeal swellings, causing the mucosa of the lateral pharyngeal wall or soft palate to bulge. These are most often retromandibular parotid tumors or neurogenic tumors (eg, neurilemmoma, neurofibroma, or paraganglioma).

The oropharynx is richly supplied with lymphatics. Posterior pharyngeal wall cancers drain bilaterally to jugular chain nodes (levels II, III, and IV) and the retropharyngeal nodes of Ranvier. Cancers of the tonsillar region drain primarily to the upper and mid jugular chain nodes and to the submandibular nodes (levels I, II, and III). Posterior triangle lymph nodes (level V) become involved following involvement of the jugular chain nodes. The overall incidence of cervical lymph node involvement from cancer of the oropharynx is approximately 70%. Bilateral cervical lymph node metastases are common (50%).

Clinical Findings

Patients with cancer of the oropharynx usually present with ulcerating cancers. Cervical lymph node metastases are a common presenting sign. Approximately 70% of patients with tongue base cancers present with advanced cancer, compared with only 35% of patients with cancer of the oral tongue. Tongue base cancers can spread laterally to involve the mandible, anteriorly to involve the oral tongue, and inferiorly to involve the vallecula and supraglottic larynx. Cancers of the tonsillar region readily extend to the mandible. They can also infiltrate the pterygoid muscles, producing trismus. This is an important presenting symptom, and it may limit access for examination. Referred otalgia is common with deeply infiltrating cancers.

T STAGE: OROPHARYNGEAL CANCER

T1	Tumor 2 cm or less in greatest dimension
T2	Tumor more than 2 cm but not more than 4 cm in greatest dimension
T3	Tumor more than 4 cm in greatest dimension
T4	Tumor invades adjacent structures (eg, through cortical bone, into deep [extrinsic] muscle of tongue, maxillary sinus, skin)

Treatment

A. PRIMARY CANCER

Treatment for cancer of the oropharynx must be individualized. For small cancers (T1 and T2), surgery or radiation therapy gives similar results. For these cancers, surgical access can be achieved through the open mouth or by splitting the lower lip and jaw and retracting the mandible laterally (mandibular swing procedure). Excision of a soft palate cancer is readily accomplished, but when the muscular continuity of the soft palate is completely disrupted, regurgitation of food into the nasal cavity occurs. Therefore, small cancers are usually treated with radiation therapy and surgery is reserved for advanced or recurrent cancer. For more advanced cancers, the choices for therapy are (1) surgery combined with postoperative radiation therapy and (2) initial radiation therapy followed by surgery in the event of recurrence. Combined therapy offers the best chance of local cancer control. Total glossectomy may be necessary to encompass large cancers of the tongue base. Tongue base cancers that extend beyond the vallecula require glossectomy and laryngectomy to remove the cancer completely and to prevent subsequent aspiration pneumonia. Operative defects can be repaired with skin grafts, pedicled myocutaneous flaps (pectoralis major flap), or free flaps (radial forearm and osteomyocutaneous fibular free flaps). Temporary tracheotomy is mandatory in these circumstances.

B. MANAGEMENT OF NECK METASTASES

Cervical lymph node metastases are treated by radical or modified neck dissection (Table 16–2). If the neck is clinically free of cancer, an elective supraomohyoid neck dissection or radiation therapy is appropriate. If the primary cancer is treated by radiation therapy, the cervical lymph nodes at risk are included in the radiation field. If the primary cancer is treated surgically, an elective neck dissection is appropriate. If postoperative radiation therapy is planned for the primary cancer site, it is reasonable to include the neck in the radiation field instead of performing an elective neck dissection. Initial (induction, neoadjuvant) chemotherapy using cisplatin, fluorouracil, and paclitaxel, singly or in combination, gives response rates of up to 80%, but these responses are rarely of long duration.

Prognosis

The 5-year survival rates for cancer of the oropharynx with appropriate treatment are as follows: stage I, 75%; stage II, 65%; stage III, 45%; and stage IV, less than 30%. Quality of life is a major consideration in the treatment of oropharyngeal cancers, since swallowing and speech are often adversely affected by treatment.

Forastiere AA et al: Radiotherapy and concurrent chemotherapy: a strategy that improves locoregional control and survival in oropharyngeal cancer. J Natl Cancer Inst 1999;91:2065.

Harrison LB et al: Long term results of primary radiotherapy with/without neck dissection for squamous cell cancer of the base of tongue. Head Neck 1998;20:668.

CANCER OF THE HYPOPHARYNX

Anatomy

The hypopharynx extends from the hyoid bone superiorly to the lower border of the cricoid cartilage inferiorly. It is composed of four subsites: (1) the piriform sinuses, situated lateral to the larynx; (2) the postcricoid area, lying immediately behind the larynx; (3) the posterior pharyngeal wall; and (4) the marginal area where the medial wall of the piriform sinus and the false vocal cord meet superiorly at the aryepiglottic fold. Laterally, the piriform sinuses are bounded by the alae of thyroid cartilage and the thyrohyoid membrane. The hypopharynx, lined by stratified squamous epithelium, has a muscular wall consisting of the middle and inferior constrictor muscles. The retropharyngeal space posterior to the hypopharynx, which contains lymphatics and loose areolar tissue, separates the visceral compartment of the neck from the prevertebral muscles with their overlying prevertebral fascia.

Pathology

Over 95% of hypopharyngeal cancers are squamous carcinomas, which usually present as infiltrating ulcerative lesions. The incidence of poorly differentiated cancer is higher in the hypopharynx than in other regions. The size of these cancers can be deceptive on clinical evaluation because of submucosal lymphatic extension. Minor salivary gland cancers and lymphomas occasionally occur in the hypopharynx, where they usually present as submucosal tumors. Benign hypopharyngeal lesions include webs, strictures, and pharyngoesophageal (Zenker's) diverticula.

Cancer of the hypopharynx has a high propensity for lymphatic invasion, with most patients having cervical lymph node metastases at the time of initial presentation. The hypopharynx—especially the piriform sinus—must always be examined in an adult with cervical lymph node metastases and no obvious primary cancer site. Occult cervical lymph node metastases (ie, clinically negative but histologically positive) are also common, causing the overall incidence of cervical lymph node metastases at presentation to be approximately 75%. The principal cervical lymph node groups involved are the upper, mid, and lower jugular nodes (levels II, III, and IV); the retropharyngeal nodes of Ranvier; and, less frequently, the cervical lymph nodes along the spinal accessory nerve in the posterior triangle (level V).

Clinical Findings

The most common site for hypopharyngeal cancer is the piriform sinus, accounting for 60% of cases. The postcricoid region is affected in 25% of patients and the posterior pharyngeal wall in 15%. Postcricoid lesions are frequently circumferential and cause dysphagia, while piriform sinus lesions tend to remain silent for a long time. Patients with hypopharyngeal cancer are typically men in their fifth to eighth decades with a history of excessive alcohol and tobacco use.

The chief symptoms of hypopharyngeal cancer are pain, dysphagia, and weight loss. Pain can be localized to the site of the cancer or can be referred to the ipsilateral ear. About 25% of patients, especially those with lesions of the piriform sinus, present with palpable cervical lymphadenopathy and no other symptoms. Advanced cancers can invade the larynx and cause vocal cord paralysis and hoarseness. Direct laryngopharyngoscopy and biopsy are necessary to confirm the diagnosis and assess the extent of the cancer.

T STAGE: HYPOPHARYNGEAL CANCER

T1 Tumor limited to one subsite of the hypopharynx

T2 Tumor invades more than one subsite of the hypopharynx or an adjacent site, without fixation of the hemilarynx

T3 Tumor invades more than one subsite of the hypopharynx or an adjacent site, with fixation of the hemilarynx

T4 Tumor invades adjacent structures (eg, cartilage or soft tissues of the neck)

Treatment

The goals of treatment are to cure the cancer and maintain functional continuity of the upper aerodigestive tract. Intensive nutritional therapy is necessary if long-standing dysphagia has resulted in cachexia. Patients with cancer of the hypopharynx also commonly have pulmonary disease that must be assessed and managed preoperatively.

A. PRIMARY CANCER

Surgical resection of hypopharyngeal cancers usually requires laryngopharyngectomy. Small (T1, T2) cancers of the piriform sinuses are curable with radiation therapy. Small (T1 and T2) cancers of the posterior pharyngeal wall can be treated with larynx-preserving local excision. Jejunal and tubed radial forearm free flaps permit excellent hypopharyngeal reconstruction. If a cancer extends to or arises in the cervical esophagus, laryngopharyngectomy and esophagectomy may be required. In this circumstance, a gastric pull-up procedure provides for upper aerodigestive tract continuity.

B. MANAGEMENT OF NECK METASTASES

The incidence of cervical lymph node metastases is so high with hypopharyngeal cancers that some form of neck treatment is appropriate for all patients. Treatment of both sides of the neck is frequently indicated. Radical or modified neck dissection is indicated for clinically evident cervical lymph node metastases. For the clinically negative neck, when the primary cancer is treated with radiation therapy, the neck is also treated with radiation therapy. If the primary cancer is treated surgically, elective neck dissection is performed. If postoperative radiation therapy will be given to the primary cancer site, radiation therapy can also be given to the neck, making an elective neck dissection unnecessary.

Prognosis

In patients with cancer of the hypopharynx, distant metastases appear in 25% of patients—a much higher incidence than with cancers of the oral cavity and oropharynx. The 5-year survival rates for patients with cancer of the hypopharynx receiving appropriate treatment are subsite-specific. Generally, patients with hypopharyngeal cancers do worse than patients with oropharyngeal cancers.

Roye GD et al: CD44 expression in dysplastic epithelium and squamous cell carcinoma of the esophagus. Int J Cancer 1996;69:254.

CANCER OF THE LARYNX

Anatomy

The larynx is composed of three anatomic subsites. The supraglottic larynx extends from the epiglottis superiorly to the false cords inferiorly. Sites within the supraglottic larynx include the epiglottis (both lingual and laryngeal surfaces), aryepiglottic folds, arytenoids and false cords. The glottic larynx consists of the true vocal cords (including the anterior commissure) superiorly and tissues within 5 mm of the inferior surface of the true vocal cords inferiorly. The subglottic larynx extends from the glottis superiorly to the inferior border of the cricoid cartilage inferiorly. Subglottic cancers are uncommon, accounting for less than 1% of all laryngeal cancers. Subglottic extension of a glottic cancer is more common.

Pathology

Squamous cell carcinoma of the supraglottic larynx accounts for 35% of laryngeal cancers. Fifty percent of these patients will present with cervical lymph node metastases. Lymphatic channels drain to the upper, mid, and lower jugular nodes (levels II, III, and IV). Local spread of cancer is usually in a superior or lateral direction. Inferior spread to the anterior commissure is less common.

Cancer of the glottic larynx accounts for nearly 65% of laryngeal cancers. It tends to be well differentiated, to grow slowly, and to metastasize late. Because the true cords have very limited lymphatic drainage, cervical lymph node metastases occur in only 10% of cases. Cervical lymph node metastases usually occur when the cancer infiltrates beyond the limits of the true cord. Submucosal extension occurs early and can lead to involvement of the anterior commissure and the contralateral vocal cord. The cancer can extend laterally, resulting in cartilage destruction, or superiorly, with involvement of the false vocal cords and aryepiglottic folds (transglottic carcinoma). Subglottic extension can also occur.

Subglottic cancers or subglottic extensions of a glottic cancer are associated with a high incidence of cervical lymph node metastases. Lymphatics from the sub-glottic larynx drain to the mid and lower jugular lymph nodes (levels III and IV) and to the prelaryngeal (cricothyroid or delphian) node. Subsequently, the pre-tracheal and paratracheal lymph nodes can be involved.

Clinical Findings

The initial presenting symptoms of cancer of the larynx depend upon the site involved. Supraglottic cancers tend to present late with symptoms of dysphagia, odynophagia, hemoptysis, or referred otalgia. Stridor and hoarseness are late findings. Palpable cervical lym-phadenopathy is a common presenting sign. Glottic cancers often present early with hoarseness, and palpa-ble lymphadenopathy is uncommon. Late symptoms include dysphagia, odynophagia, stridor, or cough. Subglottic cancer presents with dyspnea, stridor, or pal-pable cervical lymphadenopathy.

T STAGE: LARYNGEAL CANCER

Supraglottis

T1	Tumor limited to one subsite of the supraglottis with normal vocal cord mobility
T2	Tumor invades more than one subsite of the supra-glottis or glottis, with normal vocal cord mobility
T3	Tumor limited to the larynx with vocal cord fixation and/or invades the postcricoid area, medial wall of the piriform sinus, or pre-epiglottic tissues
T4	Tumor invades through the thyroid cartilage and/or extends to other tissues beyond the larynx (eg, to the oropharynx or soft tissues of the neck)

Glottis

T1	Tumor limited to the vocal cord(s) (may involve ante-rior or posterior commissures) with normal mobility
	T1a: Tumor limited to one vocal cord
	T1b: Tumor involves both vocal cords
T2	Tumor extends to the supraglottis and/or subglottis, and/or with impaired vocal cord mobility
T3	Tumor limited to the larynx with vocal cord fixation
T4	Tumor invades through the thyroid cartilage and/or extends to other tissues beyond the larynx (eg, to the oropharynx or soft tissues of the neck)

Subglottis

T1	Tumor limited to the subglottis
T2	Tumor extends to the vocal cord(s) with normal or im-pared vocal cord mobility
T3	Tumor limited to the larynx with vocal cord fixation
T4	Tumor invades through the thyroid cartilage and/or extends to other tissues beyond the larynx (eg, to the oropharynx or soft tissues of the neck)

Treatment

T1 and T2 cancers of the supraglottic and glottic larynx respond well to radiation therapy. Survival rates are similar to those achieved with surgery, but without the attendant morbidity. Elective radiation therapy to the neck is given to patients with supraglottic carcino-mas. T3 and T4 cancers of the supraglottic and glottic larynx are treated with a combination of cisplatin-based chemotherapy and radiation therapy in an effort to avoid the morbidity associated with total laryngectomy. Patients are reevaluated following initial chemotherapy and radiation therapy. If there is complete disappear-ance of the cancer and biopsies are negative, surgery is avoided. In this way, nearly two-thirds of patients can be spared laryngectomy. Survival rates for patients re-ceiving initial chemotherapy and radiation therapy are the same as those for patients receiving total laryngec-tomy.

Surgical options for supraglottic and glottic cancer include partial laryngectomy or total laryngectomy. Partial laryngectomy is appropriate for patients with T1 and T2 cancers. Vertical partial laryngectomy re-moves the ipsilateral vocal cord and overlying laryngeal cartilage. The procedure can be extended superiorly to include the ipsilateral false cord or posteriorly to in-clude the ipsilateral arytenoid cartilage. It is an appro-priate procedure for patients with reduced cord mobil-ity due to cancer bulk but not for patients with reduced cord mobility due to invasion of the intrinsic musculature. Horizontal partial laryngectomy is indi-cated for patients with cancers arising above the level of the true cords. All patients will have some degree of aspiration following this procedure, but careful patient selection can minimize the long-term consequences. Total laryngectomy is appropriate therapy for some pa-tients with T3 laryngeal cancers and for most patients with T4 cancers. In this situation, **wide field laryn-gectomy** includes removal of the bilateral level II, III, and IV cervical lymph nodes. Ipsilateral thyroid lobec-tomy is performed to facilitate paratracheal lymph node dissection.

The presence of cervical lymph node metastases is an indication for radical or modified neck dissection. Elective neck dissection or radiation therapy is not indi-cated for T1 and T2 glottic cancers but is indicated for all supraglottic cancers and for T3 and T4 glottic can-cers. If the primary cancer is treated by surgery, an elec-tive neck dissection is appropriate unless adjuvant radi-ation therapy to the primary cancer site is planned. In that case, elective neck radiation therapy can be given and the neck dissection deferred. If the primary cancer is treated with radiation therapy, elective neck radiation therapy is appropriate and operative dissection can be deferred.

Prognosis

Five-year survival rates for supraglottic cancer with appropriate treatment are as follows: stage I, 90–95%; stage II, 75–80%; stage III, 50%; stage IV, 20–40%.

Five-year survival rates for glottic cancer with appropriate treatment are as follows: stage I, 80–95%; stage II, 70–80%; stage III, 50–70%; stage IV, 20–50%.

Mendenhall WM et al: Definitive radiotherapy for T3 squamous cell carcinoma of the glottic larynx. J Clin Oncol 1997; 15:2394.

Samant S et al: Concomitant radiation therapy and targeted cisplatin chemotherapy for the treatment of advanced piriform sinus carcinoma: disease control and preservation of organ function. Head Neck 1999;21:595.

CANCER OF THE NASAL CAVITY, NASOPHARYNX, & PARANASAL SINUSES

Anatomy

The nasal cavity is divided into right and left nasal fossae by the nasal septum. Each fossa has an anterior opening (naris or nostril), a posterior opening (choana), and bony projections called turbinates protruding from the lateral walls. Posterior to the nasal cavity is the nasopharynx. Its roof is formed by the skull base, which slopes downward and backward, while the inferior limit is a posterior extension of the plane of the hard palate. The lateral wall is composed of the torus tubularis, the auditory tube orifice, and Rosenmüller's fossa. The paranasal sinuses consist of the maxillary and ethmoid sinuses bilaterally, the frontal sinus, and the sphenoid sinus. Each maxillary sinus shares a common wall with the orbit above, the nasal cavity medially, the oral cavity inferiorly, and the infratemporal fossa posteriorly.

The mucosa of the nasal cavity consists of ciliated pseudostratified columnar epithelium (respiratory mucosa) except in the region of the superior turbinate and the adjacent lateral wall and septum, which is lined by specialized nonciliated epithelium (olfactory mucosa). The sinuses are lined by respiratory epithelium, and melanocytes are scattered throughout the region. The nasopharynx is lined by respiratory epithelium in early life, but squamous metaplasia occurs with aging so that about 60% of the respiratory mucosa is replaced by squamous epithelium in the first decade of life. Initially, this squamous epithelium is nonkeratinizing, but after age 50 more keratinization occurs.

Pathology

The most common cancer of the nasal cavity and paranasal sinuses is squamous cell carcinoma. The maxillary antrum is the most common site, while cancers of the nasal cavity are rare. Adenocarcinoma, sarcoma, melanoma, lymphoma, and minor salivary gland cancers also occur. Esthesioneuroblastoma is an uncommon cancer that arises from olfactory mucosa at the superior aspect of the nasal cavity. It readily invades the ethmoid sinuses and can involve the orbit. In the nasopharynx, squamous carcinomas, 80% of which are nonkeratinizing, also predominate. Lymphoepithelioma, a subgroup of nonkeratinizing squamous carcinoma, is poorly differentiated, lacks squamous or glandular differentiation, and has a lymphocytic component. It is highly radiosensitive.

Cancers of the skin of the vestibule of the nose can drain to parotid, submandibular, or upper jugular nodes (levels I and II). Nasal cavity and maxillary sinus cancers rarely metastasize to the regional lymph nodes unless they are advanced and have invaded adjacent structures. The nasopharynx is richly supplied with lymphatics, and cancers in this region readily drain bilaterally to upper and mid jugular lymph nodes and to posterior triangle lymph nodes (levels II, III, and V). Cervical lymph node metastases occur in 80% of patients with this cancer. Palpable cervical lymphadenopathy is the initial manifestation of 50% of patients with nasopharyngeal cancer. Unlike other squamous cell carcinomas, cancers of the nasopharynx can metastasize to the posterior triangle (level V) in the absence of jugular lymph node involvement.

Clinical Findings

Cancers of the nasal cavity, paranasal sinuses, and nasopharynx are frequently advanced at presentation. Early symptoms such as nasal obstruction, nasal discharge, and sinus congestion are so commonly associated with benign conditions that they are not frequently investigated for the presence of a cancer. Hemorrhage can occur. Bone invasion and involvement of adjacent soft tissue structures are common. Along with the tonsillar fossa, the tongue base, and the piriform sinus, the nasopharynx is an important site of clinically occult primary cancer. Cancers of the maxillary sinus can invade the hard palate and enter the oral cavity. They can also invade the orbital floor, causing visual symptoms and proptosis. Anterior invasion through the skin can occur. In advanced maxillary sinus cancers, cervical lymph node metastases can be the initial manifestation. Cranial nerve symptoms result from invasion of the skull base.

Diagnosis

Diagnosis and assessment of the extent of cancer are more difficult for cancers in this area than for those elsewhere in the upper aerodigestive tract. Histologic examination of an adequate tissue biopsy specimen is always required. CT scanning is performed to delineate the extent of the cancer, though it can be difficult to differentiate between cancer and edematous mucosa. MRI is helpful in making this differentiation.

T STAGE: MAXILLARY SINUS CANCER

T1 Tumor limited to antral mucosa with no erosion or destruction of bone

T2 Tumor with erosion or destruction of the infrastructure, including the hard palate or middle nasal meatus

T3 Tumor invades any of the following: skin of cheek, posterior wall of maxillary sinus, floor or medial wall of orbit, anterior ethmoid sinus

T4 Tumor invades orbital contents and/or any of the following: cribriform plate, posterior ethmoid or sphenoid sinuses, nasopharynx, soft palate, pterygomaxillary or temporal fossas or base of skull

---

Treatment

Radiation is the principal treatment method for cancer of the nasopharynx. Undifferentiated cancers respond better than well-differentiated ones, and treatment is more successful in younger patients. A dose of 7000 cGy is usually required for the primary cancer. Both sides of the neck are treated because of the high incidence of bilateral cervical lymph node metastases.

Cancers of the maxillary sinus are treated by maxillectomy. For advanced (T3, T4) maxillary sinus cancers, surgery and postoperative radiation therapy provide for the best local control. Orbital exenteration is necessary for maxillary cancers that invade the periorbital tissues. Because the incidence of cervical lymph node metastases is low with cancers of the paranasal sinuses, prophylactic neck dissection or radiation therapy is not necessary. Resectable cancers of the upper nasal cavity and ethmoid sinuses require craniofacial excision, which entails frontal craniotomy to assess the extent of the intracranial extension of the cancer.

Prognosis

Five-year survival rates for nasopharyngeal cancer with appropriate treatment are as follows: stage I, 85%; stage II, 75%; stage III, 45%; stage IV, 10%. One-third of patients die of distant metastases.

Five-year survival rates for maxillary sinus cancer with appropriate treatment are as follows: stage I, 85%; stage II, 65%; stage III, 40%; stage IV, 15–20%.

SALIVARY GLAND TUMORS

Anatomy

The paired major salivary glands consist of the parotid and submandibular glands. Minor salivary glands are widely distributed in the mucosa of the lips, cheeks, hard and soft palate, uvula, floor of mouth, tongue, and peritonsillar region; a few are found in the nasopharynx, paranasal sinuses, larynx, trachea, bronchi, and lacrimal glands.

Pathology

A variety of site-specific and systemic diseases can affect the salivary glands. These are summarized in Table 16–3. Tumors of salivary gland tissue constitute about 5% of head and neck tumors and affect major salivary glands five times more often than minor salivary glands. The incidence of malignancy among salivary gland tumors varies inversely with the size of the gland. About 15% of parotid tumors, 50% of submandibular gland tumors, and 90% of minor salivary gland tumors are malignant.

Since 70% of salivary gland tumors occur in the parotid and 85% of these are benign, the majority of salivary gland tumors are benign. These tumors are thought to originate from two cell types: intercalated

Table 16–3. Diseases of the salivary glands.

Disease Category	Disease Entity
Inflammatory disease	Actinomycosis Acute bacterial sialoadenitis Cat scratch disease Mumps Tuberculosis
Obstructive salivary disease	Kussmaul's disease Sialolithiasis Sjögren's disease Stricture
Neoplasia of the salivary glands Benign tumors	Mixed tumor Monomorphic adenomas Oncocytoma Warthin's tumor
Malignant tumors	Acinic cell carcinoma Adenocarcinoma Adenoidcystic carcinoma Malignant mixed tumor Mucoepidermoid carcinoma Squamous cell carcinoma Undifferentiated carcinoma

and excretory duct cells. Myoepithelial cells are present in many salivary gland tumors but rarely present as the principal cell type. The differential diagnosis of a swelling in the parotid region includes parotitis, a primary parotid tumor, upper jugular chain lymph node enlargement, a tumor of the tail of the submandibular gland, an enlarged preauricular or parotid lymph node, a branchial cleft cyst, an epithelial inclusion cyst, or a mesenchymal tumor.

The most common benign salivary gland tumor is the benign mixed tumor or pleomorphic adenoma, which accounts for 70% of parotid tumors and 50% of all salivary gland tumors. Mixed tumors are more common in women than in men, with the peak incidence in the fifth decade. They are slow-growing and lobular and may become very large without interfering with facial nerve function. Although mixed tumors are benign, they will recur after surgery unless they are completely removed. Enucleation is inadequate surgery. When tumor recurs in the parotid region, the facial nerve is at greater risk from damage during reoperation than it was during the initial procedure. Malignant transformation in a benign tumor is uncommon but can occur (malignant mixed carcinoma).

Warthin's tumor (papillary cystadenoma lymphomatosum), the next most common benign tumor, accounts for about 5% of parotid tumors. Warthin's tumors are usually cystic, typically occur in men in the sixth and seventh decades, and are bilateral in about 10% of cases. They occur almost exclusively in the parotid gland and have a typical histologic appearance, consisting of a papillary-cystic pattern with a marked lymphoid component. Oncocytomas are benign tumors composed of large oxyphilic cells called oncocytes. On electron microscopy, the cytoplasm of the oxyphilic cells is packed with mitochondria. Monomorphic tumors are rare benign salivary gland tumors that are usually epithelial but occasionally myoepithelial in origin. They are most commonly seen in the minor salivary glands of the lip.

Mucoepidermoid carcinoma is the most common parotid cancer. These tumors are categorized as high-grade, intermediate-grade, or low-grade cancers. Acinic cell cancers are derived from serous acinar cells and are found almost exclusively in the parotid gland. Adenoid cystic carcinomas, which are uncommon in the parotid, have a great propensity for perineural invasion and local recurrence. Patients with this cancer tend to have protracted illness, with recurrences appearing 15 years or more after treatment. Patients with distant metastases from adenoid cystic carcinoma can survive for 5 or more years. Less common cancers include cancer arising in a mixed tumor and primary squamous cancer, which accounts for approximately 1% of salivary gland cancers and must be differentiated from mucoepidermoid carcinoma and metastatic squamous carcinoma in a parotid

lymph node. Among minor salivary gland cancers, adenoid cystic carcinoma is the most common cancer, followed by adenocarcinoma and mucoepidermoid carcinoma. Approximately 70% of all minor salivary gland cancers occur in the oral cavity, principally on the hard palate.

Diagnosis

In most cases, local excision with a margin of normal tissue is the appropriate form of biopsy for a major salivary gland tumor. In the parotid region, this requires identification of the facial nerve. For submandibular tumors, the entire submandibular triangle is cleared. In contrast, minor salivary gland tumors have a higher likelihood of being malignant, and an incisional biopsy is performed initially so that definitive treatment can be planned. In the parotid region, the presence of pain, recent rapid enlargement of a preexisting nodule, skin involvement, or facial nerve paralysis suggests cancer. Enlarged cervical lymph nodes in association with a salivary gland tumor are considered a manifestation of cancer until proved otherwise. Fine-needle aspiration is indicated if accurate diagnosis will allow for better treatment planning.

T STAGE: MAJOR SALIVARY GLAND CANCER

T1 Tumor 2 cm or less in greatest dimension

T2 Tumor more than 2 cm but not more than 4 cm in greatest dimension

T3 Tumor more than 4 cm but not more than 6 cm in greatest dimension

T4 Tumor more than 6 cm in greatest dimension

Treatment

Benign salivary gland tumors are excised. Parotid surgery requires a preauricular incision carried onto the neck to allow adequate exposure of the gland and facial nerve. The aim of the operation is to completely excise the tumor with an adequate margin of normal tissue. The minimum adequate operation is removal of the portion of the parotid that lies superficial to the facial nerve. Enucleation is avoided because it greatly increases the likelihood of recurrence and nerve damage. When a tumor arises in the parotid gland deep to the facial nerve, the portion of the parotid gland superficial to the facial nerve is removed, the facial nerve is then elevated, and finally the tumor deep to the nerve is removed along with the remaining parotid tissue. Benign tumors of the submandibular gland require total removal of the gland for diagnosis and treatment.

Surgical treatment for parotid cancer depends on the extent of the cancer. Unless the facial nerve is paralyzed or found to be directly invaded by cancer at surgery, it is preserved. When the facial nerve must be divided, it is repaired if it was functioning normally prior to surgery. The facial nerve can be reconstructed using a nerve graft, eg, the greater auricular or sural nerves. Recovery of function can take many months.

For low-grade salivary gland cancers, complete excision is sufficient treatment. For high-grade cancers, postoperative radiation therapy is indicated for the primary cancer site and regional lymph nodes. Clinically involved lymph nodes are removed by a radical or modified neck dissection. Elective neck dissections are generally not indicated, though removal of level II cervical lymph nodes requires minimal additional surgery after parotidectomy or after removal of the contents of the submandibular triangle.

Prognosis

The prognosis for salivary gland cancer depends on the stage, the histologic grade, the cancer site, the patient's age, and the adequacy of surgical removal. The most important prognostic factor is the cancer stage. The next most important factor is the histologic grade of the cancer. Low-grade cancers such as acinic cell cancers and low-grade mucoepidermoid cancers usually present as stage I or stage II cancers and have an excellent prognosis, with 10-year survival rates of about 80%. On the other hand, the 10-year survival rate after treatment of high-grade stage III and stage IV cancers—such as adenocarcinoma, squamous cell carcinoma, and high-grade mucoepidermoid carcinoma—is about 30%.

Anderson J et al: Prognostic factors in minor salivary gland cancer. Head Neck 1995;17:1.

Carrau RL et al: Management of tumors of the parapharyngeal space. Oncology 1997;11:633.

Johns MM et al: Allelotype of salivary gland tumors. Cancer Res 1996;56:1151.

Kelley DJ et al: Management of the neck in parotid carcinoma. Am J Surg 1996;172:695.

Spiro RH: Management of malignant tumors of the salivary glands. Oncology 1998;12:671.

RECONSTRUCTION

The primary aim of head and neck cancer surgery is complete eradication of the cancer. This is most likely to be achieved at the initial attempt, since treatment of recurrences is less successful. Unfortunately, surgery that achieves a good therapeutic result can be cosmetically and functionally unacceptable. Direct wound closure, skin grafting, or tissue transfer can repair surgical defects. Direct wound closure is ideal for small defects of the skin and of the mucosa of the oral cavity and oropharynx. Direct closure of large defects in the oral cavity and oropharynx can create distortion, such as tongue tethering, and is avoided. Skin grafts can be used to close defects of the skin or mucosa of the oral cavity and oropharynx that are not amenable to direct closure.

Tissue to close larger surgical defects can be obtained in several ways, including local rotational cutaneous flaps (forehead and deltopectoral flaps) for closure of defects of the skin of the face, neck, and chest, and rotational flaps of buccal or tongue mucosa for closure of defects in the oral cavity. Tissue can also be transferred from more distant sites using myocutaneous flaps (pectoralis major and latissimus dorsi flaps) and vascularized free flaps (radial forearm and osteomyocutaneous fibular flaps). Each of these techniques has its particular advantages and disadvantages, and the reconstructive procedure must be tailored to the patient and the site and extent of the operative defect.

Jaw reconstruction poses special technical difficulties, but vascularized free flaps such as the osteomyocutaneous fibular free flap appear to be most reliable. If a segment of the horizontal or vertical ramus of the mandible is resected, placement of a mandibular bar with or without transfer of harvested iliac crest bone can provide for a good result. Occasionally in the elderly or debilitated patient, only primary closure of the soft tissues is accomplished. The cosmetic and functional result is usually quite acceptable. Removal of the anterior part of the mandibular arch destroys the contour of the chin and creates the so-called "Andy Gump deformity," which severely affects eating, speech, and cosmetic appearance. Such defects are reconstructed with an osteomyocutaneous fibular free flap when the operative risk is acceptable.

Synthetic prostheses are especially useful following amputation of the nose or ear or after orbital exenteration. Excellent function can be achieved with dental obturators for patients with defects in the hard palate and upper alveolar ridges.

Urken ML: Composite free flaps in oromandibular reconstruction. Arch Otolaryngol Head Neck Surg 1991;117:724.

RADIATION THERAPY

Radiation can be used as definitive treatment with curative intent, as a postoperative adjunct to surgery, or for palliation.

Definitive Radiation Therapy

Squamous cell carcinomas are sensitive to radiation therapy, especially if they are small and only superficially invasive. T1 and T2 cancers of the oral cavity and oropharynx can be treated with surgery or radiation therapy. In some cases, radiation therapy has the advantage of avoiding the disfiguring side effects of surgery. However, mucositis, subsequent xerostomia, and the possibility of osteoradionecrosis of the mandible are disadvantages. Large oral cancers respond poorly to radiation therapy. Surgery with postoperative radiation therapy, if indicated, is the best treatment for these cancers. In the oropharynx, radiation therapy is excellent treatment for small cancers (T1, T2), especially for tonsillar cancers; because the response rate is good and radiation therapy can also treat occult cervical lymph node metastases. Large cancers of the tonsil (T3, T4) require surgery combined with radiation therapy. The surgical treatment of tongue base cancers larger than 3 cm can require total glossectomy and laryngectomy, a procedure with considerable morbidity. Radiation therapy may be the best initial treatment for these cancers, with surgery reserved for persistent cancer.

Nasopharyngeal cancers are responsive to radiation therapy. Surgical resection is usually not possible. A common side effect of radiation therapy in this area is dysfunction of the auditory tube and subsequent otitis media. A myringotomy tube can alleviate this problem. Radiation therapy is excellent treatment for early (T1 or T2) laryngeal cancers and has the advantage of preserving speech. Five-year survival rates range from 70% to 90% depending on the extent of the cancer.

Cervical lymph node metastases can be treated by radiation therapy alone if the lymph nodes measure less than 3 cm in diameter. If lymph nodes remain palpable after treatment, neck dissection is necessary. In general, clinically apparent metastatic cervical lymph nodes are best treated initially by a radical or modified neck dissection.

For most squamous cell carcinomas, radiation therapy is given in fractions of 180–200 cGy 5 days a week for approximately 6 weeks. Doses of 6000–7000 cGy are delivered to the primary cancer. When there is no palpable cervical lymphadenopathy but a high likelihood that the cervical lymph nodes harbor occult metastases, elective radiation therapy to a dose of 5000 cGy to the neck is added. Changes in fraction size and timing have been used to decrease cancer cell regeneration during treatment. Current radiation therapy protocols involve (1) accelerated fractionation, giving two or three fractions per day and shortening the overall duration of treatment; (2) hyperfractionation, giving two or three smaller fractions per day but maintaining the overall treatment duration; (3) accelerated hyperfractionation, reducing overall treatment time through a combination of greater fraction number and smaller fraction size; and (4) concomitant boost, giving a second daily dose radiation to a reduced "field within a field" during the course of conventional radiation therapy.

Adjuvant Radiation Therapy

Radiation therapy is often combined with surgery to improve local and regional control of squamous cell carcinoma. Preoperative radiation therapy (4500–5000 cGy) has been used but has the disadvantage of producing edema and increased vascularity of the operative field, with prolonged wound healing. Postoperative radiation therapy (5000–6000 cGy) is more often employed. Adjuvant radiation therapy is selective, since it is reserved for patients known from surgical or histologic findings to be at high risk of recurrence. Examples of such patients include those with a cancer of high histologic grade or poor differentiation, those with microscopic cancer at the margins of resection or macroscopic residual cancer, and those with perineural extension of cancer. Treatment commences after 4–6 weeks of wound healing.

Palliative Radiation Therapy

In some instances, when primary cancers or cervical lymph node metastases are not resectable, radiation therapy is given in high doses (eg, 6000 cGy or more) with palliation as the goal of treatment.

Adverse Effects of Radiation Therapy

The main acute complications of radiation therapy are skin reaction and mucositis. Long-term complications include fibrosis and vascular sclerosis, xerostomia, and osteoradionecrosis. Patients with carious teeth or advanced periodontal disease must have their teeth extracted before radiation therapy. Those who retain their teeth must maintain excellent dental hygiene. Surgical procedures in a previously irradiated field are technically more difficult. Cancers that have previously been treated by radiation therapy tend to respond poorly to subsequent chemotherapy.

Douglas JG, Laramore GE: Neutron radiotherapy for head and neck cancer. Adv Oncol 1998;14:24.

Spencer SA et al: Concomitant chemotherapy and reirradiation as management for recurrent cancer of the head and neck. Am J Clin Oncol 1999;22:1.

CHEMOTHERAPY

For patients with advanced squamous cell carcinoma (stage III or IV), surgery and radiation therapy have generally been used sequentially to obtain local and regional control of the cancer. Because many of these patients still develop recurrent cancer, chemotherapy has been used in protocol settings in an effort to improve long-term outcomes.

Induction Chemotherapy

Patients with advanced squamous cell carcinoma who respond to chemotherapy respond better to radiation therapy and live longer. This suggests that if those who respond to initial (induction, neoadjuvant) chemotherapy are subsequently given radiation therapy, surgery might be unnecessary. In a prospective, randomized trial, patients with stage III or stage IV laryngeal cancer were treated with either induction fluorouracil and cisplatin chemotherapy followed by radiation therapy or with surgery followed by radiation therapy. Patients not responding to chemotherapy were treated with surgery plus radiation therapy. The results showed no difference in survival between the two groups, but almost two-thirds of the patients treated with induction chemotherapy and radiation therapy avoided surgery and maintained laryngeal function. Induction chemotherapy followed by radiation therapy for T3 and some T4 laryngeal cancer has become standard therapy at some centers.

Concomitant Chemotherapy

Another strategy under investigation is concomitant chemotherapy and radiation therapy. Chemotherapy is utilized to control microscopic systemic metastases and to enhance the locoregional effects of radiation therapy. When used in this setting, several single agents have been shown to improve cancer-free survival (bleomycin, cisplatin, fluorouracil), though the benefits are small and are offset by the toxicity of the regimen.

Chemotherapy With Reirradiation

Patients with recurrent cancer after primary or adjuvant radiation therapy can benefit from reirradiation combined with fluorouracil and hydroxyurea chemotherapy. Survival is prolonged by 1 or 2 years compared with historical controls.

Adelstein DJ et al: Mature results of a phase III randomized trial comparing concurrent chemoradiotherapy with radiation therapy alone in patients with stage III and IV squamous cell carcinoma of the head and neck. Cancer 2000;88:876.

Brockstein BE et al: Concomitant and rapidly alternating chemoradiotherapy for head and neck cancer. Adv Oncol 1998;14:8.

El-Sayed S et al: Adjuvant and adjunctive chemotherapy in the management of squamous cell carcinoma of the head and neck region: a meta-analysis of prospective and randomized trials. J Clin Oncol 1996;14:838.

Kies MS et al: Induction chemotherapy followed by concurrent chemoradiation for advanced head and neck cancer: improved disease control and survival. J Clin Oncol 1998;16:2715.

Lippman SM et al: Single and combination chemotherapy for recurrent and/or metastatic head and neck squamous cell carcinoma. Adv Oncol 1998;14:16.

CHEMOPREVENTION

Chemoprevention can be defined as the introduction of selected synthetic and natural substances into the diet for the purpose of reducing cancer incidence. Since the early 1960s, vitamin A (retinol) and its derivatives (retinoids) have been used to treat oral leukoplakia, a premalignant lesion of the oral cavity. Several studies have documented resolution of disease. A clinical trial comparing 13-*cis*-retinoic acid (isotretinoin) and placebo in patients with a prior squamous cell carcinoma who had no clinically evident cancer following surgery or radiation therapy was undertaken to investigate isotretinoin's chemopreventive efficacy. After a follow-up of more than 4 years, there was a statistically significant reduction in the rate of development of second primary cancers in the group treated with isotretinoin. Other less toxic compounds such as fenretinide are also being investigated.

Beenken S et al: Modulation of transforming growth factor-α (TGF-α) by 13-cis retinoic acid in patients with dysplastic oral leukoplakia. Head Neck 1999;21:566.

Beenken SW et al: Retinoid modulation of biomarkers in oral leukoplakia/dysplasia. J Cell Biochem 1994;19:270.

Brenner SE et al: Prevention of second primary tumors with isotretinoin in patients with squamous cell carcinoma of the head and neck: long-term follow-up. J Natl Cancer Inst 1993;86:140.

Hong WK et al: Prevention of second primary tumors with isotretinoin in squamous cell carcinoma of the head and neck. N Engl J Med 1990;323:795.

Lippman SM et al: Retinoid chemoprevention studies in upper aerodigestive tract and lung carcinogenesis. Cancer Res 1994;54(Suppl):2025s.

Preventing and controlling oral and pharyngeal cancer: recommendations from a National Strategic Planning Conference. MMWR Morb Mortal Wkly Rep 1998;47(RR-14):1.

Reed JC: Fenretinide: the death of a tumor cell. J Natl Cancer Inst 1999;91:1099.

Shin DM et al: Biomarkers in upper aerodigestive tract tumorigenesis: a review. Cancer Epidemiol Biomarkers Prev 1994;3:697.

Thyroid & Parathyroid

Orlo H. Clark, MD

■ I. THE THYROID GLAND

EMBRYOLOGY & ANATOMY

See Figure 17–1. The main anlage of the thyroid gland develops as a median entodermal downgrowth from the first and second pharyngeal pouches. During its migration caudally, it contacts the ultimobranchial bodies developing from the fourth pharyngeal pouches. When it reaches the position it occupies in the adult, just below the cricoid cartilage, the thyroid divides into two lobes. The site from which it originated persists as the foramen cecum at the base of the tongue. The path the gland follows may result in thyroglossal remnants (cysts) or ectopic thyroid tissue (lingual thyroid). A pyramidal lobe is frequently present. Agenesis of one thyroid lobe may occur.

The normal thyroid weighs 15–25 g and is attached to the trachea by loose connective tissue. It is a highly vascularized organ that derives its blood supply principally from the superior and inferior thyroid arteries. A thyroid ima artery may also be present.

PHYSIOLOGY

The function of the thyroid gland is to synthesize, store, and secrete the hormones thyroxine (T_4) and triiodothyronine (T_3). Iodide is absorbed from the gastrointestinal tract and actively trapped by the acinar cells of the thyroid gland. It is then oxidized and combined with tyrosine in thyroglobulin to form monoiodotyrosine (MIT) and diiodotyrosine (DIT). These are coupled to form the active hormones T_4 and T_3, which initially are stored in the colloid of the gland. Following hydrolysis of the thyroglobulin, T_4 and T_3 are secreted into the plasma, becoming almost instantaneously bound to plasma proteins. Most T_3 in euthyroid individuals, however, is produced by extrathyroidal conversion of T_4 to T_3.

The function of the thyroid gland is regulated by a feedback mechanism that involves the hypothalamus and pituitary. Thyrotropin-releasing factor (TRF), a tripeptide amide, is formed in the hypothalamus and stimulates the release of thyrotropin (TSH), a glycoprotein, from the pituitary. Thyrotropin binds to TSH receptors on the thyroid plasma membrane, stimulating increased adenylyl cyclase activity; this increases cAMP production and thyroid cellular function. Thyrotropin also stimulates the phosphoinositide pathway and—along with cAMP—may stimulate thyroid growth.

Cavalieri RR: The effects of nonthyroid disease and drugs on thyroid function tests. Med Clin North Am 1991;75:27.

Clark OH et al: Thyroid growth factors and oncogenes. Cancer Treat Res 1992;87.

Farid NR et al: Molecular basis of thyroid cancer. Endocr Rev 1994;15:202.

EVALUATION OF THE THYROID

In a patient with enlargement of the thyroid (goiter), the history (including the family history) and examination of the gland are most important and are complemented by the selective use of thyroid function tests. The surgeon must develop a systematic method of palpating the gland to determine its size, contour, consistency, nodularity, and fixation and to examine for displacement of the trachea and the presence of palpable cervical lymph nodes. The thyroid gland moves cephalad with deglutition, whereas adjacent lymph nodes do not.

Thyroid function is assessed by highly sensitive TSH assays that can differentiate between patients with hypothyroidism (increased TSH levels), euthyroidism, and hyperthyroidism (decreased TSH levels). In most cases, therefore, serum T_3, T_4, and other variables do not need to be measured. A free T_4 level is helpful in some patients with suspected hyper- or hypothyroidism, and free T_4 along with the TSH level can identify the occasional patient with low TSH and low free T_4 level. A serum T_3 level is useful for diagnosing T_3 toxicosis (high T_3 and low TSH), or the euthyroid sick, low T_3 syndrome (low T_3 and normal or slightly increased TSH).

Radioactive iodine (RAI) uptake is useful for differentiating between hyperthyroidism and increased secretion of thyroid hormone (low TSH and increased radioactive iodine uptake) on the one hand and subacute thyroiditis (low TSH and low radioactive iodine uptake) on the other. Patients with the latter "leak" thyroid hormone from the gland which suppresses serum

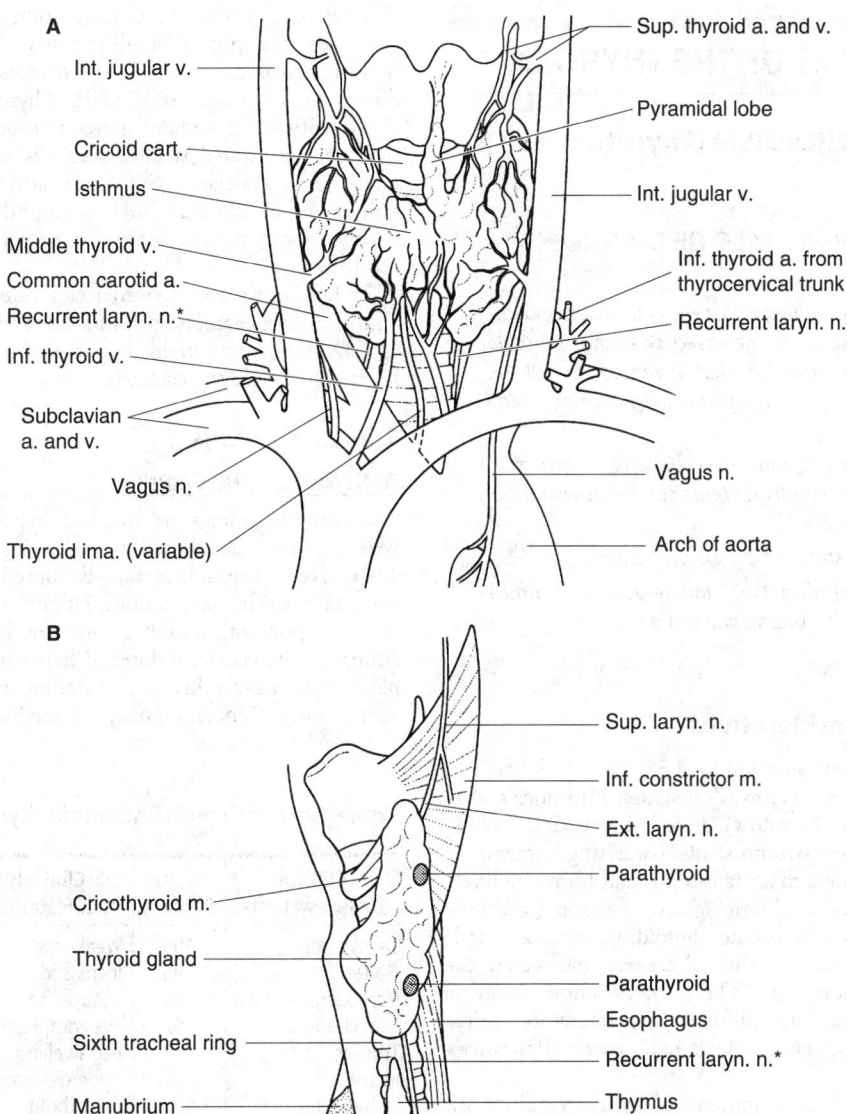

A

Int. jugular v.

Cricoid cart.

Isthmus

Middle thyroid v.

Common carotid a.

Recurrent laryn. n.*

Inf. thyroid v.

Subclavian
a. and v.

Vagus n.

Thyroid ima. (variable)

Sup. thyroid a. and v.

Pyramidal lobe

Int. jugular v.

Inf. thyroid a. from
thyrocervical trunk

Recurrent laryn. n.

Vagus n.

Arch of aorta

B

Cricothyroid m.

Thyroid gland

Sixth tracheal ring

Manubrium

Sup. laryn. n.

Inf. constrictor m.

Ext. laryn. n.

Parathyroid

Parathyroid

Esophagus

Recurrent laryn. n.*

Thymus

Figure 17–1. Thyroid anatomy.

* The recurrent laryngeal nerve runs in the tracheoesophageal groove on the left and has a slightly more oblique course on the right before it enters the larynx just posterior to the cricothyroid muscle at the level of the cricoid cartilage.

TSH levels and, consequently, iodine uptake by the thyroid. Patients with Graves' disease have increased levels of thyroid-stimulating immunoglobulins that increase iodine uptake despite low TSH levels.

■ DISEASES OF THE THYROID

HYPERTHYROIDISM (Thyrotoxicosis)

 ESSENTIALS OF DIAGNOSIS

- *Nervousness, weight loss with increased appetite, heat intolerance, increased sweating, muscular weakness and fatigue, increased bowel frequency, polyuria, menstrual irregularities, infertility.*
- *Goiter, tachycardia, atrial fibrillation, warm moist skin, thyroid thrill and bruit, cardiac flow murmur; gynecomastia.*
- *Eye signs: stare, lid lag, exophthalmos.*
- *TSH low or absent; TSI, iodine uptake, T_3, and T_4 increased; T_3 suppression test abnormal.*

General Considerations

Hyperthyroidism is caused by the increased secretion of thyroid hormone (**Graves' disease, Plummer's disease,** iodine [**jodbasedow**], amiodarone toxicity, TSH-secreting pituitary tumors, hCG-secreting tumors) or by other disorders that increase thyroid hormone levels without increasing thyroid gland secretion (factitious hyperthyroidism, subacute thyroiditis, struma ovarii, and, rarely, metastatic thyroid cancers that secrete excess thyroid hormone). The most common causes of hyperthyroidism are diffusely hypersecretory goiter (Graves' disease) and nodular toxic goiter (Plummer's disease).

In all forms, the symptoms of hyperthyroidism are due to increased levels of thyroid hormone in the bloodstream. The clinical manifestations of thyrotoxicosis may be subtle or marked and tend to go through periods of exacerbation and remission. Some patients ultimately develop hypothyroidism spontaneously or as a result of treatment. Graves' disease is an autoimmune disease—often with a familial predisposition—, whereas the etiology of Plummer's disease is unknown. Most cases of hyperthyroidism are easily diagnosed on the basis of the signs and symptoms; others—eg, mild or **apathetic hy-**

perthyroidism,—which occurs most commonly in the elderly—may be recognized only with difficulty.

Thyrotoxicosis has been described with a normal T_4 concentration, normal or elevated radioiodine uptake, and normal protein binding, but with increased serum T_3 by RIA (**T_3 toxicosis**). **T_4** pseudothyrotoxicosis is occasionally seen in critically ill patients and is characterized by increased levels of T_4 and decreased levels of T_3 due to failure to convert T_4 to T_3. Thyrotoxicosis associated with toxic nodular goiter is usually less severe than that associated with Graves' disease and is only rarely if ever associated with the extrathyroidal manifestations of Graves' disease such as exophthalmos, pretibial myxedema, thyroid acropathy, or periodic hypocalcemic paralysis.

If left untreated, thyrotoxicosis causes progressive and profound catabolic disturbances and cardiac damage. Death may occur in thyroid storm or because of heart failure or severe cachexia.

Clinical Findings

A. SYMPTOMS AND SIGNS

The clinical findings are those of hyperthyroidism as well as those related to the underlying cause (Table 17–1). Nervousness, increased diaphoresis, heat intolerance, tachycardia, palpitations, fatigue, and weight loss in association with a nodular, multinodular, or diffuse goiter are the classic findings in hyperthyroidism. The patient may have a flushed and staring appearance. The skin is warm, thin, and moist, and the hair is fine.

Table 17–1. Clinical findings in thyrotoxicosis.*

Clinical Manifestations	Percent	Clinical Manifestations	Percent
Tachycardia	100	Weakness	70
Goiter	98	Increased appetite	65
Nervousness	99		
Skin changes	97	Eye complaints	54
Tremor	97	Leg swelling	35
Increased sweating	91	Hyperdefecation (without diarrhea)	33
Hypersensitivity to heat	89		
		Diarrhea	23
Palpitations	89	Atrial fibrillation	10
Fatigue	88	Splenomegaly	10
Weight loss	85	Gynecomastia	10
Bruit over thyroid	77	Anorexia	9
Dyspnea	75	Liver palms	8
Eye signs	71	Constipation	4
		Weight gain	2

*Data from Williams RH: *J Clin Endocrinol Metab* 1946:6:1.

In Graves' disease, there may be exophthalmos, pretibial myxedema, or vitiligo, virtually never seen in single or multinodular toxic goiter. The Achilles reflex time is shortened in hyperthyroidism and prolonged in hypothyroidism. The patient on the verge of thyroid storm has accentuated symptoms and signs of thyrotoxicosis, with hyperpyrexia, tachycardia, cardiac failure, neuromuscular excitation, delirium, or jaundice.

B. Laboratory Findings

Laboratory tests reveal a suppressed TSH and an elevation of T_3, free T_4, and RAI. A history of medications is important, since certain drugs and organic iodinated compounds affect some thyroid function tests, and iodide excess may result in either iodide-induced hypothyroidism or iodine-induced hyperthyroidism (jodbasedow). In mild forms of hyperthyroidism, the usual diagnostic laboratory tests are likely to be only slightly abnormal. In these difficult to diagnose cases, two additional tests are helpful: the T_3 suppression test and the thyrotropin-releasing hormone (TRH) test. In the T_3 suppression test, hyperthyroid patients fail to suppress the thyroidal uptake of radioiodine when given exogenous T_3. In the TRH test, serum TSH levels fail to rise in response to administration of TRH in hyperthyroid patients.

Other findings include a high thyroid-stimulating immunoglobulin (TSI) level, low serum cholesterol, lymphocytosis, and occasionally hypercalcemia, hypercalciuria, or glycosuria.

Differential Diagnosis

Anxiety neurosis, heart disease, anemia, gastrointestinal disease, cirrhosis, tuberculosis, myasthenia and other muscular disorders, menopausal syndrome, pheochromocytoma, primary ophthalmopathy, and thyrotoxicosis factitia may be clinically difficult to differentiate from hyperthyroidism. Differentiation is especially difficult when the thyrotoxic patient presents with minimal or no thyroid enlargement. Patients may also have painless or spontaneously resolving thyroiditis and are hyperthyroid because of increased release of thyroid hormone from the thyroid gland. This condition, however, is self-limited, and definitive treatment with antithyroid drugs, radioactive iodine, or surgery is not necessary.

Anxiety neurosis is perhaps the condition most frequently confused with hyperthyroidism. Anxiety is characterized by persistent fatigue usually unrelieved by rest, clammy palms, a normal sleeping pulse rate, and normal laboratory tests of thyroid function. The fatigue of hyperthyroidism is often relieved by rest, the palms are warm and moist, tachycardia persists during sleep, and thyroid function tests are abnormal.

Organic disease of nonthyroidal origin that may be confused with hyperthyroidism must be differentiated largely on the basis of evidence of specific organ system involvement and normal thyroid function tests.

Other causes of exophthalmos (eg, orbital tumors) or ophthalmoplegia (eg, myasthenia) must be ruled out by ophthalmologic, ultrasonographic, CT or MRI scans, and neurologic examinations.

Treatment

Hyperthyroidism may be effectively treated by antithyroid drugs, radioactive iodine, or thyroidectomy. Treatment must be individualized and depends on the patient's age and general state of health, the size of the goiter, the underlying pathologic process, and the patient's ability to obtain follow-up care.

A. Antithyroid Drugs

The principal antithyroid drugs used in the USA are propylthiouracil (PTU), 300–1000 mg orally daily, and methimazole, 30–100 mg orally daily. These agents interfere with organic binding of iodine and prevent coupling of iodotyrosines in the thyroid gland. One advantage over thyroidectomy and radioiodine in the treatment of Graves' disease is that drugs inhibit the function of the gland without destroying tissue; therefore, there is a lower incidence of subsequent hypothyroidism. This form of treatment may be used either as definitive treatment or in preparation for surgery or radioactive iodine treatment. When propylthiouracil is given as definitive treatment, the goal is to maintain the patient in a euthyroid state until a natural remission occurs. Reliable patients with small goiters are good candidates for this regimen. A prolonged remission after 18 months of treatment occurs in 30% of patients, some of whom eventually become hypothyroid. Side effects include rashes and fever (3–4%) and agranulocytosis (0.1–0.4%). Patients must be warned to stop the drug and see the physician if sore throat or fever develops.

B. Radioiodine

Radioiodine (^{131}I) may be given safely after the patient has been treated with antithyroid medications and has become euthyroid. Radioiodine is indicated for patients who are over 40 or are poor risks for surgery and for patients with recurrent hyperthyroidism. It is less expensive than operative treatment and is effective. To date, radioiodine treatment at doses necessary to treat hyperthyroidism has not been associated with an increase in leukemia or the induction of congenital anomalies. However, an increased incidence of benign thyroid tumors and rare cases of malignant thyroid tumors have been noted to follow treatment of hyperthyroidism with radioiodine. In young patients, the radiation hazard is certainly increased, and the chance of developing hypothyroidism is virtually 100%. After the first year of treatment with radioiodine, the incidence of hypothyroidism increases about 3% per year.

Hyperthyroid children and pregnant women should not be treated with radioiodine.

C. SURGERY

1. Indications for subtotal thyroidectomy—The main advantages of subtotal thyroidectomy are rapid control of the disease and a lower incidence of hypothyroidism than can be achieved with radioiodine treatment. Surgery is often the preferred treatment (1) in the presence of a very large goiter or a multinodular goiter with relatively low radioactive iodine uptake; (2) if there is a thyroid nodule that may be malignant; (3) for patients with ophthalmopathy; (4) for the treatment of pregnant patients or children; (5) for the treatment of women who wish to become pregnant within 1 year after treatment; (6) for patients with amiodarone-induced hyperthyroidism; and (7) for the treatment of psychologically or mentally incompetent patients or patients who are for any reason unable to maintain adequate long-term follow-up evaluation.

2. Preparation for surgery—The risk of thyroidectomy for toxic goiter is small since the introduction of the combined preoperative use of iodides and antithyroid drugs. Propylthiouracil or another antithyroid drug is administered until the patient becomes euthyroid and is continued until the time of operation. Two to 5 drops of potassium iodide solution or Lugol's iodine solution are then given for 10–15 days before surgery in conjunction with the propylthiouracil to decrease the friability and vascularity of the thyroid, thereby technically facilitating thyroidectomy.

An occasional untreated or inadequately treated hyperthyroid patient may require an emergency operation for some unrelated problem such as acute appendicitis and thus require immediate control of the hyperthyroidism. Such a patient should be treated in a manner similar to one in thyroid storm, since **thyroid storm** or hyperthyroid crises may be precipitated by surgical stress or trauma. Treatment of hyperthyroid patients requiring emergency operation or those in thyroid storm is as follows: Prevent release of preformed thyroid hormone by administration of Lugol's iodine solution or with ipodate sodium; give the β-adrenergic blocking agent propranolol to antagonize the peripheral manifestations of thyrotoxicosis; and decrease thyroid hormone production and extrathyroidal conversion of T_4 to T_3 by giving propylthiouracil. The combined use of propranolol and iodide has been demonstrated to lower serum thyroid hormone levels. Other important considerations are to treat precipitating causes (eg, infec-

tion, drug reactions); to support vital functions by giving oxygen, sedatives, intravenous fluids, and corticosteroids; and to reduce fever. Reserpine may be useful in the patient in whom nervousness is a prominent symptom, and a cooling blanket—not aspirin—should be used in patients requiring operation.

3. Subtotal thyroidectomy—The treatment of hyperthyroidism by subtotal thyroidectomy eliminates both the hyperthyroidism and the goiter. As a rule, all but about 5 g of thyroid are removed, sparing the parathyroid glands and the recurrent laryngeal nerves.

The death rate associated with the procedure is extremely low—less than 0.1% in a recent collected review. Subtotal thyroidectomy thus provides safe and rapid correction of the thyrotoxic state. The frequency of recurrent hyperthyroidism and hypothyroidism depends on the amount of thyroid removed and on the natural history of the hyperthyroidism. Given an accomplished surgeon and good preoperative preparation, injuries to the recurrent laryngeal nerves and parathyroid glands occur in less than 2% of cases. Adequate exposure and avoidance of injury to the recurrent laryngeal nerves and parathyroid glands are essential.

Ocular Manifestations of Graves' Disease

The pathogenesis of the ocular problems in Graves' disease remains unclear. Evidence originally supporting the role of either long-acting thyroid stimulator (LATS) or exophthalmos-producing substance (EPS) has not been authenticated.

The eye complications of Graves' disease may begin before there is any evidence of thyroid dysfunction or after the hyperthyroidism has been appropriately treated. Usually, however, the ocular manifestations develop concomitantly with the hyperthyroidism. Relief of the eye problems is often difficult to accomplish until coexisting hyperthyroidism or hypothyroidism is controlled.

The eye changes of Graves' disease vary from no signs or symptoms to loss of sight. Mild cases are characterized by upper lid retraction and stare with or without lid lag or proptosis. These cases present only minor cosmetic problems and require no treatment. When moderate to severe eye changes occur, there is soft tissue involvement with proptosis, extraocular muscle involvement, and finally optic nerve involvement. Some cases may have marked chemosis, periorbital edema, conjunctivitis, keratitis, diplopia, ophthalmoplegia, and impaired vision. Ophthalmologic consultation is required.

Treatment of the ocular problems of Graves' disease includes maintaining the patient in a euthyroid state without increase in TSH secretion, protecting the eyes from light and dust with dark glasses and eye shields, elevating the head of the bed, using diuretics to decrease periorbital and retrobulbar edema, and giving methylcellulose or guanethidine eye drops. High doses of glucocorticoids are beneficial in certain patients, but their effectiveness is variable and unpredictable. If exophthalmos progresses despite medical treatment, lateral tarsorrhaphy, retrobulbar irradiation, or surgical decompression of the orbit may be necessary. Total thyroid removal or ablation has been recommended, but whether it has a beneficial effect is controversial. Graves' disease is more likely to worsen after radioiodine treatment than after thyroidectomy. It is important that patients with ophthalmopathy be made aware of the natural history of the disease and also that they be kept euthyroid, since hyper- and hypothyroidism may produce visual deterioration. Operations to correct diplopia should be deferred until after the ophthalmopathy has stabilized.

Franklyn JA et al: Comparison of second and third generation methods for measurement of serum thyrotropin in patients with overt hyperthyroidism, patients receiving thyroxine therapy and those with nonthyroidal illness. J Clin Endocr Metab 1994;78:1368.

Franklyn JA et al: Mortality after the treatment of hyperthyroidism with radioactive iodine. N Engl J Med 1998;338: 712.

Goldstein R et al: Followup of solitary autonomous thyroid nodules treated with 131 I. N Engl J Med 1983;309:1473.

Ljunggren JG et al: Quality of life aspects and costs in treatment of Graves' hyperthyroidism with antithyroid drugs, surgery, or radioiodine: results from a prospective randomized study. Thyroid 1998;8:653.

McDougal IR: Radionucleotide therapy for thyroid disease. West J Med 1992;157:62.

McIver B et al: The pathogenesis of Graves' disease. Endocrinol Metab Clin North Am 1998;27:73.

Menegaux F et al: The surgical treatment of Graves' disease. Surg Gynecol Obstet 1993;176:277.

Nicoloff JT: Thyroid storm and myxedema coma. Med Clin North Am 1985;69:1005.

Nygaard B et al: Long-term follow-up of thyroid scintigraphs after ^{131}I therapy of solitary autonomous thyroid nodules. Thyroid 1994;4:167.

Sawin CT et al: Low serum thyrotropin concentrations as a risk factor for atrial fibrillation in older persons. N Engl J Med 1994; 331:1249.

Sridama V et al: Long-term follow-up study of compensated low-dose ^{131}I therapy for Graves' disease. N Engl J Med 1984; 311:426.

Weetman AP et al: Autoimmune therapy disease: further developments in our understanding. Endocr Rev 1994;15:788.

EVALUATION OF THYROID NODULES & GOITERS

Thyroid Nodules

The problems facing the clinician when confronted by a patient with a nodular goiter or thyroid nodule are whether the lesion is symptomatic and whether it is be-

nign or malignant. The differential diagnosis includes benign goiter, intrathyroidal cysts, thyroiditis, and benign and malignant tumors. The history should specifically emphasize the duration of swelling, recent growth, local symptoms (dysphagia, pain, or voice changes), and systemic symptoms (hyperthyroidism, hypothyroidism, or those from possible tumors metastatic to the thyroid). The patient's age, sex, place of birth, family history, and history of radiation to the neck are most important. Low-dose therapeutic radiation (6.5–2000 cGy) in infancy or childhood is associated with an increased incidence of thyroid cancer (about 10%) in later life. A thyroid nodule is more likely to be a cancer in a man than in a woman and in a young patient than in an old one. In certain geographic areas, endemic goiter is common, making benign nodules more common. Thyroid cancer is familial in about 25% of patients with medullary thyroid cancer (familial medullary thyroid cancer, MEN 2a and 2b) and in about 7% of patients with papillary cancer or Hürthle cell cancer. Papillary thyroid cancer occurs more often in patients with Cowden's syndrome, Gardner's syndrome, or Carney's syndrome.

The clinician must systematically palpate the thyroid to determine whether there is a solitary thyroid nodule or if it is a multinodular gland and whether there are palpable lymph nodes. A solitary hard thyroid nodule is likely to be malignant, whereas most multinodular goiters are benign.

In many patients, the possibility of cancer is difficult to exclude without microscopic examination of the gland itself. Percutaneous needle biopsy is the most cost-effective diagnostic test for most patients. Cytologic results are classified as malignant, benign, indeterminate or suspicious, and inadequate specimen (Figure 17–2). False-positive diagnoses of cancer are rare, but about 20% of biopsy specimens reported as indetermi-

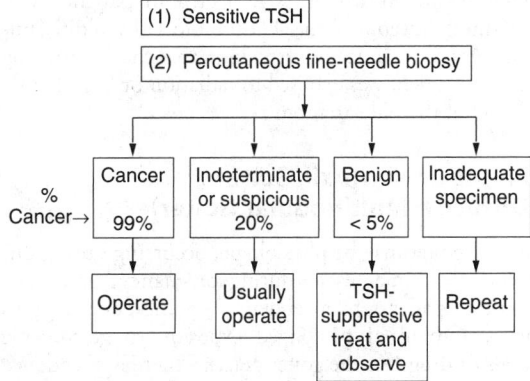

Figure 17–2. Evaluation of thyroid nodule.

nate and 5% of those reported as benign are actually malignant. If the specimen is reported as inadequate, biopsy should be repeated. Needle biopsy should in general not be performed in patients with a history of irradiation to the neck or familial thyroid cancer because radiation-induced tumors are often multifocal, and a negative biopsy may therefore be unreliable. The radioiodine scan is helpful in determining whether a follicular neoplasm by cytologic examination is functioning (warm or hot) or nonfunctioning (cold). Hot solitary thyroid nodules may cause hyperthyroidism but are rarely malignant, whereas cold solitary thyroid nodules have an incidence of cancer of about 20% and should be removed. Thyroid carcinoma is uncommon (1%) in multinodular goiters, but if there is a dominant nodule or one that enlarges, it should be biopsied or removed. Patients with thyroid nodules who received x-ray treatments to the head and neck in infancy and childhood and those with a family history of thyroid cancer have a 40% chance of having thyroid cancer. Thyroid cancer occurs in nearly 50% of the children with solitary cold thyroid nodules; therefore, thyroidectomy is usually indicated. Ultrasound differentiates solid and cystic lesions and may detect enlarged lymph nodes. About 15% of cold solitary lesions are cystic. A chest x-ray including the neck is helpful in demonstrating tracheal displacement, calcification of the thyroid nodule, or the presence of pulmonary metastases. CT or MRI scans are usually not necessary but are helpful when the limits of the tumor cannot be defined, such as in patient with large, invasive, or substernal goiters or tumors.

The principal indications for surgical removal of a nodular goiter are (1) suspicion of cancer, (2) symptoms of pressure, (3) hyperthyroidism, (4) substernal extension, and (5) cosmetic deformity. Solitary hard thyroid nodules or nodules that are cold on radioiodine scan and solid by ultrasound or are suspicious for cancer on aspiration biopsy cytology should be removed. Nonoperative treatment is indicated in patients with multinodular goiters and Hashimoto's thyroiditis unless there is a clinically suspicious area that is growing or if the patient was exposed to radiation or has a family history of thyroid carcinoma.

Simple or Nontoxic Goiter (Diffuse & Multinodular Goiter)

Simple goiter may be physiologic, occurring during puberty or the menses or during pregnancy; or it may occur in patients from endemic (iodine-poor) regions or as a result of prolonged exposure to goitrogenic foods or drugs. As the goiter persists, there is a tendency to form nodules. Goiter may also occur early in life as a consequence of a congenital defect in thyroid hormone production. It is generally assumed that nontoxic goiter represents a compensatory response to inadequate thyroid hormone production, although thyroid growth immunoglobulins may also be important. Nontoxic diffuse goiter usually responds favorably to thyroid hormone administration.

Symptoms are usually awareness of a neck mass and dyspnea, dysphagia, or symptoms caused by interference with venous return. In diffuse goiter, the thyroid is symmetrically enlarged and has a smooth surface without areas of encapsulation. However, most patients have multinodular glands by the time they seek medical care. Thyroid function is usually normal, though the sensitive TSH may be suppressed and the radioiodine uptake increased. Surgery is indicated to relieve the pressure symptoms of a large goiter for substernal goiter or to rule out cancer when there are localized areas of hardness or rapid growth. Aspiration biopsy cytology is helpful in these patients.

Berghout A et al: The long-term outcome of thyroidectomy for sporadic non-toxic goiter. Clin Endocrinol 1989;31:193.

Burguera B et al: Thyroid incidentalomas. Prevalence, diagnosis, significance and management. Endocrinol Metab Clin North Am 2000;29:87.

Cochand-Priollet B et al: The diagnostic value of fine needle aspiration biopsy under ultrasonography in nonfunctioning thyroid nodules: a prospective study comparing cytologic and histologic findings. Am J Med 1994:97;152.

Greenspan FS: The problem of the nodular goiter. Med Clin North Am 1991;75:195.

LaRosa GL et al: Levothyroxine and potassium iodide are both effective in treating benign solitary solid cold nodules of the thyroid 1995;122:1.

Mazzaferri EL: Management of a solitary thyroid nodule. N Engl J Med 1993;328;553.

Ross DS: Thyroid hormone suppressive therapy of sporadic nontoxic goiter. Thyroid 1992;2:263.

Takasu N et al: Disappearance of thyrotropin-blocking antibodies and spontaneous recovery from hypothyroidism in autoimmune thyroiditis. N Engl J Med 1992;326:513.

Wong CK et al: Thyroid nodules. Rational management. World J Surg 2000;24:934.

INFLAMMATORY THYROID DISEASE

The inflammatory diseases of the thyroid are termed acute, subacute, or chronic thyroiditis, which can be either suppurative or nonsuppurative.

Acute suppurative thyroiditis is uncommon and is characterized by the sudden onset of severe neck pain accompanied by dysphagia, fever, and chills. It usually follows an acute upper respiratory tract infection; can be diagnosed by percutaneous aspiration, smear, and culture; and is treated by surgical drainage. The organisms are most often streptococci, staphylococci, pneumococci, or coliforms. It may also be associated with a piriform sinus fistula. A barium swallow is therefore recommended in persistent or recurrent cases.

Subacute thyroiditis, a noninfectious disorder, is characterized by thyroid swelling, head and chest pain, fever, weakness, malaise, palpitations, and weight loss. Some patients with subacute thyroiditis have no pain (silent thyroiditis), in which case the condition must be distinguished from Graves' disease. In subacute thyroiditis, the erythrocyte sedimentation rate and serum gamma globulin are almost always elevated, and radioiodine uptake is very low or absent with increased or normal thyroid hormone levels. The illness is usually self-limited, and aspirin and corticosteroids relieve symptoms. These patients eventually become euthyroid.

Hashimoto's thyroiditis, the most common form of thyroiditis, is usually characterized by enlargement of the thyroid with or without pain and tenderness. It is much more common in women (about 15% of women in the USA) and occasionally causes dysphagia or hypothyroidism.

Hashimoto's thyroiditis is an autoimmune disease. Serum titers of antimicrosomal and antithyroglobulin antibodies are elevated. Appropriate treatment for most patients consists of giving thyroid hormone. Operation is indicated for marked pressure symptoms, for suspected malignant tumor, and for cosmetic reasons. In patients with pressure or choking symptoms, surgical division of the isthmus provides relief. If the thyroid is large or asymmetric and fails to regress after treatment with exogenous thyroid hormone, or if it contains a discrete nodule, percutaneous needle biopsy or thyroidectomy is recommended. Needle biopsy is helpful in confirming the diagnosis.

Riedel's thyroiditis is a rare condition that presents as a hard woody mass in the thyroid region with marked fibrosis and chronic inflammation in and around the gland. The inflammatory process infiltrates muscles and causes symptoms of tracheal compression. Hypothyroidism is usually present, and surgical treatment is required to relieve tracheal or esophageal obstruction.

Baker JR: Autoimmune endocrine diseases. JAMA 1997;278: 1931.

Miyauchi A et al: Piriform sinus fistula: an underlying abnormality common in patients with autosuppurative thyroiditis. World J Surg 1990;14:400.

Nordyke RA et al: The superiority of antimicrosomal over antithyroglobulin antibodies for detecting Hashimoto's thyroiditis. Arch Intern Med 1993;153:862.

Sheigmasa C et al: Chronic thyroiditis with painful tender thyroid enlargement and transient thyrotoxicosis. J Clin Endocrinol Metab 1990;70:385.

Singer PA: Thyroiditis: acute, subacute and chronic. Med Clin North Am 1991;75:61.

BENIGN TUMORS OF THE THYROID

Benign thyroid tumors are adenomas, involutionary nodules, cysts, or localized thyroiditis. Most adenomas are of the follicular type. Adenomas are usually solitary and encapsulated and compress the adjacent thyroid. The major reasons for removal are a suspicion of cancer, functional overactivity producing hyperthyroidism, and cosmetic disfigurement.

MALIGNANT TUMORS OF THE THYROID

 ESSENTIALS OF DIAGNOSIS

- *History of irradiation to the neck in some patients.*
- *Painless or enlarging nodule, dysphagia, or hoarseness.*
- *Firm or hard, fixed thyroid nodule; cervical lymphadenopathy.*
- *Normal thyroid function; nodule stippled with calcium (x-ray), cold (radioiodine scan), solid (ultrasound); positive or suspicious cytology.*
- *Family history of thyroid cancer.*

General Considerations

An appreciation of the classification of malignant tumors of the thyroid is important, because thyroid tumors demonstrate a wide range of growth and malignant behavior. At one end of the spectrum is **papillary adenocarcinoma,** which usually occurs in young adults, grows very slowly, metastasizes through lymphatics, and is compatible with long life even in the presence of metastases (Figure 17–3). At the other extreme is **undifferentiated carcinoma,** which appears late in life and is nonencapsulated and invasive, forming large infiltrating tumors composed of small or large anaplastic cells. Most patients with anaplastic thyroid carcinoma succumb as a consequence of local recurrence, pulmonary metastasis, or both. Between these two extremes are follicular, Hürthle cell, and medullary carcinomas, sarcomas, lymphomas, and metastatic tumors. The prognosis depends on the histologic pattern, the age and sex of the patient, the extent of tumor spread at the time of diagnosis, whether the tumor takes up radioiodine, and other factors.

Figure 17–3. Survival rates after thyroidectomy for papillary, mixed papillary-follicular, follicular, medullary, and undifferentiated thyroid cancer.

The cause of most cases of thyroid carcinoma is unknown, although persons who received low-dose (6.5–2000 cGy) therapeutic radiation to the thymus, tonsils, scalp, and skin in infancy, childhood, and adolescence have an increased risk of developing thyroid tumors. Children are most susceptible to radiation exposure such as occurred with the Chernobyl nuclear accident, but adults up to 50 years of age who were exposed to the atomic blast at Hiroshima had an increased incidence of benign and malignant thyroid tumors. The incidence of thyroid cancer increases for at least 30 years after irradiation.

Types of Thyroid Cancer

A. PAPILLARY ADENOCARCINOMA

Papillary adenocarcinoma accounts for 85% of cancers of the thyroid gland. The tumor usually appears in early adult life and presents as a solitary nodule. It then spreads via intraglandular lymphatics within the thyroid gland and then to the subcapsular and pericapsular lymph nodes. Eighty percent of children and 20% of adults present with palpable lymph nodes. The tumor may metastasize to lungs or bone. Microscopically, it is composed of papillary projections of columnar epithelium. Psammoma bodies are present in about 60% of cases. A mixed papillary-follicular or a follicular variant of papillary carcinoma is sometimes found. The rate of growth may be stimulated by TSH.

B. FOLLICULAR ADENOCARCINOMA

Follicular adenocarcinoma accounts for approximately 10% of malignant thyroid tumors. It appears later in life than the papillary form and may be rubbery or even soft on palpation. Follicular tumors are encapsulated. Microscopically, follicular carcinoma may be difficult to distinguish from normal thyroid tissue. Capsular (invasion through the capsule) and vascular invasion distinguish follicular carcinomas from follicular adenomas. Follicular thyroid cancers only occasionally (7%) metastasize to the regional lymph nodes, but they have a greater tendency to spread by the hematogenous route to the lungs, skeleton, and liver. Metastases from this tumor often demonstrate an avidity for radioactive iodine after total thyroidectomy. Skeletal metastases from follicular carcinomas may appear 10 years after resection of the primary lesion. Hürthle cells carcinoma is a variant of follicular carcinoma. It is more likely to be multifocal and involve lymph nodes than follicular carcinoma. Like follicular carcinoma, it makes thyroglobulin, but it does not usually take up radioiodine. The prognosis is not as good for either follicular or Hürthle cell cancers as with the papillary type (Figure 17–3).

C. MEDULLARY CARCINOMA

Medullary carcinoma accounts for approximately 7% of malignant tumors of the thyroid. It contains amyloid and is a solid, hard, nodular tumor that does not take up radioiodine and secretes calcitonin. Medullary carcinomas arise from cells of the ultimobranchial bodies. Familial medullary carcinoma occurs in about 25% of patients, but it also occurs with pheochromocytomas—often bilateral—and hyperparathyroidism (MEN 2a) and with pheochromocytomas. Marfanoid habitus, amyloidosis, and Hirschsprung's disease also occur in patients with familial medullary cancer. All patients with medullary thyroid cancer should be screened for an *RET* point mutation on chromosome 10 because 10% of patients without a positive family history have de novo mutations. For patients detected by family genetic screening, most experts recommend prophylactic total thyroidectomy prior to age 6.

D. UNDIFFERENTIATED CARCINOMA

This rapidly growing tumor occurs principally in women beyond middle life and accounts for 1% of all thyroid cancers. This tumor occasionally evolves from a papillary or follicular neoplasm. It is a solid, quickly enlarging, hard, irregular mass diffusely involving the gland and invading the trachea, muscles, and neurovascular structures early. The tumor may be painful and somewhat tender, may be fixed on swallowing, and may cause laryngeal or esophageal obstructive symptoms. Microscopically, there are three major types: giant cell, spindle cell, and small cell. Mitoses are frequent. Cervical lymphadenopathy and pulmonary metastases are common. Local recurrence after surgical treatment is the rule. Combination treatment with external radiation therapy, chemotherapy, and surgery offers palliation to some patients but is rarely curative (Figure 17–3).

Treatment

The treatment of differentiated thyroid carcinoma is operative removal. For papillary carcinoma, acceptable operations are total lobectomy with isthmectomy, near-total thyroidectomy, and total thyroidectomy—followed by 10-year survival rates of over 80%. Subtotal or partial lobectomy is contraindicated because the incidence of tumor recurrence is greater and survival is shorter. Total thyroidectomy is recommended by the author for papillary (> 1.5 cm), follicular, Hürthle cell, and medullary carcinomas if the operation can be done without producing permanent hypoparathyroidism or injury to the recurrent laryngeal nerves. Total thyroidectomy is preferred over other operations because of the high incidence of multifocal tumor within the gland, a clinical recurrence rate of about 7% in the contralateral lobe if it is spared, and the ease of assessment for recurrence by serum thyroglobulin assay or radioiodine scan during follow-up examinations.

A functional modified radical neck dissection preserving the sternocleidomastoid muscle and spinal accessory nerve is performed if lymph nodes in the lateral neck are clinically involved.

Medullary carcinoma is associated with such a high incidence of nodal involvement that a bilateral central neck node cleanout should be done in all patients as well as concomitant ipsilateral modified radical neck dissection for primary tumors more than 1.5 cm in diameter and when the central neck nodes are involved. When serum calcitonin or CEA levels remain elevated after thyroidectomy, laparoscopy should be done to evaluate for the common miliary metastases on the surface of the liver. If the liver is clear, then central neck dissection and bilateral functional neck dissections should be considered, including removal of nodes from the superior mediastinum.

Metastatic deposits of follicular and papillary carcinoma should be treated with ^{131}I after total thyroidectomy or thyroid ablation with radioactive iodine. All patients with thyroid cancer should be maintained indefinitely on suppressive doses of thyroid hormone. For follow-up, it is helpful to measure serum levels of thyroglobulin (a tumor marker for differentiated thyroid cancer), which are usually increased in patients with residual tumor after total thyroidectomy. For **undifferen-**

tiated carcinoma, malignant lymphoma, or **sarcoma,** the tumor should be excised as completely as possible and then treated by radiation and chemotherapy. Doxorubicin (Adriamycin), vincristine, and chlorambucil are the most effective agents. Carcinomas of the kidney, breast, and lung and other tumors sometimes metastasize to the thyroid, but they rarely present as a solitary nodule.

Alsanea O et al: Is familial non-medullary thyroid carcinoma more aggressive than sporadic thyroid cancer? A multicenter series. Surgery 2000;128:1043.

Clark OH et al: Management of patients with differentiated thyroid cancer will have positive serum thyroglobulin levels and negative radioiodine. Thyroid 1994;4:501.

Clark OH: Thyroid cancer: predisposing conditions, growth factors, signal transduction and oncogenes. Aust N Z J Surg 1998;68:469.

Jossart G et al: Well differentiated thyroid cancer. Curr Probl Surg 1994;31:933.

Kebebew E et al: Differentiated thyroid cancer: "complete" rational approach. World J Surg 2000;24:942.

Lips CJ et al: Clinical screening as compared with DNA analysis in families with multiple endocrine neoplasia type 2A. N Engl J Med 1994;331:828.

Maxon HR 3d et al: Radioiodine-131 therapy for well differentiated thyroid cancer: a quantitative radiation dosimetric approach. Outcome and validation in 85 patients. J Nucl Med 1992;33:1132.

Mazzaferri EL et al: Using recombinant human TSH in the management of well-differentiated thyroid cancer: current strategies and future directions. Thyroid 2000;10:767.

Mazzaferri EL et al: Long-term impact of initial surgical and medical therapy on papillary and follicular thyroid cancer. Am J Med 1994;97:418.

O'Riordain DS et al: Medullary thyroid carcinoma in multiple endocrine neoplasia types 2A and 2B. Surgery 1994;116:1017.

Ordonez NG et al: Anaplastic thyroid carcinoma. Am J Clin Pathol 1991;96:15.

Perrier ND et al: Classification and treatment of follicular thyroid neoplasms and discordance between and within medical specialties. Surgery 1999;126:1063.

Pittas AG et al: Bone metastases from thyroid carcinoma: clinical characteristics and prognostic variables in one hundred forty-six patients. Thyroid 2000;10:261.

Robbins J et al: Thyroid cancer: a lethal endocrine neoplasm. Ann Intern Med 1991;115:133.

■ II. THE PARATHYROID GLANDS

EMBRYOLOGY & ANATOMY

Phylogenetically, the parathyroids appear rather late, being first seen in amphibia. They arise from pharyngeal pouches III and IV and may be arrested as high as the level of the hyoid bone during their descent to the posterior capsule of the thyroid gland. Four parathyroid glands are present in 85% of the population, and about 15% have more than four glands. Occasionally, one or more may be incorporated into the thyroid gland or thymus and hence are intrathyroidal or mediastinal in location. Parathyroid III, which normally assumes the inferior position, may be found in the anterior mediastinum, usually in the thymus. The upper parathyroids (parathyroid IV) usually remain in close association with the upper portion of the lateral thyroid lobes but may be loosely attached by a long vascular pedicle and migrate caudally along the esophagus into the posterior mediastinum. The parathyroid glands may lie in front of or behind the internal jugular vein and common carotid artery.

The normal parathyroid gland has a distinct yellowish-brown color, is ovoid, tongue-shaped, polypoid, or spherical, and averages $2 \times 3 \times 7$ mm. The total mean weight of four normal parathyroids is about 150 mg. These encapsulated glands are usually supplied by a branch of the inferior thyroid artery but may be supplied by the superior thyroid or, rarely, the thyroid ima arteries. The vessels can be seen entering a hilum-like structure, a feature that differentiates parathyroid glands from fat.

Mansberger AR Jr et al: Surgical embryology and anatomy of the thyroid and parathyroid glands. Surg Clin North Am 1993;73:727.

PHYSIOLOGY

Parathyroid hormone (PTH), vitamin D, and probably calcitonin play vital roles in calcium and phosphorus metabolism in bone, kidney, and gut. Specific radioimmunoassays are available to measure PTH, vitamin D, and calcitonin. Ionized calcium, the physiologically important fraction, can now be accurately measured. Total serum calcium concentration is composed of approximately 48% ionized calcium, 46% protein-bound calcium, and 6% calcium complexed to organic anions. Total serum calcium varies directly with plasma protein concentrations, but calcium ion concentrations are unaffected.

PTH and calcitonin work in concert to modulate fluctuations in plasma levels of ionized calcium. When the ionized calcium level falls, the parathyroids secrete more PTH and the parafollicular cells within the thyroid secrete less calcitonin. The rise in PTH and fall in calcitonin produce increased bone resorption and increased resorption of calcium in the renal tubules. More calcium enters the blood, and ionized calcium levels return to normal.

In the circulation, immunoreactive PTH is heterogeneous, consisting of the intact hormone and several hormonal fragments. The amino terminal (N-terminal) fragment is biologically active, whereas the carboxyl terminal (C-terminal) fragment is biologically inert. Measurement of intact PTH by immunoassay is best for screening for hyperparathyroidism and for selective venous catheterization to localize the source of PTH production. PTH-related peptide (PTHrP) that is secreted by nonparathyroid malignant tumors does not cross-react with intact PTH assays.

Because PTH levels rise in normal subjects if ionized calcium levels are low, calcium and PTH must be determined from samples drawn simultaneously to diagnose hyperparathyroidism. The combination of increased PTH levels and hypercalcemia without hypocalciuria is almost always pathognomonic of hyperparathyroidism.

Lunghall S et al: Disturbances of basal and stimulated serum levels of intact parathyroid hormone in primary hyperparathyroidism. Surgery 1991;110:47.

Picotte SL et al: Regulation of parathyroid hormone secretion. Endocr Rev 1991;12:291.

Watson PH et al: Parathyroid hormone regulation of syntheses and secretion. Clin Invest Med 1993;16:58.

■ DISEASES OF THE PARATHYROIDS

PRIMARY HYPERPARATHYROIDISM

 ESSENTIALS OF DIAGNOSIS

- *Increased fatigue, weakness, arthralgias, nausea, vomiting, dyspepsia, constipation, polydipsia, polyuria, nocturia, psychiatric disturbances, renal colic, bone, and joint pain. ("Stones, bones, abdominal groans, psychic moans, and fatigue overtones.") Some patients are asymptomatic.*

- *Nephrolithiasis and nephrocalcinosis, osteopenia, osteoporosis, osteitis fibrosa cystica, peptic ulcer disease, gout, chondrocalcinosis, pancreatitis.*

- *Hypertension, band keratopathy, neck masses.*

- *Serum calcium, PTH, chloride, usually increased; serum phosphate low or normal; uric acid and alkaline phosphatase sometimes increased; urine calcium increased, normal, or, rarely, decreased; urine phosphate increased; tubular reabsorption*

of phosphate decreased, osteocalcin and deoxypyridinoline crosslinks increased.

- *X-rays: subperiosteal resorption of phalanges,*
  demineralization of the skeleton (osteopenia or
  osteoporosis), bone cysts, and nephrocalcinosis
  or nephrolithiasis.

General Considerations

Primary hyperparathyroidism is due to excess PTH secretion from a single parathyroid adenoma (83%), multiple adenomas (6%), hyperplasia (10%), or carcinoma
(1%). Once thought to be rare, primary hyperparathyroidism is now found in 0.1–0.3% of the general population and is the most common cause of hypercalcemia
in unselected patients. It is uncommon before puberty;
its peak incidence is between the third and fifth
decades, and it is two to three times more common in
women than in men.

Overproduction of parathyroid hormone results in
mobilization of calcium from bone and inhibition of the
renal reabsorption of phosphate, thereby producing hypercalcemia and hypophosphatemia. This causes a wasting of calcium and phosphorus, with osseous mineral loss
and **osteoporosis.** Other associated or related conditions
that offer clues to the diagnosis of hyperparathyroidism
are nephrolithiasis, nephrocalcinosis, osteitis fibrosa cystica, peptic ulcer, pancreatitis, hypertension, and gout or
pseudogout. Hyperparathyroidism also occurs in both
multiple endocrine neoplasia (MEN) type 1, known as
Werner's syndrome, and MEN type 2, known as **Sip-**
ple's syndrome. The former is characterized by tumors
of the parathyroid, pituitary, and pancreas (hyperparathyroidism, pituitary tumors, and functioning or nonfunctioning islet cell pancreatic tumors) that may cause
Zollinger-Ellison syndrome (gastrinoma), hypoglycemia
(insulinoma), glucagonoma, lipoma, somatostatinoma,
and pancreatic polypeptide tumors (PPomas). Other tumors in MEN 1 syndrome include adrenocortical tumors, carcinoid tumors, and multiple lipomas. MEN 2a
consists of hyperparathyroidism in association with
medullary carcinoma of the thyroid and pheochromocytoma. MEN 2b patients have a marfanoid habitus and
multiple neuromas but rarely have hyperparathyroidism.

Parathyroid adenomas range in weight from 65 mg
to over 35 g, and the size usually parallels the degree of
hypercalcemia. Microscopically, these tumors may be of
chief cell, water cell, or, rarely, oxyphil cell type.

Primary parathyroid hyperplasia involves all of the
parathyroid glands. Microscopically, there are two
types: chief cell hyperplasia and water-clear cell (wasser-
helle) hyperplasia. Hyperplastic glands vary considerably in size but are usually larger than normal (65 mg).

Parathyroid carcinoma is rare but is more common
in patients with profound hypercalcemia. Parathyroid
cancers are palpable in half the patients and should be
suspected in patients at operation when the parathyroid
gland is hard, has a whitish or irregular capsule, or is invasive. Parathyromatosis is a rare condition causing hypercalcemia due to multiple embryologic rests or, more
commonly, due to seeding when a parathyroid tumor
has ruptured or a tumor capsule has been breached.

Clinical Findings

A. SYMPTOMS AND SIGNS

Historically, the clinical manifestations of hyperparathyroidism have changed. Forty years ago, the diagnosis was based on bone pain and deformity (osteitis
fibrosa cystica), and in later years on the renal complications (nephrolithiasis and nephrocalcinosis). At present, over two-thirds of patients are detected by routine
screening, and some are asymptomatic. After successful
surgical treatment, many patients thought to be asymptomatic become aware of improvement in unrecognized
preoperative symptoms such as muscle fatigability,
weakness, psychiatric disturbances, constipation, polydipsia and polyuria, and bone and joint pain. Hyperparathyroidism should be suspected in all patients with
hypercalcemia and the above symptoms, especially if associated with nephrolithiasis, nephrocalcinosis, hypertension, peptic ulcer, pancreatitis, or gout. Patients
with primary hyperparathyroidism appear to have a
shortened life expectancy that improves after successful
parathyroidectomy.

B. LABORATORY FINDINGS, IMAGING STUDIES, AND DIFFERENTIAL DIAGNOSIS (APPROACH TO THE HYPERCALCEMIC PATIENT)

1. Laboratory findings—See Table 17–2. Hyperparathyroidism and cancer are responsible for about 90%
of all cases of hypercalcemia. Hyperparathyroidism is the
most common cause of hypercalcemia detected by undi-
rected methods such as routine screening, whereas cancer
is the most common cause of hypercalcemia in hospitalized patients. Other causes of hypercalcemia are listed in
Table 17–3. In many patients the diagnosis is obvious,
while in others it may be exceedingly difficult. At times,
more than one reason for hypercalcemia may exist in the
same patient, such as cancer or sarcoidosis plus hyperparathyroidism. A careful history must be obtained documenting (1) the duration of any symptoms possibly
related to hypercalcemia; (2) symptoms related to malignant disease; (3) conditions associated with hyperparathyroidism, such as renal colic, peptic ulcer disease,
pancreatitis, hypertension, or gout; or (4) possible excess
use of milk products, antacids, baking soda, or vitamins.

Table 17–2. Laboratory evaluation of hypercalcemia.

Essential	Selective
Blood Tests	
Calcium	Creatine and BUN
Phosphate	Chloride
PTH (intact or two-site assay)	Uric acid
Alkaline phosphatase	pH
	Protein electrophoresis or albumin: globulin ratio
	25-Dihydroxyvitamin D and 1,25-dihydroxyvitamin D
Radiographic or Nuclear Medicine Procedures	
Chest x-ray	Sestamibi scan of neck and
Abdominal plain films	ultrasound of neck
Ultrasound of kidneys	
Bone density (hip, lumbar spine, wrist)	
Urine Tests	
24-hour urinary calcium[1]	Urinalysis
	Deoxypyridinoline cross-links
	Osteocalcin

[1]When urine calcium is < 100 mg/24 h, a diagnosis of benign familial hypocalciuric hypercalcemia must be considered.

In patients with a recent cough, wheeze, or hemoptysis, epidermoid carcinoma of the lung should be considered. Hematuria might suggest hypernephroma, bladder tumor, or renal lithiasis. Chest roentgenograms and intravenous urograms should be performed as appropriate. A long history of renal stones or peptic ulcer disease suggests that hyperparathyroidism is likely.

The most important tests for the evaluation of hypercalcemia are, in order of importance, serum calcium, parathyroid hormone, phosphate, chloride, protein electrophoretic pattern, alkaline phosphatase, creatinine; uric acid, and urea nitrogen; urinary calcium; blood hematocrit and pH; serum magnesium; and erythrocyte sedimentation rate. Measurement of nephrogenous cAMP, 1,25-hydroxy vitamin D levels, and tubular reabsorption of phosphate are helpful in selected patients when other tests are equivocal.

A high serum calcium and a low serum phosphate suggest hyperparathyroidism, but about half of patients with hyperparathyroidism have normal serum phosphate concentrations. Patients with vitamin D intoxication, sarcoidosis, malignant disease without metastasis, and hyperthyroidism may also be hypophosphatemic, but patients with breast cancer and hypercalcemia are only rarely so. In fact, if hypophosphatemia and hyper-

Table 17–3. Causes of hypercalcemia.

	Approximate Frequency (%)
Cancer	45
Breast cancer	
Metastatic	
PTH-related peptide secreting (lung, kidney)	
Multiple myeloma	
Leukemias	
Others	
Endocrine disorders	46
Hyperparathyroidism	
Hyperthyroidism	
Addison's disease, pheochromocytoma	
Hypothyroidism, VIPoma	
Increased intake	4
Milk-alkali syndrome	
Vitamin D and A overdosage	
Thiazides, lithium, aluminum	
Granulomatous diseases	3
Sarcoidosis, tuberculosis, etc	
Benign familial hypocalciuric hypercalcemia and other disorders	2
Paget's disease	
Immobilization	
Idiopathic hypercalcemia of infancy	
Aluminum intoxication	
Dysproteinemias	
Rhabdomyolysis	

calcemia are present in association with breast cancer, concomitant hyperparathyroidism is probable. Measurement of **serum parathyroid hormone** has its greatest value in this situation, since the PTH level is low or nil in patients with hypercalcemia due to *all* causes other than primary or ectopic hyperparathyroidism, or familial hypocalciuric hypercalcemia. In general, serum PTH levels should be measured in all cases of persistent hypercalcemia without an obvious cause and in normocalcemic patients who are suspected of having hyperparathyroidism. Determination of intact serum PTH levels is best since it is sensitive and is not influenced by tumors that secrete parathyroid-related peptide. Nonparathyroid tumors that secrete pure PTH are extremely rare.

An elevated serum chloride concentration is a useful diagnostic clue found in about 40% of hyperparathyroid patients. PTH acts directly on the proximal renal tubule to decrease the resorption of bicarbonate, which leads to increased resorption of chloride and a mild hyperchloremic renal tubular acidosis. Other causes of hypercalcemia do not give increased serum chloride concentrations. Calculation of the **serum chloride to phosphate ratio** takes advantage of slight increases in serum chloride and slight decreases in serum phosphate concentrations. A ratio above 33 suggests hyperparathyroidism.

Serum protein electrophoretic patterns are helpful for excluding multiple myeloma and sarcoidosis. Hypergammaglobulinemia is rare in hyperparathyroidism but is not uncommon in patients with multiple myeloma and sarcoidosis. Roentgenograms of the skull or site of bone pain in patients with elevated alkaline phosphatase levels will often reveal typical "punched-out" bony lesions, and the diagnosis of myeloma can be firmly established by bone marrow examination. Sarcoidosis can be difficult to diagnose, because it may exist for several years with few clinical findings. A chest x-ray revealing a diffuse fibronodular infiltrate and prominent hilar adenopathy is suggestive, and the demonstration of noncaseating granuloma in lymph nodes is diagnostic. The **hydrocortisone suppression test** (150 mg of hydrocortisone per day for 10 days) reduces the serum calcium concentration in most cases of sarcoidosis and vitamin D intoxication and in many patients with carcinoma and multiple myeloma but only rarely in patients with hyperparathyroidism. It is therefore a useful diagnostic maneuver if these conditions are considered. Hydrocortisone suppression is used to treat the hypercalcemic crises that may occur with these disorders.

Serum alkaline phosphate levels are elevated in about 10% of patients with primary hyperparathyroidism and may also be increased in patients with Paget's disease and cancer. When the serum alkaline phosphatase level is elevated, serum 5'-nucleotidase, which parallels liver alkaline phosphatase, should be measured to determine if the increase is from bone, which suggests parathyroid disease, or liver. A 24-hour urine calcium level is helpful for diagnosing hypercalcemic patients who have low urinary calcium levels resulting from benign familial hypocalciuric hypercalcemia. These patients do not benefit from parathyroidectomy.

2. Bone studies—Bone densitometry and radiographic examination of bone frequently reveals osteopenia or osteoporosis, but overt skeletal changes such as subperiosteal resorption or brown tumor are found in only 10% of patients with hyperparathyroidism. Dual photon bone density studies of the femur, lumbar spine, and radius help document osteopenia that occurs in about 70% of female patients with hyperparathyroidism. Bone changes of osteitis fibrosa cystica are rare on x-ray unless the serum alkaline phosphatase concentration is increased. Primary and secondary hyperparathyroidism produce subperiosteal resorption of the phalanges and bone cysts (Figure 17–4). A ground-glass appearance of the skull with loss of definition of the tables and demineralization of the outer aspects of the clavicles are less frequently seen. In patients with markedly elevated serum alkaline phosphatase levels without subperiosteal resorption on x-ray, Paget's disease or cancer must be suspected. A 24-hour urine test for deoxypyridinoline cross-link assay or osteocalcin detects increased bone loss.

3. Differential diagnosis—The differentiation between hyperparathyroidism due to primary parathyroid disease and that due to ectopic hyperparathyroidism or nonparathyroid cancer is can now usually be determined by measuring intact PTH (increase in primary hyperparathyroidism) and PTHrP (increased in nonparathyroid malignant tumors). The most common tumors causing ectopic hyperparathyroidism are squamous cell carcinoma of the lung, renal cell carcinoma, and bladder cancer. Less commonly it is due to hepatoma or to cancer of the ovary, stomach, pancreas, parotid gland, or colon. Recent onset of symptoms, increased sedimentation rate, anemia, serum calcium greater than 14 mg/dL, and increased alkaline phosphatase activity without osteitis fibrosa cystica suggest **malignancy-associated hypercalcemia;** mild hypercalcemia with a long history of nephrolithiasis or peptic ulcer suggests primary hyperthyroidism. Documented hypercalcemia of 6 months or longer essentially rules out malignancy-associated hypercalcemia.

In **milk-alkali syndrome,** a history of excessive ingestion of milk products, calcium-containing antacids, and baking soda is often obtained. These patients be-

Figure 17–4. Subperiosteal resorption of radial side of second phalanges.

come normocalcemic after discontinuing these habits. Patients with milk-alkali syndrome usually have renal insufficiency and low urinary calcium concentrations and are usually alkalotic rather than acidotic. Because of the high incidence of ulcer disease in hyperparathyroidism, milk-alkali syndrome may occasionally coexist with that disorder.

Hyperthyroidism, another cause of hypercalcemia and hypercalciuria, can usually be differentiated because manifestations of thyrotoxicosis rather than hypercalcemia bring the patient to the physician. Occasionally, an elderly patient with apathetic hyperthyroidism may be hypercalcemic. A sensitive TSH test should be evaluated in hypercalcemic patients whose PTH levels are not increased. Treatment of hyperthyroidism with antithyroid medications causes serum calcium to return to normal levels within 8 weeks.

Normal subjects taking **thiazide diuretics** may develop a transient increase in serum calcium levels, usually less than 1 mg/dL. Larger rises in serum calcium induced by thiazides have been reported in patients with primary hyperparathyroidism and idiopathic juvenile osteoporosis. Most patients who have hypercalcemia while taking thiazides have another reason for the increase. The best way to evaluate these patients is to switch them to a nonthiazide antihypertensive agent or diuretic and to measure the PTH level. Thiazide-induced hypercalcemia is not associated with increased serum PTH in patients without hyperparathyroidism.

Benign familial hypocalciuric hypercalcemia is one of the few conditions that causes chronic hypercalcemia and mildly elevated PTH levels. It can be difficult to distinguish from primary hyperparathyroidism. The best way to diagnose this disorder is to document a low urinary calcium and a family history of hypercalcemia, especially in children.

Other miscellaneous causes of hypercalcemia are Paget's disease, immobilization (especially in Paget's disease or in young patients), dysproteinemias, idiopathic hypercalcemia of infancy, aluminum intoxication, and rhabdomyolysis (Table 17–3).

C. APPROACH TO THE NORMOCALCEMIC PATIENT WITH POSSIBLE HYPERPARATHYROIDISM

Renal failure, hypoalbuminemia, pancreatitis, deficiency of vitamin D or magnesium, and excess phosphate intake may cause serum calcium levels to be normal in hyperparathyroidism. Correction of these disorders results in hypercalcemia if hyperparathyroidism is present. The incidence of normocalcemic hyperparathyroidism in patients with hypercalciuria and recurrent nephrolithiasis (idiopathic hypercalciuria) is not known. Because the serum calcium concentration may fluctuate, it should be measured on more than three separate occasions. The serum calcium should be

determined the day the sample is obtained, because the calcium level decreases with refrigeration or freezing. Determination of serum ionized calcium is also useful, since it may be increased in patients with normal total serum calcium levels.

If a patient has elevated serum levels of ionized calcium and PTH, the diagnosis of normocalcemic hyperparathyroidism has been confirmed. There are three major causes of hypercalciuria and nephrolithiasis: (1) increased absorption of calcium from the gastrointestinal tract (absorptive hypercalciuria), (2) increased renal leakage of calcium (renal hypercalciuria), and (3) primary hyperparathyroidism. Patients with absorptive hypercalcemia absorb too much calcium from the gastrointestinal tract and therefore have low serum PTH levels. Patients with renal hypercalciuria lose calcium from leaky renal tubules and have increased PTH levels. They can be distinguished from patients with normocalcemic hyperparathyroidism by their response to treatment with thiazides. In renal leak hypercalcemia, serum PTH levels become normal because thiazides correct the excessive loss of calcium, whereas in primary hyperparathyroidism increased serum PTH levels persist and the patient often becomes hypercalcemic.

Natural History of Untreated & Treated Hyperparathyroidism

Patients with untreated hyperparathyroidism have an increased risk of dying prematurely, mainly from cardiovascular and malignant disease. There is decreased respiratory muscular capacity and increased frequency of hypertrophic cardiomyopathy even in hyperparathyroid patients without hypertension. Hyperparathyroid patients have more hypertension, nephrolithiasis, osteopenia, peptic ulcer disease, gout, renal dysfunction, and pancreatitis. After successful parathyroidectomy, previously hyperparathyroid patients still have an increased risk of premature death. Younger patients and those with less severe disease, however, return to a normal survival curve sooner than do older patients or those with more severe hyperparathyroidism. Most patients with hyperparathyroidism—even those with normocalcemic hyperparathyroidism—have symptoms and associated conditions. In 80% of patients, these clinical manifestations improve or disappear after parathyroidectomy.

Treatment

The only successful treatment of primary hyperparathyroidism is parathyroidectomy. The author feels that virtually all patients with either asymptomatic or symptomatic hyperparathyroidism benefit from the operation both symptomatically and metabolically. There are no convincing data to support a plan of medical observation, and considerable data support an active surgical approach. Once associated conditions such as hypertension and renal dysfunction become well-established, they seem to progress despite correction of the primary hyperparathyroidism. Thus, it is better to intervene early while it is still possible to correct these problems. In all patients, however, the diagnosis should be established, and short delays to clarify the diagnosis are justified.

A. MARKED HYPERCALCEMIA (HYPERCALCEMIC CRISIS)

The initial treatment in patients with marked hypercalcemia and acute symptoms is hydration and correction of hypokalemia and hyponatremia. While the patient is being hydrated, assessment of the underlying problem is essential so that more specific therapy may be started. Milk and alkaline products, estrogens, thiazides, and vitamins A and D should be immediately discontinued. Furosemide is useful to increase calcium excretion in the rehydrated patient. Etidronate, plicamycin, and calcitonin are usually effective for short periods in treating hypercalcemia regardless of cause. Glucocorticoids are very effective in vitamin D intoxication and sarcoidosis and in many patients with cancer, including those with peptide-secreting tumors, but are less effective when there is extensive bone disease. As mentioned previously, hyperparathyroid patients only occasionally respond to glucocorticoid administration.

In patients with marked hypercalcemia, once the diagnosis of hyperparathyroidism is established, cervical exploration and parathyroidectomy should be performed in a vigorously hydrated patient, since this is the most rapid and effective method of reducing serum calcium.

B. LOCALIZATION

Preoperative localization of parathyroid tumors can now be accomplished in about 75% of patients with ultrasonography and sestamibi scans. These studies, however, are helpful in only about 35% of patients with parathyroid hyperplasia (Figure 17–5). Localization studies are essential in patients with persistent or recurrent hyperparathyroidism and can direct a focused exploration in patients with sporadic primary hyperparathyroidism. An experienced surgeon can find the tumors in about 95% of patients who have not had previous parathyroid or thyroid surgery without preoperative tests. Selective venous catheterization with parathyroid hormone immunoassay is also recommended for patients who have had an unsuccessful previous operation when the noninvasive localization tests are negative or equivocal. This study helps localize the tumor in about 80% of patients. Digital subtraction angiography is useful, while arteriography is now rarely used.

C. OPERATION

Three approaches are now acceptable for patients with sporadic primary hyperparathyroidism. The bilateral approach is safe and does not require preoperative tests. A unilateral approach can be elected when one or more localization tests identify a solitary parathyroid tumor. At operation, a normal and abnormal parathyroid should be identified on the side of the localized tumor. A focal operation can be done in similar patients and the operation completed when the intraoperative PTH level decreases by more than 50% 10 minutes after the parathyroid tumor is removed. Endoscopic parathyroidectomy remains an experimental procedure.

In over 80% of cases, the parathyroid tumor is found attached to the posterior capsule of the thyroid gland. The parathyroid glands are usually symmetrically placed, and lower parathyroid glands are situated anterior to the recurrent laryngeal nerve, whereas the upper parathyroid glands lie posterior to the recurrent laryngeal nerve, where it enters the cricothyroid muscle. Parathyroid tumors may also lie cephalad to the superior pole of the thyroid gland, along the great vessels of the neck in the tracheoesophageal area, in thymic tissue, in the substance of the thyroid gland itself, or in the mediastinum. Care must be taken not to traumatize the parathyroid gland or tumors, since color is useful in distinguishing them from surrounding thyroid, thymus, lymph node, and fat. Furthermore, rupture of the parathyroid gland may result in parathyromatosis (seeding of parathyroid tissue) and possible recurrent hyperparathyroidism. Two helpful maneuvers for localizing parathyroid tumors at operation are following the course of a branch of the inferior thyroid artery and gently palpating for the parathyroid tumor. One should attempt to identify four parathyroid glands when a bilateral approach is elected, though there may be more than four or fewer than four.

If a probable parathyroid adenoma is found, it is removed and the diagnosis confirmed by frozen section or by a greater than 50% decrease in PTH. It seems unwise to remove a grossly normal parathyroid gland intentionally, both because this has no beneficial effect and because the gland may be needed to maintain normal function after all the hyperfunctioning tissue is removed. If two adenomas are found, both are removed, and both normal glands are marked and biopsied but not removed.

The presence of a normal parathyroid gland at operation indicates that the tumor removed is an adenoma rather than parathyroid hyperplasia, since in hyperplasia all the parathyroid glands are involved. A compressed rim of normal parathyroid tissue is also suggestive of an adenoma. When all parathyroid glands are hyperplastic, the most normal gland should be subto-

Figure 17–5. Parathyroid adenomas. **A:** Sestamibi scan of right lower parathyroid adenoma. **B:** Longitudinal ultrasound scan of left lower parathyroid adenoma. **C:** Transverse ultrasound scan of left lower parathyroid adenoma.

314

tally resected, leaving a 50 mg remnant, and confirmed histologically before removal of the remaining glands. The upper thymus and perithymic tract should be removed in patients with hyperplasia, because a fifth parathyroid gland is present in 15% of cases.

If exploration fails to reveal a parathyroid tumor, a missing lower gland is often in the thymus (anterior mediastinum), whereas a missing upper gland is usually paraesophageal (or in the posterior mediastinum). One should therefore perform a thymectomy, thyroid lobectomy, or partial thyroidectomy on the side that has only one parathyroid gland, since tumors may be found within the thymus or intrathyroidally. If thyroid nodules are present and clinically a problem, they should be treated as nodular goiter and possible thyroid cancer. Differentiated thyroid carcinoma occurs in 3% of patients with hyperparathyroidism and more frequently in patients with a history of radiation exposure.

The recurrence rate of hyperparathyroidism after the removal of a single adenoma in most medical centers is 5% or less. In patients with multiple endocrine neoplasia and familial hyperparathyroidism, recurrent hyperparathyroidism is more common; therefore, extra care should be taken to remove all abnormal parathyroid tissue and to carefully mark the remaining parathyroid tissue. These hyperparathyroid patients are candidates for possible prophylactic subtotal parathyroidectomy. Total parathyroidectomy with autotransplantation to the forearm is recommended by some surgeons for patients with multiple endocrine neoplasia or familial hyperparathyroidism. The author prefers subtotal parathyroidectomy leaving a well-marked parathyroid remnant because not all parathyroid autografts function effectively.

Exploration of the mediastinum via a sternal split at the initial operation is necessary in only 1–2% of cases and is only recommended in patients with a serum calcium level above 13.5 mg/dL. If cervical exploration was nonproductive or if localization studies suggest a mediastinal tumor, the patient should be allowed to recover from the initial operation and return in 6–8 weeks for mediastinal exploration. Preoperative localization tests are useful before reoperation. Angiographic ablation is worthwhile in occasional patients with mediastinal parathyroid adenomas not easily removed via a cervical incision.

D. POSTOPERATIVE CARE

Following removal of a parathyroid adenoma or hyperplastic glands, the serum calcium concentration falls to normal or below normal in 24–48 hours. Patients with severe skeletal depletion ("hungry bones"), long-standing hyperparathyroidism, or high calcium levels may develop paresthesias, carpopedal spasm, or even seizures. If the symptoms are mild and serum calcium falls

slowly, oral supplementation with calcium is all that is required. When marked symptoms develop, it is necessary to give calcium gluconate intravenously. If the response is not rapid, the serum magnesium concentration should be determined and magnesium given if low. Treatment with calcitriol, 1 μg daily, is sometimes required. (See section on Hypoparathyroidism, below.)

E. REOPERATION

Reexploration for persistent or recurrent hyperparathyroidism or after a previous thyroidectomy presents formidable problems and an increased risk of complications. First ascertain that the diagnosis is correct and that the patient does not have benign familial hypocalciuric hypercalcemia or hypercalcemia due to another cause such as a malignant tumor. Ultrasound, CT or MRI, and sestamibi scanning should be done first. If these studies are unsuccessful or equivocal, digital subtraction angiography and highly selective venous catheterization with parathyroid hormone immunoassay are recommended. Most such patients have a parathyroid tumor that can be removed through a cervical incision, making mediastinal exploration unnecessary. The success rate of parathyroidectomy performed by experienced surgeons is 95% or better at an initial operation versus a success rate of about 75% with surgeons less experienced at this procedure. The success rate for patients requiring an experienced surgeon is about 90%. This success rate is lower in patients with negative or equivocal localization tests and in patients with parathyromatosis and parathyroid cancer.

Barney RE et al: Health status improvement after surgical correction of primary hyperparathyroidism in patients with high and low preoperative calcium levels. Surgery 1999;125:608.

Carty SE et al: Concise parathyroidectomy: the impact of preoperative SPECT 99m Tc sestamibi scanning and intraoperative parathormone assay. Surgery 1997;122:1107.

Chou FF et al: Neuromuscular recovery after parathyroidectomy in primary hyperparathyroidism. Surgery 1995;117:18.

Clark OH: "Asymptomatic" primary hyperparathyroidism: is parathyroidectomy indicated? Surgery 1994;116:947.

Clark OH: Changing surgical approaches to patients with primary hyperparathyroidism. Curr Surg 2000;57: 546.

Eng C: Editorial: dissecting the genetics of hyperparathyroidism—new clues from an old friend. J Clin Endocrinol Metab 2000; 85:1752.

Gordon LL et al: The validity of quick intraoperative parathyroid hormone assay: an evaluation in seventy-two patients based on gross morphologic criteria. Surgery 1999;126:1030.

Hedback G et al: Parathyroid adenoma weight and the risk of death after treatment for primary hyperparathyroidism. Surgery 1995;117:134.

Miccoli P et al: Video-assisted versus conventional parathyroidectomy in primary hyperparathyroidism: a prospective randomized study. Surgery 1999;126:1117.

Palmer M et al: Survival and renal function in persons with untreated hypercalcemia: a population-based cohort study with 14 years follow-up. Lancet 1987;1:59.

Rodriguez J et al: Localization procedures in patients with persistent or recurrent hyperparathyroidism. Arch Surg 1994;129:870.

Silverberg SJ et al: A 10-year prospective stud of primary hyperparathyroidism with or without parathyroid surgery. N Engl J Med 1999;341:1249.

Sokol LJ et al: Intraoperative parathyroid hormone analysis: a study of 200 consecutive cases. Clin Chem 2000;46:1662.

Tezelman S et al: Double parathyroid adenomas. Clinical and biochemical characteristics before and after parathyroidectomy. Ann Surg 1993;218:300.

Thompson GS et al: Parathyroid imaging with technetium-99m-sestamibi: an initial institutional experience. Surgery 1994;116:966.

Udelsman R et al: One hundred consecutive minimally invasive parathyroid explorations. Ann Surg 2000;232:331.

Utiger RD. Treatment of primary hyperparathyroidism (editorial). N Engl J Med 1999;341:1301.

Wagner PK et al: Replantation of cryopreserved human parathyroid tissue. World J Surg 1991;6:751.

SECONDARY & TERTIARY HYPERPARATHYROIDISM

In secondary hyperparathyroidism, there is an increase in parathyroid hormone secretion in response to low plasma concentrations of ionized calcium, usually owing to renal disease and malabsorption. This results in chief cell hyperplasia. When secondary hyperparathyroidism occurs as a complication of renal disease, the serum phosphorus level is usually high, whereas in malabsorption, osteomalacia, or rickets it is frequently low or normal. Secondary hyperparathyroidism with renal osteodystrophy is a frequent if not universal complication of hemodialysis and peritoneal dialysis. Factors that play a role in renal osteodystrophy are (1) phosphate retention secondary to a decrease in the number of nephrons; (2) failure of the diseased or absent kidneys to hydroxylate 25-dihydroxyvitamin D to the biologically active metabolite 1,25-dihydroxyvitamin D, with decreased intestinal absorption of calcium; (3) resistance of the bone to the action of parathyroid hormone; and (4) increased serum calcitonin concentrations. The resulting skeletal changes are identical with those of primary hyperparathyroidism but are often more severe.

Most patients with secondary hyperparathyroidism may be treated medically. Maintaining relatively normal serum concentrations of calcium and phosphorus during hemodialysis and treatment with calcitriol (orally or intravenously) have decreased the incidence of bone disease dramatically.

Occasionally, a patient with secondary hyperparathyroidism develops relatively autonomous hyperplastic parathyroid glands (**tertiary hyperparathyroidism**). In most patients after successful renal transplantation, the serum calcium concentration returns to normal, and one should wait at least 6 months after surgery before considering parathyroidectomy for persistent mild hypercalcemia. In some patients, however, profound hypercalcemia develops. In general, surgical therapy for so-called tertiary hyperparathyroidism should be withheld until all medical approaches, including treatment with vitamin D, calcium supplementation, and phosphate binders, have been exhausted. Indications for operation include (1) a calcium × phosphate product > 70, (2) severe bone disease and pain, (3) pruritus, and (4) extensive soft tissue calcification with tumoral calcinosis and (5) calciphylaxis. Most patients with secondary hyperparathyroidism requiring parathyroidectomy have very high serum PTH levels, whereas patients with aluminum bone disease may be hypercalcemic with bone pain but PTH levels are normal or only slightly increased. In the rare patient in whom subtotal parathyroidectomy or total parathyroidectomy with autotransplantation is indicated, all but about 50 mg of parathyroid tissue should be removed, or fifteen 1-mm slices of parathyroid tissue should be transplanted into individual muscle pockets in the forearm. Some parathyroid tissue should also be cryopreserved in case the transplanted tissue does not function. These patients usually respond with dramatic relief of symptoms. A few patients may continue to have bone pain due to osteomalacia thought to be secondary to aluminum toxicity. Profound hypocalcemia frequently results following subtotal parathyroidectomy for renal osteodystrophy, both because of "hungry bones" and because of decreased parathyroid hormone secretion.

Clark OH: Secondary hyperparathyroidism. In: *Endocrine Surgery of the Thyroid and Parathyroid Glands.* Clark OH (editor). Mosby, 1985.

Delmez JA et al: Recent advances in the pathogenesis and therapy of uremic secondary hyperparathyroidism. J Clin Endocrinol Metab 1991;72:735.

Dubost C et al: Comparison of subtotal parathyroidectomy with total parathyroidectomy and autotransplantation. *Surgery of the Thyroid and Parathyroid Glands.* Churchill Livingstone, 1983.

Duh QY et al: Calciphylaxis in secondary hyperparathyroidism. Arch Surg 1991;126:1213.

Pasieka JL et al: A prospective surgical outcome study assessing the impact of parathyroidectomy on symptoms in patients with secondary and tertiary hyperparathyroidism. Surgery 2000;128:531.

Quarles LD et al: Prospective trial of pulse oral versus intravenous calcitriol treatment of hyperparathyroidism in ESRD. Kidney Int 1994;45:1710.

HYPOPARATHYROIDISM

ESSENTIALS OF DIAGNOSIS

- *Paresthesias, muscle cramps, carpopedal spasm, laryngeal stridor, convulsions, malaise, muscle and abdominal cramps, tetany, urinary frequency, lethargy, anxiety, psychoneurosis, depression, and psychosis.*
- *Surgical neck scar. Positive Chvostek and Trousseau signs.*
- *Brittle and atrophied nails, defective teeth, cataracts.*
- *Hypocalcemia and hyperphosphatemia, low or absent urinary calcium, low or absent circulating parathyroid hormone.*
- *Calcification of basal ganglia, cartilage, and arteries as seen on x-ray.*

General Considerations

Hypoparathyroidism, although uncommon, occurs most often as a complication of thyroidectomy, especially when performed for carcinoma or recurrent goiter. Idiopathic hypoparathyroidism, an autoimmune process associated with autoimmune adrenocortical insufficiency, is also unusual, and hypoparathyroidism after ^{131}I therapy for Graves' disease is rare. Neonatal tetany may be associated with maternal hyperparathyroidism.

Clinical Findings

A. SYMPTOMS AND SIGNS

The manifestations of acute hypoparathyroidism are due to hypocalcemia. Low serum calcium levels precipitate tetany. Latent tetany may be indicated by mild or moderate paresthesias with a positive Chvostek or Trousseau sign. The initial manifestations are paresthesias, circumoral numbness, muscle cramps, irritability, carpopedal spasm, convulsions, opisthotonos, and marked anxiety. Dry skin, brittleness of the nails, and spotty alopecia including loss of the eyebrows are common. Since primary hypoparathyroidism is rare, a history of thyroidectomy is almost always present. Generally speaking, the sooner the clinical manifestations appear postoperatively, the more serious the prognosis. After many years, some patients become adapted to a low serum calcium concentration, so that tetany is no longer evident.

B. LABORATORY FINDINGS

Hypocalcemia and hyperphosphatemia are demonstrable. The urine phosphate is low or absent, tubular resorption of phosphate is high, and the urine calcium is low.

C. IMAGING STUDIES

In chronic hypoparathyroidism, x-rays may show calcification of the basal ganglia, arteries, and external ear.

Differential Diagnosis

A good history is most important in the differential diagnosis of hypocalcemic tetany. Occasionally, tetany occurs with alkalosis and hyperventilation. Symptomatic hypocalcemia occurring after thyroid or parathyroid surgery is due to parathyroid removal or injury by trauma or devascularization or is secondary to "hungry bones." Other major causes of hypocalcemic tetany are intestinal malabsorption and renal insufficiency. These conditions may also be suggested by a history of diarrhea, pancreatitis, steatorrhea, or renal disease. Laboratory abnormalities include decreased concentrations of serum proteins, cholesterol, and carotene and increased concentrations of stool fat in malabsorption and an increased blood urea nitrogen and creatinine in renal failure. Serum parathyroid hormone concentrations are low in hypocalcemia secondary to idiopathic or iatrogenic hypoparathyroidism. Consequently, serum calcium concentrations and urinary calcium, phosphorus, and hydroxyproline levels are decreased, whereas serum phosphate concentrations are increased. In hypocalcemia secondary to malabsorption and renal failure, serum PTH concentrations are elevated and the serum alkaline phosphatase concentration is normal or increased.

Treatment

The aim of treatment is to raise the serum calcium concentration, to bring the patient out of tetany, and to lower the serum phosphate level so as to prevent metastatic calcification. Most postoperative hypocalcemia is transient; if it persists longer than 2–3 weeks or if treatment with calcitriol (I,25-dihydroxyvitamin D) is required, the hypoparathyroidism may be permanent.

A. ACUTE HYPOPARATHYROID TETANY

Acute hypoparathyroid tetany requires emergency treatment. Make certain an adequate airway exists. Reassure the anxious patient to avoid hyperventilation and resulting alkalosis. Give calcium gluconate, 10–20 mL of 10% solution slowly intravenously, until tetany disappears. Fifty milliliters of 10% calcium gluconate may then be added to 500 mL of 5% dextrose solution and administered by intravenous drip at a rate of 1 mL/kg/h. Adjust the rate of infusion so that hourly determinations of serum calcium are normal. Calcitriol (1,25-dihydroxyvitamin D) is very helpful for managing acute hypocalcemia because of its rapid onset of action (compared to other vitamin D preparations) and its short duration of action. Hypomagnesemia may be found in some cases of tetany not responding to calcium treatment. In such cases, magnesium (as magnesium sulfate) should be given in a dosage of 4–8 g/d intramuscularly or 2–4 g/d intravenously.

B. CHRONIC HYPOPARATHYROIDISM

Once tetany has responded to intravenous calcium, change to oral calcium (gluconate, lactate, or carbonate) three times daily or as necessary. The management of the hypoparathyroid patient is difficult, because the difference between the controlling and intoxicating dose of vitamin D may be quite small. Episodes of hypercalcemia in treated patients are often unpredictable and may occur in the absence of symptoms. Vitamin D intoxication may develop after months or years of good control on a given therapeutic regimen. Dihydrotachysterol is useful in the exceptional case when the usual measures fail to control the hypocalcemia. Frequent serum calcium determinations are necessary to regulate the proper dosage of vitamin D and to avoid vitamin D intoxication. The dose of vitamin D required to correct hypocalcemia may vary from 25,000 to 200,000 IU/d. Phosphorus should also be limited in the diet; in most patients, simple elimination of dairy products is sufficient. In some patients, aluminum hydroxide gel may be necessary to bind phosphorus in the gut to increase fecal losses.

PSEUDOHYPOPARATHYROIDISM & PSEUDOPSEUDO-HYPOPARATHYROIDISM

Pseudohypoparathyroidism is an X-linked autosomal syndrome due to a defective renal adenylyl cyclase system. It is characterized by the clinical and chemical features of hypoparathyroidism associated with a round face; a short, thick body; stubby fingers with short metacarpal and metatarsal bones; mental deficiency; and x-ray evidence of calcification. It is also associated with thyroid and ovarian dysfunction. There is evidence of increased bone resorption and osteitis fibrosa cystica despite the hypocalcemia that accompanies the syndrome. Patients with pseudohypoparathyroidism do not respond to intravenous administration of 200 units of parathyroid hormone with phosphaturia (Ellsworth-Howard test) and have increased serum concentrations of PTH. This condition is usually controlled with smaller amounts of vitamin D than idiopathic hypoparathyroidism, and resistance to therapy is uncommon.

Pseudopseudohypoparathyroidism is also a genetically transmitted disease with the same physical findings of pseudohypoparathyroidism but with normal serum calcium and phosphorus concentrations. Patients with this condition may become hypocalcemic during periods of stress, such as pregnancy and rapid growth; this suggests that a genetic defect is common with pseudohypoparathyroidism.

Abugassa S et al: Bone mineral density in patients with chronic hypoparathyroidism. J Clin Endocrinol Metab 1993;76:1617.

Bergenfelz A et al: Functional recovery of the parathyroid glands after surgery for primary hyperparathyroidism. Surgery 1994; 116:827.

Jan de Beur SM et al: Pseudohypoparathyroidism 1b: exclusion of parathyroid hormone and its receptors as candidate disease genes. J Clin Endocrinol Metab 2000;85:2239.

Juppner H et al: The gene responsible for pseudohypoparathyroidism type 1b is paternally imprinted and maps in four unrelated kindreds to chromosome 20q13.3. Proc Natl Acad Sci U S A 1998;95:1179.

Lebowitz MR et al: Hypocalcemia. Semin Nephrol 1992;12:146.

Lin CK et al: Prevalence of three mutations in the Gs alpha gene among 24 families with pseudohypoparathyroidism type Ia. Biochem Biophys Res Com 1992;189:343.

Murray TM et al: Pseudohypoparathyroidism with osteitis fibrosa cystica: direct demonstration of skeletal responsiveness to parathyroid hormone in cells cultured from bone. J Bone Min Res 1993;8:83.

Stirling HF et al: Plasma cyclic AMP response to intravenous parathyroid hormone in pseudohypoparathyroidism. Acta Paed Scand 1991;80:333.

Breast

18

Armando E. Giuliano, MD

■ CARCINOMA OF THE FEMALE BREAST

ESSENTIALS OF DIAGNOSIS

- *Higher incidence in women who have delayed childbearing, those with a family history of breast cancer, and those with a personal history of breast cancer or some types of mammary dysplasia.*
- *Early findings: Single, nontender, firm to hard mass with ill-defined margins; mammographic abnormalities and no palpable mass.*
- *Later findings: Skin or nipple retraction; axillary lymphadenopathy; breast enlargement, redness, edema, pain; fixation of mass to skin or chest wall.*
- *Late findings: Ulceration; supraclavicular lymphadenopathy; edema of arm; bone, lung, liver, brain, or other distant metastases.*

COMMON SIGNS & SYMPTOMS

The most common sign and symptom of breast disease is a palpable mass. This is usually found by the patient and may lead to the diagnosis of either benign or malignant disease. A palpable mass may be smooth and rubbery (fibroadenoma, tense cyst) or firm and irregular (carcinoma). While many patients complain of breast pain, this is not commonly associated with a serious disease and usually is due to underlying fibrocystic changes in a premenopausal woman. However, some patients who complain of pain are found to have a malignancy. Most commonly, patients have diffuse nodularity associated with pain leading to the clinical diagnosis of fibrocystic disease. Benign and malignant breast disease may present as nipple discharge or even erosion or an eczema-like rash of the nipple. Most nipple discharge is associated with benign duct ectasia or

cysts. A bloody discharge can be a sign of a malignancy but is usually a sign of a benign intraductal papilloma. Nipple erosion or even an eczema-like rash can be related to an underlying malignancy, as in Paget's disease. More diffuse skin changes can also be seen in benign and malignant conditions. Erythema and edema may signify underlying mastitis or advanced or inflammatory carcinoma. Breast tenderness is associated most commonly with fibrocystic disease, but when accompanied by erythema and edema it signifies mastitis. Local skin dimpling (indentation) or nipple retraction may be a sign of benign fibrocystic disease or a past mastitis but may signify an underlying malignancy. Rarely, a malignancy may present with palpable adenopathy and no abnormality within the breast itself.

A malignancy may be very obvious, presenting with a mass, adenopathy, and skin involvement, or may be a subtle thickening in a portion of the breast with no other identifiable abnormality. While the overwhelming majority of patients with complaints related to their breasts will have benign conditions, most breast symptoms and signs may be due to an associated or underlying malignancy and warrant workup and follow-up care.

DIAGNOSTIC TESTS

The most reliable diagnostic test for breast cancer is **open excisional biopsy.** When the sample is properly taken by the surgeon and examined by the pathologist, such a test should give no false-negative and no false-positive results.

Large-needle (core needle) biopsy is an accepted diagnostic technique in which a core of tissue is removed with a large cutting needle. As in the case of any needle biopsy, the main problem is sampling error due to improper positioning of the needle, giving rise to a false-negative test result.

Fine-needle aspiration cytology is a useful technique whereby cells from a breast tumor are aspirated with a small (usually 22-gauge) needle and examined by the pathologist. This technique can be performed easily with no morbidity and is much less expensive than excisional or open biopsy. The main disadvantages are that it requires a pathologist skilled in the cytologic diagnosis of breast cancer and that it is subject to sampling problems, particularly because deep lesions may be missed. The incidence of false-positive diagnoses is extremely low, perhaps 1–2%. The rate of false-negative diagnoses with fine-needle aspiration biopsy is as high as 10% in some series. Most experienced clinicians would not leave a dominant mass in the breast even when fine-needle aspiration cytology is negative unless the clinical diagnosis, breast imaging studies, and cytologic studies were all in agreement.

Ultrasonography is performed chiefly to differentiate cystic from solid lesions and is not diagnostic of malignancy. Ultrasonography may show an irregular mass within a cyst in the rare case of intracystic carcinoma. If a tumor is palpable and clinically feels like a cyst, an 18-gauge needle can be used to aspirate the fluid and make the diagnosis of cyst. If a cyst is aspirated and the fluid is nonbloody, it does not have to be examined cytologically. If the mass does not recur, no further diagnostic test is necessary. Nonpalpable mammographic densities that appear benign should be investigated with ultrasound to determine whether the lesion is cystic or solid.

When a suspicious abnormality is identified by mammography alone and cannot be palpated by the clinician, the patient should undergo **mammographic localization biopsy.** This is performed by obtaining a mammogram in two perpendicular views and placing a needle or hook-wire near the abnormality so that the surgeon can use the metal needle or wire as a guide during operation to locate the lesion. After mammography confirms the position of the needle in relation to the lesion, an incision is made and the subcutaneous tissue is dissected until the needle is identified. Using the films as a guide, the abnormality can then be localized and excised. It often happens that the abnormality cannot even be palpated through the incision—this is the case with microcalcifications—and it is thus essential to obtain a mammogram of the specimen to document that the lesion was excised. At that time, a second marker needle can further localize the lesion for the pathologist.

Computerized stereotactic imaging can localize abnormalities and guide needle biopsy without surgery. Under mammographic guidance, a biopsy needle can be inserted into the lesion in the mammographer's suite, and a core of tissue for histologic examination or cells for cytology can be examined. Stereotactic core needle biopsies are as accurate as mammographic localization biopsies and are preferable to mammographic localization and surgical resection for accessible lesions.

INCIDENCE & RISK FACTORS

The breast is the most common site of cancer in women, and cancer of the breast is second only to lung cancer as a cause of death from cancer among women. The probability of developing breast cancer increases throughout life. The mean and the median age of women with breast cancer is between 60 and 61 years.

There will be about 182,000 new cases of breast cancer and about 42,000 deaths from this disease in women in the USA in 2000. At the present rate of incidence, the American Cancer Society predicts that one of every eight or nine American women will develop breast cancer during her lifetime. Women whose mothers or sisters had breast cancer are more likely to develop the disease than others. Risk is increased in patients whose mothers' or sisters' breast cancers occurred before menopause or was bilateral and in those with a family history of breast cancer in two or more first-degree relatives. However, there is no history of breast cancer among female relatives in over 90% of breast cancer patients. Nulliparous women and women whose first full-term pregnancy was after age 35 have a slightly higher incidence of breast cancer than multiparous women. Late menarche and artificial menopause are associated with a lower incidence of breast cancer, whereas early menarche (under age 12) and late natural menopause (after age 50) are associated with a slight increase in risk of developing breast cancer. Mammary dysplasia (fibrocystic disease of the breast), when accompanied by proliferative changes, papillomatosis, or atypical epithelial hyperplasia, is associated with an increased incidence of cancer. A woman who has had cancer in one breast is at increased risk of developing cancer in the other breast. Women with cancer of the uterine corpus have a breast cancer risk significantly higher than that of the general population, and women with breast cancer have a comparably increased endometrial cancer risk. In the USA, breast cancer is more common in whites than in nonwhites. The incidence of the disease among nonwhites (mostly blacks), however, is increasing, especially in younger women. In general, rates reported from developing countries are low, whereas rates are high in developed countries, with the notable exception of Japan. Some of the variability may be due to underreporting in the developing countries, but a real difference probably exists. Dietary factors, particularly increased fat content, may account for some differences in incidence. Oral contraceptives do not appear to increase the risk of breast cancer. There is some evidence that administration of estrogens to postmenopausal women may result in a slightly increased risk of breast cancer, but only with higher, long-term doses of estrogens. Other studies suggest that women with a family history of breast cancer who take postmenopausal estrogens or those who take estradiol or unconjugated estrogens do slightly increase their risk of breast cancer. Alcohol consumption may increase the risk of breast cancer slightly.

Women who are at greater than normal risk of developing breast cancer (Table 18–1) should be identified by their physicians, taught the techniques of breast self-examination, and followed carefully. Screening pro-

Table 18–1. Factors associated with increased risk of breast cancer.[1]

Race	White
Age	Older
Family history	Breast cancer in mother, sister, or daughter (especially bilateral or premenopausal)
Previous medical history	Endometrial cancer Some forms of mammary dysplasia Cancer in other breast
Menstrual history	Early menarche (under age 12) Late menopause (after age 50)
Pregnancy	Late first pregnancy

[1]Normal lifetime risk in white women = 1 in 8 or 9.

grams involving periodic physical examination and mammography of asymptomatic high-risk women increase the detection rate of breast cancer and improve the survival rate by as much as 30%. Unfortunately, most women who develop breast cancer do not have significant identifiable risk factors, and analysis of epidemiologic data has failed to identify women who are not at significant risk and would not benefit from screening. Therefore, virtually all women over about age 35 are at sufficient risk of breast cancer so that they could benefit from screening. The cost-benefit ratio of screening programs to society as a whole is unclear. Less expensive screening techniques such as single-view mammography and the use of mobile vans are being investigated in an attempt to reduce the cost of widespread screenings. Recently, the National Surgical Adjuvant Breast Project (NSABP) compared tamoxifen with placebo for patients who show no evidence of breast cancer but who are at high risk for its occurrence. Women who received tamoxifen for 5 years had about a 50% reduction in noninvasive and invasive cancers compared with women taking placebo. However, women above the age of 50 who received the drug had an increased incidence of endometrial cancer and deep venous thrombosis. Unfortunately, no survival data will be produced from this trial. The estrogen replacement raloxifene, effective in preventing osteoporosis, may also prevent breast cancer. Several large studies to examine this hypothesis are under way.

EARLY DETECTION OF BREAST CANCER

Screening Programs

A number of mass screening programs consisting of physical and mammographic examination of the breasts of asymptomatic women have been conducted. Such programs frequently identify more than six asymptomatic cancers per 1000 women. About 80% of these women have negative axillary lymph nodes at the time of surgery, whereas only about 50% of patients found in the course of usual medical practice have uninvolved axillary nodes. Detecting breast cancer before it has spread to the axillary nodes greatly increases the chance of survival, and about 85% of such women will survive at least 5 years.

Both physical examination and mammography are necessary for maximum yield in screening programs, since about 35–50% of early breast cancers can be discovered only by mammography and another 40% can be detected only by palpation. About one-third of the abnormalities detected on screening mammograms will be found to be malignant when biopsy is performed. Women 20–40 years of age should have a breast examination as part of routine medical care every 2–3 years. Women over age 40 should have yearly breast examinations. The sensitivity of mammography varies from approximately 60% to 90%. This sensitivity depends on several factors, including patient age (breast density), tumor size, location, and mammographic appearance. In young women with dense breasts, mammography is less sensitive than in older woman with fatty breasts, in whom mammography can detect nearly 90% of malignancies. Smaller tumors, particularly those without calcifications, are more difficult to detect, especially in dense breasts. The lack of sensitivity in young women is leading to questions concerning the value of mammography for screening in women 40–50 years of age. The specificity of mammography varies from about 30% to 40% for nonpalpable mammographic abnormalities to 85% to 90% for clinically evident malignancies.

In February 1993, the National Cancer Institute held an international workshop on screening for breast cancer. The purpose was to review recent clinical screening trials. The conference examined only randomized studies and focused on clinical evidence related to the efficacy of breast cancer screening in various age groups. Of eight randomized trials considered, only the Health Insurance Plan Project (HIP) demonstrated a benefit of screening in women between 40 and 49 years of age. This was seen between 10 and 18 years after entry into the study and resulted in a 25% decrease in breast cancer deaths. Several other trials showed a 13% decrease in the mortality rate of breast cancer in this age group after 12 years of follow-up, but the differences were not statistically significant. In a meta-analysis of five trials, the breast cancer death rates in women aged 40–49 were the same whether the women screened or not. The value of screening in women aged 50–69 is undisputed. The evidence for those older than 70 is inconclusive, partly because few women over 70 have been screened. Therefore, doubt exists about screening in women under 50 because of concerns about the potentially harmful effects of x-rays in a large population of young women. Nevertheless, in practice screening among younger women is popular.

Currently, the National Cancer Institute states that there is no agreement on the role of screening mammography for women aged 40–49. The American College of Radiology and the American Cancer Society continue to recommend a screening mammogram by age 40 and then every 1–2 years until age 50, whereupon the study should be performed every year. They no longer urge a baseline examination at age 35. These recommendations seem reasonable, but such a policy may be too costly to justify.

Large trials will be required to determine conclusively the value of mammography in young women. Screening should be performed in those over age 70 after consideration of the patient's overall health. Women under 50 should be counseled individually.

Ductography is useful to evaluate the cause of nipple discharge. In this study, the radiologist injects contrast medium into the discharging duct and obtains a mammogram. The injected duct may contain a filling defect (most commonly an intraductal papilloma) or may have a dilated or cystic appearance in patients with duct ectasia or fibrocystic disease. Malignancy may appear as an abrupt obstruction or filling defect.

Other modalities of breast imaging have been investigated. Automated breast ultrasonography is very useful in distinguishing cystic from solid lesions but should be used only as a supplement to physical examination and mammography in screening for breast cancer. Diaphanography (transillumination of the breasts) and thermography are of no proved screening value and should not be performed.

Self-Examination

All women over age 20 should be advised to examine their breasts monthly. Premenopausal women should perform the examination 7–8 days after the menstrual period. The breasts should be inspected initially while standing before a mirror with the hands at the sides, overhead, and pressed firmly on the hips to contract the pectoralis muscles. Masses, asymmetry of breasts, and slight dimpling of the skin may become apparent as a result of these maneuvers. Next, in a supine position, each breast should be carefully palpated with the fingers of the opposite hand. Physicians should instruct women in the technique of self-examination and advise them to report at once for medical evaluation if a mass or other abnormality is noted.

Some women discover small breast lumps more readily when their skin is moist while bathing or showering.

Most women do not practice self-examination, and its value is controversial. Clearly, however, it is not harmful and may be beneficial.

Mammography

Mammography is the most useful technique for the detection of early breast cancer. The two methods of mammography in common use are ordinary film screen radiography and xeroradiography. From the standpoint of diagnosing breast cancer, the two methods give comparable results. Using film screen techniques, it is now possible to perform a high-quality mammogram while delivering less than 0.4 cGy to the mid breast per view, and for this reason film screen mammography has largely replaced the xeromammographic technique, which delivers more radiation.

Mammography is the only reliable means of detecting breast cancer before a mass can be palpated in the breast. Slowly growing breast cancers can be identified by mammography at least 2 years before reaching a size detectable by palpation.

Calcifications are the most easily recognized mammographic abnormality. The most common mammographic abnormalities associated with carcinoma of the breast are clustered polymorphic microcalcifications. Such calcifications are usually at least five to eight in number, aggregated in one part of the breast and differing from each other in size and shape, often including branched or V- or Y-shaped configurations. There may be an associated mammographic mass density or, at times, only a mass density with no calcifications. Such a density usually has irregular or ill-defined borders and may lead to architectural distortion within the breast. A small mass or architectural distortion, particularly in a dense breast, may be subtle and difficult to detect.

Indications for mammography are as follows: (1) to evaluate each breast when a diagnosis of potentially curable breast cancer has been made, and at yearly intervals thereafter; (2) to evaluate a questionable or ill-defined breast mass or other suspicious change in the breast; (3) to search for an occult breast cancer in a woman with metastatic disease in axillary nodes or elsewhere from an unknown primary; (4) to screen women prior to cosmetic operations or prior to biopsy of a mass, to examine for an unsuspected cancer; (5) to screen at regular intervals women who are at high risk for developing breast cancer (see below); and (6) to follow those women with breast cancer who have been treated with breast-conserving surgery and radiation.

Patients with a dominant or suspicious mass must undergo biopsy despite mammographic findings. The mammogram should be obtained prior to biopsy so that other suspicious areas can be noted and the contralateral breast can be checked. Mammography is never a substitute for biopsy, because it may not reveal clinical cancer in a very dense breast, as may be seen in young women with mammary dysplasia, and may not reveal medullary type cancers.

CLINICAL FINDINGS & DIAGNOSIS

The patient with breast cancer usually presents with a lump in the breast. When the history is taken, special note should be made of breast cancer risk factors, the temporal relationship of mass to menstrual cycle, and previous breast problems. Clinical evaluation should include assessment of the local lesion and a search for evidence of metastases in regional nodes or distant sites. After the diagnosis of breast cancer has been confirmed by biopsy, additional studies are often needed to complete the search for distant metastases or an occult primary in the other breast. Then, before any decision is made about treatment, all the available clinical data are used to determine the extent or stage of the patient's disease.

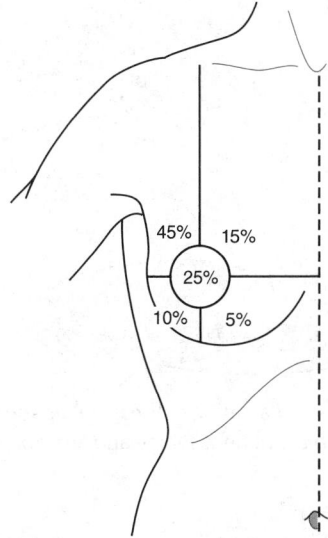

Figure 18–1. Frequency of breast carcinoma at various anatomic sites.

Symptoms

The presenting complaint in about 70% of patients with breast cancer is a lump (usually painless) in the breast. About 90% of breast masses are discovered by the patient herself. Less frequent symptoms are breast pain; nipple discharge; erosion, retraction, enlargement, or itching of the nipple; and redness, generalized hardness, enlargement, or shrinking of the breast. Rarely, an axillary mass or swelling of the arm may be the first symptom. Back or bone pain, jaundice, or weight loss may be the result of systemic metastases, but these symptoms are rarely seen on initial presentation.

Signs

The relative frequency of carcinoma in various anatomic sites in the breast is shown in Figure 18–1.

Inspection of the breast is the first step in physical examination and should be carried out with the patient sitting, arms at sides and then overhead. Abnormal variations in breast size and contour, minimal nipple retraction, and slight edema, redness, or retraction of the skin can be identified. Asymmetry of the breasts and retraction or dimpling of the skin can often be accentuated by having the patient raise her arms overhead or press her hands on her hips in order to contract the pectoralis muscles. Axillary and supraclavicular areas should be thoroughly palpated for enlarged nodes with the patient sitting (Figure 18–2). Palpation of the breast for masses or other changes should be performed

with the patient both seated and supine with the arm abducted (Figure 18–3). Some authorities recommend palpation with a rotary motion of the examiner's fingers as well as a horizontal stripping motion.

Breast cancer usually consists of a nontender, firm or hard lump with poorly delineated margins (caused

Figure 18–2. Palpation of axillary region for enlarged lymph nodes.

Figure 18–3. Palpation of breasts. Palpation is performed with the patient supine and arm abducted.

by local infiltration). Slight skin or nipple retraction is an important sign. Minimal asymmetry of the breast may be noted. Very small (1–2 mm) erosions of the nipple epithelium may be the only manifestation of Paget's carcinoma. Watery, serous, or bloody discharge from the nipple is an occasional early sign but is more often associated with benign disease.

A lesion smaller than 1 cm in diameter may be difficult or impossible for the examiner to feel and yet may be discovered by the patient. She should always be asked to demonstrate the location of the mass; if the physician fails to confirm the patient's suspicions, the examination should be repeated in several months, preferably 1–2 weeks after the onset of menses. During the premenstrual phase of the cycle, increased innocuous nodularity may suggest neoplasm or may obscure an underlying lesion. If there is any question regarding the nature of an abnormality under these circumstances, the patient should be asked to return after her period. Thirty-five to 50 percent of women with cancers detected during organized screening programs have them detected by mammography only and not physical examination.

The following are characteristic of advanced carcinoma: edema, redness, nodularity, or ulceration of the skin; the presence of a large primary tumor; fixation to the chest wall; enlargement, shrinkage, or retraction of the breast; marked axillary lymphadenopathy; supraclavicular lymphadenopathy; edema of the ipsilateral arm; and distant metastases.

Metastases tend to involve regional lymph nodes, which may be clinically palpable. With regard to the axilla, one or two movable, nontender, not particularly firm lymph nodes 5 mm or less in diameter are frequently present and are generally of no significance. Firm or hard nodes larger than 5 mm in diameter usu-

ally contain metastases. Axillary nodes that are matted or fixed to skin or deep structures indicate advanced disease (at least stage III). Histologic studies show that microscopic metastases are present in about 30% of patients with clinically negative nodes. On the other hand, if the examiner thinks that the axillary nodes are involved, that impression will be borne out by histologic section in about 85% of cases. The incidence of positive axillary nodes increases with the size of the primary tumor. Noninvasive cancers do not metastasize.

In most cases no nodes are palpable in the supraclavicular fossa. Firm or hard nodes of any size in this location or just beneath the clavicle (infraclavicular nodes) are suggestive of metastatic cancer and should be biopsied. Ipsilateral supraclavicular or infraclavicular nodes containing cancer indicate that the tumor is in an advanced stage (stage IV). Edema of the ipsilateral arm, commonly caused by metastatic infiltration of regional lymphatics, is also a sign of advanced (stage IV) cancer.

Laboratory Findings

A consistently elevated sedimentation rate may be the result of disseminated cancer. Liver or bone metastases may be associated with elevation of serum alkaline phosphatase. Hypercalcemia is an occasional important finding in advanced cancer of the breast. Carcinoembryonic antigen (CEA) and CA 15-3 or CA 27-29 may be used as markers for recurrent breast cancer.

Imaging for Metastases

Chest radiographs may show pulmonary metastases. CT scanning of the liver and brain is of value only when metastases are suspected in these areas. Bone scans utilizing technetium Tc 99m-labeled phosphates or phosphonates are more sensitive than skeletal x-rays in detecting metastatic breast cancer. Bone scanning has not proved to be of clinical value as a routine preoperative test in the absence of symptoms, physical findings, or abnormal calcium or alkaline phosphatase levels. The frequency of abnormal findings on bone scan parallels the status of the axillary lymph nodes on pathologic examination. Bone scan should be performed for patients with symptoms and for those with elevated calcium or alkaline phosphatase levels. Positron emission tomography (PET) may prove to be an effective single scan for bone and soft tissue or visceral metastases in patients with signs or symptoms of metastatic disease.

Biopsy

The diagnosis of breast cancer depends ultimately upon examination of tissue or cells removed by biopsy. Treatment should never be undertaken without an unequivocal histologic or cytologic diagnosis of cancer. The safest course is biopsy examination of all suspicious masses found on physical examination and, in the absence of a mass, of suspicious lesions demonstrated by mammography. About 60% of lesions thought to be definitely cancer prove on biopsy to be benign, and about 30% of lesions believed to be benign are found to be malignant. These findings demonstrate the fallibility of clinical judgment and the necessity for biopsy. Dominant masses or suspicious nonpalpable mammographic findings must be biopsied. A breast mass should not be followed without histologic diagnosis, except perhaps in the premenopausal woman with a nonsuspicious mass

presumed to be fibrocystic disease. A lesion such as this could be observed through one or two menstrual cycles. However, if the mass does not completely resolve during this time, it must be biopsied. Figures 18–4 and 18–5 present algorithms for management of breast masses in pre- and postmenopausal patients.

The simplest method is needle biopsy, either by aspiration of tumor cells (fine-needle aspiration cytology) or by obtaining a small core of tissue with a Vim-Silverman or other special needle. A nondiagnostic needle biopsy or fine-needle aspiration should be followed by open biopsy, because false-negative needle biopsies may occur in 5–10% of cancers. False-positive results occur rarely (< 1%).

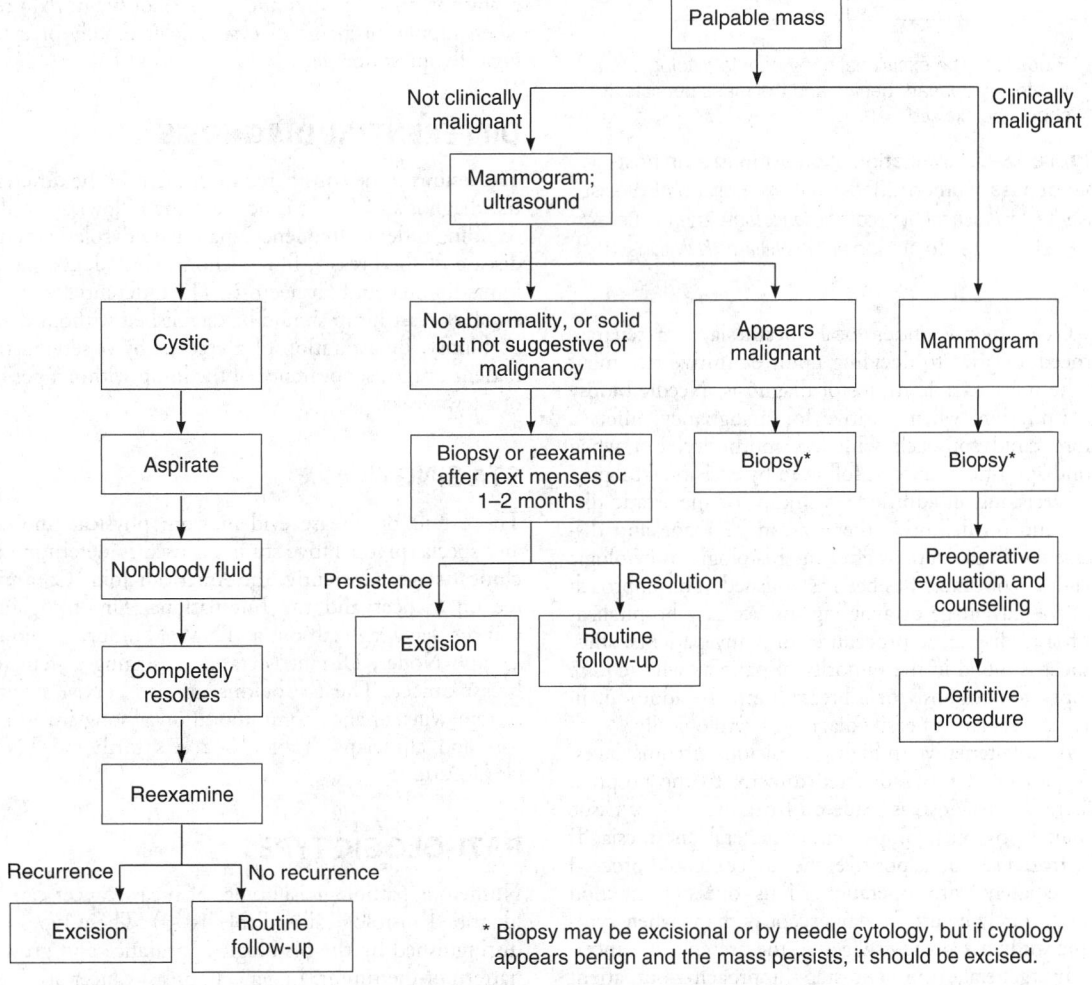

Figure 18–4. Evaluation of breast masses in premenopausal women. (Modified from Giuliano AE: Breast disease. In: *Practical Gynecologic Oncology*, 2nd ed. Berek JS, Hacker NF [editors]. Lippincott Williams & Wilkins, 1994.)

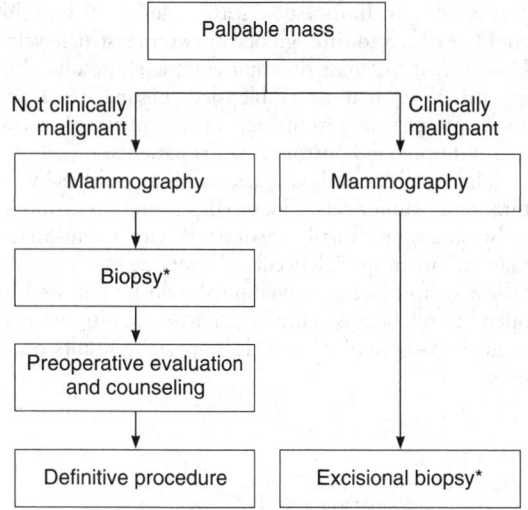

* Biopsy may be excisional or by needle cytology, but if cytology appears benign and the mass persists, it should be excised.

Figure 18–5. Evaluation of breast masses in post-menopausal women. (Modified from Giuliano AE: Breast disease. In: *Practical Gynecologic Oncology*, 2nd ed. Berek JS, Hacker NF [editors]. Lippincott Williams & Wilkins, 1994

Open biopsy under local anesthesia as a separate procedure prior to deciding upon definitive treatment is the most reliable means of diagnosis. Needle biopsy or aspiration, when positive for malignancy, offers a more rapid approach with less morbidity, but when nondiagnostic it must be followed by excisional biopsy.

Decisions on additional workup for metastatic disease and on definitive therapy can be made and discussed with the patient after the histologic or cytologic diagnosis of cancer has been established. This approach has the advantage of avoiding unnecessary hospitalization and diagnostic procedures in many patients, since cancer is found in the minority of patients who require biopsy for diagnosis of a breast lump. In addition, in situ cancers are not easily diagnosed cytologically.

As an alternative in highly suspicious circumstances, the patient may be admitted directly to the hospital, where the diagnosis is made on frozen section of tissue obtained by open biopsy under general anesthesia. If the frozen section is positive, the surgeon could proceed immediately with operation. This one-step method should rarely be used today except perhaps when cytologic study has already suggested the presence of cancer.

In general, the two-step approach—outpatient biopsy followed by definitive operation at a later date—is preferred in the diagnosis and treatment of breast cancer, because patients can be given time to adjust to the diagnosis of cancer, can carefully consider alternative forms of therapy, and can seek a second opinion if they wish. Studies have shown no adverse effect from the short (1–2 weeks) delay of the two-step procedure, and this is the current recommendation of the National Cancer Institute.

At the time of the initial biopsy of breast cancer, it is important for the physician to preserve a portion of the specimen for determination of estrogen and progesterone receptors.

Other Cytology

Cytologic examination of nipple discharge or cyst fluid may be helpful on rare occasions. As a rule, mammography (or ductography) and breast biopsy are required when nipple discharge or cyst fluid is bloody or cytologically questionable.

DIFFERENTIAL DIAGNOSIS

The lesions to be considered most often in the differential diagnosis of breast cancer are the following, in descending order of frequency: mammary dysplasia (cystic disease of the breast), fibroadenoma, intraductal papilloma, lipoma, and fat necrosis. The differential diagnosis of a breast lump should be established without delay by biopsy, by aspiration of a cyst, or by observing the patient until disappearance of the lump within a period of a few weeks.

STAGING

The extent of disease evident from physical findings and special preoperative studies is used to determine its clinical stage. Currently, the American Joint Committee on Cancer and the International Union Against Cancer have agreed on a TNM (Tumor, Regional Lymph Nodes, Distant Metastases) staging system for breast cancer. The use of this uniform TNM staging system will enhance communication among investigators and clinicians. Table 18–2 sets forth the TNM classification.

PATHOLOGIC TYPES

Numerous pathologic subtypes of breast cancer can be identified histologically (Table 18–3). These types are distinguished by the histologic appearance and growth pattern of the tumor. In general, breast cancer arises either from the epithelial lining of the large or intermedi-

Table 18–2. TNM staging for breast cancer.[1]

Stage	T	N	M
0	Tis	N0	M0
I	T1	N0	M0
IIA	T0	N1	M0
	T1	N1	M0
	T2	N0	M0
IIB	T2	N1	M0
	T3	N0	M0
IIIA	T0	N2	M0
	T1	N2	M0
	T2	N2	M0
	T3	N1, N2	M0
IIIB	T4	Any N	M0
	Any T	N3	M0
IV	Any T	Any N	M1

Tumor Size (T)

TX	Primary tumor cannot be assessed.
T0	No evidence of primary tumor.
Tis	Carcinoma in situ: intraductal carcinoma, lobular carcinoma in situ, or Paget's disease of the nipple with no tumor.
T1	Tumor 2 cm or less in greatest dimension.
	T1mic Microinvasion 0.1 cm or less in greatest dimension.
	T1a Tumor more than 0.1 cm but not more than 0.5 cm in greatest dimension.
	T1b Tumor more than 0.5 cm but not more than 1 cm in greatest dimension.
	T1c Tumor more than 1 cm but not more than 2 cm in greatest dimension.
T2	Tumor more than 2 cm but not more than 5 cm in greatest dimension.
T3	Tumor more than 5 cm in greatest dimension.
T4	Tumor of any size with direct extension to (a) chest wall or (b) skin, only as described below.
	T4a Extension to chest wall
	T4b Edema (including peau d'orange) or ulceration of the skin of the breast or satellite nodules confined to the same breast.
	T4c Both (T4a and T4b).
	T4d Inflammatory carcinoma (see text).

Regional Lymph Nodes (N)

NX	Regional lymph nodes cannot be assessed (eg, previously removed).
N0	No regional lymph node metastases.
N1	Metastasis to movable ipsilateral axillary lymph node(s).
N2	Metastasis to ipsilateral axillary lymph node(s) fixed to one another or to other structures.
N3	Metastasis to ipsilateral internal mammary lymph node(s).

Distant Metastases (M)

MX	Presence of distant metastasis cannot be assessed.
M0	No distant metastasis.
M1	Distant metastasis (including metastasis to ipsilateral supraclavicular lymph node[s]).

[1]From: *AJCC Cancer Staging Manual,* 5th ed. Lippincott-Raven, 1997.

Table 18–3. Histologic types of breast cancer.

	Percent Occurrence
Infiltrating ductal (not otherwise specified)	70–80
Medullary	5–8
Colloid (mucinous)	2–4
Tubular	1–2
Papillary	1–2
Invasive lobular	6–8
Noninvasive	4–6
Intraductal	2–3
Lobular in situ	2–3
Rare cancers	< 1
Juvenile (secretory)	...
Adenoid cystic	...
Epidermoid	...
Sudoriferous	...

ate-sized ducts (ductal) or from the epithelium of the terminal ducts of the lobules (lobular). The cancer may be invasive or in situ. Most breast cancers arise from the intermediate ducts and are invasive (invasive ductal, infiltrating ductal), and most histologic types are merely subtypes of invasive ductal cancer with unusual growth patterns (colloid, medullary, scirrhous, etc). Ductal carcinoma that has not invaded the extraductal tissue is intraductal or in situ ductal. Lobular carcinoma may be either invasive or in situ.

Except for the in situ cancers, the histologic subtypes have only a slight bearing on prognosis when outcomes are compared after accurate staging. Various histologic parameters, such as invasion of blood vessels, tumor differentiation, invasion of breast lymphatics, and tumor necrosis have been examined, but they too seem to have little prognostic value.

The noninvasive cancers by definition lack the ability to spread. However, in patients whose biopsies show noninvasive intraductal cancer, associated invasive ductal cancers are present in about 1–3% of cases. Some clinicians consider lobular carcinoma in situ to be a premalignant lesion that is not a true cancer. It lacks the ability to spread but is associated with subsequent development of invasive cancer in at least 20% of cases. The subsequent cancer may occur in either breast regardless of the side of the original biopsy.

SPECIAL CLINICAL FORMS OF BREAST CANCER

Paget's Carcinoma

The basic lesion is usually an infiltrating ductal carcinoma, usually well differentiated. The nipple epithelium is infiltrated, but gross nipple changes are often minimal, and a tumor mass may not be palpable. The first symptom is often itching or burning of the nipple, with superficial erosion or ulceration. The diagnosis is established by biopsy of the erosion.

Paget's carcinoma is not common (about 1% of all breast cancers), but it is important because it appears innocuous. It is frequently diagnosed and treated as dermatitis or bacterial infection, leading to unfortunate delay in detection. When the lesion consists of nipple changes only, the incidence of axillary metastases is about 5%, and the prognosis is excellent. When a breast tumor is also present, the incidence of axillary metastases rises, with an associated marked decrease in prospects for cure by surgical or other treatment.

Inflammatory Carcinoma

This is the most malignant form of breast cancer and constitutes less than 3% of all cases. The clinical findings consist of a rapidly growing, sometimes painful mass that enlarges the breast. The overlying skin becomes erythematous, edematous, and warm. Often there is no distinct mass, since the tumor infiltrates the involved breast diffusely. The diagnosis should be made when the redness involves more than one-third of the skin over the breast and biopsy shows invasion of the subdermal lymphatics. The inflammatory changes, often mistaken for an infectious process, are caused by carcinomatous invasion of the dermal lymphatics, with resulting edema and hyperemia. If the physician suspects infection but the lesion does not respond rapidly (1–2 weeks) to antibiotics, biopsy examination must be performed. Metastases tend to occur early and widely, and for this reason inflammatory carcinoma is rarely curable. Mastectomy is seldom, if ever, indicated. Radiation, hormone therapy, and anticancer chemotherapy are the measures most likely to be of value.

Breast Cancer Occurring During Pregnancy or Lactation

Only 1–2% of breast cancers occur during pregnancy or lactation. Breast cancer complicates approximately one in 3000 pregnancies. The diagnosis is frequently delayed, because physiologic changes in the breast may obscure the true nature of the lesion. This results in a tendency of both patients and physicians to misinterpret the findings and to procrastinate in deciding on biopsy. When the neoplasm is confined to the breast, the 5-year survival rate after mastectomy is about 70%. Axillary metastases are already present in 60–70% of patients, and for them the 5-year survival rate after mastectomy is only 30–40%. Pregnancy (or lactation) is not a contraindication to operation, and treatment should be based on the stage of the disease as in the nonpregnant (or nonlactating) woman. Overall survival rates have improved, since cancers are now diagnosed in pregnant women earlier than in the past. Pregnant women with breast cancer may undergo breast-conserving surgery, radiation, and chemotherapy.

Bilateral Breast Cancer

Clinically evident simultaneous bilateral breast cancer occurs in less than 1% of cases, but there is a 5–8% incidence of later occurrence of cancer in the second breast. Bilaterality occurs more often in women under age 50 and is more frequent when the tumor in the primary breast is lobular. The incidence of second breast cancers increases directly with the length of time the patient is alive after her first cancer—about 1% per year.

In patients with breast cancer, mammography should be performed before primary treatment and at regular intervals thereafter, to search for occult cancer in the opposite breast. Routine biopsy of the opposite breast is usually not warranted.

Noninvasive Cancer

Noninvasive cancer can occur within the ducts (ductal carcinoma in situ) or lobules (lobular carcinoma in situ). While ductal carcinoma in situ behaves as an early malignancy, lobular carcinoma in situ would perhaps be better called lobular neoplasia. Ductal carcinoma in situ tends to be unilateral and most likely progresses to invasive cancer. Approximately 40–60% of women who have ductal carcinoma in situ treated with biopsy alone will develop invasive cancer within the same breast. Lobular carcinoma in situ, however, appears to be more of a risk factor calling attention to the probability of developing invasive cancer in either breast. Approximately 20% of women with lobular carcinoma in situ will develop invasive cancer (usually ductal). This invasive cancer occurs with equal frequency in either breast.

The treatment of intraductal lesions is controversial. Ductal carcinoma can be treated with total mastectomy or breast conservation with wide excision with or without radiation therapy. Lobular carcinoma in situ is probably best managed with careful observation. However, patients who are unwilling to accept the increased risk of breast cancer may be offered bilateral total mas-

tectomy. Tamoxifen is effective in preventing invasive breast cancer in patients with lobular or ductal carcinoma in situ. Axillary metastases are rare.

HORMONE RECEPTOR SITES

The presence or absence of estrogen and progesterone receptors in the cytoplasm of tumor cells is of paramount importance in managing all patients with breast cancer, especially those with recurrent or metastatic disease. They are of proved value in determining adjuvant therapy and therapy for patients with advanced disease. Up to 60% of patients with metastatic breast cancer will respond to hormonal manipulation if their tumors contain estrogen receptors. However, fewer than 5% of patients with metastatic, ER-negative tumors can be successfully treated with hormonal manipulation.

Progesterone receptors may be an even more sensitive indicator than estrogen receptors of patients who may respond to hormonal manipulation. Up to 80% of patients with metastatic progesterone receptor-positive tumors seem to respond to hormonal manipulation. Receptors have no relationship to response to chemotherapy.

Some studies suggest that estrogen receptors are of prognostic significance. Patients whose primary tumors are receptor-positive have a more favorable course than those whose tumors are receptor-negative.

Receptor status is valuable not only for the management of metastatic disease but also for the selection of patients for adjuvant therapy. Adjuvant hormonal therapy (tamoxifen) for patients with receptor-positive tumors and adjuvant chemotherapy for patients with receptor-negative tumors improve survival rates even in the absence of lymph node metastases (see Adjuvant Therapy).

Estrogen and progesterone receptor assays should be done routinely for every breast cancer at the time of initial diagnosis. Tumors are examined by immunohistochemistry or paraffin sections. The value of this assay technique remains to be proved. Receptor status may change after hormonal therapy, radiotherapy, or chemotherapy. The specimen requires special handling, and the laboratory should be prepared to process the specimen correctly.

CURATIVE TREATMENT

Treatment may be curative or palliative. Curative treatment is advised for clinical stage I and stage II disease (Table 18–2). Patients with locally advanced (stage III) and even inflammatory tumors may be cured with multimodality therapy, but in most cases palliation is all that can be expected. Palliative treatment is appropriate for all patients with stage IV disease and for previously treated patients who develop distant metastases or who have unresectable local cancers.

The growth potential of tumors and host resistance factors vary over a wide range from patient to patient and may be altered during the course of the disease. The doubling time of breast cancer cells ranges from several weeks in a rapidly growing lesion to nearly a year in a slowly growing one. Assuming that the rate of doubling is constant and that the neoplasm originates in one cell, a carcinoma with a doubling time of 100 days may not reach clinically detectable size (1 cm) for about 8 years. On the other hand, rapidly growing cancers have a much shorter preclinical course and a greater tendency to metastasize to regional nodes or more distant sites by the time a breast mass is discovered.

The relatively long preclinical growth phase and the tendency of breast cancers to metastasize have led many clinicians to believe that breast cancer is a systemic disease at the time of diagnosis. Although it may be true that breast cancer cells are released from the tumor prior to diagnosis, variations in the host-tumor relationship may prohibit the growth of disseminated disease in many patients. For this reason, a pessimistic attitude concerning the management of localized breast cancer is not warranted, and many patients can be cured with proper treatment.

Choice of Primary Therapy

The extent of disease and its biologic aggressiveness are the principal determinants of the outcome of primary therapy. Clinical and pathologic staging help in assessing extent of disease (Table 18–2), but each is to some extent imprecise. Other factors such as DNA flow cytometry, tumor grade, hormone receptor assays, and oncogene amplification may be of prognostic value but are not important in determining the type of local therapy. Since about two-thirds of patients eventually manifest distant disease regardless of the form of primary therapy, there is a tendency to think of breast carcinoma as being systemic in most patients at the time they first present for treatment.

There is a great deal of controversy regarding the optimal method of primary therapy of stage I, II, and III breast carcinoma, and opinions on this subject have changed considerably in the past decade. Legislation initiated in California and Massachusetts and now adopted in numerous states requires physicians to inform patients of alternative treatment methods in the management of breast cancer.

Breast-Conserving Therapy

The results of the Milan trial and a large randomized trial conducted by the National Surgical Adjuvant Breast Project (NSABP) in the USA showed that disease-free survival rates were similar for patients treated by partial mastectomy plus axillary dissection followed by radiation therapy and for those treated by modified radical mastectomy (total mastectomy plus axillary dissection). All patients whose axillary nodes contained tumor received adjuvant chemotherapy.

In the NSABP trial, patients were randomized to three treatment types: (1) "lumpectomy" (removal of the tumor with *confirmed* tumor-free margins) plus whole breast irradiation, (2) lumpectomy alone, and (3) total mastectomy. All patients underwent axillary lymph node dissection. Some patients in this study had tumors as large as 4 cm with (or without) palpable axillary lymph nodes. The lowest local recurrence rate was among patients treated with lumpectomy and postoperative irradiation; the highest was among patients treated with lumpectomy alone. However, no statistically significant differences were observed in overall or disease-free survival among the three treatment groups. This study shows that lumpectomy and axillary dissection with postoperative radiation therapy is as effective as modified radical mastectomy for the management of patients with stage I and stage II breast cancer. A high local failure rate (nearly 40% at 8 years) was seen for lumpectomy without radiation therapy.

The results of these and other trials have demonstrated that much less aggressive surgical treatment of the primary lesion than has previously been thought necessary gives equivalent therapeutic results and may preserve an acceptable cosmetic appearance.

Tumor size is a major consideration in determining the feasibility of breast conservation. The lumpectomy trial of the NSABP randomized patients with tumors as large as 4 cm. To achieve an acceptable cosmetic result, the patient must have a breast of sufficient size to enable excision of a 4 cm tumor without considerable deformity. Therefore, large size is only a relative contraindication. Subareolar tumors are also difficult to excise without considerable deformity. Clinically detectable multifocality is a relative contraindication to breast-conserving surgery, as is fixation to the chest wall or skin or involvement of the nipple or overlying skin. However, the patient and not the surgeon should be the judge of what is cosmetically acceptable; some patients would prefer breast deformity rather than complete absence of the breast or even reconstruction.

It is important to recognize that axillary dissection is valuable in planning therapy, staging cancer, and preventing axillary recurrences. Intraoperative lymphatic mapping and excision of the sentinel lymph node draining a primary breast carcinoma is a less invasive but highly accurate alternative for identifying patients with clinically occult axillary nodal metastases. Because the sentinel node is the first regional lymph node to receive tumor cells that metastasize along the lymphatic pathway from a primary breast cancer, its tumor status should reflect the status of the entire axillary basin. Sentinel lymphadenectomy holds promise as a staging technique to replace formal level I and level II axillary lymph node dissection in selected patients with breast carcinoma, thus avoiding an unnecessary procedure that has no role in many patients with tumor-free axillae. Two large randomized trials conducted by the National Surgical Adjuvant Breast and Bowel Project (NSABP) and the American College of Surgeons Oncology Group (ACSOG) are examining intraoperative lymphatic mapping and sentinel lymphadenectomy for the management of patients with invasive breast carcinoma. Even when tumor is detected in the sentinel node, immunohistochemical examination of multiple sections of this node may indicate whether or not complete axillary lymph node dissection is necessary.

Biopsy and immunocytochemical examination of bone marrow may be as sensitive a staging procedure as axillary dissection and may identify patients at high risk of disseminated disease.

Current Recommendations

An NIH consensus statement argues that breast-conserving surgery with radiation is the preferred form of treatment for patients with early-stage breast cancer. However, this technique has still not gained wide acceptance by physicians or patients. Despite the numerous randomized trials comparing breast conserving surgery and radiation therapy to mastectomy, breast-conserving surgery appears underutilized and mastectomy remains the more common treatment. In a recent survey, only 25% of patients in the United States with stage I or II breast cancer were treated with breast-conserving surgery and radiation therapy, compared with 75% treated with mastectomy. Use of breast-conserving surgery and radiation therapy seems to vary by region of the country, ranging from 15% in the South Central United States to approximately 30% in the Pacific Region.

Modified radical mastectomy (total mastectomy plus axillary lymph node dissection) has been the standard therapy for most patients with breast cancer. This operation removes the entire breast, overlying skin, nipple, and areolar complex as well as the underlying pectoralis fascia with the axillary lymph nodes in continuity. It offers the same overall survival and local control rates as does lumpectomy with axillary dissection and postoperative radiation therapy. The major advantage of modified radical mastectomy is that radiation therapy is usually not necessary. The disadvantage, of course, is the psychologic trauma associated with breast loss. Radical mastectomy, which removes the underlying pectoralis muscle, should be performed rarely if at all. Axillary node dissection is not indicated for noninfiltrating cancers, because nodal metastases are rarely present. Radiotherapy consists of 5–6 weeks of five daily fractions to a total dose of 5000–6000 cGy. Most radiotherapists use a boost dose, but its value is uncertain.

Preoperatively, full discussion with the patient regarding the rationale for operation and various alternative forms of treatment is essential. Breast-conserving surgery and radiation should be offered whenever possible, since most patients would prefer to save the breast. Breast reconstruction should be discussed with patients who choose or require mastectomy, and the option of simultaneous mastectomy with immediate reconstruction should be discussed. Time spent preoperatively in educating the patient and her family about these matters is time well spent.

Adjuvant Therapy

Following surgery and radiation therapy, chemotherapy or hormonal therapy is advocated for most patients with curable breast cancer (Tables 18–4 and 18–5). The objective of adjuvant therapy is to eliminate the occult metastases responsible for late recurrences while they are microscopic and theoretically most vulnerable to anticancer agents.

Numerous clinical trials with various adjuvant chemotherapeutic regimens have been completed. The most extensive clinical experience to date is with the CMF regimen (cyclophosphamide, methotrexate, and fluorouracil). Cyclophosphamide can be given either orally, in a dose of 100 mg/m^2 daily for 14 days; or intravenously, in a dose of 600 mg/m^2 on days 1 and 8. Methotrexate is given intravenously, 40 mg/m^2 on days 1 and 8; and fluorouracil is given intravenously, 600 mg/m^2 on days 1 and 8. This cycle is repeated every 4 weeks. Some clinicians prefer to give the drugs on 1 day

Table 18–4. Adjuvant chemotherapy for premenopausal women. (Summary of NIH Consensus Conference June 18–21, 1990).

Nodal Involvement	Estrogen Receptors	Adjuvant Systemic Therapy
Yes	Positive	Combination chemotherapy
Yes	Negative	Combination chemotherapy
No	Positive	Tamoxifen[1]
No	Negative	Combination chemotherapy[1]

[1]Effect on overall survival not yet clearly demonstrated.

Table 18–5. Adjuvant chemotherapy for postmenopausal women. (Summary of NIH Consensus Conference June 18–21, 1990).

Nodal Involvement	Estrogen Receptors	Adjuvant Systemic Therapy
Yes	Positive	Tamoxifen
Yes	Negative	Combination chemotherapy[1]
No	Positive	Tamoxifen[1]
No	Negative	Combination chemotherapy[1]

[1]Effect on overall survival not yet clearly demonstrated.

only every 3 weeks. There appears to be no obvious advantage except that patient compliance is assured when the cyclophosphamide is give intravenously. The regimen should be continued for 6 months in patients with axillary metastases. Premenopausal women with positive axillary nodes definitely benefit from adjuvant chemotherapy. The recurrence rate in premenopausal patients who received no adjuvant chemotherapy was more than 1½ times that of those who received such therapy. No therapeutic effect with CMF has been shown in postmenopausal women with positive nodes, perhaps because therapy was modified so often in response to side effects that the total amount of drugs administered was less than planned. It has recently been suggested that anthracycline combination chemotherapy (usually doxorubicin and cyclophosphamide) appears superior to CMF. Despite the early findings, postmenopausal women benefit as well from systemic chemotherapy.

Tamoxifen can be given with few side effects even in the elderly. Tamoxifen appears to increase bone density and favorably affect lipid and lipoprotein profiles, which may explain the observed decreased mortality rate from coronary artery disease seen in patients taking tamoxifen.

The addition of hormones improves the results of adjuvant therapy. For example, tamoxifen has been shown to enhance the beneficial effects of melphalan and fluorouracil in postmenopausal women whose tumors are ER-positive. Tamoxifen alone in a dosage of 10 mg orally twice a day has been the recommended treatment for postmenopausal women with ER-positive tumors. However, a recent NSABP trial showed that tamoxifen plus chemotherapy (Adriamycin [doxorubicin] plus cyclophosphamide [AC] or prednisone plus Adriamycin plus fluorouracil [PAF]) lowered recurrence rates more than tamoxifen alone in postmenopausal women with ER-positive tumors.

The length of time adjuvant therapy must be administered remains uncertain. Several studies suggest that shorter treatment periods may be as effective as longer ones. For example, one study compared 6 versus 12 cycles of postoperative CMF and found 5-year disease-free survival rates to be comparable. One of the earliest adjuvant trials used a 6-day perioperative regimen of intravenous cyclophosphamide alone; follow-up at 15 years shows a 15% improvement in disease-free survival rates for treated patients, suggesting that short-term therapy may be effective.

Patients with negative nodes have not been treated with adjuvant therapy until recently. Several studies of adjuvant therapy in node-negative women have now been published and show a beneficial effect of adjuvant chemotherapy or tamoxifen in delaying recurrence and improving survival. A number of protocols, including CMF—cyclophosphamide, methotrexate, and fluorouracil—with leucovorin rescue as well as tamoxifen alone have increased disease-free survival times. The magnitude of this improvement is about one-third, ie, a group of women with an estimated 30% recurrence rate would have a 20% recurrence rate after adjuvant systemic therapy. Quality of life while receiving chemotherapy does not appear to be greatly altered.

A recent NIH consensus conference reexamined the standards for adjuvant therapy of breast cancer. Since the last conference on this topic in 1990, the long-term advantage of systemic therapy has been more firmly established. The panel acknowledged that in the last 10 years no new prognostic factors have been validated to aid in the selection of patients for adjuvant treatment. The use of adjuvant systemic therapy should be based on the patient's age; on the size, histopathologic grade, and hormone receptor status of the breast tumor; and on the status of the regional lymph nodes. The use of *HER2*-neu, *P53*, angiogenesis factors, and vascular invasion are of interest but as yet are not proved prognostic factors. The panel concluded that adjuvant systemic chemotherapy with drug combinations improves survival and should be used for most women who have potentially curable breast cancer regardless of other factors. The use of anthracyclines is superior to combinations without anthracyclines. Tamoxifen should be used as a systemic agent in all women whose tumors are hormone receptor-positive regardless of age, menopausal status, or other prognostic factors. HER2-neu status should not affect the choice of agents or the use of hormone therapy. The panelists note that ovarian ablation in premenopausal patients with estrogen receptor-positive tumors may produce a benefit similar to what can be achieved with adjuvant systemic chemotherapy. Taxanes have demonstrated benefit in patients with metastatic cancer but have not yet proved to be of value in node-negative patients. Adjuvant systemic therapy should not be given to women who have small, node-negative breast cancers with favorable histologic subtypes, such as mucinous or tubular carcinoma.

Important questions remaining to be answered are the timing and duration of adjuvant chemotherapy, which chemotherapeutic agents should be applied for which subgroups of patients, how best to coordinate adjuvant chemotherapy with postoperative radiation therapy, the use of combinations of hormonal therapy and chemotherapy, and the value of prognostic factors other than hormone receptors in predicting response to adjuvant therapy. Adjuvant systemic therapy is not currently indicated for patients with small tumors and those with negative lymph nodes who have favorable DNA studies and hormone receptor assays.

PALLIATIVE TREATMENT

This section covers palliative therapy of disseminated disease incurable by surgery (stage IV).

Radiotherapy

Palliative radiotherapy may be advised for locally advanced cancers with distant metastases in order to control ulceration, pain, and other manifestations in the breast and regional nodes. Irradiation of the breast and chest wall and the axillary, internal mammary, and supraclavicular nodes should be undertaken in an attempt to cure locally advanced and inoperable lesions when there is no evidence of distant metastases. A small number of patients in this group are cured in spite of extensive breast and regional node involvement. Adjuvant chemotherapy should be considered for such patients.

Palliative irradiation is of value also in the treatment of certain bone or soft tissue metastases to control pain or avoid fracture. Radiotherapy is especially useful in the treatment of isolated bony metastasis and chest wall recurrences.

Hormone Therapy

Disseminated disease may respond to prolonged endocrine therapy such as administration of hormones (eg, estrogens, androgens, progestins; see Table 18–6); ablation of the ovaries, adrenals, or pituitary; or administration of drugs that block hormone receptor sites (eg, antiestrogens) or drugs that block the synthesis of hormones (eg, aminoglutethimide). Hormonal manipulation is usually more successful in postmenopausal women. If treatment is based on the presence of estrogen receptor protein in the primary tumor or metastases, however, the rate of response is nearly equal in premenopausal and postmenopausal women. A favorable response to hormonal manipulation occurs in about one-third of patients with metastatic breast cancer. Of those whose tumors contain estrogen receptors, the response is about 60% and perhaps as high as 80% for patients whose tumors contain progesterone receptors as well. Because only 5–10% of women whose tumors do not contain estrogen receptors respond, they should not receive hormonal therapy except in unusual circumstances such as an elderly patient who could not tolerate chemotherapy.

Since the quality of life during a remission induced by endocrine manipulation is usually superior to a remission following cytotoxic chemotherapy, it is usually best to try endocrine manipulation first in cases where the estrogen receptor status of the tumor is unknown. However, if the estrogen receptor status is unknown but the disease is progressing rapidly or involves visceral

Table 18–6. Commonly used hormonal agents for management of metastatic breast cancer.

Drug	Action	Usual Oral Dose	Major Side Effects
Tamoxifen (Nolvadex)	Antiestrogen	10 mg twice daily	Hot flashes, uterine bleeding, thrombophlebitis, rash
Diethylstilbestrol (DES)	Estrogen	5 mg 3 times daily	Fluid retention, uterine bleeding, thrombophlebitis, nausea
Megestrol acetate (Megace)	Progestin	40 mg 4 times daily	Fluid retention
Aminoglutethimide (Cytadren)[1]	Aromatase inhibitor	250 mg 4 times daily	Adrenal suppression, skin rashes, neurologic reactions

[1]Used with hydrocortisone.

organs, endocrine therapy is rarely successful, and introducing it may waste valuable time.

In general, only one type of systemic therapy should be given at a time unless it is necessary to irradiate a destructive lesion of weight-bearing bone while the patient is on another regimen. The regimen should be changed only if the disease is clearly progressing but not if it appears to be stable. This is especially important for patients with destructive bone metastases, since minor changes in the status of these lesions are difficult to determine radiographically. A plan of therapy that would simultaneously minimize toxicity and maximize benefits is often best achieved by hormonal manipulation.

The choice of endocrine therapy depends on the menopausal status of the patient. Women within 1 year of their last menstrual period are considered to be premenopausal, while women whose menstruation ceased more than a year ago are postmenopausal. The initial choice of therapy is referred to as primary hormonal manipulation; subsequent endocrine treatment is called secondary or tertiary hormonal manipulation.

A. THE PREMENOPAUSAL PATIENT

1. Primary hormonal therapy—The potent antiestrogen tamoxifen is the endocrine treatment of choice in the premenopausal patient. Tamoxifen is usually given orally in a dose of 10 mg twice a day. At least two randomized clinical trials have now shown no significant difference in survival or response between tamoxifen therapy and bilateral oophorectomy. Most physicians prefer to use tamoxifen rather than perform oophorectomy, since it can be given with little morbidity and few side effects. Controversy continues about whether a response to tamoxifen is predictive of probable success with other forms of endocrine manipulation.

Bilateral oophorectomy is a reasonable alternative for primary hormonal manipulation in premenopausal women. It can be achieved rapidly and safely by surgery or, if the patient is a poor operative risk, by irradiation of the ovaries. Ovarian radiation therapy should be avoided in otherwise healthy patients, however, because of the high rate of complications and the longer time necessary to achieve results. Oophorectomy presumably works by eliminating estrogens, progestins, and androgens, which stimulate growth of the tumor. The average remission is about 12 months.

2. Secondary or tertiary hormonal therapy—Although patients who do not respond to tamoxifen or oophorectomy should be treated with cytotoxic drugs, those who respond and then relapse may subsequently respond to another form of endocrine treatment (Table 18–6). The initial choice for secondary endocrine manipulation has not been clearly defined. Adrenalectomy

or hypophysectomy induces regression in approximately 30–50% of patients who have previously responded to oophorectomy. However, these procedures are rarely performed now.

Patients who respond initially to oophorectomy but subsequently relapse should receive tamoxifen. If this treatment fails, use of aminoglutethimide or megestrol acetate should be considered. Aminoglutethimide is an inhibitor of adrenal hormone synthesis and, when combined with a corticosteroid, provides a therapeutically effective "medical adrenalectomy." Megestrol is a progestational agent. Both drugs cause less morbidity and mortality than surgical adrenalectomy; can be discontinued once the patient improves; and are not associated with the many problems of postsurgical hypoadrenalism, so that patients who require chemotherapy are more easily managed.

B. THE POSTMENOPAUSAL PATIENT

1. Primary hormonal therapy—Tamoxifen, 10 mg twice daily, is now the initial therapy of choice for postmenopausal women with metastatic breast cancer amenable to endocrine manipulation. It has fewer side effects than diethylstilbestrol, the former therapy of choice, and is just as effective. The main side effects of tamoxifen are nausea, vomiting, and skin rash. Rarely, it may induce hypercalcemia.

2. Secondary or tertiary hormonal therapy—Postmenopausal patients who do not respond to primary endocrine manipulation should be given cytotoxic drugs such as cyclophosphamide, methotrexate, and fluorouracil (CMF) or Adriamycin (doxorubicin) and cyclophosphamide (AC). Postmenopausal women who respond initially to tamoxifen but later manifest progressive disease could be given diethylstilbestrol or megestrol acetate. Some authorities use aminoglutethimide. Megestrol has fewer side effects than either aminoglutethimide or diethylstilbestrol. Androgens have many side effects and should rarely be used. In general, hypophysectomy or adrenalectomy is rarely necessary.

Chemotherapy

Cytotoxic drugs should be considered for the treatment of metastatic breast cancer (1) if visceral metastases are present (especially brain or lymphangitic pulmonary); (2) if hormonal treatment is unsuccessful or the disease has progressed after an initial response to hormonal manipulation; or (3) if the tumor is ER-negative. The most useful single chemotherapeutic agent to date is doxorubicin, with a response rate of 40–50%. Single agents are rarely used. The remissions tend to be brief, and in general, experience with single-agent chemotherapy in patients with disseminated disease has not been encouraging.

Combination chemotherapy using multiple agents has proved to be more effective, with objectively observed favorable responses achieved in 60–80% of patients with stage IV disease. Various combinations of drugs have been used, and clinical trials are continuing in an effort to improve results and reduce undesirable side effects. Doxorubicin (40 mg/m^2 intravenously on day 1) and cyclophosphamide (200 mg/m^2 orally on days 3–6) produce an objective response in about 85% of patients so treated. Other chemotherapeutic regimens have consisted of various combinations of drugs, including cyclophosphamide, vincristine, methotrexate, and fluorouracil, with response rates ranging up to 60–70%. Prior adjuvant chemotherapy does not seem to alter response rates in patients who relapse. Few new drugs or combinations of drugs have been sufficiently effective in breast cancer to warrant wide acceptance—except the taxanes, which have shown efficacy for metastatic disease and are being used in adjuvant therapy protocols.

Recently, high-dose chemotherapy and autologous bone marrow or stem cell autotransplantation have aroused widespread interest for the treatment of metastatic breast cancer. With this technique, the patient receives high doses of cytotoxic agents. These cause severe side effects, including bone marrow suppression, for which the patient subsequently undergoes autologous bone marrow transplantation. Reported complete response rates are as high as 30–35%—considerably better than what can be achieved with conventional chemotherapy. However, median survival times and overall survival rates do not appear to be significantly different from those reported with conventional chemotherapy. Recent randomized controlled trials have shown no benefit for high-dose chemotherapy compared with standard therapy. These studies remain to be confirmed.

Malignant Pleural Effusion

This condition develops at some time in almost half of patients with metastatic breast cancer (see Chapter 19).

PROGNOSIS

The stage of breast cancer is the single most reliable indicator of prognosis (Table 18–7). Patients with disease localized to the breast and no evidence of regional spread after microscopic examination of the lymph nodes have by far the most favorable prognosis. Estrogen and progesterone receptors appear to be an important prognostic variable, because patients with hormone receptor-negative tumors and no evidence of metastases

Table 18–7. Approximate survival (%) of patients with breast cancer by TNM stage.

TNM Stage	Five Years	Ten Years
0	95	90
I	85	70
IIA	70	50
IIB	60	40
IIIA	55	30
IIIB	30	20
IV	5–10	2
All	65	30

to the axillary lymph nodes have a much higher recurrence rate than do patients with hormone receptor-positive tumors and no regional metastases. The histologic subtype of breast cancer (eg, medullary, lobular, comedo) seems to have little, if any, significance in prognosis once these tumors are truly invasive. Flow cytometry of tumor cells to analyze DNA index and S-phase frequency aid in prognosis. Tumors with marked aneuploidy have a poor prognosis (Table 18–8). HER-2/*neu* oncogene amplification growth factors and cathepsin D may have some prognostic value, but few data exist as to their usefulness.

Most patients who develop breast cancer will ultimately die of that disease. The mortality rate of breast

Table 18–8. Prognostic factors in node-negative breast cancer.

Prognostic Factor	Increased Recurrence	Decreased Recurrence
Size	T3 T2	T1 T0
Hormone receptors	Negative	Positive
DNA flow cytometry	Aneuploid	Diploid
Histologic grade	High	Low
Tumor labeling index	< 3%	> 3%
S phase fraction	> 5%	< 5%
Lymphatic or vascular invasion	Present	Absent
Cathepsin D	High	Low
HER-2/*neu* oncogene	High	Low
Epidermal growth factor receptor	High	Low

cancer patients exceeds that of age-matched normal controls for nearly 20 years. Thereafter, the mortality rates are equal, although deaths that occur among breast cancer patients are often directly the result of tumor. Five-year statistics do not accurately reflect the final outcome of therapy.

When cancer is localized to the breast, with no evidence of regional spread after pathologic examination, the clinical cure rate with most accepted methods of therapy is 75–90%. Exceptions to this generalization may be related to the hormonal receptor content of the tumor, tumor size, host resistance, or associated illness. Patients with small estrogen and progesterone receptor-positive tumors and no evidence of axillary spread probably have a 5-year survival rate of nearly 90%. When the axillary lymph nodes are involved with tumor, the survival rate drops to 40–50% at 5 years and probably less than 25% at 10 years. In general, breast cancer appears to be somewhat more malignant in younger than in older women, and this may be related to the fact that fewer younger women have ER-positive tumors.

FOLLOW-UP CARE

After primary therapy, patients with breast cancer should be followed for life for at least two reasons: to detect recurrences and to observe the opposite breast for a second primary carcinoma. About 10% of patients will develop a contralateral primary malignancy. Local and distant metastases occur most frequently within the first 3 years. During this period, the patient is examined every 6 months. Thereafter, examination is done every 6–12 months until 5 years postoperatively and then usually every 12 months. Special attention is given to the remaining breast, because of the increased risk of developing a second primary. The patient should examine her own breast monthly, and a mammogram should be obtained annually. In some cases, metastases are dormant for long periods and may appear up to 10–15 years or longer after removal of the primary tumor. Estrogen and progestational agents are rarely used for a patient free of disease after treatment of primary breast cancer, particularly if the tumor was hormone receptor-positive. However, studies have failed to show an adverse effect of hormonal agents in patients who are free of disease. Indeed, even pregnancy has not been clearly associated with shortened survival of patients rendered disease-free—yet most oncologists are reluctant to advise a young patient with breast cancer that she may become pregnant.

Local Recurrence

The incidence of local recurrence correlates with tumor size, the presence and number of involved axillary nodes, the histologic type of tumor, and the presence of skin edema or skin and fascia fixation with the primary. About 8% of patients develop local recurrence on the chest wall after total mastectomy and axillary dissection. When the axillary nodes are not involved, the local recurrence rate is 5%, but the rate is as high as 25% when they are involved. A similar difference in local recurrence rate was noted between small and large tumors. Factors that affect the rate of local recurrence in patients who had partial mastectomies are not yet determined. However, early studies show that such things as multifocal cancer, in situ tumors, positive resection margins, chemotherapy, and radiotherapy are important.

Chest wall recurrences usually appear within the first 2 years but may occur as late as 15 or more years after mastectomy. Suspect nodules should be biopsied. Local excision or localized radiotherapy may be feasible if an isolated nodule is present. If lesions are multiple or accompanied by evidence of regional involvement in the internal mammary or supraclavicular nodes, the disease is best managed by radiation treatment of the entire chest wall including the parasternal, supraclavicular, and axillary areas.

Local recurrence after mastectomy usually signals the presence of widespread disease and is an indication for bone and liver scans, posteroanterior and lateral chest x-rays, and other examinations as needed to search for evidence of metastases. Most patients with locally recurrent tumor will develop distant metastases within 2 years. When there is no evidence of metastases beyond the chest wall and regional nodes, irradiation for cure or complete local excision should be attempted. Patients with local recurrence may be cured with local resection or radiation. After partial mastectomy, however, local recurrence does not have as serious a prognostic significance. However, those patients who do develop a breast recurrence have a worse prognosis than those who do not. It is speculated that the ability of a cancer to recur locally after radiotherapy is a sign of aggressiveness associated with distant disease rather than a cause of it. Completion of the mastectomy should be done for local recurrence after partial mastectomy; overall survival does not appear to be altered. Systemic chemotherapy or hormonal treatment should be used for postmenopausal women who develop disseminated disease or those in whom local recurrence occurs following total mastectomy.

Edema of the Arm

Significant edema of the arm occurs in about 5% after modified radical mastectomy and about 10–30% of patients after radical mastectomy. Edema of the arm occurs more commonly if radiotherapy has been given or if there was postoperative infection. Partial mastectomy with radiation to the axillary lymph nodes is followed by chronic edema of the arm in 10–20% of patients. To avoid this complication, many authorities advocate axillary lymph node sampling rather than complete axillary dissection. However, since axillary dissection is a more accurate staging operation than axillary sampling, we recommend axillary dissection, with removal of at least level I and II lymph nodes, in combination with partial mastectomy. Recent studies have shown that lymphatic mapping and excision of the sentinel lymph node can permit accurate staging without the risk of lymphedema. Judicious use of radiotherapy, with treatment fields carefully planned to spare the axilla as much as possible, can greatly diminish the incidence of edema.

Late or secondary edema of the arm may develop years after treatment, as a result of axillary recurrence or of infection in the hand or arm, with obliteration of lymphatic channels. Infection in the arm or hand on the dissected side should be treated promptly with antibiotics, rest, and elevation. When edema develops, careful examination of the axilla should be done to detect a regional recurrence. If there is no sign of recurrence, the swollen extremity should be treated with rest and elevation. A mild diuretic may be helpful for a few weeks. If there is no improvement, a compressor pump should be used to decrease the swelling, and the patient should then be fitted with an elastic glove or sleeve. Most patients are not bothered enough by mild edema to wear an uncomfortable glove or sleeve and will treat themselves with elevation alone. Benzopyrones have been reported to decrease lymphedema, but these agents are not approved for this use in the USA. Rarely, edema may be severe enough to interfere with use of the limb.

Breast Reconstruction

Breast reconstruction, with the implantation of a prosthesis, is usually feasible after standard or modified radical mastectomy. Reconstruction should probably be discussed with patients prior to mastectomy, because it offers an important psychologic focal point for recovery. However, most patients who are initially interested in reconstruction decide later that they no longer wish to undergo the procedure. Reconstruction is not an obstacle to the diagnosis of recurrent cancer. The most common breast reconstruction has been implantation of a silicone gel prosthesis in the subpectoral plane between the pectoralis minor and pectoralis major muscles. Recently, the Food and Drug Administration has placed a moratorium on the use of silicone gel implants because of possible leakage of silicone and associated autoimmune disorders. This remote possibility should

not prevent the cancer patient from having a reconstruction. Most plastic surgeons currently would place a saline-filled prosthesis rather than a silicone gel implant. Alternatively, autologous tissue can be used for reconstruction. The most popular autologous technique currently is the trans-rectus abdominis muscle flap (TRAM flap), which is done by rotating the rectus abdominis muscle with attached fat and skin cephalad to make a breast mound. A latissimus dorsi flap can be swung from the back but offers less fullness than the TRAM flap and is therefore less acceptable cosmetically. All patients who undergo mastectomy should be offered the option of breast reconstruction.

Risks of Pregnancy

Data are insufficient to determine whether interruption of pregnancy improves the prognosis of patients who are discovered during pregnancy to have potentially curable breast cancer and who receive definitive treatment. Theoretically, the increasingly high levels of estrogen produced by the placenta as the pregnancy progresses could be detrimental to the patient with occult metastases of hormone-sensitive breast cancer. Moreover, occult metastases are present in most patients with positive axillary nodes, and treatment by adjuvant chemotherapy would be potentially harmful to the fetus. Under these circumstances, interruption of early pregnancy seems reasonable, with progressively less rationale for the procedure as term approaches. Obviously, the decision must be highly individualized and will be affected by many factors, including the patient's desire to have the baby and the generally poor prognosis when axillary nodes are involved.

Equally problematic and important is the advice regarding future pregnancy (or abortion in case of pregnancy) to be given to women of child-bearing age who have had a mastectomy or other definitive treatment for breast cancer. Under these circumstances, one must assume that pregnancy will be harmful if occult metastases are present, although this has not been demonstrated. Patients whose tumors are ER-negative probably would not be affected by pregnancy. A number of studies have shown no adverse effect of pregnancy on survival of pregnant women who have had breast cancer.

In patients with inoperable or metastatic cancer (stage IV disease), induced abortion is usually advisable because of the possible adverse effects of hormonal treatment, radiotherapy, or chemotherapy upon the fetus.

Risk Factors & Prevention

Alberg AJ et al: Epidemiology, prevention, and early detection of breast cancer. Curr Opin Oncol 1997;9:505.

Braun S et al: Cytokeratin-positive cells in the bone marrow and survival of patients with stage I, II, or III breast cancer. N Engl J Med 2000;342:525.

Clinical practice guidelines for the use of tumor markers in breast and colorectal cancer. J Clin Oncol 1996;14:2843.

Collaborative Group on Hormonal Factors in Breast Cancer (Radcliffe Infirmary, Oxford, England): breast cancer and hormonal contraceptives: collaborative reanalysis of individual data on 53,297 women with breast cancer and 100,239 women without breast cancer from 54 epidemiological studies. Lancet 1996;347:1713.

Fisher B et al: Tamoxifen for prevention of breast cancer: report of the National Surgical Adjuvant Breast and Bowel Project P-1 Study. J Natl Cancer Inst 1998; 90:1371.

Hartmann LC et al: Efficacy of bilateral prophylactic mastectomy in women with a family history of breast cancer. N Engl J Med 1999;340:77.

JAMA patient page: Breast cancer. JAMA 1999;281:772.

Klijn JG et al: Should prophylactic surgery be used in women with a high risk of breast cancer? Eur J Cancer 1997;33:2149.

Piccirillo JF et al: Clinical symptoms and co-morbidity: significance for the prognostic classification of cancer. Cancer 1996; 77:834.

Schairer C et al: Menopausal estrogen and estrogen-progestin replacement therapy and breast cancer risk. JAMA 2000;283: 485.

Vassilopoulou-Sellin R et al: Estrogen replacement therapy after localized breast cancer: clinical outcome of 319 women followed prospectively. J Clin Oncol 1999;17:1482.

Velentgas P et al: Pregnancy after breast carcinoma: outcomes and influence on mortality. Cancer 1999;85:2424.

Younes M et al: Stratified multivariate analysis of prognostic markers in breast cancer: a preliminary report. Anticancer Res 1997;17:1383.

Screening

Audrain J et al: Genetic counseling and testing for breast-ovarian cancer susceptibility: what do women want? J Clin Oncol 1998;16:133.

Beckhardt S for the American Society of Clinical Oncology. Statement of the American Society of Clinical Oncology: genetic testing for cancer susceptibility. J Clin Oncol 1996; 14:1730.

Feig SA: Doubtful results in the Canadian national breast screening study. Breast Diseases 1996;6:354.

Flanagan FL et al: PET in breast cancer. Semin Nucl Med 1998;28: 290.

Gail M et al: Risk-based recommendations for mammographic screening for women in their forties. J Clin Oncol 1998;16: 3105.

Giuseppetti GM et al: Color doppler sonography. Eur J Radiol 1998;27(Suppl 2):S254.

Greely HT: Genetic testing for cancer susceptibility for creators of practice guidelines. Oncology (Huntingt) 1997;11(11A):171.

Kodish E et al: Genetic testing for cancer risk: how to reconcile the conflicts. JAMA 1998;279:179.

Kopans DB: Updated results of the trials of screening mammography. Surg Oncol Clin North Am 1997;6:233.

Leitch AM et al: American Cancer Society guidelines for the early detection of breast cancer: update 1997. CA Cancer J Clin 1997;47:150.

Obdeijn IM et al: MR lesion detection in a breast cancer population. J Magn Reson Imaging 1996;6:849.

Axillary Assessment

Avril N et al: Assessment of axillary lymph node involvement in breast cancer patients with positron emission tomography using radiolabeled 2-(fluorine-18)-fluoro-2-deoxy-D-glucose. J Natl Cancer Inst 1996;88:1204.

Giuliano AE et al: Prospective observational study of sentinel lymphadenectomy without further axillary dissection in patients with sentinel node-negative breast cancer. J Clin Oncol 2000; 18:2553.

Giuliano AE et al: Sentinel lymphadenectomy in breast cancer. J Clin Oncol 1997;15:2345.

Krag D et al: The sentinel node in breast cancer—a multicenter validation study. N Engl J Med 1998;339:941.

Turner R et al: Histopathologic validation of the sentinel node hypothesis for breast carcinoma. Ann Surg 1997;226:271.

Breast-Conserving Surgery

Brem RF et al: Atypical ductal hyperplasia: histologic underestimation of carcinoma in tissue harvested from impalpable breast lesions using 11-gauge stereotactically guided directional vacuum-assisted biopsy. AJR Am J Roentgenol 1999;172:1405.

Colozza M et al: Induction chemotherapy with cisplatin, doxorubicin, and cyclophosphamide (CAP) in a combined modality approach for locally advanced and inflammatory breast cancer. Long-term results. Am J Clin Oncol 1996;19:10.

Dale PS et al: Nipple-areolar preservation during breast-conserving therapy for subareolar breast carcinomas. Ann Surg 1996; 131:430.

Fish EB et al: Assessment of treatment for patients with primary ductal carcinoma in situ in the breast. Ann Surg Oncol 1998; 5:724.

Fisher ER et al: Pathologic findings from the National Surgical Adjuvant Breast Project (NSABP) eight-year update of Protocol B-17: intraductal carcinoma. Cancer 1999;86:429.

Hillner BE et al: Trade-offs between survival and breast preservation for three initial treatments of ductal carcinoma-in-situ of the breast. J Clin Oncol 1996;14:70.

Margolese RG: Surgical considerations for invasive breast cancer. Surg Clin North Am 1999;79:1031.

Mehta K et al: Long-term outcome in patients with four or more positive lymph nodes treated with conservative surgery and radiation therapy. Int J Radiat Oncol Biol Phys 1996;35:679.

Price J et al: Prevention and treatment of lymphedema after breast cancer. Am J Nurs 1997;97:34.

Schusterman MA et al: Advances in reconstruction for cancer patients. Cancer Treat Res 1997;90:71.

Silverstein MJ et al: The influence of margin width on local control of ductal carcinoma in situ of the breast. N Engl J Med 1999; 340:1455.

Solin LJ et al: Fifteen-year results of breast conserving surgery and definitive breast irradiation for the treatment of ductal carcinoma in situ of the breast. J Clin Oncol 1996;14:754.

Tartter PI et al: Factors associated with clear biopsy margins and clear re-excision margins in breast cancer specimens from candidates for breast conservation. J Am Coll Surg 1997;185: 268.

Touboul E et al: Local recurrences and distant metastases after breast-conserving surgery and radiation therapy for early stage breast cancer. Int J Radiat Oncol Biol Phys 1999;43:25.

Williams JK et al: The effects of radiation after TRAM flap breast reconstruction. Plast Reconstr Surg 1997;100:1153.

Hormone Receptors

Carmeci C et al: Analysis of estrogen receptor messenger RNA in breast carcinomas from archival specimens is predictive of tumor biology. Am J Pathol 1997;150:1563.

Raabe NK et al: Hormone receptor measurements and survival in 1335 consecutive patients with primary invasive breast carcinoma. Int J Oncol 1998;12:1091.

Adjuvant Systemic Therapy

Adjuvant systemic therapy for women with node-negative breast cancer. The Steering Committee on Clinical Practice Guidelines for the Care and Treatment of Breast Cancer. Can Med Assoc J 1998;10:158.

Adjuvant systemic therapy for women with node-positive breast cancer. The Steering Committee on Clinical Practice Guidelines for the Care and Treatment of Breast Cancer. Can Med Assoc J 1998;10(Suppl):S52.

Adjuvant therapy for breast cancer. NIH Consensus Statement 2000. http://odp.od.nih.gov/consensus/cons/114/114statement.htm

Clarke M: Tamoxifen for early breast cancer: an overview of the randomised trials. Lancet 1998;351:1451.

Hudis CA et al: Adjuvant drug therapy for operable breast cancer. Semin Oncol 1996;23:475.

Treatment of Advanced Breast Cancer

Borden EC et al: Biological therapies for breast carcinoma: concepts for improvements in survival. Semin Oncol 1999;26(4 Suppl 12):28.

Buzdar AU et al: a phase III trial comparing anastrozole (1–10 milligrams), a potent and selective aromatase inhibitor, with megestrol acetate in postmenopausal women with advanced breast carcinoma. Arimidex Study Group. Cancer 1997;79:730.

Buzdar AU et al: Arimidex: a potent and selective aromatase inhibitor for the treatment of advanced breast cancer. J Steroid Biochem Mol Biol 1997;61:145.

Colmer R et al: Paclitaxel/gemcitabine administered every two weeks in advanced breast cancer: preliminary results of a phase II trial. Semin Oncol 2000;27(1 Suppl 2):20.

Dhodapkar MV et al: Prognostic factors in elderly women with metastatic breast cancer treated with tamoxifen: an analysis of patients entered on four prospective clinical trials. Cancer 1996;77:683.

Haffty BG et al: Ipsilateral breast tumor recurrence as a predictor of distant disease: implications for systemic therapy at the time of local relapse. J Clin Oncol 1996;14:52.

Harvey HA: issues concerning the role of chemotherapy and hormonal therapy of bone metastases from breast cancer. Cancer 1997;80(8 Suppl):1646.

Pegram MD et al: Combination therapy with trastuzumab (Herceptin) and cisplatin for chemoresistant metastatic breast cancer: evidence for receptor-enhanced chemosensitivity. Semin Oncol 1999;26(4 Suppl 12):89.

Ramirez AJ et al: Do patients with advanced breast cancer benefit from chemotherapy? Br J Cancer 1998;78:1488.

Stadtmauer EA et al: Conventional-dose chemotherapy compared with high-dose chemotherapy plus autologous hematopoietic stem-cell transplantation for metastatic breast cancer. N Engl J Med 2000;342:1069.

Valero V: Combination docetaxel/cyclophosphamide in patients with advanced solid tumors. Oncology 1997;11:34.

■ CARCINOMA OF THE MALE BREAST

 ESSENTIALS OF DIAGNOSIS

- *A painless lump beneath the areola in a man usually over 50 years of age.*
- *Nipple discharge, retraction, or ulceration may be present.*

General Considerations

Breast cancer in men is a rare disease; the incidence is only about 1% of that in women. The average age at occurrence is about 60—somewhat older than the commonest presenting age in women. The prognosis, even in stage I cases, is worse in men than in women. Blood-borne metastases are commonly present when the male patient appears for initial treatment. These metastases may be latent and may not become manifest for many years. As in women, hormonal influences are probably related to the development of male breast cancer. There is a high incidence of both breast cancer and gynecomastia in Bantu men, theoretically owing to failure of estrogen inactivation by a damaged liver associated with vitamin B deficiency.

Clinical Findings

A painless lump, occasionally associated with nipple discharge, retraction, erosion, or ulceration, is the chief complaint. Examination usually shows a hard, ill-defined, nontender mass beneath the nipple or areola. Gynecomastia not uncommonly precedes or accompanies breast cancer in men. Nipple discharge is an uncommon presentation for breast cancer in men, as it is in women. However, nipple discharge in a man is an ominous finding associated with carcinoma in nearly 75% of cases.

Breast cancer staging is the same in men as in women. Gynecomastia and metastatic cancer from another site (eg, prostate) must be considered in the differential diagnosis of a breast lesion in a man. Biopsy settles the issue.

Treatment

Treatment consists of modified radical mastectomy in operable patients, who should be chosen by the same criteria as women with the disease. Irradiation is the first step in treating localized metastases in the skin, lymph nodes, or skeleton that are causing symptoms. Examination of the cancer for hormone receptor proteins may prove to be of value in predicting response to endocrine ablation. Adjuvant chemotherapy is used for the same indications as in breast cancer in women.

Since breast cancer in men is frequently a disseminated disease, endocrine therapy is of considerable importance in its management. Castration in advanced breast cancer is the most successful palliative measure and more beneficial than the same procedure in women. Objective evidence of regression may be seen in 60–70% of men who are castrated—approximately twice the proportion in women. The average duration of tumor growth remission is about 30 months, and life is prolonged. Bone is the most frequent site of metastases from breast cancer in men (as in women), and castration relieves bone pain in most patients so treated. The longer the interval between mastectomy and recurrence, the longer the tumor growth remission following castration. As in women, there is no correlation between the histologic type of the tumor and the likelihood of remission following castration.

Tamoxifen (10 mg orally twice daily) is becoming increasingly popular and should replace castration as the initial therapy for metastatic disease. However, little clinical experience is available with tamoxifen in male breast cancers. Aminoglutethimide (250 mg orally four times a day) should replace adrenalectomy in men as it has in women. Corticosteroid therapy alone has been considered to be efficacious but probably has no value when compared with major endocrine ablation.

Estrogen therapy—5 mg of diethylstilbestrol three times daily orally—may be effective as secondary hormonal manipulation after medical adrenalectomy (with aminoglutethimide). Androgen therapy may exacerbate bone pain. Castration and tamoxifen are the main therapeutic resources for advanced breast cancer in men at present. Chemotherapy should be administered for the same indications and using the same dosage schedules as for women with metastatic disease.

Prognosis

The prognosis of breast cancer is poorer in men than in women. The crude 5- and 10-year survival rates for clinical stage I breast cancer in men are about 58% and 38%, respectively. For clinical stage II disease, the 5- and 10-year survival rates are approximately 38% and 10%. The survival rates for all stages at 5 and 10 years are 36% and 17%.

Friedman LS et al: Mutation analysis of *BRCA1* and *BRCA2* in a male breast cancer population. Am J Hum Genet 1997;60: 313.

Joshi MG et al: Male breast carcinoma: an evaluation of prognostic factors contributing to a poor outcome. Cancer 1996;77:490.

Memon MA et al: Male breast cancer. Br J Surg 1997;84:433.

Pich A et al: Oncogenes and male breast carcinoma: c-erbB-2 and p53 coexpression predicts a poor survival. J Clin Oncol 2000;18:2948.

Winchester DJ: Male breast cancer. Semin Surg Oncol 1996;12: 364.

■ OTHER BREAST DISORDERS

MAMMARY DYSPLASIA (FIBROCYSTIC DISEASE)

 ESSENTIALS OF DIAGNOSIS

- *Painful, often multiple, usually bilateral masses in the breast.*
- *Rapid fluctuation in the size of the masses is common.*
- *Frequently, pain occurs or increases and size increases during premenstrual phase of cycle.*
- *Most common age is 30–50. Rare in postmenopausal women.*

General Considerations

This disorder, also known as fibrocystic disease or chronic cystic mastitis, is the most frequent lesion of the breast. It is common in women 30–50 years of age but rare in postmenopausal women; this suggests that it is related to ovarian activity. Estrogen hormone is considered a causative factor. The term "mammary dysplasia," or "fibrocystic disease," is imprecise and encompasses a wide variety of pathologic entities. These lesions are always associated with benign changes in the breast epithelium, some of which are found so commonly in normal breasts that they are probably variants of normal breast histology but have unfortunately been termed a "disease."

The microscopic findings of fibrocystic disease include cysts (gross and microscopic), papillomatosis, adenosis, fibrosis, and ductal epithelial hyperplasia. Although mammary dysplasia has generally been considered to increase the risk of subsequent breast cancer, only the variants in which proliferation of epithelial components is demonstrated represent true risk factors.

Clinical Findings

Mammary dysplasia may produce an asymptomatic lump in the breast that is discovered by accident, but pain or tenderness often calls attention to the mass. There may be discharge from the nipple. In many cases, discomfort occurs or is increased during the premenstrual phase of the cycle, at which time the cysts tend to enlarge. Fluctuation in size and rapid appearance or disappearance of a breast tumor are common in cystic disease. Multiple or bilateral masses are common, and many patients will give a history of a transient lump in the breast or cyclic breast pain.

Differential Diagnosis

Pain, fluctuation in size, and multiplicity of lesions are the features most helpful in differentiation from carcinoma. However, if a dominant mass is present, the diagnosis of cancer should be assumed until disproved by biopsy. Final diagnosis often depends on biopsy. Mammography may be helpful, but the breast tissue in these young women is usually too radiodense to permit a worthwhile study. Sonography is useful in differentiating a cystic from a solid mass.

Treatment

Because mammary dysplasia is frequently indistinguishable from carcinoma on the basis of clinical findings, suspicious lesions should be biopsied. Fine-needle aspiration cytology may be used, but if a suspicious mass that is nonmalignant on cytologic examination does not resolve over several months, it must be excised. Surgery should be conservative, since the primary objective is to exclude cancer. Simple mastectomy or extensive removal of breast tissue is rarely, if ever, indicated for mammary dysplasia.

When the diagnosis of mammary dysplasia has been established by previous biopsy or is practically certain because the history is classic, aspiration of a discrete mass suggestive of a cyst is indicated. The patient is reexamined at intervals thereafter. If no fluid is obtained or if fluid is bloody, if a mass persists after aspiration, or if at any time during follow-up a persistent lump is noted, biopsy examination should be performed.

Breast pain associated with generalized mammary dysplasia is best treated by avoiding trauma and by wearing (night and day) a brassiere that gives good support and protection. Hormone therapy is not advisable, because it does not cure the condition and has undesirable side effects. Danazol (100–200 mg twice daily orally), a synthetic androgen, has been used for patients with severe pain. This treatment suppresses pituitary gonadotropins, and androgenic effects (acne, edema, hirsutism) usually make this treatment intolerable; it should therefore be reserved for the unusual severe case.

The role of caffeine consumption in the development and treatment of fibrocystic disease is controversial. Some studies suggest that eliminating caffeine from the diet is associated with improvement. Many patients are aware of these studies and report relief of symptoms after giving up coffee, tea, and chocolate. Similarly, many women find vitamin E (400 IU daily) helpful. However, these observations have been difficult to confirm and are anecdotal.

Prognosis

Exacerbations of pain, tenderness, and cyst formation may occur at any time until the menopause, when symptoms usually subside, except in patients receiving estrogens. The patient should be advised to examine her own breasts each month just after menstruation and to inform her physician if a mass appears. The risk of breast cancer in women with mammary dysplasia showing proliferative or atypical changes in the epithelium is higher than that of women in general. Follow-up examinations at regular intervals should therefore be arranged.

Cady B et al: Evaluation of common breast problems: guidance for primary care providers. CA Cancer J Clin 1998;48:49.

Fitzgibbons PL et al: Benign breast changes and the risk for subsequent breast cancer: an update of the 1985 consensus statement. Cancer Committee of the College of American Pathologists Arch Pathol Lab Med 1998;122:1053.

Marchant DJ: Controversies in benign breast disease. Surg Oncol Clin N Am 1998;7:285.

FIBROADENOMA OF THE BREAST

This common benign neoplasm occurs most frequently in young women, usually within 20 years after puberty. It is somewhat more frequent and tends to occur at an earlier age in black than in white women. Multiple tumors in one or both breasts are found in 10–15% of patients.

The typical fibroadenoma is a round, firm, discrete, relatively movable, nontender mass 1–5 cm in diameter. The tumor is usually discovered accidentally. Clinical diagnosis in young patients is generally not difficult. In women over 30, cystic disease of the breast and carcinoma of the breast must be considered. Cysts can be identified by aspiration. Fibroadenoma does not normally occur after the menopause, but postmenopausal women may occasionally develop fibroadenoma after administration of estrogenic hormone.

Treatment is by excision under local anesthesia as an outpatient procedure, with pathologic examination of the specimen.

Cystosarcoma phyllodes is a type of fibroadenoma with cellular stroma that tends to grow rapidly. This tumor may reach a large size and if inadequately excised will recur locally. The lesion is rarely malignant. Treatment is by local excision of the mass with a margin of surrounding breast tissue. The treatment of malignant cystosarcoma phyllodes is more controversial. In general, complete removal of the tumor and a rim of normal tissue should avoid recurrence. Since these tumors may be large, simple mastectomy is sometimes necessary to achieve complete control.

Alle KM et al: Conservative management of fibroadenoma of the breast. Br J Surg 1996;83:1798.

Chilcote WA et al: Stereotactic breast biopsy: a less-invasive option. Cleve Clin J Med 1997;64:550.

Greenberg R et al: Management of breast fibroadenomas. J Gen Intern Med 1998;13:640.

Mangi AA et al: Surgical management of phyllodes tumors. Arch Surg 1999;134:487.

Reinfuss M et al: The treatment and prognosis of patients with phyllodes tumors of the breast: an analysis of 170 cases. Cancer 1996;77:910.

NIPPLE DISCHARGE

In order of increasing frequency, the following are the commonest causes of nipple discharge in the nonlactating breast: carcinoma, intraductal papilloma, and mammary dysplasia with ectasia of the ducts. The important characteristics of the discharge and some other factors to be evaluated by history and physical examination are as follows:

(1) Nature of discharge (serous, bloody, or other).

(2) Association with a mass or not.

(3) Unilateral or bilateral.

(4) Single duct or multiple duct discharge.

(5) Discharge is spontaneous (persistent or intermittent) or must be expressed.

(6) Discharge produced by pressure at a single site or by general pressure on the breast.

(7) Relation to menses.

(8) Premenopausal or postmenopausal.

(9) Patient taking contraceptive pills, or estrogen for postmenopausal symptoms.

Unilateral, spontaneous serous or serosanguineous discharge from a single duct is usually caused by an intraductal papilloma or, rarely, by an intraductal cancer. In either case, a mass may not be palpable. The involved duct may be identified by pressure at different sites around the nipple at the margin of the areola. Bloody discharge is more suggestive of cancer but is usually caused by a benign papilloma in the duct. Cytologic examination may identify malignant cells, but negative findings do not rule out cancer, which is more likely in women over age 50. In any case, the involved duct—and a mass if present—should be excised. Ductography may identify a filling defect prior to excision of the duct system.

In premenopausal women, spontaneous multiple duct discharge, unilateral or bilateral, most marked just before menstruation, is often due to mammary dysplasia. Discharge may be green or brownish. Papillomatosis and ductal ectasia are usually seen on biopsy. If a mass is present, it should be removed.

Milky discharge from multiple ducts in the nonlactating breast may occur in certain syndromes (Chiari-Frommel, Argonz-Del Castillo [Forbes-Albright]), presumably as a result of increased secretion of pituitary prolactin. Serum prolactin and TSH levels should be obtained to search for a pituitary tumor or hypothyroidism. Phenothiazines and contraceptive pills may also cause milky discharge that ceases on discontinuance of the medication.

Oral contraceptive agents may cause clear, serous, or milky discharge from a single duct, but multiple duct discharge is more common. The discharge is more evident just before menstruation and disappears on stopping the medication. If it does not and is from a single duct, exploration should be considered.

Purulent discharge may originate in a subareolar abscess and require excision of the abscess and related lactiferous sinus.

When localization is not possible and no mass is palpable, the patient should be reexamined every 2–3 months for 1 year. When unilateral discharge persists, even without definite localization or tumor, exploration must be considered. The alternative is careful follow-up at intervals of 2–3 months. Mammography should be done. Cytologic examination of nipple discharge for exfoliated cancer cells may rarely be helpful in diagnosis.

Chronic unilateral nipple discharge, especially if bloody, is an indication for resection of the involved ducts.

Jardines L: Management of nipple discharge. Am Surg 1996;62:119.

Taber SW: The clinical challenge of nipple discharge. J Ky Med Assoc 1996;94:387.

FAT NECROSIS

Fat necrosis is a rare lesion of the breast but is of clinical importance because it produces a mass, often accompanied by skin or nipple retraction, that is indistinguishable from carcinoma. Trauma is presumed to be the cause, though only about half of patients give a history of injury to the breast. Ecchymosis is occasionally seen near the tumor. Tenderness may or may not be present. If untreated, the mass associated with fat necrosis gradually disappears. As a rule, the safest course is to obtain a biopsy. The entire mass should be excised, primarily to rule out carcinoma. Fat necrosis is common after segmental resection and radiation therapy.

BREAST ABSCESS

During nursing, an area of redness, tenderness, and induration not infrequently develops in the breast. The organism most commonly found in these abscesses is *Staphylococcus aureus*. In the early stages, the infection can often be reversed while nursing is continued from that breast by administering an antibiotic such as dicloxacillin or oxacillin, 250 mg four times daily for 7–10 days. If the lesion progresses to form a localized mass with local and systemic signs of infection, an abscess is present and should be drained, and nursing should be discontinued.

A subareolar abscess may develop (rarely) in young or middle-aged women who are not lactating. These infections tend to recur after incision and drainage unless the area is explored in a quiescent interval with excision of the involved lactiferous duct or ducts at the base of the nipple. Except for the subareolar type of abscess, infection in the breast is very rare unless the patient is lactating. In the nonlactating breast, inflammatory carcinoma must always be considered. Therefore, findings suggestive of abscess in the nonlactating breast are an indication for incision and biopsy of any indurated tissue.

Schein M: Subareolar breast abscesses. Surgery 1996;120:902.

DISORDERS OF THE AUGMENTED BREAST

Since the development of the silicone breast implant in the early 1960s, augmentation mammoplasty has been performed on about 150,000 women per year, and nearly 4 million American women have breast implants. Breast augmentation is performed by placing implants usually under the pectoralis muscle or, less desirably, in the subcutaneous tissue. Most implants are made of an outer silicone shell filled with a silicone gel, saline, or a combination of the two. The most common problem with implants (15% of patients) is capsule contraction or scarring around the implant, leading to firmness and distortion of the breast, which can be painful. Some patient may require removal of the implant and capsule.

Reports suggesting an association between silicone gel prosthesis and autoimmune disease have caused many plastic surgeons to avoid this design. Implant rupture occurs in 5% of women, and bleeding of gel through the capsule may be more common. Although it has been postulated that silicone gel may serve as an adjuvant for autoimmune reactions, there are no data that prove the association Two large epidemiologic studies have shown no association between implants and an increased risk of breast cancer. Even so, the FDA has concluded that the safety and effectiveness of silicone gel breast implants has not been established and that additional studies are called for. They have advised women with ruptured implants to discuss the need for surgical removal with their physicians. They noted that in the absence of symptoms, the risk of removal was probably greater than the risk of retention. Most plastic surgeons now prefer saline-filled implants. Patients whose gel implant has ruptured or who have symptoms suggestive of an autoimmune disorder should consider having the device removed.

Breast cancer occasionally develops in a patient with augmentation mammoplasty. Diagnosis is more difficult because of the diminished ability of mammography to detect early lesions. Once a cancer develops, it should be treated in the same way as breast cancer in women without implants. These patients should be offered the option of mastectomy or breast-conserving therapy. Adjuvant treatments should be given upon the same indications as for those who have no implants.

Gabriel SE et al: Risk of connective-tissue diseases and other disorders after breast implantation. N Engl J Med 1994;330:1697.

Press RI et al: Antinuclear autoantibodies in women with silicone breast implants. Lancet 1992;340:1304.

Silver RM et al: Demonstration of silicon in sites of connective-tissue disease in patients with silicone-gel breast implants. Arch Dermatol 1993;129:63.

Thoracic Wall, Pleura, Mediastinum, & Lung

19

David Jablons, MD, Robert B. Cameron, MD, & Kevin Turley, MD

■ ANATOMY & PHYSIOLOGY

ANATOMY OF THE CHEST WALL & PLEURA

The chest wall is an airtight, expandable, cone-shaped cage. Lung ventilation occurs by generation of negative pressure within the thorax due to simultaneous expansion of the rib cage and downward diaphragmatic excursion.

The ventral wall of the bony thorax is the shortest dimension. It extends from the suprasternal notch to the xiphoid—a distance of approximately 18 cm. It is formed by the vertically aligned manubrium, sternum, and xiphoid and the costal cartilages of the first ten ribs. The sides of the chest wall consist of the upper ten ribs, which slope downward and forward from their posterior attachments. The posterior chest wall is formed by the 12 thoracic vertebrae, their transverse processes, and the 12 ribs (Figure 19–1). The upper ventral portion of the thoracic cage is covered by the clavicle and the subclavian vessels. Laterally, it is covered by the shoulder and axillary nerves and vessels; dorsally, it is covered by the scapula.

The superior aperture of the thorax (also called either the thoracic inlet or the thoracic outlet) is a 5- to 10-cm kidney-shaped opening bounded by the first costal cartilages and ribs laterally, the manubrium anteriorly, and the body of the first thoracic vertebra posteriorly. The inferior aperture of the thorax is bounded by the 12th vertebra and ribs posteriorly and the cartilages of the 7th to 12th ribs and the xiphisternal joint anteriorly. It is much wider than the superior aperture and is occupied by the diaphragm.

The blood supply and innervation of the chest wall are via the intercostal vessels and nerves (Figures 19–2 and 19–3), and the upper thorax also receives vessels and nerves from the cervical and axillary regions.

The parietal pleura is the innermost lining of the chest wall and is divided into four parts: the cervical pleura (cupula), costal pleura, mediastinal pleura, and diaphragmatic pleura. The visceral pleura is the serous layer investing the lungs and is continuous with the parietal pleura, joining it at the hilum of the lung. The potential pleural space is a capillary gap that normally contains only a few drops of serous fluid. This space may be enlarged when fluid (hydrothorax), blood (hemothorax), pus (pyothorax or empyema), or air (pneumothorax) is present.

PHYSIOLOGY OF THE CHEST WALL & PLEURA

Mechanics of Respiration

Breathing entails expansion of thoracic volume by elevation of the rib cage and descent of the diaphragm. The former predominates in men and the latter in women. In infants, because the ribs have not yet assumed their oblique contour, diaphragmatic breathing is required to provide sufficient ventilation.

Expiration is mainly passive and depends upon elastic recoil of the lungs except with deep breathing, when the abdominal musculature contracts, pulling the rib cage downward and simultaneously elevating the diaphragm by compressing the abdominal viscera against it.

Physiology of the Pleural Space

A. PRESSURE

The pleural cavity pressure is normally negative, owing to the elastic recoil of the lung and chest wall. During quiet respiration, it varies from –15 cm H_2O with inspiration to 0–2 cm H_2O during expiration. Deep breathing may cause large pressure changes (eg, –60 cm H_2O during forced inspiration to +30 cm H_2O during vigorous expiration). Because of gravity, pleural pressure at the apex is more negative when the body is erect and changes about 0.2 cm H_2O per centimeter of vertical height.

B. FLUID FORMATION AND REABSORPTION

Transudation and absorption of fluid within the pleural space normally follow the Starling equation, which depends on hydrostatic, colloid, and tissue pressures. In health, fluid is formed by the parietal pleura and ab-

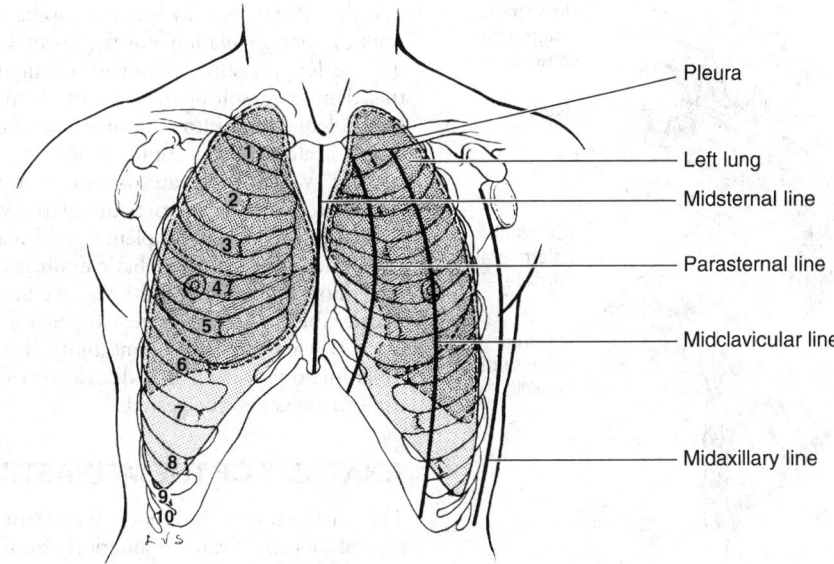

Figure 19–1. The thorax, showing rib cage, pleura, and lung fields.

sorbed by the visceral pleura (Figure 19–4). Systemic capillary hydrostatic pressure is 30 cm H_2O, and intrapleural negative pressure averages –5 cm H_2O. Together, these give a net hydrostatic pressure of 35 cm H_2O that causes fluid transudation from the parietal pleura. The colloid osmotic pressure of the systemic capillaries is 34 cm H_2O; this is opposed by 8 cm H_2O of pleural space osmotic pressure. Thus, a net 26 cm H_2O osmotic pressure draws fluid back into systemic capillaries. Systemic hydrostatic pressure (35 cm H_2O) exceeds osmotic capillary pressure (26 cm H_2O) by 9 cm H_2O; thus, there is a 9 cm H_2O net drive of fluid

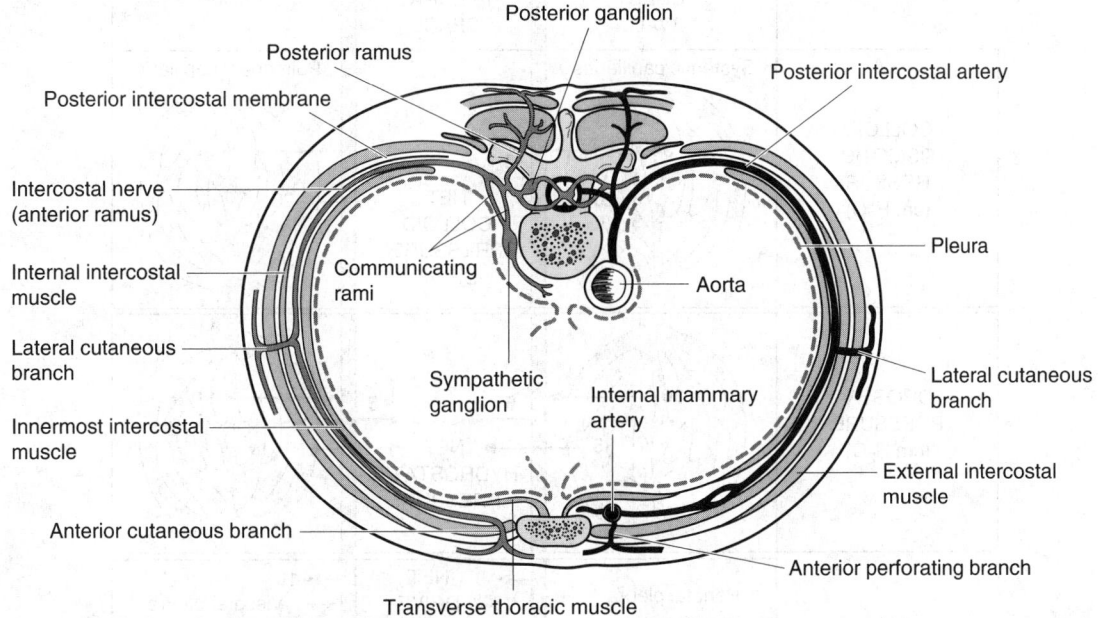

Figure 19–2. Transverse section of thorax.

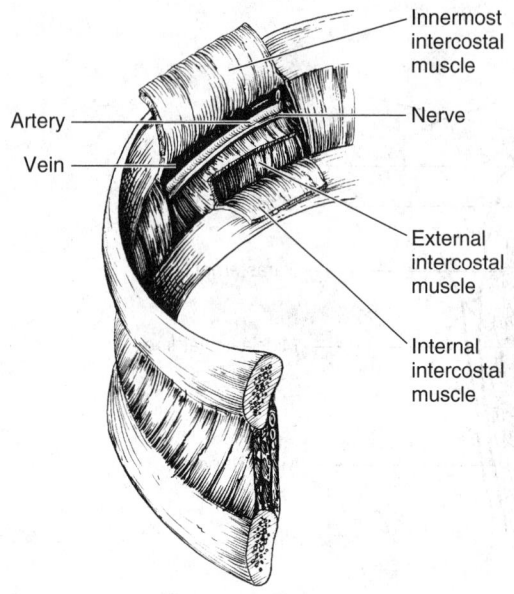

Figure 19–3. Intercostal muscles, vessels, and nerves.

into the pleural space by systemic capillaries in the chest wall. Similar calculations for the visceral pleura involving the low-pressure pulmonary circulation will show that there is a resulting net drive of 10 cm H_2O that attracts pleural fluid into pulmonary capillaries.

In health, pleural fluid is low in protein (100 mg/dL). When it increases in disease to about 1 g/dL, the net colloid osmotic pressure of the visceral pleural capillaries is equaled and pleural fluid reabsorption becomes dependent on lymphatic drainage. Thus, abnormal amounts of pleural fluid may accumulate (1) when hydrostatic pressure is increased, such as in heart failure; (2) when capillary permeability is increased, as in inflammatory or neoplastic disease; or (3) when colloid osmotic pressure is decreased.

ANATOMY OF THE MEDIASTINUM

The mediastinum is the compartment between the pleural cavities. It extends anteriorly from the suprasternal notch to the xiphoid process and posteriorly from the first to the eleventh thoracic vertebrae. Superiorly, fascial planes in the neck are in direct communication; inferiorly, the mediastinum is limited by the diaphragm, although extensions through diaphragmatic apertures communicate with retroperitoneal fascial planes.

Figure 19–4. Movement of fluid across the pleural space, showing production and absorption of pleural fluid.

In Burkell's classification (Figure 19–5), the **anterior mediastinum** contains the thymus gland, the lymph nodes, the ascending aorta and transverse aorta, the great vessels, and areolar tissue. The **middle mediastinum** contains the heart, the pericardium, the trachea, the hila of the lungs, the phrenic nerves, lymph nodes, and areolar tissue. The **posterior mediastinum** contains the sympathetic chains, the vagus nerves, the esophagus, the thoracic duct, lymph nodes, and the descending aorta.

Congenital abnormalities within the mediastinum are numerous. A defect in the anterior mediastinal pleura with communication of the right and left hemithorax is rare in humans. This retrosternal part of the anterior mediastinum is normally thin, and overexpansion of one pleural space may cause "mediastinal herniation" or a bulge of mediastinal pleura toward the opposite side.

Displacements of the mediastinum occur from masses or from accumulations of air, fluid, blood, chyle, etc, and can interfere with vital functions. Tracheal compression, vena caval obstruction, and esophageal obstructions cause clinical symptoms. The mediastinum can also be displaced laterally when pathologic processes of one hemithorax cause mediastinal shift. Fibrosis and previous pneumonectomy can shift the mediastinum toward the affected side. Open pneumothorax and massive hemothorax shift the mediastinum away from the affected side. Open pneumothorax produces alternating paradoxic mediastinal shifts with respiration and will adversely affect ventilation. Acute mediastinal displacement may produce hypoxia or reduced venous return and cause low cardiac output, tachycardia, dysrhythmias, hypotension, or cardiac arrest.

ANATOMY OF THE LUNG

See Figure 19–6 for lung anatomy.

The bronchopulmonary segments make up large lung units called lobes. The right lung has three lobes: upper, middle, and lower. The left lung consists of two lobes: upper and lower. On the left, the lingular portion of the upper lobe is the homolog of the right middle lobe. Two fissures separate the lobes on the right side. The major, or oblique, fissure divides the upper and middle lobes from the lower lobe. The minor, or horizontal, fissure separates the middle from the upper lobe. On the left side, the single oblique fissure separates the upper and lower lobes. These are the normal anatomic segments; embryologic defects such as situs inversus reverse this arrangement, and bilateral right-sided anatomy (asplenia) or bilateral

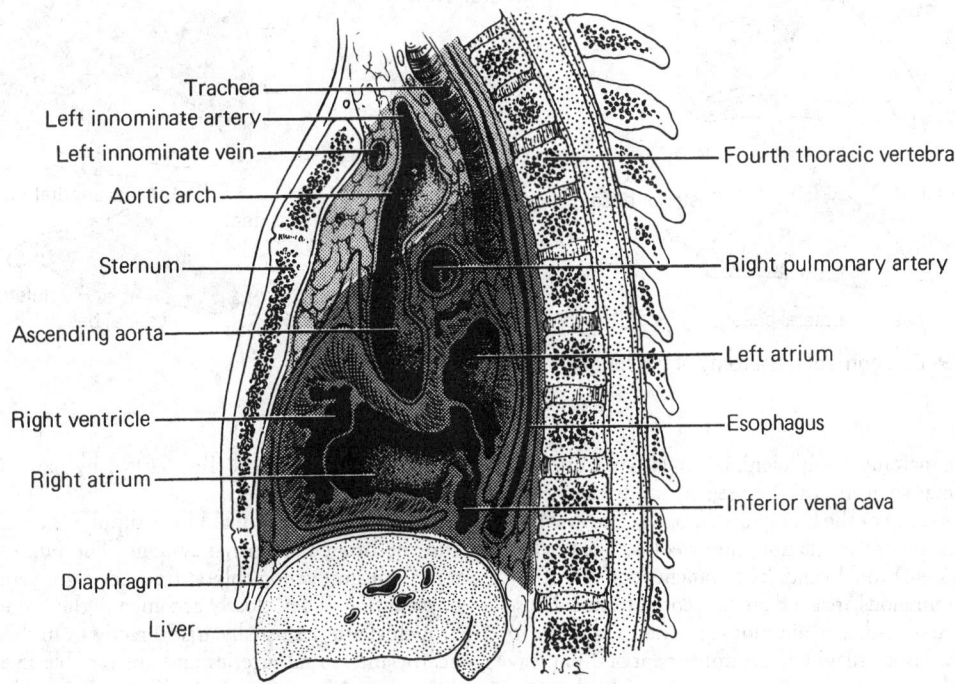

Figure 19–5. Divisions of the mediastinum (Burkell's classification). Light screening: anterior mediastinum; lower dark screening: middle mediastinum; dotted area at right: posterior mediastinum.

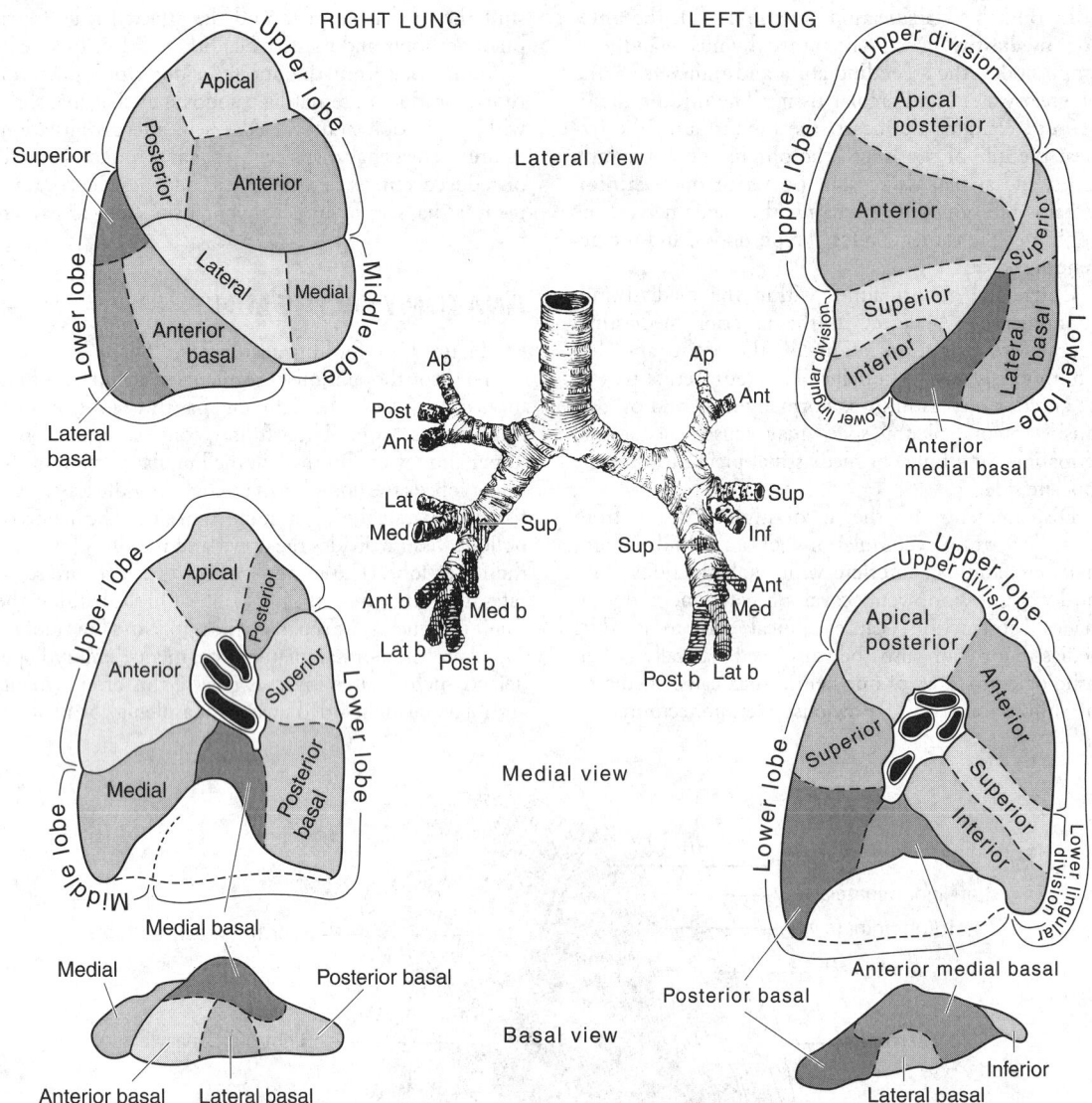

Figure 19–6. Segmental anatomy of the lungs.

left-sided anatomy (polysplenia) can also occur. The parenchymal anatomy can be seen by studying the sequential division of the bronchopulmonary tree down to the smallest unit of ventilation, the alveolus. The trachea and main stem bronchi and their branches contain a posterior membranous area and are prevented from collapsing by horseshoe-shaped anterior segments of cartilage in their walls. The cartilaginous reinforcement of the airway gradually becomes less complete as the branches become smaller, and reinforcement ceases with bronchi of 1–2 mm. The bronchopulmonary segmental anatomy is designated by numbers (Boyden) or by name (Jackson and Huber).

The lungs have a dual blood supply: the pulmonary and the bronchial arterial systems. The pulmonary arteries transmit venous blood from the right ventricle for oxygenation. They closely accompany the bronchi. The bronchial arteries usually arise directly from the aorta or nearby intercostal arteries and are variable in number. They transmit oxygenated blood at systemic arterial pressure to the bronchial wall to the level of the terminal bronchioles.

The pulmonary veins travel in the interlobar septa and do not correspond to the distribution of the bronchi or the pulmonary arteries.

THE LYMPHATIC SYSTEM

The lymphatics travel in intersegmental septa centrally as well as to the parenchymal surface to form subpleural networks. Drainage continues toward the hilum in channels that follow the bronchi and pulmonary arteries. The lymphatics eventually enter lymph nodes in the major fissures of the lungs, the hilum, and the paratracheal regions.

The direction of lymphatic drainage—irrespective of the primary site—is cephalad and usually ipsilateral, but contralateral flow may occur from any lobe. The lymphatics from the left lower lobe may be almost equally distributed to the left and right; from the left upper lobe, distribution is often to the anterior mediastinal group. Otherwise, the usual sequence of lymphatic spread of pulmonary cancer is first to the regional parabronchial nodes and then to the ipsilateral paratracheal, subcarinal, scalene, or inferior deep cervical nodes.

■ DIAGNOSTIC STUDIES

Skin Tests

Skin tests are used in the diagnosis of tuberculosis, histoplasmosis, and coccidioidomycosis. Tuberculin testing is usually done with purified protein derivative (PPD) injected intradermally. Intermediate-strength PPD should be used in patients who seem likely to have active disease. Induration of 10 mm or more at the injection site after 48–72 hours is called positive and indicates either active or arrested disease. Mumps antigen is usually placed on the opposite forearm to test for anergy. Because false-negative reactions are rare, a negative test fairly reliably rules out tuberculosis. Skin tests for histoplasmosis and coccidioidomycosis are performed in a similar way, but skin tests for fungal infections are unreliable and serologic tests should be performed instead.

Endoscopy

A. LARYNGOSCOPY

Indirect laryngoscopy is used to assess vocal cord mobility in patients suspected of having lung carcinoma, especially when there has been a voice change. It should be performed also to search for an otherwise occult source for malignant cells in sputum or metastases in cervical lymph nodes.

B. BRONCHOSCOPY

Roentgenographic evidence of bronchial obstruction, unresolved pneumonia, foreign body, suspected carcinoma, undiagnosed hemoptysis, aspiration pneumonia, and lung abscess are only a few of the indications for bronchoscopy. The procedure can be done using either the standard hollow metal (rigid) or the flexible fiberoptic bronchoscope under local or general anesthesia. Rigid bronchoscopy must be done under general anesthesia and is most often used for clearing major airways of bulky obstructing lesions such as tumors or foreign bodies. Furthermore, laser treatment of airway obstruction from endobronchial tumor typically necessitates the use of rigid bronchoscopy.

Flexible bronchoscopy is a highly effective diagnostic and therapeutic tool. Almost invariably, with proper technique it can and should be performed under local and intravenous sedation only. Washings are usually obtained for bacterial or fungal culture and cytologic examination. Visible lesions are biopsied directly, and biopsy specimens are sometimes taken from the carina even though it appears normal. Brush biopsies are obtained from specific bronchopulmonary segments. Occasionally, transcarinal needle biopsy of a subcarinal node is obtained. Thirty to 50 percent of lung tumors are visible bronchoscopically. Brushing, random biopsies, and sputum cytology may still yield a positive diagnosis of cancer or tuberculosis in the absence of a visible lesion. The yield is influenced by size, location, and histologic cell type of the lesion.

Properly performed mediastinoscopy samples nodes from at least three stations, including ipsilateral and contralateral paratracheal levels 2, 3, and 4 and subcarinal level 7.

Mediastinoscopy

Cervical mediastinoscopy is performed through a small (3–4 cm) incision one fingerbreadth above the sternal notch. The dissection is done beneath the pretracheal fascia, which allows access to mediastinal nodes and avoids major vascular structures. After palpation, the mediastinoscope can be safely inserted and nodes biopsied under direct vision. With experience and careful dissection, nodes can be biopsied directly and safely. Unclear structures can be aspirated prior to attempted biopsy.

Enlarged lymph nodes in the aorticopulmonary window are technically inaccessible by means of standard cervical mediastinoscopy. Extended cervical mediastinoscopy, however, is a technique that provides access to these aorticopulmonary window nodes. It is performed through the same small neck incision as standard mediastinoscopy except the dissection is carried laterally beside the left carotid artery toward and then over the aorta into the aorticopulmonary space. In older patients with densely calcific aortas, extended mediastinoscopy is contraindicated because of the risk of embolic phenomena from aortic manipulation.

The complications of mediastinoscopy are minimal (< 1–2%). Major bleeding complications requiring sternotomy or thoracotomy for repair are infrequent (1–2%). Other possible complications include pneumothorax, recurrent nerve injury, infection, and esophageal injury.

Mediastinoscopy is almost invariably accurate in the diagnosis of sarcoidosis. It is also useful to diagnose tuberculosis, histoplasmosis, Castleman's silicosis, metastatic carcinoma, lymphoma, and carcinoma of the esophagus. It should not be used in the investigation of primary mediastinal tumors, which should be approached by an incision permitting definitive excision.

Chamberlain Procedure

Anterior mediastinotomy (the Chamberlain procedure) is used to sample nodes and biopsy tissue in the anterior mediastinum and most commonly in the aorticopulmonary window. A small (3–4 cm.) incision is made over the second or third interspace on the appropriate side of the lesion. The mediastinum is approached through the interspace directly or after excising the costochondral cartilage using either the mediastinoscope or open technique. Careful attention is paid to preserving the mammary vessels encountered in the dissection. The mediastinum is approached extrapleurally unless lesions specifically within the thorax—effusions, tumors invading the hilum or chest wall—need to be investigated. Furthermore, if additional access is required to facilitate the dissection or to treat a complication, the incision can be converted easily to a larger anterior thoracotomy.

Complications resulting from anterior mediastinotomy are similar to those encountered with cervical mediastinoscopy and include bleeding, recurrent nerve injury, and infection, among others. Major morbidity should be less than 1–2%.

Video-Assisted Thoracoscopic Surgery (VATS)

With the advent of sophisticated video technology and optics, video-assisted thoracoscopic surgery (VATS) has evolved as an important tool in thoracic surgery. While thoracoscopic procedures have been used for many years, powerful new video cameras and improved instruments as well as increasing surgeon familiarity with minimally invasive surgery have made VATS increasingly popular and useful.

VATS plays an important role in the diagnosis and staging of thoracic malignancies (lung cancer, mesothe-

lioma, etc) as well as in the resection of isolated peripheral pulmonary nodules and bullous lung disease. Furthermore, it has been an advance in lung biopsy and pleurodesis procedures.

However, even though significant data have been generated about the use of VATS for lung cancer, most thoracic surgeons believe it is suboptimal. It can hamper the surgeon's ability to perform a complete resection and thus jeopardize the chance for cure. Full mediastinal lymph node dissections are not obtainable with standard VATS. Even for metastasectomy, concerns over pleural and chest wall seeding with VATS are documented in the literature, highlighting the need for assiduous attention to detail during these procedures. Furthermore, the inability to "feel" for subtle occult parenchymal lesions when using VATS techniques has dampened enthusiasm for its widespread acceptance in pulmonary metastasectomy.

Where VATS has been an important advance is in the treatment of benign processes, including spontaneous pneumothoraces and pleural effusions, as well for thoracic sympathectomy and thoracic vertebral discectomy.

As instruments and techniques have evolved, complications from VATS procedures—persistent air leaks, hemorrhage, tumor seeding, etc—have decreased. Overall, major complication rates of 1–2% are reported. Disadvantages of VATS include the need for general anesthesia and single lung ventilation. Faster patient recovery and decreased pain are touted as major advantages of VATS, although the qualitative differences between these approaches and formal thoracotomy using muscle-sparing incisions and thoracic epidural analgesia are less clear than initially expected.

Scalene Lymph Node Biopsy

Scalene lymph node biopsy has been largely replaced by mediastinoscopy in the evaluation of pulmonary disease since it offers the same information but is less reliable and does not evaluate nodes within the mediastinum. Furthermore, scalene lymph nodes are accessible via cervical mediastinoscopy using the mediastinoscope. In the evaluation of lung cancer, about 15% of scalene node biopsies are positive when the cervical nodes are not palpable compared with 85% when the nodes are palpable. The risk of major complications is about 5%. Deaths are rare.

Pleural Biopsy

A. NEEDLE BIOPSY

This procedure is indicated when the cause of a pleural effusion cannot be determined by analysis of the fluid or when tuberculosis is suspected. Any one of three needles can be used: Vim-Silverman, Cope, or Abrams

(Harefield). A definitive diagnosis can be obtained in 60–80% of cases of tuberculosis or cancer. The principal complication is pneumothorax. Five to 10 percent of biopsy specimens are inadequate for diagnosis.

B. OPEN BIOPSY

Open pleural biopsy is especially useful in those patients without pleural effusion or when needle biopsy has failed. The quality of the specimen and the likelihood of its representing the pathology are better with open biopsy than with needle biopsy, but open biopsy is a more extensive procedure.

Lung Biopsy

A. NEEDLE BIOPSY

The indications for percutaneous needle biopsy are not well established. It may be indicated in diffuse parenchymal disease and in some patients with localized lesions. The diagnosis of interstitial pneumonia, carcinoma, sarcoidosis, hypersensitivity lung disease, lymphoma, pulmonary alveolar proteinosis, and miliary tuberculosis has been established by this method.

Needle biopsies are done by any of three techniques: by aspiration with a cutting needle, by trephine, or by air drill. Needle biopsy of the lung is also possible by a transbronchial technique in which a modified Vim-Silverman or ultrathin needle is used.

There is controversy concerning the risks of spreading the tumor by needle biopsy in localized disease. Complications following percutaneous needle biopsy include pneumothorax (5–30%), hemothorax, hemoptysis, and air embolism. Pulmonary hypertension or cysts and bullae are contraindications. Several deaths have been reported. There is about a 60% chance of obtaining useful information.

B. OPEN BIOPSY

A limited intercostal or anterior parasternal incision is used to remove a 3- to 4-cm wedge of lung tissue in diffuse parenchymal lung disease. The site of incision is selected for accessibility and potential diagnostic value. The incision is generally made at the fifth interspace on the right at the anterior axillary line to allow for access to all three lobes for biopsy—or at the lower lobes bilaterally. The middle lobe and lingula are selected in specific cases when pathology exists only in these areas, as they generally yield results of the poorest quality. Open lung biopsy is associated with a lower death rate, fewer complications, and greater diagnostic yield than needle biopsy. It is especially useful in critically ill, immunosuppressed patients for differentiation of infectious infiltrative lesions from neoplastic infiltrative lesions. When a focal lesion is biopsied, a larger incision is used. Peripheral lesions are totally excised by wedge or seg-

mental resection, and deeply placed lesions are removed by lobectomy in suitable candidates. Thoracoscopy or VATS has become the procedure of choice for open lung biopsy in patients who can tolerate single lung ventilation.

Sputum Analysis

Exfoliative sputum cytology is most valuable for detection of lung cancer. Specimens are obtained by deep coughing or by abrasion with a brush, or bronchial washings are obtained by either bronchoscopic or percutaneous transtracheal washing techniques. Specimens should be collected in the morning and delivered to the laboratory promptly. Centrifugation or filtration can be used to concentrate the cellular elements.

In primary lung cancer, sputum cytology is positive in 30–60% of cases. Repeated sputum examination improves the diagnostic return. Examination of the first bronchoscopic washing material yields a diagnosis in 60% of cases. Postbronchoscopy sputum analysis should always be made at 6–12 and 24 hours, as findings may be positive at these times when previous tests were negative.

Newer technologies, including better sputum-inducing agents, are currently in clinical trials and appear effective. Also, more sophisticated cytologic analysis using immunohistochemistry to molecular markers (cytokeratins, hnRNP, etc) has improved accuracy and sensitivity and the ability to detect premalignant lesions.

Computed Tomography (CT Scan)

Computed tomography can accurately distinguish between aneurysmal dilation of the aorta and other lesions as the cause of a mediastinal mass. It is helpful in delineating fluid collections within the thoracic cavity and can be used to differentiate between empyema and parenchymal abscess of the lung. Metastases to the lung are more readily demonstrated by CT scan than by other techniques. Pulmonary infarcts can be detected in some cases when plain films of the chest are equivocal. CT scanning is of significant use in the staging of carcinoma, and it has proved to be of great value in defining the extent of metastatic disease. Regardless of CT findings, however, surgical staging (mediastinoscopy) is imperative in the treatment of patients with cancer.

Magnetic Resonance Imaging (MRI)

Magnetic resonance imaging uses radio waves in a magnetic field to produce images that can distinguish between tumor, cyst, normal tissues, and flowing blood. Although its major value in the thorax has been in cardiovascular imaging, it has been moderately helpful in showing invasion of lung cancer into the chest wall, vertebrae, and spinal cord as well as mediastinal structures.

Position Emission Tomography (PET)

PET has become an important tool in staging and workup of the cancer patient. PET scanners are becoming more widely available, and preliminary data suggest that PET scanning will identify unsuspected regional or distant disease in 20–30% of patients with lung cancer or esophageal cancer compared with conventional methods (CT, bone scan). Combined with CT scanning, PET scanning is highly accurate (> 90%), but by itself it has a 10–20% false-positive rate in the mediastinum. Therefore, interpretations of PET results must be accepted with caution and must be confirmed by surgical staging when inconsistent with the overall clinical picture.

■ DISEASES OF THE CHEST WALL

Anatomic developmental defects are described in Chapter 46. Neuromuscular syndromes of the inlet or shoulder are described in Chapter 35. Injuries to the chest wall are described in Chapter 14.

LUNG HERNIA

A lung hernia results from a defect in the chest wall caused by abnormal development, trauma, or surgery. Most lung hernias are thoracic in location, but cervical (defects of Sibson's fascia) or diaphragmatic herniation may occur occasionally. Lung hernias are usually asymptomatic, but some patients experience local tenderness, pain, or mild dyspnea. Operative repair rather than external support produces optimal results if symptoms are present.

CHEST WALL INFECTIONS

Infections that appear to involve only the skin and soft tissues may actually represent outward extensions of deeper infection of the ribs, cartilage, sternum, or even the pleural space (empyema necessitatis). Inadequate drainage of superficial infection can lead to inward extension into the pleural space, causing empyema.

Subpectoral abscess is caused by suppurative adenitis of the axillary lymph nodes, rib or pleural infection, or posterior extension of a breast abscess—or it may occur as a complication of chest wall surgery (eg, mastectomy, pacemaker placement). Symptoms include systemic sepsis, erythema, induration of the pectoral region, and obliteration of the normal infraclavicular depression. Shoulder movement is painful. Organisms most commonly involved include hemolytic streptococci and *Staphylococcus aureus.* Treatment involves incisional drainage along the lateral border of the pectoralis major muscle and administration of antibiotics.

Subscapular abscess may arise from osteomyelitis of the scapula but most commonly follows thoracic operations such as thoracotomy or thoracoplasty. Winging of the scapula or paravertebral induration of the trapezius muscle is usually present. A pleural communication is suggested if a cough impulse is present or if the size of the mass varies with position or direct pressure. The diagnosis is established by needle aspiration. Open drainage is indicated for pyogenic infections not involving the pleural space. Tubercular lesions should be treated by chemotherapy and needle aspiration, if possible.

Osteomyelitis of the Ribs

In the past, osteomyelitis of the ribs was often caused by typhoid fever and tuberculosis. Except in children, hematogenous osteomyelitis is a rare problem today. Thoracotomy incisions may result in osteomyelitis.

Sternal Osteomyelitis

Infection of the sternum most commonly follows median sternotomy incisions, especially in diabetics in whom bilateral internal mammary arteries have been used in coronary bypass grafting. It presents as a postoperative wound infection or mediastinitis. Treatment consists of either open drainage or a closed irrigation drainage system with antibiotics as well as systemic antibiotics. Resection of the involved sternum and a margin of adjacent normal bone may be necessary.

Gallium or PET scanning may be helpful adjuncts to making the diagnosis. Occasionally, sternal osteomyelitis will be due to tuberculosis.

Infection of the Costal Cartilages & Xiphoid

Costal cartilage infections are relatively unresponsive to antibiotic therapy because once perichondral vascularity is interrupted, the cartilage dies and remains as a foreign body to perpetuate the infection and sinus tract formation. The infection may be established during the course of septicemia, but the most common cause is direct extension of other surgical infections (eg, wound infection, subphrenic abscess). Surgical division of costal cartilages, as in a thoracoabdominal incision, may predispose to cartilage infection postoperatively if local sepsis develops. A wide variety of organisms have been implicated.

Erythema and induration with fluctance and often spontaneous drainage can occur. The course can be fulminant or may be indolent over months or years, with periodic exacerbations. Associated osteomyelitis of the sternum, ribs, or clavicle may occur.

The differential diagnosis includes local bone or cartilage tumors, Tietze's syndrome, chest wall metastasis, eroding aortic aneurysm, and bronchocutaneous fistula.

The treatment of choice includes resection of the involved cartilage and adjacent involved bony structures. Recurrence is due to underestimation of the extent of disease and inadequate resection.

Reconstruction of the Chest Wall

Chest wall reconstruction may be necessary following trauma, surgical resection, or infectious processes. Recent advances in the use of musculocutaneous flaps and the supportive use of methyl methacrylate and Marlex mesh to produce solidity below these muscular flaps have facilitated repairs. In massive chest wall defects, vascularization of the area is essential and can be accomplished by use of omental flaps as well as pectoralis, latissimus dorsi, and rectus flaps. Microsurgical techniques for repair of such defects have greatly expanded the ability of plastic surgeons to deal with extensive resectional and infective processes.

Adler BD, Padley SP, Muller NL: Tuberculosis of the chest wall: CT findings. J Comput Assist Tomogr 1993;17:271.

Mansour KA, Anderson TM, Hester TR: Sternal resection and reconstruction. Ann Thorac Surg 1993;55:838.

Pairolero PC, Arnold PG, Harris JB: Long-term results of pectoralis major muscle transposition for infected sternotomy wounds. Ann Surg 1991;213:583.

Siegman-Igra Y et al: Serious infectious complications of midsternotomy: a review of bacteriology and antimicrobial therapy. Scand J Infect Dis 1990;22:633.

Slaughter MS et al: a fifteen-year wound surveillance study after coronary artery bypass. Ann Thorac Surg 1993;56:1063.

TIETZE'S SYNDROME

Tietze's syndrome is a painful nonsuppurative inflammation of the costochondral cartilages and is of unknown cause. Recent evidence suggests that costochondritis may represent a manifestation of seronegative rheumatic disease. Local swelling and tenderness are the only symptoms; they usually disappear without therapy. The syndrome may recur.

Several recent reports have suggested the use of bone scintigraphy and chest CT for diagnosis of infected costochondritis. Bone scanning was effective in localizing and identifying inflamed costochondral junctions.

Chest CT was less sensitive in one study. Furthermore, in a small study of patients with Tietze's syndrome, transthoracic echo was able to demonstrate a dishomogeneous increase in echogenicity in the pathologically involved cartilage. Treatment is symptomatic and may include analgesics (NSAIDs) and local or systemic corticosteroids. When symptoms persist longer than 3 weeks and tumefaction suggests neoplasm, excision of the involved cartilage may be indicated and is usually curative.

Aeschlimann A, Kahn MF: Tietze's syndrome: a critical review. Clin Exper Rheumatol 1990;8:407.

MONDOR'S DISEASE (Thrombophlebitis of the Thoracoepigastric Vein)

Mondor's disease consists of localized thrombophlebitis of the anterolateral chest wall. It is more prominent in women than in men and occasionally follows radical mastectomy. There are few symptoms other than the presence of a localized tender, cord-like structure in the subcutaneous tissues of the abdomen, thorax, or axilla. The disease is self-limited and devoid of complications such as thromboembolism. The possibility of an infective origin or stasis of the interrupted venous return due to neoplasm must be ruled out.

Bejanga BI: Mondor's disease: analysis of 30 cases. J R Coll Surg Edinb 1992;37:322.

CHEST WALL TUMORS

Chest wall tumors may be simulated by enlarged costal cartilages, chest wall infection, fractures, rickets, scurvy, hyperparathyroidism, and other conditions. Most commonly, chest wall lesions present as a mass with localized or referred pain; less than 25% are asymptomatic. According to most series, approximately 60% of all chest wall masses prove to be malignant. Lesions arise from one of the three components of the chest wall, including soft tissues (muscle, nerve, fascia), bone, and cartilage.

The majority of tumors arise from bone or cartilage. Rib involvement is significantly more common than sternal presentation. Chest CT offers the most information for diagnosis and staging, especially with respect to pulmonary metastases, since most chest wall malignancies are sarcomas with a propensity for hematogenous spread to the lungs. Simple chest x-rays may initially identify a mass, especially if it is calcified. Bone scans should be obtained in all cases.

Initial diagnosis is obtained by limited incisional biopsy (transverse) if the mass is large (> 4 cm). Smaller lesions are excised en bloc, ensuring negative margins, with full knowledge that a malignancy is present in many cases. Classic teaching has been to perform en bloc wide local excisions with immediate reconstruction for all lesions at initial presentations. Progress with adjuvant multimodality therapy, however, for tumors such as rhabdomyosarcomas and Ewing's sarcoma supports the use of initial limited biopsy for tissue diagnosis to guide treatment planning.

Specific Neoplasms

A. BENIGN SOFT TISSUE TUMORS

1. Lipomas—Lipomas are the most common benign tumors of the chest wall. Occasionally they are very large and lobulated, and they may have dumbbell-shaped extensions that indent the endothoracic fascia beneath the sternum through a vertebral foramen. They may on occasion communicate with a large mediastinal or supraclavicular component.

2. Neurogenic tumors—These may arise from intercostal or superficial nerves. Solitary neurofibromas are most common, followed by neurolemmomas.

3. Cavernous hemangiomas—Hemangiomas of the thoracic wall are usually painful and occur in children. Tumors may be isolated or may involve other tissues (eg, lung), as in Rendu-Osler-Weber syndrome.

4. Lymphangiomas—This rare lesion is seen most often in children. It may have poorly defined borders that make complete excision difficult.

B. MALIGNANT SOFT TISSUE TUMORS

Malignant soft tissue tumors of the chest represent a significant percentage (40–50%) of all malignant chest wall masses, yet overall they represent only a small percentage (5%) of all malignant soft tissue sarcomas. Survival is determined by the histologic grade, the completeness of resection, and the presence and development of metastases (synchronous or metachronous). Low-grade tumors have 5-year and 10-year survivals approaching 90% and 82%, respectively. With high-grade lesions, however, 5-year survival rates are only 30–50%. The development of metastasis greatly reduces the chances of survival.

Treatment is directed at complete resection with emphasis on achieving negative margins (1–2 cm). En bloc resection techniques include raising skin flaps and reconstruction with soft tissue flaps, Marlex mesh, and methyl methacrylate to correct chest wall deformity and prevent paradoxic chest movement.

Various histologic subtypes of soft tissue sarcoma are encountered. Typically, low-grade sarcomas include desmoids or liposarcomas with low-grade features. Next most frequently seen are malignant fibrosarcoma, rhab-

domyosarcoma, and malignant fibrous histiocytoma, which are usually high-grade lesions.

Individual histologic subtype is not by itself a significant prognostic variable, but histologic grade does have that role. Metastases—either synchronous or metachronous—are commonly to the lungs (75%) and should be resected if negative margins can be achieved and adequate lung function preserved. Therapy for low-grade lesions should consist of complete resection. Incompletely resected lesions can be treated with external beam radiation therapy. High-grade lesions should be resected and patients enrolled into clinical trials evaluating the efficacy of systemic adjuvant chemotherapy. Postoperative radiotherapy is often helpful in the setting of close margins or questionable tumor soilage.

1. Fibrosarcomas—Fibrosarcoma is the most common primary soft tissue cancer of the chest wall. It occurs most frequently in young adults.

2. Liposarcomas—These tumors account for approximately one-third of all primary cancers of the chest wall. They occur more often in men.

3. Neurofibrosarcomas—These tumors involve the thoracic wall almost twice as often as other parts of the body. They often occur in patients with Recklinghausen's disease and usually originate from intercostal nerves. Overall, they are rare.

C. BENIGN SKELETAL TUMORS

1. Chondromas, osteochondromas, and myxochondromas—The combined frequency of these three cartilaginous tumors is nearly the same as that of fibrous dysplasia (ie, they comprise about 30–45% of all benign skeletal tumors). Cartilaginous tumors are usually single and occur with equal frequency in males and females between childhood and the fourth decade. The tumors are usually painless and tend to occur anteriorly along the costal margin or in the parasternal area. Wide local excision is curative.

2. Fibrous dysplasia—Fibrous dysplasia (bone cyst, osteofibroma, fibrous osteoma, fibrosis ossificans) accounts for a third or more of benign skeletal tumors of the chest wall. This cystic bone tumor can occur in any portion of the skeletal system, but approximately half involve the ribs. They may be clinically differentiated from cystic bone lesions associated with hyperparathyroidism. The tumor is usually single and may be related to trauma. Some patients complain of swelling, tenderness, or vague pain or discomfort, but the lesion is usually silent and is detected on routine chest x-ray. Treatment consists of local excision.

3. Eosinophilic granuloma—Eosinophilic granuloma may occur in the clavicle, the scapula, or (rarely) the sternum. Coexisting infiltrates of the lung are often present. This condition often represents a more benign form of Letterer-Siwe disease or Hand-Schüller-Christian disease. Fever, malaise, leukocytosis, eosinophilia, or bone pain may be present. Rib involvement presents as a swelling with cortical bone destruction and periosteal new growth. The clinical picture can resemble osteomyelitis or Ewing's sarcoma. When the disease is localized, excision will result in cure.

4. Hemangioma—Cavernous hemangioma of the ribs presents as a painful mass in infancy or childhood. The tumor appears on chest x-ray either as multiple radiolucent areas or as a single trabeculated cyst.

5. Miscellaneous—Fibromas, lipomas, osteomas, and aneurysmal bone cysts are all relatively rare lesions of the skeletal chest wall. The diagnosis is established after excisional biopsy.

D. MALIGNANT SKELETAL TUMORS

1. Chondrosarcomas—Chondrosarcomas are the most common primary malignant tumor of the chest wall (20–40%). They can involve the sternum but more commonly develop from the costochondral junctions of the ribs. The first four ribs are commonly affected. About 15–20% of all skeletal chondrosarcomas occur in the ribs or sternum. Most appear in patients 20–40 years of age. They occur most commonly at the costochondral junction of the rib cage but may occur anywhere along the rib. Local involvement of pleura, adjacent ribs, muscle, diaphragm, or other soft tissue may develop. Pain is rare, however, and most patients complain only of the mass. Chest x-ray shows destroyed cortical bone, usually with diffuse mottled calcification, and the border of the tumor is indistinct. Successful treatment necessitates wide local excision and en bloc resection to achieve negative margins. Incomplete excision carries a significantly worse prognosis. Overall survival, as in all soft tissue sarcomas, is heavily dependent on the histologic grade. Low-grade chondrosarcoma completely resected has a 60–80% 5-year survival rate. Patients with high-grade lesions who subsequently develop distant metastasis have only 20–30% 5-year survivals.

The pattern of first recurrence is important since local recurrence portends future metastatic disease and poor survival. Yet complete resection can often be curative. Therefore, even in the setting of large tumors (> 15–20 cm), resection should be considered even when it necessitates removal of more than six to eight ribs. With advances in epidural pain control and immediate reconstruction techniques, most patients will do surprisingly well. Despite large chest wall resections, most patients can be immediately extubated and will not suffer drastic changes in pulmonary function or chest wall dynamics.

2. Osteogenic sarcoma (osteosarcoma)—Osteosarcoma occurs in the second and third decades, and 60% of cases occur in men. It is more malignant than chondrosarcoma. X-ray findings consist of bone destruction and recalcification at right angles to the bony cortex, which gives the characteristic "sunburst" appearance. Osteogenic sarcoma presents commonly as an extremity lesion, with only a small percentage of cases being truncal primaries. Overall, less than 5% of all osteogenic sarcomas arise in the chest wall. Osteogenic sarcoma occurs in the second to fourth decades of life, half-again more commonly in men than in women. Typically, they are more aggressive tumors with a propensity for early metastasis to lung and bone.

Osteogenic sarcoma should be considered a systemic disease upon presentation, and treatment should consist of wide local excision and postoperative chemotherapy. The number of primary osteogenic sarcomas of the chest wall is small, and for that reason it is difficult to draw conclusions about definitive therapy. In the series with the most patients (n = 38), overall 5-year survival after complete resection and postoperative chemotherapy was only 15%.

As in all sarcomas, development of metastasis markedly decreases survival. In osteogenic sarcoma, 60–70% of resected primary cancers will ultimately develop metastasis. While prospective randomized trials of adjuvant chemotherapy are needed, most investigators agree that the current best therapy for osteogenic sarcoma of the chest wall includes resection followed by postoperative chemotherapy.

3. Myeloma (solitary plasmacytoma)—Solitary plasmacytomas of the chest wall are comparatively rare lesions. They constitute 5–20% of all chest wall tumors. Radiologically, they present as classic "punched-out" lytic lesions without evidence of new bone formation. While they are more common in men than in women and typically present in the fifth to seventh decades of life, age and sex are not significant prognostic variables.

Over three-fourths of the time, solitary chest wall plasmacytomas are harbingers of diffuse multiple myeloma. Survival is based on the development of systemic disease. Surgery plays a role in diagnosis. Incisional biopsy is performed unless the lesion is small (< 3 cm) and can be full excised. Local control and relief of pain are achieved with radiation therapy (usually 3000–4600 cGy). Once systemic disease is diagnosed, treatment consists of chemotherapy. Overall, 5-year and 10-year survivals for solitary plasmacytomas of the chest wall are 35–40% and 15–20%, respectively. Typical median survivals after treatment with radiation therapy and chemotherapy average 56 months.

4. Ewing's sarcoma (hemangioendothelioma, endothelioma)—Ewing's sarcoma accounts for 10–15%

of all primary chest wall tumors. Presentation as a primary chest lesion is not common (< 15%). Typically, Ewing's sarcoma presents as a large, warm, painful soft tissue mass usually associated with pleural effusion. Systemic symptoms such as fever, malaise, and weight loss are common. Radiologic studies demonstrate the classic "onion skin" appearance caused by widening and sclerosis of the cortex as multiple layers of new bone are produced.

Diagnosis can be made usually by fine-needle aspirate or incisional biopsy. Histologically, these tumors are unique and consist of broad sheets of small polyhedral cells with pale cytoplasm and small hyperchromatic nuclei. They stain periodic acid-Schiff-positive.

Ewing's sarcoma is commonly a disease of childhood and adolescence although in several studies, age and gender were not significant prognostic indicators. The most important prognostic indicator for survival was development of distant metastases. Current therapy after diagnosis by needle or incisional biopsy consists of chemotherapy (including cyclophosphamide, dactinomycin, doxorubicin, vincristine) followed by local radiation (5000 cGy) or surgical resection. Some data suggest that better long-term survival may be achieved by resection following chemotherapy. Overall, 5-year survivals range from 15% to 48%. Long-term survivals (10 years) are achievable by patients who do not develop metastases.

5. Lymphoma—The diagnosis and treatment of chest wall lymphomas are essentially the same as for those lesions found elsewhere in the body.

E. METASTATIC CHEST WALL TUMORS

Metastases to bones of the thorax are often multiple and are usually from tumors of the kidney, thyroid, lung, breast, prostate, stomach, uterus, or colon (Figure 19–7). Renal cell and thyroid malignancies have a high propensity for metastasizing to the sternum. Occasionally, they will present as pulsatile masses due to the excessive vascularity of the metastasis. An aneurysm of the ascending thoracic aorta, while rare, must be considered in the differential diagnosis and ruled out prior to attempts at excisional biopsy. Involvement by direct extension occurs in carcinoma of the breast and lung. Primary lung cancer with direct extension to chest wall without nodal involvement (T3 N0) carries a reasonable 5-year survival (40–50%) when treated with radical en bloc resection. Lung metastasis with direct chest wall extension should be treated with radical en bloc resection of the chest wall and underlying lung.

Brodsky JT et al: Desmoid tumors of the chest wall: a locally recurrent problem. J Thorac Cardiovasc Surg 1992;104:900.

Burt M et al: Primary bony and cartilaginous sarcomas of chest wall: results of therapy. Ann Thorac Surg 1992; 54:226.

Figure 19–7. Rib metastasis and extrapleural mass from leiomyosarcoma of the uterus.

Burt M: Primary malignant tumors of the chest wall. The Memorial Sloan-Kettering Cancer Center experience. Chest Surg Clin N Am 1994;4:137.

Burt M et al: Medical tumors of the chest wall. Solitary plasmacytoma and Ewing's sarcoma. J Thorac Cardiovasc Surg 1993; 105:89.

Perry RR et al: Survival after surgical resection for high-grade chest wall sarcomas. Ann Thorac Surg 1990;49:363.

Shamberger RC et al: Malignant small round cell tumor (Ewing) of the chest wall in children. J Pediatr Surg; 1989;29:179.

DISEASES OF THE PLEURA

The pleura can be the site of both benign and malignant diseases that may represent primary pleural processes, localized extrapleural diseases, or systemic illnesses. Perhaps the most common pleural problem is the presence of air (pneumothorax) within the pleural space. The accumulation of fluid (pleural effusion)—eg, benign sterile fluid, malignant fluid, pus, chyle, and blood—also occurs commonly. Although primary pleural tumors are uncommon, involvement of the pleura with metastatic cancer is quite common.

Pain and dyspnea are the most common symptoms of pleural disease. The pain most commonly is described as sharp, and it is characteristically worsened by respiratory movements, often inhibiting inspiration reflexively. Pleural pain is mediated through somatic intercostal nerves of the chest wall (cervical and costal pleura) and through the phrenic nerve (diaphragmatic and mediastinal pleura), causing chest wall or back pain and pain referred to the shoulder, respectively. Visceral pleura contains only sympathetic and parasympathetic nerve fibers and therefore is insensate; however, extension of visceral processes to involve the parietal pleura can produce typical pleuritic chest pain.

PLEURAL EFFUSION

Pleural effusion is the presence of fluid within the pleural space. More specific terminology may be used when the nature of the fluid is known. **Hydrothorax** is a collection of serous (most often transudative but also exudative) fluid, while pus in the pleural cavity is referred to as a **pyothorax** or **empyema**. Additional terms are used for blood (**hemothorax**) and chyle (**chylothorax**). Abnormal pleural fluid accumulates as a result of one or more of the following mechanisms: (1) increase in the pulmonary vascular hydrostatic pressure (congestive heart failure, mitral stenosis, etc), (2) decrease in the vascular colloidal osmotic pressure (hypoalbuminemia), (3) increase in the capillary permeability due to inflammation (pneumonia, pancreatitis, etc), (4) decrease in the intrapleural pressure (atelectasis), (5) decrease in the lymphatic drainage (carcinomatosis), (6) transdiaphragmatic movement of abdominal fluid through lymphatics or physical defects (ascites), and (7) rupture of a vascular or lymphatic structure (trauma, cancer, etc).

Decreased respiratory excursion, diminished breath sounds (often with a bronchial quality due to compression of underlying lung), dullness to percussion, decreased vocal and tactile fremitus, a pleural friction rub, and local tenderness are all signs that indicate the presence of pleural effusion. With long-standing and advanced disease, contraction of the hemithorax with narrowed intercostal spaces and localized bulging, swelling, or redness may occur. Chest radiographs demonstrate varying degrees of opacification of the ipsilateral hemithorax. With only 300–500 mL of fluid, blunting of the costophrenic angle may be all that is observed. If the entire hemithorax is opacified, as much as 2000–2500 mL may be present. The mediastinum may be shifted to the contralateral side in the presence of a large effusion or it may remain in the midline—particularly if proximal bronchial obstruction results in lobar or total lung atelectasis, if the mediastinum is fixed from fibrosis or tumor infiltration, if the ipsilateral lung is infiltrated with tumor, or if malignant mesothelioma is present. Occasionally, CT or ultrasonography may be required to evaluate complex, loculated, or recurrent pleural fluid collections.

Generally, serous effusions are separated into two broad categories —transudates and exudates—based on the physical characteristics of the pleural fluid. Identification of the specific type of effusion aids in determination of the cause and most often depends on examination of at least 20 mL of fluid obtained by thoracentesis. Basic tests should include total protein, lactate dehydrogenase (LDH), total and differential cell counts, glucose, pH, cytology, and Gram stain with culture. Furthermore, simultaneous serum total protein, LDH, and glucose should be measured. Effusions with total protein content less than 3 g/dL (or a fluid:serum ratio lower than 0.5), an LDH level < 200 units/dL (or a fluid:serum ratio < 0.6), and a specific gravity below 1.016 represent transudates, while all other effusions are classified as exudates. The results of these basic tests frequently allow the underlying pathologic process to be elucidated (see Table 19–1).

Specific disease processes associated with pleural effusions are described in the following paragraphs.

1. Hydrothorax

Malignancy

More than 25% of all pleural effusions are secondary to cancer, and 35% of patients with lung cancer, 23% of patients with breast cancer (12% of patients with adenocarcinomas of unknown primary site), and 10% of patients with lymphoma develop malignant pleural effusions during the course of their disease. Approximately 10% of malignant effusions are secondary to primary pleural tumors (mostly mesotheliomas). The mechanism (as noted above) is primarily through lymphatic obstruction in either the peripheral lung or central lymph node channels of the mediastinum. Malignant pleural effusions can be serous, serosanguineous, or frankly bloody and are diagnosed primarily by demonstrating malignant cells in the fluid. Cytologic confirmation is successful 50%, 65%, and 70% of the time after one, two, or three thoracenteses, respectively. Closed pleural biopsy alone is successful in only 50% of cases, but coupled with thoracentesis it can increase the diagnostic yield to 80%. Thoracoscopy with direct pleural biopsy, however, is successful in 97% of patients and should be considered in any patient with a suspicious effusion after two negative thoracenteses.

Treatment of malignant effusions is strictly palliative since most patients succumb within 3–6 months, which means that rapid diagnosis and therapy are essential. The goals of treatment are lung reexpansion and pleural symphysis. This is most readily accomplished with placement of a chest tube (20–28F) and closed tube drainage for 24–48 hours (see Figure 19–8). Generally, no more than 1 L is allowed to drain initially. Subsequently, 200–500 mL is allowed to drain every 1–2 hours until the effusion is fully drained. This controlled draining avoids the rare complication of reexpansion pulmonary edema. Once full lung expansion

Table 19–1. Differential diagnosis of pleural effusions.[1]

	Tuberculosis	Cancer	Congestive Heart Failure	Pneumonia and Other Nontuberculous Infections	Rheumatoid Arthritis and Collagen Disease	Pulmonary Embolism
Clinical context	Younger patient with history of exposure to tuberculosis.	Older patient in poor general health.	Presence of congestive heart failure.	Presence of respiratory infection.	History of joint involvement; subcutaneous nodules.	Postoperative, immobilized, or venous disease.
Gross appearance	Usually serous; often sanguineous.	Often sanguineous.	Serous.	Serous.	Turbid or yellow-green.	Often sanguineous.
Microscopic examination	May be positive for acid-fast bacilli; cholesterol crystals.	Cytology positive in 50%	...	May be positive for bacilli.	...	...
Cell count	Few have > 10,000 erythrocytes; most have > 1000 leukocytes, mostly lymphocytes.	Two-thirds bloody; 40% > 1000 leukocytes, mostly lymphocytes.	Few have > 10,000 erythrocytes or > 1000 leukocytes.	Polymorphonuclears predominate.	Lymphocytes predominate.	Erythrocytes predominate.
Culture	May have positive pleural effusion; few have positive sputum or gastric washings.	...	...	May be positive.	...	...
Specific gravity	Most > 1.016.	Most > 1.016.	Most > 1.016.	> 1.016.	> 1.016.	> 1.016.
Protein	90% 3 g/dL or more.	90% 3 g/dL or more.	75% > 3 g/dL.	3 g/dL or more.	3 g/dL or more.	3 g/dL or more.
Sugar	60% < 60 mg/dL.	Rarely < 60 mg/dL.	...	Occasionally < 60 mg/dL.	5–17 g/dL (rheumatoid arthritis).	...
Other	No mesothelial cells on cytology. Tuberculin test usually positive. Pleural biopsy positive.	If hemorrhagic fluid, 65% will be due to tumor; tends to recur after removal.	Right-sided in 55–70%.	Associated with infiltrate on x-ray.	Rapid clotting time; LE cell or rheumatoid factor may be present.	Source of emboli may be noted.

Other exudates: spgr > 1.016
   Fungal infection: Exposure in endemic area. Source fluid. Microscopy and culture may be positive for fungi. Protein 3 g/dL or more. Skin and serologic tests may be helpful.
   Trauma: Serosanguineous fluid. Protein 3 g/dL or more.
   Chylothorax: History of injury or cancer. Chylous fluid with no protein but with fat droplets.

[1]Modified from: Therapy of pleural effusion: A statement by the Committee on Therapy of the American Thoracic Society. Am Rev Respir Dis 1968;97:479.

Figure 19–8. Malignant pleural effusion (carcinoma of lung). *Left:* Posteroanterior projection before treatment. *Right:* After chest tube drainage. Note left hilar mass and osteoblastic metastasis to the first lumbar vertebra.

is obtained (regardless of the ongoing drainage), pleurodesis should be performed with an appropriate agent before loculations have formed. Different chemical, radioactive, and infectious agents have been used in the past with varying success rates, including mechlorethamine (success rate 48–57%), thiotepa (nil to 63%), fluorouracil (66%), bleomycin (50–100%), quinacrine (50–83%), tetracycline (83–100%), doxorubicin (80%), mitoxantrone (76%), talc (87–100% insufflation; 83–100% slurry), radioactive colloidal gold and chromium phosphate (50%), and *Corynebacterium parvum* (81%). Finally, mechanical pleurectomy without chemical instillation can control pleural effusions in over 99% of patients, but this requires an operative procedure (although usually only thoracoscopy). Previously, tetracycline was the most popular agent, but this option is no longer available. Doxycycline, bleomycin, and talc are now the most frequently used. Talc is inexpensive, highly effective, and easily administered either as a powder insufflated into the open chest or as a slurry instilled through a chest tube. The other two agents are less successful and are expensive (bleomycin costs $1000 per 30-unit vial). In addition, two randomized trials have proved talc to be superior to both bleomycin and tetracycline. Some hesitancy to use talc has been expressed because of the associated patient discomfort, but there have been no reports of unmanageable pain

similar to that seen previously with tetracycline instillation. Furthermore, talc no longer contains asbestos, and the induction of fibrothorax, which is a long-term theoretical concern, is not a problem in these short-lived patients. Talc is a foreign body, however, and use of antibiotics during pleurodesis for empyema prophylaxis may be prudent.

Complications following pleurodesis include pneumothorax, loculated hydrothorax, fever, infection (empyema), acute respiratory distress syndrome (particularly following bilateral simultaneous pleurodeses, which for this reason alone are contraindicated), and recurrence. Fortunately, problems are uncommon, and most patients can have their chest tubes removed within 48–72 hours following talc pleurodesis.

Cardiovascular Disease

Pleural effusions are common findings in patients with moderate to severe congestive heart failure (Figure 19–9). The heart failure may be secondary to ischemia (coronary artery disease), valvular heart disease (mitral stenosis, mitral regurgitation, etc), viral myocarditis, congenital heart disease, and other less common lesions. The effusion may be bilateral or unilateral. When unilateral, the right hemithorax is most often affected. Fluid frequently involves the interlobar fissures (most

Figure 19–9. Pleural effusion secondary to heart failure (myocarditis).

commonly the minor fissure on the right) and can form localized collections simulating mass lesions known as "pseudotumors." Other cardiovascular causes of pleural effusions include constrictive pericarditis and pulmonary venous obstruction.

Renal Disease

Hydronephrosis, nephrotic syndrome, and acute glomerulonephritis are on occasion associated with pleural effusions. Rupture of the collecting system into the pleural space can also produce a hydrothorax. In this latter case, the pleural fluid creatinine will be elevated (fluid:serum creatinine ratio significantly > 1.0).

Pancreatitis

Moderate to severe pancreatitis is associated with a pleural effusion that characteristically occurs on the left and contains fluid with an amylase concentration substantially higher than that in the serum.

Cirrhosis

Approximately 5% of patients with cirrhosis and ascites will develop a pleural effusion. In contrast to pancreatitis, nearly all of these effusions occur on the right side.

Thromboembolism

Pulmonary thromboemboli are sometimes accompanied by a pleural effusion. These effusions are typically serosanguineous and small, but they may be frankly bloody and massive. Characteristic x-ray findings are almost always present in the lung. Since the fluid is usually reabsorbed in a short period of time, drainage is seldom necessary.

2. Thoracic Empyema

Pyothorax (empyema thoracis) is the accumulation of pus within the pleural cavity. The pus is usually thick, creamy, and malodorous. If empyema occurs in the setting of underlying suppurative lung disease (ie, pneumonia, lung abscess, or bronchiectasis), it is referred to as a parapneumonic empyema (60% of cases). Other causes of thoracic empyema are surgery (20%; see Figure 19–10), trauma (10%), esophageal rupture, other chest wall or mediastinal infections, bronchopleural fistula, extension of a subphrenic or hepatic abscess, instrumentation of the pleural space (thoracentesis, chest tube placement, etc), and, rarely, hematogenous seeding from a distant site of infection.

Empyemas are divided into three phases based on their natural history: acute exudative, fibrinopurulent, and chronic organizing. The acute exudative phase is characterized by the outpouring of sterile pleural fluid (incited by pleural inflammation), which has a low viscosity, white blood cell count, and LDH concentration as well as normal glucose level and normal pH. The pleura remains mobile during this phase. A transitional or fibrinopurulent phase develops subsequently, marked by an increase in the turbidity, white content, and LDH

Figure 19–10. Postoperative loculated empyema with bronchopleural fistula. *Left:* Posteroanterior projection. *Right:* Lateral projection.

levels of the fluid. In addition, the glucose levels and pH of the fluid decrease progressively and fibrin is deposited on both pleural surfaces, thereby limiting the empyema but also fixing (trapping) the lung. The chronic organizing phase begins 7–28 days after the onset of the disease and is characterized by a pleural fluid glucose level < 40 mg/dL and a pH < 7.0. The pleural exudate becomes quite thick and the pleural fibrin deposits thicken and begin to organize, further immobilizing the lung. In patients with chronic empyema, erosion through the chest wall (empyema necessitatis), chondritis, osteomyelitis of the ribs or vertebral bodies, pericarditis, and mediastinal abscesses may occur.

The bacteriology of thoracic empyema has evolved over the years. Prior to the discovery of penicillin in the 1940s, most empyemas were caused by pneumococci and streptococci (Figure 19–11). With modern antibiotics and improved anaerobic culture techniques, however, the most common isolates from adult empyemas are now anaerobic bacteria, particularly bacteroides species as well as fusobacterium and peptococcus species.

Staphylococcus is the most common organism causing empyema (92% in children under 2 years old) and staphylococcal empyema is one of the most common complications of staphylococcal pneumonias in both adults and children (Table 19–2). Gram-negative bacteria also continue to be significant pathogens, particularly in parapneumonic empyemas. *Escherichia coli* and pseudomonas species account for 66% of aerobic gram-negative empyemas, and other organisms include *Klebsiella pneumoniae,* proteus species, *Enterobacter aerogenes,* and salmonella. Rarely, fungi (aspergillus, *Coccidioides immitis,* blastomyces, and *Histoplasma capsulatum*) and

parasites such as *Entamoeba histolytica* can cause empyemas. In a recent review, empyemas were found to contain anaerobic bacteria in only 35% of cases, aerobic bacteria in only 24%, and a combination in 41%. In addition, the average number of bacterial species isolated was 3.2 per patient.

Although patients may rarely be completely asymptomatic, most patients with thoracic empyemas present with varying symptoms depending on the underlying disease process, the extent of the pleural involvement, and the immunologic state of the patient. Patients typically complain of fever, pleuritic chest pain or a sense of chest heaviness, dyspnea, hemoptysis, and a cough usually productive of purulent sputum. Signs of thoracic empyema include anemia, tachycardia, tachypnea, diminished breath sounds with dullness to percussion on the involved side, clubbing of fingertips, and occasionally pulmonary osteoarthropathy.

Although the medical history and physical examination often suggest the presence of thoracic empyema, the plain chest radiograph is the most important noninvasive diagnostic test. Empyemas can have almost any appearance and may be associated with an underlying pneumonia, lung abscess, or pleural effusion, but most commonly they appear as posterolateral "D"-shaped densities on x-ray. In large empyemas the mediastinum may be shifted away from the affected side. Bronchoscopy should be performed on all patients to exclude the presence of endobronchial obstruction, and CT or ultrasonography may be necessary to evaluate empyemas that are loculated or that mimic a lung abscess. Thoracentesis, however, is the sine qua non for the diagnosis of thoracic empyema. Aspiration of pus

Figure 19–11. Streptococcal empyema. *Left:* Normal x-ray when patient was admitted with high fever. *Right:* Chest x-ray 3 days after admission.

Table 19–2. Incidence of various complications of staphylococcal pneumonia in adults and children (in %).

	Adults	Children
Abscess	25	50
Empyema	15	15
Pneumatocele	1	35
Effusion	30	55
Bronchopleural fistula	2	5

clearly establishes the diagnosis and allows for identification of the offending organisms. In early empyemas—particularly those partially treated with antibiotics—the pleural fluid may not be frankly purulent. In these cases, a pleural fluid pH < 7.0, glucose < 40 mg/dL, and an LDH level > 1000 units/L strongly suggests an evolving empyema even if Gram stain and cultures fail to identify organisms.

Goals for the treatment of thoracic empyemas include (1) control of the infection; (2) removal of the purulent material, with obliteration and sterilization of the pleural space and reexpansion of the lung; and (3) elimination of the underlying disease process. Options for treatment include repeated thoracentesis, closed tube thoracostomy, rib resection and open drainage, decortication and empyemectomy, thoracoplasty, and muscle flap closure. Adjunctive maneuvers reported to aid in the disruption and drainage of loculated empyemas include instillation of fibrinolytic enzymes, placement of high (–100 cm H_2O) suction, and video-assisted thoracoscopic debridement. A rational approach to empyema management is outlined in Figure 19–12). Initially, an intercostal catheter of adequate size is carefully inserted into the most dependent portion of the empyema cavity. If after 24–72 hours sepsis persists—or if there is any question as to the adequacy of drainage—a CT scan should be obtained. If, on the other hand, complete drainage and reexpansion of the lung are achieved, no further drainage procedures are necessary.

Patients with residual spaces that are inadequately drained, patients with continued sepsis, and patients thought to require prolonged tube drainage are candidates for open drainage procedures. These can usually be safely performed 10–14 days after closed-tube drainage since the pleurae fuse by that time and the risk of pneumothorax and lung collapse is eliminated. Options for open drainage include simple rib resection and open flap drainage (Eloesser procedure). Simple rib resection involves the removal of short segments (3–6 cm) of one, two, or three ribs at the most dependent portion of the empyema cavity (at or anterior to the posterior axillary line). A tube can be placed through this open-

ing and effective drainage established. A second approach involves the creation of a U-shaped flap of chest wall which is sewn to the parietal pleura after resection of short segments (3–6 cm) of one, two, or three ribs. This creates an epithelialized tract for long-term tubeless drainage of empyema cavities. The flap also acts as a one-way valve allowing fluid and air to escape during exhalation but sealing during inspiration to prevent the ingress of air. Symbas later modified the original Eloesser procedure by changing the flap to an inverted U-shaped flap with the base of the flap placed parallel to and at the level of the inferiormost aspect of the empyema cavity. This type of open drainage allows the empyema cavity to drain reliably and to be easily debrided, irrigated, and cleaned. Ultimately, through lung reexpansion, wound contraction, and granulation, the cavity often completely disappears.

Another option is early decortication and empyemectomy. This has been increasingly advocated in good-risk patients with early loculated empyemas and inadequate tube drainage or lung expansion. The procedure involves a thoracotomy with resection of both parietal and visceral pleural peels (decortication) with the intact empyema itself (empyemectomy), if possible. The best results with this approach are obtained when the underlying lung is entirely normal and reexpands fully. Posttraumatic empyema, in particular, has been amenable to this treatment.

Empyemas that occur following pulmonary resection often are more difficult to manage. If residual lung is present (resections less than pneumonectomy), the general principles outlined above still apply, although a complicating bronchopleural fistula is often present (Figure 19–13). Simple tube drainage is instituted initially followed by open drainage if necessary. Empyemas following pneumonectomy, however, pose a special problem since there is no longer any lung to obliterate the infected space. In addition, postpneumonectomy empyemas frequently are associated with bronchopleural fistulas. In these patients, specific surgical procedures designed to obliterate residual intrathoracic spaces and in many cases close remaining bronchopleural fistulas may be required (Figure 19–14). In the absence of a bronchopleural fistula, sterilization and closure of a postpneumonectomy space (without obliteration) may be attempted using an irrigation catheter inserted into the apex of the chest cavity. An antibiotic solution specific for the organisms present is then infused into the chest. The solution is allowed to drain through a dependent tube or opening created by simple rib resection. After 2–8 weeks, the catheters are removed and the cavity is closed. The success rate with this technique is quite variable and is reported to be 20–88%. For patients who fail this approach and for those patients with bronchopleural fistulas, the main

Figure 19–12. Management of empyema. (Modified and reproduced, with permission, from Shields TW: *General Thoracic Surgery*, 3rd ed. Williams & Wilkins, 1989.)

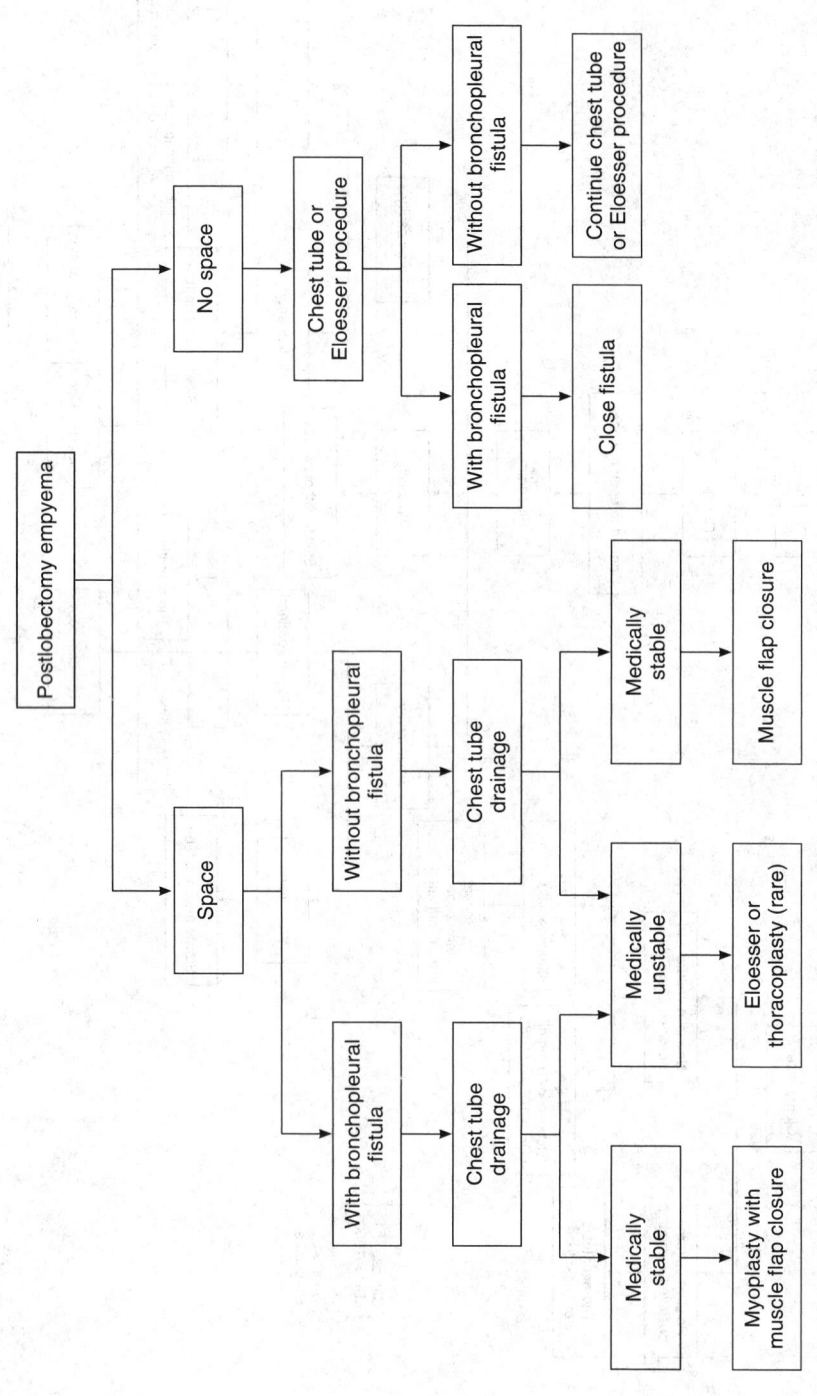

Figure 19–13. Postlobectomy empyema. (Modified and reproduced, with permission, from Shields TW: *General Thoracic Surgery,* 4th ed. Williams & Wilkins, 1994.)

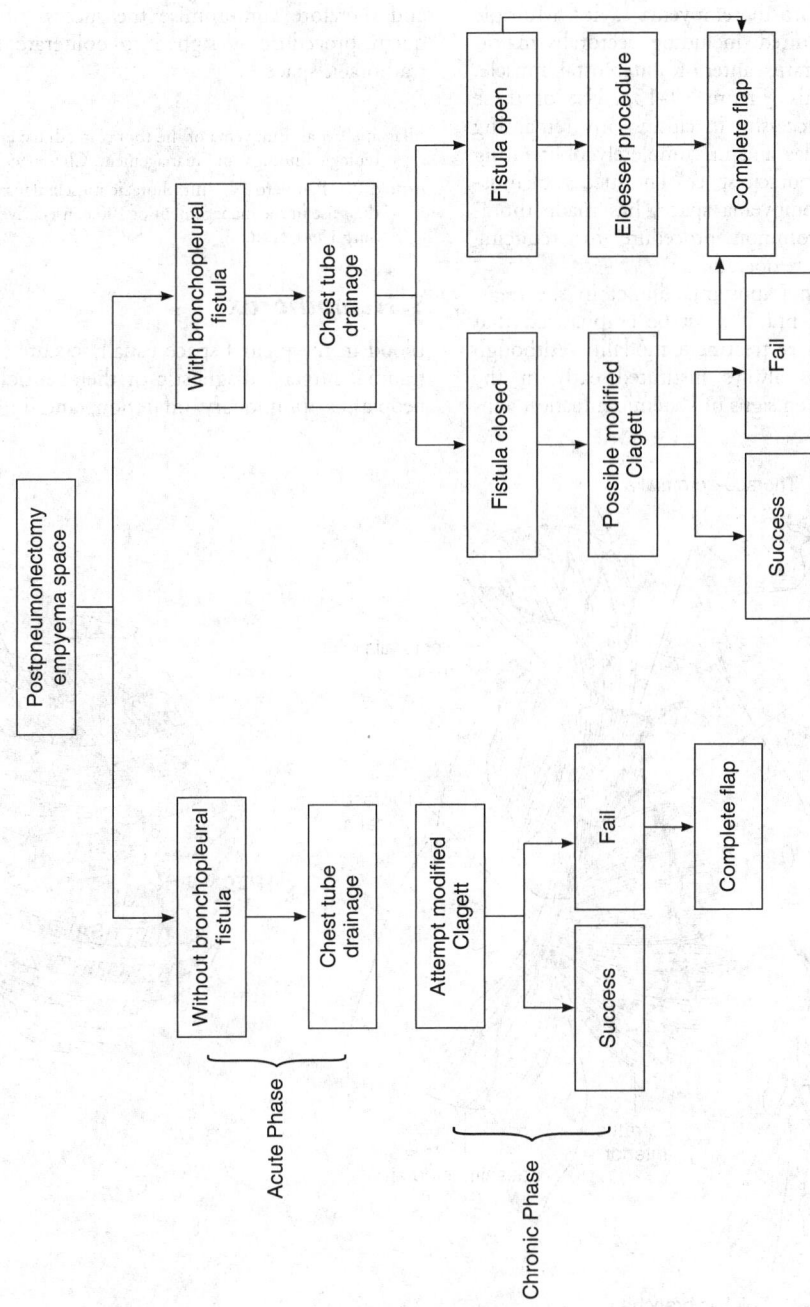

Figure 19–14. **Postpneumonectomy empyema.** (Modified and reproduced, with permission, from Shields TW: *General Thoracic Surgery*, 4th ed. Williams & Wilkins, 1994.)

goal of therapy is to obliterate the residual space and close any bronchopleural fistulas. This is most readily accomplished by the transposition of muscle with or without omentum into the empyema cavity. Multiple muscles may be required, including pectoralis major, latissimus dorsi, serratus anterior, intercostal muscle, and rectus abdominis (Figure 19–15). Use of these muscles is highly successful in closing any remaining bronchopleural fistulas and in completely obliterating the remaining intrathoracic space. The success of muscle flap closure of empyema spaces has made thoracoplasty (once a common procedure for reducing empyema spaces) a rare operation.

Antibiotics are an important adjunct in the treatment of empyemas, but it must be emphasized that drainage is the primary treatment modality. Although antibiotic therapy is always instituted early in the course of therapy when signs of systemic infection generally are present, they need not be continued once effective drainage is established. In fact, overuse of antibiotics may lead to the generation of resistant bacteria and therefore compromise the success of any subsequent procedures designed to obliterate residual intrathoracic space.

Alfageme I et al: Empyema of the thorax in adults: etiology, microbiologic findings, and management. Chest 1993;103:839.

Arnold PG, Pairolero PC: Intrathoracic muscle flaps: an account of their use in the management of 100 consecutive patients. Ann Surg 1990;211:656.

3. Hemothorax

Blood in the pleural space usually occurs secondary to trauma, surgery, diagnostic or therapeutic procedures, neoplasms, pulmonary infarction, and infections (tu-

Figure 19–15. Extrathoracic muscle flap closure of a postpneumonectomy empyema cavity. (Reproduced, with permission, from Miller JI et al: Single-stage complete muscle flap closure of the postnpneumonectomy empyema space: a new method and possible solution to a disturbing complication. Ann Thorac Surg 38:227, 1984.)

berculosis). Most hemothoraces can be treated effectively with large-bore (32–36F) closed chest tube drainage, particularly since small amounts of blood (occupying less than one-third of the hemithorax) are readily reabsorbed by the body. However, if significant blood clot has formed (occupying more than one-third of the hemithorax) or if secondary infection occurs, further measures must be taken to avoid the development of an empyema or fibrothorax with pulmonary compromise. Currently, most hemothoraces requiring more than simple tube drainage can be managed with video-assisted thoracic surgical procedures. Rarely, open thoracotomy may be required for complete decortication and evacuation.

4. Chylothorax

Accumulation of chyle within the pleural space is most often due to surgical procedures, particularly cardiothoracic and esophageal operations. Trauma, malignancy, central venous catheterization, congenital lymphatic malformations, thoracic aortic aneurysms, filariasis, and cirrhosis may also rarely cause chylothorax. Penetrating thoracic trauma can lacerate the thoracic duct at any level, but blunt thoracic trauma usually causes a shearing of the duct at the right crus of the diaphragm. This may also occur with violent coughing or hyperextension of the spine. The initial treatment of chylothorax is similar to that of a malignant pleural effusion. Closed chest tube drainage is instituted; the lung is fully reexpanded; and a low-fat diet is started. In some cases, intravenous hyperalimentation (either peripheral or central) may greatly improve the patient's condition. The irritating nature of chyle promotes pleurodesis, and in half of patients the leak will stop spontaneously. The instillation of sclerosing agents (see section on pleural effusion, above) has also been advocated to increase the chances of success. If chyle continues to drain for more than 7 days or if significant drainage continues for even a shorter period of time, serious consideration should be given to operation since patients quickly become malnourished from the large associated protein losses. Video-assisted thoracoscopic techniques are usually ideal, making open thoracotomy rarely necessary. The standard approach is via the right chest, where the thoracic duct may be identified as it emerges from beneath the diaphragm between the aorta and the azygos vein. Ligation of the tissues in this area is usually all that is needed.

PNEUMOTHORAX

Air in the pleural space (pneumothorax) can occur as a result of a breach in either the parietal (trauma, esophageal perforation, surgery, etc) or visceral pleura (bulla, fine needle aspirations, etc). Rarely, infections of the pleural space with gas-forming organisms may produce a pneumothorax. The magnitude of the pneumothorax is expressed as a percentage of the volume of the chest cavity involved. Since a chest radiograph is only a two-dimensional representation of a three-dimensional space, a relatively small separation of the pleural surfaces (eg, 1 cm) on a chest x-ray can translate into a relatively large pneumothorax (eg, 25%). A large amount of intrapleural air that causes a shift of the mediastinum toward the contralateral lung is referred to as a tension pneumothorax. A pneumothorax associated with an open chest wound may be termed an open pneumothorax or sometimes a "sucking chest wound." *Tension and open pneumothoraces are considered surgical emergencies since both seriously compromise not only ventilation but circulation as well due to decreased venous return.* A mixture of intrapleural air and blood, as frequently occurs with trauma, is called a hemopneumothorax, while a combination of pus and air— eg, in esophageal perforations—is referred to as a pyopneumothorax.

Pneumothoraces usually are classified as either spontaneous or acquired (ie, those caused by a specific event such as trauma, invasive procedures, etc). Spontaneous pneumothoraces (Figure 19–16) sometimes are divided into "primary" and "secondary" categories; however, all spontaneous pneumothoraces are secondary to some underlying pathologic process, and such a division is therefore strictly artificial. Most commonly, spontaneous pneumothoraces are caused by rupture of small subpleural blebs due to increased transpulmonary pres-

Figure 19–16. Spontaneous pneumothorax on right side.

sure most pronounced at the apex of the lung (apex of the upper lobe and superior segment of the lower lobe). Coughing, rapid falls in atmospheric pressure (> 10 millibars/24 h), rapid decompression (scuba divers), and high altitudes (jet pilots) all are associated with increased transpulmonary pressures and spontaneous pneumothorax. In addition, normal transpulmonary pressures can cause rupture of blebs in patients with connective tissue disorders such as Marfan's syndrome. Other causes of spontaneous pneumothorax include apical bullae (patients with COPD), pneumocystis pneumonia (patients with AIDS), metastatic cancer (particularly sarcomas), lymphangioleiomyomatosis, eosinophilic granuloma, rupture of the esophagus or of a lung abscess, cystic fibrosis, and menstruation (catamenial pneumothorax). Classically, however, spontaneous pneumothoraces occur in asthenic males (male:female ratio 6:1) between the ages of 16 and 24, often with a history of smoking. The true incidence is unknown since up to 20% of patients remain asymptomatic and do not seek medical attention.

Patients with pneumothoraces complain of pleuritic chest pain and dyspnea. If severe underlying cardiopulmonary disease exists or if a tension pneumothorax develops, symptoms become much more dramatic and include diaphoresis, cyanosis, weakness, and symptoms of hypotension and cardiovascular collapse. Physical examination reveals tachypnea, tachycardia, deviation of the trachea away from the involved side (tension pneumothorax), decreased breath sounds, hyperresonance, and diminished vocal fremitus on the involved side. Arterial blood gases may demonstrate hypoxia and occasionally hypocapnia from hyperventilation, and the ECG may show axis deviations, nonspecific ST segment changes, and T wave inversion. The standard test for the diagnosis of pneumothoraces is the posteroanterior (PA) and lateral chest radiograph. Exhalation accentuates the contrast between the collapsed lung and the intrapleural air as well as the magnitude of the collapse. Rarely, a CT scan may be necessary to differentiate a pneumothorax from a large bulla in patients with severe emphysema; however, this test should not be used routinely. In 5–10% of patients, a small pleural effusion may be present and can be hemorrhagic.

The treatment of spontaneous pneumothoraces varies depending on the patient's symptoms and condition, the degree of collapse, the cause, and the estimate of the chance of recurrence. Small (< 20–25%), stable, asymptomatic pneumothoraces in otherwise healthy patients can be followed (often on an outpatient basis) with the expectation of complete resolution within several weeks, since air is normally reabsorbed at a rate of 1–1.25% per day. Larger asymptomatic pneumothoraces taking longer than 2–3 weeks to resolve place the patient at risk for developing trapped lung as a result of deposition of fibrin on the visceral pleura. These patients—as well as patients with symptoms, increasing pneumothoraces, or pneumothoraces associated with pleural effusions—should have them evacuated. In highly selected patients this can be accomplished with simple aspiration as long as the immediate and 2-hour delayed chest radiographs document reexpansion. It should be emphasized, however, that some small breaks in the visceral pleural seal once the lung collapses and can reopen with reexpansion. The chance of recurrence is 20–50% with this method, and follow-up x-ray is therefore mandatory after 24 hours.

Most patients with significant pneumothoraces (> 30%) require placement of a closed-chest catheter (8–20F) for acceptable reexpansion. This catheter then can be placed either to underwater suction drainage or to a Heimlich (one-way) valve. If a Heimlich valve maintains full expansion, the patient may be treated as an outpatient; however, if a Heimlich valve fails to reexpand the lung fully or if the patient's condition is not optimal, admission to hospital and underwater chest tube suction drainage is required. Unless some contraindication exists, chest tubes should be placed in the midaxillary line at the level of the fifth intercostal space (nipple line). Placement with the use of blunt clamp dissection avoids the dangers of trocar insertion and should almost always be used. Following resolution of any air leakage, the tube may be taken off suction (water seal) and removed if the lung remains fully inflated. In patients with classic spontaneous pneumothoraces, the chance of recurrence increases with each episode. Following a single episode, the risk of a recurrent pneumothorax is 40–50%. After two episodes the risk increases to 50–75%, and with three previous episodes the risk is in excess of 80%. Currently, most first-time patients are treated initially with simple chest tube drainage; however, with subsequent recurrences, additional therapy generally is indicated. Furthermore, with the development of video-assisted thoracic surgery (VATS), some feel that a more aggressive approach should be taken even for first-time pneumothoraces.

Patients with air leaks lasting longer than 7 days, patients who do not fully reexpand their lungs, patients in high-risk occupations (scuba divers, airline pilots, etc), patients with large bullae or poor pulmonary function, and patients with bilateral or recurrent pneumothoraces are candidates for additional medical (pleurodesis) or surgical intervention. Previously, tetracycline pleurodesis was used to decrease the incidence of recurrent pneumothoraces. The use of this substance, however, was associated with significant pain and controversy. In addition, it currently is no longer available. The use of talc slurry or powder in this setting is also controversial due to the potential for long-term fibrothorax and restrictive lung disease but has been shown to reduce the recurrence rate to as low as 2%. Many other chemical agents have been used in the past, including mechlorethamine, doxycycline, iodoform, guaiacol, urea, and hypertonic glucose, with varying success rates. Since pleurodesis can make subsequent surgical procedures more difficult, the use of this treatment option continues to generate controversy.

Medically fit patients who are candidates for pleurodesis are also candidates for operation. The procedures used to prevent recurrent pneumothoraces include (1) axillary thoracotomy with apical bullectomy, mechanical pleurodesis, and partial pleurectomy; and (2) complete parietal pleurectomy. Both procedures can be performed with either open or VATS techniques. Complete parietal pleurectomy generally is avoided, since some patients may require future thoracic surgical procedures that are extremely difficult in the face of total parietal pleurectomy. Apical bullectomy, mechanical pleurodesis, and partial apical pleurectomy have been shown to reduce the recurrence rate to near zero. In addition, this procedure is easily accomplished either with VATS techniques or through a small transaxillary thoracotomy, both of which are well tolerated.

Several special situations exist that require particular expertise in treatment decisions. Patients with cystic fibrosis and severe COPD may be candidates for lung transplantation, and both pleurodesis and operation may make subsequent transplantation more dangerous. Therefore, consultation with a transplant surgeon is advisable prior to considering these therapies. AIDS patients with pneumocystis pneumonia and pneumothorax are extremely difficult to manage, having a high rate of persistent bronchopleural fistula, treatment failure, and death. For optimal management, the pulmonary surgeon should have extensive experience in the management of chest catheters.

PRIMARY PLEURAL TUMORS

Primary pleural tumors are uncommon neoplasms of two main types: diffuse malignant pleural mesotheliomas and localized fibrous tumors of the pleura (previously referred to as localized mesotheliomas). Although diffuse malignant pleural mesothelioma is the most common primary pleural tumor, involvement of the pleura with metastatic disease is far more frequent and represents the most likely cause of any newly diagnosed pleural malignancy.

1. Localized Fibrous Tumors of the Pleura

Localized fibrous tumors of the pleura arise from subpleural fibroblasts than produce an array of lesions varying from peripheral pulmonary nodules to sessile sub-

pleural masses to the more typical large pedunculated neoplasms. The visceral pleura is involved more often than the parietal pleural, and both benign (70%) and malignant (30%) variations exist. Histologically, benign tumors can exhibit three patterns—fibrous, cellular, and mixed—while malignant ones also have three distinct appearances, ie, tubulopapillary, fibrous, and dimorphic. These tumors behave more like sarcomas of the pleura than diffuse malignant mesotheliomas. Most localized fibrous tumors of the pleura are asymptomatic, discovered only incidentally on chest radiography. Extremely large tumors, however, may produce symptoms of bronchial compression with dyspnea, cough, and chest heaviness— and, rarely, symptoms of hypoglycemia from the production of an insulin-like peptide (4% of patients). On physical examination, signs of clubbing and hypertrophic pulmonary osteoarthropathy (20–35%) may be present. Chest radiography most often demonstrates a well-circumscribed mass that may move with changes in position if the tumor is pedunculated. A pleural effusion is present in 15% of cases and can be bloody, though this does not indicate unresectability. Fine-needle aspiration cytology may be suggestive; however, the diagnosis generally can be established with certainty only at surgery.

The treatment of these lesions is complete resection. Although lobectomy is usually not required for lesions involving the visceral pleura, wedge resection of the pulmonary parenchyma in the area of the tumor is recommended. For neoplasms arising from the parietal pleura, chest wall resection is prudent. Following complete surgical excision, no further therapy is indicated and the prognosis is good, with some patients surviving for over 10 years without recurrence; however, if the resection is incomplete, radiation therapy should be contemplated since the prognosis is poor, with a median survival of only 7 months.

2. Diffuse Malignant Pleural Mesothelioma

Diffuse malignant pleural mesothelioma is the most common primary tumor of the pleura. Since 1960, the disorder has been strongly linked to the use of asbestos. Thick serpentine asbestos fibers (chrysotile) generally are deposited in the proximal airways and are easily cleared with less risk of the development of tumors; however, thin needle-like amphibole fibers (crocidolite, amosite, actinolite, anthrophylite, and tremolite) and the soil silicate zeolite, found in the Anatolia region of Turkey usually lodge in the terminal airways and migrate to the pleura, thereby increasing the risk of diffuse malignant pleural mesothelioma to more than 300 times that of the general population. The latency period after exposure ranges from 15 years to 50 years. Recent research suggests that the generation of free radicals (including nitric oxide), depression of the immune system (both cellular and humoral), induction of cytokines (TNFα, IL-1α, IL-1β, and IL-6), and the production of genetic defects, eg, abnormalities of chromosomes 1, 3, 4, 6, 7, 9, 11, 17 (p53), and 22 (involves c-*sis*, which encodes for one chain of platelet-derived growth factor) all may play a role in the mechanism of asbestos-related disease.

Histologically, diffuse malignant pleural mesotheliomas are divided into four categories: (1) epithelial or tubopapillary (35–40%), which are associated with pleural effusions and a slightly better prognosis; (2) fibrosarcomatous or mesenchymal (20%), which are often "dry" mesotheliomas; (3) mixed (35–40%); and (4) undifferentiated (5–10%). The right hemithorax (60%) is affected more often than the left (35%), and 5% are bilateral.

Most patients with diffuse malignant pleural mesotheliomas complain of dyspnea on exertion and chest wall discomfort, but other symptoms, such as cough, fever (paraneoplastic), malaise, weight loss, and dysphagia also occur. Complaints of severe chest wall pain, abdominal distention, pericardial tamponade, and superior vena cava syndrome suggest advanced disease. Although most patients develop distant metastases at some time during the course of their disease, these lesions rarely become symptomatic. Chest radiographs are distinctly abnormal, showing pleural thickening, effusion (75%), and narrowing of intercostal spaces. Computed tomography often suggests the diagnosis because of diffuse irregular pleural thickening. The diagnosis generally requires substantial tissue samples and is not accessible from fine-needle aspiration cytology. Tissue can be easily obtained with a small incisional biopsy or with VATS techniques. Immunohistochemical stains for CEA, LeuM1, B72.3, and BerEP4 are usually negative, while those for vimentin and keratin are generally positive. Calretinin stain, which is specific for cells of mesothelial origin, has recently become available. This immunohistochemical marker can with near certainty determine whether an epithelial malignant tumor is either metastatic to pleura—eg, an adenocarcinoma (calretinin-negative)—or a primary malignant mesothelioma (calretinin-positive). This stain has become an important clinical tool and should be performed on all suspected cases of diffuse malignant pleural mesothelioma. Electron microscopy may also be helpful in distinguishing this disorder from metastatic adenocarcinoma, with which it is often confused. Pathologic staging of diffuse malignant pleural mesothelioma, like its treatment (see below), has been in a state of confusion. The original Butchart staging system and a more recently promulgated TNM staging system are set forth in the Table 19–3; however, neither is widely accepted or utilized.

The treatment of diffuse malignant pleural mesothelioma is controversial. Owing to the low incidence of this

Table 19–3. Staging systems for malignant mesothelioma.

BUTCHART STAGING SYSTEM

Stage I: Tumor is confined within the "capsule" of the parietal pleura—ie, involving the ipsilateral pleura, lung, diaphragm, and external surface of the pericardium within the pleural reflection only.

Stage II: Tumor invades the chest wall or mediastinum (esophagus, trachea, or great vessels). Alternatively, lymph nodes within the chest are involved with metastatic disease.

Stage III: Tumor penetrates the diaphragmatic muscle to involve the peritoneum or retroperitoneum, the pericardium to involve the internal surface or heart, and the mediastinum to involve the contralateral pleura. Alternatively, lymph nodes outside the chest are involved with metastatic disease.

Stage IV: Distant hematogenous metastatic.

TNM STAGING SYSTEM

Tumor Stage

TX: The primary tumor cannot be assessed.

T0: No evidence of primary tumor exists.

T1: The primary tumor is limited to the ipsilateral parietal or visceral pleura.

T2: Tumor invades any of the following: ipsilateral lung, endothoracic fascia, diaphragm, pericardium.

T3: Tumor invades any of the following: ipsilateral chest wall muscles, ribs, mediastinal organs or tissues.

T4: Tumor extends to any of the following: contralateral pleura or lung by direct extension, peritoneum or intra-abdominal organs by direct extension, cervical tissues.

Lymph node stage

NX: Regional lymph nodes cannot be assessed.

N0: No regional lymph node metastases are present.

N1: Metastases are present in ipsilateral bronchopulmonary or hilar lymph nodes.

N2: Metastases are present in ipsilateral mediastinal lymph nodes.

N3: Metastases are present in contralateral mediastinal, internal mammary, supraclavicular, or scalene lymph nodes.

Metastatic stage

MX: The presence of distant metastases cannot be assessed.

M0: No distant metastases exist.

M1: Distant metastases are present.

STAGE GROUPINGS

Stage I: T1–2, N0, M0

Stage II: T1–2, N1, M0

Stage III: T3, N0–1, M0; T1–3, N2, M0

Stage IV: T4, any N, M0; any T, N3, M0; any T, any N, M1

disease, its natural history has not been carefully defined with regard to various prognostic factors, and no randomized trials have been conducted to compare treatment strategies. The reported median survival for all patients ranges from 7 months to 16 months. Radiation and chemotherapy alone have had no impact on patient survival in this disease. Surgery alone has also been used in attempts to improve survival, and two major approaches have been utilized: radical pleuropneumonectomy or parietal pleurectomy with decortication. The initial experience with radical pleuropneumonectomy demonstrated only a higher associated morbidity but not a better outcome (longer survival) than what can be achieved with the less radical pleurectomy and decortication. When combined with postoperative chest wall irradiation, the latter procedure results in a median survival of up to 25 months. Other approaches have combined preoperative chemotherapy (MD Anderson), intraoperative and postoperative chemotherapy (Lung Cancer Study Group, Cleveland Clinic), photodynamic therapy (NCI), and immunotherapy with TNFα as well as IFN-α and -γ (NCI, SWOG) without any real success. Currently, the use of intraoperative radiation therapy (UCSF, MSKCC) and gene therapy are also being investigated. Although the general impression is that multimodality therapy is superior to any one therapy alone, the exact combination of treatment options for this disease is yet to be defined. It is clear, however, that new therapies are needed.

Antman KH: Natural history and epidemiology of malignant mesothelioma. Chest 1993;103:373S.

Cheng, AY: Neoplasms in the mediastinum, chest wall, and pleura. Curr Opin Oncol 1999;6:17.

Patz EF Jr et al: Malignant pleural mesothelioma: value of CT and MR imaging in predicting resectability. AJR Am J Roentgenol 199 2;159:961.

Rusch VW, Piantadosi S, Holmes EC: The role of extrapleural pneumonectomy in malignant pleural mesothelioma: a Lung Cancer Study Group trial. J Thorac Cardiovasc Surg 199 1;102:1.

Sugarbaker DJ et al: Extrapleural pneumonectomy, chemotherapy, and radiotherapy in the treatment of diffuse malignant pleural mesothelioma. J Thorac Cardiovasc Surg 1991;102:10.

■ DISEASES OF THE MEDIASTINUM

MEDIASTINITIS

Mediastinitis may be acute or chronic. There are four sources of mediastinal infection: direct contamination, hematogenous or lymphatic spread, extension of infection from the neck or retroperitoneum, and extension from the lung or pleura. The most common direct contamination is esophageal perforation. Acute mediastinitis may follow esophageal, cardiac, and other mediastinal operations. Rarely, the mediastinum is directly infected by suppurative conditions involving the ribs or vertebrae. Most direct mediastinal infections are caused by pyogenic organisms. Most mediastinal infections that invade via the hematogenous and lymphatic routes are granulomatous. Contiguous involvement of the mediastinum along fascial planes from cervical infection is frequent; this occurs less commonly from the retroperitoneum because of the influence of the diaphragm. Empyema often loculates to form a paramediastinal abscess, but extension to form a true mediastinal abscess is uncommon. Extension of mediastinal infections to involve the pleura is common.

1. Acute Mediastinitis

Esophageal perforation, the source of 90% of acute mediastinal infections, can be caused by vomiting (Boerhaave's syndrome), iatrogenic trauma (endoscopy, dilation, operation), external trauma (penetrating or blunt), cuffed endotracheal tubes, ingestion of corrosives, carcinoma, or other esophageal disease. Mediastinal infection secondary to cervical disease may follow oral surgery; cellulitis; external trauma involving the pharynx, esophagus, or trachea; and cervical operative procedures such as tracheostomy, mediastinoscopy, and thyroidectomy.

Clinical Findings

Emetogenic esophageal perforation is usually associated with a history of vomiting but in some cases is insidious in onset. Severe boring pain located in the substernal, left or right chest, or epigastric regions is the chief complaint in over 90% of cases. One-third of patients have radiation to the back, and in some cases pain in the back may predominate. Low thoracic mediastinitis can sometimes be confused with acute abdominal diseases or pericarditis. Acute mediastinitis is often associated with chills, fever, or shock. If pleural extension develops, breathing may aggravate the pain or cause radiation to the shoulder. Swallowing increases the pain, and dysphagia may be present. The patient is febrile, and tachycardia is noted. About 60% of patients have subcutaneous emphysema or pneumomediastinum. A pericardial crunching sound with systole (Hamman's sign) is often a late sign. Fifty percent of patients with esophageal perforation have pleural effusion or hydropneumothorax. Pneumothorax following esophageal endoscopy is a sine qua non of esophageal perforation. Neck tenderness and crepitation are more often found in cervical perforations.

The diagnosis may be confirmed by contrast x-ray examination of the esophagus, preferably using water-soluble media. Endoscopic visualization of the perforation is not recommended as an initial diagnostic maneuver as this may inadvertently extend the perforation. Chest CT scan with oral and intravenous contrast is helpful in determining the level of the perforation and the degree of mediastinal soilage as well as possible underlying esophageal or pulmonary pathology. The patient, however, must be clinically stable to be subjected to the rigors of these tests. For more critically ill patients, simple oral administration (or administration through a proximally placed nasogastric tube) of contrast and a simultaneous portable chest x-ray in an ICU setting can often confirm the diagnosis. Myocardial infarction is sometimes mistakenly diagnosed in patients with esophageal perforation when a predisposing cause of pneumomediastinum is not apparent.

Treatment

Surgical management of intrathoracic esophageal perforation depends on the underlying cause (iatrogenic, tumor, stricture, etc) and the amount of elapsed time from leak to diagnosis. All intrathoracic leaks should be surgically explored. Initial management includes immediate drainage of associated pleural contamination by large-bore chest tubes and decompression of the occasional pneumothorax. Broad-spectrum antibiotics, including aminoglycosides, are initiated and vigorous fluid hydration administered.

Typically, a right thoracotomy offers the most access to the intrathoracic esophagus and should be used through the sixth interspace. Even distal left-sided perforations can be managed from the right side. A left thoracotomy, however, is useful when a perforated esophagus from a distal esophageal stricture is encountered.

Treatment of an immediately recognized (< 24 hours) iatrogenic esophageal perforation in an otherwise normal esophagus includes primary two-layer closure with careful attention to complete mucosal closure by interrupted absorbable sutures. Esophageal muscle is then closed over the mucosal injury and buttressed with either a flap of parietal pleura, diaphragm, or intercostal muscle. Copious irrigation and wide drainage is performed. Occasionally, closure over a T-tube drain has been successful.

Esophageal perforations more than 48 hours old are widely drained and the esophagus either defunctionalized or resected. This depends on the degree of mediastinal soilage discovered upon exploration, the extent of sepsis, and the patient's performance status. When perforation occurs secondary to esophageal cancer or manipulation for severe reflux stricture, achalasia, or an otherwise abnormal esophagus, different surgical options exist. If the perforation is recognized immediately and the patient is not floridly septic, esophageal resection is preferred. Re-

construction (usually with a gastric pull-up) can be done at the same setting but only if the patient is stable and the degree of contamination minimal. Otherwise, reconstruction is performed at a later date when the patient has fully recovered from the septic event.

The mortality associated with esophageal perforation remains high (30–60%) despite advances in critical care, nutritional support, and operative management. The specific surgical approach—repair versus diversion or resection—must be tailored to the individual circumstances (mechanism of perforation, underlying pathology, time to diagnosis, and patient performance status) in order to achieve optimal results.

2. Chronic Mediastinitis

Chronic mediastinitis usually involves specific granulomatous processes with associated mediastinal fibrosis and cold abscesses. Histoplasmosis, tuberculosis, actinomycosis, nocardiosis, blastomycosis, and syphilis have been incriminated. Amebic abscesses and parasitic disease such as echinococcal cysts are rare causes. The infectious process is usually due to histoplasmosis or tuberculosis and involves the mediastinal lymph nodes. Esophageal obstructions may occur. Adjacent mediastinal structures may become secondarily infected. Granulomatous mediastinitis and fibrosing mediastinitis are different manifestations of the same disease. Mediastinal fibrosis is a term used synonymously with idiopathic, fibrous, collagenous, or sclerosing mediastinitis. Eighty or more cases of mediastinal fibrosis have been reported, but the cause has been determined in only 16%, and of these over 90% were due to histoplasmosis. In only 25% of 103 cases of granulomatous mediastinitis has the cause been identified. Histoplasmosis was the most common known cause (60%) and tuberculosis the second most common (25%).

About 85% of patients with mediastinal fibrosis have symptoms from entrapment of mediastinal structures as follows: superior vena caval obstruction in 82%; tracheobronchial obstruction, 9%; pulmonary vein obstruction, 6%; pulmonary artery occlusion, 6%; and esophageal obstruction, 3%. Rarely, inferior vena caval obstruction or involvement of the thoracic duct, atrium, recurrent laryngeal nerve, or stellate ganglion is found. Multiple structures may be simultaneously involved.

Seventy-five percent of patients with granulomatous mediastinitis have no symptoms, and disease is discovered by chest x-ray, which shows a mediastinal mass. The mass is in the right paratracheal region in 75% of cases. In the 25% of patients with symptoms, about half have superior vena caval obstruction and one-third have esophageal obstruction. Occasional patients have bronchial obstruction, bronchoesophageal fistula, or pulmonary venous obstruction.

A mediastinal tuberculous or fungal abscess occasionally dissects long distances to present on the chest wall paravertebrally or parasternally. Secondary rib or costal cartilage infections with multiple draining sinus tracts occur.

Clinical Findings

A. Symptoms and Signs

Granulomatous and fibrosing mediastinitis affects women two to three times more commonly than men. Women aged 20–30 years are most typically affected, though the disorder may present in the fourth to fifth decades. Esophageal involvement results in dysphagia or hematemesis. Tracheobronchial involvement may cause severe cough, hemoptysis, dyspnea, wheezing, and episodes of obstructive pneumonitis. Pulmonary vein obstruction—the most common serious manifestation—produces congestive heart failure resembling advanced mitral stenosis and is usually fatal. Although not diagnostic, the respective skin tests in cases due to histoplasmosis or tuberculosis are strongly positive.

B. Imaging Studies

X-ray findings demonstrate a right paratracheal or anterior mediastinal mass. There may be spotty or subcapsular calcifications. Classically, histoplasmosis presents with hilar node calcification or so-called "popcorn" granuloma appearance. Calcification can also occur in thymoma or teratoma located in the anterior mediastinum. Chest CT (with intravenous and oral contrast) is most effective in defining the extent of mediastinal fibrosis and impingement on vital structures.

Treatment

Specific antimicrobial therapy is indicated when an infecting organism is identified. Patients with symptomatic mediastinal masses and fibrosis can require resection for relief of obstruction.

Prognosis

The prognosis following surgical excision of granulomatous mediastinal masses is good. Operative procedures do not appear to activate fibrosing mediastinitis, but success in treatment has been unpredictable. Most patients with fibrosing mediastinitis—whether treated or not—survive but have persistent symptoms.

Cherveniakov A, Cherveniakov P: Surgical treatment of acute purulent mediastinitis. Eur J Cardiothorac Surg 1992;6:407.

Gottlieb LJ et al: Rigid internal fixation of the sternum in postoperative mediastinitis. Arch Surg 1994;129:489.

Karworde SV et al: Mediastinitis in heart transplantation. Ann Thorac Surg 1992;54:1034.

Marty-Ane CH et al: Descending neurotizing mediastinitis. Advantage of mediastinal drainage with thoracotomy. J Thorac Cardiovasc Surg 1994;57:55.

Ringelman PR et al: Long-term results of flap reconstruction in median sternotomy wound infection. Plast Reconstr Surg 1994;93:1208.

SUPERIOR VENA CAVAL SYNDROME

Superior vena caval obstruction produces a distinctive clinical syndrome. Malignant tumors are the cause in 80–90% of cases; lung cancer accounts for about 90%. The incidence of superior vena caval syndrome in lung cancer patients is 3–5%. The male:female ratio is about 5:1. Other primary mediastinal tumors that may cause superior vena caval obstruction include thymoma, Hodgkin's disease, and lymphosarcoma. Metastatic tumors from the breast or thyroid or from melanoma also occasionally cause superior vena caval obstruction. Benign tumors are an unusual cause, but substernal goiter, any large benign mediastinal masses, and atrial myxoma have been implicated. Thrombotic conditions, either idiopathic or associated with polycythemia, mediastinal infection, or indwelling catheters, are unusual causes. The association of superior vena caval obstruction with chronic mediastinitis is discussed in the preceding section. Trauma may produce acute venous obstruction (eg, traumatic asphyxia, mediastinal hematoma).

The clinical manifestations depend on the abruptness of onset, the location of the obstruction, the completeness of occlusion, and the availability of collateral pathways. Venous pressure measured in the arms or head varies from 200 to 500 mm H_2O, and severity of symptoms is correlated with the pressure. Fatal cerebral edema can occur within minutes of an acute complete obstruction, whereas a slowly evolving one permits development of collaterals and may be only mildly symptomatic. Symptoms are milder when the azygos vein is patent. Azygous blood flow—normally about 11% of the total venous return—can increase to 35% of the venous return from the head, neck, and upper extremities. Thus, the most severe cases occur when occlusion is complete and the azygos vein is involved. The thrombus may propagate proximally to occlude the innominate and axillary veins.

Clinical Findings

Symptoms include puffiness of the face, arms, and shoulders and a blue or purple discoloration of the skin. Central nervous system symptoms include headache, nausea, dizziness, vomiting, distortion of vision, drowsiness, stupor, and convulsions. Respiratory symptoms include cough, hoarseness, and dyspnea, often due to edema of the vocal cords or trachea. Nasal congestion is often an early presenting symptom. These symptoms are made worse when the patient lies flat or bends over. In long-standing cases, esophageal varices may develop and produce gastrointestinal bleeding. The veins of the neck and upper extremities are visibly distended, and in long-standing cases there are marked collateral venous channels over the anterior chest and abdomen. Onset of symptoms in fibrosing mediastinitis may be insidious, consisting initially of early morning edema of the face and hands. Occasionally, symptoms and findings are localized to one side when the level of obstruction is above the vena cava and only the innominate vein is blocked. In this situation, symptoms are mild because communicating veins in the neck usually decompress the affected side.

The diagnosis is confirmed by measuring upper extremity venous pressure; in patients with severe symptoms, a pressure of 350 mm H_2O or more is usual. The location and extent of obstruction are best determined by venography. When patients with malignant vena caval obstruction are studied by venography, 35% have thrombosis involving the innominate or axillary veins, 15% have complete caval obstruction without thrombosis, and 50% have partial superior vena caval obstruction. If patency of the azygos vein is in question, interosseous azygography may be useful. Chest x-ray may show a right upper lobe lung lesion or right paratracheal mass. Aortography is occasionally required to exclude aortic aneurysm, though CT scan with contrast enhancement for such lesions is increasingly diagnostic. The differential diagnosis may include angioneurotic edema, congestive heart failure, and constrictive pericarditis. Effort thrombosis of the axillary vein and innominate vein obstruction from elongation and buckling of the innominate artery can be considered in unilateral cases.

Complications

In patients with partial superior vena caval obstruction, thrombosis may suddenly change mild symptoms to marked venous distention, cyanotic swelling, vocal cord edema, and impaired cerebration. Bleeding from esophageal varices is rare except in severe long-standing cases.

Treatment

Superior vena caval obstruction caused by cancer should be treated with diuretics, restriction, avoidance of upper extremity intravenous lines, head elevation, and prompt radiation therapy. Cases of superior vena cava obstruction due to tumor begin to subside by 7–10 days of treatment. Because of the possibility of thrombosis in malignant cases, the use of fibrinolytic agents has been suggested. Caution must be advised in using anticoagulants, however, because many patients have advanced disease and may harbor occult cerebral

metastases. Therefore, before starting therapy, patients should undergo CT or MRI brain scanning to prevent the occurrence of intracerebral hemorrhage. Recently, the use of intravascular expansile stents has been pioneered. Limited early experience suggests that the lumen can be reopened and that good venous drainage and decompression can be achieved by minimally invasive interventional radiologic techniques. Long-term results have not been reported, and disadvantages include the need for anticoagulation to prevent recurrent thrombosis. Preliminary experience looks promising. Chemotherapy is sometimes used alone or with radiotherapy. Most cases of malignant superior vena caval obstruction are not remediable by operation. Tissue diagnosis is important for diagnosis and for guiding therapy. Invasive procedures, however, must be tailored to the individual patient and the severity of the caval obstruction. Patients with new, severe, or rapidly progressive symptoms should receive immediate palliative radiation therapy. Patients with subacute presentations can better tolerate the time required to make the diagnosis.

Fine-needle aspiration, bronchoscopy, cervical mediastinoscopy, and anterior mediastinotomy—and even, occasionally, thoracotomy—offer possible approaches for obtaining tissue. Caution must be advised, however, in the setting of acute fulminant superior vena caval obstruction as any invasive procedure will carry a significantly higher morbidity due to bleeding from venous obstruction. In this case, attempts at invasive techniques for tissue diagnosis should be avoided. Most frequently, the disease process has been previously histologically confirmed because superior vena caval obstruction presents typically as a complication of locally advanced disease. In benign incomplete superior vena caval obstruction, surgical excision of the compressing mass can provide an excellent result. In total obstruction, such as occurs in fibrosing mediastinitis, most patients will gradually improve without treatment. There are numerous surgical procedures designed to bypass caval obstruction, replace the superior vena cava, or recanalize the vena caval lumen. These procedures have been dramatically effective in some cases, but only recently have they been sufficiently successful to warrant consideration.

Prognosis

Radiotherapy is most effective when superior vena caval obstruction is incomplete. Mean survival of patients with malignant caval obstruction from lung cancer is 6–8 months. The death rate from causes related to vena caval obstruction itself is only 1–2%.

Doty DB, Doty JR, Jones KW: Bypass of superior vena cava: fifteen years' experience with spiral vein graft for obstruction of superior vena cava caused by benign disease. J Thorac Cardio-vasc Surg 1990;99:889.

Kistler AM et al: Superior vena cava obstruction in fibrosing mediastinitis: demonstration of right-to-left shunt and venous collaterals. Nucl Med Commun 1991;12:1067.

Stea B, Kinsella T: Superior vena caval syndrome: clinical features, diagnosis, and treatment. In: *Mediastinal Surgery*. Shields T (editor). Lea & Febiger, 1991.

Urschel HC Jr et al: Sclerosing mediastinitis: improved management with histoplasmosis titer and ketoconazole. Ann Thorac Surg 1990;50:215.

MEDIASTINAL MASS LESIONS

Lesions within the mediastinum represent an interesting variety of masses, both malignant and benign, that arise from the diverse organs and tissues which occupy the central thorax. Overall, the incidence of all mediastinal masses is low, especially compared with the frequency of lesions arising within the lung—bronchogenic cancer, etc. Mediastinal malignancies constitute less than 20% of all thoracic tumors.

Mediastinal masses arise from specific structures that reside in relatively constant anatomic arrangement. The mediastinum itself is defined laterally by the mediastinal pleura of each lung; superiorly and inferiorly by the thoracic inlet and diaphragm, respectively; anteriorly by the sternum; and posteriorly by the vertebral bodies. For purposes of definition, the mediastinum is divided loosely into three main compartments: anterior (or anterosuperior), middle, and posterior. The great vessels and heart, pericardium, trachea, and esophagus define and occupy the middle compartment, which separates anterior from posterior areas. The posterior compartment extends to both sides of the vertebrae to incorporate the paravertebral sulci bilaterally. The distribution and origin of mediastinal masses are summarized in Table 19–4.

The most common mediastinal masses in children are neurogenic tumors (50–60%). In young children (< 4 years of age) they are invariably malignant (neuroblastomas). In adults, neurogenic tumors are the most common mediastinal mass. They arise in the posterior compartment (typically from nerve sheaths) and are usually benign, occasionally calcified, and well circumscribed. Anterior mediastinal masses are more frequently malignant. The most common anterior mediastinal mass is a thymoma, though lymphoma is a close second in prevalence.

Complete resection is the treatment of choice for all neurogenic tumors. A standard posterolateral thoracotomy offers optimal exposure; however, more limited incisions, including thoracoscopy, can be effective for resection of clinically benign small (< 6 cm) lesions. For lesions that cannot be completely excised, postoperative radiation may decrease local recurrence and symptoms. Incompletely excised or especially large or infiltrative

Table 19–4. Distribution of tumors and other mass lesions in the mediastinum.

All parts of mediastinum
Lymph node lesions
Middle mediastinum
Aneurysms, vascular lesions
Lipoma
Myxoma
Bronchogenic cysts
Pericardial cysts
Esophageal lesions
Pheochromocytomas
Anterior mediastinum
Thymoma
Lymphoma
Teratoma
Stem cell tumor
Thyroid
Parathyroid
Lipoma

neuroblastomas should receive combination radiation and chemotherapy in conjunction with surgery.

Although classically in adults the majority of mediastinal masses tend to be benign (cysts, neurogenic tumors, etc), recent series have demonstrated a shift toward malignant processes being more prevalent. Whether this represents a true change in tumor incidence or enhanced detection secondary to improved imaging techniques is unclear. Some general rules remain valid, however.

An extensive workup of a mediastinal lesion is usually not required for diagnosis since surgery is usually required both to establish the diagnosis and provide effective treatment. Standard posteroanterior and especially lateral chest films will often provide much useful information; however, contrast CT scanning has become the diagnostic test of choice. MRI, while helpful for assessing vascular or spinal cord extension, has not proved to be more effective than dynamic CT scanning.

Oblique or overpenetrating x-rays are sometimes helpful. Fluoroscopy may show pulsation or variation of shape or location with change of position and respiration. Tomography may reveal calcification or air-fluid levels. Barium swallow is used to evaluate intrinsic esophageal lesions or esophageal displacement by extrinsic masses. Contrast studies of the intestinal tract may reveal the stomach, colon, or small bowel in a hernia. Myelography can be of crucial importance in neurogenic tumors to explain symptoms or plan operative management. Bronchography may be useful to differentiate lung tumors mimicking a mediastinal mass.

Venography, although rarely used, is occasionally helpful to evaluate distortion, obstruction, or collateral channels. Angiocardiography and aortography help to identify aneurysms or displacement. Pulmonary arteriography may be useful to distinguish mediastinal and pulmonary tumors.

Scintiscan is important in evaluating possible substernal goiter in anterior mediastinal lesions, since goiters can almost always be removed by the standard cervical approach. Skin tests and serologic studies may be used in suspected granulomatous disease. Bone marrow examination, hormone assays, and serum tumor markers (AFP, βHCG, LDH) are important adjuncts.

Bronchoscopy and esophagoscopy are occasionally useful to identify primary lung lesions or lesions of the esophagus. Mediastinoscopy and mediastinal biopsy must be used cautiously in mediastinal tumors that are potentially curable. Excisional biopsy is imperative in lesions (eg, thymomas) that are histologically difficult to evaluate since a curable cancer might be dispersed. Mediastinoscopy is useful for the diagnosis of sarcoidosis, Castleman's disease, or disseminated lymphoma.

When substernal goiter is excluded, neurogenic tumors constitute 26% of mediastinal masses, cysts 21%, teratodermoids 16%, thymomas 12%, lymphomas 12%, and all other lesions 12%. About 25% are malignant. In children, the incidence of cancer is about the same, but teratodermoids and vascular tumors are more common.

Clinical Findings

Symptoms are more frequent in malignant than benign lesions. About one-third of patients have no symptoms. Fifty percent of patients have respiratory symptoms such as cough, wheezing, dyspnea, and recurrent pneumonias. Hemoptysis and, rarely, expectoration of cyst contents may occur. Chest pain, weight loss, and dysphagia are found with equal frequency, each in about 10% of patients. Myasthenia (15–20% with thymoma), fever, and superior vena caval obstruction are each found in about 5% of patients.

The following symptoms suggest cancer and thus imply a poorer prognosis: hoarseness, Horner's syndrome, severe pain, and superior vena caval obstruction. Malignant tumors, especially lymphomas, may produce chylothorax. Fever may be intermittent in Hodgkin's disease. Thymoma causes myasthenia, hypogammaglobulinemia, Whipple's disease, red blood cell aplasia, and Cushing's disease. Hypoglycemia is a rare complication of mesotheliomas, teratomas, and fibromas. Hypertension and diarrhea occur with pheochromocytoma and ganglioneuroma. Neurogenic tumors may produce specific neurologic findings from

cord pressure or may be associated with hypertrophic osteoarthropathy and peptic ulcer disease.

A. NEUROGENIC TUMORS

Neurogenic tumors almost always occur in the posterior mediastinum—often the superior portion—arising from intercostal or sympathetic nerves. Rarely, the vagus or phrenic nerve is involved. The most common variety of tumors (40–65%) arises from the nerve sheath (schwannoma and neurofibroma) and is usually benign. Ten percent of neurogenic tumors are malignant. Malignant tumors occur more frequently in children. Most malignant tumors (neuroblastoma, etc) arise from the nerve cells. Neurogenic tumors may be multiple or dumbbell in type, with widening of the intervertebral foramen. In these cases, MRI is necessary to determine if the mass extends within the spinal canal. Myelography may also be necessary. Dumbbell tumors have been removed in the past by a two-stage approach, though a single-stage approach is now extensively used.

Pheochromocytomas of the middle mediastinum can be localized using ^{123}I metaiodobenzylguanidine.

B. MEDIASTINAL CYSTIC LESIONS

Cysts of the mediastinum may arise from the pericardium, bronchi, esophagus, or thymus. Pericardial cysts are also called springwater or mesothelial cysts. Seventy-five percent are located near the cardiophrenic angles, and 75% of these are on the right side. Ten percent are actually diverticula of the pericardial sac that communicate with the pericardial space. Bronchogenic cysts arise close to the main stem bronchus or trachea, often just below the carina. Histologically, they contain elements found in bronchi, such as cartilage, and are lined by respiratory epithelium. Enterogenous cysts are known by several names, including esophageal cyst, enteric cyst, or duplication of the alimentary tract. They arise along the surface of the esophagus and may be embedded within its wall. They may be lined by squamous epithelium similar to the esophagus or gastric mucosa. Enterogenous cysts are occasionally associated with congenital abnormalities of the vertebrae. About 10% of cysts in the mediastinum are nonspecific, without a recognizable lining.

C. GERM CELL TUMORS

Germ cell tumors are common mass lesions of the anterior mediastinum. Historically, they are both solid and cystic, and the more differentiated ones may contain hair or teeth. Microscopically, ectodermal, endodermal, and mesodermal elements are present. These tumors occasionally rupture into the pleural space, lung, pericardium, or vascular structures.

Most germ cell tumors of the mediastinum are metastatic and present with concomitant retroperitoneal disease. Primary mediastinal extragonadal germ cell malignancies are rare, representing less than 5% of all mediastinal germ cell cancers and less than 5% of all primary mediastinal tumors. Men—in particular white males in their twenties and thirties—are most commonly affected, though extragonadal germ cell tumors can arise in women.

Because germ cells are pluripotent cells, they can give rise to several histologically distinct malignancies, including seminoma (40%), embryonal carcinomas and nongestational choriocarcinomas (20%), and yolk sac tumors (20%). Teratomas (20%) can have both benign and malignant components.

Almost all of these tumors (> 90%) produce tumor markers, including βhCG and AFP. LDH—a nonspecific tumor marker—is produced by most bulky mediastinal germ cell tumors and is often an effective indicator of tumor burden.

Much progress in treating these tumors has been made with combination chemotherapy and multimodality therapy (surgery and radiation therapy). Currently, over 50% 5-year survival is achievable for nonseminomatous and over 90% 5-year survival is typical for seminomatous mediastinal germ cell cancer. Patients should be screened and followed with AFP, βhCG, and LDH markers. Surgical resection should be offered after combination chemotherapy has been administered and only after all elevated tumor markers have normalized.

Residual mediastinal masses following chemotherapy and normalization of tumor markers should be resected. At surgery, approximately 40% will be mature teratomas (with the potential for malignant degeneration), 40% necrotic tumors, and 20% residual tumors (requiring postoperative salvage chemotherapy). Rarely is palliative debulking surgery indicated if tumor markers remain elevated after several cycles of chemotherapy. Instead, alternative chemotherapy or investigational therapy should be offered.

D. LYMPHOMAS

Lymphomas are usually associated with disseminated disease metastatic to the mediastinum. They are typically identified in the anterior compartment but can present anywhere through the mediastinum. They are the second most common mass in the anterior mediastinum. Occasionally, lymphosarcoma, Hodgkin's disease, or reticulum cell sarcoma arises as a primary mediastinal lesion.

Treatment

Treatment is tailored to the specific disease process causing the mediastinal mass. In almost all cases, tissue diagnosis is imperative for guiding appropriate therapy.

Minimally invasive techniques (FNA or core needle biopsy) or mediastinoscopy and mediastinotomy are appropriate for diagnosis of a mediastinal mass that is secondary to metastatic disease (eg, lymphomas, germ cell tumors). Mediastinal masses, however, that represent primary malignancies (thymoma, neurogenic tumors, etc) are treated usually with initial surgical resection. Surgical approaches include median sternotomy (anterior masses), posterolateral thoracotomy (posterior and middle mediastinal masses) as well as VATS or bilateral anterior thoracotomy (all mediastinal compartments). Adjuvant chemotherapy is important for malignant germ cell lesions, malignant neurogenic tumors, and bulky or advanced thymomas. Postoperative radiation therapy decreases local recurrence in higher-stage thymoma and in other incompletely resected lesions. Radiation and chemotherapy constitutes the principal therapy for primary mediastinal lymphoma.

Prognosis

Overall, the outlook for patients with mediastinal masses has improved, with advances in combined chemotherapy and multimodality therapy. Surgical morbidity and mortality remain low (1–4%). Patients with benign mediastinal lesions do significantly better (> 95% cure rates) compared with those who have malignant mediastinal masses (< 50% overall survival).

Golbey RB: Mediastinal germ cell tumors. A continuing odyssey. Chest Surg Clin N Am 1994;4:195.

Gossot D et al: Thoracoscopy or CT-guided biopsy for residual intrathoracic masses after treatment of lymphoma. Chest 2001; 120:289.

Hagberg H et al: Value of transsternal core biopsy in patients with a newly diagnosed mediastinal mass. Acta Oncol 2000; 39:195.

TUMORS OF THE THYMUS & MYASTHENIA GRAVIS

The thymic gland is the site of many neoplasms—thymomas, lymphomas, Hodgkin's granulomas, and other less common tumors. Thymoma, the most common type, may be difficult to differentiate from lymphoma even with an adequate biopsy. About 30% of patients with thymoma have myasthenia gravis, and about 15% of patients with myasthenia develop a thymoma.

Besides myasthenia, thymomas can produce a variety of paraneoplastic syndromes. These include cytopenias, red cell aplasias, and hypogammaglobulinemias as well as autoimmune disorders such as rheumatoid arthritis, lupus erythematosus, and polymyositis.

The relationship of myasthenia gravis to thymoma is interesting and incompletely understood. Myasthenia gravis is a neuromuscular disorder characterized by weakness and fatigability of voluntary muscles owing to decreased numbers of acetylcholine receptors at neuromuscular junctions. Because of the high incidence of thymic abnormalities, improvement after thymectomy, association with other autoimmune disorders, and presence in the serum of 90% of patients of an antibody against acetylcholine receptors, myasthenia gravis is thought to be the result of autoimmune processes. The disease has been induced in several species of laboratory animals by immunization with specific acetylcholine receptors. About 85% of patients with myasthenia gravis have thymic abnormalities consisting of germinal center formation in 70% and thymoma in 15%.

Thymomas may be classified according to predominant cell type into lymphocytic (25%), epithelial (25%), and lymphoepithelial (50%) varieties. Spindle cell tumors, which are sometimes associated with red cell aplasias, are considered among the epithelial tumors. Histologic subtypes, however, classically have not had prognostic significance. Recent reports demonstrate that aneuploidy and the presence of epithelial cells resembling thymic carcinoma have adverse prognostic implications. The histologic classification of thymomas is currently being revised.

Myasthenia gravis may occur in association with tumors of any cell type but is more common with the lymphocytic variety.

Malignant thymomas cannot be determined by the histologic appearance of the tumor alone. Evidence of local invasion grossly or microscopically defines a thymoma as malignant. Thymomas are staged according to the Masoaka staging system as set forth in the accompanying box.

STAGE	DESCRIPTION
I	Macroscopically, completely encapsulated; microscopically, no capsular invasion.
IIa	Macroscopic invasion into surrounding fatty tissues or mediastinal pleura (without microscopic invasion).
IIb	Microscopic evidence of capsular invasion or microscopic invasion of surrounding fatty tissues or mediastinal pleura.
III	Macroscopic invasion into a neighboring organ (pericardium, great vessels, or lung).
IVa	Pleural or pericardial dissemination.
IVb	Lymphatic or hematogenous distant metastases.

Clinical Findings

Fifty percent of thymomas are first identified in an asymptomatic patient on a chest x-ray obtained for another purpose. Symptomatic patients may present with chest pain, dysphagia, myasthenia gravis, dyspnea, or superior vena caval syndrome.

In addition to the chest x-ray, CT scans are useful in making the diagnosis in equivocal cases and in assessing the extent of the lesion. MRI is occasionally helpful to assess vascular invasion.

The diagnosis of myasthenia gravis can be made from the patient's history of easy fatigability and associated decremental response in muscular contraction to repeated stimulation of the motor nerve or from improvement in these abnormalities in response to edrophonium (Tensilon), a short-acting anticholinesterase drug.

Definitive diagnosis of thymoma is based on histologic study of a tissue sample usually after excisional biopsy or complete resection has been performed. Small, well-encapsulated anterior mediastinal masses should not be biopsied, as the procedure penetrates the tumor's capsule and can lead to tumor seeding and recurrence and may jeopardize the chance of cure of an early-stage thymoma.

Treatment

The treatment of choice for thymoma is total thymectomy. The operation is usually performed through a median sternotomy. Posterior lateral thoracotomy as well as "clamshell" (bilateral anterior thoracotomy) or "trapdoor" incisions offer excellent exposure for resection of advanced-stage thymomas. Cervical incisions, while useful for thymectomy for benign conditions (myasthenia, etc.), have no role in the surgical treatment of malignant thymoma. A careful but aggressive resection should be performed for stage III lesions when they can be removed completely without sacrificing vital structures. Postoperative radiotherapy is indicated for invasive thymoma (stage II and stage III).

En bloc resection of the thymoma and associated pericardium, pleura, or lung (including lobectomy or extrapleural pneumonectomy) or great vessel (aorta, superior vena cava) reconstruction is warranted when complete resection is possible. Incomplete resections or debulking procedures do not benefit patients. Administration of neoadjuvant therapy with platinum-based chemotherapy will frequently shrink the tumor and allow subsequent complete resection. Recently, larger thymomas (> 5–6 cm) with evidence of probable invasion are being treated with combined-agent induction chemotherapy. Response rates exceed 70%, and complete resection rates are facilitated.

Large bulky lesions with clinically apparent gross invasion of local structures, pleura, or lung should be biopsied to confirm histologically the diagnosis of thymoma. Neoadjuvant chemotherapy with platinum-based regimens has been effective in shrinking bulky high-grade thymomas, thus allowing for complete resection and greater chances of cure.

Anticholinesterase drugs (eg, neostigmine bromide) are given as initial treatment to patients with myasthenia gravis. Corticosteroids may be given in selected cases, but a high incidence of side effects makes them unsuitable for more liberal use. Early thymectomy is now recommended for all patients with symptomatic myasthenia gravis whether or not a thymoma is suspected. The course of the disease is usually improved, and subsequent development of a malignant thymoma is eliminated. Thymectomy may be postponed in the occasional patient with mild disease well controlled by anticholinesterase therapy.

Prognosis

The rates of complication and death with thymectomy are low except when there are extensive tumors. Respiratory care of patients with myasthenia gravis in the immediate postoperative period now presents little difficulty because of the availability of anticholinesterase drugs.

The stage and histologic type of the tumor are the main determinants of survival after thymectomy, though the presence of myasthenia no longer has an adverse effect.

Overall survival rates are extremely good for early-stage thymomas, and greater than 10-year survival (ie, cure) is the rule. Specifically, stage I lesions approach 100% 10-year survival rates. Stage II tumors with resection and postoperative radiation therapy have approximately 75% 10-year survival rates. Survival rates drop off precipitously, however, for patients with locally advanced stage III thymomas. Long-term (10-year) survival for these patients is less than 25%. The outlook for these patients is improving, however, as results with multimodality therapy (neoadjuvant chemotherapy, surgery followed by chemotherapy and radiation therapy) have shown significant tumor responses and enhanced resectability rates. Long-term survival data with these patients have not yet been reported.

THYMIC CARCINOMA

This tumor is a rare variant (< 15%) of thymic lesions and is histologically and biologically quite different from invasive or malignant thymoma. Thymic carcinomas tend to be very invasive and difficult to resect completely. Unfortunately, even in the setting of complete resection, recurrence is common both locally and at distant sites. Still, when at all possible, an aggressive combined-modality approach (induction chemotherapy, resection, and postoperative chemoradiotherapy) should be employed. Typically, these are young men (< age 50 years) with an otherwise excellent performance status. While a good response to induction therapy and complete resection will provide a significant disease-free interval, long-term survival is still unlikely. Better systemic agents and a molecular understanding of this cancer holds hope for significant improvements in cure rates.

Following thymectomy, about 75% of patients with myasthenia gravis are improved and 30% achieve complete remission. Younger patients benefit more from thymectomy than do those over age 40 years, but a positive effect also accrues to the latter group.

Cooper JD: Current therapy for thymoma. (Review.) Chest 1993; 103(4 Suppl):3345

Maggi G et al: Thymoma: results of 241 operated cases. Ann Thorac Surg 1991;51:152.

Morgenthaler TI et al: Thymoma. (Review.) Mayo Clin Proc 1993; 68:1110.

Park HS et al: Thymoma. A retrospective study of 87 cases. Cancer 1994;73:2491.

Rea F et al: Chemotherapy and operation for invasive thymoma. J Thorac Cardiovasc Surg 1993;106:543.

■ DISEASES OF THE LUNGS

CONGENITAL CYSTIC ANOMALIES OF THE LUNG

Congenital lesions of the lung include primarily tracheobronchial atresia, bronchogenic cysts, pulmonary dysplasia, pulmonary sequestration, congenital cystic adenomatoid malformations, and congenital lobar emphysema. Although many of these lesions present early in life with dramatic symptoms and physical findings, some may remain occult until late childhood and even into adult life. These uncommon lesions arise from aberrations in normal respiratory tract development, which begins during the fourth week of fetal life when the lung bud forms at the caudal end of a groove in the primordial pharynx. An initial phase of sequential airway branching occurs until as many as 20–25 generations are reached by the 16th week of fetal life. These branches are divided into three zones: a proximal conductive zone (branches 1–16), an intermediate transitional zone (branches 17–19), and a distal respiratory zone (branches 20–25). A second canalicular phase is then entered as capillaries develop in the distal air passages. Finally, the alveolar phase begins at approximately 26 weeks of fetal life as prototype alveolar air sacs appear complete with both type I and type II pneumocytes. The number and size of alveoli continue to increase until the total alveolar surface reaches the adult size of nearly 100 m^2.

1. Tracheobronchial Atresia

Atresia of the tracheobronchial tree can occur at any level and may involve an isolated segment or multiple diffuse areas of the airway. Tracheal atresia is associated with polyhydramnios, prematurity, esophageal atresia, and tracheoesophageal fistula. Typically, neonates present with intractable cyanosis and despite a normal-appearing larynx are unable to be intubated. Emergency tracheostomy can be life-sustaining in babies with isolated subglottic atresia; in other infants with more diffuse disease, mask ventilation can achieve some palliation through anomalous esophagobronchial connections. Diffuse airway involvement, however, is invariably fatal.

Isolated bronchial atresia results in a bronchus that ends in a blind pouch. A mucocele develops distal to the obstruction and, as a result of compression of neighboring normal bronchial structures, causes emphysematous changes in the surrounding lung. Since children frequently develop wheezing, stridor, and pulmonary infections in the involved segments, resection is almost always indicated. Like bronchial atresia, true congenital bronchial stenosis is rare, although right main stem bronchial stenosis occurs not infrequently from iatrogenic airway trauma in chronically ventilated patients.

Related anomalies of the tracheobronchial tree include anomalous tracheal or esophageal bronchi and tracheal diverticula. These rare lesions often present with symptoms of bronchial obstruction and in many cases require resection of involved lung tissue due to chronic infection and the development of bronchiectasis (see below). Similar to pulmonary sequestration, these lesions can have a dominant systemic arterial blood supply that must be kept in mind if operation is contemplated.

2. Bronchogenic Cysts

Abnormal budding of the foregut during development can result in the formation of bronchogenic cysts. These occur most commonly in the pulmonary hilum or mediastinum (primarily in the paratracheal and subcarinal areas) but can also arise in the pulmonary parenchyma. The cysts are usually single, are lined by cuboidal respiratory epithelium, and occur preferentially in the lower lobes. The cyst wall is generally thin, occasionally containing cartilage, and except for mediastinal cysts they frequently communicate with the tracheobronchial tree. Radiographically, these cysts appear as discrete round densities that often are sharply defined and air-filled. They may also present as a solitary pulmonary nodule (if completely fluid-filled) or as a pulmonary abscess with an air-fluid level (see below). In general, mediastinal bronchogenic cysts present with airway compression and parenchymal cysts are manifested by pulmonary infection. Some cysts have been noted to enlarge rapidly and rupture into the pleural space, causing tension pneumothorax. All bronchogenic cysts—regardless of location—are best treated with either simple or segmental resection. Rarely, lobectomy is required.

3. Bronchopulmonary Dysplasia

Bronchopulmonary dysplasia includes pulmonary agenesis and aplasia as well as primary and secondary pulmonary hypoplasia. Unilateral pulmonary agenesis occurs when one lung and the associated vascular structures fail to develop. Neonates with pulmonary agenesis may present with tachypnea and cyanosis, particularly if associated cardiac anomalies exist (50% of cases). Some patients, however, remain asymptomatic until childhood, when they complain of dyspnea and wheezing suggestive of asthma. Physical examination in these patients reveals marked tracheal deviation toward the side of the agenesis, and chest x-ray, barium esophagography, and chest CT may be required to exclude other diagnostic possibilities such as total lung atelectasis from foreign body aspiration, total lung sequestration, and esophageal bronchus. Once bronchopulmonary dysplasia is diagnosed, treatment is limited to supportive care. The prognosis is guarded since only one-half to two-thirds of patients survive for longer than 5 years—succumbing in part from the coexisting cardiac disease. Pulmonary aplasia is essentially identical to pulmonary agenesis except that a blind bronchial tumor stump of varying length exists and can chronically soil the normal lung with infected pooled secretions. This problem necessitates resection of the bronchial stump to prevent this potentially fatal complication.

Pulmonary hypoplasia is defined pathologically as an abnormally low radial alveolus count and low ratio of lung weight to body weight and is considered primary if no inciting cause can be identified. These neonates present with tachypnea and hypoxemia resistant to administration of supplemental oxygen due to abnormal thickening of the pulmonary arteriolar wall. Persistent fetal circulation, hypoxemia, hypercapnia, and acidosis lead to early death in over 75% of patients. Secondary pulmonary hypoplasia results from numerous fetal and maternal abnormalities that physically restrict lung growth and development. The most common of these abnormalities is congenital diaphragmatic hernia (see Chapter 46). Other conditions associated with secondary pulmonary hypoplasia include those that produce oligohydramnios and direct chest compression (eg, bilateral renal agenesis [Potter's syndrome], renal dysplasia, and amniotic fluid leaks); those with abnormal bone development and small rigid chest walls (eg, achondroplasia, chrondrodystrophia fetalis calcificans, osteogenesis imperfecta, and spondyloepiphysial dysplasia); those with decreased fetal respiratory movements (eg, phrenic nerve agenesis, abdominal masses or ascites with elevation of the diaphragm, arthrogryposis multiplex congenita, camptodactyly, and congenial myotonic dystrophy); those with intrathoracic mass lesions (eg, congenital cystic adenomatoid malformation, cystic hygroma, and esophageal duplication cysts); and those with pulmonary vascular abnormalities (eg, scimitar syndrome and pulmonary artery agenesis).

dell'Agnola CA et al: Prenatal ultrasonography and early surgery for congenital cystic disease of the lung. J Pediatr Surg 1992; 27:1414.

Eber E, Zach MS: Long term sequelae of bronchopulmonary dysplasia (chronic lung disease of infancy). Thorax 2001;56:317.

4. Pulmonary Sequestration

Pulmonary sequestrations are masses of lung parenchyma that arise through abnormal budding of the caudal embryonic foregut and consequently have no bronchial communication with the otherwise normal tracheobronchial tree. Sequestrations may occur either within normal lung tissue, termed intralobar sequestrations; or as separate masses with their own visceral pleura, referred to as extralobar sequestrations. The majority (85%) of sequestrations are of the intralobar type. Both types, however, occur in or around the right (42%) or left (58%) lower lobes and have an abnormal systemic blood supply, often from the abdominal aorta. The venous drainage of intralobar sequestrations is through the pulmonary venous system in 96%, and in some cases this may be associated with anomalous venous drainage of the normal lung. The venous drainage of extralobar sequestrations, however, is to the systemic (hemiazygos or azygos) veins. Although some sequestrations (particularly extralobar) present as asymptomatic lower lobe masses, many present with recurrent lower lobe infections due to bacterial seeding that occurs through communications with the remaining normal lung known as the pores of Kohn. In rare instances, patients may present with hemoptysis or congestive heart failure from large left-to-right shunts through the se-

questration. The diagnosis is usually suspected on chest x-ray and confirmed with a CT scan of the chest. Although angiography was formerly used to confirm the diagnosis, currently it is indicated only if questions regarding the diagnosis, arterial blood supply, or venous drainage exist despite computed tomography. Treatment consists of segmental resection or, if necessary, lobectomy. Great care must be taken to identify the nature of both the arterial blood supply and the venous drainage to avoid exsanguinating hemorrhage from division of an unrecognized systemic artery or venous infarction of the normal lung from ligation of the common draining vein. Following successful resection, the prognosis is favorable.

Campbell RE et al: Image interpretation session: 1993. Intralobar pulmonary sequestration. Radiographics 1994;14:199.

Dolkart LA et al: Antenatal diagnosis of pulmonary sequestration: a review. Obstet Gynecol Surv 1992;47:515.

Javaid A, Aamir AU: Pulmonary sequestration: a case report and review. Respir Med 1994;88:65.

Louie HW, Martin SM, Mulder DG: Pulmonary sequestration: 17-year experience at UCLA. Am Surg 1993;59:801.

Nicolette LA et al: Intralobar pulmonary sequestration: a clinical and pathological spectrum. J Pediatr Surg 1993;28:802.

5. Congenital Cystic Adenomatoid Malformation

Congenital cystic adenomatoid malformation results from an overgrowth of terminal bronchiolar structures that are lined by typical respiratory epithelium and are associated with disorganized elastic connective tissue and smooth muscle. These "solid" structures are interspersed with cysts that resemble immature alveoli with bronchial-type epithelium, polypoid luminal projections, an absence of mucoserous glands and cartilage, and occasional "intestinal" mucus-secreting cells. These lesions are classified into one of three categories based on their presentation and pathologic features. Some lesions present with a predominantly solid lung mass, occur primarily in stillborn or premature neonates, and are associated with fetal anasarca, ascites, and polyhydramnios. Intermediate lesions with mixed solid and cystic components often present at birth with severe respiratory distress secondary to a large space-occupying mass and the resulting ipsilateral and occasional contralateral pulmonary hypoplasia. A third predominantly cystic lesion frequently escapes detection at birth and presents in the older infant, child, or adult with recurrent pulmonary infections. The radiographic diagnosis of congenital cystic adenomatoid malformation can be difficult, especially in the newborn, when it can be confused with congenital diaphragmatic hernia and, less frequently, congenital lobar emphysema. A radiograph demonstrating a paucity of intestinal air in the abdomen favors the diagnosis of diaphragmatic hernia, while a chest CT scan may be required in some patients to make a correct diagnosis. The treatment of essentially all lesions is surgical resection, which may be required emergently in neonates who present with severe respiratory distress. The prognosis for the intermediate and predominantly cystic types is good following resection.

6. Congenital Lobar Emphysema

Congenital lobar emphysema is associated with hypoplastic or dysplastic bronchial cartilage in 25–79% of patients and with an increased number of alveoli ("polyalveoli") in up to 37% of affected children. The left upper lobe is most commonly involved, and the right middle lobe is next in frequency. In addition, neonates who require prolonged mechanical ventilation—eg, those with hyaline membrane disease—may develop lobar emphysema from a combination of suction catheter trauma and barotrauma. The right lower lobe is most frequently affected in these patients. Most infants present within the first 6 months of life with respiratory distress. In some patients, severe respiratory distress may occur in the neonatal period, requiring emergent evaluation and treatment. Almost all infants present with tracheal and mediastinal deviation away from the affected side, hyperresonance and decreased breath sounds on the affected side, and a chest x-ray demonstrating hyperlucency in the area of the affected lobe with compression of adjacent lung. A chest x-ray often is all that is necessary prior to operation; however, occasional patients, particularly older children, may require chest CT scans to exclude other pathology, eg, bronchogenic cysts, anomalous pulmonary vessels, and hilar lymphadenopathy. Bronchoscopy also may be necessary to rule out the presence of a foreign body acting as a ball valve. Successful therapy in all patients requires surgical resection, which almost uniformly consists of lobectomy.

Kennedy CD et al: Lobar emphysema: long-term imaging follow-up. Radiology 1991;180:189.

Stigers KB, Woodring JH, Kanga JF: The clinical and imaging spectrum of findings in patients with congenital lobar emphysema. Pediatr Pulmonol 1992;14:160.

CONGENITAL VASCULAR LESIONS OF THE LUNG

Vascular diseases of the lung include two main processes: arteriovenous malformations and vascular rings. Arteriovenous malformations are uncommon congenital lesions that develop as a result of abnormal capillary formation during the canalicular phase of development. Most arise from the pulmonary artery, but occasionally a systemic arterial source may be involved similar to that in pulmonary sequestration. Rarely, the coronary arteries may be the origin of arteriovenous malformations, with the right coronary artery involved 55% of the time. Coronary arteriovenous fistulas drain into the right ventricle (40%), right atrium (25%), pulmonary artery (20%), coronary sinus (7%), superior vena cava (1%), or left-sided heart chambers (7%). Patients are either asymptomatic or they complain of dyspnea, fatigue (congestive heart failure), and, rarely, angina (myocardial infarction). A continuous murmur and signs of rapid aortic runoff may be present on physical examination. Although the diagnosis often can be established with echocardiography and color Doppler imaging, the definitive diagnosis, shunt fraction, and preoperative "road map" for planning the specific operative repair is provided by catheterization and angiography. Operation usually is indicated for symptomatic patients and for those asymptomatic patients with large shunts.

Vascular rings occur from abnormal development of the aortic arches and major branches, with resulting compression of the trachea and esophagus. In normal fetal development, a dual system of six aortic arches regresses in such a way that the left fourth arch becomes the main left-sided aorta, the left sixth arch develops as the ductus arteriosus, and the right fourth arch persists as the right innominate artery and subclavian artery. Most vascular rings, however, are associated with a right-sided aortic arch and may be classified as complete vascular rings or incomplete rings (arterial slings). Complete vascular rings include a double aortic arch (67%, the most common complete ring), a right aortic arch with a left subclavian and left ductus arteriosus (30%), a right aortic arch with mirror image branching and a left ductus arteriosus (rare), and a left aortic arch with an aberrant right subclavian and right ductus arteriosus (very rare). Incomplete rings consist of an aberrant right subclavian artery that originates on the left side and passes posterior to the esophagus (most common incomplete ring) and an anomalous left pulmonary artery arising from the right pulmonary artery and passing between the trachea and the esophagus (pulmonary artery sling).

Most patients present with symptoms of tracheal or esophageal compression. Patients with an anomalous right subclavian artery may present later in life with swallowing symptoms (dysphagia lusoria) while those with complete vascular rings and pulmonary artery slings typically present early in life (within 6 months) with symptoms of respiratory distress (often frank stridor), particularly with neck flexion and poor feeding. The diagnosis is often suggested by characteristic findings on barium esophagraphy. Bilateral indentations imply double aortic arch. A posterior indentation points to an aberrant right subclavian artery, large right sided indentations suggest complete rings associated with a right aortic arch, and an anterior impression is typical of a pulmonary artery sling. Often, the diagnosis can be confirmed by echocardiography, but occasionally computed tomography or aortography is required. Surgical repair of these lesions is indicated once the diagnosis is established and is accomplished by dividing the vascular ring usually through a left thoracotomy. With double aortic arches, the smaller of the two arches is divided distal to the subclavian artery, while other complete rings generally are treated by division of the ligamentum arteriosum. Aberrant right subclavian arteries may be simply divided or, if necessary, reimplanted on the right side. Pulmonary artery slings require reimplantation of the left pulmonary artery and often resection of the compressed trachea which often has severe tracheomalacia and stenosis. Rarely, tracheomalacia secondary to vascular ring compression necessitates suspension of the aortic arch from the sternum.

Anend R et al: Follow-up of surgical correction of vascular anomalies causing tracheobronchial compression. Pediatr Cardiol 1994;51:58.

Lowe GM, Donaldson JS, Backer CL: Vascular rings: 10-year review of imaging. Radiographics 1996,11:637.

van Son JA et al: Surgical treatment of vascular rings: The Mayo Clinic Experience. Mayo Clin Proc 1993;68:1056.

SUPPURATIVE DISEASES OF THE LUNG

1. Lung Abscess

A lung abscess is a localized collection of pus that is contained within a cavity formed by the disintegration of the surrounding tissues. The pus consists of leukocytes and a thin fluid referred to as "liquor puris." Arbitrarily, abscesses are termed acute if the duration is less than 6 weeks and chronic if more than 6 weeks. Although the incidence of lung abscesses fell dramatically following the introduction of effective antibiotics in the 1940s and 1950s, a recent increase in the number of immunocompromised individuals secondary to organ transplantation, chemotherapy, and AIDS has resulted in a resurgence in the numbers of lung abscesses requiring treatment.

Lung abscesses may be divided into two major categories based on etiology: primary and secondary. Primary lung abscesses occur because of aspiration of oropharyngeal contents (most common), acute necrotizing pneumonia (due to S aureus, K pneumoniae), chronic pneumonia (due to fungi, tubercle bacilli) and opportunistic infection in an immunodeficient host. Conditions that predispose to aspiration include anes-

thesia (both general and monitored), neurologic disorders (cerebrovascular accidents, seizures, diabetic coma, head trauma, etc), drug ingestion (alcohol, narcotics, etc), normal sleep, poor oral hygiene (increases bacterial load), and esophageal disease (gastroesophageal reflux, achalasia, cancer, tracheoesophageal fistula). Secondary causes of lung abscesses include bronchial obstruction (cancer, foreign body, hilar lymphadenopathy), cavitating lesions (cancer, pulmonary infarct), direct extension (amebiasis, subphrenic abscess), and hematogenous dissemination (S aureus, E coli, etc). It should be noted that secondary infections of congenital or acquired cystic lesions, such as bronchogenic cysts, bullae, tuberculous cavities, and hydatid cysts, are not true pulmonary abscesses because they occur in a preformed spaced. The bacteriologic findings of lung abscesses depend somewhat on the underlying cause and the thoroughness of the laboratory. Classically, aerobic gram-positive cocci (S aureus, Streptococcus pyogenes) and facilitative gram-negative bacilli (K pneumoniae, E coli, pseudomonas species) have been incriminated: however, with more fastidious culture techniques, anaerobic bacteria (bacteroides species, Clostridium ramosum, peptostreptococci, peptococci) are now isolated in over 85% of cultures. In immunocompromised patients, more unusual organisms predominate, eg, Candida albicans, Legionella micdadei and L pneumophila, and Pneumocystis carinii.

Clinical Findings & Diagnosis

Patients with lung abscesses typically complain of cough, fever, dyspnea, and occasionally pleuritic chest pain. The symptoms are often insidious in onset and associated with malaise and weight loss if chronic. Complications include rupture into a bronchus, with initial hemoptysis followed by the production of foul-smelling, purulent sputum (and the potential for life-threatening pneumonia from aspiration of pus into normal lung); rupture into the pleural space with resulting pyopneumothorax, sepsis, and possibly empyema necessitatis; and, rarely, massive hemoptysis requiring emergent pulmonary resection. On physical examination, signs of lobar consolidation predominate; but clubbing, signs of pleural effusion, cachexia, and rarely a draining chest wound (empyema necessitatis) can be present. Laboratory studies should include a differential white blood cell count and sputum culture. Chest radiography may demonstrate an area of intense consolidation or a rounded density with or without an air-fluid level (Figure 19–17). In unusual cases, a CT scan may be required for better radiographic visualization, and in cases of suspected bronchial obstruction or in all patients with unexplained lung abscesses, bronchoscopy is indicated. Fine-needle aspiration of the ab-

Figure 19–17. Lung abscess involving the superior segment of the left lower lobe.

scess cavity for diagnostic culture has been shown to isolate the offending pathogens in 94% of patients compared with only 11% and 3% from sputum culture and bronchoalveolar lavage, respectively. In addition, early fine-needle aspiration also has been reported to change the antibiotic regimen in 43% of cases and can be life-saving in immunocompromised patients with unusual organisms.

Treatment

Antibiotic administration has been the mainstay of therapy following general resuscitation measures. The selection of antibiotics varies and depends on the underlying cause, but penicillin and clindamycin are commonly used. In immunocompromised individuals, trimethoprim-sulfamethoxazole, pentamidine, erythromycin, and amphotericin B are often indicated. Once the acute sepsis subsides (after up to 2 weeks), therapy can frequently be changed to an oral outpatient regimen and continued until complete resolution of the abscess occurs (3–5 months). Important adjuncts to antibiotic administration include chest physiotherapy, bronchoscopy (may require repeated examinations to maintain bronchial drainage), and health maintenance measures (general nutrition, dental hygiene, etc). In patients who do not respond to this initial regimen and who do not have surgical indications (see below), early percutaneous drainage has been shown to be a safe and effective procedure (mortality rate 1.5%; morbidity rate 10%). Specific proposed indications for percutaneous drainage include (1) an abscess under tension as evidenced by mediastinal shift, displacement of fissures or

downward movement of the diaphragm, (2) radiographic verification of contralateral lung contamination, (3) unremitting signs of sepsis after 72 hours of adequate antibiotic therapy, (4) abscess size > 4 cm or increasing abscess size, (5) rising fluid level, and (6) persistent ventilatory dependency. Thoracotomy today is rarely indicated in the management of lung abscess but continues to be indicated in patients with massive hemoptysis, empyema, bronchial obstruction (particularly if secondary to resectable cancer), and failure of medical therapy. Furthermore, acute rupture into the pleural space (pyopneumothorax) is still a surgical emergency. When surgery is indicated, lobectomy generally is the preferred procedure.

Prognosis

Since the appearance of effective antibiotics, the mortality rate from lung abscesses has declined from 30–50% down to 5–20%. Medical therapy alone is successful in 75–88% of patients, and those requiring operation are cured 90% of the time with a mortality rate of only 1%. In the growing population of ICU and immunocompromised patients, however, the mortality rate remains high (approximately 28%).

Bartlett JG: Antibiotics in lung abscess. Semin Respir Infect 1991; 6:103.

Groskin SA et al: Bacterial lung abscess: a review of the radiographic and clinical features of 50 cases. J Thorac Imaging 1991;6:62.

Lambiase RE et al: Percutaneous drainage of 335 consecutive abscesses: results of primary drainage with 1-year follow-up. Radiology 1992;184:167.

vanSonnenberg E et al: Lung abscess: CT-guided drainage. Radiology 1991;178:347.

2. Bronchiectasis

Bronchiectasis strictly defined is abnormal dilation of the bronchi, but common usage expands the definition to denote the clinical syndrome marked by chronic dilation of bronchi, a paroxysmal cough that produces variable amounts of fetid, mucopurulent sputum, and recurrent pulmonary infections. Bronchiectasis was at one time a common problem frequently complicated by hemoptysis, lung and brain abscesses, empyema, respiratory failure, and death. Since the introduction of vaccination programs, antibiotics, and antituberculous medications, however, it is reported commonly only in isolated geographic locations.

Although congenital diseases (Kartagener's syndrome, cystic fibrosis, Williams-Campbell syndrome, Mounier-Kuhn syndrome, immunoglobulin deficiencies, and α_1-antitrypsin deficiency) can lead to the development of bronchiectasis, most cases are related to acquired disorders and are caused by two factors: infection and bronchial obstruction. Viral and bacterial pneumonias in infancy and childhood—eg, pertussis, measles, influenza, tuberculosis, and bronchopneumonia—were common predisposing conditions that led to bronchiectasis in the past. Either a single severe bout of pneumonia or repeated moderate infections can cause progressive destruction of bronchial cilia, mucosa, musculoelastic tissue, and even cartilage. Healing with fibrosis and contraction of the peribronchial tissues subsequently produces bronchial dilation. Retention of secretions resulting from destruction of normal mucociliary action leads to repeated bouts of infection and progressive scarring and bronchial dilation. Aspirated foreign bodies, endobronchial neoplasms, and hilar lymphadenopathy (see middle lobe syndrome below) also can cause retention of secretions, infections, and progressive bronchiectasis. The presence of true established bronchiectasis, however, must be distinguished from pseudobronchiectasis, which is a cylindric bronchial dilation that is associated with acute bronchopneumonia. When left untreated, true bronchiectasis progresses, while pseudobronchiectasis reverses completely after weeks to months.

Since the original description of bronchiectasis by Laennec in 1826, the disorder has been divided into two main types based on pathologic appearance: saccular and cylindric. Saccular bronchiectasis follows most infections and bronchial obstruction while the cylindric variety is associated with posttuberculosis bronchiectasis. A third type of bronchiectasis is distinguished by alternating saccular and cylindric areas and is referred to as mixed or varicose bronchiectasis. In general, bronchiectasis involves the second-order to fourth-order branches of the segmental bronchi, and its distribution is largely characteristic of the underlying pathology. Congenital disorders, for example, are associated with diffuse bilateral bronchiectasis, while tuberculosis and granulomatous diseases are characterized by unilateral or bilateral disease, most commonly limited to the upper lobes and superior segments of the lower lobes. Furthermore, bronchiectasis following pyogenic and viral pneumonias usually involves only the lower lobes, middle lobe, and lingula, and postobstructive bronchiectasis is generally limited to the obstructed segments (see also middle lobe syndrome, below). Common pathogens in patients with bronchiectasis include *H influenzae, S aureus, K pneumoniae, E coli,* and, in the chronic setting, pseudomonas species. Mycobacteria, fungi, and legionella should also be cultured.

Clinical Findings & Diagnosis

Patients with a history of recurrent febrile episodes often complain of a chronic or intermittent cough that is productive of variable amounts of foul-smelling sputum (up to 500 mL/d). Hemoptysis occurs in 41–66%, but rarely is it massive. Bronchiectasis associated with granulomatous disease may not be associated with a productive cough (so-called "dry" bronchiectasis). Exacerbations and advanced disease are manifested by increased sputum production, fever, dyspnea, anorexia, fatigue, and weight loss. A history of sinus problems, infertility, or a family history of similar problems suggests the presence of an inherited disorder associated with bronchiectasis. Physical examination may reveal cyanosis, clubbing, pulmonary osteoarthropathy, evidence of malnutrition, and, in advanced disease, signs of cor pulmonale. Although bronchiectasis is suspected, an imaging study is usually required for confirmation. Bronchograms were at one time required, but high-resolution, fine-cut (1.5-5 mm) CT scans are now the imaging procedure of choice to document bronchial dilation, particularly with saccular disease. Even with the diagnosis of bronchiectasis, however, endobronchial neoplasm or foreign body must be excluded by flexible fiberoptic bronchoscopy.

Treatment

In nearly all patients, conservative medical therapy is indicated and generally is sufficient. This includes broad-spectrum antibiotics, bronchodilators, humidification, expectorants, mucolytics, and effective routine postural drainage. In patients with continued infection, bronchoscopy with bronchoalveolar lavage should be considered to obtain more accurate culture results. Other adjunctive therapies includes influenza and pneumococcal vaccines and, in some patients, chronic "prophylactic" antibiotic administration with trimethoprim-sulfamethoxazole, erythromycin, or ciprofloxacin. A recent advance in controlling underlying bacterial (especially pseudomonas) infection and symptoms associated with bronchiectasis has been the use of inhaled antibiotics. In the cystic fibrosis and chronic bronchiectasis population, nebulized tobramycin or gentamicin has proved effective in controlling infection, sputum production, and symptoms in a significant proportion of patients.

Patients who fail intensive medical therapy may be candidates for surgical resection if the following criteria are met: (1) the disease must be localized and completely resectable; (2) pulmonary reserve must be adequate; (3) the process must be irreversible (ie, not pseudobronchiectasis, bronchial stricture, foreign body, etc); and (4) significant symptoms must persist. Preoperative assessment requires a high-resolution fine-cut CT scan, though some surgeons still prefer a bronchogram as a "road map." Pulmonary function studies generally are not necessary since the involved segments do not function. The goals of surgery are to remove all active disease and to preserve as much functioning lung parenchyma as possible. The surgical approach includes complete segmental resection of the involved areas. Partial resection almost always ends in recurrence. Resection most commonly involves all basal segments (unilaterally or bilaterally) along with the middle lobe or lingula. With tuberculosis, however, removal of the upper lobe or lobes with or without the superior segment of the lower lobes is more likely. During surgery, meticulous maintenance of a clear airway devoid of mucopurulent secretions and blood is essential. Careful dissection of the bronchovascular structures is difficult in patients with chronic inflammation and scarring but is essential to avoid complications.

Prognosis

Although most patients are successfully treated with medical therapy, some require surgery. The results of surgical resection depend on the cause and type of pulmonary involvement. Success with elimination of symptoms occurs in up to 80% of patients with limited localized disease but only 36% of those with diffuse disease. Prognostic factors include (1) unilateral disease restricted to the basal segments, (2) young age, (3) absence of sinusitis and rhinitis, (4) history of pneumonia, and (5) no major airway obstruction. Overall morbidity and mortality rates are surprisingly low at 3–5% and < 1%, respectively.

Ip M et al: Multivariate analysis of factors affecting pulmonary function in bronchiectasis. Respiration 1993;60:45.

McGuinness G et al: Bronchiectasis: CT evaluation. AJR Am J Roentgenol 1993;160:253.

Trucksis M, Swartz MN: Bronchiectasis: a current view. Curr Clin Top Infect Dis 1991;11:170.

3. Middle Lobe Syndrome

Relapsing lateral pneumonia of the middle pulmonary lobe is typically caused by intermittent obstruction, most often extrinsic. In a patient with repeated episodes of right-sided pneumonia, this diagnosis should be entertained, but only after other causes of obstruction (bronchogenic cancer, foreign body, etc), have been ruled out.

Broncholithiasis (see below) and middle lobe syndrome have been considered to be caused by compression or erosion of the bronchus by adjacent diseased lymph nodes. Other factors, such as poor natural drainage and lack of collateral ventilation, probably explain the frequency of middle lobe.

Endobronchial tumors and foreign bodies must be excluded by bronchoscopy.

Most patients respond to intensive medical therapy, and surgery is rarely required. Indications for surgery, which usually involves middle lobectomy, include bronchiectasis, fibrosis (bronchostenosis), abscess, unresolved or intractable recurrent pneumonia, and suspicion of neoplasm.

Ring-Mrozik E et al: Clinical findings in middle lobe syndrome and other processes of pulmonary shrinkage in children (atelectasis syndrome). Eur J Pediatr Surg 1991;1:266.

4. Broncholithiasis

Broncholithiasis is defined as the presence of calculi (broncholiths) within the tracheobronchial tree. In most cases, a calcified parabronchial lymph node erodes through the bronchial wall into the lumen; however, severely inspissated mucus may calcify. Calcified lymph nodes may remain attached to the bronchial wall, lodge in a bronchus, or be expectorated (lithoptysis). The most common cause of broncholithiasis in the United States is histoplasmosis. Tuberculosis is another frequent cause in some parts of the world.

Patients with broncholithiasis often complain of hemoptysis, lithoptysis (30%), cough, sputum production, fever, chills, and pleuritic chest pain. The hemoptysis is characteristically sudden and self-limited, though rarely it may be massive. Symptoms of pneumonia may indicate bronchial obstruction from an impacted broncholith. Signs suggesting broncholithiasis include localized wheezing on physical examination, evidence of hilar calcifications or segmental atelectasis and pneumonia on chest x-ray, and bronchoscopic evidence of peribronchial disease. The diagnosis is confirmed by documentation of lithoptysis or the presence of an endobronchial "lung stone."

The complications of broncholithiasis include hemoptysis, which on occasion can be massive and life-threatening; suppurative lung diseases, eg, pneumonia and bronchiectasis; midesophageal traction diverticula; and, rarely, tracheobronchoesophageal fistula. In addition to instituting appropriate therapy for underlying pulmonary diseases, treatment is primarily directed at removal of endobronchial stones. This can be accomplished at the time of bronchoscopy if the broncholith is freely floating within the tracheobronchial tree or if it extends well into the bronchial lumen and can be removed without excessive force or traction (20% of cases). The main danger of transbronchoscopic removal of broncholiths is the real possibility of massive hemorrhage. This results during inappropriate removal of broncholiths that remain substantially attached to the parabronchial tissues. Because of intense peribronchial fibrosis in this situation, the broncholith not infrequently becomes adherent to vascular structures such as the pulmonary artery, which may be torn with vigorous attempts at broncholith removal. Nearly 80% of patients with broncholiths that remain in situ require surgical removal. The goal of surgery in this disease is preservation of lung function. The broncholith may be removed safely with bronchotomy; however, most patients require segmentectomy or lobectomy, particularly if destruction of lung parenchyma has occurred from postobstruction suppurative lung disease. Fistulas between the airway and the esophagus should be repaired with interposition of normal tissue (intercostal muscle flap, etc) between the two structures to prevent recurrence. Following surgery, the prognosis is excellent.

Conces DJ Jr, Tarver RD, Vix VA: Broncholithiasis: CT features in 15 patients. AJR Am J Roentgenol 1991;157:249.

Galdermans D et al: Broncholithiasis: present clinical spectrum. Respir Med 1990;84:155.

Igoe D, Lynch V, McNicholas WT: Broncholithiasis: bronchoscopic vs. surgical management. Respir Med 1990; 84:163.

McLean TR, Beall AC Jr, Jones JW: Massive hemoptysis due to broncholithiasis. Ann Thorac Surg 1991;52:1173.

5. Cystic Fibrosis & Mucoid Impaction of the Bronchi

Cystic fibrosis is a serious congenital disorder that may lead to bronchitis, bronchiectasis, pulmonary fibrosis, emphysema, and lung abscess. Mucoid impaction occurs in patients with asthma and bronchitis. Mucoid plugs are rubbery, semisolid, gray to greenish-yellow in color, and round, oval, or elongated in shape. There is often a history of recurrent upper respiratory infection, fever, and chest pain. Expectoration of hard mucus plugs or hemoptysis may occur.

Bronchogenic carcinoma, fungal infection, tuberculosis, bronchiectasis, abscess, bacterial pneumonia, lipoid pneumonia, pulmonary eosinophilic granuloma, and Löffler's syndrome must be ruled out.

Treatment is with expectorants, detergents, bronchodilators, antibiotics, and aerosol inhalation. The availability of acetylcysteine has largely converted this condition to a purely medical disease. Surgery is indicated when cancer cannot be ruled out, for destroyed lung, or in the treatment of abscess.

Double lung transplantation is a consideration for advanced cystic fibrosis patients with end-stage pulmonary function. Overall, survivals have improved (85% at 1 year, 50% at 5 years) due to improvements in surgical technique (bronchial anastomosis) and immunosuppressive regimens. Still, chronic bronchitis obliterans remains a major obstacle after several years and is the leading cause of eventual transplant failure.

Limited donor organ availability prevents the many eligible cystic fibrosis patients from being transplanted.

Fiel SB: Clinical management of pulmonary disease in cystic fibrosis. Lancet 1993;341:1070.

Shennib H et al: Double-lung transplantation for cystic fibrosis. The Cystic Fibrosis Transplant Study Group. Ann Thorac Surg 1992;54:27.

6. Tuberculosis

Tuberculosis markedly declined as a cause of death between 1953 and 1984, but since 1985 this disease has experienced a resurgence due to increased immigration of infected individuals and HIV infection. A reservoir of about 5000–8000 clinical cases exists, and an additional 25,000 new cases occur annually. Less than 20% of the United States population are tuberculin-positive, but tuberculosis remains a common infectious cause of death worldwide.

Several species of the genus mycobacterium may cause lung disease, but 95% of cases of lung disease are due to *Mycobacterium tuberculosis. Mycobacterium bovis* and *Mycobacterium avium* are seldom found in humans. Several "atypical" species of mycobacterium that are chiefly soil-dwellers have become clinically more important in recent years because they are less responsive to preventive and therapeutic measures. Mycobacteria are nonmotile, nonsporulating, weakly gram-positive rods classified in the order Actinomycetales. Dormant organisms remain alive for the life of the host.

The initial infection often involves pulmonary parenchyma in the midzone of the lungs. When hypersensitivity develops after several weeks, the typical caseation appears. Regional hilar lymph nodes become enlarged. Most cases arrest spontaneously at this stage. If the infection progresses, caseation necrosis develops and giant cells produce a typical tubercle. A cause of latent disease in the elderly or debilitated patient is dormant reactivation tubercles. Sites in the apical and posterior segments of the upper lobes and superior segments of the lower lobes are the usual areas of infection.

Clinical Findings

A. SYMPTOMS AND SIGNS

Patients may present with minimal symptoms, including fever, cough, anorexia, weight loss, night sweats, excessive perspiration, chest pain, lethargy, and dyspnea. Extrapulmonary disease may be associated with more severe symptoms, such as involvement of the pericardium, bones, joints, urinary tract, meninges, lymph nodes, or pleural space. Erythema nodosum is seen occasionally in patients with active disease.

B. LABORATORY FINDINGS

False-negative tests with intermediate-strength PPD are usually due to anergy, improper testing, or outdated tuberculin. Anergy is sometimes associated with disseminated tuberculosis, measles, sarcoidosis, lymphomas, or recent vaccination with live viruses (eg, poliomyelitis, measles, rubella, mumps, influenza, or yellow fever).

Immunosuppressive drugs (eg, corticosteroids, azathioprine) and disease states (eg, AIDS, organ transplantation) may also cause false-negative responses. Mumps skin tests are negative in patients taking immunosuppressive drugs.

Culture of sputum, gastric aspirates, and tracheal washings as well as pleural fluid and pleural and lung biopsies may establish the diagnosis.

Table 19–5. Antituberculosis drugs and their side effects.[1]

Drug	Dosage (Adult Daily)	Side Effects (Usual)	Monitoring	Remarks
Isoniazid	5–10 mg/kg; 300–600 mg.	Peripheral neuritis, hepatitis, hypersensitivity, convulsions.	SGOT (AST)/SGPT (ALT) (not as routine).	To prevent neuritis, give pyridoxine, 25–50 mg/d orally.
Ethambutol	15–25 mg/kg/d for 60 days, then 15 mg/kg/d.	Optic neuritis (very rare at 15 mg/kg/d).	Visual acuity, red-green color discrimination.	Ocular history and funduscopic examination before use; contraindicated with optic neuritis.
Rifampin	600 mg once daily (children, 10–20 mg/kg to a maximum of 600 mg).	Hepatotoxicity (rare under age 20; 2.5% of cases over age 50). Occasionally, thrombocytopenia, anemia, nephritis.	SGOT (AST)/SGPT (ALT).	Harmless orange staining of urine, sweat, contact lenses, etc. "Flu syndrome" if rifampin given less than twice weekly.
Streptomycin	0.5–1.5 g/d IM (children, 20–40 mg/kg/d IM).	Ototoxicity, nephrotoxicity.	Gross hearing (ticking of watch); if abnormal audiograms, BUN and creatinine.	Used mainly in very ill patients as part of triple-drug regimen.
Aminosalicylic acid	10–12 g/d.	Gastrointestinal intolerance, skin rashes, hypersensitivity.	SGOT (AST)/SGPT (ALT).	Because of poor tolerance, rarely used now.
Pyrazinamide[2]	20–35 mg/kg/d, up to 3 g/d.	Hyperuricemia, hepatotoxicity, arthralgia.	Uric acid, SGOT (AST)/SGPT (ALT).	Sometimes given as first-line drug in short-course regimen (50 mg/kg twice weekly); inexpensive.
Ethionamide[2]	0.5–1 g/d.	Gastrointestinal, hepatotoxicity, hypersensitivity (rash).	SGOT (AST)/SGPT (ALT).	Temporarily stop or reduce dose with gastrointestinal irritation and hepatotoxicity.
Cycloserine[2]	0.5–1 g/d.	Psychosis, personality changes, convulsions, rash.	Drug blood levels if poor renal function.	CNS reactions sometimes controlled by phenytoin.
Capreomycin[2]	20 mg/kg/d IM (up to 1 g/d)	Nephrotoxicity, ototoxicity, hepatotoxicity.	Same as streptomycin with SGOT(AST)/SGPT (ALT) in addition.	Sometimes given as 1 g 2 or 3 times weekly.
Viomycin[2]	1 g twice daily IM 2 or 3 times weekly.	Nephrotoxicity, ototoxicity.	As for streptomycin, plus urinalysis.	As for streptomycin.
Kanamycin[2]	0.5–1 g IM.	See streptomycin.	As for streptomycin, plus urinalysis.	Used mainly for atypical mycobacterial infections.

[1]See also Chambers HF: Antimycobacterial drugs. In: *Basic and Clinical Pharmacology*, 8th ed. Katzung BG (editor). McGraw-Hill, 2001.
[2]Used only as second-line drug in *M tuberculosis* infections, mainly for re-treatment or in drug-resistant cases. Used as first-line drug, in combinations, in atypical mycobacterial infections.

C. IMAGING STUDIES

X-ray findings include involvement of the apical and posterior segments of the upper lobes (85%) or the superior segments of the lower lobes (10%). Seldom is the anterior segment of the upper lobe solely involved, as in other granulomatous diseases such as histoplasmosis. Involvement of the basal segments of the lower lobes is uncommon except in women, blacks, and diabetics, but endobronchial disease usually involves the lower lobes, producing atelectasis or consolidation. Differing x-ray patterns correspond to the pathologic variations of the disease: the local exudative lesion, the local productive lesion, cavitation, acute tuberculous pneumonia, miliary tuberculosis, Rasmussen's aneurysm, bronchiectasis, bronchostenosis, and tuberculoma.

Differential Diagnosis

It is critical to distinguish the x-ray findings from bronchogenic carcinoma, particularly when there is tuberculoma without calcification.

Treatment

A. MEDICAL TREATMENT

Active disease should be treated with one of the chemotherapeutic regimens that have recently been shown to shorten the period of treatment while maintaining their potency. Such drugs include isoniazid, streptomycin, rifampin, and ethambutol (Table 19–5). These multiple-drug regimens are designed to prevent the emergence of resistant strains and minimize toxicity.

B. SURGICAL TREATMENT

The role of surgery in treatment of tuberculosis has diminished dramatically since chemotherapy became available. It is now confined to the following indications: (1) failure of chemotherapy, (2) performance of diagnostic procedures, (3) destroyed lung, (4) postsurgical complications, (5) persistent bronchopleural fistula, and (6) intractable hemorrhage.

Surgical resection for diagnosis may be necessary to rule out other diseases, such as cancer, or to obtain material for cultures. Patients with destroyed lobes (Figure 19–18) or cavitary tuberculosis of the right upper lobe (Figure 19–19) containing large infected foci may sometimes be candidates for resection.

The disease becomes reactivated in some patients who have had thoracoplasty, plombage, or resection, and a few will require reoperation. The most common indications for surgery after plombage therapy are pleural infection (pyogenic or tuberculous) and migration of the plombage material, causing pain or compression of other organs. Following pulmonary resection, tuberculous empyema may develop in the

Figure 19–18. Tuberculosis of the right lung with empyema and bronchopleural fistula.

postpneumonectomy space, sometimes associated with a bronchopleural fistula or bony sequestration. Persistent bronchopleural fistula after chemotherapy and closed tube drainage may require direct operative closure. Use of mussel flaps (intercostal, etc.) is highly recommended to cover any bronchial stumps, especially in the setting of pneumonectomy.

Figure 19–19. Cavitary tuberculosis of the right upper lobe.

Tuberculous empyema poses unique problems of management. Treatment depends upon whether the empyema is (1) associated with parenchymal disease, (2) mixed tuberculous and pyogenic or purely tuberculous, and (3) associated with bronchopleural fistula. The ultimate objective is complete expansion of the lung and obliteration of the empyema space. Pulmonary decortication or resection may be used for tuberculosis, but open or closed drainage is necessary when the process is complicated by pyogenic infection or bronchopleural fistula.

Prognosis

The prognosis is excellent in most cases treated medically; the death rate decreased from 25% in 1945 to less than 10% currently. Perioperative mortality for pulmonary resections for tuberculosis ranges from 10% for pneumonectomy to 3% for lobectomy and 1% for segmentectomy and subsegmental resections.

The relapse rate following modern chemotherapy is about 4%.

Horowitz MD et al: Late complications of plombage. Ann Thorac Surg 1992;53:803.

Langston HT: Thoracoplasty: the how and the why. Ann Thorac Surg 1991;52:1351.

Nolan CM: Failure of therapy for tuberculosis in human immunodeficiency virus infection. Am J Med Sci 1992; 304:168.

Pomerantz M et al: Surgical management of resistant mycobacterial tuberculosis and other mycobacterial pulmonary infections. Ann Thorac Surg 1991;52:1108.

Reed CE, Parker EF, Crawford FA Jr: Surgical resection for complications of pulmonary tuberculosis. Ann Thorac Surg 1989;48:165.

FUNGAL INFECTIONS OF THE LUNG

Pulmonary fungal infections are increasing due to the widespread use of broad-spectrum antibiotics, the use of corticosteroids and other immunosuppressive drugs, and the spread of HIV infection and AIDS. Fungal infections frequently involve the respiratory tract and include histoplasmosis, coccidioidomycosis, blastomycosis, cryptococcosis, aspergillosis, mucormycosis, and candidiasis. Although these fungal infections can occur anywhere in the world, several are noted for their characteristic endemic areas. Candidiasis rarely if ever requires operative treatment and thus will not be discussed here.

1. Histoplasmosis

Histoplasma capsulatum is a dimorphic soil fungus that is frequently found in fowl and bat excreta, pigeon roosts, chicken houses, caves, hollow trees, attics, and lofts. It is endemic in fertile river valleys, such as the Mississippi, Missouri, Ohio, St. Lawrence, and Rio Grande. Infection occurs almost exclusively after inhalation of a large number of spores and occurs with a male:female ratio of 3:1. Once in the lungs, the fungus germinates in yeast form, resulting in caseation, necrosis, fibrosis, and calcification. The diagnosis of histoplasmosis relies on high or rising serum antibody complement fixation titers (> 1:32 or fourfold rise) in the appropriate clinical setting. The histoplasmin skin test, which becomes positive 2–6 weeks following infection, is useful only for epidemiologic studies and not for the diagnosis of acute disease. Sputum culture is positive in less than 10%, but tissue cultures may be more reliable.

Most infections in immunocompetent individuals are asymptomatic. Infections are classified as acute, chronic, or disseminated. Acute infections are manifested either (1) as a flu-like syndrome with fever, chills, dry cough, headache, retrosternal discomfort, arthralgias, and a rash suggesting erythema nodosum; (2) with symptoms similar to a flu-like syndrome but limited to the lungs and occasionally accompanied by a productive cough; or (3) as an acute diffuse nodular disease with mild symptoms. Radiographic findings in these three acute syndromes typically demonstrate ill-defined upper lobe nonsegmental opacities; nonsegmental areas of consolidation that tend to change; and diffuse, discrete 3- to 4-mm nodules, respectively. Hilar adenopathy on chest x-ray is common. Physical examination can be normal or may reveal signs of pneumonia.

In contrast, chronic infections include (1) an asymptomatic solitary, discrete nodule less than 3 cm in diameter known as a histoplasmoma (most common), often with central and concentric calcifications ("target lesion") and frequently located in the lower lobes; (2) chronic cavitary histoplasmosis, which typically occurs in patients with underlying obstructive disease, characteristically mild symptoms, fibronodular upper lobe infiltrates, and centrilobular emphysematous spaces; (3) mediastinal granulomas that may result in broncholithiasis, esophageal traction diverticula, superior vena cava compression, and tracheobronchoesophageal fistulas; and (4) fibrosing mediastinitis, which can produce compression of the superior vena cava, tracheobronchial tree, or esophagus.

Disseminated disease includes an acute, subacute, and chronic form.

These infections occur in children (acute and subacute) as well as adults (subacute and chronic). Fever and abdominal pain are common. Other findings include hepatosplenomegaly, pancytopenia, meningitis, endocarditis, adrenocortical insufficiency, and oropharyngeal ulceration (chronic form).

Radiographic imaging in disseminated disease may demonstrate diffuse interstitial pneumonitis (25%) or minimal findings.

The symptoms and roentgenographic findings of histoplasmosis resemble those of tuberculosis, although the disease appears to progress more slowly. There may be cough, malaise, hemoptysis, low-grade fever, and weight loss. As many as 30% of cases coexist with tuberculosis. Pulmonary fibrosis, bulla formation, and pulmonary insufficiency occur in advanced cases of histoplasmosis. Mediastinal involvement is quite frequent and may take the form of granuloma formation, fibrosis with superior vena caval syndrome, or dysphagia. Erosion of inflammatory lymph nodes into bronchi may cause expectoration of broncholiths, hemoptysis, wheezing, or bronchiectasis. Traction diverticula of the esophagus may lead to development of tracheoesophageal fistula. Pericardial involvement may lead to constrictive pericarditis.

In lesions that present as solitary pulmonary nodules, histoplasmosis is diagnosed in about 15–20% of cases. Radiologically, early infections appear as diffuse mottled parenchymal infiltrations surrounding the hila, with enlargement of hilar lymph nodes. Cavitation indicates advanced infection and is the complication about which the surgeon is most often consulted. The diagnosis rests upon finding a positive skin test or complement fixation test and culturing the fungus from sputum or a bronchial aspirate.

Medical therapy of histoplasmosis is indicated only in cavitary and severe disease and for most infections in immunocompromised hosts. Ketoconazole (400 mg/d for 6 months) or itraconazole (200–400 mg/d for 6 months) is useful in cavitary disease, while amphotericin B (1–2 g total dose) is reserved for patients with more serious infections and infections in immunocompromised patients. Surgery is reserved for treatment of complications. Broncholithectomy with or without pulmonary resection, repair of tracheobronchoesophageal fistulas, decompression of mediastinal granulomas, and spiral saphenous vein bypass of severe symptomatic superior vena cava obstruction are typical examples.

2. Coccidioidomycosis

Coccidioides immitis is a dimorphic soil fungus that is endemic in the Sonoran life zone (Utah, Arizona, California, Nevada, and New Mexico) and is associated with creosote brush. Dry heat with brief intense rain is essential for this fungus, which is spread by strong winds. Infection occurs through inhalation of as few as one to ten arthrospores which then germinate as parasitic spherules. Spherules have a double refractile cell wall and produce endospores that cause the spherule to rupture, spreading the infection into the surrounding tissues. Caseation, suppuration, abscess formation, and fibrosis follow. The diagnosis of coccidioidomycosis relies on the detection of acutely elevated titers of IgM antibodies (by latex agglutination and confirmed by immunodiffusion tube precipitin tests) or rising serum

IgG antibody complement fixation titers (seroconversion or fourfold rise) in the appropriate clinical context. The coccidioidin and spherulin skin tests, which become positive 3–21 days following infection, are generally useful only for epidemiologic studies and not for the diagnosis of acute disease. *C immitis* grows well in culture, but it is extremely hazardous to handle and requires a laminar flow hood due to the highly infectious nature of the arthrospores. Identification of the spherules in tissue, lavage samples, and fine-needle aspirates is helpful in making the diagnosis in some patients. Although many stains can be used, including routine fungal (KOH) preparations, Pap staining is most sensitive. Gram stains, however, fail to demonstrate spherules.

Primary infection is asymptomatic in 60% of patients, while most others develop **desert fever,** with fever, productive cough, pleuritic chest pain, pneumonitis, and a rash typical of erythema nodosum or erythema multiforme. Disease that includes arthralgias is known as **desert rheumatism.** Radiographic findings demonstrate segmental or nonsegmental, homogeneous or mottled infiltrates with a predilection for the lower lobes. Physical examination is often unrevealing, but rales and rhonchi may be present. Other findings include eosinophilia (66%), hilar adenopathy (20%), and small exudative pleural effusions (2–20%). Symptomatic persistent infection associated with chest x-ray findings 6–8 weeks after primary infection is classified as one of five types: persistent pneumonia, chronic progressive pneumonia, miliary coccidioidomycosis, coccidioidal nodules, or pulmonary cavities. Persistent pneumonia manifests with symptoms of fever, productive cough, and pleuritic chest pain in association with protracted infiltrates and consolidation on chest x-ray. All findings, however, resolve within 8 months. Patients with chronic progressive pneumonia complain of fever, cough, dyspnea, hemoptysis, and weight loss, with bilateral apical nodular densities and multiple cavities lasting up to 14 years. This presentation closely resembles tuberculosis and chronic histoplasmosis. Miliary coccidioidomycosis occurs early and rapidly, associated with bilateral diffuse infiltrates. This form of disease implies the presence of impaired immunity and has an associated mortality rate of 50%. Nearly half of patients with coccidioidal nodules are asymptomatic. These nodular densities (coccidiomas) appear in the middle and upper lung fields, often within 5 cm of the hilum; range from 1 cm to 4 cm in size; and do not calcify, making it hard to distinguish them from malignancy. In endemic areas, 30–50% of all nodules are coccidiomas. Patients develop pulmonary cavities in 10–15% of cases of coccidioidomycosis. Typically, these are solitary (90%), thin-walled, located in the upper lobes (70%), less than 6 cm in size (90%), and close spontaneously within 2 years (50%). Some cavities, however, cross fissures; cause hemoptysis (25–50%), usually mild; rupture, producing a pyopneumothorax with a bronchopleural fistula; or become infected with aspergillus. Uncommonly, dissemination can occur, particularly in immunocompromised individuals, in pregnancy (third trimester), and in dark-skinned individuals (blacks, Filipinos, Spanish, etc). Although pulmonary symptoms in disseminated disease are mild, meningeal involvement is common and the mortality rate is high (50%).

Medical therapy is not indicated in asymptomatic individuals. Patients with persistent or chronic pneumonia, miliary disease, and those at risk for dissemination should be treated with antifungal therapy. Amphotericin B (0.5–2.5 g intravenously as total dose) is the standard treatment, though the newer azole compounds (fluconazole, ketoconazole, and itraconazole) may be used for long-term maintenance therapy since the relapse rate may be as high as 25–50%. Surgery is reserved for patients with coccidiomas when cancer is a concern and in patients with cavities that have an associated radiographic abnormality suggesting carcinoma (ie, thick wall) or that develop a complication, eg, hemoptysis and pyopneumothorax from rupture. Resection should include all diseased tissue and most often requires lobectomy.

3. Blastomycosis

Blastomyces dermatitidis is a dimorphic soil fungus found in warm, wet, nitrogen-rich soil in an endemic area that extends east of a line from the Texas Gulf coast to the border between Minnesota and North Dakota (except Florida and New England). Infection occurs characteristically in males (male:female ratio 6:1–15:1) from 30–60 years of age through inhalation of conidia (asexual spores). At 37 °C the conidia germinate as yeasts, producing caseation in a manner similar to tuberculosis. Rarely, infection may develop through direct skin inoculation. Risk factors include poor hygiene, exposure to dust and wood, manual labor, and poor housing conditions. Since no accurate skin or serologic tests exist, the diagnosis depends on culture or histologic identification of the yeast form. Culture of the mycelial form can be hazardous. *B dermatitidis* grows as white to tan colonies of septate hyphae at room temperature but changes to budding yeast at 37 °C. This temperature-dependent change reflects the uncoupling of oxidative phosphorylation. The yeast form can be found in sputum (33%), bronchoalveolar lavage specimens (38%), lung biopsies (21%), and in fine-needle aspirates (7%) and can be demonstrated with standard KOH preparations or many other histologic stains (but not Gram stain). The yeast, however,

does not have a large capsule (distinguishes it from *Cryptococcus neoformans*) and do not grow intracellularly (differentiates it from *Histoplasma capsulatum*).

Manifestations of blastomycosis can occur in many organ systems, including the lungs, skin, bone, genitourinary tract (prostatitis and epididymoorchitis), and central nervous system. Pulmonary infection can be asymptomatic or may present with flu-like symptoms, evidence of pneumonia, or pleurisy. Cough (36%), weight loss (20%), pleuritic pain (26%), fever (23%), hemoptysis (21%), erythema nodosum, and ulcerative bronchitis are common. Radiographic findings include homogeneous or patchy consolidation in a nonsegmental distribution with pleural effusions or thickening or cavitation (15–35%). In some patients, the appearance of pulmonary masses may mimic carcinoma. A predilection for the upper lobes has been noted; however, unlike histoplasmosis and coccidioidomycosis, in blastomycosis hilar and mediastinal adenopathy is unusual.

Limited disease in asymptomatic patients requires no specific therapy. Itraconazole, 100–200 mg/d orally for at least 2–3 months, is now the therapy of choice for nonmeningeal disease, with a response rate of over 80%. Amphotericin B (0.5–2 g), however, is indicated in patients with meningeal disease or failed therapy. Surgical resection is rarely necessary except when the possibility of malignancy cannot be excluded.

4. Cryptococcosis

Cryptococcus neoformans is an encapsulated yeast-like budding fungus. It is a saprophyte existing on the skin, nasopharynx, gastrointestinal tract, and vagina of humans as well as in pigeon excreta, grasses, trees, plants, fruits, bees, wasps, insects (cockroaches), birds, milk products, pickle brine, and soil. Cryptococcal infection generally indicates the presence of an underlying debilitating disease in an immunocompromised host. Infection occurs from inhalation of the yeast form. The diagnosis can be established by the detection of serum antigen (via complement fixation tests) in patients with appropriate clinical and radiographic findings. More commonly, however, histologic identification with India ink stains is used; routine cultures are not performed since they are extremely time-consuming and require multiple biochemical tests for differentiation of cryptococcus from other fungi. No accurate skin test exists for cryptococcosis.

The most common sites of infection are the lungs and central nervous system. Pulmonary infection may remain asymptomatic, or patients may complain of cough, pleuritic chest pain, and fever. Radiographically, cryptococcus can appear as a localized, well-defined 3- to 10-cm pleural-based mass without smooth borders; as single or multiple areas of consolidation, usually within one lobe but in nonsegmental distribution; or as a disseminated miliary nodular infiltrate. A predilection for the lower lobes has been noted. Central nervous system infection usually follows an asymptomatic pulmonary infection. Central nervous system symptoms are highly variable since many patients are severely immunocompromised and do not manifest the usual signs and symptoms of meningitis or cerebritis.

Medical therapy is indicated in most cases of pulmonary infection except for rare cases of limited localized disease. Amphotericin B (0.5–2 g) remains the treatment of choice and is often combined with flucytosine (150/mg/kg per day) for synergy. New azole compounds (eg, fluconazole, itraconazole) may be useful in long-term maintenance therapy. Surgery is rarely indicated and is useful only to exclude the possibility of malignancy or to determine the etiology of an undiagnosed diffuse pulmonary infiltrate by open lung biopsy.

5. Aspergillosis

Aspergillus species are ubiquitous dimorphic soil fungi found in soil and decaying organic matter. The most common pathogenic species include *A fumigatus* (most common), *A niger, A flavus,* and *A glaucus.* In culture, these fungi resemble an aspergillum, which is a brush used to sprinkle holy water. Aspergillosis represents the second most common (after candidiasis) opportunistic fungal infection in immunocompromised hosts and the third most common systemic fungal infection requiring hospital care. Infection occurs almost exclusively through inhalation of conidia into areas of lung with impaired mucociliary function (eg, tuberculous cavities). Although the diagnosis is supported by demonstrating immediate and delayed-type hypersensitivity skin reactions, by culturing uniform septate hyphae with dichotomous branching at 45 degrees, and by detecting specific IgG and IgE antibodies, a definitive diagnosis requires demonstration of hyphal tissue invasion or documentation of hyphae on methenamine silver stain in a suspected aspergilloma.

Infection with aspergillus species usually takes one of three forms: allergic bronchopulmonary aspergillosis, invasive aspergillosis, and aspergilloma. Allergic bronchopulmonary aspergillosis occurs in patients who are atopic (asthmatics) and in patients with cystic fibrosis. Endobronchial fungal growth leads to dilated airways filled with mucus and fungus. Continuous exposure to fungal antigens results in precipitating antibodies, increased IgE levels (indicator of disease activity), and both immediate and delayed-type hypersensitivity. Patients complain of cough, fever, wheezing, dyspnea, pleuritic pain, and hemoptysis. Chest x-ray shows homogeneous densities in a "gloved-finger," inverted Y/V, or "cluster of grapes" pattern. Five stages have been de-

fined depending on disease activity and steroid dependency: Stage 1 includes acute infection with characteristic x-ray and laboratory evidence of disease; stage 2 occurs with steroid-induced remission; stage 3 is characterized by asymptomatic exacerbations of laboratory and x-ray findings; steroid-dependent asthma with worsening laboratory tests (total IgE, precipitins, etc) is indicative of stage 4 disease; and end-stage fibrosis, bronchiectasis, and obstruction define stage 5.

Invasive aspergillosis is found exclusively in immunocompromised patients, particularly in patients with leukemia (50–70% of cases). Dissemination occurs frequently, and three types of pulmonary disease have been described: tracheobronchitis (uncommon), necrotizing bronchopneumonia, and hemorrhagic infarction (most common). In tracheobronchitis, disease is usually limited to the larger airways (bronchus more so than trachea) with little parenchymal involvement. Focal or diffuse mucosal ulceration, pseudomembranes, and intraluminal fungal plugs are common. Patients often present with cough, dyspnea, wheezing, and hemoptysis. Occasionally, patchy areas of atelectasis secondary to bronchial obstruction can be seen on chest x-ray. Necrotizing bronchopneumonia should be suspected in patients with unremitting fever, dyspnea, tachypnea, radiologic evidence of bronchopneumonia, and a poor response to standard antibiotic therapy. Finally, hemorrhagic infarction due to vascular permeation with nonthrombotic occlusion of small to medium-sized arteries and necrosis typically results in either a well-defined nodule or a wedge-shaped, pleura-based density. Symptoms are nonspecific and include fever, dyspnea, dry cough, pleuritic chest pain, and hemoptysis. Cavitation is common, and radiologic examination may reveal "round" pneumonia or "air crescents" of a mycotic lung sequestrum.

Aspergillomas ("fungus balls" or mycetomas) are divided into two types: simple, thin-walled cysts lined with ciliated epithelium and surrounded by normal parenchyma; and complex cavities associated with markedly abnormal surrounding lung tissue. Aspergillomas most often occur in the upper lobes and in the superior segments of the lower lobes. Although they may be multiple (22%), calcification and air-fluid levels are rare. Most aspergillomas—particularly complex ones—are associated with cavitary lung disease, ie, tuberculosis (most common), histoplasmosis, sarcoidosis, bronchiectasis, and others. Hemoptysis occurs in 50–80% and can present with frequent minor episodes (30% subsequently have massive bleeding), repeated moderate episodes, or a single episode of massive hemoptysis. Chest x-ray may reveal a 3- to 6-cm round, mobile density with a crescent of air.

Medical therapy (corticosteroids) is indicated in patients with allergic bronchopulmonary aspergillosis. In invasive aspergillosis, amphotericin B (0.5–2 g intravenously as total dose) has been standard therapy despite a mortality of 90%. In addition, some patients with complex aspergillomas and severe pulmonary disease are not candidates for surgical resection, and intracavitary amphotericin B becomes an option. Surgery is indicated for complications of aspergillus infection. Hemoptysis due to aspergillomas is usually best treated by surgical resection. Furthermore, hemoptysis associated with localized invasive aspergillosis (particularly once cavitation has occurred) can be treated by resection and amphotericin B with some success. Generally, wide excision (lobectomy) is required; however, in some high-risk patients with aspergillomas, cavernostomy and muscle flap closure is an alternative.

6. Mucormycosis

Infection with *Rhizopus arrhizus* (most commonly), absidia species, and rhizomucor species of the class Zygomycetes and the order Mucorales occurs in certain distinct patient populations, eg, diabetics (particularly those in ketoacidosis), leukemia patients, and patients with general immunosuppression. These fungi are ubiquitous organisms that are particularly common in decaying fruit, vegetable matter, soil, and manure. Infection occurs following inhalation of sporangiospores, which germinate in a hyphal form. The diagnosis is made by demonstrating the organism in symptomatic patients. No accurate skin or serologic tests exist. Although the fungi do grow in culture as broad irregular nonseptate hyphae that branch at angles up to 90 degrees (occasionally being confused with aspergillus species), most commonly the diagnosis is made on histologic examination. The sine qua non for mucormycosis is hyphal vascular invasion between the internal elastic membrane and the media of blood vessels, causing thrombosis, infarction, and necrosis.

In addition to pulmonary infections, mucormycosis manifests as distinct clinical syndromes such as rhinocerebral infection (direct extension into the central nervous system from paranasal sinus infection), cutaneous infection (burn patients), gastrointestinal infection (children with protein-calorie malnutrition), and disseminated infection (uremic patients receiving deferoxamine therapy). Patients with pulmonary infection complain of fever, cough, pleuritic chest pain, and hemoptysis. Frequently, this type of infection occurs in immunocompromised hosts and follows a fulminant course. Three patterns of infection are noted on chest x-ray: limited disease with involvement of a single lobe or segment, diffuse or disseminated disease with involvement of both lungs and the mediastinum, and endobronchial disease with bronchial obstruction and secondary bacterial infection. Characteristic CT findings include a halo sign (area of low attenuation around a

dense infiltrate), ring enhancement, and an air-crescent sign (area of contrast between normal lung and a radiodense cavitating lesion).

Amphotericin B is standard treatment for this disease; however, infection with these fungi remains highly lethal, with a mortality of 90%. The cause of death in these patients is often fungal sepsis, progressive pulmonary dysfunction, and hemoptysis. In the small group of patients with limited disease, aggressive surgical resection in combination with amphotericin B has lowered the mortality to only 50%. In contrast, the endobronchial form can be effectively treated with transbronchoscopic resection (using the Nd:YAG laser) in a large proportion of patients.

7. Pneumocystosis

Pneumocystis carinii is a fungal organism that has been found in the lungs of a variety of domesticated and wild mammals and is distributed worldwide in humans. Pulmonary involvement leads to progressive pneumonia and respiratory insufficiency. Disease has been seen with increasing frequency in recipients of organ transplants who are undergoing immunosuppressive therapy. Diagnosis is made by open lung biopsy. Without treatment with trimethoprim-sulfamethoxazole, the course is one of relentless progression. With improved antiviral therapy for HIV infections, the incidence of pneumocystosis has been declining.

Benfield TL et al: Prognostic markers of short-term mortality in AIDS-associated *Pneumocystis carinii* pneumonia. Chest 2001;119:844.

Boyars MC, Zwischenberger JB, Cox CS Jr: Clinical manifestations of pulmonary fungal infections. J Thorac Imaging 1992;7:12.

Johnson P, Sarosi G: Current therapy of major fungal diseases of the lung. Infect Dis Clin North Am 1991;5:635.

Ledergerber B et al: Discontinuation of secondary prophylaxis against *Pneumocystis carinii* pneumonia in patients with HIV infection who have a response to antiretroviral therapy. Eight European Study Groups. N Engl J Med 2001;344;:168.

Lopez Bernaldo de Quiros JC et al: A randomized trial of the discontinuation of primary and secondary prophylaxis against *Pneumocystis carinii* pneumonia after highly active antiretroviral therapy in patients with HIV infection. Grupo de Estudio del SIDA 04/98. N Engl J Med 2001;344:159

Russian DA, Levine SJ: *Pneumocystis carinii* pneumonia in patients without HIV infection. Am J Med Sci 2001;321:56.

SARCOIDOSIS (Boeck's Sarcoid, Benign Lymphogranulomatosis)

Sarcoidosis is a noncaseating granulomatous disease of unknown cause involving the lungs, liver, spleen, lymph nodes, skin, and bones. The highest incidence is reported in Scandinavia, England, and the United

States. The incidence in blacks is 10–17 times that in whites. Half of patients are between ages 20 and 40 years, with women more frequently affected than men.

Clinical Findings

A. SYMPTOMS AND SIGNS

Sarcoidosis may present with symptoms of pulmonary infection, but usually these are insidious and nonspecific. Erythema nodosum may herald the onset, and weight loss, fatigue, weakness, and malaise may appear later. Fever occurs in approximately 15% of cases. Pulmonary symptoms occur in 20–30% and include dry cough and dyspnea. Hemoptysis is rare. One-fifth of patients with sarcoidosis have myocardial involvement, and heart block or failure may occur. Peripheral lymph nodes are enlarged in 75%; scalene lymph nodes are microscopically involved in 80% and mediastinal nodes in 90%; and cutaneous involvement is present in 30%. Hepatic and splenic involvement can be shown by biopsy in 70% of cases. There may be migratory or persistent polyarthritis, and central nervous involvement occurs in a few patients.

B. IMAGING STUDIES

The x-ray findings in sarcoidosis are classified into five descriptive categories or stages (Table 19–6). Pulmonary disease can manifest as a reticulonodular infiltrate, an acinar pattern of opacities, or large nodules with or without mediastinal adenopathy. Mediastinal lymph node involvement characteristically includes bilateral symmetric hilar and paratracheal lymphadenopathy. Anterior or posterior mediastinal adenopathy or asymmetric hilar involvement should prompt a suspicion of other diseases, particularly Hodgkin's disease and non-Hodgkin's lymphomas. Pleural effusions and cavitation are rare and, if present, necessitate an evaluation for tuberculosis, congestive heart failure, and coincidental pneumonia.

Diagnosis

Although no single test exists to confirm absolutely the diagnosis of sarcoidosis (the diagnosis remains one of

Table 19–6. Radiographic stages of sarcoidosis.

Stage 0: No x-ray abnormality
Stage 1: Hilar and mediastinal lymph node enlargement without pulmonary abnormalities
Stage 2: Hilar and mediastinal lymph node enlargement with pulmonary abnormalities
Stage 3: Diffuse pulmonary disease without adenopathy
Stage 4: Pulmonary fibrosis

exclusion), it may be suggested by the characteristic radiographic appearance of bilateral hilar and mediastinal lymphadenopathy, by gallium 67 scanning, and by elevated serum and bronchoalveolar fluid levels of angiotensin-converting enzyme and lysozyme. Pathologic documentation of noncaseating granulomas should normally be obtained either via transbronchial biopsy or mediastinoscopy (more reliable, with > 95% success rate). Culture for mycobacteria, fungi, and other atypical infections must also be negative.

Treatment

Asymptomatic patients and those with minimal clinical disease may require no therapy. Corticosteroids have been used in patients with pulmonary impairment and symptomatic disease with good success. Despite the indolent nature of the disease and steroid therapy, long-term mortality is reported as high as 10%.

■ NEOPLASMS OF THE LUNG

PRIMARY LUNG CANCER

Lung cancer is the most common cause of cancer-related deaths in both men and women in the United States. In 2001, it is estimated that 169,500 new cases and 157,000 deaths will occur due to pulmonary malignancies. This represents 15% of all new cancer cases and 28% of all cancer-related deaths. In addition, although the incidence in males appears to have stabilized, the incidence continues to rise rapidly in females.

Tobacco smoking accounts for 85% of all lung cancer cases. The effect is greatest for cigarettes and least for pipe smoking and is directly related to the amount of tobacco smoked. Following 5–6 years of smoking cessation, the risk exponentially declines, and after 15 years approaches, but never reaches, that of nonsmokers. "Passive" exposure to cigarette smoke, on the other hand, increases the risk in nonsmokers by two to three times. Exposure to all forms of asbestos (amosite, chrysotile, and crocidolite) has been implicated in as many as 23% of lung cancers, accounting for the high incidence among shipyard workers, insulators, cement makers, truck drivers, and plumbers. The effect is particularly pronounced in smokers and is most commonly associated with squamous cell and small cell carcinoma. Recently, exposure to radon and its alpha-emitting daughter isotopes has been implicated in the increased incidence of lung cancer in both uranium miners as well as certain segments of the general population living in geographic areas naturally contaminated with high levels of radon gas. Although it has been known for some time that people with high activity of 4-debrisoquine hydroxylase, the so-called debrisoquine metabolic phenotype, have a ten-times increased risk of lung cancer, only recently has the role of genetic factors been appreciated. Chromosome deletions (particularly 11p, 13q, 17p, and 3p), tumor suppressor gene mutations (P53, Hap-1, ErbAb, etc), and constitutive, high-level expression of both growth factor genes (insulin-like and transferrin-like growth factors), epidermal growth factor receptors (HER2/*neu, EGFR1,* etc) and proto-oncogenes (c-, N- and L-*myc;* H-, N-, and K-*ras;* and c-*myb*) have all been implicated in the pathogenesis of lung cancer. Other factors such as vitamin A deficiency, air pollution; exposure to arsenic, cadmium, chromium, ether, and formaldehyde; and employment as bakers, cooks, construction workers, cosmetologists, leather workers, pitchblende miners, printers, rubber workers, and pottery workers have also been incriminated. Finally, certain diseases—eg, progressive systemic sclerosis (scleroderma)—have a defined predisposition for the development of lung cancer.

Pathology

Lung cancer occurs more commonly in the right lung than the left, and the upper lobes are involved more commonly than the lower lobes or the right middle lobe. Synchronous primary lung cancers occur in up to 7% of patients, and 10% of patients will develop a metachronous new tumor (2% per year risk post resection of early stage disease). Furthermore, patients with lung cancer are at higher risk of developing cancers of the upper respiratory tract, oral cavity, esophagus, bladder, and kidney. Lung cancers typically spread by local extension to involve the visceral and parietal pleura, chest wall, great vessels, pericardium, diaphragm, esophagus, and vertebral column. Common sites of metastatic involvement include the ipsilateral pulmonary and hilar lymph nodes, the mediastinal lymph nodes, the lung, liver, bone, brain, adrenal glands, pancreas, kidney, soft tissues, and myocardium. The exact pathologic classification of lung cancer has not been uniform despite attempts at standardization by the World Health Organization. Functionally, however, squamous cell carcinoma, large cell carcinoma, and adenocarcinoma are grouped together under the designation of non-small cell carcinomas and constitute 80% of all lung tumors. Small cell carcinoma represents 15–20%, while bronchial gland adenomas, including carcinoids, comprise the remaining 5%. The differential locations of some of these neoplasms are summarized in Table 19–7.

A. Squamous Cell Carcinoma

The major pathologic features of squamous cell carcinoma are keratinization, cellular stratification, and in-

Table 19–7. Location of lung cancer by histologic type.[1]

Histology	Central (%)	Peripheral (%)
Squamous cell carcinoma	64–81	19–36
Adenocarcinoma	5–29	71–95
Large-cell carcinoma	42–49	51–58
Small-cell carcinoma	74–83	17–26
Overall	63	37

[1]From Cameron RB: Malignancies of the lung. In: *Practical Oncology.* Cameron RB (editor). Originally published by Appleton & Lange. Copyright © 1994 by The McGraw-Hill Companies, Inc.

tercellular bridges. Squamous cell carcinomas account for about 20% of all cases of lung cancer and 70% of non-small cell tumors. Two-thirds are located centrally near the hilum and one-third peripherally. The growth rate and the rate of metastasis tend to be slower than those of other lung tumors.

B. Adenocarcinoma

Adenocarcinomas, which constitute 30% of lung cancers and 60% of non-small cell tumors, are characterized as acinar, papillary, and bronchoalveolar. Acinar adenocarcinoma is composed of glands lined by columnar cells that secrete mucin. Bronchoalveolar carcinoma is characterized by intraluminal papillary fragments that appear in alveoli or small bronchioles. Bronchoalveolar carcinoma may be spread by aerosol transmission. This incidence is increasing, perhaps as a consequence of the rise in lung cancer among women, although the exact cause remains unclear.

C. Small Cell Carcinoma

Small cell (oat cell) carcinomas have small, round nuclei with nuclear chromatin and cytoplasm. They are so biologically and clinically distinct from all other cell types that the term non-small cell lung cancer often is applied to all other cell types. Small cell carcinomas comprise 15–20% of all lung cancers. They occur centrally, metastasize early, and are the most resistant to combined-modality treatment.

D. Large Cell Carcinoma

Large cell carcinomas are composed of large polygonal spindle or oval cells arranged in sheets, nests, or clusters. Multinucleated giant cells, intracellular hyalin droplets, glycogen, and acidophilic nuclear inclusions may be present. These tumors are seen peripherally and are less common.

E. Adenosquamous Tumors

Adenosquamous tumors show both cellular features and are more biologically aggressive than other non-small cell lung cancers. Survival percentages of patients with adenosquamous tumors are significantly lower than what is reported for adenocarcinoma or squamous cell cancer.

F. Bronchial Gland Adenomas

Bronchial gland adenoma is a misnomer since the vast majority of these tumors are malignant. Included in this group are carcinoid tumors, adenoid cystic carcinomas, mucoepidermoid carcinoma, mixed tumors of the salivary gland type, and mucous gland adenoma. Carcinoid tumors are derived from Kulchitsky cells, have a vascular stroma, and tend to be located centrally in proximal airways. Although they are slow-growing, they can metastasize widely. Carcinoid syndrome is rarely associated with bronchial carcinoids, as opposed to intestinal carcinoids that metastasize to the liver. Adenoid cystic carcinomas—also referred to as cylindromas—feature groups of epithelial cells that form duct-like structures interspersed with cystic spaces. These neoplasms are locally aggressive and often extend beyond apparent gross pathologic margins. Metastases from adenoid cystic carcinomas often involve the lung, are slow-growing, and are amenable to surgical excision. Mucoepidermoid carcinomas are rare tumors characterized by the presence of squamous cells, mucus-secreting cells, and an intermediate cell type. The cells are bland and less aggressive than those of adenosquamous carcinomas. Mixed tumors of the salivary type are extremely rare infiltrating tumors that are curable with wide local excision. Finally, mucus gland adenomas (papillary or bronchial cyst adenomas) are the only true benign "adenomas" of this group with no metastatic potential. These neoplasms are rare tumors of the major bronchi and consist of numerous mucus-filled cysts lined by a well-differentiated epithelium. Generally, bronchoscopic removal can be accomplished and results in long-term cure.

Clinical Presentation

Nearly 94% of patients present with symptoms from the effects of the primary tumor, regional spread, or metastatic disease. Local effects of the primary tumor account for 27% of presenting symptoms and vary depending on the location of the tumor. Central tumors are associated with cough, hemoptysis, respiratory difficulty (wheezing, stridor, or dyspnea), pain, and pneumonia. Peripheral tumors can cause cough, chest wall pain, pleural effusions, pulmonary abscess, Horner's syndrome (ipsilateral miosis, ptosis, and anhidrosis), and Pancoast's syndrome (ipsilateral shoulder and arm pain in the C8–T1 nerve root distribution, Horner's syndrome, and a superior sulcus—usually squamous—lung cancer). Symptoms due to the effect of regional spread include hoarseness from recurrent nerve paralysis, dyspnea due to phrenic nerve paralysis, dysphagia from compression of the esophagus, superior vena cava syndrome from compression or invasion of the superior vena cava, and pericardial tamponade from invasion of the pericardium. Metastatic disease may present with symptoms of systemic illness (anorexia, weight loss, weakness, and malaise), local manifestations of distant metastases (jaundice, abdominal mass, bony pain or fracture, neurologic deficits, mental status changes, seizures, and soft tissue masses), and any one of a number of paraneoplastic syndromes associated with lung cancer (Table 19–8).

Table 19–8. Paraneoplastic syndromes associated with lung cancer.

Cardiovascular
  Thrombophlebitis
  Nonbacterial thrombotic endocarditis
  Neuromuscular
  Subacute cerebellar degeneration
  Dementia
  Limbic encephalitis
  Optic neuritis, retinopathy
  Subacute necrotic myelopathy
  Autonomic neuropathy (small cell)
  Myasthenic (Eaton-Lambert) syndrome (small cell)
  Polymyositis
Gastrointestinal
  Carcinoid syndrome (carcinoid and small cell)
  Anorexia, cachexia
Hematologic
  Erythrocytosis
  Leukocytosis
Metabolic
  Inappropriate ACTH (small cell)
  Inappropriate ADH (small cell)
  Hypercalcemia (squamous cell carcinoma)
  Inappropriate gonadotropins
Dermatologic
  Acanthosis nigricans (adenocarcinoma)
  Dermatomyositis
  Erythema gyratum
  Ichthyosis
Other
  Hypertrophic pulmonary osteoarthropathy
    (squamous cell, large cell, and adenocarcinoma)
  Nephrotic syndrome
  Fever

Diagnosis & Workup

Lung cancer is usually suspected from abnormal findings on a chest x-ray obtained in the course of a routine physical examination or, more commonly, after a complaint of pulmonary symptoms (see above). Findings vary from a small peripheral nodule to an unresolving infiltrate or even total lung atelectasis. Occasionally, the location of the abnormality can suggest certain cell types (Table 19–7; Figure 19–20). Despite the utility of chest x-rays in the diagnosis of lung cancer, prospective randomized trials at three major institutions have failed to demonstrate a survival benefit from mass screening programs incorporating chest x-rays with or without the addition of sputum cytologic examinations. Once the diagnosis of lung cancer is suspected, a definitive diagnosis can be obtained in over 90% of patients with either bronchoscopy for proximal lesions or fine-needle aspiration cytology for peripheral lesions.

Currently, CT scanning is an integral part of the assessment of patients with lung cancer. Chest CT scans should also include the upper abdomen to assess two of the most common sites of metastases (liver and adrenal glands). Injection of intravenous contrast while the scan is obtained facilitates evaluation of the mediastinum. Additional radiographic workup includes tests to evaluate other common sites of metastases, such as bone and brain. A serum alkaline phosphatase is essential, and a bone scan and brain CT scan (or preferably MRI) should be obtained if indicated by elevated alkaline phosphatase levels, neurologic symptoms, or bone pain or if advanced-stage disease (stage III or beyond) is present. Recently, positron emission tomography (PET) has evolved into an important staging test. It is most effective at assay for distant occult disease. It can be helpful for assessing mediastinal node involvement, but it is not definitive. False-positive rates as high as 15–20% have been reported. Furthermore, nodules less than 1 cm in diameter are not reliably imaged by PET scanning. Thoracentesis or thoracoscopy (or both) should be performed in any patient with evidence of a pleural effusion to exclude diffuse involvement of the pleura (T4 or stage IIIB disease), which makes the lesion incurable with surgery. Finally, most patients with non-small cell lung cancer but without metastatic disease should be evaluated with cervical mediastinoscopy and parasternal mediastinotomy (Chamberlain) if necessary to document the status of the mediastinal nodes. PET scanning is also informative but less accurate than mediastinoscopy. With small cell lung cancer; however, this usually is not necessary. The use of CT scans alone is inaccurate in 40–60% of patients with enlarged lymph nodes over 1 cm (false-positive) and 15% of patients without "significant" lymphadenopathy (false-negative). Once all the information from these staging

procedures is in hand, the patient with non-small cell lung cancer can be classified into one of three categories: (1) early lung cancer without mediastinal involvement, or stage I/II (see below); (2) locally advanced lung cancer, or stage IIIA/B, and (3) metastatic lung cancer, or stage IV. Staging is important because the therapeutic choices are determined in that way. Patients with small cell lung cancer are usually grouped into two categories: disease limited to the ipsilateral hemithorax, including supraclavicular nodes (limited disease); or disease extending beyond the thorax (extensive disease), ie, below the diaphragm or brain metastases.

Staging

By 1987, the American Joint Committee on Cancer (AJCC) and the Union Internationale Contre le Cancer (UICC) had developed a joint staging system for lung carcinoma based on data gathered primarily by Clifford Mountain of the MD Anderson Cancer Center. The lung cancer staging system is based on the tumor (T), the status of regional lymph nodes (N), and the presence or absence of distant metastases (M) as outlined in Table 19–9.

Treatment

Treatment for small cell carcinoma consists primarily of chemotherapy and radiation, though recent data indicate that for early disease (T1–T2 lesions and limited hilar adenopathy) resection may improve local control and result in increased long-term survival (as high as 50%), particularly when combined with postoperative chemotherapy. Treatment for non-small cell lung cancer, however, varies with stage. Early-stage disease (stage I/II) has historically been treated with surgery alone, though new tests may prove to be a benefit for induction chemotherapy. Locally advanced but surgically resectable disease (stage IIIA) is currently best treated with combined-modality therapy utilizing induction chemotherapy or chemoradiotherapy followed by surgery and, if necessary, postoperative radiotherapy. Locally advanced and surgically unresectable disease (stage IIIB) is generally treated with radiation therapy with or without chemotherapy. Metastatic disease (stage IV) is only poorly treated with chemotherapy. Radiotherapy in this case is reserved for symptomatic lesions. Combined-agent chemotherapy offers 2–3 months (20%) survival extension to advanced-stage patients. It has been shown to be cost-effective and is generally well-tolerated by patients with reasonable performance status. New biologic agents—so-called "targeted therapies"—are showing activity in clinical trials and should improve overall survival statistics. It is hoped

Figure 19–20. X-ray manifestations of lung cancer. ***A:*** Small epidermoid carcinoma in LUL (posteroanterior projection). ***B:*** Large coin lesions; adenocarcinoma in superior segment of LLL (lateral projection). ***C and D:*** Epidermoid carcinoma in RUL. ***E:*** Right hilar mass; small cell carcinoma. ***F:*** Large cavitary epidermoid carcinoma in RUL. ***G*** (posteroanterior projection) and ***H*** (lateral projection): Middle lobe atelectasis from bronchial carcinoid (not visible). ***I:*** Opacification of left hemithorax; large cavitary epidermoid carcinoma. ***J:*** Pancoast's tumor; poorly differentiated epidermoid carcinoma with erosion of third rib and pathologic fracture of fourth rib. ***K:*** Right phrenic nerve paralysis caused by epidermoid carcinoma. ***L:*** Pleural metastasis caused by adenocarcinoma of LLL. (LUL = left upper lobe; LLL = left lower lobe, etc.)

Table 19–9. TNM stage groupings.

Primary tumor	
TX	Primary tumor cannot be assessed, or cytologic evidence of malignant cells in sputum or bronchial washings but not visualized by imaging or bronchoscopy
T0	No evidence of primary tumor
Tis	Carcinoma in situ
T1	Tumor 3 cm or less in greatest diameter, completely surrounded by lung or visceral pleura, and without bronchoscopic evidence of involvement of more proximal than a lobar bronchus
T2	Tumor more than 3 cm in greatest diameter, invading the visceral pleura, involving the main stem bronchus but greater than 2 cm distal to the carina, or tumor associated with atelectasis or obstructive pneumonitis extending to the hilum but not involving the entire lung
T3	Tumor of any size invading the chest wall, diaphragm, mediastinal pleura, parietal pericardium, tumor involving the main stem bronchus within 2 cm of but not involving the carina, or tumor associated with atelectasis or obstructive pneumonitis of the entire lung
T4	Tumor of any size invading the mediastinum, heart, great vessels, trachea, esophagus, vertebral body, or carina, or tumor associated with a malignant pleural effusion
Regional lymph nodes (N stage)	
NX	Regional lymph nodes cannot be assessed
N0	No evidence of regional lymph node metastases
N1	Metastases in ipsilateral peribronchial or hilar lymph nodes, including by direct extension
N2	Metastases in ipsilateral mediastinal or subcarinal lymph nodes
N3	Metastases in contralateral mediastinal or hilar lymph nodes or ipsilateral or contralateral scalene or supraclavicular nodes
Distant metastases (M stage)	
MX	Presence of distant metastases cannot be assessed
M0	No evidence of distant metastases
M1	Distant metastases are present
Stage grouping	
Occult disease	TX, N0, M0
Stage 0	Tis, N0, M0
Stage IA	T1, N0, M0
Stage IB	T2 N0 M0
Stage IIA	T1 N1 M0
StageIIB	T2 N1 M0 T3 N0 M0
Stage IIIA	T1–2, N2, M0, or T3, N0–2, M0
Stage IIIB	T4, Any N, M0, or Any T, N3, M0
Stage IV	Any T, Any N, M1

that with advances in targeted and conventional therapies the current overall survival (< 15% at 5 years) of patients with lung cancer can be improved.

A. SURGICAL TREATMENT

1. Surgical staging—As noted above, almost all patients with non-small cell lung cancer limited to the thorax should undergo cervical mediastinoscopy to exclude involvement of N2 mediastinal lymph nodes (N2 or N3 disease). A possible exception is a small peripheral (T1) nodule, especially of squamous cell histology without any evidence for mediastinal adenopathy on chest CT scan. With adenocarcinoma, however, negative mediastinal nodes by CT have an 18–25% false-negative rate. For left-sided lesions, left parasternal mediastinotomy (Chamberlain) may be required to assess the status of the aorticopulmonary lymph nodes. Without pathologic confirmation of the status of mediastinal lymph nodes, CT scans have been associated with high false-positive and false-negative rates. A surgical assessment of the proximal airways is also required even if this means repeating this invasive procedure, often previously performed by the pulmonologist. Since treatment decisions are based on accurate staging and because treatment of early-stage disease (stage I/II) differs significantly from locally advanced disease (stage IIIA/B), this approach is essential. The importance of accurate staging for patients with non-small cell lung cancer cannot be overstated.

2. Indications and preoperative assessment—Surgical resection is indicated for early-stage lung cancer (stage I/II) and in combination with chemotherapy and radiation in locally advanced resectable disease (stage IIIA or resectable T4, IIIb). In addition, surgery may be indicated for patients with a single site of metastatic disease, such as a solitary brain or adrenal gland metastasis. Both relative and absolute contraindications to surgical resection are listed in Table 19–10.

Preoperative assessment is aimed at evaluating both cardiopulmonary reserve and overall patient fitness. The patient's general performance status or functional classification is probably the most accurate factor in predicting a successful outcome following surgery. Advanced age, by itself, is not a contraindication to surgery. It is the physiologic age—as manifested by functional status—not the chronologic age that is important. A thorough cardiac evaluation is also necessary, since lung cancer and cardiac disease share common risk factors (eg, smoking). Patients with cardiac symptoms, an abnormal ECG, or other findings suggestive of ischemic heart disease should be screened by a stress test (exercise treadmill, dipyridamole- or adenosine-thallium study, dobutamine echocardiogram). Sig-

Table 19–10. Medical and surgical contraindications to pulmonary resection.

Absolute	Relative
Myocardial infarction within previous 3 months	Myocardial infarction within previous 6 months
SVC syndrome (due to metastatic tumor)	SVC syndrome (due to primary tumor)
Bilateral endobronchial tumor	Recurrent laryngeal nerve paralysis (due to primary tumor in aorticopulmonary window)
Contralateral lymph node metastases (N3)	Horner's syndrome
Malignant pleural effusion	Small cell histology
Distant metastases (except solitary brain and adrenal metastases)	Metastases higher than the midtracheal lymph nodes
	Pericardial involvement
	$FEV_1 < 0.8$ L (< 50%)
	FEV_1 0.9–2.4 and insufficient pulmonary reserve for planned resection
	Main pulmonary artery involvement

nificant left main coronary artery disease should be treated with coronary artery bypass prior to any contemplated pulmonary resection, and other significant disease should be individually assessed for possible bypass or angioplasty. Furthermore, significant pulmonary hypertension and myocardial infarction within 3 months are associated with up to 20% perioperative mortality and constitute absolute contraindications to surgery. Other high-risk findings include myocardial infarction within 6 months, ventricular arrhythmias, and heart block, particularly left posterior fascicular hemiblock. Finally, the patient's pulmonary function and ability to tolerate the required pulmonary resection need to be assessed. This is accomplished with pulmonary function tests (spirometry, diffusing capacity, exercise oximetry) and with differential (quantitative) ventilation-perfusion scanning when appropriate. In a 70 kg patient, the following preoperative studies indicate high morbidity risk and are relative contraindications to resection: $FEV_1 < 0.8$ L, a predicted postoperative FEV_1 < 0.8, a predicted maximum voluntary ventilation < 50%, a $PaCO_2 > 45$ mm Hg, and a $PaO_2 < 50$ mm Hg.

3. Surgical resection—

a. **Early and locally advanced non-small cell lung cancer**—The extent of pulmonary resection is dictated by the location of the primary tumor and the presence or absence of involved hilar (interlobar) lymph nodes. Limited segmental resection for stage I/II non-small cell lung cancer (NSCLC) has been evaluated by the Lung Cancer Study Group and found to result in an increased local recurrence rate (15% versus 3%) and lower overall survival. Segmental resections, therefore, are viewed as compromise procedures only indicated in patients who cannot tolerate lobectomy. Lobectomy continues to be the standard of care for resection for NSCLC. This should include a 1 cm margin of normal proximal bronchus. Samples of interlobar (hilar) lymph nodes are submitted for immediate pathologic examination to exclude involvement that would require pneumonectomy. A "sleeve" resection of main stem bronchus can also be included in the resection, particularly with the right upper lobe. Pneumonectomy is required for proximal lesions involving the main stem bronchus or the interlobar (hilar) lymph nodes. In addition, techniques are available for more extensive resection such as intrapericardial pneumonectomy and tracheal "sleeve" pneumonectomy. The overall mortality rates following segmental resection, lobectomy, and pneumonectomy are 1.4%, 2.9%, and 6.2%, respectively, in centers with large experience. Complications following pulmonary resection include cardiac arrhythmias, hemorrhage, infection (empyema), bronchopleural fistula, respiratory insufficiency, and pulmonary embolism.

b. **Advanced (metastatic) non-small cell lung cancer**—Patients with solitary brain and adrenal metastases, especially if metachronous, are still candidates for surgical resection and have benefited by prolonged survival in a few small retrospective studies in comparison with historical controls. Systemic preoperative (induction) chemotherapy and radiotherapy, however, should be administered initially. In addition, transbronchial Nd:YAG laser resection of tumors obstructing the proximal airways can significantly palliate selected patients. In addition, improvements in the design and deployment techniques of expansile stents have been a significant advance for palliation of proximal airway obstruction. Finally, photodynamic laser therapy with photosensitizers can alleviate airway obstruction from tumors, albeit not as quickly as Nd:YAG laser ablation.

c. **Small cell lung cancer**—Resection for small peripheral tumors followed by aggressive postoperative chemotherapy may increase the local control rate and potentially the overall survival rate in the early small cell lung cancer. Survival rates as high as 50% with this approach have been reported.

B. RADIATION THERAPY

1. **Non-small cell lung cancer**—Radiation therapy can be administered with curative intent in stage I/II disease in patients who refuse or are not medically suitable candidates for surgery. The 5-year survival rate with this approach, however, is only 22–33%. With locally advanced disease (stage IIIA/B), radiation therapy (5500–6000 cGy) until recently has been the treatment of choice. Although local or nodal recurrence rates are < 30%, long-term survival is < 10% in these patients, and the type of fractionation scheme has not altered the outcome. Adjuvant radiation therapy following surgical resection has been extensively studied by the Lung Cancer Study Group and has been found to decrease local or nodal recurrences but not to prolong overall survival. A much disputed meta-analysis (the PORT study) showed a decrease in survival for stage II patients treated with postoperative radiation. Differences in radiotherapy techniques within the analysis may account for the worse outcomes. Preoperative radiation has been used with T3 lesions, particularly Pancoast tumors, with improved survival; however, there is no objective evidence that radiation must be given preoperatively. Recently, a multicenter intergroup trial (SWOG) showed a significant survival advantage for combined chemoradiotherapy (etoposide, platinum, and 4500 cGy) prior to resection for Pancoast (superior sulcus) tumors that were N1 or less. Complete resection rates were improved; 20–25% complete pathologic responses were achieved; and survival was significantly improved (45–50% at 3 years) over surgery alone or preoperative radiotherapy and surgery. Intraoperative radiation has been investigated but to date has been associated with unacceptably high morbidity. Finally, in patients with metastatic disease, therapeutic radiation is indicated in patients with symptoms of pain, neurologic symptoms, and symptoms of superior vena cava compression.

2. **Small cell lung cancer**—Multiple randomized trials comparing the combination of radiation and chemotherapy to chemotherapy alone in limited-stage small cell lung cancer have been conducted. The majority show improved local control and modest (3–4 months) prolonged survival with the combination. This was at the cost of increased morbidity, however. In extensive disease, no benefit has been demonstrated for radiation therapy outside of palliative radiation of symptomatic metastases. Prophylactic cranial irradiation may be beneficial but can cause significant cognitive deficits.

C. CHEMOTHERAPY

1. **Non-small cell lung cancer**—Although chemotherapy alone has not generally been used in the treatment of early or locally advanced NSCLC, combinations of chemotherapy and radiotherapy have been

evaluated in locally advanced unresectable disease. In some instances, no benefit to the combination was demonstrated, particularly when only single agents were used; however, improved results with both radiation and combined-agent chemotherapy have recently been documented. In the presence of metastatic disease, multiple trials of combination chemotherapy have demonstrated a modest improvement in overall survival (14 weeks or 25% improved survival) but not without some toxicity. Even so, quality of life assessments and cost analyses support the use of outpatient combined-agent chemotherapy over palliative care alone.

a. Preoperative (induction) therapy—Recently, four randomized prospective trials of preoperative (neoadjuvant, induction) chemotherapy have demonstrated longer survival following treatment with chemotherapy (platinum-based regimens) and subsequent resection. As many as 10–15% pathologic complete responses have been noted. Median survival in one study was 64 months. Although these studies were small, the findings are similar to a multitude of nonrandomized studies performed previously.

b. Postoperative adjuvant therapy—Numerous studies (randomized and nonrandomized as well as prospective and retrospective) of postoperative adjuvant chemotherapy, including those performed by the Lung Cancer Study Group, have all failed to document any meaningful increase in overall survival from the use of chemotherapy. Some increase in disease-free survival was noted in one study, but this remains an isolated finding. In one large meta-analysis, a limited 5% benefit was observed.

2. Small cell lung cancer—Combination chemotherapy currently produces 85–95% and 75–85% response rates in limited stage and extensive stage disease, respectively. Furthermore, median survival is 12–16 months and 7–11 months in each group. Three or four drugs have been shown to be optimal. One of the most effective regimens combines cyclophosphamide, doxorubicin, and vincristine. In addition, a regimen of cisplatin and etoposide has been active in salvage. The optimal duration of therapy has not been defined, but the majority of the effect appears to occur within the first four cycles.

D. IMMUNOTHERAPY

Immunotherapy using BCG, levamisole, interleukin-2, tumor necrosis factor-α, lymphokine-activated killer (LAK) cells, and tumor-infiltrating lymphocytes has not proved beneficial in any clinical studies to date.

E. TARGETED THERAPIES

Molecular-based therapies targeting overexpressed growth receptors (*EGFR1*, HER2/*neu*) by monoclonal

Table 19–11. Survival in non-small cell lung cancer.

Stage	TNM Description	Five-Year Survival
I		70–76%
a	T1, N0	80–83%
b	T2, N0	60–65%
II		30–40%
a	T1, N1	32–40%
b	T2, N1	28–35%
	T3, N0	
IIIA		10–30%
	T3, N1	30–45%
	T1–2, N2	7–30%
	T3, N2	0–5%
IIIB		<10%
	T4, any N	<10%
	Any T, N3	<10%
IV	M1	<5%
Overall		14.5%

antibody or small molecules are beginning to show clinical effectiveness. Additional agents targeting signal transduction pathways (eg, farnesyl transferase inhibitors) for the *ras* pathway as well as antisense oligonucleotide and gene therapies are all in advanced clinical testing stages and in combination with standard cytotoxic chemotherapy appear to enhance response rates.

Prognosis

A. NON-SMALL CELL LUNG CANCER

The survival of patients with NSCLC is highly dependent on the pathologic stage. Overall, the 5-year survival of patients with stages I, II, IIIA, IIIB, and IV is 43–64%, 20–40%, 15–25%, 5–7%, and < 2%, respectively. A breakdown of survival by TNM classification is set forth in Table 19–11.

B. SMALL CELL LUNG CANCER

Patients with limited-stage disease achieve a median survival of 12–16 months with 5–25% 2-year survival, while those with extensive stage disease have a median survival of only 7–11 months, with only 1–3% surviving 2 years.

Albain KS et al: Concurrent cisplatin/etoposide plus chest radiotherapy followed by surgery for stages IIIA N2 and IIIB non-small cell lung cancer: mature results of Southwest Oncology Group Phase II study 8805. J Clin Oncol 1995;13:1880.

Albain KS et al: Long-term survival after concurrent cisplatin/ etoposide (PE) plus chest radiotherapy (RT) followed by surgery in bulky stages IIIA N2 and IIIB non-small cell lung cancer (NSCLC): 6-year outcomes from Southwest Oncology Group study 8805. Proc Am Soc Clin Oncol 1999;18:467a (abst.)

Friedel G et al. Neoadjuvant chemoradiotherapy of stage III non-small cell lung cancer. Lung Cancer 2000;30:175.

Grunenwald DH et al: Benefit of surgery after chemoradiotherapy in stage IIIB (T4 and/or N3) non-small cell lung cancer. J Thorac Cardiovasc Surg 2001;122:796.

Rosell R et al: A randomized trial comparing preoperative chemotherapy plus surgery with surgery alone in patients with non-small cell lung cancer. N Engl J Med 1994;330: 153.

Roth JA et al: A randomized trial comparing perioperative chemotherapy and surgery with surgery alone in resectable stage IIIA non-small cell lung cancer. J Natl Cancer Inst 1994; 86:673.

Schiller JH et al: Comparison of four chemotherapy regimens for advanced non-small cell lung cancer. N Engl J Med 2002; 346:92.

Sugarbaker DJ et al: Results of Cancer and Leukemia Group B protocol 8935: a multiinstitutional phase II trimodality trial for IIIA N2 non-small cell lung cancer. J Thorac Cardiovasc Surg 1995;109:473.

Voltolini L et al: Results of induction chemotherapy followed by surgical resection in patients with stage IIIA (N2) non-small cell lung cancer: the importance of the nodal downstaging after chemotherapy. Eur J Cardiothorac Surg 2001;20:1106.

UNUSUAL PULMONARY NEOPLASMS

Malignant Neoplasms

Bronchial adenomas are a group of low-grade malignancies arising from the bronchial tree. Carcinoid tumors constitute 85–90% of these neoplasms, with adenoid cystic carcinoma (10%) and mucoepidermoid carcinoma (< 5%) accounting for most of the remainder. Carcinoid tumors are classified as either "typical" or "atypical," with markedly different histologic characteristics (Table 19–12). Adenoid cystic carcinomas occur in the lower trachea; infiltrate locally along submucosal and perineural tissue planes, often far beyond the boundaries of

Table 19–12. Characteristics of typical and atypical carcinoid tumors.

	Typical	**Atypical**
Incidence	90%	10%
Central location	80%	50%
Peripheral location	20%	50%
Metastases	10–15%	50–70%

gross tumor; and metastasize late. Mucoepidermoid carcinomas resemble salivary tumors, with varying numbers of three distinct cell types: mucous, squamous, and intermediate. Patients with bronchial adenomas complain of cough, recurrent pulmonary infections, hemoptysis, pain, and wheezing. Only 15% of patients are completely asymptomatic. Carcinoid syndrome is rare with pulmonary carcinoid tumors. Most bronchial adenomas are diagnosed with a combination of plain chest radiography, computed tomography, and bronchoscopy. Biopsy at the time of bronchoscopy can be associated with significant bleeding, and measures to control this must be readily available.

Surgical resection is indicated for these tumors, with lobectomy being the most common procedure. "Sleeve" and bronchoplastic resections are particularly useful to preserve pulmonary function in these patients and make standard pneumonectomy rare. Removal of adenoid cystic carcinomas requires generous margins and frozen section examination of the margins at the time of surgery. Up to 8 cm of trachea can be removed with primary anastomosis. In addition, postoperative radiation may be indicated for close margins. With the possible exception of atypical carcinoid, chemotherapy is generally not indicated in the treatment of these neoplasms.

The long-term outlook is good for patients with metastatic disease. Even patients with adenoid cystic carcinoma and distant metastases may do well for extended periods due to the slow-growing nature of this malignancy; however, lymph node and distant metastases in patients with carcinoid tumors generally carry a poor prognosis.

Benign Neoplasms

Benign neoplasms of the lung are uncommon, accounting for < 1% of all pulmonary tumors. Most are hamartomas, but fibromas, leiomyomas, neurofibromas, myoblastomas, and benign metastasizing leiomyomas also occur. Most lesions are peripheral and asymptomatic; however, central lesions can produce symptoms of cough, wheezing, hemoptysis, and recurrent pneumonia. Typically, the lesions are discovered on routine chest radiographs and appear as a 1- to 2-cm well-circumscribed, bosselated lower lung nodule with calcifications in 10–30%. Central lesions may require bronchoscopy for diagnosis, but a pathologic diagnosis is most often obtained by fine-needle aspiration biopsy or surgery. Surgical resection should be conservative and limited to wedge excision unless the lesion occupies the proximal bronchial airway and is associated with recurrent distal infections or bronchiectasis. In such cases, lobectomy is indicated.

Following resection, the prognosis is excellent.

SPECIAL PROBLEM: THE SOLITARY PULMONARY NODULE

With the frequent use of chest radiography, solitary pulmonary nodules ("coin lesions") are frequently found in patients without pulmonary symptoms. These lesions pose a diagnostic problem for clinicians since they may represent something as benign as a nipple shadow or as malignant as lung cancer (Figure 19–21). The overall incidence of cancer in coin lesions is as low as 10%. Other diagnostic possibilities include (1) infections due to mycobacteria (tuberculosis), fungi (histoplasmosis, coccidioidomycosis), and helminths (echinococcosis); (2) inflammatory nodules from rheumatoid arthritis, focal pneumonitis, and Wegener's granulomatosis; (3) congenital anomalies, such as bronchogenic cysts and arteriovenous malformations; (4) benign neoplasms, eg, hamartomas, hemangiomas, papillary tumors, fibrous tumors of the pleura; (5) malignant neoplasms of the lung; and (6) miscellaneous processes, eg, hematomas, pulmonary infarcts, pleural plaques, loculated effusions, chest wall masses, and mucoid impaction. Although certain radiographic findings may suggest malignancy or benignity, solid pathologic proof that the nodule does not represent a malignancy rests with the clinician. In general, malignant neo-

plasms are larger and grow rapidly, appear spiculated, often with surface umbilication or notching and eccentric excavation. In addition, cancers often occur in smokers (or former smokers) over the age of 40 with negative skin tests for tuberculosis, histoplasmosis, or coccidioidomycosis (although positive tests do not exclude cancer), and in nodules that lack calcium (CT Hounsfield units < 175). In contrast, benign lesions are small (< 1 cm), stable (> 2 years), and calcified ("target" or "popcorn" distribution; CT Hounsfield units > 175) and are associated with positive skin tests in 70–90% of patients. Evaluation of these patients usually includes chest CT scan, but sputum cytology, cultures, bronchoscopy, and mediastinoscopy are sometimes helpful.

With the advent of spiral CT scanning, the incidence of asymptomatic pulmonary nodules can vary from 25% to 70%. The vast majority of these lesions now identified are less than 1 cm and often as small as 2–3 mm. In one series, the incidence of lung cancer in the asymptomatic 10 pack-year smoking history population over the age of 50 years was 27% of all lesions identified, followed, and treated. Ongoing trials are assessing the efficacy and cost-effectiveness of CT screening for lung cancer. In the properly selected high-risk patient population (eg, over 60 years of age, moderate COPD, $FEV_1 < 70\%$), and an over 20 pack-year smok-

Figure 19–21. Coin lesions. ***A:*** Large-cell undifferentiated carcinoma in RUL (tomogram). ***B:*** Histoplasmosis (tomogram). ***C:*** Hamartoma. ***D:*** Solitary metastasis from epidermoid carcinoma of the cervix. ***E:*** Tuberculoma (tomogram). ***F:*** Foreign body granuloma in heroin addict (tomogram). ***G:*** Adenocarcinoma of LUL (present 6 years). ***H:*** Alveolar cell carcinoma of LUL (present 3 years). (RUL = right upper lobe; LUL = left upper lobe.)

ing history), spiral CT may prove to be cost-effective and will save lives.

Ultimately, a pathologic diagnosis must be made. In some instances, fine-needle aspiration cytology may be helpful, particularly if a tissue diagnosis of hamartoma can be made or id cultures demonstrating infectious organisms are obtained. The vast majority of solitary pulmonary nodules, however, require surgical excisional biopsy to exclude the possibility of malignancy. Currently, this is accomplished with video-assisted techniques in most patients, particularly if the lesion is in the periphery of the lung. If a benign lesion is encountered, nothing further is warranted; but if a lung cancer is diagnosed, immediate lobectomy is indicated. The prognosis following resection of a coin lesion that turns out to be a bronchogenic carcinoma is good, with a 5-year survival of as high as 80–90% for lesions < 1 cm.

Baaklini WA et al: Diagnostic yield of fiberoptic bronchoscopy in evaluating solitary pulmonary nodules. Chest 2000;117: 1049.

Gould MK et al: Accuracy of positron emission tomography for diagnosis of pulmonary nodules and mass lesions: a meta-analysis. JAMA 2001;285:914.

Midthun DE, Swensen SJ, Jett JR: Approach to the solitary pulmonary nodule. Mayo Clin Proc 1993;68:378.

Midthun DE, Swensen SJ, Jett JR: Clinical strategies for solitary pulmonary nodule. Annu Rev Med 1992;43:195.

Swanson SJ et al: Management of the solitary pulmonary nodule: role of thoracoscopy in diagnosis and therapy. Chest 1999; 116(6 Suppl):523S.

SECONDARY LUNG CANCER

Autopsy studies have demonstrated that 30% of all patients with malignancies develop pulmonary metastases, and 12% have been shown to have isolated lung disease that is totally resectable. In addition, 10% of these latter patients (1.2% of all patients) have solitary lung metastases. Most pulmonary metastases occur through hematogenous spread from the primary site; lymphatic or transbronchial spread is extremely rare. Secondary metastatic spread to the pulmonary and mediastinal lymph nodes, however, can also occur. In patients with known extrathoracic primary cancers, multiple pulmonary lesions almost always represent metastatic disease. Solitary lesions, however, may be due to benign disease (18%) or new primary lung cancer (18%) as well as metastatic disease (64%). Most patients with pulmonary metastases are asymptomatic even with extensive disease. If symptoms do develop, cough, hemoptysis, fever, dyspnea, and pain are common. The diagnosis is generally initially suggested by routine chest radiography, and CT of the chest should always be ordered to assess the lungs for other nodules. Although CT scans are more sensitive, detecting nodules as small

as 3 mm, they are also less specific (false-positive rate of 55%) than plain x-rays. Pathologic confirmation of the diagnosis is essential and usually is obtained at the time of resection. For patients who are not surgical candidates, fine-needle aspiration cytology is useful for peripheral lesions, while central lesions may require bronchoscopy for tissue diagnosis.

Medically fit patients with resectable disease are surgical candidates as long as the following criteria are fulfilled: (1) the primary tumor must be controlled or imminently controllable; (2) no other sites of disease may exist; (3) no other therapy can offer comparable results; and (4) the operative risk must be low. Since adenocarcinomas (especially breast cancer) commonly involve multiple organs, it is imperative that with this histology a full evaluation be performed, including bone scan and head CT or MRI. Solitary squamous cell nodules, however—even in the presence of a previous squamous cell carcinoma (eg, head and neck tumors)—should be addressed as a new primary (lung) cancer. Surgical resection can be accomplished through a standard posterolateral thoracotomy, median sternotomy, or bilateral anterior thoracotomies. The latter approach is particularly beneficial for bilateral disease involving the lower lobes. Video-assisted thoracoscopy has also been used, but the efficacy of this approach has not been proved.

It is not uncommon during open operations for metastatic disease to find several unsuspected nodules by direct palpation that may be missed with thoracoscopy. Wedge resection is the treatment of choice unless the lesion is a solitary squamous cell carcinoma or adenocarcinoma. These latter lesions cannot be distinguished from primary lung cancer on frozen section pathologic examination, and they must therefore be treated as primary lung cancers with lobectomy and mediastinal lymph node dissection. Occasionally, other malignant tumors identified by histologic examination may require lobectomy or rarely even pneumonectomy because of involvement of the proximal pulmonary artery or bronchus.

The success rate with surgical removal of pulmonary metastases has been greatest with testicular (51% 5-year survival) and head-neck cancers (47% 5-year survival). Other types of tumors, such as osteogenic and soft tissue sarcomas, renal cell carcinoma, and colon carcinoma, are all associated with prolonged survival in 20–35% of patients. Results of resection for melanoma are less favorable (10–15% survival benefit). Isolated, resectable pulmonary metastases from rectal cancer can have as high as a 55% 5-year survival with metastasectomy alone.

Furthermore, multiple thoracotomies over periods in excess of 10 years are not unusual with the sarcomas. Numerous studies have been conducted in attempts to identify prognostic factors that could aid in the selection of patients for resection Adverse prognostic factors have included (1) multiple or bilateral lesions, (2) more than four lesions seen on CT scan, (3) tumor doubling time < 40 days, (4) a short disease-free interval, and (5) advanced age.

Although no consensus has developed regarding the selection of candidates for surgical exploration, it is generally agreed that no single criterion should be used to exclude patients from surgical resection. In all series, long-term benefit and survival hinges on complete re-section. If complete resection is not deemed possible, resection should not be offered.

LaQuaglia MP: The surgical management of metastases in pediatric cancer. Semin Pediatr Surg 1993;2:75.

Pogrebniak HW, Pass HI: Initial and reoperative pulmonary metastasectomy: indications, technique, and results. Semin Surg Oncol 1993;9:142.

Todd TR: Pulmonary metastectomy: current indications for re-moving lung metastases. Chest 1993;103(4 Suppl):401S.

The Heart: I. Acquired Diseases

20

Scot H. Merrick, MD

The impact of acquired diseases of the cardiovascular system on the human population is enormous. In the United States alone, cardiovascular disease currently affects over 60 million people and accounts for over 40% of all deaths (Figure 20–1). A subset—coronary artery disease—affects over 12 million people and is responsible for one in every five deaths in the United States. Approximately 100 billion dollars will be spent on the care of these patients in 2001.

The spectrum of valvular heart disease is changing as the population ages, increasing the incidence of degenerative valvular disorders and decreasing the incidence of rheumatic valvular diseases. Atherosclerotic disease of the thoracic aorta, more commonly seen in the elderly, is becoming more prevalent as well.

Medical and surgical advances have resulted in a significant decrease in the death rates from cardiovascular diseases over the last decade. Notable exceptions are women and minorities. More importantly, the rate of population expansion is much greater than the development of new therapies, underscoring the need for expanded research in cardiovascular disease prevention.

■ ISCHEMIC HEART DISEASE

ANGINA PECTORIS

The right and left coronary arteries arise from the sinuses of Valsalva as the first branches of the aorta. The right coronary artery passes deep in the right atrioventricular groove (Figure 20–2) and usually terminates as the posterior descending coronary artery in the posterior interventricular groove. The right coronary artery supplies multiple right ventricular branches and the right marginal artery. In 90% of patients, the right coronary artery gives rise to the posterior descending artery (right coronary dominance) and branches into an atrioventricular nodal artery and several terminal posterolateral left ventricular branches.

The left main coronary artery is usually about 1 cm long and gives rise to the left anterior descending and left circumflex coronary arteries (Figure 20–2). The left anterior descending artery provides several diagonal branches to the anterior wall of the left ventricle and a number of perforating branches to the interventricular septum. In most patients, the left anterior descending artery wraps the apex of the heart, anastomosing with the posterior descending artery. The left anterior descending artery usually is the largest and most important of the coronary arteries. The circumflex coronary artery lies in the left atrioventricular groove (Figure 20–2) and proceeds laterally and posteriorly around the lateral aspect of the left ventricle, usually terminating in several circumflex marginal arteries. In 10% of patients, the circumflex coronary artery provides the posterior descending coronary artery (left coronary dominance).

Coronary blood flow delivers oxygen and metabolic substrates to the myocardium and simultaneously removes carbon dioxide and metabolic by-products via transcapillary exchange. Normal coronary blood flow approximates 1 mL per gram of myocardium per minute and delivers 0.1 mL of oxygen per gram per minute to the heart—a high rate of energy utilization compared with the rest of the body. The extraction of oxygen in the coronary bed averages 75% under normal conditions and increases to nearly 100% during stress. Coronary artery blood flow occurs primarily during diastole because systolic myocardial contraction increases intramyocardial vascular resistance. Normally, mean coronary resistance is three to six times the totally vasodilated value, implying an extreme vasodilator reserve. During stress, oxygen delivery increases as a result of vasodilation in response to the high baseline oxygen extraction. Assuming adequate perfusion pressure, total and regional myocardial blood flow under normal conditions is determined by autoregulation of regional arteriolar resistance modulated by local metabolic demand.

The metabolic activity of heart muscle converts the chemical energy from myocardial oxygen and substrate utilization into mechanical energy in the form of blood pressure and flow. With electrical depolarization of the myocardial cell membrane, chemomechanical alteration of the myosin cross-bridge produces sliding of myosin filaments relative to actin and shortening of the sarcomere. Over the physiologic range of sarcomere lengths (1.6–2 μm), the surface area of available cross-bridge interactions (and therefore the metabolic energy transferred into mechanical work during sarcomere contraction) is directly proportionate to end-diastolic sarcom-

Figure 20–1. Leading causes of death for all males and females in the United States, 1998. (Reprinted with permission of the American Heart Association, 2001 Heart and Stroke Statistical Update. American Heart Association, 2000.)

A	Total CVD	D	Chronic Obstructive Pulmonary Disease
B	Cancer	E	Pneumonia/Influenza
C	Accidents	F	Diabetes Mellitus

ere length. The ventricles seem to function as an integrated sum of their component sarcomeres. Mechanical energy production, in the form of pressure and flow (stroke work), is a direct linear function of end-diastolic volume (Figure 20–3) and is not influenced significantly by physiologic changes in afterload. Therefore, short-term alterations in ventricular performance can be assessed by the slope of the stroke work and end-diastolic volume relationship. This basic **Frank-Starling property** of the heart is probably a direct reflection of sarcomere and myosin cross-bridge dynamics. The clinical analog of this principle allows cardiac function to be assessed as the product of cardiac output and mean arterial pressure (circulatory energy) at a given pulmonary capillary wedge pressure. For reference, the normal cardiac hemodynamic values in the adult are presented in Table 20–1.

Pathology

Coronary atherosclerosis is a progressive disease whose earliest microscopic changes have been described in the newborn infant, and advanced lesions are present in half the hearts examined at autopsy during the second decade of life. Early lesions are characterized by intimal incorporation of lipid material, progressing to an expanding plaque surrounded by fibrosis and calcification. In the final stages, rupture of the intimal plaque

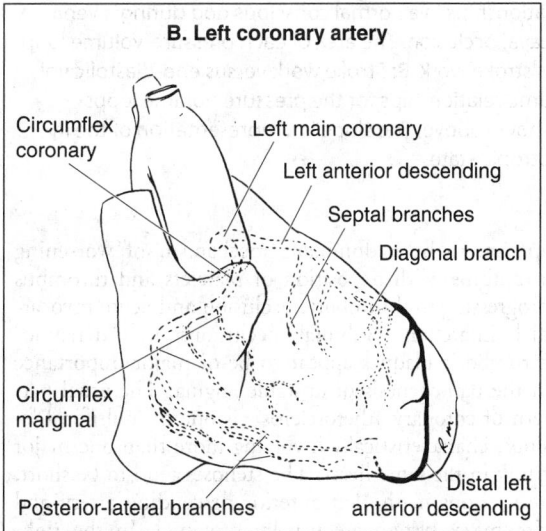

Figure 20–2. Anatomic representation of the right **(A)** and left **(B)** coronary arteries.

Figure 20–3. **A:** Left ventricular pressure-volume relationships in a normal conscious dog during a vena caval occlusion. The area of each pressure-volume loop is stroke work. **B:** Stroke work versus end-diastolic volume relationships for the pressure-volume loops shown above. The slope is a representation of the inotropic state.

appears to be a dominant mechanism of worsening symptoms, with deposition of platelets and thrombus progressing to thrombotic occlusion and acute myocardial infarction. Subtotal occlusions by "dynamic" thrombotic plaques appear to be of major importance in the pathogenesis of unstable angina. The usual pattern of coronary atherosclerosis is one of multifocal lesions, characteristically involving more than one major trunk in the same heart. The stenoses tend to be short, and lesions in the left anterior descending artery and circumflex system are usually proximal. In the right coronary artery, the disease is more diffuse and involves chiefly the proximal and middle portions of the artery;

however, the posterior descending artery and distal branches usually are spared. Type 1 diabetic patients can be an exception, often having diffuse coronary involvement.

When an atherosclerotic plaque decreases the coronary cross-sectional area by 75% (50% reduction in diameter), the resistance to flow becomes significant. The dominant point of coronary vascular resistance becomes the stenosis that limits myocardial perfusion to a fixed value. While flow may be adequate at rest, exercise or other factors that increase myocardial oxygen demand can produce relative ischemia, a fall in coronary pressure distal to the stenosis, and redistribution of blood flow away from the subendocardium. This appears to be the mechanism of exercise-induced angina pectoris. Coronary vasospasm or unstable thrombotic plaques can compound the obstructive physiology. Because of high metabolic demand and tight coupling between energy utilization and expenditure, acute coronary insufficiency—such as occurs with angina pectoris—produces an almost immediate decrement in myocardial segment shortening and work. Even when full reperfusion is accomplished after a 15-minute period of reversible ischemia, dysfunction can be prolonged, requiring 24–48 hours for complete recovery.

Risk Factors

Significant progress has been made in identifying risk factors associated with the development of coronary heart disease (see Table 20–2). Of these, cigarette smoking is the most important. In addition to the adverse effects of carbon monoxide and nicotine on the endothelial cell, cigarette smoke can increase LDL levels, reduce HDL levels, increase fibrinogen levels, and increase platelet aggregation. Exposure to secondhand smoke may increase the death rate from coronary heart disease by 30%. The risk of developing coronary heart disease is reduced 50% after 1 year of smoking abstinence; at 15 years, the risk is no different from that of never-smokers. Niacin, statins, and resins can now modify cholesterol levels effectively.

Clinical Findings

A. SYMPTOMS AND SIGNS

The most common symptom of myocardial ischemia is retrosternal chest pain, or angina pectoris, produced by a reduction in coronary blood flow. The discomfort is often described by the patient as pressure, a choking sensation, or a feeling of tightness. Early in the symptomatic course, a variety of factors such as exercise, cold exposure, eating, and emotional distress can initiate the symptoms. The pain frequently radiates down the left arm and into the left neck and occasionally to the right

Table 20–1. Normal cardiac hemodynamic values.

Site	Phasic	Mean	Oxygen Content (vol%)	Oxygen Saturation (%)
Right atrium	7/2	4	16	75
Right ventricle	20/0	5	16	75
Pulmonary artery	20/10	13	16	75
Left atrium	13/3	5–12	20	97
Left ventricle	120/5	12	20	97
Aorta	120/70	85	20	97
Heart rate (HR)	60–90 beats/min			
Forward stroke volume (SV)	73 ± 22 mL/beat			
Cardiac output (CO; HR × SV)	6 L/min			
Cardiac index (CI)	3.5 ± 1.0 L/min/m^2			
End-diastolic volume (EDV)	70 ± 30 mL/m^2			
End systolic volume (ESV)	25 ± 13 mL/m^2			
Ejection fraction (EF)	67 ± 8% (EDV–ESV/EDV)			
Systemic resistance (SVR)	900–1400 dynes•sec•cm^{-2} ((MAP–CVP)/CI) × 80			
Pulmonary resistance (PVR)	150–250 dynes•sec•cm^{-2} ((PA–CVP)/CI) × 80			

m^2 = square meter of body surface area
MAP = mean arterial pressure
CVP = central venous pressure
PA = mean pulmonary artery pressure

Table 20–2. Major risk factors for coronary heart disease.

Cigarette smoking
Serum cholesterol
    Total > 240 mg/dL
    LDL > 130 mg/dL
    HDL < 35 mg/dL
    Triglycerides > 200 mg/dL
Male gender
Diabetes mellitus
Hypertension
Family history of early heart disease
Obesity
Inactivity

LDL = low-density lipoprotein
HDL = high-density lipoprotein

arm, mandible, or ear. The severity of chest pain can be graded by the New York Heart Association (NYHA) classification, with class I indicating no symptoms; class II, symptoms with severe exertion; class III, chest pain with mild exertion; and class IV, pain at rest. While minimal anginal symptoms often are easily tolerated and compatible with a normal lifestyle (stable angina), an increasing NYHA class over a short period of time (progressive angina) worsens the prognosis. In the late stages, ischemia occurs at rest and is refractory to medical therapy (unstable angina). Unstable pain patterns imply a very poor outlook, with a high incidence of early infarction and death. Patients who develop pulmonary edema from severe ischemia and those who have angina following a myocardial infarction have a poor prognosis.

A large proportion of patients do not pursue the classic symptomatic progression and present initially with acute myocardial infarction or sudden death. Still others experience *no symptoms at all* during ischemia (silent myocardial ischemia), and coronary artery disease is only discovered in the late stage of congestive heart failure after severe ventricular damage has occurred. The physical examination is frequently unremarkable. Cardiac enlargement may be evident in patients with advanced disease, but the chest radiograph is normal in the majority. While the ECG is normal in at least half of patients, abnormal findings consist of inverted T waves, ST segment abnormalities, or Q waves on the resting ECG. Transient ST segment and T wave changes may occur during an anginal episode or exercise stress test.

B. IMAGING STUDIES

Cardiac catheterization and coronary arteriography are essential for determining the presence and extent of coronary atherosclerosis. In recent years, a trend has favored early angiography in most patients with suspected coronary disease in order to identify individual prognostic characteristics as precisely as possible. This approach has allowed a more objective application of medical therapy to low-risk subsets and selection of patients at high medical risk for elective coronary revascularization. The development of low-cost outpatient catheterization has facilitated this trend. At angiography, the major anatomic predictors of coronary death—such as the number of coronary vessels diseased and the resting left ventricular ejection fraction—are documented. While the extent of obstructive disease can be underestimated in up to 10% of patients, coronary arteriography has the highest sensitivity and specificity of any test available. Recently, electron-beam computed tomography has been used to detect and quantify the degree of coronary artery calcification. A coronary calcification scoring system can be correlated with the presence of hemodynamically significant coronary lesions. However, the expense of this study precludes its use as a primary screening tool. In patients with borderline anatomic indications for coronary revascularization, physiologic assessment with radionuclide exercise ventriculography, stress thallium scanning, or exercise echocardiography can be useful in making decisions about operative treatment. In particular, thallium scintigraphy may provide critical information about myocardial viability in patients with poor ventricular function.

Treatment

A. MEDICAL TREATMENT

Hypertension should be controlled and smoking avoided. Lipid abnormalities should be treated with drugs or diet. After bypass grafting, risk factor modification and continued medical therapy are especially important, since atherosclerotic involvement of saphenous vein grafts is a major long-term risk. When making a

choice between medical and surgical therapy, the natural history of angina pectoris should be reviewed. The annual coronary disease mortality rate is directly related to the number of vessels affected and the degree of impairment of left ventricular function (Figures 20–4 and 20–5). In current practice, adverse prognostic factors that might suggest referral for coronary revascularization include severe or progressive angina on medical therapy; refractory unstable angina; significant left main coronary disease; multivessel coronary obstruction (especially with proximal left anterior descending artery involvement); ventricular impairment with a reduced ejection fraction; multivessel coronary disease in diabetics; and ischemic cardiomyopathy. Each of these factors, individually or in combination, significantly reduces survival with medical therapy and predicts an improved longevity after coronary bypass grafting.

In patients with low-risk clinical profiles, medical management is recommended if anginal symptoms and exercise capacity can be maintained satisfactorily. Sublingual nitroglycerin, long-acting nitrate preparations, and nitroglycerin ointment can be useful. Beta-adrenergic blocking agents such as propranolol, atenolol, and timolol are effective and safe. Calcium channel blocking agents such as nifedipine, diltiazem, and verapamil are also effective. Antiplatelet agents such as aspirin have a definite therapeutic role, and short-term heparinization has been effective in preventing coronary thrombosis and infarction in patients with unstable

Figure 20–4. Survival in patients with significant lesions of one, two, and three coronary arteries and the left main coronary artery (LCA).

Figure 20–5. Survival according to ventriculographic estimates of resting left ventricular function in patients with ischemic heart disease.

angina. Patients with unstable syndromes may benefit from glycoprotein IIB/IIIA inhibitors (abciximab, tirofiban), and postinfarction patients are usually prescribed ACE-inhibitors for ventricular remodeling.

B. Surgical Treatment

It is essential that the goals and anticipated results of coronary bypass be explained objectively and in detail to patient and family. Risks and possible complications should be discussed, and all aspects of the history, physical examination, and results of cardiac catheterization should be reviewed, with emphasis on imparting knowledge about cardiac anatomy and dynamics. Complete revascularization is an important objective and is associated with a better long-term outcome. The presence of carotid bruits should be evaluated, and respiratory status, renal function, and blood coagulation should be assessed. Aspirin should be discontinued, if possible, for 1–2 weeks prior to operation because of an increased risk of postoperative bleeding. Antianginal agents should be continued until the day of operation. If further pharmacologic therapy is required for recurring angina, an intravenous nitroglycerin infusion can be employed. Intra-aortic balloon pumping is also effective for preoperative stabilization of unstable patients in the coronary care unit. Prophylactic broad-spectrum antibiotics are administered intravenously before anesthetic induction and for 24–48 hours postoperatively.

Finally, safe and effective cardiac anesthesia is essential for obtaining optimal surgical results.

1. Conventional approach—The vast majority of procedures consist of simple bypass of the obstructed coronary vessels, using either the internal mammary artery or reversed segments of saphenous vein. In most cases, after a median sternotomy incision is made, the left internal mammary artery is dissected from the chest wall. Cardiopulmonary bypass is instituted with or without mild systemic hypothermia, using aortic cannulation for arterial inflow and a single right atrial cannula for venous return to the pump. After clamping of the ascending aorta, cold potassium cardioplegia solution is infused into the aortic root to arrest and protect the heart, reducing myocardial oxygen consumption to minimal levels. The saphenous vein grafts or internal mammary arteries are then sutured to the coronary arteries beyond the stenoses (Figure 20–6), and additional volumes of cardioplegia solution are infused every 20–30 minutes to maintain myocardial temperature below 15 °C. After completion of the distal coronary anastomoses, the aorta is unclamped, proximal aorta–vein graft anastomoses are completed, and car-

Figure 20–6. Technique of end-to-side internal mammary artery–coronary anastomosis.

Table 20–3. Long-term graft patency.

Conduit	1 Year	2 Years	5 Years	10 Years
Great saphenous vein	80–90%			50%
Cephalic vein	85%	66%		
Internal mammary artery	98%			90%
Free internal mammary artery	95%		92%	
Gastroepiploic artery	95%		95%	
Radial	94%		83%	
Cryovein[1]		50%		

[1]Cryopreserved cadaver vein.

diopulmonary bypass is discontinued after adequate rewarming.

An average of three or four grafts are inserted. In general, the internal mammary artery is the graft of choice owing to its superior long-term patency. This is in part due to the preservation of a functional endothelium in this graft. At least one internal mammary artery graft is utilized in 95% of procedures, usually to the left anterior descending coronary artery, and adjunctive saphenous vein grafts are used for additional vessels. Multiple internal mammary artery procedures can be performed, using a combination of bilateral mammary artery pedicles, sequential mammary artery anastomoses, and free mammary artery grafts. At present, however, complex internal mammary artery grafting is reserved for patients with limited saphenous veins, younger patients with longer life expectancies, reoperative cases with previous vein graft failure, and patients with atherosclerotic calcification of the ascending aorta. Other arterial conduits such as the inferior epigastric artery, the gastroepiploic artery, and the radial artery are being used with increasing frequency to improve long-term patency rates. Representative patency rates for these bypass conduits are presented in Table 20–3. Graft closure within the first 30 days after surgery is usually due to technical errors, poor graft quality, or poor target vessel runoff. From 1 month to 3 years, grafts usually occlude from intimal hyperplasia. After 3 years, graft atherosclerosis is the most common reason for closure. Graft patency is adversely affected by persistent cigarette smoking and elevated LDL cholesterol.

2. Minimally invasive approach—Over the past 5 years, a number of alternative surgical methods (minimally invasive direct coronary artery bypass, MIDCAB; off-pump coronary artery bypass, OPCAB; port access) have evolved with the aim of reducing surgical morbidity, mortality, and cost. Of these, the off-pump coronary artery bypass (OPCAB) approach is the most widely used (approximately 15% of all coronary revascularization procedures) and holds the most promise. With this approach, patients undergo standard median sternotomy and graft harvesting. Cardiopulmonary bypass is eliminated, and grafts are anastomosed to target vessels on the beating heart with the assistance of a stabilizer device designed to keep the target vessel motionless. Although multivessel bypass can be achieved, lesions isolated to the left anterior descending, diagonal, and proximal right coronaries are the most appropriate. The primary advantage of the OPCAB approach is elimination of the systemic effects of cardiopulmonary bypass (hypothermia, inflammatory response, micro-emboli, etc). Incomplete revascularization and reduced early graft patency are potential problems. True reductions in morbidity, mortality, and cost await the results of randomized trials.

Transmyocardial laser revascularization has been used in patients with inoperable coronary disease. With this procedure, multiple 1 mm channels are created transmurally to provide access of left ventricular blood into ischemic myocardium. Most channels thrombose quickly; nevertheless, 70% of patients will have symptomatic improvement and better quality of life. Overall survival remains unchanged, and the exact mechanism of improvement from transmyocardial laser revascularization remains unclear.

Prognosis

As a group, patients who are treated by coronary bypass surgery have 5- and 10-year survivals of 92% and 81%, respectively. For the same intervals, freedom from recurrence of angina is 83% and 63%, respectively. The most important predictors of late cardiac mortality after surgery are diabetes, advanced age, reduced ejection fraction, and nonuse of the internal mammary graft. Successful revascularization improves resting left ventricular wall motion in a significant proportion of patients and enhances exercise ventricular performance. Fewer than 1% of patients will require repeat revascularization within 4 years of follow-up. Comprehensive morbidity and mortality data are available from the Society of Thoracic Surgeons National Cardiac Surgery Database. For isolated coronary bypass procedures, operative mortality is approximately 2.8%. Univariate predictors of adverse outcome are presented in Table 20–4. In a meta-analysis of the prospective, randomized studies comparing medical to surgical therapy, it is evident that surgery imparts

Table 20–4. Preoperative univariate predictors of mortality for coronary bypass procedures.[1]

Variable	Relative Risk
Left main disease	1.58
Female gender	1.69
NYHA class IV	1.74
Previous stroke	1.93
Peripheral vascular disease	2.22
Pulmonary hypertension	2.39
Ejection fraction 25–35%	2.92
Congestive heart failure	2.87
Age > 70	3.13
Prior CABG	3.32
Preop balloon pump	3.43
Renal failure	3.45
Acute myocardial infarction	6.12
Cardiogenic shock	7.89
Emergent operation	12.39

[1]Society of Thoracic Surgeons National Database, 1999.

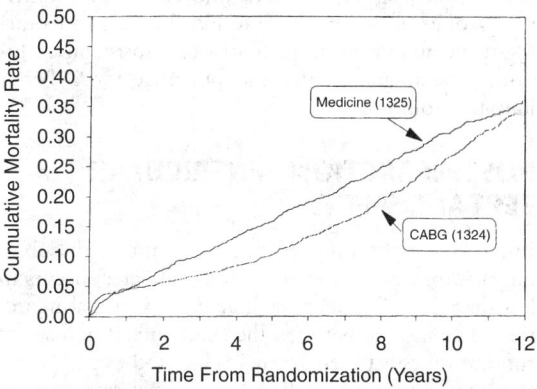

Figure 20–7. Meta-analysis of CABG versus medical survival from 7, prospective, randomized studies. (Reproduced, with permission, from Yusuf S et al: Effect of coronary artery bypass surgery on survival: overview of 10-year results from randomised trials by the Coronary Artery Graft Surgery Trialists. Lancet 1994;344:566.)

a 39% and 17% reduction in cumulative mortality at 5 and 10 years, respectively (Figure 20–7). This advantage is most evident in patients with multivessel disease, reduced ventricular function, left main coronary involvement, and NYHA class IV symptoms.

THE RELATIVE ROLES OF PTCA, CORONARY STENTS, & CORONARY BYPASS

In 1977, Gruntzig introduced percutaneous transluminal coronary angioplasty (PTCA) for dilating stenotic coronary arterial lesions. Successful dilation rates per stenosis currently exceed 90%; complication rates have fallen below 2%; and procedure-related myocardial infarction and death remain uncommon. Recent enthusiasm for balloon dilation has been accompanied by its increasing application to more complex forms of coronary disease and a marked increase in the number of procedures performed annually. In many centers, PTCA is now the most commonly used invasive therapy for coronary disease. Comparisons between PTCA and surgery remain controversial. The results of six prospective, randomized studies comparing PTCA and surgery for multi-vessel coronary disease have shown no

difference in the overall 5-year survival or nonfatal myocardial infarction rate. However, the risk of repeat revascularization is significantly higher in the PTCA patients. This is particularly evident in patients with diabetes. At 5 years, the cumulative costs for both procedures are similar. Risk-adjusted data from the New York State CABG and PTCA registries show a significant survival advantage for CABG in patients who have single-vessel or double-vessel disease with a proximal ≥ 70% stenosis of the left anterior descending coronary and in any patient with triple-vessel disease. While the addition of coronary stenting to PTCA has reduced the restenosis rate, repeat interventions are still more common when compared with surgical revascularization.

REOPERATION FOR CORONARY ARTERY DISEASE

Since the advent of coronary artery bypass, an increasing number of patients have presented for reoperation. Common reasons for reoperation include progression of atherosclerotic lesions in the native coronary arteries and atherosclerotic involvement of vein bypass grafts. Performing an internal mammary artery graft at the initial operation significantly reduces the need for reoperation. Control of postoperative hyperlipidemia should also reduce the incidence of reoperation.

The technical aspects of the second procedure are more difficult, but the operative mortality rate should be only slightly higher—generally in the range of 3%. Nevertheless, when appropriate clinical indications are present, reoperation should be undertaken with anticipation of excellent long-term results. In patients requiring reoperation for vein graft atherosclerosis and occlusion, arterial grafts offer the potential for a better long-term outcome.

POSTINFARCTION VENTRICULAR SEPTAL DEFECT

Infarction of the interventricular septum with subsequent formation of a ventricular septal defect occurs in less than 1% of patients with acute myocardial infarction. The interval between the acute infarct and septal rupture varies between 1 and 12 days and can be correlated with histologic findings of maximal cardiac muscle degeneration and weakening. Once rupture occurs, the prognosis is poor, with 24% of patients dying on the first day after rupture, 65% by the end of 2 weeks, and 81% by 2 months. The syndrome develops classically in a patient with myocardial infarction in whom shock or congestive heart failure suddenly appears.

Clinical Findings

A. SYMPTOMS AND SIGNS

A harsh holosystolic murmur is usually heard along the left sternal border, and two-thirds of patients demonstrate a palpable thrill.

B. IMAGING STUDIES

Although clinical findings may be highly suggestive, the definitive diagnosis is made by Doppler echocardiography and cardiac catheterization. The defects are often irregular, ragged tracts through the anterior apical septum with occlusion of the left anterior descending artery or through the posterior basilar septum in cases of right coronary artery occlusion. In the latter, right ventricular infarction may compound the problem.

Differential Diagnosis

The differential diagnosis includes papillary muscle dysfunction, rupture of a papillary muscle with acute mitral insufficiency, and pericardial friction rub secondary to myocardial infarction.

Treatment

Surgical correction is indicated in nearly all cases, with the possible exception of elderly patients with advanced multiorgan failure. Intervention should not be delayed, and early or even emergency operation should be the rule. A preoperative intra-aortic balloon pump is placed in most patients, and patch closure of the septal defect along with coronary bypass should be performed early

to prevent the consequences of acute right ventricular overload or multiorgan failure.

After institution of cardiopulmonary bypass and cardioplegic arrest, an incision is made in the area of infarction, and good exposure of both the left and right ventricles is obtained (Figure 20–8). A portion of the necrotic edge of the defect is resected, and a double patch technique is used for repair (Figure 20–9). Coronary bypass grafts are constructed to all diseased vessels, including the right coronary artery in cases of right ventricular infarction.

Prognosis

Fifty to 80 percent of patients should survive the operative procedure depending on the severity of preoperative shock and multiorgan failure.

LEFT VENTRICULAR ANEURYSM

Left ventricular aneurysm occurs when a large myocardial infarction progresses to a thinned-out transmural scar that bulges paradoxically beyond the normal cavitary contours during systole. While aneurysms have occurred in 2–4% of myocardial infarctions, the incidence is probably decreasing with more aggressive infarct management. Ninety percent of aneurysms involve the anteroseptal left ventricle, and 10% are posterior. Over 50% contain mural thrombus.

Clinical Findings

Patients show signs and symptoms of congestive heart failure, angina, embolization, and ventricular dysrhythmias. Clinical manifestations include a prominent apical

Figure 20–8. Operative photograph of inferior postinfarction ventricular septal defect (VSD). Infarct has been opened to expose fistula into the right ventricle.

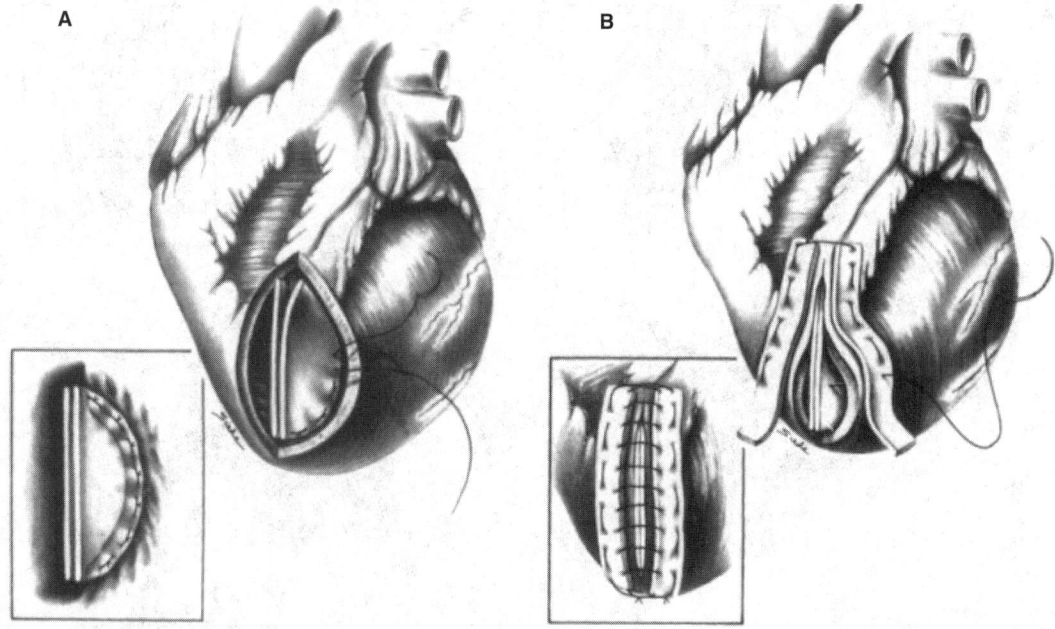

Figure 20–9. Double patch repair technique for anterior postinfarction ventricular septal defect. The ventricular septum is reconstructed by placing sheets of Teflon felt on each side of the septum *(A)* and then closing the ventricular walls to the septal patch *(B)*.

impulse, electrocardiographic evidence of an old Q wave myocardial infarction with persistent ST segment elevation, and a localized left ventricular bulge on chest x-ray.

Treatment

Surgical therapy should be considered in most cases, since the prognosis with medical management is poor. Treatment consists of aneurysm resection combined with complete coronary revascularization (Figure 20–10).

Prognosis

The prognosis without surgery is related to the acuity of symptoms, the degree of left ventricular dysfunction, and the extent of associated coronary artery disease.

Significant improvements in symptoms of congestive heart failure and angina are observed in 70–85% of patients surviving after operation, and left ventricular ejection fraction increases in the majority because of reduced end-diastolic volume. Long-term survival is improved significantly over medical therapy, with 70–80% of patients alive 5 years postoperatively. The operative mortality rate for elective cases is 5% and increases to 20% for emergency procedures. The hospital mortality rate associated with subendocardial resection for ventricular tachycardia has been 11%.

SURGERY FOR CARDIOMYOPATHY

Medical therapy for advanced heart failure carries a dismal prognosis. Approximately 60% of patients with NYHA class IV symptoms will die within 1 year. A small number of these patients may benefit from operative treatment, and the objective is to reduce ventricular chamber size, improve the shape (decrease sphericity), lower filling pressures, and eliminate mitral insufficiency. In so doing, ventricular wall stress and myocardial oxygen demand are reduced.

The type of operation depends on the underlying cause of cardiomyopathy. The two most frequent causes in the United States are ischemic and dilated (idiopathic) cardiomyopathy. The former is not actually a muscle disease but rather severe dysfunction caused by diffuse coronary artery disease. Patients with this condition may be candidates for coronary bypass if suitable target vessels are present and viable myocardium can be demonstrated by thallium scintigraphy or positron emission tomography. Many of these patients have "hibernating" myocardium, which can regain contractile function if blood supply is restored. Operative mortality is acceptable (3–10%), and published 5-year survivals range from 30% to 50%. Idiopathic dilated cardiomyopathy been treated with a number of surgical procedures (Table 20–5). Orthotopic heart transplanta-

A

B

Figure 20–10. Technique of resection *(A)* and closure *(B)* of left ventricular aneurysm.

tion offers the best long-term results in suitable candidates. Mitral valve annuloplasty can be very effective in restoring valve competence in patients with annular stretching from ventricular enlargement. Ventricular reduction surgery (Batista procedure) and dynamic cardiomyoplasty have limited application because of high operative mortality and limited survival. Biventricular pacing is a relatively simple procedure designed to restore the normal depolarization sequence in the ventricular muscle, resulting in significant increases in the ejection fraction.

American Heart Association. 2001 Heart and Stroke Statistical Update.

Bielak LF et al: Probabilistic model for prediction of angiographically defined obstructive coronary artery disease using elec-

Table 20–5. Operations for idiopathic, dilated cardiomyopathy.

Orthotopic heart transplantation
Mitral valve repair
Ventricular reduction surgery
Cardiomyoplasty
Biventricular pacemaker insertion

tron beam computed tomography calcium score strata. Circulation 2000;102:380.

Bishay ES et al: Mitral valve surgery in patients with severe left ventricular dysfunction. Eur J Cardiothorac Surg 2000;17:213.

Braile DM et al: Dynamic cardiomyoplasty: long-term clinical results in patients with dilated cardiomyopathy. Ann Thorac Surg 2000;69:1445.

Chaux AC et al: Postinfarction ventricular septal defect. Semin Thorac Cardiovasc Surg 1998;10:93.

Eagle KA et al: ACC/AHA Guidelines for Coronary Artery Bypass Graft Surgery: a Report of the American College of Cardiology/American Heart Association Task Force on Practice Guidelines (Committee to Revise the 1991 Guidelines for Coronary Artery Bypass Graft Surgery). American College of Cardiology/American Heart Association. J Am Coll Cardiol 1999;34:1262.

Favaloro RG: Landmarks in the development of coronary artery bypass surgery. Circulation 1998;98:466.

Faxon DP: Myocardial revascularization in 1997: angioplasty versus bypass surgery. Am Fam Physician 1997;56:1409.

Frazier OH et al: Transmyocardial laser revascularization. Does it have a role in the treatment of ischemic heart disease? Tex Heart Inst J 1998;25:24.

Frazier OH et al: Transmyocardial revascularization with a carbon dioxide laser in patients with end-stage coronary artery disease. N Engl J Med 1999;341:1021.

Hannan EL et al: A comparison of three-year survival after coronary artery bypass graft surgery and percutaneous transluminal coronary angioplasty. J Am Coll Cardiol 1999;33:63.

He GW: Arterial grafts for coronary artery bypass grafting: biological characteristics, functional classification, and clinical choice. Ann Thorac Surg 1999;67:277.

Kerwin WF et al: Ventricular contraction abnormalities in dilated cardiomyopathy: effect of biventricular pacing to correct interventricular dyssynchrony. J Am Coll Cardiol 2000;35:1221.

Mack MJ: Coronary surgery: off-pump and port access. Surg Clin North Am 2000;80:1575.

Mickleborough LL et al: Results of revascularization in patients with severe left ventricular dysfunction. J Thorac Cardiovasc Surg 2000;119:550.

Motwani JG, Topol EJ: Aortocoronary saphenous vein graft disease: pathogenesis, predisposition, and prevention. Circulation 1998;97:916.

Myers WO et al: CASS Registry long term surgical survival. Coronary Artery Surgery Study. J Am Coll Cardiol 1999;33:488.

Schulze, C., N. Conrad, et al: Reduced expression of systemic proinflammatory cytokines after off-pump versus conventional coronary artery bypass grafting. Thorac Cardiovasc Surg 2000;48:364.

Starling RC, McCarthy PM: Partial left ventriculectomy: sunrise or sunset? Eur J Heart Fail 1999;1:313.

Svennevig JL: Off-pump vs on-pump surgery. A review. Scand Cardiovasc J 2000;34:7.

■ VALVULAR HEART DISEASE

Developmentally, the fibrous skeleton of the heart, to which the cardiac valves attach, is derived from the endocardial cushions. The fibrous annulus of the mitral valve is a thin, incomplete ring of fibrous tissue, which is most apparent at two points: the right and left fibrous trigones (Figure 20–11). The left fibrous trigone is situated at the left anterior aspect of the mitral ring and consists of fibrous tissue joining the mitral ring to the base of the aorta. The right fibrous trigone, or central fibrous body, lies in the midline of the heart and represents the confluence of fibrous tissue from the mitral valve, the tricuspid valve, the membranous septum, and the posterior aspect of the base of the aorta.

In most patients, two mitral leaflets are evident: the anterior leaflet and the posterior leaflet (Figure 20–11). Both leaflets are approximately the shape of a trapezoid, each attaching by thin fibrous chordae tendineae to both the anterior and the posterior papillary muscles. Stated differently, the chordae from each papillary muscle fan out and attach to nearly half of both cusp margins. The edges of the leaflets have a slightly serrated appearance owing to the insertion of chordae tendineae on the ventricular surface; these serrations mark the line of closure of the normal valve.

The anatomy of the tricuspid valve apparatus is similar, except that three valve leaflets usually are evident:

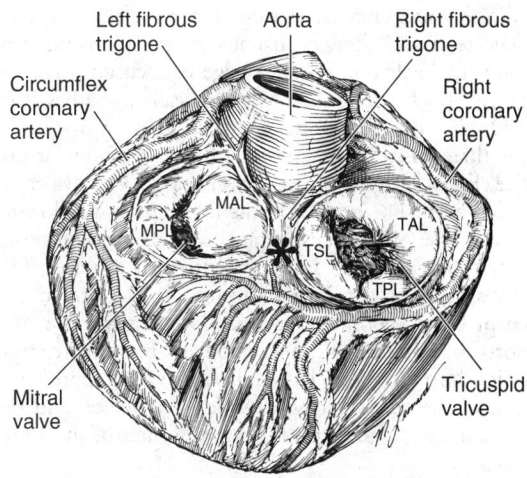

Figure 20–11. Anatomic interrelationships of the atrioventricular valves. (A, anterior leaflet; P, posterior leaflet; S, septal leaflet. The asterisk represents the area of the bundle of His.)

anterior, posterior, and septal (Figure 20–11). The anterior leaflet commonly is the largest of the three and the posterior leaflet the smallest, though many variations occur. The papillary muscles tend to be multiple but can be grouped into three components: anterior (arising from the right ventricular free wall), inferior (arising from the inferior septum), and septal (arising from the high septum in the area of the septal band). As in the mitral valve, papillary muscle groups tend to contribute chordae to multiple leaflets.

The function of the atrioventricular valves is to permit uninhibited flow of blood from the atria to the ventricles during ventricular diastole and to prevent reflux of blood into the atria during ventricular systole. The valves achieve this objective by a coordinated contraction of ventricular myocardium and the papillary muscles during the cardiac cycle. During systole, the valve is closed, and the left atrium serves as a reservoir for blood returning from the lungs. With isovolumic relaxation, left ventricular pressure falls, and when ventricular pressure becomes lower than that of the full atrium, the valve opens and initiates rapid filling of the ventricle.

The aortic valve, located between the outflow tract of the left ventricle and the ascending aorta, is usually tricuspid and is composed of a fibrous skeleton, three cusps, and the sinuses of Valsalva. The fibrous skeleton consists of three U-shaped structures that adjoin one another at the valve commissures as at the points of a crown. Beneath each commissure is the pars membranacea. The skeleton is in fibrous continuity with the anterior leaflet of the mitral valve posterolaterally and with the membranous septum anteriorly. The cusps are delicate fibrous leaflets that insert into the outline of the valve skeleton. The free edge of each cusp is concave, is thicker than the rest of the leaflet, and has at its midpoint a fibrous node. At the beginning of systole, the three cusps rapidly retract to form a triangular orifice. Eddy currents within the sinuses of Valsalva cause a slow wave-like motion of the free edge and billowing of the base of each cusp, thus preventing occlusion of the coronary ostia. During ventricular diastole, the cusps fall passively into the center of the orifice and coapt over a considerable area. The closed valve supports the ejected column of blood and prevents regurgitation into the ventricle. In a healthy valve, approximation of the cusps during diastole is complete, and the three nodes come together near the center of the aortic lumen.

The three sinuses of Valsalva are slightly dilated pockets of the aortic root between the cusps and the aortic wall. The coronary arteries arise from two of the sinuses of Valsalva. Because the aortic valve lies in an oblique plane, the origin of the left coronary artery is posterior and slightly superior to that of the right coronary artery.

A number of disease processes can affect heart valves. By far the most common include rheumatic carditis, degenerative conditions of the valve collagen, and infection. Less frequently, valves may be involved with collagen-vascular disorders, tumors, carcinoid, and Marfan's syndrome. Valvular heart disease was responsible for 89,000 hospital discharges in 1998.

MITRAL STENOSIS

The most common cause of mitral stenosis is still rheumatic fever associated with group A streptococcal pharyngitis. The early valvular lesions of rheumatic fever are characterized by an acute inflammatory infiltrate that gradually heals by organization with fibrous tissue. Chronically, the leaflets become fibrotic and thickened, so that pliability and surface area are reduced. Fusion of the anterior and posterior leaflets may be severe, and in many cases the commissures can no longer be identified. Calcification may occur in the leaflets or the fused commissures, being more common on the posteromedial aspect. The chordae are thickened, shortened, and fused by the same type of fibrosis, and occasionally the subvalvular apparatus may be calcified. The entire process transforms the mitral complex into a rigid funnel-shaped structure with a "fish mouth" opening.

The most significant effects of mitral stenosis occur on the pulmonary vasculature and right ventricle. Congestion of the pulmonary vessels is characteristic, with distention and thickening of pulmonary capillaries. In-

timal fibrosis of the pulmonary veins and arterioles also is observed, and in advanced cases medial thickening and fibrosis are common. Pulmonary hypertension progresses with time and may increase to the point of producing systemic levels of systolic blood pressure in the right ventricle and inducing functional tricuspid valve regurgitation.

Clinical Findings

A. SYMPTOMS AND SIGNS

Pulmonary venous hypertension caused by valve obstruction produces the most prominent symptom in mitral stenosis, which is dyspnea. Initially, dyspnea is observed only with effort; but with time and progressive valve obstruction dyspnea begins to occur at rest or at night and is worsened by lying flat (orthopnea). Atrial contraction augments transmitral flow significantly in mitral stenosis, so that development of atrial fibrillation increases mean left atrial pressure and reduces cardiac output by about 20%. In addition, a more rapid ventricular rate decreases diastolic filling time, further exacerbating the problem. Thus, it is common for the clinical status of a patient to deteriorate when atrial fibrillation develops. Death is due to progressive heart failure in 60–70% of patients. Systemic emboli, pulmonary emboli, and infection are the remaining causes.

On physical examination, the patient characteristically appears thin and cachectic, with a washed-out and sallow "mitral facies." Jugular venous pulsations may be prominent with fluid overload or with secondary tricuspid incompetence. If the cardiac rhythm is atrial fibrillation, irregularities in the jugular pulse and prominent v waves are observed. Peripheral edema and hepatic enlargement may be present as well as the classic "hepatojugular reflux." In the presence of pulmonary edema, respirations are rapid and shallow, the work of breathing is increased, and rales are present to varying degrees from the lung bases up the chest. A sternal heave indicates right ventricular enlargement and suggests pulmonary hypertension. In severe cases of pulmonary hypertension, the pulmonary component of the second heart sound is often palpable in the second or third left intercostal space parasternally.

Auscultation of the heart reveals accentuation of the first heart sound (S_1) in the early stages, and with development of pulmonary hypertension the pulmonary component of the second heart sound (S_2) becomes accentuated. An opening snap of the mitral valve is common and appears to be due to sudden tensing of the valve leaflets by chordae after their opening excursion. The opening snap is best heard at the apex and is associated with pliability of the valve leaflets. The mitral opening snap follows S_2 by 40–120 ms, with a shorter interval indicating severe left atrial hypertension. The diastolic murmur of mitral stenosis has a low-pitched rumbling quality, best heard at the apex with the bell of the stethoscope. Because of its low frequency, the murmur can be difficult to detect. The murmur usually commences immediately after the opening snap, and its duration is directly related to the severity of valve obstruction. In sinus rhythm, a presystolic accentuation of the murmur is characteristic, as blood flow is accelerated across the valve by atrial contraction. Presystolic accentuation is lost with development of atrial fibrillation.

B. ELECTROCARDIOGRAPHY

Ninety percent of patients in sinus rhythm exhibit a broad, notched P wave on the ECG, the so-called P mitrale. In later stages, atrial fibrillation and right ventricular hypertrophy are cardinal electrocardiographic signs.

C. IMAGING STUDIES

On x-ray, the overall cardiac silhouette may be normal, with the exception of left atrial enlargement. Pulmonary venous hypertension is accompanied by engorged, transversely oriented superior pulmonary veins. With pulmonary hypertension, the pulmonary arteries and right ventricle become enlarged, displacing the right ventricle toward the sternum on the lateral projection. Severe valvular obstruction is manifested by Kerley B lines and frank pulmonary edema.

Transthoracic echocardiography is the tool of choice in the initial evaluation, providing accurate information on valve anatomy, valve area and gradient, and pulmonary artery pressures. Ventricular function is usually normal in mitral stenosis.

Cardiac catheterization is performed in most patients but can be omitted in young patients with classic clinical and echocardiographic findings. Measurements of transvalvular gradients and calculations of valve area provide useful information about severity of the stenosis. The normal mitral orifice area is 3 cm^2/m^2 BSA, and significant mitral stenosis is suggested when the calculated area approaches 1 cm^2/m^2. Estimation of valve orifice area is subject to some error, however, particularly at low flow rates or in the presence of valvular regurgitation. Moreover, a well-diuresed patient with a contracted blood volume occasionally will exhibit a larger valve area and a lower left atrial pressure than those suggested by the clinical evaluation. Thus, it should be emphasized that catheterization findings are only supplemental, and the entire clinical picture must be considered when making therapeutic decisions.

Treatment

A. MEDICAL TREATMENT

Most would agree that asymptomatic patients should be treated medically and carefully observed. Heart rate control is helpful and anticoagulation is recommended for patients in atrial fibrillation. Survival in asymptomatic patients is > 80% at 10 years; however, once limiting symptoms occur, this number drops to 15%.

B. PERCUTANEOUS BALLOON VALVOTOMY

Symptomatic patients with moderate to severe mitral stenosis are now being considered for percutaneous valvotomy. The ideal patient has minimal valve calcification and subvalvular scarring, no valve regurgitation, and no atrial thrombus. Successful procedures commonly double the valve area. Mitral regurgitation and persistent atrial septal defect occur in 2–10%. Restenosis-free survival at 10 years is approximately 56%. However, surgical commissurotomy can achieve a larger mitral valve area, better functional recovery, and a lower incidence of late mitral regurgitation.

C. SURGICAL TREATMENT

The indications for operative treatment in mitral stenosis are similar to those for the percutaneous balloon approach. All symptomatic patients (NYHA class II or higher) should be considered for operation. Patients with significant pulmonary hypertension, episodic pulmonary edema, new-onset atrial fibrillation, or episodes of thromboembolism are operative candidates as well. Surgical procedures include open commissurotomy and valve replacement. Approximately 50% of stenotic mitral valves treated operatively can be managed with open commissurotomy. Absence of significant leaflet calcification—together with good leaflet mobility and surface area—increases the likelihood of successful repair. Complete incision of fused commissures is performed. The submitral apparatus is inspected, and fused or thickened chordae are resected. The papillary muscle heads can be split to further improve submitral outflow. If significant leaflet calcification or fibrous retraction is evident, a standard prosthetic mitral valve replacement is performed. Whenever possible, the subvalvular attachments to the mitral annulus are preserved to maintain ventricular geometry over time.

Prognosis

The operative mortality rate for isolated primary mitral valve procedures ranges from 1% to 5% depending on the severity of preoperative symptoms, the presence (or not) of severe pulmonary hypertension or right ventricular failure, and the need for mitral valve replacement. Contemporary operations significantly increase long-term survival and patient well-being. After open mitral commissurotomy or valve replacement, most patients experience improvement in symptoms, though repeat operations are necessary at a rate of 2–4% per year after valve repair. The probabilities of systemic embolization and infective endocarditis are lessened significantly by surgical therapy, and patients experiencing atrial fibrillation for less than 1 year have an excellent chance of reverting to sinus rhythm with pharmacologic therapy or cardioversion (or both).

MITRAL REGURGITATION

Competence of the mitral valve depends on an integrated function of the mitral annulus, the valve leaflets, the chordae tendineae, the papillary muscles, and the ventricular wall. Incompetence can be caused by abnormalities of any of these structures.

Rheumatic heart disease accounts for 35–45% of cases of mitral regurgitation. Involvement of the leaflets by the rheumatic process causes shortening, rigidity, and retraction of the cusps. The chordae tendineae also become fibrotic, fused, and shortened.

Idiopathic calcification of the mitral valve and annulus in the elderly can be an important cause of regurgitation and is associated with systemic hypertension, aortic stenosis, diabetes, and chronic renal failure. Calcification may involve the entire annulus and project into adjacent ventricular myocardium. Masses of calcium may protrude into the subvalvular region, immobilizing the valve or preventing leaflet coaptation, and calcium can invade the conduction system or adjacent coronary arteries.

Mitral valve prolapse is present in 3–4% of the general population and can be associated with a midsystolic click and late systolic murmur. Progressive and clinically significant mitral regurgitation develops in approximately 5% of these cases. The primary pathologic process is myxomatous degeneration of the fibrous layer of the valve leaflets and chordae tendineae, producing thinning, elongation, and redundancy. In many patients, rupture of weakened chordae can cause acute mitral regurgitation whose severity depends on the size of chordal rupture and the degree of regurgitation produced. In extreme cases, severe congestive heart failure and acute pulmonary edema may necessitate emergency treatment.

Infective endocarditis is the cause of mitral regurgitation in 5% of cases, and the mitral valve is the most common valve to become infected. Leaflet destruction or chordal rupture can result in sudden, severe incompetence.

The final category of mitral incompetence is **ischemic mitral regurgitation,** defined as moderate to severe valve incompetence precipitated by acute myocardial infarction with no primary leaflet or chordal pathology. This disorder is observed to a significant degree in 3% of patients with coronary artery disease undergoing catheterization and is quite heterogeneous from both the pathophysiologic and the clinical viewpoints. Pathologically, the majority of patients exhibit posterior papillary and annular dysfunction in which regurgitation and congestive heart failure are coincident with the onset of a large posterior wall infarction. Combinations of posterior annular dilation, papillary muscle elongation, loss of papillary muscle shortening, and preexisting congenital leaflet defects produce valve incompetence at the posterior commissural region.

Postinfarction **papillary muscle rupture** occurs more rarely and is observed in only 0.1% of coronary disease patients undergoing catheterization. Congestive heart failure associated with a new murmur usually develops several days after infarction, and the majority have severe regurgitation requiring acute intervention. The infarction usually is posterior and often is small and localized; global ejection fraction is frequently maintained.

Physiologic derangements caused by mitral regurgitation are similar to those associated with mitral stenosis. Left atrial hypertension is transmitted to the pulmonary vasculature, causing dyspnea and pulmonary edema. Pulmonary arterial hypertension, right ventricular failure, and functional tricuspid regurgitation occur by similar mechanisms. However, unlike mitral stenosis, the left ventricle is subjected to a chronic volume overload that ultimately causes myocardial failure.

Clinical Findings

A. SYMPTOMS AND SIGNS

Symptoms produced by mitral regurgitation are related to the level of pulmonary venous hypertension. Exertional dyspnea and orthopnea are common, and chronically reduced cardiac output produces easy fatigability and cardiac cachexia. Moderate to severe regurgitation can be tolerated for many years with relatively minor symptoms until irreversible left ventricular dysfunction develops. Therefore, the severity of symptoms cannot be used as the only criterion for intervention. Hemoptysis is rarely reported, and symptoms occasionally appear with the onset of atrial fibrillation, which complicates 75% of severe cases. Systemic emboli can occur in patients with atrial fibrillation but are not as common as in mitral stenosis. Infective endocarditis should be suspected if there are symptoms of malaise, fever, chills, or a new or worsening murmur or when acute decompensation occurs in a previously stable patient. Angina secondary to mitral regurgitation is rare and should suggest coexisting coronary artery disease. Patients with ischemic mitral regurgitation usually manifest either acute or chronic myocardial ischemic syndromes.

The physical signs of congestive heart failure are similar to those of mitral stenosis. The apical impulse is displaced to the left in proportion to the degree of left ventricular enlargement, and an apical systolic thrill can be palpated. With significant right ventricular enlargement, a sternal heave is evident. On auscultation, the heart sounds usually are normal with the exception of a third heart sound with congestive heart failure or an increased S_2 with pulmonary hypertension. The hallmark of mitral regurgitation is an apical high-pitched, holosystolic murmur that radiates to the axilla and back. On occasion, the murmur will radiate to the base and have a musical quality.

B. Electrocardiography

The ECG may show left ventricular hypertrophy from the chronic volume overload or biventricular hypertrophy with concomitant pulmonary arterial hypertension. In sinus rhythm, P mitrale may be present.

C. Imaging Studies

The chest radiograph illustrates left atrial enlargement in chronic cases, but because of the volume overload the left ventricle also is dilated. Right ventricular enlargement, pulmonary vascular engorgement, and Kerley B lines are common. Transesophageal echocardiography is especially helpful in the evaluation of mitral regurgitation. The site of abnormal mitral valve anatomy can usually be clearly defined along with the degree and location of mitral regurgitation jet (Figure 20–12). Increasing left ventricular end-systolic dimension can be an early sign of impending heart failure even in the absence of symptoms. Cardiac catheterization documents prominent left atrial v waves, elevated left ventricular end-diastolic pressure and increased end-diastolic volume. Pulmonary hypertension in mi-

Figure 20–12. Transesophageal echocardiogram showing "central jet" of severe ischemic mitral regurgitation.

tral incompetence has the same implications as in mitral stenosis. A reduction in cardiac index below 2 L/min/m^2 and a widened arteriovenous oxygen difference indicate severe hemodynamic impairment. Regurgitation is graded on the basis of the contrast left ventriculogram as 1–4+.

Treatment

A. Medical Therapy

The typical patient with chronic mitral regurgitation compensates by augmenting preload and reducing afterload (the left ventricle is unloaded by ejecting into the low-pressure left atrium). It is not surprising that patients can be asymptomatic for many years, but the chronic volume overload can result in significant left ventricular dysfunction. The mainstay of medical therapy is preload reduction (diuretics) and afterload reduction (ACE inhibitors). The latter can reduce the regurgitant volume and increase forward output. There are no data to suggest that this approach will benefit the asymptomatic or normotensive patient.

B. Selection of Patients for Operation

The natural history of mitral regurgitation is more variable than that of mitral stenosis because of the greater number of etiologic factors. The clinical course can range from asymptomatic, with moderate mitral regurgitation remaining stable for many years, to a fulminant progression of overwhelming congestive heart failure. There are three determinants of clinical severity: (1) the degree of regurgitation, (2) the status of left ventricular function, and (3) the cause of the valve disease.

Most patients referred for surgery are symptomatic (NYHA class II or greater). Asymptomatic patients should be referred if left ventricular dysfunction is present (ejection fraction < 60%, end-systolic dimension > 45 mm) or if significant pulmonary hypertension or new atrial fibrillation occurs. Exercise echocardiography may be useful in the equivocal patient. Significant left ventricular dysfunction (ejection fraction < 45%) have a higher operative mortality and worse long-term survival.

C. Surgical Treatment

Mitral valve incompetence can be managed by mitral valve repair or replacement. Virtually all myxomatous valves with prolapse can be repaired. Fifty percent have isolated posterior leaflet prolapse or chordal rupture, and posterior leaflet reconstruction along with Carpentier ring annuloplasty (Figure 20–13) is highly effective. Anterior leaflet reconstruction is more difficult and may require chordal transfer (from the posterior leaflet), chordal shortening, or artificial chord insertion to restore competence. In cases of ischemic mitral

Figure 20–13. Panels **A–E** represent atrial views of posterior leaflet reconstruction for isolated posterior leaflet prolapse and insertion of Carpentier annuloplasty ring.

regurgitation, ring mitral annuloplasty (Figure 20–14) combined with complete coronary revascularization is the procedure of choice. In cases of rheumatic leaflet retraction, valve calcification, or severe endocarditis, prosthetic valve replacement with preservation of the subvalvular apparatus is more appropriate.

Prognosis

Operative mortality rates for elective mitral valve procedures performed under elective conditions approximate 2–5%, and the quality and duration of life are improved. Typical 5- and 10-year survival is 80% and 65%, respectively, and is adversely affected by age and preoperative left ventricular dysfunction (Figure 20–15). Late survival after mitral valve replacement is not as good as after reparative procedures (Figure 20–16).

TRICUSPID VALVE DISEASE

Pathologic disorders of the tricuspid valve can be either functional or organic. Tricuspid regurgitation is usually functional and is secondary to right ventricular dilation

Figure 20–14. Operative photograph of semiflexible mitral ring annuloplasty for ischemic mitral regurgitation. The ring plicates the posterior annulus to restore leaflet coaptation.

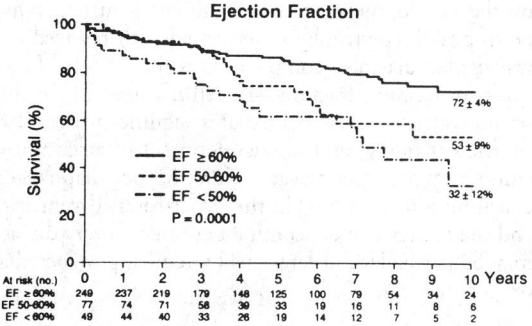

Figure 20–15. Effect of preoperative ventricular function on long-term survival after surgery for mitral regurgitation. (Reproduced with permission, from Enriquez-Sarano M et al: Echocardiographic prediction of survival after surgical correction of organic mitral regurgitation. Circulation 1994;90:830.)

and enlargement of the free-wall tricuspid annulus. The annulus in the area of the septal leaflet is spared, and the valve leaflets and chordae generally are normal. Causes of functional tricuspid regurgitation include mitral valve disease, cor pulmonale, primary pulmonary hypertension, right ventricular infarction, and congenital heart disease. In most cases, valve incompetence reflects the presence of—and in turn further aggravates—severe right ventricular failure. The main cause of organic tricuspid regurgitation is infective endocarditis.

Tricuspid stenosis is almost always rheumatic, usually accompanies mitral valve involvement, and is clinically significant in about 5% of patients with rheumatic heart disease. Pathologic changes resemble those in the mitral valve, with thickening and fusion of the leaflets

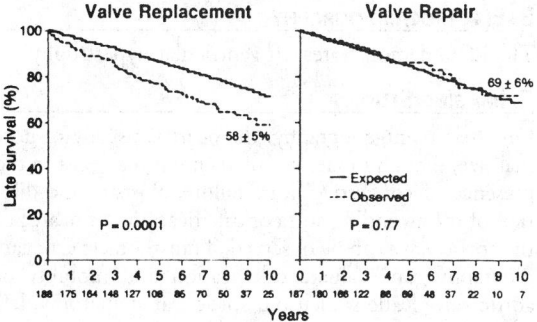

Figure 20–16. Effect of mitral valve replacement versus repair on long-term survival. (Reproduced, with permission, from Enriquez-Sarano M et al: Valve repair improves the outcome of surgery for mitral regurgitation. A multivariate analysis. Circulation 1995;91:1022.)

and chordae, producing a stenotic, fixed tricuspid orifice. Carcinoid involvement of the tricuspid valve is characterized by deposition of fibrous carcinoid plaques on the leaflets and ventricular attachments. Rarely, tumors of the right atrium (atrial myxoma) cause secondary obstruction of the tricuspid orifice. Both tricuspid stenosis and tricuspid regurgitation produce right atrial hypertension, systemic venous engorgement, and hepatic congestion. Severe fluid retention, edema, and debility are characteristic. The process can progress to hepatic failure, cardiac cirrhosis, anasarca, and renal failure.

Clinical Findings

A. SYMPTOMS AND SIGNS

Symptoms in either tricuspid stenosis or regurgitation are related to the degree of systemic venous hypertension. Fatigue and weakness are common, usually without dyspnea or other signs of pulmonary congestion. Isolated tricuspid regurgitation is well tolerated in patients with normal pulmonary artery pressure; but when combined with mitral valve disease, pulmonary hypertension, and right ventricular failure, the clinical status deteriorates rapidly.

Tricuspid valve disease is easily overlooked unless the observer is alert to that diagnostic possibility. In sinus rhythm, contraction of the right atrium against a stenotic valve produces a prominent a wave in the jugular venous pulse; with regurgitant lesions, the jugular v wave is accentuated. The liver is often enlarged and may be pulsatile, but in congestive cirrhosis the liver may be firm and fibrotic. While ascites and edema are common, the lung fields are clear despite engorged neck veins and other signs of congestive heart failure. A tricuspid opening snap may be present. Murmurs with tricuspid valve disease are similar to those observed in mitral disorders, and the two may be difficult to distinguish. Tricuspid murmurs usually are located more toward the left lower sternal border, and both the stenotic and the regurgitant varieties are augmented by inspiration. Both murmurs may be difficult to hear even when the physiologic defects are severe.

B. ELECTROCARDIOGRAPHY

In sinus rhythm, tricuspid valve disease is suggested if the lead II P wave amplitude exceeds 0.25 mV.

C. IMAGING STUDIES

The key radiographic finding is cardiomegaly, with prominence of the right atrial shadow. Echocardiography yields important information on the leaflet anatomy, the location and severity of regurgitation, and right ventricular function. At catheterization, tricuspid stenosis is confirmed by demonstrating a diastolic pressure gradient between the right atrium and right ventricle, utilizing simultaneous pressure measurements. A mean diastolic gradient of 5 mm Hg is significant in tricuspid stenosis, and values as low as 3 mm Hg may produce symptoms; the resting cardiac output is reduced. In tricuspid regurgitation, right atrial pressure is characterized by a prominent v wave, which in severe cases is described as "ventricularization" of atrial pressure. Occasionally, the atrial v wave may be normal despite severe regurgitation because of an enlarged, highly compliant venous system. Pulmonary arterial hypertension favors a functional cause in tricuspid regurgitation, whereas normal pulmonary pressures suggest organic disease.

Treatment

Rheumatic tricuspid stenosis is treated by commissurotomy or valve replacement depending on leaflet mobility, involvement of subvalvular structures, and the presence of regurgitation. Because residual gradients are tolerated poorly, valve replacement should be considered in significantly diseased valves. Because of the high thromboembolic potential of mechanical valves in the low-pressure right atrium, bioprosthetic valves or mitral allografts are preferred for tricuspid valve replacement. Symptomatic cases of carcinoid valve disease require excision of the entire tricuspid apparatus and valve replacement.

Tricuspid endocarditis is a particularly difficult problem. Many patients have septic pulmonary emboli, complicating postoperative recovery. For infections that cannot be eradicated with antibiotics, total excision of the valve has been recommended. Whenever feasible, reparative techniques or tricuspid replacement with a mitral allograft (which is very resistant to reinfection) should be considered.

Moderate to severe functional tricuspid regurgitation secondary to mitral valve disease usually is best managed by correction of the mitral valve disorder followed by tricuspid ring annuloplasty.

AORTIC STENOSIS

Aortic stenosis causes obstruction to left ventricular outflow and can be subvalvular, valvular, or supravalvular. Aortic stenosis in the adult may be due to a congenitally unicuspid or bicuspid valve, congenital subvalvular or supravalvular stenosis, rheumatic heart disease, or, most frequently, degenerative fibrosis and calcification. The cause can often be surmised from the age of the patient—congenital lesions accounting for most cases in patients under 30 years of age, rheumatic heart disease or congenital bicuspid valves in patients aged 30–65 years, and degenerative calcific stenosis in patients over 65 years of age.

Resistance to left ventricular outflow produces a pressure overload on the left ventricle that compensates by the development of concentric left ventricular hypertrophy. Hypertrophy is associated with reduced left ventricular diastolic compliance, while systolic function—or ejection fraction—is well maintained. In this setting, atrial systole contributes significantly to left ventricular filling, and the development of atrial fibrillation may precipitate heart failure. Myocardial oxygen consumption is elevated in the hypertrophied ventricle, and the presence of concomitant coronary artery disease may be particularly deleterious by reducing myocardial oxygen delivery.

Clinical Findings

A. Symptoms and Signs

Most patients remain asymptomatic for many years. The classic triad of symptoms includes angina pectoris, syncope, and congestive heart failure and usually denotes an aortic valve gradient greater than 50 mm Hg or a valve area of less than 1 cm^2. Angina pectoris is due to the imbalance between myocardial oxygen demand and delivery caused by increased myocardial oxygen consumption, and in the 25–50% of patients with coronary artery disease it is aggravated by the superimposed reduced oxygen delivery. Syncope is typically exertional and most likely related to inability of the left ventricle to increase cardiac output in the face of a fixed, high-grade obstruction. Congestive heart failure usually occurs late and is an especially ominous sign.

The pulse pressure is often narrowed, with a decreased systolic arterial pressure (parvus et tardus). A harsh midsystolic murmur is heard best at the second intercostal space and along the left sternal border. The murmur may radiate to the carotid arteries, is generally audible at the apex, and typically does not radiate into the axilla. Approximately 25–50% of patients will also have a murmur of aortic regurgitation.

B. Electrocardiography

The ECG demonstrates left ventricular hypertrophy.

C. Imaging Studies

On chest roentgenography, the heart is usually of normal size, though moderate enlargement may exist in the presence of congestive heart failure. Poststenotic dilation of the ascending aorta or calcification in the area of the aortic valve can be observed. Transthoracic echocardiography can evaluate calcification and mobility of aortic valve leaflets, bicuspid aortic leaflet anatomy, left ventricular hypertrophy, left ventricular ejection fraction, transvalvular gradients, and the presence of aortic regurgitation. Cardiac catheterization yields important information on coronary anatomy, cardiac output, transvalvular pressure gradients, overall left ventricular function, and the presence of coexisting valvular lesions. It must be emphasized that because of the compensatory pathologic alterations in preload, left ventricular compliance, and contractility, the measured ejection fraction may underestimate overall myocardial function. Mild aortic stenosis is defined as an aortic valve area of > 1.5 cm^2, moderate as aortic valve area 1–1.5 cm^2, and severe as aortic valve area ≤ 1 cm^2.

Treatment

Symptoms of angina pectoris, congestive heart failure, or syncope in a patient with aortic stenosis are associated with an average life expectancy of 1–3 years if left untreated and constitute the classic indication for aortic valve replacement. In addition, asymptomatic or minimally symptomatic patients in whom the aortic valve gradient is greater than 50 mm Hg or the aortic valve area is less than 1.0 cm^2 are also candidates for valve replacement, especially in the presence of left ventricular dysfunction or coexisting coronary artery disease. Percutaneous balloon valvotomy has a limited role in the treatment of aortic stenosis due to the high rate of restenosis within 6 months. However, patients presenting with severe heart failure may benefit from this approach as a "bridge" procedure for subsequent valve replacement. Every effort should be made to qualify patients for surgery, which offers long-term survival and a better quality of life.

Prognosis

Aortic valve replacement for elective isolated aortic stenosis is associated with a less than 5% operative mortality rate in all categories of patients. Advanced age, left ventricular dysfunction, and acute presentation increase the surgical risk. Regression of ventricular hypertrophy does occur and may continue for 10 years. Long-term survival approximates 85–90% at 5 years, and the outlook is adversely affected by preoperative left ventricular dysfunction, advanced age, and ventricular arrhythmias. Half of all late deaths are from noncardiac causes.

AORTIC INSUFFICIENCY

Aortic insufficiency is caused by abnormal coaptation of the aortic valve leaflets, allowing blood to return to the ventricle from the aorta during diastole. A common cause is rheumatic valvulitis, but varying degrees of annular dilation or annuloaortic ectasia also occur. Cystic medial necrosis, atherosclerosis, syphilitic degeneration, arthritic inflammatory diseases, and congenitally bicuspid valves are among some of the numerous causes of chronic insufficiency, while endocarditis, acute aortic dissection, and trauma account for the majority of cases of acute valve regurgitation.

Clinical Findings

A. SYMPTOMS AND SIGNS

Acute aortic regurgitation is poorly tolerated, and patients commonly present with severe pulmonary edema and failure. Signs of infective endocarditis or trauma may be present. Paradoxically, a diastolic murmur may be absent, indicating complete valve incompetence.

Patients with chronic aortic regurgitation may be asymptomatic for many years but have a reduced life expectancy once symptoms of orthopnea, paroxysmal dyspnea, and congestive failure appear. On physical examination, the pulse pressure is widened and the diastolic pressure is low (Corrigan's pulse). The apical impulse is sustained and laterally and inferiorly displaced. Characteristically, a blowing high-pitched diastolic murmur is heard best along the left lower sternal border with the patient in full expiration. A third heart sound and a diastolic rumble (Austin Flint murmur) may be audible.

B. ELECTROCARDIOGRAPHY

The ECG usually shows left ventricular hypertrophy with left axis deviation.

C. IMAGING STUDIES

Chest roentgenography usually demonstrates normal cardiac size in the acute case. In chronic regurgitation, left ventricular enlargement and pulmonary congestion are typical. Echocardiography permits estimation of left ventricular function and chamber size and the degree of regurgitation. At cardiac catheterization, supravalvular aortography is performed to define the degree of aortic insufficiency. Catheterization also identifies the coronary anatomy along with any associated abnormalities of the aortic root and annulus.

Treatment

For medically treated patients, the 5- and 10-year mortality rates in severe aortic regurgitation are 25% and 50%, respectively. Although vasodilator therapy may be useful in asymptomatic patients, this approach will not reduce the need for subsequent surgery. Aortic valve replacement is the standard operation and should be performed prior to the onset of irreversible left ventricular dilation, which not infrequently occurs prior to the onset of symptoms. The most accurate guide currently available for assessing progression toward irreversibility appears to be echocardiographic measurement of left ventricular dimensions, and significant ventricular dilation (left ventricular end-diastolic dimension > 70 mm or end-systolic dimension > 50 mm) should be used as a guide to recommending valve replacement or repair.

In selected cases of aortic regurgitation due to simple annular dilation, valve repair with subcommissural annuloplasty has been effective.

The prognosis after surgery for severe aortic regurgitation and normal ventricular function is good, with 85% of patients surviving 5 years. Abnormal preoperative ventricular function adversely affects long-term survival.

■ PROSTHETIC VALVE SELECTION

BIOLOGIC VERSUS MECHANICAL VALVES

Biologic Valves

At the present time, three types of biologic valves are used for replacement of diseased heart valves. The stented porcine bioprosthesis has been used for 25 years. Because of its low incidence of thromboembolic events, postoperative anticoagulation is not necessary for this valve, thereby reducing long-term patient morbidity. However, stented porcine valves are prone to structural failure (from leaflet calcification or leaflet-stent dehiscence), and the incidence of reoperation for this problem is approximately 40% at 10 years. Recently, introduction of the stented pericardial valve (Figure 20–17) has reduced the severity of this problem, and 80% of patients are free from structural failure at 10 years. The is no difference in prosthetic valve endocarditis occurring in porcine, pericardial or mechanical valves (about 2–10% at 10 years), and death rates from this serious complication are similar.

The stentless porcine valve (Figure 20–18) has now been approved for aortic valve replacement. This is a scalloped cylinder of porcine aortic root containing the

Figure 20–18. St. Jude Medical stentless porcine aortic valve.

native valve, with an external Dacron covering. Although somewhat more difficult to implant, this valve has a low transvalvular gradient, and faster regression of ventricular hypertrophy has been observed. Long-term durability will probably be greater than the stented valve, though calcification still remains a problem.

Human allografts have been used for aortic valve replacement for some time, and mitral allografts (Figure 20–19) have been recently introduced. Aortic allografts are virtually free from thromboembolic problems and endocarditis, and the rate of reoperation for structural failure at 10 years is low (8%). Only a handful of centers are implanting the mitral allograft, but the early results are encouraging.

Pulmonary autograft replacement of the aortic valve (Ross procedure) is another biologic option, and the outcomes are similar to those achieved with aortic allografts.

Mechanical Valves

The most commonly used mechanical valves today include the tilting disk (Medtronic-Hall) and bileaflet (St. Jude) types (Figures 20–20 and 20–21). Both mechanical prostheses offer better predictability of performance and durability than tissue valves and are easier to implant than allografts, stentless valves, or autografts. However, all patients require warfarin therapy, and valve thrombosis or thromboembolism can occur despite adequate anticoagulation. Thromboembolic rates for most mechani-

Figure 20–17. Carpentier-Edwards stented pericardial valve.

Figure 20–19. Operative photograph of mitral valve allograft.

Figure 20–21. St. Jude Medical bileaflet mechanical valve.

cal valves with adequate anticoagulation approximate 2–5% per patient year, though thromboembolism is less common with the St. Jude valve. The incidence of minor bleeding episodes is about 2–4% per year, and the incidence of major bleeding is 1–2% per year, with a mortality of 0.5% per year or less. For most mechanical valves, it is recommended that warfarin be given in doses sufficient to achieve an INR of 2.5–3.5. For isolated aortic valve replacement, the INR target can be reduced to 2.0–3.0 if low-dose aspirin is added (81 mg/d).

Acute thrombosis of mechanical valves can occur if anticoagulation is not monitored carefully, Fortunately, this occurs in less than 2% of patients over 10 years. Structural failures in the currently used valves are rare. For small annuli, (< 21 mm), the St. Jude valve offers the lowest transvalvular gradient and the largest effective orifice.

SPECIFIC INDICATIONS FOR VALVE PLACEMENT

Patient age, expected longevity, and ability to take warfarin are the major determinants of prosthetic valve recommendations. For example, young women desiring children may choose a biologic valve to reduce anticoagulation complications during pregnancy—with the understanding that the prosthesis may eventually require replacement. Young patients or those with chronic renal failure are poor candidates for porcine valves because of the accelerated calcification of these prostheses. Patients with specific contraindications to anticoagulation also are candidates for biologic valves. Many of these patients are elderly and not expected to outlive their prosthetic valves. Patients undergoing complicated valve procedures such as aortic and mitral valve replacement or valve replacement–coronary bypass combinations should receive mechanical valves because of the higher mortality rate associated with reoperation in these groups. Severe infections

Figure 20–20. Medtronic-Hall tilting disk mechanical valve.

involving the aortic root are best treated with allograft valves. Tricuspid valve replacement is performed exclusively with porcine valves because of a high incidence of mechanical valve thrombosis even with adequate anticoagulation. With the expanding application of the Maze procedure for correction of atrial fibrillation, younger patients are now being considered for biologic (allograft) valve replacement to avoid long-term anticoagulation.

■ INFECTIVE ENDOCARDITIS

Endocarditis is infection—usually bacterial—of any part of the cardiac endothelium. The valves are most frequently involved, and the resulting vegetations can cause leaflet destruction or may embolize. Abscess formation can result in heart block or persistent sepsis. Individuals with subacute endocarditis tend to have symptoms for months, and such infections are usually caused by hemolytic streptococci. Acute endocarditis, typically cause by *Staphylococcus aureus,* has a more fulminant course over days to weeks. Patients at risk for endocarditis include those with congenital or preexisting valvular defects, indwelling cardiac catheters, or prosthetic heart valves. Intravenous drug users and patients with prosthetic heart valves have the highest incidence of gram-negative and fungal infections. Infective endocarditis is now the fourth leading cause of life-threatening infection in the United States.

Clinical Findings

A. Symptoms and Signs

Classically, patients present with fever, bacteremia, peripheral emboli, and immunologic vascular phenomena. The latter include glomerulonephritis, Osler's nodes (painful, erythematous nodules usually in the pulp of the fingers), and Roth spots (retinal hemorrhages). Subungual splinter hemorrhages are a sign of peripheral emboli. Less commonly, flat, painless red spots occur on the palms and soles (Janeway lesions). Acute valvular regurgitation and heart failure may dominate the presentation.

B. Laboratory Findings

At least three sets of blood cultures spaced 1 hour apart must be positive. Culture-negative endocarditis occurs in less than 5% of cases and is usually due to prior antibiotic therapy, fastidious organisms, or fungi.

C. Electrocardiography

Electrocardiographic findings are not specific. In cases of annular abscess, prolongation of the PR interval may be seen and is an ominous finding.

D. Imaging Studies

The chest x-ray may show signs of heart failure (interstitial pulmonary edema, cardiomegaly). Parenchymal nodules (septic emboli) may be seen in right-sided heart involvement. Echocardiography should be performed in all cases to document the location and degree of valvular involvement, vegetation size, and the presence of annular abscess. Vegetations larger than 1 cm in diameter, especially if located on the mitral valve, are at higher risk for embolization. Cardiac catheterization may be contraindicated in the presence of aortic valve vegetations or abscess of the valve annulus.

Treatment

The mortality of untreated patients with infective endocarditis is virtually 100%. Appropriate parenteral antibiotic therapy for 4–6 weeks has reduced the mortality to 30–50%. Approximately 20–25% of patients will require surgery, further reducing the overall mortality to 10%. Surgery is indicated for the following situations: severe valvular regurgitation with heart failure, abscess of the valve annulus, persistent bacteremia after 7–10 days of adequate antibiotic therapy, fungal or gram-negative infections, recurrent emboli, or mobile vegetations > 1 cm. Acute, severe aortic regurgitation from endocarditis is poorly tolerated because of pulmonary edema and low coronary perfusion pressure. Surgery should be performed promptly. Because of their high resistance to infection, allograft valves are preferred for appropriate patients requiring valve replacement. Mitral valve repair, including debridement of vegetation and pericardial patch reconstruction, is possible in a small number of patients. Success in intravenous drug users is particularly frustrating, since many succumb to prosthetic valve infection or drug overdose.

Acar C et al: Homograft replacement of the mitral valve. Graft selection, technique of implantation, and results in forty-three patients. J Thorac Cardiovasc Surg 1996;111:367.

Bayer AS et al: Diagnosis and management of infective endocarditis and its complications. Circulation 1998;98:2936.

Bonow RO et al: Guidelines for the management of patients with valvular heart disease: executive summary. A report of the American College of Cardiology/American Heart Association Task Force on Practice Guidelines (Committee on Management of Patients with Valvular Heart Disease). Circulation 1998;98:1949.

Carpentier A: Cardiac valve surgery: the French correction. J Thorac Cardiovasc Surg 1983;86:323.

Doty JR et al: Aortic valve replacement with cryopreserved aortic allograft: ten-year experience. J Thorac Cardiovasc Surg 1998;115:371.

Dujardin KS et al: Mortality and morbidity of aortic regurgitation in clinical practice. A long-term follow-up study. Circulation 1999;99:1851.

Elkins RC: The Ross operation: a 12-year experience. Ann Thorac Surg 1999;68(3 Suppl):S14.

Enriquez-Sarano MA et al: Progression of mitral regurgitation: a prospective Doppler echocardiographic study. J Am Coll Cardiol 1999;34:1137.

Enriquez-Sarano M et al: Echocardiographic prediction of survival after surgical correction of organic mitral regurgitation. Circulation 1994;90:830.

Enriquez-Sarano M et al: Valve repair improves the outcome of surgery for mitral regurgitation. A multivariate analysis. Circulation 1995;91:1022.

Ferguson E et al: The surgical management of bacterial valvular endocarditis. Curr Opin Cardiol 2000;15:82.

Grigioni F et al: Ischemic mitral regurgitation: long-term outcome and prognostic implications with quantitative Doppler assessment. Circulation 2001;103:1759.

Kassai B et al: Comparison of bioprosthesis and mechanical valves, a meta-analysis of randomised clinical trials. Cardiovasc Surg 2000;8:477.

Khan JH et al: Cardiac valve surgery in octogenarians: improving quality of life and functional status. Arch Surg 1998;133:887.

Khan JH et al: Maze procedure and homograft replacement of a rheumatic mitral valve. J Heart Valve Dis 1999;8:630.

Knott-Craig CJ et al: Aortic valve replacement: comparison of late survival between autografts and homografts. Ann Thorac Surg 2000;69:1327.

Lambert AS et al: Improved evaluation of the location and mechanism of mitral valve regurgitation with a systematic transesophageal echocardiography examination. Anesth Analg 1999;88:1205.

Ling KH, Enriquez-Sarano M: Long-term outcomes of patients with flail mitral valve leaflets. Coron Artery Dis 2000;11:3.

Maselli D et al: Left ventricular mass reduction after aortic valve replacement: homografts, stentless and stented valves. Ann Thorac Surg 1999;67:966.

Moon MR et al: Treatment of endocarditis with valve replacement: the question of tissue versus mechanical prosthesis. Ann Thorac Surg 2001;71:1164.

Senthilnathan V et al: Heart valves: which is the best choice? Cardiovasc Surg 1999;7:393.

Smedira NG et al: Balloon aortic valvuloplasty as a bridge to aortic valve replacement in critically ill patients. Ann Thorac Surg 1993; 55:914.

Westaby S et al: Stentless aortic bioprostheses: compelling data from the Second International Symposium. Ann Thorac Surg 1998;65:235.

■ THORACIC AORTIC DISEASE

THORACIC AORTIC ANEURYSMS

The most common cause of thoracic aneurysms is arteriosclerosis, which causes a degenerative process in the aortic wall. Atherosclerotic aneurysms can be saccular or fusiform and occur in the ascending or descending thoracic aorta or in the arch. Another common pathophysiologic process is medial degeneration of the aortic wall, characterized by replacement of muscle cells and elastic lamina with mucoid-filled cystic spaces. In Marfan's syndrome, a defect in the fibrillin-1 gene is responsible for abnormal myofibril composition of elastic tissue. The disorder is inherited as an autosomal dominant and has many manifestations. Annuloaortic ectasia can occur in this setting and consists of enlargement of the entire aortic root, including the sinuses of Valsalva. Trauma and infection account for the remaining cases of thoracic aneurysms.

Clinical Findings

A. SYMPTOMS AND SIGNS

Thoracic aneurysms are more common in men, and a history of hypertension is usual. Symptoms, if present, are due to local pressure or obstruction of adjacent thoracic structures. In the ascending aorta, signs may include aortic regurgitation, superior vena cava obstruction, or chest pain with aneurysm expansion. In the arch of the aorta, tracheal compression may occur, while aneurysms of the descending aorta—the most common type—may be associated with recurrent laryngeal nerve compression, phrenic paralysis, dysphagia due to esophageal compression, or stridor due to tracheal compression.

B. IMAGING STUDIES

The chest radiograph may show convexity of the right cardiac border in ascending aneurysms, a prominent aortic knob in transverse aneurysms, and posterior lateral thoracic masses in descending aneurysms. Ultrafast CT scans and MR angiography are now the imaging methods of choice, defining the anatomy and extent of the aneurysm in the majority of cases. Occasionally, aortography may be useful. Because many patients have generalized atherosclerosis, screening for significant coronary artery disease is essential. This is most commonly done with thallium imaging.

Treatment

Symptoms and size are the primary determinants of intervention for thoracic aortic aneurysms. For the asymptomatic patient with an aneurysm ≤ 5.5 cm, aggressive control of blood pressure with drugs (including beta-blockers) is warranted. Any aneurysm > 5.5 cm in diameter should be considered for surgical repair, particularly if symptoms are present. Patients with Marfan's syndrome and a positive family history for rupture or dissection are at higher risk for rupture, and intervention is recommended at 5 cm. Other factors predictive of increased rupture rate include advancing age, COPD, and a growth rate > 0.1 cm per year. Dacron graft replacement is the standard operative procedure and is conducted in different ways depending on the location of the aneurysm.

A. ASCENDING AORTA AND AORTIC ARCH ANEURYSM

Ascending and arch aneurysms require cardiopulmonary bypass for graft replacement, most commonly via right atrial and femoral artery cannulation. The heart is protected during aortic cross-clamping with cold potassium cardioplegia. For aneurysms that extend proximally into the sinuses of Valsalva (annuloaortic ectasia), a composite prosthetic valve–ascending aortic graft conduit is utilized, with reimplantation of the coronary arteries into the graft (as in patients with Marfan's syndrome). More recently, preservation of the aortic valve repair and reconstruction of the aortic root with a Dacron graft (David procedure) has shown promise. For isolated ascending aortic aneurysms, Dacron graft replacement is utilized—again under cardiopulmonary bypass and cardioplegic arrest.

Replacement of a transverse arch aortic aneurysm is made more complex by the need to provide cerebral protection while aortic arch blood flow is interrupted. This may be accomplished by one of several methods. Either standard cardiopulmonary bypass with individual cannulation of arch vessels can be performed, or profound hypothermia can be induced with a period of total circulatory arrest for arch replacement. The latter approach is used most commonly. Core temperatures of 15 °C are required for safe circulatory arrest. Retrograde perfusion via the superior vena cava may be a beneficial adjunct. The brachiocephalic vessels are excised from the native aorta and anastomosed to the Dacron graft as a single button. Great care is taken to remove all air from the grafts before cerebral reperfusion is instituted.

The operative mortality rate for ascending aortic or arch reconstructions has been reduced to about 10% because of advances in myocardial and cerebral protection.

B. DESCENDING AORTA ANEURYSM

Descending aorta aneurysms occur distal to the left subclavian artery. Operation is performed through a left thoracotomy incision with one-lung anesthesia. The aorta is clamped above and below the aneurysm, which is replaced with a Dacron tube graft. A major risk in descending thoracic aneurysm repair is spinal cord ischemia with resultant paraplegia. A number of methods have been proposed for protection of the spinal cord. These include cardiopulmonary bypass—with or without deep hypothermia—or left heart bypass. The latter provides distal aortic perfusion by circulating blood from the left atrium to the femoral artery while the aorta is clamped. Heparin-coated circuits available with this method can reduce bleeding. In addition, measured drainage of cerebrospinal fluid may be useful in ischemic cord swelling. For both techniques, reimplantation of large intercostal arteries is recommended because they may provide important collaterals to the cord. Measurement of somatosensory evoked potentials may guide the reimplantation decision.

Prognosis

The operative mortality rate associated with repair of descending aortic aneurysms approximates 5–15% depending on the age of the patient and coexisting illness. The incidence of paraplegia varies with the extent of the aorta repaired and is now approximately 5–15%. The 10-year survival rate after surgery for ascending aneurysms is 50% and averages 38% for aneurysms of the descending aorta.

THORACIC AORTIC DISSECTION

Acute aortic dissection is the most common cause of aortic rupture and is often a lethal event. Approximately 2000 cases occur each year, and men are affected more commonly than women, usually in the fifth to seventh decades of life. The hallmark of this disease is degeneration of the aortic media. The pathogenesis is controversial. One theory holds that medial degeneration predisposes to rupture of the vasa vasorum, with subsequent intramural hematoma formation as a precursor to the dissection process. Another theory is that the commonly seen intimal tear allows blood to shear the weakened media. The intimal tear is located in the ascending aorta in 62% of cases, in the arch in 10%, and in the isthmus in 16%—and the remainder occur in the distal aorta. Men are more frequently affected, and hypertension is a common predisposing condition. Other causes of aortic dissection include atherosclerosis, iatrogenic injury (catheter, open heart procedures), and closed chest trauma. Patients with Marfan's syndrome and aortic coarctation are more susceptible to aortic dissection.

The DeBakey classification scheme is commonly used to describe the location and extent of aortic dissection. DeBakey type I dissections originate in the ascending aorta and extend into the distal aorta beyond the left subclavian artery; type II dissections involve the ascending aorta only, are frequently chronic, and are associated with aortic valve incompetence; and type III dissections occur distal to the left subclavian artery and commonly extend into the abdominal aorta. The Stanford scheme is simpler and is frequently used to guide therapy: any dissection occurring in the ascending aorta is classified as A; dissections involving only the descending aorta (below the isthmus) are B (Figure 20–22).

Clinical Findings

A. SYMPTOMS AND SIGNS

The most common symptom is severe chest pain, which often signifies the onset of the intimal tear and formation of the false lumen. The chest pain often is described as a severe tearing sensation that is felt anteriorly in ascending dissections and posteriorly between the scapulas in descending dissections. Hypotension may accompany the pain as a result of loss of blood into the false lumen, free rupture into the mediastinum, or leak into the pericardium. Sudden death may occur from pericardial tamponade or from extension into the aortic root with occlusion of the right or left coronary arteries. Aortic root involvement also is associated with prolapse of the aortic valve commissures and leaflets, causing aortic insufficiency and congestive heart failure.

Other manifestations, occurring as the result of obstruction (by intimal flap or false channel hematoma) of significant aortic branch vessels, include stroke, asymmetric upper extremity pulses and pressures, paraplegia, renal failure, acute mesenteric occlusion, and lower extremity arterial occlusion.

B. ELECTROCARDIOGRAPHY AND LABORATORY FINDINGS

The ECG and cardiac enzyme determinations are helpful in excluding acute myocardial infarction. This event may mimic many of the signs and symptoms of acute

Figure 20–22. DeBakey and Stanford classification schemes for acute aortic dissection. (Reproduced, with permission, from Doroghazi RM, Slater EE [editors]. *Aortic Dissection*. McGraw-Hill, 1983.)

aortic dissection or may be caused by the dissection itself if the false channel occludes one or both coronary ostia. In this situation, administration of thrombolytic therapy or angioplasty would be dangerous.

C. IMAGING STUDIES

The chest radiograph may show a widened mediastinum but is normal in up to half of patients. Cardiomegaly may reflect congestive heart failure or pericardial effusion. With contained rupture, a left pleural effusion may be evident. Ultrafast chest CT is the diagnostic procedure of choice in most centers and is highly sensitive and specific. Transesophageal echocardiography can also be performed rapidly and gives additional information about the myocardial function and aortic valve competence. However, dissections of the aortic arch and branch vessels are not well imaged. MR angiography is being used more frequently but is more time-consuming. Contrast aortography is rarely performed in acute aortic dissection but may be necessary in chronic dissection to determine branch vessel origination from the true or false channel.

Treatment & Prognosis

For the typically hypertensive patient, aggressive control of blood pressure is critical. Intravenous esmolol is commonly used to reduce dP/dT (change in pressure divided by change in time) and the aortic shear forces. Pure vasodilators, if necessary, should be added only after beta-blockade has been achieved.

A. ASCENDING DISSECTION

For patients with untreated acute Stanford type A aortic dissection, 3% die suddenly, 27% die within 24 hours, and 70% succumb by 1 week. Rupture with cardiac tamponade, acute coronary occlusion, and acute aortic regurgitation are the major causes of demise. These facts underscore the primary role of urgent surgery for this condition. Replacement of the ascending aorta is required along with resection of the intimal tear. Resuspension of the aortic valve commissures usually restores valve competence. Achieving good hemostasis can be problematic because of the fragile nature of the dissected aorta. Application of new surgical adhesives (Bioglue) may be helpful. Operative mortality for this procedure is about 5%, and the 5-year survival approximates 55%. Since the entire aorta is usually dissected, yearly imaging surveillance is needed to look for aneurysmal changes.

B. DESCENDING DISSECTION

The majority of patients presenting with acute type B aortic dissection (Figure 20–23) have a benign course. Drug therapy is the treatment of choice. However, ap-

Figure 20–23. CT scan of type B aortic dissection. Arrow points to true lumen of aorta.

proximately 20% of these acute dissection patients require surgery for rupture or significant organ ischemia from branch vessel occlusion. Operative mortality is this situation is at least 15%. Late survival is good, but 20% of patients may develop aneurysmal dilation of the descending aorta requiring operation. Therefore, yearly imaging surveillance is recommended.

Recently, endovascular aortic stent placement, with or without a fenestration procedure, has been applied to descending aortic dissection. However, control of the proximal intimal tear is not always possible, and long-term outcome studies are needed.

Coady MA et al: Natural history, pathogenesis, and etiology of thoracic aortic aneurysms and dissections. Cardiol Clin 1999;17:615.

Coady MA et al: Surgical intervention criteria for thoracic aortic aneurysms: a study of growth rates and complications. Ann Thorac Surg 1999;67:1922-6.

Coselli S LeMaire SA: Left heart bypass reduces paraplegia rates after thoracoabdominal aortic aneurysm repair. Ann Thorac Surg 1999;67:1931.

Coselli JS et al: Cerebrospinal fluid drainage in thoracoabdominal aortic surgery. Semin Vasc Surg 2000;13:308.

de Haan P et al: Spinal cord monitoring with myogenic motor evoked potentials: early detection of spinal cord ischemia as an integral part of spinal cord protective strategies during thoracoabdominal aneurysm surgery. Semin Thorac Cardiovasc Surg 1998;10:19.

Elefteriades JA et al: Management of descending aortic dissection. Ann Thorac Surg 1999;67:2002.

Greenberg R, Risher W: Clinical decision making and operative approaches to thoracic aortic aneurysms. Surg Clin North Am 1998;78:805.

Griepp RB et al: Natural history of descending thoracic and thoracoabdominal aneurysms. Ann Thorac Surg 1999;67:1927-30.

Hartnell GG: Imaging of aortic aneurysms and dissection: CT and MRI. J Thorac Imaging 2001;16:35.

Kouchoukos NT et al: Elective hypothermic cardiopulmonary bypass and circulatory arrest for spinal cord protection during operations on the thoracoabdominal aorta. J Thorac Cardiovasc Surg 1990;99:659.

Leiner T et al: Magnetic resonance angiography of an aortic dissection. Circulation 2001;103:E76.

Meszaros I et al: Epidemiology and clinicopathology of aortic dissection. Chest 2000;117:1271.

Sabik JF et al: Long-term effectiveness of operations for ascending aortic dissections. J Thorac Cardiovasc Surg 2000;119:946.

Umana JP, Mitchell RS: Endovascular treatment of aortic dissections and thoracic aortic aneurysms. Semin Vasc Surg 2000;13:290.

■ CARDIAC TUMORS

Primary tumors of the heart are rare, occurring in 0.002–0.3% of autopsy series. They can occur in any age group. Prior to the introduction of echocardiography, most tumors were diagnosed postmortem, since many patients remain asymptomatic until the tumor becomes quite large. Although most primary cardiac tumors are benign, the most common cardiac neoplasm is a metastatic lesion (Table 20–6). Most benign lesions are resectable and potentially curable. With the possible exception of lymphoma, most malignant primary and metastatic lesions are resistant to chemotherapy and radiotherapy and carry a poor prognosis.

Benign myxoma accounts for 75% of all primary benign tumors. Its physical characteristics range from a smooth, round, firm encapsulated mass to a loose conglomeration of gelatinous material, which may be friable (Figure 20–24). Most are attached by a pedicle to

Table 20–6. Types of cardiac tumors.

Primary
Benign (75%)
Myxoma
Rhabdomyoma
Papillary fibroelastoma
Fibroma
Lipoma
Teratoma
Malignant (25%)
Sarcoma (angiosarcoma, rhabdomyosarcoma, fibrosarcoma, osteogenic sarcoma, liposarcoma, lymphoma)
Teratoma
Metastatic
Carcinoma (67%) (lung, breast)
Sarcoma (20%)
Melanoma (12%)

Figure 20–24. Operative photograph of polypoid right atrial myxoma.

the fossa ovalis of the left atrial septum, though some may occur in the right atrium or ventricles. Histologically, myxomas contain various mesenchymal cells; abnormal DNA ploidy may correlate with recurrence after resection. Papillary fibroelastomas typically appear as papillary fronds attached to the aortic valve and are associated with cerebral and coronary embolization.

Clinical Findings

A. SYMPTOMS AND SIGNS

Clinical findings and presentation are dependent on the type and location of the tumor. As a general rule, malignant lesions usually present with rapidly progressive congestive heart failure from valvular or myocardial infiltration. Patients with myxoma can have protean manifestations. Systemic symptoms and signs include fever, weight loss, and anemia. Patients may also have signs of systemic embolization or mitral valve obstruction (mitral stenosis) from the tumor mass. The latter can produce a characteristic early diastolic sound or "tumor plop." Cardiac fibromas typically occur in the pediatric age group. These tumors grow slowly and tend to invade the conduction system, explaining why patients often die suddenly from arrhythmias.

B. LABORATORY AND IMAGING STUDIES

Cardiac myxoma may produce abnormalities in the sedimentation rate, gamma globulin, and liver aminotransferases. Anemia and thrombocytopenia are common to many cardiac tumors.

The diagnostic procedure of choice is transesophageal echocardiography. Occasionally, MRI and CT scans are useful for infiltrative lesions.

Treatment

Most benign lesions of the heart are resectable and potentially curable. For cardiac myxomas, it is important to resect a rim of normal tissue around the attachment stalk to reduce future recurrence. The surgeon must be careful not to embolize the tumor during manipulation. Standard cardiopulmonary bypass with cardioplegia arrest is required, and operative mortality should be less than 1%.

Surgery for cardiac sarcomas and metastatic lesions is usually for diagnostic purposes, though palliative resection may occasionally be appropriate. Rarely, orthotopic heart transplantation has been considered in patients with local disease. However, long-term survival for malignant cardiac lesions remains poor.

Araoz PA et al: CT and MR imaging of primary cardiac malignancies. Radiographics 1999;19:1421.

Lobo A et al: Intracardiac masses detected by echocardiography: case presentations and review of the literature. Clin Cardiol 2000;23:702.

Michler RE, Goldstein DJ: Treatment of cardiac tumors by orthotopic cardiac transplantation. Semin Oncol 1997; 24:534.

Schaff HV, Mullany CJ: Surgery for cardiac myxomas. Semin Thorac Cardiovasc Surg 2000;12:77.

Shapiro LM: Cardiac tumours: diagnosis and management. Heart 2001;85:218.

Vander Salm TJ: Unusual primary tumors of the heart. Semin Thorac Cardiovasc Surg 2000;12:89.

■ POSTOPERATIVE CARE

The care of patients after cardiac surgical procedures is assuming a greater role as older and sicker patients are being selected for surgical therapy. While most patients have a smooth and uncomplicated course, 5–10% experience postoperative problems, and a number of parameters are monitored to provide warning of developing complications. The fundamental goal is to provide adequate tissue perfusion. Careful physical examination after surgery is the starting point—to assess mental status, color, jugular venous pressure, pulse strength, and extremity temperature. Standard measurements include radial artery blood pressure, central venous pressure, urinary output, a continuous electrocardiographic tracing, and periodic determinations of arterial blood gases (PO_2, PCO_2) and pH. In complicated cases, cardiac function is assessed with measurements of cardiac output and pulmonary capillary wedge pressure as provided by a thermodilution Swan-Ganz catheter. Bipolar temporary atrial and ventricular pacing wires are left in most patients for control of heart rate or diagnosis of dysrhythmias. Appropriate hematologic and blood chemistry studies as well as chest radiographs are obtained periodically. Body weight is recorded daily to monitor potential fluid retention.

ANTICOAGULATION

Postoperative anticoagulation with aspirin is used routinely for most coronary bypass, valve repair, or bioprosthetic valve replacement procedures. After mechanical valve replacement, all patients should have full warfarin anticoagulation starting with the oral diet and continued indefinitely to maintain the INR at 3.0–3.5.

VENTILATORY SUPPORT

Following uncomplicated elective operations, most patients can be removed from ventilatory support and extubated within a few hours. After anesthetic recovery, criteria for early extubation include good pulmonary gas exchange, adequate ventilatory mechanics, a clear chest radiograph, absence of dysrhythmias and excess bleeding, and stable cardiac and neurologic function. Occasional patients exhibit prolonged pulmonary dysfunction requiring controlled ventilation, positive end-expiratory pressure, diuresis, and transiently increased fractional inspired oxygen. Complicated patients may benefit from prolonged mechanical ventilation by reducing the work of respiration. If pulmonary infection is suggested by radiographic infiltrates, high white blood cell counts, or positive sputum cultures, appropriate antibiotic coverage is added. As the period of required ventilatory support via an endotracheal tube approaches 2 weeks, tracheostomy should be considered. Tracheostomy is especially useful for clearing pulmonary secretions and assisting with ventilatory weaning.

MANAGEMENT OF COMPLICATIONS

Low Cardiac Output

With improving surgical techniques—and especially the introduction of cold potassium cardioplegia—postoperative low cardiac output is now uncommon in most centers. Patients judged by examination or by direct cardiac output determination (eg, cardiac index ≤ 2 L/min/m^2) to have inadequate perfusion must be treated aggressively. Therapeutic options can be categorized as alterations in preload (volume administration), inotropy (dopamine, dobutamine, etc), and afterload (vasoconstrictors, vasodilators). Inadequate heart rate can be treated with epicardial dual-chamber pacing. The most common problem is hypovolemia; volume replacement is usually accomplished with colloid solutions (blood, albumin, hetastarch), and it is not usually necessary to keep the hematocrit over 25%. Central venous pressures or pulmonary capillary wedge pressures of 15 mm Hg usually reflect adequate volume resuscitation.

Additional inotropic agents may be added if low cardiac output persists. These include epinephrine, calcium, and phosphodiesterase inhibitors (milrinone). The latter are particularly useful in situations of high pulmonary artery pressures or systemic vascular resistance. Cases of refractory low output may benefit from intra-aortic balloon counterpulsation. A small catheter is inserted percutaneously into the proximal descending aorta and helium is used to inflate a balloon on the catheter after aortic valve closure, thus augmenting coronary filling. The balloon is deflated with systole, resulting in afterload reduction.

In extreme situations, operative placement of ventricular assist devices may be indicated.

Postoperative Bleeding & Cardiac Tamponade

Cardiopulmonary bypass results in a number of hemostatic perturbations that may affect the clotting process. Residual heparin from the procedure or preoperative anticoagulants, thrombocytopenia, and altered platelet function are the most common problems. Activation of fibrinolysis and dilution of clotting factors also contribute. Most of these problems can be addressed intraoperatively. Administration of antifibrinolytics such as lysine analogs (aminocaproic acid) or serine protease inhibitors (aprotinin) during cardiopulmonary bypass has been shown to reduce postoperative bleeding in complicated patients. Criteria for excessive bleeding after open heart procedures vary widely. However, mediastinal tube outputs greater than 100 mL/h for more than 3 hours postoperatively is of concern. Prompt reexploration of the patient is always preferable to multiple blood transfusions and does not increase wound complication rates.

Cardiac tamponade can be a postoperative surgical emergency. The characteristic hemodynamic finding is elevated and equalized central venous and pulmonary wedge pressures, usually in the setting of excessive mediastinal bleeding. Low cardiac output is a sine qua non of tamponade. The urine output is low, and metabolic acidosis may be present. The chest radiograph may demonstrate mediastinal widening or blood collection. Echocardiography may be helpful in confusing cases, but if a significant question of tamponade exists, reoperation should be considered.

Atrial Dysrhythmias

Atrial dysrhythmias are common following coronary revascularization. Premature atrial contractions, atrial fibrillation, and atrial flutter reflect postoperative atrial irritability and occur in up to 40% of patients. Prophylactic treatment with beta-blocking agents or amiodarone (class III antiarrhythmic) may reduce the incidence of this complication and should be considered in most patients. Other agents that may be effective in controlling the ventricular rate in acute atrial fibrillation include intravenous digoxin, procainamide, and calcium channel blockers (verapamil). Rapid atrial pacing may be useful in converting atrial flutter. For refractory atrial fibrillation (continuing more than 48 hours after good drug therapy) or in patients with unstable signs (hypotension, ischemia), electrical cardioversion should be performed. Transesophageal echocardiography to rule out atrial thrombus has been recommended prior to cardioversion.

Ventricular Arrhythmias

Ventricular irritability manifested by frequent or multifocal premature ventricular contractions, ventricular tachycardia, or ventricular fibrillation is managed by intravenous lidocaine, procainamide, or amiodarone together with direct-current cardioversion when necessary. Short periods of closed-chest cardiac massage may be necessary, but early cardioversion should be emphasized. Polymorphic ventricular tachycardia and ventricular fibrillation are usually manifestations of significant myocardial ischemia, and problems with the quality of coronary revascularization should be considered. Significant hypokalemia, hypomagnesemia, and hypoxemia should be ruled out. Beta-blocking agents, oral procainamide, or amiodarone can be used for long-term management of persistent ventricular ectopy. Frequent unifocal premature ventricular contractions do not require therapy.

Postoperative conduction disturbances occur frequently. Right bundle branch block is the most common problem and is usually benign. Transient heart block is seen more often after valvular surgery. After 5 days of persistent complete heart block, a permanent pacemaker should be considered.

Renal Dysfunction

Postoperative renal dysfunction after heart surgery occurs in 1–5% of patients and is usually related to preoperative age, diabetic status, and renal insufficiency. The duration of cardiopulmonary bypass may also contribute to this complication. Manifestations may vary from transient oliguric tubular necrosis to permanent renal failure. Proposed mechanisms include perioperative hypotension, atheroembolism, sepsis, or administration of nephrotoxic drugs.

Therapy for renal dysfunction consists of maintaining a higher arterial perfusion pressure (especially in patients with preexisting hypertension), low-dose intravenous dopamine infusion, adequate free water hydration, and general support of cardiac output. Fluid balance and potassium intake are monitored carefully to prevent overhydration or hyperkalemia. Forced diuresis with furosemide or mannitol may reduce the severity of renal failure. Some patients may require temporary veno-venous ultrafiltration or hemodialysis. Patients with renal failure are more likely to die during their hospitalization.

Wound Infection

Sternal wound infection should occur in less than 1% of patients after cardiac surgery. Developing sternal instability, fever, leukocytosis, and wound drainage suggest the diagnosis. Severity varies from a superficial subcutaneous infection with a stable sternum to an isolated sternal infection with no mediastinal involvement to full-blown septic mediastinitis. At the first suspicion of a major wound infection, broad-spectrum antibiotics should be instituted and blood cultures obtained. The combination of diabetes and bilateral internal mammary artery harvesting predispose some patients to sternal infection. Infections producing sternal disruption should be treated with early wound debridement and pectoral or omental pedicle flaps. The mortality rate using this approach has been reduced to less than 10%, though morbidity remains high.

Myocardial Infarction

With improvements in myocardial protection and coronary grafting techniques, perioperative myocardial infarction should occur in only 1–2% of patients. Inadequate myocardial protection, incomplete revascularization, and early graft closure are the most common causes. Symptoms are often unreliable, since many patients cannot distinguish incisional pain from angina. Classic electrocardiographic changes and elevated serum troponin or CK are needed for diagnosis. Judicious anti-ischemia therapy is appropriate, and patients with possible vasospasm of arterial grafts should be treated with calcium channel blockers. Rarely, angioplasty may be used to treat acute graft closure.

Augoustides J et al: Hemodynamic monitoring of the postoperative adult cardiac surgical patient. Semin Thorac Cardiovasc Surg 2000;12:309.

De Feo M et al: Variables predicting adverse outcome in patients with deep sternal wound infection. Ann Thorac Surg 2001; 71:324.

Gorman JH et al: Circulatory management of the unstable cardiac patient. Semin Thorac Cardiovasc Surg 2000;12:316.

Milan BL et al: Management of bleeding and coagulopathy after heart surgery. Semin Thorac Cardiovasc Surg 2000;12:326.

Rho RW et al: Management of postoperative arrhythmias. Semin Thorac Cardiovasc Surg 2000;12:349.

Sirivella S et al: Mannitol, furosemide, and dopamine infusion in postoperative renal failure complicating cardiac surgery. Ann Thorac Surg 2000;69:501.

Suen WS et al: Risk factors for development of acute renal failure (ARF) requiring dialysis in patients undergoing cardiac surgery. Angiology 1998;49:789.

Sural S et al: Etiology, prognosis, and outcome of post-operative acute renal failure. Ren Fail 2000;22:87.

II. Congenital Heart Disease

Ronald K. Woods, MD, & Edward Verrier, MD

DIAGNOSIS

Whereas some newborns may have obvious symptoms and signs of heart disease, others may have complex lesions not detected for days to months. Moreover, the clinical manifestations of a particular anomaly may evolve with age—eg, progressive failure or improvement with ventricular septal defect or increase in pulmonary vasculopathy associated with lesions that cause increased pulmonary blood flow. Although certain anomalies produce certain patterns of symptoms and circulatory dysfunction, specificity is not usually adequate for planning definitive therapy.

An important aspect of postnatal diagnosis is recognition of an abnormal heart sound, murmur, or other symptom referable to the heart. Examples are feeding difficulty, lack of weight gain, frequent respiratory infections, irritability, or cyanosis. Once a clinical abnormality is recognized, an investigation must be pursued until a definitive diagnosis is established. Although most anomalies are diagnosed after birth, prenatal or fetal echocardiography may indicate the presence of an anomaly and in many cases may establish a specific diagnosis.

Chest radiography and electrocardiography should be done in all cases as part of the initial workup. For additional diagnostic screening and anatomic definition, a more specific noninvasive test such as echocardiography is essential. Two-dimensional color flow doppler echocardiography has eliminated the need to perform cardiac catheterization on every child with suspected congenital heart disease. In most cases, the decision to proceed to operation can be based on echocardiographic findings. However, cardiac catheterization remains relevant to the workup and management of several anomalies because it provides measurements of flow and resistance as well as accurate anatomic detail of the heart, great vessels, and pulmonary vasculature.

MANAGEMENT

Management of most congenital cardiac anomalies consists of surgical correction. Medication, diet, and activity regulation are important aspects of management, but the pediatrician or cardiologist should recommend a treatment program leading ultimately to surgical repair at the optimal time to prevent emergence of irreversible complications. The established success of modern care is derived from contributions of several specialties to the multidisciplinary team approach to the care of these children.

In the current era, most surgical procedures for congenital heart anomalies are considered corrective rather than palliative in that abnormal physiology is corrected—and in most cases anatomy is corrected as well. In certain cases in which initial corrective repair is considered too high-risk, it may be preferable to perform a palliative procedure initially and allow the child to grow until a more corrective procedure can be done. Most palliative procedures are designed to increase or decrease pulmonary blood flow. For example, a systemic to pulmonary artery shunt is a common means of increasing pulmonary blood flow in right heart obstructive lesions. At the other extreme, pulmonary artery banding, although used much less frequently in the current era, may be needed to decrease pulmonary blood flow—eg, in a child with a single ventricle and tricuspid atresia.

Most cardiac operations require cardiopulmonary bypass. This is usually accomplished by draining blood through cannulas placed in the right atrium or the venae cavae, through the heart-lung machine, and back to the patient through a small cannula in the aorta. Protection of the heart during the period of aortic cross-clamping or other periods of cardiac ischemia is more commonly done using various cardioplegic techniques quite similar to those described for adult cardiac operations.

Various degrees of hypothermia are employed with cardiopulmonary bypass depending on the nature of the repair and the anticipated duration of cardiac ischemia. Hypothermia decreases the metabolic rate and oxygen consumption, thereby offering additional protection against ischemia. Lower bypass pump flow rates also provide improved visualization of the operative field by decreasing the amount of blood returning to the heart. For certain types of repairs—eg, complex aortic reconstruction in small neonates—deep hypothermic circulatory arrest or low-flow deep hypothermia is considered a very useful and in some cases an essential option. Cardiopulmonary bypass is used to cool the patient to a core temperature of 15–18 °C (the brain is further cooled by packing the head in ice), at which point the bypass pump is turned off, blood can be drained to the venous reservoir of the pump, and cannulas are removed. Alternatively, flows can be maintained at much lower rates without complete circulatory arrest. With deep hypothermic arrest, most surgeons recommend reestablishing perfusion at low flows for a short time every 20 minutes. The incidence of short-term complications secondary to circulatory arrest is considered acceptably low; however, the incidence and nature of long-term neurologic sequelae are extremely difficult to characterize accurately and remain under investigation. Because of this, some surgeons advocate avoidance of circulatory arrest in favor of hypothermic continuous low-flow perfusion.

Postoperative Management

After open heart surgery, most patients are maintained with an endotracheal tube in place and controlled mechanical ventilation for 12–24 hours. Drainage catheters in the mediastinum for postoperative bleeding are usually removed the following morning. Arterial blood gases and pH are measured by intra-arterial monitoring. In most instances of complex repairs, small venous catheters are left in the major atria or pulmonary artery to accurately measure all major venous and arterial pressure changes. Prophylactic antibiotics are routinely used, usually until lines and drainage tubes are removed.

The most common complication after open heart surgery is bleeding, requiring reoperation in 2–5% of patients. This occurs because the patient is heparinized during bypass and because reversal with protamine, though efficient, is not always complete. Particularly in smaller patients, hemodilution secondary to the prime volume of the bypass pump also contributes to a dilutional coagulopathy.

The overall incidence of dysrhythmia or significant cardiac dysfunction is low. In most cases, judicious medical management is successful. Nonetheless, mechanical assistance is a recognized utility in this context, most commonly in the form of extracorporeal membrane oxygenator support. Before relying on nonsurgical management or mechanical assist devices, it is imperative to rule out a residual defect, inadequate repair, or mechanical complication of the operation.

Unlike adults, the pulmonary vasculature of newborns and older infants is quite reactive. Postoperative pulmonary artery hypertensive crises are therefore more common in this age group, particularly after repair of certain anomalies such as obstructed pulmonary veins.

Measures to reduce pulmonary vascular resistance include controlled mechanical ventilation and administration of bicarbonate to increase pH; high-dose opioid anesthesia to blunt sympathetic responses; increased fraction of inspired oxygen concentration; and, more recently, inhaled nitric oxide.

Castaneda AR et al: *Cardiac Surgery of the Neonate and Infant.* W.B. Saunders Co., 1994.

Fesslova V et al: Evolution and long term outcome in cases with fetal diagnosis of congenital heart disease: Italian multicenter study. Fetal cardiology study group of the Italian Society of Pediatric Cardiology. Heart 1999;82:594.

Kavanaugh-McHugh A et al: Transesophageal echocardiography in pediatric congenital heart disease. Cardiol Rev 2000;8:288.

Limperopoulos OT et al: Neurodevelopmental status of newborns and infants with congenital heart defects before and after open heart surgery. J Pediatr 2000;137:638.

Morris CD et al: 25-year mortality after surgical repair of congenital heart defects in childhood. A population based cohort study. JAMA 1991;266:3447.

Newburger JW et al: A comparison of the perioperative neurologic effects of hypothermic circulatory arrest versus low-flow cardiopulmonary bypass in infant heart surgery. N Engl J Med 1993;329(15):1057.

Pfammater JP et al: Pediatric open heart operations without diagnostic catheterization. Ann Thorac Surg 1999;68:532.

■ OBSTRUCTIVE CONGENITAL HEART LESIONS

Obstructive lesions impede the forward flow of blood and increase ventricular afterloads. In the absence of a ventricular septal defect, an obstructive lesion in the aortic or pulmonary valve causes the proximal ventricle to become hypertrophied. Sudden death may occur in this context. Ventricular hypertrophy is of concern because of the risk of dysrhythmias, ischemic changes in the myocardium, and potential permanent muscle damage or replacement by fibrosis.

PULMONARY STENOSIS

 ESSENTIALS OF DIAGNOSIS

- *No symptoms in patients with mild or moderately severe lesions.*
- *Cyanosis and right-sided heart failure in patients with severe lesions.*

- *High-pitched systolic ejection murmur maximal in the second left interspace. S_2 delayed and soft. Ejection click often present. Increased right ventricular impulse.*
- *No ejection click and inaudible S_2 in severe cases.*

General Considerations

Pulmonary stenosis with intact ventricular septum and a normal aortic root accounts for approximately 5–8% of cardiac anomalies. In most of these patients, the commissures are fused with a flexible tricuspid semilunar valve, producing a dome-like structure with a central opening of varying size (Figure 20–25A). Most patients with pulmonary stenosis have a patent foramen ovale; few have true atrial septal defects. In infants, severe valvular stenosis may be associated with a poorly developed right ventricle and can be an extremely serious condition requiring urgent intervention. Isolated infundibular stenosis is extremely rare and usually associated with less dramatic clinical findings since the turbulence across the infundibular area is much less than across the tight stenotic pulmonary valve (Figure 20–25B).

Clinical Findings

Infants with more severe forms of pulmonary stenosis usually feed poorly and may have hypoxic spells. Sudden death has been reported. Older children usually are asymptomatic and grow normally. A few may complain of fatigue and dyspnea on exertion. When the pulmonary stenosis physiologically worsens as the child grows, shortness of breath, dizziness, and even angina may occur.

Approximately half of the deaths caused by pulmonary stenosis occur in infants. The remainder may be asymptomatic, but the murmurs of pulmonary stenosis are easily heard and usually do not go undetected. Complete evaluation is required; if the gradient between the right ventricle and the pulmonary artery is 50 mm Hg or greater, repair is usually recommended.

Treatment

Infants with severe right ventricular failure or cyanotic spells require early intervention. In critically ill neonates, prostaglandin E_1 (alprostadil) has proved effective in maintaining pulmonary blood flow through the ductus arteriosus until the pulmonary valve obstruction is relieved. Interventional cardiology and catheter balloon dilation have essentially replaced surgery for most forms of isolated critical pulmonary stenosis. Adequate postdilation gradients with low mortality are attained in over 90% of patients. The proce-

A

Domelike stenotic valve

B

Muscular fibrous stenotic band

Figure 20–25. Pulmonary stenosis. ***A:*** Valvular pulmonary stenosis. ***B:*** Infundibular pulmonary stenosis.

dure is indicated even in the less common scenario of a minimally symptomatic newborn with systemic right ventricular pressure. Surgical valvotomy with cardiopulmonary bypass remains an acceptable approach with equivalent success. It may be necessary for cases in which catheter intervention was not successful or in the context of an extremely small annulus or marked infundibular stenosis, in which case a transannular patch—and perhaps a systemic to pulmonary artery shunt—can be performed.

Prognosis

Posttreatment mortality for critical pulmonary stenosis ranges from 3% to 10%. Restenosis rates are variable and range between 10% and 25%. Right ventricular hypertrophy regresses after relief of the valvular stenosis.

Cheung YF et al: Evolving management for critical pulmonary stenosis in neonates and young infants. Cardiol Young 2000; 10:186.

Hanley FL et al: Outcomes in critically ill neonates with pulmonary stenosis and intact ventricular septum: a multiinstitutional study. Congenital Heart Surgeons Society. J Am Coll Cardiol 1993;22:183.

Rao PS: Balloon valvuloplasty in the neonate with critical pulmonary stenosis. J Am Coll Cardiol 1996;27:473.

Rao PS: Long-term follow-up results after balloon dilatation of pulmonic stenosis, aortic stenosis, and coarctation of the aorta: a review. Prog Cardiovasc Dis 1999;42:59.

AORTIC STENOSIS

Four types of congenital aortic stenosis are generally recognized (Figure 20–26). Valvular aortic stenosis is the most common type; subaortic and supravalvular

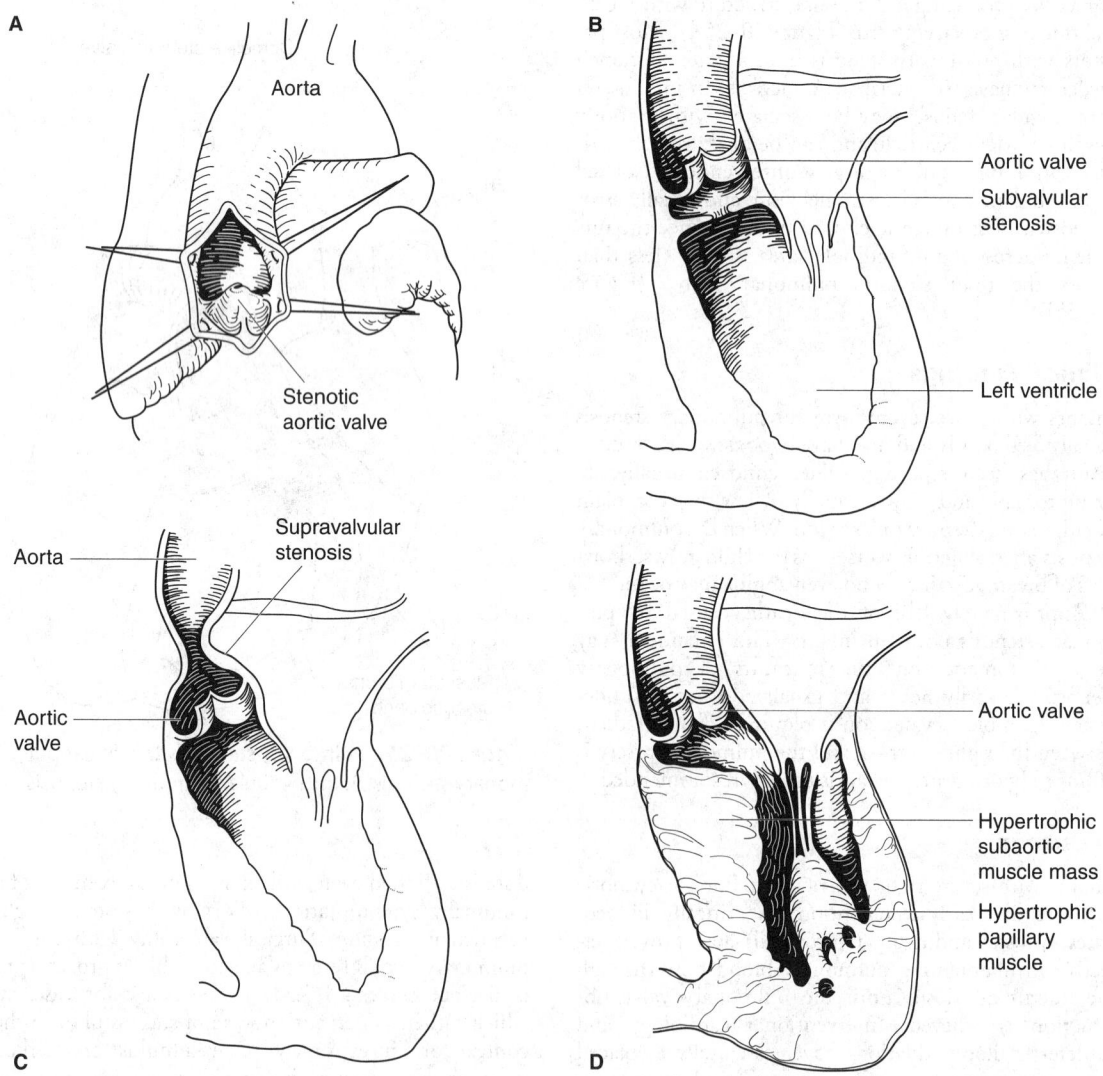

A

Aorta

Stenotic aortic valve

B

Aortic valve

Subvalvular stenosis

Left ventricle

C

Aorta

Supravalvular stenosis

Aortic valve

D

Aortic valve

Hypertrophic subaortic muscle mass

Hypertrophic papillary muscle

Figure 20–26. Types of congenital aortic stenosis. **A:** Valvular aortic stenosis. **B:** Subaortic stenosis (discrete fibrous band). **C:** Supravalvular aortic stenosis. **D:** Idiopathic hypertrophic subaortic stenosis.

aortic stenosis and asymmetric septal hypertrophy occur infrequently.

1. Valvular Aortic Stenosis

 ESSENTIALS OF DIAGNOSIS

- *Usually asymptomatic in children; angina and syncope indicate severe stenosis.*
- *May cause severe heart failure in infants.*
- *Prominent left ventricular impulse; narrow pulse pressure.*
- *Harsh systolic murmur and thrill along left sternal border; systolic ejection click.*

General Considerations

Valvular aortic stenosis accounts for approximately 5% of congenital heart anomalies and is the only type of aortic stenosis that occurs in neonates, accounting for approximately 10% of cases. The clinical characteristics of neonatal critical aortic stenosis differ from those of valvular stenosis in older children in several respects. In neonates, the valve is often unicommissural or bicommissural, and associated anomalies, including other left-sided obstructive lesions, are usually present. Profound clinical deterioration occurs after ductal closure, with severe left ventricular failure, subendocardial ischemia, and endocardial fibroelastosis. In older children, the valve is more frequently tricommissural, and associated anomalies are less common. Most children are asymptomatic, and symptoms, when present—with the exception of sudden death—typically evolve less acutely.

Clinical Findings

Children with severe stenosis develop dyspnea, angina, or syncope with effort. Newborns with aortic stenosis have severe heart failure and cyanosis and associated respiratory distress. A harsh basilar systolic murmur with thrill along the left sternal border is a common finding. The murmur may at times be inaudible because of heart failure and low cardiac output. In most cases, chest radiographs are normal or show only left ventricular hypertrophy. The ascending aorta may be dilated. In the infant, the cardiac silhouette is usually large, and pulmonary venous congestion is present. Complete evaluation including echocardiography and cardiac catheterization is indicated; in older children with isolated stenosis, echocardiography may be sufficient.

Treatment

Valvular stenosis cannot be treated medically. In neonates, clinical presentation alone is the indication to intervene in most cases. In older children, indications include a pressure gradient between the left ventricle and ascending aorta of 50 mm Hg or greater; symptoms of syncope, heart failure, and aborted sudden death; and ischemic electrocardiographic changes. Available interventions include various surgical procedures or balloon dilation. In neonates, suitability for restoration of biventricular physiology can be difficult to ascertain. After initiation of prostaglandin therapy for maintenance or restoration of ductal patency, balloon dilation is typically the initial effort to restore biventricular function in neonates. Other surgeons prefer initial surgical valvotomy with the patient supported on cardiopulmonary bypass. The success of either technique ultimately depends on selection of patients appropriate for two-ventricle physiology. For the older child, valve replacement is usually necessary. A variety of replacement options are available, including bioprostheses (stented and unstented porcine and pericardial valves; aortic homografts), pulmonary autografts (Ross procedure), or mechanical prostheses (ball valve, monocusp, bileaflet).

Prognosis

In general, surgical or balloon valvotomy of a critically stenotic valve in the neonate is not curative. Ultimately, the valve will undergo progressive thickening and calcification. Mortality ranges between 30% and 50%. Of those surviving, more than half will require repeat valvotomy or valve replacement in 5–10 years. Thus, scheduled follow-up is necessary to determine the rate and degree of restenosis. Prognosis after valve replacement in the older child is substantially better, with mortality less than 5–10%. Nonetheless, issues of growth of the patient as well as structural deterioration of the valve will necessitate eventual replacement of the valve. The pulmonary autograft (Ross procedure) is being used more frequently in children and offers growth potential and freedom from anticoagulation and synthetic surfaces. The pulmonary allograft that is used to replace the harvested autograft remains a source of concern, potentially requiring reintervention when the child is older.

2. Subaortic Stenosis

Subaortic stenosis may exist in two forms: discrete and diffuse subaortic stenosis. The discrete form is more common, consisting of a membranous or fibromuscular ring of tissue located beneath the aortic annulus. Other anomalies may coexist, particularly left-sided obstructive lesions (mitral stenosis, aortic coarctation) associated with the diffuse form. The pathophysiology of left ventricular outflow tract obstruction leads to clinical manifestations similar to those of valvular stenosis. Aortic regurgitation may be seen in 20–30% of patients. The diagnosis is typically confirmed in late childhood and is rare in neonates.

Indications for operative repair include symptoms, a gradient of 50 mm Hg or greater, or severe aortic regurgitation. Operative repair of the discrete form consists of resection of the membrane and myectomy of the septum. Fifteen-year survival is greater than 95%, with a risk of recurrent obstruction requiring reoperation of 5–10% at 15 years. Repair of the diffuse type requires more extensive modification of the outflow tract, usually with some combination of septal muscle resection, annular and outflow tract enlargement, and in some cases valve replacement, the latter procedures referred to as Konno and Ross-Konno procedures. The operative mortality and the risk of recurrence are greater for the diffuse form of stenosis and depend on the extent of the operation and the severity of associated lesions.

3. Supravalvular Aortic Stenosis

Isolated supravalvular aortic stenosis is typically in the form of an hourglass-shaped constriction of the aorta at the sinotubular junction (top of the commissures). Other forms exist, including a discrete ridge and diffuse narrowing of the entire ascending aorta (20–30% of patients). In fact, obstructive lesions can be found as well in the abdominal aorta (10% of patients) and the pulmonary vasculature or right heart outflow tract (40–70%). This distribution of lesions is due to intrinsically abnormal production of elastin in the media of vessels during development as a consequence of alterations of the elastin gene (7q11.23). It is postulated that decreased elasticity leads to increased shear stresses, leading ultimately to hyperplasia and hypertrophy of smooth muscle in the media, with decreased amounts of broken and disorganized elastin fibers. Therefore, larger arteries, subjected to greater stress, are affected more frequently. Abnormalities of the aortic valve leaflets are present in 20–40% of patients. Less commonly, the left coronary artery may demonstrate various degrees of obstruction.

Supravalvular stenosis is commonly associated with Williams-Beuren syndrome (mental retardation, distinctive facial features, and peripheral pulmonary artery stenosis). It also occurs in autosomal dominant forms and sporadic forms in which the nonvascular aspects of Williams-Beuren syndrome are absent. The various forms depend on the exact abnormality and mode of acquisition of the altered gene. In general, the dominant symptoms relate to the proximal aortic obstruction.

Various types of operative repairs are available. A synthetic or pericardial patch can be inserted to widen the area of narrowing. Another approach consists of limited resection of the stenosis, mobilization of the aorta, and tailoring the proximal and distal ends for primary anastomosis (no synthetic patch). Both techniques are associated with a low operative mortality and excellent relief of obstruction. Subsequent need for aortic valve replacement is a recognized issue. When present, obstruction of the right heart outflow tract or pulmonary vasculature has a tendency to regress with time. For severe lesions, operative repair (replacement with pulmonary allograft, pericardial patch enlargement) can be conducted at the time of aortic surgery. Balloon angioplasty is a recognized alternative; however, the durability of this approach in this particular patient population is debated.

4. Hypertrophic Obstructive Cardiomyopathy

This genetically transmitted (autosomal dominant) disease of cardiac muscle features a spectrum of ventricular hypertrophy, typically with disproportionate thickening of the septum. The myocardial sarcomeres are hypertrophied and arranged in a bizarre pattern. Stenotic septal coronary arteries are often present. The asymmetric muscle mass may or may not cause obstruction of the left ventricular outflow tract (Figure 20–26D). Mitral regurgitation is a common associated finding. Symptomatic patients nearly always have some degree of obstruction during systole. The severity of this obstruction increases during systole and is proportionate to the volume of the left ventricular cavity, the force of ventricular contraction, and the cross-sectional area of the left ventricular outflow tract during systole. Exercise or various pharmacologic agents may alter these relationships and change the degree of obstruction. The common symptoms in older children are chronic fatigue, episodes of syncope and angina, and dyspnea on exertion. Signs and symptoms of severe congestive heart failure predominate in neonates, and the mortality is extremely high. However, a morphologically similar, nongenetically transmitted form of this disease exists in over 30% of infants of diabetic mothers and typically regresses in the first few months of life.

This disease is quite variable, and the natural history is not entirely predictable. Some patients improve symptomatically with chronic beta-blockade therapy (propranolol). In the pediatric patient in whom a discrete gradient can be demonstrated, operative repair is considered superior to medical therapy. This is accomplished by incising a wide or deep trough of septal muscle under the right coronary leaflet. Extensive resection can cause left bundle branch block or complete heart block. Operative mortality is low, and the need for re-operation for recurrent obstruction is less than 10% at 5 years after repair. Associated mitral regurgitation regresses in the majority of patients after relief of the outflow tract obstruction. Dual-chamber pacing is a more recently advocated alternative but is associated with less reduction in the outflow tract gradient.

Durham LA et al: Ross procedure with aortic root tailoring for aortic valve replacement in the pediatric population. Ann Thorac Surg 1997;64:482.

Gaynor JW et al: Late outcome of survivors of intervention for neonatal aortic valve stenosis. Ann Thorac Surg 1995;60:122.

Gundry SR, Behrendt DM: Prognostic factors in valvotomy for critical aortic stenosis in infancy. J Thorac Cardiovasc Surg 1986;92:747.

Lofland GK et al: Critical aortic stenosis in the neonate: a multi-institutional study of management, outcomes, and risk factors. J Thorac Cardiovasc Surg 2001;121:10.

Lupinetti FM et al: Intermediate-term results in pediatric aortic valve replacement. Ann Thorac Surg 1999;68:521.

Lupinetti FM et al: Optimum treatment of discrete subaortic stenosis. Ann Thorac Surg 1992;54:467.

McElhinney DB et al: Issues and outcomes in the management of supravalvar aortic stenosis. Ann Thorac Surg 2000;69:562.

Mosca RS et al: Critical aortic stenosis in the neonate: a comparison of balloon valvuloplasty and transventricular dilation. J Thorac Cardiovasc Surg 1995;109:147.

Serraf A et al: Surgical treatment of subaortic stenosis: a seventeen-year experience. J Thorac Cardiovasc Surg 1999;117:669.

Stamm C et al: Congenital supravalvar aortic stenosis: a simple lesion? Eur J Cardiothorac Surg 2001;19:195.

Theodoro DA et al: Hypertrophic obstructive cardiomyopathy in pediatric patients: results of surgical treatment. J Thorac Cardiovasc Surg 1996;112:1589.

COARCTATION OF THE AORTA

 ESSENTIALS OF DIAGNOSIS

- Infants may have severe heart failure; children are usually asymptomatic.
- Absent or weak femoral pulses.
- Systolic pressure higher in upper extremities than in lower extremities; diastolic pressures are similar.
- Harsh systolic murmur heard in the back.

General Considerations

Coarctation of the aorta occurs in 0.2–0.6 per 1000 live births, accounting for 5–8% of congenital cardiovascular anomalies. It occurs two to five times more frequently in males. Fifteen to 30 percent of patients with Turner's syndrome have aortic coarctation. Ninety-eight percent of all aortic coarctations are located at or near the aortic isthmus (the segment of aorta adjacent to the ligamentum arteriosum or ductus arteriosus). Coarctation occurs in three general contexts: as an isolated lesion; with an associated ventricular septal defect; or with associated more severe intracardiac anomalies and more extensive involvement of the aortic arch. Even isolated coarctation has variable morphology and may present as hypoplasia of the isthmus and distal arch. Types of associated anomalies include patent foramen ovale and ductus arteriosus (assumed as part of the anomaly in neonates), ventricular septal defect, bicuspid aortic valve (40% patients), and Shone's syndrome. As a rule, the incidence and severity of associated lesions is inversely proportionate to the age at presentation. Associated anomalies occur in over 70% of neonates and in as few as 10–15% of older children. Theories attempting to explain the embryology and etiology of coarctation describe the effects of decreased flow through the aorta secondary to more proximal left-sided obstruction and the effects of ductal closure and ectopic ductal tissue in the wall of the aorta. No single theory offers an adequate explanation for the spectrum of coarctation morphology.

The general pathophysiology is distal arch–proximal thoracic aortic obstruction. This leads to systolic and diastolic hypertension in the proximal aorta and upper extremities. Eventually, collateral vessels develop to maintain distal perfusion. In the neonate, distal flow can be maintained by a patent ductus arteriosus. If left untreated, approximately 50% of patients with isolated coarctation will die by 30 years of age. The common causes of death include congestive heart failure, endocarditis, aortic rupture, and intracranial hemorrhage.

Clinical Findings

The hemodynamic consequences of coarctation of the aorta depend on the rate of closure of the ductus, the severity of obstruction, the development of collaterals, and the presence and severity of associated anomalies. There appear to be two distinct clinical presentations: patients who present in early infancy and those who present in later childhood. Infants with coarctation may have severe congestive heart failure and sudden cardiovascular collapse with ductal closure, necessitating maintenance of ductal patency with alprostadil.

Many older children with coarctation are asymptomatic and well-developed. Complaints of headache, pains in the calves when running, or frequent nosebleeds are common. Most of these children have hypertension in the upper extremities, and many have electrocardiographic evidence of left ventricular hypertrophy. The classic findings of notched ribs (secondary to enlarged intercostals vessels, seen in children over 4 years of age) or the "reversed 3" sign are seen less frequently in the modern era of earlier diagnosis. When the disorder is suspected, echocardiography is usually sufficient to confirm the diagnosis. Magnetic resonance imaging is another useful modality.

Treatment

With modern surgical techniques and the risk of deleterious consequences of hypertension increasing with age, most surgeons advocate correction soon after confirmation of the diagnosis. In the seriously ill neonate, administration of alprostadil (PGE_1), mechanical ventilation, and administration of bicarbonate to restore adequate organ perfusion are critical aspects of management. Options for coarctation repair include the following: (1) resection with end-to-end anastomosis; (2) extended resection with primary anastomosis; (3) various versions of subclavian flap aortoplasty with or without concomitant extended resection; (4) patch aortoplasty with polytetrafluoroethylene (Gore-Tex) or Dacron; (5) resection and interposition graft; and (6) percutaneous balloon dilation. Most authors agree that no single technique is optimal for all types of coarctation repair. General principles to consider for first-time repair include resection of the stenotic region and ductal tissue, adequate mobilization to avoid undue tension on suture lines, an attempt to avoid prosthetic material, maintenance of growth potential, and good post-repair patency with no residual pressure gradient across the repair. The timing of repair of associated anomalies is a debated issue. Although staged repair is not unreasonable (eg, banding the pulmonary artery for a ventricular septal defect at the time of coarctation repair), the recent trend is toward single-stage complete repair.

Repair is performed through a left thoracotomy. An exception is the use of median sternotomy for concomitant repair of an intracardiac anomaly. Adequate mobilization of the aorta with preservation of intercostal arteries and protection of the recurrent nerve are important considerations. Aortic cross-clamping is generally well tolerated without the extensive use of afterload reducing agents. The appropriate balance of systemic and pulmonary blood flow in the context of intracardiac shunts must be kept in mind.

Extended resection with primary repair is a preferred approach in neonates and infants. Extended mobilization of both the descending aorta and the aortic arch proximal to the innominate artery is critical to the success of this technique. A reverse subclavian flap aortoplasty is a reasonable alternative in cases of distal arch and isthmic hypoplasia. This technique entails dividing the left subclavian artery and opening the artery proximally onto the aortic arch up to the left carotid artery. The subclavian flap is then turned proximally as an insertion patch to widen the hypoplastic segment.

For the young child and a more discrete isolated coarctation, excision with primary repair is a reasonable approach. Adequate mobilization is performed to minimize anastomotic tension. For the older child or adolescent in whom adequate mobilization may be more difficult, resection with an interposition graft is another alternative, particularly for the older patient for whom growth potential is less of a concern.

The optimal management of recoarctation (gradient greater than or equal to 20 mm Hg) continues to evolve. In most cases, aortography and balloon angioplasty can be performed safely and effectively, thereby eliminating the need for reoperation. Should surgery be necessary or preferred, patch aortoplasty or a subclavian flap, combined with variable degrees of resection, is a reasonable approach.

Prognosis

Mortality is variable and depends on the severity of associated anomalies. In general, operative and 2- to 5-year survival is well over 95% but may be as low as 40–50% with an associated severe anomaly. Recurrent coarctation occurs in 5–20% of patients, usually in the first year after repair, and depends on the degree of arch hypoplasia and the technique of repair. Potential complications or morbidity include hemorrhage, damage to the recurrent laryngeal nerve, Horner's syndrome, chylothorax, paraplegia (rare), and various complications related to sacrifice of the subclavian artery (uncommon in acyanotic patients). Postoperative hypertension, another recognized morbidity, occurs in two forms. Paradoxic hypertension occurs immediately postoperatively and is often transient. A second phase of diastolic hypertension may occur 2–3 days after surgery and may persist for several days. These forms of postoperative hypertension are believed related to changes in sympathetic tone, baroreceptor sensitivity, and the renin-aldosterone system. Pressure should be carefully monitored, and hypertension should be appropriately treated. There is a recognized risk of postoperative mesenteric vasculitis that may be minimized with good blood pressure control.

Amato JJ et al: Role of extended aortoplasty related to the definition of coarctation of the aorta. Ann Thorac Surg 1991; 52:615.

Bacha EA et al: Surgery for coarctation of the aorta in infants weighing less than 2 kg. Ann Thorac Surg 2001;71:1260.

Conte S et al: Surgical management of neonatal coarctation. J Thorac Cardiovasc Surg 1995;109:663.

Dietl CA et al: Risk of recoarctation in neonates and infants after repair with patch aortoplasty, subclavian flap, and combination resection-flap procedure. J Thorac Cardiovasc Surg 1992;103:724.

Quaegebeur JM et al: Outcomes in seriously ill neonates with coarctation of the aorta: a multiinstitutional study. J Thorac Cardiovasc Surg 1994;108:841.

Rao PS et al: Role of balloon angioplasty in the treatment of aortic coarctation. Ann Thorac Surg 1991;52:621.

Sharma BK et al: Coarctation repair in neonates with subclavian-sparing advancement flap. Ann Thorac Surg 1992;54:137.

INTERRUPTED AORTIC ARCH

Absence of the aortic arch distal to the left subclavian artery (type A, 35%), between the left carotid and left subclavian artery (type B, 60%), or between the innominate and left carotid artery (type C, 5%) is an uncommon but severe form of developmental obstruction within the aorta. The distal aorta receives blood from the patent ductus that may constrict shortly after birth and thus limit flow to the lower extremities. This lesion is almost always accompanied by other intracardiac anomalies such as ventricular septal defect, truncus arteriosus, aortopulmonary window, subaortic stenosis, or transposition of the great vessels. Type B interruption is frequently associated with an aberrant right subclavian artery. Most of these patients are symptomatic in the first few days of life, require prostaglandin E_1 for hemodynamic stabilization, and require early operation for correction. Although repair may be staged, the current trend is to repair the arch as well as intracardiac anomalies during the first operation.

Jonas RA et al: Outcomes in patients with interrupted aortic arch and ventricular septal defect: a multiinstitutional study. J Thorac Cardiovasc Surg 1994;107:1099.

Luciani GB et al: One-stage repair of interrupted aortic arch, ventricular septal defect, and subaortic obstruction in the neonate: a novel approach. J Thorac Cardiovasc Surg 1996; 111:348.

Serraf A et al: Repair of interrupted aortic arch: a ten-year experience. J Thorac Cardiovasc Surg 1996;112:1150.

HYPOPLASTIC LEFT HEART SYNDROME

 ESSENTIALS OF DIAGNOSIS

- *Newborn respiratory distress with varying degrees of cyanosis and hemodynamic failure.*
- *Echocardiographic findings of atretic or stenotic aortic and mitral valves, hypoplastic left ventricle and ascending aorta.*

General Considerations

Hypoplastic left heart syndrome is a spectrum of underdevelopment of left-sided structures, including the mitral and aortic valves, the left ventricle, and the ascending aorta and aortic arch. It accounts for 5–7% of congenital cardiac anomalies and up to 25% of cardiac mortality in the first few days of life. In the more common form of this syndrome, there is atresia of the mitral and aortic valves; the left ventricle is markedly hypoplastic; and the ascending aorta measures 2–3.5 mm. The coronary arteries originate and branch normally but may be stenotic in some cases (aortic atresia, mitral stenosis). The newborn is dependent on a patent interatrial communication and ductus arteriosus. In general, other cardiac anomalies are uncommon and include ventricular septal defect and double outlet right ventricle. Autopsy data suggest that up to 25% of these children may have developmental abnormalities of the central nervous system as well as various genetically defined disorders. This syndrome is uniformly fatal without operative management. Prenatal diagnosis facilitates counseling and support of parents and is part of a well-prepared multidisciplinary approach to the care of these children.

Clinical Features

The entire cardiac output delivered from the right heart must supply systemic and pulmonary blood flow in a balance that maintains adequate oxygenation of the blood (pulmonary flow) and systemic oxygen delivery. This precarious situation is invariably disrupted by closure of the ductus or an inadequate interatrial communication. The result is respiratory failure, hemodynamic failure, metabolic acidosis, and other organ system failure (gut, kidney). Echocardiography is usually sufficient to confirm the diagnosis. Criteria to reliably distinguish between isolated aortic stenosis and hypoplastic left heart syndrome are under investigation. More so recently, prenatal echocardiographic diagnosis facilitates prenatal counseling and referral to centers with expertise in providing care for these children.

Treatment

Initial management entails resuscitation with mechanical ventilation; judicious use of fluids, pressors, and bicarbonate; and, most importantly, maintenance of ductal patency with prostaglandin infusion. If there is evidence of inadequate mixing, a balloon atrial septostomy can be performed. The fraction of inspired oxygen should be 0.21 or less, and hyperventilation should be avoided. Two types of surgical therapy are currently available for these children—staged reconstruction or transplantation (described elsewhere in this text). Staged reconstruction consists of a Norwood procedure in the neonatal period followed by a Glenn or hemi-Fontan procedure when the child is approximately 6–8 months of age (or 6–8 kg). Staged reconstruction is completed with a Fontan procedure at about 1–1.5 years of age. At the first stage, the proximal aorta and pulmonary artery are joined and the remaining aortic arch is reconstructed with pericardium or pulmonary allograft material. An atrial septostomy is also performed. Pulmonary blood flow is provided by a systemic to pulmonary artery shunt. The second stage provides relief of volume overload on the right heart by connecting the superior vena cava to the pulmonary artery and, most commonly, dividing the systemic to pulmonary artery shunt. Finally, the Fontan procedure directs inferior caval flow to the pulmonary artery, thereby completing the diversion of systemic venous return directly to the pulmonary artery. These children are followed closely, with echocardiographic and angiographic studies being performed prior to each subsequent stage to ensure suitable candidacy for each stage of repair.

Prognosis

Short-term and intermediate-term outcomes have consistently improved for these children in the past 2 decades. In general, survival at 5 years ranges from 40% to 70%, most deaths occurring soon after the first stage of repair. For those centers with dedicated programs for either staged reconstruction or transplantation, there is no significant difference in 5-year survival rates.

Iannettoni MD et al: Improving results with first-stage palliation for hypoplastic left heart syndrome. J Thorac Cardiovasc Surg 1994;107:934.

Mosca RS et al: Early results of the Fontan procedure in one hundred consecutive patients with hypoplastic left heart syndrome. J Thorac Cardiovasc Surg 2000;119:1110.

Norwood WI: Hypoplastic left heart syndrome. Ann Thorac Surg 1991;52:688.

Norwood WI et al: Fontan procedure for hypoplastic heart syndrome. Ann Thorac Surg 1992;54:1025.

Razzouk AJ et al: Transplantation as a primary treatment for hypoplastic left heart syndrome: intermediate-term results. Ann Thorac Surg 1996;62:1.

Starnes VA et al: Current approach to hypoplastic heart syndrome: palliation, transplantation, or both? J Thorac Cardiovasc Surg 1992;104:189.

Tchervenkov CI et al: Congenital Heart Surgery Nomenclature and Database Project: hypoplastic left heart syndrome. Ann Thorac Surg 2000;69:S170.

Weldner PW et al: The Norwood operation and subsequent Fontan operation in infants with complex congenital heart disease. J Thorac Cardiovasc Surg 1995;109:654.

CONGENITAL MITRAL VALVE DISEASE

Congenital mitral valve stenosis or insufficiency is an uncommon form of congenital heart disease with a wide spectrum of abnormalities and continues to be a surgical challenge. Associated anomalies are present in the majority of patients, including ventricular septal defect, atrial septal defect, and coarctation of the aorta. Insufficiency is usually associated with a dilated annulus and restricted leaflet motion due to shortened chordae and leaflet hypoplasia. In mitral stenosis, multiple levels of the valvular apparatus are typically involved, including supravalvular ring, parachute valve, commissural fusion, short chordae, and decreased interpapillary distance. Shone's anomaly is a recognized syndrome consisting of supravalvar mitral ring, parachute mitral valve, subaortic stenosis, and coarctation of the aorta.

Surgical treatment is indicated for severe symptoms. If feasible, repair—rather than replacement—is a preferred option. Replacement is more likely to be necessary in the case of severe stenosis. Regardless of the type of procedure, careful assessment should be performed to ensure adequate function before leaving the operating room (transesophageal echo, pressure tracings). Valve replacement can provide marked relief of symptoms and, indeed, may be necessary. However, replacement commits the patient to some form of anticoagulation and the need for subsequent repeat replacement when the valve is outgrown. Repair, on the other hand, is associated with a need for reintervention in 25–50% of patients. Balloon valvuloplasty has been described for stenotic lesions; however, the durability of this approach remains to be verified.

Bolling SF et al: Shone's anomaly: operative results and late outcome. Ann Thorac Surg 1990;49:887.

Sousa Uva M et al: Surgery for congenital mitral valve disease in the first year of life. J Thorac Cardiovasc Surg 1995;109:164.

Yoshimura N et al: Surgery for mitral valve disease in the pediatric age group. J Thorac Cardiovasc Surg 1999;118:99.

Zias EA et al: Surgical repair of the congenitally malformed mitral valve in infants and children. Ann Thorac Surg 1998;66:1551.

COR TRIATRIATUM

In this rare anomaly, the pulmonary veins enter an accessory venous chamber demarcated from the true left atrium by a diaphragm. There is typically an obstructive orifice connecting the chamber to the left atrium. Less commonly, the chamber connects to the right atrium. A left-sided superior vena cava is a common finding. The pathophysiology is that of pulmonary venous hypertension, pulmonary congestion, and elevated pulmonary artery pressure. Typically, respiratory compromise occurs early in life. Surgical excision of the membrane corrects the abnormality. With attentive postoperative care and control of pulmonary blood pressure, the prognosis is quite good.

Salomone G et al: Cor triatriatum: clinical presentation and operative results. J Thorac Cardiovasc Surg 1991;101:1088.

van Son JA et al: Cor triatriatum: diagnosis, operative approach, and late results. Mayo Clin Proc 1993;68:854.

Herlong JR et al: Congenital Heart Surgery Nomenclature and Database Project: pulmonary venous anomalies. Ann Thorac Surg 2000;69:S56.

■ CONGENITAL HEART LESIONS THAT INCREASE PULMONARY ARTERIAL BLOOD FLOW

Approximately 50% of all congenital heart lesions shunt blood from the systemic arterial circulation into the pulmonary circulation (left-to-right shunt). The most common lesions in this group are patent ductus arteriosus and defects of the atrial septum, atrioventricular canal, and ventricular septum. Rare lesions include ruptured sinus of Valsalva, aortopulmonary window, truncus arteriosus, some types of transposition of the great vessels, double outlet right ventricle, and other more complex lesions.

Differential compliances and pressures between right- and left-sided structures promote shunting of oxygenated blood through abnormal communications to the right heart and recirculation through the lungs. The excessive pulmonary circulation causes pulmonary vascular congestion, resulting in frequent respiratory infections, and places an additional volume load on the involved ventricle.

Increased pulmonary blood flow alone gradually increases pulmonary arterial blood pressure. Elevation of left atrial pressure from excessive flow or increased left ventricular end-diastolic pressure increases pulmonary arterial pressure, interstitial lung water, and probably pulmonary vascular resistance. If pulmonary arterioles also constrict in response to the increased blood flow, pulmonary vascular resistance increases (hyperkinetic pulmonary hypertension), and pulmonary arterial pressure may increase further unless flow decreases. Pulmonary vasoconstriction can be reversed by inhalation of oxygen, intravenous tolazoline, or nitric oxide. Lack of reversibility implies fixed pulmonary vascular obstructive disease.

Increased pulmonary blood flow and increased pulmonary arterial pressure are believed to lead to endothelial damage or activation—which, in turn, alters smooth muscle cell physiology in the media, leading to hypertrophy of the media of pulmonary arterioles (stage 1), proliferation of intima (stage 2), and, eventually, hyalinization and fibrosis of the intima (stage 3). These morphologic changes, termed pulmonary vascular obstructive disease, are acquired, but they are more likely to occur in congenital lesions producing both high pulmonary arterial pressure and large flows (ventricular septal defect, complete atrioventricular canal, truncus arteriosus) than in those producing increased pulmonary blood flow only (atrial septal defect). As the cross-sectional area of the pulmonary vascular bed decreases as a result of the morphologic changes, pulmonary vascular resistance increases and the ratio of pulmonary vascular resistance to systemic vascular resistance also increases. The amount of blood shunted from left to right decreases. When pulmonary vascular resistance equals or exceeds systemic vascular resistance, left-to-right blood flow across the lesion ceases or reverses. In Eisenmenger's syndrome, obstruction of the pulmonary vasculature reduces pulmonary blood flow and causes blood to shunt from right to left. Patients who have advanced pulmonary vascular disease (stage 3 or higher) and balanced or reversed shunts (Eisenmenger's syndrome) are not candidates for surgery other than lung or heart-lung transplantation.

Pulmonary arterial banding is a palliative operation designed to reduce pulmonary blood flow by placing an anatomically fixed resistance to blood flow across the lungs. The band constricts the main pulmonary artery downstream to the valve and adds a resistance in series to the vascular resistance of the lung. Because of dynamic changes in cardiac output and pressure and resistance within the circulation, addition of a fixed resistance (the band) cannot produce balanced pulmonary and systemic flows under all physiologic conditions. However, a good band can reduce pulmonary arterial blood flow sufficiently to alleviate ventricular failure and prevent rapid progression of pulmonary vascular disease. Unfortunately, preexisting pulmonary vascular disease may not regress after banding. Pulmonary artery banding is only palliative and is used only when other options are not available or are associated with excessive risk.

Horowitz MD et al: Pulmonary arterial banding: analysis of a 25 year experience. Ann Thorac Surg 1989;48:444.

Rabinovitch M: Pathobiology of pulmonary hypertension: impact on clinical management. Pediatr Card Surg Ann Semin Thorac Cardiovasc Surg 2000;3:63.

ATRIAL SEPTAL DEFECT, OSTIUM SECUNDUM TYPE

ESSENTIALS OF DIAGNOSIS

- *Acyanotic, asymptomatic.*
- *Right ventricular lift.*
- *S_2 widely split and fixed.*
- *Grade 1–3/6 pulmonary systolic ejection murmur.*
- *Diastolic flow murmur at the lower left sternal border.*

General Considerations

Ostium secundum defects occur in the region of the fossa ovalis and may be single or multiple. Secundum defects are the commonest and, usually, the largest of the atrial septal defects. Defects high in the atrial septum, often associated with partial anomalous pulmonary venous return, are referred to as sinus venosus defects. Anomalous venous return associated with an atrial septal defect is really more of a physiologic consideration than an anatomic one at the time of surgical repair. The lateral wall of the atrial septum is often missing, and it is difficult to say whether the right pulmonary veins actually enter the right or the left atrium. A patch is used in the repair of most of these atrial defects; it can be positioned so that the veins are not a major factor (Figure 20–27).

Heart failure from uncomplicated ostium secundum defects may occur in young children but is less common in adults. Pulmonary vascular disease is also rare, but atrial dysrhythmias are noted with increasing age. The average life expectancy in patients with untreated atrial septal defects is reduced because of right ventricular failure, dysrhythmias, and occasionally pulmonary vascular disease.

Treatment

Most ostium secundum defects should be closed. The optimal time for closure is a debated issue. Paradoxic embolism and endocarditis are small risks associated with delaying repair. Many surgeons advocate proceeding with repair in late infancy or in the second year of life. The issue has changed somewhat more recently with the availability of transluminal percutaneous devices that may be placed in children who have attained

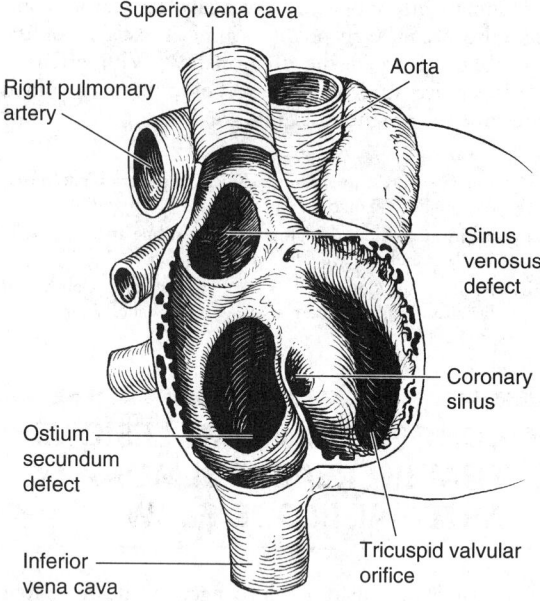

Figure 20–27. Sinus venosus and ostium secundum defects in the atrial septum as viewed from the opened right atrium.

an appropriate size (approximately 10 kg or more). In fact, a large percentage of isolated secundum defects are now closed using this technique. For the child in whom device closure is not an option, repair can easily be done on cardiopulmonary bypass using a patch of pericardium, polytetrafluoroethylene (Gore-Tex), or Dacron if primary closure is not feasible. The introduction of minimal access approaches allows surgery to be performed with a much smaller incision and potentially less morbidity. The prognosis after surgical closure is excellent. Although long-term follow-up is not yet available, short-term results of percutaneous device closure are equally promising.

Anderson RH et al: Sinus venosus defect. Am Heart J 1994; 128:365.

Berger F et al: Comparison of results and complications of surgical and Amplatzer device closure of atrial septal defects. J Thorac Cardiovasc Surg 1999;118:674.

Jacobs JP et al: Congenital Heart Surgery Nomenclature and Database Project: atrial septal defect. Ann Thorac Surg 2000; 69:S18.

Nicholson IA et al: Minimal sternotomy approach for congenital heart operations. Ann Thorac Surg 2001;71:469.

Verrier ED: Secundum atrial defects. In: *Current Therapy in Cardiothoracic Surgery,* vol 1. Grillo HC et al (editors). Bryan Decker, 1989.

ATRIOVENTRICULAR CANAL DEFECT

ESSENTIALS OF DIAGNOSIS

- *Heart failure common in infancy.*
- *Cardiomegaly, blowing pansystolic murmur, other variable murmurs.*
- *Loud S_2 with fixed splitting.*
- *Electrocardiography shows left axis deviation and a counterclockwise frontal QRS vector loop.*

General Considerations

Atrioventricular canal defect is a deficiency of tissue in the central region of the heart composed of the lower portion of the atrial septum (septum primum), the upper portion of the ventricular septum, and the adjoining components of the mitral and tricuspid valves. Normal canal development is based on proliferation of endocardial cushion tissue as well as conal tissue, which contributes to formation of the valves. Various aspects of the embryologic process can fail, thereby leading to a spectrum of defects depending on whether one or all three components are affected and to what degree. Anomalies of the atrioventricular valves can range from a cleft in the anterior mitral leaflet to a single atrioventricular valve with multiple leaflets. Partial atrioventricular canal defect, formerly called septum primum atrial septal defect, is a deficiency of only the lower aspect of the atrial septum. Transitional atrioventricular canal defect is an intermediate form in which minor deficiency occurs in the upper ventricular septum. Complete atrioventricular canal defect (Figure 20–28) consists of marked deficiency in the lower atrial septum and upper ventricular septum. Typically, the more severe valve anomalies are seen with complete defect. Associated anomalies are not uncommon and include left superior vena cava, additional muscular ventricular septal defects, anomalous pulmonary venous connections, patent ductus arteriosus, tetralogy of Fallot, and other less common complex anomalies.

Clinical Findings

The pathophysiology is that of a left-to-right shunt potentially modified by mitral regurgitation. The severity

Figure 20–28. Complete atrioventricular canal. The most common type has a divided anterior common atrioventricular leaflet. Both the mitral and tricuspid portions are attached to the interventricular septum with long, nonfused chordae tendineae. The mitral and tricuspid portions of the common posterior atrioventricular leaflet are not separated. (Modified from Rastelli GC et al: Surgical repair of the complete form of persistent common atrioventricular canal. J Thorac Cardiovasc Surg 1968;55:299.)

depends on the degree of abnormality of each structural component of the canal. For partial atrioventricular canal defect, symptoms may be minimal to absent; whereas, for complete defect life expectancy is less than 1 year because of death from congestive heart failure. Pulmonary vascular obstructive disease and progressive mitral regurgitation are recognized in the natural history of this anomaly. Certain features of this anomaly are modified or exacerbated when it occurs in a child with trisomy 21. Deficiency of valve tissue and obstruction of inflow and outflow of the left ventricle may be less common; however, these children may be more prone to earlier development of pulmonary vascular obstructive disease. Although specific electrocardiographic findings have been described, echocardiography is the best modality for delineating the anatomy. Cardiac catheterization may be needed in infants over 6 months of age in whom pulmonary vascular disease is more of a concern.

Treatment

Surgical correction is indicated, with timing dictated by the degree of the anomaly and symptoms. For complete atrioventricular canal defect, repair is generally performed by 6 months of age. Although repair may be delayed for the asymptomatic child with a partial defect, most surgeons advocate repair by 1 year of age. Mitral regurgitation is also an indication to proceed with repair regardless of age. Surgical treatment is directed by the severity of the anomaly. For partial atrioventricular canal defect, repair consists of patch closure, typically using pericardium. Transitional or complete atrioventricular canal defect requires patch closure of the septal defects (using single- or double-patch technique) and repair or reconstruction of abnormal valves (suture closure of mitral cleft with or without annuloplasty).

Prognosis

Mortality varies with the degree of defect, associated cardiac anomalies, age at the time of surgery, and postrepair status of the mitral valve. For partial defect, operative mortality is rare, and 10-year survival is greater than 98%. For complete atrioventricular canal defect, operative mortality is approximately 3–5% with over 90% 10-year survival. An important complication of repair is complete heart block, occurring in 3–5% of patients. The incidence and severity of postoperative mitral regurgitation is variable (10–40%), with approximately 10% requiring reoperation. It is expected that many of these children may need additional mitral valve work in adulthood.

Agny M et al: Repair of partial atrioventricular septal defect in children less than five years of age: late results. Ann Thorac Surg 1999;67:1412.

Anderson RH et al: The diagnostic features of atrioventricular septal defect with common atrioventricular junction. Cardiol Young 1998;8:33.

Backer CL et al: Repair of complete atrioventricular canal defects: results with the two-patch technique. Ann Thorac Surg 1995;60:530.

Jacobs JP et al: Congenital Heart Surgery Nomenclature and Database Project: atrioventricular canal defect. Ann Thorac Surg 2000;69:S36.

Najm, HK et al: Primum atrial septal defect in children: early results, risk factors, and freedom from reoperation. Ann Thorac Surg 1998;66:829.

Nicholson IA et al: Simplified single patch technique for the repair of atrioventricular septal defect. J Thorac Cardiovasc Surg 1999;118:642.

Reddy VM et al: Atrioventricular valve function after single patch repair of complete atrioventricular septal defect in infancy: how early should repair be attempted? J Thorac Cardiovasc Surg 1998;115:1032.

VENTRICULAR SEPTAL DEFECT

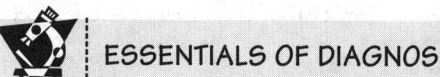 ESSENTIALS OF DIAGNOSIS

- *Asymptomatic if defect is small.*
- *Heart failure with dyspnea, frequent respiratory infections, and poor growth if the defect is large.*
- *Grade 2–6/6 pansystolic murmur maximal at the left sternal border.*
- *S_2 loud with apical diastolic flow murmur and biventricular enlargement if the defect is large.*

General Considerations

Ventricular septal defect is common, accounting for approximately 25% of congenital cardiac anomalies. These defects occur in four anatomic positions in the ventricular septum. About 85% occur in the area of the membranous septum (Figure 20–29) (perimembranous). A much smaller percentage of defects occur anterior to the crista supraventricularis (supracristal, conal, or outlet), beneath the septal leaflet of the tricuspid valve (canal or inlet), or in the muscular ventricular septum (muscular).

Ventricular septal defects are often one component of another more complex congenital heart lesion such as truncus arteriosus, atrioventricular canal defect, tetralogy of Fallot, or transposition of the great arteries. Patients with isolated perimembranous defects may have extra-

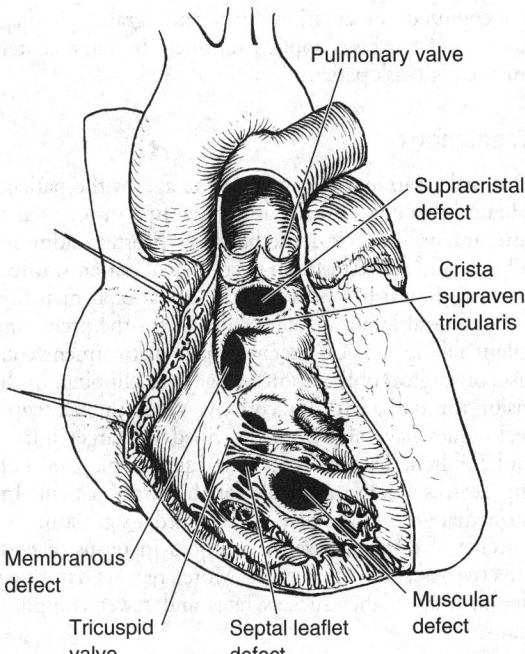

Figure 20–29. Anatomic locations of various ventricular septal defects. The wall of the right ventricle has been excised to expose the ventricular septum.

cardiac lesions such as patent ductus arteriosus or coarctation of the aorta. Patients with supracristal defects occasionally have aortic valve regurgitation.

Clinical Findings

The clinical symptoms relate to pulmonary overcirculation and congestive failure—dyspnea on exertion, poor weight gain, and easy fatigability. Infants with large defects usually fail to grow and have chronic respiratory difficulties and poor feeding habits. In general, the heart is enlarged, and the lung fields are overcirculated. Pulmonary vascular disease may develop as a result of the high pressure and large flow in the lungs. In infants, approximately one-third of defects are small and asymptomatic. Many of these defects will close spontaneously, usually after 7–8 years. About one-third of patients with large or multiple defects are symptomatic in infancy and require aggressive medical management, early diagnosis, and surgical correction. Echocardiography provides sufficient diagnostic information in the majority of cases. In the older asymptomatic infant or young child with a persistent defect, consideration may be given to catheterization to assess pulmonary artery pressure and vascular resistance.

Treatment

Indications for surgery include medically refractory symptoms in the infant, elevated pulmonary artery pressure in the asymptomatic infant or older child, the presence of a canal-type defect or a malaligned conoventricular defect, or the presence of aortic insufficiency with a supracristal defect. Optimal treatment consists of synthetic patch closure of the defect with the suture line placed away from the conduction system. The approach is through the right atrium with the child on cardiopulmonary bypass. Deep hypothermic circulatory arrest or low flow is often used in small infants. Multiple muscular defects are often difficult to close due to limited visualization. More recently, percutaneous device closure has been described and may prove useful for this difficult type of defect.

Prognosis

Operative mortality is rare and usually limited to the young infant in severe failure (3–5%). Overall, improvement in symptoms is usually quite dramatic. Pulmonary vascular resistance probably does not change significantly. Thus, earlier operation reduces the likelihood of significant pulmonary vascular disease.

Amin A et al: New device for closure of muscular ventricular septal defects in a canine model. Circulation 1999;100:320.

Anderson RH et al: The surgical anatomy of ventricular septal defect. J Card Surg 1992;7:17.

Backer CL et al: Surgical management of the conal (supracristal) ventricular septal defect. J Thorac Cardiovasc Surg 1991; 102:288.

Hardin JT et al: Primary surgical closure of large ventricular septal defects in small infants. Ann Thorac Surg 1992;53:397.

Jacobs JP et al: Congenital Heart Surgery Nomenclature and Database Project: ventricular septal defect. Ann Thorac Surg 2000;69:S25.

McGrath LB et al: Methods for repair of simple isolated ventricular septal defect. J Card Surg 1991;6:13.

Mehta AVB et al: Ventricular septal defect in the first year of life. Am J Cardiol 1992;70:364.

PATENT DUCTUS ARTERIOSUS

 ESSENTIALS OF DIAGNOSIS

- *Older patients with a small or moderately large patent ductus are asymptomatic and have a continuous murmur over the pulmonary area, loud S₂, and bounding peripheral pulses.*
- *Poor feeding, respiratory distress, and frequent respiratory infections in infants with heart failure.*

- *Murmur usually systolic, sometimes continuous.*
- *Widened pulse pressure.*

General Considerations

The ductus arteriosus is a normal component of fetal circulation, connecting the main or proximal left pulmonary artery to the aorta distal to the origin of the left subclavian artery. Elevated pulmonary vascular resistance in utero leads to the majority of flow being directed from the pulmonary artery to the aorta (right-to-left shunt), with the ductus carrying over 60% of the combined ventricular output. In utero, patency is maintained by high flow, prostaglandins (derived from the placenta), and relatively low arterial oxygen tension. In addition to diminished sensitivity to these factors as term approaches, three important events occur at birth: (1) Pulmonary resistance decreases, leading to increased pulmonary flow and decreased ductal flow; (2) the level of prostaglandin decreases as the child is removed from the placenta and increased metabolism occurs with increased flow through the lungs; and (3) the arterial oxygen tension increases. This leads to contraction of smooth muscle in the wall of the ductus with apposition of endothelial cushions (usually within 24 hours) and eventually anatomic closure (2–3 days).

For unknown reasons, closure does not always occur. The incidence of patent ductus is estimated at 2–3% of live births. The incidence increases with the degree of prematurity and may exceed 50% in infants born at 30 weeks of gestation or less. If the ductus remains open and pulmonary vascular resistance decreases, pulmonary blood flow will increase, leading to heart failure and pulmonary congestion. Patent ductus arteriosus also occurs in the context of other cardiac anomalies and may be the critical source of flow from the heart to the lungs or systemic organs.

Clinical Findings

Diagnosis is made by physical examination (wide pulse pressure, to-and-fro murmur) and confirmed by echocardiography. Approximately 5% of full-term infants with untreated patent ductus arteriosus die from heart failure and pulmonary complications in the first year of life. Another 5% have large shunts and ultimately develop pulmonary vascular disease. The remainder are usually asymptomatic, and the ductus is detected during routine examination. In the premature infant, clinical findings of heart failure must be delineated in the context of baseline pulmonary dysfunction of prematurity. Although a murmur is usually present, a widely patent ductus may be associated with minimal turbulence. Inability to wean from mechanical ventilation is

a recognized presentation. Echocardiography is diagnostic and has been applied routinely in some centers for the high-risk patient.

Treatment

Optimal treatment depends on the age of the patient. Medical therapy is usually attempted first in the premature infant using indomethacin, a prostaglandin inhibitor, and is successful in over 50% of patients. Effectiveness diminishes with age and gestational maturity. For the term infant or older child or for the premature infant failing medical therapy, optimal treatment consists of surgical obliteration by ligation, clipping, or division through a left thoracotomy. Video thoracoscopic techniques have also been described for larger infants and children. Transcatheter techniques to place occluding devices are also available for the larger patient. Intermediate-term data have not revealed a significant advantage of catheter-based techniques in terms of cost, effectiveness, or morbidity. More recent data may demonstrate higher success rates and fewer complications.

Prognosis

Operative mortality approaches zero, with recurrence of less than 1% in surgically treated cases. Complications such as injury to the recurrent laryngeal nerve, hemorrhage, and chylothorax are uncommon.

Backer CL et al: Congenital Heart Surgery Nomenclature and Database Project: patent ductus arteriosus, coarctation of the aorta, interrupted aortic arch. Ann Thorac Surg 2000; 69:S298.

Hawkins JA et al: Cost and efficacy of surgical ligation versus transcatheter coil occlusion of patent ductus arteriosus. J Thorac Cardiovasc Surg 1996;112:1634.

Laborde F et al: A new video-assisted thoracoscopic surgical technique for interruption of patent ductus arteriosus in infants and children. J Thorac Cardiovasc Surg 1993;105:278.

Mavroudis C et al: Forty-six years of patent ductus arteriosus division at Children's Memorial Hospital of Chicago. Standards for comparison. Ann Surg 1994;220:402.

AORTOPULMONARY WINDOW

Defined as a connection between the ascending aorta and the main pulmonary artery, aortopulmonary window is a rare anomaly, producing a left-to-right shunt and physical findings very similar to those of patent ductus arteriosus. Patients develop heart failure early and are prone to develop pulmonary vascular disease at an early age. Associated anomalies occur in over 50% of patients (atrial and ventricular septal defect, interrupted aortic arch). Once diagnosed, the window should be closed with a patch (synthetic or pericardial) during cardiopulmonary bypass.

McElhinney DB et al: Early and late results after repair of aortopulmonary septal defect and associated anomalies in infants < 6 months of age. Am J Cardiol 1998;81:195.

Jacobs JP et al: Congenital Heart Surgery Nomenclature and Database Project: aortopulmonary window. Ann Thorac Surg 2000;69:S44.

RUPTURED SINUS OF VALSALVA

Rupture of the thin membranous tissue between the aortic sinus of Valsalva and an intracardiac chamber causes an immediate left-to-right shunt. The murmur is usually well localized, parasternal, and continuous, with associated thrill. Most patients rapidly develop heart failure. Rupture is more common in patients with Marfan's syndrome or other autoimmune disorders. Rupture is into the right ventricle in about 70% of cases and into the right atrium in 20%. Precise anatomic diagnosis is by cardiac catheterization and echocardiography. Early operation is indicated.

Barragry TP et al: 15-30 year follow-up of patients undergoing repair of ruptured congenital aneurysms of the sinus of Valsalva. Ann Thorac Surg 1988;46:515.

Mayer ED et al: Ruptured aneurysms of the sinus of Valsalva. Ann Thorac Surg 1986;42:81.

LEFT VENTRICULAR–RIGHT ATRIAL SHUNT

A left ventricular–right atrial shunt is produced by a defect in the membranous septum near the annulus of the septal leaflet of the tricuspid valve or by a perforation or cleft of the septal leaflet. The lesion is uncommon, and the size of the shunt is variable. Symptoms of heart failure may be present in infancy or may not develop until late childhood. The systolic murmur is not diagnostic. At cardiac catheterization, blood oxygen saturation is increased in the right atrium, and on cineangiocardiograms the right atrium opacifies after injection of contrast material into the left ventricle. In symptomatic patients, the defect is closed by direct sutures from the right atrium during cardiopulmonary bypass. The operative death rate is low.

CORONARY ARTERIAL FISTULA

A fistulous communication between the right (60%) or left (40%) coronary artery and the right ventricle (90%), right atrium, or coronary sinus produces a left-to-right shunt and increased pulmonary blood flow. The involved coronary vessels are dilated, and the fistulous openings may be multiple. Many patients are asymptomatic; some develop evidence of myocardial ischemia, and others have some degree of heart failure. A continuous murmur is usually present over the heart. Angiograms are required to determine the number and location of the fistulas. The fistulous connections are ligated at operation without interrupting the coronary artery. Cardiopulmonary bypass is often required. Operative mortality is rare.

Mavroudis C et al: Coronary artery fistulas in infants and children: a surgical review and discussion of coil embolization. Ann Thorac Surg 1997;63:1235.

TOTAL ANOMALOUS PULMONARY VENOUS CONNECTION (TAPVC)

 ESSENTIALS OF DIAGNOSIS

- *Pulmonary congestion, tachypnea, cardiac failure, and variable cyanosis.*
- *Severe heart failure, cyanosis, poor pulses, acidosis in infants.*
- *Pulmonary midsystolic murmur present, with loud, fixed splitting of S_2 in some patients.*
- *Enlargement of right atrium and ventricle with severe pulmonary vascular congestion.*
- *Blood oxygen saturation similar in aorta and pulmonary artery.*
- *Pulmonary arterial and wedge pressures often elevated.*

General Considerations

The term total anomalous pulmonary venous connection (TAPVC) indicates that the pulmonary veins do not make a direct connection with the left atrium. Individual veins usually form a confluence that connects to central systemic veins, thereby draining pulmonary flow to the right atrium. The blood reaches the left atrium only through an atrial septal defect or patent foramen ovale. Mixing of blood in the right atrium leads to similar oxygen saturations in the aorta and pulmonary artery. There are three basic types of total anomalous venous return (Figure 20–30) depending on the site at which the confluence of pulmonary veins connects to the systemic venous system: (1) supracardiac (type 1)—connection to a usually left-sided vertical vein draining to the innominate vein (45%); (2) cardiac (type 2)—connection to the right atrium or coronary sinus (25%); and (3) infracardiac (type 3)—

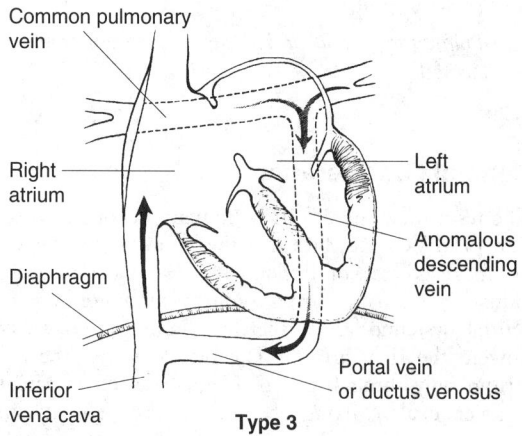

Figure 20–30. Common types of total anomalous pulmonary venous connection. ***Type 1:*** The pulmonary veins connect to a persistent left vertical vein, the innominate vein, and the right superior vena cava. ***Type 2:*** The pulmonary veins connect to the coronary sinus and the right atrium. ***Type 3:*** The pulmonary veins connect to an anomalous descending vein, a portal vein or persistent ductus venosus, and eventually the inferior vena cava.

connection to the infradiaphragmatic cava or portal vein (25%). In approximately 5% of cases venous drainage is mixed, with different pulmonary veins draining to different systemic veins. Pulmonary venous obstruction may occur with all types of drainage patterns; however, it occurs in less than 25% of patients with a supracardiac connection and in nearly all patients with an infracardiac connection. The presence of obstruction often leads to elevated pulmonary vascular resistance and is a decisive point in devising a management plan.

Clinical Findings

The presence and degree of obstruction determine the clinical presentation. If obstruction is absent, symptoms relate to the degree of pulmonary overcirculation and hypertension (poor feeding, failure to thrive, tachypnea, diaphoresis). If obstruction is severe, profound cyanosis, respiratory failure, and hypotension will develop in a few hours after birth. Echocardiography is diagnostic. Catheterization is reserved for cases in which anatomy is unclear after echocardiography or in which balloon septostomy is believed necessary to improve atrial mixing.

Treatment

All forms of TAPVC should be surgically repaired. Timing is dictated by the degree of obstruction. In fact, obstructed TAPVC is one of the few remaining surgical emergencies in pediatric cardiac surgery. Other than intubation and resuscitation, there is no indicated medical therapy. Repair of supracardiac and infracardiac drainage is accomplished by anastomosis of the pulmonary venous confluence to the left atrium and ligation of the connection to the systemic vein. Cardiopulmonary bypass or, less frequently, deep hypothermic circulatory arrest is employed for critically ill neonates with obstruction. For TAPVC with cardiac drainage, repair can be accomplished (on cardiopulmonary bypass) by unroofing the coronary sinus and patch closure of the atrial septum, leaving the coronary sinus to drain to the left atrium. After repair of obstructed TAPVC, measures are employed (alkalosis, increased oxygen tension, sedation, deep analgesia) to prevent or treat pulmonary artery hypertensive crises.

Prognosis

Hospital mortality is limited primarily to children with severe obstruction (10–15%). Pulmonary hypertension contributes substantially to this mortality. Although very uncommon, children with associated cardiac anomalies experience an exceptionally high mortality

(> 30%). Recurrence of pulmonary obstruction occurs in approximately 5–10% of patients. As this form of obstruction typically does not occur at the anastomosis, it is believed to be due to an intrinsic abnormality of the veins or to surgical trauma at the time of repair. Patients who survive without recurrent obstruction have good cardiac performance, minimal symptoms, and a good long-term prognosis.

Calderone CA et al: Surgical management of total anomalous pulmonary venous drainage: impact of coexisting cardiac anomalies. Ann Thorac Surg 1998;66:1521.

Cobanaglu A et al: Total anomalous pulmonary venous connection in neonates and young infants: repair in the current era. Ann Thorac Surg 1993;55:43.

Lacour-Gayet F et al: Surgical management of progressive pulmonary venous obstruction after repair of total anomalous pulmonary venous connection. J Thorac Cardiovasc Surg 1999;117:679.

TRUNCUS ARTERIOSUS

In truncus arteriosus, a single large truncal vessel overrides the ventricular septum and distributes all of the blood ejected from the heart. Although different patterns exist, the truncal root bifurcates, giving rise to a pulmonary trunk or separate pulmonary arteries and the aorta. A ventricular septal defect is present and is usually located directly beneath the truncal valve. Other associated anomalies include atrial septal defect (> 40%), interrupted aortic arch (10%), and abnormal origins of the coronary arteries. In most cases, pulmonary blood flow is increased and signs and symptoms of heart failure are present. Patients develop pulmonary vascular disease at a very early age. Echocardiography is usually sufficient for diagnosis; however, cardiac catheterization is indicated if there are abnormalities of the coronary arteries or truncal valve or if the child is over 3 months of age (to assess pulmonary vasculature).

Surgical correction is indicated once the diagnosis is confirmed. The only contraindication to surgery is Eisenmenger's physiology. The principles of repair include closure of the ventricular septal defect, separation of the pulmonary arteries from the truncal root, placing a valved conduit (pulmonary allograft) from the right ventricle to the pulmonary arteries, and correction of significant truncal insufficiency (Figure 20–31). Mortality is variable (5–30%), related to truncal valve insufficiency, interrupted arch, coronary anomalies, and pul-

Figure 20–31. Type 1 truncus arteriosus. **A:** The main pulmonary artery arises from the truncus arteriosus downstream to the truncal semilunar valve. A ventricular septal defect is always present. **B:** The main pulmonary artery is incised from the truncus. The ventricular septal defect is closed with a patch. A conduit of Dacron that contains a homograft aortic valve is sutured to the anterior wall of the right ventricle and the distal pulmonary artery. A conduit between the right ventricle and pulmonary artery was successfully introduced by J.W. Kirklin in 1964 during correction of severe tetralogy of Fallot.

monary vascular disease. Survivors remain at risk for the subsequent need for repair or replacement of the truncal valve and replacement of the right ventricle–pulmonary artery conduit.

Bove EL et al: Repair of truncus arteriosus in the neonate and young infant. Ann Thorac Surg 1989;47:499.

Imamura M et al: Improving early and intermediate results of truncus arteriosus repair: a new technique of truncal valve repair. Ann Thorac Surg 1999;67:1142.

Jacobs ML. Congenital Heart Surgery Nomenclature and Database Project: truncus arteriosus. Ann Thorac Surg 2000;69:S50.

Jahangiri M et al: Repair of the truncal valve and associated interrupted arch in neonates with truncus arteriosus. J Thorac Cardiovasc Surg 2000;119:508.

Rajasinghe HA et al: Long-term follow-up of truncus arteriosus repaired in infancy: a twenty-year experience. J Thorac Cardiovasc Surg 1997;113:869.

■ CONGENITAL HEART LESIONS THAT DECREASE PULMONARY ARTERIAL BLOOD FLOW

Decreased pulmonary blood flow secondary to a primary structural anomaly is more commonly due to obstructive lesions in the right heart or pulmonary artery. A classic example is tetralogy of Fallot, consisting of obstruction in the right ventricular outflow tract (infundibulum), a ventricular septal defect, right ventricular hypertrophy, and an overriding or dextroposed aorta. A variety of exceptions exist, however. For example, with transposition of the great arteries, in which the aorta arises from the right ventricle and the pulmonary artery arises from the left ventricle, pulmonary flow can be markedly reduced despite the absence of formal obstruction. Whatever the arrangement, the basic pathophysiology is that of a right-to-left shunt. Systemic return shunted to the systemic output does not circulate through the lungs, resulting in cyanosis and decreased oxygen delivery to the tissues. The degree of cyanosis is directly proportionate to the amount of the right-to-left shunt and inversely proportionate to the amount of pulmonary arterial blood flow.

Severe cyanosis stimulates red cell production, which increases the concentration of hemoglobin. This compensatory mechanism increases systemic oxygen delivery simply by increasing the amount of oxygen per unit volume of blood. The hematocrit may increase substantially (to > 70%), in which case the compensatory effects are offset by the risk of decreased flow secondary to increased viscosity and the risk of spontaneous thrombosis.

Variable cyanosis, hypoxic spells, squatting, and clubbing are frequently associated with lesions that reduce pulmonary blood flow. Several factors may alter the degree of cyanosis by altering the ratio of pulmonary and systemic resistances (exercise, acidosis, pain, and the catecholamine response decrease pulmonary blood flow).

Hypoxic spells indicate severe cerebral hypoxia and are due to acute reduction of pulmonary blood flow. The classic example is spasm of the infundibular muscle in tetralogy of Fallot, which can occur without warning. Infants and young children become unconscious for varying periods of time and occasionally die. Simple measures such as placing the child in the knee-chest position with the head down (mimics squatting, which increases pulmonary flow by increasing systemic resistance) may help. However, medical therapy may be required to reduce spasm (beta blockade), increase circulating blood volume and oxygen content (fluid and supplemental oxygen; mechanical ventilation), decrease acidosis (bicarbonate), and increase systemic resistance (norepinephrine). The phenomenon of clubbing of the fingers and toes develops in late infancy and early childhood and is due to proliferation of capillaries and small arteriovenous fistulas in the distal phalanges.

Reduced pulmonary arterial blood flow stimulates enlargement of bronchial and mediastinal arteries. These vessels connect with pulmonary arteries and, in some cases, may provide most of the pulmonary blood flow. At birth, the ductus arteriosus is patent and provides substantial flow to the pulmonary arteries of patients with obstructive right heart lesions. Unfortunately, the ductus nearly always closes during the first few hours or days after birth. The intravenous administration of alprostadil will maintain patency of the ductus for hours or days in some infants, thus allowing reversal of acidosis, reduction of cyanosis, and stabilization of the infant prior to definitive therapy.

Several palliative operations that shunt blood from the systemic to the pulmonary arterial circulation have been devised for infants and young children who have insufficient pulmonary arterial blood flow. The Blalock-Taussig operation connects the subclavian artery to the ipsilateral pulmonary artery with an end-to-side anastomosis (Figure 20–32A). The modified Blalock-Taussig shunt interposes a tube graft (3.5–6 mm), usually of polytetrafluoroethylene (Gore-Tex), between the subclavian or innominate artery and the ipsilateral pulmonary artery. The Waterston aortic to right pulmonary arterial anastomosis connects the posterior portion of the ascending aorta to the anterior wall of the right pulmonary artery (Figure 20–32B). The Potts anastomosis joins the left pulmonary artery and the descending thoracic aorta by a side-to-side anastomosis (Figure 20–32C). The Waterston and Potts aortopulmonary shunts are of mostly historical interest because

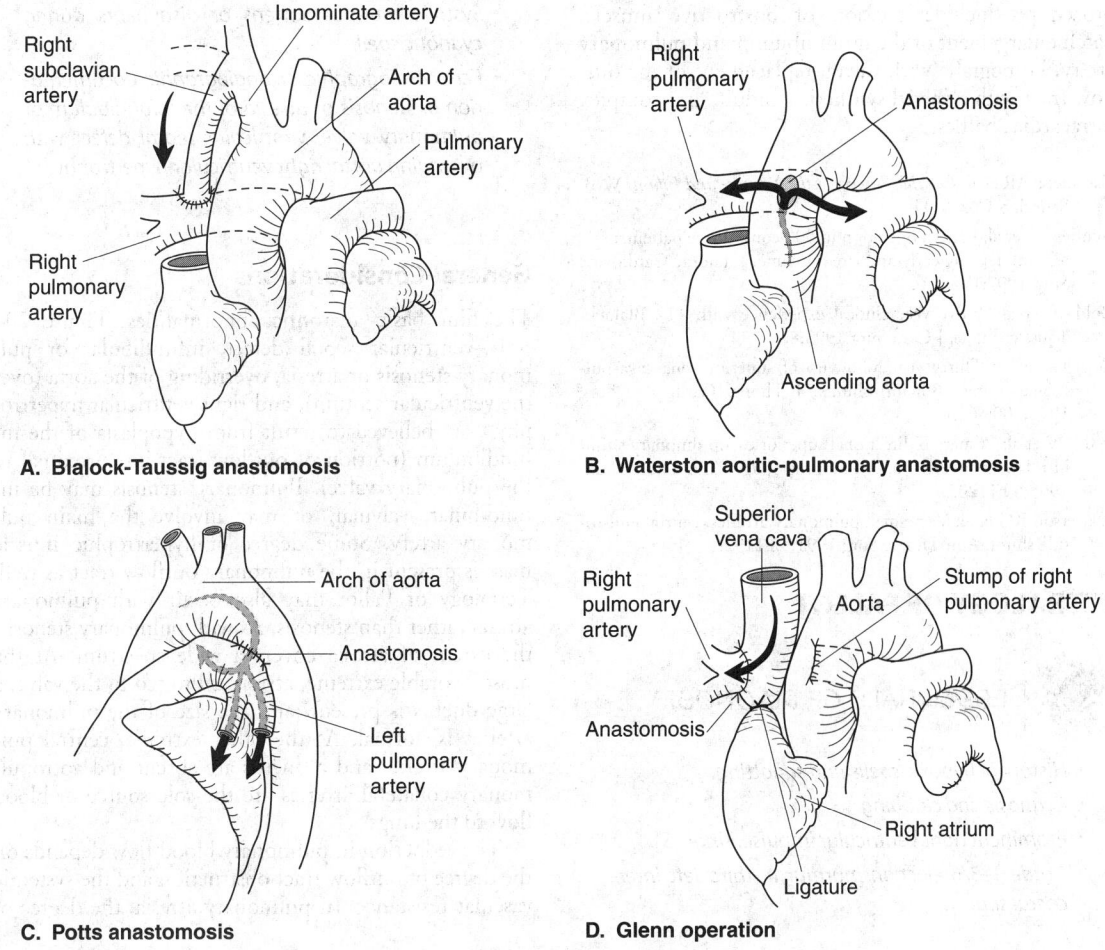

A. Blalock-Taussig anastomosis

B. Waterston aortic-pulmonary anastomosis

C. Potts anastomosis

D. Glenn operation

Figure 20–32. Palliative operations to increase pulmonary arterial blood flow. ***A:*** Blalock-Taussig subclavian-pulmonary arterial anastomosis. ***B:*** Waterston aortic to right pulmonary arterial anastomosis. ***C:*** Potts anastomosis between the left pulmonary artery and the descending thoracic aorta. ***D:*** The Glenn operation. The end of the right pulmonary artery is connected to the side of the superior vena cava, which is ligated caudad to the anastomosis.

of the difficulty of regulating flow through the shunt and the complexity of shunt take-down at the time of later correction.

Another category of options is to bypass the obstruction in the right heart by diverting part of or all the systemic venous return to the pulmonary circulation. Various connections or procedures have been described. The classic Glenn operation (Figure 20–32D) connects the superior vena cava to the right pulmonary artery in such a way that superior vena caval blood must enter the right pulmonary artery exclusively. The bidirectional Glenn operation connects the superior vena cava end-to-side to the top of the pulmonary artery, allowing flow to both lungs. Complete diversion is provided by the Fontan

procedure, in which both superior and inferior caval return are routed to the pulmonary artery. Because complete diversion is typically staged (Fontan performed a few months after the bidirectional Glenn), the modified Fontan procedure employed in recent practice refers to a variety of connections that may be used to divert flow from the inferior vena cava to the pulmonary artery. These include an intra-atrial tunnel (partial tube graft), an extracardiac tube-graft connection between the cava and pulmonary artery (with atrial disconnection oversewn), or an extracardiac pericardial connection.

A final category of surgical therapy includes various procedures that attempt to directly relieve the obstruction and reconstruct the right heart outflow tract. Such procedures include excision of obstructive muscle, patch enlargement of the infundibulum and pulmonary artery, homograft (with valve), replacement of the outflow tract with a valved synthetic conduit, and complex intracardiac baffles.

Castaneda AR et al: *Cardiac Surgery of the Neonate and Infant.* W.B. Saunders Co., 1994.

Gentles TL et al: Fontan operation in 500 consecutive patients: factors influencing early and late outcome. J Thorac Cardiovasc Surg 1997;114:376.

Gold JP et al: A five year clinical experience with 112 Blalock-Taussig shunts. J Card Surg 1993;8:9.

Kopf GS et al: Thirty year follow-up of superior vena cava-pulmonary artery (Glenn) shunts. J Thorac Cardiovasc Surg 1990;100:662.

Reddy V et al: Primary bidirectional superior cavopulmonary shunt in infants between 1 and 4 months of age. Ann Thorac Surg 1995;59:1120.

Watterson KG et al: Very small pulmonary arteries: central end-to-side shunt. Ann Thorac Surg 1991;52:1132.

TETRALOGY OF FALLOT

ESSENTIALS OF DIAGNOSIS

- *History of hypoxic spells and squatting.*
- *Cyanosis and clubbing.*
- *Prominent right ventricular impulse, single S_2.*
- *Grade 1–3/6 ejection murmur in third left intercostal space.*
- *Systolic murmur softens or disappears during cyanotic spell.*
- *Echocardiographic or angiographic documentation of stenosis or atresia of the infundibulum or pulmonary valve; ventricular septal defect with overriding aorta; right ventricular hypertrophy.*

General Considerations

The four basic anatomic abnormalities (Figure 20–33)—ventricular septal defect, infundibular or pulmonary stenosis or atresia, overriding of the aorta (over the ventricular septum), and right ventricular hypertrophy—are believed to result from hypoplasia of the infundibulum (portion of outflow tract just proximal to the pulmonary valve). Pulmonary stenosis may be infundibular, valvular, or may involve the main pulmonary artery. Some degree of hypertrophic muscle mass is present in the pulmonary outflow tract as well. Tetralogy of Fallot may also occur with pulmonary atresia rather than stenosis. As with pulmonary stenosis, the extent of atresia covers a wide spectrum. At the most favorable extreme, atresia is limited to the valve, a large ductus is present, and the size of the pulmonary arteries is normal. At the other extreme, central pulmonary arteries and a ductus are absent and aortopulmonary collateral arteries are the sole source of blood flow to the lungs.

The reduction in pulmonary blood flow depends on the degree of outflow tract obstruction and the systemic vascular resistance. In pulmonary atresia, the degree of

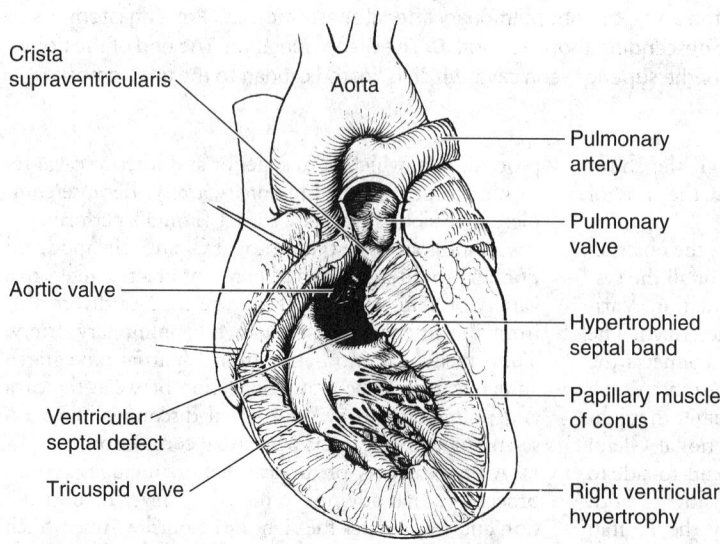

Figure 20–33. Tetralogy of Fallot. The aorta overrides the ventricular septum. A large ventricular septal defect is present, and the hypoplastic infundibulum with hypertrophied parietal and septal muscle bands obstructs blood to the pulmonary arteries.

pulmonary blood flow depends on the presence of normal pulmonary arteries and the extent of aortopulmonary collateral arteries and the degree of stenosis present in those vessels. In fact, extensive unobstructed aortopulmonary collateral arteries may lead to excessive pulmonary blood flow and congestive failure.

Clinical Findings

Symptoms are directly related to the amount of pulmonary blood flow. A patent ductus may mask the lesion and its symptoms in the early days of life. However, with ductal closure, severe pulmonary stenosis in the neonate causes severe cyanosis and acidosis. A systolic murmur is due to the pulmonary stenosis and is heard along the left sternal border. The hypoxic or cyanotic spell is the most serious symptom since it can result in cerebral hypoxia, brain injury, and even death. The diagnosis can usually be made from the cyanosis, small heart size, and diminished pulmonary blood flow seen on the chest radiograph. The ECG shows right ventricular hypertrophy. Echocardiography is usually sufficient to confirm the diagnosis. Cardiac catheterization is necessary in most forms of pulmonary atresia to define the presence and size of central pulmonary arteries (sometimes not possible) and to define the anatomy of aortopulmonary collateral arteries. One aspect of diagnosis is predicting the postrepair capability of the pulmonary vasculature to accommodate the cardiac output. If the vasculature is inadequate and the ventricular septal defect is closed, right heart failure will ensue. Various predictive parameters with variable clinical utility have been described. The McGoon ratio is the combined diameter of pulmonary arteries normalized to the diameter of the descending aorta, an acceptable value being greater than 2.0. The Nakata index is the sum of the cross-sectional areas of the right and left pulmonary arteries normalized to body surface area. Normal values exceed 300 mm_2/m_2; values less than 150 mm_2/m_2 indicate extremely small pulmonary arteries. Another estimate is provided by the normalized pulmonary annulus diameter. Values less than 2 SD below normal warrant concern.

Treatment

In general, most patients are symptomatic at the time of diagnosis, and the diagnosis is therefore an indication for repair. One-stage correction is recommended by many surgeons. This entails cardiopulmonary bypass and patch closure of the ventricular septal defect through the right atrium; a small incision in the infundibulum or proximal main pulmonary artery to resect obstructive muscle (if present); and placement of a patch (pericardium or Gore-Tex) in the infundibulum or artery to widen the outflow tract. In cases in which

patch enlargement of the infundibulum is not needed, the repair can be done entirely through the atrium. In other cases it may be necessary to extend the incision and patch insertion across the annulus. The resultant pulmonary insufficiency is usually well tolerated in the child for several years; however, untoward effects of long-standing insufficiency are just beginning to be realized in adult survivors. There are currently no ideal methods to deal with this problem at the time of initial repair. A large ventriculotomy, though, is rarely necessary, can significantly impair ventricular function, and thus should be avoided.

The palliative approach entails initial placement of a systemic to pulmonary artery shunt followed by correction (as described above) at a later age. Proponents acknowledge a lower operative mortality in the larger child as well as growth of the pulmonary vasculature induced by the shunt, thereby lowering the risk of postrepair pulmonary hypertension and right ventricular dysfunction.

Initial correction avoids the need for two operations, each with attendant risks, and eliminates the risks associated with the pathophysiology of the anomaly. However, prudent selection of therapy must consider the anatomy of the child and not be based solely on a single technique. For example, the child with pulmonary stenosis and diminutive pulmonary arteries will benefit from a modified approach that induces growth of the vasculature (reconstruction of outflow tract and shunt) yet minimizes relevant risk (such as closure of the septal defect).

Repair of tetralogy of Fallot with pulmonary atresia may also be accomplished with a single procedure or with staged procedures, depending on the degree of development of the central pulmonary vasculature and the complexity of the aortopulmonary collateral artery anatomy. Unifocalization is a term describing the process of disconnecting the collateral arteries from the aorta and joining or focalizing them to a tube of Gore-Tex or one reconstructed from pericardium. This tube (usually one on each side) may then be connected to a reconstructed right heart outflow tract if the pulmonary vasculature is deemed adequate. Alternatively, it may be connected to a systemic shunt to induce growth of the pulmonary vasculature. Closure of the ventricular septal defect is done either at a time when the pulmonary vasculature has undergone enough growth or when enough pulmonary segments have been unifocalized to allow a sufficiently low pulmonary vascular resistance (usually the equivalent of at least one lung). Some surgeons advocate repairing the septal defect with a perforated patch to allow unloading of the right heart and the ability to close the defect percutaneously with a device at a later time. This means that eventual repair of the complex case may require at least three major surgical procedures.

Prognosis

After surgery, patients with tetralogy of Fallot usually have some degree of right ventricular dysfunction due to operative trauma and the newly imposed increased volume work of the ventricle. Judicious medical management is usually successful, however. In general, mortality is less than 5% in tetralogy with stenosis and may exceed 30–45% in tetralogy with atresia. Subsequent need for reoperation on the outflow tract occurs in approximately 10–15% of patients at 10-year follow-up. Those patients reaching adulthood enjoy normal lives: More than 90% are regularly employed in all types of work; over 50% regularly participate in athletics; and less than 20% require cardiac medications. The incidence of late right ventricular dysfunction and the need for late pulmonary valve replacement is just now being recognized. A definitive statement awaits further studies and follow-up.

Di-Donato RM et al: Neonatal repair of tetralogy of Fallot with and without pulmonary atresia. J Thorac Cardiovasc Surg 1991;101:126.

Discigil B et al: Late pulmonary valve replacement after repair of tetralogy of Fallot. J Thorac Cardiovasc Surg 2001; 121:344.

Fraser CD et al: Tetralogy of Fallot: surgical management individualized to the patient. Ann Thorac Surg 2001;71:1556.

Groh MA et al: Repair of tetralogy of Fallot in infancy. Effect of pulmonary artery size on outcome. Circulation 1991;84 (5 Suppl):III206.

Karl TR et al: Tetralogy of Fallot: favorable outcome of nonneonatal transatrial, transpulmonary repair. Ann Thorac Surg 1992; 54:903.

Kirklin JW et al: Morphologic and surgical determinants of outcome events after repair of tetralogy of Fallot and pulmonary stenosis. A two institution study. J Thorac Cardiovasc Surg 1992;103:692.

Knott-Craig CJ et al: A 26-year experience with surgical management of tetralogy of Fallot: risk analysis for mortality or late reintervention. Ann Thorac Surg 1998;66:506.

Lillehei CW et al: The first open heart corrections of tetralogy of Fallot: a 26-31 year follow-up of 106 patients. Ann Surg 1986;204:490.

Norgaard MA et al: Twenty-to-thirty-seven-year follow-up after repair for tetralogy of Fallot. Eur J Cardiothorac Surg 1999; 16:125.

Pagani FD et al: The management of tetralogy of Fallot with pulmonary atresia and diminutive pulmonary arteries. J Thorac Cardiovasc Surg 1995;110:1521.

PULMONARY ATRESIA WITH INTACT VENTRICULAR SEPTUM

In pulmonary atresia with intact ventricular septum, the normally patent pulmonary valve is replaced by a diaphragm or dome of tissue that completely obstructs flow into the pulmonary artery (typically normal size). Since there is no ventricular septal defect, an atrial septal defect and patent ductus arteriosus are necessary for survival beyond the first few hours after birth. The right ventricle may be of normal size but is typically rudimentary, with the cavity obliterated by thickened muscle. Tricuspid annular size is also typically reduced and correlates with the size of the right ventricular cavity. An important associated finding in a significant number of patients is the presence of right ventricular-to-coronary artery fistulas and stenoses of coronary arteries. In fact, the suprasystemic pressure of the right ventricle may be the sole driving force for coronary flow to a major portion of the myocardium.

Cyanosis is usually present at birth. With ductal closure, the child becomes profoundly hypoxic and acidotic and will not survive unless flow is established through the ductus. The ECG shows a relative lack of normal right ventricular dominance. The chest radiograph reveals diminished flow. Diagnosis is confirmed by echocardiography. Cardiac catheterization is usually performed after the child is resuscitated to define the coronary anatomy and assess the probability of a right ventricular dependent coronary circulation.

Optimal surgical therapy depends on the degree of development of the right ventricle. Criteria to guide this decision remain inexact. In general, the procedure entails a systemic-to-pulmonary artery shunt and patch reconstruction of the right heart outflow tract. In cases in which the ventricle is deemed inadequate, a shunt alone is performed. If there is right ventricular dependent coronary circulation, the right ventricle must not be decompressed (only a shunt should be performed), as this would lead to profound myocardial ischemia. Ultimately, if growth of the ventricle and the pulmonary vasculature is adequate, the shunt can be occluded and the atrial septal defect closed, thereby establishing a two-ventricle circulation. If this is not the case, management proceeds along a single-ventricle pathway (eg, Fontan). Although the prognosis for these children is improving, 1-year mortality is in the range of 10–20% in most centers.

Bull C et al: Outcome measures for the neonatal management of pulmonary atresia with intact ventricular septum. J Thorac Cardiovasc Surg 1994;107:359.

Hawkins JA et al: Early and late results in pulmonary atresia, and intact ventricular septum. J Thorac Cardiovasc Surg 1990; 100:492.

Jahangiri M et al: Improved results with selective management in pulmonary atresia with intact ventricular septum. J Thorac Cardiovasc Surg 1999;118:1046.

Rychik J et al: Outcome after operations for pulmonary atresia with intact ventricular septum. J Thorac Cardiovasc Surg 1998; 116:924.

TRICUSPID ATRESIA

Tricuspid atresia is defined by a lack of communication between the right atrium and right ventricle. The ventricular cavity is small. A ventricular septal defect, usually restrictive to flow, connects the ventricles. An interatrial communication is invariably present. The relationship of the great arteries and their connections to the ventricles is abnormal in approximately 30% of patients. This relationship—as well as the degree of obstruction of pulmonary blood flow—provides the basis for classifying subtypes of tricuspid atresia.

A reciprocal relationship exists between the degree of obstruction to systemic and pulmonary blood flow. The clinical presentation can vary depending on the arrangement of the great vessels and the degree of restriction of the atrial and ventricular septal defects. The majority of infants suffer from some degree of reduced pulmonary blood flow and cyanosis and have no obstruction to systemic output. Diagnosis is confirmed by echocardiography; however, cardiac catheterization is often performed to determine the suitability for repair and, in cases with a restrictive atrial septal defect, to perform balloon septoplasty.

In most children, a modified Blalock-Taussig shunt is performed initially to provide adequate balanced pulmonary blood flow. A bidirectional Glenn procedure, followed later by a Fontan (modified) procedure, complete the staged repair. The underlying philosophy is to provide adequate but not excessive pulmonary blood flow and to minimize volume overload of the ventricle and the risk of developing pulmonary vascular disease. This is done by changing the source of pulmonary blood flow from arterial to venous in successive stages (Glenn and subsequent Fontan).

Castaneda AR: From Glenn to Fontan: a continuing evolution. Circulation 1992;86(5 Suppl):II80.

Cleveland DC et al: Surgical treatment of tricuspid atresia. Ann Thorac Surg 1984;38:447.

deLeval MR et al: Total cavopulmonary connection: a logical alternative to atriopulmonary connection for complex Fontan operations. J Thorac Cardiovasc Surg 1988;96:682.

Fontan F et al: Surgical repair of tricuspid atresia. Thorax 1971; 26:240.

Franklin RC et al: Tricuspid atresia presenting in infancy: survival and suitability for the Fontan operation. Circulation 1993; 87:427.

Jacobs ML et al: Fontan operation: influence of modifications on morbidity and mortality. Ann Thorac Surg 1994;58:945.

EBSTEIN'S ANOMALY

In this malformation, the septal and posterior leaflets of the tricuspid valve are small and deformed and usually displaced toward the right ventricular apex. A large portion of the right ventricle is quite thin and hypoplastic and becomes atrialized. Most patients have an associated atrial septal defect or patent foramen ovale. Cyanosis and arrhythmias in infancy are common. About half of these patients develop right heart failure, some degree of systemic desaturation, hepatomegaly, and dysrhythmias. Operative repair of this lesion without tricuspid valve replacement has been encouraging in approximately half of cases. In these cases, the atrialized portion of the ventricle may be oversewn and the tricuspid valve incompetence corrected. Newer surgical therapies are being developed to provide a functioning right ventricle and tricuspid valve. In others, tricuspid valve replacement is necessary, and in some cases the anatomic deformities are so extensive that effective surgical correction is impossible.

Danielson GK et al: Operative treatment of Ebstein's anomaly. J Thorac Cardiovasc Surg 1992;104:1497.

Dearani JA et al: Congenital Heart Surgery Nomenclature and Database Project: Ebstein's anomaly and tricuspid valve disease. Ann Thorac Surg 2000;69:S106.

Gentles TL et al: Predictors of long term survival with Ebstein's anomaly of the tricuspid valve. Am J Cardiol 1992;69:377.

Knott-Craig CJ et al: Neonatal repair of Ebstein's anomaly: indications, surgical technique, and medium-term follow-up. Ann Thorac Surg 2000;69:1505.

TRANSPOSITION OF THE GREAT ARTERIES—NORMAL VENTRICULAR ARRANGEMENT (D-TRANSPOSITION)

 ESSENTIALS OF DIAGNOSIS

- *Situs solitus, levocardia.*
- *Cyanosis from birth; hypoxic spells sometimes present.*
- *Heart failure often present.*
- *Murmurs variable; often absent and not diagnostic.*
- *Cardiac enlargement and pulmonary overcirculation on x-ray.*
- *Echocardiographic confirmation of relationship of great arteries and ventricles.*

General Considerations

Probably nowhere in pediatric cardiac surgery is the terminology potentially more confusing than in descriptions of transposition. This is due to the fact that carefully developed distinct descriptive systems of embryology and anatomy and their respective terminologies have been subsequently incorporated and combined by other authors. The original systems based on concordant or discordant connections, spatial arrangements of the great vessels, or segmental anatomic descriptions remain valid. The segmental description is probably more robust and complete and can be found in standard texts of cardiac embryology. These systems are not defined here. Rather, what follows is a simple explanation to clarify current usage of terms and their relationship to clinical anomalies.

In a general theoretical sense, the great vessels can originate from the ventricles in a number of ways—normal; both great vessels arising from the right or left ventricle; both great vessels arising in an indeterminate fashion from both ventricles in the context of a ventricular septal defect; reversal of the normal arrangement with the aorta arising from the morphologic right ventricle and vice versa; and all variations on this continuum. As a separate issue, the embryologic ventricular looping may occur levo- rather than the normal dextro- (not dextrocardia, which has nothing to do with looping), giving rise to a right-sided morphologic left ventricle and a left-sided morphologic right ventricle. Even with normal ventriculo-arterial connections, the spatial arrangement of the great vessels may differ from the usual rightward posterior aorta and leftward anterior pulmonary artery.

Malposition is the correct general term for implying any abnormal spatial arrangement of the great vessels. Letter designations indicate the position of the aorta relative to the pulmonary artery: D-, to the right; L-, to the left; and A-, anterior. Letter designation does not explicitly define ventriculo-arterial connections. On the other hand, the word "transposition" means the aorta is connected to a morphologic right ventricle regardless of whether it is a right-sided or a left-sided right ventricle. Likewise, the pulmonary artery is connected to a morphologic left ventricle. The spatial relationship of the great vessels can be D-, L-, or A-. Clinically, the more common transposition abnormality consists of normally looped ventricles and a rightward anterior aorta connected to a morphologic right ventricle, hence the term "D transposition" (Figure 20–34). However, other variations of true transposition exist that are treated correctly with an arterial switch yet do not exhibit the "D-" spatial arrangement—hence the loose or incorrect usage of "D-transposition" in this context.

As noted above, the most common spatial arrangement of the great arteries is a rightward anterior aorta. A ventricular septal defect is present in approximately 20–25% of patients, occurring more frequently in the context of unusual great arterial arrangements. Left ventricular outflow tract obstruction may also occur. It

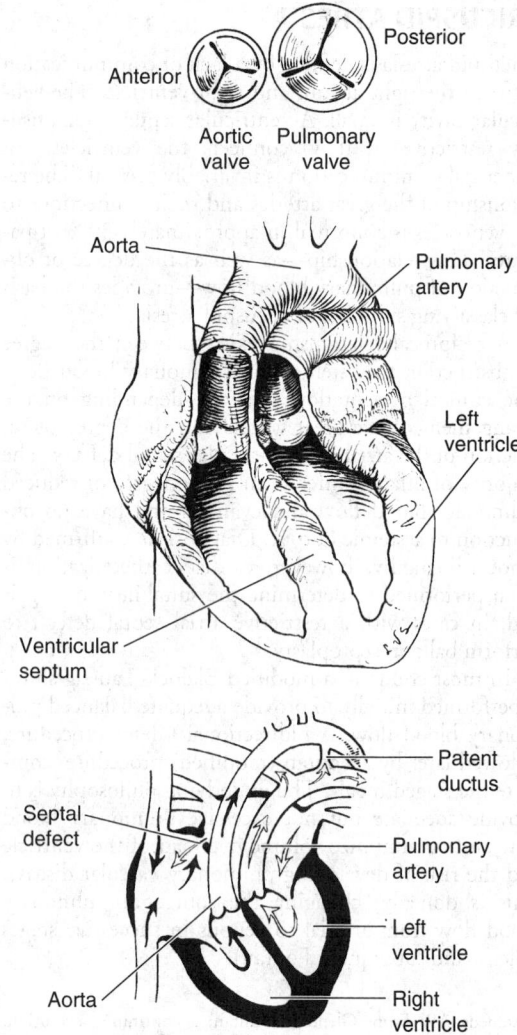

Figure 20–34. Typical transposition of the great arteries. The aorta arises from the morphologic right ventricle and is anterior to and slightly to the right of the pulmonary artery, which originates from the morphologic left ventricle. Inset at bottom illustrates the independent systemic and pulmonary circulations, which may be connected by a patent ductus arteriosus or atrial septal defect. Inset at top illustrates a common relationship of the two great arteries in typical transposition.

is more commonly dynamic in nature owing to left-ward septal displacement from higher right ventricular pressures (the systemic ventricle).

The origin and distribution of the coronary arteries are variable. Although the coronary arteries arise from the aortic sinuses facing the pulmonary artery in essentially all patients, the exact origin of the right and left arteries can vary between the two sinuses. The variant that intensifies the difficulty of the arterial switch repair is a left anterior descending artery passing between the great vessels or exhibiting a significant intramural course (passes in the wall of the aorta). In general, coronary arterial variations are more common with the side-by-side great artery arrangement and a ventricular septal defect.

The pathophysiology of transposition is related to the separation and independence of the systemic and pulmonary circulations. Some anatomic communication between the two systems must exist for the patient to survive. The common sites for mixing of blood are a ventricular septal defect, an atrial septal defect, and a patent ductus arteriosus. The degree of cyanosis is proportionate to the relative amount of oxygenated venous blood that reaches the right ventricle and aorta. In the minority of patients who have a ventricular septal defect, mixing is usually adequate; however, increased pulmonary blood flow subjects the child to the risk of rapid development of pulmonary vascular obstructive disease. Residual or induced patency of the ductus also provides good pulmonary blood flow but may lead to excessive pulmonary blood flow, pulmonary edema, and a reduced systemic output, particularly if the foramen ovale or atrial septal defect is restrictive. If mixing is inadequate or if decompression of the left atrium is needed, balloon atrial septostomy can be performed before definitive repair.

In normal development with normal anatomy, the left ventricle experiences a rapid increase in mass secondary to both volume and pressure work loads. In transposition, physiology promoting this transition is absent or directed to the right ventricle. This has relevance for timing the switch procedure, which restores normal pressure and volume loads to the left ventricle. If performed late (after 2–3 weeks of life), the risk of inadequate left ventricular adaptation may lead to failure and death.

Clinical Findings

Cyanosis is typically present at birth. Clinical deterioration occurs in 24–48 hours as the ductus closes and is manifested as worsening hypoxia and acidosis. In the child with ventricular septal defect or a large persistent ductus arteriosus, symptoms may be minimal during the first few weeks. However, with a progressive decline in pulmonary vascular resistance, signs of pulmonary overcirculation and heart failure become apparent. The ECG shows right ventricular hypertrophy and the chest radiograph reveals overcirculation and an enlarged heart. Echocardiography is usually sufficient to confirm the diagnosis as well as to demonstrate the branching pattern of the coronary arteries. Cardiac catheterization may be needed in the older infant to assess pressures and the suitability of the left ventricle for the switch procedure.

Treatment

Without treatment, about half of newborns with transposition of the great arteries die by 1 month of age and 90% die within 1 year. Repair or correction is therefore indicated. Two general types of repairs are possible. The Mustard and Senning operations create intra-atrial baffles and channels to direct the systemic venous return to the left ventricle and the pulmonary venous return to the right ventricle. This restores a series circulation and the capability to oxygenate the blood, albeit leaving the right ventricle as the systemic ventricle. Most surgeons currently advocate switching the circulation at the level of the great arteries rather than the atria. The arterial switch procedure, performed either with hypothermic low-flow cardiopulmonary bypass or with deep hypothermic circulatory arrest, disconnects the pulmonary artery and aorta and reconnects the aorta to the left ventricle and the pulmonary artery to the right ventricle (above the level of the valves). The coronary arteries are likewise transferred with the aorta. This restores a series circulation and establishes the left ventricle as the systemic ventricle.

Timing is important. The optimal sequence is prompt diagnosis, and if necessary, a balloon atrial septostomy. With stabilization of the child, the switch procedure can be performed semi-electively in the first 1-2 weeks of life. If diagnosis has occurred after this time, a two-stage approach to the switch procedure is still possible. A modified Blalock-Taussig shunt is created, and a pulmonary artery band is placed. This provides adequate pulmonary blood flow and a pressure load to acutely condition the left ventricle to function as the systemic ventricle. Approximately 1-2 weeks later, the shunt is taken down, the band removed, and the switch procedure performed. If a ventricular septal defect is present, timing is less of a concern as the left ventricle remains conditioned. The ventricular and atrial septal defects may be closed at the time of the switch procedure using standard techniques.

The Rastelli procedure is another surgical option, particularly in the context of a ventricular septal defect and left ventricular outflow tract obstruction. This entails enlargement of the ventricular septal defect and placing an intraventricular baffle between the margin of the septal defect and the aortic annulus such that the new left ventricular outflow tract is completely unobstructed. The main pulmonary artery is divided and oversewn, and an infundibulotomy is created. A pulmonary homograft is placed to connect the infundibulotomy to the distal main pulmonary artery or the bifurcation.

Prognosis

The overall results of surgery for transposition of the great arteries are excellent. In experienced centers, the switch procedure can be performed with a mortality of less than 2%. These children are truly corrected and infrequently require reintervention. Mortality and complications occur more frequently in children with left ventricular outflow tract obstruction, complicated coronary artery anatomy, and associated anomalies (eg, interrupted arch). Technical problems with the coronary transfer and coronary artery complications are a recognized contributing factor to postoperative cardiac dysfunction and death. The current experience with atrial level rearrangements is minimal. There are, however, older patients presenting with complications of the Mustard and Senning operations. Tricuspid insufficiency, atrial arrhythmias, and obstruction of the venous pathways are recognized complications. Another issue is the adult with a prior atrial level repair who presents with right ventricular failure. Criteria to direct management toward transplantation versus a double switch procedure have not been fully defined.

Alonzo-de-Begona J et al: The Mustard procedure for correction of simple transposition of the great arteries before 1 month of age. J Thorac Cardiovasc Surg 1992;104:1218.

Cochrane AD et al: Staged conversion to arterial switch for late failure of the systemic right ventricle. Ann Thorac Surg 1993; 56:854.

Ingram MT et al: Senning repair for transposition of the great arteries without patch augmentation of the septum. J Thorac Cardiovasc Surg 1988;96:485.

Kirklin JW et al: Clinical outcomes after the arterial switch operation for transposition: patient, support, procedural, and institutional risk factors. Circulation 1992;86:1501.

Kreutzer C et al: Twenty-five-year experience with Rastelli repair for transposition of the great arteries. J Thorac Cardiovasc Surg 2000;120:211.

Lupinetti FM et al: Intermediate term survival and functional results after arterial repair for transposition of the great arteries. J Thorac Cardiovasc Surg 1992;103:421.

Mee RBB: Severe right ventricular failure after Mustard or Senning operation. J Thorac Cardiovasc Surg 1986;92:385.

Turley K et al: Intermediate results from the period of the Congenital Heart Surgeons Transposition Study: 1985-1989. Congenital Heart Surgeons Society Database. Ann Thorac Surg 1995;60:505.

Wells WJ et al: Intermediate outcome after the Mustard and Senning procedures: a study by the Congenital Heart Surgeons Society. Pediatr Cardiac Surg Annu of the Semin in Thorac and Cardiovasc Surg 2000;3:186.

Wernovsky G et al: Factors influencing early and late outcome of the arterial switch operation for transposition of the great arteries. J Thorac Cardiovasc Surg 1995;109:289.

CORRECTED TRANSPOSITION OF THE GREAT ARTERIES

As noted in the previous section, commonly used transposition terminology can be confusing at times. Corrected transposition, also referred to as L-transposition, is true transposition, in that the aorta connects to a morphologic right ventricle and the pulmonary artery connects to a morphologic left ventricle. In this case, however, the ventricle has undergone leftward or levo-looping, giving rise to a right-sided morphologic left ventricle and a left-sided morphologic right ventricle. Since the aorta is commonly (though not always) to the left of the pulmonary artery, the "L-" designation is sometimes used (does not refer to the levo-ventricular loop). In this form of transposition, systemic venous blood passes through a morphologic mitral valve into a right-sided morphologic left ventricle, into the pulmonary artery and lungs, through a normal left atrium, and through a morphologic tricuspid valve into a left-sided morphologic right ventricle, to the aorta and systemic circulation. Hence, the transposition is corrected in that a series circulation which oxygenates the blood is maintained.

Associated features include a ventricular septal defect in over 75% of patients and some form of subpulmonary obstruction in less than half of patients. The coronary pattern is relatively invariant but is reversed to correspond to the ventricular arrangement. There is also a corresponding alteration of the conduction system. The conduction bundle passes on the right side of the ventricular septum (morphologically left ventricular). Rather than passing inferior to the septal defect, the conduction bundle passes superior to the defect.

Symptoms are uncommon in infancy. Congestive signs and symptoms eventually develop, however, and are often related to pulmonary stenosis and tricuspid insufficiency, which develop in a significant percentage of patients. First-, second-, or third-degree heart block is another aspect of the natural history of this disease and may be the presenting feature in infancy.

Efforts to design optimal therapy for these children are ongoing. Closure of the ventricular septal defect can be performed through the aorta or left atrium, with sutures placed on the morphologically right ventricular surface. Repair of subpulmonary obstruction remains problematic. Tricuspid insufficiency may be approached surgically through the left or right atrium, with the decision about repair or replacement based on the particular anatomy of the valve and the size of the child. The initiation of pacemaker therapy is based on standard indications. By improving the heart rate and cardiac output and lowering the ventricular volume, tricuspid function may be improved or preserved to some degree. Some surgeons advocate a double-switch procedure (atrial level and arterial level switch), typically in patients without left ventricular (subpulmonary) obstruction. Overall long-term prognosis remains inadequate, with 10-year survivals in the range of 50%.

Alva C et al: The feasibility of complete anatomical correction in the setting of discordant atrioventricular connections. Br Heart J 1999;81:539.

Karl TR et al: Senning plus arterial switch operation for discordant (congenitally corrected) transposition. Ann Thorac Surg 1997; 64:495.

Termignon J et al: "Classic" repair of congenitally corrected transposition and ventricular septal defect. Ann Thorac Surg 1996;62:199.

DOUBLE-OUTLET RIGHT VENTRICLE

In double-outlet right ventricle, both great arteries (at least 50% of the annulus of each valve) arise from the right ventricle. This is an uncommon and extremely complex anomaly with a spectrum that anatomically and clinically extends from a tetralogy-like form to a transposition-like form. Because of the rarity and complexity of this anomaly, the discussion here will be limited to brief general comments.

The location of the ventricular septal defect, which is invariably present, determines the classification. It can be subaortic, subpulmonary, noncommitted (quite proximal to the valve annuli), or doubly committed (adjacent to the annuli and flow-directed to both arteries). Subaortic obstruction occurs in approximately one-third of patients with subpulmonary defects, and subpulmonary obstruction occurs in approximately one-third of patients with subaortic defects. Great vessel arrangement and coronary artery branching can also vary. In general, a subaortic ventricular septal defect and a rightward, slightly posterior arrangement are more common. Symptoms vary depending on the location of the septal defect and the degree of outflow tract obstruction. Echocardiography is usually sufficient for diagnosis.

Optimal surgical treatment also depends on the exact anatomy. One option is the creation of an intraventricular baffle to direct left ventricular flow to the aorta in such a way as to close the septal defect and avoid subpulmonary obstruction. An arterial switch is another option if anatomy is not suitable for intraventricular baffling or for baffling combined with some type of rearrangement of the great vessels (but not switch).

Despite the complexity of this anomaly, hospital mortality is acceptably low. Ten-year survival ranges from 60% to 80%. Outflow tract reconstruction and other factors require reintervention in approximately one-third of patients.

Double outlet left ventricle is an even rarer anomaly that will not be discussed in this text.

Aoki M et al: Result of biventricular repair for double-outlet right ventricle. J Thorac Cardiovasc Surg 1994;107:338.

Musumeci F et al: Surgical treatment of double outlet right ventricle at the Brompton Hospital, 1973-1986. J Thorac Cardiovasc Surg 1988;96:278.

Planche C et al: Double-outlet right ventricle with non-committed ventricular septal defect. Eur J Cardiothorac Surg 1999; 15:747.

Serraf A et al: Anatomic repair of Taussig-Bing hearts. Circulation 1991;84 (5 Suppl):III200.

Takeuchi K et al: Surgical outcome of double-outlet right ventricle with subpulmonary VSD. Ann Thorac Surg 2001;71:49.

SINGLE VENTRICLE

The term "single ventricle" denotes a heart with one ventricular chamber that receives blood from both the tricuspid and mitral valves or a common atrioventricular valve. The anomaly accounts for 3–5% of congenital heart defects. Anomalies such as tricuspid atresia, hypoplastic left heart syndrome, double-inlet ventricles, and common ventricle are often labeled as "single ventricle" based on function and options for repair. Abnormal arrangements of the great arteries occur in approximately 85% of patients. Twenty-five to 35 percent of patients have a common atrioventricular valve, and another 25% have stenosis or regurgitation of one of the atrioventricular valves. One-third to one-half of patients have pulmonary stenosis or atresia, and another third have aortic stenosis. The lesion occurs in association with situs inversus, dextrocardia, and asplenia in approximately 20% of patients. Defects of the atrial septum, total anomalous pulmonary venous connection, and truncus arteriosus are occasionally seen with single ventricle.

Single ventricle has been subdivided into four anatomic groups on the basis of the morphology of the ventricle. In approximately 75% of patients, a dominant ventricle develops from the left ventricular portion of the ventricular loop and from the conus arteriosus and infundibulum of the right ventricle. The right ventricular contribution forms a small outflow chamber from which the great vessels originate. The diagnosis of single ventricle and specific associated lesions must be made by echocardiography and cardiac catheterization.

Clinical findings and prognosis are related to the relative amounts of pulmonary and systemic arterial blood flow. Surgical options include palliation with a shunt or pulmonary arterial band, ventricular partitioning, and staged correction toward a Fontan circulation. The most suitable anatomic types for operation are patients with an anatomic left ventricle and outflow chamber and those with a common ventricle formed from both ventricular sinuses. Prognosis has improved substantially over the past decade. Nonetheless, 1-year survival remains low, ranging between 40% and 80%.

Mayer JE et al: Factors associated with marked reduction in mortality for Fontan operations in patients with single ventricle. J Thorac Cardiovasc Surg 1992;103:444.

Mosca RS et al: Modified Norwood operation for single left ventricle and ventriculoarterial discordance: an improved surgical technique. Ann Thorac Surg 1997;64:1126.

Stein DG et al: Results of total cavopulmonary connection in the treatment of patients with a functional single ventricle. J Thorac Cardiovasc Surg 1991;102:280.

ABNORMALITIES OF SITUS & HETEROTAXIA

Situs inversus totalis is a rare anomaly in which the stomach and other abdominal organs occupy positions that are mirror images of normal (situs solitus). Except in asplenia and polysplenia (see below), the position of the viscera determines the location of the atria; thus, in situs inversus, the atria are reversed, and the morphologic left atrium is on the right. When the ventricles and atria are concordant (ventricles also reversed—formed by levo-looping), the right atrium (on the patient's left) empties into a morphologic right ventricle. If transposition is not present, the circulation is normal and the cardiac chambers and vessels are the mirror image of normal structures. Rather severe associated anomalies usually occur with situs inversus, dextrocardia, and malposition of the great arteries. If the atria and ventricles are discordant, transposition of the great arteries may result in the anomaly being "corrected."

Isolated levocardia is the remaining condition that occurs with situs inversus totalis. The heart is located in the left chest, and most patients have severe associated cardiac anomalies and agenesis of the left lung. Isolated dextrocardia is the term used to designate mirror image position of the heart when the viscera are in normal position (situs solitus). Agenesis of the right lung may occur in these patients.

Cardiac catheterization and cineangiocardiography are essential to understand the pathologic anatomy and physiology of these lesions. The diagnostic rules for locating the visceral situs, morphologic ventricles, and positions of the great vessels must be used to label each structure and chamber.

These heterotaxia variants, in which it is difficult to ascertain right or left designations, are frequently associated with abnormalities of systemic and pulmonary venous return and various splenic anomalies. In the polysplenia variant, the inferior cava is often interrupted. Blood from the lower body reaches the heart via azygous continuation of the cava. Pulmonary drainage to the side of systemic venous drainage may occur more frequently with polysplenia. In asplenia, total anomalous connections to the cava or other systemic veins may exist. Pulmonary stenosis occurs somewhat frequently. In addition, in polysplenia, the lungs, bronchi, and pulmonary vasculature on both sides tend to mimic left-sided anatomy. In general, polysplenic patients tend to demonstrate bilateral left-sided features whereas asplenic patients tend to demonstrate bilateral right-sided features. These patients are also more vulnerable to infection, particularly pneumococcal infections. Atrial isomerism, in which both atria resemble either a right or left atrium, are often seen in the splenic syndromes. Since asplenia is associated with bilateral right-sided features, right atrial isomerism is typically associated with asplenia whereas left atrial isomerism is associated with polysplenia.

Life expectancy depends upon the severity of the circulatory derangement. Some patients live to advanced age and others can be helped by specific palliative operations. A few patients are candidates for corrective repair of less severe associated lesions.

■ MISCELLANEOUS CONGENITAL HEART LESIONS

ANOMALOUS LEFT CORONARY ARTERY

Origin of the left coronary artery from the pulmonary artery causes myocardial ischemia and heart failure in infancy. The right coronary artery is normal and supplies blood to the entire myocardium and intracoronary collaterals, resulting in blood in the anomalous left coronary artery flowing retrograde into the pulmonary artery. This large coronary steal results in myocardial ischemia, dilation of the heart, and, in many cases, fibrosis. Myocardial infarction is not uncommon. The lesion is easily diagnosed by echocardiography and cardiac angiography. The symptoms are usually pallor, sweating, tachycardia, and episodic chest pain that suggests angina pectoris. Repair is indicated at the time of diagnosis and is achieved by direct anastomosis of the left coronary artery to the ascending aorta.

Barbero-Marcial M et al: Anomalous origin of the left coronary artery from the pulmonary artery with intramural aortic route: diagnosis and surgical treatment. J Thorac Cardiovasc Surg 1999;117:823.

Cochrane AD et al: Excellent long-term functional outcome after an operation for anomalous left coronary artery from the pulmonary artery. J Thorac Cardiovasc Surg 1999;117:332.

Laks, H et al: Aortic implantation of anomalous left coronary artery: an improved surgical approach. J Thorac Cardiovasc Surg 1995;109:519.

PULMONARY ARTERIOVENOUS FISTULA

In 50% of cases, this rare vascular anomaly is associated with multiple telangiectases (Rendu-Osler-Weber syndrome). Large arteriovenous fistulas that do not communicate with alveolar capillaries may occur anywhere in the lungs but are most commonly present in the lower lobes. Pulmonary arterial blood shunts through the fistula into the pulmonary veins to cause mild to moderate cyanosis. Pulmonary arterial and venous pressures are low. Occasional infants develop dyspnea, cyanosis, and right heart failure. Cyanosis, clubbing, and polycythemia are usually most pronounced in late childhood. A soft systolic or continuous murmur is occasionally present over the fistula. Chest radiographs show irregular opacified lesions in the peripheral lung fields at the site of the fistula. The lesion is confirmed by angiography or contrast-enhanced computed tomography. Excision of the fistula is indicated in symptomatic patients and in patients with solitary lesions but is not generally recommended for patients with multiple lesions. Localized resection or lobectomy is most commonly performed.

PERSISTENT LEFT SUPERIOR VENA CAVA

Persistence of a left superior vena cava that connects the left jugular and subclavian veins to the coronary sinus is usually asymptomatic. This relatively common anomaly is important to the surgeon in that an otherwise dry operative field remains obscured with venous return. If adequate right-sided venous connections exist or if an innominate vein connects a left cava to the usual right cava, the left cava may be ligated. In other cases, cannulation of the left-sided cava is necessary. Rarely, the right superior vena cava is absent; in most cases, an innominate vein and both left and right cavae are present, and each cava is adequate to carry all of the systemic venous return from the upper body.

ENDOCARDIAL FIBROELASTOSIS

This lesion is not operable, but it may occur in association with operable lesions such as coarctation of the aorta, aortic stenosis, anomalous left coronary artery, and mitral valvular disease. Hyperplasia of subendocardial elastic and collagenous tissue and proliferation of capillaries cause marked thickening of the ventricular wall and a smooth, glistening lining of the left ventricle. Trabeculae are obliterated, and papillary muscles and chordae tendineae are contracted. The disease affects principally the left ventricle and left atrium; involvement of the right heart chambers is rare. There is some evidence that the disease results from subendocardial ischemia in utero.

Fibroelastosis affects 1–2% of patients with congenital heart disease and may occur primarily without other cardiac lesions. Nearly all infants die of left heart failure within the first year. No specific therapy other than transplantation is available.

CARDIAC TUMORS

Cardiac tumors are uncommon in infancy and childhood, occurring in 0.002–0.08% of patients. In general, primary tumors are more common than tumors metastatic to the heart, though numbers vary depending on the referral patterns for specific institutions. The majority of tumors in children are benign (> 90%). Rhabdomyoma and the somewhat less common fibroma account for the majority of benign tumors. Both tumors are noted more commonly in the ventricle, particularly the septum. Rhabdomyoma appears as pale gray nodules. It may be associated with tuberous sclerosis in over 50% of cases. Fibroma is typically a solid white lesion with distinct borders but no true capsule. In infants, teratoma may be more common than fibroma. Hamartoma is another common tumor in childhood. Myxoma, the most frequently noted cardiac tumor in adults, occurs infrequently in children. Malignant tumors are rare. Malignant teratoma and various types of sarcoma account for most of these tumors.

Symptoms relate to the presence of a space-occupying lesion or to involvement of the conduction system. Therefore, when symptomatic, clinical presentation includes signs and symptoms of failure, outflow tract obstruction, and arrhythmias. Echocardiography, cardiac catheterization, and magnetic resonance imaging are all useful diagnostic modalities.

The presence of significant symptoms is an indication for surgery. Surgery, performed with the patient on cardiopulmonary bypass, should attempt complete removal of the tumor. Critical structures must be preserved, however, and excessive myocardial resection resulting in inadequate cardiac function should be avoided. For rhabdomyoma, spontaneous regression is considered the norm. Therefore, for limited symptoms, transvenous biopsy to establish the diagnosis and conservative treatment may be considered.

Chan HS et al: Primary and secondary tumors of childhood involving the heart, pericardium, and great vessels. A report of 75 cases and review of the literature. Cancer 1985;56:825.

Cooley DA et al: Primary cardiac tumors in infants and children: immediate and long-term operative results. Ann Thorac Surg 1996;62:559.

Smythe JF et al: Natural history of cardiac rhabdomyoma in infancy and childhood. Am J Cardiol 1990;66(17):1247.

■ PEDIATRIC CARDIAC TRANSPLANTATION

Cardiac transplantation is an established treatment option for infants and children with hypoplastic left heart syndrome, other complex congenital anomalies not amenable to surgical treatment, and various forms of end-stage cardiomyopathy. In certain cases, combined heart-lung transplantation is an option when end-stage cardiac disease is associated with severe pulmonary vascular obstructive disease. In 1998, the International Society for Heart and Lung Transplant recorded over 3000 pediatric cardiac transplants. In contrast to earlier years, congenital heart disease has emerged as the most common diagnosis leading to transplantation, accounting for 50–60% of transplants. Moreover, 20–30% of pediatric cardiac transplants occur in infants. Although similar in several respects to adult cardiac transplantation, there are important differences. The significant number of children with congenital anomalies imposes unique demands on explantation (usually several previous surgeries) and thoughtful preservation of certain structures needed for ultimate reconstruction with the transplanted heart. There is also a greater range of donor-recipient size mismatch and longer ischemic times associated with pediatric cardiac transplantation. Postoperative surveillance may differ as well, particularly in infants, for whom routine transvenous endomyocardial biopsy or intravenous ultrasound may be used less frequently.

The decision to transplant occurs in the context of multidisciplinary counseling and consultation and is a decision that obviously cannot be taken lightly by the family or the team. Once a patient is identified as a potential candidate, established protocols guide a thorough evaluation of ultimate suitability for transplantation. Careful analysis of native and palliated or reconstructed anatomy is imperative for successful conduct of the operation.

Immunosuppression is similar to that used in adults and is usually some form of triple therapy consisting of cyclosporine or tacrolimus (FK506), azathioprine, and corticosteroids. Induction therapy with antithymocyte globulin or monoclonal antibodies may be considered in selected cases. Prompt steroid withdrawal or a steroid-free regimen is a recognized practice in children, motivated by the deleterious effects of corticosteroids, particularly growth impairment.

Posttransplantation issues for the child are similar to those for the adult. Bleeding, graft dysfunction, rejection, posttransplant lymphoproliferative disease, and graft vasculopathy (transplant coronary artery disease) are all recognized issues. Transplant coronary artery disease has been a particularly vexing issue that has generated competing explanatory theories. One theory considers vasculopathy a consequence of inadequate immunosuppression and rejection and recommends more intense immunosuppression. At the other extreme is the theory that corticosteroids in some way promote vasculopathy, so that reduced dosage or withdrawal of steroids is recommended. Transplant coronary artery disease occurs in 10–20% of patients, is difficult if not impossible to treat effectively, and typically prompts consideration for retransplantation. Rejection is a common event, occurring with an incidence of approximately 0.5 episodes per patient year, and continues to contribute to mortality. Because of concern for rejection and transplant coronary artery disease, routine surveillance is common practice, using a combination of echocardiography, transvenous endomyocardial biopsy, and intravascular ultrasound. Infection occurs in over 50% of recipients and is another recognized contribution to mortality.

Five-year survival ranges between 60% and 75%. Recent results indicate similar survivals between patients with congenital anomalies and other forms of cardiac disease. Mortality is somewhat higher for infants and may be due to a higher incidence of early graft dysfunction. Outcome analyses do not always include pretransplant mortality. The decision to transplant necessarily invokes a period of waiting for a suitable donor, a period with a mortality that approximates 20%. This is a significant figure that should be acknowledged in the process of choosing between transplantation and another available therapeutic option.

Canter C et al: Survival and risk factors for death after cardiac transplantation in infants: a multi-institutional study. Circulation 1997;96:227.

Hsu DT et al: Heart transplantation in children with congenital heart disease. J Am Coll Cardiol 1995;26:743.

Kanter KR et al: Current results with pediatric heart transplantation. Ann Thorac Surg 1999;68:527.

Pahl E et al: Posttransplant coronary artery disease in children: a multicenter national survey. Circulation 1994;90(part 2):56.

Razzouk AJ et al: Transplantation as a primary treatment for hypoplastic left heart syndrome: Intermediate-term results. Ann Thorac Surg 1996;62:1.

DIRECTIONS IN CONGENITAL HEART SURGERY

Creative innovation, multidisciplinary team effort, and advances in hardware development will continue to promote the growth and success of pediatric cardiac surgery. Interventional pediatric cardiology has had a tremendous impact on congenital heart disease. The simultaneous combination of surgical and catheter-based techniques is a newer approach that will continue to receive attention. Cardiopulmonary bypass technology will also continue to improve. Further reduction in oxygenator prime volumes and further modification of ultrafiltration techniques for selective modulation of the inflammatory response will probably occur. Developments in mechanical assist technology will promote more widespread application to young children. Extracorporeal membrane oxygenation is commonly used in this context at the present time. Miniaturized mobile circuits that can be brought promptly to the bedside for immediate resuscitation are being used more frequently. Prenatal echocardiography, three-dimensional echocardiography, and improvements in transesophageal echocardiography will improve this already extremely versatile diagnostic modality. Prenatal intervention will continue to receive attention in selected centers. Using catheter-based techniques, it may be possible to remove or diminish simple obstructive lesions, thereby eliminating the otherwise inevitable remodeling forces that contribute to abnormal development. Information made available by the genome project will provide some degree of insight into the factors controlling cardiac embryology and development. The clinical transformation and application of this knowledge remain to be seen. Efforts in tissue engineering may ultimately provide more versatile and durable conduits. Although already under way, national and international databases will extend the power of clinical studies and provide answers in a more timely fashion.

However, as is true in other disciplines, the core of future progress is contingent upon the effectiveness and appropriate adaptability of the educational process leading to a career in pediatric cardiac surgery. Recent forces have shaped the environment of clinical surgery in such a way that the traditional sequence of training in general, adult thoracic, and pediatric thoracic (cardiac) surgery is becoming less practical. The consideration of complex issues, difficult decisions, and acceptance of certain tradeoffs will be necessary for the inevitable redesigning of surgical education in the near future.

Esophagus & Diaphragm

21

Gerard M. Doherty, MD, Carlos A. Pellegrini, MD, & Lawrence W. Way, MD

■ I. THE ESOPHAGUS

ANATOMY

The esophagus (Figure 21–1) is a muscular tube that serves as a conduit for the passage of food and fluids from the pharynx to the stomach. It originates at the level of the sixth cervical vertebra posterior to the cricoid cartilage. In the thorax, the esophagus passes behind the aortic arch and the left main stem bronchus, enters the abdomen through the esophageal hiatus of the diaphragm, and terminates in the fundus of the stomach. Its muscle fibers originate from the cricoid cartilage and pharynx above and interdigitate with those of the stomach below. About 2–4 cm of esophagus normally lie below the diaphragm. The junction between the esophagus and stomach is maintained in its normal intra-abdominal position by reflections of the peritoneum onto the stomach and of the phrenoesophageal ligament onto the esophagus. The latter is a fibroelastic membrane that lies beneath the peritoneum, on the inferior surface of the diaphragm. When it reaches the esophageal hiatus, the ligament is reflected orad onto the lower esophagus, where it inserts into the circular muscle layer above the gastroesophageal sphincter, 2–4 cm above the diaphragm.

Three anatomic areas of narrowing occur in the esophagus: (1) at the level of the cricoid cartilage (pharyngoesophageal sphincter); (2) in the mid thorax, from compression by the aortic arch and the left main stem bronchus; and (3) at the level of the esophageal hiatus of the diaphragm (gastroesophageal sphincter).

In the adult, the length of the esophagus as measured from the upper incisor teeth to the cricopharyngeus muscle is 15–20 cm; to the aortic arch, 20–25 cm; to the inferior pulmonary vein, 30–35 cm; and to the cardioesophageal junction, approximately 40–45 cm.

The musculature of the pharynx and upper third of the esophagus is skeletal in type; the remainder is smooth muscle. Physiologically, the entire organ behaves as a single functioning unit, so that no distinction can be made between the upper and lower esophagus from the standpoint of propulsive activity. As in the intestinal tract, the muscle fibers are arranged into inner circular and outer longitudinal layers.

The arterial supply to the esophagus is quite consistent. The upper end is supplied by branches from the inferior thyroid arteries. The thoracic portion receives elements from the bronchial arteries and from esophageal branches originating directly from the aorta. The intercostal arteries may also contribute. The diaphragmatic and abdominal segments are nourished by the left inferior phrenic artery and by the esophageal branches of the left gastric artery.

The venous drainage is more complex and variable. The most important veins are those that drain the lower esophagus. Blood from this region passes into the esophageal branches of the coronary vein, a tributary of the portal vein. This connection constitutes a direct communication between the portal circulation and the venous drainage of the lower esophagus and upper stomach. When the portal system is obstructed, as in cirrhosis of the liver, blood is shunted upward through the coronary vein and the esophageal venous plexus to eventually pass by way of the azygos vein into the superior vena cava. The esophageal veins may eventually form varices as they become distended from the increased blood flow and pressure.

The mucosal lining of the esophagus consists of stratified squamous epithelium that contains scattered mucous glands throughout. The esophagus has no serosal layer and, for this reason, does not heal as readily after injury or surgical anastomosis as other portions of the gastrointestinal tract.

PHYSIOLOGY

The clinical physiology of the esophagus is best studied by measuring intraluminal pressure (manometry), pH, and transit time. Manometry is performed by passing into the esophagus and stomach a bundle of fine polyethylene catheters, each of which contains a small distal opening. Continuous perfusion of these tubes with small amounts of saline solution keeps the orifices open and offers a slight resistance to squeeze. The openings are situated 1–5 cm apart and oriented radially to face the esophageal lumen. Simultaneous recordings of pressure can be made at intervals over a segment of known length. Pressures are recorded within the stomach, the gastroesophageal sphincter, the body of the esophagus,

Right common carotid artery
Innominate artery
Vagus nerve
Trachea
Azygos vein
Right bronchus
Vagus nerve plexus
Inferior vena cava
Right crus of diaphragm

Recurrent laryngeal nerve
Left common carotid artery
Left innominate vein
Vagus nerve
Arch of aorta
Left bronchus
Parietal pleura
Descending thoracic aorta
Thoracic esophagus
Mediastinal pleura
Pericardium
Diaphragm
Abdominal esophagus
Stomach

Figure 21–1. Anatomy of the esophagus.

and the upper esophageal sphincter during and after swallowing.

Esophageal pH is measured with a probe located 5 cm above the lower esophageal sphincter; a drop in pH reflects exposure to gastric juice. The number and duration of reflux episodes and the relationship of reflux to symptoms reflects the competency of the sphincter and the ability of the esophagus to clear gastric reflux.

Cineradiography is used to study the movement of liquids in relation to esophageal peristalsis. The transit time of radiolabeled food and liquid can be measured by gamma camera images.

The function of the esophagus is to transport food and fluids from the mouth to the stomach and occasionally in the reverse direction. The esophagus contains a sphincter at the junction of the pharynx and esophagus (pharyngoesophageal sphincter) and another between the esophagus and stomach (gastroesophageal sphincter). Pressures in the resting state as measured by manometry are higher in the region of these sphincters than on either side. Pressures in the mouth and pharynx are atmospheric; those within the body of the resting esophagus are slightly subatmospheric, a reflection of normal intrathoracic pressure. Pressure within the stomach is slightly greater than atmospheric.

The structures at the gastroesophageal junction normally function efficiently to prevent reflux of gastric acid and food from the stomach into the esophagus. The mechanism of gastroesophageal competence is complex and, despite intensive study, is incompletely understood at present.

The gastroesophageal sphincter comprises the lower 4 cm of esophagus, where resting pressure within the lumen normally exceeds intragastric pressure by 15–25 cm water owing to tonic contraction of the esophageal musculature. The high pressure is thought to be due mainly to thickening of the circular layer of the esophagus at this level and a special ability of these circular fibers to generate high pressures (due to different responses to neural and peptide stimulation). A small portion of the intraluminal pressure is due to the effects of extraesophageal structures (eg, diaphragmatic contraction).

Many activities transiently increase intra-abdominal pressure. Protection against reflux of gastric contents under these circumstances is aided by the presence of the intra-abdominal segment of esophagus, which is subjected to the same pressure increment, thus counterbalancing pressure increases within the stomach. Dislocation of the sphincter by a sliding hiatal hernia contributes to sphincter incompetence and gastroesophageal reflux.

Experimentally, the gastroesophageal sphincter is strengthened by gastrin and weakened by cholecystokinin, secretin, and glucagon. After a protein meal, contraction of the sphincter increases, and after a fat meal it becomes weaker; whether these effects reflect the actions of gastrin, cholecystokinin, or other hormones is unclear. Gastrin is no longer thought to be a major determinant of sphincter strength.

Cholinergic and alpha-adrenergic stimuli enhance and β-adrenergic stimuli inhibit contraction of the sphincter. A system of nonadrenergic inhibitory nerves involving vasoactive intestinal peptide (VIP) as a neurotransmitter may be responsible for sphincter relaxation.

When swallowing is begun, the tongue propels the bolus of food into the pharynx. Coordinated voluntary movement of the pharyngeal structures results in closure of the glottis and the nasopharynx. The glottis and pharynx rise during this maneuver, and the normal resting high-pressure zone at the pharyngoesophageal sphincter decreases, permitting entry of the food into the upper esophagus. After the food has traversed the pharynx and the pharyngoesophageal sphincter, the pharyngeal musculature relaxes and the high-pressure zone returns at the pharyngoesophageal sphincter. As the bolus of food enters the esophagus, a peristaltic wave begins that travels toward the stomach at a speed of 4–6 cm/s, propelling the food before it. The act of swallowing is a reflex response integrated in the medulla oblongata. The relative importance of neural and myogenic mechanisms in initiating and governing the strength, rate, and coordination of peristalsis is debated. When the subject is in the upright position, liquids and semisolid foods usually fall to the distal esophagus by gravity ahead of the slower peristaltic wave. The gastroesophageal sphincter relaxes in anticipation of the advancing food and peristalsis, thereby allowing the bolus to be transported into the stomach. After the food passes through, the sphincter regains its tone until another peristaltic wave arrives from above.

The term primary peristalsis denotes the wave of contraction initiated by swallowing that begins in the upper esophagus and travels the entire length of the organ (Figure 21–2). Local stimulation by distention at any point in the body of the esophagus will elicit a peristaltic wave from the point of stimulus. This is called secondary peristalsis and aids esophageal emptying when the primary wave has failed to clear the lumen of ingested food or when gastric contents reflux from the stomach. Tertiary waves are stationary nonpropulsive contractions that may occur in any portion of the esophagus. Tertiary waves are considered abnormal, but they are frequently present in elderly subjects who have no symptoms of esophageal disease.

Incompetence of the gastroesophageal sphincter takes place normally during vomiting. During this event, the gastroesophageal junction rises above the level of the diaphragmatic hiatus. Ascent is the result of contraction of the longitudinal musculature of the esophagus; an additional result is effacement of the mucosal rosette that ordinarily fills the lumen of the gastroesophageal junction. Expulsion of gastric contents by the violent contractions of the gastric antrum and abdominal wall then becomes possible. After vomiting has subsided, the structures resume their ordinary relationships, with the gastroesophageal junction below the level of the diaphragm.

The buccopharyngeal and esophageal structures engaged in swallowing and transmission of food to the stomach are innervated by motor fibers from the fifth, seventh, ninth, tenth, 11th, and 12th cranial nerves. Afferent sensory impulses are important in maintaining coordination of the motor activity.

Figure 21–2. Deglutition. Normal esophageal peristaltic waves and pressures during consecutive swallows. Note the orderly downward progression of the waves.

ESOPHAGEAL MOTILITY DISORDERS

UPPER ESOPHAGEAL SPHINCTER DYSFUNCTION (Cricopharyngeal Achalasia)

 ESSENTIALS OF DIAGNOSIS

- Cervical dysphagia.
- Cricopharyngeal bar on barium swallow.
- Zenker's diverticulum in some patients.

General Considerations

Upper esophageal sphincter dysfunction—the term cricopharyngeal achalasia is too precise—may cause dysphagia in a variety of situations, most of which occur in patients over age 60. It may occur as an isolated abnormality or in association with Zenker's diverticulum.

A hereditary syndrome called oculopharyngeal muscular dystrophy, consisting of ptosis and dysphagia, has been described in patients of French-Canadian ancestry. The dysphagia is the result of weak pharyngeal musculature in the face of normal upper esophageal sphincter function; it is considerably improved by upper esophageal sphincter myotomy.

Clinical Findings

A. SYMPTOMS AND SIGNS

Cervical dysphagia, more pronounced for solids than for liquids, is the main symptom of upper esophageal sphincter dysfunction. A chronic cough develops in some patients from minor aspirations of saliva and ingested food.

B. IMAGING STUDIES

Barium swallow nearly always shows a prominent cricopharyngeal bar, which is sometimes so striking as to suggest mechanical obstruction.

C. ENDOSCOPY

The findings on endoscopy are of an extrinsic constriction that allows passage of the endoscope as it is advanced.

D. MANOMETRY

Simultaneous determination of pharyngeal, cricopharyngeal, and upper esophageal pressures often reveals imperfect coordination of relaxation. Normally, the cricopharyngeal sphincter relaxes half a second before contraction of the pharyngeal musculature. In these patients, relaxation, though complete, occurs at or just after initiation of the pharyngeal contraction.

Differential Diagnosis

Esophageal neoplasms must be ruled out by endoscopy. Cervical dysphagia is occasionally the predominant complaint in reflux resulting from lower esophageal sphincter incompetence. In such cases, surgical correction of the reflux relieves the cervical dysphagia.

Treatment

Treatment consists of myotomy of the cricopharyngeus and upper 3–4 cm of the esophageal musculature. The esophagus is approached through an incision parallel to the anterior border of the sternomastoid muscle. The myotomy is made in the midline posteriorly, dividing all fibers of the muscle layers until the submucosa is reached.

Prognosis

Complications are uncommon, and relief of symptoms is usually complete and permanent postoperatively. The procedure should probably not be performed in patients with gastroesophageal reflux, because of the increased risk of aspiration.

Hila A, Castell JA, Castell DO: Pharyngeal and upper esophageal sphincter manometry in the evaluation of dysphagia. J Clin Gastroenterol 2001;33:355.

Owen W: ABC of the upper gastrointestinal tract. Dysphagia. BMJ 2001;323:850.

Wetscher GJ et al: The effect of medical therapy and antireflux surgery on dysphagia in patients with gastroesophageal reflux disease without esophageal stricture. Am J Surg 1999; 177: 189.

DIFFUSE ESOPHAGEAL SPASM

 ESSENTIALS OF DIAGNOSIS

- Dysphagia, substernal pain.
- Nervousness, intermittent symptoms.
- Fluoroscopic, cineradiographic, and manometric evidence of high-amplitude contractions.

General Considerations

Primary esophageal motility disorders are characterized by abnormal esophageal motor function, often associated with intermittent chest pain. The diagnosis is made by the characteristic findings on manometry and by eliciting the symptoms with provocative tests. Although part of a spectrum, they can be broadly classified as follows: **achalasia,** described in the next section; **nutcracker esophagus,** a syndrome of high-amplitude peristaltic waves, seen in about half of patients with motility disorders; **diffuse esophageal spasm,** characterized by nonperistaltic contractions; and **hypertensive lower esophageal sphincter,** a less common disorder. About 35% of patients with primary motility disorders have manometric features of more than one of these conditions, in which case the disorder is called **nonspecific esophageal motor disorder.** The cause of these conditions is not known, though stress can induce similar manometric findings in normal subjects, so stress and psychologic disorders might play a role. Esophageal ischemia has also been postulated. Up to a third of patients with nutcracker esophagus have abnormal gastroesophageal reflux and respond favorably to medical therapy.

Clinical Findings

A. SYMPTOMS AND SIGNS

The most common symptom is intermittent chest pain, which varies from slight discomfort to severe spasmodic pain that simulates the pain of coronary artery disease. Most patients complain of dysphagia, but weight loss is uncommon.

B. IMAGING STUDIES

The esophagogram is abnormal in 60% of patients. Fluoroscopic studies show segmental spasms, areas of narrowing, and irregular uncoordinated peristalsis described as "curling" or "corkscrew esophagus." A small hiatal hernia is frequently demonstrated; less commonly, an epiphrenic diverticulum is present.

C. MANOMETRY

Manometry is the key to the diagnosis of these disorders. In patients with diffuse esophageal spasm, swallows induce repetitive, nonperistaltic (simultaneous) contractions instead of normal peristaltic waves. Some patients also exhibit abnormally strong nonperistaltic waves (140–200 mm Hg). In about 30% of patients, the lower esophageal sphincter fails to relax in response to swallows. In nutcracker esophagus, the primary abnormality is high-amplitude (about 200 mm Hg) peristalsis. Although pressure may be high, sphincter relaxation is normal with swallowing. Why these contrac-

tions feel like angina is not known. The hypertensive lower esophageal sphincter may represent a variant of achalasia, and some patients with this disorder have been seen to progress to typical achalasia.

Provocative testing during manometry is useful. The most commonly used drug is the anticholinesterase edrophonium, which can elicit strong esophageal contractions. Elicitation of pain similar to the spontaneous symptom means that the test is positive. Bethanechol and ergonovine may be used instead of edrophonium. If the diagnosis is doubtful, manometry and pH monitoring may be performed. Manometry gives data on esophageal motor activity and its relationship to symptoms, and pH monitoring may demonstrate reflux, a common associated problem.

Differential Diagnosis

The symptoms produced by these motility disorders must be distinguished from those produced by heart disease, mediastinal masses, benign and malignant esophageal tumors, and scleroderma. Although radiologic and pressure studies are diagnostically accurate, esophagoscopy should be performed to confirm the absence of intraluminal lesions such as esophagitis that often produce esophageal spasm.

Complications

Sliding hiatal hernia and epiphrenic diverticula may be secondary complications of the uncoordinated and severe contractions of the esophagus. Regurgitation and aspiration may occur, possibly leading to repeated pneumonic infections. In general, however, the condition is usually mild and does not lead to serious complications.

Treatment

In many patients, reassurance and symptomatic therapy are sufficient. Hydralazine, long-acting nitrates, or anticholinergic agents may give some relief. A soft diet taken in five or six small feedings per day may be required, especially when dysphagia is the most prominent symptom. Peppermint oil has shown some promising effectiveness. Bougienage with mercury-weighted dilators is ineffective in diffuse spasm or nutcracker esophagus. Patients with severe pain and dysphagia refractory to medical therapy should have an esophageal myotomy extending from the gastroesophageal sphincter to the aortic arch or as high as the preoperative manometry shows abnormally elevated pressures. This procedure can be performed thoracoscopically or through a thoracotomy. The former is far easier on the patient, and the results are excellent. The open thoracotomy approach should be reserved for patients in whom thoracoscopic surgery is not feasible (eg, previous thoracotomy). Postoperative relief is associated with greatly reduced intraluminal pressures in the esophagus. Reflux esophagitis, the principal complication, may be avoided by preserving the lower esophageal sphincter. If the sphincter must be divided, a short (0.5 cm) Nissen fundoplication should also be performed. The operation is successful in 90% of cases. Persistent pain and dysphagia after surgical attempts to improve esophageal function may be treated by total thoracic esophagectomy and cervical esophagogastrostomy.

Adler DG, Romero Y: Primary esophageal motility disorders. Mayo Clin Proc 2001;76:195.

Champion JK, Delisle N, Hunt T: Comparison of thoracoscopic and laparoscopic esophagomyotomy with fundoplication for primary motility disorders. Eur J Cardiothorac Surg 1999; 16(Suppl 1):S34.

Champion JK, Delisle N, Hunt T: Laparoscopic esophagomyotomy with posterior partial fundoplication for primary esophageal motility disorders. Surg Endosc 2000;14:746.

Ellis FH Jr: Long esophagomyotomy for diffuse esophageal spasm and related disorders: an historical overview. Dis Esophagus 1998;11:210.

Pimentel M et al: Peppermint oil improves the manometric findings in diffuse esophageal spasm. J Clin Gastroenterol 2001; 33:27.

Storr M, Allescher HD: Esophageal pharmacology and treatment of primary motility disorders. Dis Esophagus 1999;12:241.

ACHALASIA

ESSENTIALS OF DIAGNOSIS

- *Dysphagia.*
- *Retention of ingested food in the esophagus.*
- *Radiologic evidence of absent primary peristalsis, dilated body of the esophagus, and a conically narrowed cardioesophageal junction.*
- *Absent primary peristalsis by manometry and cineradiography.*

General Considerations

Achalasia of the esophagus is a neuromuscular disorder in which esophageal dilation and hypertrophy occur without organic stenosis. Primary peristalsis is absent and the cardioesophageal sphincter fails to relax in response to swallowing. The circular muscle layer hypertrophies, while the longitudinal coat retains its normal thickness. There is absence, atrophy, or disintegration of the ganglion cells of Auerbach's myenteric plexuses and a reduction in nerve fibers within the wall of the esophagus in most patients. Pharmacologic studies suggest that the cholinergic innervation of the sphincter is intact but the noncholinergic, nonadrenergic inhibitory innervation, which mediates sphincter relaxation through VIP and other peptides, has been lost. The cause is unknown, but two theories exist: (1) a degenerative disease of the neurons and (2) infection of neurons by a virus (eg, herpes zoster) or other infectious agent. The latter is supported by the fact that similar findings occur in patients with **Chagas' disease** (American trypanosomiasis), a condition in which the infective organism destroys parasympathetic ganglion cells throughout the body, including the heart and the gastrointestinal, urinary, and respiratory tracts.

Achalasia affects males more often than females and may develop at any age. The peak years are from 30 to 60.

Clinical Findings

A. SYMPTOMS AND SIGNS

Dysphagia is the dominant symptom, but weight loss is not usually marked despite the functional obstruction. The dilated esophagus is able to contain large quantities of food that only gradually pass into the stomach, largely by gravity. Pain is infrequent even though shallow ulcerations may be produced in the mucosa by the retention and disintegration of ingested food. Regurgitation of retained esophageal contents is common, especially during the night while the patient sleeps in a recumbent position. Aspiration may lead to repeated bouts of pneumonia.

A variant called **vigorous achalasia** is characterized by chest pain and esophageal spasms that generate nonpropulsive high-pressure waves in the body of the esophagus. Sphincteric dysfunction is the same as in ordinary achalasia. Diffuse esophageal spasm has been observed to progress to achalasia, and vigorous achalasia may be an intermediate step in this evolution.

During esophagoscopy, the instrument can be advanced through the narrow sphincter without increased force, a feature that distinguishes achalasia from carcinoma or benign peptic stricture.

B. IMAGING STUDIES

Radiologic studies demonstrate the classic features even in early achalasia. The narrowing at the cardia has a characteristic contour. The dilated body of the esophagus blends into a smooth cone-shaped area of narrowing 3–6 cm long (Figure 21–3). On fluoroscopy the peristaltic waves are weak, simultaneous, irregular, uncoordinated, or absent. As the disease progresses, the

Figure 21–3. Achalasia of the esophagus. *Left:* Moderately advanced achalasia. Note dilated body of esophagus and smoothly tapered lower portion. *Right:* Widely patent cardioesophageal region following cardiomyotomy (Heller procedure).

esophagus dilates further and becomes tortuous and, in far-advanced cases, sigmoid in shape. The lowermost segment retains the classic long, linear narrowing even in the late stages of the disease. The column of barium is held up at the narrowed area because the sphincteric mechanism fails to relax normally.

C. MANOMETRY

Manometric studies are of value in confirming the diagnosis. In the classic form of achalasia, the motility pattern is as follows: The pharyngoesophageal sphincter has a normal action; the body of the esophagus is devoid of primary peristaltic waves, but simultaneous disorganized muscular activity may be present. Occasionally, no peristalsis of any sort can be observed. The pressure in the gastroesophageal sphincter is about twice normal (40 mm Hg), and relaxation after swallowing is incomplete or absent. Since achalasia is one of several esophageal motor disorders and since there is considerable overlap between them, features of other disorders such as diffuse esophageal spasm, high-amplitude peristaltic waves, et, are occasionally seen in manometric studies. Transition from diffuse spasm or other nonspecific motility disorders into typical achalasia over time has been documented, reinforcing the notion that these represent a group of overlapping syndromes that may have a common pathogenesis. Provocative tests may also be useful in patients with unclear features. For example, subcutaneous administration of bethanechol results in a forceful sustained contraction of the lower two-thirds of the esophagus that is often briefly painful.

This response is a manifestation of autonomic denervation of the organ and is absent in normal subjects. A positive response may also be noted in symptomatic diffuse spasm.

After successful forceful dilation or Heller myotomy of the sphincter, manometric evidence of peristalsis returns in a few patients.

Differential Diagnosis

Benign strictures of the lower esophagus and carcinoma at or near the cardioesophageal junction are important conditions to be distinguished from achalasia. Esophagoscopy should always be performed to aid in establishing the diagnosis and also to rule out other intraluminal lesions.

Rarely, an infiltrating intramural carcinoma at the cardia may produce a disorder with all of the pathophysiologic, radiologic, and clinical features of achalasia. The cause appears to be interference with neural control of esophageal motility by the neoplasm. The principal additional finding is marked weight loss.

Complications

Small mucosal ulcerations may develop from the irritation caused by retained food, but true peptic ulceration hemorrhage is rare in achalasia. Aspiration of regurgitated esophageal contents may lead to repeated episodes of pneumonitis, tracheobronchitis, and, rarely, asphyxiation. Malnutrition is usually mild to moderate, but it may be severe in neglected cases. Squamous cell carcinoma of the esophagus develops in 3–5% of patients with achalasia. The lesion occurs predominantly in the dilated portion of the esophagus, usually many years after the initial manifestations. Prolonged exposure to carcinogens from food retained in the esophagus is thought to cause inflammation and metaplasia with later development of dysplasia and cancer. There is no evidence that a Heller myotomy, pneumatic dilation, or any other treatment reduces the risk of carcinoma.

Treatment

The aim of therapy is to relieve the functional obstruction at the cardia. This can be accomplished by either forceful dilation or direct surgical division of the muscle fibers of the lower esophageal sphincter. Calcium channel blockers also decrease pressure in the lower esophageal sphincter and may improve swallowing, but because of side effects they are not practical.

Forceful dilation involves rapid pneumatic expansion of an inflatable bag placed at the esophagogastric junction. It is accompanied by pain and is thought to disrupt some of the sphincteric musculature. Usually, three or four dilations with balloons of 3–4.2 cm are required to obtain the desired symptomatic and manometric result. A successful dilation is associated with about a 60% decrease in lower esophageal sphincter pressure. After dilation, most patients experience immediate relief of dysphagia, but long-term results are good in only 50%. Persistent dysphagia or reflux esophagitis develops in the remainder. Esophageal perforation, which complicates about 7% of cases, usually presents no clear-cut symptoms in the first few hours. Consequently, patients treated by dilation should routinely be examined by esophagography shortly thereafter and should remain overnight in the hospital for observation. Perforation, demonstrated by free flow of contrast into the mediastinum or pleural space, is a life-threatening problem that requires immediate operation. Dilation is contraindicated in advanced achalasia with megaesophagus because the risk of perforation is especially high in this situation.

An alternative approach—and the procedure of choice for those with advanced disease or failed dilation—is extramucosal cardiomyotomy (Heller myotomy). This procedure can be performed through a thoracoscopic or laparoscopic approach. Using electrocautery, the muscular layer of the esophagus is divided longitudinally for a distance of 6–8 cm, extending distally about 0.5 cm onto the stomach. All muscular fibers must be divided to avoid recurrent dysphagia. The patient may resume eating on the first postoperative day and can usually be discharged the next day. The results are good to excellent in 90% of patients. In the remainder, some dysphagia remains, usually as a result of the poor esophageal peristalsis.

Heller myotomy can also be performed through open laparotomy or thoracotomy, but the videoscopic approach is technically straightforward and gives a much milder postoperative course. Some surgeons regularly add an antireflux procedure (eg, Nissen or Lind fundoplication) to a Heller myotomy. This can be done in conjunction with a laparoscopic but not a thoracoscopic myotomy. A definite need for this extra step has not been proved, and opinion is divided. Perforation complicating forceful dilation is best managed by immediate operation, with closure of the perforation and a myotomy on the opposite side of the esophagus.

The results of therapy can be gauged by measuring the rate of esophageal passage of a technetium Tc 99m-labeled solid meal. The decrease in transit time postoperatively is proportionate to the reduction in lower esophageal sphincter pressure.

Prognosis

Relief of obstructive symptoms can be obtained by forceful dilation or by surgery in at least 85–90% of pa-

tients. A properly performed Heller procedure overcomes the functional obstruction and uncommonly leads to esophageal reflux. The addition of vagotomy and gastric drainage operations to the myotomy procedure is unnecessary. It may be wise to perform esophagoscopy periodically on all patients, since successful therapy for dysphagia does not lessen the increased risk of esophageal carcinoma seen in this disease.

Ben-Meir A et al: Quality of life before and after laparoscopic Heller myotomy for achalasia. Am J Surg 2001;181:471.

Camacho-Lobato L et al: Vigorous achalasia: original description requires minor change. J Clin Gastroenterol 2001;33:375.

Finley RJ et al: Laparoscopic Heller myotomy improves esophageal emptying and the symptoms of achalasia. Arch Surg 2001;136:892.

Patti MG et al: Effects of previous treatment on results of laparoscopic Heller myotomy for achalasia. Dig Dis Sci 1999;44:2270.

Patti MG et al: Laparoscopic Heller myotomy and Dor fundoplication for achalasia: analysis of successes and failures. Arch Surg 2001;136:870.

Raymond L, Lach B, Shamji FM: Inflammatory aetiology of primary oesophageal achalasia: an immunohistochemical and ultrastructural study of Auerbach's plexus. Histopathology 1999;35:445.

Yamamura MS: Laparoscopic Heller myotomy and anterior fundoplication for achalasia results in a high degree of patient satisfaction. Arch Surg 2000;135:902.

ESOPHAGEAL MANIFESTATIONS IN SCLERODERMA & OTHER SYSTEMIC DISEASES

Scleroderma and several other systemic diseases occasionally involve the esophagus, and when the esophageal symptoms overshadow other manifestations of the disease, the diagnosis may be difficult.

Esophageal dysfunction is common in patients with scleroderma. The initial symptoms are usually those of reflux: regurgitation, heartburn, and, occasionally, bleeding. Dysphagia may also occur but is a less common complaint until esophagitis progresses to stricture formation. The esophageal symptoms usually appear in patients with the characteristic skin changes and Raynaud's syndrome. However, the motility defects may antedate other findings of the disease.

The principal abnormality is atrophy and fibrosis of the esophageal musculature, resulting in progressively weakening function. The changes affect the smooth muscle portion of the esophagus and are most marked at the gastroesophageal sphincter. The motility disorder can be recognized by manometry and cineradiography. On manometry, the resting pressure of the lower esophageal sphincter is low (eg, 5 mm Hg), and primary peristaltic waves have low amplitude or are absent. The most noticeable radiographic abnormality is a patulous cardia with free reflux. A shortened esophagus and strictures can often be seen. pH monitoring shows substantial reflux and poor clearance of the refluxed material. Esophageal shortening may draw the sphincter above the diaphragmatic hiatus, producing a hiatal hernia. Gastric emptying of solids should be measured, even if an abnormality is not suspected from the patient's history, since delayed emptying commonly contributes to the severity of reflux. In about 40% of patients, associated intestinal involvement produces a form of pseudo-obstruction with malabsorption and delayed transit. Similar esophageal changes may also occur in rheumatoid arthritis, Sjögren's syndrome, Raynaud's disease, and systemic lupus erythematosus. Related motor abnormalities are occasionally seen in alcoholism, diabetes mellitus, myxedema, multiple sclerosis, and amyloidosis.

Medical management should always be tried first. It should include dietary (small, frequent, nonfatty meals), mechanical (elevation of the head of the bed), and behavioral (avoid smoking, etc) measures. The drug of choice for esophagitis in patients with scleroderma is omeprazole. Nothing has been found that will delay the deterioration of esophageal function in scleroderma, but in other diseases, specific treatment for the underlying disorder is often of benefit. Strictures can often be managed with repeated dilations. A Roux-en-Y gastrojejunostomy is the best means to correct markedly delayed gastric emptying. If intestinal function is good enough to sustain nutrition, esophageal reflux may be treated by a Nissen fundoplication or a Collis-Nissen procedure, which are at least temporarily successful in the majority of patients even in the face of stricture formation. The late results of these operations are less satisfactory, however, and esophageal replacement (eg, by a colon interposition) will be required in many cases.

Carola F, Bianchi P, Basilisco G: Intraesophageal pH monitoring during acid infusion in patients with systemic sclerosis. Dig Dis Sci 1999;44:1716.

Ling TC, Johnston BT: Esophageal investigations in connective tissue disease: which tests are most appropriate? J Clin Gastroenterol 2001;32:33.

Marie I et al: Esophageal involvement and pulmonary manifestations in systemic sclerosis. Arthritis Rheum 2001;45:346.

Sridhar KR et al: Prevalence of impaired gastric emptying of solids in systemic sclerosis: diagnostic and therapeutic implications. J Lab Clin Med 1998;132:541.

ESOPHAGEAL DIVERTICULA

Diverticula of the esophagus are commonly associated with motor dysfunction. They are acquired lesions that result from the protrusion of mucosa and submucosa through a weakness or defect in the musculature (pul-

sion type) or from the pulling outward of the esophageal wall from inflamed and scarred peribronchial mediastinal lymph nodes (traction type). The latter are small incidental lesions of no clinical significance and will not be discussed further.

1. Pharyngoesophageal (Zenker's) Diverticulum

 ESSENTIALS OF DIAGNOSIS

- *Dysphagia, pressure symptoms, and gurgling sounds in the neck.*
- *Regurgitation of undigested food, halitosis.*
- *Manual emptying of the diverticulum by the patient.*

General Considerations

Pharyngoesophageal pulsion diverticulum is the most common of the esophageal diverticula and is three times more frequent in men than in women. It arises posteriorly in the midline of the neck—above the cricopharyngeus muscle and below the inferior constrictor of the pharynx. Between these two muscle groups is a weakened area through which the mucosa and submucosa gradually evaginate as a result of the high pressures generated during swallowing. Zenker's diverticulum is rarely seen in patients below age 30; most patients are over 60. Although its mouth is in the midline, the sac projects laterally, usually into the left paravertebral region. The body of the esophagus often shows abnormal motility patterns in patients with Zenker's diverticulum, and an associated hiatal hernia is common.

Clinical Findings

A. SYMPTOMS AND SIGNS

Dysphagia is the most common symptom and is related to the size of the diverticulum. Undigested food is regurgitated into the mouth, especially when the patient is in the recumbent position, and the patient may manually massage the neck after eating to empty the sac. Swelling of the neck, gurgling noises after eating, halitosis, and a sour metallic taste in the mouth are common symptoms.

B. IMAGING STUDIES

Fluoroscopic examination demonstrates a smoothly rounded outpouching arising posteriorly in the midline of the neck (Figure 21–4).

Figure 21–4. Large pharyngoesophageal diverticulum. Note origin in midline *(arrow, left)* and compression of esophagus *(bracket, right).*

C. MANOMETRY AND pH STUDIES

Esophageal manometry and pH measurements will show if the diverticulum is associated with an abnormal response of the cricopharyngeus muscle to swallowing (delayed opening of the sphincter) and the amount of gastroesophageal reflux. Abnormal reflux is present in about one-third of patients. Introduction of the probes is tricky, as they tend to enter the diverticulum, and care must be exercised to avoid a perforation.

Differential Diagnosis

The dysphagia produced by pharyngoesophageal diverticula must be distinguished from that produced by malignant lesions, although carcinoma at this level is uncommon. Achalasia of the cricopharyngeus muscle may produce symptoms similar to those of Zenker's diverticulum. Cervical esophageal webs must also be considered, and a web may occur in association with a diverticulum. The radiologic discovery of a smoothly rounded blind pouch is diagnostic of diverticulum. Esophagoscopy may be hazardous because the instrument may enter the ostium of the diverticulum instead of the true esophageal lumen. Since the diverticulum is composed only of mucosa and submucosa, it is easily perforated.

Regurgitation and aspiration may produce tracheobronchial irritation and pneumonitis. This usually occurs while the patient is in the recumbent position, as during sleep. Food may become trapped in the diverticulum and, rarely, may lead to perforation, mediastinitis, or a paraesophageal abscess. Retained food may ulcerate the mucosa and cause bleeding. Rarely, a fistula may form between the diverticulum and the trachea as a result of infection. Pulmonary infection is the most frequent serious complication, and many patients are first seen after experiencing repeated episodes of pneumonitis.

Treatment

Surgical therapy is the treatment of choice. When done under general anesthesia, it is important to protect the airway immediately upon induction to prevent aspiration of contents that may have collected in the diverticulum. The open approach consists of excision of the diverticulum and myotomy of the cricopharyngeal muscle (upper esophageal sphincter). Instead of excising the diverticulum, another option is to invert it into the esophageal lumen while closing the point of inversion so the change in position is permanent. For small diverticula (eg, 1–2 cm), myotomy alone is sufficient. For large diverticula, excision alone may be sufficient, but if myotomy is not performed, some patients still complain of dysphagia. A more recently applied option uses an oropharyngeally placed ligating and dividing stapler to divide and seal the septum between the diverticulum and the cervical esophagus. If the patient also has significant gastroesophageal reflux, this should be corrected before the upper sphincter is divided, in order to avoid aspiration.

Prognosis

The prognosis is excellent. Complications are rare, and the patient is usually able to eat the day after the procedure.

Feeley MA et al: Zenker's diverticulum: analysis of surgical complications from diverticulectomy and cricopharyngeal myotomy. Laryngoscope 1999;109:858.

Peracchia A et al: Minimally invasive surgery for Zenker diverticulum: analysis of results in 95 consecutive patients. Arch Surg 1998;133:695.

Rocco G et al: Results of reoperation on the upper esophageal sphincter. J Thorac Cardiovasc Surg 1999;117:28.

Schramm VL Jr, Imola MJ: Management of nasopharyngeal salivary gland malignancy. Laryngoscope 2001;111:1533.

Thaler ER: Feasibility and outcome of endoscopic staple-assisted esophagodiverticulostomy for Zenker's diverticulum. Laryngoscope 2001;111:1506.

2. Epiphrenic Diverticulum

 ESSENTIALS OF DIAGNOSIS

- *Dysphagia and a sensation of pressure in the lower esophagus after eating.*
- *Intermittent vomiting, substernal pain.*
- *Typical radiologic contour.*
- *Disturbed motility of the lower esophagus.*
- *Associated hiatal hernia on occasion.*

General Considerations

Epiphrenic pulsion diverticula are usually located just above the diaphragm but may occur as high as the mid thorax. They are usually associated with motility disturbances and are frequently larger than diverticula that arise elsewhere in the esophagus. Esophagitis may develop at the ostium. Peridiverticular localized mediastinitis may be seen, especially if ulceration of the mucosa occurs.

Dysphagia and regurgitation are the predominant symptoms, but aspiration and pulmonary symptoms are also seen. Manometric studies demonstrate simultaneous repetitive contractions (or sometimes high-amplitude, prolonged contractions) in the body of the esophagus and in many cases abnormal lower esophageal sphincter function (ie, high resting pressure, incomplete relaxation with swallowing, or an exaggerated postglutition pressure rise).

Diagnosis

The appearance on x-ray films and on fluoroscopy is so distinctive that a definitive diagnosis can usually be made. Associated conditions such as benign or malignant stenoses, webs, hiatal hernia, achalasia and other motility disorders must be ruled out. Esophageal manometry should be performed in every case.

Complications

Esophagitis, periesophagitis, and occasional bleeding from ulceration are the most frequent complications. Tracheobronchial aspiration of regurgitated esophageal contents is uncommon. Perforation occurs rarely.

Treatment

Most patients have minor symptoms that do not require surgery. Surgery is indicated when symptoms become severe. The operation should consist of thoracotomy (or thoracoscopy if feasible), diverticulectomy, and longitudinal myotomy placed opposite the diverticulum on the esophageal circumference. The myotomy should include the abnormal lower esophageal sphincter and should extend proximally to the level where esophageal function becomes manometrically normal. A Belsey or loose Nissen fundoplication is also performed to prevent reflux.

Prognosis

Surgery is successful in 80–90% of cases.

Thomas ML et al: Oesophageal diverticula. Br J Surg 2001;88:629.

Tobin RW: Esophageal rings, webs, and diverticula. J Clin Gastroenterol 1998;27:285.

HIATAL HERNIA & ESOPHAGEAL REFLUX

1. Paraesophageal Hiatal Hernia

 ESSENTIALS OF DIAGNOSIS

- *Often asymptomatic.*
- *Symptoms from mechanical obstruction: dysphagia, incarceration, stasis gastric ulcer.*

General Considerations

There are two types of esophageal hiatal hernia: paraesophageal and sliding. Sliding hiatal hernia is discussed below. Symptoms usually develop in adult life. Obesity, aging, and general weakening of the musculofascial structures set the stage for enlargement of the esophageal hiatus.

In the paraesophageal type of diaphragmatic hernia (Figures 21–5 and 21–6), all or part of the stomach herniates into the thorax immediately adjacent and to the left of an undisplaced gastroesophageal junction

Figure 21–5. Paraesophageal hernia.

(Figure 21–6). Since the gastroesophageal sphincteric mechanism functions normally in most of these cases, reflux of gastric contents is uncommon. Rarely, paraesophageal hernia occurs in association with the sliding type, and gastroesophageal reflux may occur along with other symptoms of an otherwise pure parae-

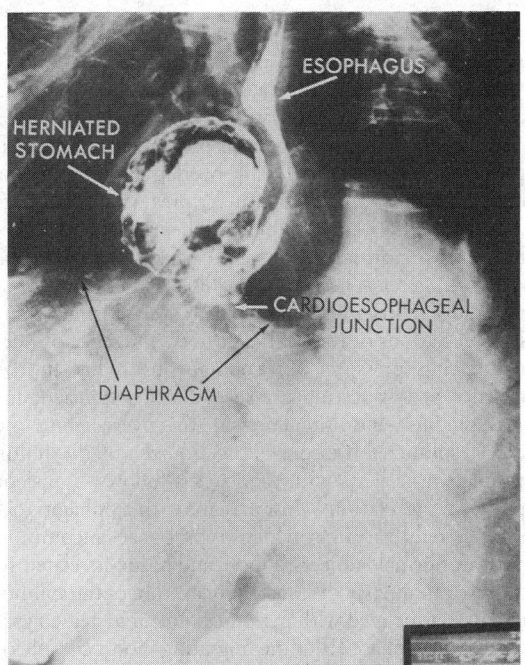

Figure 21–6. Paraesophageal hernia. Note that the cardioesophageal junction remains in its normal anatomic position below the diaphragm.

sophageal type. Paraesophageal hernia accounts for less than 10% of hernias of the esophageal hiatus.

Clinical Findings

Symptoms from an uncomplicated paraesophageal hernia usually develop in adult life and consist of gaseous eructations, a sense of pressure in the lower chest after eating, and, occasionally, palpitations due to cardiac dysrhythmias. All of these are pressure phenomena caused by enlargement of the herniated gastric pouch by food displacing the fundic air bubble. As noted, heartburn due to gastroesophageal reflux is uncommon.

Complications

The most frequent complications of paraesophageal hernia are hemorrhage, incarceration, obstruction, and strangulation. The herniated portion of the stomach often becomes congested, and bleeding occurs from erosions of the mucosa. Obstruction may occur, most often at the esophagogastric junction as a result of torsion and angulation at this point—especially if a large portion (or all) of the stomach herniates into the chest. In paraesophageal hiatal hernia—in contrast to the sliding type—other viscera such as the small and large intestine and spleen may also enter the mediastinum along with the stomach.

Treatment

Since complications are frequent even in the absence of symptoms, operative repair is indicated in most cases. The usual method is to return the herniated stomach to the abdomen and fix it there by sutures to the posterior rectus sheath (anterior gastropexy). The enlarged hiatus is closed snugly around the gastroesophageal junction with interrupted sutures. It is unnecessary to excise the hernia sac. With rare exceptions, this operation can be performed with laparoscopically.

Prognosis

The results of surgical management are excellent.

Hashemi M, Sillin LF, Peters JH: Current concepts in the management of paraesophageal hiatal hernia. J Clin Gastroenterol 1999;29:8.

Luketich JD et al: Laparoscopic repair of giant paraesophageal hernia: 100 consecutive cases. Ann Surg 2000;232:608.

Watson DI et al: Importance of dissection of the hernial sac in laparoscopic surgery for large hiatal hernias. Arch Surg 1999; 134:1069.

2. Reflux Esophagitis Sliding Hiatal Hernia

 ESSENTIALS OF DIAGNOSIS

- *Heartburn, often worse on recumbency.*
- *Regurgitation ("water brash").*
- *Sliding hiatal hernia on upper gastrointestinal series.*
- *Endoscopic biopsy evidence of esophagitis.*
- *Decreased resting pressure in lower esophageal sphincter.*
- *Abnormal esophageal acid exposure on prolonged pH monitoring.*

General Considerations

Small amounts of gastric contents reflux normally through the cardia, most commonly after meals and often in association with belching. The refluxed material triggers secondary peristalsis, which rapidly clears the esophagus. Esophagitis develops when the frequency of these episodes or the volume of reflux increases beyond a certain point or when the esophagus is unable to clear refluxed material readily. Inflammation worsens in direct relationship to the length of time the esophagus is exposed to refluxed material. Esophagitis, which is usually limited to the distal 7–10 cm of the esophagus, is caused primarily by acid and pepsin. The

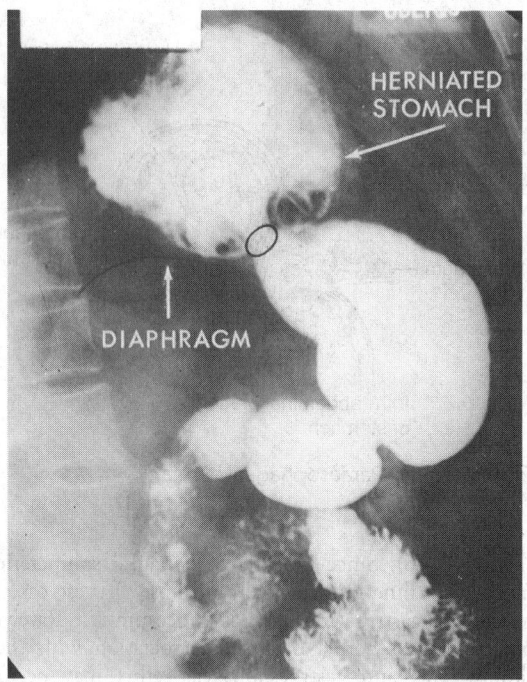

Figure 21–8. Large sliding hiatal hernia. Diaphragmatic hiatus is circled.

esophagus is particularly sensitive to bile acids, however, which may also play a role, especially in patients with previous gastric surgery.

The principal barrier to reflux is the lower esophageal sphincter. There is considerable overlap in the values for resting lower esophageal sphincter pressures in patients with reflux and normal subjects. The episodes of reflux that occur in normal persons follow transient relaxations of the sphincter. Three abnormalities of sphincter function allow reflux in patients with esophagitis: (1) transient relaxations of the sphincter in the presence of normal resting pressure; (2) spontaneous reflux in the presence of low resting pressure; and (3) transient increases in intra-abdominal pressure that overwhelm a low resting sphincter pressure. Three-fourths of the reflux episodes in patients with esophagitis follow a transient sphincteric relaxation. Most patients with esophagitis experience reflux at night while sleeping—an uncommon event in normal subjects. Nighttime reflux is related to increased frequency of transient relaxation of the sphincter and is associated with periodic bouts of increased gastric motility (phase III of the migrating motor complex). The chance of developing esophagitis is greater during the night because the refluxed material is primarily composed of acid and pepsin (no food in the stomach), esophageal peristalsis is decreased (delaying clearance),

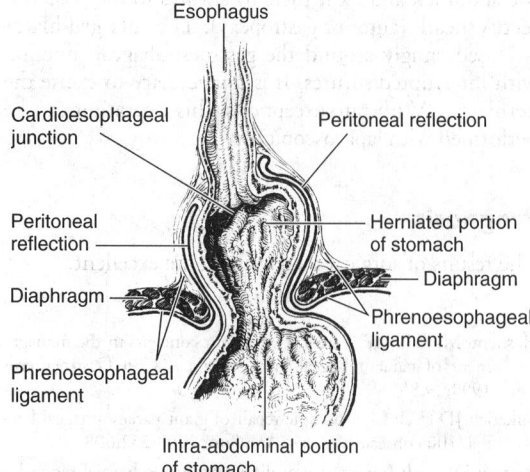

Figure 21–7. Sliding esophageal hernia.

and there is less saliva available to neutralize the acid. As the inflammation of the esophageal wall worsens, peristalsis is further compromised, causing further esophageal acid exposure and damage.

Most patients (80%) with clinically significant reflux have a sliding hiatal hernia (Figure 21–7 and 21–8). In these patients, the cardioesophageal junction and the fundus of the stomach are displaced upward into the posterior mediastinum, exposing the lower esophageal sphincter to intrathoracic pressure. Normally, the intraabdominal position of the lower esophagus causes it to be exposed to higher external pressures, and loss of this position accounts for the close association of reflux and hiatal hernia. In summary, sphincter competence is a function of sphincter pressure, sphincter length, and the length exposed to intra-abdominal pressure.

Clinical Findings

A. SYMPTOMS AND SIGNS

Retrosternal and epigastric burning pain—heartburn—occurs after eating and while sleeping or lying in a recumbent position. This distress is relieved partially or completely by drinking water or other liquids, by antacids, or, in many instances, by standing or sitting. The pain is sometimes similar to that of angina pectoris. Patients with severe regurgitation often report that bitter or sourtasting fluid may regurgitate as far as the throat and mouth (water brash), especially when they are supine. Nausea and vomiting are uncommon in adults but are the most common symptoms in infants, who usually present with failure to thrive. This is the result of postprandial regurgitation leading to vomiting. Anemia is another common presentation in this age group. Pulmonary symptoms (eg, wheezing, dyspnea) may occur as the result of aspiration, and when heartburn is not prominent (especially in infants and children), esophageal reflux may be overlooked as a cause of the disease.

Dysphagia may be a prominent complaint and results from the inflammatory edema (stricture formation) in the lower esophagus. Dysphagia indicates a more advanced stage of the disease and a greater likelihood that complications will develop.

B. Imaging Studies

The diagnosis of sliding esophageal hiatal hernia is made by the radiographic demonstration of a portion of the stomach protruding upward through the esophageal hiatus (Figure 21–8). Fluoroscopic observations while the stomach is full of barium are insensitive (40%) but relatively specific (85%) for diagnosing reflux. Only the most severe cases of esophagitis produce changes in the wall of the esophagus that can be seen on x-ray. X-rays are also useful to evaluate peptic strictures of the esophagus and esophageal ulceration, two complications of reflux.

C. SPECIAL EXAMINATIONS

Special examinations are needed (1) to diagnose abnormal reflux, (2) to quantify and characterize the amount of reflux, (3) to determine the extent of damage to the esophageal mucosa, and (4) to diagnose associated lesions and exclude cancer. Esophagoscopy (and biopsies) are particularly useful to determine the presence and degree of esophagitis and to diagnose associated upper gastrointestinal disease (eg, Barrett's epithelium, duodenal ulcer). One must be cautious, however, in interpreting the semiquantitative visual grading of esophagitis, for there is substantial inter-observer variation, particularly with the lower grades (Table 21–1).

Esophageal motility studies aid in the evaluation of gastroesophageal reflux by providing information on sphincter function and esophageal peristalsis. Mean resting pressure in the lower esophageal sphincter is lower in patients with reflux esophagitis (15 mm Hg) than in control subjects (30 mm Hg), but there is enough overlap so that abnormal reflux can only be diagnosed with certainty if resting pressure is below 6 mm Hg. Patients with more severe esophagitis have lower resting pressures than do those with less severe esophagitis. The normal amplitude of peristaltic contractions in the distal body of the esophagus averages 100 ± 40 mm Hg. Most patients with reflux have abnormal esophageal peristalsis: low amplitude and decreased velocity of propagation of the peristaltic wave. The defect is usually limited to the lower third of the esophagus, and it worsens with more severe esophagitis. Lack of peristalsis suggests the presence of another disease (eg, achalasia) or an associated condition (eg, scleroderma) that may require special treatment.

Prolonged monitoring of pH in the lower esophagus is the most sensitive method of establishing the presence of abnormal reflux. A pH probe is placed 5 cm above the manometrically identified lower esophageal sphincter, and a continuous recording of esophageal pH is stored in a small recorder attached to the patient's belt

Table 21–1. Endoscopic grading system for esophagitis.

Grade 1	Reddening of the mucosa without ulceration
Grade 2	Linear ulcerations lined with granulation tissue that bleeds easily when touched
Grade 3	Ulcerations have coalesced to leave islands of epithelium
Grade 4	Stricture

over a 24-hour period. The patient is asked to register any symptoms and is encouraged to live as normal a life as possible during the recording time. Computer analysis of the record provides a fairly accurate measurement of total esophageal acid exposure, frequency of reflux episodes, and time of day reflux occurred (Table 21–2). A relationship between reflux and symptoms can also be determined. This has virtually eliminated the need for the Bernstein test (infusion of acid in the esophagus to determine whether or not pain is elicited). Prolonged pH monitoring has demonstrated that most patients who have esophagitis reflux predominantly at night.

An accurate **scintigraphic technique** has been described for quantifying gastroesophageal reflux. It may be used for diagnosis or for assessing response to surgical therapy.

If sphincter function as measured manometrically seems good, the possibility of delayed gastric emptying should be suspected as a contributing factor. This should be assessed by measuring the rate of passage from the stomach of a technetium Tc 99m-labeled solid meal; symptoms are unreliable and barium x-rays and liquid emptying tests grossly insensitive.

Differential Diagnosis

Sliding esophageal hiatal hernia has been called the great masquerader of the upper abdomen. Other conditions may present symptoms that mimic those of hiatal hernia, and vice versa. The symptoms caused by a variety of abdominal and intrathoracic diseases are often difficult to differentiate from each other and from those of an uncomplicated sliding hernia. Cholelithiasis, diverticulitis, peptic ulcer, achalasia, and coronary artery disease are common examples. Since esophageal pain may be referred upward into the neck, shoulders, or

Table 21–2. Normal values for ambulatory 24-hour pH monitoring.

Percentage of total time pH < 4.0	4.5%
Percentage of upright time pH < 4.0	8.4%
Percentage of supine time pH < 4.0	3.5%
Number of episodes of reflux < 4.0	47
Number of episodes > 5 minutes	3½
Longest episode (minutes)	20
Composite score[1]	14.7

[1]The composite score indicates the extent to which the patient's values deviate from the normal means of the six variables. It allows one to express in a single figure the degree of the patient's abnormality. Calculation of the composite score is explained in Stein HJ et al: Outpatient physiologic testing and surgical management of foregut motility disorders. Curr Probl Surg 1992; 24:495.

arms, angina pectoris must be considered. The special examinations described above are particularly helpful in the differential diagnosis and in ascertaining the origin of symptoms in patients with associated diseases (cholelithiasis, angina pectoris, etc).

Complications

As indicated above, esophagitis due to reflux is the most common complication. Small, shallow ulcerations may develop. Areas of denuded epithelium at the cardia are occasionally replaced by columnar epithelium (Barrett's esophagus). This complication is associated with worse reflux and may lead to the development of adenocarcinoma. Aspiration of refluxed material may result in pneumonia, and rarely in pulmonary abscess. Aspiration of small amounts of regurgitated material or the presence of acid in the esophagus through reflex pathways has been thought to be responsible for the development of asthma.

Treatment

A. Medical Treatment

At least half of sliding esophageal hiatal hernias are asymptomatic and require no treatment. The great majority of patients with esophagitis can be managed by a conservative program.

Every effort must be made to enlist the aid of gravity in preventing reflux at night. The patient should not lie down after meals and should not eat a late meal before bedtime. The head of the patient's bed should be elevated on 4- to 6-inch blocks; attempting to sleep propped up on pillows almost never succeeds.

Frequent small meals keep gastric contents neutralized and avoid gastric distention. Meals low in fat and high in protein increase lower esophageal sphincter tone and decrease reflux. Prokinetic drugs such as cisapride and metoclopramide enhance healing of esophagitis, presumably by increasing sphincter tone and peristalsis of the esophagus and stomach.

Mild to moderate forms of esophagitis respond well to 8–12 weeks of treatment with H_2 receptor blockers. These drugs are less useful in severe esophagitis. Omeprazole is substantially better than cimetidine or ranitidine, achieving complete remission of symptoms and healing of esophagitis in 80–85% of patients. The problem with these drugs is that recurrences are the rule when they are discontinued, probably because neither sphincter pressure nor esophageal peristalsis is improved. The addition of a prokinetic agent does not appear to improve the outcome. Antacids do not add to the effects of H_2 blockers but may be used when side effects preclude their use. In this case, they should be used according to the principles outlined in Chapter 24.

B. Surgical Treatment

Surgery is indicated in the 15% of patients who have persistent or recurrent symptoms despite good medical therapy, in those with complete mechanical incompetence of the sphincter (pressure < 6 mm Hg), and in patients who present with or develop strictures during treatment. Antireflux operations can nearly always be performed laparoscopically.

The objectives are to restore the gastroesophageal junction and lower 5 cm of the esophagus to their normal intra-abdominal position and to buttress the gastroesophageal sphincter. In addition, the hiatal opening is narrowed by several sutures posteriorly that approximate the crura. The most effective procedure is Nissen fundoplication (Figure 21–9A), which involves wrapping part of the fundus completely around the lower 3–4 cm of esophagus and suturing it in place so the gastroesophageal sphincter passes through a short tunnel of

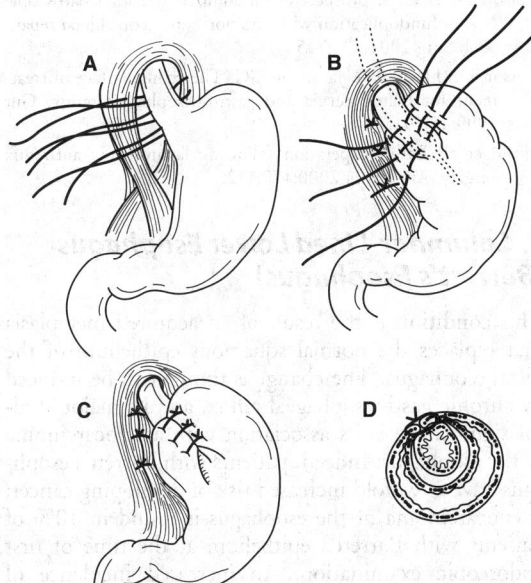

Figure 21–9. **A:** Dissection of the hiatus and lower mediastinum to mobilize the distal esophagus and restore about 6 cm to the abdominal position. **B:** Closure of the diaphragmatic crura behind the esophagus. **C:** Wrapping of the esophagus with the previously dissected fundus of the stomach. **D:** The transverse cut shows the gastric wrap around the distal esophagus. Note how increases in intragastric pressure would be transmitted to the esophagus, facilitating closure of the distal esophagus. The radius of this area of the esophagus is reduced, and the sphincter is prevented from dilating further because of the wrap.

stomach (Figure 21–9B). The wrap should be made relatively loose with a No. 56F dilator in the esophagus. The top of the wrap should be sutured to the side of the esophagus to prevent axial slipping. Figure 21–10 shows the radiographic appearance of the esophagogastric junction before and after this operation. The Lind fundoplication is similar except that the fundus is wrapped only 270 degrees around the esophagus. It is useful when peristalsis in the body of the esophagus is weak.

When the hernia cannot be reduced, the condition is called **acquired short esophagus.** Treatment involves constructing a tubular extension of the esophagus along the lesser curvature of the stomach (Collis procedure) with a GIA stapler. The resulting neofundus can be wrapped around the esophageal extension (Collis-Nissen). This is a rare operation. The alternative tactic of making a Nissen wrap in the chest has been associated with frequent complications unless the esophageal hiatus is surgically enlarged to prevent stasis in the thoracic portion of the stomach.

A procedure to reduce gastric acidity should not routinely be added to the hiatal hernia repair but should be reserved for patients with known peptic ulcer disease. A parietal cell vagotomy combined with a Nissen fundoplication is probably best in such cases but is rarely indicated.

Mild strictures can be managed by dilations with orally passed bougies (eg, Hurst or Maloney dilators) and an intensive medical regimen for the esophagitis. If this approach fails to result in improvement, surgery should be considered. Hiatal hernia repair plus occasional dilations will provide relief in most cases. Rigid strictures that cannot be successfully dilated are best treated by excising the stricture and interposing a segment of colon between normal esophagus and the antrum of the stomach.

When there have been one or more complicated operations around the gastroesophageal junction that have failed, it may be impossible to perform a safe dissection in this area or to mobilize the tissues enough to accomplish fundoplication. Delayed gastric emptying is often found to be a major contributing factor to reflux in these cases, occasionally as a result of unintentional vagotomy from the previous operations. The best treatment for many of these patients is vagotomy, antrectomy, and a Roux-en-Y gastrojejunostomy, which decreases acid secretion, accelerates gastric emptying, and prevents bile and pancreatic juice from gaining access to the esophagus.

Prognosis

About 90% of patients experience a good result following surgery; the remaining 10% have persistent or recurrent reflux. Relief of symptoms is accompanied by

Figure 21–10. Esophagogram before and after Nissen fundoplication in the same patient. **A:** Wide-open reflux of barium occurs through an incompetent sphincter associated with a sliding hiatal hernia. **B:** Three months after surgery, the fundic wrap is evident. Note contrast passing through a small channel surrounded by the wrap. The slightly impregnated transverse folds around this channel represent fundal mucosa of the wrap.

an increase in resting pressure in the lower esophageal sphincter of about 10 mm Hg. Recurrence of symptoms is more frequent than an anatomic recurrence. The latter may be due to inadequate technical repair initially; to excessive tension on the point of fixation of the cardioesophageal junction due to shortening of the esophagus; or to weakening of the musculofascial structures by aging, atrophy, or obesity.

Awad CG, Filipi CJ: The short esophagus: pathogenesis, diagnosis, and current surgical options. Arch Surg 2001;136:113.

Hunter JG et al: Laparoscopic fundoplication failures: patterns of failure and response to fundoplication revision. Ann Surg 1999;230:595.

Mattioli S et al: Clinical and surgical relevance of the progressive phases of intrathoracic migration of the gastroesophageal junction in gastroesophageal reflux disease. J Thorac Cardiovasc Surg 1998;116:267.

Schowengerdt CG: Standard acid reflux testing revisited. Dig Dis Sci 2001;46:603.

Watson DI et al: A prospective randomized trial of laparoscopic Nissen fundoplication with anterior vs posterior hiatal repair. Arch Surg 2001;136:745.

Watson DI, Devitt PG, Jamieson GG: The changing face of treatment for hiatus hernia and gastro-oesophageal reflux. Gut 1999;45:791.

Yau P et al: Early reoperation following laparoscopic antireflux surgery. Am J Surg 2000;179:172.

3. Columnar-Lined Lower Esophagus (Barrett's Esophagus)

This condition is the result of an acquired metaplasia that replaces the normal squamous epithelium of the distal esophagus. The change is thought to be induced by chronic gastroesophageal reflux, and its major clinical significance is its association with adenocarcinoma of the esophagus. Indeed, patients with Barrett's esophagus have a twofold increased risk of developing cancer; adenocarcinoma of the esophagus is found in 10% of patients with Barrett's epithelium at the time of first endoscopic examination. An increased incidence of other tumors (eg, colon cancer) has also been noted. The condition is more prevalent among men aged 50–70 years.

Barrett's esophagus is found in 10–15% of patients with reflux esophagitis, and it represents a more virulent form of gastroesophageal reflux. For example, lower esophageal sphincter pressure averages 5 mm Hg (compared with an average of 10 mm Hg for all patients with reflux); 24-hour pH monitoring reveals greater esophageal acid exposure than observed in uncomplicated esophagitis; and acid clearing of the distal esophagus is disproportionately impaired. As a result, damage to the esophagus is greater: ulcers and strictures are present in the majority of patients. In fact, 45% of patients with benign esophageal strictures have Barrett's esophagus. Ulcers in association with Barrett's epithelium are particularly worrisome because they have a tendency to penetrate adjacent organs, including the trachea, aorta, and heart. Barrett's esophagus in children is also associated with abnormal gastroesophageal reflux.

Limited extension of columnar epithelium above the gastroesophageal junction is relatively common in normal subjects. In order to qualify for the diagnosis of Barrett's, this epithelium must extend at least 3 cm above the gastroesophageal junction. The abnormal epithelium may be patchy when confined to the lower 10 cm of esophagus, but when it extends more proximally it is confluent from the gastroesophageal junction to the point of transition to squamous epithelium. Histologically, the epithelium may be one of three types: intestinal (the most common), junctional, or gastric fundic. The intestinal type does not absorb lipids, as does normal intestinal epithelium, and the gastric fundic type, although it contains parietal cells, is atrophic and not a source of significant amounts of acid.

Heartburn, regurgitation, and—with stricture formation—dysphagia are the most common symptoms. Heartburn is milder than in the absence of Barrett's changes, presumably because the metaplastic epithelium is less sensitive than squamous epithelium. The diagnosis is often suggested by the esophagoscopic finding of a pink epithelium in the lower esophagus instead of the shiny gray-pink squamous mucosa, but every case should be verified by biopsy. Radiographic findings consist of hiatal hernia, stricture, or ulcer or a reticular pattern to the mucosa—changes of low sensitivity and specificity.

Treatment is the same as for reflux esophagitis in general: antacids, H_2-blocking agents, elevation of the head of the bed, and avoidance of smoking and ulcerogenic beverages or drugs. Antireflux surgery (eg, Nissen fundoplication), is commonly indicated because of the severity of gastroesophageal reflux or the development of ulcers or strictures. Some strictures may require periodic postoperative dilation. Resection is required on rare occasions to treat a nondilatable stricture or to control bleeding. The abnormal epithelium rarely regresses after medical or surgical therapy.

Because of the substantially increased risk of cancer, routine endoscopy and biopsy should be performed every 6–12 months, especially in patients with intestinal metaplasia. Biopsies should be obtained at multiple levels looking for carcinoma (which is not always identifiable by gross examination) and for dysplasia. High-grade dysplasia is clearly associated with carcinoma, but the histologic diagnosis is difficult. Flow cytometry can now identify abnormalities of DNA content, such as aneuploidy or increased G_2/tetraploid fractions, that are associated with high-grade dysplasia and increased risk of cancer. Transmission electron microscopy may detect abnormalities in cytoplasmic organelles that have similar implications. Patients who are found to have high-grade dysplasia or the abnormalities described should be considered for resection of the entire portion of esophagus lined with Barrett's mucosa.

Campos GM et al: Predictive factors of Barrett esophagus: multivariate analysis of 502 patients with gastroesophageal reflux disease. Arch Surg 2001;136:1267.

Castell DO: Medical, surgical, and endoscopic treatment of gastroesophageal reflux disease and Barrett's esophagus. J Clin Gastroenterol 2001;33:262.

Fitzgerald RC et al: Rigorous surveillance protocol increases detection of curable cancers associated with Barrett's esophagus. Dig Dis Sci 2001;46:1892.

Hofstetter WL et al: Long-term outcome of antireflux surgery in patients with Barrett's esophagus. Ann Surg 2001;234:532.

Morris CD et al: Prevention of the neoplastic progression of Barrett's oesophagus by endoscopic argon beam plasma ablation. Br J Surg 2001;88:1357.

Oberg S et al: Endoscopic surveillance of columnar-lined esophagus: frequency of intestinal metaplasia detection and impact of antireflux surgery. Ann Surg 2001;234:619.

Spechler SJ et al: Long-term outcome of medical and surgical therapies for gastroesophageal reflux disease: follow-up of a randomized controlled trial. JAMA 2001;285:2331.

OTHER SURGICAL DISORDERS OF THE ESOPHAGUS

PERFORATION OF THE ESOPHAGUS

ESSENTIALS OF DIAGNOSIS

- *History of recent instrumentation of the esophagus or severe vomiting.*
- *Pain in the neck, chest, or upper abdomen.*
- *Signs of mediastinal or thoracic sepsis within 24 hours.*
- *Contrast radiographic evidence of an esophageal leak.*
- *Crepitus and subcutaneous emphysema of the neck in some cases.*

General Considerations

Esophageal perforations can result from iatrogenic instrumentation (eg, endoscopy, balloon dilation), severe vomiting, external trauma, and other rare causes. The subsequent clinical manifestations are influenced by the site of the perforation (ie, cervical or thoracic) and, in the case of thoracic perforations, whether or not the mediastinal pleura has been ruptured. Morbidity resulting from esophageal perforation is principally due to cervical or mediastinal and thoracic infection. Immediately after injury, the tissues are contaminated by esophageal fluids, but infection has not become established; surgical closure of the defect will usually prevent the development of serious infection. If more than 24 hours have elapsed between injury and surgical treatment, infection will have occurred. At this time, the esophageal defect usually breaks down if it is surgically closed, and measures to treat mediastinitis and empyema may not be adequate to avoid a fatal outcome. Although serious infection usually occurs if surgical repair is delayed, a few cases of minor instrumental perforations can be managed by antibiotics without operation.

A. INSTRUMENTAL PERFORATIONS

Instrumental perforations are most likely to occur in the cervical esophagus. The esophagoscope may press the posterior wall of the esophagus against osteoarthritic spurs of the cervical vertebrae, causing contusion or laceration. The cricopharyngeal area is the most common site of injury. Perforations of the thoracic esophagus may occur at any level but are most common at the natural sites of narrowing, ie, at the level of the left main stem bronchus and at the diaphragmatic hiatus.

B. SPONTANEOUS (EMETOGENIC) PERFORATION (BOERHAAVE'S SYNDROME)

Spontaneous perforation usually occurs in the absence of preexisting esophageal disease, but 10% of patients have reflux esophagitis, esophageal diverticulum, carcinoma, etc. Most cases follow a bout of heavy eating and drinking. The rupture usually involves all layers of the esophageal wall and most frequently occurs in the left posterolateral aspect 3–5 cm above the gastroesophageal junction. The tear results from excessive intraluminal pressure, usually caused by violent retching and vomiting. Cases have also been associated with childbirth, defecation, convulsions, heavy lifting, and forceful swallowing. The overlying pleura is also torn, so that the chest as well as the mediastinum is contaminated with esophageal contents. The second most common site of perforation is at the midthoracic esophagus on the right side at the level of the azygos vein.

Clinical Findings

A. SIGNS AND SYMPTOMS

The principal early manifestation is pain, which is felt in the neck with cervical perforations and in the chest or upper abdomen with thoracic perforations. The pain may radiate to the back. With cervical perforations, pain followed by crepitus in the neck, dysphagia, and gradually developing signs of infection is the extent of the syndrome. Thoracic perforations, which communicate with the pleural cavity in about 75% of cases, are usually accompanied by tachypnea, hyperpnea, dyspnea, and the early development of hypotension. With perforation into the chest, pneumothorax is produced followed by hydrothorax and, if not promptly treated, empyema. The left chest is involved in 70% and the right chest in 20%; involvement is bilateral in 10%. The rate of fluid accumulation in the chest may be as high a 1 L/h, which results in hypovolemia and a shift of the mediastinum to the right. Escape of air into the mediastinum may result in a "mediastinal crunch," which is produced by the heart beating against air-filled tissues (Hamman's sign). If the pleura remains intact, mediastinal emphysema appears more rapidly, and pleural effusion is slow to develop.

B. IMAGING STUDIES

X-ray studies are important to demonstrate that perforation has occurred and to locate the site of the injury. In perforations of the cervical esophagus, x-rays show air in the soft tissues, especially along the cervical spine. The trachea may be displaced anteriorly by air and fluid. Later, widening of the superior mediastinum may be seen. With thoracic perforations, mediastinal widening and pleural effusion with or without pneumothorax are the usual findings. Mediastinal emphysema, seen in about 40% of cases, takes at least an hour to develop.

An esophagogram using water-soluble contrast medium should be performed promptly in every patient suspected of having an esophageal perforation (Figure 21–11). The patient should be studied in the decubitus as well as the upright position. If a leak is not seen, the examination should be repeated using barium.

C. SPECIAL STUDIES

Thoracentesis will reveal cloudy or purulent fluid depending on how much time has passed since the contamination first occurred. The amylase content of the fluid is elevated, and serum amylase levels may also be high as a result of absorption of amylase from the pleural cavity.

Treatment

Antibiotics should be given immediately. Early surgery is appropriate for all but a few cases, and every effort should be made to operate before the perforation is 24 hours old. For lesions treated within this time limit, the operation should consist of closure of the perforation and external drainage. External drainage alone may suf-

Figure 21–11. Extravasation of contrast material through instrumental perforation of upper thoracic esophagus. Note loculi of air and fluid anterior to esophagus, indicating that mediastinitis has already developed.

fice for small cervical perforations, which may be difficult to find. Patients with achalasia in whom perforation has resulted from balloon dilation of the lower esophageal sphincter should have the tear in the esophagus repaired and a Heller myotomy performed on the opposite side of the esophagus. Definitive therapy (eg, resection) should also be performed in patients with other surgical conditions, such as esophageal carcinoma.

Primary repair has a high failure rate if the perforation is older than 24 hours. The classic recommendation in this situation has been to isolate the perforation (ie, to minimize further contamination) by performing a temporary cervical esophagostomy, ligating the cardia, and constructing a feeding jejunostomy. Probably a better approach is to resect the site of the perforation, bringing the proximal end of esophagus out through the neck and closing the distal end. The mediastinum is drained and a feeding jejunostomy created. Later, the esophagostomy is taken down and colon interposed to bridge the gap at the site of resection. Blunt esophagectomy may be feasible as emergency treatment of instrumental perforation in a patient with lye stricture.

Spontaneous incomplete rupture of the esophagus is seen occasionally. This lesion may be the result of increased intraluminal pressure or may be idiopathic, but the tear is usually located in the mid esophagus. In incomplete rupture, the tear is confined to the mucosal layer; it dissects distally in the submucosal plane, often as far as the gastroesophageal junction. The manifestations consist of chest pain, dyspnea, odynophagia, and, sometimes, bleeding. An esophagogram demonstrates an intramural tract of barium (which may give a double-lumen appearance) and sometimes encroachment on the esophageal lumen by an intramural hematoma. Treatment is with antibiotics and total parenteral nutrition.

Nonoperative management consisting of antibiotics alone may be all that is necessary in a few selected cases of instrumental perforation. This approach should be confined to patients without thoracic involvement (eg, pneumothorax or hydrothorax) whose esophagogram demonstrates just a short extraluminal sinus tract without wide mediastinal spread (ie, the contamination is limited) and who have no systemic signs of sepsis (eg, hypotension and tachypnea).

Prognosis

The survival rate is 90% when surgical treatment is accomplished within 24 hours. The rate drops to about 50% when treatment is delayed.

Dresner SM et al: Spontaneous oesophageal perforation during vaginal delivery. J R Soc Med 2001;94:90.

Younes Z, Johnson DA: The spectrum of spontaneous and iatrogenic esophageal injury: perforations, Mallory-Weiss tears, and hematomas. J Clin Gastroenterol 1999;29:306.

INGESTED FOREIGN OBJECTS

Most cases of ingested foreign objects occur in children who swallow coins or other small objects. In adults, the problem most often consists of esophageal meat impaction or, less commonly, lodged bones or toothpicks. Dentures, which interfere with the ability to judge the size and consistency of a food bolus, and esophageal disease, such as a benign stricture, are the principal predisposing factors in adults. Prisoners and mentally defective persons occasionally swallow foreign objects intentionally.

About 90% of swallowed foreign objects pass into the stomach and from there into the intestine and are eventually passed without incident. Ten percent hang up in the esophagus. If they traverse the esophagus, objects whose dimensions exceed 2×5 cm tend to remain in the stomach. Ten percent of ingested foreign objects require endoscopic removal, and 1% require surgery.

About 10% of ingested foreign objects enter the tracheobronchial tree.

The history usually defines the problem adequately. The patient with a foreign object in the esophagus may or may not experience dysphagia or chest pain.

Specific Kinds of Ingested Foreign Objects

A. Coins

Pennies and dimes usually pass into the stomach, but larger coins will lodge in the esophagus at or just beyond the cricopharyngeus. It is important to know if a swallowed coin has remained in the esophagus, and whether or not the patient has symptoms is an unreliable basis for making the determination. Therefore, anteroposterior and lateral chest x-rays should be obtained to determine whether the coin is in the esophagus or trachea. Small children should be x-rayed from the base of the skull to the anus in order to find any additional coins in the gut.

Coins in the esophagus should be removed promptly, since serious complications (eg, esophagoaortic fistula) may occur if treatment delay exceeds 24 hours. The procedure is best accomplished with a grasping forceps passed through a flexible endoscope. Sedation is adequate for older children or adults, but general endotracheal anesthesia is required in order to protect the airway of infants and young children. A smooth foreign body too large to grasp with a forceps can be removed by passing a dilating balloon beyond it and then withdrawing the endoscope and balloon as a unit. If the object is small enough (< 20 mm), it may be pushed into the stomach.

Another popular technique for extracting coins is to pass a Foley catheter into the esophagus under radiologic control and withdraw the coin with the inflated balloon. Although usually successful, this method has the disadvantage of providing incomplete protection of the airway.

Once a coin has passed into the stomach, it can be observed by periodic x-rays for as long as a month before the conclusion is reached that spontaneous elimination is unlikely and endoscopic removal is indicated.

B. Meat Impaction

Meat is the most common foreign object that lodges in the esophagus of adults, and many affected patients have underlying esophageal disease. The site of meat impaction is usually at the cricopharyngeus muscle or cervical esophagus, where it may exert pressure anteriorly on the trachea and produce respiratory obstruction.

No x-rays (especially barium studies) are indicated, for they make the endoscopist's task more difficult. If obstruction is complete and the patient cannot handle saliva, endoscopy should be performed as an emergency to prevent aspiration. If the clinical findings are minor, however, endoscopy can be postponed for up to 12 hours (but no longer) to see whether the food will pass spontaneously.

Meat can usually be removed as a single piece using a polypectomy snare passed through a flexible endoscope. If the meat has begun to fragment, a rigid endoscope makes the job of piecemeal removal easier. In some cases, a meat bolus can be pushed into the stomach, which is safe so long as it passes with minimal pressure. After the esophagus has been cleared, it should be checked endoscopically for underlying disease. An esophageal stricture should be dilated if the esophageal wall is not acutely inflamed as a result of the meat impaction.

Attempts to digest meat in the esophagus with topical papain are not advised. The enzyme actually has little effect on the meat, and it may damage the esophageal wall. Gas-forming agents (which push the object) and glucagon (which relaxes the esophagus) have been recommended for this purpose, but these methods are less effective than flexible endoscopy.

C. Sharp and Pointed Objects

Bones, safety pins, hat pins, razor blades, toothpicks, nails, and many others constitute this group of foreign objects. The general principles of management are (1) to remove sharp or pointed objects endoscopically by grasping and pulling a blunt side (eg, the hinge of an open safety pin) if there is one with forceps; (2) to remove a piece of glass or a razor blade by pulling it into the lumen of a rigid esophagoscope; or (3) to operate if neither of these methods appears to be safe. Sharp or pointed objects in the stomach should be removed surgically, since 25% of them will perforate the intestine, usually near the ileocecal valve, if they exit the pylorus.

D. Button Batteries

These small batteries are swallowed by children, just like coins, but unlike coins they are highly corrosive and should be removed urgently before a serious complication such as an esophagotracheal or esophagoaortic fistula develops.

E. Cocaine Packets

Cocaine smugglers may swallow small packets of cocaine in balloons or condoms. Rupture of just one of these packets can be fatal, so attempts at endoscopic removal are unsafe. If it appears that the packets will pass spontaneously, the patient may be watched; otherwise, surgical removal is indicated.

F. Foreign Bodies in the Pharynx and Cricopharyngeus

Foreign objects at this level should be removed using sedation and direct laryngoscopy. Most are fish bones.

Complications

Aspiration and esophageal ulceration are the most common complications. Perforation of the esophagus or other portions of the gut requires surgical repair. It is estimated that about 1500 people die in the USA each year from complications of ingested foreign bodies.

Arana A et al: Management of ingested foreign bodies in childhood and review of the literature. Eur J Pediatr 2001;160:468.

Sapru A et al: Esophageal foreign body causing recurrent respiratory symptoms. Gastrointest Endosc 1998;48:218.

Soprano JV, Mandl KD: Four strategies for the management of esophageal coins in children. Pediatrics 2000;105:e5.

Younger RM, Darrow DH: Handheld metal detector confirmation of radiopaque foreign bodies in the esophagus. Arch Otolaryngol Head Neck Surg 2001;127:1371.

CORROSIVE ESOPHAGITIS

ESSENTIALS OF DIAGNOSIS

- *History of ingestion of caustic liquids or solids.*
- *Burns of the lips, mouth, tongue, and oropharynx.*
- *Chest pain and dysphagia.*

General Considerations

Ingestion of strong solutions of acid or alkali or of solid substances of similar nature produces extensive chemical burns, often leading to corrosive esophagitis. The injury usually represents a suicide attempt in adults and accidental ingestion in children. Strong alkali produces "liquefaction necrosis," which involves dissolution of protein and collagen, saponification of fats, dehydration of tissues, thrombosis of blood vessels, and deep penetrating injuries. Acids produce a "coagulation necrosis" involving eschar formation, which tends to shield the deeper tissues from injury. Depending upon the concentration and the length of time the irritant remains in contact with the mucosa, sloughing of the mucous membrane, edema and inflammation of the submucosa, infection, perforation, and mediastinitis may develop.

Ingested lye in solid form tends to adhere to the mucosa of the pharynx and proximal esophagus. Severe acute esophageal necrosis is rare, and the main clinical problems are early edema and late stricture formation, principally of the proximal esophagus. Liquid caustics commonly produce much more extensive esophageal necrosis, and occasionally even tracheoesophageal and esophagoaortic fistulas. If the patient survives the acute phase, a lengthy nondilatable stricture often develops.

Ingestion of strong acid characteristically produces greatest injury to the stomach, with the esophagus remaining intact in over 80% of cases. The result may be immediate gastric necrosis or late antral stenosis.

Nearly all severe injuries are caused by strong alkali. Weak alkali and acid are associated with less extensive lesions.

Clinical Findings

A. SYMPTOMS AND SIGNS

Systemic symptoms roughly parallel the severity of the caustic burn. The most common finding is inflammatory edema of the lips, mouth, tongue, and oropharynx; in the absence of visible injury in this area, severe esophageal damage is rare. Patients with serious esophageal burns often experience chest pain and dysphagia and drooling of large amounts of saliva. Pain on attempted swallowing may be intense. If the damage is severe, the patient often appears toxic, with high fever, prostration, and shock. The absence of toxicity does not rule out severe injury, however. Tracheobronchitis accompanied by coughing and increased bronchial secretions is frequently noted. Stridor may be present, and in a few patients respiratory obstruction progresses rapidly and requires tracheostomy for relief. Complete esophageal obstruction due to edema, inflammation, and mucosal sloughing may develop within the first few days.

B. ESOPHAGOSCOPY

A determination of the extent of injury by esophagoscopy contributes substantially to therapeutic decisions. Esophagoscopic examination should be performed after the initial resuscitation, usually within 12 hours of admission. The scope is inserted far enough to gauge the most serious degree of burn, which is classified as first-, second-, or third-degree as defined in Table 21–3.

Treatment

Classic treatment for caustic injuries of the esophagus was the administration of antibiotics and corticosteroids and observation for late stricture formation. The advent of strong liquid alkalis in the marketplace, however, has resulted in more severe full-thickness injuries, which are too often fatal or cause lengthy nondilatable strictures when treated in this fashion. Furthermore, the evidence now indicates that corticosteroids really have little or no effect on stricture formation. Early surgery is now recommended for patients with second- and third-degree burns.

Table 21–3. Endoscopic grading of corrosive burns of esophagus and stomach.[1]

Grade	Definition	Endoscopic Findings
First-degree	Superficial mucosal injury	Mucosal hyperemia and edema; superficial mucosal desquamation.
Second-degree	Full-thickness mucosal involvement. No or partial-thickness muscular injury.	Sloughing of mucosa. Hemorrhage, exudate, ulceration, pseudomembrane formation, and granulation tissue when examined late.
Third-degree	Full-thickness esophageal or gastric injury with extension into adjacent tissues.	Sloughing of tissues with deep ulceration. Complete obliteration of esophageal lumen by edema; charring and eschar formation; full-thickness necrosis; perforation.

[1]Reproduced, with permission, from Estrera A et al: Corrosive burns of the esophagus and stomach: a recommendation for an aggressive surgical approach. Ann Thorac Surg 1986;41:276.

Patients with first-degree burns do not require aggressive therapy and may be discharged from the hospital after a short period of observation. Patients with second- or third-degree burns are best treated by early laparotomy, at which time the distal esophagus and stomach are inspected and a full-thickness biopsy of the gastric wall is taken to further grade the lesion. It is not possible to distinguish between a minor third-degree injury and extensive full-thickness third-degree necrosis from the esophagoscopic findings alone. This must be done from external appearances at laparotomy.

Second-degree and minor spotty third-degree injuries are treated by inserting an esophageal stent (a Silastic tube) and a jejunostomy feeding tube. If any question remains about the viability of the tissues, a second-look operation should be performed 36 hours later. Antibiotics and corticosteroids are given, and the stent is left in place for 3 weeks, at which time an esophagogram is performed. If barium passes freely alongside the stent, it is removed. If it does not, the stent is left in place for another week, and x-rays are repeated. Periodic esophagograms are obtained in late follow-up to look for stricture formation, which is treated early in its development by dilations.

Third-degree burns involving extensive esophagogastric necrosis require emergency esophagogastrectomy, esophagostomy, and feeding jejunostomy. Esophagec-

tomy is best performed by the blunt technique using a laparotomy and cervical incision. It is sometimes necessary to resect adjacent organs (eg, transverse colon) that have also been damaged. Reconstruction by substernal colon interposition is performed 6–8 weeks later.

Prognosis

Early and proper management of caustic burns provides satisfactory results in most cases. The ingestion of strong acid or alkaline solutions with extensive immediate destruction of the mucosa produces profound pathologic changes which may result in fibrous strictures that require dilations and, in some cases, esophagectomy and colon interposition.

Avanoglu A, Ergun O, Mutaf O: Management of instrumental perforations of the esophagus occurring during treatment of corrosive strictures. J Pediatr Surg 1998;33:1393.

Cury EK et al: Thoracoscopic esophagectomy in children. J Pediatr Surg 2001;36:E17.

de Jong AL et al: Corrosive esophagitis in children: a 30-year review. Int J Pediatr Otorhinolaryngol 2001;57:203.

Huang YC et al: Balloon dilation of double strictures after corrosive esophagitis. J Pediatr Gastroenterol Nutr 2001;32:496.

Kim YT, Sung SW, Kim JH: Is it necessary to resect the diseased esophagus in performing reconstruction for corrosive esophageal stricture? Eur J Cardiothorac Surg 2001;20:1.

Samad L, Ali M, Ramzi H: Button battery ingestion: hazards of esophageal impaction. J Pediatr Surg 1999;34:1527.

TUMORS OF THE ESOPHAGUS

1. Benign Tumors of the Esophagus

 ESSENTIALS OF DIAGNOSIS

- Dysphagia often present but frequently mild.
- Sense of pressure in thorax or neck.
- Radiographic demonstration of intra- or extraluminal mass, smooth in outline.

General Considerations

Benign growths may arise in any layer of the esophagus. Inflammatory polyps or granulomas are occasionally associated with esophagitis and may be mistakenly interpreted as neoplastic lesions. Papillomas arising from the mucosa are either sessile or pedunculated; although they are usually small lesions, occasionally they become large enough to produce obstruction. They may slough off spontaneously into the esophageal lumen.

Leiomyoma is the most common benign lesion of the esophagus. Leiomyomas are benign tumors that originate in the smooth muscle of the esophagus. As they grow, they narrow the esophageal lumen. The mucosa overlying the tumor is generally intact, but occasionally it may become ulcerated as a result of pressure necrosis by an enlarging lesion. Leiomyomas are not associated with the development of cancer. Other tumors such as fibromas, lipomas, fibromyomas, and myxomas are rare.

Congenital cysts or reduplications of the esophagus (the second most common benign lesion after leiomyoma) may occur at any level, although they are most common in the lower esophagus.

Clinical Findings

Many benign lesions are asymptomatic and are discovered incidentally during upper gastrointestinal fluoroscopic examination. Cysts and leiomyomas may be large enough to appear as a density, usually round or ovoid, in the mediastinum on routine chest x-rays. Benign tumors or cysts grow slowly and become symptomatic only after enough encroachment of the esophageal lumen has occurred. Barium swallow in a patient with leiomyoma shows a smoothly rounded, often spherical mass that causes extrinsic narrowing of the esophageal lumen (Figure 21–12). The overlying mucosa is almost always intact. Peristalsis is not affected by leiomyomas but is often abnormal in the presence of cysts or reduplications. Spasm of the musculature adjacent to the cyst or duplication is the most common abnormality of peristalsis. Dilation of the esophagus proximal to any of the benign lesions is rare. Intraluminal growths can be recognized at esophagoscopy, and a specific tissue diagnosis should always be obtained. Intramural lesions such as leiomyomas should not be biopsied, because (1) there is a risk of hemorrhage and (2) an adhesion develops between the tumor and the mucosa, making the lesion difficult to shell out during surgery and resulting in an otherwise avoidable mucosal opening.

Differential Diagnosis

Leiomyomas, cysts, and reduplications can be distinguished from cancerous growths by their classic radiographic appearance. Intraluminal papillomas, polyps, or granulomas may be indistinguishable radiographically from early carcinoma, so their exact nature must be confirmed histologically.

Complications

Cysts and duplications derive their arterial supply directly from the aorta. Hemorrhage into these lesions may occur, especially following infection, although this complication is uncommon. Adhesions that form between the cystic lesions and the adjacent esophagus often produce progressive dysphagia. Pedunculated intraluminal tumors may cause sudden obstruction by torsion of their pedicles, which is followed by edema, infection, and bleeding. In the upper esophagus, pedunculated polypoid growths may be regurgitated upward into the hypopharynx and occasionally may fall into the glottic chink and produce laryngeal obstruction.

Bleeding may occur from ulcerations of the mucosa overlying a leiomyoma. Symptoms related to benign lesions of the esophagus are usually due to the presence of the lesion itself; the severity of the dysphagia is accentuated by the development of swelling, infection, hemorrhage, or obstruction.

Treatment

Small polypoid intraluminal lesions may be removed completely with biopsy forceps during esophagoscopy. Some intramural lesions can also be removed endoscopically or, in the cases of cysts, injected through the endoscope after endosonographic localization. However, most intramural lesions, such as leiomyomas, should be resected if symptomatic. This can be accomplished in most cases thoracoscopically. A cervical approach is used for lesions in the cervical esophagus.

Figure 21–12. Leiomyoma of esophagus. Note smooth, rounded density causing extrinsic compression of esophageal lumen.

Bonavina L et al: Surgical therapy of esophageal leiomyoma. J Am Coll Surg. 1995;181:257.

Takada N et al: Utility of endoscopic ultrasonography in assessing the indications for endoscopic surgery of submucosal esophageal tumors. Surg Endosc 1999;13:228.

Tamura K et al: Thoracoscopic resection of a giant leiomyoma of the esophagus with a mediastinal outgrowth. Ann Thorac Cardiovasc Surg 1998;4:351.

2. Carcinoma of the Esophagus

 ESSENTIALS OF DIAGNOSIS

- *Progressive dysphagia, initially during ingestion of solid foods and later for liquids.*
- *Progressive weight loss and inanition.*
- *Classic radiographic outlines: irregular mucosal pattern with narrowing, with shelf-like upper border or concentrically narrowed esophageal lumen.*
- *Definitive diagnosis established by endoscopic biopsy or cytology.*

General Considerations

Carcinoma of the esophagus constituted about 1% of all malignant lesions and 6% of those of the gastrointestinal tract in the USA in 2001. Blacks have a fivefold higher incidence of squamous cell carcinoma than whites, but the incidence of adenocarcinoma among blacks is one-third that of whites. Both lesions are more common among men, with a male-to-female ratio of 7:10 for adenocarcinoma and 3:4 for squamous cell tumors. The peak incidence is between ages 50 and 60 years. Heavy alcohol or tobacco use is thought to predispose to esophageal carcinoma in the USA. Although some adenocarcinomas of the cardia represent an upward extension of a gastric tumor, true adenocarcinoma of the esophagus, primarily related to Barrett's epithelium, has been increasing in frequency in the USA and accounts for up to 40% of cases in some series. Twenty percent of esophageal tumors occur in the upper third, 30% in the middle third, and 50% in the lower esophagus. Squamous cell lesions predominate in the mid esophagus; adenocarcinomas are more common in the lower third.

The carcinoma usually appears as a fungating growth extending irregularly into the esophageal lumen and spanning a distance of 5 cm in the average case. Ulceration of its central portion is common. Annular lesions with extensive infiltration of the esophageal wall produce obstruction earlier than those that involve only a portion of the circumference of the esophagus. Regardless of cell type, the tumors disseminate by direct invasion into surrounding mediastinal structures, through the blood-stream by local vascular involvement, and by lymphatic dissemination. Direct intramural extension from the gross margin of the lesion is greater proximally than distally. It reaches 3 cm in 65% of cases; 6 cm in 20%; and 9 cm in 10%. In 15% of patients, there are additional islands of tumor within 5 cm of the gross margin of the lesion, suggesting a multicentric origin. Metastases to lymph nodes in the neck, mediastinum, or celiac area of the abdomen are present at the time of diagnosis in 80% of cases regardless of the site of the primary lesion. Lymph node metastases are present in 50% of cases with a primary tumor of less than 5 cm and in 90% of those with a larger tumor. Extramural extension of the tumor with involvement of other structures, such as the trachea, left main stem bronchus, or aorta is relatively common and carries an ominous prognosis. Lung, bone, liver, and adrenal glands are frequent sites of distant metastases. About 5% of patients have a second primary neoplasm of the stomach, oral cavity, pharynx, larynx, or skin. Flow cytometric analysis of nuclear DNA has shown that tumors with the aneuploid pattern have a higher frequency of lymph node metastasis and a higher recurrence rate after surgery. Other karyometric measurements, including total nuclear DNA content and nuclear area, also have prognostic significance. For example, the greater the area, the more likely it is that the tumor will have transmural penetration. Similarly, high levels of epidermal growth factor receptors are associated with a poor prognosis in patients with squamous cell carcinoma.

In certain well-circumscribed areas of the world (eg, Caspian littoral of Iran; southeastern South Africa; and northern provinces of China), the incidence of esophageal carcinoma exceeds 100 cases per 100,000 population. The cause in these areas is still unknown. In northern China, silica particles have been detected in millet bran used in bread making and in the esophageal walls of affected patients. The presence of nitrosamines in drinking water, fungal contamination of food, and malnutrition are probably of etiologic importance in some regions of the world. Other premalignant states are chronic iron deficiency, esophageal stasis (eg, achalasia), Barrett's esophagus, reflux esophagitis, and congenital tylosis of the esophagus.

Clinical Findings

A. SYMPTOMS AND SIGNS

Dysphagia is the most prominent symptom, and as a result, loss of weight is often striking. Solid foods initially cause difficulty; later, even liquids may be difficult to swallow. Weight loss, weakness, anemia, and inanition are almost always present. Pain, a major complaint in 30% of patients at presentation, may be related to swallowing; if pain is constant, the tumor has probably invaded somatic structures. Regurgitation and aspiration are common, especially at night when the patient is recumbent. Coughing related to swallowing indicates either a high lesion or the presence of a tracheoesophageal fistula. Hoarseness most often reflects spread to the recurrent laryngeal nerves.

B. IMAGING STUDIES

Chest x-rays may show pneumonitis, pleural effusion, or a lung abscess. A column of air in the esophageal lumen, absent in a normal esophagus, may be visible on plain films, or an air-fluid level may be present.

Barium swallow demonstrates narrowing of the esophageal lumen at the site of the lesion and dilation proximally, although the magnitude of the dilation is not as great as in benign conditions such as achalasia. The tumor appears as an irregular mass of variable size and length whose upper border is roughly horizontal and resembles a "shelf." Annular lesions appear as constricting bands with a narrowed lumen that contains an irregular mucosal outline (Figure 21–13). Angulation of the axis of the esophagus above and below the tumor may be seen, a finding that strongly suggests spread of the lesion to extraesophageal sites.

CT scans are useful to diagnose liver metastasis and, to a lesser degree, mediastinal and celiac axis nodal in-volvement. Esophageal endosonography is more accurate in the determination of wall penetration and mediastinal invasion.

C. ESOPHAGOSCOPY AND BRONCHOSCOPY

Esophagoscopy with biopsy provides accurate tissue diagnosis in 95% of cases. However, the mucosa immediately proximal to a very stenotic lesion may be so redundant, edematous, and inflamed that the tumor may not be directly visible at esophagoscopy. In this case, cellular material should be obtained by esophageal washings or brushings.

Because lesions of the upper and mid esophagus may invade the tracheobronchial tree, bronchoscopy is always indicated in the assessment of growths at these levels. Positive findings include distortion of the bronchial lumen, blunting of the carina, or intrabronchial tumor.

Differential Diagnosis

The fungating type of esophageal cancer presents a typical radiographic picture consisting of an irregular mucosal contour and the uppermost "shelf." Annular carcinomas may be mistaken for benign strictures, especially if most of the growth is intramural. Benign papillomas,

Figure 21–13. Two common types of esophageal carcinoma.

polyps, or granulomatous masses can be distinguished from early carcinomas only on histologic examination.

Complications

Cancer of the esophagus rarely bleeds massively, although anemia due to occult bleeding is frequent. The most common complications result from invasion of important mediastinal structures such as the trachea, major bronchi, and pericardium. Fatal hemorrhage, tracheal obstruction, and cardiac dysrhythmias may result. A fistula may develop between the esophagus and the tracheobronchial tree and lead to aspiration pneumonitis, purulent bronchitis, and pulmonary abscess formation.

Treatment

Esophageal carcinoma is treated by surgery, radiotherapy, chemotherapy, or a combination of these methods. It is important to stage the lesion as accurately as possible before deciding on the treatment plan. Resectability of the primary lesion must first be determined. Nonresectability is suggested by direct spread to the tracheobronchial tree or aorta as seen on bronchoscopy or CT scans or by noting angulation of the esophageal axis. The presence of a tracheoesophageal fistula or hoarseness associated with vocal cord paralysis has a similar significance. Primary tumors larger than 10 cm are rarely resectable. Overall, about 50% of tumors are resectable at the time of presentation and about 75% following preoperative radiotherapy and chemotherapy. As long as the patient is a suitable candidate for major surgery and distant organ metastases are absent, the primary tumor should be resected if possible. If life expectancy is longer than a few months, resection is usually recommended regardless of the chance for cure, because it provides the best palliation.

Preoperative radiation therapy may convert an unresectable growth to a resectable one, but adjuvant radiotherapy has not increased the overall cure rate. Radiation therapy combined with chemotherapy, with or without radiosensitizing agents, has been used with the hope of enhancing local tumor control and effecting simultaneous destruction of systemic micrometastases. For example, fluorouracil, cisplatin, and mitomycin C or vincristine sulfate have been given in combination with 2500–3000 cGy directed at the primary lesion in several trials. This therapy produced complete remission in 20–35% of patients. In most trials, patients were subjected to esophagectomy following chemotherapy and radiation. Overall median survival was 18–24 months, with responders doing better than nonresponders. Even among those with complete responses, however, most tumors recurred, usually in distant sites. Because dysphagia was relieved in many patients by the combination of chemotherapy and radiation, some have proposed that esophagectomy adds little to the chemotherapy-radiation combination. The ultimate impact of these protocols on patient survival is unclear.

The patient must stop smoking, and respiratory therapy should be instituted to optimize pulmonary function. Patients who have lost more than 10% of their body weight are usually given total parenteral nutrition or supplemental enteral tube feedings before surgery, but evidence is lacking that this decreases complications.

For tumors of the lower third of the esophagus, most surgeons prefer to perform the resection through a laparotomy followed by a right thoracotomy. The limited access afforded by the left chest approach results in a less generous esophagectomy and a higher incidence of residual tumor at the esophageal margin. The resection should include the celiac lymph nodes and left gastric vessels, the stomach proximal to the left gastric artery, and the lower esophagus to a point above the azygos vein. The spleen is preserved in patients with squamous cell carcinoma but should probably be removed in those with adenocarcinoma. A pyloroplasty is performed. The site of gastric transection is closed, the stomach is pulled up into the chest, and an esophagogastrostomy is performed at a convenient spot on the anterior surface of the gastric remnant.

For tumors of the middle and upper thirds of the esophagus, less stomach need be resected, but the esophagectomy should extend to the cervical esophagus, and the anastomosis should be performed through a separate (third) incision in the neck. Whenever possible, at least 10 cm of grossly uninvolved esophagus should be resected proximal to an esophageal cancer, and the margins of transection should be checked by frozen sections during surgery. Patients with Barrett's esophagus are at high risk of developing recurrent cancer if any portion of the columnar-lined epithelium is left behind.

If the tumor does not involve the trachea, bronchi, or aorta, esophagectomy can be performed without a thoracotomy through simultaneous abdominal and cervical incisions. The esophagus is shelled out by blunt dissection, and the stomach is brought up to the cervical esophagus through the posterior mediastinum. This procedure has been criticized on theoretic grounds as being inadequate treatment for cancer, but the reported survival rates are similar to those achieved with more aggressive operations. Patients (especially those with chronic pulmonary disease) tolerate esophagectomy without thoracotomy better than other operations for removing the esophagus. Tumors of the lower esophagus lend themselves better to this operation than do those in the mid esophagus. The presence of any mediastinal extension beyond what can be directly controlled from the abdomen increases the chance of massive intraoperative bleeding or laceration of the membranous trachea.

If the lesion is unresectable, radiation therapy may be used. Radiotherapy relieves dysphagia in about two-thirds of the patients, but the relief is transient in half of those who do respond. Irradiation or chemotherapy should not be the initial therapy in patients with tracheobronchial involvement with or without a tracheoesophageal fistula, because patients without a fistula often develop one following treatment. Therefore, patients with an unresectable tumor who are able to withstand a major operation are best treated by a preliminary substernal gastric bypass with a cervical esophagogastrostomy. The esophagus is closed above and below the fistula or may be drained by a Roux-en-Y esophagojejunostomy. After the patient has recovered from the esophagogastrostomy, the primary tumor is treated by radiotherapy. Colon is rarely used to bypass an esophageal carcinoma, because the operation is more complex than gastric bypass and the death rate is higher.

The dose of x-ray should be between 4500 and 6000 cGy. Patients treated with doses at the higher end of this range are more likely to experience complications, such as pulmonary fibrosis, esophageal bleeding, or esophageal perforation.

Palliation may be attempted with intubation of the tumor in patients too weak to withstand a major operation. The tube is inserted by laparotomy (eg, Celestin tube, Mousseau-Barbin tube) or esophagoscopy (eg, Souttar tube). Unfortunately, the quality of palliation achieved with tube stents is generally very poor. The tube has a tendency to become dislodged or blocked with food, thus aggravating pain. Furthermore, concomitant radiotherapy increases the complications (eg, bleeding, perforation) of tubes. Therefore, intubation should be reserved for patients with extensive disease and a life expectancy limited to 1–2 months.

In some patients with unresectable tumors, dysphagia can be relieved by endoscopic laser therapy. With this technique, a core of tumor is vaporized, opening the lumen without perforating the esophagus. Treatment needs to be repeated every 6–8 weeks, and most patients are able to swallow only liquids and semiliquid diets. Success is greatest with lesions of the body of the esophagus 5 cm or less in length. Greatest technical difficulties are encountered with cervical lesions and angulated lesions at the cardioesophageal junction. When technically feasible, endoscopic laser therapy is preferable to Celestin tube intubation.

Patients with malignant tracheoesophageal fistulas cannot be cured, but palliation is a realistic goal. Aspiration of saliva and swallowed liquids produces incessant coughing, and dysphagia is usually pronounced. Nevertheless, the tumor is rarely widespread in these patients. The best treatment is probably substernal gastric bypass with a cervical esophagogastric anastomosis. Both ends of the thoracic esophagus are closed. The fistula is usually large enough to accommodate the small amount of esophageal secretion. Celestin tubes are of little value.

Prognosis

The operative death rate following resection or bypass averages 5–8%. After potentially curative resection, survival for 1 year is 70%; for 2 years, 30%; and for 5 years, 20%. About 50% of patients who have no lymph node involvement are cured. The 5-year survival rate after curative resection is about 30% for patients with squamous cell carcinoma and 10% for patients with adenocarcinoma. Surgery is much more successful in restoring and maintaining swallowing than is radiotherapy or intubation. Survival of patients following insertion of a Celestin tube averages 1 month.

DeCamp MM Jr, Swanson SJ, Jaklitsch MT: Esophagectomy after induction chemoradiation. Chest 1999;116(6 Suppl):466S.

Geh JI, Crellin AM, Glynne-Jones R: Preoperative (neoadjuvant) chemoradiotherapy in oesophageal cancer. Br J Surg 2001; 88:338.

Hagen JA et al: Curative resection for esophageal adenocarcinoma: analysis of 100 en bloc esophagectomies. Ann Surg 2001; 234:520.

Lehnert T: Multimodal therapy for squamous carcinoma of the oesophagus. Br J Surg 1999;86:727.

Lerut T et al: Treatment of esophageal carcinoma. Chest 1999;116 (6 Suppl):463S.

Lew JI et al: Long-term survival following induction chemoradiotherapy and esophagectomy for esophageal carcinoma. Arch Surg 2001;136:737.

Lowe VJ, Naunheim KS: Current role of positron emission tomography in thoracic oncology. Thorax 1998;53:703.

Morales TG, Sampliner RE: Barrett's esophagus: update on screening, surveillance, and treatment. Arch Intern Med 1999 Jul 12;159:1411.

Tamim WZ et al: Neoadjuvant chemoradiotherapy for esophageal cancer: is it worthwhile? Arch Surg 1998;133:722.

Wijnhoven BP, Tilanus HW, Dinjens WN: Molecular biology of Barrett's adenocarcinoma. Ann Surg 2001;233:322.

ESOPHAGEAL BANDS, WEBS, OR RINGS

Congenital bands or webs may develop at any level but are most frequent in the subcricoid region. Others form in the lower esophageal segment. These bands cause dysphagia and may be treated by endoscopic dilation in which the thin, web-like band is usually fractured, followed by complete relief of symptoms. Resection and primary anastomosis are occasionally necessary for the more fibrous unyielding concentric bands. The latter are more likely to be in the lower esophagus.

A narrow mucosal ring (**Schatzki's ring**) may develop at the lower end of the esophagus. Most patients are relatively free from symptoms unless the ring is less than 12 mm in diameter. Dysphagia may be severe, however. In most cases, the ring is located at the squamocolumnar junction and occurs in a patient with gastroesophageal reflux. Being confined to the mucosa, it differs from an inflammatory (peptic) stricture, which involves all layers of the esophagus. Endoscopy often fails to reveal the smooth concentric narrowing, since the overlying mucosa is intact. Esophagitis may be present but usually is not. Repair of an associated hiatal hernia is insufficient to control the dysphagia; the ring must be dilated or excised. In most cases, the ring can be ruptured by rapidly inflating a balloon in its lumen, as is done for achalasia. Afterward, the patient should be treated for esophagitis.

Buckley K et al: Schatzki ring in children and young adults: clinical and radiologic findings. Pediatr Radiol 1998;28:884.

Scolapio JS et al: A randomized prospective study comparing rigid to balloon dilators for benign esophageal strictures and rings. Gastrointest Endosc 1999;50:13.

Uygur-Bayramicli O, Tuncer K, Dolapcioglu C: Plummer-Vinson syndrome presenting with an esophageal stricture. J Clin Gastroenterol 1999;29:291.

■ II. THE DIAPHRAGM

The diaphragm (Figure 21–14) is a musculotendinous dome-shaped structure attached posteriorly to the first, second, and third lumbar vertebrae, anteriorly to the lower sternum, and laterally to the costal arches. It separates the abdominal and the thoracic cavities. The diaphragm allows the passage of various normal structures through anatomic foramina. The aortic hiatus lies posteriorly at the level of the 12th thoracic vertebra, and through it pass the aorta, the thoracic duct, and the azygos venous system. The esophageal hiatus lies immediately anteriorly and slightly to the left at the level of the tenth thoracic vertebra and is separated from the aortic hiatus by the decussation of the right crus of the diaphragm. Through this hiatus pass the esophagus and the vagus nerves. At the level of the ninth thoracic vertebra and slightly to the right of the esophageal hiatus is the vena caval foramen, which allows passage of the inferior vena cava and small branches of the phrenic nerve. The phrenic arteries arising directly from the aorta supply the diaphragm along with the lower inter-

Figure 21–14. Inferior surface of diaphragm.

costal arteries and the terminal branches of the internal mammary arteries.

PARASTERNAL OR RETROSTERNAL (FORAMEN OF MORGAGNI) HERNIA & PLEUROPERITONEAL (FORAMEN OF BOCHDALEK) HERNIA

Failure of fusion of the sternal and costal portions of the diaphragm anteriorly in the midline creates a defect (foramen of Morgagni) through which hernias can occur. Normally, the diaphragm becomes fused, allowing only the internal mammary arteries and their superior epigastric branches, along with lymphatics, to pass through this area. Posterolaterally, failure of fusion of the pleuroperitoneal canal creates a defect though which viscera may herniate to produce a foramen of Bochdalek hernia (Figure 21–15).

Although both types of hernia are congenital, symptoms in the Morgagni hernia usually do not develop until middle life or later. On the other hand, the Bochdalek hernia may cause severe respiratory distress at birth, requiring an emergency operation. In both types in the adult, complications are not common and many cases are asymptomatic. Routine chest films show a retrosternal solid mass, a retrosternal air-filled viscus, or similar findings in the posterolateral thorax if a Bochdalek hernia is present.

Parasternal (Morgagni) hernias

Pleuroperitoneal (Bochdalek) hernias

Figure 21–15. Sites of congenital diaphragmatic herniation.

Elective surgical repair is indicated in most instances to prevent complications. An emergency operation may become necessary in the newborn infant who develops progressive cardiorespiratory insufficiency. Repair of the defect by a transabdominal approach is preferable, and the results are excellent.

Jastaniah S et al: Bochdalek hernia in adulthood: a case report and review of recent literature. Indian J Chest Dis Allied Sci 1998;40:281.

Schumpelick V et al: Surgical embryology and anatomy of the diaphragm with surgical applications. Surg Clin North Am 2000;80:213.

TRAUMATIC DIAPHRAGMATIC HERNIA

Traumatic rupture of the diaphragm may occur as a result of penetrating wounds or severe blunt external trauma. Lacerations usually occur in the tendinous portion of the diaphragm, most often on the left side. The liver provides protection to diaphragmatic injury on the right side except from penetrating wounds. Abdominal viscera may immediately herniate through the defect in the diaphragm into the pleural cavity or may gradually insinuate themselves into the thorax over a period of months or years.

Clinical Findings

Diaphragmatic ruptures present in two ways. In the acute form, the patient has recently experienced blunt trauma or a penetrating wound to the chest, abdomen, or back. The clinical manifestations are essentially those of the associated injuries, but occasionally, massive herniation of abdominal viscera through the diaphragm causes respiratory insufficiency. In the chronic form, the diaphragmatic tear is unrecognized at the time of the original injury. Some time later, symptoms appear from herniation of viscera: pain, bowel obstruction, etc. Respiratory symptoms in such cases are rare.

Plain films of the chest may show a radiopaque area and occasionally an air-fluid level if hollow viscera have herniated. If the stomach has entered the chest, the abnormal path of a nasogastric tube may be diagnostic. Ultrasonography, CT scan, and MRI may demonstrate the diaphragmatic rent. Barium study of the colon may show irregular patches of barium in the colon above the diaphragm or a smooth colonic outline if the colon does not contain feces.

Differential Diagnosis

Traumatic rupture of the diaphragm must be differentiated from atelectasis, space-consuming tumors of the lower pleural space, pleural effusion, and intestinal obstruction due to other causes.

Complications

Hemorrhage and obstruction may occur. If herniation is massive, progressive cardiorespiratory insufficiency may threaten life. The most severe complication is strangulating obstruction of the herniated viscera.

Treatment

For acute ruptures, a transabdominal (most commonly) or transthoracic route is used depending on the procedure required to treat ancillary injuries. When the diaphragmatic tear is the only injury, it is usually fixed by laparotomy. Chronic injuries can be repaired by either approach. Asymptomatic tears of the diaphragm with herniated viscera should be repaired, because the risk of strangulating obstruction is high.

Prognosis

Surgical repair of the rent in the diaphragm is curative, and the prognosis is excellent. The diaphragm supports sutures well, so that recurrence is practically unknown.

Grover SB, Ratan SK: Simultaneous dual posttraumatic diaphragmatic and abdominal wall hernias. J Trauma 2001;51:583.

Meyer G et al: Laparoscopic repair of traumatic diaphragmatic hernias. Surg Endosc 2000;14:1010.

Reina A et al: Traumatic intrapericardial diaphragmatic hernia: case report and literature review. Injury 2001;32:153.

TUMORS OF THE DIAPHRAGM

Primary tumors of the diaphragm are not common. The majority are benign lipomas. Pericardial cysts develop in the interval between the heart and the diaphragm and are usually unilocular and on the right side. Fibrosarcoma, the most common primary malignant diaphragmatic tumor, is extremely rare.

Benign tumors are usually asymptomatic. Since their benign nature cannot be established except by histologic study, all lesions of this type should be excised through an appropriate thoracotomy.

The Acute Abdomen

Gerard M. Doherty, MD, & John H. Boey, MD

The term "an acute abdomen" denotes any sudden spontaneous nontraumatic disorder whose chief manifestation is in the abdominal area and for which urgent operation may be necessary. Because there is frequently a progressive underlying intra-abdominal disorder, undue delay in diagnosis and treatment adversely affects outcome.

The approach to a patient with an acute abdomen must be orderly and thorough. An acute abdomen must be suspected even if the patient has only mild or atypical complaints. The history and physical examination should suggest the probable causes and guide the choice of initial diagnostic studies. The clinician must then decide if in-hospital observation is warranted; if additional tests are needed; if early operation is indicated; or if nonoperative treatment would be more suitable.

All clinicians should be thoroughly familiar with the presenting picture of the most common causes of an acute abdomen (Table 22–1). Moreover, they should be familiar with the disease patterns specific to the region and locality where they practice. Other chapters in this book provide detailed descriptions of specific diseases and their management.

HISTORY

Abdominal Pain

History taking by an experienced physician is an active process whereby a cluster of diagnostic possibilities is considered in order to systematically eliminate less likely conditions. Pain is the most common and predominant presenting feature of an acute abdomen. Careful consideration of the location, the mode of onset and progression, and the character of the pain will suggest a preliminary list of differential diagnoses.

A. LOCATION OF PAIN

Because of the complex dual visceral and parietal sensory network subserving the abdominal area, pain is not as precisely localized as in the extremities. Fortunately, some general patterns do emerge that provide clues to diagnosis. Visceral sensation is mediated primarily by afferent C fibers located in the walls of hollow viscera and in the capsules of solid organs. Unlike cutaneous pain, **visceral pain** is elicited either by distention, by

inflammation or ischemia stimulating the receptor neurons, or by direct involvement (eg, malignant infiltration) of sensory nerves. The centrally perceived sensation is generally slow in onset, dull, poorly localized, and protracted. Different visceral structures are associated with different sensory levels in the spine (Table 22–2). Because of this, increased wall tension due to luminal distention or forceful smooth muscle contraction (colic) produces diffuse deep-seated pain felt in the mid epigastrium, periumbilical area, lower abdomen, or flank areas (Figure 22–1). Visceral pain is most often felt in the midline because of the bilateral sensory supply to the spinal cord.

By contrast, **parietal pain** is mediated by both C and A delta nerve fibers, the latter being responsible for the transmission of more acute, sharper, better-localized pain sensation. Direct irritation of the somatically innervated parietal peritoneum (especially the anterior and upper parts) by pus, bile, urine, or gastrointestinal secretions leads to more precisely localized pain. The cutaneous distribution of parietal pain corresponds to the T6–L1 areas. Parietal pain is more easily localized than visceral pain because the somatic afferent fibers are directed to only one side of the nervous system. Abdominal parietal pain is conventionally described as occurring in one of the four abdominal quadrants or in the epigastric or central abdominal area.

Abdominal pain may be referred or may shift to sites far removed from the primarily affected organs (Figure 22–2). The term **referred pain** denotes noxious (usually cutaneous) sensations perceived at a site distant from that of a strong primary stimulus. Distorted central perception of the site of pain is due to the confluence of afferent nerve fibers from widely disparate areas within the posterior horn of the spinal cord. For example, pain due to subdiaphragmatic irritation by air, peritoneal fluid, blood, or a mass lesion is referred to the shoulder via the C4-mediated (phrenic) nerve. Pain may also be referred to the shoulder from supradiaphragmatic lesions such as pleurisy or lower lobe pneumonia, especially in young patients. Although more often perceived in the right scapular region, referred biliary pain may mimic angina pectoris if it is perceived in the anterior chest or left shoulder areas. Posterolateral right flank pain may be seen in retrocecal appendicitis.

Table 22–1. Common causes of the acute abdomen.[1]

Gastrointestinal tract disorders
  *Nonspecific abdominal pain
  *Appendicitis
  *Small and large bowel obstruction
  *Perforated peptic ulcer
  Incarcerated hernia
  Bowel perforation
  Meckel's diverticulitis
  Boerhaave's syndrome
  *Diverticulitis
  Inflammatory bowel disorders
  Mallory-Weiss syndrome
  Gastroenteritis
  Acute gastritis
  Mesenteric adenitis
  Parasitic infections
Liver, spleen, and biliary tract disorders
  *Acute cholecystitis
  Acute cholangitis
  Hepatic abscess
  Ruptured hepatic tumor
  Spontaneous rupture of the spleen
  Splenic infarct
  Biliary colic
  Acute hepatitis
Pancreatic disorders
  *Acute pancreatitis
Urinary tract disorders
  *Ureteral or renal colic
  Acute pyelonephritis
  Acute cystitis
  Renal infarct
Gynecologic disorders
  Ruptured ectopic pregnancy
  Twisted ovarian tumor
  Ruptured ovarian follicle cyst
  *Acute salpingitis
  Dysmenorrhea
  Endometriosis
Vascular disorders
  Ruptured aortic and visceral
    aneurysms
  Acute ischemic colitis
  Mesenteric thrombosis
Peritoneal disorders
  Intra-abdominal abscesses
  Primary peritonitis
  Tuberculous peritonitis
Retroperitoneal disorders
  Retroperitoneal hemorrhage

[1]The most common causes are marked with an asterisk. Conditions in italic type often require urgent operation.

Table 22–2. Sensory levels associated with visceral structures.

Structures	Nervous System Pathways	Sensory Level
Liver, spleen, and central part of diaphragm	Phrenic nerve	C3–5
Peripheral diaphragm, stomach, pancreas, gallbladder, and small bowel	Celiac plexus and greater splanchnic nerve	T6–9
Appendix, colon, and pelvic viscera	Mesenteric plexus and lesser splanchnic nerve	T10–11
Sigmoid colon, rectum, kidney, ureters, and testes	Lowest splanchnic nerve	T11–L1
Bladder and rectosigmoid	Hypogastric plexus	S2–4

Spreading or shifting pain parallels the course of the underlying condition. The site of pain at onset should be distinguished from the site at presentation. Beginning classically in the epigastric or periumbilical region, the incipient visceral pain of acute appendicitis (due to distention of the appendix) later shifts to become sharper parietal pain localized in the right lower quadrant when the overlying peritoneum becomes directly inflamed (Figure 22–2). In perforated peptic ulcer, pain almost always begins in the epigastrium, but as the leaked gastric contents track down the right paracolic gutter, pain may descend to the right lower quadrant with even diminution of the epigastric pain.

The location of pain serves only as a rough guide to the diagnosis—"typical" descriptions are reported in only two-thirds of cases. This great variability is due to atypical pain patterns, a shift of maximum intensity away from the primary site, or advanced or severe disease. In cases presenting late with diffuse peritonitis, generalized pain may completely obscure the precipitating event. Pain confined to either upper quadrant may be evaluated by anatomic consideration of acute conditions that affect the underlying organs.

B. MODE OF ONSET AND PROGRESSION OF PAIN

The mode of onset of pain reflects the nature and severity of the inciting process. Onset may be explosive (within seconds), rapidly progressive (within 1–2 hours), or gradual (over several hours). Unheralded, excruciating generalized pain suggests an intra-abdominal catastrophe such as a perforated viscus or rupture of an aneurysm, ectopic pregnancy, or abscess. Accompanying systemic signs (tachycardia, sweating, tachypnea, shock) soon supersede the abdominal disturbances and

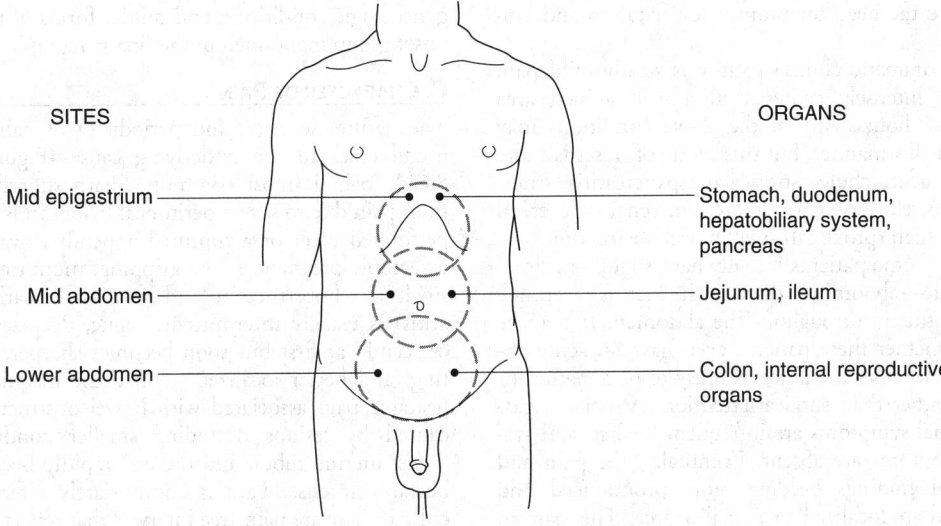

SITES

Mid epigastrium

Mid abdomen

Lower abdomen

ORGANS

Stomach, duodenum,
hepatobiliary system,
pancreas

Jejunum, ileum

Colon, internal reproductive
organs

Figure 22–1. Visceral pain sites.

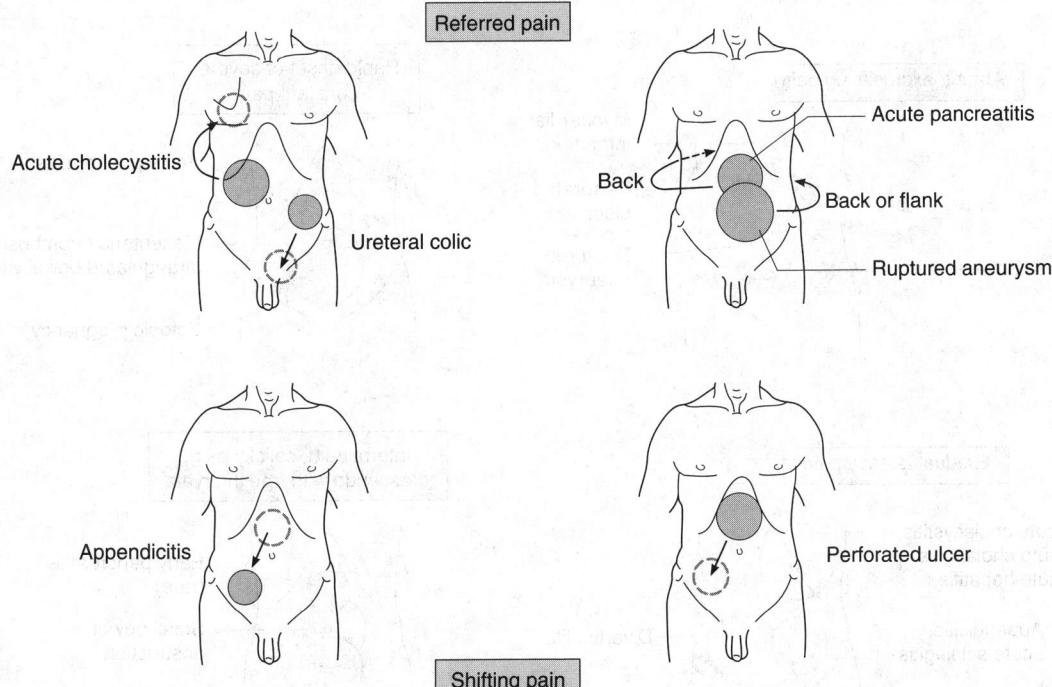

Referred pain

Acute cholecystitis

Ureteral colic

Acute pancreatitis

Back

Back or flank

Ruptured aneurysm

Appendicitis

Perforated ulcer

Shifting pain

Figure 22–2. Referred pain and shifting pain in the acute abdomen. Solid circles indicate the site of maximum pain; dashed circles indicate sites of lesser pain.

underscore the need for prompt resuscitation and laparotomy.

A less dramatic clinical picture is steady mild pain becoming intensely centered in a well-defined area within 1–2 hours. Any of the above conditions may present in this manner, but this mode of onset is more typical of acute cholecystitis, acute pancreatitis, strangulated bowel, mesenteric infarction, renal or ureteral colic, and high (proximal) small bowel obstruction.

Finally, some patients initially have slight—at times only vague—abdominal discomfort that is fleetingly present diffusely throughout the abdomen. It may be unclear whether these patients even have an acute abdomen or whether the illness is likely to be a matter for medical rather than surgical attention. Associated gastrointestinal symptoms are infrequent at first, and systemic symptoms are absent. Eventually, the pain and abdominal findings become more pronounced and steady and are localized to a smaller area. This pattern may reflect a slowly developing condition or the body's defensive efforts to cordon off an acute process. This broad category includes acute appendicitis (especially retrocecal or retroileal), incarcerated hernias, low (distal) small bowel and large bowel obstructions, uncomplicated peptic ulcer disease, walled-off (often malignant) visceral perforations, some genitourinary and gynecologic conditions, and milder forms of the rapid-onset group mentioned in the first paragraph.

C. CHARACTER OF PAIN

The nature, severity, and periodicity of pain provide useful clues to the underlying cause (Figure 22–3). Steady pain is most common. Sharp superficial constant pain due to severe peritoneal irritation is typical of perforated ulcer or a ruptured appendix, ovarian cyst, or ectopic pregnancy. The gripping, mounting pain of small bowel obstruction (and occasionally early pancreatitis) is usually intermittent, vague, deep-seated, and crescendo at first but soon becomes sharper, unremitting, and better localized. Unlike the disquieting but bearable pain associated with bowel obstruction, pain caused by lesions occluding smaller conduits (bile ducts, uterine tubes, and ureters) rapidly becomes unbearably intense. Pain is appropriately referred to as **colic** if there are pain-free intervals that reflect intermittent smooth muscle contractions, as in ureteral colic. In the strict sense, the term "biliary colic" is a misnomer because biliary pain does not remit. The reason is that the gallbladder and bile duct, in contrast to the ureters and intestine, do not have peristaltic movements. The "aching discomfort" of ulcer pain, the "stabbing, breathtaking" pain of acute pancreatitis and mesenteric

Figure 22–3. The location and character of pain are helpful in the differential diagnosis of the acute abdomen.

infarction, and the "searing" pain of ruptured aortic aneurysm remain apt descriptions. Despite the use of such descriptive terms, the quality of visceral pain is not a reliable clue to its cause.

Agonizing pain denotes serious or advanced disease. Colicky pain is usually promptly alleviated by analgesics. Ischemic pain due to strangulated bowel or mesenteric thrombosis is only slightly assuaged even by narcotics. Nonspecific abdominal pain is usually mild, but mild pain may also be found with perforated ulcers that have become localized and in mild acute pancreatitis. An occasional patient will deny pain but complain of a vague feeling of abdominal fullness that feels as though it might be relieved by a bowel movement. This visceral sensation (**gas stoppage sign**) is due to reflex ileus induced by an inflammatory lesion walled off from the free peritoneal cavity, as in retrocecal or retroileal appendicitis.

Past episodes of pain and factors that aggravate or relieve pain should be noted. Pain caused by localized peritonitis, especially when it affects upper abdominal organs, tends to be exacerbated by movement or deep breathing.

The clinician should be familiar with the pathophysiology and salient features of the common causes of acute abdomen. The location, character, and severity of the pain in relation to its duration of onset along with the presence or absence of systemic symptoms help to differentiate rapidly progressive (and usually more serious) surgical conditions (eg, intestinal ischemia) from more indolent or medical causes (eg, ruptured ovarian cysts).

Other Symptoms Associated With Abdominal Pain

Anorexia, nausea and vomiting, constipation, or diarrhea often accompanies abdominal pain, but since these are nonspecific symptoms, they do not have much diagnostic value.

A. VOMITING

When sufficiently stimulated by secondary visceral afferent fibers, the medullary vomiting centers activate efferent fibers to induce reflex vomiting. Hence, pain in the acute surgical abdomen usually precedes vomiting, whereas the reverse holds true in medical conditions. Vomiting is a prominent symptom in upper gastrointestinal diseases such as Boerhaave's syndrome, Mallory-Weiss syndrome, acute gastritis, and acute pancreatitis. Severe uncontrollable retching provides temporary pain relief in moderate attacks of pancreatitis. The absence of bile in the vomitus is a feature of pyloric stenosis. Where associated findings suggest bowel obstruction, the onset and character of vomiting may indicate the level of the lesion. Recurrent vomiting of bilestained fluid is a typical early sign of proximal small bowel obstruction. In distal small or large bowel obstruction, prolonged nausea precedes vomiting, which may become feculent in late cases. Disorders that induce vomiting in younger patients may give rise only to anorexia or nausea in older patients. Although vomiting may present in either acute appendicitis or nonspecific abdominal pain, coexisting nausea and anorexia are more suggestive of the former condition.

B. CONSTIPATION

Reflex ileus is often induced by visceral afferent fibers stimulating efferent fibers of the sympathetic autonomic nervous system (splanchnic nerves) to reduce intestinal peristalsis. Hence, paralytic ileus undermines the value of constipation in the differential diagnosis of an acute abdomen. Constipation itself is hardly an absolute indicator of intestinal obstruction. However, **obstipation** (the absence of passage of both stool and flatus) strongly suggests mechanical bowel obstruction if there is progressive painful abdominal distention or repeated vomiting.

C. DIARRHEA

Copious watery diarrhea is characteristic of gastroenteritis and other medical causes of an acute abdomen. Blood-stained diarrhea suggests ulcerative colitis, Crohn's disease, or bacillary or amebic dysentery. It is also common with ischemic colitis but often absent in intestinal infarction due to superior mesenteric artery occlusion.

D. OTHER SPECIFIC SYMPTOMS

These are extremely helpful if present. **Jaundice** suggests hepatobiliary disorders; **hematochezia** or **hematemesis,** a gastroduodenal lesion or Mallory-Weiss syndrome; **hematuria,** ureteral colic or cystitis. The passage of blood clots or necrotic mucosal debris may be the sole evidence of advanced intestinal ischemia.

Other Relevant Aspects of the History

A. GYNECOLOGIC HISTORY

The menstrual history is crucial to the diagnosis of ectopic pregnancy, mittelschmerz (due to a ruptured ovarian follicle), and endometriosis. A history of vaginal discharge or dysmenorrhea may denote pelvic inflammatory disease.

B. DRUG HISTORY

Anticoagulants have been implicated in retroperitoneal and intramural duodenal and jejunal hematomas; oral contraceptives in the formation of benign hepatic adenomas and in mesenteric venous infarction. Corticosteroids, in particular, may mask the clinical signs of even advanced peritonitis. Pyloric perforation has been caused by "crack" smoking.

C. FAMILY HISTORY

This often provides the best information about medical causes of an acute abdomen (see below).

D. TRAVEL HISTORY

This may raise the possibility of amebic liver abscess or hydatid cyst, malarial spleen, tuberculosis, *Salmonella typhi* infection of the ileocecal area, or dysentery.

E. OPERATION HISTORY

Any history of a previous abdominal, groin, vascular, or thoracic operation may be relevant to the current illness. Particular attention to the mode of operation (laparoscopic, open, endovascular) and any anatomic reconstructions may clarify aspects of the current complaint. If possible within the time constraints imposed by the urgency of the current problem, operative notes and pathology reports should be obtained and reviewed.

PHYSICAL EXAMINATION

The tendency to concentrate on the abdomen should be resisted in favor of a methodical and complete general physical examination. A systematic approach to the abdominal examination is outlined in Table 22–3. One should search for specific signs that confirm or rule out differential diagnostic possibilities (Table 22–4).

(1) **General observation:** General observation affords a fairly reliable indication of the severity of the clinical situation. Most patients, although uncomfortable, remain calm. The writhing of patients with visceral pain (eg, intestinal or ureteral colic) contrasts with the rigidly motionless bearing of those with parietal pain (eg, acute appendicitis, generalized peritonitis). Diminished responsiveness or an altered sensorium often precedes imminent cardiopulmonary collapse.

Table 22–3. Steps in physical examination of the acute abdomen.

1. Inspection	7. Punch tenderness
2. Auscultation	Costal area
3. Cough tenderness	Costovertebral area
4. Percussion	8. Special signs
5. Guarding or rigidity	9. External hernias and male
6. Palpation	genitalia
One-finger	10. Rectal and pelvic examina-
Rebound tenderness	tion
Deep	

Table 22–4. Physical findings in various causes of acute abdomen.

Condition	Helpful Signs
Perforated viscus	Scaphoid, tense abdomen; diminished bowel sounds (late); loss of liver dullness; guarding or rigidity.
Peritonitis	Motionless; absent bowel sounds (late); cough and rebound tenderness; guarding or rigidity.
Inflamed mass or abscess	Tender mass (abdominal, rectal, or pelvic); punch tenderness; special signs (Murphy's, psoas, or obturator).
Intestinal obstruction	Distention; visible peristalsis (late); hyperperistalsis (early) or quiet abdomen (late); diffuse pain without rebound tenderness; hernia or rectal mass (some).
Paralytic ileus	Distention; minimal bowel sounds; no localized tenderness.
Ischemic or strangulated bowel	Not distended (until late); bowel sounds variable; severe pain but little tenderness; rectal bleeding (some).
Bleeding	Pallor, shock; distention; pulsatile (aneurysm) or tender (eg, ectopic pregnancy) mass; rectal bleeding (some).

(2) **Systemic signs:** Systemic signs usually accompany rapidly progressive or advanced disorders associated with an acute abdomen. Extreme pallor, hypothermia, tachycardia, tachypnea, and sweating suggest major intra-abdominal hemorrhage (eg, ruptured aortic aneurysm or tubal pregnancy). Given such findings, one must proceed rapidly with the subsequent examination and tests in order to exclude extra-abdominal causes and to institute treatment.

(3) **Fever:** Constant low-grade fever is common in inflammatory conditions such as diverticulitis, acute cholecystitis, and appendicitis. High fever with lower abdominal tenderness in a young woman without signs of systemic illness suggests acute salpingitis. Disorientation or extreme lethargy combined with a very high fever (> 39 °C) or swinging fever or with chills and rigors signifies impending septic shock. This is most often due to advanced peritonitis, acute cholangitis, or pyelonephritis. However, fever is often mild or absent in elderly, chronically ill, or immunosuppressed patients with a serious acute abdomen.

(4) **Examination of the acute abdomen**

(a) **Inspection:** The abdomen should be thoughtfully inspected before palpation. A tensely distended abdomen with an old surgical scar suggests both the presence and the cause (adhesions) of small bowel obstruction. A scaphoid contracted abdomen is seen with perforated ulcer; visible peristalsis occurs in thin patients with advanced bowel obstruction; and soft doughy fullness is seen in early paralytic ileus or mesenteric thrombosis.

(b) Auscultation: Auscultation of the abdomen should also precede palpation. Peristaltic rushes synchronous with colic are heard in mid small bowel obstruction and in early acute pancreatitis. These tend to last longer but occur less frequently than in normal patients or in those with acute cholecystitis. They differ from the high-pitched hyperperistaltic sounds unrelated to the crampy pain of gastroenteritis, dysentery, and fulminant ulcerative colitis. An abdomen that is silent except for infrequent tinkly or squeaky sounds characterizes late bowel obstruction or diffuse peritonitis. Except for these more extreme patterns, the many auscultatory variants heard in paralytic ileus and other conditions render them largely useless for specific diagnosis.

(c) Coughing to elicit pain: The patient should be asked to cough and point to the area of maximal pain. Peritoneal irritation so demonstrated may be confirmed afterward without causing unnecessary pain by rigorous testing for rebound tenderness. Unlike the parietal pain of peritonitis, colic is visceral pain and is seldom aggravated by deep inspiration or coughing.

(d) Percussion: Percussion serves several purposes. Tenderness on percussion is akin to eliciting rebound tenderness; both reflect peritoneal irritation and parietal pain. With a perforated viscus, free air accumulating under the diaphragm may efface normal liver dullness. Tympany near the midline in a distended abdomen denotes air trapped within distended bowel loops. Free peritoneal fluid may be detected by demonstrating shifting dullness.

(e) Palpation: Palpation is performed with the patient resting in a comfortable supine position. Incisional and periumbilical hernias are noted. **Guarding** is assessed by placing both hands over the abdominal muscles and depressing the fingers gently. Properly performed, this maneuver is comforting to the patient. If there is voluntary spasm, the muscle will be felt to relax when the patient inhales deeply through the mouth. With true involuntary spasm, however, the muscle will remain taut and rigid ("board-like") throughout respiration. Except for rare neurologic disorders—and, for unknown reasons, renal colic—only peritoneal inflammation (by reflex afferent stimulation of efferent motor fibers) produces rectus muscle rigidity. Unlike peritonitis, renal colic induces spasm confined to the ipsilateral rectus muscle.

Tenderness that connotes localized peritoneal inflammation is the most important finding in patients with an acute abdomen. Its extent and severity are determined first by one- or two-finger palpation, beginning away from the area of cough tenderness and gradually advancing toward it. Tenderness is usually well demarcated in acute cholecystitis, appendicitis, diverticulitis, and acute salpingitis. If there is poorly localized tenderness unaccompanied by guarding, one should suspect gastroenteritis or some other inflammatory intestinal process without peritonitis. Compared with the degree of pain, unexpectedly little and only vague tenderness is elicited in uncomplicated hollow viscus obstruction, walled-off or deep-seated perforations (eg, retrocecal or retroileal appendicitis or diverticular phlegmons), and in very obese patients.

When the patient raises his or her head from the bed or examination table, the abdominal muscles will be tensed. Tenderness persists in abdominal wall conditions (eg, rectus hematoma), whereas deeper peritoneal pain due to intraperitoneal disease is lessened (Carnett's test). Hyperesthesia may be demonstrable in abdominal wall disorders or localized peritonitis, but it is more prominent in herpes zoster, spinal root compression, and other neuromuscular problems. Trigger point sensitivity, lateral costal rib tip tenderness, and pain exacerbated by spinal motion reflect parietal abdominal wall conditions that subside dramatically after infiltration with local anesthetic agents.

Abdominal masses are usually detected by deep palpation. Superficial lesions such as a distended gallbladder or appendiceal abscess are often tender and have discrete borders. If one suspects that abdominal guarding is masking an acutely inflamed gallbladder, the right subcostal area should be palpated while the patient inhales deeply. Inspiration will be arrested abruptly by pain (**Murphy's sign**), or the gallbladder fundus may be felt as it strikes the examining fingers during descent of the diaphragm.

Deeper masses may be adherent to the posterior or lateral abdominal wall and are often partially walled off by overlying omentum and small bowel. As a result, their borders are ill-defined, and only dull pain may be elicited by palpation. Examples include pancreatic phlegmon and ruptured aortic aneurysm.

Even if a mass cannot be directly felt, its presence may be inferred by other maneuvers. A large psoas abscess arising from a perinephric abscess or perforated Crohn's enteritis may cause pain when the hip is passively extended or actively flexed against resistance (**iliopsoas sign**). Similarly, internal and external rotation of the flexed thigh may exert painful pressure (**obturator sign**) on a loop of the small bowel entrapped within the obturator canal (obturator hernia). **Punch tenderness** over the lower costal ribs indicates an inflammatory condition affecting the diaphragm, liver, or spleen or its adjacent structures. While this may suggest a hepatic, splenic, or subphrenic abscess, it is also common in acute cholecystitis, acute hepatitis, or splenic infarct. **Costovertebral angle tenderness** is common in acute pyelonephritis. Since they are not invariably present, these special signs are helpful only in conjunction with a compatible history and related physical findings.

(f) Inguinal and femoral rings; male genitalia: The inguinal and femoral rings in both sexes and the genitalia in male patients should be examined next.

(g) Rectal examination: A rectal examination should be performed in most patients with an acute abdomen. Diffuse tenderness is nonspecific, but right-sided rectal tenderness accompanied by lower abdominal rebound tenderness is indicative of peritoneal irritation due to pelvic appendicitis or abscess. Other useful findings include a rectal tumor, blood-stained stool, or occult blood (detected by guaiac testing). Rectal examination may be dispensed with in children diagnosed as having appendicitis because of marked right lower quadrant tenderness, guarding, or rigidity.

(h) Pelvic examination: An acute abdomen is incorrectly diagnosed more often in women than in men, particularly in younger age groups. A pelvic examination is vital in women with a vaginal discharge, dysmenorrhea, menorrhagia, or left lower quadrant pain. A properly performed pelvic examination is invaluable in differentiating among acute pelvic inflammatory diseases that do not require operation and acute appendicitis, twisted ovarian cyst, or tubo-ovarian abscess (see Chapter 42).

INVESTIGATIVE STUDIES

The history and physical examination by themselves provide the diagnosis in two-thirds of cases of an acute abdomen. Supplementary laboratory and radiologic examinations are indispensable for diagnosis of many surgical conditions, for exclusion of medical causes ordinarily not treated by operation, and for assistance in preoperative preparation. Even in the absence of a specific diagnosis, there may already be enough information on which to base a rational decision about management. Additional studies are worthwhile only if they are likely to significantly alter or improve therapeutic decisions. A more liberal use of diagnostic studies is justified in elderly or seriously ill patients, in whom the history and physical findings may be less reliable and an early diagnosis vital to ensure a successful outcome.

The availability and reliability of certain studies vary in different hospitals. The invasiveness, risks, and cost-effectiveness of a test should be weighed when the physician selects diagnostic studies. Test results must always be interpreted within the clinical context of each case. Basic studies should be obtained in all but the most desperately ill patients. Other less vital tests may be requested later as indicated (Table 22–5).

Laboratory Investigations

A. BLOOD STUDIES

Hemoglobin, hematocrit, and white blood cell and differential counts taken on admission are highly informa-

Table 22–5. General principles of timing of diagnostic studies in an acute abdomen.

	Immediate	Same Day[1]	Next Day[1]
Blood	Hematocrit, white blood cell count, urea, creatinine, cross-matching,[1] arterial gases.[1]	Clotting studies, amylase, liver function tests.	Specific tests.
Urine	Microscopy, dipstick testing, culture.[1]		Specific tests.
Stool	Occult blood.	Warm smear, culture.	
Radiography and ultrasound	Chest, abdomen.	Ultrasonography or CT scan, angiography, water-soluble upper gastrointestinal series, HIDA scan (see Chapter 27).	Repeat abdominal films; barium enema or small bowel follow-through, intravenous urogram, and PTC (see Chapter 27); liver-spleen, gallium, and technetium scans.
Endoscopy		Proctosigmoidoscopy, upper endoscopy.	ERCP (see Chapter 27), colonoscopy laparoscopy.
Other		Paracentesis, culdocentesis.	

[1]When indicated.

tive. Only a rising or marked leukocytosis (> 13,000/μL), especially in the presence of a shift to the left on the blood smear, is indicative of serious infection. Moderate leukocytosis, commonly encountered in medical as well as surgical inflammatory conditions, is nonspecific and may be even absent in elderly or debilitated patients with infections. A low white blood cell count (< 8000/μL) is a feature of viral infections such as mesenteric adenitis or gastroenteritis and nonspecific abdominal pain.

A specimen of clotted blood for cross-matching should be sent whenever urgent surgery is anticipated. An additional tube of clotted blood may be reserved in case of such need.

Serum electrolytes, urea nitrogen, and creatinine are important, especially if hypovolemia is expected (ie, due to shock, copious vomiting or diarrhea, tense abdominal distention, or delay of several days after onset of symptoms). Arterial blood gas determinations should be obtained in patients with hypotension, generalized peritonitis, pancreatitis, possible ischemic bowel, and septicemia. Unsuspected metabolic acidosis may be the first clue to serious disease.

A raised serum amylase level corroborates a clinical diagnosis of acute pancreatitis. Moderately elevated values must be interpreted with caution, since abnormal levels frequently accompany strangulated or ischemic bowel, twisted ovarian cyst, or perforated ulcer. Moreover, a normal or even low amylase value may be seen in hemorrhagic pancreatitis or pseudocyst. Cloudy (lactescent) serum in a patient with abdominal pain suggests pancreatitis even though the serum amylase is normal.

In patients with suspected hepatobiliary disease, liver function tests (serum bilirubin, alkaline phosphatase, AST, ALT, albumin, and globulin) are useful to differentiate medical from surgical hepatic disorders and to gauge the severity of underlying parenchymal disease.

Clotting studies (platelet counts; prothrombin time and partial thromboplastin time) and a peripheral blood smear should be requested if the history hints at a possible hematologic abnormality (cirrhosis, petechiae, etc). The erythrocyte sedimentation rate, often nonspecifically raised in the acute abdomen, is of dubious diagnostic value; a normal value does not exclude serious surgical illness.

Antibody titers for amebic, typhoid, or viral disease and other special blood tests may pinpoint a specific disease, but therapeutic decisions often cannot await their results.

B. Urine Tests

Urinalysis is easily performed and may reveal useful information. Dark urine or a raised specific gravity re-

flects mild dehydration in patients with normal renal function. Hyperbilirubinemia may give rise to tea-colored urine that froths when shaken. Microscopic hematuria or pyuria can confirm ureteral colic or urinary tract infection and obviate a needless operation. Initial antibiotic treatment should be adjusted after culture and sensitivity reports are available. Dipstick testing (for albumin, bilirubin, glucose, and ketones) may reveal a medical cause of an acute abdomen. Pregnancy tests should be ordered if there is a history of a missed period.

C. Stool Tests

Gastrointestinal bleeding is not a common feature of the acute abdomen. Nonetheless, testing for occult fecal blood should be routinely performed. A positive test points to a mucosal lesion that may be responsible for large bowel obstruction or chronic anemia, or it may reflect an unsuspected carcinoma.

Warm stool smears for bacteria, ova, and animal parasites may demonstrate amebic trophozoites in patients with bloody or mucous diarrhea. Stool samples for culture should be taken in patients with suspected gastroenteritis, dysentery, or cholera.

Imaging Studies

A. Plain Chest X-Ray Studies

An erect chest x-ray is essential in all cases of an acute abdomen. Not only is it vital for preoperative assessment, but it may also demonstrate supradiaphragmatic conditions that simulate an acute abdomen (eg, lower lobe pneumonia or ruptured esophagus). An elevated hemidiaphragm or pleural effusion may direct attention to subphrenic inflammatory lesions.

B. Plain Abdominal X-Ray Studies

Plain supine films of the abdomen should be obtained only selectively. In general, erect (or lateral decubitus) views contribute little additional information except in suspected intestinal obstruction. Even though radiologic abnormalities are present in up to 40% of patients, these are diagnostic only half the time. Plain films are indicated in patients who have appreciable abdominal tenderness or distention, abnormal bowel sounds, a history of abdominal surgery, suspected foreign body ingestion, or who have a depressed sensorium or who are in a high-risk category. They are helpful in patients with possible intestinal obstruction or ischemia, perforated viscus, renal or ureteral calculi, or acute cholecystitis. They are seldom of value in patients suspected to have appendicitis or urinary tract infection. They are inappropriate in pregnant patients, unstable individuals in whom clear-cut physical signs mandating laparotomy already exist, or patients with only mild, resolving nonspecific pain. Maximal information is obtained by an experienced radiologist apprised of the clinical situation. However, the surgeon who is familiar with the clinical details should review all x-rays.

One should observe the gas pattern of the hollow viscera; free or abnormal air patterns under the diaphragm, within the biliary radicles, or outside the bowel wall; the outline of solid organs and the peritoneal fat lines; and radiopaque densities.

An abnormal bowel gas pattern suggests paralytic ileus, mechanical bowel obstruction, or pseudo-obstruction. A diffuse gas pattern with air outlining the rectal ampulla suggests paralytic ileus, especially if bowel sounds are absent. Gaseous distention is the rule in bowel obstruction. Air-fluid levels are usually seen in distal small bowel obstruction and a distended cecum with small bowel dilation in large bowel obstruction. Along with the clinical findings, the distinctive radiologic appearances of colonic dilation in toxic megacolon or volvulus establish the diagnosis (see Figure 31–15). Adynamic ileus associated with long-standing acute appendicitis or with an atypical appendix location often produces a pattern that suggests localized right lower quadrant ileus. This radiologic picture in a patient without previous abdominal surgery should influence the diagnostic decision toward appendicitis or other ileocecal disease (tumor, inflammatory disorders). "Thumbprint" impressions on the colonic wall are noted in about half of patients with ischemic colitis. A displaced gastric or colonic air shadow may be the only sign of subcapsular splenic hematoma.

Free gas under the hemidiaphragm must be looked for specifically. Its presence in approximately 80% of perforated ulcers corroborates the clinical diagnosis. Massive pneumoperitoneum is observed in free colonic perforations.

Biliary tree air designates a biliary-enteric communication, such as a spontaneous or surgically created choledochoduodenal fistula or gallstone ileus. Air delineating the portal venous system characterizes pylephlebitis. Air between loops of small bowel may arise from a small localized perforation.

Obliteration of the psoas muscle margins or enlargement of the kidney shadows indicates retroperitoneal disease.

Radiopaque densities of characteristic appearance and location may confirm a clinical suspicion of biliary, renal staghorn, or ureteral calculi; appendicitis; or aortic aneurysm. Whereas pelvic phleboliths are readily distinguishable, a migrant gallstone may be mistaken for a calcified mesenteric lymph node if the accompanying small bowel distention or biliary tree air is overlooked in gallstone ileus.

C. ANGIOGRAPHY

Angiographic studies are indicated if intra-abdominal intestinal ischemia or ongoing hemorrhage is suspected. They should precede any gastrointestinal contrast study that might obscure film interpretation. Selective visceral angiography is a reliable method of diagnosing mesenteric infarction. Emergency angiography may confirm a ruptured liver adenoma or carcinoma or an aneurysm of the splenic artery or other visceral artery. In patients with massive lower gastrointestinal bleeding, angiography may identify the bleeding site, may suggest the likely diagnosis (eg, vascular ectasia, polyarteritis nodosa), and may even be therapeutic if embolization can be performed. Angiography is of little value in ruptured aortic aneurysm or if frank peritoneal findings (peritonitis) are present. It is contraindicated in unstable patients with severe shock or sepsis and seldom warranted if other findings or tests already dictate the need for laparotomy or laparoscopy.

D. CONTRAST X-RAY STUDIES

Gastrointestinal contrast studies should not be requested routinely or be regarded as screening studies. They are helpful only if a specific condition being considered can be verified or treated by a contrast x-ray examination. For suspected perforations of the esophagus or gastroduodenal area without pneumoperitoneum, a water-soluble contrast medium (eg, meglumine diatrizoate [Gastrografin]) is preferred. If there is no clinical evidence of bowel perforation, a barium enema may identify the level of a large bowel obstruction or even reduce a sigmoid volvulus or intussusception. Only if there is no likelihood of large bowel obstruction should a barium small bowel follow-through study be used to study a partial small bowel obstruction or to look for an intramural duodenal (or jejunal) hematoma that is best managed conservatively.

An emergency intravenous urogram is seldom necessary to evaluate nontraumatic causes of hematuria. It should be performed electively after microscopic examination of a stained and centrifuged urine specimen and cystoscopic examination. Ultrasonography and HIDA scans have replaced intravenous cholangiography in the evaluation of jaundiced patients and those suspected of having acute cholecystitis.

E. ULTRASONOGRAPHY

Ultrasonography is useful in evaluating upper abdominal pain that does not resemble ulcer pain or bowel obstruction and in investigating abdominal masses. Ultrasonography has a diagnostic sensitivity of about 80% for acute appendicitis and is most useful in pregnant patients and those presenting with features suggestive of atypical appendicitis or in young women with mid or lower abdominal pain. Color Doppler studies can distinguish avascular cysts and twisted masses from inflammatory and infectious processes. CT scanning may be more useful if excessive bowel gas, so common in elderly and ill patients, precludes satisfactory ultrasound examination. It is particularly helpful in pancreatic and retroperitoneal lesions and any severe localized infections (eg, acute diverticulitis).

F. CT Scan

Urgent or emergent CT scan of the abdomen is now generally routinely available. This has proved extremely useful in the evaluation of abdominal complaints for patients who do not already have clear indications for laparotomy or laparoscopy. CT is helpful in identifying small amounts of free intraperitoneal gas and sites of inflammatory diseases that may prompt (appendicitis, tubo-ovarian abscess) or postpone (diverticulitis, pancreatitis, hepatic abscess) operation.

G. Radionuclide Scans

Liver-spleen scans, HIDA scans, and gallium scans may be useful for localizing intra-abdominal abscesses. However, their utility has been greatly decreased by the routine availability of urgent CT scans. Radionuclide blood pool or Tc-sulfur colloid scans may identify sources of slow or intermittent intestinal bleeding. Technetium pertechnetate scans may reveal ectopic gastric mucosa in Meckel's diverticulum. Tc-99m hexamethylpropyleneamineoxide (HMPAO) scanning may help in patients with vague signs of appendicitis. It has a sensitivity rate of 85%, specificity of 93%, and accuracy rate of 89%. It may also suggest other causes of intra-abdominal inflammation.

Endoscopy

Proctosigmoidoscopy is indicated in any patient with suspected large bowel obstruction, grossly bloody stools, or a rectal mass. Minimal air should be used for bowel insufflation. Besides reducing a sigmoid volvulus, colonoscopy may also locate the source of bleeding in cases of lower gastrointestinal hemorrhage that has subsided. Gastroduodenoscopy and ERCP are usually done electively to evaluate less urgent inflammatory conditions (eg, gastritis, peptic disease) in patients without alarming abdominal signs.

Paracentesis

In patients with free peritoneal fluid, aspiration of blood, bile, or bowel contents is a strong indication for urgent laparotomy. On the other hand, infected ascitic fluid may establish a diagnosis in spontaneous bacterial peritonitis, tuberculous peritonitis, or chylous ascites (see Chapter 23), which rarely require surgery. Culdocentesis may be useful for suspected ruptured corpus luteum cyst.

Peritoneal cytology (obtained by direct aspiration through a fine catheter) or diagnostic peritoneal lavage may disclose tumor or an acute intra-abdominal inflammatory problem. These investigations should be used selectively after imaging studies in patients with equivocal findings and in those who would poorly tolerate a negative laparotomy.

Laparoscopy

Laparoscopy is now a therapeutic as well as a diagnostic modality. In young women, it may distinguish a nonsurgical problem (ruptured graafian follicle, pelvic inflammatory disease, tubo-ovarian disease) from appendicitis. In obtunded, elderly, or critically ill patients, who often have deceptive manifestations of an acute abdomen, it may facilitate earlier treatment in those with positive findings while eliminating the added morbidity of a laparotomy in negative cases. Where appendicitis is confirmed, laparoscopic appendectomy may be performed. Increasingly, surgeons must acquire new laparoscopic skills in order to deal with other acute intra-abdominal conditions (eg, adhesive bowel obstruction) that previously demanded a formal laparotomy.

DIFFERENTIAL DIAGNOSIS

The age and gender of the patient help in the differential diagnosis: Mesenteric adenitis mimics acute appendicitis in the young; gynecologic disorders complicate the evaluation of lower abdominal pain in women of childbearing age; and malignant and vascular diseases are more common in the elderly. Causes of an acute abdomen reflect the disease patterns of the indigenous population, and an awareness of common causes within the physician's locale will improve diagnostic accuracy. The clinical picture in early cases is often unclear. The following observations should be borne in mind:

(1) Any patient with acute abdominal pain persisting for over 6 hours should be regarded as having a surgical problem requiring in-hospital evaluation. Well-localized pain and tenderness usually indicate a surgical condition. Systemic hypoperfusion in conjunction with generalized abdominal pain is seldom due to a medical problem.

(2) Acute cholecystitis, appendicitis, bowel obstruction, cancer, and acute vascular conditions are the most common causes of the surgical acute abdomen in older patients. In children, appendicitis accounts for one-

third of all cases and nonspecific abdominal pain for nearly all the remainder.

(3) Acute appendicitis and intestinal obstruction are the most frequent final diagnoses in cases erroneously believed at first to be nonsurgical. Appendicitis should always remain a foremost concern if sepsis or an inflammatory lesion is suspected. It is the commonest cause of bizarre peritoneal findings that produce ileus or intestinal obstruction. Half of children with appendicitis present with a marked facial flush (due to high serotonin levels). The presence of the gas stoppage sign or x-ray findings of right lower quadrant ileus should raise the possibility of retrocecal or retroileal appendicitis. Appendicitis is less likely in previously healthy individuals if the history exceeds 3 days' duration and the patient has no fever, appreciable tenderness, ileus, or leukocytosis.

Pelvic appendicitis, with mild abdominal pain, vomiting, and frequent loose stools, simulates gastroenteritis. The initial abdominal signs may be mild and the rectal and pelvic examinations unremarkable. A low white blood cell count or lymphocytosis favors gastroenteritis.

Atypical presentations of appendicitis are encountered during pregnancy. Maternal illness and fetal death in such cases are caused mainly by complications following delayed diagnosis. Appendectomy is well tolerated during pregnancy, and removal of a normal appendix is more frequently tolerated than observation of the perforation.

(4) Salpingitis, dysmenorrhea, ovarian lesions, and urinary tract infections complicate the evaluation of the acute abdomen in young women. Many diagnostic errors can be avoided by taking a careful menstrual history and performing a pelvic examination and urinalysis. Ultrasound study and pregnancy tests are helpful in appropriate cases. Compared with patients with appendicitis, patients with acute salpingitis tend to present with a longer history of pain, often related to the menstrual cycle, and to have higher fever, bilateral pelvic signs, and a markedly elevated white blood cell count.

(5) Unusual types or atypical manifestations of intestinal obstruction, especially early cases, are easily missed. Emesis, abdominal distention, and air-fluid levels on x-ray may be negligible in Richter's hernia, proximal or closed-loop small bowel obstructions, and early cecal volvulus.

Intestinal obstruction in an elderly woman who has not had a previous operation suggests an incarcerated femoral hernia or, rarely, an obturator hernia or gallstone ileus. There may be no pain or tenderness in the area of the hernia. Carefully examine the inguinofemoral region; repeat the rectal and pelvic examinations; and check for an obturator sign. Transient mild upper abdominal pain followed several days later by signs of intestinal obstruction is typical of gallstone ileus. Look for a radiopaque stone and air outlining the biliary tree on the plain abdominal x-ray.

(6) Elderly or cardiac patients with severe unrelenting diffuse abdominal pain but without commensurate peritoneal signs or abnormalities on plain abdominal films may have intestinal ischemia. Arterial blood pH should be measured and visceral angiography performed early.

(7) Medical causes of the acute abdomen should be excluded before exploratory laparotomy is considered (Table 22–6). Upper abdominal pain may be encountered in myocardial infarction, acute pulmonary conditions (pneumothorax, lower lobe pneumonia, pleurisy, empyema, infarction), and acute hepatitis. Generalized or migratory abdominal discomfort may be felt in acute rheumatic fever, polyarteritis nodosa and other types of diffuse vasculitis, acute intermittent porphyria, and acute pleurodynia. Sharp flank pain, often accompanied by rectus spasm and cutaneous hyperesthesia, may be caused by osteoarthritis with thoracic or spinal nerve compression. Likewise, acute bursitis and hip joint disorders may produce pain radiating into the lower quadrants. Exquisite tingling or pinpricking sensations along a flank dermatome are characteristic of preeruptive herpes zoster.

Medical conditions usually can be distinguished from surgical ones by a careful assessment of the history and physical examination. The family history may fur-

Table 22–6. Medical causes of an acute abdomen for which surgery is not indicated.

Endocrine and metabolic disorders	Infections and inflammatory disorders
Uremia	Tabes dorsalis
Diabetic crisis	Herpes zoster
Addisonian crisis	Acute rheumatic fever
Acute intermittent porphyria	Henoch-Schönlein purpura
Acute hyperlipoproteinemia	Systemic lupus erythematosus
Hereditary Mediterranean fever	Polyarteritis nodosa
Hematologic disorders	**Referred pain**
Sickle cell crisis	Thoracic region
Acute leukemia	Myocardial infarction
Other dyscrasias	Acute pericarditis
Toxins and drugs	Pneumonia
Lead and other heavy metal poisoning	Pleurisy
Narcotic withdrawal	Pulmonary embolus
Black widow spider poisoning	Pneumothorax
	Empyema
	Hip and back

nish the first clue. The history is usually atypical in some aspects, and thoughtful scrutiny will disclose details such as unusual or exaggerated symptoms—or concomitant extra-abdominal complaints—that point to the true cause. Despite the apparent severity of pain, localized abdominal tenderness with involuntary guarding is seldom present. Fever and associated systemic signs may be disproportionate to the degree of pain. Laboratory and x-ray studies will verify the diagnosis and avoid an operation.

(8) Beware of acute cholecystitis, acute appendicitis, and perforated peptic ulcer in patients already hospitalized for an illness affecting another organ system. Their presentation is often atypical, leading to delayed diagnosis and complications.

(9) Exploration is most often undertaken without benefit for salpingitis, mesenteric adenitis, gastroenteritis, pyelonephritis, and acute viral hepatitis.

(10) Nonspecific abdominal pain, comprising one-third of all cases, is the most common cause of the acute abdomen, especially in children. Generally mild, short-lived, and seldom associated with other serious symptoms, it resolves without specific treatment. Most cases represent undiagnosed viral and mild bacterial infections, irritable bowel syndrome, gynecologic problems, abdominal wall pain, psychosomatic pain, or worm infection.

INDICATIONS FOR SURGICAL EXPLORATION

The need for operation is apparent when the diagnosis is certain, but surgery sometimes must be undertaken before a precise diagnosis is reached. Table 22–7 lists some indications for urgent laparotomy or laparoscopy. Among patients with acute abdominal pain, those over age 65 more often require operation (33%) than do younger patients (15%).

A liberal policy of exploration is advisable in patients with inconclusive but persistent right lower quadrant tenderness. Pain in the left upper quadrant infrequently requires urgent laparotomy, and its cause can usually await elective confirmatory studies.

PREOPERATIVE MANAGEMENT

After initial assessment, parenteral analgesics for pain relief should not be withheld. In moderate doses, analgesics neither obscure useful physical findings nor mask their subsequent development. Indeed, abdominal masses may become obvious once rectus spasm is relieved. Pain that persists in spite of adequate doses of narcotics suggests a serious condition often requiring operative correction.

Table 22–7. Indications for urgent operation in patients with an acute abdomen.

Physical findings
  Involuntary guarding or rigidity, especially if spreading
  Increasing or severe localized tenderness
  Tense or progressive distention
  Tender abdominal or rectal mass with high fever or hypotension
  Rectal bleeding with shock or acidosis
  Equivocal abdominal findings along with—
    Septicemia (high fever, marked or rising leukocytosis, mental changes, or increasing glucose intolerance in a diabetic patient)
    Bleeding (unexplained shock or acidosis, falling hematocrit)
    Suspected ischemia (acidosis, fever, tachycardia)
    Deterioration on conservative treatment
Radiologic findings
  Pneumoperitoneum
  Gross or pregressive bowel distention
  Free extravasation of contrast material
  Space-occupying lesion on scan, with fever
  Mesenteric occlusion on angiography
Endoscopic findings
  Perforated or uncontrollably bleeding lesion
Paracentesis findings
  Blood, bile, pus, bowel contents, or urine

Resuscitation of acutely ill patients is outlined in Chapter 2. Medications should be restricted to only essential requirements. Particular care should be given to use of cardiac drugs and corticosteroids and to control of diabetes. Antibiotics are indicated for some infectious conditions or as prophylaxis during the perioperative period (see Chapter 9).

A nasogastric tube should be inserted in patients likely to undergo surgery and for those with hematemesis or copious vomiting, suspected bowel obstruction, or severe paralytic ileus. This precaution may prevent aspiration in patients suffering from drug overdose or alcohol intoxication, patients who are comatose or debilitated, or elderly patients with impaired cough reflexes. However, since the tube interferes with coughing and is uncomfortable, it should be removed once it is safe to do so.

A urinary catheter should be placed in patients with systemic hypoperfusion. In some elderly patients, it eliminates the cause of pain (acute bladder distention) or unmasks relevant abdominal signs.

Informed consent for surgery may be difficult to obtain when the diagnosis is uncertain. It is prudent to discuss with the patient and family the possibility of multiple staged operations; temporary or permanent stomal openings; impotence or sterility; and postoperative intubation for mechanical ventilation. Whenever the exact diagnosis is uncertain—especially in young or frail or severely ill patients—a frank preoperative discussion of the diagnostic dilemma and reasons for laparotomy or laparoscopy will reduce postoperative anxieties and misunderstanding.

REFERENCES

Eskelinen M et al: Contributions of history-taking, physical examination, and computer assistance to diagnosis of acute small-bowel obstruction. A prospective study of 1333 patients with acute abdominal pain. Scand J Gastroenterol 1994;29:715.

Hoekstra HJ et al: Gastrointestinal complications in lung transplant survivors that require surgical intervention. Br J Surg 2001;88:433.

Kraemer M et al: Acute appendicitis in late adulthood: incidence, presentation, and outcome. Results of a prospective multicenter acute abdominal pain study and a review of the literature. Langenbecks Arch Surg 2000;385:470.

Mindelzun RE et al: The acute abdomen: current CT imaging techniques. Semin Ultrasound CT MR 1999;20:63.

Rao PM et al: Effect of computed tomography of the appendix on treatment of patients and use of hospital resources. N Engl J Med 1998;338:141.

Siewert B et al: CT of the acute abdomen: findings and impact on diagnosis and treatment. AJR Am J Roentgenol 1994;163:1317.

Silliman CC et al: Indications for surgical intervention for gastrointestinal emergencies in children receiving chemotherapy. Cancer 1994;74:203.

Simic O et al: Incidence and prognosis of abdominal complications after cardiopulmonary bypass. Cardiovasc Surg 1999;7:419.

Urban BA et al: Targeted helical CT of the acute abdomen: appendicitis, diverticulitis, and small bowel obstruction. Semin Ultrasound CT MR 2000;21:20.

Vander Velpen GC et al: Diagnostic yield and management benefit of laparoscopy: a prospective audit. Gut 1994;35:1617.

Whitney TM et al: Emergent abdominal surgery in AIDS: experience in San Francisco. Am J Surg 1994;168:239.

Peritoneal Cavity

Gerard M. Doherty, MD, & John H. Boey, MD

■ THE PERITONEUM & ITS FUNCTIONS

The peritoneal cavity is lined by the **parietal peritoneum,** a mesothelial lining. This lining is called the **visceral peritoneum** where it is reflected onto the enclosed abdominal organs. Its relationship to intraperitoneal structures defines discrete compartments within which abscesses may form (see Intra-abdominal Abscesses). The peritoneal surface area is a semipermeable membrane with an area comparable to that of the cutaneous body surface. Nearly 1 m^2 of the total 1.7 m^2 area participates in fluid exchange with the extracellular fluid space at rates of 500 mL or more per hour. Normally, there is less than 50 mL of free peritoneal fluid, a transudate with the following characteristics: specific gravity below 1.016; protein concentration less than 3 g/dL; white blood cell count less than 3000/µL; complement-mediated antibacterial activity; and lack of fibrinogen-related clot formation. The circulation of peritoneal fluid is directed toward lymphatics in the undersurface of the diaphragm. There, particulate matter—including bacteria up to 20 µm in size—is cleared via stomas in the diaphragmatic mesothelium and lymphatics and discharged mainly into the right thoracic duct.

The peritoneal cavity is normally sterile. Small numbers of bacteria can be efficiently disposed of, but peritonitis ensues if the defense mechanisms are overwhelmed by massive or continued contamination. In response to tissue damage, mast cells in the delicate mesothelial lining discharge histamine and other vasoactive substances that enhance vascular permeability. The resulting fibrinogen-rich plasma exudate supplies complement and opsonic proteins that promote bacterial destruction. Tissue thromboplastin released by injured mesothelial cells converts fibrinogen into fibrin, which may in turn lead to collagen deposition and formation of fibrous adhesions. In health, this reaction is limited by a plasminogen activator in the cell lining, but the plasminogen activator is inactivated by injury or infection. Bacterial lipopolysaccharide (endotoxin) and cytokines can stimulate production of tumor necrosis factor (TNF). TNF, in turn, mediates the release of plasminogen activator inhibitor produced by inflamed peritoneal mesothelial cells, which can lead to persistence of fibrin. Fibrin clots segregate bacterial deposits, a source of endotoxins that contribute to sepsis, but segregation may also inadvertently shield bacteria from bacteria-clearing mechanisms.

The **omentum** is a well-vascularized pliable, mobile double fold of peritoneum and fat that participates actively in the control of peritoneal inflammation and infection. Its composition is well suited to sealing off a leaking viscus (eg, perforated ulcer) or area of infection (eg, resulting from a ruptured appendix) and for carrying a collateral blood supply to ischemic viscera. Its bacteria scavenger functions include absorption of small particles and delivery of phagocytes that destroy unopsonized bacteria.

■ DISEASES & DISORDERS OF THE PERITONEUM

ACUTE SECONDARY BACTERIAL PERITONITIS

Pathophysiology

Peritonitis is an inflammatory or suppurative response of the peritoneal lining to direct irritation. Peritonitis can occur after perforating, inflammatory, infectious, or ischemic injuries of the gastrointestinal or genitourinary system. Common examples are listed in Table 23–1. **Secondary peritonitis** results from bacterial contamination originating from within viscera or from external sources (eg, penetrating injury). It most often follows disruption of a hollow viscus. Extravasated bile and urine, although only mildly irritating when sterile, are markedly toxic if infected and provoke a vigorous peritoneal reaction. Gastric juice from a perforated duodenal ulcer remains mostly sterile for several hours, during which time it produces a chemical peritonitis with large fluid losses; but if left untreated, it evolves within 6–12 hours into bacterial peritonitis. Intraperitoneal fluid dilutes opsonic proteins and impairs phagocytosis. Furthermore, when hemoglobin is present in the peritoneal cavity, *Escherichia coli* growing within the cavity can

Table 23–1. Common causes of peritonitis.

Severity	Cause	Mortality Rate
Mild	Appendicitis Perforated gastroduodenal ulcers Acute salpingitis	< 10%
Moderate	Diverticulitis (localized perforations) Nonvascular small bowel perforation Gangrenous cholecystitis Multiple trauma	< 20%
Severe	Large bowel perforations Ischemic small bowel injuries Acute necrotizing pancreatitis Postoperative complications	20–80%

elaborate leukotoxins that reduce bactericidal activity. Limited, localized infection can be eradicated by host defenses, but continued contamination invariably leads to generalized peritonitis and eventually to septicemia with multiple organ failure (see Chapter 9).

Factors that influence the severity of peritonitis include the type of bacterial or fungal contamination, the nature and duration of the injury, and the host's nutritional and immune status. The grade of peritonitis varies with the cause. Clean (eg, proximal gut perforations) or well-localized (eg, ruptured appendix) contaminations progress to fulminant peritonitis relatively slowly (eg, 12–24 hours). In contrast, bacteria associated with distal gut or infected biliary tract perforations quickly overwhelm host peritoneal defenses. This degree of toxicity is also characteristic of postoperative peritonitis due to anastomotic leakage or contamination. Conditions that ordinarily cause mild peritonitis may produce life-threatening sepsis in an immunocompromised host.

Causative organisms. Systemic sepsis due to peritonitis occurs in varying degrees depending on the virulence of the pathogens, the bacterial load, and the duration of bacterial proliferation and synergistic interaction. Except for spontaneous bacterial peritonitis, peritonitis is almost invariably polymicrobial; cultures usually contain more than one aerobic and more than two anaerobic species. The microbial picture reflects the bacterial flora of the involved organ. As long as gastric acid secretion and gastric emptying are normal, perforations of the proximal bowel (stomach or duodenum) are generally sterile or associated with relatively small numbers of gram-positive organisms. Perforations or ischemic injuries of the distal small bowel (eg, strangulated hernia) lead to infection with aerobic bacteria in about 30% of cases and anaerobic organisms in

about 10% of cases. Fecal spillage, with a bacterial load of 10^{12} or more organisms per gram, is extremely toxic. Positive cultures with gram-negative and anaerobic bacteria are characteristic of infections originating from the appendix, colon, and rectum. The predominant aerobic pathogens include the gram-negative bacteria *E coli,* streptococci, proteus, and the enterobacter-klebsiella groups. Besides *Bacteroides fragilis,* anaerobic cocci and clostridia are the prevalent anaerobic organisms. Synergism between fecal anaerobic and aerobic bacteria increases the severity of infections.

Clinical Findings

By estimating the severity of peritonitis from clinical and laboratory findings, the need for specific organ-supportive care and surgery can be determined.

See Chapter 22 for details of radiologic and other investigations.

A. Symptoms and Signs

The clinical manifestations of peritonitis reflect the severity and duration of infection and the age and general health of the patient. Physical findings can be divided into (1) abdominal signs arising from the initial injury and (2) manifestations of systemic infection. Acute peritonitis frequently presents as an acute abdomen. **Local findings** include abdominal pain, tenderness, guarding or rigidity, distention, free peritoneal air, and diminished bowel sounds—signs that reflect parietal peritoneal irritation and resulting ileus. **Systemic findings** include fever, chills or rigors, tachycardia, sweating, tachypnea, restlessness, dehydration, oliguria, disorientation, and, ultimately, refractory shock. Shock is due to the combined effects of hypovolemia and septicemia with multiple organ dysfunction. *Recurrent unexplained shock is highly predictive of serious intraperitoneal sepsis.*

The findings in abdominal sepsis are modified by the patient's age and general health. Physical signs of peritonitis are subtle or difficult to interpret in both very young and very old patients as well as in those who are chronically debilitated, immunosuppressed, or receiving corticosteroids and in postoperative patients. Paracentesis or diagnostic peritoneal lavage may be occasionally useful in equivocal cases and in senile or confused patients. A white blood cell count of greater than 200 cells/μL is indicative of peritonitis, with virtually no false-positive and minimal false-negative errors. Delayed recognition is a major cause of the high mortality rate of peritonitis.

B. Laboratory Findings

Laboratory studies gauge the severity of peritonitis and guide therapy. Blood studies should include a complete blood cell count, cross-matching, arterial blood gases, electrolytes, a blood clotting profile, and liver and renal function tests. Samples for culture of blood, urine, sputum, and peritoneal fluid should be taken before antibiotics are started. A positive blood culture is usually present in toxic patients.

Differential Diagnosis

Specific kinds of infective (eg, gonococcal, amebic, candidal) and noninfective peritonitis may be seen. In the elderly, systemic diseases (eg, pneumonia, uremia) may produce intestinal ileus so striking that it resembles bowel obstruction or peritonitis.

Familial Mediterranean fever (periodic peritonitis, familial paroxysmal polyserositis) is a rare genetic condition that affects individuals of Mediterranean genetic background. Its exact cause is unknown. Patients present with recurrent bouts of abdominal pain and tenderness along with pleuritic or joint pain. Fever and leukocytosis are common. Colchicine prevents but does not treat acute attacks. Provocative testing by infusion of metaraminol (10 mg) induces abdominal pain within 2 days.

Laparoscopy has superseded laparotomy in suspect individuals. Free fluid and inflamed peritoneal surfaces are found, but smears and cultures are negative. The appendix should be removed to simplify diagnosis in subsequent episodes. Amyloidosis with renal failure is a late complication that is preventable by long-term colchicine therapy.

Treatment

Fluid and electrolyte replacement, operative control of sepsis, and systemic antibiotics are the mainstays of treatment of peritonitis.

A. PREOPERATIVE CARE

1. Intravenous fluids—The massive transfer of fluid into the peritoneal cavity must be replaced by an appropriate amount of intravenous fluid. If systemic toxicity is evident or if the patient is old or in fragile health, a central venous pressure (or pulmonary artery wedge pressure) line and bladder catheter should be inserted; a fluid balance chart should be kept; and serial body weight measurements should be taken to monitor fluid requirements. Sufficient balanced or lactated Ringer's solution must be infused rapidly enough to correct intravascular hypovolemia promptly and to restore blood pressure and urine output to satisfactory levels. Potassium supplements are withheld until tissue and renal perfusion are adequate and urine is produced. Blood is reserved for anemic patients or those with concomitant bleeding.

2. Care for advanced septicemia—Cardiovascular agents and mechanical ventilation in an intensive care unit are essential in patients with advanced septicemia. An arterial line for continuous blood pressure recording and blood sampling is helpful. Cardiac monitoring with a Swan-Ganz catheter is essential if inotropic drugs are used. (See Chapters 9, 10, and 13 for details of fluid resuscitation and the management of septic shock.)

3. Antibiotics—Loading doses of intravenous antibiotics directed against the anticipated bacterial pathogens should be given after fluid samples have been obtained for culture. Initial antibiotics employed include third-generation cephalosporins, ampicillin-sulbactam, ticarcillin-clavulanic acid, aztreonam or imipenem-cilastatin for gram-negative coliforms, and metronidazole or clindamycin for anaerobic organisms. The choice of single-, double- or triple-drug therapy is of less importance than adequate coverage of both anticipated aerobic and anaerobic organisms. Inadequate initial drug dosing and scheduling contribute to treatment failures. Aminoglycosides should be used judiciously because renal impairment is often a feature of peritonitis and because lowered intraperitoneal pH may impair their in vivo activity.

Empirically chosen antibiotics should be modified postoperatively by culture and sensitivity results if there is persistent or subsequent infection (seen in 15–20% of patients). Antibiotics are continued until the patient has remained afebrile with a normal white count and a differential count of less than 3% bands.

B. OPERATIVE MANAGEMENT

1. Control of sepsis—The objectives of surgery for peritonitis are to remove all infected material, correct the underlying cause, and prevent late complications. Except in early, localized peritonitis, a midline incision offers the best surgical exposure. Materials for aerobic and anaerobic cultures of fluid and infected tissue are obtained immediately after the peritoneal cavity is entered. Occult pockets of infection are located by thorough exploration, and contaminated or necrotic material is removed. Routine radical debridement of all peritoneal and serosal surfaces does not increase survival rates. The primary disease is then treated. This may require resection (eg, ruptured appendix or gallbladder), repair (eg, perforated ulcer), or drainage (eg, acute pancreatitis). Attempts to reanastomose resected bowel in the presence of extensive sepsis or intestinal ischemia often lead to leakage. Temporary stomas are safer, and these can be taken down several weeks later after the patient has recovered from the acute illness. Surgical wounds should seldom be closed primarily. They should be left open in grossly soiled cases or delayed primary closure employed in those with less contamination.

2. Peritoneal lavage—In diffuse peritonitis, lavage with copious amounts (> 3 L) of warm isotonic crystalloid solution removes gross particulate matter as well as blood and fibrin clots and dilutes residual bacteria. The addition of antiseptics or antibiotics to the irrigating solution is generally useless or even harmful because of induced adhesions (eg, tetracycline, povidone-iodine). Antibiotics given parenterally will reach bactericidal levels in peritoneal fluid and may afford no additional benefit when given by lavage. Furthermore, lavage with aminoglycosides can produce respiratory depression and complicate anesthesia because of the neuromuscular blocking action of this group of drugs. After lavage is completed, all fluid in the peritoneal cavity must be aspirated because it may hamper local defense mechanisms by diluting opsonins and removing surfaces upon which phagocytes destroy bacteria.

3. Peritoneal drainage—Drainage of the free peritoneal cavity is ineffective and often undesirable. Not only are drains quickly isolated from the rest of the peritoneal cavity, but they still act as a channel for exogenous contamination. Prophylactic drainage in diffuse peritonitis does not prevent abscess formation and may even predispose to abscesses or fistulas. Drainage is useful for residual focal infection or when continued contamination is present or likely to occur (eg, fistula). It is indicated for localized inflammatory masses that cannot be resected or for cavities that cannot be obliterated. Soft sump drains with continuous suction through multiple side perforations are effective for large volumes of fluid. Smaller volumes of fluid are best handled with closed drainage systems (eg, Jackson-Pratt drains). Large cavities with thick walls may be drained by several large Penrose drains placed in a dependent position.

To achieve more effective peritoneal drainage in severe peritonitis, some surgeons have previously left the entire abdominal wound open to widely expose the peritoneal cavity. Besides requiring intensive nursing and medical support to cope with massive protein and fluid losses (averaging 9 L the first day), there are serious complications such as spontaneous fistulization, wound sepsis, segmental colonic necrosis, and large incisional hernias. Consequently, this method is seldom employed now.

An alternative method is to reexplore the abdomen every 1–3 days until all loculations have been adequately drained. The wound may be closed temporarily with a sheet of polypropylene (Marlex) mesh that contains a nylon zipper or Velcro to avoid a tight abdominal closure and to facilitate repeated opening and closing. Another option is to use a plastic sheet may be used (Bogota bag). Exploration may even be performed in the intensive care unit without general anesthesia.

Available data suggest that this method should be restricted to selected patients with long-standing (more than 48 hours) extensive intraperitoneal sepsis associated with multiple organ failure (high sepsis scores). One prospective study failed to demonstrate a significant difference in mortality rates between the conventional closed (31%) and open (44%) techniques.

4. Management of abdominal distention—Abdominal distention caused by ileus frequently accompanies peritonitis, and decompression of the intestine is often ineffective in reliably decreasing the distention. An alternative approach is to close the abdomen temporarily with a sheet of plastic (Bogota bag) to avoid further distention, increased intra-abdominal pressure, and respiratory or renal problems (abdominal compartment syndrome). A **gastrostomy** may be advantageous if prolonged nasogastric decompression is expected, especially in elderly patients or those with chronic respiratory disease. A central TPN line or needle jejunostomy catheter (for proximal gut lesions) is placed when prolonged nutritional support is anticipated.

C. POSTOPERATIVE CARE

Intensive care monitoring, often with ventilatory support, is mandatory in unstable and frail patients. Achieving hemodynamic stability to perfuse major organs is the immediate objective, and this may entail the use of cardiac inotropic agents besides fluid and blood product supportive measures. Antibiotics are given for 10–14 days, depending on the severity of peritonitis. A favorable clinical response is evidenced by well-sustained perfusion with good urine output, reduction in fever and leukocytosis, resolution of ileus, and a returning sense of well-being. The rate of recovery varies with the duration and degree of peritonitis.

The early removal of all nonessential catheters (arterial, central venous, urinary, and nasogastric) reduces the risk of secondary infected foci. Drains should be removed or advanced once drainage diminishes and becomes more serous in nature. Excessive or prolonged suction may produce fistulas or bleeding even within a few days.

Growing awareness of the association between proximal gut colonization with candida, *Streptococcus faecalis,* pseudomonas, and coagulase-negative staphylococci and secondary nosocomial infections and subsequent multiple organ failure has encouraged early gut feeding and discontinuation of unnecessary antibiotics whenever feasible.

Complications

Postoperative complications are frequent and may be divided into local and systemic problems. Deep wound infections, residual abscesses and intraperitoneal sepsis, anastomotic breakdown, and fistula formation usually become manifest toward the end of the first postoperative week. Persistent high or swinging fever, inability to wean off cardiac inotropes, generalized edema with unexplained continued high fluid requirements, increased abdominal distention, prolonged mental apathy and weakness, or general failure to improve despite intensive treatment may be the sole indicators of residual intra-abdominal infection. This should prompt a thorough examination of the patient for infected catheters and an abdominal CT scan. Percutaneous catheter drainage of localized abscesses or open reexploration is undertaken as needed (see next section).

Uncontrolled sepsis leads inexorably to sequential multiple organ failure affecting the respiratory, renal, hepatic, clotting, and immune systems. Supportive measures, including mechanical ventilation, transfusions, total parenteral nutrition, and hemodialysis, are ineffectual unless primary septic foci are eliminated by combined surgical and antibiotic therapy.

Prognosis

The overall mortality rate of generalized peritonitis is about 40% (Table 23–1). Factors contributing to a high mortality rate include the type of primary disease and its duration, associated multiple organ failure before treatment, and the age and general health of the patient. Mortality rates are consistently below 10% in patients with perforated ulcers or appendicitis; in young patients; in those having less extensive bacterial contamination; and in those diagnosed and operated upon early. Patients with distal small bowel or colonic perforations or postoperative sepsis tend to be older, to have concurrent medical illnesses and greater bacterial contamination, and to have a greater propensity to renal and respiratory failure; their mortality rates are about 50%. Markedly poor physiologic indices (eg, APACHE II or Mannheim Peritonitis Index), reduced cardiac status, and low preoperative albumin levels identify high-risk patients who require intensive treatment to reduce a daunting mortality rate.

INTRA-ABDOMINAL ABSCESSES

1. Intraperitoneal Abscesses

Pathophysiology

An intra-abdominal abscess is a collection of infected fluid within the abdominal cavity. Gastrointestinal perforations, postoperative complications, penetrating trauma, and genitourinary infections are the most common causes. An abscess forms by one of two modes: It may develop (1) adjacent to a diseased viscus (eg, with perforated appendix, Crohn's enterocolitis, or divertic-

ulitis) or (2) as a result of external contamination (eg, postoperative subphrenic abscesses). In one-third of cases, the abscess occurs as a sequela of generalized peritonitis. Interloop and pelvic abscesses form if extravasated fluid gravitating into a dependent or localized area becomes secondarily infected (Figure 23–1).

Bacteria-laden fibrin and blood clots and neutrophils contribute to the formation of an abscess. The pathogenic organisms are similar to those responsible for peritonitis, but anaerobic organisms occupy an important role. Experimentally, mixed aerobic *(E coli)* and anaerobic *(B fragilis)* infections, especially in conjunction with adjuvants (eg, feces or barium), reduce intraperitoneal O_2 and pH, thereby fostering anaerobic proliferation and abscess formation.

Sites of Abscesses

The areas in which abscesses commonly occur are defined by the configuration of the peritoneal cavity with its dependent lateral and pelvic basins (Figure 23–1), together with the natural divisions created by the transverse mesocolon and the small bowel mesentery. The supracolic compartment, located above the transverse mesocolon, broadly defines the subphrenic spaces (Figure 23–2A). Within this area, the subdiaphragmatic (suprahepatic) and subhepatic areas of the subphrenic space may be distinguished. **The subdiaphragmatic space** on each side occupies the concavity between the hemidiaphragms and the domes of the hepatic lobes. The inferior limits of its posterior recess are the attachments of the coronary and triangular ligaments on the dorsal—not superior—aspect of the diaphragm. Anteriorly, the lower limits are defined on the right by the transverse colon and on the left by the anterior stomach surface, omentum, transverse colon, spleen, and phrenicocolic ligament. Although each subdiaphragmatic space is continuous over the convex liver surface, inflammatory adhesions may delimit an abscess in an anterior or posterior position (Figure 23–2B). The falciform ligament separates the right and left subdiaphragmatic divisions.

The **right subhepatic division** (Figure 23–2B) of the subphrenic space is located between the undersurfaces of the liver and gallbladder superiorly and the right kidney and mesocolon inferiorly. The anterior bulge of the kidney partitions this space into an anterior (gallbladder fossa) and posterior (Morison's pouch) section.

The **left subhepatic space** also has an anterior and posterior part (Figure 23–2C). The smaller anterior subhepatic space lies between the undersurface of the left lobe and the anterior surface of the stomach. Left subdiaphragmatic collections often extend into this anterior subhepatic area. The posterior subhepatic space is the lesser sac, which is situated behind the lesser omentum and stomach and lies anterior to the pancreas, duo-

Psoas muscle

Perinephric space

Anterior retroperitoneal space

Anterior and posterior renal fasciae

Figure 23–1. Lateral *(top)* and cross-sectional *(bottom)* views of the abdomen, showing fluid gravitating to the dependent areas of the peritoneal cavity. The retroperitoneal compartments are also outlined.

denum, transverse mesocolon, and left kidney. It extends posteriorly to the attachment of the left triangular ligament superiorly on to the hemidiaphragm. The lesser sac communicates with both the right subhepatic and right paracolic spaces through the narrow foramen of Winslow.

The **infracolic compartment,** below the transverse mesocolon, includes the pericolic and pelvic areas (Figure 23–3). The diagonally aligned root of the small bowel mesentery divides the midabdominal area between the fixed right and left colons into right and left infracolic spaces. Each lateral paracolic gutter and lower quadrant area communicates freely with the pelvic cavity. However, while right paracolic collections may track upward into the subhepatic and subdiaphragmatic spaces, the phrenicocolic ligament hinders fluid migration along the left paracolic gutter into the left subdiaphragmatic area.

The most common abscess sites are in the lower quadrants, followed by the pelvic, subhepatic, and subdiaphragmatic spaces (Table 23–2).

Clinical Findings

A. SYMPTOMS AND SIGNS

An intraperitoneal abscess should be suspected in any patient with a predisposing condition. Fever, tachycar-

dia, and pain may be mild or absent, especially in patients receiving antibiotics. A deep-seated or posteriorly situated abscess may exist in seemingly well individuals whose only symptom is persistent fever. Not infrequently, prolonged ileus or a sluggish recovery in a patient who has had recent abdominal surgery or peritoneal sepsis, rising leukocytosis, or nonspecific radiologic abnormality provides the initial clue. A mass is seldom felt except late in patients with lower quadrant or pelvic lesions. Irritation of contiguous structures may produce lower chest pain, dyspnea, referred shoulder pain or hiccup, or basilar atelectasis or effusion in subphrenic abscesses; or diarrhea or urinary frequency in pelvic abscesses. The diagnosis is more difficult in postoperative, chronically ill, confused, or diabetic patients and in those receiving immunosuppressive drugs, a group particularly susceptible to septic complications.

Sequential multiple organ failure—principally respiratory, renal, or hepatic failure—or stress gastrointestinal bleeding with disseminated intravascular coagulopathy is highly suggestive of intra-abdominal infection.

B. LABORATORY FINDINGS

A raised leukocyte count, abnormal liver or renal function test results, hyperglycemia, and abnormal arterial blood gases are nonspecific signs of infection. Serial postoperative measurement of serum lysozyme (derived

A

Subdiaphragmatic space

Right posterior
subhepatic
space

Anterior
subhepatic
space

B

Coronary
ligament

Posterior
subhepatic
space

Subdiaphragmatic
space

Anterior
subhepatic
space

C

Left
triangular
ligament

Posterior
subhepatic
space
(lesser sac)

Figure 23–2. Subphrenic spaces. *A:* Anterior view. *B:* Right lateral view. *C:* Left lateral view.

from phagocytic cells) is a promising but not widely available test that appears to be highly specific for intra-abdominal pus. Persistently positive blood cultures point strongly to an intra-abdominal focus. A cervical smear demonstrating gonococcal infection is of specific value in diagnosing tubo-ovarian abscess.

C. IMAGING STUDIES

1. X-ray studies—Plain x-rays may suggest an abscess in up to one-half of cases. In subphrenic abscesses, the chest x-ray may show pleural effusion, a raised hemidiaphragm, basilar infiltrates, or atelectasis. Abnormalities on plain abdominal films include an ileus pattern, soft tissue mass, air-fluid levels, free or mottled gas pockets, effacement of properitoneal or psoas outlines, and displacement of viscera. Many of these findings are vague or nonspecific, but they may suggest the need for a CT scan. Barium contrast studies interfere with and have been largely superseded by other imaging techniques. A water-soluble upper gastrointestinal series may reveal an unsuspected perforated viscus or outline perigastric and lesser sac abscesses.

2. Ultrasonography—Real-time ultrasonography is sensitive (about 80% of cases) in diagnosing intra-ab-

dominal abscesses. The findings consist of a sonolucent area with well-defined walls containing fluid or debris of variable density. Bowel gas, intervening viscera, skin incisions, and stomas interfere with ultrasound examinations, limiting their efficacy in postoperative patients. Nevertheless, the procedure is readily available, portable, and inexpensive, and the findings are specific when correlated with the clinical picture. Ultrasonography is most useful when an abscess is clinically suspected, especially for lesions in the right upper quadrant and the paracolic and pelvic areas.

3. CT scan—CT scan of the abdomen, the best diagnostic study, is highly sensitive (over 95% of cases) and specific. Neither gas shadows nor exposed wounds interfere with CT scanning in postoperative patients, and the procedure is reliable even in areas poorly seen on ultrasonography. Abscesses appear as cystic collections with density measurements of between 0 and 15 attenuation units. Resolution is increased by contrast media (eg, sodium diatrizoate) injected intravenously or instilled into hollow viscera adjacent to the abscess. One drawback of CT scan is that diagnosis may be difficult in areas with multiple thick-walled bowel loops or if a pleural effusion overlies a subphrenic abscess, so that occasionally

Right subdiaphragmatic abscess

Right subhepatic abscess

Right paracolic abscess

Right lower quadrant abscess

Phrenicocolic ligament

Left paracolic abscess

Pelvic abscess

Figure 23–3. The infracolic peritoneal compartment and common abscess sites. Note how paracolic fluid on the right side can migrate up into the subphrenic spaces, whereas collections on the left side are prevented from doing so by the phrenicocolic ligament.

Table 23–2. Common sites and causes of intraperitoneal abscesses.

Site	Cause
Right lower quadrant	Appendicitis, perforated ulcer, regional enteritis
Left lower quadrant	Colorectal perforation (diverticulitis, carcinoma, inflammatory bowel diseases)
Pelvis	Appendicitis, colorectal perforation, gynecologic sepsis, postoperative complications
Subphrenic region	Postoperative complications following gastric or hepatobiliary surgery or splenectomy, perforated ulcer, acute cholecystitis, appendicitis, pancreatitis (lesser sac)
Interloop	Postoperative bowel perforation

a very large abscess is missed. CT- or ultrasonography-guided needle aspiration can distinguish between sterile and infected collections in uncertain cases.

4. Radionuclide scan—Gallium-67 citrate and indium 111-labeled autologous leukocyte scans have been superseded by CT scanning and largely relegated to a secondary role because they cannot provide a same-day answer, are of limited value in leukopenic individuals, and are subject to false-positive errors due to nonpyogenic inflammatory conditions, bowel accumulation of labeled leukocytes, or surgically placed foreign bodies in postoperative patients. Some of these shortcomings have been overcome with Tc-99m hexamethylpropyleneamineoxide (HMPAO)-labeled leukocyte scans, which can be performed within 2 hours. In leukopenic patients, radiopharmaceutical imaging with indium 111-labeled human nonspecific immunoglobulin G is an improvement. Radionuclide scanning has an overall sensitivity of about 80%. It may be helpful if peritoneal sepsis is clinically uncertain or if the site of a suspected abscess has not been localized. Occasionally, an unsuspected extra-abdominal source is disclosed.

5. Magnetic resonance imaging—The scanning time, patient inaccessibility during scan acquisition, and upper respiratory motion have limited the usefulness of MRI in the investigation of upper abdominal abscesses. CT scan is generally preferable.

Treatment

Treatment consists of prompt and complete drainage of the abscess, control of the primary cause, and adjunctive use of effective antibiotics. Depending upon the abscess site and the condition of the patient, drainage may be achieved by operative or nonoperative methods. **Percutaneous drainage** is the preferred method for single, well-localized, superficial bacterial abscesses that do not have fistulous communications or contain solid debris. Following CT scan or ultrasonographic delineation, a needle is guided into the abscess cavity; infected material is aspirated for culture; and a suitably large drainage catheter is inserted.

Postoperative irrigation is vital to remove debris and ensure catheter patency. This technique is not appropriate for multiple or deep (especially pancreatic) abscesses or for patients with ongoing contamination, fungal infections, or thick purulent or necrotic material. Percutaneous drainage can be performed in about 75% of cases. The success rate exceeds 80% in simple abscesses but is often less than 50% in more complex ones. It is heavily influenced by the availability of appropriate equipment and the experience of the radiologist performing the drainage. Complications include septicemia, fistula formation, bleeding, and peritoneal contamination.

Open drainage is reserved for abscesses for which percutaneous drainage is inappropriate or unsuccessful. These include many cases where there is a persistent focus of infection (eg, diverticulitis or anastomotic dehiscence) that needs to be controlled. In cases without evidence of continued soiling, the direct extraserous route has the advantage of establishing dependent drainage without contaminating the rest of the peritoneal cavity. Only light general anesthesia or even local anesthesia is necessary, and surgical trauma is minimized. Right anterior subphrenic abscesses can be drained by a subcostal incision (Clairmont incision, Figure 23–4). Posterior subdiaphragmatic and subhepatic lesions can be decompressed posteriorly through the bed of the resected twelfth rib (Nather-Ochsner incision, Figure 23–4) or by a lateral extraserous method (DeCosse incision). Most lower quadrant and flank abscesses can be drained through a lateral extraperitoneal approach. Pelvic abscesses can often be detected on pelvic or rectal examination as a fluctuant mass distorting the contour of the vagina or rectum. If needle aspiration directly through the vaginal or rectal wall returns pus, the abscess is best drained by making an incision in that area. In all cases, digital or direct exploration must

Figure 23–4. Extraperitoneal approaches to the right subphrenic spaces. An abscess in the anterior subhepatic space usually requires transperitoneal drainage. Posterior abscesses may also be drained laterally.

ensure that all loculations are broken down. Penrose and sump drains are used to allow continued drainage postoperatively until the infection has resolved. Serial sonograms or imaging studies help document obliteration of the abscess cavity.

Transperitoneal exploration is indicated if the abscess cannot be localized preoperatively, if there are several or deep-lying lesions, if an enterocutaneous fistula or bowel obstruction exists, or if previous drainage attempts have been unsuccessful. This is especially likely in postoperative patients with multiple abscesses and persistent peritoneal soiling. The need to achieve complete drainage fully justifies the greater stress of laparotomy and the small possibility that infection might be spread to other uninvolved areas. Laparoscopy alone is often inadequate, especially in critically toxic patients without a localized focus.

Satisfactory drainage is usually evidenced by improving clinical findings within 3 days after starting treatment. Failure to improve indicates inadequate drainage, another source of (or ongoing) sepsis, or organ dysfunction. Additional localizing studies and repeated percutaneous or operative drainage should be undertaken urgently (ie, within 24–48 hours, depending on the seriousness of the case). Failure to acknowledge adequate progress delays essential studies and incurs higher mortality.

Prognosis

The mortality rate of serious intra-abdominal abscesses is about 30%. Deaths are related to the severity of the underlying cause, delay in diagnosis, multiple organ failure, and incomplete drainage. Right lower quadrant and pelvic abscesses are usually caused by perforated ulcers and appendicitis in younger individuals. They are readily diagnosed and treated, and the mortality rate is less than 5%. Diagnosis is often delayed in older patients; this increases the likelihood of multiple organ failure. Decompensation of two major organ systems is associated with a mortality rate of over 50%. Shock is an especially ominous sign. Subphrenic, deep, and multiple abscesses frequently require operative drainage and are associated with a mortality rate of over 40%. An untreated residual abscess is nearly always fatal.

Barkhausen J et al: Impact of CT in patients with sepsis of unknown origin. Acta Radiol 1999;40:552.

Eddy V et al: Abdominal compartment syndrome. The Nashville experience. Surg Clin North Am 1997;77:801.

Farthmann EH et al: Epidemiology and pathophysiology of intraabdominal infections (IA). Infection 1998;25:329.

2. Retroperitoneal & Retrofascial Abscesses

Pathophysiology

The large retroperitoneal space, extending from the diaphragm to the pelvis, is divided into anterior and posterior compartments (Figure 23–1). The **anterior portion** includes structures between the posterior peritoneum and the perinephric fascia (pancreas; parts of the duodenum and the ascending and descending colon). The **posterior portion** contains the adrenals, kidneys, and perinephric spaces. The compartment posterior to the transversalis fascia is involved in retrofascial abscesses.

Abscesses occur less commonly in the retroperitoneum than in the peritoneal cavity. Retroperitoneal abscesses arise chiefly from injuries or infections in adjacent structures: gastrointestinal tract abscesses due to appendicitis, pancreatitis, penetrating posterior ulcers, regional enteritis, diverticulitis, or trauma; genitourinary tract abscesses due to pyelonephritis; and spinal column abscesses due to osteomyelitis or disk space infections.

Psoas abscesses may be primary or secondary. Primary psoas abscesses, which occur without associated disease of other organs, are caused by hematogenous spread of *Staphylococcus aureus* from an occult source and are predominantly seen in children and young adults. They are more common in underdeveloped countries. Secondary psoas abscesses result from spread of infection from adjacent organs, principally from the intestine, and are therefore most often polymicrobial. The most common cause is Crohn's disease.

The pyogenic bacteria *(E coli,* bacteroides, proteus, klebsiella) have replaced *Mycobacterium tuberculosis* as the major causative organism. Surprisingly, only a single causative organism is involved in over one-half of cases. A positive blood culture—especially with *Bacteroides*—is an ominous finding.

Clinical Findings

Although they may be symptomless, retroperitoneal abscesses tend to develop in patients with obvious acute illnesses. Fever and abdominal or flank pain are prominent features, sometimes accompanied by anorexia, weight loss, and nausea and vomiting. The clinical findings in patients with psoas abscess consist of hip pain, flexion of the hip with pain on extension, and a positive iliopsoas sign. Abdominal, thigh, and back pain may also occur. The diagnosis is apt to be overlooked when pain in the hip aggravated by walking is the major complaint. The differential diagnosis includes retroperitoneal tumors and hematomas. Radionuclide scanning, bowel contrast studies, and urograms are the common preliminary investigations, but CT scanning most accurately delineates these lesions. Gas bubbles are diagnostic of an abscess. Awareness of the overall clinical picture is essential for CT scanning to differentiate retroperitoneal abscesses from neoplasms or hematomas. Abscesses are confined to specific compartments, whereas malignant lesions, by contrast, frequently violate peritoneal and fascial barriers and can invade bone.

Treatment

Failure to institute prompt and adequate drainage in addition to systemic antibiotics leads to a fatal outcome. Apart from multiloculated pancreatic abscesses, many retroperitoneal abscesses are amenable to percutaneous CT scan-guided needle aspiration and catheter drainage. Drainage by catheter, however, has a lower success rate for retroperitoneal than intraperitoneal abscesses for the following reasons: (1) Retroperitoneal abscesses often dissect along planes, giving a stellate instead of globular shape; (2) they often contain necrotic debris that will not pass through catheters; and (3) they often invade adjacent muscle (eg, psoas abscess). Operation is indicated if there is no clinical improvement after 2 days of percutaneous drainage. An extraperitoneal approach via the flank is preferred for upper retroperitoneal and perirenal abscesses—and one via the perineum presacrally between the anus and the coccyx for pelvic lesions. Transperitoneal exploration may be unavoidable for deep anterior retroperitoneal abscesses. Resection of necrotic or diseased organs, debridement of the affected compartment, and thorough drainage should be accomplished. In general, retroperitoneal abscesses are difficult to drain completely, and residual or recurrent abscesses are common (especially with regional enteritis). Psoas abscesses may invade the spine or ipsilateral hip to cause osteomyelitis or may track across the midline to cause a contralateral psoas abscess.

The surgical mortality rate is about 25%. Failure of the fever to subside within 3 days indicates inadequate drainage and persistent sepsis that will prove fatal if not corrected promptly.

PRIMARY PERITONITIS

Primary ("spontaneous") peritonitis occurring in the absence of gastrointestinal perforation is caused mainly by hematogenous spread but occasionally by transluminal or direct bacterial invasion of the peritoneal cavity. Impairment of the hepatic reticuloendothelial system and compromised peripheral destruction of bacteria by neutrophils promotes bacteremia, which readily infects ascitic fluid that has reduced bacterium-killing capacity. Primary peritonitis is most closely associated with cirrhosis and advanced liver disease with a low ascitic fluid protein concentration. It is also seen in patients with the nephrotic syndrome or systemic lupus erythematosus, or after splenectomy during childhood. Recurrence is common in cirrhosis and often proves fatal.

Clinical Findings

The clinical presentation simulates secondary bacterial peritonitis, with abrupt onset of fever, abdominal pain, distention, and rebound tenderness. However, one-fourth of patients have minimal or no peritoneal symptoms. Most have clinical and biochemical manifestations of advanced cirrhosis or nephrosis. Leukocytosis, hypoalbuminemia, and a prolonged prothrombin time are characteristic findings. The diagnosis hinges upon examination of the ascitic fluid, which reveals a white blood cell count greater than 500/µL and more than 25% polymorphonuclear leukocytes. A blood-ascitic fluid albumin gradient greater than 1.1 g/dL, a raised serum lactic acid level (> 33 mg/dL), or a reduced ascitic fluid pH (< 7.31) supports the diagnosis. Bacteria are seen on gram-stained smears in only 25% of cases. Culture of ascitic fluid inoculated immediately into blood culture media at the bedside usually reveals a single enteric organism, most commonly E coli, klebsiella, or streptococci, but Listeria monocytogenes has been reported in immunocompromised hosts.

Treatment

Antibiotic prophylaxis is of no proved value. Systemic antibiotics with third-generation cephalosporins (eg, ce-

fotaxime) or a beta-lactam-clavulanic acid combination along with supportive treatment are begun once the diagnosis has been established. The 50% average mortality rate is due to peritonitis in only about a third of cases. Multiple organ failure as indicated by gastrointestinal bleeding, hepatic encephalopathy, and renal failure are ominous signs.

Troidle L et al: Differing outcomes of gram-positive and gram-negative peritonitis. Am J Kidney Dis 1998;32:623.

TUBERCULOUS PERITONITIS

Pathophysiology

Tuberculosis peritonitis is encountered in 0.5% of new cases of tuberculosis. It presents as a primary infection without active pulmonary, intestinal, renal, or uterine tube involvement. Its cause is reactivation of a dormant peritoneal focus derived from hematogenous dissemination from a distant nidus or breakdown of mesenteric lymph nodes. Some cases occur as a systemic manifestation of extra-abdominal infection. Multiple small, hard, raised, whitish tubercles studding the peritoneum, omentum, and mesentery are the distinctive finding. A cecal tuberculoma, matted lymph nodes, or omental involvement may form a palpable mass.

The disease affects young persons, particularly women, and is more prevalent in countries where tuberculosis is still endemic. AIDS patients are especially susceptible to development of extrapulmonary tuberculosis.

Clinical Findings

Chronic symptoms (lasting more than a week) include abdominal pain and distention, fever, night sweats, weight loss, and altered bowel habits. Ascites is present in about half of cases, especially if the disease is of long standing, and may be the primary manifestation. A mass may be felt in a third of cases. The differential diagnosis includes Crohn's disease, carcinoma, hepatic cirrhosis, and intestinal lymphoma. One-fourth of patients have acute symptoms suggestive of acute bowel obstruction or peritonitis that mimics appendicitis, cholecystitis, or a perforated ulcer.

Detection of an extra-abdominal site of tuberculosis, evident in half of cases, is the single most useful diagnostic clue. Pleural effusion is present in up to 50% of patients. Paracentesis, laparoscopy, or peritoneal biopsy is applicable only in patients with ascites. The peritoneal fluid is characterized by a protein concentration above 3 g/dL with less than 1.1 g/dL serum-ascitic fluid albumin difference and lymphocyte predominance among white blood cells. Definitive diagnosis is possible in 80% of cases by culture (often taking several weeks) and direct smear. A PPD skin test is useful only when positive (about 80% of cases). Hematologic and biochemical studies are seldom helpful, and leukocytosis is uncommon. The sedimentation rate is elevated in many cases. The presence of high-density ascites or soft tissue masses on ultrasonography or CT scan supports the diagnosis. Young patients from endemic areas who present with classic symptoms or who have suggestive imaging findings should undergo diagnostic laparoscopy, which may obviate laparotomy.

Treatment

In chronic cases, nonoperative therapy is preferable if the diagnosis can be established. Most patients presenting with acute symptoms are diagnosed only by laparotomy. In the absence of intestinal obstruction or perforation, only a biopsy of a peritoneal or omental nodule should be taken. Obstruction due to constriction by a tuberculous lesion usually develops in the distal ileum and cecum, although multiple skip areas along the small bowel may exist. Localized short segments of diseased bowel are best treated by resection with primary anastomosis. Multiple strictured areas may be managed either by side-to-side bypass or a stricturoplasty of partially narrowed segments.

Combination antituberculosis chemotherapy should be started once the diagnosis is confirmed or considered likely. A favorable response is the rule, but isoniazid and rifampin must be continued for 18 months postoperatively.

GRANULOMATOUS PERITONITIS

Pathophysiology

Talc (magnesium silicate), cornstarch glove lubricants, gauze fluffs, and cellulose fibers from disposable surgical fabrics may elicit a vigorous granulomatous (probably a delayed hypersensitivity) response in some patients 2–6 weeks after laparotomy. The condition is uncommon now that surgeons wipe clean their gloves before handling abdominal viscera. Less rarely, granulomatous peritonitis may develop as a hypersensitivity reaction to other foreign material (eg, intestinal ascariasis or food particles from a perforated ulcer). This process should be distinguished from congenital peritoneal encapsulation or abdominal cocoon.

Clinical Findings

Besides abdominal pain, which is often out of proportion to the low-grade fever, there may be nausea and vomiting, ileus, and other systemic complaints. Abdominal tenderness is usually diffuse but mild. Free abdominal fluid, if detectable, should be tapped and in-

spected for the diagnostic Maltese cross pattern of starch particles.

Treatment

Reoperation achieves little and should be avoided if the diagnosis can be made. Most patients undergo reexploration because they present an erroneous impression of postoperative bowel obstruction or peritoneal sepsis. The diffuse hard, white granulomatous masses studding the peritoneum and omentum are easily mistaken for cancer or tuberculosis unless a biopsy specimen is taken to demonstrate foreign body granulomas.

If granulomatous peritonitis is suspected, the response to treatment with corticosteroids or other anti-inflammatory agents is often so dramatic as to be diagnostic in itself. After clinical improvement, intravenous methylprednisolone can be replaced by oral prednisone for 2–3 weeks. The disease is self-limited and does not predispose to late intestinal obstruction.

ASCITES*

1. Chylous Ascites

The accumulation of free chyle in the peritoneal cavity is a rare form of ascites. Most patients are adults—many of them elderly women—with occult cancer, often a lymphoma or adenocarcinoma (of the pancreas or stomach), causing lymphatic obstruction. Chylous ascites resulting from external trauma or operative mishap (portosystemic decompression, abdominal aneurysmectomy and retroperitoneal lymphadenectomy procedures) has a more favorable prognosis. About 15% of cases occur in young children (usually < 1 year old) with congenital lymphatic anomalies.

Clinical Findings

The typical presentation is of abdominal distention and pain along with vague constitutional symptoms. Physical findings—besides ascites—include concomitant pleural effusion and peripheral edema. The combination of fever, night sweats, and lymphadenopathy should arouse suspicion of a lymphoma. The discovery of milky ascitic fluid on paracentesis suggests the correct diagnosis. Only a rough correlation exists between the gross appearance of the fluid and its triglyceride content (> 200 mg/dL, with a mean level of 1500 mg/dL). The fluid leukocyte count (mostly lymphocytes) averages 1000/μL. Hypoalbuminemia, lymphocytopenia, and anemia are frequently present.

---

*Cirrhotic ascites is discussed in Chapter 25.

Conventional radiologic investigations, particularly CT scan of the abdomen, may be helpful. Lymph node biopsy, where applicable, and laparotomy have the highest diagnostic value.

Treatment

Treatment of spontaneous chylous ascites is largely supportive rather than operative. Symptomatic relief can be obtained by intermittent abdominal and pleural tapping. Repeated punctures seldom arrest the chylous leakage and are not without hazard. Dietary measures should begin with a low-fat diet supplemented by medium-chain triglycerides, the latter being transported via the portal rather than the lymphatic circulation. Two-thirds of pediatric cases resolve spontaneously on expectant management within a month or so as collaterals develop. If dietary measures fail, oral findings should be halted and total parenteral nutrition instituted. In adults, the most hopeful situation is if an underlying cancer (which is rarely amenable to curative resection) producing the chylous ascites regresses with chemotherapy or irradiation. Spontaneous improvement is the rule in posttraumatic cases.

Except for resectable congenital chylous cysts, surgery has little to offer. In refractory traumatic cases, intraoperative lymphangiography or perioperative injection of lipophilic dyes at times identifies a leaking site that can be plicated. At operation, the root of the small bowel mesentery around the superior mesenteric vessels should be carefully examined, as a discrete tear is more common at this site. Peritoneovenous shunting has been successful in some postoperative cases. Other surgical endeavors such as bowel resection and retroperitoneal dissection are uniformly futile.

2. Malignant Ascites

Ascites due to advanced cancer is a distressing complication that often necessitates in-hospital care. Peritoneal implants stimulate production of ascitic fluid while impeding its resorption by diaphragmatic lymphatics. Malignant ascites also occurs in the absence of free peritoneal tumor cells if there is advanced venous or lymphatic obstruction. A positive cytologic diagnosis is obtained in 60–90% of cases and supported by a high LDH (> 500 IU/L) or CEA content. DNA aneuploidy on flow cytometry analysis is confirmatory in cytology-negative cases.

Since this is often a preterminal condition, conservative management is preferred, with diuretics (especially spironolactone), paracentesis if warranted by the symptoms, and chemotherapy.

Peritoneovenous shunting (preferably with the Denver shunt) should be considered in symptomatic patients who have ascites refractory to conservative methods and an expected survival time of at least 2 months. Shunting is not effective for viscous or loculated ascites, heavily bloodstained ascites, or ascites with an unusually high cell count. The procedure is most suitable in patients with breast, gastric, or ovarian adenocarcinoma or cytology-negative ascites. Complications include shunt obstruction, disseminated intravascular coagulation, fluid overload, and sepsis. Surprisingly, dissemination of the tumor is rare. About half of the patients derive substantial benefits but few survive beyond 6 months.

Arroyo V et al: Complications of cirrhosis. II. Renal and circulatory dysfunction. Lights and shadows in an important clinical problem. J Hepatol 2000;32(1 Suppl):157.

Dugernier T et al: Ascites fluid in severe acute pancreatitis: from pathophysiology to therapy. Acta Gastroenterol Belg 2000; 63:264.

Heneghan MA et al: Pathogenesis of ascites in cirrhosis and portal hypertension. Med Sci Monit 2000;6:807.

Uriz J et al: Pathophysiology, diagnosis and treatment of ascites in cirrhosis. Baillieres Best Pract Res Clin Gastroenterol 2000; 14:927.

PERITONEAL ADHESIONS

Tissue ischemia, mechanical or thermal trauma, infection, radiation injury, and foreign body reaction predispose to adhesion formation. The peritoneal injury underlying these noxious stimuli evokes a serosanguineous inflammatory reaction that leads to fibrin deposition. Ordinarily, local plasminogen activators initiate lysis of the fibrin strands within 3 days of their formation. Metamorphosis of mesodermal cells regenerates a single layer of new mesothelium as early as 5 days after injury. Inadequate fibrinolysis due to reduced mesothelial plasminogen activator activity allows fibroblastic proliferation to produce fibrous adhesions. Adhesions are now the most prevalent cause of acute and recurrent small bowel obstruction (see Chapter 30) and a persistent bane of abdominal and especially pelvic surgery. However, adhesions may also provide useful vascular bridges that promote tissue healing, such as in ischemic areas of a bowel anastomosis.

Adhesions develop in two-thirds of patients after laparotomy, especially after extensive procedures, pelvic operations, or multiple abdominal operations. Spontaneous adhesions, presumably related to subclinical inflammation, are also found in one-quarter of patients on postmortem examination. Postoperative adhesions are most heavily distributed near the operative site. The omentum, small bowel, colon, and rectum (in descending order of frequency) are involved most often. Short obese female patients seem to have a greater tendency to form adhesions.

Prevention & Treatment

Precise operative technique with avoidance of serosal trauma will reduce but not eliminate adhesion formation. Ischemic tissue trauma caused by crushing, cautery, and mass ligation should be minimized. Reperitonealization of the pelvic floor under tension has been shown to promote rather than hinder adhesion formation. Indeed, well-vascularized peritoneal edges will resurface adjacent denuded areas with epithelium within 2 weeks. The use of an omental flap or synthetic absorbable or nonabsorbable material (eg, Goretex) appears useful after extensive pelvic dissections. Abdominal packs, moist or dry, should be used sparingly, because they produce abrasive serosal tears. Blood and foreign bodies alone induce only a slight peritoneal reaction, but this becomes extensive when there are accompanying serosal injuries. Precise hemostasis is vital, because unclotted blood in the peritoneal cavity acts as an additional source of fibrin, and platelets themselves stimulate serosal inflammation. Starch glove powder, lint gauze fluffs, and cellulose fibers from disposable drapes provoke a rigorous foreign body reaction, and care should be taken to prevent such contamination. The differences between similar types of nonreactive suture material are less critical than the manner in which they are employed: A large number of coarse sutures creates more adhesions than well-placed finer sutures. Laparoscopic procedures tend to produce fewer adhesions than laparotomy.

Hyaluronic acid-carboxymelthylcellulose film (Sprafilm) decreases the formation of intraperitoneal adhesions and is particularly useful in patients likely to need early reoperation, such as those with a temporary bowel diversion.

Beck DE: The role of Seprafilm bioresorbable membrane in adhesion prevention. Eur J Surg Suppl 1997;(577):49.

TUMORS OF THE PERITONEUM & RETROPERITONEUM

Most tumors affecting the peritoneum are secondary implants from primary intraperitoneal cancers. Some unusual peritoneal and retroperitoneal lesions present with abdominal masses or ascites that may be confused with carcinomatosis or chronic inflammatory peritonitis.

Peritoneal Mesothelioma

These rare primary neoplasms are derived from the mesodermal lining of the peritoneum. The malignant variety develops most commonly in men, with a long latent period (averaging 40 years) after prolonged asbestos exposure. Pleural malignant mesotheliomas outnumber peritoneal ones by a ratio of 3:1. Patients present typically with weight loss, crampy abdominal pain, a large mass or distention due to ascites, and a history of asbestos contact. Fewer than half of these patients have asbestosis demonstrated on plain chest films. In contrast to peritoneal carcinomatosis, mesotheliomas are associated with less ascites than the degree of abdominal distention would suggest, and cytologic studies of ascitic fluid are rarely positive. CT scan of the lower thorax and abdomen will demonstrate ascites, peritoneal and mesenteric thickening, pleural plaques, and soft tissue masses involving the omentum and peritoneum. Multiple fine-needle aspiration biopsies guided by ultrasonography, CT scan, or laparoscopy can establish the diagnosis. Electron microscopy is confirmatory in equivocal cases.

Patients usually undergo laparotomy either for diagnosis or because of bowel obstruction. Localized masses should be resected to avoid subsequent obstruction. Metastases to the liver and lung occur late. Encouraging results have been reported with long-term survival following cytoreductive surgery and intraperitoneal cisplatin-based combination chemotherapy. Long-term survivors (beyond 1 year) have been reported with combined treatment by surgical debulking, intraperitoneal cisplatin-doxorubicin, and whole-abdomen irradiation. One should differentiate malignant mesotheliomas from cystic mesotheliomas and well-differentiated papillary mesotheliomas in women, which are less malignant and carry a better prognosis even though they tend to recur locally.

Pseudomyxoma Peritonei

This unusual disease is caused by a low-grade mucinous cystadenocarcinoma of the appendix or ovary that secretes large amounts of mucus-containing epithelial cells. It should be distinguished from benign appendiceal mucocele, which may also have local mucinous deposits but carries a favorable outlook. Patients seldom complain until advanced stages of disease, at which time they have abdominal distention and pain and, in many instances, intermittent or chronic partial small bowel obstruction. Weight loss and other features of cancer are uncommon. The shed neoplastic cells spread freely to two main areas: the upper abdominal sites of peritoneal fluid resorption (undersurface of diaphragm and omentum) and the dependent peritoneal areas (pelvis and lateral abdominal gutters). Distant metastases and visceral involvement are rare. Ultrasonography and CT scans show a distinctive peritoneal scalloping of the liver margin, calcified plaques, ascites, and low-density masses.

At laparotomy, the surgeon should remove as much of the primary lesion and gelatinous material as possible. The omentum also should be resected and existing or impending bowel obstruction relieved. This often necessitates right hemicolectomy. If there is no apparent primary tumor, the appendix and, in women, both ovaries should be removed. Some surgeons advocate radical peritonectomy (including splenectomy, cholecystectomy, appendectomy, sigmoid colectomy, and hysterectomy) to eliminate potential areas of microscopic spread. Whether the higher morbidity incurred is justified remains debated.

Current therapy favors very early intraperitoneal fluorouracil-based adjuvant chemotherapy. Systemic chemotherapy is generally useless. Adjuvant intracavitary radiotherapy has also been advocated, especially for patients with residual disease. Reexploration should be undertaken either as a planned second-look laparotomy or to debulk residual tumor responsible for recurrent obstruction or debilitating mucous ascites. Two-thirds of patients eventually succumb to local or regional disease. The survival rate is about 50% at 5 years and 30% at 10 years.

Sebbag G et al: Results of treatment of 33 patients with peritoneal mesothelioma. Br J Surg 2000;87:1587.

Sugarbaker PH: Management of peritoneal-surface malignancy: the surgeon's role. Langenbecks Arch Surg 1999;384:576.

Cysts of the Mesentery & Retroperitoneum

These rare developmental lesions are usually ectopic pockets of lymphatic tissue or, more rarely, mucinous ovarian cystadenomas. Patients—one-third of whom are children—present with an asymptomatic abdominal mass, chronic pain, or an acute abdomen. The mass is often large, smooth, round, compressible, and more mobile transversely than longitudinally. CT or ultrasonographic scans along with contrast studies of the gastrointestinal and urinary tracts reveal the cystic nature and location of the mass. The differential diagnosis includes pancreatic pseudocysts, enteric duplication (in children), inflammatory cysts, and retroperitoneal tumors. Laparotomy or laparoscopy reveals the cyst, which contains serous fluid if it is in the mesocolon; chylous fluid if it is in the small bowel mesentery; or blood-stained fluid. Most lesions are benign, and enucleation suffices. Segmental resection may be necessary for cysts that impinge upon the bowel wall or its blood supply. Recurrences are more frequent with retroperitoneal cysts, because they may not be amenable to complete excision, and marsupialization may be required instead.

Mesenteric Lipodystrophy (Mesenteric Panniculitis)

There are fewer than 200 reported cases of mesenteric lipodystrophy, in which chronic fat degeneration and

fibrosis affecting the root of the mesentery produce diffuse mesenteric thickening or masses. Its cause is unknown, but it may be a localized form of Weber-Christian disease.

The patient, often an elderly man, has recurrent abdominal pain, weight loss, or symptoms of partial intestinal obstruction. A hard irregular abdominal mass, usually in the left upper quadrant, is felt in over half of patients. CT or ultrasound examination and barium follow-up studies can outline the lesion. CT scanning shows the characteristic features of nonhomogeneous masses of fat and soft tissue density. MRI may suggest the fibrous nature of the lesion and delineates vascular involvement. The diagnosis is usually made only by biopsy at laparotomy, but resection is neither feasible nor indicated. An occasional patient will require a side-to-side intestinal bypass to relieve obstruction.

The process subsides spontaneously in most cases. A more serious variant (**retractile mesenteritis**) associated with obstruction of the mesenteric lymphatics and veins often proves fatal. Corticosteroids, cyclophosphamide, and azathioprine should be reserved for such cases and for patients with clinical deterioration. Lymphoma occurs in 15% of cases on follow-up.

RETROPERITONEAL FIBROSIS

This uncommon entity is characterized by extensive fibrotic encasement of retroperitoneal tissues. Over two-thirds of cases are idiopathic and the rest secondary to drugs (eg, methysergide, beta-adrenergic blocking agents), retroperitoneal hemorrhage, perianeurysmal inflammation, irradiation, urinary extravasation, or cancer. The fibrosis represents an allergic reaction to insoluble lipid (ceroid) that has leaked from atheromatous plaques, especially those within the aorta. The urinary tract may be involved with a diagnostic triad of hydronephrosis and hydroureter (usually bilateral), medial deviation of the ureters, and extrinsic ureteric compression near the L4–5 level. Desmoplastic involvement of the small and large bowel may give rise to obstructive symptoms. Most patients are men over age 50 who present with renal failure or obstructive uropathy. Pain in the low back or flank is common. Pyuria is present in most patients. The diagnosis is suggested by a CT scan that shows the fibrotic process and any coexisting aneurysmal changes in the aorta. MRI may distinguish fibrosis from lymphoma or metastatic carcinoma. Withdrawal of suspect drugs is usually followed by gradual improvement.

Severe urinary obstruction should be decompressed by ureteric stents or nephrostomy. Prednisone (30–60 mg daily) and immunosuppression have been tried but with inconclusive benefits. These agents should be started early postoperatively before marked fibrosis develops. Tamoxifen has produced regression of desmoid tumors. If surgery becomes necessary, a thick rubbery or fibrotic plaque containing chronic inflammatory cells is found at exploration. Multiple biopsy specimens should be taken to exclude cancer. Ureterolysis should be attempted, and there may be some advantage to wrapping omentum around the freed ureters to reduce the risk of subsequent entrapment. Laparoscopic ureterolysis may occasionally be feasible. The outlook is good as long as there is no underlying cancer.

Amis ES Jr: Retroperitoneal fibrosis. AJR Am J Roentgenol 1991; 157:321.

Marzano A et al: Treatment of idiopathic retroperitoneal fibrosis using cyclosporin. Ann Rheum Dis 2001;60:427.

McDougal WS et al: Treatment of idiopathic retroperitoneal fibrosis by immunosuppression. J Urol 1991;134:112.

DISORDERS INVOLVING THE OMENTUM

Infection

The omentum plays an important role in protecting against spreading peritonitis. In chronic infections such as tuberculosis, it may become infected and appear as a rolled-up thickened, inflamed mass. Nonspecific inflammation of the omentum, often a sequela of previous torsion, causes vague abdominal pain.

Torsion & Infarction

Primary (spontaneous) torsion of the omentum may develop if a free portion is fixed by an adhesion or trapped within a hernia. Rotation around the pedicle occludes the blood supply and leads to ischemic necrosis. Infarction may also be secondary to abdominal trauma or vascular conditions such as polyarteritis nodosa. Paraesophageal omental herniation may predispose to a hiatal hernia and may mimic a mediastinal lipoma.

Clinically, torsion presents as acute abdominal pain with nausea and vomiting. Tenderness is confined to the involved area, usually on the right side but away from McBurney's point. A mobile, tender mass is noted in one-third of cases. These features may suggest acute appendicitis or cholecystitis but are not typical of those diseases. The clinical findings usually mandate surgical exploration, which reveals serosanguineous fluid, a normal appendix, and the hemorrhagic necrotic segment of omentum. Resection of the affected portion is curative.

Tumors & Cysts of the Omentum

The omentum is frequently involved secondarily by intra-abdominal malignant tumors, especially gastrointestinal and ovarian adenocarcinomas. Primary cysts or vascular anomalies, usually incidentally discovered at laparotomy, are readily resected.

Stomach & Duodenum

24

Gerard M. Doherty, MD, & Lawrence W. Way, MD

■ I. STOMACH

The stomach receives food from the esophagus and has four functions: (1) It acts as a reservoir that permits eating reasonably large quantities of food at intervals of several hours. (2) Food contained in the stomach is mixed, triturated, and delivered into the duodenum in amounts regulated by its chemical nature and texture. (3) The first stages of protein and carbohydrate digestion are carried out in the stomach. (4) A few substances are absorbed across the gastric mucosa.

ANATOMY

The anatomy of the stomach may be seen in Figures 24–1, 24–2, and 24–3.

The **cardia** is located at the gastroesophageal junction. The **fundus** is the portion of the stomach that lies cephalad to the gastroesophageal junction. The **corpus** is the capacious central part; division of the corpus from the pyloric antrum is marked approximately by the angular incisure, a crease on the lesser curvature just proximal to the "crow's-foot" terminations of the nerves of Latarjet (Figure 24–3). The **pylorus** is the boundary between stomach and the duodenum.

The **cardiac gland area** is the small segment located at the gastroesophageal junction. Histologically, it contains principally mucus-secreting cells, though a few parietal cells are sometimes present. The **oxyntic gland area** is the portion containing parietal (oxyntic) cells and chief cells (Figure 24–2). The boundary between this region and the adjacent pyloric gland area is reasonably sharp, since the zone of transition spans a segment of only 1–1.5 cm. The **pyloric gland** area constitutes the distal 30% of the stomach and contains the G cells that manufacture gastrin. Mucous cells are common in the oxyntic and pyloric gland areas.

As in the rest of the gastrointestinal tract, the muscular wall of the stomach is composed of an outer longitudinal and an inner circular layer. An additional incomplete inner layer of obliquely situated fibers is most prominent near the lesser curvature but is of less substance than the other two layers.

Blood Supply

The blood supply of the stomach and duodenum is illustrated in Figure 24–3. The left gastric artery supplies the lesser curvature and connects with the right gastric artery, a branch of the common hepatic artery. In 60% of persons, a posterior gastric artery arises off the middle third of the splenic artery and terminates in branches on the posterior surface of the body and the fundus. The greater curvature is supplied by the right gastroepiploic artery (a branch of the gastroduodenal artery) and the left gastroepiploic artery (a branch of the splenic artery). The mid portion of the greater curvature corresponds to a point at which the gastric branches of this vascular arcade change direction. The fundus of the stomach along the greater curvature is supplied by the vasa brevia, branches of the splenic and left gastroepiploic arteries.

The blood supply to the duodenum is from the superior and inferior pancreaticoduodenal arteries, which are branches of the gastroduodenal artery and the superior mesenteric artery, respectively. The stomach contains a rich submucosal vascular plexus. Venous blood from the stomach drains into the coronary, gastroepiploic, and splenic veins before entering the portal vein. The lymphatic drainage of the stomach, which largely parallels the arteries, partially determines the direction of spread of gastric neoplasms.

Nerve Supply

The parasympathetic nerves to the stomach are shown in Figure 24–3. As a rule, two major vagal trunks pass through the esophageal hiatus in close approximation to the esophageal muscle. The nerves are originally located to the right and left of the esophagus and stomach during embryonic development. When the foregut rotates, the lesser curvature turns to the right and the greater curvature to the left, and corresponding shifts in location of the vagal trunks follow. Hence, the right vagus supplies the posterior and the left the anterior

533

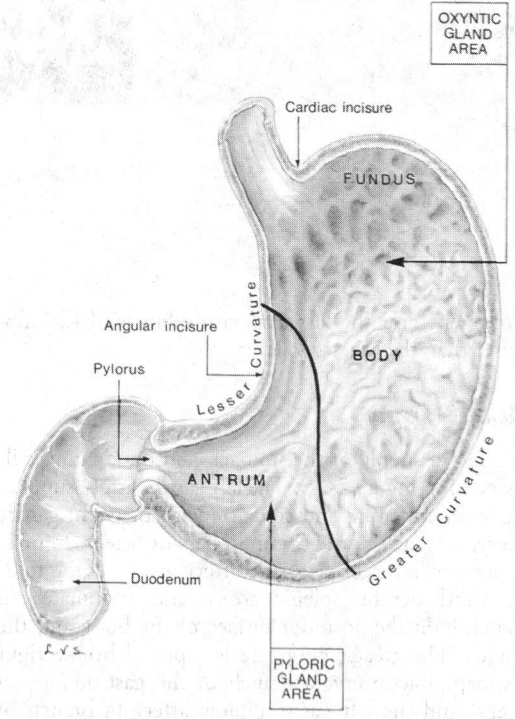

OXYNTIC
GLAND
AREA

Cardiac incisure

FUNDUS

Angular incisure

Pylorus

Lesser Curvature

BODY

ANTRUM

Greater Curvature

Duodenum

L.v.s.

PYLORIC
GLAND
AREA

Figure 24–1. Names of the parts of the stomach. The line drawn from the lesser to the greater curvature depicts the approximate boundary between the oxyntic gland area and the pyloric gland area. No prominent landmark exists to distinguish between antrum and body (corpus). The fundus is the portion craniad to the esophagogastric junction.

gastric surface. About 90% of the vagal fibers are sensory afferent; the remaining 10% are efferent.

In the region of the gastroesophageal junction, each trunk bifurcates. The anterior trunk sends to the liver a division that travels in the lesser omentum. The bifurcation of the posterior trunk gives rise to fibers that enter the celiac plexus and supply the parasympathetic innervation to the remainder of the gastrointestinal tract as far as the mid transverse colon. Both trunks, after giving rise to their extragastric divisions, send some fibers directly onto the surface of the stomach and others along the lesser curvature (anterior and posterior nerves of Latarjet) to supply the distal part of the organ. As shown in Figure 24–3, a variable number of vagal fibers ascend with the left gastric artery after having passed through the celiac plexus.

The preganglionic motor fibers of the vagal trunks synapse with ganglion cells in Auerbach's plexus (plexus myentericus) between the longitudinal and circular muscle layers. Postganglionic cholinergic fibers are distributed to the cells of the smooth muscle layers and the mucosa.

The adrenergic innervation to the stomach consists of postganglionic fibers that pass along the arterial vessels from the celiac plexus.

PHYSIOLOGY

Motility

Storage, mixing, trituration, and regulated emptying are accomplished by the muscular apparatus of the stomach. Peristaltic waves originate in the body and pass toward the pylorus. The thickness of the smooth muscle increases in the antrum and corresponds to the stronger contractions that can be measured in the distal stomach. The pylorus behaves as a sphincter, though it normally allows a little to-and-fro movement of chyme across the junction.

An electrical pacemaker situated in the fundal musculature near the greater curvature gives rise to regular (3/min) electrical impulses (pacesetter potential, basic electrical rhythm) that pass toward the pylorus in the outer longitudinal layer. Every impulse is not always followed by a peristaltic muscular contraction, but the impulses determine the maximal peristaltic rate. The frequency of peristalsis is governed by a variety of stimuli mentioned below. Each contraction follows sequential depolarization of the underlying circular muscle resulting from arrival of the pacesetter potential.

Peristaltic contractions are more forceful in the antrum than the body and travel faster as they progress distally. Gastric chyme is forced into the funnel-shaped antral chamber by peristalsis; the volume of contents delivered into the duodenum by each peristaltic wave depends on the strength of the advancing wave and the extent to which the pylorus closes. Most of the gastric contents that are pushed into the antral funnel are propelled backward as the pylorus closes and pressure within the antral lumen rises. Five to 15 mL enter the duodenum with each gastric peristaltic wave.

The volume of the empty gastric lumen is only 50 mL. By a process called receptive relaxation, the stomach can accommodate about 1000 mL before intraluminal pressure begins to rise. Receptive relaxation is an active process mediated by vagal reflexes and abolished by vagotomy. Peristalsis is initiated by the stimulus of distention after eating. Various other factors have positive or negative influences on the rate and strength of contractions and the rate of gastric emptying. Vagal reflexes from the stomach have a facilitating influence on peristalsis. The texture and volume of the meal both play a role in the regulation of emptying; small particles are emptied more rapidly than large ones, which the

Gastric pit

Epithelial cell

Epithelium

Parietal cell

Mucous cell

Gland

Zymogen
(chief) cell

A

B

Figure 24–2. Histologic features of the mucosa in the oxyntic gland area. Each gastric pit drains three to seven tubular gastric glands. ***A:*** The neck of the gland contains many mucous cells. Oxyntic (parietal) cells are most numerous in the mid portion of the glands; peptic (chief) cells predominate in the basal portion. ***B:*** Drawing from photomicrograph of the gastric mucosa.

organ attempts to reduce in size (trituration). The osmolality of gastric chyme and its chemical makeup are monitored by duodenal receptors. If osmolality is greater than 200 mosm/L, a long vagal reflex (the enterogastric reflex) is activated, delaying emptying. Gastrin causes delay in emptying. Gastrin is the only circulating gastrointestinal hormone to have a physiologic effect on emptying.

Gastric Juice

The output of gastric juice in a fasting subject varies between 500 and 1500 mL/d. After each meal, about 1000 mL are secreted by the stomach.

The components of gastric juice are as follows:

A. MUCUS

Mucus is a heterogeneous mixture of glycoproteins manufactured in the mucous cells of the oxyntic and pyloric gland areas. Mucus provides a weak barrier to the diffusion of H^+ and probably protects the mucosa. It also acts as a lubricant and impedes diffusion of pepsin.

B. PEPSINOGEN

Pepsinogens are synthesized in the chief cells of the oxyntic gland area (and to a lesser extent in the pyloric area) and are stored as visible granules. Cholinergic stimuli, either vagal or intramural, are the most potent pepsigogues, though gastrin and secretin are also effective. The precursor zymogen is activated when pH falls below 5.00, a process that entails severance of a polypeptide fragment from the larger molecule. Pepsin cleaves peptide bonds, especially those containing phenylalanine, tyrosine, or leucine. Its optimal pH is about 2.00. Pepsin activity is abolished at pH greater than 5.00, and the molecule is irreversibly denatured at pH greater than 8.00.

C. INTRINSIC FACTOR

Intrinsic factor, a mucoprotein secreted by the parietal cells, binds with vitamin B_{12} of dietary origin and greatly enhances absorption of the vitamin. Absorption occurs by an active process in the terminal ileum.

Intrinsic factor secretion is enhanced by stimuli that evoke H^+ output from parietal cells. Pernicious anemia is characterized by atrophy of the parietal cell mucosa,

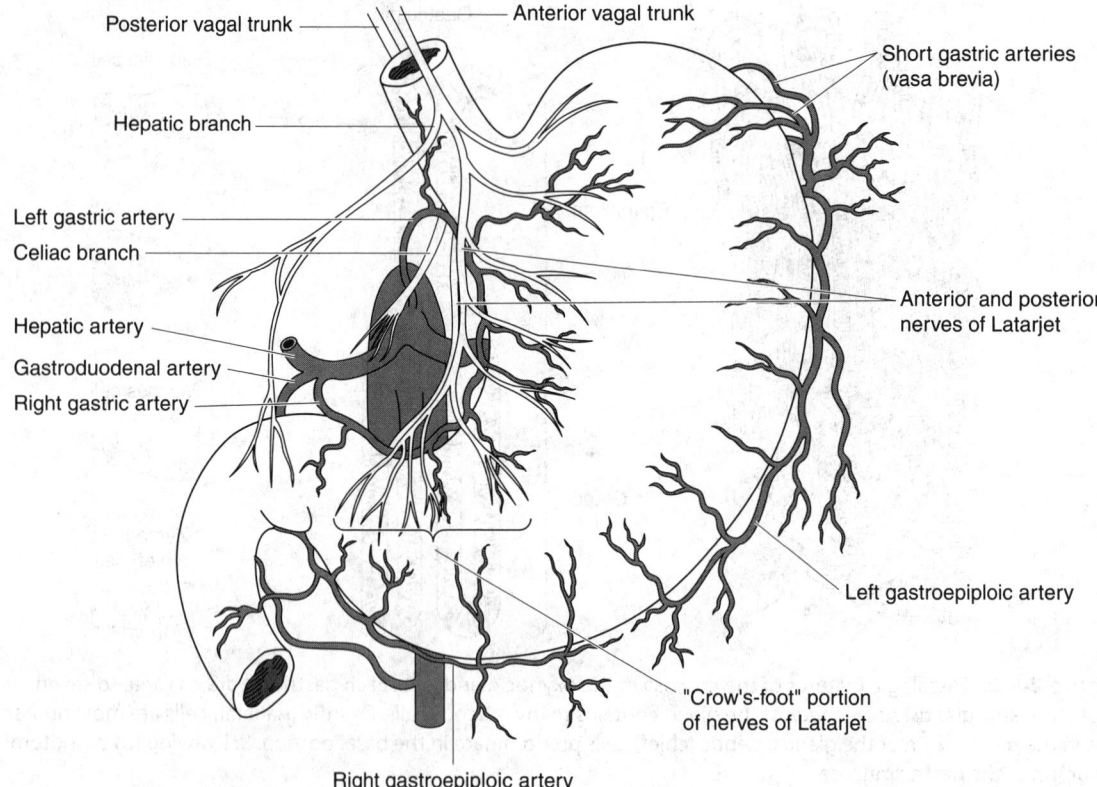

Figure 24–3. Blood supply and parasympathetic innervation of the stomach and duodenum.

deficiency in intrinsic factor, and anemia. Subclinical deficiencies in vitamin B_{12} have been described after operations that reduce gastric acid secretion, and abnormal Schilling tests in these patients can be corrected by the administration of intrinsic factor. Total gastrectomy creates a dependence on parenteral administration of vitamin B_{12}.

D. BLOOD GROUP SUBSTANCES

Seventy-five percent of people secrete blood group antigens into gastric juice. The trait is genetically determined and is associated with a lower incidence of duodenal ulcer than in nonsecretors.

E. ELECTROLYTES

The unique characteristic of gastric secretion is its high concentration of hydrochloric acid, a product of the parietal cells. As the concentration of H^+ rises during secretion, that of Na^+ drops in a reciprocal fashion. K^+ remains relatively constant at 5–10 meq/L. Chloride concentration remains near 150 meq/L, and gastric juice maintains its isotonicity at varying secretory rates.

The Parietal Cell & Acid Secretion

Many of the key events in acid secretion by gastric parietal cells are illustrated in Figure 24–4. The onset of secretion is accompanied by striking morphologic changes in the apical membranes. Resting parietal cells are characterized by an infolding of the apical membrane, called the secretory canaliculus, which is lined by short microvilli. Multiple membrane-bound tubulovesicles and mitochondria are present in the cytoplasm. With stimulation, the secretory canaliculus expands, the microvilli become long and narrow and filled with microfilaments, and the cytoplasmic tubulovesicles disappear. The proton pump mechanism for acid secretion is located in the tubulovesicles in the resting state and in the secretory canaliculus in the stimulated state.

The basal lateral membrane contains the receptors for secretory stimulants and transfers HCO_3^- out of the cell to balance the H^+ output at the apical membrane. Active uptake of Cl^- and K^+ conduction also occur at the basal lateral membrane. Separate membrane-bound receptors exist for histamine (H_2 receptor), gastrin, and acetylcholine. The intracellular second messengers are

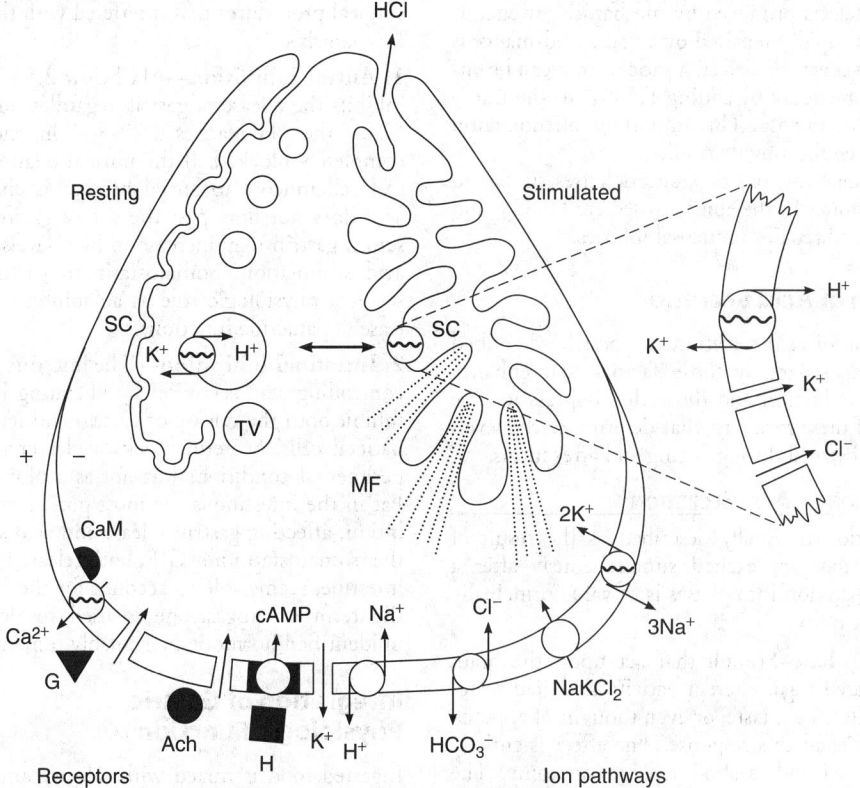

Figure 24–4. Diagram of a parietal cell, showing the receptor systems and ion pathways in the basal lateral membrane and the apical membrane transition from a resting to a stimulated state. Ach, acetylcholine; CaM, calmodulin; G, gastrin; H, histamine; MF, microfilaments; SC, secretory canaliculus; TV, tubulovesicles. (Redrawn and reproduced, with permission, from Malinowska DH, Sachs G: Cellular mechanisms of acid secretion. Clin Gastroenterol 1984;13:309.)

thought to be cAMP for histamine and Ca^{2+} for gastrin and acetylcholine.

Acid secretion at the apical membrane is accomplished by a membrane-bound H^+/K^+-ATPase (the proton pump); H^+ is secreted into the lumen in exchange for K^+.

Mucosal Resistance in the Stomach & Duodenum

The healthy mucosa of the stomach and duodenum is provided with mechanisms that allow it to withstand the potentially injurious effects of high concentrations of luminal acid. Disruption of these mechanisms may contribute to acute or chronic ulceration.

The surface of the gastric mucosa is coated with mucus and secretes HCO_3^- in addition to H^+. Protected by the blanket of mucus, the surface pH is much higher than the luminal pH. HCO_3^- secretion is stimulated by cAMP, prostaglandins, cholinomimetics, glu-

cagon, CCK, and by as yet unidentified paracrine hormones. Inhibitors of HCO_3^- secretion include nonsteroidal anti-inflammatory agents, alpha-adrenergic agonists, bile acids, ethanol, and acetazolamide. Increases in luminal H^+ result in increased HCO_3^- secretion, probably mediated by tissue prostaglandins.

Gastric mucus is a gel composed of high-molecular-weight glycoproteins and 95% water. Since it forms an unstirred layer, it helps the underlying mucosa to maintain a higher pH than that of gastric juice, and it also acts as a barrier to the diffusion of pepsin. At the surface of the layer of mucus, peptic digestion continuously degrades mucus, while below it is continuously being replenished by mucous cells. Gastric acid is thought to enter the lumen through thin spots in the mucus overlying the gastric glands. Secretion of mucus is stimulated by luminal acid and perhaps by cholinergic stimuli. The layer of mucus is damaged by exposure to nonsteroidal anti-inflammatory agents and is enhanced by topical prostaglandin E_2.

Mucosal defects produced by mechanical or chemical trauma are rapidly repaired by adjacent normal cells that spread to cover the defect, a process that can be enhanced experimentally by adding HCO_3^- to the nutrient side of the mucosa. This important phenomenon has not yet been thoroughly studied.

The duodenal mucosa possesses defenses similar to those in the stomach: the ability to secrete HCO_3^- and mucus and rapid repair of mucosal injuries.

Regulation of Acid Secretion

The regulation of acid secretion can best be described by considering separately those factors that enhance gastric acid production and those that depress it. The interaction of these forces is what determines the levels of secretion observed during fasting and after meals.

A. STIMULATION OF ACID SECRETION

Acid production is usually described as the result of three phases that are excited simultaneously after a meal. The separation into phases is of value principally for descriptive purposes.

1. Cephalic phase–Stimuli that act upon the brain lead to increased vagal efferent activity and acid secretion. The sight, smell, taste, or even thought of appetizing food may elicit this response. The effect is entirely vagally mediated and is abolished by vagotomy. The vagal stimuli have a direct effect on the parietal cells to increase acid output.

2. Gastric phase—Food in the stomach (principally protein hydrolysates and hydrophobic amino acids) stimulates gastrin release from the antrum. Gastric distention has a similar but less intense effect.

The presence of food in the stomach excites long vagal reflexes, impulses that pass to the central nervous system via vagal afferents and return to stimulate the parietal cells.

A third aspect of the gastric phase involves the sensitizing effect of distention of the parietal cell area to gastrin that is probably mediated through local intramural cholinergic reflexes.

3. Intestinal phase—The role of the intestinal phase in the stimulation of gastric secretion has been incompletely investigated. Various experiments have shown that the presence of food in the small bowel releases a humoral factor, named entero-oxyntin, that evokes acid secretion from the stomach.

B. INHIBITION OF ACID SECRETION

Without systems to limit secretion, unchecked acid production could become a serious clinical problem. Examples can be found (eg, Billroth II gastrectomy with retained antrum) where acid production rose after surgical procedures that interfered with these inhibitory mechanisms.

1. Antral inhibition—pH below 2.50 in the antrum inhibits the release of gastrin regardless of the stimulus. When the pH reaches 1.20, gastrin release is almost completely blocked. If the normal relationship of parietal cell mucosa to antral mucosa is changed so that acid does not flow past the site of gastrin production, serum gastrin may increase to high levels, with marked acid stimulation. Somatostatin in gastric antral cells serves a physiologic role as an inhibitor of gastrin release (a paracrine function).

2. Intestinal inhibition—The intestine participates in controlling acid secretion by liberating hormones that inhibit both the release of gastrin and its effects on the parietal cells. Secretin blocks acid secretion under experimental conditions but not as a physiologic action. Fat in the intestine is the most potent method of inhibition, affecting gastrin release and acid secretion. Neither somatostatin nor GIP, both released by food in the intestine, seems able to account for the inhibition, and the term enterogastrone is used to denote the still unidentified hormone presumably responsible.

Integration of Gastric Physiologic Function

Ingested food is mixed with salivary amylase before it reaches the stomach. The mechanisms stimulating gastric secretion are activated. Serum gastrin levels increase from a mean fasting concentration of about 50 pg/mL to 200 pg/mL, the peak occurring about 30 minutes after the meal. Food in the lumen of the stomach is exposed to high concentrations of acid and pepsin at the mucosal surface. Food settles in layers determined by sequence of arrival, but fat tends to float to the top. The greatest mixing occurs in the antrum. Antral contents therefore become more uniformly acidic than those in the body of the organ, where the central portion of the meal tends to remain alkaline for a considerable time, allowing continued activity of the amylase.

Peptic digestion of protein in the stomach is only about 5–10% complete. Carbohydrate digestion may reach 30–40%. A lipase originating from the tongue initiates the first stages of lipolysis in the stomach.

The gastric contents are delivered to the duodenum at a rate determined by the volume and texture of the meal, its osmolality and acidity, and its content of fat. A meal of lean meat, potatoes, and vegetables leaves the stomach within 3 hours. A meal with a very high fat content may remain in the stomach for 6–12 hours.

Calam J, Baron JH: ABC of the upper gastrointestinal tract: pathophysiology of duodenal and gastric ulcer and gastric cancer. BMJ 2001;323:980.

PEPTIC ULCER

Peptic ulcers result from the corrosive action of acid gastric juice on a vulnerable epithelium. Depending on circumstances, they may occur in the esophagus, the duodenum, the stomach itself, the jejunum after surgical construction of a gastrojejunostomy, or the ileum in relation to ectopic gastric mucosa in Meckel's diverticulum. When the term peptic ulcer was first used, it was thought that the most important factor was the peptic activity in gastric juice. Since then, evidence has implicated acid as the chief injurious agent; in fact, it is axiomatic that if gastric juice contains no acid, a (benign) peptic ulcer cannot be present. Appreciation of the role of acid has led to the emphasis on therapy with antacids and H_2 blocking agents for the medical therapy of ulcers and to operations that reduce acid secretion as the major surgical approach. In the case of duodenal and gastric ulcers, *Helicobacter pylori* must colonize and weaken the mucosa before acid is able to do the damage, and therapy directed against this organism has a more definitive effect on the disease.

It has been estimated that about 2% of the adult population in the USA suffers from active peptic ulcer disease, and about 10% of the population will have the disease during their lifetime. Men are affected three times as often as women. Duodenal ulcers are ten times more common than gastric ulcers in young patients, but in the older age groups the frequency is about equal. Probably as a result of a declining prevalence of *H pylori* infection, the incidence has declined to less than half what it was 20 years ago.

In general terms, the ulcerative process can lead to four types of disability: (1) **Pain** is the most common. (2) **Bleeding** may occur as a result of erosion of submucosal or extraintestinal vessels as the ulcer becomes deeper. (3) Penetration of the ulcer through all layers of the affected gut results in **perforation** if other viscera do not seal the ulcer. (4) **Obstruction** may result from inflammatory swelling and scarring and is most likely to occur with ulcers located at the pylorus or gastroesophageal junction, where the lumen is narrowest.

The clinical features and prognosis of duodenal ulcer and gastric ulcer are sufficiently different to be dealt with separately here.

DUODENAL ULCER

 ESSENTIALS OF DIAGNOSIS

- *Epigastric pain relieved by food or antacids.*
- *Epigastric tenderness.*
- *Normal or increased gastric acid secretion.*
- *Signs of ulcer disease on upper gastrointestinal x-rays or endoscopy.*
- *Evidence of* Helicobacter pylori *infection.*

General Considerations

Duodenal ulcers may occur in any age group but are most common in the young and middle-aged (20–45 years). They appear in men more often than women. About 95% of duodenal ulcers are situated within 2 cm of the pylorus, in the duodenal bulb.

Considerable evidence implicates *H pylori* as the principal cause of duodenal ulcer disease. This microaerophilic gram-negative curved bacillus can be found colonizing patches of gastric metaplasia within the duodenum in 90% of patients with this disease. The bacilli remain on the surface of the mucosa rather than invading it. They are thought to render the duodenum more vulnerable to the injurious effects of acid and pepsin by releasing urease or other toxins.

The epidemiology of peptic ulcer disease reflects the prevalence of *H pylori* infection in different populations. In areas of the world where peptic ulcer is uncommon (eg, rural Africa), human infection is rare. Duodenal ulcer disease has emerged as a major clinical entity in Western society only since the latter part of the 19th century. The incidence reached a peak about 30 years ago and then declined to reach a lower plateau a few years ago. These changes are thought to be explained by variations in *H pylori* infection resulting from public health factors. Within countries like the USA, the distribution of *H pylori* is explainable by a fecal-oral theory of transmission. The prevalence of infection is higher among lower socioeconomic groups. Interestingly, only a minority of infected persons develop ulcers. *H pylori* also has an important role in the etiology of gastric ulcer, gastric cancer, and gastritis. The 10% of duodenal ulcers that are not associated with helicobacter infection are caused by nonsteroidal anti-inflammatory drugs and other agents.

Gastric acid secretion is characteristically higher than normal in patients with duodenal ulcer compared with normal subjects, but only one-sixth of the duodenal ulcer population have secretory levels that exceed the normal range (ie, acid secretion in normal subjects and those with duodenal ulcer overlap considerably), so the disease cannot be explained simply as a manifestation of increased acid production. Whether acid secretion increases in response to helicobacter infection is doubted. One possibility is that the patches of metaplastic gastric epithelium in the duodenum on which helicobacter take up residence result from the action of acid. Then the colonized patches undergo ulceration.

Chronic liver disease, chronic lung disease, and chronic pancreatitis have all been implicated as increasing the possibility of duodenal ulceration.

Clinical Findings

A. SYMPTOMS AND SIGNS

Pain, the presenting symptom in most patients, is usually located in the epigastrium and is variably described as aching, burning, or gnawing. Radiologic survey studies indicate, however, that some patients with active duodenal ulcer have no gastrointestinal complaints.

The daily cycle of the pain is often characteristic. The patient usually has no pain in the morning until an hour or more after breakfast. The pain is relieved by the noon meal, only to recur in the later afternoon. Pain may appear again in the evening, and in about half of cases it arouses the patient during the night. Food, milk, or antacid preparations give temporary relief.

When the ulcer penetrates the head of the pancreas posteriorly, back pain is noted; concomitantly, the cyclic pattern of pain may change to a more steady discomfort, with less relief from food and antacids.

Varying degrees of nausea and vomiting are common. Vomiting may be a major feature even in the absence of obstruction.

The abdominal examination may reveal localized epigastric tenderness to the right of the midline, but in many instances no tenderness can be elicited.

B. ENDOSCOPY

Gastroduodenoscopy is useful in evaluating patients with an uncertain diagnosis, those with bleeding from the upper intestine, and those who have obstruction of the gastroduodenal segment and for assessing response to therapy.

C. DIAGNOSTIC TESTS

1. Gastric analysis—A gastric analysis may be indicated in certain cases. The standard gastric analysis consists of the following: (1) Measurement of acid production by the unstimulated stomach under basal fasting conditions; the result is expressed as H^+ secretion in meq/h and is termed the **basal acid output (BAO).** (2) Measurement of acid production during stimulation by histamine or pentagastrin given in a dose maximal for this effect. The result is expressed as H^+ secretion in meq/h and is termed the **maximal acid output (MAO).**

Interpretation of the results is outlined in Table 24–1.

2. Serum gastrin—Depending on the laboratory, normal basal gastrin levels average 50–100 pg/mL, and levels over 200 pg/mL can almost always be considered high.

Table 24–1. Mean values for acid output during gastric analysis for normals and patients with duodenal ulcer. The upper limits of normal are: Basal, 5 meq/h; maximal, 30 meq/h.

		Mean Acid Output (meq/h)	
	Sex	Normal	Duodenal Ulcer
Basal	Male	2.5	5.5
	Female	1.5	3
Maximal (pentagastrin)	Male	30	40
	Female	20	30

Gastrin concentrations may rise in hyposecretory and hypersecretory states. In the former conditions (eg, atrophic gastritis, pernicious anemia), the cause is higher antral pH with loss of antral inhibition for gastrin release. More important clinically is elevated gastrin levels with concomitant hypersecretion, where the high gastrin level is responsible for the increased acid and resulting peptic ulceration. The best-defined clinical condition in this category is Zollinger-Ellison syndrome (gastrinoma).

A fasting serum gastrin determination should be obtained in patients with peptic ulcer disease that is unusually severe or refractory to therapy.

D. RADIOGRAPHIC STUDIES

On an upper gastrointestinal series, the changes induced by duodenal ulcer consist of duodenal deformities and an ulcer niche. Inflammatory swelling and scarring may lead to distortion of the duodenal bulb, eccentricity of the pyloric channel, or pseudodiverticulum formation. The ulcer itself may be seen either in profile or, more commonly, en face.

Differential Diagnosis

The most common diseases simulating peptic ulcer are (1) chronic cholecystitis, in which cholecystograms show either nonfunctioning of the gallbladder or stones in a functioning gallbladder; (2) acute pancreatitis, in which the serum amylase is elevated; (3) chronic pancreatitis, in which ERCP shows an abnormal pancreatic duct; (4) functional indigestion, in which x-rays are normal; and (5) reflux esophagitis.

Complications

The common complications of duodenal ulcer are hemorrhage, perforation, and duodenal obstruction. Each of these is discussed in a separate section. Less common complications are pancreatitis and biliary obstruction.

Prevention

Prevention of ulcer disease entails avoidance of *H pylori* infection.

Treatment

Acute duodenal ulcer can be controlled by suppressing acid secretion in most patients, but the long-term course of the disease (ie, frequency of relapses and of complications) is unaffected unless *H pylori* infection is eradicated. Surgical therapy is recommended principally for the treatment of complications: bleeding, perforation, or obstruction.

A. MEDICAL TREATMENT

The goals of medical therapy are (1) to heal the ulcer and (2) to cure the disease. Treatment in the first category is aimed at decreasing acid secretion or neutralizing acid. The principal drugs consist of H_2 receptor antagonists (eg, cimetidine, ranitidine) and proton pump blockers (eg, omeprazole). One of the H_2 receptor antagonists is usually the first choice, and when given in therapeutic doses, it will bring about healing of the ulcer in 80% of patients within 6 weeks. Omeprazole is reserved for patients whose ulcers are refractory to H_2 antagonists or for those with Zollinger-Ellison syndrome. Antacids may be used alternatively as primary therapy or on an as-needed basis to treat ulcer pain. Antacids are just as effective as H_2 receptor antagonists but slightly more difficult to administer.

After the ulcer has healed, discontinuation of therapy results in an 80% recurrence rate within 1 year, which may be avoided by chronic nighttime administration of a single dose of H_2 receptor antagonists. A better approach is to treat the *H pylori* infection along with the ulcer, since eradication of *H pylori* eliminates recurrent ulceration unless the infection recurs—an uncommon event. At present, the optimal daily regimen consists of the following combination of drugs: lansoprazole, 30 mg twice daily for 14 days; amoxicillin, 1 g twice daily for 14 days; and clarithromycin, 500 mg twice daily for 14 days.

B. SURGICAL TREATMENT

If medical treatment has been optimal, a persistent ulcer may be judged intractable, and surgical treatment is indicated. This is now uncommon.

The surgical procedures that can cure peptic ulcer are aimed at reduction of gastric acid secretion. Excision of the ulcer itself is not sufficient for either duodenal or gastric ulcer; recurrence is nearly inevitable with such procedures.

The surgical methods of treating duodenal ulcer are vagotomy (several varieties) and antrectomy plus vago-

tomy. All of these procedures can be performed laparoscopically. With rare exceptions, one of the vagotomy operations is sufficient (Figure 24–5).

1. Vagotomy—Truncal vagotomy consists of resection of a 1- or 2-cm segment of each vagal trunk as it enters the abdomen on the distal esophagus. The resulting vagal denervation of the gastric musculature produces delayed emptying of the stomach in many patients unless a drainage procedure is performed. The method of drainage most often selected is **pyloroplasty (Heineke-Mikulicz procedure;** Figure 24–6); **gastrojejunostomy** is used less often. Neither procedure gives a superior functional result, and pyloroplasty is less time-consuming.

Vagal denervation of just the parietal cell area of the stomach is called **parietal cell vagotomy** or **proximal gastric vagotomy.** The technique spares the main nerves of Latarjet (Figures 24–3 and 24–5) but divides all vagal branches that terminate on the proximal two-thirds of the stomach. Since antral innervation is preserved, gastric emptying is relatively normal, and a drainage procedure is unnecessary. Nevertheless, parietal cell vagotomy plus pyloroplasty gives better results (ie, fewer recurrent ulcers) than parietal cell vagotomy alone. Parietal cell vagotomy appears to have about the same effectiveness as truncal or selective vagotomy for curing the ulcer disease, but dumping and diarrhea are much less frequent. It is probably the procedure of choice for intractable and perforated duodenal ulcers and is relatively less useful for obstructing and bleeding ulcers.

The vagotomy procedures have the advantages of technical simplicity and preservation of the entire gastric reservoir capacity. The principal disadvantage is recurrent ulceration in about 10% of patients. The recurrence rate after parietal cell vagotomy is about twice as high in patients with prepyloric ulcer, and most surgeons use a different operation for an ulcer in this location.

2. Antrectomy and vagotomy—This operation entails a distal gastrectomy of 50% of the stomach, with the line of gastric transection carried high on the lesser curvature to conform with the boundary of the gastrin-producing mucosa.

The terms antrectomy and hemigastrectomy are loosely synonymous. The proximal remnant may be reanastomosed to the duodenum (**Billroth I resection**) or to the side of the proximal jejunum (**Billroth II resection**). The Billroth I technique is most popular, but there is no conclusive evidence that the results are superior. When creating a Billroth II (gastrojejunostomy) reconstruction, the surgeon may bring the jejunal loop up to the gastric remnant either anterior to the transverse colon or posteriorly through a hole in the trans-

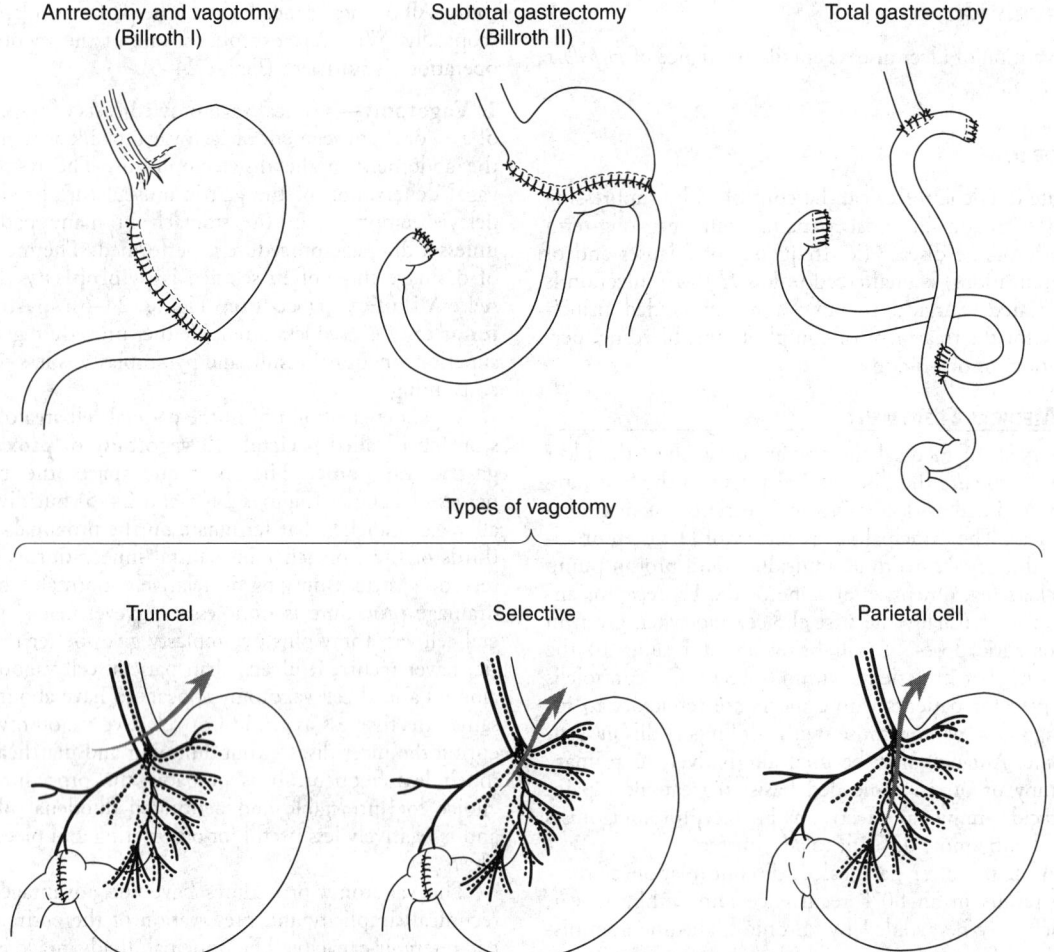

Antrectomy and vagotomy
(Billroth I)

Subtotal gastrectomy
(Billroth II)

Total gastrectomy

Types of vagotomy

Truncal

Selective

Parietal cell

Figure 24–5. Various types of operations currently popular for treating duodenal ulcer disease. Total gastrectomy is reserved for Zollinger-Ellison syndrome. The choice among the other procedures should be individualized according to principles discussed in the text.

verse mesocolon. Since either method is satisfactory, an antecolic anastomosis is elected in most cases because it is simpler. Truncal vagotomy is performed as described in the preceding section; antrectomy by itself will not prevent a high recurrence rate. In most instances, the surgeon will be able to remove the ulcerated portion of duodenum in the course of resection.

Vagotomy and antrectomy is associated with a low incidence of marginal ulceration (2%) and a generally good overall outcome, but the risk of complications is higher than after vagotomy without resection.

3. Subtotal gastrectomy—This operation consists of resection of two-thirds to three-fourths of the distal stomach. After subtotal gastrectomy for duodenal ulcer,

a Billroth II reconstruction is preferable. Subtotal gastrectomy is largely of historical interest.

Complications of Surgery for Peptic Ulcer

A. EARLY COMPLICATIONS

Duodenal stump leakage, gastric retention, and hemorrhage may develop in the immediate postoperative period.

B. LATE COMPLICATIONS

1. Recurrent ulcer (marginal ulcer, stomal ulcer, anastomotic ulcer)—Recurrent ulcers form in about 10% of duodenal ulcer patients treated by vagotomy

Figure 24–6. Heineke-Mikulicz pyloroplasty. A longitudinal incision has been made across the pylorus, revealing an active ulcer in the duodenal bulb. The insert shows the transverse closure of the incision that widens the gastric outlet. The accompanying vagotomy is not shown.

and pyloroplasty or parietal cell vagotomy; and in 2–3% after vagotomy and antrectomy or subtotal gastrectomy. These figures were accumulated before the emergence of effective treatment against *H pylori,* however, and are likely to be lower with current management. Recurrent ulcers nearly always develop immediately adjacent to the anastomosis on the intestinal side.

The usual complaint is upper abdominal pain, which is often aggravated by eating and improved by antacids. In some patients, the pain is felt more to the left in the epigastrium, and left axillary or shoulder pain is occasionally reported. About a third of patients with stomal ulcer will experience major gastrointestinal hemorrhage. Free perforation is less common (5%).

Diagnosis and treatment are essentially the same as for the original ulcer.

2. Gastrojejunocolic and gastrocolic fistula—A deeply eroding ulcer may occasionally produce a fistula between the stomach and colon. Most examples have resulted from recurrent peptic ulcer after an operation that included a gastrojejunal anastomosis.

Severe diarrhea and weight loss are the presenting symptoms in over 90% of cases. Abdominal pain typical of recurrent peptic ulcer often precedes the onset of the diarrhea. Bowel movements number 8–12 or more a day; they are watery and often contain particles of undigested food.

The degree of malnutrition ranges from mild to very severe. Laboratory studies reveal low serum proteins and manifestations of fluid and electrolyte depletion.

Appropriate tests may reflect deficiencies in both water-soluble and fat-soluble vitamins.

An upper gastrointestinal series reveals the marginal ulcer in only 50% of patients and the fistula in only 15%. Barium enema unfailingly demonstrates the fistulous tract.

Initial treatment should replenish fluid and electrolyte deficits. The involved colon and ulcerated gastrojejunal segment should be excised and colonic continuity reestablished. Vagotomy, partial gastrectomy, or both are required to treat the ulcer diathesis and prevent another recurrent ulcer. Results are excellent in benign disease. In general, the outlook for patients with a malignant fistula is poor.

3. Dumping syndrome—Symptoms of the dumping syndrome are noted to some extent by most patients who have an operation that impairs the ability of the stomach to regulate its rate of emptying. Within several months, however, dumping is a clinical problem in only 1–2% of patients. Symptoms fall into two categories: cardiovascular and gastrointestinal. Shortly after eating, the patient may experience palpitations, sweating, weakness, dyspnea, flushing, nausea, abdominal cramps, belching, vomiting, diarrhea, and, rarely, syncope. The degree of severity varies widely, and not all symptoms are reported by all patients. In severe cases, the patient must lie down for 30–40 minutes until the discomfort passes.

Diet therapy to reduce jejunal osmolality is successful in all but a few cases. The diet should be low in carbohydrate and high in fat and protein content. Sugars and carbohydrates are least well tolerated; some patients are especially sensitive to milk. Meals should be taken dry, with fluids restricted to between meals. This dietary regimen ordinarily suffices, but anticholinergic drugs may be of help in some patients; others have reported improvement with supplemental pectin in the diet, and the use of somatostatin analogues offers some promise.

4. Alkaline gastritis—Reflux of duodenal juices into the stomach is an invariable and usually innocuous situation after operations that interfere with pyloric function, but in some patients, it may cause marked gastritis. The principal symptom is postprandial pain, and the diagnosis rests on endoscopic and biopsy demonstration of an edematous inflamed gastric mucosa. Since a minor degree of gastritis is found in most patients after Billroth II gastrectomy, the endoscopic findings are to some degree nonspecific. Persistent severe pain is an indication for surgical reconstruction. Roux-en-Y gastrojejunostomy with a 40-cm efferent jejunal limb is the treatment of choice.

5. Anemia—Iron deficiency anemia develops in about 30% of patients within 5 years after partial gastrectomy. It is caused by failure to absorb food iron bound in an organic molecule. Before this diagnosis is accepted, the patient should be checked for blood loss, marginal ulcer, or an unsuspected tumor. Inorganic iron—ferrous sulfate or ferrous gluconate—is indicated for treatment and is absorbed normally after gastrectomy.

Vitamin B_{12} deficiency and megaloblastic anemia appear in a few cases after gastrectomy.

6. Postvagotomy diarrhea—About 5–10% of patients who have had truncal vagotomy require treatment with antidiarrheal agents at some time, and perhaps 1% are seriously troubled by this complication. The diarrhea may be episodic, in which case the onset is unpredictable after symptom-free intervals of weeks to months. An attack may consist of only one or two watery movements or, in severe cases, may last for a few days. Other patients may continually produce 3–5 loose stools per day.

Most cases of postvagotomy diarrhea can be treated satisfactorily with constipating agents.

7. Chronic gastroparesis—Chronic delayed gastric emptying is seen occasionally after gastric surgery. Prokinetic agents (eg, metoclopramide) are often helpful, but some cases are refractory to any therapy except a completion gastrectomy and Roux-en-Y esophagojejunostomy (ie, total gastrectomy).

Donahue PE: Parietal cell vagotomy versus vagotomy-antrectomy: ulcer surgery in the modern era. World J Surg 2000;24:264.

Erstad BL: Proton-pump inhibitors for acute peptic ulcer bleeding. Ann Pharmacother 2001;35:730.

Jamieson GG: Current status of indications for surgery in peptic ulcer disease. World J Surg 2000;24:256.

Logan RP, Walker MM: ABC of the upper gastrointestinal tract: epidemiology and diagnosis of Helicobacter pylori infection. BMJ 2001;323:920.

Macintyre IM: Peptic ulcer surgery—an obituary. Proc R Coll Physicians Edinb 2000;30:158.

Macintyre IM: Peptic ulcer surgery—an obituary. (Part 2.) Proc R Coll Physicians Edinb 2000;30:245.

Peterson WL, Cook DJ: Antisecretory therapy for bleeding peptic ulcer. JAMA 1998;280:877.

Peura D: Helicobacter pylori: rational management options. Am J Med 1998;105:424.

Zittel TT, Jehle EC, Becker HD: Surgical management of peptic ulcer disease today–indication, technique and outcome. Langenbecks Arch Surg 2000;385:84.

ZOLLINGER-ELLISON SYNDROME (Gastrinoma)

 ESSENTIALS OF DIAGNOSIS

- *Peptic ulcer disease (often severe) in 95%.*
- *Gastric hypersecretion.*
- *Elevated serum gastrin.*
- *Non-B islet cell tumor of the pancreas or duodenum.*

General Considerations

Zollinger-Ellison syndrome is manifested by gastric acid hypersecretion caused by a gastrin-producing tumor (gastrinoma). Although the normal pancreas does not contain appreciable amounts of gastrin, most gastrinomas occur in the pancreas; others are found submucosally in the duodenum and rarely in the antrum or ovary. The gastrin-producing lesions (called **apudomas** from the theory of their histogenesis) in the pancreas are non-B islet cell carcinomas (60%), solitary adenomas (25%), and hyperplasia or microadenomas (10%); the remaining cases (5%) are due to solitary submucosal gastrinomas in the first or second portion of the duodenum. About one-third of patients have the multiple endocrine neoplasia type I syndrome (MEN 1), which is characterized by a family history of endocrinopathy and the presence of tumors in other glands, especially the parathyroids and pituitary. Patients with MEN 1 usually have multiple benign gastrinomas. Those without MEN 1 usually have solitary gastrinomas that are often malignant. The tumors may be as small as 2–3 mm and are often difficult to find. In about one-third of cases, the tumor cannot be located at laparotomy.

The diagnosis of cancer can be made only with findings of metastases or blood vessel invasion, because the histologic pattern is similar for benign and malignant tumors. In most patients with malignant gastrinomas, the illness caused by hypergastrinemia (ie, severe peptic ulcer disease) is a greater threat to health than the illness caused by malignant growth and spread.

Clinical Findings

A. Symptoms and Signs

Symptoms associated with gastrinoma are principally a result of acid hypersecretion—usually from peptic ulcer disease. Some patients with gastrinoma have severe diarrhea from the large amounts of acid entering the duodenum, which can destroy pancreatic lipase and produce steatorrhea, damage the small bowel mucosa, and overload the intestine with gastric and pancreatic secretions. About 5% of patients present with diarrhea only.

Ulcer symptoms are often refractory to large doses of antacids or standard doses of H_2 blocking agents. Hemorrhage, perforation, and obstruction are common complications. Marginal ulcers appear after surgical procedures that would cure the ordinary ulcer diathesis.

B. Laboratory Findings

Hypergastrinemia in the presence of acid hypersecretion is almost pathognomonic for gastrinoma. Gastrin levels are normally inversely proportionate to gastric acid output; therefore, diseases that result in increased gastric pH may cause a rise in serum gastric concentration (eg, pernicious anemia, atrophic gastritis, gastric ulcer, postvagotomy state). Serum gastrin levels should be measured in any patient with suspected gastrinoma or ulcer disease severe enough to warrant consideration of surgical treatment. H_2 receptor blocking agents, omeprazole, or antacids may increase serum gastrin concentrations and should be avoided for several days before gastrin measurements are made. It is often helpful to measure gastric acid secretion to rule out H^+ hyposecretion as a cause of hypergastrinemia.

The normal gastrin value is less than 200 pg/mL. Patients with gastrinoma usually have levels exceeding 500 pg/mL and sometimes 10,000 pg/mL or higher. Very high gastrin levels (eg, > 5000 pg/mL) or the presence of alpha chains of hCG in the serum usually indicates cancer. Patients with borderline gastrin values (eg, 200–500 pg/mL) and acid secretion in the range associated with ordinary duodenal ulcer disease should have a secretin provocative test. Following intravenous administration of secretin (2 units/kg as a bolus), a rise in the gastrin level of >150 pg/mL within 15 minutes is diagnostic.

Marked basal acid hypersecretion (> 15 meq H^+ per hour) occurs in most Zollinger-Ellison patients who have an intact stomach. In a patient who has previously undergone gastrectomy, a basal acid output of 5 meq/h or more is highly suggestive. Since the parietal cells are already under near maximal stimulation from hypergastrinemia, there is little increase in acid secretion following an injection of pentagastrin, and the ratio of basal to maximal acid output (BAO/MAO) characteristically exceeds 0.6.

Hypergastrinemia and gastric acid hypersecretion may be seen in gastric outlet obstruction, retained antrum after a Billroth II gastrojejunostomy, and in antral gastrin cell hyperactivity (hyperplasia). These conditions may be differentiated from gastrinoma by use of the secretin test. Because associated hyperparathyroidism is so common, serum calcium concentrations should be measured in all patients with gastrinoma.

Serum levels of neuron-specific enolase, β-hCG, and chromogranin-A are often elevated in patients with functioning apudomas. Although they are probably of no physiologic importance, the high levels of these peptides may be useful in diagnosing apudomas and following the results of therapy.

C. Imaging Studies

An upper gastrointestinal series usually shows ulceration in the duodenal bulb, though ulcers sometimes appear in the distal duodenum or proximal jejunum. The presence of ulcers in these distal ("ectopic") locations is nearly diagnostic of gastrinoma. The stomach contains prominent rugal folds, and secretions are present in the lumen despite overnight fasting. The duodenum may be dilated and exhibit hyperactive peristalsis. Edema may be detected in the small bowel mucosa. The barium flocculates in the intestine, and transit time is accelerated. A CT or MR scan will often demonstrate the pancreatic tumors. Somatostatin-receptor scintigraphy is extremely sensitive for detection of gastrinoma primary and metastatic sites. Transhepatic portal vein blood sampling to find gradients of gastrin production has been supplanted by the intra-arterial secretin test. Infusion of secretin into the artery supplying a functional gastrinoma causes an increase in hepatic vein gastrin levels. This invasive test is usually reserved for difficult situations.

Treatment

A. Medical Treatment

Initial treatment should consist of H_2 blocking agents (eg, cimetidine, 300–600 mg, four times daily; ranitidine, 300–450 mg, four times daily). The dose should be adjusted to keep gastric H[+] output below 5 meq in the hour preceding the next dose. Although the response to H$_2$ blocking agents is usually excellent at first. With time, the dose must be increased in order to maintain the same level of control, and control eventually becomes unsatisfactory even at high doses. Omeprazole, a proton pump blocker, is indicated sooner or later in nearly all patients.

A combination of streptozocin, fluorouracil, and doxorubicin is the most effective chemotherapeutic regimen for advanced cancer.

B. Surgical Treatment

Resection is the ideal treatment for gastrinoma and is appropriate in all patients with apparently localized disease and no other significant limitations to their survival. Surgical cure may be possible when there are resectable metastases in peripancreatic lymph nodes or the liver. Overall, about 70% of patients have immediate biochemical cure, and about 30% of patients remain disease-free after 5 years.

Every patient with sporadic Zollinger-Ellison syndrome should be considered a candidate for tumor resection. The preoperative workup should include a CT or MR scan of the pancreas and somatostatin-receptor scintigraphy. Regardless of other findings, exploratory laparotomy is then recommended in the absence of evidence of unresectable metastatic disease. If the tumor is found in the pancreas, it is enucleated if possible. Operative ultrasound may help in the examination of the pancreas. Most lesions will be found either in the head of the pancreas or in the duodenum. All patients should have longitudinal duodenotomy and palpation of the duodenal mucosa to identify the frequent primary tumors in this site.

Prognosis

Since H$_2$ blocking agents become less effective with time, omeprazole is eventually required in medically treated patients. Because it is usually multifocal, the disease can rarely be cured surgically in patients with MEN 1. Malignant gastrinomas cause death from growth of metastases.

Alexander HR et al: Prospective study of somatostatin receptor scintigraphy and its effect on operative outcome in patients with Zollinger-Ellison syndrome. Ann Surg 1998;228:228.

Brentjens R, Saltz L: Islet cell tumors of the pancreas: the medical oncologist's perspective. Surg Clin North Am 2001;81:527.

Doherty GM et al: Lethality of multiple endocrine neoplasia type I. World J Surg 1998;22:581.

Lairmore TC et al: Duodenopancreatic resections in patients with multiple endocrine neoplasia type 1. Ann Surg 2000;231:909.

Lim JH et al: Prospective study of the utility of somatostatin-receptor scintigraphy in the evaluation of patients with multiple endocrine neoplasia type 1. Surgery 1998;124:1037.

Lowney JK et al: Pancreatic islet cell tumor metastasis in multiple endocrine neoplasia type 1: correlation with primary tumor size. Surgery 1998;124:1043.

Norton JA et al: Surgery to cure the Zollinger-Ellison syndrome. N Engl J Med 1999;341:635.

Norton JA et al: Surgical treatment of localized gastrinoma within the liver: a prospective study. Surgery 1998;124:1145.

Norton JA: Intraoperative methods to stage and localize pancreatic and duodenal tumors. Ann Oncol 1999;10(Suppl 4):182.

Pisegna JR: The effect of Zollinger-Ellison syndrome and neuropeptide-secreting tumors on the stomach. Curr Gastroenterol Rep 1999;1:511.

GASTRIC ULCER

 ESSENTIALS OF DIAGNOSIS

- *Epigastric pain.*
- *Ulcer demonstrated by x-ray.*
- *Acid present on gastric analysis.*

General Considerations

The peak incidence of gastric ulcer is in patients aged 40–60 years, or about 10 years older than the average for those with duodenal ulcer. Ninety-five percent of gastric ulcers are located on the lesser curvature, and 60% of these are within 6 cm of the pylorus. The symptoms and complications of gastric ulcer closely resemble those of duodenal ulcer.

Gastric ulcers may be separated into three types with different causes and different treatments. **Type I ulcers,** the most common variety, are found in patients who on the average are 10 years older than patients with duodenal ulcers and who have no clinical or radiographic evidence of previous duodenal ulcer disease; gastric acid output is normal or low. The ulcers are usually located within 2 cm of the boundary between parietal cell and pyloric mucosa, but always in the latter. As noted above, 95% are on the lesser curvature, usually near the incisura angularis.

Antral gastritis is universally present, being most severe near the pylorus and gradually diminishing. This is associated in most cases with the presence of *H pylori* beneath the mucus layer, on the luminal surface of epithelial cells, and gastric ulcer disease is probably the result of infection with this organism.

Type II ulcers are located close to the pylorus (prepyloric ulcers) and occur in association with (most often following) duodenal ulcers. The risk of cancer is very low in these gastric ulcers. Acid secretion measured by gastric analysis is in the range associated with duodenal ulcer.

Type III ulcers occur in the antrum as a result of chronic use of nonsteroidal anti-inflammatory agents.

One must always consider whether the ulcer seen on x-ray or by endoscopy represents an ulcerated malignant tumor rather than a simple benign ulcer. Efforts must be expended during the *initial* stage of the workup to establish this distinction. Despite the generally discouraging results of surgery for gastric adenocarcinoma, those whose tumors are difficult to distinguish from benign ulcer have a 50–75% chance of cure after gastrectomy.

Clinical Findings

A. SYMPTOMS AND SIGNS

The principal symptom is epigastric pain relieved by food or antacids, as in duodenal ulcer. Epigastric tenderness is a variable finding. Compared with duodenal ulcer, the pain in gastric ulcer tends to appear earlier after eating, often within 30 minutes. Vomiting, anorexia, and aggravation of pain by eating are also more common with gastric ulcer.

Achlorhydria is defined as no acid (pH > 6.00) after pentagastrin stimulation. Achlorhydria is incompatible with the diagnosis of benign peptic ulcer and suggests a malignant gastric ulcer. About 5% of malignant gastric ulcers will be associated with this finding.

B. GASTROSCOPY AND BIOPSY

Gastroscopy should be performed as part of the initial workup to attempt to find malignant lesions. The rolled-up margins of the ulcer that produce the meniscus sign on x-ray can often be distinguished from the flat edges characteristic of a benign ulcer. Multiple (preferably six) biopsy specimens and brush biopsy should be obtained from the edge of the lesion. False-positives are rare; false-negatives occur in 5–10% of malignant ulcers.

C. IMAGING STUDIES

Upper gastrointestinal x-rays will show an ulcer, usually on the lesser curvature in the pyloric area. In the absence of a tumor mass, the following suggest that the ulcer is malignant: (1) the deepest penetration of the ulcer is not beyond the expected border of the gastric wall; (2) the meniscus sign is present, ie, a prominent rim of radiolucency surrounding the ulcer, caused by heaped-up edges of tumor; and (3) cancer is more common (10%) in ulcers greater than 2 cm in diameter. Coexistence of duodenal deformity or ulcer favors a diagnosis of benign ulcer in the stomach.

Differential Diagnosis

The characteristic symptoms of gastric ulcer are often clouded by numerous nonspecific complaints. Uncomplicated hiatal hernia, atrophic gastritis, chronic cholecystitis, irritable colon syndrome, and undifferentiated functional problems are distinguishable from peptic ulcer only after appropriate radiologic studies and sometimes not even then.

Gastroscopy and biopsy of the ulcer should be performed to rule out malignant gastric ulcer.

Complications

Bleeding, obstruction, and perforation are the principal complications of gastric ulcer. They are discussed separately elsewhere in this chapter.

Treatment

A. MEDICAL TREATMENT

Medical management of gastric ulcer is the same as for duodenal ulcer. The patient should be questioned regarding the use of ulcerogenic agents, which should be eliminated as far as possible.

Repeat endoscopy should be obtained to document the rate of healing. After 4–16 weeks (depending on the initial size of the lesion and other factors), healing usually has reached a plateau. In order to cure the disease and avoid recurrent ulcers, *H pylori* must be eradicated. The success of therapy in this regard can be checked by serologic testing for *H pylori* antibodies.

B. SURGICAL TREATMENT

Before the significance of *H pylori* in the etiology of gastric ulcer was appreciated, the most effective surgical treatment was distal hemigastrectomy (including the ulcer); somewhat less effective but still useful in high-risk patients was vagotomy and pyloroplasty. Parietal cell vagotomy for prepyloric ulcers was followed by a high (eg, 30%) recurrence rate, but parietal cell vagotomy plus pyloroplasty worked well.

Intractability to medical therapy has now become a rare indication for surgery in gastric ulcer disease, since H_2 receptor antagonists or omeprazole can bring the condition under control, and treatment of *H pylori* infection can almost eliminate the problem of recurrence. Consequently, surgery will be needed principally for complications of the disease: bleeding, perforation, or obstruction.

Calam J, Baron JH: ABC of the upper gastrointestinal tract: pathophysiology of duodenal and gastric ulcer and gastric cancer. BMJ 2001;323:980.

Miller JS, Hendren SK, Liscum KR: Giant gastric ulcer in a body packer. J Trauma 1998;45:617.

Pai R, Tarnawski A: Signal transduction cascades triggered by EGF receptor activation: relevance to gastric injury repair and ulcer healing. Dig Dis Sci 1998;43(9 Suppl):14S.

Peskar BM, Maricic N: Role of prostaglandins in gastroprotection. Dig Dis Sci 1998;43(9 Suppl):23S.

UPPER GASTROINTESTINAL HEMORRHAGE

Upper gastrointestinal hemorrhage may be mild or severe but should always be considered an ominous manifestation that deserves thorough evaluation. Bleeding is the most common serious complication of peptic ulcer, portal hypertension, and gastritis, and these conditions taken together account for most episodes of upper gastrointestinal bleeding in the average hospital population.

The major factors that determine the diagnostic and therapeutic approach are the amount and rate of bleeding. Estimates of both should be made promptly and monitored and revised continuously until the episode has been resolved. It is important to know at the outset that bleeding stops spontaneously in 75% of cases; the remainder includes those who will require surgery, experience complications, or die.

Hematemesis or melena is present except when the rate of blood loss is minimal. **Hematemesis** of either bright-red or dark blood indicates that the source is proximal to the ligament of Treitz. It is more common from bleeding that originates in the stomach or esophagus. In general, hematemesis denotes a more rapidly bleeding lesion, and a high percentage of patients who vomit blood require surgery. Coffee-ground vomitus is due to vomiting of blood that has been in the stomach long enough for gastric acid to convert hemoglobin to methemoglobin.

Most patients with **melena** (passage of black or tarry stools) are bleeding from the upper gastrointestinal tract, but melena can be produced by blood entering the bowel at any point from mouth to cecum. The conversion of red blood to dark depends more on the time it resides in the intestine than on the site of origin. The black color of melenic stools is probably caused by hematin, the product of oxidation of heme by intestinal and bacterial enzymes. Melena can be produced by as little as 50–100 mL of blood in the stomach. When 1 L of blood was instilled into the upper intestine of experimental subjects, melena persisted for 3–5 days, which shows that the rate of change in character of the stool is a poor guide to the time bleeding stops after an episode of hemorrhage.

Hematochezia is defined as the passage of bright-red blood from the rectum. Bright-red rectal blood can be produced by bleeding from the colon, rectum, or anus. However, if intestinal transit is rapid during brisk bleeding in the upper intestine, bright-red blood may be passed unchanged in the stool.

Tests for Occult Blood

Normal subjects lose about 2.5 mL of blood per day in their stools, presumably from minor mechanical abrasions of the intestinal epithelium. Between 50 and 100 mL of blood per day will produce melena. Tests for occult blood in the stool should be able to detect amounts between 10 and 50 mL/d. False-positive results may be due to dietary hemoglobin, myoglobin, or peroxidases of plant origin. Iron ingestion does not give positive reactions. The various tests using guaiac, benzidine, phenolphthalein, or orthotoluidine have similar specificities. The sensitivity of the guaiac slide test (Hemoccult) is in the desired range, and this is the best test available at present.

Initial Management

In an apparently healthy patient, melena of a week or more suggests that the bleeding is slow. In this type of patient, admission to the hospital should be followed by a deliberate but nonemergency workup. However, patients who present with hematemesis or melena of less than 12 hours' duration should be handled as if exsanguination were imminent. The approach entails a simultaneous series of diagnostic and therapeutic steps with the following initial goals: (1) Assess the status of the circulatory system and replace blood loss as necessary. (2) Determine the amount and rate of bleeding. (3) Slow or stop the bleeding by ice-water lavage. (4) Discover the lesion responsible for the episode. The last step may lead to more specific treatment appropriate to the underlying condition.

The patient should be admitted to the hospital and a history and physical examination performed. Experienced clinicians are able to make a correct diagnosis of the cause of bleeding from clinical findings in only 60% of patients. Peptic ulcer, acute gastritis, esophageal varices, esophagitis, and Mallory-Weiss tear account for over 90% of cases (see Table 24–2). Questions concerning the symptoms and predisposing factors should be asked. The patient should be questioned about salicylate intake and any history of a bleeding tendency.

Of the diseases commonly responsible for acute upper gastrointestinal bleeding, only portal hypertension is associated with diagnostic clues on physical examination. However, gastrointestinal bleeding should not be automatically attributed to esophageal varices in a patient with jaundice, ascites, splenomegaly, spider angiomas, or hepatomegaly; over half of cirrhotic patients who present with acute hemorrhage are bleeding from gastritis or peptic ulcer.

Table 24–2. Causes of massive upper gastro-intestinal hemorrhage. Note that cancer is rarely the cause.

	Relative Incidence	
Common causes		45%
Peptic ulcer		
Duodenal ulcer	25%	
Gastric ulcer	20%	
Esophageal varices		20%
Gastritis		20%
Mallory-Weiss syndrome		10%
Uncommon causes		5%
Gastric carcinoma		
Esophagitis		
Pancreatitis		
Hemobilia		
Duodenal diverticulum		

Blood should be drawn for cross-matching, hematocrit, hemoglobin, creatinine, and tests of liver function. An intravenous infusion should be started and, in the massive bleeder, a large-bore nasogastric tube inserted. In cases of melena, the gastric aspirate should be examined to verify the gastroduodenal source of the hemorrhage, but about 25% of patients with bleeding duodenal ulcers have gastric aspirates that test negatively for blood. The tube must be larger than the standard nasogastric tube (16F) so the stomach can be lavaged free of liquid blood and clots. After its contents have been removed, the stomach should be irrigated with copious amounts of ice water or saline solution until blood no longer returns. If the patient was bleeding at the time the nasogastric tube was inserted, iced saline irrigation usually stops it. The large tube can then be exchanged for a standard nasogastric tube attached to continuous suction so further blood loss can be measured.

It is common to give H_2 receptor antagonists or omeprazole, though controlled trials have shown no benefit. If bleeding continues or if tachycardia or hypotension is present, the patient should be monitored and treated as for hemorrhagic shock.

In acute rapid hemorrhage, the hematocrit may be normal or only slightly low. A very low hematocrit without obvious signs of shock indicates more gradual blood loss.

All of the above tests and procedures can be performed within 1 or 2 hours after admission. By this time, in most instances, bleeding is under control, blood volume has been restored to normal, and the patient is being adequately monitored so that recurrent bleeding can be detected promptly. When this stage is reached, additional diagnostic tests should be performed.

Diagnosis of Cause of Bleeding

Once the patient is stabilized, endoscopy should be the first study. In general, endoscopy should be performed within 24 hours after admission, and under these circumstances the source of bleeding can be demonstrated in about 80% of cases. Longer delays will give a lower diagnostic yield. Two lesions are seen in about 15% of patients. An upper gastrointestinal series should be performed if endoscopy is equivocal or unavailable. Although the diagnostic information provided by endoscopy does not appear to have resulted in decreased blood loss or improved outcome, endoscopic therapy, in the form of sclerosis of varices or injection of a bleeding ulcer, may do so. Having the diagnosis will also help in planning subsequent treatment, including the surgical approach if surgery becomes necessary.

Rarely, selective angiography will have diagnostic or therapeutic usefulness. For diagnosis, it is most helpful when other studies fail to demonstrate the cause of bleeding. Infusion through the angiographic catheter of vasoconstrictors (eg, vasopressin) and embolization of the bleeding vessel with Gelfoam may be able to halt the bleeding in special cases.

Later Management

Although a precise diagnosis of the cause of the bleeding may be valuable in later management, the patient must not be allowed to slip out of clinical control during the search for definitive diagnostic information. *The decision for emergency surgery depends more on the rate and duration of bleeding than on its specific cause.*

The need for transfusion should be determined on a continuing basis, and blood volume must be maintained. Blood pressure, pulse, central venous pressure, hematocrit, hourly urinary volume, and amount of blood obtained from the gastric tube or from the rectum all enter into this assessment. Many studies have shown the tendency to underestimate blood loss and inadequately transfuse massively bleeding patients who truly need aggressive therapy. Continued slow bleeding is best monitored by serial determinations of the hematocrit.

The following criteria define patients with a very low risk of serious bleeding: age less than 75 years, no unstable comorbid illness, no ascites evident on physical examination, normal prothrombin time, and, within 1 hour after admission, a systolic blood pressure above 100 mm Hg and nasogastric aspirate free of fresh blood. Patients with all six of these findings may be spared emergency endoscopy and discharged from the hospital early to undergo outpatient workup.

Several factors are associated with a worse prognosis with continued medical management of the bleeding episode. These are not absolute indications for laparotomy, but they should alert the clinician that emergency surgery may be required.

High rates of bleeding or amounts of blood loss predict high failure rates with medical treatment. Hematemesis is usually associated with more rapid bleeding and a greater blood volume deficit than melena. The presence of hypotension on admission to the hospital or the need for more than four units of blood to achieve circulatory stability implies a worse prognosis; if bleeding continues and subsequent transfusion requirements exceed 1 unit every 8 hours, continued medical management is usually unwise. The level of serum fibrin degradation products, indicating endogenous fibrinolysis, correlates with the severity of hemorrhage and the death rate. This may be a useful prognostic test, and the results could be used as a guide for the administration of fibrinolytic inhibitors in therapy. Evidence for or against this view is not yet available.

Total transfusion requirements also correlate with death rates. Death is uncommon when fewer than seven units of blood have been used, and the death rate rises progressively thereafter.

In general, bleeding from a gastric ulcer is more dangerous than bleeding from gastritis or duodenal ulcer, and patients with gastric ulcer should always be considered for early surgery. Regardless of the cause, if bleeding recurs after it has once stopped, the chances of success without operation are low. Most patients who rebleed in the hospital should have surgery.

Patients over age 60 tolerate continued blood loss less well than younger patients, and their bleeding should be stopped before secondary cardiovascular, pulmonary, or renal complications arise.

In 85% of patients, bleeding stops within a few hours of admission. About 25% of patients rebleed once bleeding has stopped. Rebleeding episodes are concentrated within the first 2 days of hospitalization, and if the patient has had no further bleeding for a period of 5 days, the chance of rebleeding is only 2%. Rebleeding is most common in patients with varices, peptic ulcer, anemia, or shock. About 10% of patients require surgery to control bleeding, and most of these patients have bleeding ulcers or, less commonly, esophageal varices. The death rate is 30% among patients who rebled and 3% among those who do not. The mortality rate is also high in the elderly and in patients who are already hospitalized at the onset of bleeding. Analyses of large series of patients suggest that a number of those who died would not have done so if operations had been performed earlier and more often.

Dallal HJ, Palmer KR: ABC of the upper gastrointestinal tract: upper gastrointestinal haemorrhage. BMJ 2001;323:1115.

Palmer KR: Intravenous omeprazole after endoscopic treatment of bleeding peptic ulcers. Gut 2001;49:610.

Peterson WL, Cook DJ: Antisecretory therapy for bleeding peptic ulcer. JAMA 1998;280:877.

Spiegel BM, Vakil NB, Ofman JJ: Endoscopy for acute nonvariceal upper gastrointestinal tract hemorrhage: is sooner better? A systematic review. Arch Intern Med 2001;161:1393.

Van Dam J, Brugge KR: Endoscopy of the upper gastrointestinal tract. N Engl J Med 1999;341:1738.

HEMORRHAGE FROM PEPTIC ULCER

Approximately 20% of patients with peptic ulcer will experience a bleeding episode, and this complication is responsible for about 40% of the deaths from peptic ulcer. Peptic ulcer is the most common cause of massive upper gastrointestinal hemorrhage, accounting for over half of all cases. Chronic gastric and duodenal ulcers have about the same tendency to bleed, but the former produce more severe episodes. Bleeding ulcers are more common in persons with blood group O, though the reason for this association is not known.

Bleeding ulcers in the duodenum are usually located on the posterior surface of the duodenal bulb. As the ulcer penetrates, the gastroduodenal artery is exposed and may become eroded. Since no major blood vessels lie on the anterior surface of the duodenal bulb, ulcerations at this point are not as prone to bleed. Patients with concomitant bleeding and perforation usually have two ulcers, a bleeding posterior ulcer and a perforated anterior one. Postbulbar ulcers (those in the second portion of the duodenum) bleed frequently, though ulcers are much less common in this site than near the pylorus.

In some patients, the bleeding is sudden and massive, manifested by hematemesis and shock. In others, chronic anemia and weakness due to slow blood loss are the only findings. The diagnosis is unreliable when based on clinical findings, so endoscopy should be performed early (ie, within 24 hours) in most cases.

In the preceding section, the management of acute upper gastrointestinal hemorrhage, the selection of diagnostic tests, and the factors suggesting the need for operation were discussed. Most patients (75%) with bleeding peptic ulcer can be successfully managed by medical means alone. Initial therapeutic efforts usually halt the bleeding. H_2 blockers and proton pump inhibitors decrease the risk of bleeding but have no effect on active bleeding.

After 12–24 hours have passed and the bleeding has clearly stopped, a patient who feels hungry should be fed. Twice-daily hematocrit readings should be ordered as a check on slow continued blood loss. Stools should be tested daily for the presence of blood; they will usually remain guaiac-positive for several days after bleeding stops.

Rebleeding in the hospital has been attended by a death rate of about 30%. A policy of early surgery for those who rebleed would improve this figure. Patients who are over age 60, present with hematemesis, are actively bleeding at the time of endoscopy, or whose admission hemoglobin is below 8 g/dL have a higher risk of rebleeding. About three times as many patients with gastric ulcer (30%) rebleed compared with those with duodenal ulcer. Most instances of rebleeding occur within 2 days from the time the first episode has stopped. In one study, only 3% of patients who stopped bleeding for this long bled again.

Endoscopic Therapy

Treatments administered through the endoscope may stop active bleeding or prevent rebleeding. Effective methods include injection into the ulcer of epinephrine, epinephrine plus 1% polidocanol (a sclerosing agent), or ethanol; or cautery using the heater probe, monopolar electrocautery, or the Nd:YAG laser. At least two modalities should be available to the endoscopist in the event one is unsuitable for a specific case or fails to work. Except for the laser, all are inexpensive. The indications for treatment are (1) active bleeding at the time of endoscopy and (2) the presence of a visible vessel in the base of the ulcer. Endoscopic therapy decreases transfusion requirements (by about half) and the rate of rebleeding (by about three-quarters) compared with sham-treated controls. When treatment fails the first time, it may often be repeated with a good chance of success. It is important, however, not to allow the patient to deteriorate during nonoperative attempts at halting the bleeding.

Emergency Surgery

Less than 10% of patients bleeding from a peptic ulcer require emergency surgery. Selection of those most likely to survive with surgical compared with medical treatment rests on the rate of blood loss and the other factors associated with a poor prognosis.

The overall death rate is significantly less after vagotomy and pyloroplasty than after gastrectomy for bleeding ulcer, and rebleeding occurs with about equal frequency after either procedure.

During laparotomy, the first step is to make a pyloroplasty incision if the endoscopic diagnosis is a bleeding duodenal ulcer. If a duodenal ulcer is found, the bleeding vessel should be suture-ligated and the duodenum and antrum inspected for additional ulcers. The pyloroplasty incision should then be closed and a truncal vagotomy performed. If the posterior wall of the duodenal bulb has been destroyed by a giant duodenal ulcer, a gastrectomy and Billroth II gastrojejunostomy may be preferable, since this somewhat uncommon ulcer is especially prone to bleed again if left in continuity with the stomach. Gastric ulcers can be handled by either gastrectomy or vagotomy and pyloroplasty. A thorough search should always be made for second ulcers or other causes of bleeding.

Prognosis

The death rate for an acute massive hemorrhage is about 15%. Careful study of the causes of death suggests that this figure could be improved by (1) more precise blood replacement—since undertransfusion is the cause of some complications and deaths; and (2) earlier surgery in selected patients who fall into serious-risk categories—since the tendency has been to perform surgery on too few patients too late in the illness. Patients who stop bleeding should be treated as outlined in the section on duodenal ulcer.

Rockall TA: Management and outcome of patients undergoing surgery after acute upper gastrointestinal haemorrhage. Steering Group for the National Audit of Acute Upper Gastrointestinal Haemorrhage. J R Soc Med 1998;91:518.

MALLORY-WEISS SYNDROME

Mallory-Weiss syndrome is responsible for about 10% of cases of acute upper gastrointestinal hemorrhage. The lesion consists of a 1- to 4-cm longitudinal tear in the gastric mucosa near the esophagogastric junction; it usually follows a bout of forceful retching. The disruption extends through the mucosa and submucosa but not usually into the muscularis mucosae. About 75% of these lesions are confined to the stomach; 20% straddle the esophagogastric junction; and 5% are entirely within the distal esophagus. Two-thirds of patients have a hiatal hernia.

The majority of patients are alcoholics, but the tear may appear after severe retching for any reason. Several cases have been reported following closed chest cardiac compression.

Clinical Findings

Typically, the patient first vomits food and gastric contents. This is followed by forceful retching and then bloody vomitus. Rapid increases in gastric pressure, sometimes aggravated by hiatal hernia, cause the tear. Actual rupture of the distal esophagus can also be produced by vomiting (Boerhaave's syndrome), but the difference seems to depend on vomiting of food in rupture and nonproductive retching in gastric mucosal tear.

Esophagogastroscopy is the most practical means of making the diagnosis.

Treatment & Prognosis

Initially, the patient is handled according to the general measures prescribed for upper gastrointestinal hemorrhage. In about 90% of patients, the bleeding stops spontaneously after ice-water lavage of the stomach. Patients who are still bleeding vigorously by the time endoscopy is performed are likely to require surgery. The bleeding can sometimes be controlled by endoscopic therapy (eg, electrocautery). If bleeding persists, surgical repair of the tear will be required.

If the diagnosis has been made before laparotomy, the surgeon should make a long, high gastrotomy after the abdomen is opened. The tear may be difficult to expose adequately. The search must be thorough, since in about 25% of patients there are two tears. A running polyglycolic acid (not catgut) suture should be used to oversew the lesion. Postoperative recurrence is rare.

Kortas DY: Mallory-Weiss tear: predisposing factors and predictors of a complicated course. Am J Gastroenterol 2001;96:2863.

Younes Z, Johnson DA: The spectrum of spontaneous and iatrogenic esophageal injury: perforations, Mallory-Weiss tears, and hematomas. J Clin Gastroenterol 1999;29:306.

PYLORIC OBSTRUCTION DUE TO PEPTIC ULCER

The cycles of inflammation and repair in peptic ulcer disease may cause obstruction of the gastroduodenal junction as a result of edema, muscular spasm, and scarring. To the extent that the first two factors are involved, the obstruction may be reversible with medical treatment. Obstruction is usually due to duodenal ulcer and is less common than either bleeding or perforation. The few gastric ulcers that obstruct are close to the pylorus. Obstruction due to peptic ulcer must be differentiated from that caused by a malignant tumor of the antrum or of the pancreas. Malignancy is becoming the more common cause, and it may be difficult to identify.

Clinical Findings

A. SYMPTOMS AND SIGNS

Most patients with obstruction have a long history of symptomatic peptic ulcer, and as many as 30% have been treated for perforation or obstruction in the past. The patient often notes gradually increasing ulcer pains over weeks or months, with the eventual development of anorexia, vomiting, and failure to gain relief from antacids. The vomitus often contains food ingested several hours previously, and absence of bile staining reflects the site of blockage. Weight loss may be marked if the patient has delayed seeking medical care.

Dehydration and malnutrition may be obvious on physical examination but are not always present. A succussion splash can often be elicited from the retained gastric contents. Peristalsis of the distended stomach may be visible on gross inspection of the abdomen, but this sign is relatively rare. Most patients have upper abdominal tenderness. Tetany may appear with advanced alkalosis.

B. LABORATORY FINDINGS

Anemia is found in about 25% of patients. Prolonged vomiting leads to a unique form of metabolic alkalosis with dehydration. Measurement of serum electrolytes shows hypochloremia, hypokalemia, hyponatremia, and increased bicarbonate. Vomiting depletes the patient of Na^+, K^+, and Cl^-; the latter is lost in excess of Na^+ and K^+ as HCl. Gastric HCl loss causes extracellular HCO_3^- to rise, and renal excretion of HCO_3^- increases in an attempt to maintain pH. Large amounts of Na^+ are excreted in the urine with the HCO_3^-. Increasing Na^+ deficit evokes aldosterone secretion, which in turn brings about renal Na^+ conservation at the expense of more renal loss of K^+ and H^+. GFR may drop and produce a prerenal azotemia. The eventual result of the process is a marked deficit of Na^+, Cl^-, K^+, and H_2O. Treatment involves replacement of water and NaCl until a satisfactory urine flow has been established. KCl replacement should then be started. Details of management are found in Chapter 9.

C. SALINE LOAD TEST

This is a simple means of assessing the degree of pyloric obstruction and is useful in following the patient's progress during the first few days of nasogastric suction.

Through the nasogastric tube, 700 mL of normal saline (at room temperature) is infused over 3–5 minutes, and the tube is clamped. Thirty minutes later, the stomach is aspirated and the residual volume of saline recorded. Recovery of more than 350 mL indicates obstruction. It must be recognized that the results of a saline load test do not predict how well the stomach will handle solid food. Solid emptying can be measured with technetium Tc 99m-labeled chicken liver.

D. IMAGING STUDIES

Plain abdominal x-rays may show a large gastric fluid level. An upper gastrointestinal series should not be performed until the stomach has been emptied, because dilution of the barium in the retained secretions makes a worthwhile study impossible.

E. ENDOSCOPY

Gastroscopy is usually indicated to rule out the presence of an obstructing neoplasm.

Treatment

A. MEDICAL TREATMENT

A large (32F) Ewald tube should be passed and the stomach emptied of its contents and lavaged until clean. After the stomach has been completely decompressed, a smaller tube should be inserted and placed on suction for several days to allow pyloric edema and spasm to subside and to permit the gastric musculature to regain its tone. A saline load test may be performed at this point to provide a baseline for later comparison. If chronic obstruction has produced severe malnutrition, total parenteral nutrition should be instituted.

After decompression of the stomach for 48–72 hours, the saline load test should be repeated. If this indicates sufficient improvement, the tube should be withdrawn and a liquid diet may be started. Gradual resumption of solid foods is permitted as tolerated.

B. SURGICAL TREATMENT

If 5–7 days of gastric aspiration do not result in relief of the obstruction, the patient should be treated surgically. Persistence of nonoperative effort beyond this point in the absence of progress rarely achieves the result hoped for. Failure of the obstruction to resolve completely (eg, if the patient can take only liquids) and recurrent obstruction of any degree are indications for surgery.

Surgical treatment may consist of a truncal or parietal cell vagotomy and drainage procedure (Figure 24–5). Truncal vagotomy and gastrojejunostomy is the easiest to perform laparoscopically.

Prognosis

About two-thirds of patients with acute obstruction fail to improve sufficiently on medical therapy and require operation to relieve the blockage. Patients who respond to medical treatment should be treated as outlined in the section on duodenal ulcer.

Jamieson GG: Current status of indications for surgery in peptic ulcer disease. World J Surg 2000;24:256.

PERFORATED PEPTIC ULCER

Perforation complicates peptic ulcer about half as often as hemorrhage. Most perforated ulcers are located anteriorly, though occasionally gastric ulcers perforate into the lesser sac. The 15% death rate correlates with increased age, female sex, and gastric perforations. The diagnosis is overlooked in about 5% of patients, most of whom do not survive.

Anterior ulcers tend to perforate instead of bleed because of the absence of protective viscera and major blood vessels on this surface. In less than 10% of cases, acute bleeding from a posterior "kissing" ulcer complicates the anterior perforation, an association that carries a high death rate. Immediately after perforation, the peritoneal cavity is flooded with gastroduodenal secretions that elicit a chemical peritonitis. Early cultures show either no growth or a light growth of streptococci or enteric bacilli. Gradually, over 12–24 hours, the process evolves into bacterial peritonitis. Severity of illness and occurrence of death are directly related to the interval between perforation and surgical closure.

In an unknown percentage of cases, the perforation becomes sealed by adherence to the undersurface of the liver. In such patients, the process may be self-limited, but a subphrenic abscess will develop in many.

Clinical Findings

A. SYMPTOMS AND SIGNS

The perforation usually elicits a sudden, severe upper abdominal pain whose onset can be recalled precisely. The patient may or may not have had preceding chronic symptoms of peptic ulcer disease. Perforation rarely is heralded by nausea or vomiting, and it typically occurs several hours after the last meal. Shoulder pain, if present, reflects diaphragmatic irritation. Back pain is uncommon.

The initial reaction consists of a chemical peritonitis caused by gastric acid or bile and pancreatic enzymes. The peritoneal reaction dilutes these irritants with a thin exudate, and as a result the patient's symptoms may temporarily improve before bacterial peritonitis occurs. The physician who sees the patient for the first time during this symptomatic lull must not be misled into interpreting it as representing bona fide improvement.

The patient appears severely distressed, lying quietly with the knees drawn up and breathing shallowly to minimize abdominal motion. Fever is absent at the start. The abdominal muscles are rigid owing to severe involuntary spasm. Epigastric tenderness may not be as marked as expected because the board-like rigidity protects the abdominal viscera from the palpating hand. Escaped air from the stomach may enter the space between the liver and abdominal wall, and upon percussion the normal dullness over the liver will be tympanitic. Peristaltic sounds are reduced or absent. If delay in treatment allows continued escape of air into the peritoneal cavity, abdominal distention and diffuse tympany may result.

The above description applies to the typical case of perforation with classic findings. In as many as one-third of patients, the presentation is not as dramatic, diagnosis is less obvious, and serious delays in treatment may result from failure to consider this condition and to obtain the appropriate abdominal x-rays. Many of these atypical perforations occur in patients already hospitalized for some unrelated illness, and the significance of the new symptom of abdominal pain is not appreciated. The only way to improve this record is to routinely obtain abdominal films on patients with abdominal pain of recent onset.

Lesser degrees of shock with minimal abdominal findings occur if the leak is small or rapidly sealed. A small duodenal perforation may slowly leak fluid that runs down the lateral peritoneal gutter, producing pain and muscular rigidity in the right lower quadrant and thus raising a problem of confusion with acute appendicitis.

Perforations may be sealed by omentum or by the liver, with the later development of a subhepatic or subdiaphragmatic abscess.

B. Laboratory Findings

A mild leukocytosis in the range of 12,000/μL is common in the early stages. After 12–24 hours, this may rise to 20,000/μL or more if treatment has been inadequate. The mild rise in the serum amylase value that occurs in many patients is probably caused by absorption of the enzyme from duodenal secretions within the peritoneal cavity. Direct measurement of fluid obtained by paracentesis may show very high levels of amylase.

C. Imaging Studies

Plain x-rays of the abdomen reveal free subdiaphragmatic air in 85% of patients. Films should be taken with the patient both supine and upright. A film in the left lateral decubitus position may be a more practical way to demonstrate free air in the uncomfortable patient. If the findings are questionable, 400 mL of air can be insufflated into the stomach through a nasogastric tube and the films repeated. Free air in the abdomen in a patient with sudden upper abdominal pain should clinch the diagnosis.

If no free air is demonstrated and the clinical picture suggests perforated ulcer, an emergency upper gastrointestinal series should be performed. If the perforation has not sealed, the diagnosis is established by noting escape of the contrast material from the lumen. Barium is more reliable than water-soluble contrast media, and, contrary to previous views, does not appear to aggravate infection or to be difficult to remove.

Differential Diagnosis

The differential diagnosis includes acute pancreatitis and acute cholecystitis. The former does not have as explosive an onset as perforated ulcer and is usually accompanied by a high serum amylase level. Acute cholecystitis with perforated gallbladder could mimic perforated ulcer closely but free air would not be present with ruptured gallbladder. Intestinal obstruction has a more gradual onset and is characterized by less sever pain that is crampy and accompanied by vomiting.

The simultaneous onset of pain and free air in the abdomen in the absence of trauma usually means perforated peptic ulcer. Free perforation of colonic diverticulitis and acute appendicitis are other rare causes.

Treatment

The diagnosis is often suspected before the patient is sent for confirmatory x-rays. Whenever a perforated ulcer is considered, the first step should be to pass a nasogastric tube and empty the stomach to reduce further contamination of the peritoneal cavity. Blood should be drawn for laboratory studies, and intravenous antibiotics (eg, cefazolin, cefoxitin) should be started. If the patient's overall condition is precarious owing to delay in treatment, fluid resuscitation should precede diagnostic measures. X-rays should be obtained as soon as the clinical status will permit.

The simplest surgical treatment, laparoscopy (or laparotomy) and suture closure of the perforation solves the immediate problem. The closure most often consists of securely plugging the hole with omentum (Graham-Steele closure) sutured into place rather than bringing together the two edges with sutures. All fluid should be aspirated from the peritoneal cavity, but drainage is not indicated. Reperforation is rare in the immediate postoperative period.

About three-fourths of patients whose perforation is the culmination of a history of chronic symptoms continue to have clinically severe ulcer disease after simple closure. This has gradually led to a more aggressive treatment policy involving a definitive ulcer operation for most patients with acute perforation, eg, parietal cell vagotomy plus closure of the perforation or truncal vagotomy and pyloroplasty. Now that ulcer disease can be cured by eradicating *H pylori*, the value of anything more than simple closure will have to be reexamined.

Concomitant hemorrhage and perforation are most often due to two ulcers, an anterior perforated one and a posterior one that is bleeding. Perforated ulcers that also obstruct obviously cannot be treated by suture closure of the perforation alone. Vagotomy plus gastroenterostomy or pyloroplasty should be performed. Perforated anastomotic ulcers require a vagotomy or gastrectomy, since in the long run, closure alone is nearly always inadequate.

Nonoperative treatment of perforated ulcer consists of continuous gastric suction and the administration of antibiotics in high doses. Although this has been shown to be effective therapy, with a low death rate, it is occasionally accompanied by a peritoneal and subphrenic abscess, and side effects are greater than with laparoscopic closure.

Prognosis

About 15% of patients with perforated ulcer die, and about a third of these are undiagnosed before surgery. The death rate of perforated ulcer seen early is low. Delay in treatment, advanced age, and associated systemic diseases account for most deaths.

Donovan AJ, Berne TV, Donovan JA: Perforated duodenal ulcer: an alternative therapeutic plan. Arch Surg 1998;133:1166.

Hernandez-Diaz S, Rodriguez LA: Association between non-steroidal anti-inflammatory drugs and upper gastrointestinal tract bleeding/perforation: an overview of epidemiologic studies published in the 1990s. Arch Intern Med 2000;160:2093.

Memon MA, Fitzgibbons RJ Jr: The role of minimal access surgery in the acute abdomen. Surg Clin North Am 1997;77:1333.

Millat B, Fingerhut A, Borie F: Surgical treatment of complicated duodenal ulcers: controlled trials. World J Surg 2000;24:299.

Svanes C: Trends in perforated peptic ulcer: incidence, etiology, treatment, and prognosis. World J Surg 2000;24:277.

STRESS GASTRODUODENITIS, STRESS ULCER & ACUTE HEMORRHAGIC GASTRITIS

The term stress ulcer has been used to refer to a heterogeneous group of acute gastric or duodenal ulcers that develop following physiologically stressful illnesses. There are four major etiologic factors associated with such lesions: (1) shock, (2) sepsis, (3) burns, and (4) central nervous system tumors or trauma.

Etiology

A. STRESS ULCER

Acute ulcers following major surgery, mechanical ventilation, shock, sepsis, and burns (Curling's ulcers) have enough common features to suggest they evolve by a similar pathogenetic mechanism

Hemorrhage is the major clinical problem, though perforation occurs in about 10% of cases. Despite the predilection of stress ulcers to develop in the parietal cell mucosa, in about 30% of patients the duodenum is affected, and sometimes both stomach and duodenum are involved. Morphologically, the ulcers are shallow, discrete lesions with congestion and edema but little inflammatory reaction at their margins. Gastroduodenal endoscopy performed early in traumatized or burned patients has shown acute gastric erosions in the majority of patients within 72 hours after the injury (Figures 24–7 and 24–8). Such studies illustrate how frequently the disease process remains subclinical; clinically appar-

Figure 24–7. Scanning electron photomicrograph of the surface epithelium of a normal subject showing individual cells and numerous gastric pits. (Reduced from × 350.) (Courtesy of Jeanne M. Riddle.)

ent ulcers develop in about 20% of susceptible patients. Clinically evident bleeding is usually seen 3–5 days after the injury, and massive bleeding generally does not appear until 4–5 days later.

Decreased mucosal resistance is the first step, which may involve the effects of ischemia (with production of toxic superoxide and hydroxyl radicals) and circulating toxins, followed by decreased mucosal renewal, decreased production of endogenous prostanoids, and thinning of the surface mucus layer. Decreased gastric mucosal blood flow also plays a role by decreasing the

Figure 24–8. Scanning electron photomicrograph of the surface epithelium of a patient with acute gastric mucosal erosions, showing a patch of cellular defoliation. Lesions such as this may account for back diffusion of H⁺. (Reduced from × 1145.) (Courtesy of Jeanne M. Riddle.)

supply of blood buffers available to neutralize hydrogen ions that are diffusing into the weakened mucosa. Experimental evidence has implicated platelet-activating factor, released by endotoxin, as a possible mediator of gut ulceration in sepsis. The mucosa is thus rendered more vulnerable to acid-pepsin ulceration and lysosomal enzymes. Acid hypersecretion may be involved to some extent, since burn patients who manifest serious bleeding have higher gastric acid output than patients with a more benign course. Disruption of the gastric mucosal barrier to back diffusion of acid has been found in less than half of patients and is now thought to be a manifestation of the disease rather than a cause.

B. CUSHING'S ULCERS

Acute ulcers associated with central nervous system tumors or injuries differ from stress ulcers because they are associated with elevated levels of serum gastrin and increased gastric acid secretion. Morphologically, they are similar to ordinary gastroduodenal peptic ulcers. Cushing's ulcers are more prone to perforate than other kinds of stress ulcers.

C. ACUTE HEMORRHAGIC GASTRITIS

This disorder may share some causative factors with the above conditions, but the natural history is different and the response to treatment considerably better. Most of these patients can be controlled medically. When surgery is required for alcoholic gastritis, a high proportion of patients are cured by pyloroplasty and vagotomy.

Clinical Findings

Hemorrhage is nearly always the first manifestation. Pain rarely occurs. Physical examination is not contributory except to reveal gross or occult fecal blood or signs of shock.

Prevention

H_2 receptor antagonists given prophylactically to critically ill patients decrease the incidence of stress erosions and overt bleeding. The drug may be given orally (eg, ranitidine, 150 mg through a nasogastric tube every 12 hours) or intravenously (eg, cimetidine, 50–100 mg/h). Sucralfate is also effective. Patients receiving total parenteral nutrition appear to be protected by this therapy and experience no increased benefit from H_2 antagonists. A concern that decreasing gastric acidity with H_2 blocking agents would increase the rate and severity of nosocomial pneumonia (from gastric bacterial overgrowth) has not been justified by experience.

Treatment

Initial management should consist of gastric lavage with chilled solutions and measures to combat sepsis if present. H_2 receptor blockers are of no value in the actively bleeding patient, but they probably decrease the rate of rebleeding once bleeding has stopped.

Some success has been reported with the selective infusion of vasoconstricting agents (eg, vasopressin) into the left gastric artery through a percutaneously placed catheter. In the sickest patients, if facilities and trained personnel are available, this technique should probably be attempted before operation is considered.

Perform laparotomy if the nonoperative regimen fails to halt the bleeding. Surgical treatment should consist of vagotomy and pyloroplasty, with suture of the bleeding points, or vagotomy and subtotal gastrectomy. There is a trend toward the first of these options, particularly in the sickest patients. When it occurs, rebleeding is nearly always from an ulcer left behind at the initial procedure. Rarely, total gastrectomy has had to be used because of the extent of ulceration and severity of bleeding or because of rebleeding after a lesser operation.

Felig DM, Carafa CJ: Stress ulcers of the stomach. Gastrointest Endosc 2000;51:596.

Phillips JO et al: A randomized, pharmacokinetic and pharmacodynamic, cross-over study of duodenal or jejunal administration compared to nasogastric administration of omeprazole suspension in patients at risk for stress ulcers. Am J Gastroenterol 2001;96:367.

GASTRIC CARCINOMA

There are about 20,000 new cases of carcinoma of the stomach in the USA annually. The incidence has dropped to one-third of what it was 30 years ago. This may reflect changes in the prevalence of *H pylori* infection, which has a role in the etiology of this disease. *H pylori* is known to be a cause of chronic atrophic gastritis, which in turn is a recognized precursor of gastric adenocarcinoma. Epidemiologic studies have linked gastric *H pylori* infection with a 3.6- to 18-fold (all patients versus women) increase in the risk of developing carcinoma of the body or antrum (not the cardia), and the risk is proportionate to serum levels of *H pylori* antibodies.

The present incidence in American males is ten new cases per 100,000 population per year. The highest rate, 63 per 100,000 males, is seen in Costa Rica; in eastern and central European countries, it is about 35 per 100,000 per year. Epidemiologic studies suggest that the incidence of gastric carcinoma is related to low dietary intake of vegetables and fruits and high intake of starches. Carcinoma of the stomach is rare under age

40, from which point the risk gradually climbs. The mean age at discovery is 63. It is about twice as common in men as in women.

Gastric epithelial cancers are nearly always adenocarcinomas. Squamous cell tumors of the proximal stomach involve the stomach secondarily from the esophagus. Five morphologic subdivisions correlate loosely with the natural history and outcome.

1. Ulcerating carcinoma (25%)—This consists of a deep, penetrating ulcer-tumor that extends through all layers of the stomach. It may involve adjacent organs in the process. The edges are shallow by contrast with overhanging edges noted in benign ulcers.

2. Polypoid carcinomas (25%)—These are large, bulky intraluminal growths that tend to metastasize late.

3. Superficial spreading carcinoma (15%)—Also known as early gastric cancer, superficial spreading carcinoma is confined to the mucosa and submucosa. Metastases are present in only 30% of cases. Even when metastases are present, the prognosis after gastrectomy is much better than for the more deeply invading lesions of advanced gastric cancer. In Japan, screening programs have been so successful that early gastric cancer now constitutes 30% of surgical cases, and survival rates have improved accordingly.

4. Linitis plastica (10%)—This variety of spreading tumor involves all layers with a marked desmoplastic reaction in which it may be difficult to identify the malignant cells. The stomach loses its pliability. Cure is rare because of early spread.

5. Advanced carcinoma (35%)—This largest category contains the big tumors that are found partly within and partly outside the stomach. They may originally have qualified for inclusion in the preceding groups but have outgrown that early stage.

Gastric adenocarcinomas can also be classified by degree of differentiation of their cells. In general, rate and extent of spread correlate with lack of differentiation. Some tumors are found histologically to excite an inflammatory cell reaction at their borders, and this feature indicates a relatively good prognosis. Tumors whose cells form glandular structures (intestinal type) have a somewhat better prognosis than tumors whose cells do not (diffuse type); the diffuse type is often associated with a substantial stromal component. The intestinal type of tumor accounts for a much larger proportion of cases in countries such as Japan and Finland where gastric cancer is especially common. The gradual decline in incidence in these areas is due principally to decreased occurrence of the intestinal type of tumor. Signet ring carcinomas, which contain more than 50% signet ring cells, have become increasingly more common and now constitute one-third of all cases. They behave as the diffuse type of cancer and occur more frequently in women, in younger patients, and in the distal part of the stomach. Previous *H pylori* infection is not associated with the development of any specific histologic type of gastric cancer.

Extension occurs by intramural spread, direct extraluminal growth, and lymphatic metastases. Pathologic staging, which correlates closely with survival, is illustrated in Figure 24–9. Three-fourths of patients have metastases when first seen. Within the stomach, proximal spread exceeds distal spread. The pylorus acts as a partial barrier, but tumor is found in 25% of cases in the first few centimeters of the bulb.

Early gastric cancer, defined as a primary lesion confined to the mucosa and submucosa with or without lymph node metastases, is associated with an excellent prognosis (5-year survival rate of 90%) after resection. In Japan, mass screening programs detect about 30% of patients with this lesion, whereas in the USA, only 10% of patients have early gastric cancer.

Forty percent of tumors are in the antrum, predominantly on the lesser curvature; 30% arise in the body and fundus, 25% at the cardia, and 5% involve the entire organ. Frequency of location has gradually changed, so that proximal lesions are more common now than 10–20 years ago. Benign ulcers develop at the greater curvature and cardia less commonly than malignant ones. Ulcers at these points are particularly suspect for neoplasm.

Clinical Findings

A. SYMPTOMS AND SIGNS

The earliest symptom is usually vague postprandial abdominal heaviness that the patient does not identify as a pain. Sometimes the discomfort is no different from other vague dyspeptic symptoms that have been intermittently present for years, but the frequency and persistence are new.

Anorexia develops early and may be most pronounced for meat. Weight loss, the most common symptom, averages about 6 kg. True postprandial pain suggesting a benign gastric ulcer is relatively uncommon, but if it is present one may be misled if subsequent x-rays show an ulcer. Vomiting may be present and becomes a major feature if pyloric obstruction occurs. It may have a coffee-ground appearance owing to bleeding by the tumor. Dysphagia may be the presenting symptom of lesions at the cardia.

An epigastric mass can be felt on examination in about one-fourth of cases. Hepatomegaly is present in 10% of cases. The stool will be positive for occult blood in half of patients, and melena is seen in a few. Otherwise, abnormal physical findings are confined to signs

STAGE   I   II   III   IV

Mucosa

Submucosa

Muscularis propria

Serosa

Positive lymph nodes

Positive lymph nodes plus distant metastases or involvement of contiguous structures

Figure 24–9. Staging system for gastric carcinoma. The darkly shadowed areas represent cancers with different depths of mucosal penetration

of distant spread of the tumor. Metastases to the neck along the thoracic duct may produce a Virchow node. Rectal examination may reveal a Blumer shelf, a solid peritoneal deposit anterior to the rectum. Enlarged ovaries (Krukenberg tumors) may be caused by intraperitoneal metastases. Further dissemination may involve the liver, lungs, brain, or bone.

B. LABORATORY FINDINGS

Anemia is present in 40% of patients. Carcinoembryonic antigen (CEA) levels are elevated in 65%, usually indicating extensive spread of the tumor.

C. IMAGING STUDIES

An upper gastrointestinal series is diagnostic for many tumors, but the overall false-negative rate is about 20%. Major diagnostic problems are posed by ulcerating tumors, a few of which may not be distinguishable radiologically from benign peptic ulcers. The differential features are listed in the section on gastric ulcer, but x-rays alone will not establish a diagnosis of benign ulcer. All patients with a newly discovered gastric ulcer should undergo gastroscopy and gastric biopsy.

D. GASTROSCOPY AND BIOPSY

Large gastric carcinomas can usually be identified as such by their gross appearance at endoscopy. All gastric lesions, whether polypoid or ulcerating, should be examined by taking multiple biopsy and brush cytology specimens during endoscopy. False results are seen occasionally as a result of sampling error, and a minimum of six biopsies is necessary for greatest accuracy.

Treatment

Surgical resection is the only curative treatment. About 85% of patients are operable, and in 50% the lesions are amenable to resection; of the resectable lesions, half are potentially curable (ie, no signs of spread beyond the limits of resection).

The surgical objective should be to remove the tumor, an adjacent uninvolved margin of stomach and duodenum, the regional lymph nodes, and, if necessary, portions of involved adjacent organs. The proximal margin should be a minimum of 6 cm from the gross tumor. If the tumor is located in the antrum, a curative resection would entail distal gastrectomy with en bloc removal of the omentum, a 3- to 4-cm cuff of duodenum and the subpyloric lymph nodes, and, in some instances, excision of the left gastric artery and nearby lymph nodes. Reconstruction after gastrectomy may be by either a Billroth I or II procedure, but the latter is preferable because postoperative growth of residual tumor near the pylorus may obstruct a gastroduodenal anastomosis early.

Total gastrectomy with splenectomy is required for tumors of the proximal half of the stomach and for extensive tumors (eg, linitis plastica). Whether or not the spleen should be removed in such cases is a subject of debate. Alimentary continuity is most often reestablished by a Roux-en-Y esophagojejunostomy. Construction of an intestinal pouch as a substitute food reservoir (eg, Hunt-Lawrence pouch) is of no nutritional value, and it increases the risks of immediate complications.

Esophagogastrectomy plus splenectomy with intrathoracic esophagogastrostomy is the operation usually performed for tumors of the cardia. The procedure is usually done through two separate incisions: first, a laparotomy for the gastric part, and then a right posterolateral thoracotomy for the anastomosis.

Japanese surgeons have devised a more detailed staging system than the one used in most other countries and have also recommended more aggressive lymphadenectomy as a matter of routine in the resection of gastric cancers. The results of resections as reported from Japan are better than those obtained by the standard operations described above, so attempts are being made to determine whether the difference is due to the more radical operations. Most Western surgeons are skeptical, and radical lymphadenectomy (eg, clearing all nodal levels up to and including the para-aortic nodes) is not recommended at present.

The propensity for proximal submucosal spread must be appreciated at surgery. It is often advisable to perform a frozen section at the proximal margin before constructing the anastomosis. If tumor is found, the gastrectomy should be extended.

Palliative resection is usually indicated if the stomach is still movable and life expectancy is estimated to be more than 1–2 months. Palliative gastrectomy is usually performed to remove an antral lesion and prevent obstruction, but in selected cases, total gastrectomy is appropriate palliative treatment if the operation can be done safely and the amount of extragastric tumor is minimal. Whenever technically feasible, palliative gastrectomy is preferable to palliative gastrojejunostomy.

Adjuvant chemotherapy after curative surgery has not been of value with the regimens tested to date. For advanced disease, doxorubicin or fluorouracil alone, each of which results in a 20% response rate, is as good as a combination of chemotherapeutic agents.

Prognosis

In the USA, the overall 5-year survival rate is about 12%. The 5-year survival rate for patients with early gastric cancer is about 90%. The 5-year survival rates in relation to the extent of spread are stage I, 70%; stage II, 30%; stage III, 10%; and stage IV, 0%.

Death from tumor may follow dissemination to other organs or may be the result of progressive gastric obstruction and malnutrition.

Ceelen WP et al: Hyperthermic intraperitoneal chemoperfusion in the treatment of locally advanced intra-abdominal cancer. Br J Surg 2000;87:1006.

De Vivo R et al: The role of chemotherapy in the management of gastric cancer. J Clin Gastroenterol 2000;30:364.

Gastric cancer and *Helicobacter pylori:* a combined analysis of 12 case control studies nested within prospective cohorts. Gut 2001;49:347.

Hardman MJ et al: Barrier formation in the human fetus is patterned. J Invest Dermatol 1999;113:1106.

Hulscher JB et al: Prospective analysis of the diagnostic yield of extended en bloc resection for adenocarcinoma of the oesophagus or gastric cardia. Br J Surg 2001;88:715.

Huntsman DG et al: Early gastric cancer in young, asymptomatic carriers of germ-line E-cadherin mutations. N Engl J Med 2001;344:1904.

Kalmar K et al: Comparison of quality of life and nutritional parameters after total gastrectomy and a new type of pouch construction with simple Roux-en-Y reconstruction: preliminary results of a prospective, randomized, controlled study. Dig Dis Sci 2001;46:1791.

Kelly S et al: A systematic review of the staging performance of endoscopic ultrasound in gastro-oesophageal carcinoma. Gut 2001;49:534.

Lee HK et al: Influence of the number of lymph nodes examined on staging of gastric cancer. Br J Surg 2001;88:1408.

Macdonald JS et al: Chemoradiotherapy after surgery compared with surgery alone for adenocarcinoma of the stomach or gastroesophageal junction. N Engl J Med 2001;345:725.

Yasuda K et al: Risk factors for complications following resection of large gastric cancer. Br J Surg 2001;88:873.

GASTRIC POLYPS

Gastric polyps are single or multiple benign tumors that occur predominantly in the elderly. Those located in the distal stomach are more apt to cause symptoms. Whenever gastric polyps are discovered, gastric cancer must be ruled out.

Gastric polyps can be classified histologically as hyperplastic, adenomatous, or inflammatory. Other polypoid lesions, such as leiomyomas and carcinoid tumors, are discussed elsewhere. Hyperplastic polyps, which constitute 80% of cases, consist of an overgrowth of normal epithelium; they are not true neoplasms and have no relationship to gastric cancer. About 30% of adenomatous polyps contain a focus of adenocarcinoma, and adenocarcinoma can be found elsewhere in the stomach in 20% of patients with a benign adenomatous polyp. The incidence of cancer in an adenomatous polyp rises with increasing size. Lesions with a stalk and those less than 2 cm in diameter are usually not malignant. About 10% of benign adenomatous polyps undergo malignant change during prolonged follow-up.

Anemia may develop from chronic blood loss or deficient iron absorption. Over 90% of patients are achlorhydric after maximal stimulation. Vitamin B_{12} absorption is deficient in 25%, although megaloblastic anemia is present in only a few. Exfoliative cytologic examination of specimens obtained by endoscopy and brush biopsy should be performed in all patients.

Excision with a snare through the endoscope can be performed safely for most polyps. Otherwise, laparotomy is indicated for polyps greater than 1 cm in diameter or when cancer is suspected. Single polyps may be excised through a gastrotomy and a frozen section performed. If the polyp is found to be carcinoma, an appropriate type of gastrectomy is indicated. Partial gastrectomy should be performed for multiple polyps in the distal stomach. If 10–20 polyps are distributed throughout the stomach, the antrum should be removed and the fundic polyps excised. Total gastrectomy may be required for symptomatic diffuse multiple polyposis.

These patients should be followed because they have an increased risk of late development of pernicious anemia or gastric cancer. Recurrent polyps are uncommon.

Abraham SC et al: Hyperplastic polyps of the stomach: associations with histologic patterns of gastritis and gastric atrophy. Am J Surg Pathol 2001;25:500.

Karheuser A et al: Familial adenomatous polyposis associated with multiple adrenal adenomas in a patient with a rare 3′ APC mutation. J Med Genet 1999;36:65.

Ohkusa T et al: Disappearance of hyperplastic polyps in the stomach after eradication of *Helicobacter pylori*. A randomized, clinical trial. Ann Intern Med 1998;129:712.

GASTRIC LYMPHOMA & PSEUDOLYMPHOMA

Lymphoma is the second most common primary cancer of the stomach but constitutes only 2% of the total number, 95% being adenocarcinomas. Almost all are non-Hodgkin's lymphomas and are generally classified as B cell mucosa-associated lymphoid tissue (MALT) lymphomas. They are further subclassified as low-grade or high-grade based on nuclear pattern. About 20% of patients manifest a second primary cancer in another organ.

The principal symptoms are epigastric pain and weight loss, similar to those of carcinoma. Characteristically, the tumor has attained bulky proportions by the time it is discovered; by comparison with adenocarcinoma of the stomach, the symptoms from a gastric lymphoma are usually mild in relation to the size of the lesion. A palpable epigastric mass is present in 50% of patients. Barium x-ray studies will demonstrate the lesion, although it usually is mistaken for adenocarcinoma or, in 10% of cases, for benign gastric ulcer. Gastroscopy with biopsy and brush cytology provides the correct diagnosis preoperatively in about 75% of cases. If a pathologic diagnosis has not been made, the surgeon may incorrectly judge the lesion to be inoperable carcinoma because of its large size. Preoperative staging should include a CT scan and bone marrow biopsy.

Treatment of low-grade gastric lymphoma consists of long-term chemotherapy with cyclophosphamide. Surgical resection followed by total abdominal radiotherapy may be the treatment of choice for high-grade lymphomas, but the subject is debated. Intraoperative staging should consist of needle biopsies of both lobes of the liver and biopsies of celiac and para-aortic lymph nodes. Splenectomy should be performed only if the spleen is directly invaded. Extension into the duodenum or esophagus should not lead to resection of these organs but to postoperative adjunctive therapy. The 5-year disease-free survival rate is 50%. Survival correlates with stage of disease, extent of penetration of the gastric wall, and histologic grade of the tumor. Most recurrences appear within 2 years of surgery. Because two-thirds of recurrences are outside the abdomen, patients at high risk of recurrence should receive postoperative chemotherapy also.

Gastric pseudolymphoma consists of a mass of lymphoid tissue in the gastric wall, often associated with an overlying mucosal ulcer. It is thought to represent a response to chronic inflammation. The lesion is not malignant, though the presentation, which includes pain, weight loss, and a mass on barium studies, cannot be distinguished from that of a malignant lesion.

Treatment of gastric pseudolymphoma consists of resection. The distinction from lymphoma is made on histologic examination of the specimen, which shows mature germinal centers in pseudolymphoma. No additional therapy is indicated postoperatively.

Crump M, Gospodarowicz M, Shepherd FA: Lymphoma of the gastrointestinal tract. Semin Oncol 1999;26:324.

Kolve ME, Fischbach W, Wilhelm M: Primary gastric non-Hodgkin's lymphoma: requirements for diagnosis and staging. Recent Results Cancer Res 2000;156:63.

Steinbach G et al: Antibiotic treatment of gastric lymphoma of mucosa-associated lymphoid tissue. An uncontrolled trial. Ann Intern Med 1999 Jul 20;131:88.

Yamashita H et al: When can complete regression of low-grade gastric lymphoma of mucosa-associated lymphoid tissue be predicted after *Helicobacter pylori* eradication? Histopathology 2000;37:131.

GASTRIC LEIOMYOMAS & LEIOMYOSARCOMAS

Leiomyomas are common submucosal growths that are usually asymptomatic but may cause intestinal bleeding. Leiomyosarcomas may grow to a large size and most often present with bleeding. Radiologically, the tumor usually contains a central ulceration caused by necrosis from outgrowth of its blood supply. In most cases the tumor arises from the proximal stomach. It may grow into the gastric lumen, remain entirely on the serosal surface, or even become pedunculated within the abdominal cavity. Spread is by direct invasion or blood-borne metastases. CT scans provide useful information on the amount of extragastric extension. Leiomyomas should be removed by enucleation or wedge resection. After the more radical resections required for leiomyosarcomas, the 5-year survival rate is 20%. If technically possible, complete resection of metastases (eg, peritoneal, hepatic) in addition to the primary may improve the outcome. The results are affected by tumor size, DNA ploidy pattern, and tumor grade. Lesions that exhibit ten or more mitoses in a high-powered field rarely can be cured. The tumor is resistant to radiotherapy.

MÉNÉTRIER'S DISEASE

Ménétrier's disease, a form of hypertrophic gastritis, consists of giant hypertrophy of the gastric rugae; high, normal, or low acid secretion; and excessive loss of protein from the thickened mucosa into the gut, with resulting hypoproteinemia. The etiology may involve altered expression of TGFα. Clinical manifestations include edema, diarrhea, anorexia, weight loss, and skin rash. Chronic blood loss may also be a problem. Indigestion may respond to antacids, but this treatment does not improve the gastric pathologic process or secondary hypoproteinemia. The hypertrophic rugae present as enormous filling defects on upper gastrointestinal series and are frequently misinterpreted as carcinoma. The protein leak from the gastric mucosa may respond to atropine (and other anticholinergic drugs), hexamethonium bromide, eradication of *H pylori,* or H$_2$ blocking agents or omeprazole. Rarely, total gastrectomy is indicated for severe intractable hypoproteinemia, anemia, or inability to exclude cancer. Medical management is best for most patients, though the gastric abnormalities and hypoproteinemia may persist. Some cases gradually evolve into atrophic gastritis. In children the disease characteristically is self-limited and benign. There is an increased risk of adenocarcinoma of the stomach in adults with Ménétrier's disease.

Badov D et al: *Helicobacter pylori* as a pathogenic factor in Menetrier's disease. Am J Gastroenterol 1998;93:1976.

Burdick JS et al: Treatment of Menetrier's disease with a monoclonal antibody against the epidermal growth factor receptor. N Engl J Med 2000;343:1697.

Madsen LG et al: Menetrier's disease and *Helicobacter pylori:* normalization of gastrointestinal protein loss after eradication therapy. Dig Dis Sci 1999;44:2307.

PROLAPSE OF THE GASTRIC MUCOSA

This uncommon lesion occasionally accompanies small prepyloric gastric ulcers. Episodes of vomiting and abdominal pain simulate peptic ulcer disease. X-ray shows prolapse of antral folds into the duodenum. One must be alert to the presence of gastric or duodenal ulcer as the underlying cause.

Antrectomy with a Billroth I anastomosis is occasionally required. Generally, conservative treatment suffices.

GASTRIC VOLVULUS

The stomach may rotate about its longitudinal axis (organo-axial volvulus) or a line drawn from the mid lesser to the mid greater curvature (mesenterioaxial volvulus). The former is more common and is often associated with a paraesophageal hiatal hernia. In other patients, eventration of the left diaphragm allows the colon to rise and twist the stomach by pulling on the gastrocolic ligament.

Acute gastric volvulus produces severe abdominal pain accompanied by a diagnostic triad (Brochardt's triad): (1) vomiting followed by retching and then inability to vomit, (2) epigastric distention, and (3) inability to pass a nasogastric tube. The situation calls for immediate laparotomy to prevent death from acute gastric necrosis and shock. An emergency upper gastrointestinal series will show a block at the point of the volvulus. The death rate is high.

Chronic volvulus is more common than acute. It may be asymptomatic or may cause crampy intermittent pain. Cases associated with paraesophageal hiatal hernia should be treated by repair of the hernia and anterior gastropexy. When cases are due to eventration of the diaphragm, the gastrocolic ligament should be divided the entire length of the greater curvature. The colon rises to fill the space caused by the eventration, and the stomach will resume its normal position, to be fastened by a gastropexy.

GASTRIC DIVERTICULA

Gastric diverticula are uncommon and usually asymptomatic. Most are pulsion diverticula consisting of mucosa and submucosa only, located on the lesser curvature within a few centimeters of the esophagogastric junction. Those in the prepyloric region generally possess all layers and are more likely to be symptomatic. A few patients have symptoms from hemorrhage of inflammation within a gastric diverticulum, but for the most part these lesions are incidental findings on upper gastrointestinal series. Radiologically, they can be confused with a gastric ulcer.

BEZOAR

Bezoars are concretions formed in the stomach. Trichobezoars are composed of hair and are usually found in young girls who pick at their hair and swallow it. Phytobezoars consist of agglomerated vegetable fibers. Pressure by the mass can create a gastric ulcer that is prone to bleed or perforate.

The postgastrectomy state predisposes to bezoar formation because pepsin and acid secretion are reduced and the triturating function of the antrum is gone. Orange segments or other fruits that contain a large amount of cellulose have been implicated in most cases. Improper mastication of food is a contributing factor that can sometimes be obviated by providing the patient with properly fitted dentures. The fruit may remain in the stomach or pass into the small intestine and cause obstruction. Some surgeons routinely warn postgastrectomy patients to avoid citrus fruits.

Large semisolid bezoars of *Candida albicans* have also been found in postgastrectomy patients. Some can be fragmented with the gastroscope. The patient should also be treated with oral nystatin.

Patients with symptomatic gastric bezoars may complain of abdominal pain. Ulceration and bleeding are associated with a death rate of 20%.

Nearly all gastric bezoars can be broken up and dispersed by endoscopy. Neglected lesions with complications (ie, bleeding or perforation) require gastrectomy.

■ II. DUODENUM

DUODENAL DIVERTICULA

Diverticula of the duodenum are found in 20% of autopsies and 5–10% of upper gastrointestinal series. Symptoms are uncommon, and only 1% of those found by x-ray warrant surgery.

Duodenal pulsion diverticula are acquired outpouchings of the mucosa and submucosa, 90% of which are on the medial aspect of the duodenum. They are rare before age 40. Most are solitary and within 2.5 cm of the ampulla of Vater. There is a high incidence of gallstone disease of the gallbladder in patients with juxtapapillary diverticula. Diverticula are not seen in the first portion of the duodenum, where diverticular configurations are due to scarring by peptic ulceration or cholecystitis.

A few patients have chronic postprandial abdominal pain or dyspepsia caused by a duodenal diverticulum. Treatment is with antacids and anticholinergics.

Serious complications are hemorrhage or perforation from inflammation, pancreatitis, and biliary obstruction. Bile acid-bilirubinate enteroliths are occasionally formed by bile stasis in a diverticulum. Enteroliths can precipitate diverticular inflammation or biliary obstruction and, rarely, have caused bowel obstruction after entering the intestinal lumen.

Surgical treatment is required for complications and, rarely, for persistent symptoms. Excision and a two-layer closure are usually possible after mobilization of the duodenum and dissection of the diverticulum from the pancreas. Removal of the diverticulum and closure of the defect are superior to simple drainage in the case of perforation. If biliary obstruction appears in a patient whose bile duct empties into a diverticulum, excision might be more hazardous than a side-to-side choledochoduodenostomy.

The rare wind sock type of intraluminal diverticulum usually presents with vague epigastric pain and postprandial fullness, though intestinal bleeding or pancreatitis is occasionally seen. The diagnosis can be made by barium x-ray studies. The diverticulum can be excised through a nearby duodenotomy. In some cases, the narrow diverticular outlet can be enlarged endoscopically.

Lobo DN et al: Periampullary diverticula and pancreaticobiliary disease. Br J Surg 1999;86:588.

DUODENAL TUMORS

Tumors of the duodenum are rare. Carcinoma of the ampulla of Vater is discussed in Chapter 27.

1. Malignant Duodenal Tumors

Most malignant duodenal tumors are adenocarcinomas, leiomyosarcomas, or lymphomas. They appear in the descending duodenum more often than elsewhere. Pain, obstruction, bleeding, obstructive jaundice, and an abdominal mass are the modes of presentation. Duodenal carcinomas, particularly those in the third and fourth portions of the duodenum, are often missed on barium x-ray studies. Endoscopy and biopsy will usually be diagnostic if the examiner is suspicious enough and can reach the lesion.

If possible, adenocarcinomas and leiomyosarcomas should be resected. Pancreaticoduodenectomy is usually necessary if the tumor is localized. Unresectable lesions should be treated by radiotherapy. Biopsy and radiotherapy are recommended for lymphoma.

After curative resections, the 5-year survival rate is 30%. The overall 5-year survival rate is 18%.

2. Benign Duodenal Tumors

Brunner's gland adenomas are small submucosal nodules that have a predilection for the posterior duodenal wall at the junction of the first and second portions. Sessile and pedunculated variants are seen. Symptoms are due to bleeding or obstruction. Leiomyomas may also be found in the duodenum and ordinarily are asymptomatic.

Carcinoid tumors of the duodenum are often endocrinologically active, producing gastrin, somatostatin, or serotonin. Simple excision is the treatment of choice.

Heterotopic gastric mucosa, presenting as multiple small mucosal nodules, is an occasional endoscopic finding of no clinical significance.

Villous adenomas of the duodenum may give rise to intestinal bleeding or may obstruct the papilla of Vater and cause jaundice. As in the colon, the risk of malignant change is high—about 50%. Small pedunculated villous adenomas may be snared during endoscopy, but sessile tumors must be locally excised via laparotomy. Tumors that contain malignant tissue should be treated by a Whipple procedure.

Alarcon FJ et al: Familial adenomatous polyposis: efficacy of endoscopic and surgical treatment for advanced duodenal adenomas. Dis Colon Rectum 1999;42:1533.

Bakaeen FG et al: What prognostic factors are important in duodenal adenocarcinoma? Arch Surg 2000;135:635.

Bouvet M et al: Factors influencing survival after resection for periampullary neoplasms. Am J Surg 2000;180:13.

Isomoto H et al: Clinical and endoscopic features of adult T-cell leukemia/lymphoma with duodenal involvement. J Clin Gastroenterol 2001;33:241.

Kaklamanos IG et al: Extent of resection in the management of duodenal adenocarcinoma. Am J Surg 2000;179:37.

Ryder NM et al: Primary duodenal adenocarcinoma: a 40-year experience. Arch Surg 2000;135:1070.

Wallace MH et al: Randomized, placebo-controlled trial of gastric acid-lowering therapy on duodenal polyposis and relative adduct labeling in familial adenomatous polyposis. Dis Colon Rectum 2001;44:1585.

SUPERIOR MESENTERIC ARTERY OBSTRUCTION OF THE DUODENUM

Rarely, obstruction of the third portion of the duodenum is produced by compression between the superior mesenteric vessels and the aorta. It most commonly appears after rapid weight loss following injury, including burns. Patients in body casts are particularly susceptible.

The superior mesenteric artery normally leaves the aorta at an angle of 50–60 degrees, and the distance between the two vessels where the duodenum passes between them is 10–20 mm. These measurements in patients with superior mesenteric artery syndrome average 18 degrees and 2.5 mm. Acute loss of mesenteric fat is thought to permit the artery to drop posteriorly, trapping the bowel like a scissors.

Skepticism exists regarding the frequency of this condition in adults who have not experienced acute loss of weight. Most often the patient in question is a thin, nervous woman whose complaints of dyspepsia and occasional emesis are more properly explained on a functional basis. When a clear-cut example is encountered, it may actually represent a form of intestinal malrotation with duodenal bands.

The patient complains of epigastric bloating and crampy pain relieved by vomiting. The symptoms may remit in the prone position. Anorexia and postprandial pain lead to additional malnutrition and weight loss.

Upper gastrointestinal x-rays demonstrate a widened duodenum proximal to a sharp obstruction at the point where the artery crosses the third portion of the duodenum. When the patient moves to the knee-chest position, the passage of barium is suddenly unimpeded. Further verification can be provided if angiography shows an angle of 25 degrees or less between the superior mesenteric artery and the aorta. However, this procedure is not recommended for routine evaluation of obvious cases.

Many patients whose superior mesenteric artery makes a prominent impression on the duodenum are asymptomatic, and in ambulatory patients one should hesitate to attribute vague chronic complaints to this finding.

Involvement of the duodenum by scleroderma leads to duodenal dilatation and hypomotility and an x-ray and clinical picture highly suggestive of superior mesenteric artery syndrome. In the latter, increased duodenal peristalsis should be demonstrable proximal to the arterial blockage, whereas diminished peristalsis characterizes scleroderma. Patients with duodenal scleroderma usually have dysphagia from concomitant esophageal involvement.

Malrotation with duodenal obstruction by congenital bands can mimic this syndrome.

Postural therapy may suffice. The patient should be placed prone when symptomatic or in anticipation of postprandial difficulties. Ambulatory patients should be instructed to assume the knee-chest position, which allows the viscera and the artery to rotate forward off the duodenum.

Chronic obstruction may require section of the suspensory ligament and mobilization of the duodenum, or a duodenojejunostomy to bypass the obstruction. Patients with various forms of malrotation should be treated by mobilizing the duodenojejunal flexure, which releases the duodenum from entrapment by congenital bands.

Diwakaran HH, Stolar CG, Prather CM: Superior mesenteric artery syndrome. Gastroenterology 2001;121:516, 746.

Richardson WS, Surowiec WJ: Laparoscopic repair of superior mesenteric artery syndrome. Am J Surg 2001;181:377.

REGIONAL ENTERITIS OF THE STOMACH & DUODENUM

The proximal intestine and stomach are rarely involved in regional enteritis, though this disease has now been reported in every part of the gastrointestinal tract from the lips to the anus. Most patients with Crohn's disease in the stomach or duodenum have ileal involvement as well.

Pain can in many instances be relieved by antacids. Intermittent vomiting from duodenal stenosis or pyloric obstruction is frequent. The x-ray finding of a cobblestone mucosa or stenosis would be suggestive when associated with typical changes in the ileum. The endoscopic appearance is fairly characteristic, and biopsy with the peroral suction device usually gives an adequate specimen for histologic confirmation of the diagnosis.

Medical treatment is nonspecific and consists principally of corticosteroids during exacerbations. Surgery may be indicated for disabling pain or obstruction. If the disease is localized to the stomach, a partial gastrectomy can be performed. Duodenal involvement most often requires a gastrojejunostomy to bypass the obstruction. Vagotomy should also be performed to prevent development of a marginal ulcer. Recurrent Crohn's disease involving the anastomosis is an occasional late complication, but it can usually be managed successfully by reoperation.

Internal fistulas involving the stomach or duodenum usually represent extensions from primary disease in the ileum or colon. Surgical treatment consists of resection of the diseased ileum or colon and closure of the fistulous opening in the upper gut.

Mansari OE et al: Adenocarcinoma complicating Crohn's disease of the duodenum. Eur J Gastroenterol Hepatol 2001;13: 1259.

Reynolds HL Jr, Stellato TA: Crohn's disease of the foregut. Surg Clin North Am 2001;81:117.

Worsey MJ et al: Strictureplasty is an effective option in the operative management of duodenal Crohn's disease. Dis Colon Rectum 1999;42:596.

Yamamoto T et al: Gastroduodenal fistulas in Crohn's disease: clinical features and management. Dis Colon Rectum 1998;41: 1287.

Liver & Portal Venous System

25

Gerard M. Doherty, MD, & Lawrence W. Way, MD

SURGICAL ANATOMY

Segments

The liver develops as an embryologic outpouching from the duodenum by a process described in Chapter 26. The liver is one of the largest organs in the body, representing 2% of the total body weight. In classic descriptions, the liver was characterized as having four lobes: right, left, caudate, and quadrate. However, these traditional lobes do not describe the true segmental anatomy of the liver, which is depicted in Figure 25–1. The main lobar fissure can be thought of as represented by an oblique plane passing posteriorly from the gallbladder bed to the vena cava, dividing the anatomic right and left lobes. This primary division is to the right of the falciform ligament. The right lobe is subdivided into anterior and posterior segments by the right segmental fissure. The left lobe is subdivided into medial and lateral segments by the left segmental fissure, marked by the position of the falciform ligament.

The relationship of the liver to the other abdominal organs is shown in Figure 25–2.

Portal Circulation

The portal vein is formed by the confluence of the splenic and superior mesenteric veins at the level of the second lumbar vertebra behind the head of the pancreas (Figure 25–3). It runs for 8–9 cm to the hilum of the liver, where it divides into lobar branches. The left gastric vein usually enters the portal vein on its anteromedial aspect just cephalad to the margin of the pancreas, in which case it usually must be ligated during the surgical construction of a portacaval shunt; in 25% of cases, the left gastric vein joins the splenic vein. Other small venous tributaries from the pancreas and duodenum are less constant but must be anticipated during surgical mobilization of the portal vein.

The inferior mesenteric vein generally drains into the splenic vein several centimeters to the left of the junction with the superior mesenteric vein; not uncommonly, it empties directly into the superior mesenteric vein.

In the hepatoduodenal ligament, the portal vein lies dorsal and slightly medial to the common bile duct. A large lymph node is often encountered lateral to the vein and must be dissected off before a shunt can be performed.

Venous Blood Supply

The anatomy of venous blood supply is shown in Figure 25–4. Both the portal and hepatic venous systems lack valves. The portal vein terminates in the porta hepatis by dividing into right and left lobar branches. The right lobar branch immediately follows the course of the segmental ducts and arteries. The left lobar branch has two portions: the transverse part and the umbilical part. The former is a short segment coursing through the porta hepatis. The latter descends into the umbilical fossa and supplies the medial and lateral segments of the left lobe.

The hepatic veins represent the final common pathway for the central veins of the lobules of the liver. There are three major hepatic veins: left, right, and middle. The middle hepatic vein lies in the major lobar fissure and drains blood from the medial segment of the left lobe and the inferior portion of the anterior segment of the right lobe. The left hepatic vein drains the lateral segment of the left lobe, and the right hepatic vein drains the posterior segment and much of the anterior segment of the right lobe. Several small accessory veins enter the inferior vena cava directly from the posterior segment of the right lobe and must be carefully ligated during a right hemihepatectomy. The middle hepatic vein usually joins the left hepatic vein before they meet the inferior vena cava.

Arterial Blood Supply

The common hepatic artery arises from the celiac axis, ascends in the hepatoduodenal ligament, and gives rise to the right gastric and gastroduodenal arteries before dividing into right and left branches in the hilum. The hepatic artery supplies approximately 25% of the 1500 mL of blood that enters the liver each minute; the remaining 75% is supplied by the portal vein. In 10% of individuals, the common hepatic artery has an anomalous origin. In the most common variants, the common hepatic or the right hepatic artery arises from the superior mesenteric artery. The left hepatic originates from the left gastric artery in 15% of subjects. The common hepatic artery divides to follow the segmental

565

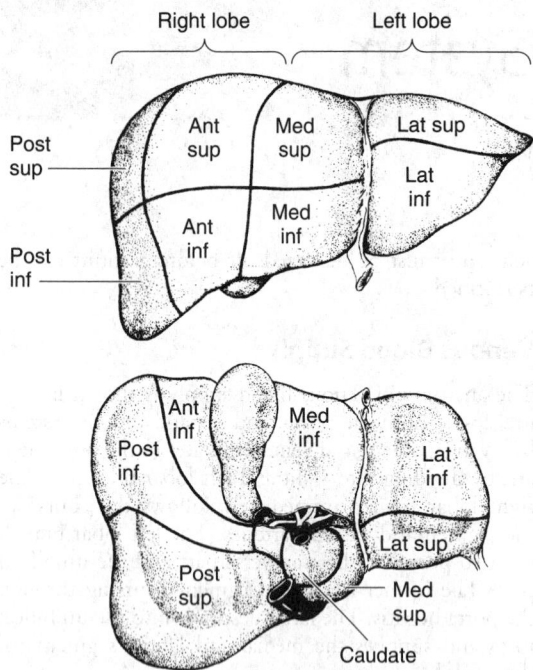

Figure 25-1. Segmental anatomy of the liver. The major lobar fissure, separating the right and left lobes, passes from the inferior vena cava through the gallbladder bed.

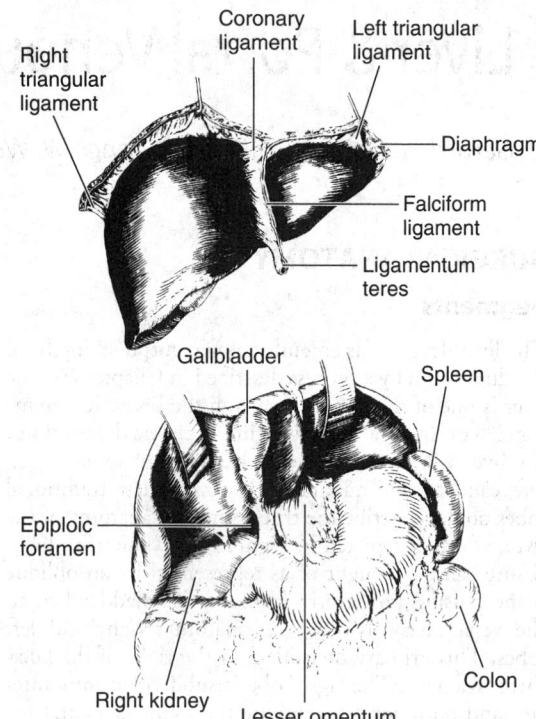

Figure 25-2. Relationships of the liver to adjacent abdominal organs.

ducts. Once they enter the liver and divide, the various segmental branches are termed end-arteries, since they do not communicate with each other via collaterals.

Biliary Drainage

Segmental bile ducts drain each segment. The right anterior and right posterior segmental ducts unite to form the right hepatic duct, and the left lateral and left medial segmental ducts form the left hepatic duct. These lobar ducts join outside the parenchyma to form the common hepatic duct. Anatomic variations are common. In over 25% of specimens, the duct from the right posterior segment joins the left hepatic duct independently. Variations are far less common on the left side.

Lymphatics

Superficial lymphatics arise from superficial portions of the lobules and pass beneath the capsule to enter the posterior mediastinum via the diaphragm and the suspensory ligaments of the liver. Some enter the porta hepatis and others enter the coronary chain. Other lym-

phatics arise deep in the liver lobules and pass either with the hepatic veins along the vena cava or with the portal veins into the porta hepatis.

PHYSIOLOGY

Total hepatic blood flow (about 1500 mL/min; 30 mL/min per kg body weight) constitutes 25% of the cardiac output, though the liver accounts for only 2.5% of body weight. About 30% of the hepatic volume is blood (12% of total blood volume). Two-thirds of the flow enters through the portal vein and one-third through the hepatic artery. Pressure in the portal vein is normally 10–15 cm H_2O (7–11 mm Hg). The liver derives half of its oxygen from hepatic arterial blood and half from portal venous blood.

Portal venous and hepatic arterial blood becomes pooled after entering the periphery of the hepatic sinusoid (Figure 25-5). Hepatic arterial flow increases or decreases reciprocally with changes in portal flow. The regulatory mechanism for hepatic arterial flow involves an adenosine washout phenomenon: adenosine is released into the space of Mall surrounding the hepatic arterial re-

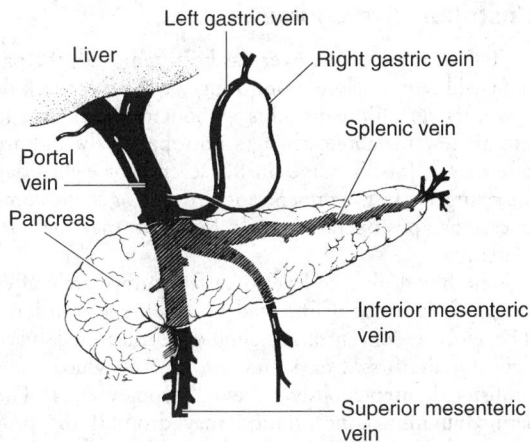

Figure 25–3. Anatomic relationships of portal vein and branches.

Figure 25–5. Vascular anatomy of the liver lobule.

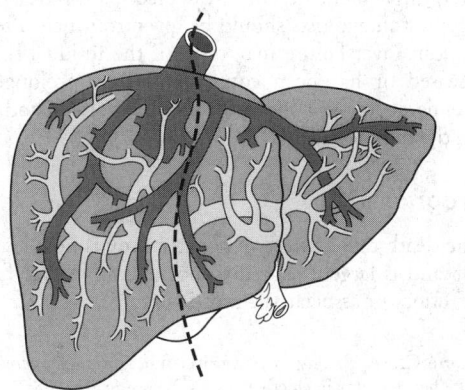

Figure 25–4. Anatomy of the veins of the liver. The major lobar fissure is represented by the dashed line. Branches of the hepatic artery and biliary ducts follow those of the portal vein. The darker vessels represent the hepatic veins and vena cava; the lighter system represents the portal vein and its branches.

sistance vessels. High concentrations of adenosine dilate the vessels, which increases flow and washes out the adenosine. Blood flow within the liver is uniform, as demonstrated by an even distribution of microspheres injected into the hepatic artery or portal vein.

Sudden occlusion of the portal vein results in an immediate 60% rise in hepatic arterial flow. In a matter of weeks, total flow gradually returns toward normal. On the other hand, sudden reductions in hepatic arterial supply are not immediately met by significant increases in portal vein flow. In both normal subjects and cirrhotics, total hepatic flow and portal pressure drop following hepatic arterial occlusion. Arterial collaterals develop over the ensuing months, and arterial perfusion is ultimately restored.

HEPATIC RESECTION

The indications for resection of portions of the liver include primary and secondary malignant tumors, benign tumors, traumatic ruptures, cysts, and abscesses. Removal of as much as 80–85% of the normal liver is consistent with survival. Liver function may be decreased for several weeks after extensive resection, but the extraordinary regenerative capacity of the liver rapidly provides new functioning hepatocytes. Within 24 hours after partial hepatectomy, cell replication becomes active and continues until the original weight of the organ is restored. Considerable regeneration occurs within 10 days, and the process is essentially complete by 4–5 weeks. Excised lobes are not re-formed as such. Rather, the growth consists of formation of new lobules and expansion of residual lobules. The stimuli for hepatic regeneration are thought to include the following: hepatocyte growth factor, TGFα, heparin binding growth factor, hepatopoietin B, and disinhibition by TGFβ$_1$ (ie, decreased levels of this inhibitor of hepatic growth).

Preoperative Evaluation

Since liver function is compromised after major hepatic resection, the decision to perform such operations must take into account the preoperative functional status. Cirrhosis is a relative contraindication for partial hepatectomy because the limited reserve of the residual cirrhotic liver is usually insufficient to meet essential metabolic demands and the cirrhotic liver has little capacity for regeneration. These factors prohibit resection of some primary hepatic tumors that develop in cirrhotics.

Extent of Hepatic Resection

Based upon the labor anatomy, hepatic resections are classified as segmental or nonsegmental. Wedge resections and resectional debridement of devitalized tissue are examples of the latter. Major lobar resections must be planned in accordance with the segmental vascular anatomy. The terminology and extent of the common types of resections are depicted in Figure 25–6. The operation entails removal of a lobe or segment with its afferent and efferent vessels while avoiding injury to vessels and bile ducts supplying the residual tissue. An extended right hepatectomy—the most extensive—removes all but 15–20% of the hepatic mass.

Most elective hepatic lobectomies can be performed through an abdominal incision, though some surgeons prefer a thoracoabdominal approach for right lobectomies. The key to technical success is hemostasis.

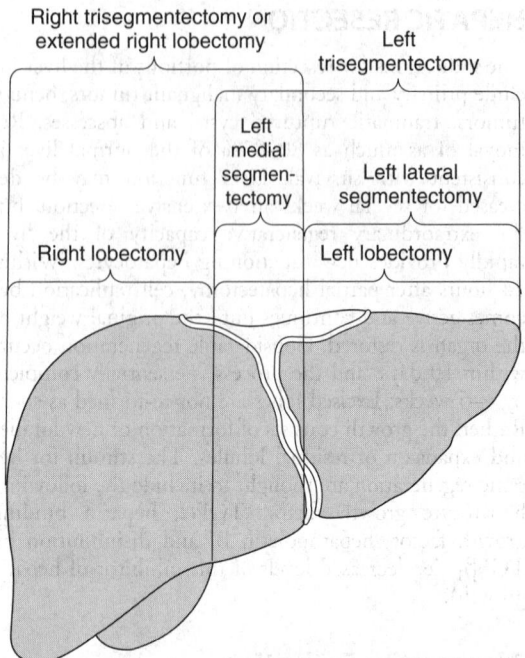

Figure 25–6. Terminology of various segmental resections of the liver. Lobectomy is sometimes referred to as hemihepatectomy.

Postoperative Course

If 50% or more of the liver has been removed, the patient will require close monitoring for the first week or two after operation. Patients without cirrhosis usually exhibit few metabolic changes postoperatively and are often ready for discharge on the seventh or eighth day after surgery. In the presence of cirrhosis or septic complications, postoperative liver function may be impaired.

The blood glucose level may fall immediately after surgery if it is not maintained by parenteral infusions. The glucose concentration should be measured twice daily for the first 2 days and 5% or 10% glucose administered intravenously to avoid hypoglycemia. The serum albumin concentration may drop. If the prothrombin level falls, vitamin K should be given. Low concentrations of fibrinogen and factor IX usually improve spontaneously and require no treatment.

Occasionally, the serum bilirubin will rise several days after resection, but it usually returns to normal within 1–2 weeks. The alkaline phosphatase usually remains normal. AST and serum LDH rise for several days and then return to normal levels.

Complications

Postoperative fever may be due to pulmonary complications or perihepatic abscess formation, but in many cases no cause can be identified, and convalescence in the latter patients may be otherwise unmarred. Abscesses formed in the space created by the resection can usually be drained by percutaneous catheters.

Because partial hepatectomy is attended by a relatively high incidence of stress ulcers, prophylactic H_2 receptor antagonists should be given routinely after operation. Liver failure may result if the residual tissue is diseased or has been compromised by prolonged ischemia during the operation. Ascites, varices, and coma are the manifestations.

Prognosis

The death rate of elective hepatectomy is now less than 5% and is largely related to postoperative liver failure, infection, or associated conditions.

Ettorre GM et al: Postoperative liver function after elective right hepatectomy in elderly patients. Br J Surg 2001;88:73.

Jackson PG et al: Predictors of outcome in 100 consecutive laparoscopic antireflux procedures. Am J Surg 2001;181:231.

Nagino M et al: Liver regeneration after major hepatectomy for biliary cancer. Br J Surg 2001;88:1084.

Nuzzo G et al: Liver resections with or without pedicle clamping. Am J Surg 2001;181:238.

Papadimitriou JD et al: The impact of new technology on hepatic resection for malignancy. Arch Surg 2001;136:1307.

Strasberg SM: Terminology of liver anatomy and liver resections: coming to grips with hepatic Babel. J Am Coll Surg 1997; 184:413.

Takayama T et al: Randomized comparison of ultrasonic vs clamp transection of the liver. Arch Surg 2001;136:922.

Yamashita Y et al: Bile leakage after hepatic resection. Ann Surg 2001;233:45.

■ DISEASES & DISORDERS OF THE LIVER

HEPATIC TRAUMA

Based on the mechanism of injury, liver trauma is classified as penetrating or blunt. Penetrating wounds, constituting more than half of cases, are due to bullets, knives, etc. In civilian practice, most of these tend to be clean wounds—dangerous because of abdominal bleeding but not producing much devitalization of liver substance. In contrast, high-velocity missiles, in addition to piercing the liver, shatter the parenchyma for a variable distance from the track of the missile.

Blunt trauma can be inflicted by a direct blow to the upper abdomen or lower right rib cage or can follow sudden deceleration, as occurs with a fall from a great height. Most often a consequence of automobile accidents, direct blunt trauma tends to produce explosive bursting wounds or linear lacerations of the hepatic surface, often with considerable parenchymal destruction. The stellate, bursting type of injury tends to affect the posterior superior segment of the right lobe because of its relatively vulnerable location, convex surface, fixed position, and concentration of hepatic mass. Damage to the left lobe is much less common than damage to the right. Injuries that involve shearing forces can tear the hepatic veins where they enter the liver substance, producing an exsanguinating retrohepatic injury in an area difficult to surgically expose and repair. The staging system described in Table 25–1 is used to categorize liver injuries and provide a common language in order to allow comparisons of results of treatment between institutions.

The principal surgical goals are to stop bleeding and debride devitalized liver. Because some degree of liver failure is common postoperatively, efforts should be made during each step to maintain adequate oxygenation of blood and perfusion of the liver by avoiding hypoxemia and hypovolemia.

Table 25–1. Liver Injury Scale.[1]

Grade	Type	Description
I	Hematoma	Subcapsular, nonexpanding, < 10% surface area.
	Laceration	Capsular tear, nonbleeding; < 1 cm deep in parenchyma.
II	Hematoma	Subcapsular, onexpanding, 10–50% surface area; intraparenchymal, non-expanding, < 2 cm in diameter.
	Laceration	Capsular tear, active bleeding; 1–3 cm deep into the parenchyma, < 10 cm long.
III	Hematoma	Subcapsular, > 50% surface area or expanding; ruptured subcapsular hematoma with active bleeding; intraparenchymal hematoma > 2 cm or expanding.
	Laceration	> 3 cm deep into the parenchyma.
IV	Hematoma	Ruptured intraparenchymal hematoma with active bleeding.
	Laceration	Parenchymal disruption involving > 50% of hepatic lobe.
V	Laceration	Parenchymal disruption involving > 50% of hepatic lobe.
	Vascular	Juxtahepatic venous injuries; ie, retrohepatic vena cava or major hepatic veins.
VI	Vascular	Hepatic avulsion.

[1]Increase by one grade when there are two or more injuries to the liver. Grading applied based on best available evidence, whether from x-rays, operative findings, or autopsy findings.

Clinical Findings

A. SYMPTOMS AND SIGNS

The clinical manifestations of liver injury are those of hypovolemic shock, ie, hypotension, decreased urinary output, low central venous pressure, and, in some cases, abdominal distention.

B. LABORATORY FINDINGS

The rate of blood loss is usually so rapid that anemia does not develop. Leukocytosis greater than $15,000/\mu L$ is common following rupture of the liver from blunt trauma.

C. IMAGING TECHNIQUES

CT scans should be obtained in most stable patients suspected of having a hepatic injury. The scans demonstrate the extent of the injury and provide a rough estimate of the amount of blood loss. The findings are useful for triaging, since minor injuries rarely require surgical treatment whereas extensive ones usually do. One must exercise caution, however, in using CT estimates of injury grade, since they correlate poorly (ie, they both understage and overstage) with what is found at surgery.

Sonography has not been helpful other than as the rapid abdominal abdominal sonogram to identify fluid in the abdomen. It does not help to define the injury. Angiography is diagnostic in hemobilia.

Treatment

Patients with stable minor injuries may be managed expectantly unless symptoms or signs of bleeding appear. The CT findings in patients who may be considered for nonoperative management include contained subcapsular or intrahepatic hematoma, unilobar fracture, absence of devitalized liver, minimal intraperitoneal blood, and absence of injuries to other intra-abdominal organs. Serial CT scans should be obtained to verify the assumption that the lesion is stable rather than expanding.

Most patients have CT or clinical evidence of active bleeding or a major injury, however, and require prompt exploration.

Most lacerations have stopped bleeding by the time operation is performed. In the absence of active hemorrhage, these wounds should be drained but not sutured. Active bleeding should be managed by clipping or direct suture of identifiable vessels, not by mass ligatures. Subcapsular hematomas often overlie an active bleeding site or parenchyma in need of debridement and should be explored even though the injury appears to be tamponaded and of limited severity. Blunt injuries associated with substantial amounts of parenchymal destruction may be particularly difficult to manage. Rarely, a very severe pulverizing injury requires formal lobectomy.

Temporary occlusion of the hepatic artery and portal vein with a vascular clamp (Pringle's maneuver) for periods of 15–20 minutes may permit more accurate ligation of bleeding vessels in the wound. If this is unsuccessful, the bleeding area should be packed; the packing is removed under general anesthesia 2–3 days later. Absorbable gauze mesh (eg, polyglycolic acid) can sometimes be wrapped around an injured lobe and sutured in a way that maintains pressure and tamponades the bleeding. In a few cases, control of arterial hemorrhage requires ligation of the hepatic artery or one of the accessible lobar branches in the hilum.

The most difficult problems involve lacerations of the major hepatic veins behind the liver. Temporary clamping of the inflow vessels may or may not slow blood loss enough to allow inspection and suturing of the bleeding point. For persistent bleeding, the abdominal incision should be extended into a median sternotomy to improve exposure. An ancillary technique, which is used only rarely, is to place a tube through the atrial appendage into the inferior vena cava past the origin of the hepatic veins. Appropriately placed ligatures around the cava permit total isolation of the liver circulation without interrupting venous return from the lower extremities to the heart. Lobectomy, usually of the right lobe, may be required to manage these retrohepatic injuries.

Nevertheless, the great majority of patients who come to surgery require only drainage of the hepatic wound. Suture ligation of bleeding hepatic vessels and debridement of devitalized tissue are indicated in about 30% and 10% of cases, respectively. The other procedures are indicated even less often.

Penetrating injuries that involve the hepatic flexure of the colon as well as the liver are apt to result in subhepatic sepsis if managed by primary colonic anastomosis. After the liver is repaired and the injured colon is resected, a temporary ileostomy and mucous fistula may avoid this complication.

Postoperative Complications

With present techniques, hemorrhage at laparotomy is rarely uncontrollable except with retrohepatic venous injuries. Patients who rebleed from the liver wound after initial suture ligation should be treated by reexploration, packing, or, rarely, lobectomy. Angiography and CT scanning may provide useful diagnostic information preoperatively in such patients.

Subhepatic sepsis develops in about 20% of cases; it is more frequent if lobectomy has been done.

Hemobilia may be responsible for gastrointestinal bleeding in the postoperative period and can be diagnosed by selective angiography. Treatment consists of embolization through the arteriography catheter.

Bleeding from stress ulcers is common after hepatic trauma, so patients with liver injuries should be given H_2 receptor antagonists after operation.

Prognosis

The death rate of 10–15% following hepatic trauma depends largely on the type of injury and the extent of associated injury to other organs. About one-third of patients admitted in shock cannot be saved. Only 1% of penetrating civilian wounds are lethal, whereas a 20% death rate attends blunt trauma. The death rate in blunt hepatic injury is 10% when only the liver is injured. If three major organs are damaged, the death rate is close to 70%. Bleeding causes more than half of deaths.

Carrillo EH et al: Non-operative management of blunt hepatic trauma. Br J Surg 1998;85:461.

Chen RJ et al: Factors determining operative mortality of grade V blunt hepatic trauma. J Trauma 2000;49:886.

Chen RJ et al: Factors determining operative mortality of grade V blunt hepatic trauma. J Trauma 2000;49:886.

David Richardson J et al: Evolution in the management of hepatic trauma: a 25-year perspective. Ann Surg 2000;232:324.

Leone RJ Jr, Hammond JS: Nonoperative management of pediatric blunt hepatic trauma. Am Surg 2001;67:138.

Pryor JP, Stafford PW, Nance ML: Severe blunt hepatic trauma in children. J Pediatr Surg 2001;36:974.

SPONTANEOUS HEPATIC RUPTURE

Spontaneous rupture of the liver is not common. Most cases of ruptured normal liver are due to preeclampsia-eclampsia, and most cases of ruptured diseased liver are due to hepatic tumors. Hepatic rupture should be suspected in any pregnant or postpartum patient (especially if hypertensive) who complains of acute discomfort in the upper abdomen. Spontaneous rupture has also been reported in association with hepatic hemangioma, gallstone obstruction, typhoid fever, malaria, tuberculosis. syphilis, polyarteritis nodosa, and diabetes mellitus. The diagnosis can be made by ultrasound or CT scanning. Rupture of the liver in the newborn is related to birth trauma in larger infants after difficult deliveries. The common course is intrahepatic hemorrhage expanding to capsular rupture.

Treatment consists of emergency surgery as for traumatic rupture (see above).

Chiappa A et al: Emergency liver resection for ruptured hepatocellular carcinoma complicating cirrhosis. Hepatogastroenterology 1999;46:1145.

Risseeuw JJ et al: Liver rupture postpartum associated with preeclampsia and HELLP syndrome. J Matern Fetal Med 1999;8:32.

PRIMARY LIVER CANCER

Primary hepatic cancer is uncommon in the USA. However, the incidence is high and is increasing in parts of Asia and Africa. In some regions, hepatoma is the single most frequent abdominal tumor. The etiologic factors in these high-risk areas are environmental or cultural, since persons of similar racial background in the USA are at only slightly greater risk than Caucasians. About 9000 cases—distributed equally between men and women—occur in the USA each year. Most arise in persons over age 50, but a few are found in children, mainly under 2 years of age.

Chronic hepatitis B and C virus (HBV and HCV) infection is the principal etiologic factor worldwide. Patients chronically seropositive for HBsAg constitute a high-risk group for development of hepatoma, which in some cases may be detected early by screening for serum alpha-fetoprotein levels. Hepatitis B virus DNA has been detected integrated into the genome of host hepatocytes and hepatoma cells, but whether it has any direct oncogenic effect is unknown. Cirrhosis from almost any cause (eg, alcoholism, hemochromatosis, α_1-antitrypsin deficiency, or primary biliary cirrhosis) is associated with an increased risk of hepatocellular carcinoma. Widespread infection with liver flukes (*Clonorchis sinensis*) is at least partly responsible for the higher incidence of these tumors in Asia. Certain fungus metabolites called aflatoxins have been shown experimentally to be capable of producing liver tumors. These substances are present in staple foods (eg, ground nuts and grain) in some parts of Africa where hepatomas are common.

Three main cellular types of primary liver cancer are recognized: hepatocellular carcinoma (hepatoma), cholangiocellular carcinoma (cholangiocarcinoma), and a mixed form (hepatocholangioma). In children, the hepatocellular tumor is sometimes termed a hepatoblastoma because of its cellular similarly to fetal liver and the occasional presence of hematopoiesis.

Hepatomas constitute about 80% of primary hepatic cancers. Their gross morphology allows separation into three classes: a **massive** form, characterized by a single predominant mass clearly demarcated from the surrounding liver, occasionally with small satellite nodules; a **nodular** form, composed of multiple nodules, often distributed throughout the liver; and a **diffuse** variety, characterized by infiltration of tumor throughout the remaining parenchyma. About 50% of resectable tumors are surrounded by a fibrous capsule, a structure that develops as a result of compression and collagenization of adjacent liver stroma. Encapsulated tumors exhibit a lower incidence of direct liver invasion, tumor microsatellites, and venous permeation compared with nonencapsulated ones, and the finding is a favorable sign. An uncommon variety of the massive type, **fibrolamellar hepatoma,** contains numerous fibrous septa and may resemble focal nodular hyperplasia. Fibrolamellar hepatoma occurs in a younger age group (average 25 years) and is not associated with cirrhosis or hepatitis B virus infection.

In 70% of patients, tumor has spread outside the liver when hepatoma is first diagnosed. Metastases are almost invariably present with the nodular or diffuse forms, but 40% of the massive type are confined to the liver. The hilar and celiac lymph nodes are most commonly involved. Metastases to lung and the peritoneal surface also occur frequently. The portal or hepatic veins are often invaded by tumor, and venous occlusion may occur in either case.

Microscopically, there is usually little stroma between the malignant cells, and the tumor has a soft consistency. The tumor may be highly vascularized, a feature that sometimes produces massive intraperitoneal hemorrhage following spontaneous rupture. Hepatocellular function occurs in some, as indicated by the presence of bile pigment between or in the tumor cells.

Cholangiocarcinomas make up about 15% of primary liver cancers. They are usually well-differentiated adenocarcinomas that spread invasively in the liver substance. Extrahepatic metastases are the rule by the time the tumor is detected.

The mixed tumors resemble hepatomas in their pathologic and clinical behavior.

Angiosarcoma of the liver, a rare fatal tumor, has been seen in workers intensively exposed to vinyl chloride for prolonged periods in polymerization plants.

Clinical Findings

A. SYMPTOMS AND SIGNS

The diagnosis is often difficult. Early cases present with right upper quadrant pain, which may be associated with referred pain in the right shoulder. Weight loss is usually present, and jaundice is evident in about one-third of cases.

Hepatomegaly or a mass is palpable in many patients. An arterial bruit or a friction rub may be audible over the liver. Intermittent fever may be a presenting feature. Ascites or gastrointestinal bleeding from varices indicates advanced disease, and ascites fluid with blood in it should always suggest hepatoma.

The patterns of presentation are as follows: (1) pain with or without hepatomegaly; (2) sudden deterioration of the condition of a cirrhotic patient owing to the appearance of hepatic failure, bleeding varices, or ascites; (3) sudden, massive intraperitoneal hemorrhage; (4) acute illness with fever and abdominal pain; (5) distant metastases; and (6) no clinical findings.

B. LABORATORY FINDINGS

The serum bilirubin is elevated in one-third of patients. In another 25%, serum alkaline phosphatase is increased but the serum bilirubin is normal. Since many of these patients have cirrhosis, the significance of these alterations is often difficult to assess. About 75% of patients are positive for HBsAg or hepatitis C.

C. LIVER SCAN

CT scans, ultrasound scans, and MRI scans demonstrate the principal lesion in 80% of patients. MRI scans are the best way to show extension into the hepatic veins. CT portography is superior to ordinary contrast-enhanced CT scans.

D. ANGIOGRAPHY

Hepatomas are usually supplied by the hepatic artery, and 80% are more vascular than adjacent parenchyma. In some cases, the center of the tumor has become necrotic, and only the peripheral areas are hypervascular. Cholangiocarcinomas usually appear less vascular than adjacent tissue. Hemangiomas can be recognized by a characteristic picture of patchy vascular pooling.

The venous phase of a superior mesenteric arterial injection may show invasion or occlusion of the portal vein by tumor.

Angiography may be equivocal in small tumors, which may be demonstrated with greater certainty by a selective injection of iodized oil (Lipiodol) followed 1–2 weeks later by CT scans. Normal liver clears the contrast medium, but hepatomas cannot do so and remain opacified.

E. LIVER BIOPSY

The diagnosis can be established by percutaneous core biopsy or aspiration biopsy in most patients if the biopsy site is selected according to the scan. Percutaneous biopsy is risky, however (rate of fatal hemorrhage is 0.4%), because these tumors are so vascular.

F. SCREENING

Attempts have been made to detect hepatocellular carcinomas early at a surgically more favorable stage by screening patients with chronic liver disease with periodic hepatic ultrasound examinations. These programs appear to have been worthwhile in Asia, with about two-thirds of detected lesions being under 2 cm in diameter, a majority of which are resectable. A similar effort in Italy, however, was disappointing. The explanation may be that the disease simply follows a more aggressive course in Europe than in Asia.

G. TUMOR MARKERS

Alpha-fetoprotein (AFP), a glycoprotein normally present only in the fetal circulation, is present in high concentrations in the serum of many patients with primary hepatomas and testicular tumors. Increased levels may also be seen rarely as a product of tumors elsewhere in the body, such as the lung, stomach, pancreas, and biliary tree.

The upper limit of normal in the serum is 20 ng/mL; values above 200 ng/mL are suggestive of hepatoma. Levels in the intermediate range may occur with other kinds of liver disease, such as cirrhosis and chronic hepatitis, where they represent a manifestation of liver cell proliferation. As imaging methods have improved, the diagnosis of liver cancer is being made earlier and the frequency of AFP levels above 200 ng/mL in newly diagnosed cases has declined to about 25%. In general, whether or not AFP levels are abnormal is related to the size of the tumor, whereas the absolute level, which may exceed 10,000 ng/mL, is related to lack of differentiation histologically. Consequently, the prognosis is worse when AFP levels are high.

Differential Diagnosis

The clinical picture is usually nonspecific. Because of weight loss and weakness, liver cancer is most often confused with other abdominal carcinomas. Once hepatomegaly and a filling defect in the liver are found, it must be determined whether the liver harbors a primary neoplasm or a metastasis. Arteriography, biopsy, and serum AFP levels establish the diagnosis in most cases. However, it may be difficult to distinguish hepatic cancer from benign tumors or cysts or, if the patient is febrile, from liver abscess.

When complications develop suddenly in a cirrhotic patient, the possibility of hepatoma must always be considered. Portacaval shunts have been performed for recent variceal hemorrhage in cirrhotic patients without the physician suspecting that a hepatoma was responsible for the portal hypertension.

In rare instances, primary hepatocellular cancer is associated with metabolic or endocrine abnormalities such as erythrocytosis, hypercalcemia, hypoglycemic attacks, Cushing's syndrome, or virilization.

Complications

Sudden intra-abdominal hemorrhage may occur from spontaneous bleeding. Obstruction of the portal vein may produce portal hypertension, and obstruction of the hepatic veins may produce the Budd-Chiari syndrome. Liver failure is a common cause of death.

Treatment

A. PARTIAL HEPATECTOMY

Resection of the tumor offers the only possibility of cure. The operation should usually begin with a diagnostic laparoscopy, for this may reveal previously undetected spread of tumor within the liver or abdominal cavity that militates against resection. The criteria of resectability are that (1) the tumor must be confined to the liver (ie, distant metastases or extension into the hepatic or portal veins must be absent) and (2) the lesion must be entirely encompassed by local excision, lobectomy, or extended lobectomy. Small lesions, particularly in cirrhotics, may be removed by local excision. About 25% of patients with primary liver cancer meet these requirements.

If visible tumor is left behind or if the margins of resection are less than 0.5 cm, progressive disease is the rule. After what is thought to be a complete resection, the outlook is worse with any of the following: (1) age over 50 years, (2) coexistent hepatocellular disease (ie, cirrhosis), (3) vascular invasion, (4) portal vein thrombosis, (5) tumor located deep in the liver, (6) intracapsular infiltration of tumor cells, (7) bilobar involvement, and

(8) more than one deposit of tumor. In general, however, cirrhosis constitutes the major obstacle. Any but the most limited resection is apt to trigger acute liver failure in cirrhotic patients, but in addition to this immediate concern, there is a late risk of death from bleeding esophageal varices or liver failure, and a high rate (> 75%) of new tumors developing in the residual liver. This is why liver transplantation has been tried for this group.

Overall, the rate of tumor recurrence is about 50% (though it is higher, as mentioned above, in patients with cirrhosis). The 5-year survival rate for patients with cirrhosis is close to zero, but for those without cirrhosis, it is about 40%. The results are still better (5-year survival about 60%) for fibrolamellar carcinomas.

After surgery, the patient should be followed by imaging studies and AFP measurements, and a localized recurrence should be considered for repeat resection or palliative therapy if technically feasible.

B. LIVER TRANSPLANTATION

Liver transplantation is of theoretic advantage because it should overcome the following problems: (1) lesions that are unresectable because of size or multifocal distribution (2) the inability of a cirrhotic liver to tolerate any but the most limited resection and (3) the likelihood in many cases that an undetectable second tumor is located remote from the index lesion. The results of liver transplantation have been good for fibrolamellar carcinoma and hemangioblastoma: 5-year survival rates for each are about 50%. There have been no survivors among those with hemangiosarcoma.

In patients with clinically apparent hepatomas complicating cirrhosis, 5-year survival is about 35%, good enough to encourage further efforts. The results are almost twice as good for patients with just one locus of tumor. Therefore, although the logistical problems and expense are enormous, transplantation is presently the best treatment for hepatoma in a cirrhotic liver.

The immunosuppressive therapy required to support the transplant is thought to impair the host's defenses against the tumor: Calculated tumor doubling time for lesions in transplanted patients was 37 days compared with 274 days in patients treated by hepatic resection (no immunosuppression).

C. ETHANOL INJECTION

Using ultrasound guidance, 95% ethanol (5–20 mL) is injected through a 22-gauge needle into the neoplasm, which results in complete necrosis of the lesion in 75% of patients and partial (90%) necrosis in 20%. The patient is followed and re-treatment given for residual or new primary tumors. In one multi-institutional series from Italy, survival 1, 2, and 3 years after treatment for patients with solitary tumors was 90%, 80%, and 63%, respectively.

D. Radiofrequency Ablation

Using ultrasound guidance, a radiofrequency ablation probe is introduced into the liver lesion percutaneously, at laparotomy or laparoscopy. Electrical energy is used to destroy the lesion by producing heat. Initial experiences are promising.

E. Arterial Chemoembolization

This approach takes advantage of the fact that primary liver cancers obtain their blood supply almost exclusively from the hepatic artery, whereas the rest of the liver is supplied more by the portal vein than by the artery. The strategy is to combine selective hepatic arterial injection of cancer chemotherapeutic agents with embolization, the latter to produce ischemia and slow the washout of the drugs. Patients with Child class C cirrhosis or thrombosis of the portal vein are not suitable candidates.

A variety of techniques have been used. Embolization is usually performed with Gelfoam, which dissolves after a few weeks, allowing repeated treatment. Doxorubicin, mitomycin, and cisplatin in various combinations are the drugs most often given. Lipiodol, which lodges in the tumor, has occasionally been used as a carrier for the drugs. A reduction in tumor size of 50% or more is seen in about 25% of patients. The best 3-year survival rates are around 50%. Histologic studies of tumors resected shortly after treatment reveal viable neoplastic cells in the tumor capsule, which receives blood from the portal vein as well as the hepatic artery.

Prognosis

Most patients with unresectable lesions succumb within a year after diagnosis. Patients generally die from the effects of the expanding hepatic neoplasm rather than from metastases.

Akriviadis EA et al: Hepatocellular carcinoma. Br J Surg 1998; 85:1319.

Baffis V et al: Use of interferon for prevention of hepatocellular carcinoma in cirrhotic patients with hepatitis B or hepatitis C virus infection. Ann Intern Med 1999;131:696.

Bergsland EK, Venook AP: Hepatocellular carcinoma. Curr Opin Oncol 2000;12:357.

Grasso A et al: Radiofrequency ablation in the treatment of hepatocellular carcinoma—a clinical viewpoint. J Hepatol 2000; 33:667.

Krinsky GA, Lee VS, Theise ND: Focal lesions in the cirrhotic liver: high resolution ex vivo MRI with pathologic correlation. J Comput Assist Tomogr 2000;24:189.

Mor E et al: Treatment of hepatocellular carcinoma associated with cirrhosis in the era of liver transplantation. Ann Intern Med 1998;129:643.

Trevisani F et al: Randomized control trials on chemoembolization for hepatocellular carcinoma: is there room for new studies? J Clin Gastroenterol 2001;32:383.

Tung-Ping Poon R, Fan ST, Wong J: Risk factors, prevention, and management of postoperative recurrence after resection of hepatocellular carcinoma. Ann Surg 2000;232:10.

METASTATIC NEOPLASMS OF THE LIVER

Metastatic cancer is 20 times more common than primary tumors in the liver. Cancers of the breast, lung, pancreas, stomach, large intestine, kidney, ovary, and uterus account for about 75% of cases. Spread to the liver may be via the systemic circulation, portal vein, or, less often, the lymphatics. The cirrhotic liver, which often gives rise to primary hepatic tumors, is less susceptible than normal liver to implantation of metastases.

Over 90% of patients with hepatic metastases have tumor implants in other organs. The lung is most commonly involved and contains tumor in 30% of cases. About 20% of patients with hepatic metastases have gross tumor deposits demonstrable on hepatic section that cannot be seen or felt from the surface of the liver during laparotomy.

Clinical Findings

A. Symptoms and Signs

Weight loss, fatigue, and anorexia are the presenting general complaints. Right upper abdominal pain, ascites, and jaundice are the usual symptoms. Fever without demonstrable infection is present in 15% of cases and bears only a loose relationship to leukocytosis.

In 60% of cases, physical examination reveals hepatomegaly or a palpable metastatic tumor in the upper abdomen. Either may be tender. Portal hypertension may be manifested by abdominal venous collaterals or splenomegaly. A friction rub is sometimes heard over the liver.

B. Laboratory Findings

Laboratory investigation reveals a hematocrit between 30% and 36%. The serum bilirubin is elevated in almost half of patients, and half of these have values over 4 mg/dL. The alkaline phosphatase is also usually increased.

The diagnosis can be established in most cases by percutaneous liver biopsy or fine-needle aspiration for malignant cells, especially if scans are used to direct the site of the biopsy.

C. Imaging Studies

The detection of liver metastases usually relies on CT or ultrasound scans. MRI provides useful additional information, however, and it may be superior to CT scans. CT portography is superior to ordinary contrast-enhanced CT. Where available, MRI and CT portography should both be performed if the patient is being considered for resection of hepatic metastases or insertion of a hepatic artery infusion pump. During surgery the liver should be further examined by ultrasound to check for lesions that might have been missed by preoperative studies.

Treatment

Little effective treatment is available for the average patient with diffuse metastases throughout the liver or with combined hepatic and extrahepatic disease.

A. Hepatic Resection

Partial hepatectomy—either wedge resection or lobectomy—is indicated for the 5% of patients with liver metastases from colorectal cancer whose disease is resectable. If all gross tumor can be removed, about 25% of patients are cured. The only absolute requirements are that no extrahepatic disease be present and that resection be technically feasible. The following indicate a worse prognosis after resection: (1) original tumor stage Dukes C compared with Dukes B; (2) four or more liver lesions; (3) over 25% of the mass of the liver replaced by tumor; (4) less than 1 year since resection of the colon primary; and (5) 1 cm or less margin of resection. Variables that do not influence the outcome include (1) lobectomy versus wedge resection; (2) histologic pattern of the tumor; (3) bilateral rather than unilateral disease; (4) site of the primary tumor within the large intestine; and (5) the gender of the patient. The mortality rate for resection of hepatic metastases is about 2% in hospitals where this operation is performed frequently.

When the disease returns following a resection that removed all detectable tumor, the median time to recurrence is 9 months. The initial recurrence in about half of these patients is confined to the liver. Another resection may be performed if the criteria listed above are once again met, which amounts to perhaps 30% of cases. The chances of permanently eradicating the disease by a second resection is about 15%.

Other tumors that occasionally produce disease localized to one lobe of the liver and amenable to curative resection include pancreatic islet cell carcinomas, renal cell carcinomas, and carcinoids. Debulking liver resections may provide palliation of the carcinoid syndrome even when it is impossible to remove all the tumor. Partial hepatectomy is also sometimes worthwhile to extirpate a tumor invading directly from a contiguous organ. Hepatic resection of apparently solitary metastases from cancers of the breast, pancreas, stomach, female pelvic organs, and lung has been fruitless.

B. Radiofrequency Ablation

Radiofrequency energy has been used to destroy metastases to the liver from a variety of tumor types. Trials are currently ongoing to define the role of this therapy.

C. Chemotherapy

In as many as 30% of cases, the liver is the only evident site of metastases from colorectal cancer. If the lesion cannot be resected, local chemotherapy of these lesions can be given by placing a catheter in the hepatic artery connected to an implantable infusion pump (Infusaid pump), which allows the delivery of much higher concentrations of drug to the tumor than is possible with systemic administration. This regimen is not used for metastases from other kinds of tumors. The pump is primed with floxuridine, which is delivered by continuous infusion (0.3 mg/kg/d) for 14-day periods alternating with 14-day rests. The discovery of extrahepatic lesions at laparotomy for pump placement is considered an absolute contraindication to proceeding with this approach. Treatment is continued until toxicity or relapse occurs, or rarely until the response is complete. Toxicity consists mainly of gastroduodenal erosions (caused by unintentional perfusion of these areas), chemical hepatitis, or chemical sclerosing cholangitis. Extrahepatic lesions that appear during therapy are treated by concomitant systemic chemotherapy. Survival is related principally to the initial amount of liver involvement by tumor, objective response to treatment (which is seen in about 50% of patients), and extent of weight loss. Median survival of patients with less than 30% of liver replaced by tumor is 24 months, compared with 10 months if the extent of replacement exceeds 30%. There is a general feeling that hepatic artery infusion therapy improves survival, but the objective evidence is inconclusive. Cure is not a realistic objective.

Hepatic artery infusion chemotherapy may be a useful adjunctive therapy, after complete tumor resection or radiofrequency ablation. Studies of this option are under way.

Systemic chemotherapy (eg, with fluorouracil) does not improve survival, though it is often prescribed.

D. Miscellaneous

Hepatic artery ligation or angiographic embolization of the tumor has been of benefit in a few patients with hepatic metastases from specific tumor types, such as carcinoid and islet cell tumors.

Prognosis

Survival varies with the extent of disease, ranging from 3 months for patients with extensive hepatic replacement by multiple lesions to 2–3 years for patients with small solitary lesions. Survival is slightly longer in patients with metastases from colonic cancer than in patients with metastases from pancreatic or gastric tumors.

Cady B et al: Surgical margin in hepatic resection for colorectal metastasis: a critical and improvable determinant of outcome. Ann Surg 1998;227:566.

DeMatteo RP et al: Results of hepatic resection for sarcoma metastatic to liver. Ann Surg 2001;234:540.

Gruenberger T et al: Reduction in recurrence risk for involved or inadequate margins with edge cryotherapy after liver resection for colorectal metastases. Arch Surg 2001;136:1154.

Harmon KE et al: Benefits and safety of hepatic resection for colorectal metastases. Am J Surg 1999;177:402.

Heslin MJ et al: Colorectal hepatic metastases: resection, local ablation, and hepatic artery infusion pump are associated with prolonged survival. Arch Surg 2001;136:318.

Kokudo N et al: Anatomical major resection versus nonanatomical limited resection for liver metastases from colorectal carcinoma. Am J Surg 2001;181:153.

Lambert LA, Colacchio TA, Barth RJ Jr: Interval hepatic resection of colorectal metastases improves patient selection. Arch Surg 2000;135:473.

Nagakura S, Shirai Y, Hatakeyama K: Computed tomographic features of colorectal carcinoma liver metastases predict posthepatectomy patient survival. Dis Colon Rectum 2001;44:1148.

Primrose JN: Treatment of colorectal metastases: surgery, cryotherapy, or radiofrequency ablation. Gut 2002;50:1.

Scudamore CH et al: Radiofrequency ablation followed by resection of malignant liver tumors. Am J Surg 1999;177:411.

Strasberg SM et al: Survival of patients evaluated by FDG-PET before hepatic resection for metastatic colorectal carcinoma: a prospective database study. Ann Surg 2001;233:293.

Taylor I, Gillams AR: Colorectal liver metastases: alternatives to resection. J R Soc Med 2000;93:576.

BENIGN TUMORS & CYSTS OF THE LIVER*

Hemangiomas

Hemangioma is the most common benign hepatic tumor, and—except for the skin and mucous membranes—the liver is the most common location for hemangiomas. Women are affected more often than men in a ratio of 6:1. Histologically, hepatic hemangiomas are of the cavernous type. Most are small solitary subcapsular growths that are found incidentally during laparotomy or at autopsy. Those greater than 4 cm in diameter may cause abdominal pain or a palpable mass. Rare patients have presented with hemorrhagic shock resulting from spontaneous rupture. Large congenital hemangiomas of the liver may be associated with others in the skin. Occasionally, a hemangioma may behave as an arteriovenous fistula and produce cardiac hypertrophy and congestive heart failure.

Large-bore needle biopsy is hazardous, but aspiration biopsy with a fine needle is safe. Nevertheless, biopsy is rarely indicated, since the diagnosis can be made with certainty in most cases by scintigraphy, contrast-enhanced CT scans, MRI, or angiography. CT scans show a vascular lesion with delayed clearing of the contrast medium. Similar features are seen with technetium-labeled red blood cell scintigrams. Arteriograms demonstrate puddling of contrast medium within the tumor that clears slowly.

Symptomatic hemangiomas should be excised by lobectomy or enucleation. Even large lesions can be safely removed with modest blood loss if they are confined to one lobe. Radiotherapy or embolization via a catheter in the hepatic artery may be tried in patients who are poor candidates for surgery. It has been suggested that exogenous estrogens may contribute to the occasional recurrence of giant hemangiomas, so they should probably be proscribed.

The natural history of asymptomatic hemangiomas, whether large or small, is benign. If discovered as an incidental finding during laparotomy, a hemangioma should not be biopsied or removed, because of potential difficulties with hemostasis.

Bykov S et al: The role of hepatobiliary scintigraphy in the follow-up of benign liver tumors secondary to oral contraceptive use. Clin Nucl Med 2001;26:946.

Cherqui D et al: Laparoscopic liver resections: a feasibility study in 30 patients. Ann Surg 2000;232:753.

Popescu I et al: Liver hemangioma revisited: current surgical indications, technical aspects, results. Hepatogastroenterology 2001;48:770.

Terkivatan T et al: Indications and long-term outcome of treatment for benign hepatic tumors: a critical appraisal. Arch Surg 2001;136:1033.

Cysts

Hepatic cysts are usually solitary unilocular lesions that produce no symptoms. The occasional large cyst may present as an upper abdominal mass or discomfort. Polycystic liver disease is associated in about half of cases with polycystic renal disease. The possibility of echinococcosis (see Chapter 9) should always be considered in patients with just one or two cysts.

Most solitary cysts have a serous lining. Solitary cysts lined with cuboidal epithelium are classified as cystadenomas and should be resected, since they are premalignant. Multilocular (septated) cysts (if not echinococcal) are usually neoplastic. There are few indications for aspirating hepatic cysts, because simple cysts reaccumulate fluid quickly; neoplastic cysts must be ex-

---

*Echinococcal cysts are discussed in Chapter 9.

cised; and parasitic cysts might be ruptured and the parasite thus allowed to spread. On the other hand, it may be possible to eliminate a small cyst by aspiration of the contents followed by an injection into the lumen of 20–100 mL of absolute alcohol.

Large symptomatic cysts are difficult to eradicate with alcohol injections, and serious superinfection of the cyst cavity may occur. The simplest method of treatment consists of laparoscopic excision of the superficial portion (about 20–40%) of the cyst wall. A tongue of omentum is fixed so it lies in the residual cyst cavity as an ancillary measure to prevent the edges from coapting. The operation is curative in nearly all patients.

Multiple cysts do not usually require treatment, but large polycystic livers that cause discomfort or are associated with obstructive jaundice can be managed by surgically unroofing the cysts on the surface of the liver and creating windows between superficial cysts and adjacent deep cysts. The opened cysts are allowed to drain into the abdominal cavity. Postoperatively, the liver shrinks to about half its previous size. In some cases, the liver returns to its original size quickly; in others, it remains smaller.

Cowles RA, Mulholland MW: Solitary hepatic cysts. J Am Coll Surg 2000;191:311.

Hansen P, Ludemann R, Swanstrom LL: Minimally invasive approaches to hepatic surgery. Hepatogastroenterology 2001; 48:37.

Inaba Y et al: Focal attenuation differences in pericystic liver tissue as seen on CT hepatic arteriography and CT arterial portography: observation using a unified helical CT and angiography system. Abdom Imaging 1999;24:360.

Hepatic Adenoma

Hepatic adenomas occur almost exclusively in women and appear to be related to the widespread use of oral contraceptives. Mestranol-containing compounds have been associated with a disproportionate number of cases, but mestranol has been in use longer than the other agents.

The tumors are soft, yellow-tan, well-circumscribed masses that measure 2–15 cm in diameter. Most of those that cause symptoms are in the 8- to 15-cm range. Two-thirds of hepatic adenomas are solitary; the remainder are multiple. A few are pedunculated. Transition from benign hepatic adenoma to hepatocellular carcinoma may occur, with liver cell dysplasia as an intermediate step. Histologically, hepatic adenomas consist of an encapsulated homogeneous mass of normal-appearing hepatocytes without bile ducts or central veins. Hemorrhage may be present.

About half of patients are asymptomatic. Most of those with symptoms present with right upper quad-

rant pain or acute intra-abdominal hemorrhage and shock. These complications are due to spontaneous hemorrhage into the substance of the tumor, which may rupture into the peritoneal cavity. There is a strong association of acute bleeding episodes with menstruation. Patients with symptoms usually have a palpable mass in the liver.

Liver function tests and AFP levels are usually normal. Hepatic CT and ultrasound scans show a focal defect. On hepatic angiography, the lesions range from avascular to hypervascular and cannot usually be distinguished from malignant hepatoma. Aspiration biopsy is safe, but core needle biopsy is risky because of the danger of bleeding.

Symptomatic hepatic adenomas should be resected; in acutely bleeding patients, this may be lifesaving. Some may be removed by wedge resection, but deep-seated or large lesions usually require partial hepatectomy. Hepatic adenomas may regress when oral contraceptive agents are discontinued, and expectant management is appropriate for asymptomatic or mildly symptomatic lesions smaller than about 6 cm. The tumor should be followed by periodic ultrasound or CT scan and resection recommended if it enlarges. The possibility that the tumor may be a hepatoma must always be kept in mind, because there is no completely reliable means of making the differentiation. In fact, even at laparotomy it may be difficult to distinguish between hepatoma and hepatic adenoma by gross inspection or frozen section examination. Large hepatic adenomas should be removed without a period of expectant management, because they are more likely to bleed or be malignant.

Most patients recover without sequelae after surgical removal; recurrence is rare. Oral contraceptives should be proscribed permanently in all cases. Radiotherapy and chemotherapy are of no value.

Focal Nodular Hyperplasia

Focal nodular hyperplasia is a benign lesion with no malignant potential. It is found in women twice as often as in men. The average age is about 40 years, but the tumor can occur at any age. The use of oral contraceptive agents may stimulate the development or growth of this tumor.

Grossly, the tumor is a well-circumscribed, firm, tan, usually subcapsular mass measuring 2–3 cm in diameter. In patients with symptoms, the lesions average 4–7 cm in diameter and occasionally are multiple. Eighty percent are solitary. The appearance on cut section is pathognomonic, consisting of a central stellate scar with radiating fibrous septa that compartmentalize the lesion into lobules. Histologically, there are nodular aggregations of normal-appearing hepatocytes without central veins or portal triads. Bile duct proliferation is present in the nodules.

Most patients with focal nodular hyperplasia are asymptomatic. The few with symptoms present with a right upper quadrant mass, discomfort, or both. Unlike hepatic adenomas, these lesions rarely grow or bleed, and the natural history of asymptomatic lesions is benign. A few patients with diffuse focal nodular hyperplasia develop portal hypertension.

Hepatic function tests and AFP levels are usually normal. Hepatic scintiscans usually do not show a filling defect; CT scans demonstrate the tumor and usually the central stellate scar. The arteriographic pattern is one of hypervascularity.

Patients taking oral contraceptives should have these drugs withdrawn. Symptomatic lesions should be removed; asymptomatic ones (the majority) should be left undisturbed. Focal nodular hyperplasia can be reliably identified on examination of frozen sections.

Bioulac-Sage P, Balabaud C, Wanless IR: Diagnosis of focal nodular hyperplasia: not so easy. Am J Surg Pathol 2001;25:1322.

Leconte I et al: Focal nodular hyperplasia: natural course observed with CT and MRI. J Comput Assist Tomogr 2000 Jan-Feb;24:61.

Terkivatan T et al: Indications and long-term outcome of treatment for benign hepatic tumors: a critical appraisal. Arch Surg 2001;136:1033.

Terkivatan T et al: Treatment of ruptured hepatocellular adenoma. Br J Surg 2001;88:207.

PORTAL HYPERTENSION

Etiology

The causes of portal hypertension are listed in Table 25–2. In all but a few instances, the basic lesion is increased resistance to portal flow. Those associated with increased resistance can be subclassified according to the site of the block as prehepatic, hepatic, and posthepatic. Cirrhosis accounts for about 85% of cases of portal hypertension in the USA, and the most common form is that due to alcoholism. Postnecrotic cirrhosis is next in frequency, followed by biliary cirrhosis. The other intrahepatic causes of portal hypertension are relatively rare in this country, although in some parts of the world hepatic schistosomiasis constitutes the largest single group. Idiopathic portal hypertension occurs with greater frequency in southern Asia.

Next to cirrhosis, extrahepatic portal venous occlusion is the most common cause of portal hypertension in the USA. These patients are generally younger than the cirrhotics, and many are children. Posthepatic obstruction due to Budd-Chiari syndrome or constrictive pericarditis is rare.

Table 25–2. Causes of portal hypertension.

I. Increased resistance to flow
  A. Prehepatic (portal vein obstruction)
    1. Congenital atresia or stenosis
    2. Thrombosis of portal vein
    3. Thrombosis of splenic vein
    4. Extrinsic compression (eg, tumors)
  B. Hepatic
    1. Cirrhosis
      a. Portal cirrhosis (nutritional, alcoholic, Laennec's)
      b. Postnecrotic cirrhosis
      c. Biliary cirrhosis
      d. Others (Wilson's disease, hemochromatosis)
    2. Acute alcoholic liver disease
    3. Congenital hepatic fibrosis
    4. Idiopathic portal hypertension (hepatoportal sclerosis)
    5. Schistosomiasis
  C. Posthepatic
    1. Budd-Chiari syndrome
    2. Constrictive pericarditis
II. Increased portal blood flow
  A. Arterial-portal venous fistula
  B. Increased splenic flow
    1. Banti's syndrome
    2. Splenomegaly (eg, tropical splenomegaly, myeloid metaplasia)

Pathophysiology

Since pressure in the portal venous system is determined by the relationship $P = F \times R$, portal hypertension could result either from increased volume of portal blood flow or increased resistance to flow. In practice, however, all but a few cases are caused by increased resistance, though the site of the resistance varies in different diseases. A pathophysiologic classification of the causes of portal hypertension is given in Table 25–2.

Portal venous pressure normally ranges from 7 to 10 mm Hg. In portal hypertension, portal pressure exceeds 10 mm Hg, averaging around 20 mm Hg and occasionally rising as high as 50–60 mm Hg.

In alcoholic liver disease, the abnormal resistance is predominantly at the postsinusoidal position, as shown by the results of wedged hepatic vein pressure studies.*

---

*A catheter wedged in a tributary of the hepatic vein permits estimation of the pressure in the afferent veins to the sinusoid. The gradient between the wedged pressure and that in the hepatic vein reflects resistance at any point between the wedged position and the periphery of the sinusoid. The current view holds that the site of principal resistance in normal persons is in reasonably large hepatic veins. In cirrhosis, it is probably in the sinusoids as well as the hepatic veins.

The causes of increased resistance in this disease are thought to be (1) distortion of the hepatic veins by regenerative nodules and (2) fibrosis of the hepatic veins and perisinusoidal areas.

Even in the absence of cirrhosis, acute alcoholism can raise portal pressure by producing centrilobular swelling and fibrosis. Sinusoidal resistance to flow is also increased by engorgement of adjacent hepatocytes with fat and resultant distortion and narrowing of the vascular pathway. Cases have been documented where the elevated portal pressure dropped with resolution of the pathologic changes.

Schistosomiasis alone produces a presinusoidal block as a consequence of deposition of parasite ova in small portal venules. However, many patients with schistosomiasis who have bleeding varies or other complications of liver disease also harbor chronic hepatitis B infection, which produces concomitant cirrhosis.

Fluctuations in the level of portal hypertension also occur in conjunction with changes in blood volume, and patients with ascites are especially sensitive. Administration of colloid solutions to a patient with a normal or expanded blood volume could theoretically aggravate the clinical manifestations of portal hypertension.

Budd-Chiari syndrome is produced by restriction to flow through the hepatic veins or the inferior vena cava above the liver. The resulting sinusoidal hypertension produces prominent ascites and hepatomegaly.

Banti's syndrome was defined as liver disease secondary to primary splenic disease and was incorrectly considered to explain the average case of portal hypertension now known to result from cirrhosis and other kinds of hepatic disease.

The average portal flow in cirrhotic patients with complications of portal hypertension is about 30% of normal, ranging from 0 to 700 mL/min. Hepatic arterial flow is usually reduced by a similar proportion. The range of portal flow rates in different patients may vary greatly; in a few, blood in the portal vein moves only sluggishly, and in rare instances the direction of flow may even be reversed so that the portal vein functions as an outflow tract from the liver. These states of low flow predispose to spontaneous thrombosis of the portal vein, a complication of cirrhosis that usually renders the portal vein unsuitable for a shunt.

The obstacle to flow through the liver stimulates expansion of collateral channels between the portal and systemic venous systems. As the pathologic process develops, portal pressure increases until a level of about 40 cm H_2O (30 mm Hg) is reached. At this point, increasing hepatic resistance, even to the point of occlusion of the portal vein, diverts a greater fraction of portal flow through the collaterals without significant increments in portal pressure.

The type of collateral that develops depends partly on the cause of the portal hypertension. In extrahepatic portal vein thrombosis (without liver disease), collaterals (hepatopetal) in the diaphragm, in the hepatocolic and hepatogastric ligaments, etc, transport blood into the liver around the occluded vein. In both cirrhosis and portal vein thrombosis, collaterals (hepatofugal) appear that carry blood around the liver into the systemic circulation, and it is these that produce esophageal and gastric varices. Other common spontaneous collaterals are through a recanalized umbilical vein to the abdominal wall, from the superior hemorrhoidal vein into the middle and inferior hemorrhoidal veins, and through numerous small veins (of Retzius) connecting the retroperitoneal viscera with the posterior abdominal wall.

Isolated thrombosis of the splenic vein causes localized splenic venous hypertension and gives rise to large collaterals from spleen to gastric fundus. From there, the blood returns to the main portal system through the coronary vein. In this condition, gastric varices are often present without esophageal varices.

Of the many large collaterals that form as a result of portal hypertension, spontaneous bleeding is rare except from those at the gastroesophageal junction; the reason for this bleeding is only vaguely understood. Compared with adjacent areas of the esophagus and stomach, this segment is especially rich in submucosal veins, which expand disproportionately in patients with portal hypertension. The cause of variceal bleeding is most probably rupture of one of these veins due to sudden increases in hydrostatic pressure. Esophagitis is not present.

Increased flow may contribute to portal hypertension in patients with traumatic arterial-portal venous fistulas and perhaps in some cases of giant splenomegaly, as in myeloid metaplasia or tropical splenomegaly. When an arteriovenous fistula occurs, portal hypertension and its clinical manifestations usually do not appear for several months, because sinusoidal capacity is so great that the immediate rise in portal pressure is only moderate. With time, however, sinusoidal sclerosis develops, resistance increases, and portal pressure gradually reaches high levels and stimulates variceal formation. Even in cirrhosis, the increased splenic blood flow accompanying "congestive" splenomegaly may occasionally be great enough so that splenic artery ligation or splenectomy decreases portal pressure.

Debernardi-Venon W et al: CO_2 wedged hepatic venography in the evaluation of portal hypertension. Gut 2000;46:856.

Krige JE, Beckingham IJ: ABC of diseases of liver, pancreas, and biliary system. Portal hypertension—1: varices. BMJ 2001; 322:348.

Krige JE, Beckingham IJ: ABC of diseases of liver, pancreas, and biliary system: portal hypertension—2. Ascites, encephalopathy, and other conditions. BMJ 2001;322:416.

CIRRHOSIS

The death rate from cirrhosis exceeds 23,000 per year in the USA. The incidence of the disease is increasing, and at present it is the third most common cause of death in men in the fifth decade of life.

The alcoholic person satisfies caloric needs from dietary alcohol to the exclusion of other important nutrients such as protein, vitamins, and minerals. Alcohol exerts direct toxic effects on the liver that are magnified in the presence of protein deficiency, but it is not known why only 15% of alcoholics develop cirrhosis. Alcohol induces a specific cytochrome P450 in the liver (ie, P450 2E1) that participates in the metabolism of alcohol. Acetaldehyde production is increased, which has a host of deleterious effects—antibody formation, decreased DNA repair, enzyme inactivation, and alterations in microtubules, mitochondria, and plasma membranes. Acetaldehyde also promotes glutathione depletion, toxicity mediated by free radicals, lipid peroxidation, and hepatic collagen synthesis. Hepatic steatosis and alcoholic hepatitis are stages of alcoholic liver injury that precede cirrhosis. Alcoholic hyalin, a glycoprotein, accumulates in centrilobular hepatocytes of patients with alcoholic hepatitis. There is some evidence that immunologic responses to alcoholic hyalin may be important in the pathogenesis of cirrhosis.

Collagen deposition in cirrhosis results from primary increased fibroblastic activity as well as from repair following hepatocellular necrosis. The ultimate result is a liver containing regenerative nodules and connective tissue septa linking portal fields with central canals.

The natural history of cirrhosis is not fully known. Once the diagnosis has been established, about 30% or more of patients are dead within a year. In newly diagnosed cirrhotics, the chances of dying within the subsequent 2–3 years are influenced by the status of liver function (as reflected by the Child-Pugh classification), the presence of large varices, and the absolute height of the portal pressure. A group of cirrhotics with varices followed by the Boston Interhospital Liver Group experienced a 1-year death rate of 66%. Cirrhotics without varices may benefit substantially by returning to a nutritious diet and abstaining from alcohol. Bleeding occurs in about 40% of all patients with cirrhosis, and the initial episode of variceal hemorrhage is fatal to 50–80%. At least two-thirds of those who survive their initial hemorrhage will bleed again, and the risk of dying from the second is about the same as from the first episode. It is principally for such patients that portacaval shunts are recommended.

Menon KV, Gores GJ, Shah VH: Pathogenesis, diagnosis, and treatment of alcoholic liver disease. Mayo Clin Proc 2001; 76:1021.

Menon KV, Kamath PS: Managing the complications of cirrhosis. Mayo Clin Proc 2000;75:501.

ACUTELY BLEEDING VARICES

About half of patients with massive bleeding from varices die as a result of the acute event. This high death rate reflects not only the amount and rate of hemorrhage but also the frequent presence of severely compromised liver function and other systemic disease that may or may not be related to alcoholism. Malnutrition, pulmonary aspiration and infection, and coronary artery disease are frequent coexistent factors. The alcoholic patient often does not cooperate during therapy, and if delirium tremens ensues, even physical control of the patient may present a major challenge.

Clinical Findings

A. SYMPTOMS AND SIGNS

The initial management of the patient with massive gastrointestinal hemorrhage is discussed in Chapter 24. It must be emphasized that bleeding from varices cannot be accurately diagnosed on clinical grounds alone even though the history or the appearance of the patient may strongly suggest the presence of cirrhosis or portal hypertension. Most patients with bleeding varices have alcoholic cirrhosis, and the diagnosis may seem obvious in a patient with hepatomegaly, jaundice, and vascular spiders who admits to a recent alcoholic binge. Splenomegaly, the most constant physical finding, is present in 80% of patients with portal hypertension regardless of the cause. Ascites is frequently present. Massive ascites and hepatosplenomegaly in a nonalcoholic would suggest the rare Budd-Chiari syndrome. If cirrhosis or varices have been documented on previous examinations, hematemesis later may point toward bleeding varices.

B. LABORATORY FINDINGS

Most alcoholics with acute upper gastrointestinal bleeding have compromised liver function. The bilirubin is usually elevated, and the serum albumin is often below 3 g/dL. The leukocyte count may be elevated. Anemia may be a reflection of chronic alcoholic liver disease or hypersplenism as well as acute hemorrhage. The development of a hepatoma by a cirrhotic sometimes is first manifested by bleeding varices; CT scan and determination of serum alpha-fetoprotein will make the diagnosis. The prothrombin time and partial thromboplastin time may be abnormal.

C. SPECIAL EXAMINATIONS

1. Esophagogastroscopy—Emergency esophagogastroscopy is the most useful procedure for diagnosing bleeding varices and should be scheduled as soon as the patient's general condition is stabilized by blood transfusion and other supportive measures. Varices appear as three or four large, tortuous submucosal bluish vessels running longitudinally in the distal esophagus. The bleeding site may be identified, but sometimes the lumen fills with blood so rapidly that the lesion is obscured.

2. Upper gastrointestinal series—A barium swallow outlines the varices in about 90% of affected patients, but barium studies are neither as sensitive nor as specific as endoscopy, and they are difficult and dangerous in the bleeding patient.

Treatment of Acute Bleeding

The general goal of treatment is to control the bleeding as quickly and reliably as possible using methods with the fewest possible side effects. The methods currently in use for acute variceal bleeding are listed in Table 25–3.

The patient's condition is stabilized to the extent possible by following the general guidelines for treating upper gastrointestinal bleeding described in Chapter 24. Other therapy should include measures to treat or prevent encephalopathy, parenteral vitamin K to correct a prolonged prothrombin time, and electrolytes (especially potassium) as required to restore electrolyte balance.

Acute endoscopic sclerotherapy is the first treatment recommended by most experts. Vasopressin or propranolol may or may not be included in the initial resuscitative regimen. Balloon tamponade is no longer used as a routine—as it once was—but is reserved for special situations when simpler methods fail.

These measures are successful in stopping the bleeding in about 90% of cases, but the early rebleeding rate is about 30%. When bleeding continues and if the patient is a good operative risk, emergency shunt is the preferred treatment.

Death rates rise rapidly in patients receiving more than ten units of blood, and in general, patients still bleeding after six units—or those whose bleeding is still unchecked 24 hours after admission—should be considered for operation. Whether or not the bleeding is brought under control, the mortality rate among patients who present with acutely bleeding varices is high (about 35%) as a result of liver failure and other complications.

SPECIFIC MEASURES

1. Acute endoscopic sclerotherapy or ligation—Via fiberoptic endoscopy, 1–3 mL of sclerosant solution is injected into the lumen of each varix, causing it to become thrombosed. Variations in the kind of endoscope, different sclerosant solutions, whether or not the varices are physically compressed, etc, appear to have little influence on the outcome. Endoscopy is usually repeated within 48 hours and then once or twice again at weekly intervals, at which time any residual varices are injected.

Sclerotherapy controls acute bleeding in 80–95% of patients, and rebleeding during the same hospitalization is about half (25% versus 50%) the rebleeding rate of patients treated with a combination of vasopressin and balloon tamponade. Even though controlled trials show improvement in the control of bleeding, the evidence is conflicting on whether this results in increased patient survival.

A somewhat similar effect can be achieved by endoscopic rubber band ligation of the varices. The varix is lifted with a suction tip, and a small rubber band is slipped around the base. The varix necroses to leave a superficial ulcer. A controlled trial has reported rubber band ligation to be more effective in controlling bleeding (eg, fewer episodes of rebleeding; lower mortality rate) than sclerotherapy.

2. Vasopressin and terlipressin (triglycyl lysine vasopressin)—Vasopressin and terlipressin lower portal blood flow and portal pressure by a direct constricting action on splanchnic arterioles. Acute bleeding is controlled in about 80% of patients—when used in conjunction with balloon tamponade, in about 95% of patients. Cardiac output, oxygen delivery to the tissues, hepatic blood flow, and renal blood flow are also decreased—effects that occasionally produce complications such as myocardial infarction, cardiac arrhythmias, and intestinal necrosis. These unwanted side effects may sometimes be prevented without interfering with the decrease in portal pressure by simultaneous administration of nitroglycerin or isoproterenol.

Although the results are somewhat contradictory, controlled trials generally indicate that vasopressin plus

Table 25–3. Measures to control acute bleeding from esophageal varices.

Noninterventional
1. Vasopressin, terlipressin
2. Somatostatin analogs
3. Balloon tamponade

Interventional, nonsurgical
4. Endoscopic sclerotherapy
5. Transphepatic embolization and sclerotherapy

Surgical
6. Emergency portasystemic shunts
7. Esophageal transection and reanastomosis
8. Esophagogastric devascularization
9. Suture ligation of varices

nitroglycerin is superior to vasopressin alone and that vasopressin alone is superior to placebo in controlling active variceal bleeding. Survival is not increased, however. Vasopressin is given as a peripheral intravenous infusion (at about 0.4 units/min), which is safer than bolus injections. The nitroglycerin can be given intravenously or sublingually. Terlipressin, a synthetic vasopressin analog, undergoes gradual conversion to vasopressin in the body and is safe to give by intravenous bolus injection (2 mg intravenously every 6 hours). It may cause fewer cardiac side effects than vasopressin.

3. Octreotide acetate—Somatostatin and the synthetic longer-lasting analog octreotide have the same effect on the splanchnic circulation as vasopressin but without significant side effects. These drugs are as effective as vasopressin in controlling acute variceal bleeding and are now the first choice for the pharmacologic control of acutely bleeding varices. Octreotide is given as an initial bolus of 100 μg followed by a continuous infusion of 25 μ/h for 24 hours.

4. Balloon tamponade—(Figure 25–7.) Tubes designed for tamponade have two balloons that can be inflated in the lumen of the gut to compress bleeding varices. There are three or four lumens in the tube: two are for filling the balloons and the third permits aspiration of gastric contents. A fourth lumen in the Minnesota tube is used to aspirate the esophagus orad to the esophageal balloon. The main effect is due to traction

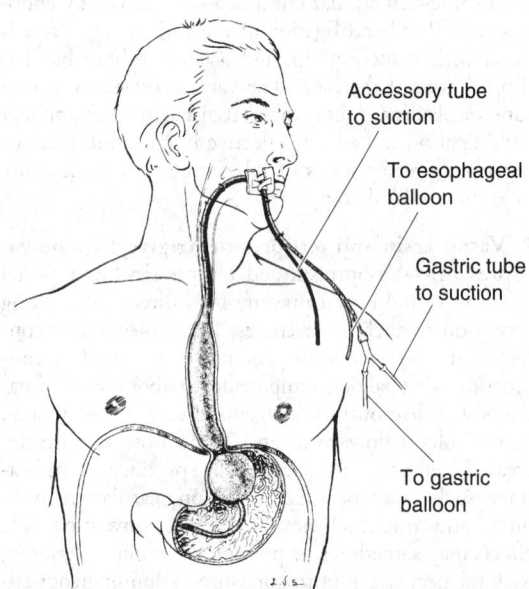

Figure 25–7. Sengstaken-Blakemore tube with both gastric and esophageal balloons inflated.

applied to the tube, which forces the gastric balloon to compress the collateral veins at the cardia of the stomach. Inflating the esophageal balloon probably contributes little, since barium x-rays suggest that it does not actually compress the varices.

The most common serious complication is aspiration of pharyngeal secretions and pneumonitis.

Another serious hazard is the occasional instance of esophageal rupture caused by inflation of the esophageal balloon. To avoid this risk, the instructions packaged with the tube must be followed carefully.

About 75% of actively bleeding patients can be controlled by balloon tamponade. When bleeding has stopped, the balloons are left inflated for another 24 hours. They are then decompressed, leaving the tube in place. If bleeding does not recur, the tube should be withdrawn.

5. Transjugular intrahepatic portasystemic shunt (TIPS)—This is a minimally invasive way of creating a shunt between the portal vein and the hepatic vein through the liver. A catheter is introduced through the jugular vein and, under radiologic control, positioned in the hepatic vein. From this point, the portal vein is accessed through the liver, the tract is dilated, and the channel is kept open by inserting an expandable metal stent, which is left in place. This technique is of great value in controlling portal hypertension and variceal bleeding and can be used to stop acute bleeding or to prevent rebleeding in a patient who has recovered from an acute episode. The shunts remain open in most patients for up to a year, at which point intimal overgrowth and thrombosis occlude a gradually increasing number.

TIPS has its greatest usefulness as a bridge to transplantation. With current materials, it should probably not be regarded as definitive therapy, though the shunt will usually remain patent for many months. Thus, patients with advanced liver disease are the principal candidates for TIPS, whereas those with less severe disease should be considered for propranolol therapy or a standard shunt operation.

6. Surgery—The operative procedures to control active bleeding are emergency portasystemic shunt and variceal ligation or esophageal transection.

a. Emergency portacaval shunt—An emergency portasystemic shunt has a 95% rate of success in stopping variceal bleeding. The death rate of the operation is related to the status of the patient's liver function (eg, Child-Pugh classification) (Table 25–4) as well as the rate and amount of bleeding and its effects on cardiac, renal, and pulmonary function. Some patients with advanced liver disease—especially those with severe encephalopathy and ascites—are so unlikely to survive that surgery is unwarranted for them despite continued

Table 25–4. Child-Pugh classification of functional status in liver diseases.

Class: Risk:	A Low	B Moderate	C High
Ascites	Absent	Slight to moderate	Tense
Encephalopathy	None	Grades I–II	Grades III–IV
Serum albumin (g/dL)	> 3.5	3.0–3.5	< 3.0
Serum bilirubin (mg/dL)	< 2.0	2.0–3.0	> 3.0
Prothrombin time (seconds above control)	< 4.0	4.0–6.0	> 6.0

bleeding. On the other hand, patients with good liver function usually recover after an emergency shunt. The only relevant controlled trial showed that the death rate in acutely bleeding Child's C patients was insignificantly lower after endoscopic sclerotherapy (44%) than after emergency portacaval shunt (50%).

For active bleeding, an end-to-side portacaval shunt or H-mesocaval shunt is most commonly performed.

The distal splenorenal (Warren) shunt is usually too time-consuming for use in emergency operations. The central splenorenal shunt is more complicated than an end-to-side portacaval shunt and has no specific advantages. A side-to-side portacaval shunt might be preferable in an acutely bleeding patient with severe ascites, and it or a variant (eg, H-mesocaval shunt) would be required for someone with Budd-Chiari syndrome.

Hepatic failure is the cause of death in about two-thirds of those who succumb after an emergency portacaval shunt. Renal failure, which is often accompanied by ascites, is another potentially lethal problem. Metabolic alkalosis and delirium tremens are common postoperatively in alcoholics. Antacids should be given for 1–2 weeks after surgery to prevent stress ulceration.

b. Esophageal transection—Varices may be obliterated by firing the end-to-end stapler in the distal esophagus after tucking a full-thickness ring of tissue into the cartridge with a circumferential tie. This procedure has gained popularity in the past decade, and in many surgical units it is the first choice for therapy when nonsurgical methods fail. If transection is performed, it must be done as soon as it is recognized that a second attempt at sclerotherapy or band ligation has failed. As a last-ditch effort—after many units of blood have been transfused—death from liver failure is all but

certain. The results (eg, survival) are better in patients with nonalcoholic cirrhosis. Stapled transection has replaced the older technique of direct suture ligation of the varices. Transection must be viewed as an emergency measure to stop persistent bleeding—not as definitive treatment—because varices recur months later in many patients.

Cales P et al: Early administration of vapreotide for variceal bleeding in patients with cirrhosis. French Club for the Study of Portal Hypertension. N Engl J Med 2001;344:23.

Gerbes AL et al: Transjugular intrahepatic portosystemic shunt (TIPS) for variceal bleeding in portal hypertension: comparison of emergency and elective interventions. Dig Dis Sci 1998;43:2463.

Mercado MA et al: Comparative study of 2 variants of a modified esophageal transection in the Sugiura-Futagawa operation. Arch Surg 1998;133:1046.

Orozco H et al: A comparative study of the elective treatment of variceal hemorrhage with beta-blockers, transendoscopic sclerotherapy, and surgery: a prospective, controlled, and randomized trial during 10 years. Ann Surg 2000;232:216.

Shibata D et al: Transjugular intrahepatic portosystemic shunt for treatment of bleeding ectopic varices with portal hypertension. Dis Colon Rectum 1999;42:1581.

Woods JE, Kiely JM: Short-term international medical service. Mayo Clin Proc 2000;75:311.

NONBLEEDING VARICES

Patients with varices that have never bled have a 30% chance of bleeding; and of those who bleed, 50% die. For patients who do not bleed during the first year after diagnosis of varices, the risk of bleeding subsequently decreases by half and continues to drop thereafter. Patients who have bled once from esophageal varices have a 70% chance of bleeding again, and about two-thirds of repeat bleeding episodes are fatal.

Evaluation

A. SEVERITY OF HEPATIC DISEASE AND OPERATIVE RISK

The immediate death rate of an elective shunt procedure can be predicted from the patient's hepatic function as reflected by the Child-Pugh classification (Table 25–4). In addition to operative death rate, the figures also correlate with the death rate in the first postshunt year. Thereafter, survival curves of the different risk classes become reasonably parallel.

The severity of histopathologic changes in liver biopsies correlates with the immediate surgical death rate, the most ominous findings being hepatocellular necrosis, polymorphonuclear leukocyte infiltration, and the presence of Mallory bodies. The extent of histologic change also correlates with the more easily obtained data in the Child-Pugh classification (ie, severe changes occur in class C patients), so results of biopsies have no independent predictive value.

B. PORTAL FLOW AND PRESSURE MEASUREMENTS

Measurements of pressure and flow in the splanchnic vasculature have been used for diagnosis and as a guide to therapy and prognosis in portal hypertension. Portal pressure can be measured directly at surgery or preoperatively by any of the following techniques: (1) Wedged hepatic venous pressure (WHVP), which accurately reflects free portal pressure when portal hypertension is caused by a postsinusoidal (or sinusoidal) resistance, as in cirrhosis. The measurement obtained with the catheter in the wedged position should be corrected by subtracting the free hepatic venous pressure (FHVP). This is the most commonly used technique. (2) Direct measurement of splenic pulp pressure by a percutaneously placed needle. (3) Percutaneous transhepatic catheterization of the intrahepatic branches of the portal vein. This is the method of choice in patients thought to have presinusoidal block or Budd-Chiari syndrome. (4) Catheterization of the umbilical vein through a small incision, the catheter being threaded into the portal system. With each of these methods, one may also obtain anatomic information by performing angiography through the catheter.

It is not customary in the average case to measure portal pressure preoperatively, however, since the information obtained does not influence management of the average case.

Duplex ultrasonography is an accurate noninvasive means of assessing the amount and direction of flow in the portal vein. Preoperatively, duplex ultrasonography is useful to determine patency of the portal vein and direction of flow. Because of spontaneous thrombosis, about 10% of patients with cirrhosis have a portal vein unsuitable for a portacaval shunt. If flow in the portal vein is reversed (hepatofugal), a selective shunt is not recommended, because it compromises the ability of portal tributaries to serve as an outflow tract for liver blood. Duplex ultrasonography can also be used to follow changes in portal perfusion after shunt operations.

C. PORTAL ANGIOGRAPHY

The portal venous anatomy is often studied preoperatively by angiographic techniques. The objectives are to determine the patency, location, and size of the veins tentatively chosen for a shunt, to demonstrate the presence of varices, and to estimate the degree of prograde portal flow. Some of this information can now be obtained less invasively by duplex ultrasonography. When a splenorenal shunt is contemplated, the left renal vein should be opacified, either by injection of the renal artery or renal vein.

Treatment

The treatment options consist of expectant management, endoscopic sclerotherapy, propranolol, portasystemic shunts, devascularization of the esophagogastric junction, and miscellaneous rarely used operations. The treatment of patients with varices that have never bled is usually referred to as "prophylactic" therapy (eg, "prophylactic" sclerotherapy or "prophylactic" propranolol). By convention, procedures performed on patients who have bled previously are referred to as "therapeutic" (eg, "therapeutic" shunts).

A. PROPHYLACTIC THERAPY

Prophylactic therapy could theoretically be of value since the mortality rate of variceal bleeding is high (50%), the risk of bleeding in patients with varices is relatively high (30%), and varices can often be diagnosed before the initial episode of bleeding. In patients who have never bled before, the following have been shown to be related to the risk of bleeding: Child-Pugh classification, the size of the varices, and the presence of red wale markings (longitudinal dilated venules resembling whip marks) on the varices. This information can be used to identify and consider for prophylactic propranolol those patients who have a 65% chance of bleeding within a year.

B. THERAPY OF PATIENTS WHO HAVE BLED PREVIOUSLY

As noted earlier, patients who recover from an episode of variceal bleeding have about a 70% chance of bleeding again. Much effort is being expended in attempts to ascertain the best treatment regimen for these patients. The methods of greatest interest include endoscopic sclerotherapy, propranolol, and various kinds of portasystemic shunts.

1. Endoscopic sclerotherapy—The technique of endoscopic sclerotherapy was described earlier in this chapter. Chronic sclerotherapy has been disappointing as a method for preventing future bleeding, and most have come to think of it principally as a way to stop acute bleeding when bleeding recurs.

2. Propranolol—Propranolol, a β-adrenergic blocking agent, decreases cardiac output and splanchnic blood flow and consequently portal blood pressure. Chronic propranolol therapy, 20–160 mg twice daily (a dose that reduces resting pulse rate by 25%), decreases by about 40% the frequency of rebleeding from esophageal or gastric varices, deaths from rebleeding, and overall mortality. The benefits are greater in Child's A and B than in Child's C cirrhotics. The addition of chronic sclerotherapy to the propranolol regimen does not improve the outcome. Abstinence from alcohol may not be critical to success, as was initially thought.

C. SURGERY

The objective of the surgical procedures used to treat portal hypertension is either to obliterate the varices or to reduce blood flow and pressure within the varices (Table 25–5). A more recent option is liver transplantation.

1. Liver transplantation—Any relatively young patient with cirrhosis who has survived an episode of variceal hemorrhage should be considered a candidate for liver transplantation, since any other form of ther-

Table 25–5. Surgical procedures for esophageal varices.

A. Direct variceal obliteration
1. Variceal suture ligation
   a. Transthoracic
   b. Transabdominal
2. Esophageal transection and reanastomosis
   a. Suture technique
   b. Staple technique
3. Variceal sclerosis
   a. Esophagoscopic
   b. Transhepatic
4. Variceal resection
   a. Esophagogastrectomy
   b. Subtotal esophagectomy
B. Reduction of variceal blood flow and pressure
1. Portasystemic shunts
   a. End-to-side
   b. Side-to-side
      1. Side-to-side portacaval
      2. Mesocaval
      3. Central splenorenal
      4. Renosplenic
2. Selective shunts
   a. Distal splenorenal (Warren)
   b. Left gastric vena caval (Inokuchi)
3. Reduction of portal blood flow
   a. Splenectomy
   b. Splenic artery ligation
4. Reduction of proximal gastric blood flow
   a. Esphagogastric devascularization
   b. Gastric transection and reanastomosis (Tanner)
5. Stimulation of additional portasystemic venous collaterals
   a. Omentopexy
   b. Splenic transposition
C. Measures to preserve hepatic blood flow after portacaval shunt
1. Arterialization of portal vein stump

---

apy carries a much higher (about 80%) mortality rate within the subsequent year or two as a result of repeated bleeding or complications of hepatic failure. Obviously, continued alcoholism will serve as an absolute contraindication to transplantation in most patients. The good transplantation candidates, however, should not be subjected to portasystemic shunts or other procedures if it appears that they will come to transplantation in the near future. In general, Child's class A patients are candidates for portal decompression; Child's class C patients are candidates for a transplant. A transjugular intrahepatic shunt (see previous section) is an excellent way to control bleeding while the patient is being prepared for a transplant.

2. Portasystemic shunts—Portasystemic shunts can be grouped into those that shunt the entire portal system (total shunts) and those that selectively shunt blood from the gastrosplenic region while preserving the pressure-flow relationships in the rest of the portal bed (selective shunts). All of the shunt operations commonly used today reduce the incidence of rebleeding to less than 10%, compared with about 75% in unshunted patients. Unfortunately, the price of this achievement is an operative mortality rate of 5–20% (depending on the Child-Pugh classification [Table 25–4]), decreased liver function, and an increase in encephalopathy (at least with total shunts). Therefore, since shunts have these drawbacks in addition to the ability to prevent bleeding, experimental trials are needed to pinpoint their place within an overall treatment strategy.

In one well-designed trial, patients who had bled previously were randomized to chronic sclerotherapy or a distal splenorenal shunt (Warren shunt). Patients randomized to chronic sclerotherapy who had recurrent episodes of bleeding during treatment (ie, treatment failures, which amounted to 30% of the sclerotherapy group) were then treated surgically (ie, shunted). The results showed that 2-year survival was better among those originally randomized to sclerotherapy (90%) than among those originally assigned to the shunt group (60%). This trial supports a general treatment plan consisting initially of sclerotherapy and reserving portasystemic shunts for the patients in whom sclerotherapy fails to control bleeding adequately.

The choice of what kind of shunt to use has been the subject of much debate and several randomized trials. The principal question in recent years has been whether encephalopathy and survival are better with a selective shunt (eg, a distal splenorenal shunt) than with a total shunt (eg, a mesocaval or an end-to-side portacaval shunt). The results are conflicting, but in general they support the contention that there is about half as much severe encephalopathy following selective shunts.

None of the trials have shown any particular shunt to be associated with longer survival than other shunts.

a. Types of portasystemic shunts—Figure 25–8 depicts the various shunts in use at this time. Although they differ technically, physiologically there are only three different types: end-to-side, side-to-side, and selective.

(1) Total shunts—The end-to-side shunt completely disconnects the liver from the portal system. The portal vein is transected near its bifurcation in the liver hilum and anastomosed to the side of the inferior vena cava. The hepatic stump of the vein is oversewn. Postoperatively, the wedged hepatic venous pressure (sinusoidal pressure) drops slightly, reflecting the inability of the hepatic artery to compensate fully for the loss of portal inflow. The side-to-side portacaval, mesocaval, mesorenal, and central splenorenal shunts are all physiologically similar, since the shunt preserves continuity between the hepatic limb of the portal vein, the portal system, and the anastomosis. Flow through the hepatic limb of the standard side-to-side shunt is nearly always away from the liver and toward the anastomosis. The extent to which hepatofugal flow is produced by the other types of "side-to-side" shunts listed above is not known.

The end-to-side portacaval shunt gives immediate and permanent protection from variceal bleeding and is somewhat easier to perform than a side-to-side portacaval or central splenorenal shunt. Encephalopathy may be slightly more common after side-to-side than end-to-side portacaval shunts. Side-to-side shunts are required in patients with Budd-Chiari syndrome or refractory ascites (when the latter is treated by a portasystemic shunt).

The mesocaval shunt interposes a segment of prosthetic graft or internal jugular vein between the inferior vena cava and the superior mesenteric vein where the latter passes in front of the uncinate process of the pancreas. The mesocaval shunt is particularly useful in the presence of severe scarring in the right upper quadrant or portal vein thrombosis, and in some cases it may be technically easier than a conventional side-to-side portacaval shunt if a side-to-side type of shunt is necessary. In most cases, portal flow to the liver is lost after this shunt. Evidence has been presented, however, that by limiting the diameter of the prosthetic graft to 8 mm (compared with 12- to 20-mm grafts), prograde flow is preserved in the portal vein, which decreases the incidence of postoperative encephalopathy while still preventing variceal hemorrhage.

(2) Selective shunts—Selective shunts lower pressure in the gastroesophageal venous plexus while preserving blood flow through the liver via the portal vein.

The distal splenorenal (Warren) shunt involves anastomosing the distal (splenic) end of the transected splenic vein to the side of the left renal vein, plus ligation of the major collaterals between the remaining portal and isolated gastrosplenic venous system. The latter step involves division of the gastric vein, the right gastroepiploic vein, and the vessels in the splenocolic ligament. The operation is more difficult and time-consuming than conventional shunts and except for the experienced operator is probably too complex for emergency portal decompression. If mobilization of the splenic vein is hazardous, the renal vein may be transected and its caval end joined to the side of the undisturbed splenic vein. The segment of splenic vein between the anastomosis and the portal vein is then ligated. Surprisingly, this seems to have little permanent effect on renal function as long as the remaining tributaries are preserved on the oversewn renal vein stump.

In contrast to total shunts, the Warren shunt does not improve ascites and should not be performed in pa-

Figure 25–8. Types of portacaval anastomoses: *A:* Normal. *B:* Side-to-side. *C:* End-to-side. *D:* Mesocaval. *E:* Central splenorenal. *F:* Distal splenorenal (Warren). The H-mesocaval shunt is not illustrated

tients whose ascites has been difficult to control. Preoperative angiography should be performed to determine if the splenic vein and left renal vein are large enough and close enough together for performance of this shunt. Recent pancreatitis may preclude safe dissection of the splenic vein from the undersurface of the pancreas.

Another type of selective shunt (Inokuchi shunt) consists of joining the left gastric vein to the inferior vena cava by a short segment of autogenous saphenous vein. The procedure has not become popular, perhaps because of its technical complexity.

Selective shunts tend to become less selective over several years as new collaterals develop between the high- and low-pressure regions of the portal system. This is accompanied by a gradual decrease in portal pressure (measured by WHVP) and evolution of the procedure into a version of side-to-side total shunt. The enlargement postoperatively of small venous tributaries entering the distal splenic vein from the pancreas suggests that this is the path by which nonselectivity develops. It is possible that this can be avoided by mobilizing the splenic vein all the way to the hilum (dividing these small vessels) before performing the splenorenal anastomosis.

b. Choice of shunt—Our current approach to shunt selection is as follows: The distal splenorenal shunt is the first choice for elective portal decompression. If ascites is present or the anatomy is unfavorable, an end-to-side portacaval shunt is preferred. Side-to-side shunts would be done for patients with severe ascites or Budd-Chiari syndrome. We reserve the H-mesocaval and central splenorenal shunts for special anatomic situations in which the above operations are unsuitable. An end-to-side shunt or H-mesocaval shunt is performed for emergency decompression.

Portacaval and distal splenorenal shunts are often followed by a rise in platelet count in patients with secondary hypersplenism. Even though the response is unpredictable, however, hypersplenism rarely produces clinical manifestations, so it does not have to be taken into account in making a choice of shunt. A central splenorenal shunt, in which splenectomy is performed, should not be considered preferable to other kinds of shunt just because the patient has a low platelet count.

c. Results of portasystemic shunts—Over 90% of portasystemic shunts remain patent, and the incidence of recurrent variceal bleeding is less than 10%. The 5-year survival rate after a portacaval shunt for alcoholic liver disease averages 45%. Some degree of encephalopathy develops in 15–25% of patients. Severe encephalopathy is seen in about 20% of alcoholics following a total shunt; its occurrence is not related to the severity of preshunt encephalopathy.

D. Devascularization Operations

The objective of devascularization is to destroy the venous collaterals that transport blood from the high-pressure portal system into the veins in the submucosa of the esophagus.

The Sugiura procedure is done in two stages. In the first stage, performed through a thoracotomy, the dilated venous collaterals between esophagus and adjacent structures are divided, and the esophagus at the level of the diaphragm is transected and reanastomosed. The second stage, a laparotomy, is performed immediately after the thoracotomy if the patient is actively bleeding, but for elective cases it is deferred 4–6 weeks. The upper two-thirds of the stomach is devascularized, selective vagotomy and pyloroplasty are performed, and the spleen is removed. It is possible in some cases to perform the entire operation through the left chest. An analogous operation has been described that consists of splenectomy, gastroesophageal devascularization, and resection of a 5-cm segment of the gastroesophageal junction. Continuity of the gut is restored by an end-to-side esophagogastrostomy, and pyloroplasty is performed.

In the reports from Japan, where these operations originated, there was a 5% operative death rate, a 2–4% rate of variceal rebleeding, and an 80% 5-year survival rate. The new operations of this type performed in alcoholic patients in North America have had poor results, owing to a high rate (40%) of late rebleeding.

E. Miscellaneous Operations

Attempts have also been made to decrease portal pressure by decreasing splanchnic inflow through splenectomy or splenic artery ligation. Diseases characterized by marked splenomegaly may rarely be associated with portal hypertension as a consequence of increased splenic blood flow, which has been known to reach levels as high as 1000 mL/min. Splenic blood flow may occasionally be increased enough in patients with cirrhosis to contribute significantly to the portal hypertension. However, splenectomy or splenic artery ligation in cirrhosis most often gives only a transient decrease in portal pressure, and over half of patients having these operations bleed again. Some workers have suggested that the absolute size of the splenic artery (a crude index of splenic flow) correlates with the clinical effectiveness of splenic artery ligation, a good result being predictable if the diameter of the artery is 1 cm or greater.

de Franchis R: Updating consensus in portal hypertension: report of the Baveno III Consensus Workshop on definitions, methodology and therapeutic strategies in portal hypertension. J Hepatol 2000;33:846.

Gentilini P et al: Ascites and hepatorenal syndrome during cirrhosis: two entities or the continuation of the same complication? J Hepatol 1999;31:1088.

Krige JE, Beckingham IJ: ABC of diseases of liver, pancreas, and biliary system. Portal hypertension—1: varices. BMJ 2001; 322:348.

Lebrec D: Drug therapy for portal hypertension. Gut 2001;49:441.

Sarin SK et al: Comparison of endoscopic ligation and propranolol for the primary prevention of variceal bleeding. N Engl J Med 1999;340:988.

Suzuki H, Stanley AJ: Current management and novel therapeutic strategies for refractory ascites and hepatorenal syndrome. QJM 2001;94:293.

Vlachogiannakos J et al: Angiotensin converting enzyme inhibitors and angiotensin II antagonists as therapy in chronic liver disease. Gut 2001;49:303.

EXTRAHEPATIC PORTAL VENOUS OCCLUSION

Idiopathic portal vein thrombosis (in the absence of liver disease) accounts for most cases of portal hypertension in childhood and for a few cases in adults. Neonatal septicemia, omphalitis, umbilical vein catheterization for exchange transfusion, and dehydration have all been incriminated as possible causes, but collectively they can be implicated in less than half of cases. The causes of portal vein thrombosis in adults include hepatic tumors, cirrhosis, trauma, pancreatitis, pancreatic pseudocyst, myelofibrosis, thrombotic states (eg, protein C deficiency), and sepsis.

Although clinical manifestations may be delayed until adulthood, 80% of patients present between 1 and 6 years of age with variceal bleeding. About 70% of hemorrhages are preceded by a recent upper respiratory tract infection. Some of these children first come to medical attention because of splenomegaly and pancytopenia. Failure to recognize the underlying problem has occasionally led to splenectomy, with the result that portal decompression using the splenic vein is precluded. Ascites is uncommon except transiently after bleeding. Liver function is either normal or only slightly impaired, which probably accounts for the low incidence of overt encephalopathy. There is an increased frequency of neuropsychiatric problems, which may be a subtle form of encephalopathy.

Because the patient's general condition and liver function are good, the death rate for sudden massive bleeding is about 20%, much below the rate in other types of portal hypertension. The diagnosis can be confirmed radiologically by percutaneous mesenteric angiography. Wedged hepatic venous pressure is normal.

Bleeding episodes in children under age 8 are usually self-limited and often do not require endoscopic sclerotherapy, administration of vasopressin, or Sengstaken tube tamponade. In general, however, the bleeding episodes are self-limited and uncommonly fatal, so emergency operations are rarely necessary.

The thrombosed portal vein is unsuitable for a shunt. A cavomesenteric shunt is best for young children, whose vessels are small. In older individuals, treatment should be started with sclerotherapy; if that fails to control the bleeding, a distal splenorenal shunt is preferred. Splenectomy alone has no permanent effect and sacrifices the splenic vein, which might be needed later for a shunt. Because shunts in small children have a high rate of spontaneous thrombosis, variceal bleeding is preferably managed without a shunt until the child is 8–10 years of age and the vessels are larger. Nevertheless, using silk sutures and precise technique, some surgeons have obtained a high rate of anastomotic patency even in the very young. Patients with encephalopathy and hepatic dysfunction many years after a total shunt may be improved if they are converted to a selective shunt.

Splenectomy alone is never indicated in this disease, either for hypersplenism or in an attempt to reduce portal pressure, because the rebleeding rate is 90% and fatal postsplenectomy sepsis is not uncommon. If it is not possible to construct an adequate shunt, expectant management is the best regimen. Repeated severe hemorrhages should be treated by transendoscopic sclerosis. Esophagogastrectomy with colon interposition is a last resort.

Janssen HL et al: Extrahepatic portal vein thrombosis: aetiology and determinants of survival. Gut 2001;49:720.

Sheen CL et al: Clinical features, diagnosis and outcome of acute portal vein thrombosis. QJM 2000;93:531.

Valla DC, Condat B: Portal vein thrombosis in adults: pathophysiology, pathogenesis and management. J Hepatol 2000; 32:865.

van't Riet M et al: Diagnosis and treatment of portal vein thrombosis following splenectomy. Br J Surg 2000;87:1229.

SPLENIC VEIN THROMBOSIS

Isolated thrombosis of the splenic vein is a rare cause of variceal bleeding that can be cured by splenectomy. The splenic venous blood, blocked from its normal route, flows through the short gastric vessels to the gastric fundus and then into the left gastric vein, continuing toward the liver. As the blood traverses the stomach, large gastric varices are produced that may rupture and bleed. Characteristically, the collateral pattern does not involve the esophagus, so esophageal varices are uncommon.

The principal causes of this syndrome are pancreatitis, pancreatic pseudocyst, neoplasm, and trauma. Splenomegaly is present in two-thirds of patients. Diagnosis can be made by selective splenic arteriography that opacifies the venous phase. Splenectomy is curative. Many cases of splenic vein thrombosis are unaccompanied by bleeding varices, and in such cases, no therapy is required.

de Franchis R: Updating consensus in portal hypertension: report of the Baveno III Consensus Workshop on definitions, methodology and therapeutic strategies in portal hypertension. J Hepatol 2000;33:846.

Gentilini P et al: Ascites and hepatorenal syndrome during cirrhosis: two entities or the continuation of the same complication? J Hepatol 1999;31:1088.

Krige JE, Beckingham IJ: ABC of diseases of liver, pancreas, and biliary system. Portal hypertension—1: varices. BMJ 2001; 322:348.

Lebrec D: Drug therapy for portal hypertension. Gut 2001;49:441.

Mercado MA et al: Results of surgical treatment (modified Sugiura-Futagawa operation) of portal hypertension associated to complete splenomesoportal thrombosis and cirrhosis. HPB Surg 1999; 11:157.

Sakorafas GH et al: The significance of sinistral portal hypertension complicating chronic pancreatitis. Am J Surg 2000;179:129.

Sakorafas GH, Tsiotou AG: Splenic-vein thrombosis complicating chronic pancreatitis. Scand J Gastroenterol 1999;34:1171.

Sarin SK et al: Comparison of endoscopic ligation and propranolol for the primary prevention of variceal bleeding. N Engl J Med 1999;340:988.

Stein M, Link DP: Symptomatic spleno-mesenteric-portal venous thrombosis: recanalization and reconstruction with endovascular stents. J Vasc Interv Radiol 1999;10:363.

Suzuki H, Stanley AJ: Current management and novel therapeutic strategies for refractory ascites and hepatorenal syndrome. QJM 2001;94:293.

Vlachogiannakos J et al: Angiotensin converting enzyme inhibitors and angiotensin II antagonists as therapy in chronic liver disease. Gut 2001;49:303.

BUDD-CHIARI SYNDROME

Budd-Chiari syndrome is a rare disorder resulting from obstruction of hepatic venous outflow. Most cases are caused by spontaneous thrombosis of the hepatic veins, often associated with polycythemia vera or the use of birth control pills. Some patients present with idiopathic membranous stenosis of the inferior vena cava located between the hepatic veins and right atrium, which is usually associated with thrombosis of one or both hepatic veins. Most patients with this lesion are HBsAg-positive, and many have malignancies (eg, hepatocellular carcinoma). It was originally thought that these lesions were congenital, but they are now known to consist of stenosis resulting from thrombosis and scar formation.

The posthepatic (postsinusoidal) obstruction raises sinusoidal pressure, which is transmitted upstream to cause portal hypertension. Because the parenchyma is relatively free of fibrosis, filtration across the sinusoids and hepatic lymph formation increase greatly, producing marked ascites.

Symptoms usually begin with a mild prodrome consisting of vague right upper quadrant abdominal pain, postprandial bloating, and anorexia. After weeks or months, a more florid picture develops consisting of gross ascites, hepatomegaly, and hepatic failure. At this stage the AST is usually markedly increased, the serum bilirubin is slightly elevated, and the alkaline phosphatase is inconsistently abnormal.

Except in patients with membranous obstruction of the vena cava, liver scan usually demonstrates absent function through most of the liver except for a small central area representing the caudate lobe, whose venous outflow is spared (it goes directly to the vena cava through multiple small tributaries). CT scans show pooling of intravenous contrast media in the periphery of the liver; patent hepatic veins cannot be seen on ultrasound scans. An enlarged azygos vein may be seen on chest x-rays of patients with caval obstruction. Liver biopsy reveals grossly dilated central veins and sinusoids, pericentral necrosis, and replacement of hepatocytes by red blood cells. Centrilobular fibrosis develops late. The clinical diagnosis should be confirmed by venography, which shows the hepatic veins to be obstructed, usually with a beak-like deformity at their orifice. The inferior vena cava should be opacified to verify that it is patent—a requirement for a successful portacaval shunt. The x-rays may show compression of the intrahepatic cava by the congested liver.

A side-to-side portacaval or mesocaval shunt should be constructed when the obstruction is confined to the hepatic veins. Focal membranous obstruction of the suprahepatic cava may be treated by excision of the lesion with or without the addition of a patch angioplasty. Some cases may be managed nonsurgically by percutaneous transluminal balloon dilation of the stenosis.

Occlusion of the inferior vena cava by thrombosis or compression from the liver requires a mesoatrial shunt using a prosthetic vascular graft. Because the incidence of graft thrombosis is relatively high, it may be advisable to perform a second-stage side-to-side portacaval shunt a few months after mesoatrial shunt decompression of the liver in patients with hepatic vein thrombosis whose vena cava was originally blocked by a congested liver. Development of hepatocellular carcinoma is common in patients with membranous obstruction of the vena cava. The postoperative results are excellent in patients without malignant neoplasms.

Liver transplantation is indicated in patients with advanced hepatic decompensation either from cirrhosis or as part of the acute syndrome. The results are excellent, and the risk of later hepatocellular carcinoma is eliminated.

Michl P et al: Successful treatment of chronic Budd-Chiari syndrome with a transjugular intrahepatic portosystemic shunt. J Hepatol 2000;32:516.

Olzinski AT, Sanyal AJ. Treating Budd-Chiari Syndrome: making rational choices from a myriad of options. J Clin Gastroenterol. 2000;30:155.

Orloff MJ et al: A 27-year experience with surgical treatment of Budd-Chiari syndrome. Ann Surg 2000;232:340.

ASCITES

Ascites in hepatic disease results from (1) increased formation of hepatic lymph (from sinusoidal hypertension), (2) increased formation of splanchnic lymph, (3) hypoalbuminemia, and (4) salt and water retention by the kidneys. Before therapy is started, paracentesis should be performed and the following examinations made on a sample of ascitic fluid: (1) Culture and leukocyte count: Spontaneous bacterial peritonitis is common and may be clinically silent. A white count above 250/μL is highly suggestive of infection. (2) LDH levels: A ratio of LDH in ascites to serum that exceeds 0.6 suggests the presence of cancer or infection. (3) Serum amylase: A high level indicates pancreatic disease. (4) Albumin: The ratio of serum to ascites albumin concentrations is above 1.1 in liver disease and below 1.1 in malignant ascites.

Medical Treatment

In general, the intensity of medical therapy required to control ascites can be predicted from the pretreatment 24-hour urine Na$^+$ output as follows: A Na$^+$ output above 5 meq/24 h will require strong diuretics; 5–25 meq/24 h, mild diuretics; and above 25 meq/24 h, no diuretics. Initial treatment is usually with spironolactone, 200 mg/d. The objective is to stimulate a weight loss of 0.5–0.75 kg/d, except in patients with peripheral edema who can mobilize fluid faster. If spironolactone alone is insufficient, another drug such as furosemide should be added. A loop diuretic (eg, furosemide, ethacrynic acid) should be given only in combination with a distally acting diuretic (eg, spironolactone, triamterene). Alternatively, massive ascites may be treated by one or more large (eg, 5-L) paracenteses accompanied by an intravenous infusion of albumin. If albumin is not given, the incidence of renal and electrolyte complications is high. Salt or water restriction is no longer recommended except in the most refractory cases.

Surgical Treatment

A. PORTACAVAL SHUNT

A history of ascites that has been easy to control need not influence the choice of shunt operation intended to treat variceal bleeding. When ascites has been severe, however, a side-to-side shunt (eg, side-to-side portacaval, H-mesocaval, central splenorenal) may be considered, because it reduces sinusoidal as well as splanchnic venous pressure. A side-to-side portacaval shunt is indicated rarely just to treat ascites—eg, in patients in whom several LeVeen shunts have thrombosed—although the incidence of severe postoperative encephalopathy is high under these circumstances.

B. PERITONEAL-JUGULAR SHUNT (LEVEEN SHUNT)

Refractory ascites can be treated with a LeVeen shunt—a subcutaneous Silastic catheter that transports ascitic fluid from the peritoneal cavity to the jugular vein. A small unidirectional valve sensitive to a pressure gradient of 3–5 cm H$_2$O prevents backflow of blood. A modification called the Denver shunt contains a small chamber that can be used as a pump to clear the line by external pressure. In practice, Denver shunts become blocked more often than LeVeen shunts.

In patients with ascites due to cirrhosis, use of a LeVeen shunt should be confined to those who fail to respond to high doses of diuretics (eg, 400 mg of spironolactone and 400 mg of furosemide daily) or who repeatedly develop encephalopathy or azotemia during diuretic therapy.

Peritoneovenous shunts may also be used for ascites associated with cancer. The best results occur in patients whose ascitic fluid contains no malignant cells. A LeVeen shunt is of benefit in Budd-Chiari syndrome but is ineffective for chylous ascites. Because the incidence of complications and early shunt thrombosis is high, a LeVeen shunt is relatively contraindicated if the ascitic fluid is grossly bloody, contains many malignant cells, or has a high protein concentration (> 4.5 g/dL). The incidence of tumor embolization is low (5%).

The ascitic fluid should be cultured a few days before the shunt is inserted. Antibiotics are given pre- and postoperatively. The operation is best performed under general anesthesia but can be done with local anesthesia.

Postoperatively, the patient is outfitted with an abdominal binder and instructed to perform respiratory exercises against mild pressure to increase abdominal pressure and flow through the shunt. Dietary salt should not be restricted. A functioning LeVeen shunt is unable by itself to eliminate ascites, but it renders the patient much more responsive to diuretics. Therefore, furosemide should be administered postoperatively.

An average of 10 kg of weight is lost during the first 10 days after the operation, and eventually the abdomen assumes a normal configuration. Nutrition and serum albumin levels often improve postoperatively. Urinary sodium excretion increases promptly, and renal function may improve in patients with the hepatorenal syndrome. Serious complications and deaths are most common in patients with advanced hepatorenal syndrome or a serum bilirubin level greater than 4 mg/dL.

Although some patients eventually bleed from varices following insertion of a LeVeen shunt, the risk of bleeding is not increased by the shunt, which actually decreases portal pressure. Thus, a previous episode of variceal bleeding is not a contraindication for this procedure. Disseminated intravascular coagulation (DIC), manifested by increased fibrin split products, decreased platelet count, etc, occurs in more than half of cases but presents a clinical problem in only a few. The frequency and severity of DIC may be minimized by emptying most of the ascitic fluid from the abdomen during operation and partially replacing it with Ringer's lactate solution. Lethal septicemia may occur if the ascitic fluid is infected at the time the shunt is inserted.

In about 10% of cases, the valve becomes thrombosed and must be replaced.

Hydrothorax, usually on the right side, may develop in patients with cirrhosis and ascites. The fluid reaches the chest through a pinhole opening in the membranous portion of the diaphragm, a pathway that can be demonstrated by aspirating the thoracic fluid, injecting technetium Tc 99m colloid into the ascites fluid, and observing rapid accumulation of the label in the chest. Treatment consists of a peritoneovenous shunt and injection of a sclerosing agent into the pleural cavity after it has been tapped dry. If a leak persists, it may be closed surgically by thoracotomy.

Aslam N, Marino CR: Malignant ascites: new concepts in pathophysiology, diagnosis, and management. Arch Intern Med 2001;161:2733.

Ben-Ami H et al: Acute transient chylous ascites associated with acute biliary pancreatitis. Am J Med Sci 1999;318:122.

Helton WS et al: Transjugular intrahepatic portasystemic shunt vs surgical shunt in good-risk cirrhotic patients: a case-control comparison. Arch Surg 2001;136:17.

Kaser S et al: Transjugular intrahepatic portosystemic shunt (TIPS) augments hyperinsulinemia in patients with cirrhosis. J Hepatol 2000;33:902.

Krige JE, Beckingham IJ: ABC of diseases of liver, pancreas, and biliary system: portal hypertension-2. Ascites, encephalopathy, and other conditions. BMJ 2001;322:416.

Rossle M et al: A comparison of paracentesis and transjugular intrahepatic portosystemic shunting in patients with ascites. N Engl J Med 2000;342:1701.

Suzuki H, Stanley AJ: Current management and novel therapeutic strategies for refractory ascites and hepatorenal syndrome. QJM 2001;94:293.

Zervos EE, Rosemurgy AS: Management of medically refractory ascites. Am J Surg 2001;181:256.

HEPATIC ENCEPHALOPATHY

Central nervous system symptoms may be seen in patients with chronic liver disease and are especially prone to develop after portacaval shunt. Portal-systemic encephalopathy, ammonia intoxication, hepatic coma, and meat intoxication are terms used to refer to this condition. The manifestations range from lethargy to coma—from minor personality changes to psychosis—from asterixis to paraplegia. Hypothermia and hyperventilation may precede coma.

Pathogenesis

Hepatic encephalopathy is a reversible metabolic neuropathy that results from the effects of toxins absorbed from the gut on the brain. Increased exposure of the brain to these toxins is the result of decreased detoxification by the liver due to diminished function and spontaneous or surgically created shunts of portal venous blood around the liver and increased permeability of the blood-brain barrier. The toxins form from the action of colonic bacteria on protein within the gut. Potential aggravating factors include gastrointestinal hemorrhage, constipation, azotemia, hypokalemic alkalosis, infection, excessive dietary protein, and sedatives (Table 25–6). Four main theories concerning mediation of this syndrome currently attract the most attention.

A. AMINO ACID NEUROTRANSMITTERS

Gamma-aminobutyric acid (GABA), the principal inhibitory neurotransmitter in the brain, produces a state similar to hepatic encephalopathy when given experimentally. It is synthesized in the brain and by bacteria within the colon, is degraded by the liver, and is found in increased levels in the serum of patients with hepatic encephalopathy. The passage of GABA across the blood-brain barrier is increased in hepatic encephalopathy. Experiments also indicate the presence of increased numbers of GABA receptors in encephalopathy and in-

Table 25–6. Factors contributing to encephalopathy.

A. Increased systemic toxin levels
  1. Extent of portal-systemic venous shunt
  2. Depressed liver function
  3. Intestinal protein load
  4. Intestinal flora
  5. Azotemia
  6. Constipation
B. Increased sensitivity of central nervous system
  1. Age of patient
  2. Hypokalemia
  3. Alkalosis
  4. Diuretics
  5. Sedatives, narcotics, tranquilizers
  6. Infection
  7. Hypoxia, hypoglycemia, myxedema

---

creased GABA-ergic tone, perhaps due to a benzodiazepine receptor agonist ligand on the receptor complex (GABA/benzodiazepine receptor). This has raised the possibility of treating encephalopathy with benzodiazepine antagonists, and the drug flumazenil has shown promise in preliminary trials.

B. Ammonia

Ammonia is produced in the colon by bacteria and is absorbed and transported in portal venous blood to the liver, where it is extracted and converted to glutamine. Ammonia concentrations are elevated in the arterial blood and cerebrospinal fluid of patients with encephalopathy, and experimental administration of ammonia produces central nervous system symptoms.

C. False Neurotransmitters

According to this theory, cerebral neurons become depleted of normal neurotransmitters (norepinephrine and dopamine), which are partially replaced by false neurotransmitters (octopamine and phenylethanolamine). The result is inhibition of neural function. Serum levels of branched-chain amino acids (leucine, isoleucine, valine) are decreased and levels of aromatic amino acids (tryptophan, phenylalanine, tyrosine) are elevated in patients with encephalopathy. Because these two classes of amino acids compete for transport across the blood-brain barrier, the aromatic amino acids have increased access to the central nervous system, where they serve as precursors for false neurotransmitters. Trials of therapy with supplements of branched-chain amino acids have given conflicting results.

D. Synergistic Neurotoxins

This theory postulates that ammonia, mercaptans, and fatty acids, none of which accumulate in brain in amounts capable of producing encephalopathy, have synergistic effects that produce the full-blown syndrome.

Prevention

Encephalopathy is a major side effect of portacaval shunt and is to some extent predictable. Elderly patients are considerably more susceptible. Alcoholics fare better than those with postnecrotic or cryptogenic cirrhosis, apparently owing to the invariable progression of liver dysfunction in the latter. Good liver function partially protects the patients from encephalopathy. If the liver has adapted to complete or nearly complete diversion of portal blood before operation, a surgical shunt is less apt to depress liver function further. For example, patients with thrombosis of the portal vein (complete diversion and normal liver function) rarely experience encephalopathy after portal-systemic shunt.

Encephalopathy is less common after a distal splenorenal (Warren) shunt than after other kinds of shunts.

Increased intestinal protein whether of dietary origin or from intestinal bleeding aggravates encephalopathy by providing more substrate for intestinal bacteria. Constipation allows more time for bacterial action on colonic contents. Azotemia results in higher concentration of blood urea, which diffuses into the intestine, is converted to ammonia, and is then reabsorbed. Hypokalemia and metabolic alkalosis aggravate encephalopathy by shifting ammonia from extracellular to intracellular sites where the toxic action occurs.

Laboratory Findings

Arterial ammonia levels are usually high. The presence of high levels of glutamine in the cerebrospinal fluid may help distinguish hepatic encephalopathy from other causes of coma. Electroencephalography is more sensitive than clinical evaluation in detecting minor involvement. The changes are nonspecific and consist of slower mean frequencies. Studies performed at different times can be compared to assess the effects of therapy.

Treatment

Acute encephalopathy is treated by controlling precipitating factors, halting all dietary protein intake, cleansing the bowel with purgatives and enemas, and administering antibiotics (neomycin or ampicillin) or lactulose. Neomycin may be given orally or by gastric tube (two to four times daily) or rectally as an enema (1% solution one or two times daily). At least 1600 kcal of carbohydrate should be provided daily, along with therapeutic amounts of vitamins. Blood volume must be maintained to avoid prerenal azotemia. After the patient responds to initial therapy, dietary protein may be started at 20 g/d and increased by increments of 10–20 g every 2–5 days as tolerated.

Chronic encephalopathy is treated by restriction of dietary protein, avoidance of constipation, and elimination of sedatives, diuretics, and tranquilizers. To avoid protein depletion, protein intake must not be chronically reduced below 50 g/d. Vegetable protein in the diet is tolerated better than is animal protein. Lactulose, a disaccharide unaffected by intestinal enzymes, is the drug of choice for long-term control. When given orally (20–30 g three or four times daily), it reaches the colon, where it stimulates bacterial anabolism (which increases ammonia uptake) and inhibits bacterial enzymes (which decreases the generation of nitrogenous toxins). Its effect is independent of colonic pH. A related compound outside the United States, lactitol (β-galactoside sorbitol), is also effective and appears to work faster. As a powder, it is easier to use than liquid lactulose. Intermittent courses of oral neomycin or metronidazole may be given if lactulose therapy and preventive measures are inadequate.

Butterworth RF: Hepatic encephalopathy: a neuropsychiatric disorder involving multiple neurotransmitter systems. Curr Opin Neurol 2000;13:727.

Gill RQ, Sterling RK: Acute liver failure. J Clin Gastroenterol 2001;33:191.

Lockwood AH: Early detection and treatment of hepatic encephalopathy. Curr Opin Neurol 1998;11:663.

Menon KV, Kamath PS: Managing the complications of cirrhosis. Mayo Clin Proc 2000;75:501.

HEPATIC ABSCESS

Hepatic abscesses may be bacterial, parasitic, or fungal in origin. In the USA, pyogenic abscesses are the most common and amebic abscesses (see Chapter 9) the next most common. Unless otherwise specified, these remarks refer to bacterial abscesses.

Cases are about evenly divided between those with a single abscess and those with many abscesses. About 90% of right lobe abscesses are solitary, while only 10% of left lobe abscesses are solitary.

In most cases, the development of a hepatic abscess follows a suppurative process elsewhere in the body. Many abscesses are due to direct spread from biliary infections such as empyema of the gallbladder or protracted cholangitis. Abdominal infections such as appendicitis or diverticulitis may spread through the portal vein to involve the liver with abscess formation. About 40% of patients have an underlying malignancy. Other cases develop after generalized sepsis from bacterial endocarditis, renal infection, or pneumonitis. In 25% of cases, no antecedent infection can be documented ("cryptogenic" abscesses). Rare causes include secondary bacterial infection of an amebic abscess, hydatid cyst, or congenital hepatic cyst.

In most cases, the organism is of enteric origin. *Escherichia coli, Klebsiella pneumoniae,* bacteroides, enterococci (eg, *Streptococcus faecalis*), anaerobic streptococci (eg, peptostreptococcus), and microaerophilic streptococci are most common. Staphylococci, hemolytic streptococci, or other gram-positive organisms are usually found if the primary infection is bacterial endocarditis or pneumonitis.

Clinical Findings

A. SYMPTOMS AND SIGNS

When liver abscess develops in the course of another intra-abdominal infection such as diverticulitis, it is accompanied by increasing toxicity, higher fever, jaundice, and a generally deteriorating clinical picture. Right upper quadrant pain and chills may appear.

In other cases, the diagnosis is much less obvious, since the illness develops insidiously in a previously healthy person. In these, the first symptoms are usually malaise and fatigue, followed after several weeks by fever. Epigastric or right upper quadrant pain is present in about half of cases. The pain may be aggravated by motion or may be referred to the right shoulder.

The course of fever is often erratic, and spikes to 40–41 °C are common. Chills are present in about 25% of cases. The liver is usually enlarged and may be tender to palpation. If tenderness is severe, the condition may be confused with cholecystitis.

Jaundice is unusual in solitary abscesses unless the patient's condition is seriously worsening. It is often present in patients with multiple abscesses and primary disease in the biliary tree and in general is a bad prognostic sign.

B. LABORATORY FINDINGS

Leukocytosis is pre-sent in most cases and is usually over 15,000/μL. A small group of patients—including some of the most seriously ill—fail to develop leukocytosis. Anemia is present in most. The average hematocrit is 33%.

Serum bilirubin is usually normal except in patients with multiple abscesses or biliary obstruction or when hepatic failure has supervened. Alkaline phosphatase is often elevated even in the presence of a normal bilirubin.

C. IMAGING STUDIES

X-ray changes present in the right lung in about one-third of cases consist of basilar atelectasis or pleural effusion. The right diaphragm may be elevated and less mobile than the left.

Plain films of the abdomen are usually normal or show only hepatomegaly. In a few patients, an air-fluid level in the region of the liver reveals the presence and location of the abscess. Distortion of the contour of the stomach on upper gastrointestinal series may be seen with large abscesses involving the left lobe.

Ultrasound and CT scans are the most useful diagnostic tests, providing accurate information regarding the presence, size, number, and location of abscesses within the liver. CT scans have the added advantage of being able to demonstrate abscesses or neoplasms elsewhere in the abdomen. The radioisotope liver scintiscan is able to demonstrate most liver abscesses but given no information about the rest of the abdomen.

Differential Diagnosis

In many cases, early findings may be so vague that hepatic abscess is not even considered. The multiple other causes of malaise, weight loss, and anemia would enter into the differential diagnosis. With spiking fevers, one must consider all the causes of fever of unknown origin. Failure to entertain the idea of hepatic abscess and to obtain the necessary scans leads to most errors in diagnosis.

Once imaging tests have demonstrated the abscess, the responsible organisms must be identified. Amebiasis should be considered in every case of solitary abscess. Compared with amebic abscesses, pyogenic liver abscesses are seen more often in patients older than 50 years and are associated with jaundice, pruritus, sepsis, a palpable mass, and elevated bilirubin and alkaline phosphatase levels. Patients with amebic abscesses more often have been to an endemic area and have abdominal pain and tenderness, diarrhea, hepatomegaly, and positive serologic tests for amebiasis.

Complications

Intrahepatic spread of infection may create multiple additional abscesses and is responsible for some failures after treatment of an apparently solitary abscess. As the untreated abscess expands, rupture may occur into the pleural or peritoneal cavity, usually with catastrophic results. Septicemia and septic shock are common terminal complications of diffuse hepatic infection. Hepatic failure may develop in addition to uncontrolled sepsis, or it may predominate over signs of infection.

Hemobilia may follow bleeding from the vascular wall into the abscess cavity. In this case, hepatic artery embolization or ligation may be required to control bleeding.

Treatment

Antibiotics should be started promptly. Initial coverage, before culture results are available, should be adequate for *E coli, K pneumoniae*, bacteroides, enterococci, and anaerobic streptococci and consequently would usually include an aminoglycoside, clindamycin or metronidazole, and ampicillin. The regimen may be modified later according to the results of cultures.

About 80% of patients with liver abscesses are adequately treated by suction catheters inserted percuta-

neously under ultrasound or CT guidance. Whether the patient has a single abscess or multiple abscesses, this is usually the most appropriate initial therapy. The catheters can be removed in 1–2 weeks after output becomes nonpurulent and scant.

In about 40% of patients, the catheters do not drain well following initial placement and must be repositioned. The principal advantage of percutaneous drainage is lower morbidity (not lower mortality). It is easier to provide thorough drainage surgically, so when difficulties are encountered with percutaneous drainage, laparotomy should be performed promptly. Surgical therapy may also be called for in patients whose underlying disease requires an operation.

In many cases, multiple abscesses cannot be drained satisfactorily. Rarely, multiple abscesses are confined to a single lobe and can be cured by lobectomy. Biliary obstruction or other causes of sepsis must also be corrected.

Prognosis

The overall mortality rate of 15% is more closely related to the underlying disease than to any other factor. The mortality rate is about 40% in patients with malignant disease. Pleural effusion, leukocytosis over 20,000/μL, hypoalbuminemia, and polymicrobial infection correlate with a poor outcome. In the USA, whether the abscess is solitary or multiple no longer has a major influence on survival, but where benign biliary disease remains a major cause of this disease, multiple hepatic abscesses are associated with a worse prognosis. Death is rare in patients with a cryptogenic liver abscess.

Dharmarajan TS et al: Pyogenic liver abscess: a geriatric problem. J Am Geriatr Soc 2000;48:1022.

Johannsen EC, Sifri CD, Madoff LC: Pyogenic liver abscesses. Infect Dis Clin North Am 2000;14:547.

Molle I et al: Increased risk and case fatality rate of pyogenic liver abscess in patients with liver cirrhosis: a nationwide study in Denmark. Gut 2001;48:260.

Narayanan S et al: Crohn's disease presenting as pyogenic liver abscess with review of previous case reports. Am J Gastroenterol 1998;93:2607.

Biliary Tract

Gerard M. Doherty, MD, & Lawrence W. Way, MD

EMBRYOLOGY & ANATOMY

The anlage of the biliary ducts and liver consists of a diverticulum that appears on the ventral aspect of the foregut in 3 mm embryos. The cranial portion becomes the liver; a caudal bud forms the ventral pancreas; and an intermediate bud develops into the gallbladder. Originally hollow, the hepatic diverticulum becomes a solid mass of cells that later recanalizes to form the ducts. The smallest ducts—the bile canaliculi—are first seen as a basal network between the primitive hepatocytes that eventually expands throughout the liver (Figure 26–1). Numerous microvilli increase the canalicular surface area. Bile secreted here passes through the interlobular ductules (canals of Hering) and the lobar ducts and then into the hepatic duct in the hilum. In most cases, the common hepatic duct is formed by the union of a single right and left duct, but in 25% of individuals, the anterior and posterior divisions of the right duct join the left duct separately. The origin of the common hepatic duct is close to the liver but always outside its substance. It runs about 4 cm before joining the cystic duct to form the common bile duct. The common duct begins in the hepatoduodenal ligament, passes behind the first portion of the duodenum, and runs in a groove on the posterior surface of the pancreas before entering the duodenum. Its terminal 1 cm is intimately adherent to the duodenal wall. The total length of the common duct is about 9 cm.

In 80–90% of individuals, the main pancreatic duct joins the common duct to form a common channel about 1 cm long. The intraduodenal segment of the duct is called the hepatopancreatic ampulla, or ampulla of Vater.

The gallbladder is a pear-shaped organ adherent to the undersurface of the liver in a groove separating the right and left lobes. The fundus projects 1–2 cm below the hepatic edge and can often be felt when the cystic or common duct is obstructed. It rarely has a complete peritoneal covering, but when this variation does occur, it predisposes to infarction by torsion. The gallbladder holds about 50 mL of bile when fully distended. The neck of the gallbladder tapers into the narrow cystic duct, which connects with the common duct. The lumen of the cystic duct contains a thin mucosal septum, the spiral valve of Heister, that offers mild resistance to bile flow. In 75% of persons, the cystic duct enters the common duct at an angle. In the remainder, it runs parallel to the hepatic duct or winds around it before joining the common duct (Figure 26–2).

In the hepatoduodenal ligament, the hepatic artery is to the left of the common duct and the portal vein is posterior and medial. The right hepatic artery usually passes behind the hepatic duct and then gives off the cystic artery before entering the right lobe of the liver, but variations are common.

The mucosal epithelium of the bile ducts varies from cuboidal in the ductules to columnar in the main ducts. The gallbladder mucosa is thrown into prominent ridges when the organ is collapsed, and these flatten during distention. The tall columnar cells of the gallbladder mucosa are covered by microvilli on their luminal surface. Wide channels, which play an important role in water and electrolyte absorption, separate the individual cells.

The walls of the bile ducts contain only small amounts of smooth muscle, but the termination of the common duct is enveloped by a complex sphincteric muscle. The gallbladder musculature is composed of interdigitated bundles of longitudinal and spirally arranged fibers.

The biliary tree receives parasympathetic and sympathetic innervation. The former contains motor fibers to the gallbladder and secretory fibers to the ductal epithelium. The afferent fibers in the sympathetic nerves mediate the pain of biliary colic.

PHYSIOLOGY

Bile Flow

Bile is produced at a rate of 500–1500 mL/d by the hepatocytes and the cells of the ducts. Active secretion of bile salts into the biliary canaliculus is responsible for most of the volume of bile and its fluctuations. Na^+ and water follow passively to establish isosmolality and electrical neutrality. Lecithin and cholesterol enter the canaliculus at rates that correlate with variations in bile salt output. Bilirubin and a number of other organic anions—estrogens, sulfobromophthalein, etc—are actively secreted by the hepatocyte by a different transport system from that which handles bile salts.

The columnar cells of the ducts add a fluid rich in HCO_3^- to that produced in the canaliculus. This in-

Figure 26–1. Scanning electron photomicrograph of a hepatic plate with adjacent sinusoids and sinusoidal microvilli and a bile canaliculus running in the center of the liver cells. Although their boundaries are indistinct, about four hepatocytes constitute the section of the plate in the middle of the photograph. Occasional red cells are present within the sinusoids. (Reduced from × 2000.)(Courtesy of Dr James Boyer.)

volves active secretion of Na^+ and HCO_3^- by a cellular pump stimulated by secretin, VIP, and cholecystokinin. K^+ and water are distributed passively across the ducts (Figure 26–3).

Between meals, bile is stored in the gallbladder, where it is concentrated at rates of up to 20% per hour. Na^+ and either HCO_3^- or Cl^- are actively transported from its lumen during absorption. The changes in composition brought about by concentration are shown in Figure 26–4.

Three factors regulate bile flow: hepatic secretion, gallbladder contraction, and choledochal sphincteric resistance. In the fasting state, pressure in the common bile duct is 5–10 cm H_2O, and bile produced in the liver is diverted into the gallbladder. After a meal, the gallbladder contracts, the sphincter relaxes, and bile is forced into the duodenum in squirts as ductal pressure intermittently exceeds sphincteric resistance. During contraction, pressure within the gallbladder reaches 25 cm H_2O and that in the common bile duct 15–20 cm H_2O.

Cholecystokinin (CCK) is the major physiologic stimulus for postprandial gallbladder contraction and relaxation of the sphincter, but vagal impulses facilitate its action. CCK is released into the bloodstream from the mucosa of the small bowel by fat or lipolytic products in the lumen. Amino acids and small polypeptides are weaker stimuli, and carbohydrates are ineffective. Bile flow during a meal is augmented by turnover of bile salts in the enterohepatic circulation and stimulation of ductal secretion by secretin, VIP, and CCK. Motilin stimulates episodic partial gallbladder emptying in the interdigestive phase.

Bile Salts & the Enterohepatic Circulation

Bile salts, lecithin, and cholesterol comprise about 90% of the solids in bile, the remainder consisting of bilirubin, fatty acids, and inorganic salts. Gallbladder bile contains about 10% solids and has a bile salt concentration between 200 and 300 mmol/L (Figure 26–4).

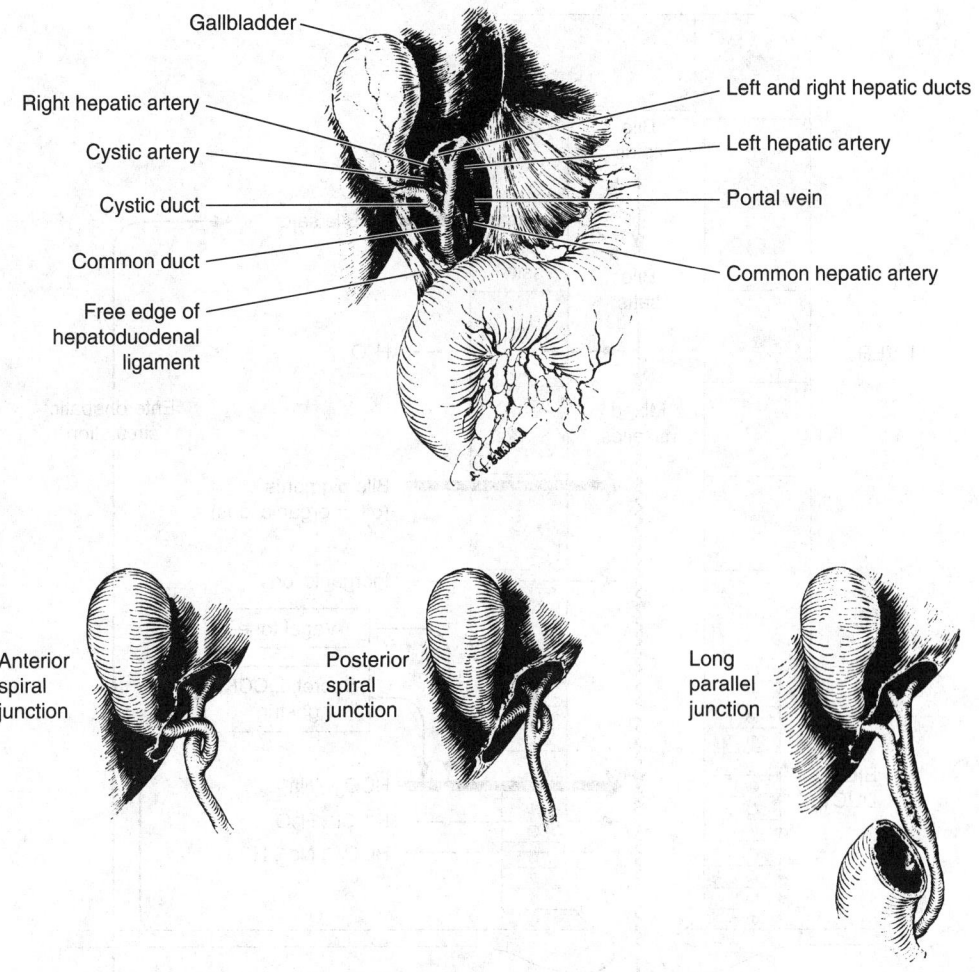

Gallbladder

Right hepatic artery

Cystic artery

Cystic duct

Common duct

Free edge of hepatoduodenal ligament

Left and right hepatic ducts

Left hepatic artery

Portal vein

Common hepatic artery

Anterior spiral junction

Posterior spiral junction

Long parallel junction

Figure 26–2. Anatomy of the gallbladder and variations in anatomy of the cystic duct.

Bile salts are steroid molecules formed from cholesterol by hepatocytes. The rate of synthesis is under feedback control and can be increased a maximum of about 20-fold. Two **primary** bile salts—cholate and chenodeoxycholate—are produced by the liver. Before excretion into bile, they are conjugated with either glycine or taurine, which enhances water solubility. Intestinal bacteria alter these compounds to produce the **secondary** bile salts, deoxycholate and lithocholate. The former is reabsorbed and enters bile, but lithocholate is insoluble and is excreted in the stool. Bile is composed of 40% cholate, 40% chenodeoxycholate, and 20% deoxycholate, conjugated with glycine or taurine in a ratio of 3:1.

The functions of bile salts are (1) to induce the flow of bile, (2) to transport lipids, and (3) to bind calcium ions in bile. The importance of the last of these is unknown. Bile acid molecules are amphipathic—ie, they have hydrophilic and hydrophobic poles. In bile, they form multimolecular aggregates called micelles in which the hydrophilic poles become aligned to face the aqueous medium. Water-insoluble lipids, such as cholesterol, can be dissolved within the hydrophobic centers of bile salt micelles. Molecules of lecithin, a water-insoluble but polar lipid, aggregate into hydrated bilayers that form vesicles in bile, and they also become incorporated into bile acid micelles to form mixed micelles. Mixed micelles have an increased lipid-carrying capacity compared with pure bile acid micelles. Cholesterol in bile is transported within the phospholipid vesicles and the bile salt micelles.

Figure 26–3. Bile formation. Solid lines into the ductular lumen indicate active transport; dotted lines represent passive diffusion.

Bile salts remain in the intestinal lumen throughout the jejunum, where they participate in fat digestion and absorption (Figure 26–5). Upon reaching the distal small bowel, they are reabsorbed by an active transport system located in the terminal 200 cm of ileum. Over 95% of bile salts arriving from the jejunum are transferred by this process into portal vein blood; the remainder enter the colon, where they are converted to secondary bile salts. The entire bile salt pool of 2.5–4 g circulates twice through the enterohepatic circulation during each meal, and six to eight cycles are made each day. The normal daily loss of bile salts in the stool amounts to 10–20% of the pool and is restored by hepatic synthesis.

Arias IM et al: The biology of the bile canaliculus. Hepatology 1993;17:318.

Gustafsson U, Sahlin S, Einarsson C: Biliary lipid composition in patients with cholesterol and pigment gallstones and gallstone-free subjects: deoxycholic acid does not contribute to

Figure 26–4. Changes in gallbladder bile composition with time. (Courtesy of J Dietschy.)

Figure 26–5. Enterohepatic circulation of bile salts. (Courtesy of M Tyor.)

formation of cholesterol gallstones. Eur J Clin Invest 2000; 30:1099.

Hofmann AF: The continuing importance of bile acids in liver and intestinal disease. Arch Intern Med 1999;159:2647.

Kullak-Ublick GA: Regulation of organic anion and drug transporters of the sinusoidal membrane. J Hepatol 1999;31:563.

Sahin M et al: Effect of octreotide (Sandostatin 201-995) on bile flow and bile components. Dig Dis Sci 1999;44:181.

Bilirubin

About 250–300 mg of bilirubin is excreted each day in the bile, 75% of it from breakdown of red cells in the reticuloendothelial system and 25% from turnover of hepatic heme and hemoproteins. First, heme is liberated from hemoglobin, and the iron and globin are removed for reuse by the organism. Biliverdin, the first pigment formed from heme, is reduced to unconjugated bilirubin, the indirect-reacting bilirubin of the van den Bergh test. Unconjugated bilirubin is insoluble in water and is transported in plasma bound to albumin.

Unconjugated bilirubin is extracted from blood by hepatocytes, where it is conjugated with glucuronic acid to form bilirubin diglucuronide, the water-soluble direct bilirubin. Conjugation is catalyzed by glucuronyl transferase, an enzyme on the endoplasmic reticulum. Bilirubin is transported within the hepatocyte by cytosolic binding proteins, which rapidly deliver the molecule to the canalicular membrane for active secretion into bile. Within bile, conjugated bilirubin is largely transported in association with mixed lipid micelles.

After entering the intestine, bilirubin is reduced by intestinal bacteria to several compounds known as urobilinogens, which are subsequently oxidized and converted to pigmented urobilins. The term urobilinogen is often used to refer to both urobilins and urobilinogens.

DIAGNOSTIC EXAMINATION OF THE BILIARY TREE

Plain Abdominal Film

The posteroanterior supine view of the abdomen will show gallstones in the 10–15% of cases where they are radiopaque. The bile itself sometimes contains sufficient calcium (milk of calcium bile) to be seen. An enlarged gallbladder can occasionally be identified as a soft tissue mass in the right upper quadrant indenting an air-filled hepatic flexure.

In several types of biliary disease, the diagnosis may be suggested by air seen in the bile ducts on a plain film. This usually signifies the presence of a biliary-intestinal fistula (from disease or surgery) but also occurs rarely in severe cholangitis, emphysematous cholecystitis, and biliary ascariasis.

Oral Cholecystography

Tyropanoate sodium or iopanoic acid is taken orally the night before the examination, along with a light meal. The drug is absorbed, bound to albumin in portal blood, extracted by hepatocytes, and secreted in bile. Opacification occurs only with concentration in the gallbladder and on the average is optimal 10 hours after tyropanoate ingestion. Posteroanterior and oblique supine views and an upright or lateral decubitus film are obtained.

Oral cholecystograms are unsatisfactory if the contrast agent is inefficiently absorbed from the intestine or poorly excreted by the liver. Absorption is often impaired in acute abdominal illnesses with ileus, vomiting, or diarrhea. If the bilirubin level is over 3 mg/dL, hepatic excretion will probably be inadequate. False-negative results are obtained in 5% of tests. A normal gallbladder may not opacify for several weeks after severe trauma or a major illness.

Nonopacification occurs in 20% of patients after the usual single-dose regimen. When a second dose is given and x-rays repeated the following day, opacification is obtained in 25% of these patients. Persistent nonopacification is a highly reliable (> 95% true positive) indication of gallbladder disease. Instead of performing a double-dose oral cholecystogram as the next step when a single dose fails to opacify, it is simpler to obtain an ultrasound scan.

Percutaneous Transhepatic Cholangiography (THC, PTC)

Percutaneous transhepatic cholangiography is performed by passing a fine needle through the right lower rib cage and the hepatic parenchyma and into the lumen of a bile duct. Water-soluble contrast material is injected, and x-ray films are taken.

The technical success is related to the degree of dilatation of the intrahepatic bile ducts. THC is especially valuable in demonstrating the biliary anatomy in patients with benign biliary strictures, malignant lesions of the proximal bile duct, or when ERCP (see below) has been unsuccessful. Failure of the contrast medium to enter a duct does not prove that obstruction is absent. THC should not be done in patients with cholangitis until the infection has been controlled with antibi-

otics. Virtually all patients should be premedicated with antibiotics regardless of whether they have cholangitis—septic shock has been produced by sudden inoculation of organisms from bile into the systemic circulation. Otherwise, the contraindications are the same as for percutaneous liver biopsy.

Endoscopic Retrograde Cholangiopancreatography (ERCP)

ERCP involves cannulating the sphincter of Oddi under direct vision through a side-viewing duodenoscope. It requires special training involving more than familiarity with the use of fiberoptic endoscopes. Usually it is possible to opacify the pancreatic as well as the bile ducts. This method of cholangiography is especially applicable to patients with an abnormal clotting mechanism who would not be candidates for transhepatic puncture of the ducts. It is usually the preferred method of examining the biliary tree in patients with presumed choledocholithiasis or obstructing lesions in the periampullary region.

Ultrasound

Ultrasonography is both sensitive and specific in detecting gallbladder stones and dilatation of bile ducts. In the investigation of gallbladder disease, false-positive diagnoses for stones are rare, and false-negative reports owing to small stones or a contracted gallbladder occur in only 5% of patients examined by real time ultrasound. Ultrasound usually misses stones in the common duct.

Dilatation of bile ducts in a jaundiced patient indicates bile duct obstruction, but it is fairly common for the ducts to be normal in the presence of obstruction. When ultrasound shows dilated ducts, THC will nearly always be technically successful.

The ultrasonographer occasionally reports that the gallbladder contains "sludge." This material is sonographically opaque, does not cast an acoustic shadow, and forms a dependent layer in the gallbladder. On clinical analysis, it is a fine precipitate of calcium bilirubinate. Sludge may accompany gallstone disease or may be a solitary finding. It is seen in a variety of clinical settings, many of which are characterized by gallbladder stasis (eg, prolonged fasting). By itself, sludge is not an indication for cholecystectomy.

Radionuclide Scan (HIDA Scan)

Technetium 99m-labeled derivatives of iminodiacetic acid (IDA) are excreted in high concentration in bile and produce excellent gamma camera images. Following intravenous injection of the radionuclide, imaging of the bile ducts and gallbladder normally appears within 15–30 minutes and of the intestine within 60 minutes. In patients with acute right upper quadrant pain and tenderness, a good image of the bile duct accompanied by no image of the gallbladder indicates cystic duct obstruction and strongly supports a diagnosis of acute cholecystitis. The test is easy to perform and is occasionally a useful method of confirming this diagnosis.

JAUNDICE

Jaundice is categorized as prehepatic, hepatic, or posthepatic, depending upon the site of the underlying disease. Hemolysis, the most common cause of prehepatic jaundice, involves increased production of bilirubin. Less common causes of prehepatic jaundice are Gilbert's disease and the Crigler-Najjar syndrome.

Hepatic parenchymal jaundice is subdivided into hepatocellular and cholestatic types. The former includes acute viral hepatitis and chronic alcoholic cirrhosis. Some cases of intrahepatic cholestasis may be indistinguishable clinically and biochemically from cholestasis due to bile duct obstruction. Primary biliary cirrhosis, toxic drug jaundice, cholestatic jaundice of pregnancy, and postoperative cholestatic jaundice are the most common forms.

Extrahepatic jaundice most often results from biliary obstruction by a malignant tumor, choledocholithiasis, or biliary stricture. Pancreatic pseudocyst, chronic pancreatitis, sclerosing cholangitis, metastatic cancer, and duodenal diverticulitis are less common causes.

The cause of jaundice can be ascertained in the majority of patients from clinical and laboratory findings alone. In the remainder, THC or ERCP and ultrasound or CT scans will be necessary. The indications for these tests are discussed in later sections.

History

The age, sex, and parity of the patient and possible deleterious habits should be noted. Most cases of infectious hepatitis occur in patients under age 30. A history of drug addiction may suggest serum hepatitis transmitted by shared hypodermic equipment. Chronic alcoholism can usually be documented in patients with cirrhosis, and acute jaundice in alcoholics usually follows a recent binge. Obstructing gallstones or tumors are more common in older people.

Patients with jaundice due to choledocholithiasis may have associated biliary colic, fever, and chills and may report previous similar attacks. The pain in malignant obstruction is deep-seated and dull and may be affected by changes in position. Pain in the region of the liver is frequently experienced in the early stages of viral hepatitis and acute alcoholic liver injury. The patient

with extrahepatic obstruction may report that stools have become lighter in color and the urine dark.

Cholestatic diseases are often accompanied by pruritus—a source of severe discomfort in some cases. Pruritus may precede jaundice, but usually it appears at about the same time. The itching is most severe on the extremities and is aggravated by warm, humid weather. The cause remains obscure; itching does not correlate with bile salt levels in the skin, as was once believed. Cholestyramine, an anion exchange resin, usually provides relief by binding bile salts in the intestinal lumen and preventing their reabsorption.

Physical Examination

Hepatomegaly is common in both hepatic and posthepatic jaundice. In some cases, palpation of the liver may suggest cirrhosis or metastatic cancer, but impressions of this kind are unreliable. Secondary stigmas of cirrhosis usually accompany acute alcoholic jaundice; liver palms, spider angiomas, ascites, collateral veins on the abdominal walls, and splenomegaly suggest cirrhosis. A nontender, palpable gallbladder in a jaundiced patient suggests malignant obstruction of the common duct (Courvoisier's law), but absence of a palpable gallbladder is of little significance in ruling out cancer.

Laboratory Tests

In hemolytic disease, the increased bilirubin is principally in the unconjugated indirect fraction. Since unconjugated bilirubin is insoluble in water, the jaundice in hemolysis is acholuric. The total bilirubin in hemolysis rarely exceeds 4–5 mg/dL, because the rate of excretion increases as the bilirubin concentration rises, and a plateau is quickly reached. Greater values suggest concomitant hepatic parenchymal disease.

Jaundice due to hepatic parenchymal disease is characterized by elevations of both conjugated and unconjugated serum bilirubin. An increase in the conjugated fraction always signifies disease within the hepatobiliary system. The direct bilirubin predominates in about half of cases of hepatic parenchymal disease.

Both intrahepatic cholestasis and extrahepatic obstruction raise the direct bilirubin fraction, though the indirect fraction also increases somewhat. Since direct bilirubin is water-soluble, bilirubinuria develops. With complete extrahepatic obstruction, the total bilirubin rises to a plateau of 25–30 mg/dL, at which point loss in the urine equals the additional daily production. Higher values suggest concomitant hemolysis or decreased renal function. Obstruction of a single hepatic duct does not usually cause jaundice.

In extrahepatic obstruction caused by neoplasms, the serum bilirubin usually exceeds 10 mg/dL, and the average concentration is about 18 mg/dL. Obstructive jaundice due to common duct stones often produces transient bilirubin increases in the range of 2–4 mg/dL, and the level rarely exceeds 15 mg/dL. Serum bilirubin values in patients with alcoholic cirrhosis and acute viral hepatitis vary widely in relation to the severity of the parenchymal damage.

In extrahepatic obstruction, modest rises of AST levels are common, but levels as high as 1000 units/L are seen (though rarely) in patients with common duct stones and cholangitis. In the latter patients, the high values last for only a few days and are associated with increases in LDH concentrations. In general, AST levels above 1000 units/L suggest viral hepatitis.

Serum alkaline phosphatase comes from three sites: liver, bone, and intestine. In normal subjects, liver and bone contribute about equally, and the intestinal contribution is small. Hepatic alkaline phosphatase is a product of the epithelial cells of the cholangioles, and increased alkaline phosphatase levels associated with liver disease are the result of increased enzyme production. Alkaline phosphatase levels go up with intrahepatic cholestasis, cholangitis, or extrahepatic obstruction. Since the elevation is from overproduction, it may occur with focal hepatic lesions in the absence of jaundice. For example, a solitary hepatic metastasis or pyogenic abscess in one lobe or a tumor obstructing only one hepatic duct may fail to obstruct enough hepatic parenchyma to cause jaundice but usually is associated with increased alkaline phosphatase. In cholangitis with incomplete extrahepatic obstruction, serum bilirubin levels may be normal or mildly elevated, but serum alkaline phosphatase may be very high.

Bone disease may complicate the interpretation of abnormal alkaline phosphatase levels (Figure 26–6). If one suspects that the increased serum enzyme may be from bone, serum calcium, phosphorus, and 5′-nucleotidase or leucine aminopeptidase levels should be determined. These last two enzymes are also produced by cholangioles and are elevated in cholestasis, but their serum concentrations remain unchanged with bone disease.

Changes in serum protein levels may reflect hepatic parenchymal dysfunction. In cirrhosis, the serum albumin falls and the globulins increase. Serum globulins reach high values in some patients with primary biliary cirrhosis. Biliary obstruction generally produces no changes unless secondary biliary cirrhosis has developed.

Diagnosis

The principal diagnostic objective is to distinguish surgical (obstructive) from nonsurgical jaundice. The history, physical examination, and basic laboratory data allow an accurate diagnosis to be made in most cases without invasive tests (eg, liver biopsy, cholangiograms).

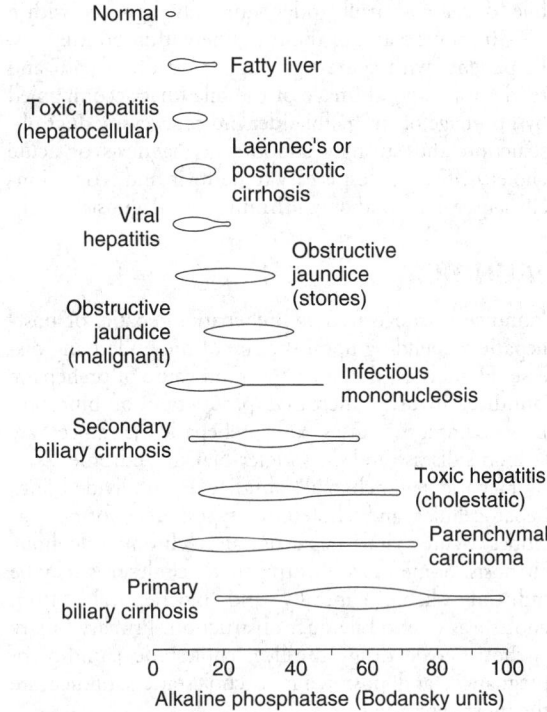

Figure 26–6. Range of alkaline phosphatase values in various hepatobiliary disorders.

Since most jaundiced patients are not critically ill when first seen, diagnosis and therapy may be conducted in a stepwise fashion, with each test selected according to the information available at that point. Only severe or worsening cholangitis requires urgent intervention. If the jaundice is mild and recent, it often passes within 24–48 hours, at which time an oral cholecystogram or ultrasound scan can be ordered to verify gallstone disease.

In patients with persistent jaundice, the first test will usually be an ultrasound scan, which may show dilated intrahepatic bile ducts (indicating ductal obstruction) or gallbladder stones. The lesion may be further delineated by ERCP or THC. ERCP is preferable when the lower end of the duct is thought to be obstructed (eg, suspected carcinoma of the pancreas or other periampullary tumors). THC is usually preferred for proximal lesions (eg, biliary stricture, neoplasm of the bifurcation of the hepatic ducts), because it gives better opacification of the ducts proximal to the obstruction and therefore provides more information that can be used in planning surgery. If the clinical presentation suggests neoplastic obstruction, a CT scan could be selected in preference to an ultrasound scan, because CT gives better definition of mass lesions while also demonstrating the presence and general location of bile duct obstruction.

If ultrasound or CT scans suggest biliary obstruction, a decision must be made about whether cholangiograms are indicated. In general, patients with gallstone disease do not require preoperative cholangiograms, whereas cholangiograms would be routine in patients with neoplastic obstruction, benign biliary stricture, or rare or unknown causes of obstructive jaundice.

PATHOGENESIS OF GALLSTONES

More than 20 million people in the USA have gallstones in their gallbladders; about 300,000 operations are performed annually for this disease, and at least 6000 deaths result from its complications or treatment. The incidence of gallstones rises with age, so that between 50 and 65 years of age about 20% of women and 5% of men are affected (Figure 26–7).

The gallstones in 75% of patients are composed predominantly (70–95%) of cholesterol and are called cholesterol stones. The remaining 25% are pigment stones. Regardless of composition, all gallstones give rise to similar clinical sequelae.

Cholesterol Gallstones

Cholesterol gallstones result from secretion by the liver of bile supersaturated with cholesterol. Influenced by various factors present in bile, the cholesterol precipitates from solution and the newly formed crystals grow to macroscopic stones. Except when the common bile duct is dilated or partially obstructed, the stones in this disease form almost exclusively within the gallbladder. Those found in the ducts usually reach that location after passing through the cystic duct.

The incidence of cholesterol gallstone disease is highest in American Indians, lower in Caucasians, and lowest in blacks, with a twofold gradient from one group to the next. More than 75% of American Indian women over age 40 are affected. Before puberty, the disease is rare but of equal frequency in both sexes. Thereafter, women are more commonly affected than men until after menopause, when the discrepancy lessens. Hormonal effects are also reflected in the increased incidence of gallstones with multiparity and the increased cholesterol saturation of bile and greater incidence of gallstones following ingestion of oral contraceptives. Obesity is the other major risk factor. The relative risk rises proportionately to the

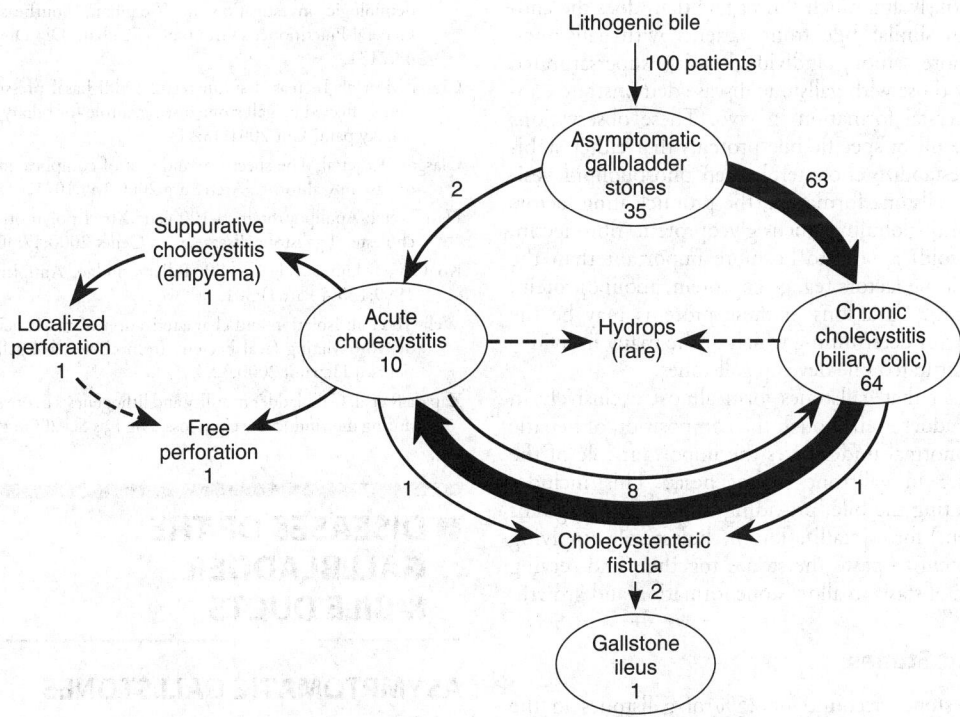

Figure 26–7. The natural history of gallbladder stones. The numbers approximate the percentage of patients in each category. Note that most patients with acute cholecystitis have previously had biliary colic.

extent of overweight due to a progressively increasing output of cholesterol in bile.

As noted previously, cholesterol is insoluble and in bile must be transported within bile salt micelles and phospholipid (lecithin) vesicles. When the amount of cholesterol in bile exceeds the cholesterol holding capacity, cholesterol crystals begin to precipitate from the phospholipid vesicles.

The secretion of bile salt and cholesterol into bile is linked. Bile salt elutes cholesterol from the hepatocyte membrane during passage into the bile canaliculus. At higher bile salt output levels, the amount of cholesterol relative to bile salt entering bile decreases. This means that during low bile flow (eg, during fasting), bile holding capacity for cholesterol is more saturated than during high bile flow. In fact, almost half of persons in Western cultures have bile supersaturated with cholesterol in the morning after an overnight fast. The bile salt pool in patients with cholesterol gallstone disease is about half the size of that of normal subjects, but this is a result of the gallstone disease (eg, gallstones displace bile in the gallbladder) and not a cause.

The occurrence of cholesterol gallstone disease requires cholesterol supersaturation of bile, but that in itself is not sufficient. Cholesterol in supersaturated bile from individuals without gallstone disease precipitates spontaneously at a much slower rate than does the cholesterol in similar bile from patients with gallstones. Furthermore, among individuals with supersaturated bile, only those with gallstone disease demonstrate cholesterol crystal formation in vivo. These observations are the result of specific bile proteins that either stabilize or destabilize cholesterol-laden phospholipid vesicles. For gallstone formation, the pronucleating factors (eg, immunoglobulin, mucus glycoprotein, fibronectin, orosomucoid) appear to be more important than the antinucleating factors (eg, glycoprotein, apolipoprotein, cytokeratin). Variations in these proteins may be the critical factor determining which of the many individuals with saturated bile develop gallstones.

The fact that gallstones form almost exclusively in the gallbladder even though the composition of hepatic bile is abnormal underscores the important role of the gallbladder in gallstone pathogenesis. This includes concentrating the bile, providing nidi (eg, small grains of pigment) for crystallization of cholesterol, supplying mucoprotein to paste the stones together, and serving as an area of stasis to allow stone formation and growth.

Pigment Stones

Pigment stones account for 25% of gallstones in the USA and 60% of those in Japan. Pigment stones are black to dark brown, 2–5 mm in diameter, and amorphous. They are composed of a mixture of calcium bilirubinate, complex bilirubin polymers, bile acids, and other unidentified substances. About 50% are radiopaque, and in the USA they constitute two-thirds of all radiopaque gallstones. The incidence is similar in men and women and in blacks and whites. Pigment stones are rare in American Indians.

Predisposing factors are cirrhosis, bile stasis (eg, a strictured or markedly dilated common duct), and chronic hemolysis. Some patients with pigment stones have increased concentrations of unconjugated bilirubin in their bile. Scanning electron microscopy demonstrates that about 90% of pigment stones are composed of dense mixtures of bacteria and bacterial glycocalix along with pigment solids. This suggests that bacteria have a primary role in pigment gallstone formation, and it also helps to explain why patients with pigment gallstone disease have sepsis more often than do those with cholesterol gallstone disease. It seems likely that bacterial β-glucuronidase is responsible for deconjugating the soluble bilirubin-diglucuronide to insoluble unconjugated bilirubin, which subsequently becomes agglomerated by glycocalix into macroscopic stones.

Beckingham IJ: ABC of diseases of liver, pancreas, and biliary system. Gallstone disease. BMJ 2001;322:91.

Caroli-Bosc FX et al: Cholelithiasis and dietary risk factors: an epidemiologic investigation in Vidauban, Southeast France. General Practitioner's Group of Vidauban. Dig Dis Sci 1998; 43:2131.

Cicala M et al: Increased sphincter of Oddi basal pressure in patients affected by gall stone disease: a role for biliary stasis and colicky pain? Gut 2001;48:414.

Glasgow RE et al: The spectrum and cost of complicated gallstone disease in California. Arch Surg 2000;135:1021.

Han T etal: Apolipoprotein B-100 gene Xba I polymorphism and cholesterol gallstone disease. Clin Genet 2000;57:304.

Ko CW, Sekijima JH, Lee SP: Biliary sludge. Ann Intern Med 1999;130(4 Part 1):301.

Wells JE et al: Isolation and characterization of cholic acid 7alpha-dehydroxylating fecal bacteria from cholesterol gallstone patients. J Hepatol 2000;32:4.

Zapata R et al: Gallbladder motility and lithogenesis in obese patients during diet-induced weight loss. Dig Dis Sci 2000;45:421.

■ DISEASES OF THE GALLBLADDER & BILE DUCTS

ASYMPTOMATIC GALLSTONES

Data on the prevalence of gallstones in the USA indicate that only about 30% of people with cholelithiasis come to surgery. Symptoms of gallstone disease generally do not change in severity. Each year, about 2% of patients with asymptomatic gallstones develop symptoms, usually biliary colic rather than one of the complications of gallstone disease. Patients with chronic colic tend to have symptoms of the same level of severity and frequency. The present practice of operating only on symptomatic patients, leaving the millions without symptoms alone, seems appropriate. A question is often raised about what to advise the asymptomatic patient found to have gallstones during the course of unrelated studies. The presence of either of the following portends a more serious course and should probably serve as a reason for prophylactic cholecystectomy: (1) large stones (> 2 cm in diameter), because they produce acute cholecystitis more often than small stones; and (2) a calcified gallbladder, because it so often is associated with carcinoma. However, most asymptomatic patients have no special features. If coexistent cardiopulmonary or other problems increase the risk of surgery, operation should not be considered. For the average asymptomatic patient, it is not reasonable to make a strong recommendation for cholecystectomy. The tendency, however, is to operate on younger patients and temporize in the elderly.

Beckingham IJ: ABC of diseases of liver, pancreas, and biliary system. Gallstone disease. BMJ 2001;322:91.

GALLSTONES & CHRONIC CHOLECYSTITIS (Biliary Colic)

 ESSENTIALS OF DIAGNOSIS

- *Episodic abdominal pain.*
- *Dyspepsia.*
- *Gallstones on cholecystography or ultrasound scan.*

General Considerations

Chronic cholecystitis is the most common form of symptomatic gallbladder disease and is associated with gallstones in nearly every case. In general, the term cholecystitis is applied whenever gallstones are present regardless of the histologic appearance of the gallbladder. Repeated minor episodes of obstruction of the cystic duct cause intermittent biliary colic and contribute to inflammation and subsequent scar formation. Gallbladders from symptomatic patients with gallstones who have never had an attack of acute cholecystitis are

of two types: (1) In some, the mucosa may be slightly flattened, but the wall is thin and unscarred and, except for the stones, appears normal. (2) Others exhibit obvious signs of chronic inflammation, with thickening, cellular infiltration, loss of elasticity, and fibrosis. The clinical history in these two groups cannot always be distinguished, and inflammatory changes may also be found in patients with asymptomatic gallstones.

Clinical Findings

A. SYMPTOMS AND SIGNS

Biliary colic, the most characteristic symptom, is caused by transient gallstone obstruction of the cystic duct. The pain usually begins abruptly and subsides gradually, lasting for a few minutes to several hours. The pain of biliary colic is usually steady—not intermittent, like that of intestinal colic. In some patients, attacks occur postprandially; in others, there is no relationship to meals. The frequency of attacks is quite variable, ranging from nearly continuous trouble to episodes many years apart. Nausea and vomiting may accompany the pain.

Biliary colic is usually felt in the right upper quadrant, but epigastric and left abdominal pain are common, and some patients experience precordial pain. The pain may radiate around the costal margin into the back or may be referred to the region of the scapula. Pain on top of the shoulder is unusual and suggests direct diaphragmatic irritation. In a severe attack, the patient usually curls up in bed, changing position frequently in order to be more comfortable.

During an attack, there may be tenderness in the right upper quadrant, and, rarely, the gallbladder is palpable.

Fatty food intolerance, dyspepsia, indigestion, heartburn, flatulence, nausea, and eructations are other symptoms associated with gallstone disease. Because they are also frequent in the general population, their presence in any given patient may only be incidental to the gallstones.

B. LABORATORY FINDINGS

An ultrasound scan of the gallbladder should usually be the first test. Gallstones can be demonstrated in about 95% of cases, and a positive reading for gallstones is almost never in error. An oral cholecystogram should be obtained if the ultrasound study is equivocal, if the patient is a candidate for lithotripsy or ursodiol therapy, or if symptoms are highly suggestive and an ultrasound study has been read as normal.

About 2% of patients with gallstone disease have normal ultrasound studies and oral cholecystograms. Therefore, if the clinical suspicion of gallbladder disease is high and these two tests are negative, the patient should be studied by ERCP (to opacify the gallbladder in the search for stones) or duodenal intubation and examination of duodenal bile for cholesterol crystals or bilirubinate granules.

Differential Diagnosis

Gallbladder colic may be strongly suggested by the history, but the clinical impression should always be verified by an ultrasound study. Biliary colic may simulate the pain of duodenal ulcer, hiatal hernia, pancreatitis, and myocardial infarction.

An ECG and a chest x-ray should be obtained to investigate cardiopulmonary disease. It has been suggested that biliary colic may sometimes aggravate cardiac disease, but angina pectoris or an abnormal ECG should rarely be indications for cholecystectomy.

Right-sided radicular pain in the T6–T10 dermatomes may be confused with biliary colic. Osteoarthritic spurs, vertebral lesions, or tumors may be shown on x-rays of the spine or may be suggested by hyperesthesia of the abdominal skin.

An upper gastrointestinal series may be indicated to search for esophageal spasm, hiatal hernia, peptic ulcer, or gastric tumors. In some patients, the irritable colon syndrome may be mistaken for gallbladder discomfort. Carcinoma of the cecum or ascending colon may be overlooked on the assumption that postprandial pain in these conditions is due to gallstones.

Complications

Chronic cholecystitis predisposes to acute cholecystitis, common duct stones, and adenocarcinoma of the gallbladder. The longer the stones have been present, the higher the incidence of all of these complications. Complications are infrequent, however, and the presence of gallstones is not reason enough for prophylactic cholecystectomy in a person with asymptomatic or mildly symptomatic disease.

Treatment

A. Medical Treatment

Avoidance of offending foods may be helpful.

1. Dissolution–Cholesterol gallstones in the gallbladder can be dissolved in some cases by chronic treatment with ursodiol, which reduces the cholesterol saturation of bile by inhibiting cholesterol secretion. The resulting undersaturated bile slowly dissolves the solid cholesterol in the gallstones.

Unfortunately, bile salt therapy has marginal efficacy. The gallstones must be small (eg, < 5 mm) and devoid of calcium (ie, nonopaque on CT scans), and the gallbladder must opacify on oral cholecystography

(an indication of unobstructed flow of bile between bile duct and gallbladder). About 15% of patients with gallstones are candidates for treatment. Dissolution is achieved within 2 years in about 50% of highly selected patients. Stones recur, however, in 50% of cases within 5 years. In general, dissolution therapy—alone or in conjunction with lithotripsy—is used only rarely.

2. Lithotripsy and dissolution–Extracorporeal shock wave lithotripsy (ESWL) involves focusing shock waves, which pass through tissue and fluids, upon the gallstones. The stones are fragmented by explosion of small air bubbles within interstices of the solid material.

Lithotripsy is of little therapeutic value because the fragments remain in the gallbladder unless they can be dissolved. Consequently, candidates for lithotripsy must also use ursodiol therapy. Complete elimination of gallbladder stones is attained within 9 months in about 25% of appropriately selected patients. Because of the many drawbacks of this form of treatment, it has not been approved by the FDA in the United States.

B. Surgical Treatment

Cholecystectomy is indicated in most patients with symptoms. The procedure can be scheduled at the patient's convenience, within weeks or months after diagnosis. Active concurrent disease that increases the risk of surgery should be treated before operation. In some chronically ill patients, surgery should be deferred indefinitely.

Cholecystectomy is most often performed laparoscopically, but when the laparoscopic approach is contraindicated (eg, too many adhesions) or unsuccessful, it may be performed through a laparotomy. The difference consists of 4 fewer days in the hospital and several fewer weeks off work when done laparoscopically. Regardless of how it is done, operative cholangiography is usually included to look for common duct stones. If stones are found, common duct exploration is performed (see under choledocholithiasis).

Prognosis

Serious complications and deaths related to the operation itself are rare. The operative death rate is about 0.1% in patients under age 50 and about 0.5% in patients over age 50. Most deaths occur in patients recognized preoperatively to have increased risks. The operation relieves symptoms in 95% of cases.

Beyer AJ 3rd, Delcore R, Cheung LY: Nonoperative treatment of biliary tract disease. Arch Surg 1998;133:1172.

Binmoeller KF, Schafer TW: Endoscopic management of bile duct stones. J Clin Gastroenterol 2001;32:106.

Calland JF et al: Outpatient laparoscopic cholecystectomy: patient outcomes after implementation of a clinical pathway. Ann Surg 2001;233:704.

Fletcher DR et al: Complications of cholecystectomy: risks of the laparoscopic approach and protective effects of operative cholangiography: a population-based study. Ann Surg 1999; 229:449.

Gadacz TR: Update on laparoscopic cholecystectomy, including a clinical pathway. Surg Clin North Am 2000;80:1127.

Maxwell JG et al: Cholecystectomy in patients aged 80 and older. Am J Surg 1998;176(6):627.

Montori A et al: Endoscopic and surgical integration in the approach to biliary tract disease. J Clin Gastroenterol 1999; 28:198.

Moonka R et al: The presentation of gallstones and results of biliary surgery in a spinal cord injured population. Am J Surg 1999; 178:246.

Sakuramoto S et al: Preoperative evaluation to predict technical difficulties of laparoscopic cholecystectomy on the basis of histological inflammation findings on resected gallbladder. Am J Surg 2000;179:114.

Stuart SA et al: Routine intraoperative laparoscopic cholangiography. Am J Surg 1998;176(6):632.

Tocchi A et al: The need for antibiotic prophylaxis in elective laparoscopic cholecystectomy: a prospective randomized study. Arch Surg 2000;135:67.

Traverso LW: Risk factors for intraoperative injury during cholecystectomy: an ounce of prevention is worth a pound of cure. Ann Surg 1999;229:458.

Yerdel MA et al: Direct trocar insertion versus Veress needle insertion in laparoscopic cholecystectomy. Am J Surg 1999; 177:247.

ACUTE CHOLECYSTITIS

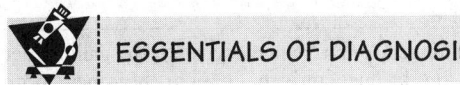 ESSENTIALS OF DIAGNOSIS

- *Acute right upper quadrant pain and tenderness.*
- *Fever and leukocytosis.*
- *Palpable gallbladder in one-third of cases.*
- *Nonpacified gallbladder on radionuclide excretion scan.*
- *Sonographic Murphy sign.*

General Considerations

In 80% of cases, acute cholecystitis results from obstruction of the cystic duct by a gallstone impacted in Hartmann's pouch. The gallbladder becomes inflamed and distended, creating abdominal pain and tenderness. The natural history of acute cholecystitis varies, depending on whether the obstruction becomes relieved, the extent of secondary bacterial invasion, the age of the patient, and the presence of other aggravating factors such as diabetes mellitus. Most attacks resolve spontaneously without surgery or other specific therapy, but

some progress to abscess formation or free perforation with generalized peritonitis.

The pathologic changes in the gallbladder evolve in a typical pattern. Subserosal edema and hemorrhage and patchy mucosal necrosis are the first changes. Later, PMNs appear. The final stage involves development of fibrosis. Gangrene and perforation may occur as early as 3 days after onset, but most perforations occur during the second week. In cases that resolve spontaneously, acute inflammation has largely cleared by 4 weeks, but some residual evidence of inflammation may last for several months. About 90% of gallbladders removed during an acute attack show chronic scarring, although many of these patients deny having had any previous symptoms.

The cause of acute cholecystitis is still partially conjectural. Obstruction of the cystic duct is present in most cases, but in experimental animals, cystic duct obstruction does not result in acute cholecystitis unless the gallbladder is filled with concentrated bile or bile saturated with cholesterol. There is also evidence that trauma from gallstones releases phospholipase from the mucosal cells of the gallbladder. This is followed by conversion of lecithin in bile to lysolecithin, which is a toxic compound that may cause more inflammation. Bacteria appear to have a minor role in the early stages of acute cholecystitis, even though most complications of the disease involve suppuration.

About 20% of cases of acute cholecystitis occur in the absence of cholelithiasis (acalculous cholecystitis). Some of these are due to cystic duct obstruction by another process such as a malignant tumor. Rarely, acute acalculous cholecystitis results from cystic artery occlusion or primary bacterial infection by *E coli,* clostridia, or, occasionally, *Salmonella typhi.* Most cases occur in patients hospitalized with some other illness; acute acalculous cholecystitis is particularly common in trauma victims (civilian or military) and in patients receiving total parenteral nutrition. Small-vessel occlusion occurs early, and unless treatment is given promptly, the disease progresses rapidly to gangrenous cholecystitis and septic complications, at which point the death rate is high.

Clinical Findings

A. SYMPTOMS AND SIGNS

The first symptom is abdominal pain in the right upper quadrant, sometimes associated with referred pain in the region of the right scapula. In 75% of cases, the patient will have had previous attacks of biliary colic, at first indistinguishable from the present illness. However, in acute cholecystitis, the pain persists and becomes associated with abdominal tenderness. Nausea and vomiting are present in about half of patients, but the vomiting is rarely severe. Mild icterus occurs in 10% of cases. The temperature usually ranges from 38 to 38.5 °C. High fever and chills are uncommon and should suggest the possibility of complications or an incorrect diagnosis.

Right upper quadrant tenderness is present, and in about a third of patients the gallbladder is palpable (often in a position lateral to its normal one). Voluntary guarding during examination may prevent detection of an enlarged gallbladder. In others, the gallbladder is not enlarged because scarring of the wall restricts distention. If instructed to breathe deeply during palpation in the right subcostal region, the patient experiences accentuated tenderness and sudden inspiratory arrest (Murphy's sign).

B. Laboratory Findings

The leukocyte count is usually elevated to 12,000–15,000/μL. Normal counts are common, but if the count goes much above 15,000, one should suspect complications. A mild elevation of the serum bilirubin (in the range of 2–4 mg/dL) is common, presumably owing to secondary inflammation of the common duct by the contiguous gallbladder. Bilirubin values above this range would most likely indicate the associated presence of common duct stones. A mild increase in alkaline phosphatase may accompany the attack. Occasionally, the serum amylase concentration transiently reaches 1000 units/dL or more.

C. Imaging Studies

A plain x-ray of the abdomen may occasionally show an enlarged gallbladder shadow. In 15% of patients, the gallstones contain enough calcium to be seen on the plain film.

Ultrasound scans show gallstones, sludge, and thickening of the gallbladder wall, and the ultrasonographer can determine even better than the clinician whether the point of maximum tenderness is over the gallbladder (ultrasonographic Murphy's sign). This last finding is often absent, however, when the gallbladder is gangrenous. Usually, ultrasound is the only test needed to make the diagnosis of acute cholecystitis.

If additional diagnostic information is desirable (eg, if ultrasound is equivocal or negative), a radionuclide excretion scan (eg, HIDA scan) should be performed. This test cannot demonstrate gallstones, but if the gallbladder is imaged, acute cholecystitis is ruled out except in rare cases of acalculous cholecystitis (the test is positive in most cases of acute acalculous cholecystitis). Imaging of the duct but not the gallbladder supports the diagnosis of acute cholecystitis. A few false positives are seen in advanced gallstone disease without acute inflammation and in acute biliary pancreatitis.

Differential Diagnosis

The differential diagnosis includes other common causes of acute upper abdominal pain and tenderness. An acute peptic ulcer with or without perforation might be suggested by a history of epigastric pain relieved by food or antacids. Most cases of perforated ulcer demonstrate free air under the diaphragm on x-ray. An emergency upper gastrointestinal series may help.

Acute pancreatitis can be confused with acute cholecystitis, especially if cholecystitis is accompanied by an elevated amylase level. Furthermore, HIDA scans fail to outline the gallbladder in most cases of acute biliary pancreatitis. Sometimes the two diseases coexist, but pancreatitis should not be accepted as a second diagnosis without specific findings.

Acute appendicitis in patients with a high cecum may closely simulate acute cholecystitis.

Severe right upper quadrant pain with high fever and local tenderness may develop in acute gonococcal perihepatitis (Fitz-Hugh-Curtis syndrome). Clues to the proper diagnosis may be found in tenderness in the adnexa, vaginal discharge that shows gonococci on a Gram-stained smear, and a disparity between the patient's high fever and her general lack of toxicity.

Complications

The major complications of acute cholecystitis are empyema, gangrene, and perforation.

A. Empyema

In empyema (suppurative cholecystitis), the gallbladder contains frank pus, and the patient becomes more toxic, with high spiking fever (39–40 °C), chills, and leukocytosis greater than 15,000/μL. Parenteral antibiotics should be given, and percutaneous cholecystostomy or cholecystectomy should be performed.

B. Perforation

Perforation may take any of three forms: (1) localized perforation with pericholecystic abscess; (2) free perforation with generalized peritonitis; and (3) perforation into an adjacent hollow viscus, with the formation of a fistula. Perforation may occur as early as 3 days after the onset of acute cholecystitis or not until late in the second week. The total incidence of perforation is about 10%.

1. Pericholecystic abscess—Pericholecystic abscess, the most common form of perforation, should be suspected when the signs and symptoms progress, especially when accompanied by the appearance of a palpable mass. The patient often becomes toxic, with fever to 39 °C and a leukocyte count above 15,000/μL, but sometimes there is no correlation between the clinical signs and the development of local abscess. Cholecystectomy and drainage of the abscess can be performed safely in many of these patients, but if the patient's condition is unstable, percutaneous cholecystostomy is preferable.

2. Free perforation—Free perforation occurs in only 1–2% of patients, most often early in the disease when gangrene develops before adhesions wall off the gallbladder. The diagnosis is made preoperatively in less than half of cases. In some patients with localized pain, sudden spread of pain and tenderness to other parts of the abdomen suggests the diagnosis. Whenever it is suspected, free perforation must be treated by emergency laparotomy. Abdominal paracentesis may be misleading and has proved to be of little diagnostic usefulness. Cholecystectomy should be performed if the patient's condition will permit; otherwise, cholecystostomy is done. The death rate depends partly on whether the cystic duct remains obstructed or the stone becomes dislodged after perforation. The former leads to a purulent peritonitis that is lethal in 20% of cases. In the latter, a true bile peritonitis ensues and over 50% of patients die. The earlier operation is performed, the better the prognosis.

3. Cholecystenteric fistula—If the acutely inflamed gallbladder becomes adherent to adjacent stomach, duodenum, or colon and necrosis develops at the site of one of these adhesions, perforation may occur into the lumen of the gut. The resulting decompression often allows the acute disease to resolve. If the gallbladder stones discharge through the fistula and if they are large enough, they may obstruct the small intestine (gallstone ileus; see below). Rarely, patients vomit gallstones that have entered the stomach through a cholecystogastric fistula. In most patients, the acute attack subsides and the cholecystenteric fistula is clinically unsuspected.

Cholecystenteric fistulas do not usually cause symptoms unless the gallbladder is still partially obstructed by stones or scarring. Neither oral nor intravenous cholangiograms will opacify the gallbladder or the fistula, but the latter may be shown on upper gastrointestinal series, where it must be differentiated from a fistula due to perforated peptic ulcer. Malabsorption and steatorrhea have been reported in isolated cases of cholecystocolonic fistulas. Steatorrhea in this situation could be due either to absence of bile in the proximal bowel following diversion into the colon or, more rarely, to excess bacteria in the upper intestine.

Symptomatic cholecystenteric fistulas should be treated by cholecystectomy and closure of the fistula. The majority are discovered incidentally during cholecystectomy for symptomatic gallbladder disease.

Treatment

Intravenous fluids should be given to correct dehydration and electrolyte imbalance, and a nasogastric tube should be inserted. For acute cholecystitis of average severity, parenteral cefazolin (2–4 g daily) should be given. Parenteral penicillin (20 million units daily), clindamycin, and an aminoglycoside should be given for severe disease. Single-drug therapy using imipenem is a good alternative.

There are two schools of thought about the treatment of acute cholecystitis. Since the disease resolves with antibiotics and supportive care in about 60% of cases, one approach is to manage the patient expectantly, with a plan to perform elective cholecystectomy after recovery, reserving surgery during the acute attack for those with severe or worsening disease. (This approach is untenable in acute acalculous cholecystitis.)

The preferred plan is to perform cholecystectomy in all patients unless there are specific contraindications to operation (eg, serious concomitant disease). Four controlled trials have supported this approach with the following data: (1) the incidence of technical complications is no greater with early surgery; (2) early surgery reduces the total duration of illness by approximately 30 days, length of hospitalization by 5–7 days, and direct medical costs by several thousand dollars; and (3) the death rate is slightly lower with early surgery because of earlier treatment for some patients whose condition would have worsened during expectant management. Since these trials were completed, the average case appears to have become more severe, and the arguments against expectant management are now even more compelling.

The following are the major factors that affect the decision (Figure 26–8): (1) whether the diagnosis is established; (2) the general health of the patient as modified by coexistent disease or the present illness; and (3) signs of local complications of acute cholecystitis. The diagnosis should be clear-cut and the patient optimally prepared; if perforation or empyema is suspected, emergency surgery is indicated.

In about 30% of cases, the diagnosis of acute cholecystitis is established but the general condition of the patient is unsatisfactory. If possible, surgery should be postponed in these cases until the ancillary disease is controlled. Expectant management cannot be rigidly adhered to, however, if the manifestations of cholecystitis worsen.

About 10% of patients require emergency treatment. These are generally clinical situations in which the disease appears to have become complicated or is about to. High fever (39 °C), marked leukocytosis (> 15,000/μL), or chills suggest suppurative progression. Acalculous acute cholecystitis should automatically be placed in this category. When the patient's general condition is poor, percutaneous catheter cholecystostomy is the preferable treatment. Patients in better overall health should be treated by cholecystectomy.

The sudden appearance of generalized abdominal pain may indicate free perforation. Appearance of a mass

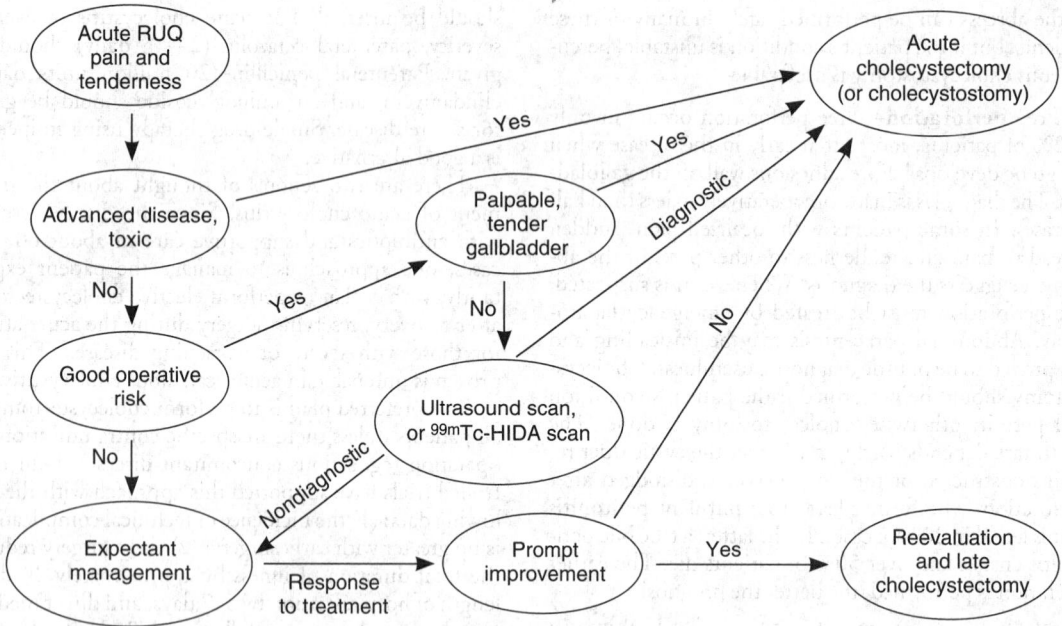

Figure 26–8. Scheme for the management of acute cholecystitis.

while the patient is under observation may be a sign of local perforation and abscess formation. Changes of this sort are indications for emergency surgery.

Cholecystectomy is the preferable operation in acute cholecystitis, and it can be performed laparoscopically in about 50% of patients. Operative cholangiography should be performed in most cases, and the common bile duct explored if appropriate indications are present (see section on choledocholithiasis). Patients with severe acute cholecystitis who are in poor condition for emergency cholecystectomy should be treated by percutaneous cholecystostomy. Percutaneous cholecystostomy may also be the preferred therapy for acute acalculous cholecystitis. A catheter inserted under ultrasound or CT guidance is allowed to drain the gallbladder of its bile or pus. The resulting decompression controls the acute disease, including any local infection, but the gallstones cannot be removed. Therefore, cholecystectomy should be performed after the patient recovers in order to avoid recurrent attacks. Cholecystectomy is definitive therapy in the patient with acalculous cholecystitis. At one time, cholecystostomy was performed surgically, but most hospitals now have radiologists skilled in the simpler percutaneous method.

Prognosis

The overall death rate of acute cholecystitis is about 5%. Nearly all of the deaths are in patients over age 60

or those with diabetes mellitus. In the older age group, secondary cardiovascular or pulmonary complications contribute substantially to the death rate. Uncontrolled sepsis with peritonitis and intrahepatic abscesses are the most important local conditions responsible for death.

Common duct stones are present in about 15% of patients with acute cholecystitis, and some of the more seriously ill patients have simultaneous cholangitis from biliary obstruction. Acute pancreatitis may also complicate acute cholecystitis, and the combination carries a greater risk.

Patients who develop the suppurative forms of gallbladder disease such as empyema or perforation are less likely to recover. Earlier admission to the hospital and early cholecystectomy reduce the chances of these complications.

Berber E et al: Selective use of tube cholecystostomy with interval laparoscopic cholecystectomy in acute cholecystitis. Arch Surg 2000;135:341.

Borzellino G et al: Emergency cholecystostomy and subsequent cholecystectomy for acute gallstone cholecystitis in the elderly. Br J Surg 1999;86:1521.

Davis CA, Landercasper J, Gundersen LH, Lambert PJ: Effective use of percutaneous cholecystostomy in high-risk surgical patients: techniques, tube management, and results. Arch Surg 1999;134:727.

Eldar S et al: The impact of patient delay and physician delay on the outcome of laparoscopic cholecystectomy for acute cholecystitis. Am J Surg 1999;178:303.

Geoghegan JG, Keane FB: Laparoscopic management of complicated gallstone disease. Br J Surg 1999;86:145.

Greenwald JA et al: Standardization of surgeon-controlled variables: impact on outcome in patients with acute cholecystitis. Ann Surg 2000;231:339.

Kim KH et al: Percutaneous gallbladder drainage for delayed laparoscopic cholecystectomy in patients with acute cholecystitis. Am J Surg 2000;179:111.

Laycock WS et al: Variation in the use of laparoscopic cholecystectomy for elderly patients with acute cholecystitis. Arch Surg 2000;135:457.

Lillemoe KD: Surgical treatment of biliary tract infections. Am Surg 2000;66:138.

Lobe TE: Cholelithiasis and cholecystitis in children. Semin Pediatr Surg 2000;9:170.

Svanvik J: Laparoscopic cholecystectomy for acute cholecystitis. Eur J Surg 2000;(Suppl 585):16.

EMPHYSEMATOUS CHOLECYSTITIS

Emphysematous cholecystitis is a rare condition in which bubbles of gas from anaerobic infection appear in the lumen of the gallbladder, its wall, the pericholecystic space, and, on occasion, the bile ducts. Clostridia species are the most commonly implicated organisms, but other gas-forming anaerobes such as *E coli* or anaerobic streptococci may be found. Three times as many men as women are affected, and 20% of patients have diabetes mellitus. In contrast to the usual form of acute cholecystitis, the disease probably is a bacterial infection from the earliest moment. In many cases, the gallbladder contains no stones.

The disease begins with sudden and rapidly progressive right upper quadrant pain. Fever and leukocytosis reach high levels quickly, and the patient is considerably more toxic than is usually the case in acute cholecystitis. On examination, a mass can usually be found in the right upper quadrant.

Plain films of the abdomen show tissue emphysema outlining the gallbladder and, in some cases, an air-fluid level in the lumen. The clinical and x-ray pictures are characteristic enough so that the diagnosis is usually obvious. If the changes on plain films are equivocal, a CT scan may bring them out.

The patient should be treated with high doses of antibiotics effective against clostridia and the other species mentioned above. Emergency surgical treatment should follow the initial resuscitative measures. Cholecystectomy can be safely performed in most cases, but the most critically ill might fare better with cholecystostomy. The types of complications are the same as in other forms of acute cholecystitis, but illness is more severe and death rates are higher.

Danse EM, Laterre PF: Images in clinical medicine. Emphysematous cholecystitis. N Engl J Med 1999;341):1126.

Garcia-Sancho Tellez L et al: Acute emphysematous cholecystitis. Report of twenty cases. Hepatogastroenterology 1999;46:2144.

Zeebregts CJ et al: Percutaneous drainage of emphysematous cholecystitis associated with pneumoperitoneum. Hepatogastroenterology 1999;46:771.

GALLSTONE ILEUS

Gallstone ileus is mechanical intestinal obstruction caused by a large gallstone lodged in the lumen. It is seen most often in women, and the average age is about 70.

Clinical Findings

A. SYMPTOMS

The patient usually presents with obvious small bowel obstruction, either partial or complete. The obstructing gallstone enters the intestine through a cholecystenteric fistula located in the duodenum, colon, or, rarely, the stomach or jejunum. The gallbladder may contain one or several stones, but stones that cause gallstone ileus are almost always 2.5 cm or more in diameter. The lumen in the proximal bowel will allow most of these large calculi to pass caudally until the ileum is reached. Obstruction of the large intestine may follow passage of a gallstone through a fistula at the hepatic flexure or may occur even after the stone has traversed the entire small bowel.

B. SIGNS

In most patients, the findings on physical examination are typical of distal small bowel obstruction. Obstruction of the duodenum or jejunum may give a perplexing clinical picture because of the lack of distention. Right upper quadrant tenderness and a mass may be present in some cases, but the distended abdomen may be difficult to examine accurately.

C. IMAGING STUDIES

In addition to dilated small intestine, plain films of the abdomen may show a radiopaque gallstone, and unless one is alert to the possibility of gallstone ileus, the ectopic stone can be a puzzling finding. In about 40% of cases, careful examination of the film will reveal gas in the biliary tree, a manifestation of the cholecystenteric fistula. When the clinical picture is unclear, an upper gastrointestinal series should be obtained, which will demonstrate the cholecystoduodenal fistula and verify intestinal obstruction.

Treatment

The proper treatment is emergency laparotomy and removal of the obstructing stone through a small enterotomy. The proximal intestine must be carefully inspected for the presence of a second calculus that might cause a postoperative recurrence. The gallbladder should be left undisturbed at the original operation.

Once the patient has recovered, an elective cholecystectomy should be scheduled if the patient complains of chronic gallbladder symptoms. On this basis, interval cholecystectomy will be required in about 30% of patients. The fistula itself is rarely the source of trouble and closes spontaneously in most patients.

Prognosis

The death rate of gallstone ileus remains about 20%, largely because of the poor general condition of elderly patients at the time of laparotomy. In many cases, the patient has developed cardiac or pulmonary complications during a preoperative delay when the diagnosis was unclear.

Lobo DN, Jobling JC, Balfour TW: Gallstone ileus: diagnostic pitfalls and therapeutic successes. J Clin Gastroenterol 2000; 30:72

Scarpa F et al: Gallstone ileus: diagnostic pitfalls and therapeutic successes. J Clin Gastroenterol 2000;30:72.

CHOLANGITIS (Bacterial Cholangitis)

Bacterial infection of the biliary ducts always signifies biliary obstruction, since in the absence of obstruction even heavy bacterial contamination of the ducts fails to produce symptoms or pathologic changes. The block to flow may be partial or, less commonly, complete. The principal causes are choledocholithiasis, biliary stricture, and neoplasm. Less common causes are chronic pancreatitis, ampullary stenosis, pancreatic pseudocyst, duodenal diverticulum, congenital cyst, and parasitic invasion. Iatrogenic cholangitis may complicate transhepatic or T tube cholangiography. Not all obstructing lesions are followed by cholangitis, however. For example, biliary infection develops in only 15% of patients with neoplastic obstruction. The likelihood of cholangitis is greatest when the obstruction occurs after the duct has acquired a resident bacterial population.

With obstruction, ductal pressure rises, and bacteria proliferate and escape into the systemic circulation via the hepatic sinusoids. Experimentally, the incidence of positive blood cultures with ductal infection is directly proportionate to the absolute height of the pressure in the duct.

The symptoms of cholangitis (sometimes referred to as Charcot's triad) are biliary colic, jaundice, and chills and fever, though a complete triad is present in only 70% of cases. Laboratory findings include leukocytosis and elevated serum bilirubin and alkaline phosphatase levels. The predominant organisms in bile (in approximately decreasing frequency) are *E coli*, klebsiella, pseudomonas, enterococci, and proteus. *Bacteroides fragilis* and other anaerobes (eg, *Clostridium perfringens*) can be detected in about 25% of cases, and their presence correlates with multiple previous biliary operations (often including a biliary enteric anastomosis), severe symptoms, and a high incidence of postoperative suppurative complications. Anaerobes are nearly always seen in the company of aerobes. Two species of bacteria can be cultured in about 50% of cases. Bacteremia probably occurs in most cases, and blood cultures obtained at the appropriate time contain the same organisms as the bile. Early in an attack, an ultrasound scan will often give useful diagnostic information. Further workup (THC, ERCP, etc) can proceed later after the acute manifestations are brought under control. Cholangiography is dangerous during active cholangitis.

The term **suppurative cholangitis** has been used for the most severe form of this disease, when manifestations of sepsis overshadow those of hepatobiliary disease. The diagnostic pentad of suppurative cholangitis consists of abdominal pain, jaundice, fever and chills, mental confusion or lethargy, and shock. The diagnosis is often missed because the signs of biliary disease are overlooked.

Most cases of cholangitis can be controlled with intravenous antibiotics. A cephalosporin antibiotic (eg, cefazolin, cefoxitin) is the drug of choice in the average mild to moderately severe case. If disease is severe or progressively worsens, an aminoglycoside plus clindamycin or metronidazole should be added to the regimen.

For patients with severe cholangitis or unremitting cholangitis despite antibiotic therapy, the bile duct must be promptly decompressed. Most cases of severe acute cholangitis are associated with choledocholithiasis, where the best treatment consists of emergency endoscopic sphincterotomy. In the uncommon case where this is unsuccessful, laparotomy is indicated in order to decompress the bile duct. Cholangitis accompanying neoplastic obstruction may be managed by insertion of a transhepatic drainage catheter into the bile duct. A cholangiogram should not be obtained because the procedure could worsen sepsis.

Urgent intervention (eg, endoscopic sphincterotomy, percutaneous transhepatic drainage, or operative decompression) is required in about 10% of patients with acute cholangitis. The remaining 90% are eventually treated by elective surgery or endoscopic sphincterotomy following antibiotic therapy and a thorough diagnostic evaluation.

Elsakr R et al: Antimicrobial treatment of intra-abdominal infections. Dig Dis 1998;16:47.

Hanau LH, Steigbigel NH: Acute (ascending) cholangitis. Infect Dis Clin North Am 2000;14:521.

Poon RT et al: Management of gallstone cholangitis in the era of laparoscopic cholecystectomy. Arch Surg 2001;136:11.

Raraty MG, Finch M, Neoptolemos JP: Acute cholangitis and pancreatitis secondary to common duct stones: management update. World J Surg 1998;22:1155.

CHOLEDOCHOLITHIASIS

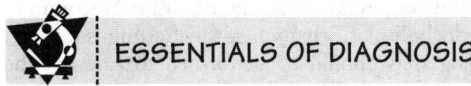

ESSENTIALS OF DIAGNOSIS

- *Biliary pain.*
- *Jaundice.*
- *Episodic cholangitis.*
- *Gallstones in gallbladder or previous cholecystectomy.*

General Considerations

Approximately 15% of patients with stones in the gallbladder are found to harbor calculi within the bile ducts. Common duct stones are usually accompanied by others in the gallbladder, but in 5% of cases, the gallbladder is empty. The number of duct stones may vary from one to more than 100.

There are two possible origins for common duct stones. The evidence suggests that most cholesterol stones develop within the gallbladder and reach the duct after traversing the cystic duct. These are called secondary stones. Pigment stones may have a similar pedigree or, more often, develop de novo within the common duct. These are called primary common duct stones. About 60% of common duct stones are cholesterol stones and 40% are pigment stones. The latter are, on the average, associated with more severe clinical manifestations.

Patients may have one or more of the following principal clinical findings, all of which are caused by obstruction to the flow of bile or pancreatic juice: biliary colic, cholangitis, jaundice, and pancreatitis (Figure 26– 9). It seems likely, however, that as many as 50% of patients with choledocholithiasis remain asymptomatic.

The common duct may dilate to 2–3 cm proximal to an obstructing lesion, and truly huge ducts develop in patients with biliary tumors. In choledocholithiasis or biliary stricture, the inflammatory reaction restricts dilation, so the dilatation is less marked. Dilation of the ductal system within the liver can also be limited by cirrhosis.

Biliary colic is the result of rapid rises in biliary pressure whether the block is in the common duct or neck of the gallbladder. Gradual occlusion of the duct—as in

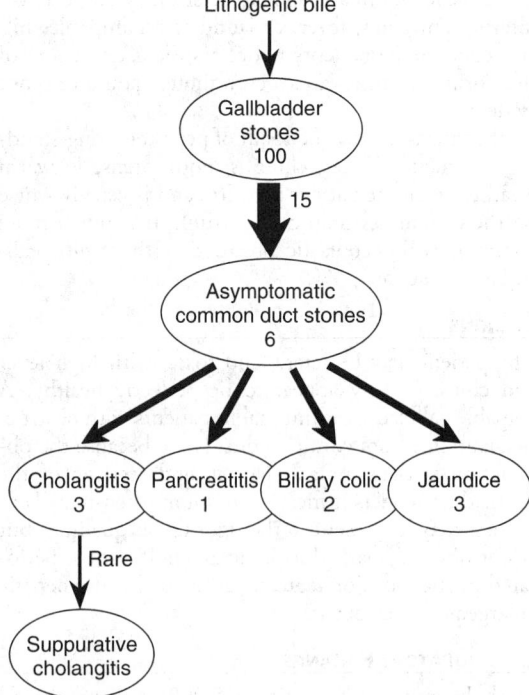

Figure 26–9. The natural history of common duct stones. Of every 100 patients with gallbladder stones, 15 will have common duct stones, which will produce the spectrum of syndromes illustrated. Note that the individual syndromes overlap, indicating that they may appear together in various combinations

cancer—rarely produces the same kind of pain as gallstone disease.

Clinical Findings

A. SYMPTOMS

Choledocholithiasis may be asymptomatic or may produce sudden toxic cholangitis, leading to a rapid demise. The seriousness of the disease parallels the degree of obstruction, the length of time it has been present, and the extent of secondary bacterial infection (see Cholangitis, above). Biliary colic, jaundice, or pancreatitis may be isolated findings or may occur in any combination along with signs of infection (cholangitis).

Biliary colic from common duct obstruction cannot be distinguished from that caused by stones in the gallbladder. The pain is felt in the right subcostal region, epigastrium, or even the substernal area. Referred pain to the region of the right scapula is common.

Choledocholithiasis should be strongly suspected if intermittent chills, fever, or jaundice accompanies biliary colic. Some patients notice transient darkening of their urine during an attack even though jaundice is not evident.

Pruritus is usually the result of persistent long-standing obstruction. The itching is more intense in warm weather when the patient perspires and is usually worse on the extremities than on the trunk. It is much more common with neoplastic obstruction than with gallstone obstruction.

B. Signs

The patient may be icteric and toxic, with high fever and chills, or may appear to be perfectly healthy. A palpable gallbladder is unusual in patients with obstructive jaundice from common duct stone because the obstruction is transient and partial, and scarring of the gallbladder renders it inelastic and nondistensible. Tenderness may be present in the right upper quadrant but is not often as marked as in acute cholecystitis, perforated peptic ulcer, or acute pancreatitis. Tender hepatic enlargement may occur.

C. Laboratory Findings

In cholangitis, leukocytosis of 15,000/µL is usual, and values above 20,000/µL are common. A rise in serum bilirubin often appears within 24 hours after the onset of symptoms. The absolute level usually remains under 10 mg/dL, and most are in the range of 2–4 mg/dL. The direct fraction exceeds the indirect, but the latter becomes elevated in most cases. Bilirubin levels do not ordinarily reach the high values seen in malignant tumors because the obstruction is usually incomplete and transient. In fact, fluctuating jaundice is so characteristic of choledocholithiasis that it fairly reliably differentiates between benign and malignant obstruction.

The serum alkaline phosphatase level usually rises and may be the only chemical abnormality in patients without jaundice. When the obstruction is relieved, the alkaline phosphatase and bilirubin levels should return to normal within 1–2 weeks, with the exception that the former may remain elevated longer if the obstruction was prolonged.

Mild increases in AST and ALT are often seen with extrahepatic obstruction of the ducts; rarely, AST levels transiently reach 1000 units.

D. Imaging Studies

Radiopaque gallstones may be seen on plain abdominal films or CT scans. Ultrasound scans will usually show gallbladder stones and, depending on the degree of obstruction, dilatation of the bile duct. Ultrasound and CT scans are insensitive in the search for stones in the common duct. ERCP is indicated if the patient has had a previous cholecystectomy. If cholecystectomy has not been performed, cholangiography should be part of operative management. Some clinicians choose preoperative ERCP for patients scheduled for cholecystectomy in order to clear the common bile duct. If ERCP is not technically successful, the surgeon will be forced to convert to open common bile duct exploration to clear the duct of stones.

Bilirubin values above 10 mg/dL are so uncommon in choledocholithiasis that when this finding is present, cholangiography should be performed to rule out the possibility of neoplastic obstruction.

Differential Diagnosis

The workup should consider the same possibilities in differential diagnosis as for cholecystitis.

Serum amylase levels above 500 units/dL can result from acute pancreatitis, acute cholecystitis, or choledocholithiasis. Other manifestations of pancreatic disease should be documented before an unqualified diagnosis of pancreatitis is accepted.

Alcoholic cirrhosis or acute alcoholic hepatitis may present with jaundice, right upper quadrant tenderness, and leukocytosis. The differentiation from cholangitis may be impossible from clinical data. A history of a recent binge suggests acute liver disease. A percutaneous liver biopsy may be specific.

Intrahepatic cholestasis from drugs, pregnancy, chronic active hepatitis, or primary biliary cirrhosis may be difficult to distinguish from extrahepatic obstruction. ERCP would be appropriate to make the distinction, particularly if other studies (eg, ultrasound scan) failed to provide evidence of gallstone disease. If jaundice has persisted for 4–6 weeks, a mechanical cause is probable. Since most patients improve during this interval, persistent jaundice should never be assumed to be the result of parenchymal disease unless a normal cholangiogram rules out obstruction of the major ducts.

Intermittent jaundice and cholangitis after cholecystectomy are compatible with biliary stricture, and the distinction require ERCP.

Biliary tumors usually produce intense jaundice without biliary colic or fever, and once it begins, the jaundice rarely remits.

Complications

Long-standing ductal infection can produce intrahepatic abscesses. Hepatic failure or secondary biliary cirrhosis may develop in unrelieved obstruction of long duration. Since the obstruction is usually incomplete and intermittent, cirrhosis develops only after several years in untreated disease. Acute pancreatitis, a fairly common complication of calculous biliary disease, is discussed in Chapter 27. Rarely, a stone in the common duct may erode through the ampulla, resulting in gallstone ileus. Hemorrhage (hemobilia) is also a rare complication.

Treatment

Patients with acute cholangitis should be treated with systemic antibiotics and other measures as described in the preceding section; this usually controls the attack within 24–48 hours. If the patient's condition worsens or if marked improvement is not observed within 2–4 days, endoscopic sphincterotomy or surgery and common bile duct exploration should be performed.

The typical patient presents with mild cholangitis and evidence on ultrasound scans of gallbladder stones. Laparoscopic cholecystectomy is indicated and, depending on the experience of the surgeon, laparoscopic exploration of the common duct if an operative cholangiogram or laparoscopic ultrasound demonstrates the expected common duct stones. Laparoscopic common duct exploration is usually accomplished through the cystic duct (which may have to be dilated), but when the common duct is enlarged (> 1.5 cm), it may be accomplished through a choledochotomy incision, just as in open surgery. Eventually, nearly all cases of common duct stones should be manageable by laparoscopic techniques, but at this stage the requisite laparoscopic skills are not available in most hospitals. If the surgeon thinks the common duct stones cannot be removed laparoscopically, it is probably best to remove the gallbladder laparoscopically and the common duct stones by endoscopic sphincterotomy. If the stones cannot be removed by sphincterotomy, a second (open) operation may be necessary.

There is also a lack of consensus regarding the importance of operative cholangiography or ultrasound during cholecystectomy when there are no clues suggesting stones in the duct. In such cases the chances of finding a stone are only 3–5%, and some consider the effort unwarranted. On the other hand, operative cholangiograms also provide confirmation of the biliary anatomy, which contributes to avoidance of bile duct injuries, and the natural history of the few overlooked stones is worrisome. Therefore, we side with those who perform operative cholangiography liberally in such cases.

When the common duct is explored through the cystic duct and gallstones are removed, the cystic duct must be ligated, but a drainage catheter is not usually left within the common duct. When the common duct is explored through a choledochotomy (either during a laparoscopic or open operation), a T tube is usually left in the duct, and cholangiograms are taken a week or so postoperatively. Any residual stones discovered on these postoperative x-rays can be extracted 4–6 weeks later through the T tube tract.

Patients with common duct stones who have had a previous cholecystectomy are best treated by **endoscopic sphincterotomy.** Using a side-viewing duodenoscope, the ampulla is cannulated, and a 1-cm incision is made in the sphincter with an electrocautery wire. The opening created in the sphincter permits stones to pass from the duct into the duodenum. Endoscopic sphincterotomy is unlikely to be successful in patients with large stones (eg, > 2 cm), and it is contraindicated in the presence of stenosis of the bile duct proximal to the sphincter. Laparotomy and common duct exploration are required in a few cases.

Stones in the intrahepatic branches of the bile duct can usually be removed without difficulty during common duct exploration. In some cases, however one or more of the intrahepatic ducts have become packed with stones, and the associated chronic inflammation has produced stenosis of the duct near its junction with the common hepatic duct. It is often impossible in these cases to clear the duct of stones, and if the disease involves only one lobe (usually the left lobe), hepatic lobectomy is indicated.

Binmoeller KF, Schafer TW: Endoscopic management of bile duct stones. J Clin Gastroenterol 2001;32:106.

Lauter DM, Froines EJ: Laparoscopic common duct exploration in the management of choledocholithiasis. Am J Surg 2000;179:372.

Prat F et al: Prediction of common bile duct stones by noninvasive tests. Ann Surg 1999;229:362.

Rosenthal RJ, Rossi RL, Martin RF: Options and strategies for the management of choledocholithiasis. World J Surg 1998;22:1125.

Soetikno RM, Montes H, Carr-Locke DL: Endoscopic management of choledocholithiasis. J Clin Gastroenterol 1998;27:296.

Soper NJ: Intraoperative detection: intraoperative cholangiography vs. intraoperative ultrasonography. J Gastrointest Surg 2000;4:334.

Suc B et al: Surgery vs endoscopy as primary treatment in symptomatic patients with suspected common bile duct stones: a multicenter randomized trial. French Associations for Surgical Research. Arch Surg 1998;133:702.

Tranter SE, Thompson MH: Potential of laparoscopic ultrasonography as an alternative to operative cholangiography in the detection of bile duct stones. Br J Surg 2001;88:65.

Wu JS, Dunnegan DL, Soper NJ: The utility of intracorporeal ultrasonography for screening of the bile duct during laparoscopic cholecystectomy. J Gastrointest Surg 1998;2:50.

POSTCHOLECYSTECTOMY SYNDROME

This term has been used to signify the heterogeneous group of disorders affecting patients who continue to complain of symptoms after cholecystectomy. It is not really a syndrome, and the term is confusing.

The usual reason for incomplete relief after cholecystectomy is that the preoperative diagnosis of chronic cholecystitis was incorrect. The only symptom entirely characteristic of chronic cholecystitis is biliary colic. When a calculous gallbladder is removed in the hope that the patient will gain relief from dyspepsia, fatty food intolerance, belching, etc, the operation may leave the symptoms unchanged.

The presenting symptom may be dyspepsia or pain. An organic cause for the symptoms is more likely to be discovered in patients with severe episodic pain than in those with other complaints. Abnormal liver function studies, jaundice, and cholangitis are other manifestations that indicate residual biliary disease. Patients with suspicious findings should be studied by ERCP or THC. Choledocholithiasis, biliary stricture, and chronic pancreatitis are the most common causes of symptoms. Evidence is accumulating to implicate sphincter of Oddi dysmotility as a cause of pain in some patients. The diagnosis may be possible by biliary manometry, but experience is still too meager to justify acceptance of this entity without question. Relief of pain may follow endoscopic sphincterotomy. Stenosis of the hepatobiliary ampulla, a long cystic duct remnant, and neuromas have been blamed for continued symptoms, but well-verified cases are uncommon.

CARCINOMA OF THE GALLBLADDER

Carcinoma of the gallbladder is an uncommon neoplasm that occurs in elderly patients. It is associated with gallstones in 70% of cases, and the risk of malignant degeneration correlates with the length of time gallstones have been present. The tumor is twice as common in women as in men, as one would expect from the association with gallstones.

Most primary tumors of the gallbladder are adenocarcinomas that appear histologically to be scirrhous (60%), papillary (25%), or mucoid (15%). Dissemination of the tumor occurs early by direct invasion of the liver and hilar structures and by metastases to the common duct lymph nodes, liver, and lungs. In an occasional case, where carcinoma is an incidental finding after cholecystectomy for gallstone disease, the tumor is confined to the gallbladder as a carcinoma in situ or an early invasive lesion. Most invasive carcinomas, however, have spread by the time of surgery, and spread is virtually certain if the tumor has progressed to the point where it causes symptoms.

Clinical Findings

A. SYMPTOMS AND SIGNS

The most common presenting complaint is of right upper quadrant pain similar to previous episodes of biliary colic but more persistent. Obstruction of the cystic duct by tumor sometimes initiates an attack of acute cholecystitis. Other cases present with obstructive jaundice and, occasionally, cholangitis due to secondary involvement of the common duct.

Examination usually reveals a mass in the region of the gallbladder, which may not be recognized as a neoplasm if the patient has acute cholecystitis. If cholangitis is the principal symptom, a palpable gallbladder would be an unusual finding with choledocholithiasis alone and should suggest gallbladder carcinoma.

B. IMAGING STUDIES

Oral cholecystograms almost never opacify except in patients with small incidental cancers. CT and ultrasound scans may demonstrate the extent of disease, but more often they show only gallstones.

The correct diagnosis is made preoperatively in only 10% of cases.

Complications

Obstruction of the common duct may produce multiple intrahepatic abscesses. Abscesses in or next to the tumor-laden gallbladder are frequent.

Prevention

The incidence of gallbladder cancer has decreased in recent years as the frequency of cholecystectomy has increased. It has been estimated that one case of gallbladder cancer is prevented for every 100 cholecystectomies performed for gallstone disease.

Treatment

If a localized carcinoma of the gallbladder is recognized at laparotomy, cholecystectomy should be performed along with en bloc wedge resection of an adjacent 3–5 cm of normal liver and dissection of the lymph nodes in the hepatoduodenal ligament. If a small invasive carcinoma overlooked during cholecystectomy for gallstone disease is later discovered by the pathologist, reoperation is indicated to perform a wedge resection of the liver bed plus regional lymphadenectomy. Some surgeons also recommend that the common duct be included routinely (ie, even in the absence of gross invasion) in the lymph node dissection for any lesion that involves the full thickness of the gallbladder wall. In the few cases where cancer has not penetrated the muscularis mucosae, cholecystectomy alone should suffice. More extensive hepatectomies (eg, right lobectomy) are not worthwhile. Lesions that invade the bile duct and produce jaundice should be resected if possible. When not, a stent should be inserted endoscopically or percutaneously. There is little that surgery can offer in cases with hepatic metastases or more distant spread.

Prognosis

Radiotherapy and chemotherapy are not effective palliative measures. About 85% of patients are dead within a year after diagnosis.

The 10% of patients who presently survive more than 5 years consist of those whose carcinoma was an incidental finding during cholecystectomy for symptomatic gallstone disease and those in whom an aggressive resection has removed all gross tumor.

Baillie J: Tumors of the gallbladder and bile ducts. J Clin Gastroenterol 1999;29:14.

Bismuth H, Majno PE: Hepatobiliary surgery. J Hepatol 2000; 32(1 Suppl):208.

Kondo S et al: Regional and para-aortic lymphadenectomy in radical surgery for advanced gallbladder carcinoma. Br J Surg 2000;87:418.

Mainprize KS, Gould SW, Gilbert JM: Surgical management of polypoid lesions of the gallbladder. Br J Surg 2000;87:414.

Scott TE et al: A case-control assessment of risk factors for gallbladder carcinoma. Dig Dis Sci 1999;44:1619.

Sugiyama M, Atomi Y, Yamato T: Endoscopic ultrasonography for differential diagnosis of polypoid gall bladder lesions: analysis in surgical and follow up series. Gut 2000;46:250.

MALIGNANT TUMORS OF THE BILE DUCT

 ESSENTIALS OF DIAGNOSIS

- *Intense cholestatic jaundice and pruritus.*
- *Anorexia and dull right upper quadrant pain.*
- *Dilated intrahepatic bile ducts on ultrasound or CT scan.*
- *Focal stricture on transhepatic or retrograde endoscopic cholangiogram.*

General Considerations

Primary bile duct tumors are not more common in patients with cholelithiasis, and men and women are affected with equal frequency. Tumors appear at an average age of 60 years but may appear at any time between 20 and 80 years of age. More young people have been seen with this disease in recent years. Ulcerative colitis is a common associated condition, and in occasional cases bile duct cancer develops in a patient with ulcera-

tive colitis who has been known to have sclerosing cholangitis for several years. Chronic parasitic infestation of the bile ducts in the Orient may be responsible for the greater incidence of bile duct tumors in that area.

Most malignant biliary tumors are adenocarcinomas located in the hepatic or common bile duct. The histologic pattern varies from typical adenocarcinoma to tumors composed principally of fibrous stroma and few cells. The acellular tumors may be mistaken for benign strictures or sclerosing cholangitis if adequate biopsies are not obtained. About 10% are bulky papillary tumors, which tend to be less invasive and less apt to metastasize.

At presentation, metastases are uncommon, but the tumor has often grown into the portal vein or hepatic artery.

Clinical Findings

A. SYMPTOMS AND SIGNS

The illness presents with gradual onset of jaundice or pruritus. Chills, fever, and biliary colic are usually absent, and except for a deep discomfort in the right upper quadrant the patient feels well. Bilirubinuria is present from the start, and light-colored stools are usual. Anorexia and weight loss develop insidiously with time.

Icterus is the most obvious physical finding. If the tumor is located in the common duct, the gallbladder may distend and become palpable in the right upper quadrant. The tumor itself is never palpable. Patients with tumors of the hepatic duct do not develop palpable gallbladders. Hepatomegaly is common. If obstruction is unrelieved, the liver may eventually become cirrhotic, and splenomegaly, ascites, or bleeding varices become secondary manifestations.

B. LABORATORY FINDINGS

Since the duct is often completely obstructed, the serum bilirubin is usually over 15 mg/dL. Serum alkaline phosphatase is also increased. Fever and leukocytosis are not common, since the bile is sterile in most cases. The stool may contain occult blood, but this is more common with tumors of the pancreas or hepatopancreatic ampulla than those of the bile ducts.

C. IMAGING STUDIES

Ultrasound or CT scans usually detect dilated intrahepatic bile ducts. THC or ERCP clearly depicts the lesion, and both are indicated in most cases. THC is of greater value, since it better demonstrates the ductal anatomy on the hepatic side of the lesion. With tumors involving the bifurcation of the common hepatic duct (Klatskin tumors), it is important to determine the proximal extent of the lesion (ie, whether the first branches of the lobar ducts are also involved). ERCP is of value with proximal tumors because if it shows concomitant obstruction of the cystic duct, the diagnosis will most often prove to be gallbladder cancer invading the common duct (not a primary common duct neoplasm). The typical pattern with distal bile duct cancers consists of stenosis of the bile duct with sparing of the pancreatic duct. Adjacent stenoses of both ducts (the double-duct sign) indicate primary cancer of the pancreas. MR cholangiopancreatography may be useful if high-quality studies are available.

Occasionally, bile samples obtained at the time of THC will show malignant cells on cytologic study, but this is not a particularly useful test since the diagnosis of cancer must be presumed from the cholangiographic findings and a negative cytologic study is unreliable. Angiography may suggest invasion of the portal vein or encasement of the hepatic artery. False positives may occur, however.

Differential Diagnosis

The differential diagnosis must consider other causes of extrahepatic and intrahepatic cholestatic jaundice. Choledocholithiasis is characterized by episodes of partial obstruction, pain, and cholangitis, which contrast with the unremitting jaundice of malignant obstruction. Bilirubin concentrations rarely surpass 15 mg/dL and are usually below 10 mg/dL in gallstone obstruction, whereas bilirubin levels almost always exceed 10 mg/dL and are usually above 15 mg/dL in neoplastic obstruction. A rapid rise of the bilirubin level to above 15 mg/dL in a patient with sclerosing cholangitis should suggest superimposed neoplasm. Dilatation of the gallbladder may occur with tumors of the distal common duct but is rare with calculous obstruction.

The combination of an enlarged gallbladder with obstructive jaundice is usually recognized as being due to tumor. If the gallbladder cannot be felt, primary biliary cirrhosis, drug-induced jaundice, chronic active hepatitis, metastatic hepatic cancer, and common duct stone must be ruled out. In general, any patient with cholestatic jaundice of more than 2 weeks' duration whose diagnosis is uncertain should be studied by THC or ERCP. The finding of focal bile duct stenosis in the absence of previous biliary surgery is almost pathognomonic of neoplasm.

Treatment

Patients without evidence of metastases or other signs of advanced cancer (eg, ascites) are candidates for laparotomy. The 30% of patients who do not qualify may be treated by insertion of a tube stent into the bile duct transhepatically under radiologic control or from the duodenum under endoscopic control. The tube is positioned so that holes above and below the tumor reestablish flow of bile into the duodenum. If both lobar ducts are blocked by a tumor at the bifurcation of the common hepatic duct, it is usually necessary to place a transhepatic tube into only one lobar duct. If the lesion blocks the takeoff of the segmental ducts, stents are rarely beneficial.

Laparotomy is indicated in most cases, however, with the objective of removing the tumor. Preoperative decompression of the bile duct with a percutaneous catheter to relieve jaundice does not lower the incidence of postoperative complications. At operation, which may be immediately preceded by diagnostic laparoscopy, the extent of the tumor should be determined by external examination of the bile duct and the adjacent portal vein and hepatic artery.

Tumors of the distal common duct should be treated by radical pancreaticoduodenectomy (Whipple procedure) if it appears that all tumor would be removed. Secondary involvement of the portal vein is the usual reason for unresectability of tumors in this location. Mid common duct or low hepatic duct tumors should also be removed if possible. If the tumor cannot be excised, bile flow should be reestablished into the intestine by a cholecystojejunostomy or Roux-en-Y choledochojejunostomy. The choice is based on technical considerations.

Tumors at the hilum of the liver should be resected if possible and a Roux-en-Y hepaticojejunostomy performed. The anastomosis is usually between hilum and bowel rather than between individual bile ducts and bowel. A curative operation nearly always requires resection of either the right or the left lobe of the liver and, in all cases, the caudate lobe. Extension into the lobar and segmental ducts and secondary involvement of the hepatic artery and portal vein are the most common reasons for inability to resect the tumor. Subtotal resections offer little in the way of palliation.

Postoperative radiotherapy is commonly recommended.

Prognosis

The average patient with adenocarcinoma of the bile duct survives less than a year. The overall 5-year survival rate is 15%. Following a thorough radical operation, 5-year survival is about 40%. Biliary cirrhosis, intrahepatic infection, and general debility with terminal pneumonitis are the usual causes of death. Palliative resections and stents may improve the length and quality of survival in this disease even though surgical cure is uncommon. Limited experience with liver transplantation for this disease has been discouraging: tumor has recurred postoperatively in most patients.

Ahrendt SA, Nakeeb A, Pitt HA: Cholangiocarcinoma. Clin Liver Dis 2001;5:191.

Burke EC et al: Hilar cholangiocarcinoma: patterns of spread, the importance of hepatic resection for curative operation, and a presurgical clinical staging system. Ann Surg 1998;228:385.

Chamberlain RS, Blumgart LH: Hilar cholangiocarcinoma: a review and commentary. Ann Surg Oncol 2000;7:55.

Jarnagin WR: Cholangiocarcinoma of the extrahepatic bile ducts. Semin Surg Oncol 2000;19:156.

Kosuge T et al: Improved surgical results for hilar cholangiocarcinoma with procedures including major hepatic resection. Ann Surg 1999;230:663.

Lillemoe KD, Cameron JL: Surgery for hilar cholangiocarcinoma: the Johns Hopkins approach. J Hepatobiliary Pancreat Surg 2000;7:115.

Molmenti EP et al: Hepatobiliary malignancies. Primary hepatic malignant neoplasms. Surg Clin North Am 1999;79:43.

BENIGN TUMORS & PSEUDOTUMORS OF THE GALLBLADDER

Various unrelated lesions appear on the cholecystogram as projections from the gallbladder wall. The differentiation from gallstones is based upon observing whether a shift in position of the projections follows changes in posture of the patient, since stones are not fixed. Cancer should be suspected in any polypoid lesion that exceeds 1 cm in diameter.

Polyps

Most of these are not true neoplasms but cholesterol polyps, a local form of cholesterosis. Histologically, they consist of a cluster of lipid-filled macrophages in the submucosa. They easily become detached from the wall when the gallbladder is handled at surgery. It is not known whether cholesterol polyps are important in the genesis of gallstones. Some patients experience gallbladder pain, but whether this is related to the presence of the polyps per se or is a manifestation of functional gallbladder disease has not been established.

Inflammatory polyps have also been reported, but they are quite rare.

Adenomyomatosis

On cholecystography, this entity presents as a slight intraluminal convexity that is often marked by central umbilication. It is usually found in the fundus but may occur elsewhere. It is unclear whether adenomyomatosis is an acquired degenerative lesion or a developmental abnormality (ie, hamartoma). The following synonyms for this lesion appear in the literature: adenomatous hyperplasia, cholecystitis glandularis proliferans, and diverticulosis of the gallbladder. Although the condition is probably asymptomatic in many cases, adenomyomatosis can cause abdominal pain. Cholecystectomy should be performed in such patients.

Adenomas

These appear as pedunculated adenomatous polyps, true neoplasms that may be papillary or nonpapillary histologically. In a few cases they have been found in association with carcinoma in situ of the gallbladder.

BENIGN TUMORS OF THE BILE DUCTS

Benign papillomas and adenomas may arise from the ductal epithelium. Only 90 cases have been reported to date. The neoplastic propensity of the ductal epithelium is widespread, so the tumors are often multiple, and recurrence is common after excision. The affected duct must be radically excised for permanent cure to result.

BILE DUCT INJURIES & STRICTURES

 ESSENTIALS OF DIAGNOSIS

- *Episodic cholangitis.*
- *Previous biliary surgery.*
- *Transhepatic cholangiogram often diagnostic.*

General Considerations

Benign biliary injuries and strictures are caused by surgical trauma in about 95% of cases. The remainder result from external abdominal trauma or, rarely, from erosion of the duct by a gallstone. Prevention of injury to the duct depends on a combination of technical skill, experience, and a thorough knowledge of the normal anatomy and its variations in the hilum of the liver. The number of bile duct injuries has risen sharply in the past few years along with the shift from open to laparoscopic cholecystectomy.

The most common lesion consists of excision of a segment of the common duct as a result of mistaking it for the cystic duct. Partial transection, occlusion with metal clips, injury to the right hepatic duct, and leakage from the cystic duct are other examples. A full discussion of how these injuries occur and how they can be prevented is beyond the scope of this text.

A clean incision of the duct without additional damage is best managed by opening the abdomen and suturing the incision with fine absorbable suture material.

Clinical Findings

A. Symptoms

Manifestations of injury to the duct may or may not be evident in the postoperative period. Following laparoscopic surgery, bile ascites, manifested by abdominal distention, bloating, and pain plus mild jaundice, is the usual presentation, since the duct is usually open to the abdomen. The symptoms are relatively mild and may for a time be thought to represent only ileus until a worsening picture requires further investigation.

Injuries following open cholecystectomy more often present with intermittent cholangitis or jaundice as a consequence of a biliary stricture. The first clear-cut symptoms may not be evident for weeks or months after surgery.

B. Signs

Findings are not distinctive. Bile ascites produces abdominal distention and ileus and, rarely, true bile peritonitis with toxicity. The right upper quadrant may be tender but usually is not. Jaundice is usually present during an attack of cholangitis.

C. Laboratory Findings

The serum alkaline phosphatase concentration is elevated in cases of stricture. The serum bilirubin fluctuates in relation to symptoms but usually remains well below 10 mg/dL.

Blood cultures are usually positive during acute cholangitis.

D. Imaging Studies

Bile ascites can be suspected on ultrasound or CT scan. Fluid should be aspirated, and if it is bile, the diagnosis is clear. THC and ERCP are necessary to depict the anatomy. After laparoscopic cholecystectomy, the most common pattern is a blocked (by a metal clip) lower duct and an upper duct draining freely into the abdomen. With a stricture, the findings most often consist of focal narrowing of the common hepatic duct within 2 cm of the bifurcation and mild to moderate dilatation of the intrahepatic ducts.

Differential Diagnosis

Choledocholithiasis is the condition that most often must be differentiated from biliary stricture because the clinical and laboratory findings can be identical. A history of trauma to the duct would point toward stricture as the more likely diagnosis. The final distinction must often await radiologic or surgical findings. THC or ERCP should be definitive.

Other causes of cholestatic jaundice may have to be ruled out in some cases.

Complications

Complications develop quickly if the leak is not controlled. Bile peritonitis and abscesses may form. With stricture, persistent cholangitis may progress to multiple intrahepatic abscesses and a septic death.

Treatment

Bile duct injuries should be surgically repaired in all but a few patients who are likely to improve with a nonoperative approach. Excision of the damaged duct and Roux-en-Y hepaticojejunostomy is indicated for most acute and chronic injuries. The entire biliary tree must be outlined by cholangiograms preoperatively. The key to success is the thoroughness of the dissection and the ability ultimately to suture healthy duct to healthy bowel. This, in turn, depends on the experience of the surgeon with this particular operation.

When a definitive repair is technically impossible, the stricture may be dilated with a transhepatic balloon-tipped catheter. This is particularly applicable to patients with portal hypertension, whose hepatic hilum contains numerous venous collaterals that make operation hazardous.

Prognosis

The death rate from biliary injuries is about 5%, and severe illness is frequent. If the stricture is not repaired, episodic cholangitis and secondary liver disease are inevitable.

Surgical correction of the stricture should be successful in about 90% of cases. Experience at centers with a special interest in this problem indicates that good results can be obtained even if several previous attempts did not relieve the obstruction. There is essentially no place for liver transplantation in this disease.

Nealon WH, Urrutia F: Long-term follow-up after bilioenteric anastomosis for benign bile duct stricture. Ann Surg 1996; 223:639.

Savader SJ et al: Laparoscopic cholecystectomy-related bile duct injuries: a health and financial disaster. Ann Surg 1997; 225:268.

Strasberg SM, Eagon CJ, Drebin JA: The "hidden cystic duct" syndrome and the infundibular technique of laparoscopic cholecystectomy—the danger of the false infundibulum. J Am Coll Surg 2000;191:661.

Strasberg SM, Hertl M, Soper NJ: An analysis of the problem of biliary injury during laparoscopic cholecystectomy. J Am Coll Surg 1995;180:101.

Strasberg SM, Picus DD, Drebin JA: Results of a new strategy for reconstruction of biliary injuries having an isolated right-sided component. J Gastrointest Surg 2001;5:266.

Yeh TS et al: Value of magnetic resonance cholangiopancreatography in demonstrating major bile duct injuries following laparoscopic cholecystectomy. Br J Surg 1999;86:181.

UNCOMMON CAUSES OF BILE DUCT OBSTRUCTION

Congenital Choledochal Cysts

About 30% of congenital choledochal cysts produce their first symptoms in adults, usually presenting with jaundice, cholangitis, and a right upper quadrant mass. Diagnosis can be made by THC or ERCP. The optimal surgical procedure is excision of the cyst and construction of a Roux-en-Y hepaticojejunostomy. If this is not technically possible or if the patient's condition will not permit a prolonged operation, the cyst should be emptied of precipitated biliary sludge and a cystenteric anastomosis constructed. Congenital cysts of the biliary tree have a high incidence of malignant degeneration, which is another argument for excision rather than drainage.

Vercruysse R, Van den Bossche MR: Choledochal cyst in adults. Acta Chir Belg 1998;98:220.

Watanatittan S, Niramis R: Choledochal cyst: review of 74 pediatric cases. J Med Assoc Thai 1998;81:586.

Caroli's Disease

Caroli's disease, another form of congenital cystic disease, consists of saccular intrahepatic dilatation of the ducts. In some cases, the biliary abnormality is an isolated finding, but more often it is associated with congenital hepatic fibrosis and medullary sponge kidney. The latter patients often present in childhood or as young adults with complications of portal hypertension. Others have cholangitis and obstructive jaundice as initial manifestations. There is no definitive surgical solution to the problem except in rare cases with isolated involvement of one hepatic lobe, where lobectomy is curative. Intermittent antibiotic therapy for cholangitis is the usual regimen.

Hara H et al: Surgical treatment for congenital biliary dilatation, with or without intrahepatic bile duct dilatation. Hepatogastroenterology 2001;48:638.

Parada LA et al: Clonal chromosomal abnormalities in congenital bile duct dilatation (Caroli's disease). Gut 1999;45:780.

Waechter FL et al: The role of liver transplantation in patients with Caroli's disease. Hepatogastroenterology 2001;48:672.

Hemobilia

Hemobilia presents with the triad of biliary colic, obstructive jaundice, and occult or gross intestinal bleeding. Most cases in Western cultures follow several weeks after hepatic trauma with bleeding from an intrahepatic branch of the hepatic artery into a duct. It is seen with less frequency now, because the general principles of management of hepatic trauma are better understood. In the Orient, hemobilia usually follows ductal parasitism (*Ascaris lumbricoides*) or Oriental cholangiohepatitis. Other causes are hepatic neoplasms, rupture of a hepatic artery aneurysm, hepatic abscess, and choledocholithiasis. The diagnosis may be suspected from a technetium 99m-labeled red blood cell scan, but an arteriogram is usually required for diagnosis and planning of therapy. Sometimes the bleeding can be stopped by embolizing the lesion with stainless steel coils, Gelfoam, or autologous blood clot infused through a catheter selectively positioned in the hepatic artery. If this is unsuccessful, either direct ligation of the bleeding point in the liver or proximal ligation of an upstream branch of the hepatic artery in the hilum is required.

Green MH et al: Haemobilia. Br J Surg 2001;88:773.

Pancreatitis

Pancreatitis can cause obstruction of the intrapancreatic portion of the bile duct by inflammatory swelling, encasement with scar, or compression by a pseudocyst. The patient may present with painless jaundice or cholangitis. Occasionally, a distended gallbladder can be felt on abdominal examination. Differentiation from choledocholithiasis and secondary acute pancreatitis depends on biliary x-rays or surgical exploration if the jaundice persists. Jaundice due to inflammation alone rarely lasts more than 2 weeks; persistent jaundice following an attack of acute pancreatitis suggests the development of a pseudocyst, underlying chronic pancreatitis with obstruction by fibrosis, or even an obstructing neoplasm.

Biliary obstruction from chronic pancreatitis may have few or no clinical manifestations. Jaundice is usually present, but the average peak bilirubin level is only 4–5 mg/dL. Some patients with functionally significant stenosis have persistently elevated alkaline phosphatase levels as the only abnormality; when surgical decompression of the bile duct is not performed, these patients often develop secondary biliary cirrhosis within a year or so. Diagnosis of stricture is made by ERCP, which shows a long stenosis of the intrapancreatic portion of the duct, proximal dilatation, and either a gradual or abrupt tapering of the lumen at the pancreatic border, occasionally accompanied by ductal angulation. If cholangiograms show stenosis and if alkaline phosphatase or bilirubin levels remain more than twice normal for longer than 2 months, the stenosis is functionally significant and unlikely to resolve and requires surgical correction. Choledochoduodenostomy is done in most cases. Cholecystoduodenostomy is unreliable because the cystic duct is often too narrow to provide continued biliary decompression.

Patients with obstructive jaundice and pseudocyst usually respond to surgical drainage of the pseudocyst. However, occasionally they do not respond, because chronic scarring—not the cyst—is the cause of obstruction. Procedures to drain both the bile duct and the pseudocyst are indicated if operative cholangiograms demonstrate persistent bile duct obstruction after the cyst has been decompressed.

Ampullary Dysfunction & Stenosis

Stenosis of the hepatopancreatic ampulla (ampullary stenosis) has been implicated as a cause of pain and other manifestations of ampullary obstruction and is often considered as a cause of postcholecystectomy complaints. Some cases are idiopathic, whereas others may be the result of trauma from gallstones. If the patient has secondary manifestations of biliary obstruction (eg, jaundice, increased alkaline phosphatase concentration, cholangitis) in the absence of gallstones or some other obstructing lesion, and cholangiography shows dilatation of the common duct, ampullary stenosis is a plausible explanation. However, the diagnosis is more often proposed as a reason for upper abdominal pain without these more objective findings. Ampullary dysfunction is postulated in these cases.

Sphincter of Oddi dysfunction may be the cause of biliary-like pain and is often considered in patients who remain uncomfortable after cholecystectomy. The pathogenesis of the symptoms is thought to be similar to that of esophageal dysmotility and the irritable bowel syndrome. The patients typically experience severe, intermittent upper abdominal pain that lasts for 1–3 hours, sometimes following a meal.

Residual gallstone and pancreatic disease must first be ruled out. Ampullary dysfunction can then be diagnosed by sphincter of Oddi manometry. Patients are placed in one of three groups depending on the presence of three objective manifestations of biliary obstruction: abnormal liver function tests, prolonged (> 45 minutes) common bile duct emptying of contrast media after ERCP; and a common duct greater than 12 mm in diameter. Patients in group I have all three findings; patients in group II have one or two findings; and patients in group III have none of the findings.

Group I patients are thought to have enough evidence of disease that sphincterotomy should be performed without manometry. Group I patients have abnormal motility so rarely that they should not be considered further for sphincterotomy. Thus, motility studies are most often of value in determining which of the group II patients will improve after sphincterotomy.

The abnormalities sought on the motility studies include an elevated (> 40 mm Hg) basal sphincter pressure and a paradoxic rise in sphincter pressure in response to CCK. The former is most reliable. About 50% of group II patients have elevated sphincter pressures, and these are the ones who benefit from sphincterotomy.

A scintigraphic test may be just as accurate. The patient is given a bolus of CCK followed by ^{99m}Tc-DISIDA. Gamma camera images of the liver and bile duct are obtained for 60 minutes. A scoring system (score: 0–12) is based on the rate of passage of the imaging agent past various relevant points (eg, appearance and clearance through the liver, bile duct, and bowel). The normal range is 0–5; abnormal is 6–12.

Sphincter of Oddi dysfunction is an uncommon explanation for abdominal pain, and it is appropriate to remain skeptical unless the objective findings of biliary obstruction are clear-cut. In well-selected cases, however, endoscopic sphincterotomy is truly beneficial.

Chen JW, Saccone GT, Toouli J: Sphincter of Oddi dysfunction and acute pancreatitis. Gut 1998;43:305.

Rosenblatt ML et al: Comparison of sphincter of Oddi manometry, fatty meal sonography, and hepatobiliary scintigraphy in the diagnosis of sphincter of Oddi dysfunction. Gastrointest Endosc 2001;54:697.

Silverman WB et al: Hybrid classification of sphincter of Oddi dysfunction based on simplified Milwaukee criteria: effect of marginal serum liver and pancreas test elevations. Dig Dis Sci 2001;46:278.

Thomas PD et al: Use of (99m)Tc-DISIDA biliary scanning with morphine provocation for the detection of elevated sphincter of Oddi basal pressure. Gut 2000;46:838.

Toouli J et al: Manometry based randomised trial of endoscopic sphincterotomy for sphincter of Oddi dysfunction. Gut 2000;46:98.

Duodenal Diverticula

Duodenal diverticula usually arise on the medial aspect of the duodenum within 2 cm of the orifice of the bile duct, and in some individuals the duct empties directly into a diverticulum. Even in the latter circumstance, duodenal diverticula are usually innocuous. Occasionally, distortion of the duct entrance or obstruction by enterolith formation in the diverticulum produces symptoms. Either choledochoduodenostomy or Roux-en-Y choledochojejunostomy is usually a safer method of reestablishing biliary drainage than attempts to excise the diverticulum and reimplant the duct.

Ascariasis

When the worms invade the duct from the duodenum, ascariasis can produce symptoms of ductal obstruction. Air may sometimes be seen within the ducts on plain films. Antibiotics should be used until cholangitis is controlled, and anthelmintic therapy (mebendazole, albendazole, or pyrantel pamoate) should then be given. The acute symptoms usually subside with antibiotics, but if they do not, endoscopic sphincterotomy should be performed and attempts made to extricate the worms. If this is unsuccessful and the patient remains acutely ill, the duct should be emptied surgically.

Recurrent Pyogenic Cholangitis (Oriental Cholangiohepatitis)

Oriental cholangiohepatitis is a type of chronic recurrent cholangitis prevalent in coastal areas from Japan to Southeast Asia. In Hong Kong it is the third most common indication for emergency laparotomy and the most frequent type of biliary disease. The disease is currently thought to result from chronic portal bacteremia, with portal phlebitis antedating the biliary disease. *E coli* causes secondary infection of the bile ducts, which initiates pigment stone formation within the ducts.

Biliary obstruction from the stones gives rise to recurrent cholangitis, which, unlike gallstone disease in Western countries, may be unaccompanied by gallbladder stones. The gallbladder is usually distended during an attack and may contain pus.

Chronic recurrent infection often leads to biliary strictures and hepatic abscess formation. The strictures are usually located in the intrahepatic bile ducts, and for some unknown reason the left lobe of the liver is more severely involved. Intrahepatic gallstones are common, and their surgical removal may be difficult or impossible. Acute abdominal pain, chills, and high fever are usually present, and jaundice develops in about half of cases. Right upper quadrant tenderness is usually marked, and in about 80% of cases the gallbladder is palpable. ERCP or THC is the best way to study the biliary tree and can help in determining the need for surgery and the type of procedure.

Systemic antibiotics should be given for acute cholangitis. Surgical treatment consists of cholecystectomy, common duct exploration, and removal of stones. Sphincteroplasty should also be performed to allow any residual or recurrent stones to escape from the duct. A Roux-en-Y choledochojejunostomy is indicated for patients with strictures, markedly dilated ducts (eg, > 3 cm), or recurrent disease after a previous sphincteroplasty.

The results of surgery are good in 80% of patients. Chronic intrahepatic stones and infection, which often involve only one lobe, may require hepatic lobectomy.

Although many patients are cured, prolonged illness from repeated infection is almost unavoidable once strictures have appeared or the intrahepatic ducts have become packed with stones.

Cosenza CA et al: Current management of recurrent pyogenic cholangitis. Am Surg 1999;65:939.

Harris HW et al: Recurrent pyogenic cholangitis. Am J Surg 1998;176:34.

Kim M et al: MR imaging findings in recurrent pyogenic cholangitis. AJR Am J Roentgenol 1999;173:1545.

Park MS et al: Recurrent pyogenic cholangitis: comparison between MR cholangiography and direct cholangiography. Radiology 2001;220:677.

Sclerosing Cholangitis

Sclerosing cholangitis is a rare chronic disease of unknown cause characterized by nonbacterial inflammatory narrowing of the bile ducts. About 60% of cases occur in patients with ulcerative colitis, and sclerosing cholangitis develops in about 5% of patients with that disorder. Other less commonly associated conditions are thyroiditis, retroperitoneal fibrosis, and mediastinal fibrosis. The disease chiefly affects men 20–50 years of age. In most cases, the entire biliary tree is affected by the inflammatory process, which causes irregular partial obliteration of the lumen of the ducts. The narrowing may be confined, however, to the intrahepatic or extrahepatic ducts, though it is almost never so short as to resemble a posttraumatic or focal malignant stricture. The woody-hard duct walls contain increased collagen and lymphoid elements and are thickened at the expense of the lumen.

The clinical onset usually consists of the gradual appearance of mild jaundice and pruritus. Symptoms of bacterial cholangitis (eg, fever and chills) are uncommon in the absence of previous biliary surgery. Laboratory findings are typical of cholestasis. The total serum bilirubin averages about 4 mg/dL and rarely exceeds 10 mg/dL. ERCP is usually diagnostic, demonstrating ductal stenoses and irregularity, which often gives a beaded appearance. Liver biopsy may show pericholangitis and bile stasis, but the changes are nonspecific.

The complications of sclerosing cholangitis include gallstone disease and adenocarcinoma of the bile duct. The latter is most common in patients with ulcerative colitis. Furthermore, patients with ulcerative colitis and sclerosing cholangitis appear to be at greater risk for colonic mucosal dysplasia and colon cancer than those with ulcerative colitis not associated with sclerosing cholangitis.

Ursodiol (ursodeoxycholic acid), 10 mg/kg/d, improves liver function tests and symptoms. Cholestyramine will give relief from pruritus. Percutaneous transhepatic balloon dilatation can be of value to treat dominant strictures. In cases where the disease is largely confined to the distal extrahepatic duct and the proximal ducts are dilated, a Roux-en-Y hepaticojejunostomy may be indicated. For patients with severe intrahepatic involvement, hepatic transplantation should be considered.

The natural history of sclerosing cholangitis is one of chronicity and unpredictable severity. Some patients seem to obtain nearly complete remission after treatment, but this is not common. Bacterial cholangitis may develop after operation if adequate drainage has not been established. In these cases, antibiotics will be required at intervals. Most patients experience the grad-

ual evolution of secondary biliary cirrhosis after many years of mild to moderate jaundice and pruritus. Liver transplantation is indicated when the disease becomes advanced. The results are good.

Ghosh S, Shand A, Ferguson A: Ulcerative colitis. BMJ 2000; 320:1119.

Kim WR et al: A revised natural history model for primary sclerosing cholangitis. Mayo Clin Proc 2000;75:688.

Kubicka S et al: K-ras mutations in the bile of patients with primary sclerosing cholangitis. Gut 2001;48:403.

Ryder SD, Beckingham IJ: ABC of diseases of liver, pancreas, and biliary system. Other causes of parenchymal liver disease. BMJ 2001;322:290.

van Hoogstraten HJ et al: Ursodeoxycholic acid therapy for primary sclerosing cholangitis: results of a 2-year randomized controlled trial to evaluate single versus multiple daily doses. J Hepatol 1998;29:417.

Pancreas

Gerard M. Doherty, MD, & Lawrence W. Way, MD

EMBRYOLOGY

The pancreas arises in the fourth week of fetal life from the caudal part of the foregut as dorsal and ventral pancreatic buds. Both anlagen rotate to the right and fuse near the point of origin of the ventral pancreas. Later, as the duodenum rotates, the pancreas shifts to the left. In the adult, only the caudal portion of the head and the uncinate process are derived from the ventral pancreas. The cranial part of the head and all of the body and tail are derived from the dorsal pancreas. Most of the dorsal pancreatic duct joins with the duct of the ventral pancreas to form the main pancreatic duct (**duct of Wirsung**); a small part persists as the accessory duct (**duct of Santorini**). In 5–10% of people, the ventral and dorsal pancreatic ducts do not fuse, and most regions of the pancreas drain through the duct of Santorini and the orifice of the minor papilla. In this case, only the small ventral pancreas drains with the common bile duct through the papilla of Vater.

ANATOMY

The pancreas is a thin elliptic organ that lies within the retroperitoneum in the upper abdomen (Figures 27–1 and 27–2). In the adult, it is 12–15 cm long and weighs 70–100 g. The gland can be divided into three portions—head, body, and tail. The head of the pancreas is intimately adherent to the medial portion of the duodenum and lies in front of the inferior vena cava and superior mesenteric vessels. A small tongue of tissue called the uncinate process lies behind the superior mesenteric vessels as they emerge from the retroperitoneum. Anteriorly, the stomach and the first portion of the duodenum lie partly in front of the pancreas. The common bile duct passes through a posterior groove in the head of the pancreas adjacent to the duodenum. The body of the pancreas is in contact posteriorly with the aorta, the left crus of the diaphragm, the left adrenal gland, and the left kidney. The tail of the pancreas lies in the hilum of the spleen. The main pancreatic duct (the duct of Wirsung) courses along the gland from the tail to the head and joins the common bile duct just before entering the duodenum at the ampulla of Vater. The accessory pancreatic duct (the duct of Santorini) enters the duodenum 2–2.5 cm proximal to the ampulla of Vater (Figure 27–1).

The blood supply of the pancreas is derived from branches of the celiac and superior mesenteric arteries (Figure 27–2). The superior pancreaticoduodenal artery arises from the gastroduodenal artery, runs parallel to the duodenum, and eventually meets the inferior pancreaticoduodenal artery, a branch of the superior mesenteric artery, to form an arcade. The splenic artery provides tributaries that supply the body and tail of the pancreas. The main branches are termed the dorsal pancreatic, pancreatica magna, and caudal pancreatic arteries. The venous supply of the gland parallels the arterial supply. Lymphatic drainage is into the peripancreatic nodes located along the veins.

The innervation of the pancreas is derived from the vagal and splanchnic nerves. The efferent fibers pass through the celiac plexus from the celiac branch of the right vagal nerve to terminate in ganglia located in the interlobular septa of the pancreas. Postganglionic fibers from these synapses innervate the acini, the islets, and the ducts. The visceral afferent fibers from the pancreas also travel in the vagal and splanchnic nerves, but those that mediate pain are confined to the latter. Sympathetic fibers to the pancreas pass from the splanchnic nerves through the celiac plexus and innervate the pancreatic vasculature.

PHYSIOLOGY

Exocrine Function

The external secretion of the pancreas consists of a clear, alkaline (pH 7.0–8.3) solution of 1–2 L/d containing digestive enzymes. Secretion is stimulated by the hormones secretin and cholecystokinin (CCK) and by parasympathetic vagal discharge. Secretin and cholecystokinin are synthesized, stored, and released from duodenal mucosal cells in response to specific stimuli. Acid in the lumen of the duodenum causes the release of secretin, and luminal digestion products of fat and protein cause the release of cholecystokinin.

The water and electrolyte secretion is formed by the centroacinar and intercalated duct cells principally in response to secretin stimulation. The secretion is modified by exchange processes and active secretion in the ductal collecting system. The cations sodium and potassium are present in the same concentrations as in plasma.

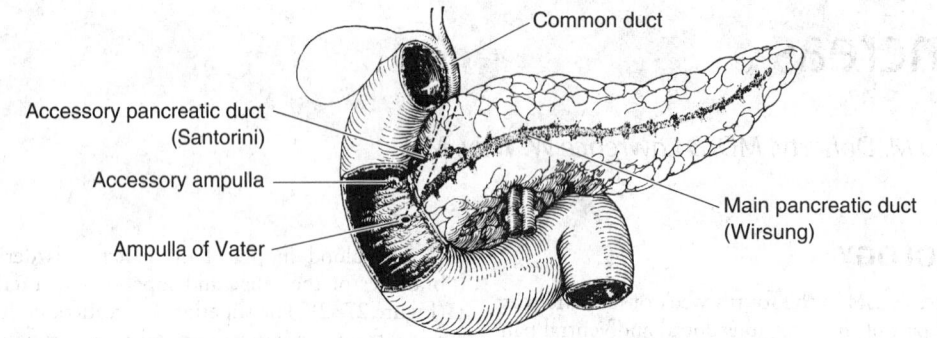

Figure 27–1. Anatomic configuration of pancreatic ductal system. (Courtesy of W Silen.)

The anions bicarbonate and chloride vary in concentration according to the rate of secretion: with increasing rate of secretion, the bicarbonate concentration increases and chloride concentration falls, so that the sum of the two is the same throughout the secretory range. Pancreatic juice helps neutralize gastric acid in the duodenum and adjusts luminal pH to the level that gives optimal activity of pancreatic enzymes.

Pancreatic enzymes are synthesized, stored (as zymogen granules), and released by the acinar cells of the gland, principally in response to cholecystokinin and vagal stimulation. Pancreatic enzymes are proteolytic, lipolytic, and amylolytic. Lipase and amylase are stored and secreted in active forms. The proteolytic enzymes are secreted as inactive precursors and are activated by the duodenal enzyme enterokinase. Other enzymes se-

creted by the pancreas include ribonucleases and phospholipase A. Phospholipase A is secreted as an inactive proenzyme activated in the duodenum by trypsin. It catalyzes the conversion of biliary lecithin to lysolecithin.

Turnover of protein in the pancreas exceeds that of any other organ in the body. Intravenously injected amino acids are incorporated into enzyme protein and may appear in the pancreatic juice within 1 hour. Three mechanisms prevent autodigestion of the pancreas by its proteolytic enzymes: (1) The enzymes are stored in acinar cells as zymogen granules, where they are separated from other cell proteins. (2) The enzymes are secreted in an inactive form. (3) Inhibitors of proteolytic enzymes are present in pancreatic juice and pancreatic tissue.

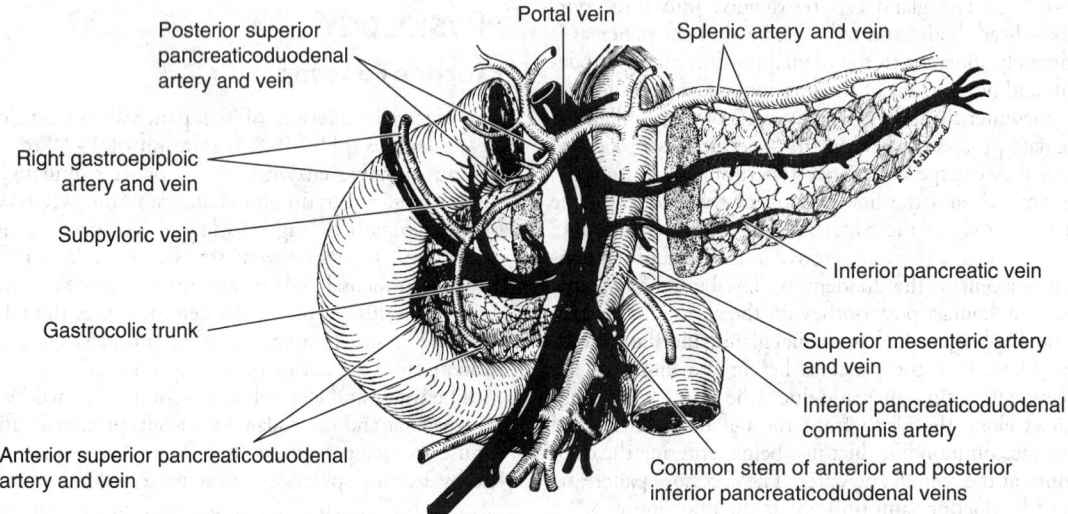

Figure 27–2. Arterial supply and venous drainage of the pancreas. (Courtesy of W Silen.)

Endocrine Function

The function of the endocrine pancreas is to facilitate storage of foodstuffs by release of insulin after a meal and to provide a mechanism for their mobilization by release of glucagon during periods of fasting. Insulin and glucagon, as well as pancreatic polypeptide and somatostatin, are produced by the islets of Langerhans.

Insulin, a polypeptide (MW 5734) consisting of 51 amino acid residues, is formed in the beta cells of the pancreas via the precursor proinsulin. Insulin secretion is stimulated by rising or high serum concentrations of metabolic substrates such as glucose, amino acids, and perhaps short-chain fatty acids. The major normal stimulus for insulin release appears to be glucose. The release and synthesis of insulin are stimulated by activation of specific glucoreceptors located on the surface membrane of the beta cell. Insulin release is also stimulated by calcium, glucagon, secretin, cholecystokinin, vasoactive intestinal polypeptide (VIP), and gastrin, all of which sensitize the receptors on the beta cell to glucose. Epinephrine, tolbutamide, and chlorpropamide release insulin by acting on the adenylyl cyclase system.

Glucagon, a polypeptide (MW 3485) consisting of 29 amino acid residues, is formed in the α cells of the pancreas. The release of glucagon is stimulated by a low blood glucose concentration, amino acids, catecholamines, sympathetic nervous discharge, and cholecystokinin. It is suppressed by hyperglycemia and insulin.

The principal functions of insulin are to stimulate anabolic reactions involving carbohydrates, fats, proteins, and nucleic acids. Insulin decreases glycogenolysis, lipolysis, proteolysis, gluconeogenesis, ureagenesis, and ketogenesis. Glucagon stimulates glycogenolysis from the liver and proteolysis and lipolysis in adipose tissue as well as in the liver. With the increase in lipolysis, there is an increase in ketogenesis and gluconeogenesis. Glucagon increases cAMP in the liver, heart, skeletal muscle, and adipose tissue. The short-term regulation of gluconeogenesis depends on the balance between insulin and glucagon. Studies on insulin and glucagon suggest that the hormones exert their effects via receptors on the cell membrane. Before entering the systemic circulation, blood draining from the islets of Langerhans perfuses the pancreatic acini, and this exposure to high levels of hormones is thought to influence acinar function.

ANNULAR PANCREAS

Annular pancreas is a rare congenital condition in which a ring of pancreatic tissue from the head of the pancreas surrounds the descending duodenum. The abnormality usually presents in infancy as duodenal obstruction with postprandial vomiting. There is bile in the vomitus if the constriction is distal to the entrance of the common bile duct. X-rays show a dilated stomach and proximal duodenum (double bubble sign) and little or no air in the rest of the small bowel.

After correction of fluid and electrolyte imbalance, the obstructed segment should be bypassed by a duodenojejunostomy or other similar procedure. No attempt should be made to resect the obstructing pancreas, because a pancreatic fistula or acute pancreatitis often develops postoperatively.

Occasionally, annular pancreas will present in adult life with similar symptoms.

PANCREATITIS

Pancreatitis is a common nonbacterial inflammatory disease caused by activation, interstitial liberation, and autodigestion of the pancreas by its own enzymes. The process may or may not be accompanied by permanent morphologic and functional changes in the gland. Much is known about the causes of pancreatitis, but despite the accumulation of much experimental data, understanding of the pathogenesis of this disorder is still incomplete.

In **acute pancreatitis,** there is sudden upper abdominal pain, nausea and vomiting, and elevated serum amylase. **Chronic pancreatitis** is characterized by chronic pain, pancreatic calcification on x-ray, and exocrine (steatorrhea) or endocrine (diabetes mellitus) insufficiency. Attacks of acute pancreatitis often occur in patients with chronic pancreatitis. **Acute relapsing pancreatitis** is defined as multiple attacks of pancreatitis without permanent pancreatic scarring, a picture most often associated with biliary pancreatitis. The unsatisfactory term **chronic relapsing pancreatitis,** denoting recurrent acute attacks superimposed on chronic pancreatitis, will not be used in this chapter. Alcoholic pancreatitis often behaves in this way. The term **subacute pancreatitis** has also been used by some to denote the minor acute attacks that typically appear late in alcoholic pancreatitis.

Etiology

Most cases of pancreatitis are caused by gallstone disease or alcoholism; a few result from hypercalcemia, trauma, hyperlipidemia, and genetic predisposition; and the remainder are idiopathic. Important differences exist in the manifestations and natural history of the disease as produced by these various factors.

A. BILIARY PANCREATITIS

About 40% of cases of pancreatitis are associated with gallstone disease, which, if untreated, usually gives rise to additional acute attacks. For unknown reasons, even repeated attacks of acute biliary pancreatitis seldom produce chronic pancreatitis. Eradication of the biliary disease nearly always prevents recurrent pancreatitis. The etiologic mechanism most likely consists of transient obstruction of the ampulla of Vater and pancreatic duct by a gallstone. Choledocholithiasis is found in only 25% of cases, but because over 90% of patients excrete a gallstone in feces passed within 10 days after an acute attack, it is assumed that most attacks are caused by a gallstone or biliary sludge traversing the common duct and ampulla of Vater. Other possible steps in pathogenesis initiated by passage of the gallstone are discussed below.

B. Alcoholic Pancreatitis

In the USA, alcoholism accounts for about 40% of cases of pancreatitis. Characteristically, the patients have been heavy users of hard liquor or wine; the condition is relatively infrequent in countries where beer is the most popular alcoholic beverage. Most commonly, 6 years or more of alcoholic excess precede the initial attack of pancreatitis, and even with the first clinical manifestations, signs of chronic pancreatitis can be detected if the gland is examined microscopically. Thus, alcoholic pancreatitis is often considered to be synonymous with chronic pancreatitis no matter what the clinical findings.

Acetaldehyde, an ethanol metabolite, has been implicated as a mediator, since it can generate toxic oxygen metabolites under the influence of xanthine oxidase. In experimental studies, alcohol decreases incorporation of phosphate into parenchymal phospholipids, decreases zymogen synthesis, and produces ultrastructural changes in acinar cells. Acute administration of alcohol stimulates pancreatic secretion and induces spasm in the sphincter of Oddi. This has been compared to experiments that produce acute pancreatitis by combining partial ductal obstruction and secretory stimulation. If the patient can be persuaded to stop drinking, acute attacks may be prevented, but parenchymal damage continues to occur owing to persistent ductal obstruction and fibrosis.

C. Hypercalcemia

Hyperparathyroidism and other disorders accompanied by hypercalcemia are occasionally complicated by acute pancreatitis. With time, chronic pancreatitis and ductal calculi appear. It is thought that the increased calcium concentrations in pancreatic juice that result from hypercalcemia may prematurely activate proteases. They may also facilitate precipitation of calculi in the ducts.

D. Hyperlipidemia

In some patients—especially alcoholics—hyperlipidemia appears transiently during an acute attack of pan-

creatitis; in others with primary hyperlipidemia (especially those associated with elevated chylomicrons and very low density lipoproteins), pancreatitis seems to be a direct consequence of the metabolic abnormality. Hyperlipidemia during an acute attack of pancreatitis is usually associated with normal serum amylase levels, because the lipid interferes with the chemical determination for amylase; urinary output of amylase may still be high. One should inspect the serum of every patient with acute abdominal pain, because if it is lactescent, pancreatitis will almost always be the correct diagnosis. If a primary lipid abnormality is present, dietary control reduces the chances of additional attacks of pancreatitis as well as other complications.

E. Familial Pancreatitis

In this condition, attacks of abdominal pain usually begin in childhood. The genetic defect appears to be transmitted as a non-X-linked dominant with variable penetrance. Some affected families also have aminoaciduria, but this is not a universal finding. Diabetes mellitus and steatorrhea are uncommon. Chronic calcific pancreatitis develops eventually in most patients, and many patients become candidates for operation for chronic pain. Pancreatic carcinoma is more frequent in patients with familial pancreatitis.

F. Protein Deficiency

In certain populations where dietary protein intake is markedly deficient, the incidence of chronic pancreatitis is high. The reason for this association is obscure, especially in view of the observation that pancreatitis afflicts alcoholics with higher dietary protein and fat intake than those who consume less protein and fat.

G. Postoperative (Iatrogenic) Pancreatitis

Most cases of postoperative pancreatitis follow common bile duct exploration, especially if sphincterotomy was performed. Two practices, now largely abandoned, were often responsible: (1) use of a common duct T tube with a long arm passing through the sphincter of Oddi, and (2) dilation of the sphincter to 5–7 mm during common duct exploration. Operations on the pancreas, including pancreatic biopsy, are another cause. A few cases follow gastric surgery or even operations remote from the pancreas. Pancreatitis is particularly common after cardiac surgery with cardiopulmonary bypass, where the risk factors are preoperative renal failure, valve surgery, postoperative hypotension, and (particularly) the perioperative administration of calcium chloride (> 800 mg calcium chloride per square meter of body surface area). Pancreatitis may also complicate endoscopic retrograde pancreatography or endoscopic sphincterotomy.

Rarely, pancreatitis follows Billroth II gastrectomy, owing to acute obstruction of the afferent loop and reflux of duodenal secretions under high pressure into the pancreatic ducts. The condition has been recreated experimentally in dogs (Pfeffer loop preparation).

H. DRUG-INDUCED PANCREATITIS

Drugs are probably responsible for more cases of acute pancreatitis than is generally suspected. The most commonly incriminated drugs are corticosteroids, estrogen-containing contraceptives, azathioprine, thiazide diuretics, and tetracyclines. Pancreatitis associated with use of estrogens is usually the result of drug-induced hypertriglyceridemia. The mechanisms involved in the case of other drugs are unknown.

I. OBSTRUCTIVE PANCREATITIS

Chronic partial obstruction of the pancreatic duct may be congenital or may follow healing after injury or inflammation. Over time, the parenchyma drained by the obstructed duct is replaced by fibrous tissue, and chronic pancreatitis develops. Sometimes there are episodes of acute pancreatitis as well.

Pancreas divisum may predispose to a kind of obstructive pancreatitis. If this anomaly is present and further narrowing of the opening of the minor papilla occurs (eg, by an inflammatory process), the orifice may be inadequate to handle the flow of pancreatic juice. The diagnosis of pancreas divisum may be made by ERCP. If a patient with the anomaly is found to have documented episodes of acute pancreatitis and no other cause is found, it is reasonable to assume that the anomaly is the cause.

Surgical sphincteroplasty of the minor papilla or the insertion of a stent has been proposed as treatment, but results have been suboptimal. This may be due to the presence of irreversible parenchymal changes and the persistence of chronic inflammation. In patients with obvious changes of chronic pancreatitis, surgical treatment should consist of pancreatic resection or drainage (see p 631).

J. IDIOPATHIC PANCREATITIS AND MISCELLANEOUS CAUSES

In about 15% of patients, representing the third largest group after biliary and alcoholic pancreatitis, there is no identifiable cause of the condition. If investigated in greater than usual detail (eg, duodenal drainage examination for cholesterol crystals), many of these patients will be found to have gallstones or biliary sludge undetectable by ultrasound scans. Recent data have linked mutations of the cystic fibrosis gene to idiopathic pancreatitis.

Viral infections and scorpion stings may cause pancreatitis.

Pathogenesis

The concept that pancreatitis is due to enzymatic digestion of the gland is supported by the finding of proteolytic enzymes in ascitic fluid and increased amounts of phospholipase A and lysolecithins in pancreatic tissue from patients with acute pancreatitis. Experimentally, pancreatitis can be created readily if activated enzymes are injected into the pancreatic ducts under pressure. Trypsin has not been found in excessive amounts in pancreatic tissue from affected humans, possibly because of inactivation by trypsin inhibitors. Nevertheless, although the available evidence is inconclusive, the autodigestion theory is almost universally accepted. Other proposed factors are vascular insufficiency, lymphatic congestion, and activation of the kallikrein-kinin system.

For many years, trypsin and other proteases were held to be the principal injurious agents, but recent evidence has emphasized phospholipase A, lipase, and elastase as perhaps of greater importance. Trypsin ordinarily does not attack living cells, and even when trypsin is forced into the interstitial spaces, the resulting pancreatitis does not include coagulation necrosis, which is so prominent in human pancreatitis.

Phospholipase A, in the presence of small amounts of bile salts, attacks free phospholipids (eg, lecithin) and those bound in cellular membranes to produce extremely potent lyso- compounds. Lysolecithin, which would result from the action of phospholipase A on biliary lecithin, or phospholipase A itself, plus bile salts, is capable of producing severe necrotizing pancreatitis. Trypsin is important in this scheme, because small amounts are needed to activate phospholipase A from its inactive precursor.

Elastase, which is both elastolytic and proteolytic, is secreted in an inactive form. Because it can digest the walls of blood vessels, elastase has been thought to be important in the pathogenesis of hemorrhagic pancreatitis.

If autodigestion is the final common pathway in pancreatitis, earlier steps must account for the presence of active enzymes and their reaction products in the ducts and their escape into the interstitium. The following are the most popular theories that attempt to link the known etiologic factors with autodigestion:

A. OBSTRUCTION-SECRETION

In animals, ligation of the pancreatic duct generally produces mild edema of the pancreas that resolves within a week. Thereafter, atrophy of the secretory apparatus occurs. On the other hand, partial or intermittent ductal obstruction, which more closely mimics what seems to happen in humans, can produce frank pancreatitis if the gland is simultaneously stimulated to secrete. The major shortcoming of these experiments has been the difficulty encountered in attempting to cause severe pancreatitis in this way. However, since the human pancreas manufactures ten times as much phospholipase A as does the dog or rat pancreas, the consequences of obstruction in humans conceivably could be more serious.

B. COMMON CHANNEL THEORY

Opie, having observed pancreatitis in a patient with a gallstone impacted in the ampulla of Vater, speculated that reflux of bile into the pancreatic ducts might have initiated the process. Flow between the biliary and pancreatic ducts requires a common channel connecting these two systems with the duodenum. Although these ducts converge in 90% of humans, only 10% have a common channel long enough to permit biliary-pancreatic reflux if the ampulla contained a gallstone. Experimentally, pancreatitis produced by pancreatic duct obstruction alone is similar in severity to pancreatitis following obstruction of a common channel, so biliary reflux is discounted as an etiologic factor in this disease.

C. DUODENAL REFLUX

The above theories do not explain activation of pancreatic enzymes, a process that normally takes place through the action of enterokinase in the duodenum. In experimental animals, if the segment of duodenum into which the pancreatic duct empties is surgically converted to a closed loop, reflux of duodenal juice initiates severe pancreatitis (Pfeffer loop). Pancreatitis associated with acute afferent loop obstruction after Billroth II gastrectomy is probably the result of similar factors. Other than in this specific example, there is no direct evidence for duodenal reflux in the pathogenesis of pancreatitis in humans.

D. BACK DIFFUSION ACROSS THE PANCREATIC DUCT

Just as the gastric mucosa must serve as a barrier to maintain high concentrations of acid, so must the epithelium of the pancreatic duct prevent diffusion of luminal enzymes into the pancreatic parenchyma. Experiments in cats have shown that the barrier function of the pancreatic duct is vulnerable to several injurious agents, including alcohol and bile acids. Furthermore, the effects of alcohol can occur even after oral ingestion, because alcohol is secreted in the pancreatic juice. Injury to the barrier renders the duct permeable to molecules as large as MW 20,000, and enzymes from the lumen may be able to enter the gland and produce pancreatitis.

The studies by Steer and his coworkers have shown that a very early event in several forms of experimental pancreatitis, including that due to pancreatic duct obstruction, consists of zymogen activation within acinar cells by lysosomal hydrolases (eg, cathepsin B). This may represent the long-sought unifying explanation. Other factors must be postulated, however, to account for the variations in severity of the disease. In biliary pancreatitis, transient obstruction of the ampulla of Vater by a gallstone is most likely the first event. Alcoholic pancreatitis probably has several causes, including partial ductal obstruction, secretory stimulation, acute effects on the ductal barrier, and toxic actions of alcohol on parenchymal cells.

E. SYSTEMIC MANIFESTATIONS

Severe acute pancreatitis may be complicated by multiple organ failure, principally respiratory insufficiency (acute respiratory distress syndrome [ARDS]), myocardial depression, renal insufficiency, and gastric stress ulceration. The pathogenesis of these complications is similar in many respects to that of multiple organ failure in sepsis, and in fact, sepsis due to pancreatic abscess formation is a contributing factor in some of the most severe cases of acute pancreatitis. During acute pancreatitis, pancreatic proteases, bacterial endotoxins, and other active agents are liberated into the systemic circulation. The concentrations of serum factors able to complex with the proteases (eg, α_2-macroglobulin) decrease in proportion to the severity of the illness, and complexed α_2-macroglobulin, which normally is cleared rapidly by macrophages, accumulates. These circulating complexes, which retain proteolytic activity, are thought to contribute to systemic toxicity. The endotoxin probably originates from bacteria that translocate through an abnormally permeable intestinal mucosa. Within the circulation, the proteases and the endotoxin activate the complement system (especially C5) and kinins. Complement activation leads to granulocyte aggregation and accumulation of aggregates in the pulmonary capillaries. The granulocytes release neutrophil elastase, superoxide anion, hydrogen peroxide, and hydroxide radicals, which in concert with bradykinin exert local toxic effects on the pulmonary epithelium that result in increased permeability. Arachidonate metabolites (eg, PGE_2, PGI_2, leukotriene B_4) may also be involved in some way. Analogous events are thought to occur in other organs.

Brady M et al: Cytokines and acute pancreatitis. Baillieres Best Pract Res Clin Gastroenterol 1999;13:265.

Chen JW, Saccone GT, Toouli J: Sphincter of Oddi dysfunction and acute pancreatitis. Gut 1998;43:305.

Cohn JA et al: Relation between mutations of the cystic fibrosis gene and idiopathic pancreatitis. N Engl J Med 1998; 339:653.

Cushman R: Apples, oranges, forests, and trees. J Health Polit Policy Law 1999;24:763.

Eckerwall G, Andersson R: Early enteral nutrition in severe acute pancreatitis: a way of providing nutrients, gut barrier protection, immunomodulation, or all of them? Scand J Gastroen-terol 2001;36:449.

Etemad B, Whitcomb DC: Chronic pancreatitis: diagnosis, classifi-cation, and new genetic developments. Gastroenterology 2001;120:682.

Halangk W et al: Role of cathepsin B in intracellular trypsinogen activation and the onset of acute pancreatitis. J Clin Invest 2000;106:773.

Layer P, Keller J: Pancreatic enzymes: secretion and luminal nutri-ent digestion in health and disease. J Clin Gastroenterol 1999;28:3.

Miskovitz P: Role of selectins in acute pancreatitis. Crit Care Med 2001;29:686.

Okazaki K et al: Recent concept of autoimmune-related pancreati-tis. J Gastroenterol 2001;36:293.

Opie EL: The theory of retrojection of bile into the pancreas. Rev Surg 1970;27:1.

Saluja AK, Steer MLP6: Pathophysiology of pancreatitis. Role of cytokines and other mediators of inflammation. Digestion 1999;60(Suppl 1):27.

Sharer N et al: Mutations of the cystic fibrosis gene in patients with chronic pancreatitis. N Engl J Med 1998;339:645.

Steer ML: How and where does acute pancreatitis begin? Arch Surg 1992;127:1350.

Vaccaro MI et al: Lipopolysaccharide directly affects pancreatic aci-nar cells: implications on acute pancreatitis pathophysiology. Dig Dis Sci 2000;45:915.

Whitcomb DC, Ulrich CD 2nd: Hereditary pancreatitis: new in-sights, new directions. Baillieres Best Pract Res Clin Gas-troenterol 1999;13:253.

1. Acute Pancreatitis

 ESSENTIALS OF DIAGNOSIS

- Abrupt onset of epigastric pain, frequently with back pain.
- Nausea and vomiting.
- Elevated serum or urinary amylase.
- Cholelithiasis or alcoholism (many patients).

General Considerations

While edematous and hemorrhagic pancreatitis are manifestations of the same pathologic processes and the general principles of treatment are the same, hemor-rhagic pancreatitis has more complications and a higher death rate. In edematous pancreatitis, the glandular tis-sue and surrounding retroperitoneal structures are en-gorged with interstitial fluid, and the pancreas is infil-trated with inflammatory cells that surround small foci of parenchymal necrosis. Hemorrhagic pancreatitis is characterized by bleeding into the parenchyma and sur-rounding retroperitoneal structures and extensive pan-creatic necrosis. In both forms, the peritoneal surfaces may be studded with small calcifications representing areas of fat necrosis.

Clinical Findings

A. SYMPTOMS AND SIGNS

The acute attack frequently begins following a large meal and consists of severe epigastric pain that radiates through to the back. The pain is unrelenting and usu-ally associated with vomiting and retching. In severe cases, the patient may collapse from shock.

Depending on the severity of the disease, there may be profound dehydration, tachycardia, and postural hy-potension. Myocardial function is depressed in severe pancreatitis, presumably because of circulating factors that affect cardiac performance. Examination of the ab-domen reveals decreased or absent bowel sounds and tenderness that may be generalized but more often is lo-calized to the epigastrium. Temperature is usually nor-mal or slightly elevated in uncomplicated pancreatitis. Clinical evidence of pleural effusion may be present, es-pecially on the left. If an abdominal mass is found, it probably represents a swollen pancreas (phlegmon) or, later in the illness, a pseudocyst or abscess. In 1–2% of patients, bluish discoloration is present in the flank (**Grey Turner's sign**) or periumbilical area (**Cullen's sign**), indicating hemorrhagic pancreatitis with dissec-tion of blood retroperitoneally into these areas.

B. LABORATORY FINDINGS

The hematocrit may be elevated as a consequence of dehydration or low as a result of abdominal blood loss in hemorrhagic pancreatitis. There is usually a moder-ate leukocytosis, but total white blood cell counts over 12,000/μL are unusual in the absence of suppurative complications. Liver function studies are usually nor-mal, but there may be a mild elevation of the serum bilirubin concentration (usually < 2 mg/dL).

The serum amylase concentration rises to more than 2½ times normal within 6 hours after the onset of an acute episode and generally remains elevated for several days. Values in excess of 1000 IU/dL occur early in the attack in 95% of patients with biliary pancreatitis and 85% of patients with acute alcoholic pancreatitis. Those with the most severe disease are more apt to have amy-lase levels below 1000 IU/dL.

Elevated serum lipase is detectable early and for sev-eral days after the acute attack. Since the lipase level tends to be higher in alcoholic pancreatitis and the amylase level higher in gallstone pancreatitis, the li-pase/amylase ratio has been suggested as a means to help distinguishing the two.

Elevated amylase levels may occur in other acute abdominal conditions, such as gangrenous cholecystitis, small bowel obstruction, mesenteric infarction, and perforated ulcer, though levels rarely exceed 500 IU/dL. Episodes of acute pancreatitis may occur without rises in serum amylase; this is the rule if hyperlipidemia is present. Furthermore, high levels may return to normal before blood is drawn.

The methods most commonly used for measuring amylase in the serum detect pancreatic amylase, salivary amylase, and macroamylase. However, hyperamylasemia is sometimes present in patients with abdominal pain when the elevated amylase levels consist entirely of salivary amylase or macroamylase and the pancreas is not inflamed.

Urine amylase excretion is also increased and is of diagnostic value. Excretion of more than 5000 units/24 h is abnormal. The urinary clearance of amylase increases during acute pancreatitis owing to a decrease in tubular reabsorption of amylase (normally 75% of filtered amylase). This was once thought to be specific, and the amylase-to-creatinine clearance ratio was used as a diagnostic test for acute pancreatitis. However, the increased amylase clearance results from overload of the tubular reabsorptive pathway with various urine proteins and is a nonspecific effect of tissue damage seen in many acute illnesses or following trauma.

In severe pancreatitis, the serum calcium concentration may fall as a result of calcium being complexed with fatty acids (liberated from retroperitoneal fat by lipase) and impaired reabsorption from bone owing to the action of calcitonin (liberated by high levels of glucagon). Relative hypoparathyroidism and hypoalbuminemia have also been implicated.

C. IMAGING STUDIES

In about two-thirds of cases, a plain abdominal film is abnormal. The most frequent finding is isolated dilation of a segment of gut (**sentinel loop**) consisting of jejunum, transverse colon, or duodenum adjacent to the pancreas. Gas distending the right colon that abruptly stops in the mid or left transverse colon (**colon cutoff sign**) is due to colonic spasm adjacent to the pancreatic inflammation. Both of these findings are relatively nonspecific. Glandular calcification may be evident, signifying chronic pancreatitis. An upper gastrointestinal series may show a widened duodenal loop, swollen ampulla of Vater, and, occasionally, evidence of gastric irritability. Chest films may reveal pleural effusion on the left side.

A CT scan of the pancreas using intravenous contrast media should be obtained in any patient with acute pancreatitis whose illness is not resolving after 48–72 hours. The radiologic findings may be consistent with any of the following: relatively normal appearing pancreas, pancreatic **phlegmon**, pancreatic phlegmon

with extension of the inflammatory process to adjacent extrapancreatic spaces, pancreatic **necrosis**, or pancreatic pseudocyst or **abscess** formation.

Occasionally, radiopaque gallstones will be apparent on plain x-rays. Ultrasound study may demonstrate gallstones early in the attack and may be used as a baseline for sequential examinations of the pancreas.

Several weeks after the pancreatitis has subsided, ERCP may be of value in patients with a tentative diagnosis of idiopathic pancreatitis (ie, those who have no history of alcoholism and no evidence of gallstones on ultrasound and oral cholecystogram). This examination demonstrates gallstones or changes of chronic pancreatitis in about 40% of such patients.

Differential Diagnosis

To some extent, acute pancreatitis is a diagnosis of exclusion, for other acute upper abdominal conditions such as acute cholecystitis, penetrating or perforated duodenal ulcer, high small bowel obstruction, acute appendicitis, and mesenteric infarction must always be seriously considered. In most cases, the distinction is possible on the basis of the clinical picture, laboratory findings, and CT scans. The critical point is that the diseases with which acute pancreatitis is most likely to be confused are often lethal if not treated surgically. Therefore, diagnostic laparotomy is indicated if they cannot be ruled out on clinical grounds.

Chronic hyperamylasemia occurs rarely without any relation to pancreatic disease. Some cases are associated with renal failure, chronic sialadenitis, salivary tumors, ovarian tumors, or liver disease, but often there is no explanation. Analysis of serum amylase isoenzymes is the only way to determine whether the amylase originates from salivary glands or pancreas. **Macroamylasemia** is a chronic hyperamylasemia in which normal amylase (usually salivary) is bound to a large serum glycoprotein or immunoglobulin molecule and is therefore not excreted into urine. The diagnosis rests on the combination of hyperamylasemia and low urinary amylase. Macroamylasemia has been found in patients with other diseases such as malabsorption, alcoholism, and cancer. Many patients have abdominal pain, but the relationship of the pain and the macroamylasemia is uncertain.

Complications

The principal complications of acute pancreatitis are abscess and pseudocyst formation. These are discussed in separate sections. Gastrointestinal bleeding may occur from adjacent inflamed stomach or duodenum, ruptured pseudocyst, or peptic ulcer. Intraperitoneal bleeding may occur spontaneously from the celiac or splenic artery or from the spleen following acute splenic vein thrombosis.

Involvement of the transverse colon or duodenum by the inflammatory process may result in partial obstruction, hemorrhage, necrosis, or fistula formation.

Early identification of patients at greatest risk of complications allows them to be managed more aggressively, which appears to decrease the mortality rate. The criteria of severity that have been found to be reliable are based either on the systemic manifestations of the disease as reflected in the clinical and laboratory findings or on the local changes in the pancreas as reflected by the findings on CT scan. Ranson used the former approach to develop the staging criteria listed in Table 27–1. Just the single finding of fluid sequestration (ie, fluid administered minus urine output) exceeding 2 L/d for more than 2 days is a reasonably accurate dividing line between severe (life-threatening) and mild-to-moderate disease. The local changes in the pancreas as shown on CT scans may be even more revealing. The presence of any of the following indicates a high risk of local infection in the pancreatic bed: involvement of extrapancreatic spaces in the inflammatory process, pancreatic necrosis (areas in the pancreas that do not enhance with intravenous contrast media), and early signs of abscess formation (eg, gas bubbles in the tissue).

Treatment

A. MEDICAL TREATMENT

The goals of medical therapy are reduction of pancreatic secretory stimuli and correction of fluid and electrolyte derangements.

1. Gastric suction—Oral intake is withheld, and a nasogastric tube is inserted to aspirate gastric secretions, although the latter has no specific therapeutic effect.

Table 27–1. Ranson's criteria of severity of acute pancreatitis.[1]

Criteria present initially
Age > 55 years
White blood cell count > 16,000/μL
Blood glucose > 200 mg/dL
Serum LDH > 350 IU/L
AST (SGOT) > 250 IU/dL
Criteria developing during first 24 hours
Hematocrit fall > 10%
BUN rise > 8 mg/dL
Serum Ca^{2+} < 8 mg/dL
Arterial Po_2 < 60 mm Hg
Base deficit > 4 meq/L
Estimated fluid sequestration > 600 mL

[1]Morbidity and mortality rates correlate with the number of criteria present. Mortality rates correlate as follows: 0–2 criteria present = 2%; 3 or 4 = 15%; 5 or 6 = 40%; 7 or 8 = 100%.

Oral feeding should be resumed only after the patient appears much improved, appetite has returned, and serum amylase levels have dropped to normal. Premature resumption of eating may result in exacerbation of disease.

2. Fluid replacement—Patients with acute pancreatitis sequester fluid in the retroperitoneum, and large volumes of intravenous fluids are necessary to maintain circulating blood volume and renal function. Patients with severe pancreatitis should receive albumin to combat the capillary leak that contributes to the pathophysiology. In severe hemorrhagic pancreatitis, blood transfusions may also be required. The adequacy of fluid replacement is the single most important aspect of medical therapy. In fact, undertreatment with fluids may actually contribute to the progression of pancreatitis. Fluid replacement may be judged most accurately by monitoring the volume and specific gravity of urine.

3. Antibiotics—Antibiotics are not useful in mild cases of acute pancreatitis. However, recent studies have shown benefit of antibiotics that penetrate pancreatic tissue for patients with severe pancreatitis. Imipenem is the most commonly used antibiotic. Antibiotics should also be used for treatment of specific operative complications.

4. Calcium and magnesium—In severe attacks of acute pancreatitis, hypocalcemia may require parenteral calcium replacement in amounts determined by serial calcium measurements. Recognition of hypocalcemia is important because it may produce cardiac dysrhythmias. Hypomagnesemia is also common, especially in alcoholics, and magnesium should also be replaced as indicated by serum levels.

5. Oxygen—Hypoxemia severe enough to require therapy develops in about 30% of patients with acute pancreatitis. It is often insidious, without clinical or x-ray signs, and out of proportion to the severity of the pancreatitis. The most pronounced examples accompany severe pancreatitis, often in association with hypocalcemia. The basic lesion, a form of adult respiratory distress syndrome, is poorly understood. Pulmonary changes include decreased vital capacity and an oxygen diffusion defect.

Hypoxemia must be suspected in every patient, and arterial blood gases should be measured every 12 hours for the first few hospital days. Supplemental oxygen therapy is indicated for Pao_2 levels below 70 mm Hg. An occasional patient requires endotracheal intubation and mechanical ventilation. Diuretics may be useful in decreasing lung water and improving arterial oxygen saturation.

6. Peritoneal lavage—Peritoneal lavage has been employed in severe refractory cases to remove toxins in the peritoneal fluid that would otherwise have been absorbed into the systemic circulation. Some patients appear to improve in response to this therapy although controlled trials have not substantiated its efficacy. Severe pancreatitis that fails to show clinical improvement after 24–48 hours of standard inpatient treatment is the usual indication for peritoneal lavage. The technique involves infusing and withdrawing 1–2 L of lactated Ringer's solution through a peritoneal dialysis catheter every hour for 1–3 days. Meta-analysis of the existing data shows no benefit; this treatment is not recommended outside of a clinical trial.

7. Nutrition—Total parenteral nutrition avoids pancreatic stimulation and should be used for nutritional support in any severely ill patient who will be unable to eat for more than 1 week. Elemental diets ingested orally or given by tube into the small intestine do not avoid secretory stimulation. Neither form of nutrition directly affects recovery of the pancreas.

8. Other drugs—Octreotide, H_2 receptor blockers, anticholinergic drugs, glucagon, and aprotinin have shown no beneficial effects in controlled trials.

B. ENDOSCOPIC SPHINCTEROTOMY

Biliary pancreatitis is caused by a gallstone becoming lodged in the ampulla of Vater. In most cases, the stone passes into the intestine but occasionally it becomes impacted in the ampulla, which results in more severe disease. Less than 10% of cases of biliary pancreatitis are severe (ie, three or more three Ranson criteria), but in severe cases, endoscopic sphincterotomy performed within 72 hours of the onset of the disease has been shown to decrease the incidence of concomitant biliary sepsis and lower the mortality rate from the pancreatitis.

C. SURGICAL TREATMENT

Surgery is generally contraindicated in uncomplicated acute pancreatitis. However, when the diagnosis is uncertain in a patient with severe abdominal pain, diagnostic laparotomy is not thought to aggravate pancreatitis.

When laparotomy has been performed for diagnosis and mild to moderate pancreatitis is found, cholecystectomy and operative cholangiography should be performed if gallstones are present, but the pancreas should be left undisturbed. For *severe* edematous pancreatitis, the gastrocolic omentum should be divided and the pancreas inspected. Although some surgeons place drains and irrigating catheters in the region of the pancreas, we prefer to keep foreign bodies out of this area.

The diagnosis of biliary pancreatitis can usually be suspected on the basis of ultrasound studies of the gallbladder early in the acute attack. Cholecystectomy should be performed on these patients during hospitalization for the acute attack soon after the attack re-

solves. A longer delay (even a few weeks) is associated with a high incidence (80%) of recurrent pancreatitis. Since life-threatening attacks are uncommon in gallstone pancreatitis, operation (common duct exploration; sphincteroplasty) or endoscopic therapy (sphincterotomy) early in an attack is rarely justified. However, when the attack is especially severe, elective cholecystectomy should be deferred up to several months to allow complete recovery from pancreatitis.

It is currently thought that debridement of dead peripancreatic tissue, which is often (40% of cases) colonized by bacteria, reduces the mortality rate of acute severe necrotizing pancreatitis. Historical controls place the mortality rate at 50–80% in the absence of operative treatment and 10–40% among patients subjected to necrosectomy. The diagnosis of necrotizing pancreatitis is suspected from the clinical findings; patients treated surgically have three or more Ranson criteria and average about 4½ criteria. Contrast-enhanced CT scans obtained early in the course of the disease are studied for the presence of nonenhancing areas, which indicate lack of vascular perfusion and reflect the presence of necrotic peripancreatic fat or pancreatic parenchyma. Percutaneous needle aspiration of these areas is used to detect the presence of bacterial colonization. A distinction is made between these cases of "infected necrotizing pancreatitis" and "pancreatic abscess," which may appear later in the course of the disease. Patients with infected necrotizing pancreatitis and severe clinical findings benefit most from surgical therapy, but laparotomy may be undertaken just because of a deteriorating condition in patients with necrotizing pancreatitis in the absence of bacterial colonization. At surgery, all peripancreatic spaces are opened and any necrotic tissue is removed by gentle blunt dissection. A T-tube is inserted if there is bile duct obstruction, and cholecystectomy is performed for gallstone disease. Two large drains are placed within the debrided spaces and are used postoperatively for sterile lavage. About 8 L of fluid are infused through this system daily for an average of 2 weeks. Other than CT evidence of necrotic tissue with or without infection, there are presently no other criteria in general use that call for pancreatic surgery in patients with severe pancreatitis.

Surgery for complications of acute pancreatitis, such as abscess, pseudocyst, and pancreatic ascites, is discussed below.

Prognosis

The death rate associated with acute pancreatitis is about 10%, and nearly all deaths occur in a first attack and among patients with three or more Ranson criteria of severity. Respiratory insufficiency and hypocalcemia indicate a poor prognosis. The death rate associated with severe necrotizing pancreatitis is 50% or more, but surgical therapy lowers the figure to about 20%. Persistent fever or hyperamylasemia 3 weeks or longer after an attack of pancreatitis usually indicates the presence of a pancreatic abscess or pseudocyst.

Abu-Zidan FM, Bonham MJ, Windsor JA: Severity of acute pancreatitis: a multivariate analysis of oxidative stress markers and modified Glasgow criteria. Br J Surg 2000;87:1019.

Beckingham IJ, Bornman PC: ABC of diseases of liver, pancreas, and biliary system. Acute pancreatitis. BMJ 2001;322:595.

Bornman PC, Beckingham IJ: ABC of diseases of liver, pancreas, and biliary system. Chronic pancreatitis. BMJ 2001;322:660.

Brivet FG, Emilie D, Galanaud P: Pro- and anti-inflammatory cytokines during acute severe pancreatitis: an early and sustained response, although unpredictable of death. Parisian Study Group on Acute Pancreatitis. Crit Care Med 1999; 27:749.

Chang L et al: Preoperative versus postoperative endoscopic retrograde cholangiopancreatography in mild to moderate gallstone pancreatitis: a prospective randomized trial. Ann Surg 2000;231:82.

Dervenis C, Bassi C: Evidence-based assessment of severity and management of acute pancreatitis. Br J Surg 2000;87:257.

Frakes JT: Biliary pancreatitis: a review. Emphasizing appropriate endoscopic intervention. J Clin Gastroenterol 1999;28:97.

Gumaste V: Prophylactic antibiotic therapy in the management of acute pancreatitis. J Clin Gastroenterol 2000;31:6.

Hamano H et al: High serum IgG4 concentrations in patients with sclerosing pancreatitis. N Engl J Med 2001;344:732.

Nealon WH, Matin S: Analysis of surgical success in preventing recurrent acute exacerbations in chronic pancreatitis. Ann Surg 2001;233:793.

Platell C, Cooper D, Hall JC: A meta-analysis of peritoneal lavage for acute pancreatitis. J Gastroenterol Hepatol 2001;16:689.

Schmid SW et al: The role of infection in acute pancreatitis. Gut 1999;45:311.

Toh SK, Phillips S, Johnson CD: A prospective audit against national standards of the presentation and management of acute pancreatitis in the South of England. Gut 2000;46:239.

Uhl W et al: Acute gallstone pancreatitis: timing of laparoscopic cholecystectomy in mild and severe disease. Surg Endosc 1999;13:1070.

Williams M, Simms HH: Prognostic usefulness of scoring systems in critically ill patients with severe acute pancreatitis. Crit Care Med 1999;27:901.

Windsor JA, Hammodat H: Metabolic management of severe acute pancreatitis. World J Surg 2000;24:664.

2. Pancreatic Pseudocyst

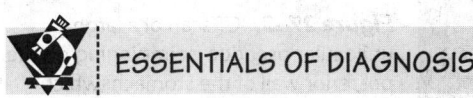

ESSENTIALS OF DIAGNOSIS

- *Epigastric mass and pain.*
- *Mild fever and leukocytosis.*
- *Persistent serum amylase elevation.*
- *Pancreatic cyst demonstrated by ultrasound or CT scan.*

General Considerations

Pancreatic pseudocysts are encapsulated collections of fluid with high enzyme concentrations that arise from the pancreas. They are usually located either within or adjacent to the pancreas in the lesser sac, but pancreatic pseudocysts have also been found in the neck, mediastinum, and pelvis. The walls of a pseudocyst are formed by inflammatory fibrosis of the peritoneal, mesenteric, and serosal membranes, which limits spread of the pancreatic juice as the lesion develops. The term pseudocyst denotes absence of an epithelial lining, whereas true cysts are lined by epithelium.

Two different processes are involved in the pathogenesis of pancreatic pseudocysts. Many occur as complications of severe acute pancreatitis, where extravasation of pancreatic juice and glandular necrosis form a sterile pocket of fluid that is not reabsorbed as inflammation subsides. Superinfection of such collections leads to pancreatic abscess instead of pseudocyst. In other patients, usually alcoholics or trauma victims, pseudocysts appear without preceding acute pancreatitis. The mechanism in these cases consists of ductal obstruction and formation of a retention cyst that loses its epithelial lining as it grows beyond the confines of the gland. In posttraumatic pseudocyst, symptoms usually do not appear until several weeks after the injury. Some are iatrogenic, eg, occurring during splenectomy; others follow an external blow to the abdomen.

Pseudocysts develop in about 2% of cases of acute pancreatitis. The cysts are single in 85% of cases and multiple in the remainder.

Clinical Findings

A. SYMPTOMS AND SIGNS

A pseudocyst should be suspected when a patient with acute pancreatitis fails to recover after a week of treatment or when, after improving for a time, symptoms return. Since it is now fairly routine to obtain a CT scan early in an attack of severe acute pancreatitis, the early stages of pseudocyst formation are often demonstrated radiographically before specific clinical findings appear. The first clinical manifestation is usually a palpable tender mass in the epigastrium, consisting of a swollen pancreas and contiguous viscera (a phlegmon). With time, the mass may subside, but if it persists it most likely represents a pseudocyst.

In other cases, the pseudocyst develops insidiously without an obvious attack of acute pancreatitis.

Regardless of the type of prodromal phase, pain is the most common finding. Fever, weight loss, tenderness, and a palpable mass are present in about half of patients. A few have jaundice, a manifestation of obstruction of the intrapancreatic segment of the bile duct.

B. LABORATORY FINDINGS

An elevated serum amylase and leukocytosis are present in about half of patients. When present, elevated bilirubin levels reflect biliary obstruction. Of those patients with acute pancreatitis whose serum amylase remains elevated for as long as 3 weeks, about half will have a pseudocyst.

C. IMAGING STUDIES

CT scan (Figure 27–3) is the diagnostic study of choice. The size and shape of the cyst and its relationship to other viscera can be seen. Acute pseudocysts are often irregular in shape; chronic pseudocysts are most often circular or nearly so. An enlarged pancreatic duct may be demonstrated in patients with chronic pancreatitis. A dilated common bile duct would suggest biliary obstruction, either from the cyst or from underlying chronic pancreatitis.

The gallbladder should be studied by ultrasound to look for gallstones, especially in patients with acute pancreatitis. Although ultrasound can also demonstrate pseudocysts, the amount of important detail obtained is less than that from CT scans, and consequently the role of ultrasound is mainly to follow changes in size of an acute pseudocyst already imaged by CT scans, so the amount of x-ray exposure can be kept to a minimum.

ERCP should be performed if there are thought to be significant abnormalities of the bile or pancreatic duct as suggested by CT scans or the results of liver function tests. Either duct may be dilated and in need of surgical drainage in conjunction with drainage of the pseudocyst. ERCP usually opacifies the pseudocyst as well, but the information is not usually of major value in planning treatment, so ERCP is not obtained routinely.

An upper gastrointestinal series will often reveal a mass in the lesser sac that distorts the stomach or duodenum, but this is not particularly useful information. The principal indication for an upper gastrointestinal series is to search for a site of gastric or duodenal obstruction in patients who are vomiting.

With wide use of sensitive imaging studies in the diagnosis of pancreatic disease, small asymptomatic pseudocysts are often demonstrated. The natural his-

Figure 27–3. CT scan of a large unilocular pseudocyst impinging on the posterior wall of the stomach (which contains contrast media). A cyst in this location is usually best drained into the stomach.

tory of these subclinical lesions is benign, and there is no indication for prophylactic surgical treatment.

Differential Diagnosis

Pancreatic pseudocysts must be distinguished from pancreatic abscess and acute pancreatic phlegmon. Patients with an abscess exhibit signs of infection.

Rarely, patients with pseudocyst present with weight loss, jaundice, and a nontender palpable gallbladder and are first thought to have pancreatic carcinoma. CT scans show that the lesion is fluid-filled, which suggests the correct diagnosis.

Neoplastic cysts—either cystadenoma or cystadenocarcinoma—account for about 5% of all cases of cystic pancreatic masses and may be indistinguishable preoperatively from pseudocyst. The correct diagnosis can be made from the gross appearance supplemented by a biopsy obtained at operation.

Complications

A. INFECTION

Infection is a rare complication resulting in high fever, chills, and leukocytosis. Drainage is required as soon as the diagnosis is suspected. Some lesions can be drained externally via a catheter placed percutaneously using ultrasound guidance. Internal drainage of infected pseudocysts adherent to the stomach can be achieved surgically by cystogastrostomy; otherwise, drainage should be external, because the suture line of a Roux-en-Y cystojejunostomy may not heal.

B. RUPTURE

Sudden perforation into the free peritoneal cavity produces severe chemical peritonitis, with board-like abdominal rigidity and severe pain. Rapid enlargement of the pseudocyst is sometimes noted before it ruptures. The treatment is emergency surgery with irrigation of the peritoneal cavity and a drainage procedure for the pseudocyst. The wall of a ruptured pseudocyst is usually too flimsy to hold sutures securely, so most ruptured cysts must be drained externally. Rupture of a pseudocyst occurs in less than 5% of cases, but even with prompt treatment it may be fatal.

C. HEMORRHAGE

Bleeding may occur into the cyst cavity or an adjacent viscus into which the cyst has eroded. Intracystic bleeding may present as an enlarging abdominal mass with anemia resulting from blood loss. If the cyst has eroded into the stomach, there may be hematemesis, melena, and blood in the nasogastric aspirate. The rapidity of the blood loss often produces hemorrhagic shock, which may preclude arteriography. If time permits, however,

emergency arteriography should be performed to delineate the site of bleeding, which is usually a false aneurysm of an artery in the cyst wall, and to embolize it if possible. If embolization successfully occludes the bleeding vessel, several weeks should elapse to ensure that bleeding will not recur, and at that point the pseudocyst should be drained surgically in the same fashion as a nonbleeding pseudocyst. If the bleeding cannot be stopped by embolization, emergency surgery should be performed. Usually all that can be done is to open the cyst and suture ligate the bleeding vessel in the cyst wall, followed by external or internal drainage of the cyst. Sometimes it is possible to excise the cyst, which is desirable because doing so more certainly avoids the risk of recurrent hemorrhage.

Treatment

The principal indications for treating pancreatic pseudocysts are to improve symptoms and to prevent complications. Recent data indicate that the natural history of these lesions is more benign than previously thought—that in the absence of symptoms or radiographic evidence of enlargement (and irrespective of cyst size), expectant management is not unreasonable, and that a few untreated cysts resolve spontaneously even after being stable for months. Expectant management is especially important in the first 6–12 weeks of existence of cysts that have arisen during an attack of acute pancreatitis. The chances of spontaneous resolution are about 40%; catheter drainage at this stage is meddlesome; and internal drainage of the cyst by surgery may be difficult or even impossible. Thereafter, for cysts greater than 5 cm, treatment is usually recommended over expectant management (in the absence of contraindications, such as serious concomitant disease), because most cysts can be promptly eliminated by percutaneous catheter drainage or surgical drainage into the stomach or intestine. This obviates the need for prolonged follow-up with repeated ultrasound or CT scans and avoids the risks, albeit low, of complications. Patients who present with a symptomatic pseudocyst and no history of recent acute pancreatitis may be treated without the 6- to 12-week delay, because their cyst wall is tough (mature) enough to hold sutures and allow an anastomosis with the gut. Jaundice in a patient with a pseudocyst is usually caused by pressure from the cyst on the bile duct. Draining the pseudocyst usually relieves the obstruction, but an operative cholangiogram should be obtained to make sure.

A. EXCISION

Excision is the most definitive treatment but is usually confined to chronic pseudocysts in the tail of the gland. This approach is recommended especially for cysts that follow trauma, where the head and body of the gland are normal. Most cysts should be drained either externally or internally into the gut.

B. EXTERNAL DRAINAGE

External drainage is best for critically ill patients or when the cyst wall has not matured sufficiently for anastomosis to other organs. A large tube is sewn into the cyst lumen, and its end is brought out through the abdominal wall. External drainage is complicated in a third of patients by a pancreatic fistula that sometimes requires surgical drainage but on the average closes spontaneously in several months. The incidence of recurrent pseudocyst is about four times greater after external drainage than after drainage into the gut.

C. INTERNAL DRAINAGE

The preferred method of treatment is internal drainage, where the cyst is anastomosed to a Roux-en-Y limb of jejunum (cystojejunostomy), to the posterior wall of the stomach (cystogastrostomy), or to the duodenum (cystoduodenostomy). The interior of the cyst should be inspected for evidence of a tumor and biopsy performed as appropriate. Cystogastrostomy is preferable for cysts behind and densely adherent to the stomach. This may well be done laparoscopically in the future. To accomplish free, dependent drainage, Roux-en-Y cystojejunostomy provides better drainage of cysts in various other locations. Cystoduodenostomy is indicated for cysts deep within the head of the gland and adjacent to the medial wall of the duodenum—lesions that would be difficult to drain by any other technique. The procedure consists of making a lateral duodenotomy, opening into the cyst through the medial wall of the duodenum, and then closing the lateral duodenotomy. Following internal drainage, the cyst cavity becomes obliterated within a few weeks. Even after cystogastrostomy, an unrestricted diet can be allowed within a week after surgery, and x-rays taken at this time usually show only a small residual cyst cavity.

D. NONSURGICAL DRAINAGE

External drainage can be established by a percutaneous catheter placed into the cyst under radiographic or ultrasound control. This is the preferred method for infected pseudocysts. In some centers, it is also used for the majority of uncomplicated pseudocysts as the primary mode of therapy. About two-thirds of cysts so treated are permanently eradicated. It may also be useful to shrink a truly huge pseudocyst (eg, one that occupies half of the abdominal cavity), because it is technically difficult to obtain adequate internal drainage of these lesions into the gut. Occasionally, a sterile cyst may become infected when a narrow catheter is inserted into it. This is more likely when the cyst lumen contains debris that is not drained effectively by this technique. Chronic external pancreatic fistula is a potential complication of this method.

Two other drainage techniques have been tried: (1) Passing a catheter percutaneously through the anterior abdominal wall, the anterior wall of the stomach, and through the posterior stomach into the cyst. After several weeks, the catheter is removed, and a chronic tract remains from cyst to gastric lumen. (2) Using a fiberoptic gastroscope to make a small incision through the back wall of the stomach into the cyst. Because of questions about efficacy and safety, neither method is widely used.

Prognosis

The recurrence rate for pancreatic pseudocyst is about 10%, and recurrence is more frequent after treatment by external drainage. Serious postoperative hemorrhage from the cyst occurs rarely—most often after cystogastrostomy. In most cases, however, surgical treatment of pseudocysts is uncomplicated and definitively solves the immediate problem. Many patients later experience chronic pain as a manifestation of underlying chronic pancreatitis.

Cooperman AM: Surgical treatment of pancreatic pseudocysts. Surg Clin North Am 2001;81:411.

Heider R et al: Percutaneous drainage of pancreatic pseudocysts is associated with a higher failure rate than surgical treatment in unselected patients. Ann Surg 1999;229:781.

Heider R, Behrns KE: Pancreatic pseudocysts complicated by splenic parenchymal involvement: results of operative and percutaneous management. Pancreas 2001;23:20.

Mori T et al: Laparoscopic pancreatic cystgastrostomy. J Hepatobiliary Pancreat Surg 2000;7:28.

Neff R: Pancreatic pseudocysts and fluid collections: percutaneous approaches. Surg Clin North Am 2001;81:399.

Vidyarthi G, Steinberg SE: Endoscopic management of pancreatic pseudocysts. Surg Clin North Am 2001;81:405.

3. Pancreatic Abscess

Pancreatic abscess, which complicates about 5% of cases of acute pancreatitis, is invariably fatal if it is not treated surgically. It tends to develop in severe cases accompanied by hypovolemic shock and pancreatic necrosis and is an especially frequent complication of postoperative pancreatitis. Abscess formation follows secondary bacterial contamination of necrotic pancreatic debris and hemorrhagic exudate. The organisms may spread to the pancreas hematogenously as well as directly through the wall of the transverse colon. It is unknown whether prophylactic antibiotics given early in the course of severe acute pancreatitis decrease the incidence of abscess.

Clinical Findings

An abscess should be suspected when a patient with severe acute pancreatitis fails to improve and develops rising fever or when symptoms return after a period of recovery. In most cases, there is improvement for a while before signs of infection appear 2–4 weeks after the attack began. Epigastric pain and tenderness and a palpable tender mass are clues to diagnosis. In many cases, the findings are not especially striking—ie, the temperature is only modestly elevated and the patient does not appear septic. Vomiting or jaundice may be present, but in some cases fever and leukocytosis are the only findings. The serum amylase may be elevated but usually is normal. Characteristically, the serum albumin is below 2.5 g/dL and the alkaline phosphatase is elevated. Pleural fluid and diaphragmatic paralysis may be evident on chest x-rays. An upper gastrointestinal series may show deformity of the stomach or duodenum by a mass, but it usually does not, and the changes are nonspecific in any case. Diagnostic CT scans will usually indicate the presence of a fluid collection in the area of the pancreas. Gas in the collection on plain films or CT scans is virtually diagnostic. Percutaneous CT scan-guided aspiration may be used to aid in diagnosis and obtain a specimen for Gram stain and culture.

In general, the diagnosis is difficult, treatment is often instituted late, illness is severe, and death rates are high.

Treatment

The collection of pus must be drained. Percutaneous catheter drainage may be helpful as a first step in order to decrease toxicity or to obtain a specimen for culture. In some cases, catheter drainage will prove to be definitive, but most often the infected retroperitoneal space is honeycombed and contains necrotic debris that cannot pass through the catheter, so surgical debridement is necessary. It is best to consider catheter drainage as a preparatory step for surgery rather than a curative treatment, for that is the usual relationship. Otherwise, there may be a tendency to delay surgery for too long as futile efforts are repeatedly made to manipulate the catheters into better positions. In fact, the two measures—surgical debridement and catheter drainage—are complementary.

Preoperatively, the patient should be given broad-spectrum antibiotics, since the organisms are usually a mixed flora, most often *Escherichia coli, Bacteroides, Staphylococcus, Klebsiella, Proteus, Candida albicans,* etc. Necrotic debris should be removed and external drainage instituted.

Postoperative hemorrhage (immediate or delayed) from the abscess cavity occurs occasionally.

Prognosis

The death rate is about 20%, a consequence of the severity of the condition, incomplete surgical drainage, and the inability in some cases to make the diagnosis.

Baril NB et al: Does an infected peripancreatic fluid collection or abscess mandate operation? Ann Surg 2000;231:361.

Beger HG, Rau B, Isenmann R: Prevention of severe change in acute pancreatitis: prediction and prevention. J Hepatobiliary Pancreat Surg 2001;8:140.

Kang CY et al: Development of HIV/AIDS vaccine using chimeric gag-env virus-like particles. Biol Chem 1999;380:353.

Tsiotos GG, Sarr MG: Management of fluid collections and necrosis in acute pancreatitis. Curr Gastroenterol Rep 1999;1:139.

Venu RP et al: Endoscopic transpapillary drainage of pancreatic abscess: technique and results. Gastrointest Endosc 2000;51(4 Part 1):391.

4. Pancreatic Ascites & Pancreatic Pleural Effusion

Pancreatic ascites consists of accumulated pancreatic fluid in the abdomen without peritonitis or severe pain. Since many of these patients are alcoholic, they are often thought at first to have cirrhotic ascites. The syndrome is most often due to chronic leakage of a pseudocyst, but a few cases are due to disruption of a pancreatic duct. The principal causative factors are alcoholic pancreatitis in adults and traumatic pancreatitis in children. Marked recent weight loss is a major clinical manifestation, and unresponsiveness of the ascites to diuretics is an additional diagnostic clue. The ascitic fluid, which ranges in appearance from straw-colored to blood-tinged, contains elevated protein (> 2.9 g/dL) and amylase levels. Once this condition is suspected, definitive diagnosis is based on chemical analysis of the ascitic fluid and endoscopic retrograde pancreatography. The latter procedure frequently demonstrates the point of fluid leak and allows a rational surgical approach if operation is required.

Initial therapy should consist of a period of intravenous hyperalimentation and somatostatin. This often cures the problem. If considerable improvement has not occurred within 2–3 weeks, surgery should be performed. A preoperative ERCP is essential to demonstrate the site of the leak. If it is not entirely obvious from the films taken during ERCP, a CT scan should be performed immediately afterward, while contrast media is still in the pancreatic duct. The greater sensitivity of the CT scan will be enough to reveal the tiny trickle from the pancreatic duct into the abdomen. The operation involves suturing a Roux-en-Y limb of jejunum to the site of the leak on the surface of the pancreas or a pancreatic pseudocyst. With appropriate therapy, the outlook is excellent. The death rate is low in patients treated before debilitation becomes severe.

Chronic pleural effusions of pancreatic origin represent a variant in which the pancreatic fistula drains into the chest. The diagnosis is made by measuring high concentrations of amylase (usually > 3000 IU/dL) in the fluid. A CT scan of the pancreas and retrograde pancreatogram should be obtained. Medical therapy consists of draining the fluid with a chest tube, somatostatin, and total parenteral nutrition. If after several weeks the fistula persists or if it recurs after the tube has been removed, the source of the leak on the pancreas should either be drained into a Roux-en-Y limb of jejunum or excised as part of a distal pancreatectomy.

Dugernier T, Laterre PF, Reynaert MS: Ascites fluid in severe acute pancreatitis: from pathophysiology to therapy. Acta Gastroenterol Belg 2000;63:264.

Kaman L et al: Internal pancreatic fistulas with pancreatic ascites and pancreatic pleural effusions: recognition and management. Aust N Z J Surg 2001;71:221.

Takeo C, Myojo S: Marked effect of octreotide acetate in a case of pancreatic pleural effusion. Curr Med Res Opin 2000; 16:171.

5. Chronic Pancreatitis

 ESSENTIALS OF DIAGNOSIS

- *Persistent or recurrent abdominal pain.*
- *Pancreatic calcification on x-ray in 50%.*
- *Pancreatic insufficiency in 30%; malabsorption and diabetes mellitus.*
- *Most often due to alcoholism.*

General Considerations

Chronic alcoholism causes most cases of chronic pancreatitis, but a few are due to gallstones, hypercalcemia, hyperlipidemia, duct obstruction from any cause, or inherited predisposition (familial pancreatitis). Direct trauma to the gland, either from an external blow or from surgical injury, can produce chronic pancreatitis if a ductal stricture develops during the healing process. In such cases, disease is often localized to the segment of gland drained by the obstructed duct. Although gallstone disease may cause repeated attacks of acute pancreatitis, this uncommonly leads to chronic pancreatitis.

There is evidence that pancreatic juice normally contains a specific protein responsible for maintaining calcium carbonate in solution. Levels of this protein are

decreased in patients with chronic pancreatitis, a situation that allows calcium carbonate to precipitate and form calculi. Pressure within the duct is increased in patients with chronic pancreatitis (about 40 cm H_2O) compared with normal subjects (about 15 cm H_2O). This is a result of increased viscosity of pancreatic juice, partial obstruction by calculi, and impaired distensibility of the gland because of diffuse fibrosis (eg, a compartment syndrome). Sphincteric pressure remains in the normal range. The increased pressure causes dilation of the duct in the patient whose pancreas has not yet become fixed by scarring. It may also impair nutrient blood flow, causing further functional damage. Pathologic changes in the gland include destruction of parenchyma, fibrosis, dedifferentiation of acini, calculi, and ductal dilation.

Clinical Findings

A. SYMPTOMS AND SIGNS

Chronic pancreatitis may be asymptomatic, or it may produce abdominal pain, malabsorption, diabetes mellitus, or (usually) all three manifestations. The pain is typically felt deep in the upper abdomen and radiating through to the back, and it waxes and wanes from day to day. Early in the course of the disease, the pain may be episodic, lasting for days to weeks and then vanishing for several months before returning again. Attacks of acute pancreatitis may occur, superimposed on the pattern of chronic pain. Many patients become addicted to the narcotics prescribed for pain.

B. LABORATORY FINDINGS

Abnormal laboratory findings may result from (1) pancreatic inflammation, (2) pancreatic exocrine insufficiency, (3) diabetes mellitus, (4) bile duct obstruction, or (5) other complications such as pseudocyst formation or splenic vein thrombosis.

1. Amylase—In acute exacerbations, serum and urinary amylase levels may be elevated, but most often they are not, perhaps because pancreatic fibrosis has destroyed so much of the enzyme-forming capacity of the parenchyma.

2. Tests of exocrine pancreatic function—The secretin and cholecystokinin stimulation tests are the most sensitive tests to detect exocrine malfunction but are difficult to perform.

3. Diabetes mellitus—About 75% of patients with calcific pancreatitis and 30% of those with noncalcific pancreatitis have insulin-dependent diabetes. Most of the rest have either abnormal glucose tolerance curves or abnormally low serum insulin levels after a test meal. The margin of reserve is such that partial pancreatectomy is quite likely to convert a patient who does not require insulin into one who does require it postoperatively.

4. Biliary obstruction—Elevated bilirubin or alkaline phosphatase levels may result from fibrotic entrapment of the lower end of the bile duct. The differential diagnosis of biliary obstruction in these patients must consider acute pancreatic inflammation, pseudocyst, or pancreatic neoplasm.

5. Miscellaneous—Splenic vein thrombosis may produce secondary hypersplenism or gastric varices.

C. IMAGING STUDIES

Endoscopic retrograde pancreatography is helpful in establishing the diagnosis of chronic pancreatitis, in ruling out pancreatic pseudocyst and neoplasm, and in preoperative planning for patients thought to be candidates for surgery. The typical findings are ductal stones and irregularity, with dilation and stenoses and, occasionally, ductal occlusion. The discovery of small unsuspected pseudocysts is common. Retrograde cholangiography should be performed simultaneously to determine whether the common bile duct is narrowed by the pancreatitis, to determine whether biliary calculi are present, and to aid the surgeon in avoiding injury to the bile duct during operation.

Complications

The principal complications of chronic pancreatitis are pancreatic pseudocyst, biliary obstruction, duodenal obstruction, malnutrition, and diabetes mellitus. Adenocarcinoma of the pancreas occurs with greater frequency in patients with familial chronic pancreatitis than in the general population.

Treatment

A. MEDICAL TREATMENT

Malabsorption and steatorrhea are managed with support and measures. Controlled trials have shown that administering pancreatic enzymes has little effect on the pain.

Patients with chronic pancreatitis should be urged to discontinue the use of alcohol. Abstention from alcohol will reduce chronic or episodic pain in more than half of cases even though damage to the pancreas is irreversible. Psychiatric treatment may be beneficial. Diabetes in these patients usually requires insulin.

B. SURGICAL TREATMENT

Surgical therapy is principally of value to relieve chronic intractable pain. It is essential that every effort be made to eliminate alcohol abuse. The best surgical

candidates are those whose pain persists after alcohol has been abandoned.

Surgical treatment in most cases involves a procedure that facilitates drainage of the pancreatic duct or resects diseased pancreas—or that serves both purposes. The choice of operation can usually be made preoperatively based on the findings of a retrograde pancreatogram and CT scans. Coincidental bile duct obstruction is common and should be treated by simultaneous choledochoduodenostomy.

1. Drainage procedures—A dilated ductal system reflects obstruction, and when dilation is present, procedures to improve ductal drainage usually relieve pain. Calcific alcoholic pancreatitis most often falls into this category.

The usual finding is an irregular, widely dilated duct (1–2 cm in diameter) with points of stenosis ("chain of lakes" appearance) and ductal calculi. For such patients, a longitudinal pancreaticojejunostomy (**Puestow procedure**) is appropriate (Figure 27–4). The duct is opened anteriorly from the tail into the head of the gland and anastomosed side-to-side to a Roux-en-Y segment of proximal jejunum. Pain improves postopera-

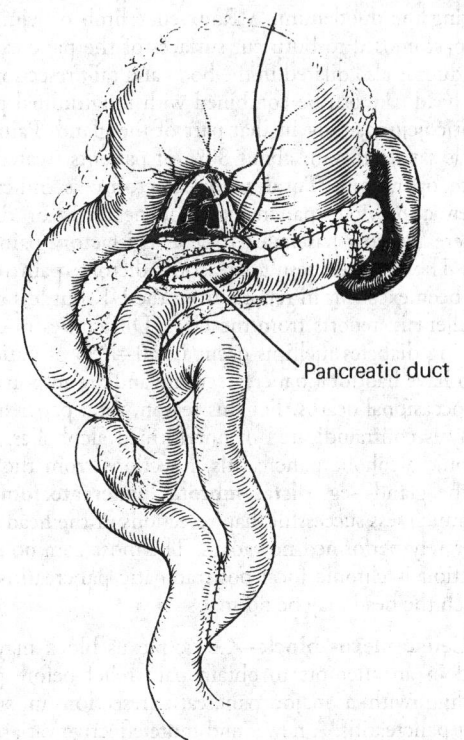

Pancreatic duct

Figure 27–4. Longitudinal pancreaticojejunostomy (Puestow) for chronic pancreatitis.

tively in about 80% of patients, but improvement of pancreatic insufficiency is uncommon. This procedure, however, has a low rate of success when the pancreatic duct is narrow (ie, < 8 mm).

Sphincteroplasty and distal (caudal) pancreaticojejunostomy (**Du Val procedure**) are other drainage techniques that were used more often in the past. The latter is only of historical interest, but surgical sphincteroplasty plus extraction of pancreatic ductal calculi continuous in use. Attempts are currently being made to accomplish something similar by subjecting pancreatic calculi to external shock wave lithotripsy, followed by endoscopic sphincterotomy and stone extraction. Another experimental method involves decompression of the duct by an endoscopically placed stent. Questions of safety and efficacy have tempered the early enthusiasm for these procedures.

2. Pancreatectomy—In the absence of a dilated duct, pancreatectomy is the best procedure, and the extent of resection can often be determined from a CT scan and pancreatogram. In patients with small ducts, the most severe disease is usually located in the head of the gland, and **pancreaticoduodenectomy** (Whipple procedure) is the operation of choice. A variant of this procedure involves resection of the head of the gland while preserving the duodenum. A Roux-en-Y limb of jejunum is anastomosed to both cut surfaces of the pancreas. If the duct is also dilated in the body and tail, resection of the head can also be combined with longitudinal pancreaticojejunostomy in that part of the gland. Pain relief is satisfactory in about 80% of patients treated by these operations. **Total pancreatectomy** is indicated when a previous pancreaticoduodenectomy or distal pancreatectomy has failed to give satisfactory pain relief. The reported results are contradictory; pain relief has been excellent in reports from the UK but less than excellent in reports from the USA. Difficulties in controlling diabetes mellitus occur in 30–40% of patients who have had total pancreatectomy and are responsible for occasional deaths. For this reason, total pancreatectomy is contraindicated in unreformed alcoholics. For chronic alcoholic pancreatitis, resections from the left of the gland—eg, **distal subtotal pancreatectomy**— are much less successful than resections of the head and are rarely performed nowadays. The most common indication is chronic focal posttraumatic pancreatitis, in which the head may be normal.

3. Celiac plexus block—Celiac plexus block may be used in an attempts to obtain pain relief before proceeding with a major pancreatic resection in small duct pancreatitis. A newer and more effective variant of this approach consists of **thoracoscopic splanchnicectomy**—resection of segments of the greater and lesser splanchnic nerves as they enter the thorax from the abdomen. When performed thoracoscopically, the procedure is relatively minor, and it interrupts the pain afferents with greater certainty.

Prognosis

Longitudinal pancreaticojejunostomy relieves pain in about 80% of patients with a dilated duct. Weight gain is common but less predictable. The results of pancreaticoduodenectomy are good in 80% of patients, but removal of the distal pancreas is less successful. Total pancreatectomy, which is principally reserved for failures of other operations, gives satisfying relief in 30–90% of patients depending on the series. The reasons for these widely differing results are not known. Celiac plexus block is of lasting benefit to no more than 30% of patients. In some patients, pain subsides with advancing pancreatic insufficiency.

Except in advanced cases with continuous pain, alcoholics who can be persuaded to stop drinking often experience relief from pain and recurrent attacks of pancreatitis. In familial pancreatitis, the progress of the disease is inexorable, and many of these patients require surgery. The results of longitudinal pancreaticojejunostomy are excellent in familial pancreatitis. Narcotic addiction, diabetes, and malnutrition are serious problems in many patients.

Adamek HE et al: Long term follow up of patients with chronic pancreatitis and pancreatic stones treated with extracorporeal shock wave lithotripsy. Gut 1999;45:402.

Apte MV, Keogh GW, Wilson JS: Chronic pancreatitis: complications and management. J Clin Gastroenterol 1999;29:225.

Berney T et al: Long-term metabolic results after pancreatic resection for severe chronic pancreatitis. Arch Surg 2000; 135:1106.

Bornman PC, Beckingham IJ: ABC of diseases of liver, pancreas, and biliary system. Chronic pancreatitis. BMJ 2001;322:660.

Izbicki JR et al: Extended drainage versus resection in surgery for chronic pancreatitis: a prospective randomized trial comparing the longitudinal pancreaticojejunostomy combined with local pancreatic head excision with the pylorus-preserving pancreatoduodenectomy. Ann Surg 1998;228:771.

Jimenez RE et al: Outcome of pancreaticoduodenectomy with pylorus preservation or with antrectomy in the treatment of chronic pancreatitis. Ann Surg 2000;231:293.

McCutcheon AD: Neurological damage and duodenopancreatic reflux in the pathogenesis of alcoholic pancreatitis. Arch Surg 2000;135:278.

Pitchumoni CS: Chronic pancreatitis: pathogenesis and management of pain. J Clin Gastroenterol 1998;27:101.

Sakorafas GH et al: Pancreatoduodenectomy for chronic pancreatitis: long-term results in 105 patients. Arch Surg 2000; 135:517.

Whitcomb DC: Hereditary pancreatitis: new insights into acute and chronic pancreatitis. Gut 1999;45:317.

PANCREATIC INSUFFICIENCY
(Steatorrhea; Malabsorption)

Pancreatic exocrine insufficiency may follow pancreatectomy or pancreatic disease, especially chronic pancreatitis. Many patients with varying degrees of pancreatic insufficiency have no symptoms and require no treatment, whereas others may benefit greatly from a rational medical regimen.

Malabsorption and steatorrhea do not appear until more than 90% of pancreatic exocrine function is lost; with 2–10% of normal function, steatorrhea is mild to moderate; with less than 2% of normal function, steatorrhea is severe. On a diet containing 100 g of fat per day, normal subjects excrete 5–7 g/d, and the efficiency of assimilation is similar over a wide range of fat intake. Total pancreatectomy causes about 70% fat malabsorption. If the pancreatic remnant is normal, subtotal resections may have little effect on absorption.

Pancreatic insufficiency affects fat absorption more than that of protein or carbohydrate, because protein digestion is aided by gastric pepsin and carbohydrate digestion by salivary and intestinal amylase. Malabsorption of vitamins is rarely a significant problem. Water-soluble B vitamins are absorbed throughout the small intestine, and fat-soluble vitamins, although dependent on micellar solubilization by bile salts, do not require pancreatic enzymes for absorption. Vitamin B_{12} malabsorption has been detected in some patients with pancreatic insufficiency, but it is rarely a clinical problem, and vitamin B_{12} replacement is unnecessary.

Thus, the principal problem in otherwise uncomplicated pancreatic insufficiency is fat malabsorption and accompanying caloric malnutrition.

Tests of Pancreatic Exocrine Function

A. SECRETIN OR CHOLECYSTOKININ TEST

Pancreatic juice is obtained by peroral duodenal intubation, and the response to an intravenous injection of secretin or cholecystokinin is measured. The results vary, depending on the dose and preparation of hormone used. Both tests (using purified hormones or the synthetic octapeptide of cholecystokinin) seem to be reliable. Pancreatic fluid should normally have a bicarbonate concentration greater than 80 meq/L and bicarbonate output above 15 meq/30 min.

B. PANCREOLAURYL TEST

Fluorescein dilaurate is given orally with breakfast, and urinary fluorescein excretion is measured. Release and absorption of fluorescein depend on the action of pancreatic esterase. The test is relatively specific, but considerable exocrine insufficiency is required for a positive result. It is currently the most widely used test of exocrine function because it is inexpensive and easy to do.

C. PABA EXCRETION (BENTIROMIDE) TEST

The patient ingests 1 g of the synthetic peptide bentiromide (Bz-Ty-PABA), and urinary excretion of aromatic amines (PABA) is measured. Cleavage of the peptide to liberate PABA depends on intraluminal chymotrypsin activity. Patients with chronic pancreatitis excrete about 50% of the normal amount of PABA.

D. FECAL FAT BALANCE TEST

The patient ingests a diet containing 75–100 g fat each day for 5 days. The amounts of dietary fat should be measured and should be the same each day. Excretion of less than 7% of ingested fat is normal. Clinically significant steatorrhea is present when fat malabsorption exceeds about 25%. Total pancreatectomy results in about 70% fat malabsorption.

Examination of a stool specimen for fat globules (obviously much simpler than the fat balance test) is specific and relatively sensitive for fat malabsorption.

Treatment

The diet should aim for 3000–6000 kcal/d, emphasizing carbohydrate (400 g or more) and protein (100–150 g). Patients with steatorrhea may or may not have diarrhea, and dietary restriction of fat is important mainly to control diarrhea. Patients with diarrhea may be restricted to 50 g of fat and the amount increased until diarrhea appears. Permissible fat intake averages 100 g/d distributed equally among four meals.

Pancrelipase replacement may be accomplished with pancreatic extracts containing 30,000–50,000 units of lipase distributed throughout each of four daily meals. Lesser amounts are much less effective; an hourly dosage regimen probably has no advantages.

If enzymes alone do not improve the malabsorption enough, the problem is probably due to destruction of lipase by gastric acid. This can be largely alleviated by adding an H2 receptor blocking agent to the enzyme regimen. A preparation of enzymes as enteric-coated microspheres (Pancrease) is less vulnerable to low pH and may be more effective in refractory cases.

Medium-chain triglycerides (MCT), which can be obtained as a powder or an oil, may be used as a caloric supplement. This product is more rapidly hydrolyzed and the fatty acids more readily absorbed than are long-chain triglycerides, which make up 98% of the fat in a normal diet. Unfortunately, MCT oil is relatively unpalatable and is frequently associated with nausea and vomiting, bloating, and diarrhea, which limit patient acceptance.

DiMagno EP: Gastric acid suppression and treatment of severe exocrine pancreatic insufficiency. Best Pract Res Clin Gastroenterol 2001;15:477.

Durie PR: Pancreatic aspects of cystic fibrosis and other inherited causes of pancreatic dysfunction. Med Clin North Am 2000;84:609.

Layer P, Keller J: Pancreatic enzymes: secretion and luminal nutrient digestion in health and disease. J Clin Gastroenterol 1999;28:3.

Tsiotos GG et al: Long-term outcome of necrotizing pancreatitis treated by necrosectomy. Br J Surg 1998;85:1650.

ADENOCARCINOMA OF THE PANCREAS

An estimated 29,200 patients will develop pancreatic cancer in the United States in 2001, and 28,900 will die of the disease. These nearly equal numbers illustrate the dismal prognosis generally associated with pancreatic carcinoma. The death rate per 100,000 people has been basically unchanged since the mid 1960s at about 10/100,000 for men and 27/100,000 for women. After tumors of the lung and colon, pancreatic carcinoma is the third leading cause of death due to cancer in men between ages 35 and 54. Factors associated with an increased risk of pancreatic cancer are cigarette smoking, dietary consumption of meat (especially fried meat) and fat, previous gastrectomy (> 20 years earlier), and race (in the USA but not Africa, blacks are more susceptible than whites).

The peak incidence is in the fifth and sixth decades. In two-thirds of cases, the tumor is located in the head of the gland; the remainder occur in the body or tail. Ductal adenocarcinoma, mainly of a poorly differentiated cell pattern, accounts for 80% of the cancers; the remainder are islet cell tumors and cystadenocarcinomas, tumors that are discussed later in this chapter. Pancreatic adenocarcinoma is characterized by early local extension to contiguous structures and metastases to regional lymph nodes and the liver. Pulmonary, peritoneal, and distant nodal metastases occur later.

Clinical Findings

A. SYMPTOMS AND SIGNS

1. Carcinoma of the head of the pancreas—About 75% of patients with carcinoma of the head of the pancreas present with weight loss, obstructive jaundice, and deep-seated abdominal pain. Back pain occurs in 25% of patients and is associated with a worse prognosis. In general, smaller tumors confined to the pancreas are associated with less pain. Weight loss averages about 20 lb (44 kg). Hepatomegaly is present in half of patients but does not necessarily indicate spread to the liver. A palpable mass, which is found in 20%, nearly always signifies surgical incurability. Jaundice is unrelenting in most patients but fluctuates in about 10%. Cholangitis occurs in only 10% of patients with bile duct obstruction. A palpable nontender gallbladder in a jaundiced patient suggests neoplastic obstruction of the common duct (**Courvoisier's sign**), most often due to pancreatic cancer; this finding is present in about half of cases. Jaundice is often accompanied by pruritus, especially of the hands and feet.

2. Carcinoma of the body and tail of the pancreas—Since carcinomas of the body and tail of the pancreas are remote from the bile duct, less than 10% of patients are jaundiced. The presenting complaints are weight loss and pain, which sometimes occurs in excruciating paroxysms. In the few patients with jaundice or hepatomegaly, metastatic involvement has usually occurred. Migratory thrombophlebitis develops in 10% of cases. Once considered relatively specific as a clue to pancreatic cancer, this complication is now known to affect patients with other types of malignant disease.

The diagnosis of pancreatic carcinoma may be extremely difficult. The typical patient who presents with abdominal pain, weight loss, and obstructive jaundice rarely presents a problem, but those with just weight loss, vague abdominal pain, and nondiagnostic x-rays are occasionally labeled psychoneurotics until the existence of cancer becomes obvious. If back pain predominates, orthopedic or neurosurgical causes may be sought at first. One characteristic feature is the tendency for the patient to seek relief of pain by assuming a sitting position with the spine flexed. Recumbency, on the other hand, aggravates the discomfort and sometimes makes sleeping in bed impossible. Sudden onset of diabetes mellitus is an early manifestation in 25% of patients.

B. LABORATORY FINDINGS

Elevated alkaline phosphatase and bilirubin levels reflect either common duct obstruction or hepatic metastases. The bilirubin level with neoplastic obstruction averages 18 mg/dL, much higher than that generally seen with benign disease of the bile ducts. Only rarely are serum aminotransferase levels markedly elevated. Repeated examination of stool specimens for occult blood gives a positive reaction in many cases.

Serum levels of the tumor marker CA 19-9 are elevated in most patients with pancreatic cancer, but the sensitivity in resectable (< 4 cm) lesions is probably too low (50%) for this to serve as a screening tool. Elevated levels also occur with other gastrointestinal cancers. The greatest usefulness of CA 19-9 measurements may be in following the results of treatments. After complete resection of a tumor, elevated levels drop to normal, but they rise again with recurrence.

C. IMAGING STUDIES

Nearly all patients should have a CT scan.

1. CT scan—CT scans show a pancreatic mass in 95% of cases, usually with a central zone of diminished attenuation, and in over 90% of patients with a mass there are signs of extension beyond the boundaries of the pancreas. The upstream pancreatic duct is noted to be dilated in 70% of patients, and the bile duct is dilated in 60% (principally in those with jaundice). The presence of both bile duct and pancreatic duct dilation is strong evidence for pancreatic cancer even in the absence of a mass. Findings suggesting unresectability include local tumor extension (eg, behind the pancreas; into the liver hilum), contiguous organ invasion (eg, duodenum, stomach), distant metastases, involvement of the superior mesenteric or portal vessels, or ascites. In general, size of the mass is only loosely related to resectability. CT scans using modern dynamic scanning techniques are as accurate as angiography in assessing vascular involvement.

2. ERCP—In patients with a typical clinical history and a pancreatic mass on CT, ERCP is unnecessary. In the absence of a mass, an ERCP is indicated. It is the most sensitive test (95%) for detecting pancreatic cancer, though specificity in differentiating between cancer and pancreatitis is low. Consequently, a pancreatogram should be obtained early in cases where the existence of a pancreatic lesion is suspected but unproved. The findings consist of stenosis or obstruction of the pancreatic duct. Adjacent lesions of the bile duct and pancreatic duct ("double-duct sign") are highly suggestive of neoplastic disease, especially if the biliary involvement is focal. Although ERCP is useful to distinguish between the various kinds of periampullary tumors, that information rarely alters management.

3. Upper gastrointestinal series—An upper gastrointestinal series is not sensitive in detecting pancreatic cancer, but it provides information about patency of the duodenum that may be useful in deciding whether a gastrojejunostomy will have to be performed. The classic findings consist of widening of the duodenal sweep, narrowing of the lumen, and the "reversed-3 sign," named for the duodenal configuration.

4. Other studies—Angiography has not proved reliable in detecting or staging pancreatic neoplasms, and ultrasound is a poor second to CT scans for imaging.

D. ASPIRATION BIOPSY

Percutaneous aspiration biopsy of pancreatic mass lesions is positive in 85% of malignant tumors. The procedure is relatively safe, but there is a risk of spreading a localized (resectable) tumor, so it is contraindicated in patients who are candidates for surgery. Aspiration biopsy in them should be performed, if desired, during laparotomy. Percutaneous aspiration biopsy is principally of value to verify a presumptive diagnosis of adenocarcinoma of the pancreas in patients with radiographic evidence of unresectability. In these cases, cytologic proof is important, for treatment decisions should not be made solely on the basis of the indirect evidence provided by CT scans and other imaging tests. There is too great a risk of misdiagnosing something unusual, such as a retroperitoneal lymphoma or sarcoma, and administering inappropriate treatment.

Differential Diagnosis

The other periampullary neoplasms—carcinoma of the ampulla of Vater, distal common bile duct, or duodenum—may also present with pain, weight loss, obstructive jaundice, and a palpable gallbladder. Preoperative cholangiography and gastrointestinal x-rays may suggest the correct diagnosis, but laparotomy is sometimes required.

Complications

Obstruction of the splenic vein by tumor may cause splenomegaly and segmental portal hypertension with bleeding gastric or esophageal varices.

Treatment

Pancreatic resection for pancreatic cancer is appropriate only if all gross tumor can be removed with a standard resection. The lesion is considered resectable if the following areas are free of tumor: (1) the hepatic artery near the origin of the gastroduodenal artery; (2) the superior mesenteric artery where it courses under the body of the pancreas; and (3) the liver and regional lymph nodes. Since the pancreas is so close to the portal vein and the superior mesenteric vessels, these structures may be involved early. About 20% of cancers of the head of the pancreas can be resected, but because of local and distant spread, this is rarely possible for lesions of the body and tail.

A histologic diagnosis can usually be made at operation by aspiration biopsy. With small lesions of the head of the gland, it may be difficult to obtain a specimen for histologic diagnosis because much of the palpable mass may consist of inflamed pancreatic tissue. Occasionally, histologic diagnosis is impossible, and clinical decisions must rest on indirect evidence.

For curable lesions of the head, pancreaticoduodenectomy (**Whipple operation**) is required (Figure 27–5). This involves resection of the common bile duct, the gallbladder, the duodenum, and the pancreas to the mid body. There is an increasing tendency to preserve the

Figure 27–5. Pancreaticoduodenectomy (Whipple procedure). ***A***: Preoperative anatomic relationships showing a tumor in the head of the pancreas. ***B***: Postoperative reconstruction showing pancreatic, biliary, and gastric anastomoses. A cholecystectomy and bilateral truncal vagotomy are also part of the procedure. In many cases, the distal stomach and pylorus can be preserved, and vagotomy is then unnecessary

antrum and pylorus. Involvement of a short (< 1.5 cm) segment of the portal vein is not a contraindication to a curative resection. This is managed by a partial or circumferential resection of the affected area.

When the procedure is performed by surgeons who do it frequently, the operative mortality rate is less than 5%. When it is performed by less experienced surgeons, the mortality rate is 20–30%. Postoperative deaths are due to complications such as pancreatic and biliary fistulas, hemorrhage, and infection.

In an attempt to increase the cure rate, total pancreatectomy has been given a trial on the theory that many pancreatic cancers are multicentric. However, total pancreatectomy produces a brittle type of diabetes mellitus that compromises the quality of life, and cure rates were not higher.

For unresectable lesions, cholecystojejunostomy or choledochojejunostomy provides relief of jaundice and pruritus. A cholangiogram should be obtained to verify patency between the cystic and common bile ducts unless it is grossly obvious. Percutaneous or endoscopically placed biliary stents may also provide effective palliation and are preferable to surgical biliary decompression if the lesion is known to be unresectable. Gastrojejunostomy is required if the tumor blocks the duodenum. If laparotomy has been performed, gastrojejunostomy should be considered regardless of the presence of duodenal obstruction, because with time this often develops before other life-threatening complications.

Laparoscopy is a useful first step in patients scheduled for a possible Whipple procedure. If metastases are seen that militate against a curative resection, laparoscopic gastrojejunostomy or cholecystojejunostomy (or both) can be performed. If not, one should proceed with the laparotomy. About 15% of patients thought to have localized disease from preoperative studies are found to be unresectable at laparoscopy.

Gemcitabine-based chemotherapy has clear benefits in patients with metastatic disease. Its uses in combination with radiation therapy and as adjuvant therapy are being defined.

Prognosis

The mean survival following palliative therapy is 7 months. Following a Whipple procedure, survival averages about 18 months. Factors associated with tumor recurrence and shorter survival include lymph node involvement, tumor size over 2.5 cm, blood vessel invasion, and amount of blood transfused. If tumor cells extend to the margins of the resected specimen, long-term survival is rare. If the margins are clear, about 20% of patients live more than 5 years. Overall 5-year survival is about 10%, but only 60% of these patients are actually free of tumor.

Balci NC, Semelka RC: Radiologic diagnosis and staging of pancreatic ductal adenocarcinoma. Eur J Radiol 2001;38:105.

Bodner WR, Hilaris BS, Mastoras DA: Radiation therapy in pancreatic cancer: current practice and future trends. J Clin Gastroenterol 2000;30:230.

Bornman PC, Beckingham IJ: ABC of diseases of liver, pancreas, and biliary system. Pancreatic tumours. BMJ 2001;322:721.

Crane CH et al: Combining gemcitabine with radiation in pancreatic cancer: understanding important variables influencing the therapeutic index. Semin Oncol 2001;28(3 Suppl 10):25.

Farnell MB, Nagorney DM, Sarr MG: The Mayo clinic approach to the surgical treatment of adenocarcinoma of the pancreas. Surg Clin North Am 2001;81:611.

Kozuch P et al: Treatment of metastatic pancreatic adenocarcinoma: a comprehensive review. Surg Clin North Am 2001; 81:683.

Madura JA et al: Adenosquamous carcinoma of the pancreas. Arch Surg 1999;134:599.

Mangray S, King TC: Molecular pathobiology of pancreatic adenocarcinoma. Front Biosci 1998;3:D1148.

Molinari M, Helton WS, Espat NJ: Palliative strategies for locally advanced unresectable and metastatic pancreatic cancer. Surg Clin North Am 2001;81:651.

Rose DM et al: [18]Fluorodeoxyglucose-positron emission tomography in the management of patients with suspected pancreatic cancer. Ann Surg 1999;229:729.

Sohn TA, Yeo CJ: The molecular genetics of pancreatic ductal carcinoma: a review. Surg Oncol 2000;9:95.

CYSTIC NEOPLASMS

Cystic neoplasms of the pancreas usually present with abdominal pain, a mass, or jaundice and are diagnosed from the findings on CT scans.

Cystadenomas can be classified as serous or mucinous. Serous cystadenomas, which are usually microcystic adenomas, are well-circumscribed lesions consisting of multiple small cysts ranging in size from microscopic to about 2 cm. The cut surface has the appearance of a sponge. The multicystic nature of the lesion is usually—but not always—evident on CT scans, which may also show a few calcifications. The epithelium, which is flat to cuboidal, has no malignant potential. Treatment usually entails excision, but in the rare case where this is too hazardous, the lesion may be left in place with the knowledge that complications are rare. An occasional serous cystadenoma will consist of one or more large cysts (ie, macrocystic).

Mucinous cystadenomas (macrocystic adenomas), which are much more common in women than in men, are unilocular or, more often, multilocular lesions that have a smooth lining with papillary projections. The septate appearance on CT scans is characteristic. The cystic spaces measure 2–20 cm in diameter and contain mucus. The lining consists of tall columnar and goblet cells, which are often arranged in a papillary pattern. In time, most mucinous cystadenomas will evolve into cystadenocarcinomas, so total excision is the required treatment.

Cystadenocarcinomas invariably present as a focus of malignancy within an existing mucinous cystadenoma. The tumors are often quite large (eg, 10–20 cm) at the time of diagnosis. Metastases occur in about 25% of cases. Complete excision results in a 5-year survival rate of 70%.

An uncommon lesion, referred to as solid-and-papillary or papillary-cystic neoplasm of the pancreas, occurs almost exclusively in young women (under age 25 years). The tumor is usually large. It may be locally invasive, but metastases are uncommon, and cure is to be expected after resection.

Balci NC, Semelka RC: Radiologic features of cystic, endocrine and other pancreatic neoplasms. Eur J Radiol 2001;38:113.

Balcom JH 4th et al: Cystic lesions in the pancreas: when to watch, when to resect. Curr Gastroenterol Rep 2000;2:152.

Le Borgne J, de Calan L, Partensky C: Cystadenomas and cystadenocarcinomas of the pancreas: a multiinstitutional retrospective study of 398 cases. French Surgical Association. Ann Surg 1999;230:152.

Sarr MG et al: Clinical and pathologic correlation of 84 mucinous cystic neoplasms of the pancreas: can one reliably differentiate benign from malignant (or premalignant) neoplasms? Ann Surg 2000;231:205.

Sarr MG et al: Cystic neoplasms of the pancreas: benign to malignant epithelial neoplasms. Surg Clin North Am 2001;81:497.

Shima Y et al: Diagnosis and management of cystic pancreatic tumours with mucin production. Br J Surg 2000;87:1041.

Verdolini K et al: Laryngeal adduction in resonant voice. J Voice 1998;12:315.

Vihtelic TS, Doro CJ, Hyde DR: Cloning and characterization of six zebrafish photoreceptor opsin cDNAs and immunolocalization of their corresponding proteins. Vis Neurosci 1999; 16:571.

Wilentz RE et al: Pathologic examination accurately predicts prognosis in mucinous cystic neoplasms of the pancreas. Am J Surg Pathol 1999;23:1320.

ADENOMA & ADENOCARCINOMA OF THE AMPULLA OF VATER

Adenoma and adenocarcinoma of the ampulla of Vater account for about 10% of neoplasms that obstruct the distal bile duct. One-third are adenomas and two-thirds adenocarcinomas. Since a remnant of benign adenoma can be found in a majority of adenocarcinomas, it is suspected that malignant change in an adenoma gives rise to most carcinomas. The presenting symptom is most often jaundice or occasionally gastrointestinal bleeding. Weight loss and pain are more common with carcinoma than with adenoma, but the differences are not great enough to allow a distinction to be made on this basis alone.

CT and ultrasound scans reveal dilation of the biliary tree and pancreatic duct. Gallstones are an incidental finding in 20% of patients, and when common duct stones are present, they may incorrectly be held responsible for the biliary obstruction. The most important diagnostic study is ERCP. In 75% of cases, tumor is visible on duodenoscopy as an exophytic papillary lesion, an ulcerated tumor, or an infiltrating mass. An adequate biopsy usually can be obtained of these lesions. In 25% of cases, there is no intraduodenal growth, and endoscopic sphincterotomy is necessary to display the tumor. It is best to wait 10–14 days to biopsy these tumors because of transient artifacts that result from the sphincterotomy. ERCP also demonstrates dilation of the biliary and pancreatic ducts. It has become common to perform a sphincterotomy whenever possible, not only to facilitate performance of a biopsy but also to decompress the biliary tree and allow jaundice to subside in anticipation of subsequent surgical therapy. The value of this step has not been established.

Although some adenomas have been successfully treated by snare excision or, preferably, by neodymium:YAG laser destruction, local resection or pancreaticoduodenectomy is preferable because of the significant chance that an invasive carcinoma will be undertreated at a time that it is curable. These nonsurgical methods should be reserved for patients who are poor candidates for resection.

Treatment of adenocarcinoma consists of pancreaticoduodenectomy as for pancreatic carcinoma. The operative mortality rate is less than 5%, and the 5-year survival rate is about 50%. The presence of metastases in resectable peripancreatic lymph nodes is not a contraindication to pancreaticoduodenectomy, for the 5-year survival rate under these circumstances is still a respectable 25%. Local excision is an alternative for noninfiltrating papillary adenocarcinomas in patients who are too poor a risk for pancreaticoduodenectomy, but this operation is not as successful as pancreaticoduodenectomy. Endoscopic sphincterotomy alone or with retrograde stent placement (the combination is usually required) is indicated when there is definite evidence (eg, hepatic metastases) that the tumor is incurable. Survival averages less than a year with this approach, however.

Bakaeen FG et al: What prognostic factors are important in duodenal adenocarcinoma? Arch Surg 2000;135:635.

Crucitti A et al: Ampullary carcinoma: prognostic significance of ploidy, cell-cycle analysis and proliferating cell nuclear antigen (PCNA). Hepatogastroenterology 1999;46:1187.

Howe JR et al: Factors predictive of survival in ampullary carcinoma. Ann Surg 1998;228:87.

Lee JH et al: Outcome of pancreaticoduodenectomy and impact of adjuvant therapy for ampullary carcinomas. Int J Radiat Oncol Biol Phys 2000;47:945.

Roberts RH et al: Pancreaticoduodenectomy of ampullary carcinoma. Am Surg 1999;65:1043.

PANCREATIC ISLET CELL TUMORS

Islet cell tumors may be functioning (ie, hormone-producing) or nonfunctioning, malignant or nonmalignant. More than half are functioning; less than half are malignant. Insulinoma, the most common functioning islet cell neoplasm, arises from beta cells and produces insulin and symptoms of hypoglycemia. Tumors of the δ or α_1 cells produce gastrin and the Zollinger-Ellison syndrome. Alpha$_2$ cell neoplasms may produce excess glucagon and hyperglycemia. Non-beta islet cell tumors may secrete serotonin, ACTH, MSH, and kinins (and evoke the carcinoid syndrome). Some produce pancreatic cholera, a severe diarrheal illness.

1. Nonfunctioning Islet Cell Tumors

Most of these lesions are malignant tumors of the head of the gland, which present with abdominal and back pain, weight loss, and, in many cases, a palpable abdominal mass. Jaundice is seen occasionally. CT scans reveal a pancreatic mass, and angiography typically shows it to be hypervascular. The histologic pattern on biopsy specimens is diagnostic of islet cell tumor, but whether or not the lesion is malignant rests on evidence of invasiveness or metastases, not the appearance of the cells. Immunohistochemical staining of the tissue is positive for chromogranin and neuron-specific enolase (markers of APUD tumors). Metastases are present at the time of diagnosis in 80% of patients. Resection of all gross tumor (eg, by a Whipple procedure), the preferred treatment, is possible in less than half of patients because of local extension or distant metastases. A combination of streptozocin and doxorubicin is the most effective chemotherapeutic regimen. The 5-year disease-free survival rate is about 15%.

Bartsch DK et al: Management of nonfunctioning islet cell carcinomas. World J Surg 2000;24:1418.

Jensen RT: Carcinoid and pancreatic endocrine tumors: recent advances in molecular pathogenesis, localization, and treatment. Curr Opin Oncol 2000;12:368.

Somogyi L, Mishra G: Diagnosis and staging of islet cell tumors of the pancreas. Curr Gastroenterol Rep 2000;2:159.

2. Insulinoma

Insulinomas have been reported in all age groups. About 75% are solitary and benign. About 10% are malignant, and metastases are usually evident at the time of diagnosis. The remaining 15% are manifestations of multifocal pancreatic disease—either adenomatosis, nesidioblastosis, or islet cell hyperplasia.

The symptoms (related to cerebral glucose deprivation) are bizarre behavior, memory lapse, or unconsciousness. Patients may be mistakenly treated for psychiatric illness. There may be profuse sympathetic discharge, with palpitations, sweating, and tremulousness. Hypoglycemic episodes are usually precipitated by fasting and are relieved by food, so weight gain is common. The classic diagnostic criteria (**Whipple's triad**) are present in most cases: (1) hypoglycemic symptoms produced by fasting, (2) blood glucose below 50 mg/dL during symptomatic episodes, and (3) relief of symptoms by intravenous administration of glucose.

The most useful diagnostic test and the only one indicated in all but a few patients is demonstration of fasting hypoglycemia in the presence of inappropriately high levels of insulin. The patient is fasted, and blood samples are obtained every 6 hours for glucose and insulin measurements. The fast is continued until hypoglycemia or symptoms appear or for a maximum of 72 hours. If hypoglycemia has not developed after 70 hours, the patient should be exercised for the final 2 hours. Although insulin levels are not always elevated in patients with insulinoma, they will be high relative to the blood glucose concentration. A ratio of plasma insulin to glucose greater than 0.3 is diagnostic. Ratios should be calculated before and during the fast. Proinsulin, which constitutes more than 25% of total insulin (the upper limit of normal) in about 85% of patients with insulinomas, should also be measured. Proinsulin levels greater than 40% suggest a malignant islet cell tumor.

Drugs that release insulin (tolbutamide, glucagon, leucine, arginine, calcium) were used in the past as provocative tests. No provocative tests are currently used.

Localization of the tumor is important but may be difficult. In about 10% of cases, the tumor is so small or located so deeply that it is difficult or impossible to find at laparotomy. High-resolution CT and MR scans are successful in demonstrating about 40% of tumors. Endoscopic (gastroscopic) ultrasound examination of the pancreas may be able to show a much higher percentage. The most important examination is intraoperative ultrasound, which can identify a pancreatic tumor in nearly all cases. It is more sensitive than any preoperative test.

In patients who have had previous resection or significant upper abdominal surgery, exploration with intraoperative ultrasound may be difficult. Invasive preoperative testing may then be useful. Angiography gives a yield of about 50%. Transhepatic portal venous sampling has proved an accurate preoperative localizing method, demonstrating the position in the pancreas in about 95% of lesions. However, this test is time-consuming and somewhat invasive, involving entering the portal vein with a catheter passed percutaneously through the liver and testing blood at various sites within the portal, superior mesenteric, and splenic veins for insulin levels. The point where insulin concentrations rise sharply indicates the site of the tumor. An alternative invasive localizing test uses arteriography with selective calcium infusion into arteries supplying the pancreas. Blood samples from the hepatic veins reveal an increase in insulin level when calcium is infused into an artery supplying the tumor.

Differential Diagnosis

Fasting hypoglycemia may be a manifestation of some nonpancreatic, non-islet cell tumors. Clinically, the condition is identical to that resulting from insulinoma, but the cause is rarely secretion of insulin by the tumors, as serum insulin levels are normal. Most non-islet cell tumors associated with hypoglycemia are large and readily detected on physical examination. The majority are of mesenchymal origin (eg, hemangiopericytoma, fibrosarcoma, leiomyosarcoma) and are located in the abdomen or thorax, but hepatoma, adrenocortical carcinoma, and a variety of other lesions may also produce hypoglycemia. The principal means by which these tumors produce hypoglycemia are the following: (1) secretion by the tumor of insulin-like growth factor II (IGF-II), an insulin-like peptide that normally mediates the effects of growth hormone; and (2) inhibition of glycogenolysis or gluconeogenesis. Rapid utilization of glucose by the tumor, replacement of liver tissue by metastases, and secretion of insulin are other postulated mechanisms that are probably uncommon.

Surreptitious self-administration of insulin is seen occasionally, most often in an individual with access to insulin on the job. If insulin injections have been given for as long as 2 months, insulin antibodies will be detectable in the patient's serum. Circulating C peptide levels are normal in these patients but elevated in most patients with insulinoma. Sulfonylurea ingestion can be detected by measuring the drug in plasma.

Treatment

Surgery should be done promptly, because with repeated hypoglycemic attacks, permanent cerebral damage occurs and the patient becomes progressively more obese. Moreover, the tumor may be malignant. Medical treatment is reserved for surgically incurable lesions.

A. MEDICAL TREATMENT

Diazoxide is administered to suppress insulin release. For incurable islet cell carcinomas, streptozocin is the best chemotherapeutic agent. Sixty percent of patients live up to 2 additional years. Toxicity is considerable; streptozocin is not recommended as a routine adjunct to surgical therapy.

B. SURGICAL TREATMENT

At surgery, the entire pancreas must be palpated carefully because the tumors are usually small and difficult to find. The gland should also be examined intraoperatively with ultrasound, which may be able to locate a tumor that cannot be felt, or to demonstrate signs of invasion (ie, irregular borders) that indicate malignancy—something that cannot be detected by palpation. When the tumor is found, it may be enucleated if it is superficial or resected as part of a partial pancreatectomy if it is deep-seated or invasive. Insulinomas in the head of the gland can nearly always be enucleated.

In the past, the tumor could not be detected in about 5% of cases by these methods. The traditional recommendation was to resect the distal half of the pancreas and have the pathologist slice the specimen into thin sections and look for the tumor. If the tumor was found, the operation was concluded; if it was not found, additional pancreas would be resected until an 80% distal pancreatectomy had been performed. Since the tumors are evenly distributed, this strategy is 80% successful in removing the tumor. Intraoperative monitoring of blood glucose is often done as a means of determining if the tumor has been excised, but it is unreliable. With the use of operative ultrasound scanning, however, no more than 1–2% of insulinomas remain occult, and blind distal pancreatectomy is rarely even considered.

Patients with insulinoma associated with MEN-1 usually have multiple (average of three) lesions. Because persistence of the disease is much more likely in this condition following the standard surgical approach, the operation recommended here is distal pancreatectomy plus enucleation of any lesions found in the head of the gland.

For islet cell hyperplasia, nesidioblastosis, or multiple benign adenomas, distal subtotal pancreatectomy usually decreases insulin levels enough that medical management is simplified. For islet cell carcinomas, resection of both primary and metastatic lesions is warranted if technically feasible.

Patients with sporadic insulinomas lead a normal life after the tumor has been removed. The outcome is less predictable in patients with MEN-1, who may have several insulin-producing tumors.

Dolan JP, Norton JA: Occult insulinoma. Br J Surg 2000;87:385.

Grant CS: Insulinoma. Surg Oncol Clin N Am 1998;7:819.

Grant CS: Surgical aspects of hyperinsulinemic hypoglycemia. Endocrinol Metab Clin North Am 1999;28:533.

Service FJ: Classification of hypoglycemic disorders. Endocrinol Metab Clin North Am 1999;28:501.

3. Pancreatic Cholera (WDHA Syndrome: Watery Diarrhea, Hypokalemia, & Achlorhydria)

Most cases of pancreatic cholera are caused by a non-beta islet cell tumor of the pancreas that secretes VIP (vasoactive intestinal polypeptide) and peptide histidine isoleucine. The syndrome is characterized by profuse watery diarrhea, massive fecal loss of potassium, low serum potassium, and extreme weakness. Gastric acid secretion is usually low or absent even after stimulation with betazole or pentagastrin. Stool volume averages about 5 L/d during acute episodes and contains over 300 meq of potassium (20 times normal). Severe metabolic acidosis frequently results from loss of bicarbonate in the stool. Many patients are hypercalcemic, possibly from secretion by the tumor of a parathyroid hormone-like substance. Abnormal glucose tolerance may result from hypokalemia and altered sensitivity to insulin. Patients who complain of severe diarrhea must be studied carefully for other causes before the diagnosis of WDHA syndrome is entertained seriously. Chronic laxative abuse is a frequent explanation.

CT scan is the best initial imaging test; somatostatin receptor scintigraphy is also very useful for localization. Approximately 80% of the tumors are solitary, located in the body or tail, and can be removed easily. About half of the lesions are malignant, and three-fourths of those have metastasized by the time of exploration. Even if all of the tumor cannot be removed, resection of most of it alleviates symptoms in about 40% of patients even though the average survival is only 1 year. Streptozocin has produced remissions in several cases, but nephrotoxicity may limit its effectiveness. Treatment with long-acting somatostatin analogs decreases VIP levels, controls diarrhea, and may even reduce tumor size. The effect persists indefinitely in most patients, but in a few it is transient.

Jensen RT: Overview of chronic diarrhea caused by functional neuroendocrine neoplasms. Semin Gastrointest Dis 1999;10: 156–72.

Soga J, Yakuwa Y: Vipoma/diarrheogenic syndrome: a statistical evaluation of 241 reported cases. J Exp Clin Cancer Res 1998;17:389–400.

4. Glucagonoma

Glucagonoma syndrome is characterized by migratory necrolytic dermatitis (usually involving the legs and perineum), weight loss, stomatitis, hypoaminoacidemia, anemia, and mild to moderate diabetes mellitus. Scotomas and changes in visual acuity have been reported in some cases. The age range is 20–70 years, and the condition is more common in women. The diagnosis may be suspected from the distinctive skin lesion; in fact, the presence of a prominent rash in a patient with diabetes mellitus should be enough to raise suspicions. Glucagonoma should also be suspected in any patient with new onset of diabetes after age 60. Confirmation of the diagnosis depends on measuring elevated serum glucagon levels. CT scans demonstrate the tumor and sites of spread. Angiography is not essential but reveals a hypervascular lesion.

Glucagonomas arise from α_2 cells in the pancreatic islets. Most are large at the time of diagnosis. About 25% are benign and confined to the pancreas. The remainder have metastasized by the time of diagnosis, most often to the liver, lymph nodes, adrenal gland, or vertebrae. A few cases have been the result of islet cell hyperplasia.

Severe malnutrition should be corrected preoperatively with a period of total parenteral nutrition and treatment with somatostatin analogs. Surgical removal of the primary lesion and resectable secondaries is indicated if technically feasible. If the tumor is confined to the pancreas, cure is possible. Even if it is not possible to remove all the tumor deposits, considerable palliation may result from subtotal removal, so surgery is indicated in almost every case. Low-dose heparin therapy should be administered pre- and postoperatively because of a high risk of deep venous thrombosis and pulmonary embolism. Streptozocin and dacarbazine are the most effective chemotherapeutic agents for unresectable lesions. Somatostatin therapy normalizes serum glucagon and amino acid levels, clears the rash, and promotes weight gain. The clinical course generally parallels changes in serum levels of glucagon in response to therapy.

Bernstein M et al: Amino acid, glucose, and lipid kinetics after palliative resection in a patient with glucagonoma syndrome. Metabolism 2001;50:720.

Chastain MA: The glucagonoma syndrome: a review of its features and discussion of new perspectives. Am J Med Sci 2001; 321:306.

El Rassi Z et al: Necrolytic migratory erythema, first symptom of a malignant glucagonoma: treatment by long-acting somatostatin and surgical resection. Report of three cases. Eur J Surg Oncol 1998;24:562.

Metz DC: Diagnosis of non-Zollinger-Ellison syndrome, non-carcinoid syndrome, enteropancreatic neuroendocrine tumours. Ital J Gastroenterol Hepatol 1999;31(Suppl 2):S153.

5. Somatostatinoma

Somatostatinomas are characterized by diabetes mellitus (usually mild), diarrhea and malabsorption, and dilation of the gallbladder (usually with cholelithiasis). Serum calcitonin and IgM concentrations may be elevated. The syndrome results from secretion of somatostatin by an islet cell tumor of the pancreas, half of which are malignant and accompanied by hepatic metastases. The lesion is usually large and readily demonstrated by CT scan. The diagnosis may be made by recognizing the clinical syndrome and measuring increased concentrations of somatostatin in the serum. Often, however, the somatostatin syndrome is unsuspected until histologic evidence of metastatic islet cell carcinoma has been obtained. When the disease is localized, resection is able to cure about 50% of cases. Enucleation is inappropriate for these tumors. Chemotherapy with streptozocin, dacarbazine, or doxorubicin is the best treatment for unresectable tumors. Small somatostatin-rich tumors of the duodenum or ampulla of Vater have also been reported, but none of these lesions have been associated with high serum levels of somatostatin or the clinical syndrome.

Metz DC: Diagnosis of non-Zollinger-Ellison syndrome, non-carcinoid syndrome, enteropancreatic neuroendocrine tumours. Ital J Gastroenterol Hepatol 1999;31(Suppl 2):S153.

Soga J, Yakuwa Y: Somatostatinoma/inhibitory syndrome: a statistical evaluation of 173 reported cases as compared to other pancreatic endocrinomas. J Exp Clin Cancer Res 1999;18:13.

Tanaka S et al: Duodenal somatostatinoma: a case report and review of 31 cases with special reference to the relationship between tumor size and metastasis. Pathol Int 2000;50:146.

Spleen

Gerard M. Doherty, MD, Douglas L. Fraker, MD, & David C. Hohn, MD

ANATOMY

The spleen is a dark purplish, highly vascular, coffee bean-shaped organ of mesodermal origin situated in the left upper quadrant of the abdomen at the level of the eighth to eleventh ribs between the fundus of the stomach, the diaphragm, the splenic flexure of the colon, and the left kidney (Figure 28–1). The adult spleen weighs 100–150 g, measures about $12 \times 7 \times 4$ cm, and usually cannot be palpated. It is attached to adjacent viscera, the abdominal wall, and the diaphragm by peritoneal folds or "ligaments." The gastrosplenic ligament carries the short gastric vessels. The other ligaments are avascular except in patients with portal hypertension or myelofibrosis.

The splenic capsule consists of peritoneum overlying a 1- to 2-mm fibroelastic layer that contains a few smooth muscle cells. The fibroelastic layer sends into the pulp numerous fibrous bands (trabeculae) that form the framework of the spleen. Corrosion cast studies demonstrate that the spleen consists of specific segments based on arterial supply numbering between two and six separated by an avascular plane.

The splenic artery enters the hilum of the spleen, branches into the trabecular arteries, and then branches into the central arteries that course through the surrounding white pulp and send radial branches to the peripheral marginal zone and the more distant red pulp. The white pulp consists of lymphatic tissue including T cells adjacent to the central artery (periarteriolar lymphoid sheets: PALS), with a surrounding area containing lymphoid follicles rich in B cells interspersed with dendritic and reticular cells important in antigen presentation. The vascular spaces of the marginal zone between the red and white pulp channel blood into the splenic Billroth cords and out to the associated sinuses. The red pulp vascular structures have a noncontiguous basement membrane that filters cells such as senescent erythrocytes into the macrophage-lined sinuses.

Accessory spleens (spleniculi) are seen in 10–15% of the normal population located primarily in the gastrosplenic, gastrocolic, and lienorenal ligaments but which can also be found throughout the peritoneal cavity in the omentum, bowel mesentery, and pelvis. Accessory spleens probably result from a failure of infusion of splenic embryologic tissues. Ordinarily of no significance, they may play a role in recurrence of certain hematologic disorders for which splenectomy is performed. Removal of accessory spleens may lead to remission of disease in these patients. Patients who fail to respond to initial splenectomy should undergo scanning with technetium 99m-labeled red cells or indium 111-labeled platelets to identify potential sites of missed accessory spleens.

Ectopic spleen (wandering spleen) is an unusual condition in which a long splenic pedicle allows the spleen to move within the peritoneum. It often resides in the lower abdomen or pelvis, where even a normal-sized spleen can be felt as a mass. The condition is 13 times more common in women than in men. Diagnostic radionuclide scan can diagnose the mass as a spleen. Acute torsion of the pedicle occurs occasionally, necessitating emergency splenectomy, and elective removal of pelvic spleens is recommended.

PHYSIOLOGY

The primary function of the spleen is filtration of the blood for clearance of cells, microorganisms, and other particulate matter as well as related immune and hematologic storage functions.

The spleen receives 5% of the total cardiac output, or approximately 150–300 mL/min, such that each red cell averages 1000 passes through the spleen each day. Normal blood cells pass rapidly through the spleen, while abnormal and senescent cells are retarded and entrapped. As they travel through the hypoxic, acidotic, glucose-deprived splenic cords and sinuses of the red pulp, senescent erythrocytes pass into the vascular spaces and are phagocytosed by macrophages in a process called "culling." Part of the membrane of erythrocytes can be removed through the gaps between endothelial cells lining the vascular spaces in a similar process called pitting. In the presence of splenomegaly and other disease states, the flow patterns of the spleen become more circuitous as the red pulp volume expands, so that even normal cells may be trapped.

The adult spleen produces monocytes, lymphocytes, and plasma cells. Production of other blood elements occurs in patients with myeloid metaplasia and in the fetal spleen.

The spleen is considered to be a secondary organ of the immune system and represents the largest single col-

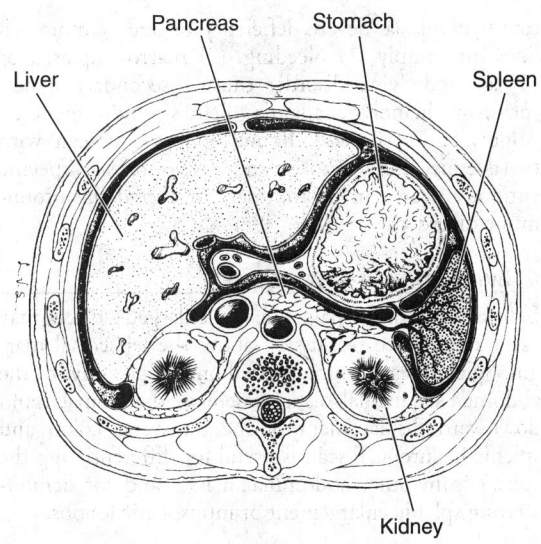

Liver

Pancreas

Stomach

Spleen

Kidney

Figure 28–1. Normal anatomic relations of the spleen.

lection of lymphoid tissue in the body. The white pulp of the spleen contains the various cellular components needed to generate an immune response with structural and functional relationships similar to those of lymph nodes. Lymphocytes and circulating antigen-presenting cells enter the white pulp via the marginal zone capillaries and traverse the T cell–rich PALS before passing through bridging channels into the red pulp. Primary follicles or germinal centers with secondary follicles at the periphery of the white pulp are sites of B cell expansion and immunoglobulin production. Blood passing through the spleen is exposed to all the key cellular components necessary for both humoral and cellular immune responses. Moreover, the concentration of macrophages in the red pulp vascular spaces facilitates opsonization of particles coated with IgG and plays an important role in autoimmune hematologic diseases as well as explaining the increased risk of sepsis that follows splenectomy in children under 2 years of age. Even in adults, splenectomy leads to a slight but definite reduction in immune function.

Normally, about 30% of the total platelet pool is sequestered in the spleen. Splenomegaly typically involves expansion of the red pulp, which increases this sequestration to between 80% and 95% of the platelet cell mass. Storage of erythrocytes and granulocytes in the spleen is limited in humans, but newly formed reticulocytes released from the bone marrow concentrate in the spleen to undergo a maturational process.

Skandalakis PN et al: The surgical anatomy of the spleen. Surg Clin North Am 1993;73:747.

HYPERSPLENISM

In the past, the term hypersplenism has been used to denote the syndrome characterized by splenic enlargement, deficiency of one or more blood cell lines, normal or hyperplastic cellularity of deficient cell lines in the marrow, and increased turnover of affected cells. If the defect was not corrected by splenectomy, the diagnosis was considered incorrect.

Increased understanding of the pathophysiology of specific disorders has shown that hypersplenism is not synonymous with splenomegaly. Some disorders in which there is spleen-dependent destruction of blood elements do not manifest all features of hypersplenism. For example, splenomegaly is rarely a feature of immune thrombocytopenic purpura, and splenectomy is not always curative. Conversely, other conditions that enlarge the spleen may not result in destruction or sequestration of blood elements with resultant cytopenias. In disorders with known pathogenesis, the recent trend has been to classify them as separate disease entities rather than as hypersplenic conditions.

The defects in hypersplenism are exaggerations of normal splenic functions primarily associated with the red pulp. The principal cause of cytopenias in hypersplenism is increased sequestration and destruction of blood cells in the spleen. Etiologic factors include (1) splenic enlargement, (2) intrinsic defects in blood cells, or (3) autoimmune destruction of blood cells. The hyperplastic spleen is not selective in its hyperfunction. For example, even though the splenomegaly may have been induced by sequestration of abnormal red cells (eg, hemolytic anemia), platelets and leukocytes may also be destroyed more rapidly than normal.

Primary hypersplenism is a diagnosis of exclusion reached after a careful search (including pathologic examination of the spleen) for conditions that can produce secondary hypersplenism. True primary hypersplenism is exceedingly rare; most cases diagnosed as primary hypersplenism involve intrinsic defects in the blood cells or the presence of unrecognized blood cell antibodies. What appears to be primary hypersplenism may be an early manifestation of lymphoma or leukemia, since these cancers develop in some patients after splenectomy.

Secondary hypersplenism occurs in association with splenomegaly of known cause. It is most often due to congestive splenomegaly caused by portal hypertension (cirrhosis or portal or splenic vein obstruction), by hematologic or neoplastic diseases involving the spleen (eg, lymphoma, myeloid metaplasia, leukemia), or by inflammatory, metabolic, or autoimmune disorders (Table 28–1).

About 60% of patients with cirrhosis develop splenomegaly and 15% develop hypersplenism. The hyper-

Table 28–1. Disorders associated with secondary hypersplenism.

Congestive splenomegaly (cirrhosis, portal or splenic vein obstruction)
Neoplasm (leukemia, metastatic carcinoma)
Inflammatory disease (sarcoid, lupus erythematosus, Felty's syndrome)
Acute infections with splenomegaly
Chronic infection (tuberculosis, brucellosis, malaria)
Storage diseases (Gaucher's disease, Letterer-Siwe disease, amyloidosis)
Chronic hemolytic diseases (spherocytosis, thalassemia, glucose-6-phosphate dehydrogenase deficiency, elliptocytosis)
Myeloproliferative disorders (myelofibrosis with myeloid metaplasia)

splenism of cirrhosis is seldom of clinical significance; the anemia and thrombocytopenia are usually mild and rarely are indications for splenectomy.

If portal decompression is indicated for bleeding esophageal varices, any procedure that lowers the portal pressure tends to improve the thrombocytopenia and anemia and reduce the size of the spleen. It is rare for hypersplenism to develop after a successful portal-systemic shunt. In the rare case of portal hypertension caused by massive splenomegaly and huge splenic blood flow, splenectomy alone will cure the hypersplenism and portal hypertension.

Clinical Findings

A. SYMPTOMS AND SIGNS

The clinical findings depend largely on the underlying disorder or are secondary to the depletion of circulating blood elements caused by the hypersplenism. Manifestations of hypersplenism usually develop gradually, and the diagnosis often follows a routine physical or laboratory examination. Some patients experience left upper quadrant fullness, discomfort (can be severe), or early satiety. Others have hematemesis due to gastroesophageal varices.

Purpura, bruising, and diffuse mucous membrane bleeding are unusual symptoms despite the presence of thrombocytopenia. Recurrent infections and chronic leg ulcers are sometimes seen in patients with Felty's syndrome and severe leukopenia.

B. LABORATORY FINDINGS

Patients with primary hypersplenism usually exhibit pancytopenia of moderate degree and generalized mar-

row hyperplasia. Severe deficiency of one or more cell lines may imply (1) bleeding, (2) marrow aplasia, or (3) an underlying disorder causing secondary hypersplenism (hemolytic anemia, Felty's syndrome, etc). Abnormalities of red cell morphology are seen with thalassemia, elliptocytosis, and myelofibrosis. Specific antibody titers can be routinely measured in autoimmune disorders.

C. EVALUATION OF SPLENIC SIZE

Before it becomes palpable, an enlarged spleen may cause dullness to percussion above the left costal margin. Splenomegaly is manifested on supine x-rays of the abdomen by medial displacement of the stomach and downward displacement of the transverse colon and splenic flexure. CT scan is useful for differentiating the spleen from other abdominal masses and for demonstrating splenic enlargement or intrasplenic lesions.

D. EVALUATION OF SPLENIC FUNCTION

Reduced red cell or platelet survival can be measured by labeling the patient's cells with ^{51}Cr or the platelets with indium-111 and measuring the rate of disappearance of radioactivity from the blood. The spleen's role in producing the anemia or thrombocytopenia can be determined by measuring the ratio of radioactivity that accumulates in the liver and spleen during destruction of the tagged cells; a spleen/liver ratio greater than 2:1 indicates significant splenic pooling and suggests that splenectomy would be beneficial.

Differential Diagnosis

Leukemia and lymphoma are diagnosed by marrow aspiration, lymph node biopsy, and examination of the peripheral blood (white count and differential). In hereditary spherocytosis there are spherocytes, osmotic fragility is increased, and platelets and white cells are normal. The hemoglobinopathies with splenomegaly are differentiated on the basis of hemoglobin electrophoresis or the demonstration of an unstable hemoglobin. Thalassemia major becomes apparent in early childhood, and the blood smear morphology is characteristic. In myelofibrosis, the bone marrow shows proliferation of fibroblasts and replacement of normal elements. In idiopathic thrombocytopenic purpura, the spleen is normal or only slightly enlarged. In aplastic anemia, the spleen is not enlarged and the marrow is fatty.

Treatment & Prognosis

The course, response to treatment, and prognosis of the hypersplenic syndromes differ widely depending on the underlying disease and its response to treatment and will be discussed for each particular disorder below.

The indications for splenectomy are given in Table 28–2. Splenectomy should be performed for primary hypersplenism. In secondary hypersplenism, the severity and prognosis of the primary disease and the risk of surgery must be considered. Splenectomy may decrease transfusion requirements, decrease the incidence and number of infections, prevent hemorrhage, and reduce pain.

The course of congestive splenomegaly due to portal hypertension depends upon the degree of venous ob-

Table 28–2. Indications for splenectomy.

Splenectomy always indicated
  Primary splenic tumor (rare)
  Hereditary spherocytosis (congenital hemolytic anemia)
Splenectomy usually indicated
  Primary hypersplenism
  Chronic immune thrombocytopenic purpura
  Splenic vein thrombosis causing gastric varices
  Splenic abscess (rare)
Splenectomy sometimes indicated
  Splenic injury
  Autoimmune hemolytic disease
  Elliptocytosis with hemolysis
  Nonspherocytic congenital hemolytic anemias
  Hodgkin's disease (for staging)
  Thrombotic thrombocytopenic purpura
  Idiopathic myelofibrosis
  Splenic artery aneurysm
  Wiscott-Aldrich syndrome
  Gaucher's disease
  Mastocytosis-aggressive disease
Splenectomy rarely indicated
  Chronic leukemia
  Splenic lymphoma
  Macroglobulinemia
  Thalassemia major
  Sickle cell anemia
  Congestive splenomegaly and hypersplenism due to portal hypertension
  Felty's syndrome
  Hairy cell leukemia
  Chédiak-Higashi syndrome
  Sarcoidosis
Splenectomy not indicated
  Asymptomatic hypersplenism
  Splenomegaly with infection
  Splenomegaly associated with elevated IgM
  Hereditary hemolytic anemia of moderate degree
  Acute leukemia
  Agranulocytosis

struction and liver damage. The hypersplenism is rarely a major problem and is almost always overshadowed by variceal bleeding or liver dysfunction.

■ DISORDERS POTENTIALLY AMENABLE TO SPLENECTOMY

Disorders treated by splenectomy can be categorized as hereditary hematologic disorders, autoimmune diseases, metabolic diseases, neoplastic diseases, infection, vascular conditions, or trauma (Table 28–1).

In the category of hematologic conditions are inherited defects expressed within the erythrocyte causing increased clearance via the normal filtration function of the red pulp of the spleen. Shortened erythrocyte life span leads to anemia, and the increased red cell destruction can result in splenic enlargement as well as secondary complications such as formation of pigmented gallstones.

HEREDITARY DISORDERS
1. Hereditary Spherocytosis

 ESSENTIALS OF DIAGNOSIS

- *Malaise, abdominal discomfort.*
- *Jaundice, anemia, splenomegaly.*
- *Spherocytosis, increased osmotic fragility of red cells, negative Coombs test.*

General Considerations

Hereditary spherocytosis (congenital hemolytic jaundice, familial hemolytic anemia), the commonest congenital hemolytic anemia (affecting 1:5000 individuals) is transmitted as an autosomal dominant trait. It is caused by a variety of genetic defects related to abnormal cellular structural proteins, primarily spectrin and ankyrin, which alter binding of the cytoskeleton to the cellular membrane, causing a decreased cellular plasticity with membrane loss. The normal shape of the erythrocyte is changed from a biconcave disk into a sphere, and the decreased membrane-to-cell volume ratio causes a lack of deformability which delays passage through the channels of the splenic red pulp. Significant cell destruction occurs only in the presence of the spleen. Hemolysis is largely relieved by splenectomy.

The condition is seen in all races but is more frequent in whites than in blacks. When discovered early in infancy, it may resemble hemolytic disease of the newborn due to ABO incompatibility. In occasional instances the diagnosis is not made until later in adult life, but it is usually discovered in the first 3 decades.

Clinical Findings

A. SYMPTOMS AND SIGNS

The principal manifestations are splenomegaly, mild to moderate anemia, and jaundice. The patient may complain of easy fatigability. The spleen is almost always enlarged and may cause fullness and discomfort in the left upper quadrant. However, most patients are diagnosed during a family survey at a time when they are asymptomatic.

Periodic exacerbations of hemolysis can occur. The rare hypoplastic crises, which often follow acute viral illnesses, may be associated with profound anemia, headache, nausea, abdominal pain, pancytopenia, and hypoactive marrow.

B. LABORATORY FINDINGS

The red cell count and hemoglobin are moderately reduced. Some of the asymptomatic patients detected by family surveys have normal red cell counts when first seen. The red cells are usually normocytic, but microcytosis may occur. Macrocytosis may present during periods of marked reticulocytosis. Spherocytes in varying numbers, sizes, and shapes are seen on a Wright-stained smear. The reticulocyte count is increased to 5–20%.

The indirect serum bilirubin and stool urobilinogen are usually elevated, and serum haptoglobin is usually decreased to absent. The Coombs test is negative. Osmotic fragility is increased; hemolysis of 5–10% of cells may be observed at saline concentrations of 0.6%. A more accurate reflector of fragility is the cryohemolysis test, which has a sensitivity and specificity of almost 95% for spherocytosis. Occasionally, the osmotic fragility is normal but the incubated fragility test (defibrinated blood incubated at 37 °C for 24 hours) will show increased hemolysis. Autohemolysis of defibrinated blood incubated under sterile conditions for 48 hours is usually greatly increased (10–20%, compared to a normal value of < 5%). The addition of 10% glucose before incubation will decrease the abnormal osmotic fragility and autohemolysis. Infusion of the patient's own blood labeled with ^{51}Cr shows a greatly shortened red cell life span and sequestration in the spleen. Normal red cells labeled with ^{51}Cr have a normal life span when transfused into a spherocytic patient, indicating that splenic function is normal.

Differential Diagnosis

At present there is no pathognomonic test for hereditary spherocytosis, although the cryohemolysis test is very promising. Spherocytes in large numbers may occur in autoimmune hemolytic anemias, in which osmotic fragility and autohemolysis may be increased but are usually not improved by incubation with glucose. The positive Coombs test, negative family history, and sharply reduced survival of normal donor red cells are diagnostic of autoimmune hemolysis. Spherocytes are also seen in hemoglobin C disease, in some alcoholics, and in some severe burns.

Complications

Pigment gallstones occur in about 85% of adults with spherocytosis but are uncommon under age 10. On the other hand, gallstones in a child should suggest congenital spherocytosis.

Chronic leg ulcers unrelated to varicosities are a rare complication but, when present, will heal only after the spleen is removed.

Treatment

Splenectomy is the sole treatment for hereditary spherocytosis and is indicated even when the anemia is fully compensated and the patient is asymptomatic. The longer the hemolytic process persists, the greater the potential risk of complications such as hypoplastic crises and cholelithiasis. At operation, the gallbladder should be inspected for stones and accessory spleens should be sought. When there is associated cholelithiasis, cholecystectomy should be performed along with the splenectomy. Unless the clinical manifestations are severe, splenectomy should be delayed in children until age 6 to avoid the risk of increased infection due to loss of reticuloendothelial function. For children under age 5 with severe disease and high transfusion requirements, a partial (80%) splenectomy may correct symptoms while maintaining the normal immune functions of the spleen.

Prognosis

Splenectomy cures the anemia and jaundice in all patients. The membrane abnormality, spherocytosis, and increased osmotic fragility persist, but red cell life span becomes almost normal. An overlooked accessory spleen is an occasional cause of failure of splenectomy. The presence of Howell-Jolly bodies in red cells makes the presence of accessory spleens unlikely.

Iglauer A et al: Cryohemolysis test as a diagnostic tool for hereditary spherocytosis. Ann Hematol 1999;78:555.

Garbaz M et al: A 5' splice region G→C mutation in exon 3 of the human beta-spectrin gene leads to decreased levels of beta-spectrin mRNA and is responsible for dominant hereditary spherocytosis (spectrin Guemene-Penfao). Br J Haematol 1998;100:90.

Marchetti M et al: Prophylactic splenectomy and cholecystectomy in mild hereditary spherocytosis: analyzing the decision in different clinical scenarios. J Intern Med 1998;244:217.

2. Hereditary Elliptocytosis

This autosomal dominant genetic disorder, also known as ovalocytosis, is usually of little clinical significance. Normally, up to 15% oval or elliptic red blood cells can be seen on a peripheral blood smear. In elliptocytosis, at least 25% and up to 90% of circulating erythrocytes are elliptic. As with hereditary spherocytosis, this disease is due to a variety of genetic defects in cytoskeletal proteins such as spectrin. The predominant abnormality is that this structural protein exists as a dimer instead of a tetramer, leading to change in the erythrocyte's shape, decreased plasticity, and a shortened life span of the cell.

Most affected individuals are asymptomatic; about 10% have clinical manifestations consisting of moderate anemia, slight jaundice, and a palpable spleen.

Symptomatic patients should have splenectomy, and cholecystectomy if gallstones are present. The red cell defect persists after splenectomy, but the hemolysis and anemia are cured.

Bruce LJ et al: Erythroid band 3 variants and disease. Baillieres Best Pract Res Clinical Haematol 1999;12:637.

Silveira P et al: Red blood cell abnormalities in hereditary elliptocytosis and their relevance to variable clinical expression. Am J Clin Pathol 1997;108:391.

3. Hereditary Nonspherocytic Hemolytic Anemia

This is a heterogeneous group of rare hemolytic anemias caused by inherited intrinsic red cell defects that lead to oxidative hemolysis. Included in the group are pyruvate kinase deficiency and glucose 6-phosphate dehydrogenase (G6PD) deficiency. They are usually manifested in early childhood with anemia, jaundice, reticulocytosis, erythroid hyperplasia of the marrow, and normal osmotic fragility. As with other hemolytic anemias, there may be associated cholelithiasis.

Multiple blood transfusions are often required. Splenectomy, while not curative, may ameliorate some of these conditions, especially pyruvate kinase deficiency. In G6PD deficiency, splenectomy is not beneficial, and treatment consists of avoidance of dietary oxidants.

Baronciani L et al: Hematologically important mutations: red cell pyruvate kinase. Blood Cells Mol Dis 1998;24:273.

4. Thalassemia Major (Mediterranean Anemia; Cooley's Anemia)

In the most common form of this autosomal dominant disorder, a structural defect in the β-globin chain causes excess α chains to precipitate on the inner surface of the membrane of the erythrocyte and produces abnormal red cells (eg, target cells). Heterozygotes usually have mild anemia (thalassemia minor); however, starting early in infancy, homozygotes have severe chronic anemia accompanied by jaundice, hepatosplenomegaly (often massive), retarded body growth, and enlargement of the head. The peripheral blood smear reveals target cells, nucleated red cells, and a hypochromic microcytic anemia. Gallstones are present in about 25% of patients. A characteristic feature is the persistence of fetal hemoglobin (Hb F).

Since the anemia of thalassemia is due to both increased destruction of red cells and decreased hemoglobin production, splenectomy does not cure the anemia, as in spherocytosis, but it may reduce transfusion requirements by removing an enlarged, uncomfortable spleen. Treatment is by iron chelation and transfusion.

Weatherall DJ: The thalassemias. BMJ 1997; 314:1675.

AUTOIMMUNE DISORDERS

The production of IgG autoantibodies specific for cell membrane proteins on erythrocytes causes autoimmune hemolytic anemia; on platelets, it causes idiopathic thrombocytopenic purpura (ITP) and may cause neutropenia in Felty's syndrome. Macrophages express Fc receptors for IgG, and antibody-coated cells that pass through the splenic sinuses of the red pulp come into contact with these phagocytic cells. Furthermore, the microenvironment of the red pulp with slow flow of blood with a high cellular content through circuitous spaces facilitates opsonization of cells in the spleen. Production of autoantibodies in the white pulp germinal centers may also enhance cellular destruction, particularly in ITP. Understanding this pathophysiologic mechanism is important, since autoimmune hemolytic anemia caused by IgM autoantibodies (ie, cold agglutinin hemolytic anemia) does not respond to splenectomy because macrophages do not have Fc receptors for IgM. This mechanism also explains why treatment with high-dose intravenous immune globulin is beneficial in these diseases because it blocks the macrophage Fc receptor.

1. Acquired Hemolytic Anemia

 ESSENTIALS OF DIAGNOSIS

- *Fatigue, pallor, jaundice.*
- *Splenomegaly.*
- *Persistent anemia and reticulocytosis.*

General Considerations

The **autoimmune hemolytic anemias** have also been classified according to the optimal temperature at which autoantibodies react with the red cell surface (warm or cold antibodies). This classification is particularly useful, since patients with cold antibodies will not benefit from splenectomy but those with warm antibodies may.

Although hemolysis without demonstrable antibody (Coombs test-negative) may occur in uremia, cirrhosis of the liver, cancer, and certain infections, in most cases the red cell membranes are coated with either immunoglobulin or complement (Coombs test-positive). The antibody in IgG autoimmune hemolytic anemia is specifically directed against the Rh locus on the erythrocyte. Initiation of this disease is either idiopathic (40–50%) or secondary to drug exposure, connective tissue disorders, or lymphoproliferative disorders. Cold agglutinin hemolytic anemia is due typically to an IgM directed against the I red cell antigen, and hemolysis occurs intravascularly by complement fixation and not within the spleen.

About 20% of cases of secondary immune hemolytic anemia are due to drug use, and hemolysis is usually mediated by warm antibodies. Penicillin, quinidine, hydralazine, and methyldopa have been most commonly implicated in this syndrome (Table 28–3).

Clinical Findings

A. SYMPTOMS AND SIGNS

Autoimmune hemolytic anemia may be encountered at any age but is most common after age 50; it occurs twice as often in women. The onset is usually acute, consisting of anemia, mild jaundice, and sometimes fever. The spleen is palpably enlarged in over 50% of patients, and pigment gallstones are present in about 25%. Rarely, a sudden severe onset produces hemoglobinuria, renal tubular necrosis, and a 40–50% death rate.

B. LABORATORY FINDINGS

Hemolytic anemia is diagnosed by demonstrating a normocytic normochromic anemia, reticulocytosis (over 10%),

Table 28–3. Disorders associated with immune hemolysis.

Immune drug reaction (penicillin, quinidine, hydralazine, methylodopa, cimetidine)
Collagen vascular disease (lupus erythematosus, rheumatoid arthritis)
Tumors (lymphoma, myeloma, leukemia, dermoid cysts, ovarian teratoma)
Infection (*Mycoplasma*, malaria, syphilis, viremia)

erythroid hyperplasia of the marrow, and elevation of serum indirect bilirubin. Stool urobilinogen may be greatly increased, but there is no bile in the urine. Serum haptoglobin is usually low or absent. The direct Coombs test is positive because the red cells are coated with immunoglobulins or complement (or both).

Treatment

Associated diseases must be carefully sought and appropriately treated. For drug-induced secondary hemolytic anemia, further exposure to the offending agent must be terminated. Corticosteroids produce a remission in about 75% of patients, but only 25% of remissions are permanent. Transfusion should be avoided if possible, since cross-matching may be extremely difficult, requiring washed red cells and saline-active antisera.

Splenectomy is indicated for patients with warm-antibody hemolysis who fail to respond to 4–6 weeks of high-dose corticosteroid therapy, for patients who relapse after an initial response when steroids are withdrawn, and for patients in whom steroid therapy is contraindicated (eg, those with active pulmonary tuberculosis). Patients who require chronic high-dose steroid therapy should also be considered for splenectomy, since the risks of long-term steroid administration are substantial.

Splenectomy is effective because it removes the principal site of red cell destruction. Occasionally, splenectomy discloses the presence of an underlying disorder such as lymphoma. About half of patients who fail to respond to splenectomy will respond to azathioprine or cyclophosphamide. Plasmapheresis has been employed as salvage therapy in patients with refractory hemolytic anemia.

Prognosis

Relapses may occur after splenectomy but are less frequent if the initial response was good. The ultimate prognosis in the secondary cases depends upon the underlying disorder.

Beutler E et al: Hemolytic anemia. Semin Hematol 1999;36:38.

2. Immune Thrombocytopenic Purpura (Idiopathic Thrombocytopenic Purpura, ITP)

ESSENTIALS OF DIAGNOSIS

- Petechiae, ecchymoses, epistaxis, easy bruising.
- No splenomegaly.
- Decreased platelet count, prolonged bleeding time, poor clot retraction, normal coagulation time.

General Considerations

Immune thrombocytopenic purpura is a hemorrhagic syndrome with diverse causes which can occur in an acute or chronic form and is characterized by marked reduction in the number of circulating platelets, abundant megakaryocytes in the bone marrow, and a shortened platelet life span. It may be idiopathic or secondary to a lymphoproliferative disorder, drugs or toxins, bacterial or viral infection (especially in children), systemic lupus erythematosus, or other conditions. An increased incidence of immune thrombocytopenic purpura has also been identified in homosexual males and appears to be associated with the acquired immunodeficiency syndrome (AIDS). Although responses to corticosteroids and to splenectomy in these patients are comparable to the responses observed in other patients with immune thrombocytopenic purpura, splenectomy should be reserved for those with signs of blood loss, since surgical complications are high and survival may be short. These patients may also have associated opportunistic infections, making corticosteroid treatment more hazardous.

The pathogenesis of both primary and secondary disorders involves a circulating antiplatelet IgG autoantibody usually directed against a membrane protein which is the fibrinogen receptor (glycoprotein IIb/IIIa). In this disorder, the spleen is primarily the site of platelet destruction and may also be a significant source of autoantibody production. Splenomegaly, present in only 2% of cases, is usually a manifestation of another underlying disease such as lymphoma or lupus erythematosus. Five to 15 percent of HIV-positive patients have thrombocytopenia independent of the immunologic state of their disease that is clinically indistinguishable from typical chronic ITP. The precise pathophysiologic mechanism in relation to HIV infection is not known.

Clinical Findings

A. SYMPTOMS AND SIGNS

The onset may be acute, with ecchymoses or showers of petechiae, and may be accompanied by bleeding gums, vaginal bleeding, gastrointestinal bleeding, and hematuria. Central nervous system bleeding occurs in 3% of patients. The acute form is most common in children, usually occurring before 8 years of age, and often begins 1–3 weeks after a viral upper respiratory illness.

The chronic form, which may start at any age, is more common in women. It characteristically has an insidious onset, often with a long history of easy bruisability and menorrhagia. Showers of petechiae may occur, especially over pressure areas. Cyclic remissions and exacerbations may continue for several years.

B. LABORATORY FINDINGS

The platelet count is moderately to severely decreased (always below 100,000/μL), and platelets may be absent from the peripheral blood smear. Although white and red cell counts are usually normal, iron deficiency anemia may be present as a result of bleeding. The bone marrow shows increased numbers of large megakaryocytes without platelet budding.

The bleeding time is prolonged, capillary fragility (Rumpel-Leede test) greatly increased, and clot retraction poor. Partial thromboplastin time, prothrombin time, and coagulation time are normal. Specific determinations of antiplatelet antibody titers can now be routinely assessed to aid in diagnosis.

It is now recognized that splenic sequestration studies using ^{51}Cr-tagged platelets correlate poorly with response to splenectomy and are of little value.

Differential Diagnosis

Other causes of nonimmunologic thrombocytopenia must be ruled out, such as leukemia, aplastic anemia, and macroglobulinemia. Thrombocytopenia and purpura may be caused by ineffective thrombocytopoiesis (eg, pernicious anemia, preleukemic states) or by nonimmune platelet destruction (eg, septicemia, disseminated intravascular coagulation, or other causes of hypersplenism).

Treatment

Treatment of immune thrombocytopenic purpura depends on the age of the patient, the severity of the disease, the duration of the thrombocytopenia, and the clinical variant. Secondary immune thrombocytopenias are best managed by treating the underlying primary disorder (eg, if it is drug-induced, the drug should be stopped).

Patients with mild or no symptoms need no specific therapy but should avoid contact sports, elective surgery, and all unessential medications. Corticosteroids are indicated in patients with moderate to severe purpura of short duration. Usually, 60 mg of prednisone (or equivalent) is required daily; this is continued until the platelet count returns to normal and then is gradually tapered after 4–6 weeks. Corticosteroids produce a response in 70–80%, but sustained remissions in only 20% of adults.

Splenectomy is the most effective form of therapy and is indicated for patients who do not respond to corticosteroids, for those who relapse after an initial remission on steroids, and for steroid-dependent patients. Corticosteroid therapy is not necessary in the immediate preoperative period unless bleeding is severe or the patient was receiving steroids before the operation. If indicated, platelet transfusions are given intraoperatively only after ligation of the splenic artery or removal of the spleen, since platelets from earlier transfusions would be rapidly sequestered in the spleen. For temporary treatment of the thrombocytopenia, intravenous immunoglobulin (IGIV) is effective.

Splenectomy produces a sustained remission in about 80% of patients. As with corticosteroids, success rates are better with acute than chronic immune thrombocytopenic purpura. The platelet count usually rises promptly following splenectomy (eg, it may double in 24 hours) and reaches a peak after 1–2 weeks. If the platelet count remains elevated after 2 months, the patient can be considered cured. When corticosteroids and splenectomy have failed, immunosuppressive drugs (azathioprine, vincristine) will achieve a remission in 25% of cases.

The benefit of splenectomy for HIV-associated ITP has been less clear. The risk of infection and the overall shortened survival in this population argue against splenectomy. However, in HIV patients without AIDS, clinically significant thrombocytopenia responds completely in 70% and there is partial improvement in 20% following splenectomy. Splenectomy does not appear to alter the overall natural history of HIV infection.

Prognosis

Acute immune thrombocytopenic purpura in children under age 16 has an excellent prognosis; approximately 80% of patients have a complete and permanent spontaneous remission. This occurs rarely in adults. Splenectomy is successful in about 80% of patients, but more often in idiopathic cases than in those secondary to another disorder.

George JN et al: Idiopathic thrombocytopenic purpura: diagnosis and management. Am J Med Sci 1998;316:87.

Lilleyman JS: Management of childhood idiopathic thrombocytopenic purpura. Br J Haematol 1999;105:871.

Silver RM: Management of idiopathic thrombocytopenic purpura in pregnancy. Clin Obstet Gynecol 1998;41:436.

3. Felty's Syndrome

Approximately 1% of patients with rheumatoid arthritis have splenomegaly and neutropenia—a triad known as Felty's syndrome. High levels of IgG have been identified on the surface of neutrophils with evidence of increased of granulopoiesis in the bone marrow. Pathologic analysis of the spleen in Felty's syndrome patients shows a larger proportionate increase in the white pulp as opposed to most conditions of splenomegaly. There is evidence of excess accumulation of neutrophils in both the T cell zone of the white pulp as well as the cord and sinuses of the red pulp.

Patients with severe neutropenia have clinical symptoms of recurring infections in Felty's syndrome. Symptomatic patients who have evidence of IgG on the surface of neutrophils should be considered for splenectomy. Neutropenia will improve in 60–70% of these patients, but relapse of neutropenia as well as recurrent infections in the presence of normal neutrophil counts may occur, and these untoward events have dampened enthusiasm for splenectomy in this disease.

Logue GL et al: Failure of splenectomy in Felty's syndrome. N Engl J Med 1981;304:580.

4. Thrombotic Thrombocytopenic Purpura

Thrombotic thrombocytopenic purpura (TTP) is a rare disease with a pentad of clinical features: (1) fever, (2) thrombocytopenic purpura, (3) hemolytic anemia, (4) neurologic manifestations, and (5) renal failure. The cause is unknown, but autoimmunity to endothelial cells or a primary platelet defect has been implicated, and its occurrence in patients with the AIDS has been reported. It is most common between ages 10 and 40 years.

The thrombocytopenia is probably due to a shortened platelet life span. The microangiopathic hemolytic anemia is produced by passage of red cells over damaged small blood vessels containing fibrin strands. Rigid red cells are trapped and fragmented in the spleen, whereas those that escape the spleen may be more vulnerable to damage and destruction in the abnormal microvasculature. The anemia is often severe, and it may be aggravated by hemorrhage secondary to thrombocytopenia. Hepatomegaly and splenomegaly occur in 35% of cases.

Treatment & Prognosis

Until recently, there was no effective therapy for this disorder, and mortality rates as high as 95% were reported. Most patients died of renal failure or cerebral bleeding. Plasmapheresis with plasma exchange has recently emerged as an effective form of treatment which is superior to simple plasma infusion. The plasma supernatant after cryoprecipitation may be more effective than whole plasma. When combined with other therapies, including corticosteroids, dextran, splenectomy, and antiplatelet drugs, prolonged remission can be achieved in most patients.

Allford SL et al: Current understanding of the pathophysiology of thrombotic thrombocytopenic purpura. J Clin Path 2000; 53:497.

Rock GA: Management of thrombotic thrombocytopenic purpura. Br J Haematology 2000;109:496.

METABOLIC DISORDERS

Metabolic disorders amenable to splenectomy are rare inherited diseases that include as a component either the destruction of blood elements within the spleen or splenic enlargement with hypersplenism. Either of these aspects of these diseases may be corrected by splenectomy.

1. Gaucher's Disease

Gaucher's disease is an autosomal recessive disorder characterized by a deficiency in beta-glucosidase, a lysosomal enzyme that degrades the sphingolipid glucocerebroside. There is an increased incidence of this disorder in Ashkenazi Jews. Three types of this disease exist, and the one amenable to splenectomy is type I, or the adult type. Pathologically, Gaucher's disease results in lipid accumulation within the white pulp of the spleen, the liver, or the bone marrow. Predominant symptoms relate to massive splenomegaly from either the direct effects of the size of the spleen or secondary to cytopenias from hypersplenism.

Treatment & Prognosis

Treatment by total splenectomy alleviates the symptoms but results in accelerated hepatic and bone disease as well as a significant increased risk of postsplenectomy infections. Treatment with partial or subtotal splenectomy has been studied over the past 10 years for both adults and children with Gaucher's disease. Removing most of the spleen corrects the symptoms of splenomegaly, but leaving a splenic remnant provides a site for further deposition of lipid that protects the liver and bone. The major problem with partial splenectomy is the eventual recurrence and enlargement of the splenic remnant accompanied by recurrent symptoms. The goal of subtotal splenectomy in Gaucher's disease is to leave a small fragment approximately the size of

the fist of the patient. Replacement therapy with recombinant glucocerebrosidase enzyme has recently become available, but the cost of chronic treatment is prohibitive.

Cohen IJ et al: Long-term follow-up of partial splenectomy in Gaucher's disease. Am J Surg 1992;164:345.

Morgenstern L et al: Subtotal splenectomy for Gaucher's disease: a follow-up study. Am Surg 1993;59:860.

Zer M et al: Subtotal splenectomy in Gaucher's disease: towards a definition of critical splenic mass. Br J Surg 1992;79:742.

2. Wiskott-Aldrich Syndrome

Wiskott-Aldrich syndrome is an X-linked disease characterized by thrombocytopenia, combined B and T immunodeficiency, eczema, and a propensity to develop malignancies. Thrombocytopenia is the major feature of this rare disorder, with most patients presenting with bloody diarrhea, epistaxis, and petechiae at a young age. Platelet counts typically range between 20,000/μL and 40,000/μL, and the platelets that are present are between one-fourth and one-half of normal size. The spleen sequesters and destroys platelets in this disease, releasing "microplatelets" back into the circulation. The genetic defect in this disorder may be related to an abnormal adhesion molecule affecting immune as well as platelet cell-to-cell interaction.

Treatment & Prognosis

Splenectomy in Wiskott-Aldrich syndrome was at one time withheld since the postoperative course was characterized by severe and fatal infections due to the underlying immune defect of this disorder combined with loss of the immune function of the spleen. However, splenectomy does normalize platelet shape, size, and numbers, and the use of prophylactic antibiotics after splenectomy has significantly increased survival rates. The optimal treatment of Wiskott-Aldrich syndrome is an HLA-matched sibling bone marrow transplantation. However, splenectomy with antibiotics results in better survival than an unmatched bone marrow transplantation. Patients who do not undergo bone marrow transplantation or splenectomy typically do not survive past the age of 5 years.

Muller CA et al: Splenectomy and/or bone marrow transplantation in the management of the Wiskott-Aldrich syndrome: long-term follow-up in 62 cases. Blood 1993;82:2961.

3. Chédiak-Higashi Syndrome

Chédiak-Higashi syndrome is a rare autosomal recessive disease characterized by immunodeficiency that increases the susceptibility to bacterial and viral infections and is manifested by recurrent fever, nystagmus, and photophobia. Most patients experience widespread infiltration of tissues with histiocytes similar to a lymphoma. Secondary hepatosplenomegaly with lymphadenopathy, leukopenia, and bleeding complications occur in the accelerated phase of Chédiak-Higashi syndrome. Standard treatment includes chemotherapy, steroids, and ascorbic acid, but these patients have a poor prognosis. Splenectomy has been used in the accelerated phase with beneficial results.

Harfi HA et al: Chédiak-Higashi syndrome: clinical, hematologic, and immunologic improvement after splenectomy. Ann Allergy 1992:69,147.

4. Sarcoidosis

Sarcoidosis is a granulomatous disease of unknown origin that can involve virtually any organ or area of the body. Pulmonary disease is most common, but autopsy studies have shown that the spleen is the second most common site, with enlargement by noncaseating granulomas in 50–60% of patients. However, most patients do not have massive splenomegaly. When this does occur, patients can have significant cytopenias related to hypersplenism as well as the constitutional symptoms and hypercalcemia of sarcoidosis. In this subgroup of patients, splenectomy is indicated as a potential curative procedure for each of these symptoms.

Kruithoff KL et al: Giant splenomegaly and refractory hypercalcemia due to extrapulmonary sarcoidosis. Arch Intern Med 1993;153,2793.

NEOPLASTIC DISEASES

Neoplastic diseases in which splenectomy may play a role in management include chronic lymphocytic leukemia (CLL), hairy cell leukemia, and Hodgkin's or non-Hodgkin's lymphoma. Splenectomy may be indicated for hypersplenism, for diagnosis, or for primary surgical removal of the predominant or only site of disease. Lymphoma is discussed in detail in Chapter 47.

Related neoplastic disorders of idiopathic myelofibrosis and mastocytosis are also discussed as variants of neoplastic diseases in which splenectomy is occasionally indicated.

1. Chronic Lymphocytic Leukemia

Chronic lymphocytic leukemia (CLL) is a low-grade neoplasm of B cell lineage characterized by accumulations of populations of lymphocytes that are mature morphologically but functionally incompetent. The clinical manifestations and natural history are variable, but initially the disease tends to be indolent. In more

advanced stages, splenomegaly, which is frequently massive, is a common characteristic of CLL. Most symptoms related to the spleen are from thrombocytopenia and anemia due to secondary hypersplenism (80–90% of splenic symptoms). Ten to 20 percent of patients may have symptoms primarily related to pressure from the size of the enlarged spleen.

Other causes of cytopenia in CLL relate to decreased cellular production from the bone marrow. Bone marrow failure can be due to replacement with leukemic cells or to depletion of the bone marrow as a toxic effect of prior antitumor chemotherapy.

Splenectomy in patients with CLL corrects thrombocytopenia in 70–85% of cases and anemia in 60–75% of cases. The median duration of benefit for both platelets and red cell populations is well over 1 year. Patients with smaller spleens preoperatively, lower preoperative platelet counts, and extensive prior chemotherapy are less likely to respond to splenectomy. However, a positive bone marrow aspirate for leukemic cells is not a contraindication to splenectomy in CLL. Patients who do not have a good performance status should not undergo splenectomy, since patients in terminal stages have unacceptable operative morbidity.

Coad JE et al: Splenectomy in lymphoproliferative disorders: a report on 70 cases and review of the literature. Leuk Lymphoma 1993;10:245.

Delpero JR et al: Splenectomy for hypersplenism in chronic lymphocytic leukaemia and malignant non-Hodgkin's lymphoma. Br J Surg 1990;77:443.

Neal TF Jr et al: Splenectomy in advanced chronic lymphocytic leukemia: a single institution experience with 50 patients. Am J Med 1992;93:435.

Thiruvengadam R et al: Splenectomy in advanced chronic lymphocytic leukemia. Leukemia 1990;4:758.

2. Hairy Cell Leukemia

Hairy cell leukemia is a low-grade lymphoproliferative disorder with characteristic "hairy cells"—ie, B lymphocytes with irregular cytoplasmic protrusions—which infiltrate the bone marrow and spleen. Patients are typically male, and onset of the disease is in the fifth or sixth decade of life. Symptoms relate to pancytopenia, with anemia requiring transfusions; and to neutropenia, characterized by increased susceptibility to infections and increased bleeding tendencies. Some patients may have symptoms from splenomegaly, which is present in 80% of patients at the time of diagnosis of hairy cell leukemia. The cytopenias are due to a combination of bone marrow replacement and secondary hypersplenism.

The initial standard therapy for hairy cell leukemia was splenectomy, but recent advances in pharmacotherapy have superseded this surgical approach. Splenectomy is successful in improving cell counts in 80–90% of patients, but the duration of improvement is short-lived, with the majority of patients relapsing within 6–12 months. Chronic therapy with alpha interferon produced a higher proportion of responses of longer duration than splenectomy. First line therapy is now treatment with purine nucleoside analogs (fludarabine, pentostatin, or cladribine), with a complete response rate of 80–90%. It has never been shown that splenectomy offers survival benefit in this indolent disease, and the operation should be reserved for palliation of splenomegaly in patients who have failed treatment with purine analogs and alpha interferon.

Pettit AR et al: Hairy-cell leukaemia: biology and management. Br J Hematol 1999;106:2.

Saven A, Piro L: Newer purine analogues for the treatment of hairy-cell leukemia. N Engl J Med 1994;330:691.

Smalley RV et al: Splenectomy vs alpha interferon: a randomized study in patients with previously untreated hairy cell leukemia. Am J Hematol 1992;41:13.

3. Idiopathic Myelofibrosis (Agnogenic Myeloid Metaplasia)

Myelofibrosis is a myeloproliferative disorder of unknown cause that is closely related to polycythemia vera and myelogenous leukemia. It appears to be a clonal disorder or a neoplasm originating from a stem cell that results in extensive bone marrow fibrosis, extramedullary hematopoiesis in the spleen and liver, and a leukoerythroblastic blood reaction.

The bone marrow is usually almost completely replaced by fibrous tissue, although in some cases it is hyperplastic and fibrosis is minimal. Extramedullary hematopoiesis develops mainly in the spleen, liver, and long bones. Symptoms are attributable to anemia (weakness, fatigue, dyspnea) and to splenomegaly (abdominal fullness and pain, which may be severe). Pain over the spleen from splenic infarcts is common. Spontaneous bleeding, secondary infection, bone pain, and a hypermetabolic state are frequent. Portal hypertension develops in some cases as a result of fibrosis of the liver, greatly increased splenic blood flow, or both.

Hepatomegaly is present in 75% of cases and splenomegaly with a firm and irregular spleen in all cases. Striking changes in the peripheral blood are referable to the combination of extramedullary hematopoiesis and hypersplenism. Patients are uniformly anemic, and red cells vary greatly in size and shape, many of them distorted and fragmented. The white count is usually high (20,000–50,000/µL). The platelet count may be elevated, but values less than 100,000/µL are seen in 30% of cases due to secondary hypersplenism. Bone marrow aspirates frequently result in a dry tap because marrow is replaced with fibrosis. It was once incorrectly thought that the spleen performed a crucial function of extramedullary hematopoiesis in this disease and that splenectomy could be lethal. In fact, many patients with myeloid metaplasia feel better if the massive spleen is removed, and their hypersplenism is often corrected.

About 30% of patients are asymptomatic at the time of initial diagnosis and require no therapy. When anemia and splenomegaly produce symptoms, transfusions, androgenic steroids, antimetabolites, and radiation therapy are indicated. Splenectomy is indicated in the following situations: (1) major hemolysis unresponsive to medical management, (2) severe symptoms of massive splenomegaly, (3) life-threatening thrombocytopenia, and (4) portal hypertension with variceal hemorrhage. This is one of the rare occasions when portal hypertension may be cured by splenectomy.

Splenectomy in myeloid metaplasia is associated with an 8–13% death rate and frequent complications often related to postsplenectomy hepatic morbidity. Splenectomy best relieves symptoms of splenomegaly and portal hypertension, but only about 50% of patients get relief from anemia and thrombocytopenia. Younger patients with normal platelet counts and symptoms are the best candidates for splenectomy in idiopathic myelofibrosis.

Barosi G et al: The Italian Consensus Conference on Diagnostic Criteria for Myelofibrosis with Myeloid Dysplasia. Br J Haematol 1999;104:730.

Reilly JT: Pathogenesis of idiopathic myelofibrosis: present status and future directions. Br J Haematol 1994;88:1.

Teffer A: Myelofibrosis with myeloid metaplasia. N Engl J Med 2000;342:1255.

4. Systemic Mast Cell Disease

Systemic mast cell disease, or mastocytosis, is a rare condition characterized by mast cell infiltration of a number of tissues, including the spleen. There are two types: indolent and aggressive. In indolent systemic mass cell disease, there is no need for consideration of splenectomy. The aggressive type is associated with hematologic diseases with characteristics of lymphoma. Splenomegaly may occur, with the predominant symptoms resulting from thrombocytopenia due to hypersplenism. In this subgroup of patients with aggressive disease, splenectomy improves platelet counts and is associated with longer median survival time than for patients with aggressive disease who do not undergo splenectomy.

Austen KF: Systemic mastocytosis. N Engl J Med 1992;326:639.

5. Cysts & Tumors of the Spleen

Parasitic cysts are almost always echinococcal (see Chapter 9). They may be asymptomatic, but usually the patient notices splenomegaly. Calcification of the cyst wall may be seen on x-ray. Eosinophilia may be found, and serologic tests may confirm the diagnosis. The treatment of choice is splenectomy.

Other cysts are dermoid, epidermoid, endothelial, and pseudocysts. The latter are thought to be late results of infarction or trauma. Splenectomy may be indicated to exclude tumor; however, partial splenectomy or observation has been advocated.

The rare primary tumors of the spleen include lymphoma, sarcoma, hemangioma, and hamartoma. Hamartomas may be confused grossly with splenic lymphoma at laparotomy. These lesions are usually asymptomatic until splenomegaly causes abdominal discomfort or a palpable mass. The benign vascular tumors of the spleen (angiomas) can produce hypersplenism. Spontaneous rupture with massive hemorrhage can occur. Splenectomy is indicated if the tumor appears to be limited to the spleen. Inflammatory pseudotumors are benign lesions composed of a mixture of inflammatory cells and a granulomatous reaction that can occur in a variety of organs, including the spleen. Constitutional symptoms of lethargy, weight loss, and fatigue occur and can be alleviated by splenectomy.

The spleen is a common site for metastases in advanced cancers, especially of the lung and breast and melanoma. Splenic metastases are common autopsy findings but are rarely clinically significant.

Du Plessis DG et al: Mucinous epithelial cysts of the spleen associated with pseudomyxoma peritonei. Histopathology 1999; 35:551.

Hayes TC et al: Symptomatic splenic hamartoma: case report and literature review. Pediatrics 1998;101:918.

Ooi LL et al: Splenic abscesses from 1987 to 1995. Am J Surg 1997;174:87.

Scott GC et al: CT patterns of nodular hepatic and splenic sarcoidosis: a review of the literature. J Comput Assist Tomogr 1997;21:369.

INFECTIONS OF THE SPLEEN (Splenic Abscess)

Splenic abscesses are uncommon but are important because the death rate ranges between 40% and 100%. They may be caused by hematogenous seeding of the spleen with bacteria from remote sepsis such as endocarditis, by direct spread of infection from adjacent structures, or by splenic trauma resulting in a secondarily infected splenic hematoma. Splenic abscess is a complication of intravenous drug abuse. In 80% of cases, one or more abscesses exist in organs other than the spleen, and the splenic abscess develops as a terminal manifestation of uncontrolled sepsis in other organs. Enteric organisms are found in over two-thirds of splenic abscesses, with staphylococci and nonenteric streptococci comprising the majority of the remainder. In some patients, unexplained sepsis, progressive splenic enlargement, and abdominal pain are the presenting manifestations. The spleen may not be palpable, because of left upper quadrant tenderness and guarding. A left pleural effusion combined with unexplained leukocytosis in a septic patient suggests a splenic abscess. The finding of gas in the spleen on plain abdominal x-ray is pathognomonic of splenic abscess, but CT scan is the optimal way to define and diagnose a splenic abscess.

Most splenic abscesses remain localized, periodically seeding the bloodstream with bacteria, but spontaneous rupture and peritonitis may occur. Splenectomy is essential for cure if sepsis is localized to the spleen. Percutaneous drainage of large, solitary juxtacapsular abscesses may occasionally be feasible but is associated with an extremely high mortality rate and should be reserved for patients unable to withstand an operation.

Phillips GS et al: Splenic abscess: another look at an old disease. Arch Surg 1997;132:1331.

SPLENOSIS (Splenic Autotransplantation)

In splenosis, multiple small implants of splenic tissue grow in scattered areas on the peritoneal surfaces throughout the abdomen. They arise from dissemination and autotransplantation of splenic fragments following traumatic rupture of the spleen. Splenic implants or intentional autotransplants are capable of cell culling, and some immunologic function appears to be exhibited in cases of intentional autotransplantation. Aggressive attempts at surgical excision are not warranted. Splenosis is usually an incidental finding discovered much later during laparotomy for an unrelated problem. However, the implants stimulate formation of adhesions and may be a cause of intestinal obstruction. They must be distinguished from peritoneal nodules of metastatic carcinoma and from accessory spleens. Histologically, they differ from accessory spleens by the absence of elastic or smooth muscle fibers in the delicate capsule.

Pisters PWT et al: Autologous splenic transplantation for splenic trauma. Ann Surg 1994;219:225.

Timens W et al: Splenic autotransplantation and the immune system. Ann Surg 1993;215:256.

Zoli G et al: Splenic autotransplantation after splenectomy: tuftsin activity correlates with residual splenic function. Br J Surg 1994;81:716.

■ SPLENECTOMY

Preoperative preparation of patients undergoing elective splenectomy should correct coagulation abnormalities and deficits in red cell mass, treat infections, and control immune reactions. Because platelets are removed so rapidly from the circulation, they usually are not given for thrombocytopenia until after the splenic artery has been ligated. Antibodies in the patient's serum may complicate cross-matching of blood. Many patients with autoimmune disorders require corticosteroid coverage in the perioperative period. For emergency splenectomy, hypovolemia should be corrected by whole blood transfusions. For elective cases, prophylactic vaccination with a polyvalent pneumococcal vaccine that protects against a common encapsulated offending organism in postsplenectomy infection is recommended. Elective splenectomy is now most commonly performed as a laparoscopic procedure. This reduces the recovery period and is significantly better tolerated by most patients.

Details of surgical technique are not within the scope of this text, but it should be noted that there are two approaches to open splenectomy (Figure 28–2). In one, which is of value chiefly in traumatic rupture of the spleen, the organ is immediately mobilized and the splenic artery is secured from behind as it enters the hilum. In the other, which is of vital importance in the removal of massively enlarged spleens, the organ is left in situ. The gastrocolic ligament is opened, and the splenic artery is ligated as it courses along the upper edge of the pancreas. This permits blood to leave the spleen through the splenic vein while all other attachments (ie, the short gastric vessels and colic attachments) are divided before the spleen is delivered. This method permits the removal of massively enlarged vascular spleens with practically no loss of blood.

Splenorrhaphy is operative repair of the spleen following trauma. The principles of splenorrhaphy are to debride the devitalized tissue and to attempt to approximate the normal contour of the spleen with capsular sutures or external wraps of material. Partial splenic resections may be performed for trauma or for disease states in which splenic debulking is indicated. Partial splenectomy for Gaucher's disease, large cysts, or benign tumors has been reported using automatic stapling devices as well as microwave coagulators.

Massive splenomegaly is defined as a spleen weight of greater than 1500 g or eight to ten times the normal size. Disease processes leading to massive splenomegaly include lymphoma, leukemia, and metabolic storage diseases. The morbidity and mortality rates of splenectomy for massive splenomegaly are increased primarily as a result of the risk of severe and rapid intraoperative blood loss. The operative approach in these cases is initial ligation of the splenic artery through the lesser sac at the superior border of the pancreas. Next, ligation of the short gastric vessels along the greater curvature all the way to the gastroesophageal junction is performed, allowing the stomach and left lobe of the liver to be retracted away from the spleen.

Figure 28–2. *A*: Anterior approach to splenic artery. *B:* Mobilization of spleen with posterior exposure of splenic artery.

Only after decreasing the splenic arterial inflow by the above maneuvers should mobilization of the lateral and superior attachments be performed, leading to removal of the massive spleen.

The technique for laparoscopic splenectomy has been developed and may be utilized for elective resections in which there is minimal splenic enlargement. Laparoscopic splenectomy is performed using four or five ports. Midline ports for the cannula as well as for retraction of the stomach away from the splenic hilum are placed. Left subcostal ports are used as operating sites for dissection of the splenic hilum. An angled laparoscope is required for visualization of the superior and lateral attachments of the spleen. Vessels are divided with clips, sutures, or stapling devices. Clinical conditions such as idiopathic thrombocytopenic purpura and hereditary spherocytosis are the most common indications for laparoscopic splenectomy as the spleen is of normal size. Search via the laparoscope for accessory spleens is important in these procedures for a successful outcome.

Danforth DN et al: Splenectomy for the massively enlarged spleen. Am Surg 1991;56:108.

Katkouda N et al: Laparoscopic splenectomy: outcome and efficacy in 103 consecutive patients. Ann Surg 1998;228:568.

HEMATOLOGIC EFFECTS OF SPLENECTOMY

Absence of the spleen in a normal adult usually has few clinical consequences. Red cell count and indices do not change, but red cells with cytoplasmic inclusions may appear, eg, Heinz bodies, Howell-Jolly bodies, and siderocytes. Granulocytosis occurs immediately after splenectomy but is replaced in several weeks by lymphocytosis and monocytosis. Platelets are usually increased, occasionally markedly so, and may stay at levels of 400,000–500,000/μL for over a year. Even more striking thrombocytosis (eg, 2–3 million/μL) may develop after splenectomy for hemolytic anemia. A platelet count of over a million is not an indication for anticoagulants, but antiplatelet agents such as aspirin may help prevent thrombosis.

Horowitz J et al: Postsplenectomy leukocytosis: physiologic or an indicator of infection? Am Surg 1992;58:387.

Rutherford EJ et al: The white blood cell response to splenectomy and bacteraemia. Injury 1994;25:289.

POSTSPLENECTOMY SEPSIS & OTHER POSTSPLENECTOMY PROBLEMS

Complications related to splenectomy per se are relatively few, with atelectasis, pancreatitis, and postopera-

tive hemorrhage being the most common. If splenectomy is done for thrombocytopenia, secondary bleeding may occur even though the platelet count usually rises promptly. Platelet transfusions should be given if primary hemostasis is abnormal (ie, oozing occurs) and the platelet count remains low. Thromboembolic complications may be more common following splenectomy, but this complication does not correlate with the degree of thrombocytosis. The risk of portal vein thrombosis is small but important, since this complication may be lethal if not recognized. Symptoms include fever, abdominal pain, diarrhea, and abnormal liver function tests. Treatment consists of anticoagulation plus antibiotics.

Individuals are more susceptible to fulminant bacteremia after splenectomy. This is a result of the following changes that occur after splenectomy: (1) decreased clearance of bacteria from the blood, (2) decreased levels of IgM, and (3) decreased opsonic activity. The risk is greatest in young children, especially in the first 2 years after surgery (80% of cases) and when the disorder for which splenectomy was required was a disease of the reticuloendothelial system. In general, the younger the patient undergoing splenectomy and the more severe the underlying condition, the greater the risk for developing overwhelming postsplenectomy infection. There is a low but significant risk of infection even in otherwise normal adults following splenectomy. Most of these infections occur after the first year, and nearly half occur more than 5 years after splenectomy. Lethal sepsis is very rare in adults. There is a distinct clinical syndrome: mild, nonspecific symptoms are followed by high fever and shock from sepsis, which may rapidly lead to death. *Streptococcus pneumoniae, Haemophilus influenzae,* and meningococci are the most common pathogens. Disseminated intravascular coagulation is a common complication. Awareness of this fatal complication has led to efforts to avoid splenectomy or to perform partial splenectomy or splenic repair for ruptured spleens (analogous to surgical management of liver trauma) to maintain adequate splenic function. Splenic autotransplantation may also achieve partial restoration of splenic function after splenectomy.

The risk of fatal sepsis is less after splenectomy for trauma than for hematologic disorders, probably due to splenic autotransplantation. Prophylactic vaccination against pneumococcal sepsis should be used in all surgically or functionally asplenic patients. Since splenic function may be important in the immune response to vaccine, early administration of polyvalent pneumococcal vaccine (Pneumovax) is advisable. The vaccine provides protection in adults and older children for 4–5 years, after which revaccination is advisable. Since the vaccine is only effective against about 80% of organisms, some authorities have recommended a 2-year course, treatment until age 16, or lifelong prophylaxis with penicillin following splenectomy. Others have advocated use of ampicillin to provide coverage for *H influenzae* as well as pneumococci. Antibiotic prophylaxis is essential in children under 2 years of age and should be continued until at least age 6. In general, splenectomy should be deferred until age 6 unless the hematologic problem is especially severe.

Brigden ML et al: Prevention and management of overwhelming postsplenectomy infection—an update. Crit Care Med 1999; 27:836.

Eber SW et al: Frequency of very late fatal sepsis after splenectomy for hereditary spherocytosis: impact of insufficient antibody response to pneumococcal infection. Ann Hematol 1999; 78:524.

Foss Abrahamsen A et al: Systemic pneumococcal disease after staging splenectomy for Hodgkin's disease 1969-1980 without pneumococcal vaccine protection: a follow-up study 1994. Eur J Haematol 19997;58:73.

Park A et al: Laparoscopic vs open splenectomy. Arch Surg 1999; 134:1263.

Appendix

Lawrence W. Way, MD

ANATOMY & PHYSIOLOGY

In infants, the appendix is a conical diverticulum at the apex of the cecum, but with differential growth and distention of the cecum, the appendix ultimately arises on the left and dorsally approximately 2.5 cm below the ileocecal valve. The taeniae of the colon converge at the base of the appendix, an arrangement that helps in locating this structure at operation. The appendix is fixed retrocecally in 16% of adults and is freely mobile in the remainder.

The appendix in youth is characterized by a large concentration of lymphoid follicles that appear 2 weeks after birth and number about 200 or more at age 15. Thereafter, progressive atrophy of lymphoid tissue proceeds concomitantly with fibrosis of the wall and partial or total obliteration of the lumen.

If the appendix has a physiologic function, it is probably related to the presence of lymphoid follicles. Reports of a statistical relationship between appendectomy and subsequent carcinoma of the colon and other neoplasms in humans are not supported by controlled studies.

Schumpelick V et al: Appendix and cecum. Embryology, anatomy, and surgical applications. Surg Clin North Am 2000;80:295.

ACUTE APPENDICITIS

ESSENTIALS OF DIAGNOSIS

- Abdominal pain.
- Anorexia, nausea and vomiting.
- Localized right lower quadrant abdominal tenderness.
- Low-grade fever.
- Leukocytosis.

General Considerations

Approximately 7% of people in Western countries have appendicitis at some time during their lives, and about 200,000 appendectomies for acute appendicitis are performed annually in the United States. The incidence has been steadily dropping over the past 25 years, however, while the incidence in developing countries—which in the past has been quite low—has been rising in proportion to economic gains and changes in lifestyle.

Obstruction of the proximal lumen by fibrous bands, lymphoid hyperplasia, fecaliths, calculi, or parasites has long been considered to be the major cause of acute appendicitis, though that theory is doubted by many experts. Evidence of temporal and geographic clustering of cases has suggested a primary infectious etiology. A fecalith or calculus is found in only 10% of acutely inflamed appendices.

As appendicitis progresses, the blood supply is impaired by bacterial infection in the wall and distention of the lumen by pus; gangrene and perforation occur at about 24 hours, though the timing is highly variable. Gangrene implies microscopic perforation and bacterial peritonitis (which may be localized by adhesions from nearby viscera).

Clinical Findings

Acute appendicitis has protean manifestations. It may simulate almost any other acute abdominal illness and in turn may be mimicked by a variety of conditions. Progression of symptoms and signs is the rule—in contrast to the fluctuating course of some other diseases.

A. SYMPTOMS AND SIGNS

Typically, the illness begins with vague midabdominal discomfort followed by nausea, anorexia, and indigestion. The pain is persistent and continuous but not severe, with occasional mild cramps. There may be an episode of vomiting, and within several hours the pain shifts to the right lower quadrant, becoming localized and causing discomfort on moving, walking, or coughing. The patient may feel constipated.

Examination at this point shows localized tenderness to one-finger palpation and perhaps slight muscular guarding. Rebound or percussion tenderness (the latter provides the same information more humanely) may be elicited in the same area. Peristalsis is normal or slightly reduced. Rectal and pelvic examinations are likely to be negative. The temperature is only slightly elevated (eg, 37.8 °C) in the absence of perforation.

Contrary to traditional teaching, tenderness on rectal examination is not a sign of acute appendicitis. If present, it more often points to another cause of the symptoms. Another common misconception is that inflammation in a retrocecal appendix produces an atypical syndrome. This too is incorrect; the clinical findings in this situation are the same as for ordinary (antececal) appendicitis.

Rarely, the cecum may lie on the left side of the abdomen, and appendicitis may be mistaken for sigmoid diverticulitis. An inflamed appendix in the right upper quadrant may mimic acute cholecystitis or perforated ulcer. Even when the cecum is normally situated, a long appendix may reach to other parts of the abdomen, and acute appendicitis in these circumstances may be very confusing indeed.

A couple of general points are worth remembering: (1) People with early (nonperforated) appendicitis often do not appear ill and may even apologize for taking your time. Finding localized tenderness over McBurney's point is the cornerstone of diagnosis. (2) A rule that will help considerably with atypical cases is never to place appendicitis lower than second in the differential diagnosis of acute abdominal pain in a previously healthy person.

B. LABORATORY FINDINGS

The average leukocyte count is 15,000/μL, and 90% of patients have counts over 10,000/μL. In three-fourths of patients, the differential white count shows more than 75% neutrophils. It must be emphasized, however, that one patient in ten with acute appendicitis has a leukocyte count indistinguishable from normal, and many have normal differential cell counts. Appendicitis in patients infected with HIV produces the same syndrome as in other people, but the white blood cell count is usually normal.

The urine is usually normal, but a few leukocytes and erythrocytes and occasionally even gross hematuria may be noted, particularly in retrocecal or pelvic appendicitis.

C. IMAGING STUDIES

Localized air-fluid levels, localized ileus, or increased soft tissue density in the right lower quadrant is present in 50% of patients with early acute appendicitis. Less common findings are a calculus, an altered right psoas shadow, or an abnormal right flank stripe. The finding on plain films of a calculus in the right lower quadrant coupled with pain in this area strong supports a diagnosis of appendicitis. Although perforated peptic ulcer is by far the most common cause of free intraperitoneal air, free air is also a rare manifestation of perforated appendicitis. In general, however, the findings on plain films are nonspecific and rarely of help in diagnosis. A suggestion that barium enema may contribute to the diagnosis has not been supported by experience.

A spiral CT examination of the appendix may be of help in diagnosis. An enlarged appendix with periappendiceal fat stranding, found in 90% of cases, is the most common CT finding of acute appendicitis. Other criteria are less reliable. CT scans are of greatest value in patients with less than typical clinical and laboratory findings, where a positive study would be an indication for appendectomy. In the face of typical right lower quadrant pain and tenderness plus signs of inflammation (eg, fever, leukocytosis), a CT scan would be superfluous and, if negative, even misleading. Ultrasound imaging is much less reliable than CT. When appendicitis is accompanied by a right lower quadrant mass, an ultrasound or CT scan should be obtained to differentiate between a periappendiceal phlegmon and an abscess.

D. APPENDICITIS DURING PREGNANCY

Appendicitis is the most common nonobstetric surgical disease of the abdomen during pregnancy. Pregnant women develop appendicitis with the same frequency as do nonpregnant women of the same age, and the cases are equally distributed through the three trimesters of pregnancy. By far the most common presentation is right lower quadrant pain and tenderness—the classic syndrome—but the enlarged uterus occasionally will have pushed the appendix into the right upper quadrant, which gives rise to pain in this location. Fever is less common than with appendicitis in the absence of pregnancy. Leukocytosis is typical, but it too may be absent. The main problem is to recognize the possibility of appendicitis and perform appendectomy promptly. Delay in operation runs a higher than usual risk of perforation and diffuse peritonitis, because omentum is less available to wall off the infection. The mother is in greater jeopardy of serious abdominal infection, and the fetus is more vulnerable to premature labor with complications. Laparoscopic appendectomy (specifically the pneumoperitoneum) is well tolerated by the mother and fetus, but the frequency of technical complications is higher than with the open approach. Appendectomy during pregnancy is often followed by preterm labor but rarely by preterm delivery. Early appendectomy has decreased the maternal death rate to under 0.5% and the fetal death rate to under 10%.

Diagnosis & Differential Diagnosis

The clinical diagnosis of appendicitis rests on a combination of localized pain and tenderness accompanied by signs of inflammation, such as fever, leukocytosis, and elevated C-reactive protein levels. Migration of pain from the periumbilical area to the right lower quadrant is also diagnostically significant. In the absence of signs of inflammation, the diagnosis is less certain (ie, falsely positive), and in this situation a CT scan might be of value. The best strategy in equivocal cases is to observe the patient for a period of 6 hours or more. During this time, patients with appendicitis experience increasing pain and signs of inflammation and those without appendicitis generally improve. False-positive diagnoses often involve cases where the surgeon has accorded more significance to the patient's pain than to the presence or absence of inflammatory signs. Anorexia, nausea, and rectal tenderness are not indicative of appendicitis. During the past 15 years, the overall false- positive rate for the diagnosis of appendicitis has dropped from 15% to 10% without an accompanying rise in the number of perforations. Thus, diagnostic accuracy appears to be improving.

The diagnosis of acute appendicitis is particularly difficult in the very young and in the elderly. These are the groups where diagnosis is most often delayed and perforation most common. Infants manifest only lethargy, irritability, and anorexia in the early stages, but vomiting, fever, and pain are apparent as the disease progresses. Classic symptoms may not be elicited in aged patients, and the diagnosis is often not considered by the examining physician. The course of appendicitis is more virulent in the elderly, and suppurative complications occur earlier.

The highest incidence of false-positive diagnosis (20%) is in women between ages 20 and 40 and is attributable to pelvic inflammatory disease and other gynecologic conditions. Compared with appendicitis, pelvic inflammatory disease is more often associated with bilateral lower quadrant tenderness, left adnexal tenderness, onset of illness within 5 days of the last menstrual period, and a history that does not include nausea and vomiting. Cervical motion tenderness is common in both diseases.

Complications

The complications of acute appendicitis include perforation, peritonitis, abscess, and pylephlebitis.

A. Perforation

Delay in seeking medical care appears to be the principal reason for perforations; the disease has just been allowed to progress according to its natural history. Perforation is accompanied by more severe pain and higher fever (average, 38.3 °C) than in appendicitis. It is unusual for the acutely inflamed appendix to perforate within the first 12 hours. The appendicitis has progressed to perforation by the time of appendectomy in about 50% of patients under age 10 or over age 50. Nearly all deaths occur in the latter group.

The acute consequences of perforation vary from generalized peritonitis to formation of a tiny abscess that may not appreciably alter the symptoms and signs of appendicitis. Perforation in young women increases the subsequent risk of tubal infertility about fourfold.

B. Peritonitis

Localized peritonitis results from microscopic perforation of a gangrenous appendix, while spreading or generalized peritonitis usually implies gross perforation into the free peritoneal cavity. Increasing tenderness and rigidity, abdominal distention, and adynamic ileus are obvious in patients with peritonitis. High fever and severe toxicity mark progression of this catastrophic illness in untreated patients. Peritonitis is discussed in Chapter 23.

C. Appendiceal Abscess (Appendiceal Mass)

Localized perforation occurs when the periappendiceal infection becomes walled off by omentum and adjacent viscera. The clinical presentation consists of the usual findings in appendicitis plus a right lower quadrant mass. An ultrasound or CT scan should be performed; if an abscess is found, it is best treated by percutaneous ultrasound-guided aspiration. Opinion differs about how very small abscesses and phlegmons should be handled. Some surgeons prefer a regimen consisting of antibiotics and expectant management followed by elective appendectomy 6 weeks later. The purpose is to avoid spreading the localized infection, which usually resolves in response to the antibiotics. Other surgeons recommend immediate appendectomy, which considerably shortens the duration of the illness. The trend is in favor of the latter approach, since it is more expeditious and appears to be just as safe.

When the surgeon encounters an unsuspected abscess during appendectomy, it is usually best to proceed and remove the appendix. If the abscess is large and further dissection would be hazardous, drainage alone is appropriate.

Appendicitis recurs in only 10% of patients whose initial treatment consisted of antibiotics or antibiotics plus drainage of an abscess. Therefore, when the presence of ancillary conditions increases the risks of surgery, interval appendectomy may be postponed unless symptoms recur.

D. Pylephlebitis

Pylephlebitis is suppurative thrombophlebitis of the portal venous system. Chills, high fever, low-grade jaundice, and, later, hepatic abscesses are the hallmarks of this grave condition. The appearance of shaking chills in a patient with acute appendicitis demands vigorous antibiotic therapy to prevent the development of pylephlebitis.

CT scanning is the best means of detecting thrombosis and gas in the portal vein. In addition to antibiotics, prompt surgery is indicated to treat appendicitis or other primary sources of infection (eg, diverticulitis).

Prevention

In the past it was common to perform an incidental appendectomy in people under age 50 during the course of an abdominal operation for another illness—as long as the exposure was adequate and there were no specific contraindications. The declining lifetime risk of appendicitis now calls this practice into question. A related question concerns the appropriate course when a laparoscopy is performed for presumptive appendicitis and the appendix looks normal. The trend in this case is to leave the appendix intact—not to remove it prophylactically or on the assumption that the visual assessment may be inaccurate.

Treatment

With few exceptions, the treatment of appendicitis is surgical (ie, appendectomy). The operation can be done open (see Figure 29–1) or laparoscopically. The results of clinical trials comparing the two methods show no clear-cut advantage of one method over the other, though patients treated laparoscopically return to work a few days earlier. A laparoscopic approach is desirable when the preoperative diagnosis is uncertain because the morbidity is less if the appendix is found to be uninflamed and an appendectomy is not done.

Prophylactic antibiotics are indicated preoperatively. A single-drug regimen, usually a cephalosporin, is as effective as more aggressive multiple-drug combinations. The practice of routinely culturing abdominal fluid is of no practical value even when the appendix has perforated. The organisms obtained are the usual fecal flora.

Abdominal drains are called for only to treat established abscesses, not for diffuse inflammation or abdominal fluid.

If a patient with appendicitis cannot be taken to a modern surgical facility for care, treatment should consist of antibiotics alone. The complication-free success rate of this approach is high.

Prognosis

Although a death rate of zero is theoretically attainable in acute appendicitis, deaths still occur, some of which are avoidable. The death rate in simple acute appendicitis is approximately 0.1% and has not changed significantly since 1930. Progress in pre- and postoperative care—particularly the emphasis on fluid replacement before operation—has reduced the death rate from perforation to about 5%. Nonetheless, postoperative infections still occur in 30% of cases of gangrenous or perfo-

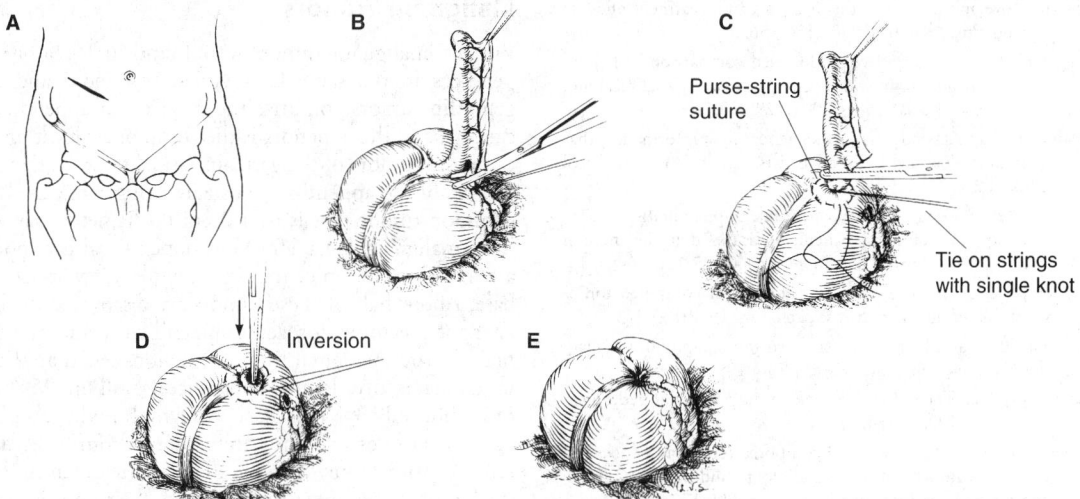

Figure 29–1. Technique of appendectomy. ***A:*** Incision. ***B:*** After delivery of the tip of the cecum, the mesoappendix is divided. ***C:*** The base is clamped and ligated with a simple throw of the knot. The next step—inversion of the stump—is optional. ***D:*** A clamp is placed to hold the knot during inversion with a purse-string suture of fine silk. ***E:*** The loosely tied inner knot on the stump assures that there is no closed space for the development of a stump abscess.

rated appendix. Although most of these patients survive, many near fatalities require prolonged hospitalization. The substantial increase in tubal infertility that follows perforation in young women is also avoidable by early appendectomy.

Andersson RE et al: Repeated clinical and laboratory examinations in patients with an equivocal diagnosis of appendicitis. World J Surg 2000;24:479.

Andersson RE et al. Diagnostic value of disease history, clinical presentation, and inflammatory parameters of appendicitis. World J Surg 1999;23:133.

Andersson RE et al. Why does the clinical diagnosis fail in suspected appendicitis? Eur J Surg 2000;166:796.

Asfar S et al. Would measurement of C-reactive protein reduce the rate of negative exploration for acute appendicitis? J R Coll Edinb 2000;45:21.

Bilik R et al: Is abdominal cavity culture of any value in appendicitis? Am J Surg 1998;175:267.

Blomqvist PG et al. Mortality after appendectomy in Sweden, 1987–1996. Ann Surg 2001;233:455.

Carr NJ: The pathology of acute appendicitis. Ann Diagn Pathol 2000;4:46.

Gronroos JM et al: Leucocyte count and C-reactive protein in the diagnosis of acute appendicitis. Br J Surg 1999;86:501.

Kokoska ER et al. Perforated appendicitis in children: risk factors for the development of complications. Surgery 1998; 124:619.

Kraemer M et al. Perforating appendicitis: is it a separate disease? Acute Abdominal Pain Study Group. Eur J Surg 1999; 165:473.

Lee SL et al: Computed tomography and ultrasonography do not improve and may delay the diagnosis and treatment of acute appendicitis. Arch Surg 2001;136:556.

Long KH et al. A prospective randomized comparison of laparoscopic appendectomy with open appendectomy: clinical and economic analyses. Surgery 2001;129:390.

Mourad J et al: Appendicitis in pregnancy: new information that contradicts long-held clinical beliefs. Am J Obstet Gynecol 2000;182:1027.

Rucinski J et al. Gangrenous and perforated appendicitis: a meta-analytic study of 2532 patients indicates that the incision should be closed primarily. Surgery 2000;127:136.

Schuler JG et al. Is there a role for abdominal computed tomographic scans in appendicitis? Arch Surg 1998;133:373.

Stroman DL et al. The role of computed tomography in the diagnosis of acute appendicitis. Am J Surg 1999;178:485.

Watters JM et al. The influence of age on the severity of peritonitis. Can J Surg 1996;39:142.

Weyant MJ et al Interpretation of computed tomography does not correlate with laboratory or pathologic findings in surgically confirmed acute appendicitis. Surgery 2000;128:145.

CHRONIC APPENDICITIS

Chronic abdominal pain is a common problem, and when the complaints are confined to the right lower quadrant, the question of chronic appendicitis is usually raised. Patients with genuine chronic appendicitis experience pain that lasts for 3 weeks or more. The history usually includes an acute illness at some time in the past, compatible with acute appendicitis, which was managed nonoperatively. On examination, the appendix is chronically inflamed or fibrotic. The symptoms resolve with appendectomy.

Chronic intermittent pain in the right lower quadrant is most often caused by something other than appendicitis, such as Crohn's disease or renal disease. Barium x-rays are sometimes helpful, particularly in children. In many patients, the diagnosis is not obvious. Appendectomy relieves symptoms occasionally, but laparotomy for chronic abdominal pain is generally unproductive in the absence of objective findings (eg, localized tenderness, palpable mass, leukocytosis).

Mattei P et al: Chronic and recurrent appendicitis are uncommon entities often misdiagnosed. J Am Coll Surg 1994;178:385.

TUMORS OF THE APPENDIX

Benign tumors, including carcinoids, were found in 4.6% of 71,000 human appendix specimens examined microscopically. Benign neoplasms may arise from any cellular element and are usually incidental findings. Occasionally, a neoplasm obstructs the appendiceal lumen and produces acute appendicitis. No treatment other than appendectomy is indicated.

Malignant Tumors

Primary malignant tumors were found in 1.4% of appendices in the same large series. Carcinoid and argentaffin tumors comprise the majority of appendiceal cancers, and the appendix is the commonest location of carcinoid tumors of the gastrointestinal tract. Carcinoid tumors of the appendix are usually benign, but the uncommon tumor that is over 2 cm in diameter may exhibit malignant behavior. Most appendiceal carcinoids are found in the tip of the organ, while a few are at the base. About half of these tumors are discovered during an appendectomy for acute appendicitis, and the remainder are incidental findings. Lesions less than 2 cm in diameter invade the appendiceal wall in 25% of cases, but only 3% metastasize to lymph nodes, and hepatic metastases and the carcinoid syndrome are truly rare. Appendectomy alone is adequate treatment unless the lymph nodes are visibly involved, the tumor is more than 2 cm in diameter, mucinous elements are present in the tumor (adenocarcinoid), or the mesoappendix or base of the cecum is invaded. Right hemicolectomy is recommended for these more aggressive lesions.

Adenocarcinoma of the colonic type can arise in the appendix and spread rapidly to regional lymph nodes or implant on ovaries or other peritoneal surfaces. Ten percent of patients have widespread metastases when first seen. Adenocarcinoma is virtually never diagnosed preoperatively; about half of cases present as acute appendicitis, and 15% have formed appendiceal abscesses. Right hemicolectomy should be performed if disease is localized to the appendix and regional lymph nodes. The 5-year survival rate is 60% after right hemicolectomy and only 20% after appendectomy alone, but the latter group includes patients with distant metastases at the time of diagnosis.

Mucocele

Mucocele of the appendix is a cystic, dilated appendix filled with mucin. Simple mucocele is not a neoplasm and results from chronic obstruction of the proximal lumen, usually by fibrous tissue. If the appendiceal contents distally are sterile, mucous cells continue to secrete until distention of the lumen thins the wall and interferes with nutrition of the lining cells; histologically, simple mucocele is lined by flattened cuboidal epithelium or no epithelium at all. Simple mucocele is cured by appendectomy.

Less commonly, mucocele is caused by a neoplasm—cystadenoma, or adenocarcinoma grade 1 in the older terminology. This lesion may arise de novo or (perhaps) in a preceding simple mucocele. In cystadenoma, the lumen is filled with mucin but the wall is lined by columnar epithelium with papillary projections. Tumor does not infiltrate the appendiceal wall and does not metastasize, although it may recur locally after appendectomy. Cystadenoma is believed to undergo malignant change in some instances. Appendectomy is adequate treatment.

Carr NJ et al: Epithelial noncarcinoid tumors and tumor-like lesions of the appendix. A clinicopathologic study of 184 patients with a multivariate analysis of prognostic factors. Cancer 1995;75:757

Connor SJ et al: Appendiceal tumors: retrospective clinicopathologic analysis of appendiceal tumors from 7,970 appendectomies. Dis Colon Rectum 1998;41:75.

Deans GT et al: Neoplastic lesions of the appendix. Br J Surg 1995; 82:299

Gouzi JL et al: Indications for right hemicolectomy in carcinoid tumors of the appendix. The French Associations for Surgical Research. Surg Gynecol Obstet 1993;176:543

Kim SH et al: Mucocele of the appendix: ultrasonographic and CT findings. Abdom Imaging, 1998;23:292.

Nitecki SS et al: The natural history of surgically treated primary adenocarcinoma of the appendix. Ann Surg 1994;219:51.

Roggo A et al: Carcinoid tumors of the appendix. Ann Surg 1993; 217:385

Soweid AM et al: Diagnosis and management of appendiceal mucoceles. Dig Dis 1998;16:183.

Sugarbaker PH et al: Results of treatment of 385 patients with peritoneal surface spread of appendiceal malignancy. Ann Surg Oncol 1999;6:727.

Small Intestine

30

Andrew A. Shelton, MD, Theodore R. Schrock, MD, & Mark Lane Welton, MD

The small intestine is the portion of the alimentary tract extending from the pylorus to the cecum. The structure, function, and diseases of the duodenum are discussed in Chapter 24; the jejunum and ileum are described in this chapter.

ANATOMY

Gross Anatomy

The small intestine in an adult is 5–6 m long from the ligament of Treitz to the ileocecal valve. The upper two-fifths of the small intestine distal to the duodenum are termed the **jejunum** and the lower three-fifths the **ileum.** There is no sharp demarcation between the jejunum and the ileum; however, as the intestine proceeds distally, the lumen narrows, the mesenteric vascular arcades become more complex, and the circular mucosal folds become shorter and fewer (Figure 30–1). In general, the jejunum resides in the left side of the peritoneal cavity and the ileum occupies the pelvis and right lower quadrant.

The small bowel is attached to the posterior abdominal wall by the mesentery, a reflection from the posterior parietal peritoneum. This peritoneal fold arises along a line originating just to the left of the midline and passing obliquely to the right lower quadrant. Although the mesentery joins the intestine along one side, the peritoneal layer of the mesentery envelops the bowel and is called the visceral peritoneum, or serosa.

The mesentery contains fat, blood vessels, lymphatics, lymph nodes, and nerves. The arterial blood supply to the jejunum and ileum derives from the superior mesenteric artery. Branches within the mesentery anastomose to form arcades (Figure 30–1), and small straight arteries travel from these arcades to enter the mesenteric border of the gut. The antimesenteric border of the intestinal wall is less richly supplied with arterial blood than the mesenteric side, so when blood flow is impaired, the antimesenteric border becomes ischemic first. Venous blood from the small intestine drains into the superior mesenteric vein and then enters the liver through the portal vein.

Submucosal lymphoid aggregates (Peyer's patches) are much more numerous in the ileum than in the jejunum. Lymphatic channels within the mesentery drain through regional lymph nodes and terminate in the cisterna chyli.

Parasympathetic nerves from the right vagus and sympathetic fibers from the greater and lesser splanchnic nerves reach the small intestine through the mesentery. Both types of autonomic nerves contain efferent and afferent fibers, but intestinal pain appears to be mediated by the sympathetic afferents only.

Microscopic Anatomy

The wall of the small intestine consists of four layers: mucosa, submucosa, muscularis, and serosa.

A. MUCOSA

The absorptive surface of the mucosa is multiplied by circular mucosal folds termed plicae circulares (valvulae conniventes) that project into the lumen; they are taller and more numerous in the proximal jejunum than in the distal ileum (Figure 30–1). On the surface of the plicae circulares are delicate villi less than 1 mm in height, each containing a central lacteal, a small artery and vein, and fibers from the muscularis mucosae that lend contractility to the villus. Villi are in turn covered by columnar epithelial cells that have a brush border consisting of microvilli 1 μm in height (Figure 30–2). The presence of villi multiplies the absorptive surface about 8 times, and microvilli increase it another 14–24 times; the total absorptive area of the small intestine is 200–500 m².

The major cell types in the epithelium of the small intestine are absorptive enterocytes, mucous cells, Paneth cells, endocrine cells, and M cells. Absorptive enterocytes are responsible for absorption; they arise from continually proliferating undifferentiated cells in the crypts of Lieberkühn (Figure 30–3) and migrate to the tips of villi over a 3- to 7-day period. Peptide growth factors regulate this process. The life span of enterocytes in humans is 5–6 days.

Mucous cells originate in crypts and migrate to the tips of villi also; mature mucous cells are termed goblet cells. Paneth cells are found only in the crypts; their function is unknown but may be secretory. Endocrine cells have abundant cytoplasmic granules that contain 5-hydroxytryptamine and various peptides. Enterochromaffin cells are the most numerous; N cells (containing neurotensin), L cells (glucagon), and other cells con-

674

Figure 30–1. Blood supply and luminal surface of the small bowel. The arterial arcades of the small intestine increase in number from one or two in the proximal jejunum to four or five in the distal ileum, a finding that helps to distinguish proximal from distal bowel at operation. Plicae circulares are more prominent in the jejunum.

taining motilin and cholecystokinin are also present. M cells are thin membranous cells that cover Peyer's patches. They have the ability to sample luminal antigens such as proteins and microorganisms. Mucosal T lymphocytes of several phenotypes play an important role in mucosal cell-mediated immunity. Mast cells in the lamina propria are closely applied to nerve fibers, thus providing an anatomic basis for communication between these two structures in disease processes such as inflammation.

B. OTHER LAYERS

The submucosa is a fibroelastic layer containing blood vessels and nerves. Submucosa is the strongest component of bowel wall and must be included in intestinal sutures. The muscularis consists of an inner circular layer and an outer longitudinal coat of smooth muscle. The serosa is the outermost covering of the intestine.

Dignass AU et al: Fibroblast growth factors modulate intestinal epithelial cell growth and maturation. Gastroenterology 1994; 106:1254.

Kagnoff MF: Immunology of the intestinal tract. Gastroenterology 1993;105:1275.

PHYSIOLOGY

The principal function of the small intestine is absorption.

Motility

Smooth muscles of the small intestine undergo spontaneous oscillations of membrane potential; these cyclic changes are termed pacesetter potentials or electrical control activity. Each segment of intestine has a characteristic frequency of pacesetter potentials; it is highest proximally, and it decreases progressively from duodenum to ileum. In intact intestine, higher-frequency pacesetter potentials can drive adjacent distal intestine so that both segments have the same frequency (said to be phase-locked). In humans, the duodenum determines the frequency of pacesetter potentials for the entire small intestine.

As pacesetter potentials spread distally, they bring the onset of action potentials and muscular contractions into phase. One type of muscular contraction (nonpropagating, or stationary) causes segmentation, which mixes chyme with digestive juices, repeatedly exposes the mixture to the absorptive surface, and moves chyme slowly in an aboral direction. Another type of muscular contraction (propagating) is peristaltic. Normal peristalsis is a short, weak propulsive movement that travels at about 1 cm/s for a distance of 10–15 cm before subsiding. Mean transit time for a solid meal is 4 hours from mouth to colon.

The enteric nervous system is a dominant regulator of all aspects of motility of the small intestine. The two major types of nerve plexuses in the enteric nervous system are the myenteric plexus, mainly responsible for control of peristaltic activity, and the submucosal plexus, which regulates secretion and absorption. The enteric nervous system contains four types of neurons: motor, secretory, sensory, and interneurons (which provide communication between neurons in the intestinal wall). Neurotransmitters found in the enteric nervous system include cholinergic, adrenergic, serotonergic, and peptidergic substances. Among the numerous peptides secreted by neurons in the enteric nervous system are cholecystokinin, vasoactive intestinal peptide (VIP), somatostatin, neurotensin, enkephalin, galanin, and substance P. In general, intestinal action potentials and muscular contractions are stimulated by substance P and galanin, and motility is inhibited by VIP, somatostatin, neurotensin, and enkephalin. Nitric oxide medi-

Figure 30–2. Scanning electron microscopic photo of small intestinal villi from the human terminal ileum. (Reduced from × 320.) **Inset:** Detail of a villous surface showing a mucous (goblet) cell surrounded by polygonal columnar cells. (Reduced from × 2100.) Epithelial cell borders are visible (white arrows). The pebbled columnar cell surface represents closely packed microvilli seen end-on. (Courtesy of Robert L. Owen, MD, and Albert L. Jones, MD.)

ates neural inhibition in circular muscle of human small intestine.

Peristalsis is initiated by stretch of the intestinal wall by a food bolus, and a dual reflex is set in motion. The circular smooth muscle orad to the bolus contracts; this reflex is mediated by enteric neurons with acetylcholine and substance P as neurotransmitters. Simultaneous relaxation of the intestinal circular muscle below is mediated by enteric neurons using VIP as the neurotransmitter. Relaxation of gut sphincters, including the ileocecal valve, is mediated by VIP, and contraction of sphincters is effected by cholinergic or adrenergic neurons (or both).

The interdigestive migrating myoelectric complex (MMC) originates every 1½–2 hours in the stomach and duodenum of fasting mammals. It is an aborally progressive front of action potentials and muscular contractions consisting of three successive phases: a quiescent phase 1 with slow waves only, phase 2 with in-creasing action potential activity, and phase 3 with action potentials on every slow wave. The MMC progresses aborally until it reaches the colon, and then another burst of potentials and contractions begins proximally. The MMC has been called the "intestinal housekeeper" because it cleans up remnants of the preceding meal and gets rid of microorganisms that escaped destruction by gastric acid. The MMC is controlled by the enteric nervous system; motilin and 5-hydroxytryptamine may play regulatory roles. The MMC is abolished by ingestion of food, and some features are altered by major abdominal operations or peritonitis.

Numerous peptides have been found to act in the brain to alter gastrointestinal motility. Hypothalamic hormones (eg, corticotropin-releasing factor and thyrotropin-releasing hormone), calcitonin, and nearly all of the enteric nervous system neurotransmitters have central nervous system actions that affect motility, at

Figure 30–3. Schematic representation of villi and crypts of Lieberkühn.

least in animals. Exogenous opioids, including codeine and loperamide, exert antidiarrheal action by inhibition or disruption of the pattern of circular muscle contraction; some of these effects may be mediated in the central nervous system. The vagus plays an important role in many of these phenomena.

Paralytic (adynamic) ileus is routine after abdominal operations, and it also accompanies inflammatory conditions in the abdomen, intestinal ischemia, ureteral colic, pelvic fractures, and back injuries. Abdominal surgery abolishes gastrointestinal motility for a period of time that varies with the type of operation; the MMC returns within 3 hours after cholecystectomy, but it may take up to 6 days following colon resection. The small intestine recovers in 12–24 hours, and the colon may not regain normal motility until the sixth postoperative day. The clinical manifestations of postoperative ileus do not correlate well with the myoelectric parameters, however, and the pathophysiology of ileus remains incompletely understood. Recent data suggest that corticotropin-releasing factor is an important mediator of postoperative ileus.

Orocecal transit time is an important indicator of small bowel function. Transit may be accelerated in patients with diarrhea and delayed in constipation; a variety of disease states are responsible. Orocecal transit time can be measured by the lactulose breath hydrogen test. An ingested solution of lactulose reaches the cecum in about 90 minutes; colonic fermentation of lactulose produces hydrogen, which is detected in the breath. Several techniques of gamma scintigraphy, including the use of isotopically labeled pellets, are alternative methods of estimating small bowel transit time.

Digestion, Secretion, & Absorption

With a few exceptions (eg, iron, calcium), the normal small intestine absorbs indiscriminately without regard to body composition. Absorption of fat, carbohydrate, and protein is just as complete in the obese patient as in the slender individual. The enteric nervous system regulates secretion and absorption in the small intestine; VIP is one mediator, and neuropeptide Y may be another.

A. WATER AND ELECTROLYTES

Ingested fluid and salivary, gastric, biliary, pancreatic, and intestinal secretions present a total of 5–9 L of water to the absorptive surface of the small intestine each day, and 1–2 L are discharged from the ileum into the colon. Water is absorbed throughout the intestine, but the major site of absorption after a meal is in the upper tract.

The net flow of water and electrolytes across the intestinal mucosa is equal to the difference between absorption and secretion. The villi are mainly absorbing structures, and secretion of water and electrolytes is localized to the crypts. Much of the transfer of water and small solutes occurs via paracellular "shunt" pathways. The intercellular tight junctions between cells are actually rather loose, and it is through these "pores" that water moves passively in response to osmotic and hydrostatic pressures in the lumen and in the interstitial fluid. The pores are larger in the jejunum (0.7–0.9 nm) than in the ileum (0.3–0.4 nm). Hypertonic solutions in the duodenum and upper jejunum are rapidly brought into osmotic equilibrium with blood, and as the osmotic pressure of luminal contents is increased further by breakdown of large molecules into smaller ones, still more water enters the lumen. Net absorption of water accompanies active transport of ions and small molecules such as glucose and amino acids. If the lumen contains nonabsorbable solute, water is retained to maintain isotonicity.

Three mechanisms are responsible for sodium and chloride absorption in the small intestine: (1) active electrogenic transport of sodium, which establishes an electrical gradient for passive absorption of chloride, mostly through the paracellular pathway; (2) sodium absorption directly coupled to the absorption of water-soluble organic solutes such as hexoses, amino acids, and triglycerides, with passive absorption of chloride; and (3) neutral sodium chloride cotransport, in which a carrier at the mucosal membrane mediates the one-for-one entry of both ions into the cell. The ileum has low permeability to chloride, so that active absorption processes are needed for chloride in that part of the gut.

Potassium diffuses passively along electrical and concentration gradients. Calcium diffuses passively and also is actively transported, a process stimulated by vitamin D. Calcium absorption is most efficient in the duodenum, but because intestinal contents are in the jejunum and ileum longer, most calcium is absorbed in these areas. Magnesium is absorbed by all segments of the intestine, but relatively poorly. Iron is absorbed in the duodenum and jejunum, primarily as the ferrous ion.

Bicarbonate is absorbed by secretion of hydrogen ions in exchange for sodium ions; one bicarbonate ion is released into the interstitial fluid for every hydrogen ion secreted, and CO_2 is generated in the intestinal lumen. Phosphate is absorbed in all portions of the small bowel.

Epithelial transport of water and electrolytes is under partial control of the enteric nervous system. Ingestion of a meal increases the magnitude of jejunal water and electrolyte absorption by neuroendocrine mechanisms that have not been clarified. Intramural nervous reflexes elicited by luminal stimuli increase fluid secretion from the crypts. The afferent part of these reflexes is not well understood, but acetylcholine and perhaps substance P and VIP are secretory neurotransmitters on the efferent side. Absorption and secretion are influenced by other polypeptides such as somatostatin, corticosteroids, prostaglandins, neuropeptide YY, cAMP, various drugs, and bacterial toxins.

B. CARBOHYDRATE

The polysaccharides starch and glycogen and the disaccharides sucrose and lactose comprise about half the calories ingested by humans. Digestion of starch is begun by salivary amylase and is completed by pancreatic amylase in the duodenum and upper jejunum. The products of hydrolysis are further hydrolyzed by contact with enzymes contained in the brush border of intestinal epithelial cells. The monosaccharides glucose, galactose, and fructose are actively transported against a concentration gradient by a carrier-mediated mechanism that is dependent on and coupled to the absorption of sodium. Monosaccharides are delivered directly into portal blood from the intestinal mucosa.

Although the entire small intestine has the capacity for carbohydrate digestion and absorption, under normal circumstances most absorption of monosaccharides occurs in the duodenum and proximal jejunum. About 10% of dietary starch passes unabsorbed into the colon.

Fiber is insoluble matrix substance of plant cells and is mostly indigestible by human enzymes. It is composed of the carbohydrates cellulose and hemicellulose and the noncarbohydrate lignin. Dietary fiber increases the osmotic load to the distal small intestine and colon and therefore increases stool mass.

C. PROTEIN

Protein is denatured and partially digested in the stomach, but these steps are not essential. Pancreatic enzymes digest protein to form free amino acids and oligopeptides; oligopeptides are attacked by carboxypeptidases and aminopeptidases in the brush border, liberating amino acids, dipeptides, and tripeptides. Amino acids are absorbed by means of an active, carrier-mediated transport mechanism. Dipeptides and tripeptides are actively absorbed into columnar cells, where they are hydrolyzed completely to constituent amino acids. More than 80% of protein absorption occurs in the proximal 100 cm of jejunum. Absorption of ingested protein is virtually complete, and the protein excreted in feces is derived from bacteria, desquamated cells, and mucoproteins.

Important changes occur in the intestine during critical illness, eg, following trauma or abdominal surgery. The intestinal epithelial barrier to absorption of bacteria and endotoxins may be compromised, permitting translocation of bacteria into the circulation. Furthermore, glutamine extraction from the circulation by the small intestine is impaired in septic patients. Glutamine is the preferred fuel for oxidative metabolism by the enterocyte, and diminished uptake of this mucosal nutrient may be significant. In stressed states, glutamine deficiency is associated with mucosal atrophy.

D. FAT

Dietary fat is largely in the form of triglycerides, which are water-insoluble oil droplets until attacked by pancreatic lipase. Colipase, a protein in pancreatic juice, helps lipase adhere to the surface of these oil droplets as the triglycerides are partially hydrolyzed to fatty acids and 2-monoglycerides. These products of digestion are also water-insoluble, and their efficient absorption depends on the presence of bile acids. When the concentration of bile acids exceeds a certain level (the critical micellar concentration), they spontaneously aggregate to form micelles. Bile acids in micelles are arranged with the fat-soluble portion of the molecule toward the center of the aggregate and the water-soluble portion at the periphery; hydrophobic molecules such as fatty acids, monoglycerides, cholesterol, and fat-soluble vitamins are carried in the centers of the micelles.

Micelles release monoglycerides and fatty acids to enter the mucosal cells, where triglycerides are resynthesized, aggregated with phospholipid and cholesterol, and delivered to the lymph as chylomicrons. Medium-chain triglyceride is a synthetic substance that is hydrolyzed to water-soluble fatty acids which do not require bile acids for absorption. Also, these fatty acids are not reesterified to triglycerides in the mucosal cells; they pass directly into portal blood.

Normally, most of the ingested fat is digested and absorbed in the duodenum and proximal jejunum. Conjugated bile acids are actively absorbed in the distal ileum and returned via portal blood to the liver, where they again are secreted into the bile. Disease or resection of the terminal ileum disrupts this enterohepatic circulation, and increased amounts of bile acids enter the colon, where they induce net secretion of water and electrolytes and cause diarrhea (cholerrheic diarrhea). Malabsorbed fatty acids contribute to diarrhea by an effect similar to that of castor oil.

E. VITAMINS

Vitamin B_{12} (cyanocobalamin) is a water-soluble cobalt compound that requires a special mechanism for absorption, because of its large molecular weight. Dietary vitamin B_{12} complexes with intrinsic factor, a mucoprotein secreted by the gastric parietal cells. The complex dissociates at the surface of cells in the distal ileum, and vitamin B_{12} enters the cells, perhaps by receptor-mediated endocytosis. Folic acid, thiamin, and ascorbic acid are also absorbed by active transport. Other water-soluble vitamins diffuse passively across the mucosa.

Fat-soluble vitamins—notably vitamins A, D, E, and K—are dissolved in mixed micelles and absorbed like other lipids. Since they are totally nonpolar lipids, the absence of bile seriously impairs their absorption.

Agarwal R, Afzalpurkar R, Fordtran JS: Pathophysiology of potassium absorption and secretion by the human intestine. Gastroenterology 1994;107:548.

Ahluwalia NK et al: Human small intestinal contractions and aboral traction forces during fasting and after feeding. Gut 1994;35:625.

Ducerf C, Cuchamp C, Pouyet M: Postoperative electromyographic profile in human jejunum. Ann Surg 1992;215:237.

Fine KD et al: Mechanism by which glucose stimulates the passive absorption of small solutes by the human jejunum in vivo. Gastroenterology 1994;107:389.

Frantzides CT et al: Small bowel myoelectric activity in peritonitis. Am J Surg 1993;165:681.

Gleeson D: Acid-base transport systems in gastrointestinal epithelia. Gut 1992;33:1134.

Gorard DA, Libby GW, Farthing MJG: 5-Hydroxytryptamine and human small intestinal motility: effect of inhibiting 5-hydroxytryptamine reuptake. Gut 1994;35:496.

Inoue Y, Copeland EM, Souba WW: Growth hormone enhances amino acid uptake by the human small intestine. Ann Surg 1994;219:715.

Otterson MF, Sarr MG: Normal physiology of small intestinal motility. Surg Clin North Am 1993;73:1173.

Sanderson IR, Walker WA: Uptake and transport of macromolecules by the intestine: possible role in clinical disorders (an update). Gastroenterology 1993;104:622.

Stark ME et al: Nitric oxide mediates inhibitory nerve input in human and canine jejunum. Gastroenterology 1993;104:398.

von der Ohe MR, Camilleri M: Measurement of small bowel and colonic transit: indications and methods. Mayo Clin Proc 1992;67:1169.

BLIND LOOP SYNDROME

The normal concentration of bacteria in the small intestine is about 10^5/mL. Mechanisms that limit bacterial populations include the continual flow of luminal contents, resulting from peristalsis, the interdigestive migrating myoelectric complex, gastric acidity, local effects of immunoglobulins, and the prevention of reflux of colonic contents by the ileocecal valve. Disturbance of any of these mechanisms can lead to bacterial overgrowth and the blind loop (contaminated small bowel, intestinal bacterial overgrowth) syndrome. Strictures, diverticula, fistulas, or blind (poorly emptying) segments of intestine are anatomic lesions that cause stagnation and permit bacterial proliferation. In many patients, stasis of intestinal contents is the result of a functional abnormality of motility (eg, scleroderma). Bacterial overgrowth is observed in patients with immunodeficiency syndromes.

Steatorrhea, diarrhea, megaloblastic anemia, and malnutrition are the hallmarks of the blind loop syndrome. Steatorrhea is the consequence of bacterial deconjugation and dehydroxylation of bile salts in the proximal small bowel. Deconjugated bile salts have a higher critical micellar concentration, and micelle formation is inadequate to solubilize ingested fat in preparation for absorption. The presence of partially digested triglycerides in the distal ileum inhibits jejunal motility ("ileal brake" reflex); nevertheless, the unabsorbed fatty acids enter the colon, where they increase net secretion of water and electrolytes, and diarrhea results. Hypocalcemia occurs because calcium is bound to unabsorbed fatty acids in the intestinal lumen. Macrocytic anemia is due to malabsorption of vitamin B_{12}, largely because of binding of the vitamin by anaerobic bacteria. Malabsorption of carbohydrate and protein is due partly to bacterial catabolism and partly to impaired absorption of these nutrients because of direct damage to the small intestinal mucosa. All of these mechanisms contribute to malnutrition in blind loop syndrome.

Quantitative culture of upper intestinal aspirates is valuable if properly performed; bacterial counts of more than 10^5 per milliliter are generally abnormal. Endoscopic biopsies of duodenum can be helpful in patients with suspected small intestinal malabsorption. Laboratory studies reveal impaired absorption of orally administered vitamin B_{12} (Schilling test), D-xylose, and ^{14}C triolein. Fecal fat measurement is an obsolete procedure. A large variety of breath tests have been studied, but most have proved to be unreliable. The ^{14}C-D-xylose breath test is the best of these methods available at present. Anaerobic bacteria in the small bowel metabolize xylose, releasing $^{14}CO_2$, which is detected in the breath.

Surgical treatment of the underlying neoplasm, fistula, blind loop, diverticula, or other lesion is carried out whenever possible. A majority of patients do not have a problem that is amenable to surgical correction, however, and treatment consists of broad-spectrum antibiotics and drugs to control diarrhea. It may be necessary to use different antibiotics in sequence, guided by culture results and response to therapy. Damage to enterocytes appears to be reversible with treatment. Octreotide (somatostatin analog) may reduce bacterial overgrowth and improved abdominal symptoms in patients with scleroderma according to a recent report.

Hughes JP et al: Scintigraphic demonstration of a blind loop following surgery for Crohn's disease: the value of Tc-99m HMPAO white cell scanning. Clin Nucl Med 1994;19:469.

Ladas SD et al: Effect of forceps size and mode of orientation on endoscopic small bowel biopsy evaluation. Gastrointest Endosc 1994;40:51.

Patel MC et al: Blind loop syndrome: diagnosis by In-111-labeled leukocyte scintigraphy. Clin Nucl Med 1999;24:623.

Rubesin SE, Rubin RA, Herlinger H: Small bowel malabsorption: clinical and radiologic perspectives. How we see it. Radiology 1992;184:297.

Strocchi A et al: Detection of malabsorption of low doses of carbohydrate: accuracy of various breath H_2 criteria. Gastroenterology 1993;105:1404.

Takahashi M et al: Use of the conjugate of disulphated ursodeoxycholic acid with *p*-aminobenzoic acid for the detection of intestinal bacteria. Gut 1993;34:823.

SHORT BOWEL SYNDROME

 ESSENTIALS OF DIAGNOSIS

- *Extensive small bowel resection.*
- *Diarrhea.*
- *Steatorrhea.*
- *Malnutrition.*

General Considerations

The absorptive capacity of the small intestine is normally far in excess of need. The short bowel syndrome may develop after extensive resection of the small intestine for trauma, mesenteric thrombosis, regional enteritis, radiation enteropathy, strangulated small bowel obstruction, or neoplasm. Necrotizing enterocolitis and congenital atresia are the most common pediatric causes.

The ability of a patient to maintain nutrition after massive small bowel resection depends on the extent and site of resection, the presence or absence of the ileocecal valve and the colon, the absorptive function of the intestinal remnant, adaptation of remaining bowel, and the nature of the underlying disease process and its complications. When 3 m or less of the small intestine remain, serious nutritional abnormalities develop. With 2 m or less remaining, function is clinically impaired in most patients, and many patients with 1 m or less of normal bowel require parenteral nutrition at home indefinitely. Some patients with a very short small bowel are net absorbers, and others are net secretors—ie, they put out more intestinal fluid than they take orally.

If the jejunum is resected, the ileum is able to take over most of its absorptive function. Because transport of bile salts, vitamin B_{12}, and cholesterol is localized to the ileum, resection of this region is poorly tolerated (Figure 30–4). Bile salt malabsorption causes diarrhea, and steatorrhea occurs if 100 cm or more of distal ileum is resected. Abdominal gamma counting after oral administration of 23-selena-25-homocholyltaurine (^{75}SeHCAT) is a test of bile acid absorption in the distal ileum. Steatorrhea and diarrhea are more pronounced if the ileocecal valve is removed because this sphincter retards transit into the colon; it also helps prevent reflux of bacteria from the colon. Blind loop syndrome due to bacterial overgrowth in the shortened small bowel (see above) compounds the problems. Patients who undergo colectomy in addition to extensive small bowel resection are among the most difficult to manage.

Calcium oxalate urinary tract calculi form in 7–10% of patients who have extensive ileal resection (or disease) and an intact colon. This condition, called **enteric hyperoxaluria,** results from excessive absorption of oxalate from the colon. Two synergistic mechanisms are responsible: (1) Unabsorbed fatty acids combine with calcium, preventing the formation of insoluble calcium oxalate and allowing oxalate to remain available for absorption. (2) Unabsorbed fatty acids and bile acids increase the permeability of the colon to oxalate.

D-Lactic acidosis may result from colonic fermentation of unabsorbed carbohydrate; symptoms of confusion, loss of memory, slurred speech, unsteady gait, and inappropriate behavior resemble those associated with alcoholic intoxication. Treatment includes correction of the acidosis with bicarbonate infusion, thiamine replacement, and antibiotics to reduce colonic flora.

Generalized transport of water, electrolytes, sugars, proteins, fats, vitamins; most absorption occurs proximally.

Localized transport of bile salts, cholesterol, vitamin B_{12}; absorption in ileum only.

RESECTION OF JEJUNUM

Generalized transport work load assumed by ileum. Localized transport unaffected. No malabsorption.

RESECTION OF ILEUM

Generalized transport continues. Localized transport lost. Malabsorption of vitamin B_{12}, cholesterol, bile salts, and fats.

Figure 30–4. The consequences of complete resection of jejunum or ileum are predictable in part from the loss of regionally localized transport processes.

Some patients develop gastric hypersecretion after extensive small bowel resection. It is more marked after proximal resection, and it improves with time. The outpouring of gastric juice may damage the mucosa of the upper intestine, inactivate lipase and trypsin by lowering intraluminal pH, and present an excessive solute load to the intestinal remnant. The increased acid production results from loss of inhibitory hormones normally secreted by the small intestine. Elevated basal and postprandial serum gastrin levels have been detected in some cases.

Clinical Course

During the immediate postoperative period, more than 2 L of daily fluid and electrolyte losses from diarrhea are characteristic. The diarrhea is less severe after a few weeks, and eventually a reasonably normal existence is possible in most cases. The progression of a patient from strict dependence on intravenous feeding to nutritional maintenance by oral intake is possible because of intestinal **adaptation,** a compensatory increase of absorptive capacity in the intestinal remnant. The mucosa becomes hyperplastic, the villi lengthen and the crypts become deeper, the wall thickens, and the intestine elongates and dilates. The intensity of these responses is proportionate to the amount of intestine removed, the segment remaining (greater after proximal than after distal small bowel resection), and the presence of a luminal stream. Nutritional support is essential, and although nutrition must be provided intravenously at first, food in the lumen of the intestine is required for full adaptation. Short-chain fatty acids and long-chain triglycerides, sugars, and proteins are all important trophic nutrients. Glutamine is the principal fuel utilized by the small intestine, and gut glutamine extraction is increased in the first week after massive small bowel resection in animals, but it is not clear whether glutamine needs to be provided to patients to aid in adaptation. Circulating peptide factors no doubt are important. Enteroglucagon, epidermal growth factor (urogastrone), neurotensin, and insulin-like growth factors are implicated as trophic agents, and somatostatin and transforming growth factor-β (TGFβ) may play inhibitory roles.

Treatment

A. General Measures

Treatment of severe short bowel syndrome may be divided into three stages:

1. Stage 1 (intravenous feeding)—During this stage, which lasts 1–3 months, diarrhea is massive and patients should receive nothing by mouth. Careful intravenous fluid and electrolyte therapy and parenteral nutrition must be given. Catheter sepsis is a common complication in this setting. Other important measures include reduction of gastric secretion with intravenous H_2 blockers, control of diarrhea (eg, with loperamide), and protection of perianal skin from irritation. Somatostatin has limited value in reduction of fecal output.

2. Stage 2 (intravenous and oral feeding)—Oral feedings should not be initiated until diarrhea subsides to less than 2.5 L/d. Intravenous nutrition should continue while oral intake begins. Oral rehydration solutions that are used for diarrheal diseases in developing countries are applicable to short bowel syndrome as well. An oral solution of sodium and potassium salts and glucose takes advantage of the phenomenon of cotransport whereby sodium ions are absorbed with the hexose molecules across the intestinal epithelium. Other liquid diets are best tolerated if they are isotonic. Liquid polymeric diets are the next step, and then a more liberal selection of food is allowed. A diet with normal fat content is more palatable and just as effective as a low-fat diet.

Milk may aggravate diarrhea, because total intestinal lactase activity is severely reduced after extensive resection; cheese is tolerated because lactose has been digested in this product. There may be some advantage in making breakfast the largest meal of the day, because as a result of gallbladder filling during the overnight fast, morning may be the time when the greatest amount of bile salts are present in the proximal intestine.

3. Stage 3 (complete oral feeding)—After a few months, complete dependence on oral intake may be expected in patients with 1–2 m of remaining small bowel, but full adaptation may require up to 2 years. Maintenance of body weight at levels 20% or more below normal, acceptable bowel habits, and return to productive life are reasonable expectations in many patients. Chronic parenteral nutrition at home is required if oral intake is not tolerated.

Patients with extensive ileal resection require parenteral vitamin B_{12} (1000 μg intramuscularly every 2–3 months) for life. Hyperoxaluria often can be prevented by a diet low in fat and oxalate; supplementary oral calcium or citrate may be helpful. An organic hydrocolloid charged with calcium that has the ability to bind oxalate and reduce urinary oxalate excretion is under study. Oral cholestyramine to minimize diarrhea is usually rejected by patients; loperamide (Imodium) is well tolerated. Pancreatic enzyme supplements may reduce diarrhea also. Deficiencies in magnesium, vitamins D, A, and K, and water-soluble vitamins should be prevented. Osteomalacia is common, and x-rays are falsely negative in many cases; the diagnosis can only be made by bone biopsy. Blind loop syndrome may require treatment. H_2 receptor antagonists or omeprazole reduce acid secretion and improve absorption in the early stages but probably are not needed long-term. The incidence of cholelithiasis is increased in patients with short bowel syndrome, and symptoms should be investigated. Interestingly, the stones may be composed of pigment rather than cholesterol.

B. Adjunctive Surgical Procedures

Surgical procedures to slow intestinal transit, reduce gastric acidity, or increase the absorptive surface are not recommended routinely. Reversed segments, recirculating loops, and construction of valve mechanisms have been tried in the hope of slowing transit and improving absorption. None of these methods have a clearly established role. By enhancing bacterial growth, damaging additional bowel, and obstructing the intestine, they are likely to make matters worse. An implantable pacing unit to slow intestinal transit is under study. Gastric hyperacidity is controlled by H_2 receptor antagonists, and operation is rarely necessary for this problem. A method of lengthening the small intestine by longitudinal division of the bowel and its mesentery has been described for certain pediatric situations. In vivo growth of neomucosa on patches of colonic serosa that are sutured into the wall of the small intestine is promising but experimental. Transplantation of the small intestine has not reached the stage of clinical utility.

Chris Anderson-Hill D, Heimburger DC: Medical management of the difficult patient with short-bowel syndrome. Nutrition 1993;9:536.

Georgeson K et al: Sequential intestinal lengthening procedures for refractory short bowel syndrome. J Pediatr Surg 1994;29:316.

Hines OJ et al: Up-regulation of Na⁺, K⁺ adenosine triphosphatase after massive intestinal resection. Surgery 1994;116:401.

Inoue Y et al: Effect of total parenteral nutrition on amino acid and glucose transport by the human small intestine. Ann Surg 1993;217:604.

Jeppesen PB: Glucagon-like peptide 2 improves nutrient absorption and nugtritional sgtatus in short-bowel patients with no colon. Gastroengterology 2001;120:806.

Ko TC et al: Glutamine is essential for epidermal growth factor-stimulated intestinal cell proliferation. Surgery 1993;114:147.

Kurkchubasche AG, Rowe MI, Smith SD: Adaptation in short-bowel syndrome: reassessing old limits. J Pediatr Surg 1993;28:1069.

Nightingale JM, Lennard-Jones JE: The short bowel syndrome: what's new and old? Dig Dis 1993;11:12.

Nightingale JMD et al: Oral salt supplements to compensate for jejunostomy losses: comparison of sodium chloride capsules, glucose electrolyte solution, and glucose polymer electrolyte solution. Gut 1992;33:759.

Playford RJ et al: Effect of luminal growth factor preservation on intestinal growth. Lancet 1993;341:843.

Rodriguez DJ, Clevenger FW: Successful enteral refeeding after massive small bowel resection. West J Med 1993;159:192.

Shanbhogue LKR, Molenaar JC: Short bowel syndrome: metabolic and surgical management. Br J Surg 1994;81:486.

Thompson JS: Surgical considerations in the short bowel syndrome. Surg Gynecol Obstet 1993;176:89.

van der Hulst RRWJ et al: Glutamine and the preservation of gut integrity. Lancet 1993;341:1363.

Veenendaal RA et al: Clinical aspects of small-bowel transplantation. Scand J Gastroenterol Suppl 2000;(232):65.

OBSTRUCTION OF THE SMALL INTESTINE

 ESSENTIALS OF DIAGNOSIS

Complete proximal obstruction:

- *Vomiting.*
- *Abdominal discomfort.*
- *Abnormal oral contrast x-rays.*

Complete mid or distal obstruction:

- *Colicky abdominal pain.*
- *Vomiting.*
- *Abdominal distention.*
- *Constipation-obstipation.*
- *Peristaltic rushes.*
- *Dilated small bowel on x-ray.*

General Considerations

Obstruction is the most common surgical disorder of the small intestine.

Mechanical obstruction implies a physical barrier that impedes aboral progress of intestinal contents; it may be complete or partial. **Simple obstruction** occludes the lumen only; **strangulation obstruction** impairs the blood supply also and leads to necrosis of the intestinal wall. Most simple obstructions occur at only one point. Closed loop obstruction, in which the lumen is occluded in at least two places (eg, in a volvulus), is commonly associated with strangulation. Ileus is a term whose definition includes mechanical obstruction, but in the USA it usually refers to **paralytic ileus** (adynamic ileus), a disorder in which there is neurogenic failure of peristalsis to propel intestinal contents but no mechanical obstruction.

A. ETIOLOGY

1. Adhesions—Adhesions are by far the most common cause of mechanical small bowel obstruction (Table 30–1). Congenital bands are seen in children, but adhesions acquired from abdominal operations or inflammation are much more frequent in adults. Surgical glove dusting powders evoke an inflammatory response and contribute to adhesion formation.

2. Neoplasms—Intrinsic small bowel neoplasms can progressively occlude the lumen or serve as a leading point in intussusception. Symptoms may be intermittent, onset of obstruction is slow, and signs of chronic

Table 30–1. Causes of obstruction of the small intestine in adults.

Causes	Relative Incidence (%)
Adhesions	60
External hernia	10
Neoplasms	20
Intrinsic	3
Extrinsic	17
Miscellaneous	10

anemia are present. Neoplasms extrinsic to small bowel may entrap loops, and strategically situated lesions of the colon—particularly those near the ileocecal valve—may present as small bowel obstruction.

3. Hernia—Incarceration of an external hernia is uncommon since prophylactic repair of hernias became routine. Inguinal, femoral, or umbilical hernias may have been present for years, or the patient may be unaware of the defect before the onset of obstructive symptoms. An incarcerated hernia may be overlooked by the examining surgeon, particularly if the patient is obese or if the hernia is of the femoral type, and a careful search for external hernias must be made during evaluation of every patient with acute abdominal illness. Internal hernias into the obturator foramen, foramen epiploicum (Winslow), or other anatomic defects are rare, but internal herniation is one of several mechanisms by which acquired adhesions produce obstruction. Surgical defects—lateral to an ileostomy, for example—also provide sites for internal herniation of small bowel loops.

4. Intussusception—Invagination of one loop of intestine into another is rarely encountered in adults and is usually caused by a polyp or other intraluminal lesion. Intussusception is more often seen in children; an organic lesion is not required, and the syndrome of colicky pain, passage of blood per rectum, and a palpable mass (the intussuscepted segment) is characteristic.

5. Volvulus—Volvulus results from rotation of bowel loops about a fixed point, often the consequence of congenital anomalies or acquired adhesions. Onset of obstruction is abrupt, and strangulation develops rapidly. Malrotation of the intestine is a cause of volvulus in infants and rarely in adults.

6. Foreign bodies—Bezoars and ingested foreign bodies may pass into the intestine and block the lumen.

7. Gallstone ileus—Passage of a large gallstone into the intestine through a cholecystenteric fistula may produce obstruction of the small bowel. Gallstone ileus is discussed in Chapter 26.

8. Inflammatory bowel disease—Inflammatory bowel disease often causes obstruction when the lumen is narrowed by inflammation or fibrosis of the wall.

9. Stricture—Stricture due to ischemia or radiation injury or surgical trauma can result in mechanical obstruction.

10. Cystic fibrosis—Cystic fibrosis causes chronic partial obstruction of the distal ileum and right colon in adolescents and adults. It is equivalent to meconium ileus in newborns.

11. Hematoma—Hematoma may develop spontaneously in the intestinal wall in a patient taking anticoagulants.

B. PATHOPHYSIOLOGY

The small bowel proximal to a point of obstruction distends with gas and fluid. Swallowed air is the major source of gaseous distention, at least in the early stages, because nitrogen is not well absorbed by mucosa. When bacterial fermentation occurs later on, other gases are produced; the partial pressure of nitrogen within the lumen is lowered, and a gradient for diffusion of nitrogen from blood to lumen is established.

Enormous quantities of fluid from the extracellular space are lost into the gut and from the serosa into the peritoneal cavity. Fluid fills the lumen proximal to the obstruction, because the bidirectional flux of salt and water is disrupted and net secretion is enhanced. Mediator substances (eg, endotoxin, prostaglandins) released from proliferating bacteria in the static luminal contents are responsible. Somatostatin effectively inhibits secretion in animal models of intestinal obstruction, but it has no defined role in humans. Reflexly induced vomiting accentuates the fluid and electrolyte deficit. Hypovolemia leads to multi-organ system failure and is the cause of death in patients with nonstrangulating obstruction.

Audible peristaltic rushes are manifestations of attempts by the small bowel to propel its contents past the obstruction. The vomitus becomes feculent—particularly with distal obstruction—as the illness progresses. Bacterial translocation from lumen to mesenteric nodes and the bloodstream occurs even in simple obstruction. Abdominal distention elevates the diaphragm and impairs respiration, so that pulmonary complications are frequent.

Strangulation is a threat early in the course of closed loop obstruction but must be feared in any complete mechanical obstruction. Incarcerated inguinal hernia and volvulus are examples of obstructing mechanisms that occlude the vascular supply as well as the intestinal lumen. Strangulation rarely if ever results just from progressive distention. Venous drainage is more apt to be interrupted than arterial inflow when the mesentery is trapped. Gangrenous intestine bleeds into the lumen and into the peritoneal cavity, and eventually it perforates. The luminal contents of strangulated intestine are a toxic mixture of bacteria, bacterial products, necrotic tissue, and blood. Some of this fluid may enter the circulation by way of intestinal lymphatics or by absorption from the peritoneal cavity; septic shock is the result.

Clinical Findings

A. SIMPLE OBSTRUCTION

1. Symptoms and signs—(Figure 30–5.) Proximal (high) small bowel obstruction usually presents as profuse vomiting that seldom becomes feculent even in prolonged obstruction. Abdominal pain is variable and often is described as upper abdominal discomfort rather than cramping pain.

Obstruction of the mid or distal small intestine causes cramping periumbilical or poorly localized abdominal pain. Each episode of cramps has a crescendo-decrescendo pattern, lasts for a few seconds to a few minutes, and recurs every few minutes. Between cramps, the patient may be entirely free of pain. Vomiting follows the onset of pain after an interval that varies with the level of obstruction; it may not occur until several hours later. The more distal the obstruction, the more likely it is that vomitus will become feculent. Gas and feces present in the colon may be expelled after the onset of pain, but obstipation always occurs eventually in complete obstruction.

Vital signs may be normal in the early stages, but dehydration is noted with continued loss of fluid and electrolytes. Temperature is normal or mildly elevated. Abdominal distention is minimal to absent in proximal obstruction but is pronounced in more distal obstruction. Peristalsis in dilated loops of small bowel may be visible beneath the abdominal wall in thin patients. Mild tenderness may be elicited. Peristaltic rushes, gurgles, and high-pitched tinkles are audible in coordination with attacks of cramping pain in distal obstruction. Incarcerated hernias should be sought. Rectal examination is usually normal.

2. Laboratory findings—In the early stages, laboratory findings may be normal; with progression of disease, there are hemoconcentration, leukocytosis, and electrolyte abnormalities that depend on the level of obstruction and the severity of dehydration. Serum amylase is often elevated.

3. Imaging studies—Supine and upright plain abdominal films reveal a ladder-like pattern of dilated small bowel loops with air-fluid levels (Figure 30–6). These features may be minimal or absent in early obstruction, proximal obstruction, or closed loop obstruction or in some cases when fluid-filled loops contain lit-

High	Middle	Low
Frequent vomiting. No distention. Intermittent pain but not classic crescendo type.	Moderate vomiting. Moderate distention. Intermittent pain (crescendo, colicky) with free intervals.	Vomiting late, feculent. Marked distention. Variable pain; may not be classic crescendo type.

Figure 30–5. Small bowel obstruction. Variable manifestations of obstruction depend upon the level of blockage of the small bowel.

tle gas. The colon is often devoid of gas unless the patient has been given an enema, has undergone sigmoidoscopy, or has only a partial obstruction. Opaque gallstones and air in the biliary tree should be looked for. Administration of contrast media orally confirms the presence of mechanical obstruction and its completeness. Enteroclysis gives more detail about the level and cause of obstruction, and it may diagnose closed loop obstruction. CT scan is useful in patients with a history of abdominal malignancy and in some other situations.

B. STRANGULATION OBSTRUCTION

Although certain clinical features should make the surgeon suspicious of strangulation, no historical, physical, or laboratory findings entirely exclude the possibility of strangulation in complete small bowel obstruction. At least one-third of strangulation obstructions are unsuspected before operation, which underscores the need for early operation whenever obstruction is complete. Newer tools may have an impact on this problem in the future. Computer-assisted prediction of strangulation

has shown promise, and enteroclysis may detect closed-loop obstruction before strangulation can occur.

1. Symptoms and signs—Shock that appears early in the course of obstruction suggests a strangulated closed loop. When strangulation supervenes in simple obstruction, high fever may develop, previously cramping abdominal pain may become a severe continuous ache, vomitus may contain gross or occult blood, and abdominal tenderness and rigidity may appear.

2. Laboratory findings—Marked leukocytosis not accounted for by hemoconcentration alone should suggest strangulation. Increased plasma levels of malondialdehyde may be diagnostic

3. Imaging studies—Intraperitoneal fluid is seen as widened spaces between adjacent loops of dilated bowel and is often found in simple obstruction as well as in strangulation. Thumbprinting, loss of mucosal pattern, and gas within the bowel wall or within intrahepatic branches of the portal vein may be seen in strangulation. Air-fluid levels outside the bowel indicate perfora-

Figure 30–6. Small bowel obstruction. Note dilated loops of small bowel in a ladder-like pattern. Air-fluid levels are not obvious, because the patient is supine.

tion. Abdominal ultrasonography has diagnosed up to 90% of patients with strangulation in one study.

Differential Diagnosis

Pain from paralytic ileus is usually not severe but is constant and diffuse, and the abdomen is distended and mildly tender. If ileus has resulted from an acute intraperitoneal inflammatory process (eg, acute appendicitis), there should be symptoms and signs of the primary problem as well as the ileus. Plain films show gas mainly in the colon in uncomplicated postoperative ileus; gas in the small bowel suggests peritonitis. Small bowel x-rays may be required in order to distinguish ileus from mechanical obstruction in postoperative patients.

Obstruction of the large intestine is characterized by obstipation and abdominal distention; pain is less often colicky, and vomiting is an inconstant symptom. X-rays usually make the diagnosis by demonstrating colonic dilation proximal to the obstructing lesion. If the ileocecal valve is incompetent, the distal small bowel will be dilated, and a barium enema may be needed to determine the level of obstruction. This subject is covered in detail in Chapter 31.

Acute gastroenteritis, acute appendicitis, and acute pancreatitis can mimic simple intestinal obstruction. Strangulation obstruction may be confused with acute hemorrhagic pancreatitis or mesenteric vascular occlusion.

Intestinal pseudo-obstruction is a diverse group of disorders in which there are symptoms and signs of intestinal obstruction without evidence for an obstructing lesion. Acute pseudo-obstruction of the colon carries the risk of cecal perforation and is discussed in Chapter 31. Chronic or recurrent pseudo-obstruction affecting the small bowel with or without colonic involvement is often idiopathic. In other cases, pseudo-obstruction is associated with scleroderma, myxedema, lupus erythematosus, amyloidosis, drug abuse (eg, phenothiazine ingestion), radiation injury, or progressive systemic sclerosis. Several variations of familial visceral *myopathy* have been identified with seemingly distinct patterns of intestinal pseudo-obstruction. Patients with familial visceral *neuropathy* have degeneration of axons and neurons of the myenteric plexus of the gastrointestinal tract, and pseudo-obstruction results.

Patients with chronic pseudo-obstruction have recurrent attacks of vomiting, cramping abdominal pain, and abdominal distention. In some patients the esophagus, stomach, small bowel, colon, and urinary bladder all have abnormal motility, but in others one or more of these organs may be spared. Treatment is directed at the underlying disease if there is one. Management of idiopathic pseudo-obstruction is largely supportive, but cisapride may be effective in the neuropathic variety.

Treatment

Partial small bowel obstruction can be treated expectantly as long as there is continued passage of stool and flatus. Plain abdominal x-rays show gas in the colon, and small bowel contrast x-rays prove the diagnosis. Decompression with a nasogastric or long intestinal tube is successful in 90% of such patients. Operation is required if obstruction persists for several days even though it is incomplete.

Complete obstruction of the small intestine is treated by operation after a period of careful preparation. The compelling reason for operation is that strangulation cannot be excluded with certainty, and strangulation is associated with high rates of complications and death. The surgeon must avoid being lulled into a false sense of security by the improvement in symptoms and signs that almost invariably occurs after resuscitation.

There are exceptions to the general rule that operation must be performed promptly: Incomplete obstruction, postoperative obstruction, a history of numerous previous operations for obstruction, radiation therapy, inflammatory bowel disease, and abdominal carcinomatosis are situations demanding mature judgment, and judicious nonoperative management may be in the patient's best interests. A long intestinal tube (eg,

Miller-Abbott tube) may be passed in these cases to decompress the intestine.

A. PREPARATION

Proper timing of the operation is determined by the requirements of individual patients. The risk of strangulation must be weighed against the severity of fluid and electrolyte abnormalities and the need for evaluation and treatment of associated systemic diseases.

1. Nasogastric suction—A nasogastric tube should be inserted immediately upon admission to the emergency ward in order to relieve vomiting, avoid aspiration, and reduce the contribution of further swallowed air to the abdominal distention. A few surgeons routinely attempt to pass a long intestinal tube. Endoscopy may be of use when manipulating a tube through the pylorus.

2. Fluid and electrolyte resuscitation—Depending upon the level and duration of obstruction, fluid and electrolyte deficits are mild to severe. Hemoconcentration induced by long-standing obstruction cannot be corrected by dextrose solutions alone. Fluid losses are isotonic, and resuscitation should begin with infusion of isotonic saline solution. Losses of gastrointestinal fluid also entail acid-base deficits, and since there is no neuroendocrine mechanism for correcting these deficits, the surgeon must do so. Serum electrolyte concentrations and arterial blood gas determinations are guides to electrolyte therapy; potassium is best withheld until urine output is satisfactory, but patients should not undergo operation until hypokalemia has been treated. The volume of fluid required and its exact electrolyte composition must be calculated for each patient, and careful monitoring of clinical signs and associated systemic diseases is imperative. Some patients—notably those with strangulation obstruction—require plasma or blood. Antibiotics should be given if strangulation is even remotely suspected.

B. OPERATION

Operation may commence when the patient has been rehydrated and vital organs are functioning satisfactorily. Occasionally, the toxic effects of strangulation may force operation at an earlier time.

A standard groin incision is used for patients with incarcerated inguinal or femoral hernias. Laparoscopic adhesiolysis may be performed in carefully selected patients by surgeons skilled in this procedure. Generally, however, an open procedure is performed through an incision that is partly dictated by the location of scars from previous operations.

Details of the operative procedure vary according to the cause of obstruction. Adhesive bands causing obstruction should be lysed; an obstructing tumor should be resected; and an obstructing foreign body should be removed through an enterotomy. Gangrenous intestine must be resected, but it may be difficult to determine whether obstructed bowel is viable or not. The loop should be wrapped in a warm saline-soaked pack and inspected for color, mesenteric pulsation, and peristalsis several minutes later. Intraoperative use of Doppler ultrasound is a method of determining viability of obstructed intestine. The qualitative fluorescein test may be helpful; 1000 mg of fluorescein is injected into a peripheral vein over a 30- to 60-second period, and the bowel is then inspected under ultraviolet (Wood's) light. If the loop appears nonviable, resection with end-to-end anastomosis is the safest course.

Extirpation of the obstructing lesion is not possible in some patients with carcinoma or radiation injury. Anastomosis of proximal small bowel to small or large intestine distal to the obstruction (bypass) may be the best procedure in these patients. Rarely, adhesions are so dense that the intestine cannot be freed and bypass cannot be accomplished. Prolonged decompression through a gastrostomy or jejunostomy tube and provision of nutrition via the parenteral route may allow spontaneous resolution over a period of a few weeks.

Decompression of massively dilated small bowel loops facilitates closure of the abdomen and may shorten the time for recovery of bowel function postoperatively. Decompression is accomplished by threading down a long tube passed orally or by needle aspiration through the bowel wall.

Attempts to prevent uncontrolled adhesion formation by suturing loops of bowel so that they are fixed in a suitable relation to one another (Nobel plication procedures) are unsuccessful. However, another procedure in which a long tube is inserted through a gastrostomy or jejunostomy for 10 days to provide intraluminal stenting has some proponents. Attempts to prevent adhesions by placement of various substances in the peritoneal cavity have met limited success; a 5% solution of polyethylene glycol 4000 has shown promise.

Prognosis

Nonstrangulating obstruction has a death rate of about 2%; most of these deaths occur in the elderly. Strangulation obstruction has a mortality rate of approximately 8% if operation is performed within 36 hours of the onset of symptoms and 25% if operation is delayed beyond 36 hours. Recurrent obstruction after lysis of adhesions is uncommon.

Assalia A et al: Therapeutic effect of oral Gastrografin in adhesive, partial small-bowel obstruction: a prospective randomized trial. Surgery 1994;115:433.

Balthazar EJ: George W. Holmes Lecture: CT of small-bowel obstruction. AJR Am J Roentgenol 1994;162:255.

Beck DE et al: Incidence of small-bowel obstrucgtion and adhesiolysis after open colorectal and general surgery. Dis Colon Rectum 1999;42:241.

Camilleri M, Balm RK, Zinsmeister AR: Determinants of response to a prokinetic agent in neuropathic chronic intestinal motility disorder. Gastroenterology 1994;106:916.

Cox MR et al: The operative aetiology and types of adhesions causing small bowel obstruction. Aust N Z J Surg 1993;63:848.

Dijkstra FR: Recent clinical developments in pathophysiology, epidemiology, diagnosis and treatment of intra-abdominal adhesions. Scand J Gastroenterol Suppl 2000;(232):52.

Frager D et al: CT of small-bowel obstruction: value in establishing the diagnosis and determining the degree and cause. AJR Am J Roentgenol 1994;162:37.

Francois Y et al: Postoperative adhesive peritoneal disease: laparoscopic treatment. Surg Endosc 1994;8:781.

Harlow CL et al: Diagnosis of bowel obstruction on plain abdominal radiographs: significance of air-fluid levels at different heights in the same loop of bowel. AJR Am J Roentgenol 1993;161:291.

Hass BE, Schrager RE: Small bowel obstruction due to Richter's hernia after laparoscopic procedures. J Laparoendosc Surg 1993;3:421.

Jenkins JT: Secondary causes of intestinal obstruction: rigorous preoperative evaluation is required. Am Surg 2000;66:662.

Lo CY, Lorentz TG, Lau PWK: Obturator hernia presenting as small bowel obstruction. Am J Surg 1994;167:396.

Meagher AP, Moller C, Hoffmann DC: Non-operative treatment of small bowel obstruction following appendicectomy or operation on the ovary or tube. Br J Surg 1993;80:1310.

Merrett ND et al: Bacteremia associated with operative decompression of a small bowel obstruction. J Am Coll Surg 1994; 179:33.

Miller G et al: Natural history of patients with adhesive small bowel obstruction. Br J Surg 2000;87:1240.

Ogata M et al: Abdominal ultrasonography for the diagnosis of strangulation in small bowel obstruction. Br J Surg 1994;81:421.

Sandikcioglu TG et al: Contrast radiography in small bowel obstruction: a randomized trial of barium sulfate and a nonionic low-osmolar contrast medium. Acta Radiol 1994;35:62.

Seror D et al: How conservatively can postoperative small bowel obstruction be treated? Am J Surg 1993;165:121.

Stricker B, Blanco J, Fox HE: The gynecologic contribution to intestinal obstruction in females. J Am Coll Surg 1994;178:617.

von Flue M et al: Acute and chronic presentation of intestinal nonrotation in adults. Dis Colon Rectum 1994;37:192.

Zalcman M et al: Helical CT signs in the diagnosis of intestinal ischemia in small-bowel obstruction. AJR Am J Roentgenol 2000;175:1601.

ACQUIRED INTESTINAL DIVERTICULA*

Congenital diverticula of the jejunum are rare, but acquired diverticula are found in the jejunum (or ileum) in 1.3% of radiographic studies or autopsy series

---

*Meckel's diverticulum and other congenital diverticula of the small intestine are discussed in Chapter 46.

when specifically sought. Jejunal diverticula are wide-mouthed sacs measuring 1–25 cm in diameter. Most contain all layers of the intestinal wall (true diverticula), but some consist of mucosa and submucosa herniated through thickened muscularis (false diverticula). Diverticula in the small bowel are often multiple; they diminish in frequency from the ligament of Treitz to the ileocecal valve and are associated with diverticulosis of the duodenum or colon in 30% of cases. Most symptomatic patients are over age 60.

Jejunal diverticulosis is a heterogeneous disorder associated with abnormalities of smooth muscle or the myenteric plexus. Intestinal pseudo-obstruction is a common associated problem, also reflecting the presence of an underlying motility disorder such as familial visceral myopathy or progressive systemic sclerosis.

Symptoms may be due to pseudo-obstruction or to inflammation of the diverticula. Acute intestinal bleeding and diverticulitis leading to perforation may occur. Blind loop syndrome is caused by bacterial overgrowth in the stagnant bowel with pseudo-obstruction or in large diverticula.

Barium x-rays may outline the diverticula (Figure 30–7) and reveal the underlying motility disorder. The primary cause should be sought.

Operation is required for perforation or bleeding. Symptoms of the underlying motility disorder are not improved by resection of the segment containing diverticula.

Figure 30–7. Jejunal diverticula.

Akhrass R et al: Small-bowel diverticulosis: perceptions and reality. J Am Coll Surg 1997;184:383.

Benya EC, Ghahremani GG, Brosnan JJ: Diverticulitis of the jejunum: clinical and radiological features. Gastrointest Radiol 1991;16:24.

Longo WE, Vernava Ad: Clinical implications of jejunoileal diverticular disease. Dis Colon Rectum 1992;35:381.

Sibille A, Willocx R: Jejunal diverticulitis. Am J Gastroenterol 1992;87:655.

CROHN'S DISEASE*
(Regional Enteritis)

 ESSENTIALS OF DIAGNOSIS

- *Diarrhea.*
- *Abdominal pain and palpable mass.*
- *Low-grade fever, lassitude, weight loss.*
- *Anemia.*
- *Radiographic findings of thickened, stenotic bowel with ulceration and internal fistulas.*

General Considerations

Crohn's disease is a chronic progressive granulomatous inflammatory disorder of the gastrointestinal tract. From two to nine cases per 100,000 population are detected annually in Europe and the USA. The prevalence ranges broadly from 20 to 90 per 100,000 population. There is geographic variation (more common in urban dwellers and Northern residents of the USA), and there is a relatively high incidence among Ashkenazi Jews. The peak incidence occurs between the second and fourth decades. Cigarette smoking and a high intake of sugar are independent risk factors for Crohn's disease.

A. ETIOLOGY

The cause of Crohn's disease is unknown. Theories holding that Crohn's disease is caused by bovine milk products or is the result of psychophysiologic abnormalities have been discarded. The favored hypothesis is that Crohn's disease results from the interaction of genetic and environmental factors. A genetic influence is suggested by a family history of inflammatory bowel disease in 15–20% of patients. Offspring of couples, both of whom have inflammatory bowel disease, have a high risk (36%) of developing the illness. Transmissible agents, including small viruses, cell wall-deficient pseudomonas-like bacteria, mycobacteria, chlamydiae, and yersinia, have been isolated from tissues of patients with Crohn's disease. Data thus far lack reproducibility and specificity, but this type of environmental influence is a likely candidate for an important role in the causation of Crohn's disease. Numerous immunologic abnormalities have been reported, but the importance of these changes remains conjectural.

B. PATHOLOGY

Crohn's disease may affect any part of the gastrointestinal tract from the lips to the anus and may even spill over into the larynx or extend beyond the gut to the skin. "Metastatic" skin lesions have been described. The distal ileum is the most frequent site of involvement, eventually becoming diseased in about three-fourths of patients. The small bowel alone is involved in 15–30%, both the distal ileum and the colon in 40–60%, and the large bowel alone in 25–30%. Duodenal Crohn's disease is found in 0.5–7% of patients. Discontinuous areas of disease with segments of normal bowel between ("skip lesions") occur in 15% of patients. Subtle histologic changes can be seen in "normal," grossly uninvolved intestine of patients with Crohn's disease, suggesting that the mucosa of the entire bowel may be abnormal in this disorder.

The earliest Crohn's lesion is a focal accumulation of inflammatory cells adjacent to an epithelial crypt. Candidate mediators of inflammation include plasma activating factor, leukotrienes, complement, cytokines, enterotoxin, interleukins, tumor necrosis factor, phospholipase A_2, and neurotransmitters of the enteric nervous system. In a process similar to that seen in ischemia, reactive molecules such as oxygen radicals are generated; they propagate the inflammatory response and contribute to tissue damage. Erosions, crypt abscesses, and granulomas result.

Granulomas are seen in the bowel wall in 50–70% and in mesenteric lymph nodes in 25% of patients. The number of granulomas is related to the duration of the history and the site of involvement. It has been speculated that granuloma formation reflects efforts to localize or eliminate the causative agent of Crohn's disease. Mucosal lesions appear grossly as tiny (pinpoint) hemorrhagic spots or shallow ulcers with white bases and elevated margins (aphthous ulcers). Punched out ulcers are seen with progression of the disease. The next stage is development of fissures—knife-like clefts beginning in mucosa and extending deeply into the wall. These fissures and the serpiginous or linear ulcers surrounding islands of intact mucosa overlying edematous submucosa give a cobblestone appearance to the luminal surface. Crohn's disease ultimately becomes a transmural inflammatory process with thickening of the bowel wall, and it often progresses to stricture formation. The

---
*Crohn's disease of the colon is discussed in Chapter 31.

bowel and its mesentery are foreshortened in advanced cases, and on gross inspection mesenteric fat seems to have advanced over the surface of the bowel toward the antimesenteric border.

Clinical Findings

A. SYMPTOMS AND SIGNS

Crohn's disease has many modes of presentation:

1. Diarrhea—Continuous or episodic diarrhea is noted in about 90% of patients. Stools are liquid or semisolid and characteristically contain no blood if small bowel alone is diseased. One-third of patients with colonic involvement pass blood, and a few present with bloody diarrhea resembling that seen in ulcerative colitis.

2. Recurrent abdominal pain—Mild colic initiated by meals, centered in the lower abdomen, and relieved by defecation is common. These symptoms are due to chronic partial obstruction of the small bowel, colon, or both. Some patients progress to complete obstruction, and they have severe cramping, vomiting, and abdominal distension.

3. Abdominal symptoms and constitutional effects—Episodic attacks of abdominal pain and diarrhea accompanied by lassitude, malaise, weight loss, fever, and anemia are a common syndrome. A mass is often palpable in the right lower quadrant in these patients. Occasionally, fever of unknown origin is the only clinical finding.

4. Anorectal lesions—Chronic anal fissures, large ulcers, complex anal fistulas, or pararectal abscesses are seen in 15–25% of patients with Crohn's disease confined to small bowel and in 50–75% of those with colonic involvement. These problems may appear many years before the intestinal disease. Histologic features of Crohn's disease, including granulomas, are often found in biopsies of anorectal lesions even when the only other identifiable disease is located much higher in the gastrointestinal tract.

5. Anemia—Iron deficiency anemia or macrocytic anemia due to vitamin B_{12} or folate deficiency may occur in the absence of abdominal symptoms.

6. Malnutrition—Protein-losing enteropathy, steatorrhea, chronic obstruction, and diminished dietary intake from chronic illness contribute to malnutrition and weight loss. Mineral and vitamin deficiencies (especially vitamin D deficiency) are common. Deficiencies of water-soluble and fat-soluble vitamins are common in patients with Crohn's disease of the small intestine, but clinical symptoms of vitamin deficiency are rare. Zinc deficiency has been recognized. Children afflicted

with extensive Crohn's disease fail to grow and may have severely retarded sexual maturation. Reversal of growth arrest by parenteral feeding emphasizes the importance of malnutrition as a cause of growth failure in Crohn's disease. Somatomedin C levels may be a reliable marker of nutritional adequacy.

7. Acute onset—Acute abdominal pain and right lower quadrant tenderness mimicking acute appendicitis may be found at operation to be due to acute inflammation of the distal ileum. Only 15% of such cases evolve into chronic Crohn's disease, suggesting that most patients with acute ileitis have an infectious process unrelated to Crohn's disease. This condition is discussed further in the section on acute enteritis and mesenteric lymphadenitis.

8. Systemic complications—Any of the systemic complications described below may prompt the patient to seek medical advice.

B. LABORATORY FINDINGS

Test results are nonspecific and vary greatly according to the site of intestinal involvement, the severity of disease, and the presence of complications such as abscess or fistula. The sedimentation rate may not be elevated in patients with disease of the small intestine. Hypoalbuminemia, anemia, and steatorrhea are common. Abnormal D-xylose absorption suggests extensive disease or fistula formation, since carbohydrate is normally absorbed in the jejunum. Breath tests, as described in the section on blind loop syndrome, are abnormal if the ileum is diseased or if bacterial overgrowth has occurred. Fecal markers of intestinal inflammation, including α_1-antitrypsin (α_1-antiprotease) and TNFα, may become useful clinically in the future.

C. IMAGING STUDIES

Radiographic studies contribute substantially to the diagnosis of Crohn's disease. The appearance of small bowel during a barium study is a composite of proliferative and destructive changes. The principal findings include thickened bowel wall with stricture ("string sign"), longitudinal ulceration that is shallow at first but becomes deep and undermining, deep transverse fissures resembling spicules, and cobblestone formation (Figure 30–8). Deformity of the cecum, fistulas, abscesses, and skip lesions are additional findings of importance. Enteroclysis provides excellent detail. CT scan, ultrasound, and MRI have diagnostic value in some cases.

[111]In-tagged granulocytes accumulate in Crohn's lesions over 2–3 hours and can be detected by scintiscan. Tc-99m hexamethylpropyleneamineoxime (^{99m}Tc HMPAO) white cell scintigraphy has advantages of availability and image resolution. Autologous ^{99m}Tc-

Figure 30–8. Barium x-ray showing spicules, edema, and ulcers in Crohn's disease

labeled phagocyte scanning assesses disease activity. Gamma scanning after oral administration of ^{75}Se-HCAT is a nonspecific test for the presence of diseased or dysfunctional distal ileum. Sucralfate complexed to ^{99m}Tc helps localize Crohn's disease. Other isotope tests include ^{51}Cr EDTA for intestinal permeability and ^{99m}Tc-porphyrins for assessing intestinal inflammation.

D. Endoscopy

Upper gastrointestinal endoscopy diagnoses esophageal, gastric, and duodenal lesions. Colonoscopy reveals typical changes of Crohn's disease in the colon if it is involved or in the ileum if it can be examined. Ileoscopy after colectomy is accurate for the diagnosis of Crohn's disease in the ileum.

Differential Diagnosis

A. Ulcerative Colitis

Crohn's disease of the colon may be difficult to distinguish from ulcerative colitis. This topic is covered in detail in Chapter 31.

B. Appendicitis

Acute ileitis may be the presenting manifestation, and differentiation from appendicitis may be impossible without operation.

C. Tuberculosis

Tuberculosis may affect any part of the gastrointestinal tract but is uncommon distal to the cecum. Small

bowel tuberculosis is discussed elsewhere in this chapter.

D. Lymphoma

Radiographic findings help differentiate lymphoma from Crohn's disease, but histologic examination of the tissue is occasionally required before the diagnosis is certain. Rectal or colonic biopsies that show granulomas or colitis may support the diagnosis of Crohn's disease.

E. Other Diseases

Carcinoma, amebiasis, ischemia, eosinophilic gastroenteritis, and other inflammatory conditions may simulate Crohn's disease. Enteropathy from nonsteroidal anti-inflammatory agents has recently been added to this list.

Complications

A. Intestinal

Some intestinal complications, such as obstruction, abscess, fistula, and anorectal lesions, are so common that they are regarded as part of the characteristic clinical picture. Free perforation and massive hemorrhage are uncommon. The risk of cholelithiasis is increased. Oral manifestations of Crohn's disease may cause disabling pain. Carcinoma may occur in segments of small or large bowel that are involved with Crohn's disease, especially in segments excluded from the fecal stream by surgical bypass procedures.

B. Systemic

Systemic complications such as hepatobiliary disease, uveitis, arthritis, ankylosing spondylitis, aphthous ulcers, erythema nodosum, amyloidosis, thromboembolism, and vascular disorders are found both in Crohn's disease and in ulcerative colitis. These manifestations are described more fully in Chapter 31. "Metastatic" (distant cutaneous) Crohn's disease is a cutaneous ulcer with a granulomatous reaction at a site separated from gut by normal skin. Urinary complications include cystitis, calculi, and ureteral obstruction.

Treatment

The initial treatment of Crohn's disease is nonoperative. Physical rest, relief of emotional stress, and a confiding patient-doctor relationship have favorable effects. A low-residue, milk-free, high-protein diet may provide adequate nutrition. Malnourished patients benefit from elemental or polymeric diets if standard food is not tolerated, and total or supplementary parenteral nutrition is an important adjunct. As nutrition improves, infection is more successfully treated, and complications such as fistulas may be reversed. Chronic intermittent elemental diet improves growth failure in prepubertal children. Most clinicians prefer enteral feeding over the parenteral route when conditions permit, though comparative studies are inconclusive on this issue. Preoperative total parenteral nutrition prolongs the hospital stay and does not reduce the incidence or severity of postoperative complications. Chronic parenteral nutrition at home allows some patients with extensive disease to postpone operation, but it does not reduce the necessity of operation over the long term.

Enteral nutrition alone is insufficient therapy for active Crohn's disease compared with pharmacologic treatment. The standard drugs for Crohn's disease are steroids, aminosalicylates, immunosuppressives, and antibiotics. Prednisone, prednisolone, and methylprednisolone are the most common corticosteroids for this purpose. Studies suggest that steroids are most effective for Crohn's disease of the small intestine, but they are applied to Crohn's colitis as well. Prednisone (0.25–0.75 mg/d) is superior to placebo in the control of acute disease over the short term. The utility of prednisone is limited by side effects. Sulfasalazine, an aminosalicylate, has been a cornerstone of therapy of Crohn's disease for many years. It is superior to placebo in control of acute disease, but its use is complicated by adverse reactions. The active principle of sulfasalazine is 5-aminosalicylic acid (5-ASA). Oral aminosalicylates (mesalamine in the USA, mesalazine in Europe and Canada) are now used widely and are considered to be therapeutically equivalent to sulfasalazine. Not only are they beneficial for patients with active Crohn's colitis and ileocolitis, but oral aminosalicylates also may succeed in maintaining remission of Crohn's disease, a goal that has not been achieved by any other agents to date. Azathioprine and mercaptopurine are the immunosuppressive drugs with the longest records. They are effective in Crohn's colitis and less so in ileitis; they spare steroids (allow reduction of steroid doses), help close fistulas, maintain remissions, and heal perianal disease. The disadvantage of azathioprine and mercaptopurine is their slow action, often requiring 4 months or more before effects are seen. Cyclosporine is another immunosuppressive agent that is used in inflammatory bowel disease; 59% of patients with active chronic Crohn's disease benefited from cyclosporine in a controlled trial, and the drug worked quickly—within days or weeks. Various broad-spectrum antibiotics have been tried, but only metronidazole is used regularly. Metronidazole is effective for Crohn's colitis, particularly perianal disease. Infliximab (anti-TNFα monoclonal chimeric antibody) is now FDA-approved for use in patients with active Crohn's disease. Despite medical advances in management, there is still no cure for Crohn's disease.

The indication for operation in Crohn's disease of the small bowel is obstruction in about half of cases; perforation, internal fistula, external fistula, abscess, perianal disease, and growth failure in children are other reasons for operation. Over the long term, about 70% of patients with Crohn's disease undergo definitive surgery. Conservative resection of diseased bowel with end-to-end anastomosis is the preferred surgical procedure. Extensive involvement of small bowel, either diffusely or by skip lesions, is unfavorable for curative resection. Resection is usually limited to the area responsible for the complications that prompted operation. If multiple symptomatic strictures are encountered, they can be treated by "strictureplasty," a procedure in which the bowel is incised through the stricture and the wall is sutured or stapled in such a way that the lumen is widened.

Prognosis

Crohn's disease is a chronic condition. It may progress to involve additional portions of bowel or may seem to spread no farther. Surgical procedures are palliative, not curative, but operations contribute greatly to rehabilitation of patients with refractory disease. The recurrence rate after resection of ileal or ileocolic disease increases with time; symptomatic recurrence rates range from 25% to 50% at 5 years, from 35% to 80% at 10 years, and from 45% to 85% at 15 years. The marked variability is due to differences in patient populations, type of surgical procedures, and criteria for recurrence. Extensive confluent ulcers seen endoscopically in the ileum at the anastomosis within 1 year after ileocolectomy strongly predict symptomatic recurrence. Strictureplasty is effective for obstructive lesions, and there are few postoperative complications. Reoperation is needed in about 10% of patients within a year after strictureplasty and in one-third of patients by 10 years; surprisingly, however, the strictureplasty sites are usually not the source of symptoms.

Surgery should be used to manage complications in coordination with medical therapy. This team approach enables 80–85% of patients who require surgery to lead normal lives. Community-based studies have shown that long-term survival of people with Crohn's disease is similar to that of the general population irrespective of the age at diagnosis. There is little evidence that pregnancy affects the course of Crohn's disease or that inactive Crohn's disease alters the course of pregnancy.

Alcantara M et al: Endoscopic and bioptic findings in the upper gastrointestinal tract in patients with Crohn's disease. Endoscopy 1993;25:282.

Block GE et al: Crohn's disease. Curr Probl Surg 1993;30:173.

Cameron JL et al: Patterns of ileal recurrence in Crohn's disease: a prospective randomized study. Ann Surg 1992;215:546.

Cellier C et al: Correlations between clinical activity, endoscopic severity, and biological parameters in colonic or ileocolonic Crohn's disease. A prospective multicentre study of 121 cases. The Groupe d'Etudes Therapeutiques des Affections Inflammatoires Digestives. Gut 1994;35:231.

Dixon PM, Roulston ME, Nolan DJ: The small bowel enema: a ten year review. Clin Radiol 1993;47:46.

Geier DL, Miner PBJ: New therapeutic agents in the treatment of inflammatory bowel disease. Am J Med 1992;93:199.

Halligan S et al: The distribution of small bowel Crohn's disease in children compared to adults. Clin Radiol 1994;49:314.

Hay JW, Hay AR: Inflammatory bowel disease: costs-of-illness. J Clin Gastroenterol 1992;14:309.

Heimann TM et al: Prediction of early symptomatic recurrence after intestinal resection in Crohn's disease. Ann Surg 1993; 218:294.

Heresbach D et al: Indium scanning in assessment of acute Crohn's disease: a prospective study of sensitivity and correlation with severity of mucosal damage. Dig Dis Sci 1993;38:1601.

Kennan N, Hayward M: Tc HMPAO-labelled white cell scintigraphy in Crohn's disease of the small bowel. Clin Radiol 1992; 45:331.

Kurata JH et al: Crohn's disease among ethnic groups in a large health maintenance organization. Gastroenterology 1992; 102:1940.

Kyle J: Crohn's disease in the northeastern and northern isles of Scotland: an epidemiological review. Gastroenterology 1992; 103:392.

Lavy A, Militianu D, Eidelman S: Diseases of the intestine mimicking Crohn's disease. J Clin Gastroenterol 1992;15:17.

Linn FV, Peppercorn MA: Drug therapy for inflammatory bowel disease: Part I. Am J Surg 1992;164:85.

Linn FV, Peppercorn MA: Drug therapy for inflammatory bowel disease: Part II. Am J Surg 1992;164:178.

Love JR, Irvine EJ, Fedorak RN: Quality of life in inflammatory bowel disease. J Clin Gastroenterol 1992;14:15.

Makowiec F et al: Intestinal stenosis and perforating complications in Crohn's disease. Int J Colorectal Dis 1993;8:197.

Mayberry MK et al: Perceived discrimination in education and employment by people with Crohn's disease: a case control study of educational achievement and employment. Gut 1992; 33:312.

McLeod RS et al: Prophylactic mesalamine treatment decreases postoperative recurrence of Crohn's disease. Gastroenterology 1995;109:404.

Michelassi F et al: Adenocarcinoma complicating Crohn's disease. Dis Colon Rectum 1993;36:654.

Nwokolo CU et al: Surgical resections in parous patients with distal ileal and colonic Crohn's disease. Gut 1994;35:220.

Nyhlin H, Merrick MV, Eastwood MA: Bile acid malabsorption in Crohn's disease and indications for its assessment using Se-HCAT. Gut 1994;35:90.

Olaison G, Smedh K, Sjodahl R: Natural course of Crohn's disease after ileocolic resection: endoscopically visualised ileal ulcers preceding symptoms. Gut 1992;33:331.

Prantera C et al: Oral 5-aminosalicylic acid (Asacol) in the maintenance treatment of Crohn's disease. Gastroenterology 1992; 103:363.

Probert CSJ et al: Mortality from Crohn's disease in Leicestershire, 1972–1989: an epidemiological community based study. Gut 1992;33:1226.

Ricart E et al: Infliximab for Crohn's disease in clinical practice at the Mayo Clinic: the first 100 patients. Am J Gastroenterol 2001;96:722.

Salomon P et al: How effective are current drugs for Crohn's disease? A meta-analysis. J Clin Gastroenterol 1992;14:211.

Shoenut JP et al: Comparison of magnetic resonance imaging and endoscopy in distinguishing the type and severity of inflammatory bowel disease. J Clin Gastroenterol 1994;19:31.

Smedh K et al: Intraoperative enteroscopy in Crohn's disease. Br J Surg 1993;80:897.

Stokes MA: Crohn's disease and nutrition. Br J Surg 1992;79:391.

Sutherland LR et al: Prevention of relapse of Crohn's disease. Inflamm Bowel Dis 2000;6:321.

Tjandra JJ, Fazio VW, Lavery IC: Results of multiple strictureplasties in diffuse Crohn's disease of the small bowel. Aust N Z J Surg 1993;63:95.

OTHER INFLAMMATORY & ULCERATIVE DISEASES OF THE SMALL INTESTINE

Acute Enteritis & Mesenteric Lymphadenitis

Acute inflammation of the small intestine (enteritis) often also affects the stomach (**gastroenteritis**) or the colon (**enterocolitis**). Involvement of regional lymph nodes is termed **mesenteric adenitis.** These usually self-limiting illnesses may be caused by viruses, bacteria, parasites, toxins, or unknown agents. These conditions are of importance to the surgeon when they mimic acute appendicitis or other problems that require operative treatment.

Achong DM, Oates E, Harris B: Mesenteric lymphadenitis depicted by indium 111-labeled white blood cell imaging. J Pediatr Surg 1993;28:1550.

Giannella RA: Enteric infections: 50 years of progress. Gastroenterology 1993;104:1589.

Kapikian AZ: Viral gastroenteritis. JAMA 1993;269:627.

HIV-Associated Enteropathy

Gastrointestinal infections are frequent in AIDS patients. Enteric pathogens recoverable from these patients include *Cryptosporidium*, cytomegalovirus, *Entamoeba histolytica*, *Giardia lamblia*, *Mycobacterium avium-intracellulare*, *Salmonella typhimurium*, *Shigella*, and *Campylobacter jejuni*.

Many symptomatic patients have no identifiable intestinal pathogen, and there is evidence to support the existence of an enteropathy caused by the human immunodeficiency virus itself. Intestinal perforation is a rare but devastating complication in these patients.

Kotler DP et al: Effects of enteric parasitoses and HIV infection upon small intestinal structure and function in patients with AIDS. J Clin Gastroenterol 1993;16:10.

Ullrich R et al: Gastrointestinal symptoms in patients infected with human immunodeficiency virus: relevance of infective agents isolated from gastrointestinal tract. Gut 1992;33:1080.

Yersinia Enteritis

Much attention has focused on *Yersinia enterocolitica;* this pathogen may cause acute gastroenteritis, terminal ileitis, enterocolitis, colitis, mesenteric lymphadenitis, hepatic and splenic abscesses, and autoimmune processes such as erythema nodosum and polyarthritis. *Y enterocolitica* has also been implicated in other disease (especially in women), including carditis, glomerulonephritis, Graves' disease, and Hashimoto's thyroiditis.

Acute gastroenteritis with fever, diarrhea, and sometimes vomiting is the most common clinical syndrome, especially in children. Acute mesenteric lymphadenitis and acute terminal ileitis are more frequent in adolescents and adults. These infections may cause enough abdominal pain and tenderness that appendicitis seems a likely diagnosis. If operation is performed, large inflamed lymph nodes are found in the mesentery of the distal ileum, and the bowel itself may be grossly inflamed. In these circumstances, appendectomy is usually performed. Organisms can be cultured from stool, and antibody titers may rise and then fall in some patients. *Y enterocolitica* may respond to trimethoprim-sulfamethoxazole or doxycycline, and complicated *Y enterocolitica* infections should be treated. Fatal septicemia has been reported. No patient with *Y enterocolitica* enteritis has progressed to classic Crohn's disease.

Saebø A, Lassen J: Acute and chronic gastrointestinal manifestations associated with *Yersinia enterocolitica* infection: a Norwegian 10-year follow-up study on 458 hospitalized patients. Ann Surg 1992;215:250.

Van Noyen R et al: Causative role of *Yersinia* and other enteric pathogens in the appendicular syndrome. Eur J Clin Microbiol Infect Dis 1991;10:735.

Campylobacter Enteritis

Campylobacter jejuni is a gram-negative rod that is now recognized as an important cause of human illness in all parts of the world. *C jejuni* infection is more common than infection by either salmonella or shigella. Raw milk, untreated drinking water, and undercooked poultry are recognized vehicles of transmission. Clinical features vary from mild abdominal pain, fever, emesis, and diarrhea indistinguishable from viral gastroenteritis to severe chronic or relapsing bloody diarrhea that resembles ulcerative or granulomatous colitis. *C jejuni* produces an enterotoxin that may play a role in causing diarrhea.

Darkfield or phase-contrast microscopy of stool samples may reveal the characteristic darting motility of *C jejuni* and allow for a presumptive diagnosis. Stool and occasionally blood cultures are positive. Colonoscopy may reveal colonic lesions, and x-rays show inflammation of the small bowel or colon.

Although *C jejuni* infection is self-limited in most patients and symptoms subside within a week, relapses occur in 20% of untreated patients. The appropriate antibiotic is erythromycin, ciprofloxacin, or doxycycline, depending on the results of in vitro sensitivity studies. Disease can be spread by symptomatic patients; once diarrhea subsides, transmission is unlikely.

Perkins DJ, Newstead GL: *Campylobacter jejuni* enterocolitis causing peritonitis, ileitis and intestinal obstruction. Aust N Z J Surg 1994;64:55.

Peterson MC: Clinical aspects of *Campylobacter jejuni* infections in adults. West J Med 1994;161:148.

Tuberculosis

Primary tuberculous infection of the intestine, caused by ingestion of the bovine strain of *Mycobacterium tuberculosis,* is rare in the USA. Secondary infection is due to swallowing the human tubercle bacillus. About 1% of patients with pulmonary tuberculosis have intestinal involvement. Recent immigration from endemic areas has increased the incidence. Tuberculosis is prevalent in individuals infected with HIV.

The distal ileum is the most common site of disease. The bacillus localizes in the mucosal glands and spreads to Peyer's patches, where inflammation, sloughing of tissue, and local attempts at walling off give rise to symptoms. The pathologic reaction is hypertrophic or ulcerative. Hypertrophic tuberculous enteritis results in stenosis, and the symptoms and signs are those of obstruction. The ulcerative form causes abdominal pain, alternating constipation and diarrhea, and, occasionally, progressive inanition. Free perforation, fistula formation, or hemorrhage may occur in severe untreated disease.

The diagnosis of intestinal tuberculosis can be difficult, but medical treatment should not be based on clinical suspicion alone, since carcinoma and Crohn's disease cause similar symptoms and signs. Less than half of patients in a recent study had an abnormality on chest x-ray, and none had a positive sputum. Biopsy by colonoscopy, laparoscopy, or even laparotomy is needed to demonstrate the organism.

Antituberculosis chemotherapy is the mainstay of management. Surgery is required if the diagnosis is uncertain, if disease is resistant to chemotherapy, or if complications develop. Some surgeons recommend early operation because medical treatment results in healing by fibrosis with resultant obstruction. Resection is the preferred surgical procedure, and bypass is done only if abscesses or fistulas are present. The prognosis is good if the patient is operated on in the early stages of the illness.

Al-Quorain AA et al: Abdominal tuberculosis in Saudi Arabia: a clinicopathological study of 65 cases. Am J Gastroenterol 1993;88:75.

Marshall JB: Tuberculosis of the gastrointestinal tract and peritoneum. Am J Gastroenterol 1993;88:989.

Underwood MJ et al: Presentation of abdominal tuberculosis to general surgeons. Br J Surg 1992;79:1077.

Typhoid

Salmonella typhi may cause ulcers in the distal ileum or cecum. Bleeding or perforation presents a formidable surgical challenge. Early operation offers the best hope for survival.

Mandal BK: *Salmonella typhi* and other salmonellas. Gut 1994; 35:726.

Mock CN, Amaral J, Visser LE: Improvement in survival from typhoid ileal perforation: results of 221 operative cases. Ann Surg 1992;215:244.

Enteropathy From Nonsteroidal Anti-inflammatory Drugs

Nonsteroidal anti-inflammatory drugs increase intestinal permeability within hours after ingestion, exposing the mucosa to macromolecules and toxins in the lumen. Bacterial invasion may contribute to inflammation. Perhaps 70% of patients of any age and either sex who have taken these agents for 6 months or longer develop enteropathy, with subclinical intestinal inflammation and occult blood loss. Fewer than 1% of patients develop mucosal ulceration or transmural inflammation with submucosal fibrosis and circumferential diaphragm-like strictures. These patients may have obstruction, perforation, or anemia. The differential diagnosis includes Crohn's disease, ischemia, tuberculosis, and lymphoma.

The drug should be withdrawn. Strictures require resection.

Allison MC et al: Gastrointestinal damage associated with the use of nonsteroidal antiinflammatory drugs. N Engl J Med 1992; 327:749.

Bjarnason I et al: Side effects of nonsteroidal anti-inflammatory drugs on the small and large intestine in humans. Gastroenterology 1993;104:1832.

Henry D, Dobson A, Turner C: Variability in the risk of major gastrointestinal complications from nonaspirin nonsteroidal anti-inflammatory drugs. Gastroenterology 1993;105:1078.

Radiation Enteropathy

Aggressive radiation therapy for abdominal or pelvic cancer is almost always associated with some gastrointestinal injury, because proliferating intestinal epithelial cells are extremely radiosensitive. Degeneration of cells and edema of bowel wall may produce abdominal pain, nausea and vomiting, and sometimes bloody diarrhea during therapy or a few months later. Symptoms are usually minor and transient for most patients with modern irradiation techniques.

Injury to blood vessels in the bowel wall is far more serious than the early mucosal lesion. Endothelial proliferation and fibrosis in the media may gradually obliterate the vessel lumen over months or years, producing chronic intestinal ischemia. Carcinoma arising in irradiated small intestine is a rare late complication.

The incidence of significant bowel injury is dose-related and varies from 5% after 4500 cGy to 30% after 6000 cGy. Fixation of small bowel loops in the radiation field by adhesions from previous operations greatly increases the risk of intestinal complications. Absorbable polyglycolic acid mesh can be used to keep the small bowel out of the pelvis when radiation therapy is planned following pelvic surgery. Oral glutamine protects the small bowel mucosa from some of the morbidity of irradiation in preliminary animal studies.

Symptoms necessitating operation appear as early as 1 month or as late as 30 years after completion of therapy. Operation is required for obstruction due to stricture or entrapment in pelvic fibrosis, perforation with abscess or fistula formation, or hemorrhage from ulcerated mucosa. Symptoms should not be attributed to cancer until residual cancer is proved to be present.

The objective of operation is relief of symptoms. If resection of the involved segment is not possible, bypass is performed. It is imperative that normal bowel be used for anastomoses, because suture lines in irradiated bowel are likely to disrupt. The bowel is friable despite its thickness, and care must be taken in freeing adhesions. If the distal colon and rectum are involved, diverting colostomy is the safest course. Radiation proctitis is discussed in Chapter 32.

The operative death rate is 10–15%, and the prognosis thereafter depends on the extent of involvement and the presence of untreatable fistulas, short bowel syndrome, and cancer. Only 30–45% of patients with significant intestinal complications of radiation therapy are alive 5 years after operation.

Cross MJ, Frazee RC: Surgical treatment of radiation enteritis. Am Surg 1992;58:132.

Johnson RJ, Carrington BM: Pelvic radiation disease. Clin Radiol 1992;45:4.

van Halteren HK et al: Surgical intervention for complications caused by late radiation damage of the small bowel: a retrospective analysis. Eur J Surg Oncol 1993;19:336.

Yeoh E et al: Effect of pelvic irradiation on gastrointestinal function: a prospective longitudinal study. Am J Med 1993; 95:397.

SMALL INTESTINE FISTULAS

 ESSENTIALS OF DIAGNOSIS

- *Fever and sepsis.*
- *Abdominal pain.*
- *Localized abdominal tenderness.*
- *External drainage of small bowel contents.*
- *Dehydration and malnutrition.*

General Considerations

External fistulas of the small bowel may form spontaneously as a result of disease, but about 95% are complications of surgical procedures (anastomotic dehiscence or injury to bowel during dissection). Fistulas are particularly prone to develop when the surgeon encounters extensive adhesions, inflamed intestine, or radiation enteropathy.

Fistulas can be classified according to anatomic site, characteristics of the tract (simple or complex), and volume of output (high or low). A high-output fistula produces more than 500 mL/24 h. Other descriptive terms are also used, eg, end fistula, which encompasses the entire diameter of the bowel, and lateral fistula, which arises from one side only.

Clinical Findings

A. Symptoms and Signs

Postoperative fistula formation is heralded by fever and abdominal pain until bowel contents discharge through the abdominal incision. Spontaneous fistulas from neoplasms or inflammatory disease usually develop in a more indolent manner. Most fistulas are associated with one or more abscesses, which often drain incompletely with fistulization, so that persistent sepsis is a common feature. Intestinal fluid escaping through the fistula may severely excoriate the skin and abdominal wall tissues. Fluid and electrolyte losses may be severe, especially if the fistula is large, if it is located in the upper tract, or if there is partial or complete intestinal obstruction distal to the fistula. Persistent sepsis and difficulty in nourishing the patient contribute to rapid weight loss.

B. Laboratory Findings

Routine laboratory tests reflect the severity of deficits in red cell mass, plasma volume, and electrolytes. Leukocytosis due to sepsis and hemoconcentration is common. Disease of other organs such as liver and kidneys may be detected.

C. Imaging Studies

Abscesses and intestinal obstruction may be evident on plain abdominal films. Contrast medium administered orally, per rectum, or through the fistula (fistulogram) delineates the abnormal anatomy, including intrinsic bowel disease, and demonstrates the location and number of fistulas, the length and course of fistula tracts, associated abscess cavities, and the presence of distal obstruction. Radiologists can manipulate catheters into tracts and provide detailed diagnostic information; this procedure may also be therapeutic (see below). Chest films, CT scans, ultrasound, endoscopy, and other special studies may be indicated in certain individuals.

Complications

Fluid and electrolyte losses, malnutrition, and sepsis contribute to multiple organ failure and death unless effective therapy is instituted promptly.

Treatment

A systematic approach combining diagnostic, supportive, and operative procedures is essential in the management of patients with fistulas (Table 30–2). In few other conditions is the proper timing of operative intervention more critical.

A. Fluid and Electrolyte Resuscitation

Many fistula patients are profoundly depleted of intravascular and interstitial volume, and replacement of

Table 30–2. Treatment of fistulas.

First:
  Restore blood volume and begin correction of fluids and
    electrolyte imbalance.
  Drain accessible abscesses.
  Control fistula and measure losses.
  Begin nutritional support.
Second:
  Delineate anatomy of fistulas by radiographic studies.
Third:
  Maintain caloric intake of 2000–3000 kcal or more per day,
    depending on status of nutrition and energy expenditure.
  Drain abscesses as they appear.
Fourth:
  Operate if fistula fails to close.

this fluid with isotonic saline solution takes first priority. Central venous pressure, urine output, and skin turgor are guides to the progress of volume resuscitation. Blood is sent to the laboratory for measurement of serum electrolyte concentrations and arterial blood gases. Results of these studies assist in correcting electrolyte deficits and deranged acid-base balance. Fluid should be collected from fistula output, nasogastric suction, and urine for measurement of volume and electrolyte composition. Body weight is recorded daily. Fluid and electrolyte resuscitation can usually be accomplished within the first day or two. Subsequent maintenance of homeostasis depends on accurately measuring losses and replacing them.

B. Control of Fistula

Fistula drainage fluid must be collected to avoid excoriation of skin and abdominal wall tissues and to record volume losses. An ostomy appliance may fit around the fistula or a catheter inserted by a radiologist under x-ray guidance may work best. Skilled and experienced nursing care is indispensable.

C. Control of Sepsis

Abscesses should be drained as soon as they are diagnosed. The source of sepsis is often obscure, and a continuous diligent search for abscesses must be made by repeated physical examination and imaging studies until the infection is located and treated. Blind therapy with broad-spectrum antibiotics is not a substitute for drainage of abscesses. In many cases, an incompletely drained abscess can be managed by an interventional radiologist, who passes a catheter through a fistula tract into the associated abscess cavity. Drainage is accomplished, and the fistula may close as the sump tube is gradually withdrawn over a period of weeks.

D. Delineation of Fistula

Radiographic contrast studies (see above) should be obtained as soon as feasible.

E. Nutrition

Adequate nutrition and control of sepsis make the difference between survival and death for these patients. A useful general rule is to avoid all oral intake at the outset. Nasogastric suction may be necessary temporarily. As soon as intravascular fluid and electrolytes are restored, parenteral nutrition should be instituted via a central intravenous catheter.

For many patients, total parenteral nutrition is the principal exogenous source of calories and nitrogen until the fistula heals or is closed surgically. For patients with low-output or distal fistulas, the enteral route for nutrition is preferred, and elemental or polymeric diets can be delivered into the distal gut in some patients with proximal fistulas.

F. Other Measures

H_2 receptor antagonists are useful adjuncts in patients with proximal fistulas. By reducing gastric acid secretion, fistula output is decreased and fluid and electrolyte management is simplified. Somatostatin decreases fistula output and accelerates fistula closure. The short half-life of this agent, its inhibitory effects on pancreatic insulin secretion, and rebound recurrences after fistula closure leave the value of somatostatin unclear. New somatostatin analogs may prove more useful in the future.

G. Operation

About 30% of fistulas close spontaneously; Crohn's disease, irradiated bowel, cancer, foreign body, distal obstruction, extensive disruption of intestinal continuity, and a short (< 2 cm) fistula tract are associated with failure of fistulas to heal. An experimental approach is instillation of fibrin glue into the tract directly or through an endoscope inserted into the fistula; despite promising reports, this method has not been proved safe and effective, and it is not applicable to most fistulas that come to operation. If they are going to heal spontaneously, fistulas usually close within a month after eradication of infection and institution of adequate nutritional support, and persistence much beyond a month indicates the need for surgical closure in most cases. Serum levels of short-turnover proteins, particularly transferrin, might be useful in predicting which patients are unlikely to close their fistulas. The operation should be postponed, however, until one can predict that intra-abdominal inflammation has resolved—typically 2–3 months after the last operation. The fistulous segment should be resected, associated obstruction relieved, and continuity reestablished by end-to-end anastomosis.

Prognosis

The plan of management outlined above results in survival rates of 80–95% in patients with external fistulas. Uncontrolled sepsis is the chief cause of death.

Borison DI, Bloom AD, Pritchard TJ: Treatment of enterocutaneous and colocutaneous fistulas with early surgery or somatostatin analog. Dis Colon Rectum 1992;35:635.

Kubshinoff BW et al: Serum transferrin as a prognostic indicator of spontaneous closure and mortality in gastrointestinal cutaneous fistulas. Ann Surg 1993;217:615.

Spiliotis J et al: Treatment of fistulas of the gastrointestinal tract with total parenteral nutrition and octreotide in patients with carcinoma. Surg Gynecol Obstet 1993;176:575.

Torres AJ et al: Somatostatin in the management of gastrointestinal fistulas. A multicenter trial. Arch Surg 1992;127:97.

ACUTE VASCULAR LESIONS OF THE SMALL INTESTINE & MESENTERY

Lesions producing acute or chronic ischemia or hemorrhage may result from intrinsic vascular disease, systemic illness, pharmacologic agents, and surgical procedures. Chronic occlusion may be amenable to vascular reconstruction and is discussed in Chapter 35. Acute mesenteric ischemia is discussed here.

1. Acute Mesenteric Vascular Occlusion

ESSENTIALS OF DIAGNOSIS

- Severe, diffuse abdominal pain.
- Gross or occult intestinal bleeding.
- Minimal physical findings.
- Radiographic findings (sometimes).
- Operative findings.

General Considerations

Sudden occlusion of major small bowel arteries or veins is catastrophic. It is predominantly a disease of the elderly and is highly lethal. Mesenteric **arterial emboli** account for 50% of cases of acute mesenteric ischemia; they most commonly originate from mural thrombus in an infarcted left ventricle or clot in a fibrillating left atrium in patients with mitral stenosis. **Thrombosis of a mesenteric artery** (25% of cases) is the end result of atherosclerotic stenosis, and these patients often give a history of intestinal angina before the acute thrombosis occurs. Other causes of acute arterial occlusions, such as dissecting aortic aneurysm or fusiform aortic aneurysm, are rare. Occlusions of smaller mesenteric arteries often are associated with connective tissue or other systemic disorders. Cocaine ingestion is another cause. Nonocclusive disease (see below) is responsible for about 20% of patients with acute mesenteric ischemia.

Thrombosis of mesenteric veins (5% of cases) is associated with portal hypertension, abdominal sepsis, hypercoagulable states, or trauma, or there may be no apparent underlying disease. Mesenteric venous or arterial thrombosis can occur in women taking oral contraceptives. Some venous occlusions develop peripherally and progress insidiously, causing segmental infarction that resembles strangulation obstruction. Others have acute, severe, rapidly progressive ischemia.

The consequences of major vascular occlusion depend on the vessel involved, the level of occlusion, the status of other visceral vessels, the development of collaterals, the establishment of reperfusion, and other factors. Tissue injury is caused by events related to the ischemia itself (ischemic injury) and by return of blood flow, either spontaneous or as a result of treatment (reperfusion injury). Complete interruption of oxygen supply to the intestine produces necrosis first at the tips of villi. Mucosal slough begins within 3 hours after onset of ischemia, and ulceration and bleeding soon become extensive. Full-thickness infarction of bowel wall occurs as early as 6 hours after onset in total ischemia; in partial ischemia, it may take several days for this stage to be reached. Hemorrhage into the lumen, accumulation of bloody abdominal fluid, perforation, and death from sepsis are the end results of infarction. Sepsis and multi-organ system failure may develop even in the absence of full-thickness necrosis or perforation; bacteria proliferate in the necrotic segment; the mucosal barrier is disrupted; and bacteria and their toxic products translocate into the circulation. A variety of plasma substances including tumor necrosis factor and platelet-activating factor arise at the site of intestinal injury, enter the circulation, and damage target organs such as the lung.

There is increasing recognition of the importance of reperfusion injury in the outcome of intestinal ischemia. Return of arterial blood flow from spontaneous events, lysis of clot by anticoagulants, or arterial reconstruction converts the enzyme xanthine dehydrogenase to xanthine oxidase, resulting in the release of superoxide and hydrogen peroxide. These oxygen radicals destabilize cell membranes, disrupt the mucosal barrier, and flood the systemic circulation with mediators of damage to other organs. Most of the data come from experimental animals, but there is little doubt that reperfusion injury is an important and potentially lethal phenomenon in patients. Drug prophylaxis against ischemic and reperfusion injury has not reached the stage of clinical utility.

Clinical Findings

A. SYMPTOMS AND SIGNS

The most constant symptom is severe, poorly localized abdominal pain that is often unresponsive to narcotics. Nausea and vomiting, diarrhea, and constipation are variable in occurrence.

In the early stages there is a striking paucity of abdominal findings; in fact, pain out of proportion to the objective findings is a hallmark of mesenteric vascular occlusion. Ischemia can also occur with much less severe pain, and serious illness may be recognized only when secondary toxicity develops. Later in the course, abdominal distention and tenderness occur. Shock and generalized peritonitis eventually develop, but by that time the opportunity for salvage has been lost. In some instances—particularly with a high venous occlusion—

shock is an early finding. Stool or gastric contents contain blood in 75–95% of patients later in the course. Paracentesis does not help to establish the diagnosis in the reversible stages.

B. LABORATORY FINDINGS

Striking leukocytosis is present. Serum amylase is elevated in about half of patients, and creatine kinase (BB isoenzyme) correlates with intestinal infarction. Significant base deficits may be observed. Increased inorganic phosphate levels in serum and peritoneal fluid are a sign of irreversible ischemia. Hemoconcentration and the effects of hemorrhage into the lumen or mesentery are reflected in laboratory tests in the late stages. Antithrombin III deficiency and other abnormalities of coagulation should be sought.

C. IMAGING STUDIES

Plain abdominal films allow a presumptive diagnosis of vascular occlusion to be made in about 20% of patients. Absence of intestinal gas, diffuse distention with air-fluid levels, and distention of small bowel and colon up to the splenic flexure are nonspecific but suggestive. Blunt plicae, thickened bowel wall, and small bowel loops that remain unchanged over several hours are seen occasionally. Specific findings of intestinal necrosis, including intramural gas and gas in the portal venous system, occur late. Barium studies may reveal "thumbprinting" and disordered motility (either slow or rapid). CT gives useful information in 50% of patients, though a specific diagnosis is possible in only 25% of cases. MRI may be useful. Mesenteric arteriography may be helpful but is logistically cumbersome in acutely ill patients and is not sensitive enough to rule out the diagnosis.

D. SPECIAL STUDIES

Indium 111-labeled leukocyte scans are useful for detection of infarcted bowel in some cases.

Differential Diagnosis

Acute pancreatitis and strangulation obstruction of the intestine may be difficult to distinguish from mesenteric vascular occlusion. A very high serum amylase early in the disease or a swollen pancreas on CT scan suggests pancreatitis. Differentiation from strangulation obstruction is less important, since both conditions require operation. Angiography may be definitive. Even surgeons with a special interest in this condition are unable to make an early diagnosis in more than half of cases.

Treatment

Survival depends upon diagnosis and operative treatment within 12 hours after onset of symptoms. Although acute occlusion of major arteries or veins requires operation, pre- and postoperative intra-arterial infusion of papaverine (30–60 mg/h) has been recommended if the angiogram demonstrates embolic occlusion of the superior mesenteric artery.

Acute venous thrombosis is diagnosed by the edematous mesentery and extrusion of clots when mesenteric veins are cut. Resection of all of the involved gut and its mesentery is the treatment of choice; direct mesenteric venous surgery (thrombectomy) is seldom successful. Administration of heparin postoperatively is recommended. Antithrombin III deficiency and other causes of hypercoagulability should be treated.

In arterial occlusion, there is segmental or diffuse ischemia or infarction of small bowel and colon in the distribution of the occluded vessel. Arterial pulsations are absent or reduced, and mesenteric edema is not so striking as in venous occlusion. Many methods of helping the surgeon judge viability have been suggested, but most have not proved their worth. The Doppler ultrasonic flowmeter is of some help, and the laser Doppler system is promising. The qualitative fluorescein test is not as sensitive as once believed. Quantitative fluorescence, as measured by a perfusion fluorometer, is under investigation.

Necrotic bowel should be resected unless the extent of damage is so great that satisfactory life could not be expected. With the availability of home parenteral nutrition, more patients are salvageable now than before. It is not clear how to integrate the new information about reperfusion injury into management of patients with reversibly ischemic bowel. Perhaps it is better to just resect the affected intestine, particularly in the elderly, even though vascular reconstruction may be technically possible by embolectomy, thromboendarterectomy, or arterial bypass. Vascular reconstruction was attempted in 10% or less of patients before reperfusion injury became recognized, and it is likely that even fewer patients will be treated by a direct approach to the vessels in the future.

Massive volume support and antibiotics are mandatory, and anticoagulants or drugs that inhibit platelet aggregation are given by some surgeons. A second-look operation is performed 12–24 hours later if marginally viable bowel was left in.

Percutaneous transluminal angioplasty has been used to treat acute mesenteric ischemia, but its role is yet to be defined, and abdominal operation remains the standard treatment.

Prognosis

Acute mesenteric vascular occlusion is often lethal, because diagnosis and treatment are delayed, infarction is extensive, and arterial reconstruction is difficult. The overall mortality rate of arterial occlusion is about

45%, although a recent report of deaths occurring in only 24% is encouraging. If infarction is so extensive that over half of the small bowel must be resected, the death rate is 45–85%. Reconstruction of acutely thrombosed visceral arteries is often not feasible, and patency rates are poor. In a few patients, the acute ischemic episode goes unrecognized, and the process resolves spontaneously with stricture formation. The prognosis is excellent in this situation. Acute venous thrombosis has a death rate of 30%, and if long-term anticoagulants are not used, approximately 25% of patients have another episode of thrombosis. Administration of coumarin anticoagulants for at least 3 months is recommended to minimize the possibility of recurrence.

2. Nonocclusive Intestinal Ischemia

In about one-fourth of patients with intestinal ischemia, vascular occlusion does not involve a major artery or vein (although arterial stenosis is usually present). In the presence of some other acute disease such as a cardiac dysrhythmia or sepsis, splanchnic vasoconstriction occurs, and the intestine becomes ischemic because of low perfusion pressure and flow. Arterial blood is shunted away from the villi in these circumstances, and the ischemic villi are destroyed if the condition persists.

The diagnosis is suspected when a potentially susceptible patient develops acute abdominal pain. The clinical picture is similar to that of arterial thrombosis, but the onset is less often sudden. Arteriography documents the absence of major vascular occlusion but is not otherwise diagnostic in most cases.

Direct infusion of vasodilator agents into the superior mesenteric artery may reverse splanchnic vasoconstriction in selected cases. Papaverine is the drug of choice, but other drugs are under investigation. Operation is usually required to exclude other diseases that simulate intestinal ischemia and to resect infarcted bowel.

Patchy or diffuse ischemia varies in extent and severity. Ischemia is most pronounced on the antimesenteric border, and the mucosa may be extensively involved before abnormalities are visible on the serosal surface. There are often ischemic areas in other organs such as liver and spleen. Vascular reconstruction is ineffective, and surgical procedures are limited to resection of infarcted bowel. Decisions about when to perform a primary anastomosis or second-look operation are individualized. The death rate was about 90% until recently, mainly because the underlying disease often could not be corrected. Intra-arterial vasodilator therapy has lowered this figure.

Boley SJ, Brandt LJ: Intestinal ischemia. Surg Clin North Am 1992;72:1.

Bulkley GB: Free radicals and other reactive oxygen metabolites: clinical relevance and the therapeutic efficacy of antioxidant therapy. Surgery 1993;113:479.

Gennaro M et al: Acute mesenteric ischemia after cardiopulmonary bypass. Am J Surg 1993;166:231.

Inderbitzi R et al: Acute mesenteric ischaemia. Eur J Surg 1992; 158:123.

Kaleya RN, Boley SJ: Acute mesenteric ischemia: an aggressive diagnostic and therapeutic approach. 1991 Roussel Lecture. Can J Surg 1992;35:613.

Kam DM, Scheeres DE: Fluorescein-assisted laparoscopy in the identification of arterial mesenteric ischemia. Surg Endosc 1993;7:75.

Kempczinski RF et al: Intestinal ischemia secondary to thromboangiitis obliterans. Ann Vasc Surg 1993;7:354.

Kirschner RE, Fantini GA: Role of iron and oxygen-derived free radicals in ischemia-reperfusion injury. J Am Coll Surg 1994; 179:103.

MacDonald PH et al: The use of oximetry in determining intestinal blood flow. Surg Gynecol Obstet 1993;176:451.

MacSweeney STR, Postlethwaite JC: "Second-look" laparoscopy in the management of acute mesenteric ischaemia. Br J Surg 1994;81:90.

Sheridan WG et al: Determination of a critical level of tissue oxygenation in acute intestinal ischaemia. Gut 1992;33:762.

Simpson R et al: Neutrophil and nonneutrophil-mediated injury in intestinal ischemia-reperfusion. Ann Surg 1993;218:444.

Stoney RJ, Cunningham CG: Acute mesenteric ischemia. Surgery 1993;114:489.

Wade TP, Jewell WR, Andrus CH: Mesenteric venous thrombosis: modern management and endoscopic diagnosis. Surg Endosc 1992;6:283.

3. Other Vascular Lesions

Vasculitis

Vascular lesions associated with systemic disorders such as polyarteritis nodosa and systemic lupus erythematosus may cause patchy infarction of the small intestine. Similar lesions have been seen in patients with a history of amphetamine abuse. The presenting manifestation is usually perforation with peritonitis or intraluminal bleeding, but strictures occur as well. The prognosis depends on the underlying pathologic process and the severity of peritoneal contamination. These patients are often on corticosteroid therapy and do not tolerate infection well. Survival is rare.

Kempczinski RF et al: Intestinal ischemia secondary to thromboangiitis obliterans. Ann Vasc Surg 1993;7:354.

Krant JD, Ross JM: Extracranial giant cell arteritis restricted to the small bowel. Arthritis Rheum 1992;35:603.

Kuehne SE, Gauvin GP, Shortsleeve MJ: Small bowel stricture caused by rheumatoid vasculitis. Radiology 1992;184:215.

Mesenteric Apoplexy

Mesenteric apoplexy is a rare disorder caused by spontaneous rupture of mesenteric arteries. The more general category of **abdominal apoplexy** includes spontaneous hemorrhage into the peritoneal cavity from tumors (particularly hepatomas), the spleen, or other organs. Arteriosclerotic lesions are the cause of arterial rupture in older individuals; the superior mesenteric, right colic, and branches of the celiac artery are the usual sites. Sudden hemorrhage from congenital aneurysms occurs in younger patients; the splenic artery is most commonly involved and is particularly prone to rupture during pregnancy (see Chapter 42). The typical picture is sudden onset of diffuse abdominal pain followed by hypotension. Operation is imperative.

Bellucci MJ, Burke MC, Querusio L: Atraumatic rupture of uteroovarian vessels during pregnancy: a lethal presentation of maternal shock. Ann Emerg Med 1994;23:360.

Berera T et al: Spontaneous rupture of hepatocellular carcinoma. Ital J Gastroenterol 1992;24:461.

Jacobs PP et al: Haemoperitoneum caused by a dissecting aneurysm of the gastroepiploic artery. Eur J Vasc Surg 1994;8:236.

Bleeding Lesions

Arteriovenous malformations and other bleeding lesions in the small intestine are discussed under Acute Lower Gastrointestinal Hemorrhage in Chapter 31.

GAS CYSTS (Pneumatosis Cystoides Intestinalis)

Pneumatosis cystoides intestinalis is a rare condition characterized by gas-filled cysts in the wall of the gut and sometimes in the mesentery. When the process is limited to the large intestine, the term **pneumatosis coli** is used. Cysts vary in size from microscopic to several centimeters in diameter.

Pneumatosis may be primary or secondary. About 15% of cases are primary and idiopathic; the cysts are submucosal and usually are limited to the left colon. Secondary pneumatosis comprises 85% of cases. Cysts are subserosal and may be located anywhere in the gastrointestinal tract or its mesentery. Conditions that underlie secondary pneumatosis intestinalis or pneumatosis coli include inflammatory bowel disease, infectious gastroenteritis or colitis, steroid therapy, connective tissue disorders, intestinal obstruction, diverticulitis, chronic obstructive pulmonary disease, acute leukemia, lymphoma, AIDS, and organ transplantation.

The mechanism of cyst formation may not be the same in all patients. In some, anaerobic bacterial fermentation of carbohydrates leads to excess production of hydrogen gas, which enters the intestinal wall by diffusion. Some patients have greatly diminished activity of methanogenic and sulfate-reducing bacteria, which normally consume or metabolize hydrogen. Patients with impaired pulmonary function are less able to excrete excessive hydrogen gas through the lungs, and they are more prone to develop pneumatosis. Cysts are maintained because additional hydrogen is generated with each meal, thus replacing gas that may have diffused into the bloodstream since the previous meal. High breath hydrogen levels have been reported in pneumatosis patients even during fasting.

Symptoms are absent or nonspecific. In secondary pneumatosis, symptoms are due to the underlying disease. In the primary form, patients may complain of abdominal discomfort, distention, diarrhea with mucus, or passing of excessive amounts of gas. Rarely, perforation of a cyst, hemorrhage, obstruction, or malabsorption may bring benign pneumatosis to medical attention. **Fulminant pneumatosis** is associated with acute bacterial infection and necrosis of the bowel wall. Such patients are toxic and may have underlying impaired immunologic defenses. Gas may also be seen within the intestinal wall late in intestinal infarction. Pneumoperitoneum is sometimes present.

Treatment of secondary pneumatosis intestinalis is directed toward the underlying disease. Resolution of cysts can be accomplished in either primary or secondary pneumatosis by having patients breathe oxygen by mask for several days interrupted only at mealtime. Response to hyperbaric oxygen is more rapid. Recurrence of cysts after oxygen treatment reflects continued production of hydrogen, and in these patients it is necessary to reduce the amount of gas being generated. The amount of substrate can be controlled by dietary manipulation, and the fecal flora can be suppressed by antibacterial agents such as ampicillin or metronidazole. Surgical resection of bowel involved with benign primary pneumatosis is rarely required, but underlying disease may need operative treatment in the secondary form of this condition. Fulminant pneumatosis is treated surgically, but the mortality rate is high.

Christl SU et al: Impaired hydrogen metabolism in pneumatosis cystoides intestinalis. Gastroenterology 1993;104:392.

Collins CD et al: Case report: pneumatosis intestinalis occurring in association with cryptosporidiosis and HIV infection. Clin Radiol 1992;46:410.

Hoover EL et al: Avoiding laparotomy in nonsurgical pneumoperitoneum. Am J Surg 1992;164:99.

TUMORS OF THE SMALL INTESTINE

Neoplasms of the jejunum and ileum comprise 1–5% of all tumors of the gastrointestinal tract. The terminal ileum is the favored site, followed by proximal jejunum.

Approximately 85% of patients are over age 40. There is a high correlation of small bowel tumors with primary neoplasms elsewhere.

Only 10% of small bowel tumors are symptomatic. Benign lesions are ten times as common as malignant ones. Lymphoma is now the most common primary malignant tumor of the small intestine. At least 75% of symptomatic neoplasms are malignant. Bleeding and obstruction, sometimes due to intussusception, are the most frequent symptoms.

1. Benign Tumors

Polyps

Adenomatous or villous polyps of the type seen in the colon are rare in the small bowel; they are usually solitary and cause symptoms by intussusception or bleeding.

Polypoid **hamartomas** may be solitary in patients who are free of associated anomalies. Hamartomas are multiple in 50% of cases, and 10% of these have **Peutz-Jeghers syndrome,** a familial disorder characterized by diffuse gastrointestinal polyposis and mucocutaneous pigmentation. The malignant potential of these polyps is very small. Operation is indicated only for symptoms (eg, obstruction, bleeding), at which time all polyps greater than about 1 cm should be removed. A combined surgical and endoscopic approach is the best strategy.

Familial adenomatous polyposis (familial polyposis coli, Gardner's syndrome; see Chapter 31) is characterized by multiple intestinal and colonic polyps, osteomas, and subcutaneous cysts or fibromas. The polyps are true neoplasms, and malignant degeneration of colonic polyps is common; there is a predilection for periampullary duodenal cancer as well.

Juvenile (retention) polyps may bleed or obstruct. They are more common in the colon than the small bowel and usually autoamputate before adolescence. Some pathologists regard these lesions as hamartomas.

Other Tumors

Leiomyomas, lipomas, neurofibromas, and fibromas may cause symptoms that require operation. Endometriosis can implant on the small bowel. Hemangiomas are discussed in the section on Acute Lower Gastrointestinal Hemorrhage in Chapter 31.

Ali J et al: Clinical presentations of gastrointestinal inflammatory fibroid polyps. Can J Surg 1992;35:194.

Bertoni G et al: Jejunal polyps in familial adenomatous polyposis assessed by push-type endoscopy. J Clin Gastroenterol 1993;17:343.

Buck JL et al: Peutz-Jeghers syndrome. Radiographics 1992; 12:365.

Gall JA et al: Multiple benign stromal cell tumours of the small bowel. J Clin Pathol 1993;46:869.

Gourtsoyiannis NC et al: Radiological appearances of small intestinal leiomyomas. Clin Radiol 1992;45:94.

Hizawa K et al: Cancer in Peutz-Jeghers syndrome. Cancer 1993;72:2777.

Leggett BA et al: Exclusion of APC and MCC as the gene defect in one family with familial juvenile polyposis. Gastroenterology 1993;105:1313.

Serour F et al: Primary neoplasms of the small bowel. J Surg Oncol 1992;49:29.

2. Malignant Tumors

Primary

Adenocarcinoma is often asymptomatic or causes only minimal symptoms for prolonged periods. It usually arises in the proximal jejunum, except in Crohn's disease, in which bypassed distal ileum is at greatest risk. Metastases are present in 80% of cases at the time of operation. Segmental resection of bowel and adjacent mesentery is done when possible, but metastases near the superior mesenteric artery may make the procedure difficult. Five-year survival is 25% in patients undergoing intestinal resection.

Primary small intestinal lymphomas of the Western type arise focally. These lymphomas develop in the proximal jejunum in patients with celiac disease, and in another group of patients the lymphomas arise de novo in the distal ileum. Most primary lymphomas of the small intestine involve B cell proliferation, but a few cases of primary T cell lymphoma have been reported. In the Middle East, primary small bowel lymphoma is the most common form of extranodal lymphomatous disease. **Immunoproliferative small intestinal disease** is a geographic variant in that part of the world; it is characterized by diffuse infiltration of the small intestine by abnormal lymphoid cells. The infiltrate is probably benign in the initial phase of alpha-chain disease, but the other cases are malignant. AIDS-associated non-Hodgkin's lymphomas of B cell origin can involve the small intestine; the prognosis in these patients is very poor.

Western-type lymphomas develop as a nodular, polypoid, or ulcerating mass. Lesions are multiple in 20% of patients. Obstruction, bleeding, and perforation bring the lesion to attention. Abdominal operation is often required to establish a histologic diagnosis by conservative resection of the intestinal lesion. Operation is followed by whole abdominal radiation, with or without chemotherapy, in some patients. The overall 5-year survival rate is about 40%.

Leiomyosarcoma in small bowel tends to ulcerate centrally and bleed. Other types of primary malignant neoplasm are rare.

Metastatic

Small bowel metastases are found in 50% of patients dying of malignant melanoma. Carcinomas of the cervix, kidney, breast, lung, etc, may also spread to bowel. Obstruction or hemorrhage may require operation if life expectancy is reasonably good. Significant palliation may be achieved, particularly in patients with solitary metastatic lesions.

Amer MH, El-Akkad S: Gastrointestinal lymphoma in adults: clinical features and management of 399 cases. Gastroenterology 1994;106:846.

Carbonnel F et al: Extensive small intestinal T-cell lymphoma of low-grade malignancy associated with a new chromosomal translocation. Cancer 1994;73:1286.

Chami TN et al: Angiosarcoma of the small intestine: a case report and literature review. Am J Gastroenterol 1994;89:797.

DiSario JA et al: Small bowel cancer: epidemiological and clinical characteristics from a population-based registry. Am J Gastroenterol 1994;89:699.

Greenstein AJ et al: Lymphoma in inflammatory bowel disease. Cancer 1992;69:1119.

Nakamura S et al: Diagnostic value of push-type jejunal endoscopy in primary jejunal carcinoma. Surg Endosc 1993;7:188.

Ng E-H et al: Prognostic factors influencing survival in gastrointestinal leiomyosarcomas: implications for surgical management and staging. Ann Surg 1992;215:68.

Ruskone-Fourmestraux A et al: Primary digestive tract lymphoma: a prospective multicentric study of 91 patients. Gastroenterology 1993;105:1662.

Stemmermann GN, Goodman MT, Nomura AM: Adenocarcinoma of the proximal small intestine. A marker for familial and multicentric cancer? Cancer 1992;70:2766.

Stollman N et al: Intestinal lymphomatous polyposis in a patient with AIDS: an enteroscopic view and discussion. Am J Gastroenterol 1994;89:802.

3. Carcinoid Tumors & Carcinoid Syndrome

Carcinoid tumors are apudomas that arise from enterochromaffin cells throughout the gut. Carcinoids may be associated with multiple endocrine neoplasia (MEN) type 1 and type 2. Rare familial clustering not associated with MEN has been reported. Neoplasms of other organs—most commonly the colon, lung, stomach, or breast—are present in 15% of patients. Carcinoids occur in patients 25–45 years of age.

The origin of carcinoid tumors of the gastrointestinal tract is foregut, 5%; midgut, 88%; and hindgut, 6%. Most carcinoids associated with MEN are of foregut origin. Midgut carcinoids produce serotonin and substance P; neurotensin, gastrin, somatostatin, motilin, secretin, and pancreatic polypeptide are also common. Foregut and hindgut carcinoids do not produce serotonin, but they often contain gastrin, somatostatin, pancreatic polypeptide, and glucagon.

The appendix is the most common site of carcinoid tumors, and the small intestine is the second most common location; about ten times as many originate in the ileum as in the jejunum. Multiple tumors are present in 40% of cases. Grossly, carcinoids are firm, yellowish submucosal nodules. Special stains may demonstrate argentaffin or argyrophil reactions in microscopic sections.

Carcinoid of the small bowel should be regarded as "a malignant neoplasm in slow motion." At the time of surgical diagnosis, 40% of tumors have invaded the muscularis and 45% have metastasized to lymph nodes or liver. Of primary tumors less than 1 cm in diameter, fewer than 2% metastasize, but 80% of those larger than 2 cm have spread at the time of operation. Huge metastatic deposits emanating from a minute primary are sometimes encountered.

Clinical Findings

A. SYMPTOMS AND SIGNS

Small tumors are usually asymptomatic. Overall, 30% of small bowel carcinoids cause symptoms of obstruction, pain, bleeding, or the carcinoid syndrome. Obstruction due to sclerosis and kinking of the bowel may be related to elaboration of vasoactive materials by metastases in the mesentery. Intestinal ischemia has been reported.

About 10% of patients with small bowel carcinoids present with **carcinoid syndrome,** and others develop it later. The syndrome consists of cutaneous flushing, diarrhea, bronchoconstriction, and right-sided cardiac valvular disease due to collagen deposition. Biologically active substances secreted by carcinoids are usually inactivated in the liver, but hepatic metastases or primary ovarian or bronchial carcinoids release these compounds directly into the systemic circulation, where they produce symptoms. Serotonin production in large quantities occurs in almost all cases of carcinoid syndrome; it is responsible for much of the diarrhea. A host of other vasoactive substances may participate, including amines (histamine, dopamine, 5-hydroxytryptophan, and 5-HIAA), tachykinins (kallikrein, substance P, and neuropeptide K), peptides (pancreatic polypeptide, chromogranins, neurotensin, and motilin), and prostaglandins.

B. LABORATORY FINDINGS

Some carcinoid tumors are detected by radiographic methods. Elevated urinary levels of 5-hydroxyindoleacetic acid (5-HIAA) are the diagnostic hallmark of carcinoid syndrome. An injection of pentagastrin can be used as a provocative test: Symptoms appear, and serum levels of serotonin and substance P increase.

Treatment

All accessible carcinoid tumor in small bowel, mesentery, and the peritoneal cavity should be removed. If metastases are present in the mesentery but all gross disease can be removed, a second-look operation is often recommended 6 months later.

If intestinal obstruction is the principal serious manifestation of incurable abdominal disease, it should be treated aggressively because tumor growth is so slow. Extensive enterectomy followed by chronic total parenteral nutrition may even be justified in some cases.

Localized hepatic metastases should be resected. Unresectable hepatic metastases can sometimes be palliated by hepatic artery embolization or hepatic artery infusion chemotherapy. Doxorubicin gives a 20% response rate. A combination of fluorouracil, doxorubicin, cyclophosphamide, and streptozocin gives a response rate of 30%. Suppression of tumor growth in animals is achieved by interferon, octreotide, and difluoromethylornithine in combination.

Carcinoid syndrome can be treated by various pharmacologic agents designed to block the effects of active substances. Among the agents sometimes used are phenothiazines, corticosteroids, and histamine H_1 and H_2 receptor antagonists. Cyproheptadine, an antihistamine that blocks serotonin 1, serotonin 2, and histamine H_1 receptors, is useful for the control of diarrhea. Octreotide inhibits release of gastrointestinal hormones; in carcinoid syndrome, it relieves flushing, wheezing, and severe diarrhea refractory to other measures. Interferon

has a mixed record of tumor suppression and reduction of symptoms of carcinoid syndrome.

Prognosis

Carcinoid tumors grow slowly over months and years. The overall 5-year survival rate after resection of small bowel carcinoid is 70%; 40% of patients with inoperable metastases and 20% of those with hepatic metastases survive 5 years or longer. Median survival from the time of histologic diagnosis is 14 years, and from onset of the carcinoid syndrome it is 8 years.

Ahlman H et al: Clinical efficacy of octreotide scintigraphy in patients with midgut carcinoid tumours and evaluation of intraoperative scintillation detection. Br J Surg 1994;81:1144.

Basson MD et al: Biology and management of the midgut carcinoid. Am J Surg 1993;165:288.

Delcore R, Friesen SR: Gastrointestinal neuroendocrine tumors. J Am Coll Surg 1994;178:187.

Farahvash MJ et al: Jejunized colon: a rare complication of carcinoid tumor. Am J Gastroenterol 1994;89:429.

Marshall JB, Bodnarchuk G: Carcinoid tumors of the gut: our experience over three decades and review of the literature. J Clin Gastroenterol 1993;16:123.

Moyana TN, Satkunam N: A comparative immunohistochemical study of jejunoileal and appendiceal carcinoids: implications for histogenesis and pathogenesis. Cancer 1992;70:1081.

Pyke CM et al: Carcinoid syndrome secondary to a primary tumour in a Meckel's diverticulum. Aust N Z J Surg 1993;63:732.

Søoreide O et al: Surgical treatment as a principle in patients with advanced abdominal carcinoid tumors. Surgery 1992;111:48.

von der Ohe MR et al: Motor dysfunction of the small bowel and colon in patients with the carcinoid syndrome and diarrhea. N Engl J Med 1993;329:1073.

Yoshikane H et al: Carcinoid tumors of the gastrointestinal tract: evaluation with endoscopic ultrasonography. Gastrointest Endosc 1993;39:375.

Large Intestine

31

George J. Chang, MD, Andrew Shelton, MD, Theodore R. Schrock, MD, &
Mark L. Welton, MD

ANATOMY

The colon extends from the end of the ileum to the rectum. The cecum, ascending colon, hepatic flexure, and proximal transverse colon comprise the **right colon.** The distal transverse colon, splenic flexure, descending colon, sigmoid colon, and rectosigmoid comprise the **left colon** (Figure 31–1). The ascending and descending portions are fixed in the retroperitoneal space, and the transverse colon and sigmoid colon are suspended in the peritoneal cavity by their mesocolons. The caliber of the lumen is greatest at the cecum and diminishes distally. The wall of the colon has four layers: mucosa, submucosa, muscularis, and serosa (Figure 31–2). The muscularis propria consists of an inner circular layer and an outer longitudinal layer. The longitudinal muscle completely encircles the colon in a very thin layer, and at three points around the circumference it is gathered into thick bands called taeniae coli. Sacculations (haustra) are the result of shortening of the colon by the taeniae and contractions of the circular muscle. The haustra are not fixed anatomic structures and may be observed to move longitudinally. There are fatty appendages (the appendices epiploicae) on the serosal surface. The wall of the colon is so thin that it becomes markedly distended when obstructed.

The **rectum** is 12–15 cm in length. The taeniae coli spread out at the rectosigmoid junction and are not apparent distal to that area. The upper rectum is invested by peritoneum anteriorly and laterally, but posteriorly it is retroperitoneal up to the rectosigmoid. The anterior peritoneal reflection dips low into the pelvis to approximately 7 cm above the anal verge—a fact to be noted when rectal lesions are biopsied or fulgurated; perforation into the peritoneal cavity can occur at a much lower level anteriorly than posteriorly. The anterior peritoneal reflection lies behind the bladder in males and behind the uterus (the rectouterine pouch of Douglas) in females. Tumor masses or abscesses in this location are readily palpated on digital rectal or pelvic examination. The rectum is normally capacious and distensible. When its capacity to distend is lost or impaired by surgery or disease, fecal urgency and frequency are noted.

The rectal valves of Houston are prominent spirally arranged mucosal folds within the rectum. Less than half of people have the so-called normal three valves, two on the left and one on the right. The valves are at variable distances from the anal verge in different individuals. Normally, the valves appear thin, with sharp edges, but they become thickened and blunted when inflamed. A rectal valve may hide a small lesion from endoscopic view, and during rigid sigmoidoscopy the valve must be "ironed out" so its superior surface can be examined. Because of angulation and local muscular contraction, the most difficult level to pass with the sigmoidoscope is the rectosigmoid junction.

In males, the prostate gland, the seminal vesicles, and the seminal ducts lie anterior to the rectum. The prostate usually is easily felt, but the seminal vesicles are not palpable unless distended, because the firm, unyielding rectovesical fascia of Denonvilliers intervenes. In females, the rectovaginal septum and uterus lie anterior and the uterine adnexa anterolateral to the rectum. The structures are easily palpated with one finger in the vagina and one in the rectum.

Blood Supply & Lymphatic Drainage

The arterial supply of the right colon, from the ileocecal junction to approximately the mid transverse colon, is from the superior mesenteric artery through its ileocolic, right colic, and middle colic branches.

The inferior mesenteric artery arises from the abdominal aorta and gives off the left colic and sigmoid branches before it becomes the superior hemorrhoidal artery. The vasa recta are the terminal arterial branches to the colon and run directly to the mesocolic wall or through the bowel wall to the antimesocolic border.

The colic arteries bifurcate and form arcades about 2.5 cm from the mesocolic border of the bowel, forming a pathway of communicating vessels called the **marginal artery of Drummond.** The marginal artery thus forms an anastomosis between the superior mesenteric and inferior mesenteric arteries. The configuration of the blood supply, however, varies greatly; the typical pattern is present in only 15% of individuals.

The middle hemorrhoidal artery arises on each side from the anterior division of the internal iliac artery or from the internal pudendal artery and runs inward in the lateral ligaments of the rectum. The inferior hemorrhoidal arteries derive from the internal pudendal arteries

705

Figure 31–1. The large intestine: anatomic divisions and blood supply. The veins are shown in black. The insert shows the usual configuration of the colon.

and pass through Alcock's canal. The anastomoses between the superior hemorrhoidal vessels and branches of the internal iliac arteries provide collateral circulation; this is important after surgical interruption or atherosclerotic occlusion of the vascular supply of the left colon.

The veins accompany the corresponding arteries and drain into the liver through the portal vein or into the systemic circulation by way of the hypogastric veins. Continuous lymphatic plexuses in the submucous and subserous layers of the bowel wall drain into the lymphatic channels and lymph nodes that accompany the blood vessels.

Nerve Supply

The sympathetic nerves originating in T10–12 travel in the thoracic splanchnic nerves to the celiac plexus and then to the preaortic and superior mesenteric plexuses, from which postganglionic fibers are distributed along the superior mesenteric artery and its branches to the right colon. The left colon is supplied by sympathetic fibers that arise in L1–3, synapse in the paravertebral ganglia, and accompany the inferior mesenteric artery to the colon. The parasympathetic nerves to the right colon come from the right vagus and travel with the sympathetic nerves. The parasympathetic supply to the left colon derives from S2–4. These fibers emerge from the spinal cord as the nervi erigentes, which form the pelvic plexus and send branches to the transverse, descending, and pelvic portions of the colon.

Al-Fallouji MA, Tagart RE: The surgical anatomy of the colonic intramural blood supply and its influence on colorectal anastomosis. J R Coll Surg Edinb 1985;30:380.

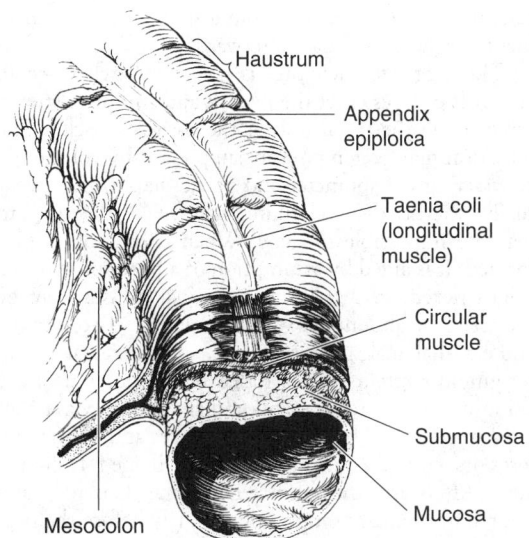

Figure 31–2. Cross section of colon. The longitudinal muscle encircles the colon but is thickened in the region of the taeniae coli.

Crowe R et al: Peptide-containing neurons in different regions of the submucous plexus of human sigmoid colon. Gastroenterology 1992;102:461.

Irving MH, Catchpole B: ABC of colorectal diseases: Anatomy and physiology of the colon, rectum, and anus. Br Med J 1992;304:1106.

Pace JL: The anatomy of the haustra of the human colon. Proc R Soc Med 1968;61:934.

Ward SM: Interstitial cells of Cajal in enteric neurotransmission. Gut 2000;47 Suppl 4:40.

PHYSIOLOGY

The primary functions of the colon are absorption, secretion, motility, and intraluminal digestion. These interrelated phenomena process ileal effluent and convert it into semisolid feces that are stored until defecation is convenient. Regional variations in function are significant. The proximal colon absorbs electrolytes and water more efficiently than do the descending colon and rectum, and motility and intraluminal digestion differ by region also. Loss of colonic function through disease or surgery results in a continuous discharge of food wastes and increases daily intestinal losses of water and electrolytes, chiefly sodium and chloride.

The small intestine digests and absorbs most nutrients from ingested foods. The role of the colon in human nutrition is not well defined. Metabolism of carbohydrate to absorbable volatile fatty acids is proba-bly important. Ureolysis—conversion of circulating urea to ammonia, which is reabsorbed and reused—may be significant. The colon also absorbs amino acids, bile acids, and vitamin K, but the contribution of the colon to homeostasis by these mechanisms has not been quantitated.

Intestinal Gas

The volume and composition of intestinal gas vary greatly among normal individuals. The small intestine contains approximately 100 mL of gas and the colon somewhat more. Some gas is absorbed through the mucosa and excreted through the lungs, and the remaining 400–1200 mL/d are discharged as flatus.

Nitrogen (N_2) comprises 30–90% of intestinal gas. Swallowed air is the principal source of intestinal N_2, but N_2 also can diffuse across the mucosa from blood to lumen when other gases are produced in sufficient volume to lower the partial pressure of N_2 and establish a gradient for diffusion. Other intestinal gases include oxygen (O_2), carbon dioxide (CO_2), hydrogen (H_2), methane (CH_4), and odoriferous trace substances such as methyl sulfide, hydrogen sulfide, indole, and skatole. H_2 and CO_2 are generated by fermentation of ingested nonabsorbed carbohydrate, especially carbohydrate present in polysaccharides (eg, fiber) and some starches. Lactose in milk provides the substrate in lactase-deficient persons. Mucus is the main endogenous source of carbohydrate in the colon; intestinal glycoproteins are 80% carbohydrate. Only about one-third of the population produces CH_4, which is also a product of colonic bacteria that use hydrogen to reduce CO_2. Stools of CH_4 producers nearly always float, even in the absence of fecal fat. CH_4, like H_2, can be measured in the breath. H_2 and CH_4 are explosive gases, and caution must be exercised when using electrocautery in the bowel lumen. Mannitol, a carbohydrate alcohol that is not absorbed by the small bowel, has been used to cleanse the bowel for colonoscopy. Since colonic bacteria ferment mannitol to produce hydrogen, this agent should not be used.

Patients with "excessive gas" may complain of abdominal pain and distention, increased flatus, and watery stools. Some of these patients have irritable bowel syndrome. "Increased" flatus may reflect extreme sensitivity of the rectum to small volumes, resulting in frequent passage of gas. Alternatively, gas may be produced in excessive quantities in symptomatic patients. Almost invariably, hydrogen is the culprit. Measurement of breath hydrogen is a potentially useful test for malabsorption states. Treatment of overproduction of gas at present is directed toward elimination of lactose, legumes, and wheat from the diet.

Motility

Motor activity of the colon occurs in three patterns, and there is marked regional variation between the right and left colon. A pacemaker in the transverse colon has been postulated, perhaps pacing the proximal colon retrograde to facilitate storage and absorption while pacing the distal colon in the aborad direction to favor propulsion. **Retrograde peristalsis (antiperistalsis)**—annular contractions moving orad—dominates in the right colon. This kind of activity churns the contents and tends to confine them to the cecum and ascending colon. As ileal effluent continually enters the cecum, some of the column of liquid stool in the right colon is displaced and flows into the transverse colon. **Segmentation** is the most common type of motor activity in the transverse and descending colon. Annular contractions divide the lumen into uniform segments, propelling feces over short distances in both directions. Segmental contractions form, relax, and re-form in different locations, seemingly at random. **Mass movement** is a strong ring contraction moving aborad over long distances in the transverse and descending colon. It occurs infrequently—perhaps only a few times daily—most commonly after meals.

The enteric nervous system coordinates and programs motility (see Chapter 30). Eating produces a group of alterations in colonic myoelectrical and motor activity collectively termed the gastrocolic response. As a result, more fluid is emptied from the ileum into the colon; mass movements are increased; and the urge to defecate is perceived. The magnitude of the gastrocolic response depends on the caloric content of the meal. Dietary fat is the principal stimulus.

Physical activities such as changes in posture, walking, and lifting are physiologically important stimuli of movement of colonic contents. Colonic motility is also affected by emotional states. Transit through the colon is speeded by a diet containing large amounts of fiber from vegetables or bran. Fiber is defined as insoluble plant cell matrix and consists of cellulose, hemicellulose, and lignin. Dietary fiber slows transit through the jejunum.

Normal colonic movements are slow, complex, and extremely variable, making it difficult to define altered motility in disease states. The fecal stream itself does not move along in anything resembling orderly laminar flow. Some of the material entering the cecum flows past feces remaining from earlier periods. Portions of the stream enter the periphery of haustra, where they may fail to progress for 24 hours or more. In most persons with normal bowel function, residue from a meal reaches the cecum after 4 hours and the rectosigmoid by 24 hours. The transverse colon is the primary site for fecal storage. Mixing of bowel content in the colon re-

sults in passage of residue from a single meal in movements for up to 3–4 days afterward.

The urge to defecate is perceived when small amounts of feces enter the rectum and stimulate stretch receptors in the rectal wall or the levator muscles. The sensation may be temporarily suppressed by voluntarily contracting the sphincter and pelvic diaphragm. Eventually, increased rectal filling may make the urge to defecate impossible to deny. When defecation is performed, it is aided by assumption of a position with the thighs flexed, so that intra-abdominal pressure can be increased by abdominal wall contraction. The internal and external anal sphincters relax, and the rectal or rectosigmoid contents are extruded by contraction of the colon and by increasing abdominal pressure via a Valsalva maneuver. The pelvic floor relaxes and the rectum loses its curves as the feces are discharged from the anus. Afterward, the sphincters resume their tone and the rectum remains empty until shortly before the next movement, when arrival of more feces from the sigmoid elicits the urge to defecate once again.

Absorption

The colon participates in maintaining the body economy by absorption of water and electrolytes, but the absorptive function of the colon is not essential to life. Although amino acids, fatty acids, and some vitamins can be absorbed slowly from the large bowel, only a small amount of these nutrients reaches the colon normally. Perhaps 10—20% of ingested starch, however, passes unabsorbed into the colon, where bacterial fermentation converts starch to short-chain volatile fatty acids (eg, acetate). Absorption of fatty acids contributes importantly to assimilation of calories. Dietary celluloses and hemicelluloses are degraded by colonic bacteria.

Approximately 1000–2000 mL of ileal effluent consisting of 90% water enters the cecum each day. This material is desiccated during transit through the colon, so that only 100–200 mL of water is excreted in the feces. Table 31–1 gives average values for the electrolyte and water composition of ileal effluent and feces; the differences provide a rough estimate of colonic absorption and secretion. Data are listed also for the estimated maximal absorptive capacity, which is greater in the right colon than in the left. This capacity depends on the rate at which fluid enters the cecum. Normally, formed feces are composed of 70% water and 30% solids. Almost half of these solids are bacteria; the remainder is food waste and desquamated epithelium.

Sodium is absorbed by an active transport mechanism that is enhanced by mineralocorticoids, glucocorticoids, and volatile fatty acids produced by bacteria. Volatile fatty acids may be essential mucosal nutrients

Table 31–1. Mean values for electrolyte and water balance in the normal colon. A plus (+) sign indicates absorption from the colonic lumen; a minus (–) sign indicates secretion into the lumen.

| | Ileal Effluent | | Fecal Fluid | | Net Colonic Absorption (per 24 h) | |
	Concentration (meq/L)	Quantity (per 24 h)	Concentration (meq/L)	Quantity (per 24 h)	Normal	Maximal Capacity
Na^+	120	180 meq	30	2 meq	+178 meq	+400 meq
K^+	6	10 meq	67	5 meq	+5 meq	–45 meq
Cl^-	67	100 meq	20	1.5 meq	+98 meq	+500 meq
HCO_3^-	40	60 meq	50	4 meq	+56 meq	
H_2O		1500 mL		100 mL	+1400 mL	+5000 mL

for normal colonic absorption of electrolytes and water. There are segmental differences in the mode of absorption of sodium and water. Normally, sodium absorption is so efficient that a person can remain in balance on as little as 5 meq in the daily diet, but colectomy increases the minimum daily requirements to 80—100 meq to offset losses from the ileostomy. Potassium enters feces by passive diffusion and by secretion in mucus. Excessive mucus production may occur in colitis or with certain tumors such as villous adenomas and may lead to substantial potassium losses in the stool. Chloride is absorbed in exchange for bicarbonate.

Bowel Habits

The frequency of defecation is influenced by social and dietary customs. The average interval between bowel movements among the population of Western countries is a little over 24 hours but may vary in normal subjects from 8–12 hours to 2–3 days. Dietary fiber content and physical activity influence stool frequency to a great extent. Many bedridden patients have infrequent, hard stools. Self-reported constipation in the general population of the USA has a prevalence of about 10% in men and 20% in women; gender differences in colonic function (slower transit and smaller fecal mass in women under controlled conditions) may be responsible for the difference in frequency of constipation. Diarrhea is reported by 5% of men and women. These complaints are more frequent with aging.

A change in bowel habits demands investigation for organic disease. Diarrhea may be debilitating and even fatal, because it is associated with loss of large amounts of water and electrolytes. Diarrhea is usually said to be present if stools contain more than 300 mL of fluid daily. Osmotic diarrhea results when excess water-soluble molecules remain in the bowel lumen, causing osmotic retention of water; this is one mechanism by

which saline laxatives act. Colonic diseases that produce diarrhea usually cause excessive fluid secretion more so than impaired absorption. Bile salts, hydroxy fatty acids, and castor oil (ricinoleic acid) are a few of the many substances that stimulate secretion of fluid by the colon by increasing mucosal cAMP. Increased secretion by the small bowel may also cause diarrhea. Loss of absorptive surface (eg, after intestinal resection) and exudative diseases are other reasons for feces to contain excess fluid. Disordered intestinal motility is not primarily responsible for increased fecal excretion of water. The physician should be alert to surreptitious laxative abuse among patients who complain of diarrhea.

Constipation means infrequent stools (less than two per week), excessive straining, or incomplete evacuation. Recent onset of this complaint in an adult should prompt a search for obstructing lesions.

Severe idiopathic constipation refractory to usual remedies is more common in women; it often begins in adolescence and worsens during the 20s or 30s, or it may be precipitated by childbirth or hysterectomy. A heterogeneous group of disorders is responsible. Slow colonic transit (colonic inertia) is one mechanism of constipation, and failure of the pelvic floor to relax during defecation (obstructed defecation) is a separate category. A classification of disorders in which constipation and obstructed defecation are symptoms is given in Table 31–2. Conditions giving rise to obstructed defecation are part of a larger group of abnormalities termed disorders of the pelvic floor.

A thorough history and physical examination may elucidate the origin of the symptoms, eg, depression, psychotropic or other drugs, or anatomic abnormalities. Further investigation of chronic idiopathic constipation requires assessment of colonic transit and study of pelvic floor function. Colonic transit is evaluated by obtaining serial plain abdominal x-rays after ingestion

Table 31–2. Classification of constipation and obstructed defecation.[1]

Constipation
Normal colon
Normal transit
Slow transit
Megacolon/megarectum
Congenital
Acquired
Obstructed defecation
Solitary rectal ulcer syndrome
Descending perineum syndrome
Rectal intussusception
Complete rectal prolapse
Anismus (inappropriate sphincter contraction)

[1]Modified from Bartolo DCG: Pelvic floor disorders: Incontinence, constipation, and obstructed defecation. Perspect Colon Rectal Surg 1988;1:1.

of tiny radiopaque markers or by scintigraphy after ingestion of radiolabeled solid pellets. Tests of pelvic floor function include defecography, anorectal manometry, electromyography, and nerve conduction studies.

Severe slow-transit constipation does not respond to dietary fiber; lactulose or an irritant laxative (eg, Senokot, Dulcolax) may be effective. Selected patients qualify for a surgical procedure (colectomy and ileorectal anastomosis). Obstructed defecation related to rectal prolapse responds to operation to repair the prolapse. Rectal intussusception should be repaired also, but relief of symptoms is less predictable. Surgical treatment of the other conditions is unsatisfactory at present.

Agarwal R, Afzalpurkar R, Fordtran JS: Pathophysiology of potassium absorption and secretion by the human intestine. Gastroenterology 1994;107:548.

Bartolo DCC et al: Working party report: defecation disorders. Am J Gastroenterol 1994;89:S154.

Bassotti G et al: Colonic motility in man: features in normal subjects and in patients with chronic idiopathic constipation. Am J Gastroenterol 1999;94:1760.

Brown SR et al: Biofeedback avoids surgery in patients with slow-transit constipation: report of four cases. Dis Colon Rectum 2001;44:737.

Francis CY, Whorwell PJ: Bran and irritable bowel syndrome: time for reappraisal. Lancet 1994;344:39.

Grotz RL et al: Discriminant value of psychological distress, symptom profiles, and segmental colonic dysfunction in outpatients with severe idiopathic constipation. Gut 1994;35:798.

Knowles CH, Scott M, Lunniss PJ: Outcome of colectomy for slow transit constipation. Ann Surg 1999;230:627.

Knowles CH, Scott SM, Lunniss PJ: Slow transit constipation: a disorder of pelvic autonomic nerves? Dig Dis Sci 2001; 46:389.

Mollen RM, Kuijpers HC, Claassen AT: Colectomy for slow-transit constipation: preoperative functional evaluation is important but not a guarantee for a successful outcome. Dis Colon Rectum 2001;44:577.

Monahan DW, Peluso FE, Goldner F: Combustible colonic gas levels during flexible sigmoidoscopy and colonoscopy. Gastrointest Endosc 1992;38:40.

Moran BJ, Jackson AA: Function of the human colon. Br J Surg 1992;79:1132.

Nordgaard I, Hansen BS, Mortensen PB: Colon as a digestive organ in patients with short bowel. Lancet 1994;343:373.

Pezim ME et al: Parameters of anorectal and colonic motility in health and in severe constipation. Dis Colon Rectum 1993; 36:484.

Pikarsky AJ et al: Long-term follow-up of patients undergoing colectomy for colonic inertia. Dis Colon Rectum 2001; 44:179.

Robertson G et al: Effects of exercise on total and segmental colon transit. J Clin Gastroenterol 1993;16:300.

Scheppach W, Luehrs H, Menzel T: Beneficial health effects of low-digestible carbohydrate consumption. Br J Nutr 2001;85 Suppl 1: S23.

Soffer EE: Constipation: an approach to diagnosis, treatment, referral. Cleve Clin J Med 1999;66:41.

Tack J, Vanden Berghe P: Neuropeptides and colonic motility: it's all in the little brain. Gastroenterology 2000;119:257.

Thakur A et al: Surgical treatment of severe colonic inertia with restorative proctocolectomy. Am Surg 2001;67:36.

MICROBIOLOGY

The colon of the fetus is sterile, and the bacterial flora is established soon after birth. The type of organisms present in the colon depends in part on dietary and environmental factors. It is estimated that stool contains up to 400 different species of autochthonous (native) bacteria.

Over 99% of the normal fecal flora is anaerobic. *Bacteroides fragilis* is most prevalent, and counts average 10^{10}/g of wet feces. *Lactobacillus bifidus,* clostridia, and cocci of various types are other common anaerobes. Aerobic fecal bacteria are mainly coliforms and enterococci. *Escherichia coli* is the predominant coliform and is present in counts of 10^7/g of feces; other aerobic coliforms include klebsiella, proteus, and enterobacter. *Streptococcus faecalis* is the principal enterococcus. *Methanobrevibacter smithii* is the predominant methane-producing organism in humans.

The fecal flora participates in numerous physiologic processes. Bacteria degrade bile pigments to give the stool its brown color, and the characteristic fecal odor is due to the amines indole and skatole produced by bacterial action. Fecal organisms deconjugate bile salts (only free bile salts are found in feces) and alter the steroid nucleus. Bacteria influence colonic motility and absorption, consume and generate intestinal gases, supply vitamin K to the host, and may be important in the defense against infection. Nutrition of colonic mucosal cells may be partially derived from fuels (eg, fatty acids) produced by bacteria. Intestinal bacteria participate in the pathophysiology of a variety of disease processes. Bacterial translocation from the small and large bowel in critically ill or traumatized patients is believed to contribute to multiple organ system failure. There is evidence that bacteria play a role in the pathogenesis of carcinoma of the large bowel.

Bourquin LD et al: Fermentation of dietary fibre by human colonic bacteria: disappearance of, short-chain fatty acid production from, and potential water-holding capacity of, various substrates. Scand J Gastroenterol 1993;28:249.

Chapman MA: The role of the colonic flora in maintaining a healthy large bowel mucosa. Ann R Coll Surg Engl 2001; 83:75.

Gibson GR, MacFarlane GT, Cummings JH: Sulphate reducing bacteria and hydrogen metabolism in the human large intestine. Gut 1993;34:437.

Pochart P et al: Pyxigraphic sampling to enumerate methanogens and anaerobes in the right colon of healthy humans. Gastroenterology 1993;105:1281.

Strocchi A et al: Methanogens outcompete sulphate reducing bacteria for H_2 in the human colon. Gut 1994;35:1098.

X-RAY EXAMINATION

Plain films of the abdomen depict the distribution of gas in the intestines, calcifications, tumor masses, and the size and position of the liver, spleen, and kidneys. In the presence of acute intra-abdominal disease, erect, lateral, and oblique projections and lateral decubitus views are helpful.

The lumen of the colon can be seen radiographically by instilling a suspension of barium sulfate through the anus (barium enema) (Figure 31–3). Adequate preparation of the bowel is imperative before barium enema examination so that the colon will be as free as possible of fecal material and gas. Although many rectal lesions can be demonstrated by barium enema, x-rays are not as accurate here as with lesions above the rectosigmoid. Proctosigmoidoscopy is the best method for inspecting the rectum. Postevacuation films reveal the mucosal pattern and small lesions.

Barium enemas are performed as single-column or double-column studies. In the double-column (air contrast) barium enema, a higher-density, more viscous barium is used. After the mucosa is first coated with barium, carbon dioxide or air is insufflated to distend the colon and provide a second contrast medium. The double-column barium enema is more sensitive for detection of small lesions, but it is more strenuous and for that reason less well tolerated by frail or elderly patients.

Arteriography is used to detect bleeding sites and is discussed in the section on massive hemorrhage. CT

Figure 31–3. X-ray of normal colon. The colon has been rendered radiopaque by a barium enema (single-column technique).

scan and sonography (external, endorectal, and endovaginal) help diagnose masses (neoplasms and abscesses). MRI is proving reliable for staging of cancers. Single-photon emission CT (SPECT), positron emission tomography (PET), and other potentially useful radiographic techniques have specialized applications. More recently, CT scan with 3D reconstruction, also known as virtual colonoscopy, is being developed. Thus far, the major limitations include the need for full bowel preparation and follow-up colonoscopy for tissue diagnosis of radiographic abnormalities.

Berlin JW et al: Staging of colorectal cancer. Semin Roentgenol 2000;35:370.

Fenlon HM et al: A comparison of virtual and conventional colonoscopy for the detection of colorectal polyps. N Engl J Med 1999;341:1496.

Freeman AH: CT and bowel disease. Br J Radiol 2001;74 (877):4.

Hageman MJHH, Goei R: Cleansing enema prior to double-contrast barium enema examination: is it necessary? Radiology 1993;187:109.

Hunerbein M et al: Preoperative evaluation of colorectal neoplasms by colonoscopic miniprobe ultrasonography. Ann Surg 2000; 232:46.

Jensen DM: What to choose for diagnosis of bleeding colonic angiomas: colonoscopy, angiography, or helical computed tomography angiography? Gastroenterology 2000;119:581.

Suri S et al: Comparative evaluation of plain films, ultrasound and CT in the diagnosis of intestinal obstruction. Acta Radiol 1999;40:422.

Vernava AM 3rd et al: Lower gastrointestinal bleeding. Dis Colon Rectum 1997;40:846.

FIBEROPTIC COLONOSCOPY & SIGMOIDOSCOPY

The flexible colonoscope permits examination of the entire colon in most individuals, and biopsies or brushings (for cytologic examination) can be obtained under direct vision. Video technology has replaced fiberoptic viewing systems.

Diagnostic colonoscopy is indicated in patients age 50 and over and repeated every 5 years if normal (Table 31–3). It is indicated also in those with a personal or family history of colorectal cancer, polyps, or specific familial cancer syndromes; after an abnormal or equivocal barium enema or episode of unexplained rectal bleeding; after abnormal sigmoidoscopy (eg, polyps); and for any patient with a diagnosis of inflammatory bowel disease. Therapeutic uses of colonoscopy include excision of polyps, control of bleeding, removal of a foreign body, detorsion of volvulus, decompression of pseudo-obstruction, dilation of strictures, and destruction of neoplasms. Relative contraindications to colonoscopy are fulminant colitis and suspected colonic perforation. Complications (mainly perforation) occur in 0.4% of diagnostic colonoscopy procedures. Success may be limited by such technical difficulties as diverticular disease, strictures, sharp flexures, redundant colon, or previous pelvic surgery. Colonoscopy is performed intraoperatively on occasion.

Table 31–3. Indications for colonoscopy.

Diagnostic indications
Age ≥ 50
Personal or family history of colorectal cancer, polyps, or specific familial cancer syndromes
Post abnormal or equivocal barium enema or episode of unexplained rectal bleeding
Post abnormal sigmoidoscopy (eg, polyps)
Inflammatory bowel disease
Therapeutic indications
Excision of polyps
Control of bleeding
Removal of a foreign body
Detorsion of volvulus
Decompression of pseudo-obstruction
Dilation of strictures
Destruction of neoplasms

Flexible sigmoidoscopy uses an instrument 65 cm long. The diagnostic yield is two to six times greater than with the rigid sigmoidoscope because two to three times more colon can be seen. Flexible sigmoidoscopy is especially suitable for screening asymptomatic patients for neoplasms; the presence of gross or occult blood may be an indication for total colonoscopy. Flexible sigmoidoscopy has few complications when performed expertly, but the technique must be learned under supervision. Flexible sigmoidoscopes have replaced the rigid variety for most but not all purposes.

Botoman VA, Pietro M, Thirlby RC: Localization of colonic lesions with endoscopic tattoo. Dis Colon Rectum 1994; 37:775.

Hull T, Church JM: Colonoscopy: how difficult, how painful? Surg Endosc 1994;8:784.

Lieberman DA et al: Use of colonoscopy to screen asymptomatic adults for colorectal cancer. Veterans Affairs Cooperative Study Group 380. N Engl J Med 2000;343:162.

Sakanoue Y et al: Intraoperative colonoscopy. Surg Endosc 1993; 7:84.

Sieg A, Hachmoeller-Eisenbach U, Eisenbach T: Prospective evaluation of complications in outpatient GI endoscopy: a survey among German gastroenterologists. Gastrointest Endosc 2001;53:620.

Winawer SJ et al: A comparison of colonoscopy and double-contrast barium enema for surveillance after polypectomy. National Polyp Study Work Group. N Engl J Med 2000; 342:1766.

■ DISEASES OF THE COLON & RECTUM

OBSTRUCTION OF THE LARGE INTESTINE

 ESSENTIALS OF DIAGNOSIS

- *Constipation or obstipation.*
- *Abdominal distention and sometimes tenderness.*
- *Abdominal pain.*
- *Nausea and vomiting (late).*
- *Characteristic x-ray findings.*

General Considerations

Approximately 15% of intestinal obstructions in adults occur in the large bowel. The obstruction may be in any portion of the colon but most commonly is in the sigmoid. Complete colonic obstruction is most often due to carcinoma; volvulus, diverticular disease, inflammatory disorders, benign tumors, fecal impaction, and miscellaneous rare problems account for the remainder (Table 31–4). Adhesive bands seldom obstruct the colon, and intussusception is uncommon in adults.

Obstruction by a lesion at the ileocecal valve produces the symptoms and signs of small bowel obstruction. The pathophysiology of more distal colonic obstruction depends on the competence of the ileocecal valve (Figure 31–4). In 10–20% of individuals, the ileocecal valve is incompetent, and colonic pressure is relieved by reflux into the ileum. If the colon is not decompressed through the ileocecal valve, a "closed loop" is formed between the valve and the obstructing point. The colon distends progressively because the ileum continues to empty gas and fluid into the obstructed segment. If luminal pressure becomes very high, circulation is impaired and gangrene and perforation can result. The wall of the right colon is thinner than that of the left colon and its luminal caliber is larger, so the cecum is at greatest risk of perforation in these circumstances (law of Laplace). In general, if the cecum acutely reaches a diameter of 10–12 cm, the risk of perforation is great.

Clinical Findings

A. SYMPTOMS AND SIGNS

Simple mechanical obstruction of the colon may develop insidiously. Deep, visceral, cramping pain from obstruction of the colon is usually referred to the hypogastrium. Lesions of the fixed portions of the colon (cecum, hepatic flexure, splenic flexure) may cause pain that is felt immediately anteriorly. Pain originating from the sigmoid is often located to the left in the lower abdomen. Severe, continuous abdominal pain suggests intestinal ischemia or peritonitis. Borborygmus may be loud and coincident with cramps. Constipation or ob-

Figure 31–4. The role of the ileocecal valve in obstruction of the colon. The obstruction is in the upper sigmoid. **A:** The ileocecal valve is competent, creating a closed loop between the obstruction and the valve. Tension in the closed loop is increased further by emptying of gas and fluid from the ileum into the colon. **B:** The ileocecal valve is incompetent. Reflux into the ileum is permitted. The colon is relieved of some of its distention, and the small bowel has become distended.

Table 31–4. Causes of colonic obstruction in adults.

Cause	Relative incidence (%)*
Carcinoma of colon	65
Diverticulitis	20
Volvulus	5
Miscellaneous	10

*Obstruction due to diverticulitis is usually incomplete; volvulus is second to carcinoma as a cause of complete obstruction.

stipation is a universal feature of complete obstruction, though the colon distal to the obstruction may empty after the initial symptoms begin. Vomiting is a late finding and may not occur at all if the ileocecal valve prevents reflux. If reflux decompresses the cecal contents into the small intestine, the symptoms of small bowel as well as large bowel obstruction appear. Feculent vomiting is a late manifestation.

Physical examination discloses abdominal distention and tympany, and peristaltic waves may be seen if the abdominal wall is thin. High-pitched, metallic tinkles associated with rushes and gurgles may be heard on auscultation. Localized tenderness or a tender, palpable mass may indicate a strangulated closed loop. Signs of localized or generalized peritonitis suggest gangrene or rupture of the bowel wall. Fresh blood may be found in the rectum in intussusception and in carcinoma of the rectum or colon. Sigmoidoscopy may disclose a neoplasm. Colonoscopy may be diagnostic and perhaps therapeutic in some patients with strictures or neoplasms.

B. Imaging Studies

The distended colon frequently creates a "picture frame" outline of the abdominal cavity. The colon can be distinguished from the small intestine by its haustral markings, which do not cross the entire lumen of the distended colon. Barium enema will confirm the diagnosis of colonic obstruction and identify its exact location. Water-soluble contrast medium should be used if strangulation or perforation is suspected. Once the obstruction is seen, the procedure should be discontinued. Barium must not be given orally in the presence of suspected colonic obstruction.

Differential Diagnosis

A. Small Versus Large Bowel Obstruction

Large bowel obstruction is frequently slow in onset, causes less pain, and may not cause vomiting in spite of considerable distention. Elderly patients with no history of abdominal surgery or prior attacks of obstruction frequently have carcinoma of the large bowel. Plain abdominal x-rays are essential to make the differential diagnosis, and barium contrast studies are often helpful.

B. Paralytic Ileus

The distinguishing features of paralytic ileus are signs of peritonitis or a history of trauma to the back or pelvis. The abdomen is silent, and abdominal cramping is not present. There may be tenderness. Plain films show a dilated colon. Contrast enema may be required to exclude an obstruction.

C. Pseudo-obstruction

Acute pseudo-obstruction of the colon (**Ogilvie's syndrome**) is massive colonic distention in the absence of a mechanically obstructing lesion. It is a severe form of ileus and arises in bedridden patients who have serious extraintestinal illness (renal, cardiac, respiratory) or trauma (eg, vertebral fracture). Aerophagia and impairment of colonic motility by drugs are contributing factors. Abdominal distention without pain or tenderness is the earliest manifestation, but later symptoms mimic those of true obstruction. Plain x-rays of the abdomen show marked gaseous distention of the colon. Although the entire colon may contain gas, the distention is typically localized to the right colon, with a cutoff at the he-

patic or splenic flexure. Contrast enema proves the absence of obstruction, but instillation of radiopaque material should cease as soon as the dilated colon is reached.

Conservative treatment with nasogastric suction and enemas succeeds in resolving colonic pseudo-obstruction in 86% of patients within 3 days. Neostigmine is effective in treating colonic pseudo-obstruction. If the cecum is markedly dilated, the risk of perforation is high, and direct intervention must be prompt. Colonoscopic decompression is the method of choice if an expert is available. Initial success is claimed in 90% of patients, but recurrence is common (25% or more). Often it is possible to place a tube into the proximal colon during colonoscopy to maintain decompression. Placement of a decompressive tube per rectum under fluoroscopic guidance has been described recently. Another alternative is cecostomy, performed either in the standard open fashion or by an endoscopic percutaneous method, similar to the technique for gastrostomy, using laparoscopic assistance.

Complications

Cecal perforation, described above, is a potentially lethal complication. Partially obstructive lesions of the colon may be complicated by acute colitis in the bowel proximal to the obstruction; it is probably a form of ischemic colitis secondary to impaired mucosal blood flow in the distended segment.

Treatment

The primary goal of treatment is decompression of the obstructed segment to prevent perforation; an operation is almost always required. Removal of the obstructing lesion is a secondary goal, but a single operation to accomplish both objectives is preferred whenever possible.

Colonoscopic balloon dilation of obstructing benign strictures or neoplasms is applicable sometimes. However, stent placement has largely replaced balloon dilation for neoplasms, particularly of distal lesions in the sigmoid colon and rectum. Laser photocoagulation of an obstructing cancer, especially in the rectum, may enlarge the lumen to permit an elective operation later under better circumstances, and occasionally a patient with advanced cancer may avoid operation entirely. Permanent diverting colostomy may be the only possible choice in a debilitated patient with unresectable obstructing rectal cancer.

Obstructing lesions of the right colon are resected in one stage, with ileotransverse colostomy if the patient's condition is good. If the patient's condition is precarious or if the colon has perforated, the bowel is resected but no anastomosis is done; an ileostomy is established, and anastomosis is performed at a second operation. Nonresectable lesions may be bypassed. Cecostomy is seldom used for obstruction in this area.

Obstructing lesions of the left colon are best treated by resection in patients who seem likely to tolerate this procedure. It is advantageous to immediately remove the lesion (often a malignant tumor) rather than delay for days or weeks after a preliminary decompressive maneuver. There are four choices of operation. Anastomosis may be postponed and a temporary end colostomy created (two-stage procedure; Figure 31–12). Alternatively, intraoperative colonic lavage can be performed by inserting a tube into the ileum or appendix and then into the cecum; a large-bore tube is inserted into the colon proximal to the obstruction to allow effluent to drain out of the sterile field. This procedure may cleanse the colon well enough so that primary anastomosis can be performed safely. Primary anastomosis with the aid of an intraluminal bypass tube (Coloshield) to prevent anastomotic leakage is another option that very few surgeons use. Total abdominal colectomy with ileorectal anastomosis in one stage is another acceptable option because it avoids the risks of anastomosing unprepared obstructed colon.

Cecostomy (Figure 31–5) is the operation of choice in patients with distal obstruction if the surgical risks prohibit definitive resection. It gives adequate decompression if the distal colon is not packed with feces and complete diversion of the fecal stream is not necessary. Cecostomy has the advantage that it does not interfere with subsequent extensive resection of the left colon. **Transverse colostomy** can provide complete fecal diversion, but a serious disadvantage is the need for three operations if this approach is elected: (1) colostomy, (2) resection of the obstructing lesion, and (3) closure of the colostomy.

Prognosis

The prognosis depends upon the age and general condition of the patient, the extent of vascular impairment of the bowel, the presence or absence of perforation, the cause of obstruction, and the promptness of surgical management. The overall mortality rate is about 20%. Cecal perforation carries a 40% mortality rate. Obstructing cancer of the colon has a worse prognosis than nonobstructing cancer because it is more likely to be locally extensive or metastatic to nodes or distant sites.

Baron TH: Expandable metal stents for the treatment of cancerous obstruction of the gastrointestinal tract. N Engl J Med 2001; 344:1681.

Bender GN, Do-Dai DD, Briggs LM: Colonic pseudo-obstruction: decompression with a tricomponent coaxial system under fluoroscopic guidance. Radiology 1993;188:395.

Figure 31–5. Cecostomy. **A:** Through a small incision overlying the cecum, a tube has been inserted through the wall of the cecum into its lumen and secured with a purse-string suture. **B:** Peritoneal closure. The cecum is fixed to the peritoneum. **Note:** A useful modification is to suture the peritoneum to the cecum circumferentially around the proposed cecostomy before the bowel is opened; this maneuver excludes the cecum from the peritoneal cavity and avoids the risk of fecal contamination of the abdomen.

Bharucha AE et al: Acute, toxic, and chronic. Curr Treat Options Gastroenterol 1999;2:517.

Boorman P et al: Endoluminal stenting of obstructed colorectal tumours. Ann R Coll Surg Engl 1999;81:251.

Chapman AH, McNamara M, Porter G: The acute contrast enema in suspected large bowel obstruction: value and technique. Clin Radiol 1992;46:273.

Fenlon HM et al: A comparison of virtual and conventional colonoscopy for the detection of colorectal polyps. N Engl J Med 1999;341:1496.

Gooszen AW et al: Operative treatment of acute complications of diverticular disease: primary or secondary anastomosis after sigmoid resection. Eur J Surg 2001;167:35.

Gooszen AW et al: Prospective study of primary anastomosis following sigmoid resection for suspected acute complicated diverticular disease. Br J Surg 2001;88:693.

Stewart J, Diament RH, Brennan TG: Management of obstructing lesions of the left colon by resection, on-table lavage, and primary anastomosis. Surgery 1993;114:502.

Suri S et al: Comparative evaluation of plain films, ultrasound and CT in the diagnosis of intestinal obstruction. Acta Radiol 1999;40:422.

Tanaka T et al: Endoscopic transanal decompression with a drainage tube for acute colonic obstruction: clinical aspects of preoperative treatment. Dis Colon Rectum 2001;44:418.

CANCER OF THE LARGE INTESTINE

 ESSENTIALS OF DIAGNOSIS

Right colon:

- *Unexplained weakness or anemia.*
- *Occult blood in feces.*
- *Dyspeptic symptoms.*
- *Persistent right abdominal discomfort.*
- *Palpable abdominal mass.*
- *Characteristic x-ray findings.*
- *Characteristic colonoscopic findings.*

Left colon:

- *Change in bowel habits.*
- *Gross blood in stool.*
- *Obstructive symptoms.*
- *Characteristic x-ray findings.*
- *Characteristic colonoscopic or sigmoidoscopic findings.*

Rectum:

- *Rectal bleeding.*
- *Alteration in bowel habits.*
- *Sensation of incomplete evacuation.*
- *Intrarectal palpable tumor.*
- *Sigmoidoscopic findings.*

General Considerations

In Western countries, cancer of the colon and rectum ranks second after cancer of the lung in incidence and death rates. An estimated 156,000 new cases of colorectal cancer are diagnosed and 65,000 people die of this disease in the USA each year. The death rate from colorectal cancer in the USA has begun to decline for the first time, perhaps related to earlier detection. The incidence increases with age, from 0.39 per 1000 persons per year at age 50 to 4.5 per 1000 persons per year at age 80. Carcinoma of the colon, particularly the right colon, is more common in women, and carcinoma of

the rectum is more common in men. The distribution of cancers of the colon and rectum is shown in Figure 31–6. An apparent "proximal shift" of cancer (increased incidence in the right colon and decreased incidence in the rectum) in recent decades is at least partially explainable by improved diagnostic accuracy for proximal lesions as a result of total colonoscopy. Multiple synchronous colonic cancers—ie, two or more carcinomas occurring simultaneously—are found in 5% of patients. Metachronous cancer is a new primary lesion in a patient who has had a previous resection for cancer. The cumulative risk of metachronous colorectal cancer was 6.3% at 18 years in one study. Ninety-five percent of malignant tumors of the colon and rectum are adenocarcinomas.

Genetic predisposition to cancer of the large bowel is well recognized in persons with familial adenomatous polyposis. In addition, at least two varieties of autosomal dominant hereditary nonpolyposis colorectal cancer (HNPCC) have been identified: (1) cancer family syndrome (Lynch syndrome II), with early onset (average age 44), proximal dominance, synchronous and metachronous cancers, and other associated extracolonic adenocarcinomas, especially endometrial carcinoma; and (2) hereditary site-specific colon cancer (HSSCC; Lynch syndrome I), which shows the same characteristics except that there are no extracolonic cancers. Perhaps 6% of patients with cancer of the colon or rectum have HNPCC. The gene responsible for this syndrome has been localized to chromosome 2p. First-degree relatives of patients with colorectal cancer have a two- to threefold increased risk of large bowel cancer

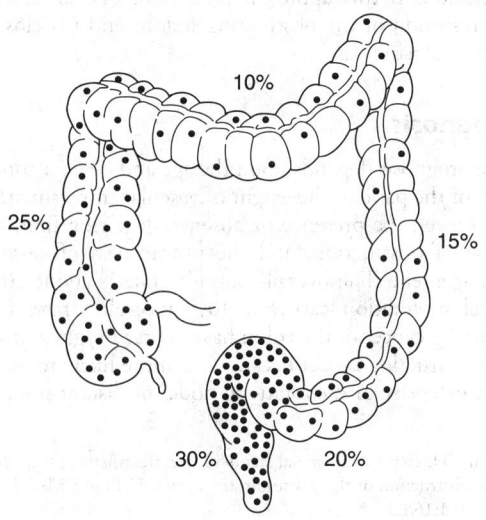

Figure 31–6. Distribution of cancer of the colon and rectum.

even in the absence of HNPCC, and it is estimated that 15–20% of cancers of the large bowel are due primarily to an inherited genetic defect.

Ulcerative colitis, Crohn's colitis, schistosomal colitis, exposure to radiation, colorectal polyps, and the presence of a ureterocolostomy are conditions that predispose to cancer of the large bowel. Association between Barrett's esophagus and colonic cancer has been reported. Women with a history of breast cancer have a small increase in risk for colorectal adenomas and cancer. Also in women, gallstones (and the consequent cholecystectomy) are associated with colorectal cancer, especially in the right colon. An association of human papillomavirus types 16 and 18 and colorectal adenocarcinoma has been reported.

A high incidence of colorectal cancer occurs in populations that are economically prosperous. This observation has focused attention on environmental factors, particularly diet, in the etiology of this tumor. Increased intake of saturated fat, increased caloric intake, decreased dietary calcium, and decreased intake of fiber are among the possible dietary influences. Dietary fat enhances cholesterol and bile acid synthesis by the liver, and the amounts of these sterols in the colon increase. Anaerobic colonic bacteria convert these compounds to secondary bile acids, which are promoters of carcinogenesis. Other possible mechanisms by which saturated fat promotes colorectal cancer include changes in immunity, effects on lipid peroxidation, and modulation of prostaglandin synthesis through arachidonic acid metabolism. Experimental studies have suggested that dietary fish oil, rich in unsaturated fatty acids of the n-3 type, is protective against colorectal cancer, and the mechanism may be inhibition of prostaglandin synthesis from arachidonic acid.

The mechanism by which dietary fiber is protective remains elusive. Effects of fiber on fecal bulk, water content, transit time, and pH are less important than once thought. Plant lignans in fiber are fermented to a group of human lignans by colonic bacteria, and these substances may be important in some way. Metabolic activity of gut microflora is altered by dietary fiber, perhaps with important inhibitory effects on tumor promoters such as bile acids. Another possible mechanism is chelation of dietary iron by the phytate content of high-fiber foods. Iron catalyzes oxidation of lipid to substances that are genotoxic, and iron has been associated with the initiating and promoting phases of carcinogenesis in experimental systems. Ingested calcium affects colonic epithelial cell proliferation topically and by absorption into the bloodstream. If these concepts are correct, the risk of colorectal cancer can be minimized by reducing dietary saturated fat and calories and increasing the intake of calcium and fermentable fiber. Populations with a high incidence of colon cancer tend to have low serum cholesterol levels, and average serum cholesterol levels are higher in groups with less cancer of the colon. In a study from Denmark, short stature and low body weight were strong predictors of rectal cancer development in men, and thin men had a higher risk of colon cancer than their obese counterparts. Cigarette smoking reportedly increases the risk of colorectal adenomas and cancer in both men and women.

Carcinogenesis in the large bowel and elsewhere is a long multistep process. Colorectal cancer involves multiple genetic alterations, ie, oncogene activation, including Ki-*ras* point mutation, c-*myc* amplification and overexpression, and c-*src* kinase activation. Tumor-suppressor gene inactivation is also important; these events may include point mutations in the *APC* gene (adenomatous polyposis coli, at chromosome 5q21), the *DCC* gene (deleted in colorectal carcinoma, on chromosome 18q), and *P53* (on chromosome 17). The *DCC* gene has been isolated. Genetic damage is initiated by carcinogenic agents. Promoters, such as bile acids, may stimulate growth of a benign neoplasm, and it may be that still other promoters cause malignant change to occur. There is evidence that female hormones are promoters, perhaps by influencing the availability of secondary bile acids in the colon. Estrogen and progesterone receptors are expressed in both normal and malignant colonic mucosa. Another series of changes, termed progression, make cancer cells more aggressive in their behavior. This sequence is the basis for an enormous amount of current research in colorectal cancer. Aspirin and other NSAIDs, particularly the cyclooxygenase-2 inhibitors, may reduce the incidence of and mortality rate from colorectal cancer, perhaps by inhibition of the series 2 prostaglandins implicated in immune suppression and the promotion of metastasis.

Cancer of the colon and rectum spreads in the following ways:

A. DIRECT EXTENSION

Carcinoma grows circumferentially and may completely encircle the bowel before it is diagnosed; this is especially true in the left colon, which has a smaller caliber than the right. It takes about 1 year for a tumor to encircle three-fourths of the circumference of the bowel. Longitudinal submucosal extension occurs with invasion of the intramural lymphatic network, but it rarely goes beyond 2 cm from the edge of the tumor unless there is concomitant spread to lymph nodes. As the lesion extends radially, it penetrates the outer layers of the bowel wall, and it may extend by contiguity into neighboring structures: the liver, the greater curvature of the stomach, the duodenum, the small bowel, the pancreas, the spleen, the bladder, the vagina, the kidneys and ureters, and the abdominal wall. Cancer of the rectum may invade the vaginal wall, bladder, prostate, or sacrum, and it may extend along the levators. Suba-cute perforation with inflammatory attachment of bowel to an adjacent viscus may be indistinguishable from actual invasion on gross examination.

B. HEMATOGENOUS METASTASIS

The tumor may invade colonic veins and be carried via portal venous blood to the liver to establish hepatic metastases. Tumor embolization also occurs through lumbar and vertebral veins to the lungs and elsewhere. Rectal cancer spreads through tributaries of the hypogastric veins. Metastases to ovaries are mostly hematogenous; they are found in 4% of women with colorectal cancer. Venous invasion occurs in 15–50% of cases even though it does not always cause distant metastases. An attempt is made to avoid producing hematogenous metastases during operation by minimizing manipulation of the tumor.

C. REGIONAL LYMPH NODE METASTASIS

This is the most common form of tumor spread (Figure 31–7). Longitudinal spread via extramural lymphatics is an important mechanism. Rectal cancer metastasizes radially along lymphatics to the pelvic side walls, where obturator nodes can become involved. The lymphatic

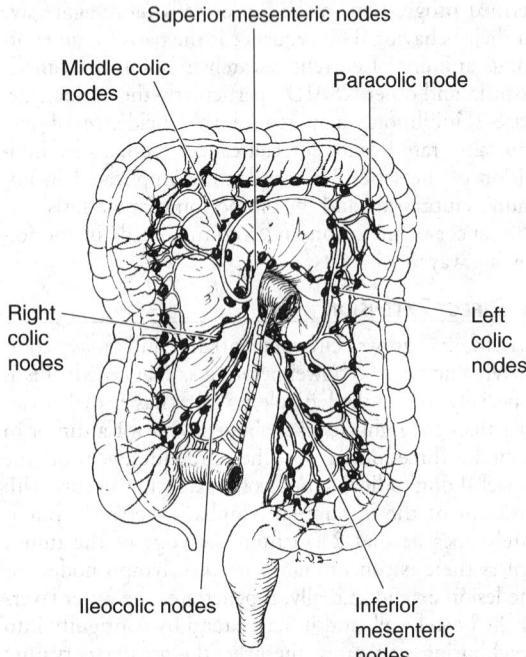

Figure 31–7. Lymphatic drainage of the colon. The lymph nodes (black) are distributed along the blood vessels to the bowel.

Superior mesenteric nodes

Middle colic nodes

Paracolic node

Right colic nodes

Left colic nodes

Ileocolic nodes

Inferior mesenteric nodes

drainage of the tumor must be removed in curative operations, and some nodal involvement will be found in over half of the specimens. Regional nodes are not necessarily involved in a progressive or orderly fashion: Positive nodes may be found at some distance from the primary site, with normal nodes intervening. The size of the lesion bears little relationship to the degree of nodal involvement. The more anaplastic the lesion, the more likely that lymph node metastasis will occur.

D. TRANSPERITONEAL METASTASIS

"Seeding" may occur when the tumor has extended through the serosa and tumor cells enter the peritoneal cavity, producing local implants or generalized abdominal carcinomatosis. Large metastatic deposits in the pelvic cul-de-sac are palpable as a hard shelf (Blumer's shelf).

E. INTRALUMINAL METASTASIS

Malignant cells shed from the surface of the tumor can be swept along in the fecal current. Implantation more distally on intact mucosa occurs rarely, if ever, but viable exfoliated cells presumably can be trapped in an anastomotic suture or staple line during operation. Most "anastomotic recurrences," however, are believed to arise from malignant cells outside the bowel wall (eg, in lymphatics in the mesocolon) that invade the intestine secondarily.

Clinical Findings

A. SYMPTOMS AND SIGNS

Adenocarcinoma of the colon and rectum has a median doubling time (the time required for the tumor to double in volume) of 130 days, suggesting that at least 5 years—and often 10–15 years—of silent growth are required before a cancer reaches symptom-producing size. During this asymptomatic phase, diagnosis depends on routine examination.

The value of routine screening of asymptomatic populations who lack high-risk factors for development of large bowel cancer is still being debated. The goals of screening are detection of early cancers and prevention of cancer by finding and removing adenomas. The American Cancer Society recommends that a fecal occult blood test using guaiac slides be obtained annually after age 50 and that flexible sigmoidoscopy be performed every 5 years beginning at age 50. There has been evidence for some time that screening for occult blood detects cancers at an earlier stage, but only recently has a survival benefit been shown in a USA prospective trial of occult blood testing followed by colonoscopy in those with positive tests. Improved survival in the screened group was related to a lower percentage of advanced cancers—the lesions that usually prove fatal. It is not clear whether the survival benefit in this study should be attributed mainly to the tests for occult blood or the colonoscopy, because the latter test alone might have achieved the same outcome. Several other controlled trials of fecal occult blood tests are currently under way. Case-control studies show that just one sigmoidoscopic examination confers protection against rectal cancer for as long as 10 years. Many questions remain about screening, and it may be years before definitive answers are available. Meanwhile, it may be prudent for practitioners to screen their average-risk patients by occult blood testing and flexible sigmoidoscopy.

Screening of patients in high-risk groups is less controversial, but questions remain about the choice and timing of various tests. Children with possible familial adenomatous polyposis should have sigmoidoscopy at puberty. Annual colonoscopy beginning at age 25 is the recommendation for members of families with Lynch syndrome. Colonoscopy every year is probably the best advice for patients with ulcerative colitis for longer than 10 years. The best method of screening for people with a history of colorectal cancer in one first-degree relative is unclear, but there is little evidence supporting colonoscopy over sigmoidoscopy with or without fecal occult blood testing. Dissatisfaction with the poor specificity of guaiac slide tests has led to development of alternative methods, including a quantitative assay specific for heme and an immunologic method using an antibody to hemoglobin. If fecal occult blood testing is positive, total colonoscopy is the single best study. If colonoscopy to the cecum in a well-prepared patient is unrevealing, further diagnostic evaluation of the lower or upper gastrointestinal tract is probably unnecessary since the yield of upper tract neoplasms in asymptomatic patients is nil.

Symptoms in patients with large bowel cancer depend upon the anatomic location of the lesion, its type and extent, and upon complications, including perforation, obstruction, and hemorrhage. Marked systemic manifestations such as cachexia are indications of advanced disease. The average delay between the onset of symptoms and definitive therapy is 7–9 months; both patients and physicians are responsible.

The **right colon** has a large caliber and a thin and distensible wall, and the fecal content is fluid. Because of these anatomic features, carcinoma of the right colon may attain large size before it is diagnosed. Patients often see a physician for complaints of fatigability and weakness due to severe anemia. Unexplained microcytic hypochromic anemia should always raise the question of carcinoma of the ascending colon. Gross blood may not be visible in the stool, but occult blood may be detected. Patients may complain of vague right abdominal discomfort, which is often postprandial and may be

mistakenly attributed to gallbladder or gastroduodenal disease. Alterations in bowel habits are not characteristic of carcinoma of the right colon, and obstruction is uncommon. In about 10% of cases, the first evidence of the disease is discovery of a mass by the patient or the physician.

The **left colon** has a smaller lumen than the right, and the feces are semisolid. Tumors of the left colon can gradually occlude the lumen, causing changes in bowel habits with alternating constipation and increased frequency of defecation (not true watery diarrhea). Partial or complete obstruction may be the initial picture. Bleeding is common but is rarely massive. The stool may be streaked or mixed with bright red or dark blood, and mucus is often passed together with small blood clots.

In **cancer of the rectum,** the most common symptom is the passage of bright red blood with bowel movements (hematochezia). Bleeding is usually persistent; it may be slight or (rarely) copious. Blood may or may not be mixed with stool or mucus. Predictions of an anal source of bleeding based on color and pattern are unreliable. *Whenever rectal bleeding occurs in a middle-aged or older individual, even in the presence of hemorrhoids, cancer must be ruled out.* There may be tenesmus (painful incomplete evacuation).

Physical examination is important to determine the extent of local disease, to identify distant metastases, and to detect diseases of other organ systems that may influence treatment. The supraclavicular areas should be carefully palpated for metastatic nodes. Examination of the abdomen may disclose a mass, enlargement of the liver, ascites, or engorgement of the abdominal wall veins if there is portal obstruction. If a mass is palpated, its location and extent of fixation are important.

Distal rectal cancers can be felt as a flat, hard, oval or encircling tumor with rolled edges and a central depression. Its extent, the size of the lumen at the site of the tumor, and the degree of fixation should be noted. Blood may be found on the examining finger. Vaginal and rectovaginal examination will yield additional information on the extent of the tumor. Retrorectal nodes may be palpable.

B. Laboratory Findings

Urinalysis, leukocyte count, and hemoglobin determination should be done. Serum proteins, calcium, bilirubin, alkaline phosphatase, and creatinine should be measured if clinically indicated.

The most familiar chemical marker for cancer of the large bowel is **carcinoembryonic antigen (CEA),** a glycoprotein found in the cell membranes of many tissues, including colorectal cancer. Some of the antigen enters the circulation and is detected by radioimmunoassay of serum; CEA is also detectable in various other body fluids, urine, and feces. Elevated serum CEA is not specifically associated with colorectal cancer; abnormally high levels are also found in sera of patients with other gastrointestinal cancers, nonalimentary cancers, and various benign diseases. CEA levels are high in 70% of patients with cancer of the large intestine, but less than half of patients with localized disease are CEA-positive. CEA does not, therefore, serve as a useful screening procedure, nor is it an accurate diagnostic test for colorectal cancer in a curable stage. CEA is helpful in detecting recurrence after curative surgical resection; if high CEA levels return to normal after operation and then rise progressively during the follow-up period, recurrence of cancer is likely. Other putative chemical markers include CA 19.9, CA 72-4, the K isozyme of lactate dehydrogenase, and plasma prolactin. None have been proved to have clinical value. Biologic and molecular markers are discussed below in the section on prognosis.

C. Imaging Studies

Chest films should be obtained routinely. Barium enema examination is the most important radiographic means of diagnosing cancer of the colon, though cancers are increasingly being diagnosed by colonoscopy, and contrast x-rays are unnecessary in those cases. Carcinoma of the left colon appears as a fixed filling defect, usually 2–6 cm long, with an annular ("apple core") configuration (Figure 31–8). Lesions of the right colon may appear as a constriction or an intraluminal mass. The bowel wall is inflexible at the site of the lesion, and the mucosal pattern is destroyed. It is important to remember that this is the typical picture of locally advanced carcinoma. Earlier stages of the disease produce less characteristic filling defects that should be investigated with the colonoscope. Artifacts (stool, spasm) can resemble carcinoma. Barium should not be administered by mouth if there is evidence of carcinoma of the colon, especially on the left side, since it may precipitate acute large bowel obstruction. X-rays are unreliable in detecting cancer of the rectum. Such growths are more accurately diagnosed by palpation and sigmoidoscopy.

CT scans are not essential in patients with cancer of the colon, but they are helpful in assessing extramural extension in patients with rectal cancer. MRI is probably even more accurate for this purpose. PET scans are experimental in colorectal cancer. Detection of liver metastases by CT scan and other methods is discussed in Chapter 25. Endorectal ultrasonography provides very accurate information about the depth of penetration of rectal cancer into or through the bowel wall. It also reveals the presence of enlarged pararectal lymph nodes but cannot at present distinguish between cancerous and reactive nodes.

Figure 31–8. Barium enema roentgenogram of an encircling carcinoma of the descending colon presenting an "apple core" appearance. Note the loss of mucosal pattern, the "hooks" at the margins of the lesion owing to undermining by the growth, the relatively short (6 cm) length of the lesion, and its abrupt ends.

Radioactively labeled monoclonal antibodies directed against tumor-associated antigens can be injected intravenously. In such patients, gamma scintiscanning (radioimmunoscintigraphy) detects tumor deposits preoperatively. A handheld gamma detecting probe can be used intraoperatively to search for radioactively labeled tumor deposits that would otherwise escape detection. This procedure, termed radioimmunoguided surgery, is still investigative.

D. Special Examinations

1. Proctosigmoidoscopy—From 50% to 65% of colorectal cancers are within the reach of a 60-cm flexible sigmoidoscope. Only 20% can be seen with a rigid sigmoidoscope. The typical cancer is raised, red, centrally ulcerated, and bleeding slightly. Mobility of the lesion can be determined by manipulation with the tip of the instrument. The size of the lumen should be noted, and the sigmoidoscope should be passed beyond the lesion to inspect the proximal bowel if possible. The tumor should be biopsied.

2. Colonoscopy—Endoscopic examination of the entire colon should be performed in every patient with suspected or known cancer of the colon or rectum if the intention is curative treatment. Preoperative colonoscopy is preferred unless obstructing cancer or other circumstances do not allow it. Increasingly today, a patient with rectal bleeding will undergo prompt total colonoscopy; a cancer is found and biopsied; synchronous lesions are excluded (or treated); and operation is planned without the need for barium enema x-rays. If barium studies are done first, colonoscopy is still necessary to prove that the defect is neoplastic and, more importantly, to detect synchronous polyps or cancers. Barium enema still has a role if colonoscopy is incomplete or if the findings do not explain the symptoms. Ultrasonography also can be performed through the colonoscope.

Differential Diagnosis

An initial erroneous diagnosis is made in as many as 25% of patients with cancer of the colon and rectum after gastrointestinal symptoms appear. Symptoms may be attributed mistakenly to disease of the upper gastrointestinal tract, particularly gallstones or peptic ulcer. Chronic anemia may be attributed to a primary hematologic disorder if fecal occult blood testing is not done. Acute pain in the right side of the abdomen owing to carcinoma can simulate appendicitis.

Most errors are made when the clinical findings are ascribed to benign disease, and patients may even be operated upon for benign anorectal conditions in the presence of undetected cancer. Cancer must be searched for in every patient with recent onset of significant rectal bleeding even if there are obvious hemorrhoids.

Carcinoma may be difficult to distinguish from diverticular disease; colonoscopy is useful in these cases. Other colonic diseases—including ulcerative colitis, Crohn's colitis, ischemic colitis, and amebiasis—usually can be diagnosed by sigmoidoscopy, colonoscopy, and barium enema. Symptoms should be attributed to irritable bowel syndrome only after neoplasm has been ruled out.

Treatment

A. Cancer of the Colon

Treatment consists of wide surgical resection of the lesion and its regional lymphatic drainage after preparation of the bowel. The primary tumor is resected even if distant metastases have occurred, since prevention of obstruction or bleeding may offer palliation for long periods.

The abdomen is explored to determine resectability of the tumor and to search for multiple primary carcinomas of the colon, distant metastases, and associated abdominal disease. Care is taken not to contribute to spread of the tumor by unnecessary palpation. The bowel is occluded tightly with an encircling tape on either side of the lesion to contain exfoliated cancer cells within the segment to be resected. The cancer-bearing portion of colon is then mobilized and removed. Most surgeons irrigate the two open ends of bowel with saline solution or dilute povidone-iodine before anastomosis in the hope that tumor cells in the lumen will be washed away or destroyed. The extent of resection of the colon and mesocolon for cancers in various locations and the methods for restoration of continuity are shown in Figure 31–9.

B. Cancer of the Rectum

For cancer of the rectum, the choice of operation depends on the height of the lesion above the anal verge, the configuration (whether polypoid or infiltrative), the gross extent of the tumor, the degree of differentiation, and the patient's size, habitus, and general condition. Preoperative staging by digital rectal examination followed by CT, MRI, endorectal ultrasound, or some combination of these tests helps tailor the treatment to the patient. Preservation of the anal sphincter and avoidance of colostomy are desirable if possible.

The principal procedures for rectal tumors are as follows:

1. Abdominoperineal resection of the rectum—The distal sigmoid, rectosigmoid, rectum, and anus are removed through combined abdominal and perineal incisions. A permanent end-sigmoid colostomy is required. The procedure is not performed in the presence of peritoneal seeding or fixation to the bony pelvis.

2. Low anterior resection of the rectum—This operation, performed through an abdominal incision, is the curative procedure of choice provided a margin of at least 2 cm of normal bowel—as estimated at operation—can be resected below the lesion. At least 10 cm of bowel proximal to the growth should also be removed along with the lymph node-bearing tissue. It is important to excise 5 cm of mesorectum distal to the tumor to minimize the chance of local recurrence from cancer in lymph nodes. The descending or sigmoid colon is anastomosed to the rectum. This type of resection is likely to fail in patients with extensive carcinoma and local spread. The end-to-end stapling device facilitates very low anastomosis, sometimes even as low as the anal canal (colon-anal anastomosis).

3. Laparoscopic-assisted resection—All types of curative resections for cancer of the colon or rectum can be carried out by laparoscopic-assisted techniques. Prospective studies comparing conventional resections with laparoscopic-assisted procedures are under way to answer questions about adequacy of mesocolon exci-

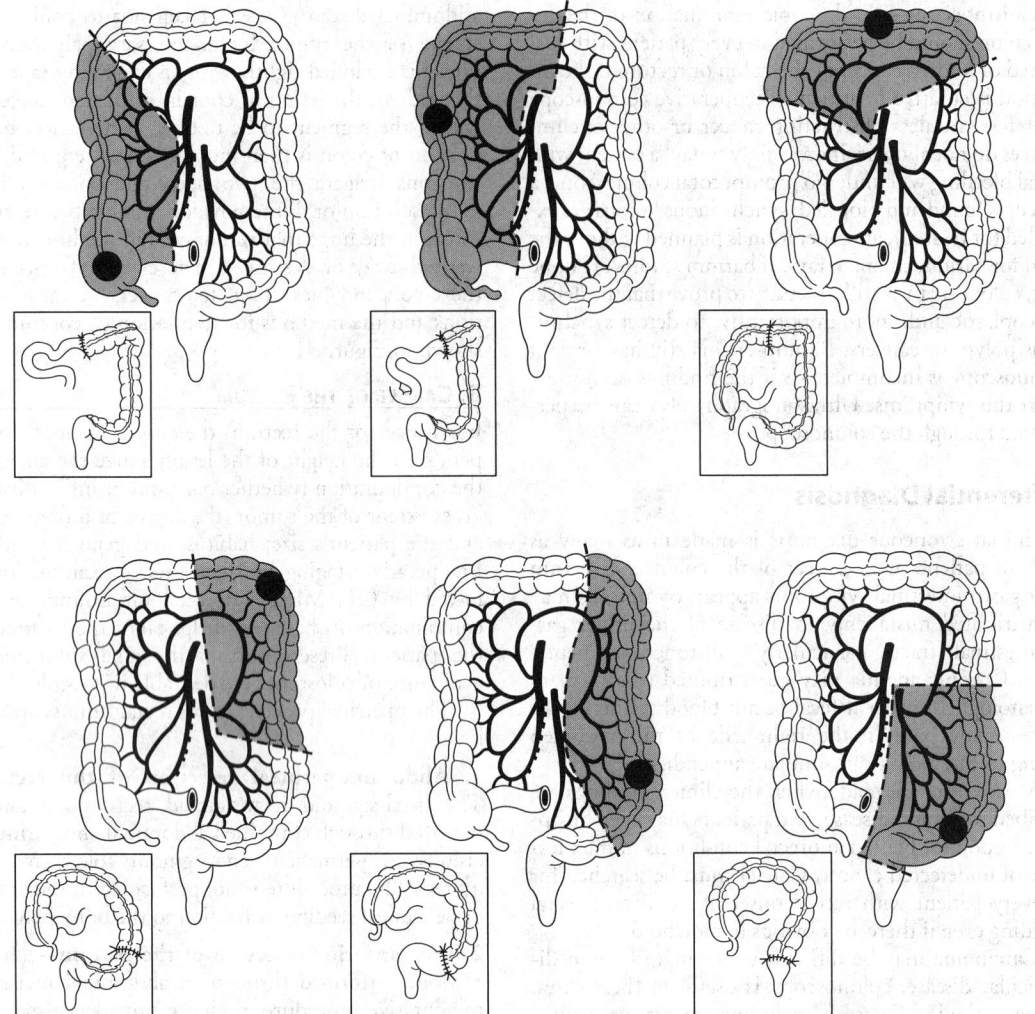

Figure 31–9. Extent of surgical resection for cancer of the colon at various sites. The cancer is represented by a black disk. Anastomosis of the bowel remaining after resection is shown in the small insets. The extent of resection is determined by the distribution of the regional lymph nodes along the blood supply. The lymph nodes may contain metastatic cancer.

sion, morbidity, cost, and survival. A staging benefit of laparoscopy has been suggested in preliminary reports.

4. Local excision—In carefully selected patients with small, well-differentiated mobile polypoid lesions, a disk of rectum containing the tumor can be excised as definitive therapy. Lymph nodes are not sampled or treated by local excision, and success is based on adherence to strict criteria that predict a low likelihood of nodal spread.

5. Palliative procedures—Unresectable rectal cancers can be palliated by fulguration (electrocoagulation) or

laser photocoagulation. Fulguration requires general anesthesia, and the laser procedure does not. Unfortunately, symptom relief—of bleeding, tenesmus, and mucus discharge—in patients with these advanced lesions is often less than anticipated. Photodynamic therapy is an experimental modality whereby a photosensitizing agent with some selectivity for cancer is administered intravenously and activated with light from a laser. Local tissue destruction occurs. Diverting colostomy is performed for obstructing rectal cancer that cannot be resected. Rarely, the Hartmann procedure is indicated in poor-risk patients—the bowel with its contained cancer is removed through the abdomen with permanent colostomy but without excision of the distal rectum, which is sutured closed.

6. Radiation therapy—Intracavitary, external, or implantation techniques are used alone or in combination with surgical excision for small rectal cancers. In some cases, the lesion responds so well that radical surgical procedures are avoided. Preoperative megavoltage radiation therapy, often given with chemotherapy to enhance the radiation effect, may shrink a rectal carcinoma, kill cells in regional lymphatics, and prevent pelvic recurrence. External radiation therapy is widely employed in patients with bulky fixed lesions that do not seem to be resectable; after such treatment, some lesions can be removed. Intraoperative radiation therapy is a promising method of treatment of local pelvic recurrences.

C. ADJUVANT THERAPY

Chemotherapy and radiation therapy have been studied extensively as adjuvants to curative resection of cancer of the large intestine. It is apparent that strategies be different for cancer of the colon and cancer of the rectum. Patients with stage I lesions in either site do not benefit from adjuvant therapy. Stage II and stage III rectal cancer patients have improved local control and survival with combined postoperative chemotherapy and radiation therapy. Patients with stage II colon cancer should enter clinical trials of adjuvant chemotherapy; irradiation is not used for cancer of the colon. Stage III colon cancer patients also should enroll in clinical trials, but if that is not possible a combination of oral levamisole and intravenous fluorouracil is acceptable. It is anticipated that molecular markers and other innovative staging techniques discussed below will help select patients for adjuvant therapy in the future.

Treatment of Complications

A. OBSTRUCTION

Obstructing cancer of the left or right colon is treated by immediate resection in good-risk patients. (See Obstruction of the Large Intestine, above.)

B. PERFORATION

An aggressive approach to perforated cancer of the colon is advisable, but anastomosis usually is delayed. The proximal end is exteriorized as a colostomy (or ileostomy), and the distal end is exteriorized or closed. Secondary anastomosis is performed after inflammation subsides.

C. DIRECT EXTENSION

When carcinoma of the colon has spread by contiguity to adjacent viscera such as the small intestine, spleen, uterus, or urinary bladder, the involved viscus—or a portion of it—should be resected en bloc with the colon.

Prognosis

Results of surgical treatment are better for cancer of the colon than for cancer of the rectum, and rectal cancer below the pelvic peritoneal reflection has a worse prognosis than cancer higher in the rectum. The stage of disease is the most important determinant of survival rates after surgical resection, however. **Clinicopathologic staging** has been the most important guide since the Dukes classification was introduced decades ago. In recent years, many centers in the USA have adopted the TNM system developed by the American Joint Committee for Cancer Staging and End Results Reporting has been adopted widely in the USA. Table 31–5 lists the definitions of TNM and the stage grouping along with the corresponding Dukes classification. Clinical data are used for determination of M, and both clinical and pathologic information is included in assessment of T and N. Laparoscopy may have a staging benefit in detecting small metastases in regional nodes, and this information may be integrated into clinicopathologic staging more widely in the future. Survival rates differ considerably in various series; actuarial rates are higher than crude survival rates. Average crude 5-year survival rates for colon and rectal cancer using the Dukes system are as follows: stage A, 80%; stage B, 60%; stage C, 30%; stage D, 5%. In the view of many experts, clinicopathologic staging is not sufficiently discriminating for the purpose of selecting patients for adjuvant therapy because lesions of similar TNM stage may have widely different potentials for local recurrence and distant metastasis. Colorectal cancers with predominantly diploid cells generally have a better prognosis than aneuploid tumors, but clinical application of the results of DNA analysis by flow cytometry have had limited success. Innovative staging techniques include immunohistology with antibodies to various transformation-related phenotypes and genotypic subset analysis for molecular markers. Allelic loss on chromosome 18q is predictive of a fatal outcome; other promising molecular markers include allelic losses on chromosomes 17p and 22q and mutations of the tumor suppressor gene *P53*. Further study is required before clinicians can base therapeutic decisions on assays of these and other molecular markers.

Approximately 10% of lesions are not resectable at the time of operation, and an additional 20% of patients have liver or other distant metastases. Hence, operation for cure can be performed on only about 70% of patients. The operative mortality rate is 2–4%. The survival rate of patients undergoing curative resection is about 55%; the overall survival rate (all stages) is about 35%.

Table 31–5. TNM classification of cancer of the colon and rectum.[1]

PRIMARY TUMOR (T)

TX	Primary tumor cannot be assessed
T0	No evidence of primary tumor
Tis	Carcinoma in situ
T1	Tumor invades submucosa
T2	Tumor invades muscularis propria
T3	Tumor invades through the muscularis propria into the subserosa, or into nonperitonealized pericolic or perirectal tissues
T4	Tumor perforates the visceral peritoneum, or directly invades other organs or structures

REGIONAL LYMPH NODES (N)

NX	Regional lymph nodes cannot be assessed
N0	No regional lymph node metastasis
N1	Metastasis in one to three pericolic or perirectal lymph nodes
N2	Metastasis in four or more pericolic or perirectal lymph nodes
N3	Metastasis in any lymph node along the course of a named vascular trunk

DISTANT METASTASIS (M)

MX	Presence of distant metastasis cannot be assessed
M0	No distant metastasis
M1	Distant metastasis

STAGE GROUPING

				Dukes
Stage 0	Tis	N0	M0	
Stage I	T1	N0	M0	A
	T2	N0	M0	A
Stage II	T3	N0	M0	B
	T4	N0	M0	B
Stage III	Any T	N1	M0	C
	Any T	N2, N3	M0	C
Stage IV	Any T	Any N	M1	

[1]Used with the permission of the American Joint Committee on Cancer (AJCC), Chicago, IL. The original source for this material is *AJCC Cancer Staging Manual,* 5th ed. Lippincott-Raven, 1997.

The prognosis is adversely affected by complications such as obstruction or perforation. The histologic features—including the degree of differentiation of the tumor, intravascular tumor cells, or malignant cells in the perineural space—also have a bearing on prognosis. Mucinous adenocarcinoma is more aggressive than nonmucinous cancer. Suggestions that colorectal cancer has a worse prognosis in patients younger than age 40 compared with older people have not been substantiated.

Studies from several countries show that low-income people have more advanced disease when diagnosed and that their stage-for-stage survival rates are worse; these observations have not been explained satisfactorily. An association of perioperative blood transfusions with poorer prognosis from colorectal cancer has been found by some but not all investigators; if it is genuine, the effect may reflect other effects—larger tumors requiring more extensive surgery and transfusions, for example—rather than some consequence of transfusion itself.

Follow-up after curative resection of cancer of the large bowel is controversial. There are good data to support the view that periodic colonoscopy to detect and remove adenomas after colonoscopic polypectomy prevents subsequent cancer, and colonoscopy at 3 years is just as beneficial as colonoscopy at 1 and 3 years after removal of the index adenoma. It is not known whether these observations can be extrapolated to follow-up after curative resection of cancer, but in the absence of data many clinicians perform surveillance colonoscopy periodically for the purpose of detecting adenomas and metachronous carcinomas. Other goals of follow-up are the diagnosis of recurrent cancer or metastatic cancer, and here it is uncertain whether the benefits outweigh the costs, mainly because so few asymptomatic recurrences detected in follow-up are treatable for cure. Perhaps the principal benefit is psychologic for both patient and physician. Follow-up programs usually involve serum CEA levels, fecal occult blood tests, chest x-rays, and CT scans in addition to colonoscopy every few years.

If recurrent cancer or metastatic cancer is discovered, the patient is evaluated for potential surgical resection of the lesions; this may be feasible in cases of hepatic or pulmonary metastases, and it may be possible to remove some local (eg, pelvic) recurrences in combination with intraoperative radiation therapy. Unfortunately, the prognosis of patients with local recurrence is poor. If recurrent cancer is suggested on the basis of rising serum CEA levels and if the responsible lesion cannot be located, a second-look laparotomy may be undertaken. Although apparently resectable cancer is found in 30% or more of patients, treatment is largely ineffective in prolonging survival.

Allison JE et al: A comparison of fecal occult-blood tests for colorectal-cancer screening. N Engl J Med 1996;334:155.

Arulampalam TH et al: Positron emission tomography and colorectal cancer. Br J Surg 2001;8:176.

Bruinvels DJ et al: Follow-up of patients with colorectal cancer. A meta-analysis. Ann Surg 1994;219:174.

Busch ORC et al: Blood transfusions and prognosis in colorectal cancer. N Engl J Med 1993;328:1372.

Chu KC et al: Temporal patterns in colorectal cancer incidence, survival, and mortality from 1950 through 1990. J Natl Cancer Inst 1994;86:997.

Gann PH et al: Low-dose aspirin and incidence of colorectal tumors in a randomized trial. J Natl Cancer Inst 1993;85:1220.

Giardiello FM et al: The use and interpretation of commercial *APC* gene testing for familial adenomatous polyposis. N Engl J Med 1997;336:823.

Gryfe R et al: Tumor microsatellite instability and clinical outcome in young patients with colorectal cancer. N Engl J Med 2000; 342:69.

Hecht JR: Dietary fat and colon cancer. Adv Exp Med Biol 1996;399:157.

Heys SD et al: Prognostic factors and survival of patients aged less than 45 years with colorectal cancer. Br J Surg 1994;81:685.

Howe GR et al: Dietary intake of fiber and decreased risk of cancers of the colon and rectum: evidence from the combined analysis of 13 case-control studies. J. Natl Cancer Inst 1992; 84:1887.

Jessup JM et al: The National Cancer Data Base. Report on colon cancer. Cancer 1996;78:918.

Lavery IC et al: Treatment of colon and rectal cancer. Surg Clin North Am 2000;80:535.

Lichtenstein P et al: Environmental and heritable factors in the causation of cancer–analyses of cohorts of twins from Sweden, Denmark, and Finland. N Engl J Med 2000;343:78.

Lieberman DA et al: Use of colonoscopy to screen asymptomatic adults for colorectal cancer. Veterans Affairs Cooperative Study Group 380. N Engl J Med 2000;343:162.

Lin KM et al: Colorectal and extracolonic cancer variations in MLH1/MSH2 hereditary nonpolyposis colorectal cancer kindreds and the general population. Dis Colon Rectum 1998; 41:428.

Macdonald JS, Astrow AB: Adjuvant therapy of colon cancer. Semin Oncol 2001;28:30.

Scholefield JH: ABC of colorectal cancer: screening. BMJ 2000; 321:1004.

Steinbach G et al: The effect of celecoxib, a cyclooxygenase-2 inhibitor, in familial adenomatous polyposis. N Engl J Med 2000;342:1946.

Watanabe T et al: Molecular predictors of survival after adjuvant chemotherapy for colon cancer. N Engl J Med 2001; 344:1196.

Winawer SJ, Zauber AG: Colonoscopic polypectomy and the incidence of colorectal cancer. Gut 2001;48:753.

Wu JS, Fazio VW: Colon cancer. Dis Colon Rectum 2000; 43:1473.

POLYPS OF THE COLON & RECTUM

 ESSENTIALS OF DIAGNOSIS

- *Family history.*
- *Sigmoidoscopic, colonoscopic, or radiologic discovery of polyps.*

General Considerations

Colorectal polyps are masses of tissue that project into the lumen. They comprise a heterogeneous group of sessile or pedunculated, benign or malignant, mucosal, submucosal, or muscular lesions. "Polyp" is a morphologic term, and no histologic diagnosis is implied. The most common epithelial polyps of the colon and rectum are listed in Table 31–6. Most adenomas are tubular, tubulovillous, or villous. Hyperplastic polyps are diminutive lesions most often found in the left colon. Hamartomas are uncommon. Polyposis, discussed later in this section, is a term reserved for the presence of many polyps in the large bowel.

Estimates of the incidence of colonic and rectal polyps in the general population range from 9% to 60%—the higher figure includes small polyps found at autopsy. Polypoid adenomas are found in about 25% of asymptomatic adults who undergo screening colonoscopy. The prevalence of adenomas is 30% at age 50 years, 40% at age 60, 50% at age 70, and 55% at age 80. The mean age is 55 years, about 5–10 years younger than the mean age of patients with colorectal cancer. Approximately 50% of polyps occur in the sigmoid or rectum. About 50% of patients with adenoma have more than one lesion, and 15% have more than two lesions. An increased incidence of adenomas in breast cancer patients has been reported.

Inflammatory polyps have no malignant potential, and cancer developing in association with hamartomas is rare. Hyperplastic polyps are not neoplastic and therefore do not become malignant. It has been suggested that hyperplastic polyps in the left colon are markers for neoplastic polyps elsewhere in the colon, but the weight of evidence is against this concept.

Table 31–6. Polyps of the large intestine.

Type	Histologic Diagnosis

Neoplastic	Adenoma
	  Tubular adenoma (adenomatous polyp)
	  Tubulovillous adenoma (villoglandular adenoma)
	  Villous adenoma (villous papilloma)
	Carcinoma

Hamartomas	Juvenile polyp Peutz-Jeghers polyp
Inflammatory	Inflammatory polyp (pseudopolyp) Benign lymphoid polyp
Unclassified	Hyperplastic polyp
Miscellaneous	Lipoma, leiomyoma, carcinoid

Adenomas are a premalignant lesion. The vast majority of adenocarcinomas of the large bowel in North America and Europe are believed to evolve from adenomas (adenoma-to-carcinoma sequence), although in Japan it appears that small cancers can arise de novo with no evidence of a benign neoplastic phase. In Western populations, both adenomas and cancer increase in incidence with age, and the distribution of adenomas and cancer in the bowel is similar. Approximately 25% of patients who have five or more adenomatous polyps have a synchronous colon cancer at the initial colonoscopy. About one-third of colonic and rectal specimens resected for cancer also harbor adenomas; if a surgical specimen contains two or more synchronous carcinomas, the incidence of associated adenomas is 75%. All gradations of malignancy—from total absence, to dysplasia, to a microscopic cytologic cancer, to invasive cancer, to a gross cancer with remnants of benign tumor at one margin—may be seen in colonic neoplasms; on the other hand, cancers that are smaller than 0.5 cm in diameter and contain no benign adenoma are extremely rare. Additional support for the malignant potential of adenomas is as follows: (1) Patients with familial adenomatous polyposis die of cancer at a young age unless the colon is removed. (2) Chemical carcinogens produce adenomas and cancers indiscriminately in the colons of experimental animals. (3) Routine removal of adenomas from the colon reduces the incidence of subsequent rectal cancer.

The malignant potential of an adenoma depends on size, growth pattern, and the degree of epithelial atypia. Cancer is found in 1% of adenomas under 1 cm in diameter, 10% of adenomas 1–2 cm in size, and up to 45% of adenomas larger than 2 cm. So-called flat adenomas, small flat or depressed tubular adenomas that tend to occur in the right colon, may be an exception to these guidelines; they may become malignant when still only a few millimeters in diameter. The three histologic patterns of adenoma are variations of one neoplastic process; about 5% of tubular adenomas, 22% of tubulovillous adenomas, and 40% of villous adenomas become malignant. The potential for cancerous transformation rises with increasing degrees of epithelial dysplasia. Sessile lesions are more apt to be malignant than pedunculated ones. It probably takes at least 5 years, and more often 10–15 years, for an adenoma to become malignant.

Clinical Findings

A. SYMPTOMS AND SIGNS

Most polyps are asymptomatic, but the larger the lesion, the more likely it is to cause symptoms. Rectal bleeding is by far the most frequent complaint. Blood is bright red or dark red depending on the location of the polyp, and bleeding is usually intermittent. Profuse hemorrhage from polyps is rare.

Alterations in bowel habits are more common in the presence of frank carcinoma, but large benign tumors may produce tenesmus, constipation, or increased frequency of bowel movements. Some polyps, notably large villous adenomas, may secrete copious amounts of mucus that are evacuated per rectum. Polypoid tumors may induce peristaltic cramps or varying degrees of intussusception, but most often obstructive symptoms are due to associated diverticular disease or irritable bowel syndrome and persist after polypectomy. Occasionally, a polyp on a very long pedicle will prolapse through the anus; this is most apt to occur with juvenile polyps.

General physical examination yields little information about the colonic polyps themselves, although other manifestations of diseases such as Peutz-Jeghers syndrome may be found. A polyp may be palpable by digital rectal examination, and proctosigmoidoscopy may disclose polyps in the rectum or sigmoid. Blood-tinged mucus strongly suggests the presence of a neoplasm situated farther proximally. Since polyps are often multiple and may occur synchronously with cancer, further investigation of the colon is mandatory even if a lesion is found by sigmoidoscopy.

B. IMAGING STUDIES (BARIUM ENEMA)

A polyp appears as a rounded filling defect with smooth, sharply defined margins. Double-column technique is recommended. Thorough cleansing of the colon and careful examination are essential if small polyps are to be demonstrated.

C. COLONOSCOPY

This is the most reliable way to diagnose colonic polyps, and polypectomy can be done at the same time. The entire colon should be examined by colonoscopy in every patient with known polyps or symptoms suggestive of their presence.

Differential Diagnosis

Artifacts seen on barium enema x-ray examination may be confused with polyps. These include bits of feces, air bubbles, diverticula, indenting appendices epiploicae, calcified lymph nodes, and others. Colonoscopy is essential in doubtful situations.

Polyps of various histologic types can be differentiated only by microscopic examination of the entire lesion, though clues may be gained from clinical and radiographic features.

Treatment

Polyps of the colon and rectum are treated because they produce symptoms, because they may be malignant when first discovered, or because they may become malignant later. In a study of untreated colonic polyps, the cumulative risk of eventual cancer at the polyp site was 2.5% at 5 years, 8% at 10 years, and 24% at 20 years.

Small polyps can be removed with an electrocautery snare passed through a rigid or flexible sigmoidoscope, but since total colonoscopy is recommended in all patients who have a polyp, it is best to wait and do the polypectomy in a well-prepared colon during that procedure.

Large, sessile, soft, velvety lesions in the rectum are usually villous adenomas; these tumors have high malignant potential and must be excised completely. With the patient anesthetized, this can be accomplished through the anus in most instances. Only if histologic sections show invasive cancer at the margins of excision is further therapy necessary. Management of villous tumors by endoscopic Nd:YAG laser photocoagulation may be useful for extensive carpet-like tumors. Excision has the advantage of permitting histologic examination of the specimen.

Pedunculated polyps and small sessile lesions in the sigmoid and above should be removed with a hot biopsy forceps or an electrocautery snare passed through the colonoscope. Colonoscopic polypectomy is usually successful, but technical obstacles occasionally seem insurmountable. Only experts should attempt colonoscopic removal of large sessile lesions, because the risk of perforation, bleeding, and incomplete excision is greater if there is no pedicle. Colonoscopic polypectomy is safer than laparotomy; the combined incidence of perforation and hemorrhage is 2%, and deaths are rare. Colonoscopy is less expensive and incurs much less disability than laparotomy.

Open or laparoscopic-assisted colonic resection should be considered if colonoscopy is unsuccessful, if the lesion is large and sessile, or if there are many polyps. Patients with HNPCC and others with multiple polyps may require total abdominal colectomy with ileorectal anastomosis.

From 2% to 4% of colonoscopically excised polyps contain invasive adenocarcinoma, and a decision must be made whether to resect the segment of colon or simply follow the patient. Carcinoma in situ is a cytologic abnormality equivalent to severe dysplasia and does not require further treatment. Only when malignant cells penetrate the muscularis mucosae is there any potential for metastasis (because there are no lymphatics in the lamina propria of the large intestine), and only these lesions should be labeled as cancers. The incidence of metastasis is low, and resection of the colon is not required if the following criteria are met: (1) Gross margin is clear at endoscopy; (2) microscopic margin is clear; (3) cancer is well-differentiated; (4) there is no lymphatic or venous invasion; and (5) cancer does not invade the stalk. Other malignant polyps of the colon should be managed by resection of involved bowel. Molecular markers may help make this determination in the future. Since rectal cancers are sometimes treated definitively by local excision, it may not be necessary to do a radical resection if the malignant polyp arose in the distal rectum.

Familial adenomatous polyposis (adenomatous polyposis coli) is a rare but important disease because colorectal cancer develops before age 40 in nearly all untreated patients. The trait is autosomal dominant. Genetic advances have been explosive. The *APC* gene ("FAP" had already been used in the genetic lexicon) was localized to chromosome 5q21 in 1991, and since then more than 100 different mutations have been identified. At present, genetic testing of at-risk individuals is still experimental, but clinical utility is anticipated soon. More than a hundred (occasionally fewer) polyps of varying size and configuration are present in the colon and rectum. A long list of benign and malignant extracolonic manifestations are associated with familial adenomatous polyposis (Table 31–7). **Gardner's syndrome** (polyposis, desmoid tumors, osteomas of mandible or skull, and sebaceous cysts) and **Turcot's syndrome** (polyposis and a medulloblastoma or glioma) are examples of familial adenomatous polyposis with variations in expression of the extracolonic mani-

Table 31–7. Extracolonic manifestations of familial adenomatous polyposis.[1]

Benign	Malignant
Endocrine adenoma	Duodenal carcinoma
Osteoma	Bile duct carcinoma
Epidermoid cyst	Pancreatic carcinoma
Hypertrophic retinal pigmentation	Desmoid tumor
	Carcinoma of the stomach
Gastric fundic gland polyp	Adrenal carcinoma
Duodenal adenoma	Medulloblastoma
Small bowel adenoma	Glioblastoma
	Thyroid carcinoma
	Small bowel carcinoma
	Carcinoid tumor of the ileum
	Osteogenic sarcoma
	Hepatoblastoma

[1]Reproduced, with permission, from Jagelman DG: The expanding spectrum of familial adenomatous polyposis. Perspect Colon Rectal Surg 1998;1:30.

festations; there is no genetic distinction among the syndromes. Congenital hypertrophy of retinal pigment epithelium is present as early as at 3 months of age in affected members of two-thirds of families with familial adenomatous polyposis; this abnormality (always bilateral, more than four lesions on each side) predicts familial adenomatous polyposis with 97% sensitivity. Polyps begin to appear at puberty. If a family lacks the retinal pigment abnormality, flexible sigmoidoscopy will need to be done from puberty until age 40 or 50 to be certain the family members do not have polyposis. Once polyposis is diagnosed, colectomy should be done. Upper gastrointestinal endoscopy is advised to look for gastroduodenal lesions.

Although total proctocolectomy eliminates the risk of cancer, it leaves the patient with a permanent ileostomy. Abdominal colectomy ("subtotal colectomy") with ileorectal anastomosis is favored by a few surgeons because an ileostomy is not required; rectal polyps regress in some patients after this procedure, and, it is hoped, cancer can be prevented by sigmoidoscopic destruction of polyps every 3 months. The long-term success rate varies in different reports, and the incidence of cancer in the remaining rectum is low. Sulindac has been reported to induce regression of rectal polyps after ileorectal anastomosis. Total colectomy and the ileoanal pouch procedure (see Ulcerative Colitis, below) is preferred for most patients, especially if there are numerous adenomas in the rectum. If the rectal mucosa is excised completely, the risk of subsequent rectal neoplasia is essentially nil. Case reports of cancer arising in the anal canal after this operation may reflect incomplete excision of susceptible mucosa at the time of ileoanal anastomosis. Prophylactic colectomy does not alter the extracolonic manifestations. Desmoid tumor is a locally invasive nonmetastasizing fibrous tumor that occurs in the mesentery or abdominal wall of some patients after the colectomy. Results of attempts to excise desmoids are poor, with 80% recurrence. Sulindac, tamoxifen, prednisolone, and progesterone have been reported to halt the growth of desmoids. Combination chemotherapy with doxorubicin and dacarbazine may be helpful, but other chemotherapeutic regimens and radiation therapy have been ineffective. Desmoids grow slowly and capriciously, but they prove fatal in 10% of patients with familial adenomatous polyposis. Upper gastrointestinal cancer occurs in up to 10% of these patients, and medulloblastoma is also a significant risk.

Hereditary flat adenoma syndrome has been described recently. It is separable from familial adenomatous polyposis and is either a variant of HNPCC or a distinct entity. Three syndromes of juvenile polyposis have been defined: (1) **juvenile polyposis coli,** (2) **generalized juvenile gastrointestinal polyposis,** and

(3) **Cronkhite-Canada syndrome** (juvenile polyposis and ectodermal lesions). The first two are inherited with an autosomal dominant pattern. Although juvenile polyps are hamartomas with a low malignant potential, the risk of gastrointestinal cancer is increased in familial juvenile polyposis patients and their relatives. Furthermore, hamartomas can coexist with adenomas, and one must not assume that a polyp is a hamartoma without proof. Colonoscopic excision is performed for large or symptomatic (bleeding, intussusception) lesions. Some juvenile polyps autoamputate. Colectomy is required in some patients with familial forms of juvenile polyposis.

Peutz-Jeghers syndrome is an uncommon autosomal dominant disease in which multiple hamartomatous polyps appear in the stomach, small bowel, and colon. Affected individuals have melanotic pigmentation of the skin and mucous membranes, especially about the lips and gums. The malignant potential of the hamartomas is small, and polyps are generally removed only if symptomatic. Carcinoma develops at an increased rate in other tissues, eg, stomach, duodenum, pancreas, small intestine, and breast.

Prognosis

Villous adenomas recur at the excision site in about 15% of cases after local removal. Tubular adenomas seldom recur, but new ones may develop, and a patient who has had any type of adenoma is at greater risk of developing adenocarcinoma than the general population. The risk of metachronous neoplasms following excision of a colorectal adenoma is greatest if there were multiple index lesions or if an adenoma was sessile, villous, or over 2 cm in diameter. The risk is somewhat higher in men than in women. In one study, the cumulative risk of developing further adenomas was linear over time, reaching about 50% by 15 years after removal of one or more colorectal adenomas; the cumulative incidence of cancer in the same population rose to 7% at 15 years. Prospective studies show that if the colon is cleared by total colonoscopy at the time of excision of the index polyp, follow-up colonoscopy at 3 years is just as effective as colonoscopy at 1 and 3 years in preventing development of ominous neoplasms.

Bond JH: Polyp guideline: diagnosis, treatment, and surveillance for patients with colorectal polyps. Practice Parameters Committee of the American College of Gastroenterology. Am J Gastroenterol 2000;95:3053.

Calland JF et al: Genetic syndromes and genetic tests in colorectal cancer. Semin Gastrointest Dis 2000;11:207.

Citarda F et al: Efficacy in standard clinical practice of colonoscopic polypectomy in reducing colorectal cancer incidence. Gut 2001;48:812.

Fahy B, Bold RJ: Epidemiology and molecular genetics of colorectal cancer. Surg Oncol 1998;7:115.

Frazier ML et al: Current applications of genetic technology in predisposition testing and microsatellite instability assays. J Clin Oncol 2000;18 (21 Suppl):70S.

Gelfand DW: Decreased risk of subsequent colonic cancer in patients undergoing polypectomy after barium enema: analysis based on data from the preendoscopic era. AJR Am J Roentgenol 1997;169:1243.

Hawk E, Lubet R, Limburg P: Chemoprevention in hereditary colorectal cancer syndromes. Cancer 1999;86 (11 Suppl):2551.

Helm JF, Sandler RS: Colorectal cancer screening. Med Clin North Am 1999;83:1403.

Lal G, Gallinger S: Familial adenomatous polyposis. Semin Surg Oncol 2000;18:314.

Lynch HT, de la Chapelle A: Genetic susceptibility to non-polyposis colorectal cancer. J Med Genet 1999;36:801.

Lynch HT, Smyrk T: An update on Lynch syndrome. Curr Opin Oncol 1998;10:349.

Macrae F: Wheat bran fiber and development of adenomatous polyps: evidence from randomized, controlled clinical trials. Am J Med 1999;106(Suppl 1A):38S.

Management of colonic polyps and adenomas. Patient Care Committee of the Society for Surgery of the Alimentary Tract (SSAT). J Gastrointest Surg 1999;3:220.

Soravia C et al: Desmoid disease in patients with familial adenomatous polyposis. Dis Colon Rectum 2000;43:363.

Spagnesi MT et al: Rectal proliferation and polyp occurrence in patients with familial adenomatous polyposis after sulindac treatment. Gastroenterology 1994;106:362.

Villavicencio RT, Rex DK: Colonic adenomas: prevalence and incidence rates, growth rates, and miss rates at colonoscopy. Semin Gastrointest Dis 2000;11:185.

Winawer SJ, Zauber AG: Colonoscopic polypectomy and the incidence of colorectal cancer. Gut 2001;48:753.

OTHER TUMORS OF THE COLON & RECTUM

Carcinoids of the large bowel are uncommon, and most of them occur in the rectum. Lesions less than 2 cm in diameter usually are asymptomatic, behave benignly, and can be managed by local excision. Larger tumors arising in the colon (mainly the right side) or rectum cause local symptoms, often metastasize, and require standard cancer operations. Carcinoid syndrome appears in less than 5% of patients with metastatic carcinoid of the large bowel.

Lymphomas are the most common noncarcinomatous malignant tumors of the large bowel. Diffuse lymphomatous polyposis is a rare gastrointestinal manifestation. Non-Hodgkin's B cell lymphoma and Kaposi's sarcoma are two AIDS-related cancers that affect the colon and rectum. Lymphoma is often aggressive, but Kaposi's sarcoma may cause few colonic or systemic symptoms.

Lipomas may be difficult to distinguish radiographically from mucosal neoplasms, but colonoscopy most often permits accurate diagnosis. Lipomas are usually asymptomatic but can cause obstruction. Removal is recommended if they cause symptoms.

Leiomyomas are much less common in the colon than in the stomach or small intestine. Colonic tumors are less apt to cause significant hemorrhage than those of the upper bowel. Some leiomyomas become malignant.

Endometriomas are masses of endometrial tissue that implant on the surface of the rectum, sigmoid colon, appendix, cecum, or distal ileum and may invade locally into the muscularis or submucosa. The ectopic tissue responds to cyclic hormonal stimulation, causing inflammation and fibrosis. Intestinal symptoms of endometriosis include altered bowel habits, rectal pain, and rectal bleeding during menstruation. Tender nodularities are palpable in the pelvis in 90% of cases. Sigmoidoscopy, fiberoptic colonoscopy, and barium enema x-rays may make the diagnosis, but diagnostic laparoscopy may be necessary to be certain of the problem. Therapeutic laparoscopy is performed if symptoms are not controlled by endocrine therapy or if cancer cannot be excluded. Endometrial lesions on peritoneal surfaces in the pelvis are destroyed by laser or cautery; colonic or rectal lesions are managed by resection of part or all of that segment of bowel. Relief of intestinal symptoms is reported in 90–100% of patients who undergo surgical treatment.

Other benign colorectal tumors include neuro-fibromas associated with Recklinghausen's disease, teratomas, enterocystomas (duplication of rectum), lymphangiomas, and cavernous hemangiomas. Adenosquamous carcinoma, primary squamous cell carcinoma, sarcomas, and primary melanoma of the colon or rectum are extremely rare malignant tumors.

Henkel A, Christensen B, Schindler AE: Endometriosis: a clinically malignant disease. Eur J Obstet Gynecol Reprod Biol 1999; 82:209.

Jerby BL et al: Laparoscopic management of colorectal endometriosis. Surg Endosc 1999;13:1125.

Kawamoto K et al: Colonic submucosal tumors: a new classification based on radiologic characteristics. AJR Am J Roentgenol 1993;160:315.

Londono-Schimmer EE, Ritchie JK, Hawley PR: Coloanal sleeve anastomosis in the treatment of diffuse cavernous haemangioma of the rectum: long-term results. Br J Surg 1994; 81:1235.

Saclarides TJ, Szeluga D, Staren ED: Neuroendocrine cancers of the colon and rectum: results of a ten-year experience. Dis Colon Rectum 1994;37:635.

Soga J: Carcinoids of the colon and ileocecal region: a statistical evaluation of 363 cases collected from the literature. J Exp Clin Cancer Res 1998;17:139.

Spread C et al: Colon carcinoid tumors. A population-based study. Dis Colon Rectum 1994;37:482.

DIVERTICULAR DISEASE OF THE COLON

Diverticula are more common in the colon than in any other portion of the gastrointestinal tract. Colonic diverticula are acquired and are classified as false because they consist of mucosa and submucosa that have herniated through the muscular coats. True diverticula containing all layers of the bowel wall are rare in the colon. Colonic diverticula are pulsion (rather than traction) diverticula, because they are pushed out by intraluminal pressure. They vary from a few millimeters to several centimeters in diameter; the necks may be narrow or wide; and some contain inspissated fecal matter. Approximately 95% of patients with diverticula have involvement of the sigmoid colon. The descending, transverse, and ascending portions of the colon are involved in decreasing order of frequency. The presence of a solitary diverticulum of the cecum and the occurrence of multiple diverticula limited to the right colon are distinct entities often seen in Asian people but seldom encountered in other populations. Giant colonic diverticulum is a very rare lesion of huge dimensions, usually arising from the sigmoid colon.

In Western countries, perhaps 50% of individuals develop diverticula—10% by age 40 years and 65% by age 80 years. Diverticular disease is more common in Western nations than in Japan or in developing countries of the tropics. The prevalence of diverticulosis is 20%; in Singapore, 70% of the cases are right-sided. Cultural factors, especially diet, play an important etiologic role. Chief among the dietary influences is the fiber content of foods.

The pathogenesis of diverticula requires defects in the colonic wall and increased pressure in the lumen relative to the serosal surface. Small openings in the circular muscle layer for penetration of nutrient blood vessels are the sites of diverticula formation in many individuals (Figure 31–10). Diverticulosis of the colon comprises a spectrum with two extremes: (1) diverticulosis associated with hypermotility and (2) simple massed diverticulosis. In the first type, colonic musculature is shortened and thickened (myochosis coli); colonic pressures are high in response to meals or pharmacologic stimuli; patients may have pain and altered bowel habits; and diverticula are limited to the sigmoid, at least initially. It is hypothesized that myochosis reflects work hypertrophy from a lifetime of fiber-deficient diet and the consequent scybalous stools. High intraluminal pressures are possible because the colon forms closed compartments when opposite walls of the thickened bowel actually touch and occlude the lumen.

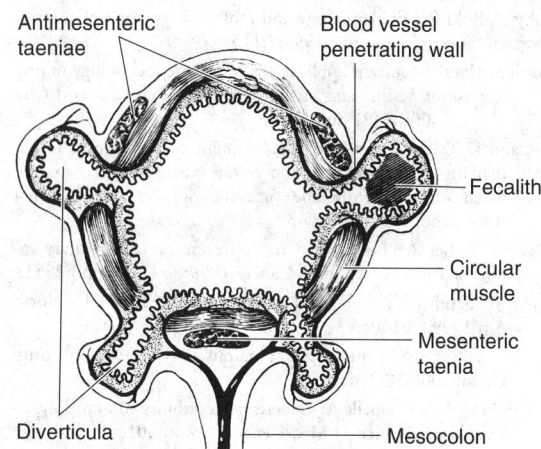

Figure 31–10. Cross section of the colon depicting the sites where diverticula form. Note that the antimesocolic portion is spared. The longitudinal layer of muscle completely encircles the bowel and is not limited to the taeniae as depicted here.

The propensity for diverticula to develop in the sigmoid is explained by the law of Laplace, which states that pressure within a tube is inversely proportionate to the radius. It had been speculated that irritable bowel syndrome was a prediverticular state, but patterns of colonic motility are different in diverticular disease and irritable bowel syndrome. Moreover, it is clear that irritable bowel syndrome can affect the esophagus and small bowel in addition to the colon, so an etiologic link to colonic diverticula now seems unlikely. The two conditions can coexist, however, and irritable bowel syndrome may be the reason for symptoms.

Patients with simple massed diverticulosis have grossly normal colonic musculature, normal pressures, often no symptoms, and diverticula throughout the colon. Presumably, the primary abnormality is weakness of the colonic wall from aging or illness. It is of interest that Ehlers-Danlos syndrome and Marfan's syndrome, both of which involve abnormal connective tissue, are associated with colonic diverticulosis.

1. Diverticulosis

Diverticulosis is the presence of multiple false diverticula.

Clinical Findings

A. SYMPTOMS AND SIGNS

Diverticulosis probably remains asymptomatic in about 80% of people and is detected incidentally on barium enema x-rays or endoscopy if it is discovered at all. Symptoms attributable to the diverticula themselves are actually complications—bleeding and diverticulitis—each described in separate sections below. Symptoms (episodic pain, constipation, diarrhea) in patients with uncomplicated diverticulosis are due to the associated motility disorder, and the diverticula are coincidental. Physical examination may disclose mild tenderness in the left lower quadrant, and the left colon is sometimes palpable as a firm tubular structure. Fever and leukocytosis are absent in patients with pain but no inflammation.

B. IMAGING STUDIES

In addition to diverticula, barium enema films may show segmental spasm and muscular thickening that narrow the lumen and give it a saw-toothed appearance.

Differential Diagnosis

Pain from the colonic muscular abnormality in the absence of inflammation can be difficult to differentiate from diverticulitis. The presence or absence of systemic signs of inflammation is the chief differential point, but the natural history of the acute episode may be the only way to make the distinction. Diverticulosis must be differentiated from other causes of rectal bleeding, especially carcinoma. Colonoscopy is essential in patients with bleeding.

Complications

Diverticulitis and massive hemorrhage are discussed below.

Treatment

A. MEDICAL TREATMENT

Asymptomatic persons with diverticulosis may be given a high-fiber diet, though it is not certain that complications of diverticulosis can be avoided by dietary changes once the diverticula have formed. Symptomatic patients also can be treated with a high-fiber diet; constipation is improved, but abdominal pain is not. Wheat bran is the least expensive source of fiber; patients should take 10–25 g daily with cereal, soup, salad, or other food. Palatable bran products are now available. Other sources of wheat fiber include whole-grain bread and breakfast cereals. Commercial bulk agents (eg, psyllium seed or hemicellulose products) are also available at greater cost. One problem in prescribing bulk agents is that different types of fiber may have dissimilar effects on the colon. Anticholinergic agents, sedatives, tranquilizers, antidepressants, and antibiotics have no value. Analgesics should be avoided, but if pain relief is neces-

sary, nonopioid medications are preferred. Education, reassurance, and a warm personal relationship between physician and patient are important to successful management.

B. SURGICAL TREATMENT

Operation is necessary for massive hemorrhage or to rule out carcinoma in some patients, but colonoscopy usually resolves the question of cancer. Colon resection for uncomplicated diverticular disease or irritable bowel syndrome is rarely necessary or advisable.

Prognosis

The natural history of diverticulosis has not been defined. Ten to 20 percent of patients with diverticulosis develop diverticulitis or hemorrhage when followed for many years. These patients are selected, however, and the incidence of complications in the population at large may be much lower. About 75% of complications of diverticular disease develop in patients with no prior colonic symptoms. Some evidence suggests that diverticulitis is more common with the hypermotility type of diverticulosis, and bleeding is the more frequent complication in simple massed diverticulosis. Irritable bowel syndrome is a chronic relapsing disorder that affects patients over long periods of their lives. There is hope that better understanding of the pathophysiologic mechanisms will soon lead to more rational therapy.

See references at end of next section.

2. Diverticulitis

 ESSENTIALS OF DIAGNOSIS

- *Acute abdominal pain.*
- *Left lower quadrant tenderness and mass.*
- *Fever and leukocytosis.*
- *Characteristic radiologic signs.*

General Considerations

Acute colonic diverticulitis is the result of perforation due to intraluminal pressure, or it begins as infection in a diverticulum. Corticosteroids or nonsteroidal anti-inflammatory drug use may contribute to this complication. With either mechanism, only one diverticulum is involved at a time, usually in the sigmoid colon. Infection limited to a tiny diverticulum may not cause symptoms, but when infection extends through the wall of the colon into peridiverticular tissue **(peridiverticulitis),** it becomes clinically significant. Peridiverticulitis implies that the diverticulum has perforated, but the process evolves slowly rather than suddenly, as may occur when intraluminal pressure causes perforation.

Microperforation of a diverticulum leads to localized inflammation in the colonic wall or paracolic tissues. Macroperforation results in more extensive bacterial contamination and more serious infection such as an abscess or generalized peritonitis. An abscess may be confined by adjacent structures or may enlarge and spread; it may resorb with antibiotic treatment or drain spontaneously into the lumen of the bowel or into an adjacent viscus to form a fistula; it may require surgical drainage; it may rupture into the peritoneal cavity and produce generalized purulent peritonitis; or it may become chronic. The other mechanism for development of generalized peritonitis is rupture of a diverticulum into the free peritoneal cavity, which contaminates the abdomen with feces. Intraluminal pressure is responsible. Fortunately, this form of diverticulitis is uncommon. Chronic colonic obstruction can result from fibrosis in response to repeated episodes of microperforation. Also, small bowel may adhere acutely to an inflamed area and cause small bowel obstruction. Cecal diverticulitis resembles appendicitis clinically.

It was once believed that nearly all perforated diverticula maintain a connection with the bowel lumen **(communicating diverticulitis).** It is now known that in many cases, the original perforation seals quickly and the paracolic infection is isolated from the colonic lumen **(noncommunicating diverticulitis).** This concept has implications for surgical treatment.

Clinical Findings

A. SYMPTOMS AND SIGNS

The acute attack consists of localized abdominal pain that is mild to severe, aching, and either steady or cramping; it resembles acute appendicitis except that it is situated in the left lower quadrant. Occasionally, pain is suprapubic, in the right lower quadrant, or throughout the lower abdomen. Constipation or increased frequency of defecation (or both in the same patient) is common, and passage of flatus may give some relief of pain. Inflammation adjacent to the bladder may produce dysuria. Nausea and vomiting depend on the location and severity of the inflammation. Physical findings characteristically include low-grade fever, mild abdominal distention, left lower quadrant tenderness, and a left lower quadrant or pelvic mass. Occult or, less commonly, gross blood is present in stools; massive hemorrhage is rare in the presence of peridiverticular inflammation. Leukocytosis is mild to moderate.

The clinical picture described above is typical, but acute diverticulitis has other modes of presentation. Free perforation of a diverticulum produces generalized peritonitis rather than localized inflammation. An acute attack of diverticulitis may go unnoticed until a complication develops, and the complication may be the reason for the patient to seek help. The course of diverticulitis may be so insidious, particularly in old people, that vague abdominal pain associated with an abscess in the groin or a colovesical fistula is the initial presentation. In some cases, pain and inflammatory signs are not marked, but a palpable mass and signs of large bowel obstruction are present, so that carcinoma of the left colon seems the more likely diagnosis. In one series of women with proved diverticulitis, 38% were initially misdiagnosed as having a gynecologic pelvic mass because gastrointestinal symptoms and signs were mild or absent.

B. IMAGING STUDIES

Plain abdominal films may show free abdominal air if a diverticulum has perforated into the general peritoneal cavity. If inflammation is localized, there is a picture of ileus, partial colonic obstruction, small bowel obstruction, or left lower quadrant mass.

CT scan is replacing water-soluble contrast enema as the initial imaging study. CT can be obtained early in the patient's course, with intravenous and usually oral contrast to enhance the image. Effacement of pericolic fat is seen in diverticulitis, and complications such as abscess or fistula may be evident. The finding of an abscess that is accessible for percutaneous drainage provides a major therapeutic advantage over contrast enemas. CT findings of perforated diverticulitis are not specific; colonoscopy and sometimes contrast enema must be obtained subsequently. Ultrasound and MRI are helpful in some cases.

Barium enema is contraindicated during the initial stages of an acute attack of diverticulitis lest barium leak into the peritoneal cavity, but water-soluble contrast media used under low pressure is safe. Barium enema can be performed a week or more after the attack began if the patient has recovered promptly. Radiographic signs include the following: (1) an abscess cavity or sinus tract outside the colonic wall communicating with the lumen; (2) an intramural abscess producing indentation of the barium column; (3) extrinsic compression by a paracolic mass; (4) intramural sinuses; and (5) fistulas. (See Figure 31–11.)

C. SPECIAL EXAMINATIONS

The rigid sigmoidoscope usually cannot be passed beyond the rectosigmoid junction because of acute angulation and fixation at that level with a decrease in size of the lumen. Erythema, edema, and spasm may be noted.

Figure 31–11. Barium enema x-ray showing upper sigmoid colon involved with diverticulitis. Note the long segment of narrowing, the spasm, and the deformity (arrow) produced by an intramural abscess.

A purulent discharge can sometimes be seen coming from above. Flexible sigmoidoscopy or colonoscopy should be avoided during an acute attack but is very helpful in evaluating strictures and other persistent abnormalities later. Small-bore upper tract instruments may be needed to examine narrow segments. Cystoscopy may reveal bullous edema of the bladder wall.

Differential Diagnosis

Free perforation of a diverticulum with generalized peritonitis often cannot be differentiated from the other causes of perforation, including foreign bodies and stercoraceous perforation. Acute diverticulitis with localized perforation may simulate appendicitis, perforated colonic carcinoma, strangulation obstruction, mesenteric vascular insufficiency, Crohn's disease, and many other conditions. One source of confusion is that diverticulitis can be precipitated by Crohn's disease, but the length of the paracolic fistulous tract is a differential point: a short tract (< 4 cm) is due to diverticulitis, and a long tract (> 8 cm) reflects either diverticulitis alone or Crohn's disease in association with diverticulitis. Differentiation from appendicitis is especially difficult when a redundant sigmoid colon lies in the right lower quadrant. A history of colonic symptoms on prior occasions, palpation of a mass, ultrasonography, CT, or water-soluble

contrast enema may be helpful in differentiating these conditions. Sigmoidoscopy may detect carcinoma, vascular insufficiency, or inflammatory disease of the colon. A difficult differential diagnosis lies between diverticulitis and carcinoma of the colon, particularly in the more silent forms of diverticulitis that present with a mass or fistula. Although barium enema and colonoscopy may clarify the issue, the diagnosis may not be known until the surgical specimen is examined by the pathologist. Persistent bleeding should not be attributed to diverticular disease until cancer has been excluded as a possibility; this nearly always requires colonoscopy.

Complications

The clinical spectrum of diverticulitis includes such complications as free perforation, abscess formation, fistulization, and partial obstruction. Colonic obstruction is usually slow in onset and incomplete; small bowel obstruction may result from the attachment of a loop of small intestine to the inflamed sigmoid.

Fistulas in males usually involve the bladder (see Colovesical Fistula, below). Fistulas may also occur to the ureter, urethra, vagina, uterus, cecum, small bowel, perineum, and abdominal wall.

Treatment

A. Expectant Treatment

Patients with acute diverticulitis may need to be hospitalized. Details of management vary with the severity of the attack. Generally, nothing is given by mouth, nasogastric suction is instituted, intravenous fluids are given, and systemic broad-spectrum antibiotics are administered. Oral nonabsorbable antibacterial drugs are of little value. Opioid pain medications should be avoided. As acute manifestations subside, oral feeding is resumed gradually, and bulk-forming agents are prescribed if there is no stricture.

Colonoscopy is performed a week or so after the attack began. Colonoscopy is mandatory in the presence of rectal bleeding or if x-rays show a possible neoplasm (stricture, mass, equivocal findings). It is recommended—even if barium x-rays reveal only diverticula—in patients with abdominal pain or change in bowel habits attributed to diverticular disease. Colonoscopy will disclose a colonic neoplasm in about 30% of such patients.

B. Surgical Treatment

Cecal diverticulitis is usually treated by right colectomy. Immediate operation for sigmoid diverticulitis is required if spreading or generalized peritonitis is present upon entry into the hospital or if peritonitis develops during the hospital stay. Abdominal pain, mass, fever, or leukocytosis that fails to improve after 3–4 days of medical therapy also indicates that intervention is necessary. Obstruction and fistula seldom become indications for urgent operation during acute diverticulitis; both of these clinical problems are discussed separately in this chapter.

Percutaneous catheter drainage of well-localized paracolic abscesses can be performed by the interventional radiologist. This technique is especially useful because it converts a potential emergency operation to an elective one when the patient is in better condition. Colonic resection will be needed eventually in most of these patients.

At laparotomy for severe acute diverticulitis, peritoneal fluid varies from turbid to purulent to grossly fecal. The sigmoid colon is involved in an inflammatory mass composed of large bowel, mesocolon, omentum, and sometimes small bowel. Except in cases of free perforation with generalized fecal peritonitis, the diseased diverticulum may not be visible. An abscess cavity may be hidden beneath colon or omentum and discovered when the bowel is mobilized; abscesses are commonly found lateral or medial to the colon, in the mesocolon, or in the pelvis. Microperforation of a diverticulum is not associated with a grossly apparent abscess. The extent of colonic inflammation, the amount of peritonitis, the patient's general condition, and the surgeon's experience and preferences determine the type of operation to be performed.

1. Primary resection with anastomosis—Resection of the diseased colon and performance of colonic anastomosis at the same time have the advantage of solving the entire problem in one operation. It is not possible to anastomose the colon safely if there is gross infection in the surgical field, because the risk of anastomotic leakage is great. Intraoperative lavage of the colon may make it possible to perform primary anastomosis if other conditions permit.

2. Primary resection without anastomosis (two-stage procedure)—The diseased bowel is removed, the proximal end of the colon is brought out as a temporary colostomy, and the distal colonic stump is closed (Hartmann procedure; Figure 31–12) or exteriorized as a mucous fistula. Intestinal continuity is restored in a second operation after the inflammation subsides. Increasingly, percutaneous drainage of abscesses avoids the need for staged procedures.

3. Three-stage procedure—The three-stage procedure consists of a first operation during which a transverse colostomy is created and the paracolic abscess is drained; a second operation during which the left colon is resected; and a third operation during which the colostomy is taken down. A variation on this theme is to suture the colonic perforation and cover it with an

Figure 31–12. Primary resection for diverticulitis of the colon. The affected segment (shaded) has been divided at its distal end. If primary anastomosis is to be done, the proximal margin (dotted line) is transected, and the bowel is anastomosed end-to-end. If a two-stage procedure will be used, a colostomy is formed at the proximal margin, and the distal stump is oversewn (Hartmann procedure, as shown), or exteriorized as a mucous fistula. The second stage consists of colostomy takedown and anastomosis.

omental patch at the first operation in addition to constructing a transverse colostomy. Although results were good in a recent Danish study, the three-stage approach is uncommonly used in the United States today).

Definitive resection for sigmoid diverticulitis should include the rectosigmoid distally to the point where the taeniae become confluent so that anastomosis is performed to the proximal rectum, which is always free of diverticula. The distal descending colon is removed, but it is unnecessary to resect additional bowel proximally; even if it is involved with diverticula, they do not become symptomatic in the absence of the sigmoid high-pressure zone. Laparoscopy-assisted resection is possible in some cases.

Prognosis

Approximately 25% of patients hospitalized with acute diverticulitis require surgical treatment. The operative mortality rate is about 5% in recent reports, compared with 25% a few years ago. Some of this improvement is attributable to the greater use of primary resection following percutaneous drainage of abscess.

Diverticulitis recurs in about one-third of medically treated cases. Most of these recurrences develop within the first 5 years. It is unknown whether recurrent attacks of diverticulitis can be prevented by increasing dietary fiber, although this measure is generally recommended. Indications for elective colon resection are recurrent diverticulitis, persistent diverticulitis (pain, tenderness, mass, dysuria), age under 50 years, and inability to rule out carcinoma. The mortality rate of elective left colectomy is 2–4%. Recurrent diverticulitis after resection is unusual (about 3–7%).

Aldoori WH et al: A prospective study of dietary fiber types and symptomatic diverticular disease in men. J Nutr 1998; 128:714.

Ambrosetti P et al: Acute left colonic diverticulitis: a prospective analysis of 226 consecutive cases. Surgery 1994;115:546.

Baevsky R: Acute diverticulitis. N Engl J Med 1998;339:1082.

Brengman ML, Otchy DP: Timing of computed tomography in acute diverticulitis. Dis Colon Rectum 1998;41:1023.

Bruce CJ et al: Laparoscopic resection for diverticular disease. Dis Colon Rectum 1996;39(10 Suppl): S1.

Carbajo Caballero MA et al: The laparoscopic approach in the treatment of diverticular colon disease. J Soc Laparoendosc Surg 1998;2:159.

Desai DC et al: The utility of the Hartmann procedure. Am J Surg 1998;175:152.

Gooszen AW et al: Operative treatment of acute complications of diverticular disease: primary or secondary anastomosis after sigmoid resection. Eur J Surg 2001;167:35.

Janower ML: Acute diverticulitis. N Engl J Med 1998;339:1081.

Kronborg O: Treatment of perforated sigmoid diverticulitis: a prospective randomized trial. Br J Surg 1993;80:505.

Lee EC et al: Intraoperative colonic lavage in nonelective surgery for diverticular disease. Dis Colon Rectum 1997;40:669.

Miura S et al: Recent trends in diverticulosis of the right colon in Japan: retrospective review in a regional hospital. Dis Colon Rectum 2000;43:1383.

Roberts P et al: Practice parameters for sigmoid diverticulitis. The Standards Task Force American Society of Colon and Rectal Surgeons. Dis Colon Rectum 1995;38:125.

Young-Fadok TM et al: Colonic diverticular disease. Curr Probl Surg 2000;37:457.

COLOVESICAL FISTULA

Colovesical fistula is the most common type of fistulous communication between the urinary bladder and the gastrointestinal tract. There is a 3:1 ratio of men to women with this condition, presumably because in women the uterus and adnexa are situated between the colon and the bladder.

Diverticulitis is the most common cause of colovesical fistula. This complication occurs in 2–4% of cases of diverticulitis, though an even higher incidence is reported from specialized referral centers. Carcinoma of the colon, cancer of other organs such as the bladder, Crohn's disease, radiation bowel injury, external trauma, foreign bodies, and iatrogenic injuries are other causes or underlying conditions.

A colovesical fistula may cause surprisingly little disturbance to the patient, and some patients remain completely asymptomatic. The appearance of a fistula from diverticulitis or colonic cancer is seldom accompanied by dramatic or sudden abdominal symptoms; more typically, refractory urinary tract infection is the presenting complaint. Fecaluria and pneumaturia may have been obvious to the patient, or it may be recollected only in response to direct questioning. The episode of diverticulitis may have gone entirely unnoticed.

Physical examination may disclose a pelvic mass or no abnormalities. Leukocytosis is absent in most cases, and routine blood chemistries are normal. Urinalysis may reveal fecaluria or infected urine. Rigid sigmoidoscopy is usually unrevealing; flexible sigmoidoscopy or colonoscopy may disclose colonic cancer or inflammation at the fistula site. Cystoscopy shows bullous edema, but the fistula is usually not visible. CT detects small amounts of air in the bladder in 90% of patients. Barium enema, sonography, and cystography may demonstrate the fistula, but small communications escape detection. In some cases, the fistula is not demonstrable because it has closed, at least temporarily.

Colovesical fistulas require surgical treatment if they persist, but there is no need for emergency or urgent operation. Patients may recover well from spontaneous drainage of a paracolic abscess through a fistula into the bladder, and operation can be delayed to be sure it is necessary and by then the conditions will be more favorable. Inability to rule out cancer may prompt earlier operation. If a fistula closes spontaneously, as it may do in up to 50% of patients with diverticulitis, requirements for resection depend on the nature of the underlying colonic disease. Some patients tolerate a colovesical fistula so well that operation is deferred indefinitely.

At operation, patients with diverticulitis or colonic carcinoma have mild to moderate inflammatory reaction around the sigmoid colon, which has dropped into the pelvis and adhered to the bladder; severe active diverticulitis with abscess or peritonitis is exceptional. If the fistula has been caused by cancer of the colon, the adherent bladder should not be separated from the colon lest tumor cells be spilled into the pelvis; a disk of bladder wall should be excised in continuity with the colon, the bladder closed primarily, and catheter drainage of the bladder provided for 7–10 days. Fortunately, most colovesical fistulas enter the bladder away from the trigone. Diverticulitis is managed by bluntly dissecting the colon from the bladder, resecting the colon, and performing a primary anastomosis. The bladder side of the fistula is sutured. It is rarely necessary to delay performance of the colonic anastomosis.

Lavery IC: Colonic fistulas. Surg Clin North Am 1996;76:1183.

Vasilevsky CA et al: Fistulas complicating diverticulitis. Int J Colorectal Dis 1998;13:57.

ACUTE LOWER GASTROINTESTINAL HEMORRHAGE

Acute hemorrhage per rectum can originate from lesions in the gastroduodenum, small bowel, colon, or anorectum. A source in the lower gastrointestinal tract is suggested by the passage of dark to bright red blood, but the color of evacuated blood is a function of the length of time it remained in the intestinal tract, and bright red blood may come from a duodenal ulcer or hemorrhoids as well as any point in between. If a patient passing bright red blood is not in shock, the bleeding site is probably in the distal small bowel or colon.

Exsanguinating hemorrhage from the colon in adults is caused by diverticular disease, angiodysplasia, solitary ulcer, ulcerative colitis, ischemic colitis, or a variety of uncommon lesions such as coagulation disorders, radiation injury, chemotherapeutic toxicity, and others. Bleeding occurs in the right colon about as often as in the left colon, probably because angiodysplasias are more prominent on the right side, but right-sided diverticula can also bleed. Bleeding lesions in the small intestine are rare and include hereditary hemorrhagic telangiectasia (Rendu-Osler-Weber syndrome).

Chronic rectal bleeding, typically seen in patients with cancer, polyps, hemorrhoids, fissures, and other conditions, does not require urgent evaluation. Anorectal examination, colonoscopy, and x-rays if indicated can be performed electively. Acute severe hemorrhage, however, is a potentially life-threatening problem, and prompt evaluation and treatment are critical. Some patients bleed rapidly, but the bleeding stops spontaneously after only a small amount of blood is lost, and these patients are never in danger. Usually, however, one cannot be sure that bleeding will not recur, so this type of bleeding must be taken seriously too, which means that aggressive evaluation is needed.

A plan of management of acute lower gastrointestinal hemorrhage is outlined in Figure 31–13. Many decisions depend on the rate of bleeding, which is difficult to include in an algorithm. Bleeding stops spontaneously in 90% of patients before transfusion requirements exceed two units.

The patient with severe rectal bleeding is resuscitated with intravenous fluids and transfusions while the diagnostic procedures are begun. Clotting parameters should be measured and deficits corrected, and associated medical conditions should be identified and treated as soon as possible. Digital rectal examination, anoscopy, and sigmoidoscopy should be performed with no attempt to prepare the bowel. If a bleeding lesion is found in the anorectum, it should be treated.

Examples include hemorrhoids, polypoid neoplasm, and ulcerative proctitis.

A nasogastric tube should be inserted and the aspirate inspected for bile, gross blood, and occult blood. Blood in the stomach is an indication of bleeding from a site proximal to the ligament of Treitz—ie, upper gastrointestinal bleeding—and esophagogastroduodenoscopy is performed. Occasionally, a patient bleeds from the duodenum but blood does not reflux back into the stomach; bile in the nasogastric aspirate would seem to eliminate this possibility, but in the absence of blood or bile, esophagogastroduodenoscopy should be done.

If esophagogastroduodenoscopy is negative and bleeding has presumably stopped or continues at a slow rate, the colon can be prepared and colonoscopy performed within a few hours. The bleeding site is identified in 25–94% of cases, depending in part on skill, experience, and, very importantly, the criteria for inclusion of a patient in this category of bleeding. Some bleeding lesions can be treated colonoscopically with a bipolar probe, heater probe, or laser. Colonoscopy with negative results probably means that bleeding has stopped. Barium enema discloses abnormalities such as diverticula but does not reveal which lesions have been bleeding.

The optimal method for evaluating patients who are bleeding rapidly is controversial, and the decision may hinge on available resources. Radionuclide "bleeding" scan after injection of ^{99m}Tc-labeled red blood cells may show whether bleeding persists. Localization of bleeding is not reliable, and enthusiasm for bleeding scans has waned recently. Angiography is seldom successful in demonstrating an active bleeding site if the bleeding scan is negative, so colonoscopy should be undertaken. Active bleeding shown on radionuclide scan should be followed by angiography.

Selective mesenteric angiography identifies the bleeding site in 14–70% of patients; here, too, enthusiasm of the angiographer is important. If the bleeding site is seen, intra-arterial infusion of vasopressin controls bleeding, at least transiently, in 35–90% of patients. Bleeding recurs after cessation of vasoconstrictor therapy in 50% of instances.

The other option for rapid bleeding is emergency colonoscopy without preliminary bowel cleansing. Blood is a cathartic, and the colon may be free of stool. Even so, colonoscopy in this situation is difficult. Experts are able to see the bleeding point in up to 50% of patients, and in 70% of cases bleeding can be localized to one region. Endoscopic therapeutic measures can be applied in up to 40% of patients, with success in half of them.

Operation is indicated for bleeding that persists or recurs despite angiographic and endoscopic therapeutic

Figure 31–13. Plan for diagnosis and treatment of acute lower gastrointestinal hemorrhage. (NG = nasogastric.)

maneuvers. Operation is advisable also in good-risk patients who have stopped bleeding if the bleeding source is known and cannot be managed in some other way (eg, colonoscopic coagulation). Operation is limited to segmental colonic resection if the bleeding site has been localized conclusively. More extensive resection is usually warranted in patients who are bleeding from the right colon and have multiple diverticula in the left colon. If the surgeon has no preoperative localizing data and intraoperative examination is unrevealing, the stomach, small bowel, and colon can be endoscoped during the procedure to search for the source of blood. If all localizing efforts fail and the colon is the likely bleeding site, total abdominal colectomy (usually with primary anastomosis) may be the only recourse. Fortunately, extensive "blind" colectomy is seldom required today.

The mortality rate from lower gastrointestinal hemorrhage is about 10–15%.

Eisen GM et al: An annotated algorithmic approach to acute lower gastrointestinal bleeding. Gastrointest Endosc 2001;53:859.

Farrell JJ, Friedman LS: Gastrointestinal bleeding in the elderly. Gastroenterol Clin North Am 2001;30:377.

Gordon RL et al: Selective arterial embolization for the control of lower gastrointestinal bleeding. Am J Surg 1997;174:24.

Jensen DM: What to choose for diagnosis of bleeding colonic angiomas: colonoscopy, angiography, or helical computed tomography angiography? Gastroenterology 2000;119:581.

Luchtefeld MA et al: Evaluation of transarterial embolization for lower gastrointestinal bleeding. Dis Colon Rectum 2000; 43:532.

The role of endoscopy in the patient with lower gastrointestinal bleeding. American Society for Gastrointestinal Endoscopy. Gastrointest Endosc 1998;48:685.

Suzman MS et al: Accurate localization and surgical management of active lower gastrointestinal hemorrhage with technetium-labeled erythrocyte scintigraphy. Ann Surg 1996;224:29.

ANGIODYSPLASIA

Angiodysplasia is an acquired condition most often affecting people over age 60. It is a focal submucosal vascular ectasia that has a propensity to bleed spontaneously. Most lesions are located in the cecum and proximal ascending colon, but in younger persons they are occasionally found in the small bowel, principally the jejunum. Multiple lesions occur in 25% of cases. Aortic stenosis is found in patients with angiodysplasias, but whether they are truly related is still being argued. Von Willebrand's disease is present in some patients, and it has been suggested that the two conditions may be reflections of a generalized tissue disorder. Bleeding is typically intermittent and is rarely massive; a typical episode requires transfusion of two to four units of blood and is not associated with hypotension. Angiodysplasia may also present clinically as melena or as iron deficiency anemia and guaiac-positive stools.

The diagnosis is made in some cases by colonoscopy, and colonoscopic therapy is often successful. Incidental angiomas should be ignored. The lesions are characterized angiographically by (1) an early-filling vein (ie, within 4–5 seconds after injection), (2) a vascular tuft, and (3) a delayed-emptying vein. It is generally thought that two of the three features should be seen for the diagnosis to be secure. Active bleeding (ie, extravasation) is rarely demonstrated by angiography. As many as 25% of persons over age 60 with no history of gastrointestinal bleeding have angiodysplasias of the cecum, so the finding of a lesion is not proof that it has caused bleeding.

The natural history of angiodysplasia is not well delineated, and in elderly, poor-risk patients who have bled only once, expectant management may be preferable to surgery if colonoscopic therapeutic methods are unsuccessful. Operation should consist of right hemicolectomy if the right colon was shown to be the bleeding site. It may be wise to resect the entire colon, with ileorectal anastomosis, in good-risk patients who also have extensive left-sided diverticulosis. In one series, 23% of patients who underwent operation for presumably bleeding colonic angiodysplasias were eventually found to have a small bowel lesion also.

Foutch PG: Colonic angiodysplasia. Gastroenterologist 1997; 5:148.

Orsi P, Guatti-Zuliani C, Okolicsanyi L: Long-acting octreotide is effective in controlling rebleeding angiodysplasia of the gastrointestinal tract. Dig Liver Dis 2001;33:330.

Rockey DC: Occult gastrointestinal bleeding. N Engl J Med 1999; 341:38.

Sharma R, Gorbien MJ: Angiodysplasia and lower gastrointestinal tract bleeding in elderly patients. Arch Intern Med 1995; 155:807.

Veyradier A et al: Abnormal von Willebrand factor in bleeding angiodysplasias of the digestive tract. Gastroenterology 2001; 120:346.

VOLVULUS

 ESSENTIALS OF DIAGNOSIS

- Colicky abdominal pain, usually with persistence of pain between spasms.
- Abdominal distention.
- Vomiting sometimes.
- Usually older age groups.
- Characteristic x-ray findings.

General Considerations

Rotation of a segment of the intestine on an axis formed by its mesentery may result in partial or complete obstruction of the lumen and may be followed by circulatory impairment of the bowel (Figure 31–14). Volvulus of the colon involves the cecum (30%), sigmoid (65%), transverse colon (3%), or splenic flexure (2%). Volvulus of the colon accounts for 5–10% of cases of large bowel obstruction in the USA and is the second most common cause of complete colonic obstruction. In certain countries where the population consumes a high-residue diet, volvulus is the most frequent cause of large bowel obstruction. Volvulus—sigmoid more often than cecal—accounts for 25% of intestinal obstructions during pregnancy; it occurs most often in the last trimester, probably because the enlarging uterus displaces the colon.

Elongation of the sigmoid and rectosigmoid is a predisposing factor in sigmoid volvulus; 50% of patients are over age 70, and many patients are mentally ill or bedridden persons who do not evacuate stool with regularity. Chagas' disease of the colon is an important cause of sigmoid volvulus in South America. Formation of cecal volvulus requires a cecum that is hypermobile owing to incomplete embryologic fixation of the ascending colon. The bowel twists about the mesentery, forming a closed-loop obstruction as the entry and exit points of the twist engage; obstruction of the lumen usually occurs when the rotation is 180 degrees. When the twist is 360 degrees, the veins are occluded, and the circulatory impairment leads to gangrene and perforation if treatment is not instituted promptly. A related

Figure 31–14. Volvulus of the sigmoid colon. The twist is counterclockwise in most cases of sigmoid volvulus.

condition called **cecal bascule** involves folding of the ascending colon so that the cecum moves anteriorly and superiorly, causing obstruction at the site of the transverse fold. Since no axial twist of the mesentery is involved in this situation, early strangulation from occlusion of the main vessels is not a factor.

Clinical Findings

A. CECAL VOLVULUS

Not only the cecum but also the terminal ileum are involved in the rotation, so the symptoms generally include those of distal small bowel obstruction. Severe intermittent colicky pain begins in the right abdomen. Pain eventually becomes continuous, vomiting ensues, and passage of gas and feces per rectum decreases to the point of obstipation. Abdominal distention is variable; occasionally, a bulging tympanitic mass may be detected. There may be a history of similar but milder attacks, and valid examples of chronic intermittent cecal volvulus exist; they can be detected and operated on electively.

The diagnosis is seldom made without x-ray examination. Plain films show a hugely dilated ovoid cecum that may change position but favors the epigastrium or left upper quadrant. In the early stages, there is a single fluid level that may be mistaken for gastric dilation, but large amounts of gas or fluid cannot be aspirated from the stomach, and the x-ray picture is not changed by this maneuver. Later, the radiologic findings of small bowel obstruction are superimposed on the cecal volvulus. The success rate of diagnosis based on plain abdominal films is extremely variable, ranging from 5% to 90%. Barium enema may show a diagnostic picture.

B. SIGMOID VOLVULUS

In volvulus of the sigmoid, there are intermittent cramp-like pains, increasing in severity as obstipation becomes complete. Abdominal distention may be marked. There may be a history of transient attacks in which spontaneous reduction of the volvulus has occurred. On a plain film of the abdomen, a single greatly distended loop of bowel that has lost its haustral markings is usually seen rising up out of the pelvis, frequently as high as the diaphragm. The distended loop may assume a "coffee bean" shape. In cecal volvulus, the concavity of the "coffee bean" points toward the right lower abdominal quadrant, and in sigmoid volvulus it points toward the left lower quadrant. On barium enema, a "bird's beak" or "ace of spades" deformity with spiral narrowing of the upper end of the lower segment is pathognomonic (Figure 31–15). Between attacks, barium enema may reveal sigmoid megacolon. The entire colon may be termed a megacolon in some cases.

Differential Diagnosis

Cecal volvulus must be differentiated from colonic pseudo-obstruction and from other causes of small bowel and colonic obstruction. Sigmoid volvulus mimics other types of large bowel obstruction. Alertness to the possibility and correct interpretation of x-rays are the essentials of diagnosis.

Complications

Early diagnosis and treatment are imperative because perforation may occur if circulation to the bowel is impaired. Delay may be due to incorrect diagnosis or to futile attempts at proximal decompression by gastric intubation.

Treatment

In cecal volvulus, decompression is advisable as soon as the patient can be prepared by replacing fluid and electrolyte deficits. Colonoscopic detorsion and decom-

Figure 31–15. Volvulus of the sigmoid colon. Barium enema taken with the patient in the supine position. Note the massively dilated sigmoid colon. The distinct vertical crease, which represents juxtaposition of adjacent walls of the dilated loop, points toward the site of torsion. The barium column resembles a "bird's beak" or "ace of spades" because of the way in which the lumen tapers toward the volvulus.

pression may be attempted if an expert is available, especially in patients who have serious associated disease that would make operation hazardous. Laparoscopic treatment by cecopexy has been reported, but most surgeons still perform open laparotomy if colonoscopic decompression is unavailable or if it fails. At laparotomy, the loop is untwisted and carefully inspected. If the bowel is viable, cecopexy (suture fixation of the bowel to the parietal peritoneum) gives good immediate results, but the long-term success rate is controversial; recurrent volvulus developed in 29% of patients after cecopexy in one review. Tube cecostomy both decompresses the cecum and fixes it, and this procedure is favored by some surgeons. Resection and anastomosis is preferred by others even if the bowel is viable, arguing that long-term results are better than with lesser procedures. Gangrenous colon or small bowel is found in about 20% of cases and requires right hemicolectomy; immediate anastomosis is performed in good-risk patients; otherwise, a temporary ileostomy is constructed, and continuity is restored later.

In many patients with sigmoid volvulus, the distended sigmoid can be decompressed by gentle insertion of a flexible colonoscope or sigmoidoscope. Decompression by passage of a tube through a rigid sigmoidoscope works well too, and some authorities argue that it should be tried first. Endoscopic decompression is contraindicated if there is evidence of strangulation or perforation. Percutaneous decompression of sigmoid volvulus has been reported, but it cannot be recommended for general use. If decompression is successful, good-risk young patients should be scheduled for elective resection as soon as the colon can be prepared, because the recurrence rate after decompression alone is 50%. No operation is indicated after endoscopic decompression of the first episode of sigmoid volvulus in patients with severe disease of other organ systems. Emergency operation is performed if strangulation or perforation is suspected or if attempts to decompress the bowel per rectum are unsuccessful. Gangrenous bowel is found in about one-third of such patients and is treated by resection. If the sigmoid is viable, most surgeons proceed with resection, deferring anastomosis to a later time if the bowel is unprepared. If the entire colon is a megacolon, total abdominal colectomy should be considered. Recurrent volvulus in nonoperated patients is managed by transrectal decompression followed by a definitive surgical procedure in all patients but those with very severe associated disease.

Prognosis

The mortality rate after emergency operation in patients with cecal volvulus is 12%; if the bowel is gangrenous, 35% of patients die after resection. Recurrence after cecopexy or resection is very unusual.

Sigmoid volvulus is fatal in about 50% of patients with perforation; mortality rates are much lower with gangrene alone, and only 5% of patients die after operation if the bowel is viable. Elective resection after endoscopic decompression has a low mortality rate, and recurrent volvulus is rare.

Feldman D: The coffee bean sign. Radiology 2000;216:178.

Grossmann EM et al: Sigmoid volvulus in Department of Veterans Affairs Medical Centers. Dis Colon Rectum 2000;43:414.

Madiba TE, Thomson SR: The management of sigmoid volvulus. J R Coll Surg Edinb 2000;45:74.

COLITIS

Colitis is a nonspecific term. Patients have diarrhea, abdominal pain, systemic symptoms, and abnormal endoscopic, radiographic, and laboratory tests. The task of the clinician is to differentiate among the various causes of colitis discussed below.

1. Idiopathic Mucosal Ulcerative Colitis

General Considerations

The age at onset of ulcerative colitis has a bimodal distribution, with the first peak between ages 15 and 30 years and a second, lower peak in the sixth to eighth decades. Females are affected slightly more often than males. The annual incidence varies from 5 to 12 per 100,000 population, and the prevalence is 50–150 per 100,000 population. The disease is found worldwide but is more common in Western countries. It is uncommon in Asia. In 15–40% of patients, there is a family history of ulcerative colitis or Crohn's disease. In the USA, Jews are more commonly affected than non-Jews, but in Israel the prevalence among new immigrants is low.

The cause of ulcerative colitis is not known. The current hypothesis is that external agents, host responses, and genetic immunologic influences interact in the pathogenesis of inflammatory bowel disease. It is possible that ulcerative colitis and Crohn's disease are different manifestations of a single disease process. The host becomes sensitized to the antigens of the inciting external agent or agents (eg, microbial, viral, or dietary). Once immunologic priming of the gut is established—perhaps during the period of microbial colonization in infancy—any insult that increases mucosal permeability to these antigens can precipitate an inflammatory reaction in the bowel wall. The types of antigens and many other factors determine the nature of the inflammatory process (eg, Crohn's disease or ulcerative colitis). Eicosanoids, metabolites of arachidonic acid, and platelet-activating factor are just two of many putative mediators of inflammation in colitis. It was reported recently that appendectomy is a protective factor against later development of ulcerative colitis. Cigarette smoking appears to decrease the risk of ulcerative colitis, but it increases the risk of Crohn's disease.

Ulcerative colitis is a diffuse inflammatory disease confined to the mucosa initially. Abscesses form in the crypts of Lieberkühn, penetrate the superficial submucosa, and by spreading horizontally cause the overlying mucosa to slough. Vascular congestion and hemorrhage are prominent. The margins of the ulcers are raised as mucosal tags that project into the lumen (pseudopolyps or inflammatory polyps). Except in the most severe forms, the muscular layers are spared; the serosal surface usually shows only dilated congested blood vessels. In fulminant disease, when the full thickness is involved, the colon may dilate or perforate. The colon is shortened, but the mesocolon remains thin—in contrast to Crohn's disease.

Ulcerative colitis involves the rectum in most patients. If confined to the rectum—as it is in one-half of cases—it is termed ulcerative proctitis. Inflammation may spread proximally to affect the left colon, and in about one-third of patients the entire colon becomes involved (pancolitis). A few centimeters of distal ileum are ulcerated in 10% of patients with pancolitis (backwash ileitis). The diseased areas are contiguous, ie, segmental disease or skip lesions are rare.

Clinical Findings

A. SYMPTOMS AND SIGNS

The cardinal symptoms are rectal bleeding and diarrhea: frequent discharges of watery stool mixed with blood, pus, and mucus accompanied by tenesmus, rectal urgency, and even anal incontinence. Nearly two-thirds of patients have cramping abdominal pain and variable degrees of fever, vomiting, weight loss, and dehydration. The onset may be insidious or acute and fulminating, and the clinical findings differ accordingly. Mild disease may be manifested only by loose or frequent stools, and, paradoxically, a few patients complain of constipation. In isolated instances, the only symptoms may be from systemic complications such as arthropathy or pyoderma. Dairy products may aggravate diarrhea.

If the disease is mild, physical examination may be normal, but in severe disease the abdomen is tender, especially in the left lower quadrant, and the colon may be distended. The anus is often fissured, tender, and spastic, and the rectal mucosa feels gritty. The gloved examining finger may be covered with blood, mucus, or pus.

Sigmoidoscopy is essential. An enema should not be given before the examination. The rectal mucosa is granular, dull, hyperemic, and friable, so that blood oozes where the mucosa is touched. The submucosal vascular pattern is lost because of edema. Gross ulcers are not visible in the rectum in ulcerative colitis because of the superficial nature of these lesions. In more advanced disease, the mucosa is purplish-red, velvety, and extremely friable. Blood mixed with mucopus is evident in the lumen. The disease is uniform in the affected bowel, and patches of normal mucosa are not seen. If the mucosa is not grossly diseased, biopsy may be helpful to confirm the diagnosis. In the recovery phase, mucosal hyperemia and edema subside and inflammatory polyps may be seen. The healing mucosa is typically dull and granular and has a neovascular pattern of telangiectatic vessels that differs from the normal pink mucosa.

B. LABORATORY FINDINGS

Anemia, leukocytosis, and an elevated sedimentation rate are usually present. Severe disease leads to hypoalbuminemia; depletion of water, electrolytes, and vitamins; and laboratory evidence of steatorrhea. Reduced plasma antithrombin III levels may contribute to thromboembolic complications. Smears of the stool should be examined for parasites, bacteria, and leukocytes, and stool should be sent for cultures.

C. IMAGING STUDIES

Barium enema examination should not be preceded by catharsis in acute cases and should not be performed at all in severely ill patients, because it may precipitate acute colonic dilation. Plain films of the abdomen should be obtained serially during fulminant attacks in order to detect colonic dilation (megacolon) if it occurs.

Barium x-rays in acute ulcerative colitis show mucosal irregularity that varies from fine serrations to rough, ragged, undermined ulcers. As the disease progresses, haustrations are gradually effaced, and the colon narrows and shortens because of muscular rigidity (Figure 31–16). Pseudopolyposis signifies severe ulceration. Widening of the space between the sacrum and rectum is due either to periproctitis or to shortening of the bowel. The presence of a stricture should always arouse suspicion of cancer, though most strictures are benign. CT and MRI can be helpful in puzzling cases.

The indium 111-labeled leukocyte scan is useful if the presence of inflammation in the colon is in question.

D. COLONOSCOPIC FINDINGS

Colonoscopy should be performed if sigmoidoscopic and radiographic findings are not diagnostic, and in fact endoscopy substitutes for barium enema in most situations. Usually the instrument need be inserted only into the sigmoid in order to make the initial diagnosis. Because of the danger of perforation, colonoscopy should be performed with great care if the disease is active, and it should not be done in the presence of colonic dilation. In chronic disease, colonoscopy with biopsies is valuable in surveillance for cancer. Strictures

Figure 31–16. Ulcerative colitis. Barium enema x-ray of colon. Note shortening of colon, loss of haustral markings ("lead pipe" appearance), and fine serrations at the edges of the bowel wall that represent multiple small ulcers.

and other x-ray abnormalities can be investigated by colonoscopy also.

Differential Diagnosis

Malignant neoplasms of the colon (including lymphomas) and diverticular disease must be considered in the differential diagnosis. Salmonellosis and other bacillary dysenteries are diagnosed by repeated stool cultures. Shigellosis may be suspected on the basis of a positive methylene blue stain for fecal leukocytes. *Campylobacter jejuni* is a common cause of bloody diarrhea; the organisms can be cultured from the stool, and serum antibody titers rise during the illness. Hemorrhagic colitis—a syndrome of bloody diarrhea and abdominal cramps but no fever—is associated with infection by *Escherichia coli* O157:H7. Legionella infections can mimic ulcerative colitis. Gonococcal proctitis is detected by culture of rectal swabs. Herpes simplex virus is the most common cause of nongonococcal proctitis in homosexual men. *Chlamydia trachomatis* infections are also common in this group; the mucosa is markedly inflamed and resembles Crohn's disease; the organism can be cultured. It is most important in every case to rule out amebiasis (see Chapter 9) by microscopic examination of stool, rectal swabs, or rectal biopsies; serologic tests confirm that clinical infection has occurred. Corticosteroids must never be given to a patient with presumed idiopathic ulcerative colitis until amebiasis has been excluded.

Rare cases of histoplasmosis, tuberculosis, cytomegalovirus disease, schistosomiasis, amyloidosis, or Behçet's disease may be very difficult to diagnose. AIDS-related gastrointestinal infections are increasingly common. Colitis caused by antibiotics is discussed separately below; the history is important in this type of disease. NSAIDs can cause mucosal inflammation and even strictures in the large intestine. Collagenous colitis may or may not be related to NSAID usage. Watery diarrhea is the main symptom of this syndrome; endoscopy is grossly normal; and biopsies show a thickened band of collagen just beneath the surface. Treatment to date has been difficult, but most patients are not seriously troubled by this condition. Ischemic colitis has a segmental pattern of involvement quite unlike the usual distribution of ulcerative colitis. Functional diarrhea can mimic colitis, but organic disease must be excluded before it can be concluded that the diarrhea is functional. Malacoplakia is a rare chronic granulomatous disease that can cause colonic strictures and may resemble colitis.

Diversion colitis is inflammation of a previously normal segment of colon or rectum following construction of a temporary colostomy, eg, in a two-stage approach to diverticulitis. Deficiency of mucosal nutrients may be responsible, and inflammation may resolve with topical application of short-chain fatty acids. Restoration of intestinal continuity also solves the problem.

The most difficult differential diagnosis is between mucosal ulcerative colitis and Crohn's colitis (Table 31–8). None of the features are specific for one or the other disease, and often the differentiation can be made only after all the data have been assembled. About 10% of cases cannot be classified (indeterminate colitis).

Complications

The following **extracolonic manifestations** may occur in association with ulcerative colitis. There is an inexact relationship between the severity of the colitis and these complications: (1) lesions of the skin and mucous membranes, eg, erythema nodosum, erythema multiforme, pyoderma gangrenosum, pustular dermatitis, and aphthous stomatitis; (2) uveitis; (3) bone and joint lesions, eg, arthralgia, arthritis, and ankylosing spondylitis; (4) hepatobiliary and possibly pancreatic lesions, eg, fatty infiltration, pericholangitis, cirrhosis, sclerosing cholangitis, bile duct carcinoma, gallstones, and pancreatic insufficiency; (5) anemia, usually due to

iron deficiency; (6) malnutrition and growth retardation; and (7) pericarditis. Sclerosing cholangitis may require liver transplantation.

Anorectal complications occur in 15–20% of patients with ulcerative colitis, a smaller percentage than in Crohn's colitis. Anal fissures are most common (about 12% of patients), and anorectal abscesses and fistulas are seen in 5% of patients.

Perforation of the colon, which occurs in about 3% of hospitalized patients, is responsible for more deaths than any other complication of ulcerative colitis. The risk of perforation is highest in the initial attack of the disease and correlates well with its extent and severity. It occurs most commonly in the sigmoid or splenic flexure and may result in a localized abscess or generalized fecal peritonitis. Any severely diseased colon may perforate, but patients with toxic dilation (megacolon) are especially vulnerable. Systemic therapy (corticosteroids and antibiotics) may mask the development of this complication.

Acute colonic dilation (toxic megacolon) occurs in approximately 3–10% of patients and in about 9% of patients coming to emergency operation. The patients are severely ill (toxic) and usually have one or more of the following contributing factors: inflammation involving the muscular coats, hypokalemia, opioid use, anticholinergic use, or barium enema examination. Toxic megacolon is diagnosed by plain abdominal x-rays or barium enemas, which show a thickened bowel wall and dilated lumen (> 6 cm in the transverse colon); often, the luminal air outlines irregular nodular pseudopolyps (Figure 31–17). Placing the patient in the knee-elbow position and use of a rectal tube are recommended medical measures to help the colon decompress. Toxic dilation also occurs in Crohn's disease and in other types of colitis such as amebiasis and salmonellosis.

Massive hemorrhage is an uncommon but life-threatening complication.

Strictures develop in 10% of patients with ulcerative colitis. They are more common in chronic disease, though they also appear in acute cases. Benign strictures are caused by thickening of the muscular coats, fibrosis, clusters of inflammatory polyps, or a combination of these processes. Carcinoma is of greatest concern.

Carcinoma of the colon or rectum begins to appear 5–8 years after onset of ulcerative colitis. By 10 years after onset, about 5% of patients have developed colorectal cancer; the cumulative incidence is 20–25% after 20 years and 30–40% by 30 years. Most of the factors previously thought to identify patients at greatest risk of cancer are unreliable (eg, age at onset, severity of first attack, and degree of activity of disease). The extent of colitis has limited usefulness as a predictor; although cancer develops earlier in the course of disease in pancolitis, left-sided colitis eventually gives rise to

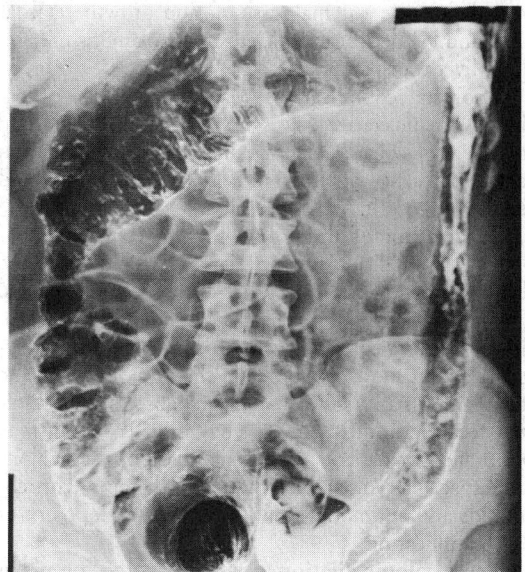

Figure 31–17. Barium enema showing acute colonic dilation in ulcerative colitis. Note dilation of the transverse colon, the multiple irregular densities in the lumen that represent pseudopolyps, and the loss of haustral markings.

carcinoma at about the same rate. Sclerosing cholangitis correlates with colorectal cancer in ulcerative colitis. Cancers in colitis tend to be multicentric, less well differentiated, and perhaps more often right-sided. Some of them are difficult to recognize grossly by endoscopy or x-ray because they are small and flat. Periodic surveillance colonoscopy and multiple biopsies are recommended to search for epithelial dysplasia. It is now believed that even low-grade dysplasia is ominous and is an indication for prophylactic colectomy. In the presence of high-grade dysplasia, the chances of finding cancer in the colon are 30–50%, and some of the cancers are advanced. There is an intensive search for a more sensitive marker, and one or more of the molecular markers may fill the need eventually. Meanwhile, the risks and benefits of colectomy should be weighed against those of repeated colonoscopy in patients with a long history of ulcerative colitis; with the availability of ileoanal anastomosis, colectomy is more appealing to physicians and their patients than in the past.

Treatment

A. CONSERVATIVE MEASURES

The goals of conservative therapy are to terminate the acute attack as rapidly as possible and to prevent re-

lapse. Management depends on the severity of the attack and the age group; children and the elderly present special problems.

1. Mild attack—Mild or insidious disease limited to the rectum and sigmoid usually can be checked with outpatient management. Reduced physical activity—even bed rest—is advisable. Diet should be free of bovine milk products and any other food that exacerbates diarrhea in the individual patient. Sulfasalazine, 2–8 g/d orally, is effective in controlling acute attacks. Patients who are allergic to sulfonamide drugs can obtain similar benefit with oral mesalamine, 2–5 g/d. Distal colitis can be treated with topical mesalamine or steroids. These agents can be delivered by suppository or foam if disease involves only 15–20 cm of distal bowel, and enemas can be used if colitis extends proximally for up to 60 cm; there are several choices of preparations. If these measures fail to relieve symptoms promptly, therapy should be intensified.

2. Severe attack—Severe or fulminating ulcerative colitis requires hospitalization. Nasogastric suction is required in patients with colonic dilation or those at risk of developing this complication. Otherwise, "bowel rest" has no special benefit, and when the danger of dilation has passed, polymeric total enteral nutrition is just as safe and effective as total parenteral nutrition in patients with acute severe ulcerative colitis.

Corticosteroids are given intravenously initially as hydrocortisone (100–300 mg/d) or prednisolone (20–80 mg/d). Broad-spectrum antibiotics (metronidazole and gentamicin or a cephalosporin) are often given to severely ill patients, though the benefit of antibiotics has not been proved. Cyclosporine (4 mg/kg/d intravenously) is effective for severe colitis refractory to steroid therapy. Toxicity is severe, however, and the long-term benefit of cyclosporine treatment is unknown. Hypokalemia is common and should be corrected. Caution should be exercised in administering anticholinergics and opioids because they may precipitate acute dilation of the colon.

3. Maintenance—Nightly mesalamine suppositories or oral mesalamine serves as maintenance therapy for patients with distal colitis. Oral mesalamine or 5-aminosalicylic acid reduces relapse rates of patients with more extensive colitis. Chronic steroid use should be avoided because of the systemic side effects even if the drug is administered topically. Immunosuppressive therapy (mercaptopurine, azathioprine) is used by some physicians to treat ulcerative colitis in patients who cannot tolerate discontinuation of corticosteroid therapy. Transdermal nicotine reportedly has a therapeutic effect on ulcerative colitis, but clinicians are understandably reluctant to use this agent until more is learned about long-term safety and efficacy.

B. Surgical Treatment

1. Indications—

a. Acute disease—Emergency operation is indicated for proved or suspected perforation of the colon. Operation on an urgent basis is required for an acute problem (toxic megacolon, hemorrhage, or fulminating colitis) treated medically at first and then surgically if the response is inadequate. There are no firm guidelines for when to switch from medical to surgical therapy in these cases. If toxic megacolon does not respond to treatment within a few hours, operation is necessary to avoid perforation. Fulminating disease without megacolon should improve in 4–5 days or less; otherwise, operation may be advisable. Prolonged medical treatment may result in the need for a staged surgical approach, whereas earlier intervention may require only one operation.

b. Chronic disease—Intractable disease is difficult to define. Frequent exacerbations, chronic continuous symptoms, malnutrition, weakness, inability to work, incapacity to enjoy a full social and sexual life—all are elements of intractable disease. Exacerbation of disease when corticosteroids are tapered—and thus inability to discontinue these drugs over months or even years—is a compelling indication for colectomy. Children with chronic colitis may have impaired growth and development. Prevention or treatment of carcinoma is an important indication for operation. Severe extracolonic manifestations such as arthritis, pyoderma gangrenosum, or hepatobiliary disease may respond to colectomy, but other problems (eg, ankylosing spondylitis) do not improve after the diseased colon is removed.

2. Surgical procedures—

Total colectomy with ileoanal anastomosis (restorative proctocolectomy, ileal pouch–anal anastomosis) is the elective operation of choice in most patients. Obesity and advanced age are limiting factors. In this procedure, the entire colon and rectum are excised, and the ileum (made into a reservoir or pouch) is brought into the pelvis and anastomosed to the anal canal just above the dentate line (Figure 31–18). Rectal mucosectomy was once routine, but many surgeons now do not strip the mucosa at all in patients with colitis; instead, the full thickness of rectum is excised to eliminate disease while preserving good rectal function. A temporary ileostomy to protect the ileoanal anastomosis for 2–3 months is no longer mandatory, but it is used if there is concern about the quality of the anastomosis or the patient's healing properties. Success is expected in 95% of patients. Pouchitis (inflammation of the reservoir, presumably from bacte-

Figure 31–18. Lateral view of the pelvis after colectomy and ileoanal anastomosis in a male. The S pouch, shown here, is one of several types of reservoirs; the J pouch and the W pouch have come to be favored by most surgeons in recent years. The pouch is anastomosed to the anal canal just above the dentate line. The distal anorectal stump as depicted is longer than is usually the practice today.

rial overgrowth) occurs in up to 40% of patients; it usually responds to antibiotics such as metronidazole.

Proctocolectomy with permanent conventional ileostomy or continent ileostomy is chosen in patients who may not be candidates for the ileoanal procedure. In an emergency operation, the rectum is preserved to minimize operative complications in an ill patient and to make it possible to do an ileoanal procedure later. This staged operation therefore consists of total abdominal colectomy (subtotal colectomy) and ileostomy with a distal mucous fistula or Hartmann procedure. Ileorectal anastomosis (ileoproctostomy, ileorectostomy) is seldom used for ulcerative colitis today.

Prognosis

The mortality rate of ulcerative colitis has dropped sharply in the last 2 decades. First attacks are seldom fatal when treated by specialists. In one large series, emergency colectomy was required in 25% of patients with severe first attacks; 60% responded rapidly to medical therapy; and 15% improved slowly on medications alone. Overall, the colitis-related mortality rate during the year after onset is about 1%. Emergency colectomy has a mortality rate of 6%; most of these deaths are due to perforation, a complication that has a fatal outcome in 40% of cases.

The long-term prognosis of ulcerative proctitis is good; about 10% of patients will develop colonic disease by 10 years, and the mortality rate is very low. If colitis involves the left colon, the prognosis is worse, and in patients with pancolitis, the likelihood of operation during the first year is about 25% and the mortality rate is 5% over 10 years. Colorectal cancer in ulcerative colitis is more often diagnosed at an advanced stage than is sporadic cancer, but the prognosis stage-for-stage is the same. Screening with colonoscopy and biopsies seems to have reduced the cancer mortality rate, but there are still too many patients who escape detection until the malignancy has progressed to incurability. The problem is lack of a sensitive marker that predicts cancer before it develops.

The operative mortality rate is less than 1% for elective colectomy. Quality of life after restorative proctocolectomy with an ileal pouch is excellent. Most patients who undergo the procedure are pleased with the outcome compared with their preoperative symptoms and treatment. In an estimated 90% of survivors, colectomy with ileostomy is consistent with normal life, but a few patients experience problems such as small bowel obstruction and ileostomy dysfunction. Altered sexual function after proctectomy occurs in about 12% of men overall, limited mostly to those over age 50. True impotence is found in 3% of men. Sexual dysfunction is common in the first few months in women.

Andersson RE et al: Appendectomy and protection against ulcerative colitis. N Engl J Med 2001;344:808.

Bernstein CN et al: Cancer risk in patients with inflammatory bowel disease: a population-based study. Cancer 2001; 91:854.

Bernstein CN et al: The prevalence of extraintestinal diseases in inflammatory bowel disease: a population-based study. Am J Gastroenterol 2001;96:1116.

Blumberg D et al: Restorative proctocolectomy: Ochsner Clinic experience. South Med J 2001;94:467.

D'Haens G et al: Intravenous cyclosporine versus intravenous corticosteroids as single therapy for severe attacks of ulcerative colitis. Gastroenterology 2001;120:1323.

Eaden JA, Abrams KR, Mayberry JF: The risk of colorectal cancer in ulcerative colitis: a meta-analysis. Gut 2001;48:526.

Farmer M et al: Association of susceptibility locus for inflammatory bowel disease on chromosome 16 with both ulcerative colitis and Crohn's disease. Dig Dis Sci 2001;46:632.

Goudet P et al: Characteristics and evolution of extraintestinal manifestations associated with ulcerative colitis after proctocolectomy. Dig Surg 2001;18:51.

Hanauer SB: Inflammatory bowel disease. N Engl J Med 1996; 334:841.

Lawrance IC, Fiocchi C, Chakravarti S: Ulcerative colitis and Crohn's disease: distinctive gene expression profiles and novel susceptibility candidate genes. Hum Mol Genet 2001; 10:445.

McIntyre PB et al: Comparing functional results one year and ten years after ileal pouch-anal anastomosis for chronic ulcerative colitis. Dis Colon Rectum 1994;37:303.

Melville DM et al: Surgery for ulcerative colitis in the era of the pouch: The St Mark's Hospital experience. Gut 1994; 35:1076.

Robinson M: Medical therapy of inflammatory bowel disease for the 21st century. Eur J Surg Suppl 1998;582:90.

Shelton AA et al: Retrospective review of colorectal cancer in ulcerative colitis at a tertiary center. Arch Surg 1996;131:806.

Thomas GA et al: Transdermal nicotine as maintenance therapy for ulcerative colitis. N Engl J Med 1995;332:988.

2. Crohn's Colitis (Granulomatous Colitis)

The general features of Crohn's disease (regional enteritis, granulomatous colitis, transmural colitis) are described in Chapter 30. Approximately 50% of patients with Crohn's disease have both small and large bowel involvement; 25% have colonic disease alone; and another 3% have anorectal involvement only. Diarrhea, cramping abdominal pain, constitutional effects, and extraintestinal manifestations are approximately the same in colonic and enteric disease. Internal fistulas and abscesses and intestinal obstruction are usually complications of small bowel disease. Anorectal complications (anal fistula, fissure, abscess, and rectal stricture) and hemorrhage are more common when the large bowel is affected, and toxic dilation is limited to patients with inflammation of the colon.

Typical anal lesions of Crohn's disease are large undermined indolent ulcers. The perianal skin has a violaceous hue, and if fistulas are present, they tend to be multiple and complex. Proctosigmoidoscopy discloses a normal rectum in 50% of patients with Crohn's colitis. Diseased mucosa is patchily involved, with irregular ulcerations separated by edematous or even normal-appearing mucosa. Biopsy may confirm the diagnosis. Radiographic features include sparing of the rectum, right colonic and ileal involvement, skip areas, transverse fissures, longitudinal ulcers, strictures, and fistulas. Features differentiating Crohn's disease from ulcerative colitis are summarized in Table 31–8. Ischemic

Table 31–8. Comparison of various features of ulcerative colitis with those of granulomatous colitis.

	Ulcerative (Mucosal) Colitis	Crohn's (Granulomatous) Colitis
Signs and symptoms		
Diarrhea	Marked.	Present; less severe.
Gross bleeding	Characteristic.	Infrequent.
Perianal lesions	Infrequent, mild.	Frequent, complex; may precede diagnosis of intestinal disease.
Toxic dilatation	Yes (3–10%).	Yes (2–5%).
Perforation	Free.	Localized.
Systemic manifestations (arthritis, uveitis, pyoderma, hepatitis	Common.	Common.
X-ray studies	Confluent, diffuse. Tiny serrations, coarse mucosa, mucosal tags. Concentric involvement. Internal fistulas very rare. Colon only except in backwash ileitis; may be limited to left side.	Skip areas. Longitudinal ulcers, transverse ridges, "cobblestone" appearance. Eccentric involvement. Internal fistula common. Any portion of intestinal tract may be involved; may be limited to ileum and right colon.
Morphology		
Gross	Confluent involvement. Rectum usually involved. Mesocolon not involved; nodes enlarged. Widespread ragged superficial ulceration. Inflammatory polyps (pseudopolyps) common. No thickening of bowel wall.	Segmental involvement with or without skip areas. Rectum often not involved. Thickened mesocolon; pronounced lymph node enlargement. Large longitudinal ulcers or transverse fissures. Inflammatory polyps not prominent. Thickened bowel wall.
Microscopic	Inflammatory reaction usually limited to mucosa and submucosa; only in severe disease are muscle coats involved; no fibrosis. Granulomas rare.	Chronic inflammation of all layers of bowel wall; damage to muscle layers usual; submucosal fibrosis. Granulomas frequent.
Natural history	Exacerbations, remissions; may be explosive, lethal.	Indolent, recurrent.
Treatment		
Response to medical treatment	Good response in 85% of cases.	Difficult to evaluate; less well controlled over long term.
Type of surgical treatment and response	Colectomy with ileoanal anastomosis; proctocolectomy with conventional or continent ileostomy. No recurrence.	Segmental colectomy; total colectomy with ileorectal anastomosis; proctocolectomy if rectum severely diseased. Recurrence common.

colitis is another disease that may be confused with Crohn's colitis, and the differential diagnosis is discussed below. *Chlamydia trachomatis* infection is diagnosed by culture of the organism. Malacoplakia is a rare chronic granulomatous disease that can cause colonic strictures, and Behçet's disease is another rare condition that can mimic inflammatory bowel disease. Tuberculosis and amebiasis must be considered also.

Frank blood in the stools is observed in about one-third of patients with granulomatous colitis, but massive hemorrhage is unusual. Acute colonic dilation (toxic megacolon) occurs in 5%; it responds to nonoperative treatment more often than it does in ulcerative colitis.

Actuarial methods suggest that the risk of colonic cancer in granulomatous colitis patients is four to twenty times that of the general population, and it appears that segments of intestine excluded from the fecal stream (eg, an isolated rectal stump or bypassed ileum) are especially vulnerable. Carcinoma can also arise in anorectal or rectovaginal fistulas. The small bowel is at risk for development of cancer in patients with regional enteritis with or without colitis. Epithelial dysplasia is associated with cancer in Crohn's disease as well as in ulcerative colitis, but this indicator is not helpful for the areas at greatest risk (eg, bypassed segments of small bowel or colon) because they cannot be examined endoscopically. Surveillance colonoscopy may be worthwhile in colonic Crohn's disease, though it has not been routine in the past.

Medical management of Crohn's disease of the small bowel is described in Chapter 30. Steroids are effective for acute attacks, but they are not advisable for maintenance therapy because of limited benefit and frequent complications. Oral 5-aminosalicylates (sulfasalazine, 4 g/d; or mesalamine, 2–5 g/d) are effective treatment for Crohn's colitis. Topical 5-aminosalicylates are beneficial for disease of the rectum and sigmoid. These agents are steroid-sparing, ie, they allow the dosage of steroids to be reduced. Metronidazole, 10–20 mg/kg/d orally in three to five doses, is used for treatment of anal complications of Crohn's disease. Abscesses and fistulas improve with less pain and drainage, but full permanent healing is unusual, and the disease worsens when the drug is discontinued. Immunosuppressants (azathioprine, mercaptopurine) are steroid-sparing drugs that seem to control Crohn's colitis well enough that surgery is delayed or avoided. There are mixed reports of effectiveness of cyclosporine in refractory Crohn's disease.

Surgical treatment is indicated for intractability, abscess or fistula, obstruction, fulminant disease, anorectal disease, hemorrhage, or cancer. Segmental colectomy with primary anastomosis is useful for limited colonic disease. Total colectomy with ileorectal anastomosis is done more frequently in Crohn's colitis than in ulcerative colitis. Proctocolectomy with ileostomy is needed if rectal disease is severe and the colon needs resection also. Diverting ileostomy or colostomy is only temporarily helpful. Perianal complications can be treated directly (eg, by fistulotomy) in carefully selected patients.

There is a high rate of recurrence at intestinal anastomoses (50–75% at 15 years). Recurrence is less common following proctocolectomy and ileostomy (about 15% at 15 years, but there is a wide disparity (3–46%) among different reports on this controversial topic). Cigarette smoking is an independent risk factor for recurrence of Crohn's disease after resection.

Surgical procedures—like medical therapy—should be regarded as palliative, not curative, in patients with Crohn's disease. Although recurrence rates are high and chronic disease is common, a productive life is usually possible with the aid of combined medical and surgical management. The mortality rate is about 15% over 30 years. Urolithiasis is a common sequela of resection for Crohn's disease.

Cellier C et al: Correlations between clinical activity, endoscopic severity, and biological parameters in colonic or ileocolonic Crohn's disease. A prospective multicentre study of 121 cases. Gut 1994;35:231.

Elton E, Hanauer SB: Review article: the medical management of Crohn's disease. Aliment Pharmacol Ther 1996;10:1.

Feagan BG et al: Low-dose cyclosporine for the treatment of Crohn's disease. N Engl J Med 1994;330:1846.

Feagan BG et al: Methotrexate for the treatment of Crohn's disease. The North American Crohn's Study Group Investigators. N Engl J Med 1995;332:292.

Guy TS, Williams NN, Rosato EF: Crohn's disease of the colon. Surg Clin North Am 2001;81:159.

McClane SJ, Rombeau JL. Anorectal Crohn's disease. Surg Clin North Am 2001;81:169.

Nwokolo CU et al: Surgical resections in parous patients with distal ileal and colonic Crohn's disease. Gut 1994;35:220.

Present DH et al: Infliximab for the treatment of fistulas in patients with Crohn's disease. N Engl J Med 1999;340:1398.

Rutgeerts P: Management of perianal Crohn's disease. Can J Gastroenterol 2000;14 Suppl C:7C.

Scott NA, Hughes LE: Timing of ileocolonic resection for symptomatic Crohn's disease: the patient's view. Gut 1994;35:656.

Slonim AE et al: A preliminary study of growth hormone therapy for Crohn's disease. N Engl J Med 2000;342:1633.

Thirlby RC, Sobrino MA, Randall JB: The long-term benefit of surgery on health-related quality of life in patients with inflammatory bowel disease. Arch Surg 2001;136:521.

3. Antibiotic-Associated Colitis

A spectrum of adverse colonic responses may develop in hospitalized patients during or after antibiotic therapy. There may be diarrhea without gross mucosal abnormality (antibiotic-associated diarrhea), gross inflammation of the mucosa, or whitish-green or yellow plaques on the inflamed mucosa (pseudomembranous colitis). It is not clear whether one or several pathologic processes are responsible. Patients may progress from mild to more severe disease. The differential diagnosis among these variations is based on endoscopic findings and the clinical picture.

Clostridium difficile is a resident of the gut in 3% of people in the general population and in about 10% of patients admitted to hospital. It is the major known cause of nosocomial antibiotic-associated diarrhea and colitis. Certain antibiotics allow the organism to proliferate, and it is then transmitted among patients and hospital personnel. Epidemics of *C difficile* infection have been noted on surgical wards. The organism can be transmitted by people caring for the patient, and gloving or hand-washing is essential. Infection with *C difficile* can be very severe in patients with AIDS.

C difficile may colonize the upper gastrointestinal tract as well as the colon, but the symptomatic infection appears at present to be colonic alone. The organism elaborates at least four toxins, including toxin A (an enterotoxin) and toxin B (a cytotoxin). Together these substances—and perhaps others—produce the symptoms and signs. Clindamycin causes watery diarrhea in 15–30% of patients and true pseudomembranous colitis in 1–10%. Lincomycin, ampicillin, cephalosporins, and penicillin are also common inciting antibiotics. Many others have been implicated, including metronidazole. Parenteral aminoglycosides seem to be an exception. Colitis may develop as early as 2 days after beginning antibiotics or as late as 3 weeks after they are discontinued.

Symptoms and signs include diarrhea (usually watery, occasionally bloody), abdominal cramps, vomiting, fever, and leukocytosis. Sigmoidoscopy in pseudomembranous colitis shows elevated plaques or a confluent pseudomembrane, and the mucosa is erythematous and edematous. Biopsies reveal acute inflammation; the pseudomembrane is made up of leukocytes, necrotic epithelial cells, and fibrin. The rectum is spared in about one-fourth of cases, and colonoscopy may be necessary to detect the presence of pseudomembranous colitis. Demonstration of *C difficile* cytotoxin in stool is sensitive and specific. Stool culture is less efficient since some strains of *C difficile* are nontoxicogenic.

Management consists first of discontinuing the inciting antibiotic agent. In most patients, the colitis resolves in 1–2 weeks after the offending agent is withdrawn, but severe symptoms or persistent diarrhea calls for additional treatment. Vancomycin (125–500 mg orally four times daily for 7–10 days) is expensive but effective—though the relapse rate is 15–20% after vancomycin is discontinued. Metronidazole, 1.5–2 g/d

orally for 7–14 days, is also effective and much less expensive. Paradoxically, however, metronidazole can also cause antibiotic-associated colitis. Bacitracin is an effective drug and, like vancomycin, is not absorbed from the gastrointestinal tract. Antidiarrheal drugs may prolong symptoms and should be avoided. Oral administration of *Saccharomyces boulardii,* a nonpathogenic yeast, has been successful in treatment of recurrent *C difficile* colitis in an experimental setting.

The outcome of pseudomembranous colitis and the other forms of antibiotic-associated colonic disease is usually excellent if the disease is recognized and treated. Untreated pseudomembranous colitis, however, may lead to severe dehydration and electrolyte imbalance, toxic megacolon, or colonic perforation. Operation is required for perforation or toxic dilation. Chronic relapsing *C difficile* diarrhea has been treated by rectal instillation of mixed colonic bacteria (bacteriotherapy).

Cappell MS, Philogene C: *Clostridium difficile* infection is a treatable cause of diarrhea in patients with advanced human immunodeficiency virus infection: a study of seven consecutive patients admitted from 1986 to 1992 to a university teaching hospital. Am J Gastroenterol 1993;88:891.

Cozart JC et al: *Clostridium difficile* diarrhea in patients with AIDS versus non-AIDS controls: methods of treatment and clinical response to treatment. J Clin Gastroenterol 1993;16:192.

Fekety R, Shah AB: Diagnosis and treatment of *Clostridium difficile* colitis. JAMA 1993;269:71.

Herman BE et al: Antibiotic-associated fulminant pseudomembranous colitis without toxic megacolon. Am J Gastroenterol 1992;87:1816.

Kelly CP, Pothoulakis C, LaMont JT: *Clostridium difficile* colitis. N Engl J Med 1994;330:257.

Marts BC et al: Patterns and prognosis of *Clostridium difficile* colitis. Dis Colon Rectum 1994;37:837.

McFarland LV et al: A randomized placebo-controlled trial of *Saccharomyces boulardii* in combination with standard antibiotics for *Clostridium difficile* disease. JAMA 1994;271:1913.

Medich DS et al: Laparotomy for fulminant pseudomembranous colitis. Arch Surg 1992;127:847.

Qamar A et al: *Saccharomyces boulardii* stimulates intestinal immunoglobulin A immune response to *Clostridium difficile* toxin A in mice. Infect Immun 2001;69:2762.

4. Ischemic Colitis

Ischemic colitis is caused by mesenteric vascular occlusion or nonocclusive mechanisms. A common precipitating event is abdominal aortic reconstruction with interruption of a vital blood supply such as the inferior mesenteric artery. An entity that resembles ischemic colitis sometimes develops proximal to obstructing colonic carcinoma. Isolated ischemia of the right colon is seen in patients with chronic heart disease, especially aortic stenosis. Ischemic colitis most often afflicts the elderly (average age 60 years), but it also occurs in younger adults in association with diabetes mellitus, systemic lupus erythematosus, or sickle cell crisis. Pancreatitis can occlude mesocolic vessels.

Ischemic colitis is categorized as reversible or irreversible. Reversible ischemia heals with nonoperative treatment, sometimes with stricture formation. Over half of the patients have a reversible injury. The severe form is fulminant from onset or may pursue an indolent course without resolution for weeks. Both of the severe forms require operation.

Patients with ischemic colitis have an abrupt onset of abdominal pain, diarrhea (commonly bloody), and systemic symptoms. The abdomen may be tender diffusely, in a localized area (eg, left lower quadrant), or not at all. Blood is seen coming from above at sigmoidoscopy; if the rectum itself is ischemic—an unusual occurrence—the mucosa is edematous, hemorrhagic, friable, and sometimes ulcerated. A grayish membrane may be present, resembling pseudomembranous colitis. The same abnormalities are seen in the ischemic segment examined with the flexible sigmoidoscope or colonoscope. Serum alkaline phosphatase is elevated in some cases. Plain abdominal x-rays are nonspecific. Barium enema x-rays show "thumbprints" or pseudotumors, typically limited to a 6- to 20-cm segment; 75% or more have involvement of the left colon. CT scan shows a thickened colonic wall and helps to exclude other conditions. Mesenteric arteriography may show major arterial occlusion or no abnormalities and is not usually recommended.

Differentiating ischemic colitis from carcinoma, ulcerative colitis, and diverticulitis should not be difficult, but Crohn's disease presents a greater diagnostic problem. Rectal bleeding—especially gross hemorrhage—is less common in Crohn's disease, and the rapid onset of ischemic colitis is also different from Crohn's disease. Radiographic findings and, in some cases, the colonoscopic appearance may be helpful, but the natural history of the acute attack is often the only way to make the distinction. Acute mesenteric ischemia may be difficult to exclude (see Chapter 30), but the more benign presentations of reversible ischemic colonic injury are not seen with ischemia of the small intestine. *C difficile* toxin is present in stool in pseudomembranous colitis.

Therapy for reversible ischemic colitis consists of intravenous fluids, antibiotics, and observation to be certain the problem is in fact reversible. Irreversible disease, whether fulminant from the beginning, becoming more severe over several days, or just failing to resolve after treatment, should be treated by operation. The diseased colon is resected; anastomosis is usually deferred if the colon is unprepared. Because patients with severe ischemia often have multiple other medical problems, the overall mortality rate is 50%.

Balthazar EJ, Yen BC, Gordon RB. Ischemic colitis: CT evaluation of 54 cases. Radiology 1999;211:381.

Houe T et al: Can colonoscopy diagnose transmural ischaemic colitis after abdominal aortic surgery? An evidence-based approach. Eur J Vasc Endovasc Surg 2000;19:304.

Hwang RF, Schwartz RW: Ischemic colitis: a brief review. Curr Surg 2001;58:192.

Hyun H, Pai E, Blend MJ: Ischemic colitis: Tc-99m HMPAO leukocyte scintigraphy and correlative imaging. Clin Nucl Med 1998;23:165.

Valentine RJ et al: Gastrointestinal complications after aortic surgery. J Vasc Surg 1998;28:404.

5. Neutropenic Colitis

Neutropenic colitis (neutropenic enterocolitis, neutropenic typhlitis, ileocecal syndrome, necrotizing enteropathy, agranulocytic colitis) occurs as colonic necrosis in neutropenic patients. Although the cecum and right colon are most often affected, all parts of the small or large bowel can be involved. Acute leukemia, aplastic anemia, and cyclic neutropenia are the underlying diseases in which this lesion occurs. Colonic perforation during treatment with interleukin-2 is probably related. The pathogenesis is not well understood, but responsible factors probably include mucosal ischemia, necrosis of intramural leukemic infiltrates, shock, hemorrhage into the bowel wall, chemotherapy, and corticosteroid therapy. *Clostridium septicum* has been implicated in some cases. The mucosa ulcerates, permitting bacterial invasion into the bowel wall, thrombosis of intramural vessels, necrosis, and perforation.

As many as 25% of patients with acute myeloblastic leukemia may develop typhlitis, and during induction chemotherapy the incidence may be much higher. Fever, watery or bloody diarrhea, abdominal discomfort and distention, and nausea are noted first. Pain and tenderness may then become localized to the right lower quadrant, and systemic toxicity increases. Careful examination and x-ray studies are required. Nasogastric suction, parenteral nutrition, and antibiotic therapy are instituted. Operation (resection of the involved segment of colon) is performed for persistent unresponsive sepsis, perforation, obstruction, severe bleeding, or abscess formation. Neutropenic colitis can recur after medical therapy.

Abbasoglu O, Cakmakci M: Neutropenic enterocolitis in patients without leukemia. Surgery 1993;113:113.

Gorbach SL: Neutropenic enterocolitis. Clin Infect Dis 1998;27:700.

Sayfan J et al: Acute abdomen caused by neutropenic enterocolitis: surgeon's dilemma. Eur J Surg 1999;165:502.

Song HK et al: Changing presentation and management of neutropenic enterocolitis. Arch Surg 1998;133:979.

■ INTESTINAL STOMAS (ILEOSTOMY & COLOSTOMY)

An intestinal stoma is an opening of the bowel onto the surface of the abdomen. It may be temporary or permanent. Esophagostomy, gastrostomy, jejunostomy, and cecostomy are usually temporary, but ileostomy, colostomy, and some urinary tract stomas are often permanent. Although "stoma" is the preferred medical term, "ostomy" is used by lay organizations devoted to the rehabilitation of these patients.

Few surgical alterations of anatomy are surrounded by as much misunderstanding as intestinal stomas, and few pronouncements by surgeons are as horrifying to patients as the indication that a stoma will be necessary. For these and other reasons, a paramedical profession, **enterostomy therapy,** has emerged. The enterostomal therapist (ET) is usually a registered nurse who has taken specialized training and is certified in the field. The enterostomal therapist provides the following services: (1) preoperative education and counseling of patient and family; (2) immediate postoperative care of the stoma; (3) training in the use of equipment and supervision of self-care; (4) fitting of a permanent appliance; (5) advice on day-to-day living with a stoma; (6) management of skin problems and odor control; (7) recognition of surgical stoma problems; (8) long-term emotional, moral, and physical support; and (9) information about the United Ostomy Association, an organization with chapters in many localities.

ILEOSTOMY

Permanent ileostomy is performed most commonly after proctocolectomy for ulcerative colitis; patients with Crohn's disease, familial polyposis, and other conditions may also require ileostomy. A temporary (loop) ileostomy often is used to divert the fecal stream for several weeks when ileoanal anastomosis is performed. An ileostomy discharges small quantities of liquid material continuously; it does not require irrigation; and an appliance must be worn at all times.

The optimal position of the stoma is in the right lower quadrant (Figure 31–19). The ileum is brought through the rectus abdominis muscle and everted upon itself, and the mucosa is sutured to the skin (surgically matured). An appliance is placed immediately; it consists of a plastic bag attached to a square sheet of protective material containing a central opening for the stoma. A reusable appliance can be fitted after a few weeks, but modern disposable appliances are so satisfac-

tory that most patients never do change to the other type. Appliances lie flat against the abdomen, adhere firmly to the skin, are inconspicuous and odor-proof, and in most cases need to be changed only every 3–5 days. They are drained at intervals during the day through an opening in the bottom of the pouch.

A **continent ileostomy** (reservoir ileostomy; Kock pouch) is designed to avoid the continual discharge of ileal effluent that necessitates construction of a protruding stoma and the wearing of an appliance at all times. A reservoir is constructed out of the distal ileum, and the outlet from the reservoir is arranged as a valve so that fluid cannot escape onto the abdominal wall. The reservoir is emptied several times a day by inserting a catheter into the stoma. Continent ileostomy is successful in 70–90% of patients. Problems with the valve, fistulas, and "pouchitis" (mucosal inflammation in the reservoir, presumably due to bacterial stasis) are causes of failure. Crohn's disease is a contraindication, because of the risk of recurrence necessitating excision of the reservoir.

Physiologic changes after ileostomy are due to the loss of the water- and salt-absorbing capacity of the colon. If the small bowel is free of disease and extensive resection has not been done, an ileostomy puts out 1–2 L of fluid per day initially (Table 31–1). The volume of effluent diminishes to between 500 and 800 mL/d after a month or two. This loss of fluid is obligatory and is not reduced by manipulations of diet. Obligatory sodium losses are about 50 meq/d greater than in patients with an intact colon, and potassium losses are also increased. Healthy ileostomy patients have low total exchangeable sodium and potassium but normal serum electrolyte concentrations. The depletion, therefore, is primarily intracellular. The patient with an ileostomy is susceptible to acute or subacute salt and water depletion manifested by fatigue, anorexia, irritability, headache, drowsiness, muscle cramps, and thirst. Gastroenteritis or diarrhea from any cause and exposure to hot weather or vigorous exercise are situations that require caution; salt and water intake must be increased in these circumstances. Ileostomy patients must never be in a position where salt and water are unavailable, eg, on long hikes in the desert. Low-salt diets and diuretics may induce salt depletion or dehydration also. Patients should be counseled to salt food liberally, but salt tablets will not be required in usual circumstances. Patients with unusually high ileostomy outputs may need supplemental potassium in the form of bananas or orange juice. Water intake in response to thirst may not be adequate to maintain hydration, and patients should consume enough water to keep the urine pale or to maintain a urine output of at least 1 L/d.

Patients must be informed about these physiologic alterations and measures to compensate for them. Oth-

Figure 31–19. Ileostomy after colectomy. **A:** A paramedian incision for colectomy is indicated by the dotted line and the site of the ileostomy by the black dot. (A midline incision is favored by many surgeons.) **B:** The ileum has been brought through the abdominal wall. **C and D:** The ileostomy stoma has been everted and its margins sutured to the edges of the wound.

erwise, instructions are simple, and patients should live normally. A low-residue diet should be advised at least initially. Certain foods (eg, fish, eggs) may cause excessive odor or gas. Ordinary physical activity, employment, and social activities are encouraged. Bathing, swimming, sexual intercourse, and pregnancy and delivery are unrestricted.

Complications (Table 31–9) are reported in about 40% of patients with conventional ileostomy; about 15% require operative correction, usually minor.

In long-term follow-up of ileostomy patients, most return to their previous occupation and consider their health to be good to excellent. Continent ileostomy is preferable to conventional ileostomy in the view of some patients who have had both types of stoma.

Sexual consequences of proctocolectomy should be discussed before and after operation. Some degree of sexual impairment occurs in 10% of men after removal of the rectum for inflammatory bowel disease. Up to three-fourths of women report dyspareunia or reduced orgasmic sensation in the first few months after proc-

tectomy and ileostomy. Infertility is more frequent among women after excision of the rectum, and cesarean delivery is necessary more often; both problems are related to pelvic fibrosis and not the ileostomy.

COLOSTOMY

Colostomies are made for the following purposes: (1) to decompress an obstructed colon; (2) to divert the fecal stream in preparation for resection of an inflammatory, obstructive, or perforated lesion or following traumatic injury; (3) to serve as the point of evacuation of stool when the distal colon or rectum is removed; and (4) to protect a distal anastomosis following resection. The colostomy may be temporary, in which event it is subsequently closed; or it may be permanent. Colostomies can be constructed by making an opening in a loop of colon (**loop colostomy**) or by dividing the colon and bringing out one end (**end [terminal] colostomy**). A colostomy is double-barreled if a loop or both ends of a colon are exteriorized and single-barreled if only one end is brought out.

Table 31–9. Ileostomy complications.

Complication	Causes and Comment
Intestinal obstruction	May be due to adhesive bands, volvulus, or para-ileostomy herniation of bowel.
Stenosis	Circumferential scar formation at the skin or subcutaneous level is usually at fault. Stenosis may cause profuse watery discharge from the ileostomy. Treatment requires a minor local procedure to release the scar.
Retraction	The stoma should protrude 2–3 cm above the skin level to avoid leakage beneath the ileostomy pouch. A flush or retracted stoma functions poorly and should be revised.
Prolapse	Uncommon if the mesentery has been sutured to the parietal peritoneum.
Para-ileostomy abscess and fistula	Perforation of the ileum by sutures, pressure necrosis from an ill-fitted appliance, or recurrent disease may cause abscess and fistula.
Skin irritation	The single most common complication of ileostomy, due to leakage of ileal effluent onto the peristomal skin. Usually minor but can be severe if neglected. Treatment is directed toward the cause of leakage, usually an ill-fitted pouch. Protection of the skin by a barrier material (eg, karaya [*Sterculia*] gum) or a variety of synthetic products will resolve the problem. Enterostomy therapists manage these problems expertly.
Offensive odors	Odor-proof appliances, commercial deodorants placed in the appliance, and attention to diet usually control the problem.
Diarrhea	Excessive output should be reported to the physician promptly, and supplemental water, salt, and potassium should be given. Codeine, diphenoxylate with atropine, or loperamide may slow the output. Recurrent intestinal disease, bowel obstruction, or ileostomy stenosis should be looked for.
Urinary tract calculi	Uric acid and calcium stones occur in about 5–10% of patients after ileostomy and are probably the result of chronic dehydration due to inadequate fluid intake. Ileostomy is associated with lower urine pH and volume and higher urine concentration of calcium, oxalate, and uric acid than in patients with intact gastrointestinal tracts.
Gallstones	Cholesterol gallstones are three times more common in ileostomy patients than in the general population. Altered bile acid absorption preoperatively may be responsible.
Ileitis	Patients who develop inflammation of the ileum just proximal to the ileostomy usually have recurrence of their original inflammatory bowel disease. Stenosis of the stoma is another cause.
Varices	Varices develop around the stoma in patients with portal hypertension. Bleeding can be troublesome.

The most common permanent colostomy is a **sigmoid (iliac) colostomy** made at the time of abdominoperineal resection for cancer of the rectum (Figure 31–20). Such a colostomy is compatible with a normal life except for the route of fecal evacuation. A sigmoid colostomy expels stool approximately once a day, but the frequency varies among individuals just as bowel habits vary in the general population. An appliance is not required, though many patients find that wearing a light pouch is reassuring. Some patients achieve a regular pattern of evacuation on their own; others require irrigation daily or every other day. Irrigation is performed by inserting a catheter into the stoma and instilling water, 500 mL at a time, by gravity flow from a reservoir held at shoulder height. A plastic olive-shaped tip on the catheter fits snugly into the stoma and greatly reduces the risk of perforation. Diet is indi-vidualized; generally, patients are able to eat the same foods they enjoyed preoperatively. Fresh fruits, fruit juices, and other foods may cause diarrhea. A properly functioning colostomy need not be dilated.

Transverse colostomy should not be constructed as a permanent stoma if it can be avoided. Unlike sigmoid colostomy, transverse colostomy is "wet"—ie, it discharges semiliquid waste frequently—and usually requires an appliance. These stomas are bulky, foul-smelling, and extremely difficult to manage. They are prone to leak under the appliance, and prolapse is common. The needs of most patients who require a permanent stoma are better served by an ileostomy than by a transverse colostomy.

The overall complication rate of colostomies is 20%, and 15% of complications require operative correction. Chronic paracolostomy hernia is a frequent complication; it develops because the abdominal wall aperture en-

Figure 31–20. Single-barreled end colostomy. The margins of the stoma are fixed to the skin with sutures.

larges with time, allowing colon, omentum, or small bowel to herniate adjacent to the colostomy. Hernia—and prolapse—are more apt to occur in obese patients. Stenosis is largely avoided by maturing the colostomy at the operating table as with ileostomy. Necrosis and retraction are due to technical errors in constructing the stoma. Paracolostomy abscess occurs occasionally regardless of precautions. Perforation is avoided by the plastic catheter tip and by keeping the irrigation reservoir at no greater than shoulder height. Less serious complications include diarrhea, fecal impaction, and skin irritation.

Leong APK, Londono-Schimmer EE, Phillips RKS: Life-table analysis of stomal complications following ileostomy. Br J Surg 1994;81:727.

Lyons AS: Ileostomy and colostomy support groups. Mt Sinai J Med 2001;68:110.

Oliveira L et al: Laparoscopic creation of stomas. Surg Endosc 1997;11:19.

Rubin MS, Schoetz DJ Jr, Matthews JB: Parastomal hernia: is stoma relocation superior to fascial repair? Arch Surg 1994; 129:413.

Rullier E et al: Loop ileostomy versus loop colostomy for defunctioning low anastomoses during rectal cancer Surgery. World J Surg 2001;25:274.

Sakai Y et al: Temporary transverse colostomy vs loop ileostomy in diversion: a case- matched study. Arch Surg 2001;136:338.

■ PREOPERATIVE PREPARATION OF THE COLON

Complications of colonic surgery such as wound infection and anastomotic dehiscence are partially related to the high bacterial content of the large bowel. It is advisable to eliminate the fecal mass and reduce the numbers of bacteria as much as possible prior to operation. Measures taken to achieve this purpose are known as the "bowel prep." Patients in good health can have preparation as an outpatient and undergo operation on the day of admission.

The fecal mass is reduced by allowing the patient only clear liquids orally for 1 day before operation. Chemically defined diets also leave a small fecal residue; because of their nutritional advantages, they are useful in patients whose colons are especially difficult to cleanse and who require prolonged periods of preparation (eg, children with Hirschsprung's disease). These liquid diets have little or no effect on fecal flora, however.

Mechanical cleansing is employed except in patients with obstructing lesions or, perhaps, severe inflammatory bowel disease. There has been a strong trend toward whole-gut lavage, which involves ingestion (or instillation through a nasogastric tube) of large quantities of fluid; the absorptive capacity of the small bowel is overwhelmed, and the colon is cleared of fecal matter. A solution containing polyethylene glycol (PEG) minimizes the risk of fluid overload and excessive dehydration. Most patients prefer this to preparation with laxatives and enemas. The original PEG solutions contained sodium sulfate as the predominant intraluminal anion. Recently, the sulfate has been deleted from some of these products in an attempt to avoid the unpleasant salty taste that some patients found disagreeable. Oral sodium phosphate compares favorably with PEG solutions.

Direct attack on the bacteria of the large bowel may be undertaken with systemic antibiotics (see Chapter 9) or oral nonabsorbable antibiotics. Oral antibiotics remain controversial despite many years of study. An important reason for disparate opinions is the difficulty of performing prospective trials in which all the variables are strictly controlled. The numbers of fecal bacteria can be reduced by giving oral neomycin and erythromycin base (1 g each at 1:00 PM, 2:00 PM, and 11:00 PM the day before operation). Metronidazole has also been shown to be effective, but an aminoglycoside or other agent effective against gram-negative pathogens should probably be added to cover against aerobic bacteria. The dose of metronidazole is 250–750 mg orally three times daily for 2 days preoperatively. Significant levels of these agents are found in the serum, and it is possible that the systemic effect is as important as the benefit from reduction of flora intraluminally.

It is agreed that some form of antibiotic prophylaxis is essential. At present, surgeons have a choice among various systemic antibiotics or one of several oral antibiotic regimens in addition to mechanical cleansing. It is unclear whether a combination of oral and systemic antibiotics compares favorably with either alone. Pseudomembranous colitis is a complication of antibiotic preparation.

Bleday R et al: Quantitative cultures of the mucosal-associated bacteria in the mechanically prepared colon and rectum. Dis Colon Rectum 1993;36:844.

Burke P et al: Requirement for bowel preparation in colorectal surgery. Br J Surg 1994;81:907.

Cohen SM et al: Prospective, randomized, endoscopic-blinded trial comparing precolonoscopy bowel cleansing methods. Dis Colon Rectum 1994;37:689.

Henderson JM et al: Single-day, divided-dose oral sodium phosphate laxative versus intestinal lavage as preparation for colonoscopy: efficacy and patient tolerance. Gastrointest Endosc 1995;42:238.

Le TH et al: Outpatient bowel preparation for elective colon resection. South Med J 1997;90:526.

Lee EC et al: Inpatient vs. outpatient bowel preparation for elective colorectal surgery. Dis Colon Rectum 1996;39:369.

Matter SE, Rice PS, Campbell DR: Colonic lavage solutions: plain versus flavored. Am J Gastroenterol 1993;88:49.

Miettinen RP et al: Bowel preparation with oral polyethylene glycol electrolyte solution vs. no preparation in elective open colorectal surgery: prospective, randomized study. Dis Colon Rectum 2000;43:669.

Platell C, Hall J: What is the role of mechanical bowel preparation in patients undergoing colorectal surgery? Dis Colon Rectum 1998;41:875.

Santos JC Jr et al: Prospective randomized trial of mechanical bowel preparation in patients undergoing elective colorectal surgery. Br J Surg 1994;81:1673.

Wolters U et al: Prospective randomized study of preoperative bowel cleansing for patients undergoing colorectal surgery. Br J Surg 1994;81:598.

Anorectum

32

Mark Lane Welton, MD

GENERAL ANATOMIC CONSIDERATIONS

The rectum, endodermal in origin, is the dorsal component of the cloaca, which is partitioned by the anorectal septum. The anal canal is an invagination of ectodermal tissue, The anorectum develops from fusion of the rectum and the anal canal, which occurs at 8 weeks, when the anal membrane ruptures. The dentate line marks the point of fusion and the transition from endodermal to ectodermal tissue.

The rectum is 12–15 cm long. It extends from the rectosigmoid junction, marked by the fusion of the tenia, to the anal canal, marked by the passage into the pelvic floor musculature (Figure 32–1). The rectum lies in the sacrum and forms three distinct curves, creating folds known as the **valves of Houston.** The proximal and distal curves are convex to the left and the middle curve is convex to the right. The middle curve roughly marks the anterior peritoneal reflection, which is 6–8 cm above the anus. The rectum gradually undergoes transition from intraperitoneal to extraperitoneal beginning 12–15 cm from the anus and becoming completely extraperitoneal 6–8 cm from the anus. The rectum is fixed posteriorly, laterally, and anteriorly by the presacral (Waldeyer's) fascia, the lateral ligaments, and Denonvilliers' fascia, respectively.

The anatomic anal canal starts at the **dentate line,** the junction of colorectal mucosa and anal mucosa, and ends at the **anal verge,** the junction of the anal mucosa with the perianal skin. However, for practical purposes, the surgical anal canal extends from the muscular diaphragm of the pelvic floor to the anal verge. The **anal canal** is a collapsed anteroposterior slit 3–4 cm long. The anal canal is supported by the surrounding **anal sphincter mechanism,** composed of the internal and external sphincters. The **internal sphincter** is a specialized continuation of the circular muscle of the rectum. It is an involuntary muscle that is normally contracted at rest. The structure and function of the **external sphincter** is the subject of some controversy, but it act as a spout on a funnel of one continuous circumferential functional muscle mass that includes the external sphincter caudally and extends cranially to the conical puborectalis and levator ani muscles. The external sphincter is composed of voluntary striated muscle. The conjoined longitudinal muscle separates the internal and external sphincters. This intersphincteric plane is created by the continuation of the longitudinal muscle of the rectum joined by fibers from the levator ani and puborectalis, forming the conjoined muscle. Some fibers from this muscle become the corrugator cutis ani and insert on the perianal skin, creating rugal folds and a puckered appearance. Other fibers traverse the internal sphincter and support the internal hemorrhoids as the mucosal suspensory ligaments.

Familiarity with the histology of the rectum and anal canal is important in order to understand the of disease processes of these areas. The rectum is composed of an innermost layer of mucosa that overlies the submucosa, two continuous sheaths of muscle—the circular and longitudinal muscles—and, in the proximal rectum, serosa. The mucosa is subdivided into three layers: (1) epithelial cells, (2) lamina propria, and (3) muscularis mucosae. The **muscularis mucosae** is a fine sheet of muscle containing a network of lymphatics. Lymphatics are essentially absent above this level, so the muscularis mucosae determines the metastatic potential of malignancies.

As the rectum enters the narrow musculature of the pelvic floor and becomes the anal canal, the tissue is thrown into folds known as the **columns of Morgagni.** At the lower end of the columns lie crypts, some of which communicate with anal glands lying in the intersphincteric plane. The epithelium of the anal canal is of three types: colorectal mucosa is present in the proximal 2–3 cm; transitional epithelium is at and just above the dentate line; and the anoderm is below the dentate line. The anoderm is squamous mucosa rich in nerve fibers. The anal verge marks the true mucocutaneous junction.

The pelvic floor is composed of the levator ani and puborectalis muscles. The levator ani two broad, thin, symmetric muscular sheets that originate from the pelvic sidewall and sacrospinous ligament, form the principal support of the pelvic viscera. The puborectalis muscle originates on the posterior aspect of the pubis, forms a sling around the rectum, and returns to the posterior aspect of the pubis. The fibers of the puborectalis are situated immediately adjacent to and below the innermost component of the levator ani muscle, where they are intimately associated with the upper postero-

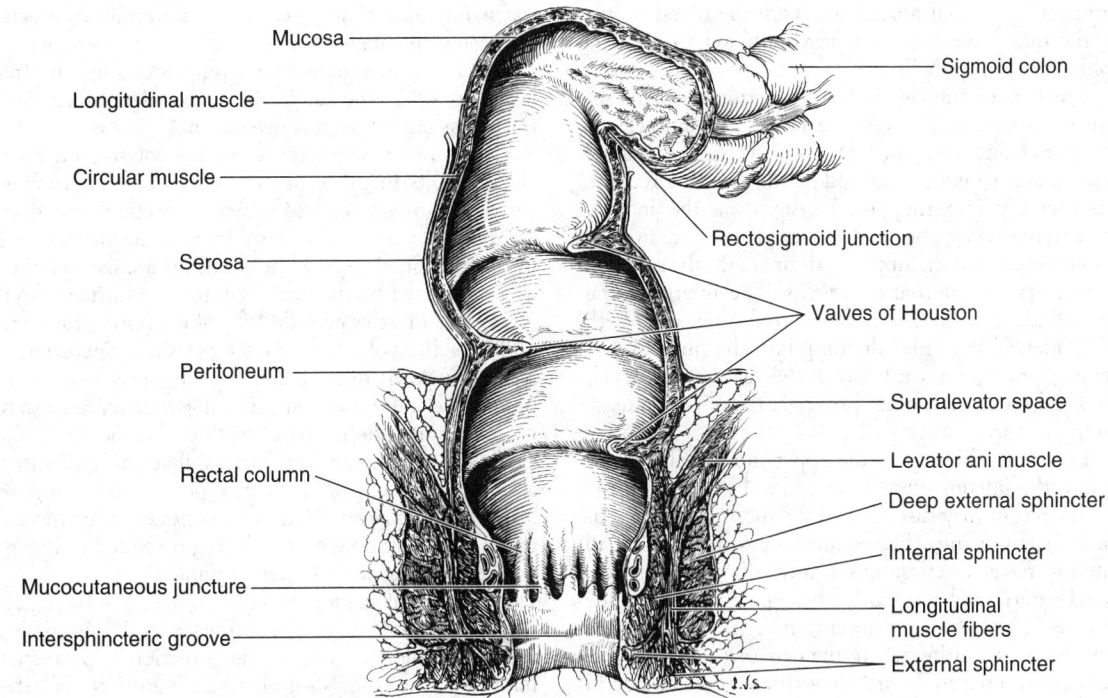

Mucosa

Longitudinal muscle

Circular muscle

Serosa

Peritoneum

Rectal column

Mucocutaneous juncture

Intersphincteric groove

Sigmoid colon

Rectosigmoid junction

Valves of Houston

Supralevator space

Levator ani muscle

Deep external sphincter

Internal sphincter

Longitudinal muscle fibers

External sphincter

Figure 32–1. Anatomy of the anorectal canal.

lateral fibers of the deep external anal sphincter. Thus, the puborectalis serves as a bridge between the broad sheet-like component of the funnel created by the levators and the narrow spout of the funnel created by the external anal sphincter. The puborectalis in the contracted state is responsible for the normal acute anorectal angle between the levators and the external sphincters. It is also responsible for the shelf that is normally palpable on digital examination as one passes from the distal narrow lumen of the anus to the more proximal capacious lumen of the rectum.

The innervation of the rectum is via the sympathetic and parasympathetic nervous systems. The sympathetic nerves originate from the lumbar segments L1–3, form the inferior mesenteric plexus, travel through the superior hypogastric plexus, and descend as the hypogastric nerves to the pelvic plexus.

The parasympathetic nerves arise from the second, third, and fourth sacral roots and join the hypogastric nerves anterior and lateral to the rectum to form the pelvic plexus, from which fibers pass to form the periprostatic plexus. Sympathetic and parasympathetic fibers pass from the pelvic and periprostatic plexuses to the rectum and internal anal sphincter as well as the prostate, bladder, and penis. Injury to these nerves can

lead to impotence, bladder dysfunction, and loss of normal defecatory mechanisms.

The internal anal sphincter is innervated with sympathetic and parasympathetic fibers. Both are inhibitory and keep the sphincter in a constant state of contraction. The external sphincters are skeletal muscles innervated by the pudendal nerve with fibers that originate from S2–4. Above the dentate line, noxious stimuli are experienced as ill-defined dull sensations conducted through afferent fibers of the parasympathetic nerves. Below the dentate line, the epithelium is exquisitely sensitive. Cutaneous sensations of heat, cold, pain, and touch are conveyed through the inferior rectal and perineal branches of the pudendal nerve.

The arterial supply of the anorectum is via the superior, middle, and inferior rectal arteries. The superior rectal artery is the terminal branch of the inferior mesenteric artery and descends in the mesorectum. It supplies the upper and middle rectum. The middle rectal arteries arise from the internal iliac arteries and enter the rectum anterolaterally at the level of the pelvic floor musculature. They supply the lower two-thirds of the rectum. Collaterals exist between the middle and superior rectal arteries. The inferior rectal arteries—branches of the internal pudendal arteries—enter posterolaterally, do not anastomose with the blood supply to the middle rectum, and provide blood to the anal sphincters and epithelium.

The venous drainage of the anorectum is via the superior, middle, and inferior rectal veins draining into the portal and systemic systems. The superior rectal veins drain the upper and middle thirds of the rectum. They empty into the portal system via the inferior mesenteric vein. The middle rectal veins drain the lower rectum and the upper anal canal into the systemic system via the internal iliac veins. The inferior rectal veins drain the lower anal canal, communicating with the pudendal veins and draining into the internal iliac veins. Communication between the venous systems allows low rectal cancers to spread via the portal and systemic systems.

Lymphatic drainage of the upper and middle rectum is into the inferior mesenteric nodes. Lymph from the lower rectum may also drain into the inferior mesenteric system or into the systems along the middle and inferior rectal arteries, posteriorly along the middle sacral artery, and anteriorly through channels in the retrovesical or rectovaginal septum. These drain to the iliac nodes and ultimately to the periaortic nodes. Lymphatics from the anal canal above the dentate line drain via the superior rectal lymphatics to the inferior mesenteric lymph nodes and laterally to the internal iliac nodes. Below the dentate line, drainage occurs primarily to the inguinal nodes but can occur to the inferior or superior rectal lymph nodes.

NORMAL FUNCTION OF THE ANORECTUM

The normal function of the anorectum is storage and release of intestinal waste products. The rectum functions mainly as a capacitance storage vessel. The normal volume of the rectum is 650–1200 mL. Resting rectal pressure is approximately 10 mm Hg. Changes in intrarectal pressure are primarily a reflection of intraabdominal pressure changes since the rectum itself has little peristaltic function.

The function of the pelvic floor is complex and poorly understood. The complexity of the interactions of the pelvic floor structures and the nature of material passed per rectum compromises the ability to study function with intraluminal monitors, as is done in the upper intestinal tract.

The levators ani form a funnel that suspends the rectum in a muscular sling which ends where the puborectalis angulates the rectum forward at the anorectal junction. The levators may contain sensory fibers that report pelvic fullness and thus may be important in the sensation of the urge to defecate. The acuity of the anorectal angle (created by the puborectalis) is critical

for maintaining continence. The puborectalis contracts, increasing the angle during Valsalva maneuvers, where continence is maintained (coughing, straining), but relaxes, to open the angle during similar efforts performed as part of normal defecation.

The internal sphincter, composed of smooth muscle, accounts for 85% of the resting tone. It is innervated by sympathetic and parasympathetic fibers. Both are inhibitory and keep the sphincter in a constant state of contraction. The external sphincters are skeletal muscles innervated by the pudendal nerve with fibers from S2–4. The muscles provide 15% of the resting tone and 100% of the voluntary squeeze pressure. The external sphincter, pelvic floor, and cricopharyngeus muscles are unique skeletal muscles in being able to maintain a state of tonic contraction. The strength of contraction in the first two is increased by factors that increase intraabdominal pressure such as erect posture, coughing, or Valsalva's maneuver. Voluntary contraction of the external sphincter doubles the resting pressure but it cannot be sustained longer than 3 minutes.

The normal hemorrhoidal pads are important participants in maintaining continence and minimizing trauma during defecation. They function as protective pillows that engorge with blood during the act of defecation, protecting the anoderm from direct trauma due to passage of stool. They also seal the anal canal and prevent leakage of gas and stool. The internal and external sphincters alone cannot close the anal canal, but when sphincter action is combined with interdigitating internal hemorrhoidal cushions, continence is achieved. Hemorrhoidal tissues become engorged when intraabdominal pressure is increased (e.g., obesity, pregnancy, lifting, and defecation).

Through complex mechanisms not clearly understood, the anal sphincters function as a unit in concert with the levator ani, the puborectalis, and the rectum, allowing defecation to be controlled. Continence is maintained when intrarectal pressures are lower than the pressures generated by the resting internal and external sphincters. In the resting state, the rectum is not completely empty but the contents are not sensed. Sensory fibers in the levators that initially signal the presence of pelvic fullness adapt and the rectum accommodates (decreases muscle tone), allowing the contents to remain. Periodically, the internal sphincter relaxes, allowing the rectal contents to drop down into the anal canal where the contents can be sensed by the anoderm. In response, the external sphincter contracts and the contents are pushed back into the rectum. This "sampling reflex," or **rectoanal inhibitory reflex,** also results from rectal distention, allowing determination of rectal contents as the rectum fills. The sampling reflex occurs up to seven times a day. Progressive distention of the rectum causes continuous inhibition of the internal sphincter and relaxation of the external sphincter, resulting in the urge to defecate. If solid waste is noted and one wishes to evacuate, a sitting or squatting position is assumed (straightening the anorectal angle), intra-abdominal pressure is increased by a Valsalva maneuver, the puborectalis relaxes, and reflex relaxation of the internal sphincter occurs as the contents enter the anal canal. As the puborectalis relaxes, the anorectal angle straightens, further shortening the anal canal and increasing the funnel shape of the musculature. The Valsalva maneuver is the principal force behind evacuation. Thus, normal defecation is a complex event involving multiple steps.

■ DYSFUNCTION OF THE ANORECTUM

INCONTINENCE

Continence is maintained through rectal compliance, anorectal sensation, anorectal reflexes, and anal sphincter function. The nature and quantity of stool and colonic transit participate as well. The incidence of fecal incontinence is difficult to determine because of underreporting and lack of a standard definition of the term. Obstetric trauma is the major cause of mechanical injury to the external sphincter and nerves. The incidence of incontinence is increased after third-degree perineal tears, multiple vaginal deliveries, and infection of an episiotomy repair. Prolonged labor may mechanically disrupt the sphincter and stretch of the pudendal nerve. Although incontinence is most common in parous women, the prevalence in men is also high.

Neurogenic causes of incontinence include pudendal nerve stretch from to prolonged labor or multiple births and a history of chronic straining to defecate. Vaginal deliveries are associated with reversible pudendal nerve injury in 80% of primigravida births. The injury may be unilateral or bilateral. If it is permanent or repeated multiple times, denervation and weakening of the external sphincter and pelvic floor result. The neuropathy and sphincter dysfunction progress with time. A weakened pelvic floor is less able to withstand increased intra-abdominal pressure, leading to further perineal descent and stretch injury.

Chronic straining at stool and a sense of incomplete evacuation are common features of the descending perineum syndrome. Straining leads to descent of the pelvic floor and straightening of the anorectal angle. This may result in folding in or prolapse of the anterior rectal wall and further obstruction of defecation. The resultant increased straining and perineal descent cause

pudendal nerve injury as the nerve is stretched over the ischial spine, leading to idiopathic fecal incontinence sometimes associated with internal rectal prolapse (intussusception).

Incontinence may result from the treatment of cryptogenic abscess or fistula disease or of perianal Crohn's disease, where the external sphincter may be divided during fistulotomy. In women, the external sphincter is a thin band of muscle anteriorly and thus especially susceptible to complete transection in this location, resulting in incontinence.

Other causes of incontinence include systemic diseases affecting either the muscular or neurologic systems (eg, scleroderma, multiple sclerosis, dermatomyositis, diabetes) and causes unrelated to the function of the sphincter itself (severe diarrhea, fecal impaction with overflow incontinence, radiation proctitis with fibrosis, and tumors of the distal colon and rectum).

Clinical Findings

A. Symptoms and Signs

Complete incontinence is lack of control of gas, liquid, and solid stool. Inability to control liquid and gas or gas alone is **partial incontinence.** Urgency, seepage, and soiling may occur regularly or intermittently, depending on the nature of the stool presenting to the rectum. Elicitation of these symptoms is important in establishing the nature of the injury. Patients who complain of soiling with urgency may have a poorly distensible rectum and normal sphincters, whereas patients complaining of inability to sense stool until it has passed may have a neurologic injury. The physical signs of incontinence may include a patulous anus, focal loss of corrugation of the anal verge, flattening and maceration of the perineum, exaggerated descent of the perineum with straining, decreased sphincter tone, diminished voluntary squeeze pressures, and loss of anal sensation.

B. Laboratory and Imaging Studies

Evaluation with anorectal manometry, transrectal ultrasound, pudendal nerve latency studies, electromyography, and defecography may all be part of the evaluation of the incontinent patient.

Anorectal manometry defines the limits of the injury by measuring the maximum resting pressure, the maximum squeeze pressure, the sphincter length and symmetry, the minimum sensory volume, the presence or absence of the rectoanal inhibitory reflex, and the ability to relax the puborectalis muscle. Maximal resting pressures normally range from 40 mm Hg to 80 mm Hg, while maximal squeeze pressures range from 80 mm Hg to l60 mm Hg. The internal sphincter gives rise to 85% of the resting maximal pressure, while the external sphincter provides 15% of the resting pressure and 100% of the maximal squeeze pressure. The sphincter is typically 3 cm long and asymmetric (longer in back), and the whole complex is shorter is women. The minimum sensory volume is about 10 mL. The rectoanal inhibitory reflex is manifested as a decrease in resting anal pressure when an air-filled balloon distends the rectum. Finally, pelvic floor function and the ability to relax the pelvic floor to achieve defecation assessed with the balloon expulsion test. This requires the patient to expel a fully inflated 60 mL latex balloon.

Transrectal ultrasound provides useful anatomic images for evaluating internal and external anal sphincter defects. Electromyographic changes correlate closely with ultrasonographic evidence of sphincter injury, allowing transrectal ultrasound to largely replace the more painful electromyography.

Pudendal nerve latency studies further define the nature of the injury. If one or both nerves are injured, surgical or nonsurgical treatment of incontinence may be predictably unsuccessful. The study is performed by inserting a gloved finger with a stimulating electrode at the fingertip in the rectum and stimulating the pudendal nerve as it traverses the ischial spine. An electrode at the base of the examining finger records the delay between stimulation and contraction of the external sphincter. The normal delay is 2 ± 0.2 s. It may be prolonged with age, after childbirth, in individuals with a history of excessive straining to defecate and perineal descent, and in systemic diseases such as diabetes and multiple sclerosis.

Defecography is useful in patients with both constipation and incontinence, as in some patients with incontinence rectal intussusception occurs during straining to defecate the intussusception produces obstruction and constipation, which is later followed by uncontrolled release of liquid stool after the straining is stopped.

Differential Diagnosis

Incontinence may result from obstructions to defecation caused by tumors or intussusception. Varying degrees of incontinence may also result from obstetric injury, either from excessive straining and pudendal nerve injury or disruption of the sphincter mechanism. Incontinence may occur immediately or after many years as the patient ages, sphincter tone decreases, and an occult injury is manifested. Chronic straining at defecation stretches the pudendal nerve over the ischial spine, leading to idiopathic fecal incontinence in the elderly. An extreme example of this is seen in rectal prolapse, where 30% of patients experience incontinence after repair because of stretch injury from chronic prolapse. Secondary effects of systemic diseases such as multiple sclerosis, dermatomyositis, and diabetes mellitus should

be considered. Incontinence may also stem from disease that overwhelms a normally functioning sphincter. Examples are severe diarrhea, fecal impaction with overflow, inflammatory bowel disease of the rectum, radiation proctitis, and fibrosis.

Treatment

An algorithm for the diagnosis and treatment of incontinence is given in (Figure 32–2). If a muscular defect is limited and there is no neurologic injury, surgical correction with an overlapping sphincter reconstruction restores continence by reestablishing a complete ring of muscle. However, if there is extensive loss of sphincter muscle or severe neurologic injury, simple overlapping repair is not as successful, and consideration must be given to muscle flap or encirclement procedures. The stimulated-gracilis, the gracilis, and the gluteal muscle flap procedures are reserved for patients with complete neurologic injury or extensive muscle loss who wish to avoid a colostomy. The stimulated-gracilis procedure is similar to the gracilis procedure with the exception that a pacemaker is used to retrain the gracilis. Reports on the success rates of these muscle wrap procedures are few. A new artificial sphincter is in trials, and early reports are promising. Incontinence from muscular weakness or decreased sensation secondary to incomplete neurologic injury may respond to retraining with biofeedback.

Anal encirclement procedures with foreign material have been reserved for the critically ill or for patients with a short life expectancy. The anal canal is encircled with either a synthetic mesh or a silver wire. Patients are given daily enemas to evacuate the rectum, providing a form of continence involving artificial obstruction and stimulated evacuation. The obstructing foreign body is prone to infection and erosion into the rectum, often necessitating its removal.

Prognosis

The incontinence associated with prolapse usually resolves after repair of the prolapse if there has not been severe nerve injury. Prior to repair, the prolapsing segment stimulates the rectoanal inhibitory reflex, decreasing internal sphincter pressure, fatiguing the external sphincter, and resulting in incontinence. The incontinence resolves after surgical repair in 70% of cases.

Cheong DM et al: Electrodiagnostic evaluation of fecal incontinence. Muscle Nerve 1995;18:612.

Falk PM et al: Transanal ultrasound and manometry in the evaluation of fecal incontinence. Dis Colon Rectum 1994;37:468.

Farouk R et al: Sustained internal sphincter hypertonia in patients with chronic anal fissure. Dis Colon Rectum 1994;37:424.

Figure 32–2. Algorithm for workup and treatment of fecal incontinence. (Reproduced, with permission, from Grendel JH, McQuaid KR, Friedman SL: *Current Diagnosis & Treatment in Gastroenterology.* Originally published by Appleton & Lange. Copyright © 1996 by The McGraw-Hill Companies, Inc.)

Hill JA et al: Pudendal neuropathy in patients with idiopathic fecal incontinence progresses with time. Br J Surg 1994;81:1492.

Johanson JF et al: Epidemiology of fecal incontinence: the silent affliction. Am J Gastroenterol 1996;91:33.

Ko CY et al: Biofeedback is effective therapy for fecal incontinence and constipation. Arch Surg 1997;132:829.

Lehur PA et al: Artificial anal sphincter: prospective clinical and manometric evaluation. Dis Colon Rectum 2000;43:1100.

Lestar B et al: The internal anal sphincter cannot close the anal canal completely. Int J Colorectal Dis 1992;7:159.

Madoff RD et al: Fecal incontinence. N Engl J Med 1992; 326:1002.

Nelson R et al: Community-based prevalence of anal incontinence. JAMA 1995;274:559.

Osterberg A et al: Results of neurophysiologic evaluation in fecal incontinence. Dis Colon Rectum 2000;43:1256.

Ryhammer AM et al: Long-term effect of vaginal deliveries on anorectal function in normal perimenopausal women. Dis Colon Rectum 1996;39:852.

Sangwan YP et al: Fecal incontinence. Surg Clin North Am J 1994; 74:1377.

Sultan AH et al: Endosonography of the anal sphincters: normal anatomy and comparison with manometry. Clin Radiol 1994;49:368.

OBSTRUCTED DEFECATION

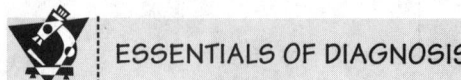

ESSENTIALS OF DIAGNOSIS

- Inability to voluntarily evacuate rectal contents.
- Normal colonic transit time.

General Considerations

Obstructed defecation may result from anal stenosis, pelvic floor dysfunction, or abnormal rectal fixation. The most common cause of anal stenosis is scarring after anal surgery. In particular, inexpertly performed hemorrhoidectomies or the circumferential Whitehead hemorrhoidectomy may lead to stenosis. Other causes include anal tumors, Crohn's disease, radiation injury, recurrent anal ulcers, infection, and trauma.

Pelvic floor dysfunction—alternatively referred to as nonrelaxing puborectalis syndrome, anismus, or paradoxic pelvic floor contraction—is a functional disorder in that the muscle is normal but control is dysfunctional. In health, the puborectalis is contracted at rest, maintaining the anorectal angle. During defecation, the muscle relaxes and evacuation occurs. In nonrelaxing puborectalis syndrome, the muscle does not relax and maintains or increases (paradoxic contraction) the anorectal angle. The patient therefore performs a Valsalva maneuver against an obstructed outlet, and elimination does not occur or is significantly diminished.

Patients who chronically strain at stool, whether from colonic inertia or pelvic floor dysfunction, may develop lengthening of the attachments of the rectum to the sacrum or descending perineum syndrome. The increased mobility that results allows for internal prolapse (intussusception), solitary rectal ulcer, and rectal procidentia. Intussusception causes outlet obstruction because the upper rectum moves away from the sacrum and telescopes into the more distal rectum.

Clinical Findings

A. SYMPTOMS AND SIGNS

Anal stenosis causes increasing difficulty with—and straining at—defecation, thin and sometimes painful bowel movements, and bloating. Patients with nonrelaxing puborectalis syndrome similarly complain of straining and anal or pelvic pain but also of constipation, incomplete evacuation, and a need to digitally evacuate rectal contents. As with nonrelaxing puborec-

talis syndrome, patients with internal intussusception complain of constipation, sensations of rectal fullness, or incomplete evacuation, but—in contrast to the above causes of obstructed defecation—they also note mucus discharge, rectal bleeding, and tenesmus.

Examination of the patient with anal stenosis may reveal postsurgical changes and a stenotic anal canal. Digital examination may be quite painful or impossible. Digital examination of the patient with nonrelaxing puborectalis syndrome may reveal a tender pelvic muscular diaphragm. During the digital examination, if the patient is directed to squeeze to mimic holding in flatus, paradoxic relaxation and a Valsalva maneuver may occur. Similarly, if the patient is asked to bear down to simulate a bowel movement he may paradoxically contract the external sphincters and puborectalis muscles. Digital examination of the patient with internal intussusception may be much the same as that for nonrelaxing puborectalis syndrome but with the additional findings of a mass. The mass is the lead point of the intussusceptum. It may be anterior and ulcerated (solitary rectal ulcer) or circumferential. The ulcer, located 4–12 cm from the anal verge, is the ischemic traumatized lead point of the internal intussusception. Sigmoidoscopy may reveal the circumferential intussusceptum or an ulcerated mass that appears malignant. Pathologic examination reveals diffuse submucosal cysts with a characteristic fibrosis pattern, distinguishing it from colorectal malignancy.

B. LABORATORY AND IMAGING STUDIES

No additional studies of the patient with anal stenosis are required, but patients with nonrelaxing puborectalis syndrome and internal intussusception should undergo defecography, colonic transit studies, anorectal manometry with the balloon expulsion test, and barium enema or colonoscopy.

The patient with nonrelaxing puborectalis syndrome will have a normal colon on barium enema or colonoscopy and a normal colonic transit time to the rectosigmoid. Cinedefecography will demonstrate persistent anterior displacement of the rectum on the lateral view. The patient will be unable to expel the balloon at completion of the anorectal manometry evaluation.

In the patient with internal intussusception, colonic transit time will be normal to the rectosigmoid, and barium enema or colonoscopy will document a normal colon. Defecography will show the intussusception. Patients with intussusception secondary to nonrelaxing puborectalis syndrome will be unable to expel the latex balloon at the completion of manometric evaluation.

Differential Diagnosis

Causes of anal pain include a fissure, thrombosed external hemorrhoids, perirectal abscess, malignancy, foreign body, and proctalgia fugax. Proctalgia fugax (levator syndrome), a diagnosis of exclusion, is suggested when a patient complains of pain that awakens him or her from sleep. The pain is generally left-sided, short-lived, and relieved by heat, anal dilation, or muscle relaxants. The patient often has a history of migraine headaches and may report that the pain is triggered by stressful events.

Complaints suggestive of obstructed defecation occur in patients with fecal impaction, rectal or anal cancer, descending perineum syndrome, rectocele, internal intussusception, and nonrelaxing puborectalis syndrome. The workup of these complex patients is outlined in (Figure 32–3).

Fecal impaction may occur as a result of nonrelaxing puborectalis syndrome, and therapy is therefore directed towards that disorder.

Treatment

A. MEDICAL TREATMENT

Mild anal stenosis may be treated successfully with gentle dilation and bulk forming agents. Nonrelaxing puborectalis syndrome is best treated with biofeedback. The puborectalis is retrained to relax during the act of defecation, which allows the act to proceed without obstruction. Mild to moderate intussusception is treated with bulk agents, modification of bowel habits, and reassurance. The patient is instructed to stimulate a bowel movement in the morning and avoid the urge to

Figure 32–3. Algorithm for workup and treatment of obstructed defecation. (Reproduced, with permission, from Grendel JH, McQuaid KR, Friedman SL: *Current Diagnosis & Treatment in Gastroenterology*. Originally published by Appleton & Lange. Copyright © 1996 by The McGraw-Hill Companies, Inc.)

defecate the remainder of the day because the fullness they sense is the proximal rectum intussuscepting into the distal rectum. With time, the urge to defecate resolves and so does the intussusception.

B. Surgical Treatment

Severe anal stenosis is treated surgically if there is no evidence of active disease (eg, Crohn's disease) and healthy tissue is available to perform the anoplasty. This can be achieved with a skin island or Y-V flap. Both procedures involve incision of the stenotic anus, mobilization of the surrounding skin, and advancement of the healthy tissue into the closure, relieving the stenosis.

Prognosis

The prognosis for anal stenosis is excellent if there is no evidence of active disease of the anus. Patients with nonrelaxing puborectalis syndrome have excellent results with biofeedback training but may require periodic retraining. Most patients with mild to moderate intussusception do quite well once they are reassured that an abnormality exists but that it is not malignant.

Glia A et al: Constipation assessed on the basis of colorectal physiology. Scand J Gastroenterol 1998;33 :1273.

Mertz H et al: Symptoms and physiology in severe chronic constipation. Am J Gastroenterol 1999;94:131.

Nyam DC et al: Long-term results of surgery for chronic constipation. Dis Colon Rectum 1997;40:273. (Published erratum appears in Dis Colon Rectum 1997;40:529.)

ABNORMAL RECTAL FIXATION

 ESSENTIALS OF DIAGNOSIS

- *Increased mobility of the rectum.*
- *Altered defecation (constipation, incontinence, or both).*
- *Digital maneuvers to defecate.*

General Considerations

Abnormal rectal fixation is a group of diseases in which the attachment of the rectum to the sacrum has lengthened, allowing the rectum to block the act of defecation, to protrude into the vagina, or to prolapse through the anus. The reason for the increased mobility appears to be related to chronic straining. This may be secondary to colonic dysmotility or nonrelaxing puborectalis syndrome.

Clinical Findings

A. Symptoms and Signs

Internal intussusception leads to complaints of rectal fullness, an urge to defecate, and, if associated with solitary rectal ulcer syndrome, complaints of rectal bleeding, mucus discharge, or tenesmus. Patients with rectal prolapse complain of mucus discharge, progressive incontinence, pain, and bleeding, and upon direct questioning they report that the rectum falls out.

Digital examination of the patient with internal intussusception may reveal a mass. This is the lead point of the intussusceptum and may be mistaken for a malignancy. The mass may be anterior and ulcerated (solitary rectal ulcer) or circumferential. The ulcer is 4–12 cm from the anal verge and is the ischemic traumatized lead point of the internal intussusception. Sigmoidoscopy may reveal the circumferential intussusceptum or an ulcerated mass that appears malignant. Pathologic examination reveals diffuse submucosal cysts with a characteristic fibrosis pattern distinguishing it from colorectal malignancy.

Physical examination of the patient with an acute rectal prolapse is not difficult. A large external mass of prolapsed tissue with concentric mucosal rings will be apparent. However, the diagnosis in a patient with a history of prolapse but without active prolapse may be more difficult. It may be necessary to give an enema, allow the patient to evacuate, and then examine the perineum. This often induces a prolapse, allowing of the diagnosis to be made in the office. An alternative is to demonstrate the prolapse on defecography. Digital examination may reveal decreased or absent sphincter tone.

B. Laboratory and Imaging Studies

Patients with internal intussusception and rectal prolapse need anorectal manometry, pudendal nerve latency studies, defecography, and barium enema or colonoscopy. Defecography will show the intussusception or prolapse and may reveal the cause. Evaluation of the entire colon with either barium enema or colonoscopy is necessary to rule out a malignancy.

Differential Diagnosis

Internal intussusception must be differentiated from adenocarcinoma. The symptoms, physical appearance, and histologic characteristics of the ulcer may be confused with malignancy.

Rectal prolapse should be distinguished from hemorrhoidal disease. Rectal prolapse is seen as uninterrupted circumferential rings of mucosa, while hemorrhoidal prolapse will be seen as prolapsing tissue with deep grooves between areas of prolapsing edematous tissue.

Complications

The complications of intussusception and prolapse include progression of intussusception to prolapse; nerve injury from prolapse or chronic straining; descending perineum syndrome; bleeding; and incontinence. A severe rectal prolapse may become so edematous that it cannot be reduced, and it may progress to ischemia and gangrene.

Treatment

A. MEDICAL TREATMENT

Treatment of mild to moderate intussusception is discussed above.

B. SURGICAL TREATMENT

There are two classes of operations for rectal prolapse: abdominal and perineal. The abdominal procedures have a lower recurrence rate and preserve the reservoir capacity of the rectum but carry more risk. The perineal procedures avoid an intra-abdominal anastomosis but remove the rectum, thereby eliminating the rectal reservoir, and have higher recurrence rates. The abdominal procedures are generally preferred in low-risk active patients under age 50 and in those who are require other abdominal procedures simultaneously.

The abdominal procedures for patients with severe intussusception or rectal prolapse with normal sphincter function are sigmoid resection with or without rectopexy and rectopexy alone. Both operations—rectopexy or resection—require complete mobilization of the entire rectum to the pelvic floor in order to avoid distal intussusception.

Rectopexy aims to secure the rectum to the sacral hollow. It may be performed with sutures or prosthetic materials such as polypropylene mesh (Marlex), Gore-Tex, polyglycolic acid or polyglactin mesh (Dexon or Vicryl), and polyvinyl alcohol sponges (Ivalon). Many studies have suggested a higher complication rate with the prosthetics, a lower continence rate, and no difference in recurrence, suggesting that suture rectopexy is preferable. Suture rectopexy is performed with heavy nonabsorbable sutures, attaching the rectum to the sacral hollow. The suture may be placed through the lateral ligaments or through the muscularis propria of the rectum.

The addition of a sigmoid resection at the time of rectopexy lowers the recurrence rate, and the incidence of postoperative constipation without increasing the morbidity. Rectopexy corrects the mobility of the rectum but does not correct the underlying disorder for patients with pelvic floor dysfunction or chronic constipation. Sigmoid resection removes the intussusceptum and the mobile portion of colon. Thus, in the constipated patient or the patient with a redundant sigmoid colon, resection is preferable to fixation alone.

Laparoscopic methods for repair of rectal prolapse are involve at fixation, usually without resection. Therefore, although no long-term follow-up data are available, the recurrence rate should be higher. Discomfort is less but, general anesthesia is still required and other benefits (eg, shorter hospital stay, faster return to work) have not been reported.

Perineal operations for rectal prolapse consist of anal encirclement, the transanal Delorme procedure, and the Altemeier procedure. Complete mechanical and antibiotic bowel preparation is necessary for all three procedures.

Anal encirclement is acceptable for patients with a very high operative risk or a limited life expectancy. The original Thiersch procedure involved placing a silver wire around the external sphincter within the ischiorectal fat. Nowadays, synthetic mesh or silicone tubes are used instead of wire. The foreign body creates an outlet obstruction, and laxatives or enemas are required for rectal evacuation. Potential complications consist of erosion of the foreign material into the rectum and infection. This operation has declined in popularity in favor of a perineal operation done with the patient under spinal or epidural anesthesia.

The Delorme procedure is essentially a mucosal proctectomy with imbrication of the prolapsing rectal wall. The dissection is started 1–2 cm above the dentate line and carried to the apex of the prolapsing segment, where the mucosa is amputated. The muscle is reefed in with four to eight heavy absorbable sutures, and the mucosa is reapproximated with sutures or a circular stapler.

The Altemeier procedure is a complete proctectomy and often a partial sigmoidectomy. The apex of the prolapsing segment is delivered and placed on traction, and a full-thickness incision is made approximately 1 cm above the dentate line. The rectum is everted. The dissection is carried into the deep cul-de-sac anteriorly. Posteriorly, the vascular supply to the rectum is taken with electrocautery or clamps when necessary. The dissection is carried up onto the midline mesorectum and sigmoid mesentery until the redundant segment of bowel has been completely mobilized. If a levatoroplasty is planned, it is most easily carried out at this time with heavy absorbable suture. A levatoroplasty plicates the pelvic floor musculature and adds to improved continence by increasing the anorectal angle. The bowel is transected proximally, excising the redundant portion, and a hand-sewn (heavy absorbable suture) or stapled anastomosis is performed.

Sphincter function returns and incontinence resolves in 65% of patients who were incontinent preoperatively, but there is no way to predict who will respond. Those who do not have return of sphincter function will not tolerate a sigmoid resection. Therefore, perineal proctectomy and posterior sphincter enhancement are recommended in these patients. The posterior reconstruction may alter the angle of the rectum or obstruct the outlet sufficiently to bring about continence. Individuals with severe intussusception and those who have rectal prolapse without sphincter dysfunction should do well with either the abdominal or the perineal approach.

Prognosis

The prognosis for patients with mild to moderate intussusception who are treated with bulking agents is excellent. Individuals with severe intussusception and those who have rectal prolapse without sphincter dysfunction should do well. Those with sphincter dysfunction have a 60–70% chance of regaining function. Long-term follow-up data on patients repaired by the perineal approach are not available, but it appears promising, especially in high-risk patients for whom an abdominal operation is undesirable.

Athanasiadis S et al: The risk of infection of three synthetic materials used in rectopexy with or without colonic resection for rectal prolapse. Int J Colorectal Dis 1996;11:42.

Darzi A et al: Stapled laparoscopic rectopexy for rectal prolapse. Surg Endosc 1995;9:301.

Graf W et al: Laparoscopic suture rectopexy. Dis Colon Rectum 1995;38:211.

Huber FT et al: Functional results after treatment of rectal prolapse with rectopexy and sigmoid resection. World J Surg 1995;19:138;discussion 143.

Jacobs LK et al: The best operation for rectal prolapse. Surg Clin North Am 1997;77:49.

Mollen RM et al: Effects of rectal mobilization and lateral ligaments division on colonic and anorectal function. Dis Colon Rectum 2000;43:1283.

Novell JR et al: Prospective randomized trial of Ivalon sponge versus sutured rectopexy for full-thickness rectal prolapse. Br J Surg 1994;81:904.

Reissman P et al: Laparoscopic-assisted perineal rectosigmoidectomy for rectal prolapse. Surg Laparosc Endosc 1995;5:217.

Wexner SD et al: Laparoscopic colorectal surgery: analysis of 140 cases. Surg Endosc 1996;10:133.

HEMORRHOIDS

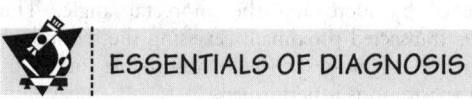 **ESSENTIALS OF DIAGNOSIS**

Internal hemorrhoids:

• *Bright red blood per rectum.*

• *Mucus discharge.*

• *Rectal fullness or discomfort.*

External hemorrhoids:

• *Sudden, severe perianal pain.*

• *Perianal mass.*

General Considerations

Hemorrhoidal tissues are part of the normal anatomy of the distal rectum and anal canal (Figure 32–1). **Internal hemorrhoids** are vascular and connective tissue cushions that originate above the dentate line and are lined with rectal or transitional mucosa. **External hemorrhoids** are vascular complexes underlying the richly innervated anoderm. Hemorrhoids function as protective pillows that become engorged with blood during the act of defecation, protecting the anal canal from direct trauma due to passage of stool. Hemorrhoidal tissues become engorged when intra-abdominal pressure is increased. This occurs with obesity, pregnancy, lifting, and defecation.

Hemorrhoidal disease may involve the internal complex, the external complex, or both. Internal hemorrhoids become symptomatic when the internal complex becomes chronically engorged or the tissue prolapses into the anal canal due to laxity of the surrounding connective tissue and dilation of the veins. The external hemorrhoids become symptomatic with thrombosis, which leads to an acute onset of severe perianal pain. When the thrombosis resolves, the overlying skin may remain enlarged, creating a skin tag.

Internal hemorrhoids develop differently in older women and younger men. In older women the principal cause appears to be chronic straining, which leads to vascular engorgement and dilatation, resulting in stretching and disruption of the supporting connective tissue surrounding the vascular channels. The most common cause of prolonged straining is the act of defecation. Contrary to popular belief, the stool may be liquid or solid. There is no correlation between hemorrhoids and constipation (infrequent passage of stool) or between hemorrhoids and portal hypertension. Hemorrhoids are not dilated vascular channels, varices, or vascular hyperplasias. The mechanism principal in younger men is increased resting pressure within the anal canal, leading to decreased venous return, venous engorgement, and disruption of the supporting tissues. No precipitating causes have been identified for external hemorrhoids.

Internal hemorrhoids are classified as follows: first-degree hemorrhoids bleed; second-degree hemorrhoids bleed and prolapse, but reduce spontaneously; third-degree hemorrhoids bleed, prolapse, and require manual reduction; and fourth-degree hemorrhoids bleed, incarcerate, and cannot be reduced.

Clinical Findings

A. SYMPTOMS AND SIGNS

Internal hemorrhoids typically cause bright red bleeding per rectum, mucus discharge, and a sense of rectal fullness or discomfort, but are painless. Infrequently, internal hemorrhoids prolapse into the anal canal, where they become incarcerated, thrombotic, and necrotic. In this instance, pain is common. Visual inspection may reveal a normal-appearing perineum, edema near the involved hemorrhoid, a prolapsed hemorrhoid, or an edematous, gangrenous, incarcerated hemorrhoid. The perineum may be macerated from chronic mucus discharge, the resulting moisture, and local irritation. Anoscopy may reveal tissue with evidence of chronic vascular dilatation, friability, mobility, and squamous metaplasia.

Acute intravascular thrombus may develop within external hemorrhoids associated with acute severe perianal pain. The pain usually peaks within 48 hours. Repeated episodes of hemorrhoidal dilation and thrombosis may lead to expansion of the overlying skin, which is seen as a skin tag on physical examination. An acutely thrombosed external hemorrhoid is a purple-black, edematous, tense subcutaneous perianal mass that is quite tender. The thrombus occasionally causes ischemia and necrosis of the overlying skin, resulting in bleeding.

B. LABORATORY AND IMAGING STUDIES

Chronic bleeding from internal hemorrhoids may rarely cause anemia. However, until all other sources of blood loss have been ruled out, anemia must not be attributed to hemorrhoids regardless of the patient's age. Barium enema or colonoscopy is necessary to rule out malignancy and inflammatory bowel disease. Defecography is helpful in the patient in whom obstructed defecation and rectal prolapse is suspected.

Differential Diagnosis

Patients with perianal diseases often come to the surgeon with an inaccurate preliminary diagnosis of "hemorrhoids." A thorough history often suggests the correct diagnosis. Painless bleeding attributed to hemorrhoids must be distinguished from rectal bleeding from colorectal malignancy, inflammatory bowel disease, diverticular disease, and adenomatous polyps. Painful bleeding associated with a bowel movement is caused by a rectal ulcer or anal fissure. Straining at stool is more often caused by obstructed defecation than hemorrhoids. Similarly, rectal prolapse must be distinguished from hemorrhoids because it is safe to band a hemorrhoid but not a prolapsed rectum. Moisture or maceration may be secondary to hemorrhoids or condylomata acuminata.

Complications

The complications of internal or external hemorrhoids are the indications for medical or surgical treatment: bleeding, pain, necrosis, mucus discharge, moisture, and, rarely, perianal sepsis.

Treatment

A. MEDICAL TREATMENT

Initial medical management is recommended for all but the most advanced cases. Dietary alterations, including elimination of constipating foods (eg, cheese), addition of bulking agents, stool softeners, and increased intake of liquids are advised. It is often beneficial to change daily routines by adding exercise and decreasing time spent on the commode.

B. SURGICAL TREATMENT

First- and second-degree hemorrhoids generally respond to medical management. Hemorrhoids that fail to respond to medical management may be treated with elastic band ligation, sclerosis, photocoagulation, cryosurgery, excisional hemorrhoidectomy, and many other local techniques that induce scarring and fixation of the hemorrhoids to the underlying tissues. The three best techniques—elastic band ligation, sclerosis, and excisional hemorrhoidectomy—are discussed here.

Elastic band ligation is safe and effective in the treatment of first-degree, second-degree, third-degree, and selected fourth-degree hemorrhoids. Hemorrhoidal tissue 1–2 cm above the dentate line is grasped, pulled into the barrel of an elastic band applicator, and two bands are placed at the base of the hemorrhoidal complex. After 7–10 days, the hemorrhoid sloughs away, removing a portion of the offending redundant tissue and leaving a scar that inhibits further prolapse and bleeding of the remaining tissue. If the band is placed in the transitional zone or below, the patient may experience severe pain, as this mucosa and skin are highly innervated. If that happens, the band should be removed immediately. Immunocompromised patients or those with unrecognized rectal prolapse have occasionally developed severe sepsis after banding, a complication heralded by inordinate pain, fever, and urinary retention. Treatment requires intravenous antibiotics, band removal, debridement of necrotic tissue, and observation. Patients are advised to avoid nonsteroidal anti-inflammatory agents and aspirin for 10 days after ligation, since significant bleeding may otherwise occur when the hemorrhoid sloughs.

Injection sclerotherapy is often tried for first-degree and second-degree hemorrhoids that continue to bleed despite medical measures. One to two milliliters of sclerosant is injected into the loose submucosal connective tissue above the hemorrhoidal complex, which causes inflammation and scarring. This inhibits prolapse and bleeding of the remaining hemorrhoidal tissue. The depth of injection is critical, since mucosal sloughing, infection, and full-thickness injury have been reported.

Excisional hemorrhoidectomy is reserved for the larger third- and fourth-degree hemorrhoids, mixed internal and external hemorrhoids not amenable to banding of the internal component, and incarcerated internal hemorrhoids requiring urgent intervention. The base of the hemorrhoid is inspected through an anoscope. The vascular pedicle is suture-ligated with 000 chromic catgut. The hemorrhoidal tissue is excised using a scalpel, scissors, cautery, or laser. Care must be taken to avoid injuring the underlying internal sphincter while dissecting free the vascular cushion and overlying mucosa. The mucosal and skin defect may be left open, may be partially closed, or may be closed with the running the suture used to control the vascular pedicle.

Severe pain, urinary retention, bleeding, and fecal impaction are the most common complications of excisional hemorrhoidectomy. The incidence of these complications can be minimized with improved postoperative pain control, limited intraoperative intravenous fluid administration, attention to surgical technique, and stool bulking agents and stool softeners. Anal stenosis is a long-term complication that may be avoided by leaving enough anoderm between excised hemorrhoidal complexes.

The acutely thrombosed external hemorrhoid may be treated with excision of the hemorrhoid or clot evacuation if the patient presents less than 48 hours after the onset of symptoms. Excision removes the clot and hemorrhoidal tissue, which decreases the chances of recurrence. However, many surgeons simply evacuate the thrombus, relieving the pressure and pain. If the patient presents over 48 hours after the symptoms begin, the thrombus will have started to organize and evacuation will be unsuccessful. Warm sitz baths, a high-fiber diet, stool softeners, and reassurance is the appropriate treatment at this point.

Prognosis

The prognosis for recurrence of hemorrhoidal disease is mostly related to success in changing the patient's bowel habits. Increasing dietary fiber, decreasing constipating foods, introducing exercise, and decreasing time spent on the toilet all decrease the amount of time spent straining in the squatting position. These behav-

ioral modifications are the most important steps in preventing recurrence.

Arbman G et al: Closed vs. open hemorrhoidectomy—is there any difference? Dis Colon Rectum 2000;43:31.

Galizia G et al: Lateral internal sphincterotomy together with haemorrhoidectomy for treatment of haemorrhoids: a randomised prospective study. Eur J Surg 2000 Mar;166:223.

Hayssen TK et al: Limited hemorrhoidectomy: results and long-term follow-up. Dis Colon Rectum 1999;42:909; discussion 914.

Ho YH et al: Randomized controlled trial of open and closed haemorrhoidectomy. Br J Surg 1997;84:1729.

Hoff SD et al: Ambulatory surgical hemorrhoidectomy—a solution to postoperative urinary retention? Dis Colon Rectum 1994;37 :1242.

Johanson JF et al: Epidemiology of fecal incontinence: the silent affliction. Am J Gastroenterol 1996;91:33.

Johanson JF: Association of hemorrhoidal disease with diarrheal disorders: potential pathogenic relationship? Dis Colon Rectum 1997;40:215.

Komborozos VA et al: Rubber band ligation of symptomatic internal hemorrhoids: results of 500 cases. Dig Surg 2000;17:71.

Konsten J et al: Hemorrhoidectomy vs. Lord's method: 17-year follow-up of a prospective, randomized trial. Dis Colon Rectum 2000;43:503.

Lee HH et al: Multiple hemorrhoidal bandings in a single session. Dis Colon Rectum 1994;37:37-41.

Loder PB et al: Haemorrhoids: pathology, pathophysiology and aetiology. Br J Surg 1994;81:946.

MacRae HM et al: Comparison of hemorrhoidal treatment modalities. A meta-analysis. Dis Colon Rectum 1995;38:687.

O'Donovan S et al: Intraoperative use of Toradol facilitates outpatient hemorrhoidectomy. Dis Colon Rectum 1994;37:793.

Pescatori M: Urinary retention after anorectal operations. Dis Colon Rectum 1999;42:964.

ANAL FISSURE & ULCER

 ESSENTIALS OF DIAGNOSIS

- *Tearing pain upon defecation.*
- *Blood on tissue or stool.*
- *Persistent perianal pain or spasm following defecation.*
- *Sphincter spasm.*
- *Disruption of anoderm.*

General Considerations

An anal fissure is a split in the anoderm. An anal ulcer is a chronic fissure. When mature, an ulcer is associated with a skin tag (**sentinel pile**) and a hypertrophied anal papilla (Figure 32–4). Fissures occur in the midline just distal to the dentate line. Two recent studies have called into question Goligher's rule that 90% are posterior, 10% anterior and less than 1% occur simultaneously in the anterior and posterior positions. Both studies found anterior fissures to be more common than expected, but the fissures were still in the midline.

Fissures result from forceful dilation of the anal canal, most commonly during defecation. The anoderm is disrupted, exposing the underlying internal sphincter muscle. The muscle goes into spasm in response to exposure and fails to relax with the next dilation (bowel movement). This leads to further tearing, deepening of the fissure, and increased muscle irritation and spasm. The persistent muscle spasm leads to relative ischemia of the overlying anoderm and inhibits healing. Ultraslow waves—low-frequency high-amplitude pressure changes—occur with increased frequency in patients with anal fissures and disappear with sphincterotomy and fissure healing, suggesting a relationship between spasm and persistent disease.

Classically, the initial insult is felt to be a firm bowel movement. The pain associated with the initial bowel movement is great and the patient therefore ignores the urge to defecate for fear of experiencing the pain again. This allows a harder stool to form which tears the anoderm more as it passes due to its size and the poor relaxation of the sphincter. A self-perpetuating cycle of pain, poor relaxation, and reinjury is the result.

Factors that may predispose to fissure formation are previous anorectal surgery (hemorrhoidectomy, fistulotomy, destruction of condylomas) resulting in scarring of the anoderm with loss of elasticity, which increases the probability that the anoderm will tear.

Hypertrophic papilla

Involved crypt

Anal fissure (ulcer)

Sentinel pile

Anal verge

Rectum

Stenotic anal canal

Figure 32–4. Diagram of the anorectum showing the fissure or ulcer triad.

Clinical Findings

A. SYMPTOMS AND SIGNS

Fissures cause pain and bleeding with defecation. The pain is often tearing or burning, worst during defecation, and subsides over a few hours. Blood is noted on the tissue and stool or dripping into the toilet water but it is not mixed in the stool. Constipation may develop because of fear of recurrent pain. Although less common, fissures may present as painless nonhealing wounds that bleed intermittently.

Although anoscopy and sigmoidoscopy cannot be performed in the initial evaluation of a patient with a fissure, they must be done later because associated anorectal malignancy or inflammatory bowel disease must be excluded. Any nonhealing midline fissure should be biopsied to exclude Crohn's disease or malignancy.

Physical examination by simple gentle traction on the buttocks will evert the anus enough to reveal a disruption of the anoderm in the midline at the mucocutaneous junction. This may be all there is in an acute fissure. In a chronic fissure, a sentinel pile may be seen at the inferior margin of the ulcer. Gentle, limited digital examination will confirm internal sphincter spasm. Anoscopy and proctosigmoidoscopy should be deferred until healing occurs, or alternatively the procedure can be performed under anesthesia. The classic triad of a proximal hypertrophied anal papilla above a fissure with the sentinel pile at the anal verge may be identified.

B. LABORATORY AND IMAGING STUDIES

Anal manometry is unhelpful. Studies have shown increased anal pressures in patients with ulcers, but patients with high pressures have not been found to be at increased risk for fissure-ulcer disease.

Differential Diagnosis

Fissure-ulcer disease occurs in the anterior or posterior midline and involves the epithelium immediately distal to the dentate line. Ulcers occurring off the midline or away from the dentate line are suspect. Crohn's disease, anal tuberculosis, anal malignancy, abscess or fistula disease, cytomegalovirus, herpes, chlamydiosis, syphilis, AIDS, and some blood dyscrasias may all mimic fissure or ulcer disease. Initial manifestations of Crohn's disease are limited to the anal canal in 10% of patients. Anal tuberculosis will be associated with a previous or concomitant history of pulmonary tuberculosis. Anal cancer may present as a painless ulcer. Nonhealing ulcers should be biopsied to rule out malignancy.

Complications

The complications are related to persistence of the disease and its associated pain, bleeding, and alteration in bowel habits. The ulcers do not become malignant.

Treatment

A. MEDICAL TREATMENT

Stool softeners, bulking agents, and sitz baths will heal 90% of anal fissures. A second episode has a 70% chance of healing with this regimen. Sitz baths after painful bowel movements soothe the muscle spasm. Patients are instructed to soak in a hot bath and contract the sphincters to identify the muscle in spasm and to then concentrate on relaxing that muscle. The effect is twofold: it decreases the pain associated with the spasm and improves blood flow to the fissure, which benefits healing. Stool softeners and bulking agents make the stool more malleable, decreasing the trauma of each successive bowel movement. Chronic (> 1 month history) or chronic-recurrent ulcers should be considered for surgery.

Botulinum toxin infiltration into the internal sphincters aids healing of anal fissures. This agent inhibits the release of acetylcholine from presynaptic nerve fibers, creating a reversible paralysis that lasts several months. This allows for improved perfusion of the disrupted anoderm and healing at rates higher than can be achieved with standard medical therapy or topical nitroglycerin ointment therapy.

0.2% nitroglycerin is also effective treatment. Nitroglycerin ointment is a nitric oxide source. Nitric oxide, an inhibitory neurotransmitter, relaxes of the internal sphincter and improve blood flow to the anoderm. The major side effect, headache, persists at the lower therapeutic range (0.2% or 0.3%), causing some to question the utility of this therapy.

B. SURGICAL TREATMENT

Lateral internal anal sphincterotomy is the procedure of choice after conservative measures have failed. This may be performed open, where an incision is made in the skin and the hypertrophied distal one-third of the internal sphincter is divided under direct vision. It may also be done closed, where a scalpel is passed in the intersphincteric plane and swept medially, dividing the internal sphincter blindly. Both techniques given similar results. It is possible to disrupt the internal sphincter with a four-finger stretch, but this is an uncontrolled disruption that is associated with a higher recurrence rate and incontinence.

Prognosis

Lateral internal anal sphincterotomy is over 90 % successful in the treatment of chronic anal fissure-ulcer disease. Fewer than 10% of patients so treated are incontinent to mucus and gas. The recurrence rate is less than 10%.

Altomare DF et al: Glyceryl trinitrate for chronic anal fissure–healing or headache? Results of a multicenter, randomized, placebo-controlled, double-blind trial. Dis Colon Rectum 2000;43:174.

Argov S et al: Open lateral sphincterotomy is still the best treatment for chronic anal fissure. Am J Surg 2000 Mar;179:201.

Brisinda G et al: A comparison of injections of botulinum toxin and topical nitroglycerin ointment for the treatment of chronic anal fissure. N Engl J Med 1999;341:65.

Cook TA et al: Oral nifedipine reduces resting anal pressure and heals chronic anal fissure. Br J Surg 1999;86:1269.

Fernández López F et al: Botulinum toxin for the treatment of anal fissure. Dig Surg 1999;16:515.

Garcia-Aguilar J et al: Open vs. closed sphincterotomy for chronic anal fissure: long-term results. Dis Colon Rectum 1996;39:440.

Hananel N et al: Re-examination of clinical manifestations and response to therapy of fissure-in-ano. Dis Colon Rectum 1997;40:229.

Jost WH: One hundred cases of anal fissure treated with botulin toxin: early and long-term results. Dis Colon Rectum 1997;40:1029.

Keck JO et al. Computer-generated profiles of the anal canal in patients with anal fissure. Dis Colon Rectum 1995;38:72.

Lund JN et al: A randomised, prospective, double-blind, placebo-controlled trial of glyceryl trinitrate ointment in treatment of anal fissure. Lancet 1997;349:11.

Lund JN et al: Aetiology and treatment of anal fissure. Br J Surg 1996;83:1335.

Maria G et al: Botulinum toxin injections in the internal anal sphincter for the treatment of chronic anal fissure: long-term results after two different dosage regimens. Ann Surg 1998;228:664.

Maria G et al: Influence of botulinum toxin site of injections on healing rate in patients with chronic anal fissure. Am J Surg 2000;179:46.

Maria G et al: A comparison of botulinum toxin and saline for the treatment of chronic anal fissure. N Engl J Med 1998;338:217.

Nelson RL: Meta-analysis of operative techniques for fissure-in-ano. Dis Colon Rectum 1999;42:1424;discussion 1428.

Nyam DC et al: Long-term results of lateral internal sphincterotomy for chronic anal fissure with particular reference to incidence of fecal incontinence. Dis Colon Rectum 1999;42:1306.

Oettle GJ: Glyceryl trinitrate vs. sphincterotomy for treatment of chronic fissure- in-ano: a randomized, controlled trial. Dis Colon Rectum 1997;40:1318.

Richard CS et al: Internal sphincterotomy is superior to topical nitroglycerin in the treatment of chronic anal fissure: results of a randomized, controlled trial by the Canadian Colorectal Surgical Trials Group. Dis Colon Rectum 2000;43:1048;

Schouten WR et al: Ischaemic nature of anal fissure. Br J Surg 1996;83:63.

■ INFECTIONS OF THE ANORECTUM

ANORECTAL ABSCESS & FISTULA

ESSENTIALS OF DIAGNOSIS

- *Severe anal pain.*
- *Palpable mass usually present on perineal or digital rectal examination.*
- *Systemic sepsis.*

General Considerations

Perirectal abscess and fistulous disease not associated with a specific systemic disease is most commonly cryptoglandular in origin. The anal canal has 6–14 glands that lie in or near the plane between the internal and external sphincters. Projections from the glands pass through the internal sphincters and drain into the crypts at the dentate line. Glands may become infected when a crypt is occluded, trapping stool and bacteria within the gland. Occlusion may follow impaction of vegetable matter or edema from trauma (firm stool or foreign body) or as a result of an adjacent inflammatory process. If the crypt does not decompress into the anal canal, an abscess may develop in the intersphincteric plane. The abscess may track within or across the intersphincteric plane. Abscesses are classified according to the space they invade (Figure 32–5). The most difficult to treat occurs when the abscess tracks proximally or circumferentially within the intersphincteric plane. Regardless of location, the extent of an abscess may be difficult to determine without examination under anesthesia.

Antibiotics given while allowing the abscess to mature are not helpful. Early surgical operative drainage is the best way to avoid the potentially disastrous complications of undrained perineal sepsis. When the abscesses are drained, either surgically or spontaneously, 50% have persistent communication with the crypt, creating a fistula from the anus to the perianal skin (fistula-in-ano). A fistula-in-ano is not a surgical emergency.

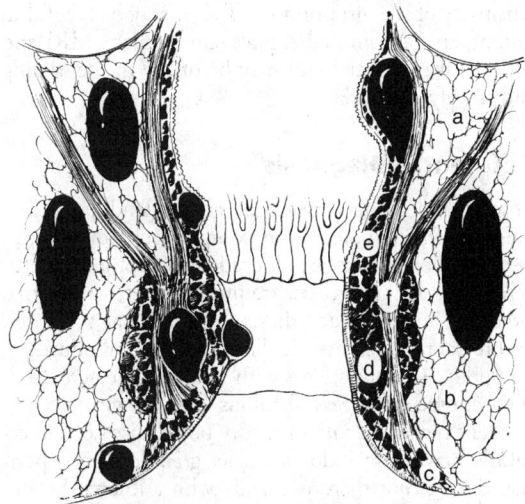

Figure 32–5. Composite diagram of acute anorectal abscesses and spaces. (a) Pelvirectal (supralevator) space. (b) Ischiorectal space. (c) Perianal (subcutaneous) space. (d) Marginal (mucocutaneous) space. (e) Submucous space. (f) Intermuscular space.

Clinical Findings

A. SYMPTOMS AND SIGNS

An anorectal abscess typically causes severe and continuous throbbing pain that may worsen with ambulation and straining. Swelling and discharge are noted less frequently. Occasional patients present with fever, urinary retention, and life-threatening sepsis. People with diabetes mellitus or immune compromise are most vulnerable. A patient with fistula-in-ano may report a history of severe pain, bloody purulent drainage associated with resolution of the pain, and subsequent chronic mucopurulent discharge.

Physical examination reveals a tender perianal or rectal mass. The size is often difficult to assess until the patient is anesthetized. An apparently small abscess may extend high into the ischiorectal or supralevator space. A fistula is present when internal and external openings are identified. A firm connecting tract is often palpable.

B. LABORATORY AND IMAGING STUDIES

No imaging studies are necessary in uncomplicated abscess fistulous disease. Sinograms, transrectal ultrasound, CT, and MRI may be useful in the evaluation of complex or recurrent disease. Transrectal ultrasound can identify branching of fistulous tracts, persistent undrained sepsis, and extent of sphincter involvement. Hydrogen peroxide injection of the tract may improve sensitivity of the ultrasound. CT scan may be helpful in finding an undiagnosed supralevator abscess. MRI and MRI with endorectal coil may be of use in identifying and classifying fistulas.

Differential Diagnosis

Abscess and fistula disease of cryptoglandular origin must be differentiated from complications of Crohn's disease, pilonidal disease, hidradenitis suppurativa, tuberculosis, actinomycosis, trauma, fissures, carcinoma, radiation injury, chlamydiosis, local dermal processes, retrorectal tumors, diverticulitis, and urethral injuries.

About 10% of patients with Crohn's disease present with anorectal abscess fistulous disease with no antecedent history of inflammatory bowel disease. Tuberculosis may cause indolent, pale, granulomatous perianal disease, but there is usually with a known history of tuberculosis. Hidradenitis suppurativa gives multiple chronic, draining fistulas, as might be seen with undiagnosed horseshoe abscess fistula disease. Pilonidal disease may extend toward the perineum; it is distinguished from cryptoglandular disease by the presence of inspissated hairs, the direction of the tract, and the presence of other openings in the sacrococcygeal area. A colonic source may be suspected in a patient with known inflammatory bowel disease or diverticular disease. Other less common causes include tumors, radiation, infections, and urologic injuries.

Complications

The complications of an undrained anorectal abscess may be severe. Unless drained, the infection may spread rapidly, and result in extensive tissue loss, sphincter injury, and even death. In contrast, a fistula-in-ano, which develops when the abscess is drained, is not a surgical emergency. A chronic fistula may be associated with recurring perianal abscess formation and, rarely, with cancer of the fistulous tract.

Treatment

Abscesses should be drained surgically. It is best done in the operating room, where anesthesia allows adequate evaluation of the extent of disease. Abscesses thought to be superficial in the office may be found to extend above the levators. Intersphincteric abscesses are treated by an internal sphincterotomy that drains the abscess and destroys the crypt. Perirectal and ischiorectal abscesses should be drained by a catheter or with adequate excision of skin to prevent premature closure and reaccumulation of the abscess. If the internal opening of the fistula is identified and external sphincter involvement is minimal, a fistulotomy may be performed when the

abscess is drained. However, the internal opening is often hard to find because of the inflammation, and drainage is all that can be achieved. In this instance, catheter drainage is preferred to skin excision since the catheter (1) establishes drainage with minimal disruption of normal perianal skin, (2) facilitates identification of the internal opening at subsequent evaluation, and (3) facilitates patient compliance by eliminating the need for packing or leaving the wound open.

Patients with chronic or recurring abscesses after apparent adequate surgical drainage often have an undrained deep postanal space abscess that communicates with the ischiorectal fossa via a horseshoe fistula. Treatment involves opening the deep postanal space and counter-draining the tract through the ischiorectal external opening. Once the postanal space heals, the counter drain may be removed.

Immunocompromised patients are a particular challenge. With moderately compromise, (e.g., diabetes mellitus) urgent drainage in the operating room is required, as these patients are prone to necrotizing anorectal infections. With severe compromise (e.g., patients receiving chemotherapy), infection may be occur without an abscess due to neutropenia. In these patients it is important to attempt to localize the process, establish drainage, localize the internal opening, and obtain a biopsy for tissue examination and culture (to rule out leukemia and to select antibiotics).

The treatment of fistulas is dictated by the course of the fistula. The Salmon-Goodsall rule is of assistance in identifying the direction of the tract (Figure 32–6). If

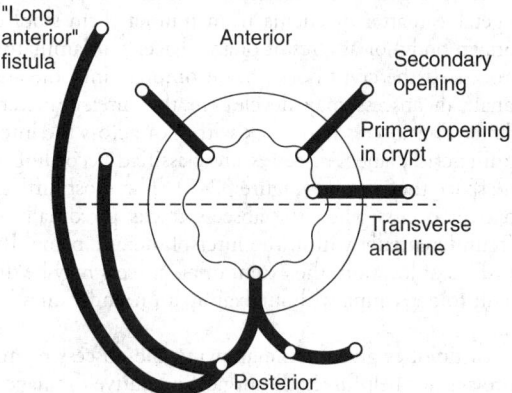

Figure 32–6. Salmon-Goodsall rule. The usual relation of the primary and secondary openings of fistulas. When there is an anterior and also a posterior opening of the same fistula, the rule of the posterior opening applies; the long anterior fistula is an exception to the rule.

the tract passes superficially and does not involve sphincter muscle, a simple incision of the tract with ablation of the gland and saucerization of the skin at the external opening is all that is necessary. A fistula that involves a small amount of sphincter may be treated similarly. A tract that passes deep or that involves an undetermined amount of muscle is best treated with a mucosal advancement flap (described in the section on rectovaginal fistulas) because immediate or delayed (as with a seton) muscle division is associated with a high rate of incontinence.

Prognosis

The prognosis for cryptoglandular abscess and fistula disease is excellent once the source of infection is identified. Fistulas persist when the source has not been identified or adequately drained, when the diagnosis is incorrect, or when postoperative care is insufficient.

Brook I et al: The aerobic and anaerobic bacteriology of perirectal abscesses. J Clin Microbiol 1997;35:2974.

Chapple KS et al: Prognostic value of magnetic resonance imaging in the management of fistula-in-ano. Dis Colon Rectum 2000;43: 511.

Cho DY: Endosonographic criteria for an internal opening of fistula-in-ano. Dis Colon Rectum 1999;42:515.

Cintron JR et al: Repair of fistulas-in-ano using fibrin adhesive: long-term follow-up. Dis Colon Rectum 2000;43:944;

Garcia-Aguilar J et al: Anal fistula surgery. Factors associated with recurrence and incontinence. Dis Colon Rectum 1996; 39:723.

Ho YH et al: Marsupialization of fistulotomy wounds improves healing: a randomized controlled trial. Br J Surg 1998; 85:105.

Jun SH et al: Anocutaneous advancement flap closure of high anal fistulas. Br J Surg 1999;86:490.

Knoefel WT et al: The initial approach to anorectal abscesses: fistulotomy is safe and reduces the chance of recurrences. Dig Surg 2000;17: 274-8.

Miller GV et al: Flap advancement and core fistulectomy for complex rectal fistula. Br J Surg 1998;85: 108-10.

Nelson RL et al: Dermal island-flap anoplasty for transsphincteric fistula-in-ano: assessment of treatment failures. Dis Colon Rectum 2000;43:681.

Park JJ et al: Repair of chronic anorectal fistulae using commercial fibrin sealant. Arch Surg 2000;135:166.

Practice parameters for treatment of fistula-in-ano—supporting documentation. The Standards Practice Task Force. The American Society of Colon and Rectal Surgeons. Dis Colon Rectum 1996;39:1363.

RECTOVAGINAL FISTULA

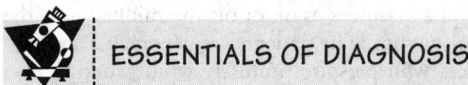

ESSENTIALS OF DIAGNOSIS

- *Passing stool and flatus through the vagina.*
- *Altered continence.*
- *Tract generally visible or palpable.*

General Considerations

Rectovaginal fistulas occur as a result of obstetric injury, Crohn's disease, diverticulitis, radiation, undrained cryptoglandular disease, foreign body trauma, surgical extirpation of anterior rectal tumors, and malignancies of the rectum, cervix, or vagina. The fistulas are classified as low, middle, or high. The location and cause of the fistula determine the operative approach.

Clinical Findings

A. SYMPTOMS AND SIGNS

Passing stool and flatus through the vagina is characteristic of rectovaginal fistulas. There may be varying degrees of incontinence. An opening in the vagina or rectum may be seen or felt on physical examination.

B. LABORATORY AND IMAGING STUDIES

A vaginogram or barium enema may identify the fistula. If the fistula is not demonstrated on radiographic or physical examination, a dilute methylene blue enema may be administered with a tampon in the vagina. If a fistula is present, it should be confirmed by methylene blue staining of the tampon.

Differential Diagnosis

The signs and symptoms of a rectovaginal fistula are fairly unmistakable. The important differential is the cause of the fistula, as this affects management, as discussed below.

Complications

The major complication of a rectovaginal fistula is impaired hygiene and incontinence.

Treatment

The cause and location of the fistula determine the treatment. Involvement of surrounding tissue by the disease process that leads to the fistula may limit the surgical options. For example, in patients with active Crohn's disease or radiation injury of the surrounding tissue, the fistula cannot be repaired with local procedures; Crohn's disease must go into remission before a fistula can be repaired. Radiation injuries require that normal healthy tissue be brought from outside the irradiated field.

Low rectovaginal fistulas (rectal opening near the dentate line and vaginal opening just above the fourchette) commonly result from obstetric injuries, trauma from foreign bodies, cryptoglandular disease, or Crohn's disease. Obstetric injuries often heal within the first 3 months. Waiting 3 months allows inflammation to resolve, which facilitates repair and allows for closure of those fistulas that will spontaneously heal. Similarly, traumatic fistulas may be repaired most easily after inflammation resolves. Fistulas secondary to cryptoglandular disease may close spontaneously once the primary process is drained.

Fistulas secondary to Crohn's disease rarely heal spontaneously. Aggressive medical therapy and surgical control of perianal sepsis are necessary to conserve the sphincters. Once the disease is in remission, local advancement flap procedures may be performed. The principle is to bring fresh, uninvolved tissue down over the fistulous tract and excise the old rectal opening. This often delays proctectomy and preserves the anal sphincter and rectum. Patients with severe disease that does not respond to local measures may require a temporary diverting colostomy. After diversion, a single focus of disease is often found and an advancement procedure may be performed while the fecal stream is diverted. Extensive destruction of the rectum or sphincters may mandate immediate proctectomy without attempts at local preservation. Early surgical intervention and conservative drainage or diversion may postpone this situation.

Midrectal fistulas from cryptoglandular disease, Crohn's disease, or obstetric injury should be treated as outlined above. Those that occur secondary to radiation are not amenable to local procedures, as the surrounding tissue is similarly affected. Transabdominal resection and coloanal anastomosis is preferred. These are particularly challenging patients. Other surgical options are beyond the scope of this chapter.

High rectal fistulas result from Crohn's disease, diverticular disease, operative injury, malignancy, and radiation. High rectovaginal fistulas are best treated via a transabdominal approach. This allows for resection of the diseased bowel that created the fistula.

Prognosis

The prognosis is determined by the cause of the fistula.

Fry RD et al: Rectovaginal fistula. Surg Ann 1995;27:113.

Hull TL et al: Surgical approaches to low anovaginal fistula in Crohn's disease. Am J Surg 1997;173:95.

Hyman N: Endoanal advancement flap repair for complex anorectal fistula. Am J Surg 1999;178:337.

Khanduja KS et al: Reconstruction of rectovaginal fistula with sphincter disruption by combining rectal mucosal advancement flap and anal sphincteroplasty. Dis Colon Rectum 1999;42:1432.

Marchesa P et al: Advancement sleeve flaps for treatment of severe perianal Crohn's disease. Br J Surg 1998;85:1695.

Ozuner G et al: Long-term analysis of the use of transanal rectal advancement flaps for complicated anorectal/vaginal fistulas. Dis Colon Rectum 1996;39:10.

Simmang CL et al: Rectal sleeve advancement: repair of rectovaginal fistula associated with anorectal stricture in Crohn's disease. Dis Colon Rectum 1998;41:787.

Tsang CB et al: Anal sphincter integrity and function influences outcome in rectovaginal fistula repair. Dis Colon Rectum 1998;41:1141.

Tsang CB et al: Rectovaginal fistulas. Therapeutic options. Surg Clin North Am 1997;77:95.

Venkatesh KS et al: Fibrin glue application in the treatment of recurrent anorectal fistulas. Dis Colon Rectum 1999;42:1136.

Yee LF et al: Use of endoanal ultrasound in patients with rectovaginal fistulas. Dis Colon Rectum 1999;42:1057.

PILONIDAL DISEASE

 ESSENTIALS OF DIAGNOSIS

- *Acute chronic recurring abscess or chronic draining sinus over the sacrococcygeal or perianal region.*
- *Pain, tenderness, purulent drainage, inspissated hair, induration.*

General Considerations

The incidence of pilonidal disease is highest in white males (3:1 male:female ratio) between ages 15 and 40 with a peak incidence between 16 and 20 years. It was once thought that pilonidal disease was a congenital condition that developed along an epithelialized tract of the natal cleft. It is now considered to be an acquired infection of natal cleft hair follicles which become distended and obstructed and rupture into the subcutaneous tissues to form a pilonidal abscess. Hair from the surrounding skin is pulled into the abscess cavity by the friction generated by the gluteal muscles during walking.

Clinical Findings

Patients with pilonidal disease may present with small midline pits or abscesses on or off the midline near the coccyx or sacrum. The patients are generally heavy hirsute males who perspire profusely while working in a hot dirty environment. The workup is limited to a physical examination unless one suspects Crohn's disease, in which case a more extensive evaluation may be necessary. Physical examination may reveal a spectrum of disease from acute suppuration and an undrained abscess or chronic draining sinuses with multiple mature tracts with hairs protruding from the pit-like openings.

Differential Diagnosis

The differential diagnosis includes cryptoglandular abscess-fistulous disease of the anus, hidradenitis suppurativa, furuncle, and actinomycosis.

Complications

Untreated pilonidal disease may result in multiple draining sinuses with chronic recurrent abscess, drainage, soiling of clothing, and, rarely, necrotizing wound infections or malignant degeneration.

Treatment

Pilonidal abscesses may be drained under local anesthesia. A probe may be inserted into the primary opening and the abscess unroofed. Granulation tissue and inspissated hair are pulled out, but definitive therapy is not required at the first procedure. Cure rates of 60–80% have been reported after primary unroofing and extraction of hair. For those that fail to heal after 3 months or develop a chronic draining sinus, definitive therapy may be considered.

Nonoperative therapy with meticulous skin care (shaving of the natal cleft, perineal hygiene) and drainage of abscesses will substantially reduce the need for surgery.

Conservative excision of midline pits with removal of hair from lateral tracts and postoperative weekly shaving has 90% success rate. Excision with open packing, marsupialization, or primary closure with or without flaps have all been advocated. Either open packing or marsupialization leaves the patient with painful wounds slow to heal, and marsupialization has a reported recurrence rate of 10%. Our preference is to excise the pilonidal disease and close the defect primarily with rotation flaps over closed suction drainage. Simple primary closure often results in dehiscence because the midline skin has a poor blood supply, the wounds are closed under tension, and there is often dead space at the base of the defect that is susceptible to infection.

Prognosis

The prognosis after surgery is excellent. Recurrent or persistent disease may occur after inadequate excision where external openings or occult tracts are missed. Inadequate postoperative hygiene with ingrowth of hair into the wound also leads to recurrence.

Abu Galala KH et al: Treatment of pilonidal sinus by primary closure with a transposed rhomboid flap compared with deep suturing: a prospective randomised clinical trial. Eur J Surg 1999;165:468.

Akinci OF et al: Simple and effective surgical treatment of pilonidal sinus: asymmetric excision and primary closure using suction drain and subcuticular skin closure. Dis Colon Rectum 2000; 43:701;

Armstrong JH et al: Pilonidal sinus disease. The conservative approach. Arch Surg 1994;129: 914;

Bozkurt MK et al: Management of pilonidal sinus with the Limberg flap. Dis Colon Rectum 1998;41:775.

Senapati A et al: Bascom's operation in the day-surgical management of symptomatic pilonidal sinus. Br J Surg 2000; 87:1067.

Spivak H et al: Treatment of chronic pilonidal disease. Dis Colon Rectum 1996;39:1136.

PRURITUS ANI

 ESSENTIALS OF DIAGNOSIS

- *Severe perianal itching, often at night.*
- *When chronic, skin becomes white, leathery, and thickened.*

General Considerations

Pruritus ani is usually idiopathic. Most patients have tried many over-the-counter preparations without relief. These agents may exacerbate the problem by keeping the perineum moist, causing further irritation, or by creating a contact dermatitis (especially local anesthetics). Poor cleansing of the perineum may lead to irritation of the exquisitely sensitive anoderm and subsequent pruritus. In contrast, frequent washing with soaps and detergents dries the skin, also leading to pruritus. Pinworms *(Enterobius vermicularis)* are the most common cause of perianal itching in children.

Clinical Findings

A. Symptoms and Signs

The patient experiences severe perianal itching, often worse at night. The skin is thickened, white, and leathery in the chronic state but may be normal to weeping in the acute stage. In children with pinworms, perianal itching is most severe at night when the pinworm deposits its eggs on the perianal skin.

B. Laboratory and Imaging Studies

The diagnosis of pinworms is made by applying cellophane tape to the perianal skin, which collects the eggs and allows them to be viewed under a microscope. Scrapings of the perianal skin viewed microscopically may reveal fungi or parasites. Biopsy and histologic evaluation may be necessary in refractory cases to rule out underlying malignancy.

Differential Diagnosis

Pruritus may be associated with other perianal lesions that distort normal anal anatomy such as hemorrhoids, fistulas, fissures, tumors of the anorectum, previous surgery, and radiation therapy. As noted above, it may be secondary to excessive cleaning or application of ointments to the perianal region. Primary dermatologic diseases such as lichen planus, atopic eczema, psoriasis, and seborrheic dermatitis may all affect the perineum. Fungal (dermatophytosis, candidiasis), parasitic (*Enterobius vermicularis,* scabies, or pediculosis) and bacterial superinfection should be considered. Other causes including contact dermatitis from local anesthetic creams or soaps, recent antibiotic usage, systemic diseases (diabetes, liver disease), dietary factors, and perianal neoplasms (Bowen's disease and extramammary Paget's disease). Pruritus may result from tight clothing, obesity, and living in a hot climate. When a specific cause cannot be found, it is considered idiopathic.

Complications

Complications include severe excoriation, ulceration, and secondary infection of the perineum.

Treatment

Identifiable causes of pruritus ani such as hemorrhoids, yeast infection, or parasites should be treated. Patients should be educated about proper perineal care, and the use of soaps and topical ointments should be discouraged. The perineum should be kept dry. Use of a blow dryer on the perineum after bathing may be helpful. Alteration in dietary habits may be necessary. Coffee, tea, cola drinks, beer, chocolate, and tomatoes cause perianal itching and should be excluded from the diet for at least 2 weeks. Symptoms should resolve with alterations in dietary and cleaning habits. After symptoms resolve, each food group may be added sequentially to identify the causative agent.

Prognosis

Relapse is common, and reeducation is often effective. In refractory cases, dermatologic and psychiatric consultation may be necessary.

PROCTITIS & ANUSITIS

Proctitis and anusitis are nonspecific terms for varying degrees of inflammation due to infectious or inflammatory diseases. The causative agent or event determines the symptoms, signs, and appropriate management. In considering these diseases, particular attention should be paid to sexual practices and sexually transmitted diseases.

1. Herpes Proctitis

Lesions appear as vesicles, which rupture to form ulcers that may become secondarily infected. Patients may present early with anal pain and vesicles or later with ulcerations, discharge, rectal bleeding, tenesmus, and even fear of defecation because of severe pain. Fever and generalized malaise are often noted. No history of anoreceptive intercourse is required, as the disease may spread by extension from the vagina. Viral culture of the vesicle or biopsy of the ulcer is diagnostic. Herpes simplex type 2 is most common.

Oral acyclovir is the treatment of choice but is not curative. It decreases the duration of outbreaks and viral shedding and increases the interval between attacks. The first episode is associated with the most pain and longest duration of ulceration. Subsequent episodes are generally shorter and not as painful.

2. Anorectal Syphilis

The chancre is an indurated, nontender perianal ulcer at the site of inoculation. Proctitis, pseudotumors, and condylomata lata may also be present. Condylomata lata are contiguous hypertrophic papules associated with secondary syphilis. Darkfield microscopy of exudate and serologic testing are the preferred methods of diagnosis. Serologic tests may initially be negative and should be repeated several months later.

Penicillin is the treatment of choice. The prognosis is good. Contacts must be sought and treated.

3. Gonococcal Proctitis

Symptoms range from none to painful defecation. Rectal bleeding and discharge, perianal excoriation, and fistulas may develop. The mucosa may appear friable and edematous. Cultures of the anus, vagina, urethra, and pharynx should be obtained and plated on Thayer-Martin medium. The gram-negative diplococcus *Neisseria gonorrhoeae* is the causative agent.

Intramuscular procaine penicillin G and oral probenecid is the treatment of choice. Resistant strains should be treated with spectinomycin. Follow-up examination and cultures should be performed to confirm adequate therapy. The prognosis is excellent.

4. Chlamydial Proctitis & Lymphogranuloma Venereum

As in gonococcal proctitis, the symptoms of chlamydial proctitis range from none to rectal pain, bleeding, and discharge. The small shallow ulcer of lymphogranuloma venereum (LGV) may go unnoticed, but the inguinal adenopathy may become quite marked. Late findings include hemorrhagic proctitis and rectal stricture. The causative agent is *Chlamydia trachomatis,* an intracellular parasite spread by anal intercourse or direct extension through the lymphatics of the rectovaginal septum. The diagnosis is made with the LGV complement fixation test. Tissue cultures are also used.

Treatment with 21 days of tetracycline is recommended, but erythromycin is an acceptable alternative. Early strictures may be dilated. Although uncommon, strictures may cause bowel obstruction and require colostomy.

5. Condylomata Acuminata

Human papilloma virus (HPV) is the cause of condylomata acuminata. Multiple types have been identified. Types HPV-6 and HPV-11 are associated with the common benign genital wart, whereas HPV-16 and HPV-18 are associated with the development of high-grade anal dysplasia and anal cancer. In the United States, condyloma acuminatum is the most common sexually transmitted viral disease, with 1 million new cases reported per year. It is the most common anorectal infection of homosexual men and is particularly prevalent in HIV-positive patients. However, the disease is not limited to men or women who practice anoreceptive intercourse. In women, the virus may track down from the vagina, and in men it may pool and track from the base of the scrotum. Immunosuppression, either from drugs after transplantation or from HIV, increases susceptibility to condylomatous disease with prevalence rates of 5% and 85%, respectively.

Clinical Findings

A. SYMPTOMS AND SIGNS

The most frequent complaint is that of a perianal growth. Pruritus, discharge, bleeding, odor, and anal pain are present to a lesser degree. Physical examination reveals the classic cauliflower-like lesion, which may be isolated, clustered, or coalescent. The warts tend to run in radial rows out from the anus. The lesions may be surprisingly large at the time of presentation.

B. LABORATORY AND IMAGING STUDIES

Anoscopy and proctosigmoidoscopy are essential because the disease extends internally in more than three-fourths of patients and because intra-anal disease is present in 95% of cases in homosexual men. Material for cultures and serologic tests for other venereal diseases may be taken from the penis, anus, mouth, and vagina.

Differential Diagnosis

These lesions must be distinguished from condylomata lata the lesions of secondary syphilis and anal squamous cell carcinoma. Condylomata are flatter, paler, and smoother than condylomata acuminata. Anal squamous cell carcinoma is generally painful and may be tender and ulcerated where condylomas are not tender or ulcerated.

Complications

Squamous cell carcinoma of the anal canal is the major complication.

Treatment & Prognosis

The extent of the disease and the risk of malignancy determine the treatment. Minimal disease is treated in the office with topical agents such as bichloracetic acid or 25% podophyllum resin in tincture of benzoin. The former is preferred and there are fewer complications (scaring) because the latter must be washed off within 4–6 hours to limit pain. The warts respond promptly to therapy. Patients should be seen at regular intervals until resolution is complete. More extensive disease may require an initial treatment session under anesthesia so that random lesions can be excised for pathologic evaluation to rule out dysplasia and the remainder coagulated. Electrocautery coagulates the lesions. Care is taken to spare surrounding skin. Follow-up evaluation may reveal residual disease, but this is often easily treated with topical agents in the office.

Laser therapy is another method of condyloma destruction. Recurrence rates are low, but the equipment is expensive.

Refractory disease may respond to excision or destruction followed by intralesional interferon or autogenous vaccine created from excisional biopsies of the lesions. Recurrence rates of only 5% have been reported for destruction and vaccination combined, but preparation of the vaccine is tedious so this technique has not gained wide acceptance.

Human papilloma viruses 16 and 18 are causally associated with squamous cell carcinomas of the anal canal. This association has led to new screening techniques to evaluate high-risk patients for occult disease. These techniques are discussed below in the section on anal cancer. Representative biopsies of clinically apparent condylomas should be sent for pathologic study because unsuspected low-grade or high-grade dysplasia or squamous cell carcinoma of the anal canal may be found.

Buschke-Löwenstein tumors are giant condylomata acuminata which are locally aggressive and exhibit malignant behavior but benign histology. Radical excision is often the only therapeutic option for either palliation or cure. Wide local excision and even surgery with adjuvant chemotherapy and radiotherapy have been used with success.

6. Chancroid

Haemophilus ducreyi causes a soft perianal ulcer that is painful, often multiple, and bleeds easily. Autoinoculation is common. Inguinal lymph nodes become fluctuant, rupture, and drain. Cultures are diagnostic.

Treatment options include azithromycin, 1 g orally in a single dose; or ceftriaxone, 250 mg intramuscularly in a single dose; or ciprofloxacin, 500 mg orally twice daily for 3 days; or erythromycin base, 500 mg orally four times daily for 7 days. All are effective.

7. Inflammatory Proctitis

Inflammatory proctitis is a mild form of ulcerative colitis that is limited to the rectum. Rectal bleeding, discharge, diarrhea, and tenesmus are common. The rectal mucosa is inflamed and friable, but the remainder of the colon appears normal on examination. The disease course is often self-limited. Only about 10% of patients ever develop colonic manifestations of ulcerative colitis. Biopsies are taken at endoscopy to rule out infectious processes and Crohn's disease.

An infectious process must be ruled out before initiating steroid therapy. Distinguishing between Crohn's disease and inflammatory proctitis may be difficult. Lack of response to appropriate therapy calls for reassessment of the patient.

Steroid retention enemas are given for 2 weeks. If there is no response, a short course of oral steroids may be given. In addition, mesalamine (5-aminosalicylic acid) may be given orally or rectally in an enema or suppository. Patients should avoid milk and milk products, fruit, and dietary fiber. The disease usually responds to these measures and resolves rapidly.

8. Radiation Proctitis

Radiation proctitis in a patient with a history of radiation to the rectum is manifested early by diarrhea, rectal bleeding, discharge, tenesmus, pain, and incontinence. Late disease may develop months to years after the injury. Symptoms of late disease are secondary to strictures, fistulas, and telangiectasias, which may present as recurrent urinary tract infections, vaginal discharge, fecal incontinence, rectal bleeding, changes in stool caliber, and constipation. The symptoms include bleeding, change in bowel habits, urinary tract infections, and vaginal discharge. Endoscopy may reveal friable edematous mucosa, telangiectasias, or strictures and may show internal openings of fistulas.

Initial therapy includes bulk-forming agents, antidiarrheals, and antispasmodics. Topical steroids, mesalamine preparations, misoprostol suppositories, and short-chain fatty acids have all been used in acute and chronic disease. Dilatation of strictures and laser coagulation of telangiectasias are useful in late disease. The key to surgical success in treating fistulas to the bladder or vagina is interposition or transposition of healthy nonirradiated tissue into the field. Only infrequently is the rectum so badly irradiated that it must be removed. The prognosis, therefore, is good.

Babb RR: Radiation proctitis: a review. Am J Gastroenterol 1996 Jul;91:1309.

Bjork M et al: Giant condyloma acuminatum (Buschke-Löwenstein tumor) of the anorectum with malignant transformation. Eur J Surg 1995;161:691.

Breese PL et al: Anal human papillomavirus infection among homosexual and bisexual men: prevalence of type-specific infection and association with human immunodeficiency virus. Sex Transm Dis 1995;22:7.

Counter SF et al: Prospective evaluation of formalin therapy for radiation proctitis. Am J Surg 1999;177:396.

El-Attar SM et al: Anal warts, sexually transmitted diseases, and anorectal conditions associated with human immunodeficiency virus. Prim Care 1999;26:81.

Fantin AC et al: Argon beam coagulation for treatment of symptomatic radiation-induced proctitis. Gastrointest Endosc 1999;49(4 Part 1):515.

Hemminki K et al: Cancer in husbands of cervical cancer patients. Epidemiology 2000;11:347.

Khan AM et al: A prospective randomized placebo-controlled double-blinded pilot study of misoprostol rectal suppositories in the prevention of acute and chronic radiation proctitis symptoms in prostate cancer patients. Am J Gastroenterol 2000;951961.

Kobal B: Herpes simplex genitalis type 2: our experiences. Clin Exp Obstet Gynec 1999;26:123.

1998 guidelines for treatment of sexually transmitted diseases. Centers for Disease Control and Prevention. MMWR Morb Mortal Wkly Rep 1998;47(RR-1):1.

Palefsky JM et al: Virologic, immunologic, and clinical parameters in the incidence and progression of anal squamous intraepithelial lesions in HIV-positive and HIV-negative homosexual men. J Acquir Immune Defic Syndr 1998;17:314.

Palefsky JM: Anal squamous intraepithelial lesions in human immunodeficiency virus-positive men and women. Semin Oncol 2000;27:471.

Palefsky JM: Anal squamous intraepithelial lesions: relation to HIV and human papillomavirus infection. J Acquir Immune Defic Syndr 1999;21(Suppl 1):S42.

Pinto A et al: Short chain fatty acids are effective in short-term treatment of chronic radiation proctitis: randomized, double-blind, controlled trial. Dis Colon Rectum 1999;42:788;

Rompalo AM: Diagnosis and treatment of sexually acquired proctitis and proctocolitis: an update. Clin Infect Dis 1999;28 (Suppl 1):S84.

Saclarides TJ et al: Formalin instillation for refractory radiation-induced hemorrhagic proctitis. Report of 16 patients. Dis Colon Rectum 1996;39:196.

Tabet SR et al: Incidence of HIV and sexually transmitted diseases (STD) in a cohort of HIV-negative men who have sex with men (MSM). AIDS 1998;12:2041.

Talley NA et al: Short-chain fatty acids in the treatment of radiation proctitis: a randomized, double-blind, placebo-controlled, cross-over pilot trial. Dis Colon Rectum 1997; 40:1046.

Taylor JG et al: KTP laser therapy for bleeding from chronic radiation proctopathy. Gastrointest Endosc 199 2000;52:353.

Wiltz OH et al: Autogenous vaccine: the best therapy for perianal condyloma acuminata? Dis Colon Rectum 1995;38:838.

FECAL IMPACTION

Fecal impaction may develop after excisional hemorrhoidectomy, in chronically debilitated patients, or from the use of constipating pain medications without stool softeners and fiber. In the hemorrhoidectomy population, preserving adequate anoderm between hemorrhoidal complexes minimizes the incidence of this complication. Postoperative pain control is essential because otherwise fear of defecation may develop. Limited use of constipating opioids, addition of nonsteroidal medications, stool bulking agents (fiber), and stool softeners will minimize the incidence of fecal impaction.

All hospitalized and postoperative patients are at risk for developing fecal impaction because of limitations on physical activity, disruption of dietary and bowel habits, and initiation of constipating medications (opioids, calcium channel blockers, etc). Thus, patients at risk who do not suffer from diarrhea should be started on stool softeners and fiber bulking agents to avoid this complication. Enemas and laxatives may be given as needed.

Patients with fecal impaction commonly present with diarrhea as only liquid stool is able to pass the obstructing inspissated fecal bolus. Some may complain of pelvic pain with episodic severe spasms from the pressure of the mass on the pelvic floor. Digital rectal examination may reveal hard, dry stool that obstructs the rectum. Abdominal examination may reveal a pelvic or abdominal mass much like a gravid uterus.

Once detected, a fecal impaction may be digitally dislodged at the bedside, but treatment in the operating room with local or regional anesthesia may be necessary to provide pelvic floor relaxation and pain control. At completion of disimpaction, sigmoidoscopy is necessary to rule out an obstructing inflammatory or malignant mass or rectal injury incurred during the procedure.

Prather CM et al: Evaluation and treatment of constipation and fecal impaction in adults. Mayo Clin Proc 1998;73:881.

Tiongco FP et al: Use of oral GoLytely solution in relief of refractory fecal impaction. Dig Dis Sci 1997;42:1454.

ANAL & PERIANAL NEOPLASMS

Tumors of the anal canal account for 1.5% of malignancies of the gastrointestinal tract, with about 3400 new cases annually in the United States. The incidence has been increasing over the last 30 years. Chronic anal irritation has historically been related to the development of anal cancer, but there is an etiologic relationship between chronic infection with the human papilloma virus and the development of anal cancer. Women are at increased risk for anal canal cancer, presumably because the virus may pool in the vagina and track down to the anus. Women also may practice anoreceptive intercourse in heterosexual relationships. Although in general women are at increased risk for anal cancer ($9:10^6$ versus $7:10^6$ women versus men, respectively), in HIV-negative and HIV-positive men who have sex with men the incidence is $36:10^5$ and $70;10^5$, respectively. Other factors associated with an increased risk for anal cancer are anogenital warts, a history of sexually transmitted disease, more than 10 sexual partners (but if one has HPV, only one is necessary), a history of cervical, vulvar, or vaginal cancer, immunosuppression (HIV-positive or transplantation), long-term corticosteroids, and cigarette smoking.

Although women are at increased risk for anal canal cancer, this is not true of anal margin carcinoma, where men are at greater risk (4:1). This difference highlights the importance of classification based on anatomic landmarks such as the dentate line, the anal verge, and the anal sphincters. These landmarks distinguish tumors of the anal margin from tumors of the anal canal. Unfortunately the literature is not clear with regard to these landmarks, and efforts have been made by the World Health Organization and the American Joint Committee on Cancer (AJCC) to establish anatomic landmarks to distinguish tumors of the anal canal from tumors of the anal margin. The found definitions is as follows the anal canal extends from the upper to the lower border of the internal anal sphincter (from the pelvic floor to the anal verge). Anal margin tumors occur outside the anal verge but presumably within a

5–6 cm radius of the anus. Tumors of the anal canal tend to be aggressive, nonkeratinizing, and associated with HPV infection. Tumors of the anal margin are generally well-differentiated keratinizing tumors that behave similarly to other squamous cell carcinomas of the skin and are treated accordingly.

Staging of anal and perianal malignancies is clinical. Physical examination with digital rectal examination, paying attention to pararectal nodes, anoscopy, bilateral groin palpation, biopsy (examination under anesthesia, if necessary), endorectal ultrasound, CT, and MRI are used as needed to assess tumor size and establish nodal and distant disease. The AJCC staging classification for anal canal and anal margin tumors is presented in Table 32–1.

TUMORS OF THE ANAL MARGIN

1. Squamous Cell Carcinoma

Patients complain of a mass, bleeding, pain, discharge, itching, and pain or tenesmus (complaints common to most lesions of this region). Typically the lesions are large and centrally ulcerated, with rolled, everted edges and have been present for over two years before detection. All chronic or nonhealing ulcers of the perineum should be biopsied to rule out squamous cell carcinoma. Squamous cell carcinoma is more common in men.

Table 32–1. Staging of anal cancer.[1]

Anal Cancer			
Tis	Carcinoma in situ		
T1	≤ 2 cm		
T2	> 2 cm to 5 cm		
T3	> 5 cm		
T4	Adjacent organ(s)		
N1	Perirectal		
N2	Unilateral internal iliac/inguinal		
N3	Perirectal and inguinal, bilateral internal iliac/inguinal		
Stage Grouping			
Stage 0	Tis	N0	M0
Stage I	T1	N0	M0
Stage II	T2	N0	M0
	T3	N0	M0
Stage IIIA	T1	N1	M0
	T2	N1	M0
	T3	N1	M0
	T4	N0	M0
Stage IIIB	T4	N1	M0
	Any T	N2, N3	M0
Stage IV	Any T	Any M	M1

[1]Adapted from: AJCC Cancer Staging Manual No. 5.

Small, well-differentiated lesions (≤ 4 cm) are treated by wide local excision. Deep lesions that involve the sphincters require abdominoperineal resection. Chemoradiation is used for less favorable lesions. Spread is to the inguinal lymph nodes, which are generally included in the radiation fields. Excision of inguinal nodal disease is reserved for palpable and symptomatic disease. Disease recurring in the skin may be treated with reexcision or abdominoperineal resection. The T stage determines survival, with reports of 100% 5-year and 10-year survivals for T1 lesions compared with 60% and 40% survival rates for T2 lesions at 5 and 10 years, respectively.

2. Basal Cell Carcinoma

Bleeding, itching, and pain are the presenting symptoms of basal cell carcinoma. The superficial, mobile lesions have raised, irregular edges and central ulceration. They are more frequent in men.

As with squamous cell carcinoma of the margin, treatment is by wide local excision when possible. Deeply invasive lesions may require abdominoperineal resection. Metastasis is rare, but the local recurrence rate is 30%. Local recurrence is are treated with reexcision.

3. Bowen's Disease

Bowen's disease (intraepithelial squamous cell carcinoma) is often associated with condylomas in young patients. Patients often complain of perianal burning, itching, or pain. Lesions are often found on routine histologic evaluation of specimens acquired during investigation of unrelated disorders. When grossly visible, the lesions appear scaly, discrete, erythematous, and sometimes pigmented. In immunocompromised patients (HIV-positive, transplantation), a Pap smear is a useful screening technique to detect of dysplasia. If the Pap smear is positive, high-resolution anoscopy with acetic acid painting may reveal otherwise occult condyloma with dysplasia.

Wide local excision with four-quadrant biopsies to establish that no residual disease persists has been the treatment of choice. Skin grafts may be necessary for larger lesions. However, there is no histologic difference between Bowen's disease and a high-grade squamous intraepithelial lesion (high-grade dysplasia), and radical skin excision ignores the intra-anal dysplastic lesions that may be even more aggressive than perianal disease. These intra-anal dysplastic lesions have been successfully managed with local excision or destruction, even in the immunocompromised host. Furthermore, fewer than 10% of patients with Bowen's disease will develop invasive squamous cell carcinoma of the anus. Therefore, the need to perform radical excision and flap procedures has been questioned.

4. Paget's Disease

Paget's disease (intraepithelial adenocarcinoma) occurs predominantly in women. Patients are usually in the seventh or eighth decade of life. Severe intractable anal pruritus of the is characteristic. On physical examination an erythematous, eczematoid rash is apparent. Biopsy of any nonhealing lesion should be taken to rule out this diagnosis. If Paget's disease is diagnosed, a thorough workup for an occult malignancy is indicated because 50% of patients have a coexistent gastrointestinal carcinoma.

Wide local excision with multiple perianal biopsies is the treatment of choice. Abdominoperineal resection may be indicated for advanced disease. Lymph node dissection should be done only be for palpable adenopathy. The role of chemoradiotherapy is less clear. The prognosis is good unless there is metastatic disease or an underlying neoplasm.

Beck DE: Paget's disease and Bowen's disease of the anus. Semin Colon Rectal Surg 1995;6:143.

Frisch M et al: Benign anal lesions, inflammatory bowel disease and risk for high-risk human papillomavirus-positive and -negative anal carcinoma. Br J Cancer 1998;78:1534.

Fuchshuber PR et al: Anal canal and perianal epidermoid cancers. J Am Coll Surg 1997185:494.

Marchesa P et al: Perianal Bowen's disease: a clinicopathologic study of 47 patients. Dis Colon Rectum 1997;40:1286.

Marchesa P et al: Long-term outcome of patients with perianal Paget's disease. Ann Surg Oncol 1997;4:475.

Peiffert D et al: Conservative treatment by irradiation of epidermoid carcinomas of the anal margin. Int J Radiat Oncol Biol Phys 1997; 39:57.

Sarmiento JM et al: Paget's disease of the perianal region—an aggressive disease? Dis Colon Rectum 1997;40:1187.

Touboul E et al: Epidermoid carcinoma of the anal margin: 17 cases treated with curative-intent radiation therapy. Radiother Oncol 1995;34:195.

TUMORS OF THE ANAL CANAL

1. Epidermoid (Squamous, Basaloid, Mucoepidermoid) Carcinoma

Clinical Findings

In most cases there is a long history of minor perianal complaints such as bleeding, itching, or discomfort. An indurated anal mass may be present. Disease may be extensive at presentation, with approximately half of the lesions extending beyond the bowel wall or perianal skin at presentation. Inguinal nodal metastases are found in 20% at diagnosis and another 15% over time.

The workup is discussed in the section on perianal cancers.

Abdominal CT and chest radiographs may reveal liver or long metastases. Endorectal ultrasound can determine the depth of invasion of the primary lesion and may identify pararectal nodes.

Treatment

Early lesions that are small, mobile, confined to the submucosa, and well differentiated may be treated with local excision. Overall reported recurrence rates with local excision alone are high, with an average survival rate of 70% at 5 years. Local excision of the most favorable lesions results in less than 10% recurrence and 5-year survival 100%. Larger lesions of the anal canal call for radiation therapy or chemoradiotherapy.

Chemoradiotherapy has now replaced surgery as first-line therapy, and surgery is advised only as a salvage procedure for persistent or recurrent disease. The Nigro regimen consisted of 30 Gy to the primary tumor and to the pelvic and inguinal nodes. Mitomycin (15 mg/m^2 as an intravenous bolus) was delivered on day 1 of radiation therapy. Two 4-day infusions of fluorouracil (5-FU) (1000 mg/m^2 per day) were given starting on days 1 and 28 of chemoradiation therapy. Excellent tumor responses with 80% disease-free survivals have been reported. Because of the morbidity associated with this two regimen the amount and type of chemotherapy and radiation have been modified. Chemotherapy has been eliminated completely in some trials but the local recurrence rate is higher. Much of the chemotherapy toxicity is related to the mitomycin, and cisplatin seems to be an effective replacement that has fewer side effects. External beam radiotherapy doses range from 30 Gy to 55 Gy; some centers use brachytherapy catheters as well.

Treatment failures occur most commonly in the pelvis at the primary site or in the locoregional lymph nodes, with disease occurring outside the pelvis in just 15% of patients. The most common site of extrapelvic failure is the liver. Salvage abdominal perineal resection for local failure with recurrent or persistent disease is associated with a 50% 5-year survival rate. Survival is related to the extent of disease at the time of failure and to nodal status before initiation of chemoradiation therapy.

Prophylactic groin dissection is not recommended, but some experts recommend that the groins be included in the radiation fields because the failure rate in the groins is 20% if they are not treated.

Prognosis

Tumor size is the single most important prognostic factor. Mobile lesions ≤ 2 cm in diameter have cure rates of 80%, but tumors 5 cm or more in diameter are associated with a 50% mortality. There are reports of excellent 5-year and 19-year survivals for T1–3 node-negative disease (88%) and T1–3 node positive disease (50%). Metastatic disease is more likely to be present with increasing depth of invasion and size and worsening histologic grade. Distant disease is uncommon at the time of diagnosis but most commonly involves the liver when present. Subsequent metastasis out of the pelvis is not uncommon, and 40% of patients die with disease that has spread to distant sites. Lymph node involvement at the time of presentation is a bad prognostic sign.

Allal AS et al: Effectiveness of surgical salvage therapy for patients with locally uncontrolled anal carcinoma after sphincter-conserving treatment. Cancer 1999;86:405.

Doci R et al: Primary chemoradiation therapy with fluorouracil and cisplatin for cancer of the anus: results in 35 consecutive patients. J Clin Oncol 1996;14:3121.

Ellenhorn JD et al: Salvage abdominoperineal resection following combined chemotherapy and radiotherapy for epidermoid carcinoma of the anus. Ann Surg Oncol 1994;1:105.

Epidermoid anal cancer: results from the UKCCCR randomised trial of radiotherapy alone versus radiotherapy, 5-fluorouracil, and mitomycin. UKCCCR Anal Cancer Trial Working Party. UK Co-ordinating Committee on Cancer Research. Lancet 1996;348:1049.

Flam M et al: Role of mitomycin in combination with fluorouracil and radiotherapy, and of salvage chemoradiation in the definitive nonsurgical treatment of epidermoid carcinoma of the anal canal: results of a phase III randomized intergroup study. J Clin Oncol 1996;14:2527.

Flam M et al: Role of mitomycin in combination with fluorouracil and radiotherapy and of salvage chemoradiation in the definitive nonsurgical treatment of epidermoid carcinoma of the anal canal: results of a phase III randomized intergroup study. J Clin Oncol 1996; 14:2527.

Klas JV et al: Malignant tumors of the anal canal: the spectrum of disease, treatment, and outcomes. Cancer 1999; 85:1686.

Myerson RJ et al: Carcinoma of the anal canal. Am J Clin Oncol 1995;18:32.

Peiffert D et al: Preliminary results of a phase II study of high-dose radiation therapy and neoadjuvant plus concomitant 5-fluorouracil with CDDP chemotherapy for patients with anal canal cancer: a French cooperative study. Ann Oncol 1997;8:575.

Pocard M et al: Results of salvage abdominoperineal resection for anal cancer after radiotherapy. Dis Colon Rectum 1998; 41:1488.

Ryan DP et al: Carcinoma of the anal canal. N Engl J Med 2000; 342:792.

Smith DE et al: Cancer of the anal canal: treatment with chemotherapy and low-dose radiation therapy. Radiology 1994;191:569.

Hernias & Other Lesions of the Abdominal Wall*

Karen E. Deveney, MD

■ I. HERNIAS

An external hernia is an abnormal protrusion of intra-abdominal tissue through a fascial defect in the abdominal wall. About 75% of hernias occur in the groin (indirect inguinal, direct inguinal, femoral). Incisional and ventral hernias comprise about 10%; umbilical 3%; and others about 3%. Generally, a hernial mass is composed of covering tissues (skin, subcutaneous tissues, etc), a peritoneal sac, and any contained viscera. Particularly if the neck of the sac is narrow where it emerges from the abdomen, bowel protruding into the hernia may become obstructed or strangulated. If the hernia is not repaired early, the defect may enlarge and operative repair may become more complicated. The definitive treatment of hernia is early operative repair.

A **reducible hernia** is one in which the contents of the sac return to the abdomen spontaneously or with manual pressure when the patient is recumbent.

An **irreducible (incarcerated) hernia** is one whose contents cannot be returned to the abdomen, usually because they are trapped by a narrow neck. The term "incarceration" does not imply obstruction, inflammation, or ischemia of the herniated organs, though incarceration is necessary for obstruction or strangulation to occur.

Though the lumen of a segment of bowel within the hernia sac may become **obstructed,** there may initially be no interference with blood supply. Compromise to the blood supply of the contents of the sac (eg, omentum or intestine) results in a **strangulated hernia,** in which gangrene of the contents of the sac has occurred. The incidence of strangulation is higher in femoral than in inguinal hernias, but strangulation may occur in other hernias as well.

An uncommon and dangerous type of hernia, a **Richter hernia,** occurs when only part of the circumference of the bowel becomes incarcerated or strangu-lated in the fascial defect. A strangulated Richter hernia may spontaneously reduce and the gangrenous piece of intestine be overlooked at operation. The bowel may subsequently perforate, with resultant peritonitis.

HERNIAS OF THE GROIN

Anatomy

All hernias of the abdominal wall consist of a peritoneal sac that protrudes through a weakness or defect in the muscular layers of the abdomen. The defect may be congenital or acquired.

Just outside the peritoneum is the **transversalis fascia,** an aponeurosis whose weakness or defect is the major source of groin hernias. Next are found the **transversus abdominis, internal oblique,** and **external oblique muscles,** which are fleshy laterally and aponeurotic medially. Their aponeuroses form investing layers of the strong **rectus abdominis muscles** above the semilunar line. Below this line, the aponeurosis lies entirely in front of the muscle. Between the two vertical rectus muscles, the aponeuroses meet again to form the **linea alba,** which is well defined only above the umbilicus. The subcutaneous fat contains Scarpa's fascia—a misnomer, since it is only a condensation of connective tissue with no substantial strength.

In the groin, an **indirect inguinal hernia** results when obliteration of the processus vaginalis, the peritoneal extension accompanying the testis in its descent into the scrotum, fails to occur. The resultant hernia sac passes through the **internal inguinal ring,** a defect in the transversalis fascia halfway between the anterior iliac spine and the pubic tubercle. The sac is located anteromedially within the spermatic cord and may extend partway along the **inguinal canal** or accompany the cord out through the subcutaneous (external) inguinal ring, a defect medially in the external oblique muscle just above the pubic tubercle. A hernia that passes fully into the scrotum is known as a **complete hernia.** The sac and the spermatic cord are invested by the **cremaster muscle,** an extension of fibers of the internal oblique muscle.

---

* See Chapter 46 for further discussion of hernias in the pediatric age group and Chapter 23 for a discussion of internal hernias.

Other anatomic structures of the groin that are important in understanding the formation of hernias and types of hernia repairs include the **conjoined tendon,** or falx inguinalis, a fusion of the medial aponeurotic transversus abdominis and internal oblique muscles that passes along the inferolateral edge of the rectus abdominis muscle and attaches to the pubic tubercle. Between the pubic tubercle and the anterior iliac spine passes the **inguinal (Poupart) ligament,** formed by the lowermost border of the external oblique aponeurosis as it rolls on itself and thickens into a cord.

Just deep and parallel to the inguinal ligament runs the iliopubic tract, a band of connective tissue that extends from the iliopsoas fascia, crosses below the deep inguinal ring, forms the superior border of the femoral sheath, and inserts into the superior pubic ramus to form the **lacunar (Gimbernat) ligament.** The lacunar ligament is about 1.25 cm long and triangular in shape. The sharp, crescentic lateral border of this ligament is the unyielding noose for the strangulation of a femoral hernia.

Cooper's ligament is a strong, fibrous band that extends laterally for about 2.5 cm along the iliopectineal line on the superior aspect of the superior pubic ramus, starting at the lateral base of the lacunar ligament.

Hesselbach's triangle is bounded by the inguinal ligament, the inferior epigastric vessels, and the lateral border of the rectus muscle. A weakness or defect in the transversalis fascia, which forms the floor of this triangle, results in a **direct inguinal hernia.** In most direct hernias, the transversalis fascia is diffusely attenuated, though a discrete defect in the fascia may occasionally occur. This **funicular** type of direct inguinal hernia is more likely to become incarcerated, since it has distinct borders.

A **femoral hernia** passes beneath the iliopubic tract and inguinal ligament into the upper thigh. The predisposing anatomic feature for femoral hernias is a small empty space between the lacunar ligament medially and the femoral vein laterally—the **femoral canal.** Because its borders are distinct and unyielding, a femoral hernia has the highest risk of incarceration and strangulation of groin hernias.

Surgeons must be familiar with the pathways of the nerves and blood vessels of the inguinal region to avoid injuring them when repairing groin hernias. The iliohypogastric nerve (T12, L1) emerges from the lateral edge of the psoas muscle and travels inside the external oblique muscle, emerging medial to the external inguinal ring to innervate the suprapubic skin. The ilioinguinal nerve (L1) parallels the iliohypogastric nerve and travels on the surface of the spermatic cord to innervate the base of the penis (or mons pubis), the scrotum (or labia majora), and the medial thigh. This nerve is the most frequently injured in anterior open inguinal hernia repairs. The genitofemoral (L1, L2) and lateral femoral cutaneous nerves (L2, L3) travel on and lateral to the psoas muscle and provide sensation to the scrotum and anteromedial thigh and to the lateral thigh, respectively. These nerves are subject to injury during laparoscopic hernia repairs. The femoral nerve (L2–L4) travels from the lateral edge of the psoas and extends lateral to the femoral vessels. It can be injured during laparoscopic or femoral hernia repairs.

The external iliac artery travels along the medial aspect of the psoas muscle and beneath the inguinal ligament, giving off the inferior epigastric artery, which borders the medial aspect of the internal inguinal ring. The corresponding veins accompany the arteries. These vessels can be injured during hernia repairs of all types.

Causes

Nearly all inguinal hernias in infants, children, and young adults are **indirect inguinal hernias.** Although these "congenital" hernias most often present during the first year of life, the first clinical evidence of hernia may not appear until middle or old age, when increased intra-abdominal pressure and dilation of the internal inguinal ring allow abdominal contents to enter the previously empty peritoneal diverticulum. An untreated indirect hernia will inevitably dilate the internal ring and displace or attenuate the inguinal floor. The peritoneum may protrude on either side of the inferior epigastric vessels to give a combined direct and indirect hernia, called a **pantaloon hernia.**

In contrast, **direct inguinal hernias** are acquired as the result of a developed weakness of the transversalis fascia in Hesselbach's area. There is some evidence that direct inguinal hernias may be related to hereditary or acquired defects in collagen synthesis or turnover. **Femoral hernias** involve an acquired protrusion of a peritoneal sac through the femoral ring. In women, the ring may become dilated by the physical and biochemical changes during pregnancy.

Any condition that chronically increases intra-abdominal pressure may contribute to the appearance and progression of a hernia. Marked obesity, abdominal strain from heavy exercise or lifting, cough, constipation with straining at stool, and prostatism with straining on micturition are often implicated. Cirrhosis with ascites, pregnancy, chronic ambulatory peritoneal dialysis, and chronically enlarged pelvic organs or pelvic tumors may also contribute. Loss of tissue turgor in Hesselbach's area, associated with a weakening of the transversalis fascia, occurs with advancing age and in chronic debilitating disease.

Classification of Groin Hernias

To facilitate comparison of results of their surgical repair, Nyhus has proposed a classification of groin hernias: types 1 and 2, indirect inguinal hernias with a normal-sized (type 1) or enlarged (type 2) internal ring but with a normal inguinal floor; type 3, either direct (type 3A), indirect with a distorted inguinal floor (type 3B), or femoral hernias (type 3C); and type 4, recurrent hernias.

Lovett J, Kirgan D, McGregor B: Inguinal herniation justifies sigmoidoscopy. Am J Surg 1989;158:615.

Nyhus LM: Individualization of hernia repair: a new era. Surgery 1993;114:1.

Skandalakis JE et al: Embryologic and anatomic basis of inguinal herniorrhaphy. Surg Clin North Am 1993;73:799.

INDIRECT & DIRECT INGUINAL HERNIAS

Clinical Findings

A. SYMPTOMS

Most hernias produce no symptoms until the patient notices a lump or swelling in the groin, though some patients may describe a sudden pain and bulge that occurred while lifting or straining. Frequently, hernias are detected in the course of routine physical examinations such as preemployment examinations. Some patients complain of a dragging sensation and, particularly with indirect inguinal hernias, radiation of pain into the scrotum. As a hernia enlarges, it is likely to produce a sense of discomfort or aching pain, and the patient must lie down to reduce the hernia.

In general, direct hernias produce fewer symptoms than indirect inguinal hernias and are less likely to become incarcerated or strangulated.

B. SIGNS

Examination of the groin reveals a mass that may or may not be reducible. The patient should be examined both supine and standing and also with coughing and straining, since small hernias may be difficult to demonstrate. The external ring can be identified by invaginating the scrotum and palpating with the index finger just above and lateral to the pubic tubercle (Figure 33–1). If the external ring is very small, the examiner's finger may not enter the inguinal canal, and it may be difficult to be sure that a pulsation felt on coughing is truly a hernia. At the other extreme, a widely patent external ring does not by itself constitute hernia. Tissue must be felt protruding into the inguinal canal during coughing in order for a hernia to be diagnosed.

Differentiating between direct and indirect inguinal hernia on examination is difficult and is of little importance since most groin hernias should be repaired regardless of type. Nevertheless, each type of inguinal

Figure 33–1. Insertion of finger through upper scrotum into the external inguinal ring.

hernia has specific features more common to it. A hernia that descends into the scrotum is almost certainly indirect. On inspection with the patient erect and straining, a direct hernia more commonly appears as a symmetric, circular swelling at the external ring; the swelling disappears when the patient lies down. An indirect hernia appears as an elliptic swelling that may not reduce easily.

On palpation, the posterior wall of the inguinal canal is firm and resistant in an indirect hernia but relaxed or absent in a direct hernia. If the patient is asked to cough or strain while the examining finger is directed laterally and upward into the inguinal canal, a direct hernia protrudes against the side of the finger, whereas an indirect hernia is felt at the tip of the finger.

Compression over the internal ring when the patient strains may also help to differentiate between indirect and direct hernias. A direct hernia bulges forward through Hesselbach's triangle, but the opposite hand can maintain reduction of an indirect hernia at the internal ring.

These distinctions are obscured as a hernia enlarges and distorts the anatomic relationships of the inguinal rings and canal. In most patients the type of inguinal hernia cannot be established accurately before surgery.

Differential Diagnosis

Groin pain of musculoskeletal or obscure origin may be difficult to distinguish from hernia. Herniography, in which x-rays are obtained after intraperitoneal injection of contrast medium, may aid in the diagnosis in cases of groin pain when no hernia can be felt even after multiple maneuvers to increase intra-abdominal pressure.

Herniation of preperitoneal fat through the inguinal ring into the spermatic cord ("lipoma of the cord") is commonly misinterpreted as a hernia sac. Its true nature may only be confirmed at operation. Occasionally, a femoral hernia that has extended above the inguinal ligament after passing through the fossa ovalis femoris may be confused with an inguinal hernia. If the examining finger is placed on the pubic tubercle, the neck of the sac of a femoral hernia lies lateral and below, while that of an inguinal hernia lies above.

Inguinal hernia must be differentiated from hydrocele of the spermatic cord, lymphadenopathy or abscesses of the groin, varicocele, and residual hematoma following trauma or spontaneous hemorrhage in patients taking anticoagulants. An undescended testis in the inguinal canal must also be considered when the testis cannot be felt in the scrotum.

The presence of an impulse in the mass with coughing, bowel sounds in the mass, and failure to transilluminate are features which indicate that an irreducible mass in the groin is a hernia.

Treatment

Inguinal hernias should always be repaired unless there are specific contraindications. The same advice applies to patients of all ages; the complications of incarceration, obstruction, and strangulation are greater threats than are the risks of operation.

Elderly patients tolerate elective repair of a groin hernia very well, especially when other medical problems are optimally controlled and local anesthetic is used. Emergency operation carries a much greater risk for the elderly than carefully planned elective operation.

If the patient has significant prostatic hyperplasia, it is prudent to solve this problem first, since the risks of urinary retention and urinary tract infection are high following hernia repair in patients with significant prostatic obstruction.

Although most direct hernias do not carry as high a risk of incarceration as indirect hernias, the difficulty in reliably differentiating them from indirect hernias makes the repair of all inguinal hernias advisable. Direct hernias of the funicular type, which are particularly likely to incarcerate, should always be repaired.

Because of the possibility of strangulation, an incarcerated, painful, or tender hernia usually requires an emergency operation. Nonoperative reduction of an incarcerated hernia may first be attempted. The patient is placed with hips elevated and given analgesics and sedation sufficient to promote muscle relaxation. Repair of the hernia may be deferred if the hernia mass reduces with gentle manipulation and if there is no clinical evi-

dence of strangulated bowel. Though strangulation is usually clinically evident, gangrenous tissue can occasionally be reduced into the abdomen by manual or spontaneous reduction en masse. It is therefore safest to repair the reduced hernia at the earliest opportunity.

At surgery, one must decide whether to explore the abdomen to make certain that the intestine is viable. If the patient has leukocytosis or clinical signs of peritonitis or if the hernia sac contains dark or bloody fluid, the abdomen should be explored.

A. Principles of Operative Treatment of Inguinal Hernia

1. Successful repair requires that any correctable aggravating factors be identified and treated (chronic cough, prostatic obstruction, colonic tumor, ascites, etc) and that the defect be reconstructed with the best available tissues that can be approximated without tension.

2. An indirect hernia sac should be anatomically isolated, dissected to its origin from the peritoneum, and ligated (Figure 33–2). In infants and young adults in whom the inguinal anatomy is normal, repair can usually be limited to high ligation, removal of the sac, and reduction of the internal ring to an appropriate size. For most adult hernias, the inguinal floor should also

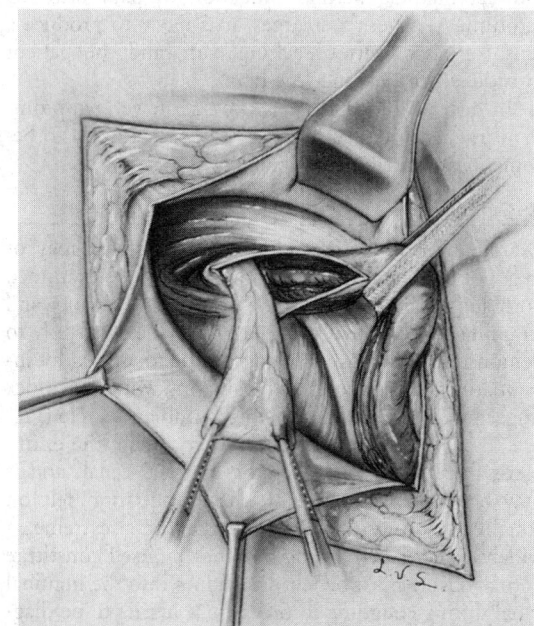

Figure 33–2. Indirect inguinal hernia. Inguinal canal opened, showing spermatic cord retracted medially and indirect hernia peritoneal sac dissected free to above the level of the internal inguinal ring.

be reconstructed. The internal ring should be reduced to a size just adequate to allow egress of the cord structures. In women, the internal ring can be totally closed to prevent recurrence through that site. To construct a solid inguinal floor in men with recurrent hernias, it may rarely be necessary to divide the cord and completely close the internal ring. The testicle may be removed or left in the scrotum.

3. In direct inguinal hernia (Figure 33–3), the inguinal canal may be so wide and its floor so weak that the repair appears to be under tension. In such cases, a vertical relaxing incision in the anterior rectus abdominis sheath has traditionally been used, though recent experience favors the use of mesh so that a tension-free repair can be accomplished.

4. Even though a direct hernia is found, the cord should always be carefully searched for a possible indirect hernia as well.

5. In patients with large hernias, bilateral repair has traditionally been discouraged since greater tension on the repair increases the recurrence rate and surgical complications. In children and adults with small hernias, bilateral hernia repair is usually recommended because it spares the patient a second anesthetic. If open

mesh repair or laparoscopic methods are used, bilateral repairs can be done with low risk of recurrence.

6. Recurrent hernia within a few months or a year of operation usually indicates an inadequate repair, such as overlooking an indirect sac or failing to repair the fascial defect securely. Any repair completed under tension is subject to early recurrence. Recurrences two or more years after repair are more likely to be caused by progressive weakening of the patient's fascia. Repeated recurrence after careful repair by an experienced surgeon suggests a defect in collagen synthesis. Because the fascial defect is often small, firm, and unyielding, recurrent hernias are much more likely to develop incarceration or strangulation than unoperated inguinal hernias, and they should nearly always be repaired again.

If recurrence is due to an overlooked indirect sac, the posterior wall is often solid and removal of the sac may be all that is required. Occasionally, a recurrence is discovered to consist of a small, sharply circumscribed defect in the previous hernioplasty, in which case closure of the defect suffices. More diffuse weakness of the posterior inguinal wall or repeated recurrences occasionally require more elaborate repair using fascia lata from the thigh or a nonabsorbable patch such as polypropylene or polytetrafluoroethylene (PTFE).

B. TYPES OF OPERATIONS FOR INGUINAL HERNIA

The goal of all hernia repairs is to eliminate the peritoneal sac (in the case of an indirect hernia) and to close the fascial defect in the inguinal floor. Traditional repairs approximated native tissues using permanent sutures. More recently, a permanent mesh has been used with greater frequency to decrease tension on the repairs.

Simple high ligation of the sac through an inguinal incision is the key to the repair of indirect hernias in infants and children. Combined with a tightening of the internal ring, it is called the **Marcy repair.**

Inguinal hernias in adults can be repaired successfully through an inguinal, preperitoneal, or abdominal approach, though inguinal repairs are most widely used today. While a given repair may be championed by a particular surgeon or group, comparative studies do not conclusively demonstrate the superiority of any one type; in fact, it seems likely that all the methods in common use give equivalent results when properly performed. Details of technique and the experience and skill of the surgeon are more likely to account for the success of the procedure than is the type of repair.

Though most methods of repairing indirect inguinal hernias in adults emphasize high ligation of the sac, as in children, elimination of the sac by reducing it may suffice. The factor common to all successful methods of inguinal hernia repairs in adults is repair of the inguinal floor. Over the past 15–20 years, mesh repairs have

Figure 33–3. Direct inguinal hernia. Inguinal canal opened and spermatic cord retracted inferiorly and laterally to reveal the hernia bulging through the floor of Hesselbach's triangle.

gradually gained in popularity and have become the most commonly employed method. Over the past decade, increased experience has been gained with laparoscopic and other minimally invasive techniques. The superiority of the newer methods has not been yet established in long-term studies.

Among the traditional autologous tissue repairs, the **Bassini repair** was the most widely used method. In this repair, the conjoined tendon is approximated to Poupart's ligament and the spermatic cord remains in its normal anatomic position under the external oblique aponeurosis. The **Halsted repair** places the external oblique beneath the cord but otherwise resembles the Bassini repair. **Cooper's ligament (Lotheissen-McVay) repair** brings the conjoined tendon farther posteriorly and inferiorly to Cooper's ligament. Unlike the Bassini and Halsted methods, McVay's repair is effective for femoral hernia but always requires a relaxing incision to relieve tension. Though the **Shouldice repair** has a low reported recurrence rate, it is not widely used, perhaps because of the more extensive dissection required and a belief that the skill of the surgeons may be as important as the method itself. In the Shouldice repair, the transversalis fascia is first divided and then imbricated to Poupart's ligament. Finally, the conjoined tendon and internal oblique muscle are also approximated in layers to the inguinal ligament.

The **preperitoneal approach** exposes the groin from between the transversalis fascia and peritoneum via a lower abdominal incision to effect closure of the fascial defect. Because it requires more initial dissection and is associated with higher morbidity and recurrence rates in less experienced hands, it has not been widely favored. For recurrent or large bilateral hernias, a preperitoneal approach using a large piece of mesh to span all areas of potential herniation has been described by Stoppa.

A desire to decrease the recurrence rate of hernias has prompted an increased use of prosthetic materials in repair of both recurrent and first-time hernias. Methods include "plugs" of mesh inserted into the internal ring and sheets of mesh to create a tension-free repair. The most widely used technique is that of Lichtenstein, an open mesh repair that allows an early return to normal activities and a low complication and recurrence rate.

The increased popularity of minimally invasive methods over the past decade has also included repair of groin hernias. Several methods have been explored, from a transabdominal intraperitoneal onlay of mesh (IPOM) to a transabdominal preperitoneal mesh technique (TAPP) to total extraperitoneal mesh placement (TEP). The high incidence of complications that occurred in early studies prompted revisions in the operative technique to avoid injury to lateral nerves. Several prospective randomized trials have subsequently been conducted comparing open with minimally invasive techniques and one type of minimally invasive technique with another. These studies generally have demonstrated decreased pain and faster return to work with the minimally invasive techniques but at increased cost of the procedure. Long-term durability of the procedures has not yet been established. Specific situations in which minimally invasive procedures may be particularly advantageous include the repair of multiply recurrent hernias after anterior open repairs, repair of bilateral hernias simultaneously, and repair in patients who must return to work particularly quickly.

C. NONSURGICAL MANAGEMENT (USE OF A TRUSS)

The surgeon is occasionally called upon to prescribe a truss when a patient refuses operative repair or when there are absolute contraindications to operation. A truss should be fitted to provide adequate external compression over the defect in the abdominal wall. It should be taken off at night and put on in the morning before the patient arises. The use of a truss does not preclude later repair of a hernia, although it may cause fibrosis of the anatomic structures, so that subsequent repair may be difficult.

Pre- & Postoperative Course

The preoperative evaluation should be completed before hospitalization. The patient usually enters the hospital on the morning of operation. The anesthetic may be general, spinal, or local. Local anesthetic is effective for most patients, and the incidence of urinary retention and pulmonary complications is lowest with local anesthesia. Recurrent hernias are more easily repaired with the patient under spinal or general anesthesia, since local anesthetic does not readily diffuse through scar tissue. In the past, the patient was routinely kept in the hospital for a few days after operation, but "come-and-go" hernia repair has been shown to be safe and effective and is now routine. A sedentary worker may return to work within a few days; heavy manual labor has traditionally not been performed for up to 4–6 weeks after hernia repair, though recent studies document no increase in recurrence when full activity is resumed as early as 2 weeks after surgery, particularly when open or laparoscopic mesh repairs have been used.

Prognosis

In addition to chronic cough, prostatism, and constipation, poor tissue quality and poor operative technique may contribute to recurrence of inguinal hernia. Because tissue is often more attenuated in direct hernias, recurrence rates are higher than for indirect hernias.

Placing the repair under tension and using absorbable suture are technical errors that lead to recurrence. Failure to find an indirect hernia, to dissect the sac high enough, or to adequately close the internal ring may lead to recurrence of indirect hernia. Postoperative wound infection is associated with increased recurrence. The recurrence rate is considerably increased in patients receiving chronic peritoneal dialysis—in one report, the rate was as high as 27%.

Recurrence rates after indirect hernia repair in adults are reported at best to be 0.6–3%, though the incidence is more probably 5–10%. Inadequate sac reduction or internal ring closure and failure to identify a femoral or direct hernia contribute to recurrence, as does inadequate repair of the inguinal canal. A wide range of figures is quoted for recurrence after repair of direct hernias, from less than 1% to as high as 28%. The point of recurrence is most often just lateral to the pubic tubercle, implicating excessive tension on the repair and adding evidence to favor mesh repairs or the use of a relaxing incision in the rectus sheath if a traditional autologous tissue method is used in the repair of a direct hernia.

Amid PK et al: Open "tension-free" repair of inguinal hernias: the Lichtenstein technique. Eur J Surg 1996;162:447.

Cheek CM et al: Trusses in the management of hernia today. Br J Surg 1995;82:1611.

Kark AE et al: 3175 primary inguinal hernia repairs: advantages of ambulatory open mesh repair using local anesthesia. J Am Coll Surg 1998;186:447.

Liem MSL et al: Comparison of conventional anterior surgery and laparoscopic surgery for inguinal hernia repair. N Engl J Med 1997;336:1541.

MacArthur DC et al: Herniography for groin pain of uncertain origin. Br J Surg 1997;84:684.

Paganini AM et al: A randomized, controlled clinical study of laparoscopic vs open tension-free inguinal hernia repair. Surg Endosc 1998;12:979.

Tschudi J et al: Controlled multicenter trial of laparoscopic transabdominal preperitoneal hernioplasty vs Shouldice herniorrhaphy. Surg Endosc 1996;10:845.

Wright DM et al: Early outcome after open versus extraperitoneal endoscopic tension-free hernioplasty: a randomized clinical trial. Surgery 1996;119:552.

Zieren J et al: Prospective randomized study comparing laparoscopic and open tension-free inguinal hernia repair with Shouldice's operation. Am J Surg 1998;178:330.

SLIDING INGUINAL HERNIA

A sliding inguinal hernia (Figures 33–4 and 33–5) is a type of indirect inguinal hernia in which the wall of a viscus forms a portion of the wall of the hernia sac. On the right side the cecum is most commonly involved, and on the left side the sigmoid colon. The development of a sliding hernia is related to the variable degree of posterior fixation of the large bowel or other sliding components (eg, bladder, ovary) and their proximity to the internal inguinal ring.

Figure 33–4. Right-sided sliding hernia, sagittal view. *Top:* Note cecum and ascending colon sliding on fascia of posterior abdominal wall. *Bottom:* Hernia has entered internal inguinal ring. Note that one-fourth of the hernia is not related to the peritoneal sac.

Clinical Findings

Though sliding hernias have no special signs that distinguish them from other inguinal hernias, they should be suspected in any large hernia that cannot be completely reduced or whenever a large scrotal hernia is seen in an elderly man. Finding a segment of colon in the scrotum on barium enema strongly suggests a sliding hernia. Recognition of this variation is of great importance at operation, since failure to recognize it may result in inadvertent entry into the lumen of the bowel or bladder.

Treatment

It is essential to recognize the entity at an early stage of operation. As is true of all indirect inguinal hernias, the sac will lie anteriorly, but the posterior wall of the sac

Figure 33–5. Right-sided sliding hernia seen in sagittal section. (After Linden in Thorek.) At arrow, the wall of the cecum forms a portion of the hernia sac.

will be formed to a greater or lesser degree by colon or bladder.

After the cord has been dissected free from the hernia sac, most sliding hernias can be reduced by a series of inverting sutures (Bevan technique) and one of the standard types of inguinal repair performed. Very large sliding hernias may have to be reduced by entering the peritoneal cavity through a separate incision (La Roque), pulling the bowel back into the abdomen, and fixing it to the posterior abdominal wall. The hernia is then repaired in the usual fashion. The laparoscopic approach may be the best one for these hernias, however, because the anatomic relationships are readily evident and the repair requires no extra steps beyond those involved in the usual laparoscopic repair.

Prognosis

Sliding hernias have a higher recurrence rate than uncomplicated indirect hernias.

The surgical complications most often encountered following sliding hernia repair are encroachment on the circulation to the large bowel, with bowel necrosis, and actual strangulation of a portion of the large bowel when attempting a high ligation of the hernia sac. Rarely, other retroperitoneal structures such as the ureter may accompany the viscus into the hernia and are at risk of injury.

Welsh DRJ et al: The Shouldice repair. Surg Clin North Am 1993; 73:451.

FEMORAL HERNIA

A femoral hernia descends through the femoral canal beneath the inguinal ligament. Because of its narrow neck, it is prone to incarceration and strangulation. Femoral hernia is much more common in women than in men, but in both sexes femoral hernia is less common than inguinal hernia. Femoral hernias comprise about one-third of groin hernias in women and about 2% of groin hernias in men.

Clinical Findings

A. SYMPTOMS

Femoral hernias are notoriously asymptomatic until incarceration or strangulation occurs. Even with obstruction or strangulation, the patient may feel discomfort more in the abdomen than in the femoral area. Thus, colicky abdominal pain and signs of intestinal obstruction frequently are the presenting manifestations of a strangulated femoral hernia, without discomfort, pain, or tenderness in the femoral region.

B. SIGNS

A femoral hernia may present in a variety of ways. If it is small and uncomplicated, it usually appears as a small bulge in the upper medial thigh just below the level of the inguinal ligament. Because it may be deflected anteriorly through the fossa ovalis femoris to present as a visible or palpable mass at or above the inguinal ligament, it can be confused with an inguinal hernia.

Differential Diagnosis

Femoral hernia must be distinguished from inguinal hernia, a saphenous varix, and femoral adenopathy. A saphenous varix transmits a distinct thrill when a patient coughs, and it appears and disappears instantly when the patient stands or lies down—in contrast to femoral hernias, which are either irreducible or reduce gradually on pressure.

Treatment

A. PRINCIPLES

The principles of femoral hernia repair are as follows: (1) complete excision of the hernia sac, (2) the use of nonabsorbable sutures, (3) repair of the defect in the transversalis fascia that is responsible for the hernia, and

(4) use of Cooper's ligament for the repair, since it gives a firm support for sutures and forms the natural line for closure of the defect.

B. TYPES OF REPAIR FOR FEMORAL HERNIA

A femoral hernia can be repaired through an inguinal, thigh, preperitoneal, or abdominal approach, though the inguinal approach is most commonly used. No matter what the approach, the hernia is often difficult to reduce. Reduction may be facilitated by carefully incising the iliopubic tract, Gimbernat's ligament, or even the inguinal ligament. Occasionally, a counterincision in the thigh is required to free attachments below the inguinal ligament.

Irrespective of the approach used, successful femoral hernia repair must close the femoral canal. The Lotheissen-McVay repair, also used for inguinal hernia, is most commonly employed.

If the hernia sac and mass reduce when the patient is given opiates or anesthesia and if bloody fluid appears in the hernia sac when it is exposed and opened, one must strongly suspect the possibility of nonviable bowel in the peritoneal cavity. In such cases, it is mandatory to open and explore the abdomen, usually through a separate midline incision.

Prognosis

Recurrence rates usually approximate the middle range for direct inguinal hernia, ie, about 5–10%.

Ballard JL et al: Ureteroinguinal hernia: a rare companion of sliding inguinal hernias. Am Surg 1991;57:720.

Bendavid R: A femoral "umbrella" for femoral hernia repair. Surg Gynecol Obstet 1987;165:153.

Berliner SD et al: The Henry operation for incarcerated and strangulated femoral hernias. Arch Surg 1992;127:314.

Glassow F: Femoral hernia: review of 2,105 repairs in a 17 year period. Am J Surg 1985;150:353.

OTHER TYPES OF HERNIAS
UMBILICAL HERNIAS IN ADULTS

Umbilical hernia in adults occurs long after closure of the umbilical ring and is due to a gradual yielding of the cicatricial tissue closing the ring. It is more common in women than in men.

Predisposing factors include (1) multiple pregnancies with prolonged labor, (2) ascites, (3) obesity, and (4) large intra-abdominal tumors.

Clinical Findings

In adults, umbilical hernia does not usually obliterate spontaneously, as in children, but instead increases steadily in size. The hernia sac may have multiple loculations. Umbilical hernias usually contain omentum, but small and large bowel may be present. Emergency repair is often necessary, because the neck of the hernia is usually quite narrow compared to the size of the herniated mass and strangulation is common.

Umbilical hernias with tight rings are often associated with sharp pain on coughing or straining. Very large umbilical hernias more commonly produce a dragging or aching sensation.

Treatment

Umbilical hernia in an adult should be repaired expeditiously to avoid incarceration and strangulation. The umbilical dimple should be preserved if possible and the fascia approximated with nonabsorbable suture. A transverse closure of the aponeurotic defect results in the strongest repair. Large umbilical hernia defects that cannot be closed without undue tension should be closed with an inlay of nonabsorbable mesh.

The presence of cirrhosis and ascites should not discourage repair of an umbilical hernia, since incarceration, strangulation, and rupture are particularly dangerous in patients with these disorders. If significant ascites exists, however, it should first be controlled medically or by peritoneovenous shunt if necessary, since morbidity and recurrence are higher after hernia repair in patients with ascites. Preoperative correction of fluid and electrolyte imbalance and improvement of nutrition will improve the outcome in these patients.

Prognosis

Factors that may lead to high rates of complication and death after surgical repair include large size of the hernia, old age or debility of the patient, and the presence of related intra-abdominal disease. In healthy individuals, surgical repair of the umbilical defects gives good results with a low rate of recurrence.

Kirkpatrick S et al: Umbilical hernia rupture in cirrhotics with ascites. Dig Dis Sci 1988;33:762.

EPIGASTRIC HERNIA

An epigastric hernia (Figure 33–6) protrudes through the linea alba above the level of the umbilicus. The hernia may develop through one of the foramina of egress of the small paramidline nerves and vessels or through an area of congenital weakness in the linea alba.

Figure 33–6. Epigastric hernia. Note closeness to midline and presence in upper abdomen. The herniation is through the linea alba.

About 3–5% of the population have epigastric hernias. They are more common in men than in women and most common between the ages of 20 and 50. About 20% of epigastric hernias are multiple, and about 80% occur just off the midline.

Clinical Findings

A. Symptoms

Most epigastric hernias are painless and are found on routine abdominal examination. If symptomatic, their presentation ranges from mild epigastric pain and tenderness to deep, burning epigastric pain with radiation to the back or the lower abdominal quadrants. The pain may be accompanied by abdominal bloating, nausea, or vomiting. The symptoms often occur after a large meal and on occasion may be relieved by reclining, probably because the supine position causes the herniated mass to drop away from the anterior abdominal wall. The smaller masses most frequently contain only preperitoneal fat and are especially prone to incarceration and strangulation. These smaller hernias are often tender. Larger hernias seldom strangulate and may contain, in addition to preperitoneal fat, a portion of the nearby omentum and, occasionally, a loop of small or large bowel.

B. Signs

If a mass is palpable, the diagnosis can often be confirmed by any maneuver that will increase intra-abdominal pressure and thereby cause the mass to bulge anteriorly. The diagnosis is difficult to make when the patient is obese, since a mass is hard to palpate; ultrasound, CT, or tangential radiographs may be needed in the very obese patient.

Differential Diagnosis

Differential diagnosis includes peptic ulcer, gallbladder disease, hiatal hernia, pancreatitis, and upper small bowel obstruction. On occasion, it may be impossible to distinguish the hernial mass from a subcutaneous lipoma, fibroma, or neurofibroma.

Another condition that must be distinguished from an epigastric hernia is **diastasis recti,** a diffuse widening and attenuation of the linea alba without a fascial defect. On examination, this condition appears as a fusiform, linear bulge between the two rectus abdominis muscles without a discrete fascial defect. Although this condition may be unsightly, repair should be avoided since there is no risk of incarceration, the fascial layer is weak, and the recurrence rate is high.

Treatment

Most epigastric hernias should be repaired, since small ones are likely to become incarcerated and large ones are often symptomatic and unsightly. The defect can usually be closed primarily. Herniated fat contents are usually dissected free and removed. Intraperitoneal herniating structures are reduced, but no attempt is made to close the peritoneal sac.

Prognosis

The recurrence rate is 10–20%, a higher incidence than with the routine inguinal or femoral hernia repair. This high recurrence rate may be partly due to failure to recognize and repair multiple small defects.

Hodgson TJ et al: Anterior abdominal wall hernias: diagnosis by ultrasound and tangential radiographs. Clin Radiol 1991; 44:185.

INCISIONAL HERNIA (Ventral Hernia)

About 10% of abdominal operations result in incisional hernias. The incidence of this iatrogenic type of hernia is not diminishing in spite of an awareness of the many causative factors.

Etiology

The factors most often responsible for incisional hernia are listed below. When more than one factor coexists in the same patient, the likelihood of postoperative wound failure is greatly increased.

(1) Poor surgical technique. Inadequate fascial bites, tension on the fascial edges, or too tight a closure are most often responsible for incisional failure.

(2) Postoperative wound infection.

(3) Age. Wound healing is usually slower and less solid in older patients.

(4) General debility. Cirrhosis, carcinoma, and chronic wasting diseases are factors that affect wound healing adversely. Any condition that compromises nutrition increases the likelihood of incision breakdown.

(5) Obesity. Fat patients frequently have increased intra-abdominal pressure. The presence of fat in the abdominal wound masks tissue layers and increases the incidence of seromas and hematomas in wounds.

(6) Postoperative pulmonary complications that stress the repair as a result of vigorous coughing. Smokers and patients with chronic pulmonary disease are therefore at increased risk of fascial disruption.

(7) Placement of drains or stomas in the primary operative wound.

(8) Intraoperative blood loss greater than 1000 mL.

(9) Failure to close the fascia of laparoscopic trocar sites over 10 mm in size.

Treatment

Small incisional hernias should be treated by early repair since they may cause bowel obstruction. If the patient is unwilling to undergo surgery or is a poor surgical risk, symptoms may be controlled by an elastic corset.

Defects too large to close easily may be left without surgical repair if they are asymptomatic, since they are unlikely to incarcerate.

A. SMALL HERNIAS

Small incisional hernias usually require only a direct fascia-to-fascia repair for satisfactory closure. Interrupted or continuous closure may be used, but the sutures should be nonabsorbable. Sutures tied too tightly or tension on the repair will predispose to recurrence.

B. LARGE HERNIAS

Although no specific diameter distinguishes a small from a large hernia, a hernia can be considered large when the fascial edges cannot be approximated without tension. In repair of large hernias, spinal or epidural anesthesia gives superior relaxation, though general anesthesia with the addition of muscle relaxants also works well.

In performing the repair, excess and scarred skin and subcutaneous tissues over the hernia are removed. The hernia sac is then carefully dissected free from the underlying muscles and fascial tissues. If there are no adherent intraperitoneal structures, the sac may be inverted and the repair done over the inverted sac. If there is incarceration or adhesion of intraperitoneal contents, the abdominal contents should be dissected free from the sac and dropped back into the abdomen. The edges of the fascial defect should be cleaned so that the closure will be to solid fascial tissue rather that to scar.

Primary closure of a large defect is not advisable, since tension on the closure increases the risk of hernia recurrence. Increasingly, repair of large or recurrent defects is performed using nonabsorbable mesh. Although a variety of techniques exist for placement of the mesh, a retrorectus inlay or sandwich technique achieves a lower recurrence rate than an edge-to-edge or onlay placement. If a large dead space persists, a closed drainage system is usually employed in the space above the fascia.. A primary fascial closure should be used only if the fascia can be brought together without tension.

Laparoscopic techniques are also currently being used to repair incisional hernias and perform adhesiolysis electively. A sheet of synthetic material, usually PTFE, is secured to the abdominal wall as an inlay graft; the intraperitoneal placement of the graft enhances the durability of the repair, though it also increases the risk of bowel adhesions or fistula formation.

The use of mesh for repair of incisional hernias does increase the risk of infection and fistula formation. Alternative methods for closure of large abdominal wall defects, such as the use of lateral counterincisions in the anterior rectus sheath to allow primary closure in the midline, are sometimes used to avoid the need for mesh.

Prognosis

The recurrence rate for first-time incisional hernia repairs varies directly with the size of the fascial defect. Small hernias have a recurrence rate of 2–5%; medium-sized hernias recur in 5–15% of cases; and large hernias, too often closed under tension, have a recurrence rate approaching 50%. Repair of recurrent incisional hernias is even less likely to succeed, with a recurrence rate exceeding 50%.

Holzman MD et al: Laparoscopic ventral and incisional hernioplasty. Surg Endosc 1997;11:32.

Israelsson LA et al: Suture technique and wound healing in midline laparotomy incisions. Eur J Surg 1996;162:605.

Leber GE et al: Long-term complications associated with prosthetic repair of incisional hernias. Arch Surg 1998;133:378.

McLanahan D et al: Retrorectus prosthetic mesh repair of midline abdominal hernia. Am J Surg 1997;173:445.

Sugerman HJ et al: Greater risk of incisional hernia with morbidly obese than steroid-dependent patients and low recurrence with prefascial polypropylene mesh. Am J Surg 1996;171:80.

Toy FK et al: Prospective, multicenter study of laparoscopic ventral hernioplasty: preliminary results. Surg Endosc 1998;12:955.

VARIOUS RARE HERNIATIONS THROUGH THE ABDOMINAL WALL

Littre's Hernia

A Littre hernia is a hernia that contains a Meckel diverticulum in the hernia sac. Although Littre first described the condition in relation to a femoral hernia, the relative distribution of Littre's hernias is as follows: inguinal, 50%; femoral, 20%; umbilical, 20%; and miscellaneous, 10%. Littre's hernias of the groin are more common in men and on the right side. The clinical findings are similar to those of Richter's hernia; when strangulation is present, pain, fever, and manifestations of small bowel obstruction occur late.

Treatment consists of repair of the hernia plus, if possible, excision of the diverticulum. If acute Meckel's diverticulitis is present, the acute inflammatory mass may have to be treated through a separate abdominal incision.

Trupo FJ et al: Meckel's diverticulum in femoral hernia: a Littre's hernia. South Med J 1987;80:655.

Spigelian Hernia

Spigelian hernia is an acquired ventral hernia through the linea semilunaris, the line where the sheaths of the lateral abdominal muscles fuse to form the lateral rectus sheath. Spigelian hernias are nearly always found above the level of the inferior epigastric vessels. They most commonly occur where the semicircular line (fold of Douglas) crosses the linea semilunaris.

The presenting symptom is pain that is usually localized to the hernia site and may be aggravated by any maneuver that increases intra-abdominal pressure. With time, the pain may become more dull, constant, and diffuse, making diagnosis more difficult.

If a mass can be demonstrated, the diagnosis presents little difficulty. The diagnosis is most easily made with the patient standing and straining; a bulge then presents in the lower abdominal area and disappears with a gurgling sound on pressure. Following reduction of the mass, the hernia orifice can usually be palpated.

Diagnosis is often made more difficult because the hernial defect may lie beneath an intact external oblique layer and therefore not be palpable. The hernia often dissects within the layers of the abdominal wall and may not present a distinct mass, or the mass may be located at a distance from the linea semilunaris. Patients with spigelian hernias should have a tender point over the hernia orifice, though tenderness alone is not sufficient to make the diagnosis. Both ultrasound and CT scan may help to confirm the diagnosis.

Spigelian hernias have a high incidence of incarceration and should be repaired. These hernias are quite easily cured by primary aponeurotic closure.

Broughton G 2nd et al: Repair of a spigelian hernia. J Am Coll Surg 1997;185:490.

Lumbar or Dorsal Hernia

Lumbar or dorsal hernias (Figure 33–7) are hernias through the posterior abdominal wall at some level in the lumbar region. The most common sites (95%) are the superior (Grynfeltt's) and inferior (Petit's) lumbar triangles. A "lump in the flank" is the common complaint, associated with a dull, heavy, pulling feeling. With the patient erect, the presence of a reducible, often tympanitic mass in the flank usually makes the diagnosis. Incarceration and strangulation occur in about 10% of cases. Hernias in the inferior lumbar triangle are most often small and occur in young, athletic women. They present as tender masses producing back-

Figure 33–7. Anatomic relationships of lumbar or dorsal hernia. (Adapted from Netter.) On the left, lumbar or dorsal hernia into space of Grynfeltt. On the right, hernia into Petit's triangle (inferior lumbar space)

ache and usually contain fat. Lumbar hernia must be differentiated from abscesses, hematomas, soft tissue tumors, renal tumors, and muscle strain.

Acquired hernias may be traumatic or nontraumatic. Severe direct trauma, penetrating wounds, abscesses, and poor healing of flank incisions are the usual causes. Congenital hernias occur in infants and are usually isolated unilateral congenital defects.

Lumbar hernias increase in size and should be repaired when found. Repair is by mobilization of the nearby fascia and obliteration of the hernia defect by precise fascia-to-fascia closure. The recurrence rate is very low.

Heniford BT et al: Laparoscopic inferior and superior lumbar hernia repair. Arch Surg 1997;132:1141.

Killeen KL et al: Using CT to diagnose traumatic lumbar hernia. AJR Am J Roentgenol 2000;174:1413.

Thor K: Lumbar hernia. Acta Chir Scand 1985;151:389.

Obturator Hernia

Herniation through the obturator canal is more frequent in elderly women and is difficult to diagnose preoperatively. The mortality rate (13–40%) of these hernias makes them the most lethal of all abdominal hernias. These hernias most commonly present as small bowel obstruction with cramping abdominal pain and vomiting. The hernia is rarely palpable in the groin, though a mass may be felt on pelvic or rectal examination. The most specific finding is a positive Howship-Romberg sign, in which pain extends down the medial aspect of the thigh with abduction, extension, or internal rotation of the knee. Since this sign is present in fewer than half of cases, diagnosis should be suspected in any elderly debilitated woman without previous abdominal operations who presents with a small bowel obstruction. Though diagnosis can be confirmed by CT scan, operation should not be unduly delayed if complete bowel obstruction is present.

The abdominal approach gives the best exposure; these hernias should not be repaired from the thigh approach. The Cheatle-Henry approach (retropubic) may also be used. Simple repair is most often possible, though bladder wall, pectineal muscle, peritoneum, or mesh has been used when the defect cannot be approximated primarily.

Naude G et al: Obturator hernia is an unsuspected diagnosis. Am J Surg 1997;174:72.

Perineal Hernia

A perineal hernia protrudes through the muscles and fascia of the perineal floor. It may be primary but is usually acquired following perineal prostatectomy, abdominoperineal resection of the rectum, or pelvic exenteration.

These hernias present as easily reducible perineal bulges and usually are asymptomatic, but may present with pain, dysuria, bowel obstruction, or perineal skin breakdown.

Repair is usually done by an abdominal approach, with an adequate fascial and muscular perineal repair. Occasionally polypropylene (Marlex) mesh or flaps using the gracilis or gluteus may be necessary, when the available tissues are too attenuated for adequate primary repair.

So JB et al: Post operative perineal hernia. Dis Colon Rectum 1997;40:954.

Interparietal Hernia

Interparietal hernias, in which the sac insinuates itself between the layers of the abdominal wall, are usually of an indirect inguinal type but, rarely, may be direct or ventral hernias. Although interparietal hernias are rare, it is essential to recognize them, because strangulation is common and the mass is easily mistaken for a tumor or abscess. The lesion usually can be suspected on the basis of the physical examination provided it is kept in mind. In most cases, extensive studies for intra-abdominal tumors have preceded diagnosis. A lateral film of the abdomen will usually show bowel within the layers of the abdominal wall in cases with intestinal incarceration or strangulation, and an ultrasound or CT scan may be diagnostic.

As soon as the diagnosis is established, operation should be performed, usually through the standard inguinal approach.

Sciatic Hernia

Sciatic hernia is the rarest of abdominal hernias and consists of an outpouching of intra-abdominal contents through the greater sciatic foramen. The diagnosis is made after incarceration or strangulation of the bowel occurs. The repair is usually made through the abdominal approach. The hernia sac and contents are reduced, and the weak area is closed by making a fascial flap from the superficial fascia of the piriformis muscle.

TRAUMATIC HERNIA

Abdominal wall hernias occur rarely as a direct consequence of direct blunt abdominal injury. The patient presents with abdominal pain. On examination, ecchymosis of the abdominal wall and a bulge are usually present. The existence of a hernia may not be obvious, however, and the patient may require CT scan to confirm it. Because of the high incidence of associated intra-abdominal injuries, laparotomy is usually required. The defect should be repaired primarily if possible.

Gill IS et al: Traumatic ventral abdominal hernia associated with small bowel gangrene: case report. J Trauma 1993;35:145.

Otero C et al: Injury to the abdominal wall musculature: the full spectrum of traumatic hernia. South Med J 1988;81:517.

Wood RJ et al: Traumatic abdominal hernia: a case report and review of the literature. Am Surg 1988;54:648.

■ II. OTHER LESIONS OF THE ABDOMINAL WALL

CONGENITAL DEFECTS

Congenital defects of the abdominal wall other than hernias or lesions of the urachus and umbilicus are rare. The important ones involving the urachus and umbilicus are discussed in Chapter 47.

TRAUMA TO THE ABDOMINAL WALL

Hematoma of the Rectus Sheath

This is a rare but important entity that may follow mild trauma to the abdominal wall or may occur secondary to disorders of coagulation, blood dyscrasia, or degenerative vascular diseases.

Abdominal pain, usually in the right lower abdomen, is a presenting sign. It may be sudden and severe in onset or slowly progressive. The key to diagnosis is the physical examination. Careful palpation will reveal an exquisitely tender mass within the abdominal wall. If the patient tenses the rectus muscles by raising the head or body, the swelling becomes more tender and distinct on palpation, in contrast to an intra-abdominal mass or tenderness that disappears when the rectus muscles are contracted (Fothergill's sign). In addition, there may be detectable discoloration or ecchymosis. If the physical signs are not diagnostic, ultrasound or CT scan can demonstrate the hematoma in the abdominal wall.

Usually, the condition can be treated without operation. The acute pain and discomfort should disappear within 2 or 3 days, although a residual mass may persist for several weeks. If pain is severe, an acceptable alternative is evacuation of the clot and control of the bleeding.

Edlow JA et al: Rectus sheath hematoma. Ann Emerg Med 1999; 34:671.

PAIN IN THE ABDOMINAL WALL

A number of conditions are characterized by pain in the abdominal wall without a demonstrable organic lesion. Pain from a diaphragmatic, supradiaphragmatic, or spinal cord lesion may be referred to the abdomen. Herpes zoster (shingles) may present as abdominal pain, in which case it will follow a dermatomal distribution.

Scars may be sensitive or painful, particularly in the first 6 months after surgery.

Entrapment of a nerve by a nonabsorbable suture may cause persistent incisional pain, sometimes quite severe. Hyperesthesia of the skin over the involved dermatome may provide a clue to the cause.

In all cases of epigastric pain in the abdominal wall, careful search should be made for a small epigastric hernia, as noted earlier.

ABDOMINAL WALL TUMORS

Tumors of the abdominal wall are quite common, but most are benign, eg, lipomas, hemangiomas, and fibromas. Musculoaponeurotic fibromatoses (desmoid tumors), which often occur in abdominal wall scars or after parturition in women, are discussed in more detail in Chapter 48. Most malignant tumors of the abdominal wall are metastatic. Metastases may appear by direct invasion from intra-abdominal lesions or by vascular dissemination. The sudden appearance of a sensitive nodule anywhere in the abdominal wall that is clearly not a hernia should arouse suspicion of an occult cancer, the lung and pancreas being the more likely primary sites.

Adrenals

Quan-Yang Duh, MD, Chienying Liu, MD, J. Blake Tyrrell, MD, & Edward G. Biglieri, MD

Operations on the adrenal glands are performed for primary hyperaldosteronism, pheochromocytoma, hyperadrenocorticism (Cushing's disease or Cushing's syndrome), and, less commonly, other adrenocortical tumors. These conditions are usually characterized by hypersecretion of one or more of the adrenal hormones.

Anatomy & Surgical Principles

The normal combined weight of the adrenals is 7–12 g. The right gland lies posterior and lateral to the vena cava and superior to the kidney (Figure 34–1). The left gland lies medial to the superior pole of the kidney, just lateral to the aorta and immediately posterior to the superior border of the pancreas. An important surgical feature is the remarkable constancy of the adrenal veins. The right adrenal vein, 2–5 mm long and several millimeters wide, connects the anterior aspect of the adrenal gland with the posterolateral aspect of the vena cava. The left adrenal vein is several centimeters long and travels inferiorly from the lower pole of the gland, joining the left renal vein after receiving the inferior phrenic vein. The adrenal arteries are small, multiple, and inconstant. They usually come from the inferior phrenic artery, the aorta, and the renal artery.

With the exception of rare nonsecreting cancers, indications for adrenal surgery result from hypersecretory states. Diagnosis and treatment begin with confirmation of a hypersecretory state (ie, measurement of excess cortisol, aldosterone, or catecholamines in blood or urine). In order to determine whether the problem originates in the adrenal, levels of the stimulator of the hormone in question (ie, ACTH or renin) must be measured. If stimulator levels are low or normal but hormone secretion is excessive, autonomous secretion is proved. The next step, except in pheochromocytoma, is to determine the degree of autonomy, a process that usually distinguishes hyperplasias (which respond to most but not all controlling mechanisms) from adenomas and adenomas from cancers. In general, cancers are under little if any feedback control. If the primary problem is not in the adrenal, as in Cushing's disease, treatment must be directed elsewhere when possible.

Adrenal masses are usually detected and localized by CT scan or MRI. Functioning tumors of the adrenal can be localized by adrenal scintigraphy, [131]I-6β-iodomethyl-norcholesterol (NP-59) for cortical tumors and ^{131}I-metaiodobenzylguanidine (MIBG) for medullary tumors. Functioning adrenal or pituitary tumors can also be localized by demonstrating a gradient of hormone levels between their venous drainage and a peripheral vein.

The major principles of adrenal surgery are as follows:

(1) Whenever possible, the surgeon must be certain of the diagnosis and the location of the lesion before undertaking the operation. Sometimes surgery must be performed based on the diagnosis alone even if a lesion cannot be pinpointed.

(2) The patient must be thoroughly prepared so he or she can withstand any metabolic problems caused by the disease or by the operation.

(3) The surgeon and consultants must be able to detect and treat any metabolic crisis that occurs during or after operation.

Surgical Approaches

Currently, almost all adrenal tumors are identified preoperatively by localization studies such as CT and MRI, so very few operations require general exploration of the abdomen. This permits the use of minimally invasive surgery for treatment.

Almost all adrenal tumors can be removed laparoscopically. Traditional open adrenalectomy is only necessary when the tumor is especially large (eg, > 12 cm, depending on the surgeon's experience) or for locally invasive adrenocortical cancer where resection of adjacent organs may be required.

Laparoscopic adrenalectomy can be performed using a transabdominal or retroperitoneal approach, but the former is preferable in most cases. This involves medial rotation of the spleen and pancreas (on the left) or the liver (on the right), using gravity to drop the viscera away from the adrenal.

The traditional open surgical approach should be used when laparoscopic expertise is not available or when required by the size and nature of the tumor. The advantages of the laparoscopic operation, however, are so great that it is otherwise strongly preferred.

The open anterior (transperitoneal) approach through a long vertical midline incision or a bilateral subcostal incision allows bilateral exploration. It permits wide ex-

Figure 34–1. Anatomy of the adrenals, showing venous return.

posure of the abdominal organs and the retroperitoneum. Unfortunately, this incision also causes more pain, ileus, and atelectasis and a much longer period of recovery. The risks of poor wound healing, such as evisceration (Table 34–1) are greater—especially for patients with Cushing's syndrome.

Table 34–1. Frequency of manifestations of hyperadrenocorticism.

	Percentage
Obesity	95%
Hypertension	70%
Glucose tolerance	80%
Centripetal distribution of fat	80%
Weakness	20%
Muscle atrophy in upper and lower extremities	70%
Hirsutism	80%
Menstrual disturbance or impotence	75%
Purple striae	50%
Plethoric facies	85%
Easy bruisability	35%
Acne	40%
Psychological symptoms	40%
Edema	20%
Headache	15%
Back pain	60%

The open posterior approach, performed through incisions on each side of the spine with the patient lying prone, is better tolerated postoperatively but provides a more limited exposure. This approach can be made through incisions varying from transpleural to those through the bed of the 11th or 12th rib. The 12th rib incision is best tolerated and is adequate for lesions smaller than 4–5 cm. Because of its shortcomings, the posterior approach has been superseded by the laparoscopic approach. An open lateral approach through the bed of the 11th rib to expose the adrenals retroperitoneally may be considered for large or invasive tumors.

■ DISEASES OF THE ADRENALS

PRIMARY HYPERALDOSTERONISM

 ESSENTIALS OF DIAGNOSIS

- *Hypertension with or without hypokalemia.*
- *Elevated aldosterone secretion and suppressed plasma renin activity.*
- *Metabolic alkalosis, relative hypernatremia.*
- *Weakness, polyuria, paresthesias, tetany, cramps due to hypokalemia.*

General Considerations

Aldosterone, the most potent mineralocorticoid secreted by the adrenal cortex, regulates the body's electrolyte composition, fluid volume, and blood pressure. Excess aldosterone increases total body sodium, decreases potassium levels, increases extracellular fluid volume (without edema), and increases blood pressure. Under normal conditions, aldosterone secretion is regulated by the renin-angiotensin system in a feedback fashion and is also stimulated transiently by ACTH.

In primary hyperaldosteronism, aldosterone levels are elevated and renin levels are decreased. In secondary hyperaldosteronism, increased aldosterone is due to increased renin secretion. Examples of secondary hyperaldosteronism include renal vascular disease, renin-secreting tumors, and cirrhosis with low intravascular volume. Among the subtypes of primary hyperaldosteronism, aldosterone-producing adenoma (aldosteronoma) and idiopathic hyperaldosteronism with adrenal hyperplasia are the most common, responsible for about 75% and 25% of cases, respectively. Unilateral primary adrenal hyperplasia, aldosterone-producing adrenocortical carcinoma, and familial hyperaldosteronism (eg, glucocorticoid-remediable hyperaldosteronism) are rare. Surgery is beneficial only in patients with aldosterone-producing adenomas and in patients with unilateral primary adrenal hyperplasia.

Primary hyperaldosteronism is characterized by hypertension, hypokalemia, increased aldosterone secretion, and suppressed plasma renin activity. Hypokalemia is not required to make the diagnosis—about 40% of patients have a normal potassium level. Primary hyperaldosteronism was once thought to be present in about 1% of patients with hypertension, but the prevalence may be as high as 8% of normokalemic hypertensives. Although rare, normotensive primary hyperaldosteronism has been described.

Aldosteronomas are usually solitary and small (0.5–2 cm). They have a characteristic chrome color when sectioned. Tumor cells typically have heterogeneous cytomorphology, resembling those of all three zones of the adrenal cortex, including hybrid cells having cytologic features of the zona glomerulosa and zona fasciculata. Hyperplasia is also often seen in glands harboring adenomas.

Clinical Findings

Aldosterone facilitates the exchange of sodium for potassium and hydrogen ions in the distal nephron. Therefore, when aldosterone secretion is chronically increased, serum potassium and hydrogen ion concentrations fall (hypokalemia and alkalosis), total body sodium rises, and hypertension results.

A. SYMPTOMS AND SIGNS

Symptoms are those of hypokalemia and depend on the severity of potassium depletion. Patients complain of a sense of malaise, muscle weakness, polyuria, polydipsia, cramps, and paresthesias. Tetany and hypokalemic paralysis occur rarely. Headaches are common. Hypertension is usually moderate to severe and may be refractory to medical therapy, but advanced retinopathy is rare. Although extracellular fluid volume is increased, edema is not seen unless renal failure occurs.

B. LABORATORY FINDINGS

1. Screening test—Primary hyperaldosteronism should be suspected in patients with hypertension and hypokalemia—either spontaneous or following the administration of diuretics—and in patients with refractory hypertension. The diagnostic evaluation should start with screening tests. A simple ambulatory test determines the ratio of plasma aldosterone (in ng/dL) to renin (in ng/mL/h). A ratio of > 20 with a plasma aldosterone concentration > 15 ng/dL suggests primary

hyperaldosteronism and warrants confirmatory biochemical studies. Hypertensive individuals without primary hyperaldosteronism usually have ratios of < 20. If the patient is taking spironolactone, the data are uninterpretable, and estrogens increase plasma aldosterone concentrations by increasing angiotensinogen. Both should be discontinued for 6 weeks before the workup. Many other medications, such as diuretics, angiotensin-converting enzyme inhibitors, prostaglandin synthetase inhibitors, cyproheptadine, and vasodilators, can also affect the renin-angiotensin-aldosterone axis and confuse the results. These medications should be discontinued for 2 weeks before the workup. Peripheral alpha-adrenergic blockers are the preferred antihypertensive agents during evaluation. In many patients, it is unwise to withdraw antihypertensive medications, and one must be content with imperfect data. Beta-blockers and calcium channel blockers cause few problems.

2. Confirmatory test—If the screening test is positive, the next step is confirmation. Failure to suppress aldosterone secretion with sodium loading will establish the diagnosis of primary hyperaldosteronism in most patients. Aldosterone can be suppressed by oral salt loading or intravenous sodium chloride infusion. The patient should consume a high-sodium diet for 3 days, supplemented with NaCl tablets (2–3 g with each meal) if necessary. A 24-hour urine sample is collected for aldosterone, sodium, and potassium determinations on the third day. Urinary aldosterone excretion > 12 μg/24 h distinguishes most patients with primary hyperaldosteronism from those with essential hypertension. If sodium intake has been as high as desired, urinary sodium excretion should exceed 200 meq/24 h. Supplemental potassium chloride should be given to avoid hypokalemia because the high-salt diet increases kaliuresis. Hypokalemia may interfere with the test results by decreasing aldosterone secretion, and it may also cause cardiac arrhythmias. Alternatively, a plasma aldosterone concentration > 10 ng/mL after an infusion of 2 L of normal saline over 4 hours is also consistent with primary hyperaldosteronism. However, the variability of aldosterone secretion throughout the day in patients with aldosteronomas makes this method less desirable than oral salt loading.

Differential Diagnosis

Once the diagnosis is established, the surgically correctable forms—aldosterone producing adenoma (aldosteronoma) and the rare unilateral primary adrenal hyperplasia—should be distinguished from idiopathic hyperaldosteronism due to bilateral adrenal hyperplasia, for which medical therapy is the best management. Aldosteronoma and idiopathic hyperaldosteronism are the most common subtypes. Compared with those with idiopathic hyperaldosteronism, patients with aldosteronoma have more severe hypertension, more severe hypokalemia, higher aldosterone secretion (> 20 ng/dL), higher 18-hydroxycorticosterone concentrations (>100 ng/dL), and are younger. Unfortunately, these features do not absolutely distinguish the two types. Combined biochemical studies and imaging studies are frequently necessary.

High-resolution thin-section CT identifies most adenomas and should be performed once the diagnosis of primary hyperaldosteronism is established. Adrenal vein sampling is indicated if the CT scan is equivocal. Adrenal vein sampling is the most certain way to differentiate aldosteronoma from idiopathic hyperaldosteronism and to diagnose and localize aldosteronoma. Nevertheless, it is technically difficult, and failure to cannulate the adrenal veins, especially the right adrenal vein, is common.

The postural stimulation test is based on the observation that aldosteronomas are usually unaffected by the renin-angiotensin system but retain sensitivity to ACTH stimulation. Therefore, the plasma aldosterone concentration follows the diurnal variation of ACTH and cortisol. In contrast, idiopathic hyperaldosteronism is characterized by enhanced sensitivity to small changes in the renin-angiotensin axis but is unaffected by ACTH. Thus, if the patient remains upright for 4 hours, plasma aldosterone levels fall and renin remains suppressed in patients with aldosteronoma. In patients with idiopathic hyperaldosteronism, plasma aldosterone increases in response to a small increase in plasma renin.

Aldosterone-secreting adrenocortical carcinoma should be suspected if the tumor is larger than 3 cm. Glucocorticoid-remediable hyperaldosteronism (familial hyperaldosteronism type 1) is inherited in an autosomal dominant fashion. The genetic defect is due to an unequal-crossing event, resulting in a chimeric gene. The mutated gene juxtaposes the promoter for expression of the 11α-hydroxylase gene, which is ACTH-responsive, with the coding sequence of the aldosterone synthase gene. This leads to aldosterone production under ACTH stimulation in the zona fasciculata. Glucocorticoid therapy reverses this type of hyperaldosteronism. These patients have a family history of onset of hypertension at an early age. The diagnosis can be established by measuring elevated 24-hour urine 18-hydroxycortisol and 18-oxocortisol levels or by genetic testing.

Tumor Localization

An aldosterone-producing adenoma can usually be demonstrated by high-resolution CT or MRI scanning, even showing most small aldosteronomas and nonfunctional adenomas. Nevertheless, a few small lesions are missed, and in this circumstance a patient with a small aldosteronoma not seen on CT may be misdiagnosed as having adrenal hyperplasia. Aldosteronomas that coexist with nonfunctional incidentalomas can be mislabeled as adrenal hyperplasia because of multinodularity or bilateral masses on CT. Small abnormalities on CT scans may represent areas of hyperplasia rather than true aldosteronomas. Therefore, unless an unequivocal unilateral tumor, preferably > 1 cm, is present on the CT scan and the contralateral gland is normal, the diagnosis and localization of aldosteronoma cannot be considered certain. The clinical features and results of the postural stimulation test may offer clues but are not always predictive. When in doubt, adrenal vein sampling should be done; it is 95% accurate in identifying an aldosteronoma. Blood is sampled from the adrenal veins and the inferior vena cava for aldosterone and cortisol levels at baseline and after ACTH infusion. Proper catheter placement is confirmed by finding high cortisol levels in adrenal venous blood compared with the inferior vena cava. Corrected aldosterone levels are calculated from the ratio of aldosterone to cortisol in the blood from each adrenal vein. A lateralization ratio of the corrected aldosterone level > 4 indicates unilateral aldosterone secretion, thereby confirming a diagnosis of aldosteronoma in most patients. Adrenal vein sampling is invasive and requires considerable skill and experience. The success rate for cannulating both adrenal veins is about 80%. Unilateral catheterization of the left adrenal vein alone does not give useful information.

Complications

Uncontrolled hypertension can lead to renal failure, stroke, and myocardial infarction. Severe hypokalemia can cause weakness and paralysis. Patients who are taking digitalis are at high risk for developing dysrhythmia from hypokalemia.

Treatment

The goal of therapy is to prevent illness associated with hypertension and hypokalemia. Treatment depends on the subtype. Unilateral adrenalectomy is recommended for patients with aldosteronoma and medical therapy for those with idiopathic hyperaldosteronism or those with aldosteronoma who are poor candidates for surgery.

A. SURGICAL TREATMENT

1. Preoperative preparation—Blood pressure and hypokalemia should be controlled before surgery. Spironolactone, a competitive aldosterone antagonist, is the ideal medication. It blocks the mineralocorticoid receptor, promotes potassium retention, restores normal potassium concentrations, and reduces the extracellular fluid volume, thereby controlling blood pressure. Furthermore, it reactivates the suppressed renin-angiotensin-aldosterone system in the contralateral adrenal gland, reducing the risk of postoperative hypoaldosteronism. Initial dosages of 200–400 mg/d may be required to control hypokalemia and hypertension. Once blood pressure is normalized and hypokalemia is corrected, the dose can be tapered and maintained at about 100–150 mg/d. Spironolactone may have antiandrogenic side effects, such as impotence, gynecomastia, menstrual irregularity, and gastrointestinal disturbances. Amiloride, 20–40 ng/d, a potassium-sparing diuretic, may be used alternatively or as a supplement to spironolactone. Other medications such as calcium channel blockers and diuretics may be required to control hypertension. These agents can be continued to the day of operation. Hypokalemia and hypertension should be controlled preoperatively, and most patients require a minimum of 1–2 weeks of treatment with spironolactone. Glucocorticoids are unnecessary for patients undergoing unilateral adrenalectomy for aldosteronoma.

2. Surgery—Because aldosteronomas are almost always small and benign, laparoscopic adrenalectomy is the procedure of choice. It can be performed safely and with equally good results by several approaches. The lateral transabdominal approach uses gravity to help medially rotate the viscera (liver on the right and spleen and pancreas on the left) and exposes the adrenal gland. It is the most versatile approach and is preferred by most surgeons. The retroperitoneal approach, either laterally or posteriorly, is used occasionally. It may be best in patients with prior upper abdominal operations, but the working space is cramped. Although some surgeons perform a subtotal resection for aldosteronoma, most excise the adrenal gland with the tumor. The surrounding adrenal tissue frequently appears hyperplastic. A few small aldosteronomas may not be visible intraoperatively, so accurate preoperative localization is important. Bilateral adrenalectomy is not indicated, since patients with idiopathic hyperaldosteronism should be treated medically, and bilateral aldosteronomas are extremely rare.

3. Postoperative care—Occasional patients may develop transient aldosterone deficiency because of suppression of the contralateral adrenal gland by the hyperfunctioning adenoma. This is rare in patients treated with spironolactone preoperatively. Symptoms include postural hypotension and hyperkalemia. Adequate sodium intake is usually sufficient for treatment; rarely, short-term fludrocortisone replacement (0.1 mg/d orally) is required.

B. MEDICAL TREATMENT

The goal is to control hypertension and hypokalemia. Spironolactone is the preferred agent, though amiloride may be better tolerated. Angiotensin-converting enzyme inhibitors and calcium channel blockers have been used with some success. A combination of antihypertensive agents may be necessary.

Prognosis

Hyperaldosteronism usually follows a prolonged and subtly changing course. Untreated hypertension may cause stroke, myocardial infarction, or renal failure.

Removal of an aldosteronoma normalizes potassium levels, but the hypertension is not always cured. About one-third of patients have persistent mild hypertension that is usually easier to control than before the operation. Essential hypertension and atherosclerosis due to chronic hypertension are contributing factors. Although most patients with idiopathic hyperaldosteronism are treated medically, adrenalectomy is indicated for those with aldosteronoma because the tumor may grow and because side effects of the medications and compliance make long-term medical treatment undesirable. The low morbidity, short hospitalization, and high success rate of laparoscopic adrenalectomy have with few exceptions made surgery preferable to long-term medical therapy.

Bravo EL: Primary aldosteronism. Issues in diagnosis and management. Endocrinol Metab Clin North Am 1994;23: 271.

Fontes RG et al: Reassessment of the predictive value of the postural stimulation test in primary aldosteronism. Am J Hypertens 1991;4:786.

Ghose RP, Hall PM, Bravo EL: Medical management of aldosterone-producing adenomas. Ann Intern Med 1999;131:105.

Gordon RD et al: High incidence of primary aldosteronism in 199 patients referred with hypertension. Clin Exp Pharmacol Physiol 1994;21:319.

Loh KC et al: Prevalence of primary aldosteronism among Asian hypertensive patients in Singapore. J Clin Endocrinol Metab 2000;85:2854.

Magill SB et al: Comparison of adrenal vein sampling and computed tomography in the differentiation of primary aldosteronism. J Clin Endocrinol Metab 2001;86;1066.

Shen WT et al: Laparoscopic vs open adrenalectomy for the treatment of primary hyperaldosteronism. Arch Surg 1999;134: 628.

Weinberger MH, Fineberg NS: The diagnosis of primary aldosteronism and separation of two major subtypes. Arch Intern Med 1993;153:2125.

Young WF: Pheochromocytoma and primary aldosteronism: diagnostic approaches. Endocrinol Metab Clin North Am 1997; 26:801.

Young WF et al: Primary aldosteronism: adrenal venous sampling. Surgery 1996;120:913.

PHEOCHROMOCYTOMA

 ESSENTIALS OF DIAGNOSIS

- *Episodic headache, excessive sweating, palpitation and visual blurring.*
- *Hypertension, frequently sustained, with or without paroxysms.*
- *Postural tachycardia and hypotension.*
- *Elevated urinary catecholamines or their metabolites, hypermetabolism, hyperglycemia.*

General Considerations

Pheochromocytomas are tumors of the adrenal medulla and related chromaffin tissues elsewhere in the body that secrete epinephrine or norepinephrine, resulting in sustained or episodic hypertension and other symptoms of excess catecholamines.

Pheochromocytoma is found in less than 0.1% of patients with hypertension and accounts for about 5% of adrenal tumors incidentally discovered by CT scanning. Most pheochromocytomas occur sporadically without other diseases, but they may be associated with various familial syndromes such as MEN 2a (medullary thyroid carcinoma, pheochromocytoma, and hyperparathyroidism), MEN 2b (medullary thyroid carcinoma, pheochromocytoma, mucosal neuromas, marfanoid habitus, and ganglioneuromatosis), Recklinghausen's disease (café au lait spots, neurofibromatosis, pheochromocytoma), von Hippel-Lindau disease (retinal hemangioma, hemangioblastoma of the central nervous system, renal cysts and carcinoma, pheochromocytoma, pancreatic cysts, and epididymal cystadenoma). Screening for these syndromes should be considered especially in young patients and in patients with multifocal tumors. Family members of patients who have been diagnosed with these syndromes also need screening to determine whether they are gene carriers and are at risk for developing the various tumors, including pheochromocytoma.

On pathologic examination, pheochromocytoma appears reddish-gray and frequently has areas of necrosis, hemorrhage, and sometimes cysts. The usual size is about 100 g or 5 cm in diameter, but they can be as small as 2–3 cm or as large as 12–16 cm. Cells are pleomorphic, showing prominent nucleoli and frequent mitoses. Cytologic findings cannot be used to determine whether a pheochromocytoma is malignant or benign. The veins and capsules may also be invaded even in clinically benign tumors. Malignancy can only be diagnosed in the presence of metastases or invasion into surrounding tissues.

Clinical Findings

A. SYMPTOMS AND SIGNS

The clinical findings of pheochromocytoma are variable, and mild cases may only come to attention because of an incidental finding of an adrenal tumor (incidentaloma) on CT or MR scans performed to evaluate other diseases. Classically, the patient has episodic hypertension associated with the triad of palpitation, headache, and sweating. The patient may also complain of anxiety, tremors, weight loss, dizziness, nausea and vomiting, abdominal discomfort, constipation, and visual blurring. Some patients have diarrhea, which may be secondary to secretion of vasoactive intestinal peptide. The physical examination may be unremarkable except during an attack, when pallor, flushing, and excess sweating may be observed. Tachycardia, postural hypotension, and hypertensive retinopathy are other signs.

Hypertension, the most common feature of pheochromocytoma, occurs in 90% of patients. More than half have sustained hypertension, which may be mild to moderate, with or without other signs and symptoms of catecholamine excess, and the diagnosis may be missed. In some cases, basal blood pressure may not be elevated, and severe hypertension occurs only while the patient is under stress, such as general anesthesia or trauma. Patients with diastolic hypertension and postural hypotension, who are not receiving antihypertensive medications, may have pheochromocytoma. Epinephrine raises blood glucose and norepinephrine decreases insulin secretion, and hyperglycemia may occur.

Traditionally, catecholamine-secreting tumors have been said to be 10% malignant, 10% familial, 10% bilateral, 10% multiple, and 10% extra-adrenal. In children, hypertension is less prominent, and about 50% have multiple or extra-adrenal tumors. Malignant tumors may be more common in extra-adrenal pheochromocytomas. Pheochromocytomas occur in 40% of patients with MEN 2; they tend to be bilateral and multiple but are rarely extra-adrenal or malignant. Screening of MEN 2 patients and family members who are *ret* proto-oncogene mutation carriers by measuring urinary catecholamine and metanephrine or plasma metanephrine levels may diagnose pheochromocytomas before they produce clinical manifestations. Plasma total metanephrine (metanephrine and normetanephrine) levels are the most sensitive test for pheochromocytoma.

B. LABORATORY FINDINGS

The diagnosis of pheochromocytoma is best made by 24-hour urine excretion of metanephrines (metanephrine and normetanephrine) and free catecholamines (Figure 34–2). Urinary output of metanephrines or free catecholamines is high in 99% of patients with pheochromocytoma. In 80% of patients, the level exceeds twice normal. Measurement of urinary vanillylmandelic acid (VMA) is less sensitive. Assays using high-pressure liquid chromatography (HPLC) reduce interference by drugs and diets, but many drugs can potentially interfere with the assays or affect the secretion and metabolism of catecholamines. Examples include acetaminophen, beta-blockers (especially labetalol), vasodilators (such as nitroglycerin), alpha-blockers, calcium channel blockers (nifedipine, verapamil), theophylline, stimulants (amphetamine, caffeine, nicotine, methylphenidate), antipsychotics (clozapine, chlorpromazine), antidepressants (fluvoxamine, venlafaxine), prochlorperazine, and methyldopa. The assay may also be affected by ethanol, bananas, radiographic dyes, drugs that contain catecholamines, and withdrawal from clonidine. These agents should be discontinued for 2 weeks before measuring urinary catecholamines and metanephrines. The interfering substances vary depending on the assays used, so a list and protocol for preparing the patient should be obtained from the specific laboratory.

Overnight urinary collection and short collection periods following a paroxysm, indexed to creatinine, have also been used. Plasma metanephrine levels are 98% sensitive and 90% specific—even better than urinary catecholamines, urinary metanephrines, and plasma catecholamines for screening—but the assays are not yet widely available. Ongoing metabolism of catecholamines to free metanephrines within the tumor may explain the superiority of using plasma metanephrine levels for diagnosis.

Plasma epinephrine and norepinephrine should only be measured under standard, controlled conditions, since their levels may be falsely elevated if the patient is under stress. The levels may be low if the tumor secretes episodically. Provocative tests—using glucagon, histamine, or tyramine—are not accurate and potentially dangerous. They are almost never indicated. Clonidine suppression tests are rarely used. Clonidine does not decrease plasma catecholamine levels in patients with pheochromocytoma, as it may in normal anxious individuals or in patients with essential hypertension.

C. LOCALIZATION OF TUMOR

Localization studies should be delayed until biochemical studies have confirmed the diagnosis of a catecholamine-secreting tumor. Ninety percent of pheochromocytomas are found in the adrenal glands and most are > 3 cm in diameter. Of the extra-adrenal pheochromocytomas, 75% are in the abdomen, 10% in the bladder, 10% in the chest, 2 % in the pelvis, and 3% in the head and neck. Both CT and MRI can local-

Figure 34–2. Scheme for evaluation of a patient with suspected pheochromocytoma.

ize most pheochromocytomas. CT scan is less expensive, but MRI avoids radiation exposure. Pheochromocytoma usually has a characteristic bright appearance on T2-weighted MRI. MIBG may be helpful for localizing extra-adrenal pheochromocytomas, and it should be considered when searching for extra-adrenal, multiple, or malignant pheochromocytomas. MIBG is more specific but less sensitive compared with CT or MRI for localization. Arteriography and fine-needle aspiration biopsy can precipitate a hypertensive crisis. They do not contribute to the diagnosis, and are not indicated. Venous sampling for catecholamines is no longer indicated.

Differential Diagnosis

The differential diagnosis includes all causes of hypertension. Hyperthyroidism and pheochromocytoma have many features in common (weight loss, tremor, and tachycardia). The diagnosis of pheochromocytoma is easier if episodic hypertension is present. Acute anxiety attacks mimic the symptoms and may precipitate hypertensive episodes, but anxiety alone rarely produces severe hypertension. Carcinoid syndrome causing episodes of flushing may also be mistaken for pheochromocytoma. The urinary 5-HIAA level is usually markedly elevated, and CT scan usually shows liver metastases in patients with carcinoid syndrome. Labile essential hypertension is not associated with elevated catecholamine levels.

Pheochromocytoma in pregnancy, if not recognized, will kill half of the fetuses and nearly half of the mothers. Hypertension in pregnancy is usually ascribed to preeclampsia-eclampsia. The diagnosis of pheochromocytoma requires the same biochemical studies; radiation (CT) and radioisotopes (MIBG) are usually not used; MRI is indicated to localize the tumor when a biochemical diagnosis has been established. Alpha- and beta-adrenergic blockers appear to be well tolerated. Timing of the operation is individualized. If recognized early, the tumor is best removed early in the second trimester. Otherwise, alpha-adrenergic blockade is continued and then followed by a planned cesarean section at term. The pheochromocytoma can be resected either at the time of cesarean section—if easily accessible through the same incision—or electively a few weeks postpartum laparoscopically.

Crisis may develop in patients with pheochromocytoma, usually precipitated by trauma, surgery, or other procedures. Crisis usually occurs when alpha-adrenergic blockade has not been instituted. These patients may develop multisystem failure, mimicking severe sepsis. If the disease is not recognized, death is the usual result. Once pheochromocytoma is diagnosed, the patient should be stabilized and alpha-adrenergic blockade

started. Emergent operation may be necessary, though—if possible—resection during the same hospitalization after the patient is stabilized is preferred.

Complications

Pheochromocytoma causes complications because of hypertension, cardiac arrhythmia, and hypovolemia. The sequelae of hypertension are stroke, renal failure, myocardial infarction, and congestive heart failure. Sudden death can result from ventricular tachycardia or fibrillation. Alpha-adrenergic stimulation by the catecholamines causes vasoconstriction and a low total blood volume. The patient is therefore unable to compensate for a sudden loss of blood volume (bleeding) or catecholamines (tumor removal) and at risk of cardiovascular collapse. Preoperative alpha-adrenergic blockade and restoration of blood volume can prevent these complications.

Treatment

A. MEDICAL TREATMENT

Treatment with alpha-adrenergic blocking agents should be started as soon as the biochemical diagnosis is established. The aims of preoperative therapy are (1) to restore the blood volume, which has been depleted by excessive catecholamines; (2) to prevent a severe crisis, with its potential complications; and (3) to allow the patient to recover from cardiomyopathy. Close control of hypertension is necessary in order to keep blood volume normal.

Phenoxybenzamine, a nonselective alpha-adrenergic antagonist, has a long duration of action and is the preferred drug. It should be started at a dosage of 10 mg per 12 hours, and the dose should be increased—as postural hypotension allows—until signs of excess catecholamine stimulation have disappeared and blood volume is clinically normal. Dosages as high as 300 mg/d may be necessary. Most patients require 10–14 days of treatment, as judged by stabilization of blood pressure and reduction of symptoms. Nasal stuffiness is usually present when alpha blockade is well established.

Metyrosine inhibits tyrosine hydroxylase and reduces catecholamine synthesis and can be added to phenoxybenzamine as preoperative therapy. Calcium channel blockers and competitive selective alpha-adrenergic blocking agents such as prazosin are effective.

Beta-adrenergic blocking agents are often useful to treat arrhythmias and tachycardia but should only be given after alpha blockade has been achieved. Otherwise, a hypertensive crisis may be precipitated because of the unopposed alpha-adrenergic effect of the catecholamines. Opioids should be avoided because they may stimulate histamine release and precipitate a crisis.

B. SURGICAL TREATMENT

The definitive treatment of pheochromocytoma is excision. It was once recommended that both adrenal glands and other areas likely to harbor extra-adrenal tumors should be examined at the time of surgery, but that practice is now outmoded even for patients clinically at risk for bilateral or multiple tumors, because CT, MRI, and MIBG scans are so sensitive in finding all lesions.

Smaller (< 5–6 cm) adrenal pheochromocytomas can be safely resected by laparoscopic adrenalectomy. Very large > 8–10 cm) and extra-adrenal tumors are technically more difficult and may require a laparotomy.

During surgery, an arterial line is necessary for continuous blood pressure monitoring. Monitoring of pulmonary artery pressure is rarely necessary in patients who are well blocked.

Nitroprusside should be immediately available to treat sudden hypertension and beta-blockers to treat the cardiac dysrhythmias that may occur when the tumor is manipulated. Manipulation of the gland is less with laparoscopic than with open adrenalectomy, which minimizes fluctuations in plasma catecholamine levels.

Very large malignant tumors may require a thoracoabdominal incision. Malignant pheochromocytomas may invade the adrenal vein or vena cava. Extra-adrenal pheochromocytomas are usually found along the abdominal aorta and in the organ of Zuckerkandl near the aortic bifurcation. However, tumors have been found in widely scattered sites such as the bladder, the vagina, the mediastinum, the neck, and even the skull and pericardium. In general, extra-adrenal tumors should be localized with MIBG, CT, or MRI preoperatively to avoid a blind exploration.

In patients with MEN 2 and bilateral pheochromocytomas, cortical-sparing subtotal adrenalectomy on the side of the smaller tumor may avoid postoperative adrenal insufficiency, though it increases the risk for recurrence. In patients with MEN 2 and a unilateral pheochromocytoma, prophylactic resection of the contralateral normal-appearing adrenal gland is contraindicated, since bilateral adrenalectomy leads to lifelong hypoadrenalism requiring cortisol replacement. These patients should be followed with biochemical evaluations, and the contralateral adrenal gland should be resected only if pheochromocytoma develops.

Many patients undergoing resection of pheochromocytoma have arrhythmias and wide variations in blood pressure and heart rate. Blood pressure will almost always fall when all functioning tissue has been removed. If the patient has been properly prepared with alpha-blockers, the changes in blood pressure will not be severe. Otherwise, intravenous infusion of large amounts of saline and catecholamine may be necessary to maintain blood pressure after the tumor is removed.

Prognosis

The outlook for patients with untreated pheochromocytoma is grim, whereas the operative mortality rate was decreased to 2% from 30% following the introduction of alpha-adrenergic blockade. Mild to moderate essential hypertension may persist after surgery. Second tumors in the remaining adrenal or metastatic tumors can occur years after excision of the primary pheochromocytoma; long-term follow-up is mandatory. Metastatic or recurrent malignant pheochromocytoma should be resected if possible to reduce the catecholamine load. Treatment with high-dose ^{131}I-MIBG may be helpful in these patients.

Ahlawat SK et al: Pheochromocytoma associated with pregnancy: case report and review of the literature. Obstet Gynecol Surv 1999;54:728.

Duh Q-Y: Editorial: Evolving surgical management for patients with pheochromocytoma. J Clin Endocrinol Metab 2001; 86:1477.

Eisenhofer G et al: Plasma normetanephrine and metanephrine for detecting pheochromocytoma in von Hippel-Lindau disease and multiple endocrine neoplasia type 2. N Engl J Med 1999;340:1872.

Gagner M et al: Is laparoscopic adrenalectomy indicated for pheochromocytomas? Surgery 1996;120:1076.

Kebebew E et al: Benign and malignant pheochromocytoma: diagnosis, treatment, and follow up. Surg Oncol Clin N Am 1998;7:765.

Lenders JW et al: Plasma metanephrines in the diagnosis of pheochromocytoma. Ann Intern Med 1995;123:101.

Peaston RT et al: Overnight excretion of urinary catecholamines and metabolites in the detection of pheochromocytoma. J Clin Endocrinol Metab 1996;81:1378.

Prys-Roberts C: Phaeochromocytoma—recent progress in its management. Br J Anaesth 2000;85:44.

van Heerden JA et al: Long-term evaluation following resection of apparently benign pheochromocytoma(s)/paraganglioma(s). World J Surg 1990;14:325.

Whalen RK et al: Extra-adrenal pheochromocytoma. J Urol 1992; 147:1.

Young WF: Pheochromocytoma and primary aldosteronism: diagnostic approaches. Endocrinol Metab Clin North Am 1997; 26:801.

HYPERADRENOCORTICISM (Cushing's Disease & Cushing's Syndrome)

 ESSENTIALS OF DIAGNOSIS

- Facial plethora, dorsocervical fat pad, supraclavicular fat pad, truncal obesity, easy bruisability,

purple striae, acne, hirsutism, impotence or amenorrhea, muscle weakness, and psychosis.
- Hypertension and hyperglycemia.

General Considerations

Cushing's syndrome is due to chronic glucocorticoid excess. It may be caused by excess ACTH stimulation or by adrenocortical tumors that secrete glucocorticoids independently of ACTH stimulation. Excess ACTH may be produced by pituitary adenomas (Cushing's disease), or extrapituitary ACTH-producing tumors (ectopic ACTH syndrome). Cushing's syndrome not dependent on ACTH is usually caused by primary adrenal diseases such as adrenocortical adenoma, macro- or micronodular hyperplasia, or carcinoma.

The natural history of Cushing's syndrome depends on the underlying disease and varies from a mild, indolent disease to rapid progression and death.

Clinical Findings

A. Symptoms and Signs

(See Table 34–1.) The classic description of Cushing's syndrome includes truncal obesity, hirsutism, moon facies, acne, buffalo hump, purple striae, hypertension, and diabetes, but other signs and symptoms are common. Weakness and depression are striking features. Weakness and other features are also seen after prolonged and excessive administration of adrenocortical steroids.

In children, Cushing's syndrome is most commonly caused by adrenal cancers, but adenomas and nodular hyperplasia have been described. Cushing's syndrome in children also causes growth retardation or arrest.

B. Pathologic Examination

The pathologic features of the adrenal gland depend on the underlying disease. Normal adrenal glands weigh 7–12 g combined. The hyperplastic adrenal glands in patients with Cushing's disease weigh below 25 g combined. In ectopic ACTH syndrome, the combined adrenal weight is greater—from 25 g to 100 g.

Adrenal adenomas in Cushing's syndrome range in weight from a few grams to over 100 g, usually over 3 cm in diameter, and are larger than aldosterone-producing adenomas. The typical cells usually resemble those of the zona fasciculata. Variable degrees of anaplasia are seen, and differentiation of benign from malignant tumors is often difficult on the basis of cytology alone. These adrenal adenomas occur in women and are very rare in men. Adrenal cancers are frequently very large—almost always over 5 cm in diameter. They are undifferentiated, invade the surrounding tissues, and metastasize via the blood stream.

Rare forms of ACTH-independent Cushing's syndrome include macronodular hyperplasia, which in some cases is due to aberrant expression of receptors in the adrenals that respond to stimuli other than ACTH. In these cases, the adrenal glands can be massively enlarged. Pigmented micronodular hyperplasia is associated with the syndrome of Carney's complex that also includes cardiac myxoma and lentigines.

Rarely, ectopic adrenal tissue can be the source of excessive cortisol secretion. It has been found in various locations, most commonly near the abdominal aorta.

Cushing's disease is most commonly caused by pituitary adenomas.

Ectopic ACTH syndrome is usually caused by small-cell lung cancers and carcinoid tumors, but tumors of the pancreas, thymus, thyroid, prostate, esophagus, colon, and ovaries—as well as pheochromocytoma and malignant melanoma—may also secrete ACTH.

C. Laboratory Findings

Since no one test is specific, a combination must be used.

Normal subjects have a circadian rhythmic of ACTH secretion that is paralleled by cortisol secretion. Levels are highest in the early morning and decline during the day to their lowest levels in the late evening. In Cushing's disease, the circadian rhythm is abolished, and total secretion of cortisol is increased. In mild cases, the plasma cortisol and ACTH levels may be within the normal range during much of the day but abnormally high in the evening.

When Cushing's syndrome is suspected, the first objective is to establish the diagnosis; the second is to establish the cause. An algorithm for the diagnosis is presented in Figure 34–3. When hyperadrenocorticism is suspected, an **overnight dexamethasone suppression test**—or measurement of 24-hour urinary free cortisol—is the first diagnostic step. Dexamethasone, 1 mg orally (equivalent to about 30 mg of cortisol), will suppress ACTH secretion and stop cortisol production. This low dose dexamethasone, however, will not suppress excessive cortisol production from autonomous adrenocortical tumors or adrenals that are being stimulated by excess ACTH in most patients. Since dexamethasone does not cross-react in the assay for plasma cortisol, suppression of endogenous circulating cortisol is easily demonstrated. The test is done as follows: At 11 PM, the patient is given 1 mg of dexamethasone by mouth. A fasting plasma cortisol is measured the following morning. Suppression of plasma cortisol to 1.8 µg/dL or less (50 nmol/L) excludes Cushing's syndrome. Higher cutoff levels have been recommended, but some patients with mild ACTH-dependent Cushing's syndrome may be suppressed so easily that the response is falsely negative and the diagnosis of

Figure 34–3. Cushing's syndrome: diagnosis and differential diagnosis.

Cushing's syndrome is missed. On the other hand, this low cutoff level increases the likelihood of a false-positive diagnosis. False-positive results are more common in patients with depression, physiologic stress, marked obesity, or renal failure and in those taking estrogens or drugs that accelerate dexamethasone metabolism, such as phenytoin, rifampin, and phenobarbital. Estrogens increase cortisol-binding globulin and elevate total plasma cortisol concentrations. In these situations, measurement of 24-hour urinary free cortisol is preferred.

The results of the dexamethasone test should be confirmed with a measurement of 24-hour urinary excretion of free cortisol. It directly measures the physiologically active form of circulating cortisol, integrates the daily variations of cortisol production, and is very sensitive and specific for the diagnosis of Cushing's syndrome. Urinary free cortisol can be measured by high-pressure liquid chromatography (HPLC) or radioimmunoassay (RIA). The upper limit of normal is usually 50 μg/24 h (135 nmol/24 h) by HPLC, and 80–120 μg/24 h (220–330 nmol/24 h) by RIA, depending on the assay.

The midnight plasma cortisol level also distinguishes Cushing's syndrome from non-Cushing states, but because it requires hospitalization it is impractical to measure. In contrast, late-night salivary cortisol sampling can be easily accomplished at home without stress. The procedure involves chewing a cotton tube for 2–3 minutes. Salivary cortisol levels correlate highly with plasma and serum free cortisol levels. The test is underutilized, mainly because it is not generally available.

If the plasma cortisol level is not suppressed by the overnight dexamethasone suppression test and the urinary free cortisol is elevated, the patient has Cushing's syndrome. The next step is to determine the cause. Plasma ACTH measurement by immunoradiometric assay (IRMA) is the most direct method. A normal to elevated ACTH level is diagnostic of hyperadrenocorticism due to pituitary adenoma or ectopic ACTH secretion. Suppressed ACTH levels are diagnostic of hyperadrenocorticism due to a primary adrenal cause such as adenoma, carcinoma, or nodular hyperplasia.

The differential diagnosis of ACTH-dependent Cushing's syndrome can be challenging. No test is perfect, and a combination of tests may be necessary. Since 90% of patients have Cushing's disease, pituitary MRI is the first test to identify the source of ACTH secretion. However, 10% of normal adults have focal pituitary lesions 3–6 mm in diameter on MRI, and many patients with Cushing's disease have no detectable lesions. Lesions smaller than 3–4 mm are more likely to represent normal variation, artifacts, volume averaging, incidental nonfunctional adenomas, or cysts. An unequivocal pituitary lesion (ie, > 4–5 mm in diameter with decreased signal intensity on gadolinium), strongly suggests Cushing's disease.

If the pituitary MRI does not show a definite lesion, the next step is inferior petrosal sinus sampling with corticotropin-releasing hormone (CRH) stimulation. Compared with other biochemical tests, such as high-dose dexamethasone suppression or CRH stimulation, petrosal sinus sampling is the most accurate way to identify an ACTH-secreting pituitary adenoma; the diagnostic accuracy is close to 100%. The test requires simultaneous bilateral venous sampling from the inferior petrosal sinuses. The inferior petrosal sinus connects the cavernous sinus with the ipsilateral internal jugular vein and drains the pituitary. A central to peripheral ACTH ratio of 2 or greater without CRH stimulation is diagnostic of pituitary adenoma. CRH, 100 μg given intravenously as a bolus injection, can increase the diagnostic sensitivity to 100%; a peak central to peripheral ACTH ratio of 3 or greater is diagnostic of pituitary adenoma. The lack of a central to peripheral ACTH gradient is diagnostic of an ectopic ACTH secreting tumor.

In Cushing's syndrome caused by primary adrenal diseases, the plasma ACTH level is completely suppressed. Adenomas are usually 3–5 cm in diameter and secrete only cortisol. Adrenal carcinomas are typically > 5 cm in diameter, are usually rapidly progressive, and cosecrete other hormones, such as adrenal androgens, deoxycorticosterone, aldosterone, and estrogens.

D. IMAGING STUDIES

For Cushing's syndrome caused by primary adrenal diseases, thin-section CT or MRI is able to detect virtually all of the adrenal tumors and hyperplasia. MRI of the sella is the imaging study of choice for pituitary adenomas. If a definitive adenoma is not seen, inferior petrosal sinus sampling with CRH stimulation can differentiate Cushing's disease from ectopic Cushing's syndrome. For ectopic Cushing's syndrome, CT or MRI of the chest and abdomen may detect nonpituitary tumors. Bronchial carcinoid tumors may be very small and difficult to find; high-resolution thin-cut CT of the chest is indicated. Occasionally, the source of an ectopic ACTH-secreting tumor cannot be determined (occult ectopic ACTH syndrome).

Complications

Severe or lethal complications may result from sustained hypercortisolism, including hypertension, cardiovascular disease, stroke, thromboembolism, infection, severe debilitating muscle wasting, and weakness. Psychosis is common. Death may also be caused by the underlying tumors, such as adrenal carcinoma, small cell lung cancer, and others causing ectopic ACTH Cushing's syndrome.

The truncal obesity and muscle weakness in patients with Cushing's syndrome predispose them to postoperative pulmonary complications. Atrophic skin and easy bruisability also predict poor wound healing.

Nelson's syndrome, due to progression of an ACTH-secreting pituitary adenoma, occurs in about 30% of cases following bilateral adrenalectomy. These tumors in patients with Nelson's syndrome are among the most aggressive of pituitary tumors, causing sellar enlargement and extrasellar extension. Plasma ACTH levels are markedly elevated. Patients are frequently hyperpigmented, hypopituitary, and have symptoms of mass effects including headaches, visual field deficits, and even blindness from optic nerve compression. Removal of feedback control from hypercortisolism at the pituitary level probably explains the aggressiveness of these tumors.

Treatment

Resection is the best treatment for cortisol-producing adrenal tumors or ACTH-producing tumors. Medical treatment may be necessary to temporarily control hypercortisolism—or for patients not cured by resection or when complete resection is impossible.

A. MEDICAL TREATMENT

Drugs are mainly used as adjuvant therapy. Hypercortisolism may be controlled with ketoconazole, metyrapone, or aminoglutethimide, all of which inhibit steroid biosynthesis. Ketoconazole is usually the first choice. A combination of drugs may be necessary to control hypercortisolism and to decrease dose-related side effects. Mifepristone (RU 486), a progesterone and glucocorticoid receptor antagonist, is also effective, but it raises cortisol and ACTH levels, making it difficult to monitor the patient.

Mitotane is a DDT derivative that is toxic to the adrenal cortex. It has been used with modest success in the treatment of adrenal hypersecretory states, especially adrenocortical carcinoma. Unfortunately, serious side effects are common at effective doses.

B. EXCISION OF PITUITARY ADENOMA

Patients with Cushing's disease are usually treated by transsphenoidal microsurgical excision of the pituitary adenomas. Relief of symptoms is rapid, and the prognosis for adequate residual pituitary-adrenal function is good. Total or subtotal hypophysectomy may be performed in older patients if a discrete tumor is not found. Pituitary procedures fail in about 15–25% of patients because of failure to find the adenoma, pituitary hyperplasia; or recurrence of adenoma. When pituitary surgery fails, the disease may respond to pituitary irradiation. In some patients, medical therapy or total adrenalectomy will be necessary. Because of the effectiveness of pituitary microsurgery, radiotherapy is usually not recommended as primary treatment for Cushing's disease.

C. ADRENALECTOMY

Compared with patients with other adrenal tumors those with severe Cushing's syndrome are at higher risk for postoperative complications such as wound infection, hemorrhage, peptic ulceration, and pulmonary embolism. Adrenalectomy, however, is usually successful in reversing the devastating effects of hypercortisolism.

Laparoscopic adrenalectomy causes less morbidity than open adrenalectomy and is preferred for benign hyperplasia or adenomas. Laparoscopic adrenalectomy for adrenocortical carcinoma is technically challenging. The notion that local recurrence may be more common after laparoscopic resection is not supported by data.

Unilateral adrenalectomy is indicated for adrenal adenomas or carcinomas that secrete cortisol. The contralateral adrenal gland and the hypothalamic-pituitary-adrenal axis will usually recover from the suppression 1–2 years after the operation.

Total bilateral adrenalectomy is indicated for selected patients with Cushing's disease or ectopic ACTH syndrome in whom the ACTH secreting tumor cannot be found or resected. It is also indicated for patients with bilateral primary adrenal disease, such as pigmented micronodular hyperplasia or massive macronodular hyperplasia.

Bilateral adrenalectomy can almost always be accomplished by the laparoscopic approach.

Subtotal resection is not recommended in patients with Cushing's syndrome, because it usually leaves inadequate adrenocortical reserve initially, and the disease frequently recurs with continuing ACTH stimulation. Total bilateral adrenalectomy with adrenal gland autotransplantation is rarely successful and offers little advantage over pharmacologic replacement.

D. POSTOPERATIVE MAINTENANCE THERAPY

After total adrenalectomy, lifelong corticosteroid maintenance therapy becomes necessary. The following schedule is commonly used: No cortisol is given until the adrenals are removed during surgery. On the first day, give 100 mg of hydrocortisone intravenously every 8 hours. On the second day, give 50 mg every 8 hours. Thereafter, the dose should be tapered as tolerated. The same tapering process is used after excision of a unilateral cortisol-secreting adenoma, because the remaining adrenal may not function normally for months.

As the hydrocortisone dose is reduced below 50 mg/d, it is often necessary to add fludrocortisone (a mineralocorticoid), 0.1 mg daily orally. The usual maintenance doses are about 20–30 mg of hydrocortisone and 0.1 mg of fludrocortisone daily. More than half the hydrocortisone dose is given in the morning.

Patients who have had a total bilateral adrenalectomy and are on maintenance therapy can develop addisonian crisis when under stress, such as general anesthesia or infection. Adrenal insufficiency causes fever, hyperkalemia, abdominal pain, and hypotension and should be promptly recognized and treated with saline infusion and cortisol.

Prognosis

The prognosis is good after resection of benign adrenal adenomas, pituitary adenomas, or benign ACTH-secreting tumors. Symptoms and signs of hypercortisolism resolve, usually over months. Short-term adrenal insufficiency after surgery requires cortisol replacement. Cushing's disease can recur after excision of a pituitary adenoma. An occult ACTH-secreting tumor may become apparent later and require removal.

Residual adrenal tissue or embryonic rests are present in up to 10% of patients after total adrenalectomy. Cushing's syndrome can then recur if stimulation with ACTH continues.

The prognosis is extremely poor in patients with adrenocortical carcinoma and in those with malignant tumors causing ectopic ACTH syndrome.

Doherty GM et al: Time to recovery of the hypothalamic-pituitary-adrenal axis after curative resection of adrenal tumors in patients with Cushing's syndrome. Surgery 1990;108:1085.

Findling JW, Raff H: Newer diagnostic techniques and problems in Cushing's disease. Endocrinol Metab Clin North Am 1999;28:191.

Hall WA et al: Pituitary magnetic resonance imaging in normal human volunteers: occult adenomas in the general population. Ann Intern Med 1994;120:817.

Kemink L et al: Residual adrenocortical function after bilateral adrenalectomy for pituitary-dependent Cushing's syndrome. J Clin Endocrinol Metab 1992;75:1211.

Oldfield EH et al: Petrosal sinus sampling with and without corticotropin-releasing hormone for the differential diagnosis of Cushing's syndrome. N Engl J Med 1991;325:897.

Papanicolaou DA et al: A single midnight serum cortisol measurement distinguishes Cushing's syndrome from pseudo-Cushing's states. J Clin Endocrinol Metab 1998;83:1163.

Raff H et al: Late-night salivary cortisol as a screening test for Cushing's syndrome. J Clin Endocrinol Metab 1998;83: 2681.

Tyrrell JB et al: Cushing's disease. Therapy of pituitary adenomas. Endocrinol Metab Clin North Am 1994;23:925.

VIRILIZING ADRENAL TUMORS

In adults, hormonally active benign adrenal adenomas usually secrete aldosterone or cortisol. Virilizing tumors in women are more likely to be caused by ovarian tumors. Virilizing adrenal tumors are rare, and virilization is usually due to hypersecretion of adrenal androgens, mainly dehydroepiandrosterone (DHEA), its sulfate derivative (DHEAS), and androstenedione, all of which are converted peripherally to testosterone and 5α-dihydrotestosterone. Very rarely, virilizing adrenal tumors secrete only testosterone.

The differentiation of benign from malignant adrenocortical tumors may be difficult when based on histologic features; some patients with histologically benign tumors may develop metastases, and others with histologically malignant tumors may never have recurrent disease. Malignancy is only definitely diagnosed from local or distant spread. Seventy percent of virilizing adrenal tumors exhibit malignant behavior. Adrenocortical carcinomas are usually large tumors with local spread or distant metastases. They often secrete multiple steroids, most commonly cortisol and androgens, leading to Cushing's syndrome and virilization.

In children, adrenocortical tumors are rare, but virilization with or without hypercortisolism is the most frequent syndrome. Virilizing adrenal tumors are less likely to be malignant in children than in adults. Histologic features of malignancy do not always predict malignant behavior. Large tumors (> 100 g) have a worse prognosis.

Signs and symptoms of virilization include hirsutism, male-pattern baldness, acne, deep voice, male musculature, irregular menses or amenorrhea, clitorimegaly, and increased libido. Rapid linear growth with advanced bone age is common in children.

CT and MRI are used to image virilizing adrenal tumors. Resection is the only successful treatment.

Virilization can also be caused by congenital adrenal hyperplasia, an autosomal recessive disorder. The mutated genes encode enzymes essential for cortisol and mineralocorticoid synthesis. 21-Hydroxylase deficiency accounts for 90% of cases. The blocked cortisol synthesis leads to stimulated ACTH secretion, accumulation of precursors, and overproduction of androgens. Administration of glucocorticoids is the mainstay of treatment. Mineralocorticoid replacement is required in the salt-wasting forms of congenital adrenal hyperplasia. Antiandrogens, aromatase inhibitors and lower-dose glucocorticoid replacement may be useful. Adrenalectomy with lifelong steroid replacement is another approach.

Del Gaudio AD et al: Virilizing adrenocortical tumors in adult women. Cancer 1993;72:1997.

Gagle PT et al: Comparison of adrenal cortical tumors in children and adults. Cancer 1986;57:2235.

Latronico AC et al: Extensive personal experience—adrenocortical tumors. J Clin Endocrinol Metab 1997;82:1317.

Lee PD et al: Virilizing adrenocortical tumors in childhood: eight cases and a review of the literature. Pediatrics 1985;76:437.

Liou LS et al: Adrenocortical carcinoma in children. Review and recent innovations. Urol Clin North Am 2000;27:403.

Merke DP et al: New approaches to the treatment of congenital adrenal hyperplasia. JAMA 1997;277:1073.

Michalkiewicz EL et al: Clinical characteristics of small functioning adrenocortical tumors in children. Med Pediatr Oncol 1997; 28:175.

Pang S: Congenital adrenal hyperplasia. Endocrinol Metab Clin North Am 1997;26:853.

FEMINIZING ADRENAL TUMORS

Estrogens are not normally synthesized by the adrenal cortex. Feminizing adrenal tumors are extremely rare and are almost always carcinomas. They are usually seen in men with feminization or in girls with precocious puberty. Vaginal bleeding may be the presenting symptom in adult women. Feminizing adrenal carcinomas frequently hypersecrete other hormones. The diagnosis is based on a finding of increased urinary or plasma estrogens. Ovarian tumors, testicular feminization, and administration of exogenous estrogen should be ruled out.

Definitive treatment is by excision of the tumor. The prognosis is guarded.

Goto T et al: Oestrogen producing adrenocortical adenoma: clinical, biochemical and immunohistochemical studies. Clin Endocrinol 1996;45:643.

ADRENOCORTICAL CARCINOMA

Adrenal cortical carcinomas are rare. Fifty percent of patients have symptoms related to hypersecretion of hormones, most commonly Cushing's syndrome and virilization. Feminizing and purely aldosterone-secreting carcinomas are rare. In some cases, hormone hypersecretion is only found by biochemical studies. A palpable abdominal mass is common. The mean diameter of adrenal carcinoma is 12 cm (range, 3–30 cm). Adrenocortical carcinoma invades the surrounding tissues, and about half of the patients have metastases (lung, liver, and elsewhere) at the time of diagnosis. In those without local spread or distant metastases, a diagnosis of carcinoma based on cytologic features may be wrong.

The median survival is 25 months, and 5-year actuarial survival is 25%. Tumor stage at the initial operation predicts the prognosis. Surgery is the only treatment that can cure or prolong survival, outcomes confined to patients with localized disease. When grossly complete resection is possible, the 5-year survival is 50%. Thus, recurrence is common despite apparent complete resection. Laparoscopic adrenalectomy is technically more difficult for adrenocortical carcinomas than for other adrenal tumors because the tumor is fragile and adjacent organs may have to be removed. Where the adrenal tumor is small, malignancy is uncertain, and the surgeon

is technically capable, starting the operation laparoscopically is acceptable, but the abdomen should be opened if there is any question about whether a better operation could be accomplished that way. For local recurrent disease, reoperation is the only effective therapy and may prolong life. Patients with distant metastases at initial presentation usually die within 1 year. Resecting the adrenal tumor in these patients may improve local symptoms but rarely increases survival.

Mitotane, an adrenolytic agent, has been used as an adjuvant to surgery in patients with adrenocortical carcinoma. It controls endocrine symptoms in 50% of patients, and the tumor regresses in some. Nevertheless, survival is not generally affected, though a few cases of prolonged remission have been reported. Dose-related side effects (eg, gastrointestinal symptoms, weakness, dizziness, and somnolence) limit its use. A variety of other chemotherapeutic agents have been tried.

Barnett CC et al: Limitations of size as a criterion in the evaluation of adrenal tumors. Surgery 2000;128:973

Bellantone R et al. Role of reoperation in recurrence of adrenal cortical carcinoma: results from 188 cases collected in the Italian National Registry for Adrenal Cortical Carcinoma. Surgery 1997;122:1212.

Decker RA et al: Eastern Cooperative Oncology Group study 1879: mitotane and adriamycin in patients with advanced adrenocortical carcinoma. Surgery 1991;110:1006.

Icard P et al: Adrenocortical carcinoma in surgically treated patients. Surgery 1992;112:972.

Icard P et al: Survival rates and prognostic factors in adrenocortical carcinoma. World J Surg 1992;16:753.

Jensen JC et al: Recurrent or metastatic disease in select patients with adrenocortical carcinoma: aggressive resection vs chemotherapy. Arch Surg 1991;126:457.

Luton JP et al: Clinical features of adrenocortical carcinoma, prognostic factors, and the effect of mitotane therapy. N Engl J Med 1990;322:1195.

Stratakis CA et al: Adrenal cancer. Endocrinol Metab Clin North Am 2000;29:15.

Wajchenberg BL et al. Adrenocortical carcinoma—clinical and laboratory observations. Cancer 2000;88:711.

INCIDENTALOMAS

Adrenal tumors have traditionally been diagnosed from clinical symptoms of excess hormone secretion. However, the increased use of ultrasonography, CT, and MRI for various diseases in the abdomen has led to the discovery of what are referred to as adrenal incidentalomas. Most are small nonfunctioning adrenal cortical adenomas; some are functioning adenomas or pheochromocytomas with subclinical secretion of hormones; and some are adrenocortical carcinomas.

Incidentalomas are found in 1–4% of CT scans and 6% of random autopsies. The incidence increases with age. Preclinical Cushing's syndrome, pheochromocytoma, and adrenocortical carcinoma each account for about 5% of cases, metastatic carcinoma for 2%, and aldosteronoma for 1% (Table 34–2). Thus, over 80% of patients have presumed nonfunctioning cortical adenomas. Simple adrenal cysts, myelolipomas, and adrenal hemorrhages can be identified by the CT characteristics alone. Adrenal cysts can be large but are rarely malignant. Adrenal hemorrhage may occur in preexisting adrenal tumors.

The major issues in managing a patient with an incidentaloma is to determine whether the tumor is hormonally active and whether it is a cancer; either would be an indication for resection. Since most incidentalomas are nonfunctioning adenomas, the workup should be selective to avoid unnecessary expense and procedures.

The workup should include a complete history and physical examination with specific reference to a history of previous malignancy and signs and symptoms of Cushing's syndrome. Hyperaldosteronism, pheochromocytoma, and virilizing or feminizing adrenocortical carcinoma should be investigated. Further laboratory studies may be indicated depending on the clinical presentation.

The management of incidentaloma depends on the functional status and size of the tumor. All functioning tumors should be excised. Large nonfunctioning tumors also should be excised because of the risk of cancer. Small nonfunctioning tumors are almost always benign adenomas; they can be followed with serial CT scans checking for changes in size.

All patients—even those who do not have hypertension—should have a 24-hour urine collection for fractionated catecholamines and metanephrines to search for pheochromocytoma; the risk of unrecognized pheochromocytoma is high, and the hypertension may be absent or episodic. Most pheochromocytomas are over 2 cm in diameter and characteristically bright on T2-weighted MRI. *Twenty-five percent of pheochromocytomas are found incidentally because of CT or MRI scans obtained for other indications.*

All patients should also have a 24-hour urine collection for cortisol and an overnight dexamethasone suppression test. These patients may subsequently become cushingoid and may experience an addisonian crisis if the tumor is resected and glucocorticoid replacement is not adequate.

Patients who are hypertensive should also have plasma aldosterone and plasma renin activity measured to screen for primary hyperaldosteronism.

If the above studies show that the tumor is nonfunctional, the size of the tumor and the patient's overall medical condition should determine the appropriate treatment. Nonfunctioning adrenal tumors larger than 5 cm in diameter should usually be removed because of the high risk of cancer (as high as one-third). Nonfunctioning adrenal tumors smaller than 3 cm are unlikely to be cancers and can be safely followed. The patient's age and overall medical condition and the CT scan findings (irregular borders and heterogeneity make cancers more likely) will usually determine whether a tumor 3–5 cm in size should be resected.

In patients with a previously treated malignancy such as lung or breast cancer, an adrenal mass larger than 3 cm is very likely a metastasis. Once the possibility of pheochromocytoma is excluded, a CT-guided FNA (fine-needle aspiration) biopsy can be used to distinguish an adrenocortical tumor from metastatic cancer. This is the only situation when the result of fine-needle aspiration biopsy influences management of an adrenal tumor. Resection of a solitary adrenal metastasis from a primary lung cancer may improve long-term survival if there are no other clinically obvious metastases. Patients with a metachronous solitary adrenal metastasis are more likely to benefit from adrenalectomy than are those with a synchronous metastasis.

Table 34–2. Adrenal incidentalomas.[1]

Tumor Types	Percentage
Preclinical Cushing's	5%
Pheochromocytoma	5%
Adrenocortical carcinoma	5%
Metastatic carcinoma	2%
Aldosterone-producing adenoma	1%
Presumed nonfunctional adenoma	82%
Total	100%

[1]Based on data reported in Endocrinol Metab Clin North Am 2000;29:159.

Bailey RH et al: The diagnostic dilemma of incidentalomas. Working through uncertainty. Emerg Med Clin North Am 2000;29:91.

Herrera MF et al: Incidentally discovered adrenal tumors: an institutional perspective. Surgery 1991;110:1014.

Khafagi FA et al: Clinical significance of the large adrenal mass. Br J Surg 1991;78:828.

Reincke M et al: Preclinical Cushing's syndrome in adrenal "incidentalomas": comparison with adrenal Cushing's syndrome. J Clin Endocrinol Metab 1992;75:826.

Ross NS et al: Hormonal evaluation of the patient with an incidentally discovered adrenal mass. N Engl J Med 1990;323:1401.

Young WF: Management approaches to adrenal incidentalomas: a review from Rochester, Minnesota. Endocrinol Metab Clin North Am 2000;29:159.

Arteries

William C. Krupski, MD

■ ATHEROSCLEROSIS

Atherosclerosis is the major degenerative disease of human arteries. It is a disease of the intima of large arteries that produces luminal narrowing, thrombosis, embolization, and occlusion associated with ischemia of the end organ. Strokes, myocardial infarctions, and ischemic gangrene with limb loss are attributable to atherosclerosis, which is undetectable until the disease becomes far-advanced. Atherosclerotic lesions are characterized by local accumulation of lipid in the vessel wall located either in the extracellular matrix or inside foam cells (lipid-filled smooth muscle cells or macrophages). The widespread prevalence of lesions in the arteries of asymptomatic individuals, the chronicity of the process, and the absence of a single etiologic factor make it impossible to explain atherogenesis or its progression simply. Atherosclerosis is most likely a nonspecific adaptation of large blood vessels to a variety of harmful stimuli; clinical consequences result when compensatory mechanisms are overwhelmed.

Several theories of atherogenesis exist. The oldest—the **lipid insudation hypothesis**—proposes that the lipid in the atherosclerotic lesion is derived from lipoproteins in the blood; it thereby links the risk factor hypercholesterolemia directly to the development of the plaque foam cell, the atheroma, and eventually the complicated lesion. The **encrustation hypothesis** states that plaque formation and progression is the consequence of repeated cycles of thrombosis and remodeling. The **monoclonal hypothesis** suggests that single cells are stimulated to enter the growth cycle and undergo several rounds of division, leading to formation of a monoclonal lesion that progresses to atherosclerotic plaque development. The mechanism of cell activation is unclear, and this theory would regard the atheroma as a type of neoplasia. The **infectious hypothesis** links infection with *Chlamydia pneumoniae* with an inflammatory response leading to atherosclerosis. The **intimal cell mass hypothesis** proposes that accumulations of smooth muscle cells found in children where atherosclerosis later develops are primordial rests, a form of stem cell capable of responding to external mitogenic stimuli such as hypercholesterolemia. The most widely popular response to injury hypothesis proposes that atherosclerosis results from continuous repair in response to continuous injury of the arterial intima. According to this theory, the endothelial lining of arteries can be damaged by factors such as hyperlipidemia, toxins from tobacco smoke, shear stress, hypertension, and hormone dysfunction. Growth factors released from platelets and arterial wall macrophages influence this process. Each hypothesis attempts to explain one or more aspects of atherogenesis. Each might be applicable at different times during plaque formation.

Atheromas most commonly occur at arterial bifurcations, at the origins of major arterial branches, and at sites where an artery passes beneath or through a fascial sling. For example, the superficial femoral artery is often most severely diseased where the vessel passes through the adductor hiatus; atherosclerosis most commonly affects the carotid bulb at the bifurcation of the common carotid artery. Although atherosclerosis is a diffuse disease, patterns of distribution vary widely. Young patients with accelerated atherosclerosis most commonly have aortoiliac arterial stenoses, while diabetics have disease involving the tibioperoneal artery. Lesions are usually symmetrically distributed on both sides of the body. Variations in symmetry may result from a local complication, such as hemorrhage or dissection within a plaque.

Multiple risk factors for atherosclerosis have been identified. These risk factors are often arbitrarily divided into major and minor categories based on their probable importance. The progress of atherosclerosis may be slowed by controlling these risk factors.

Major risk factors:
Cigarette smoking
Age
Diabetes
Hyperlipidemia (hypercholesterolemia and hypertriglyceridemia)
Hypertension
Positive family history
Homocysteinemia
Hyperfibrinogenemia
Lipoprotein(a)
Minor risk factors:
Obesity
Sedentary lifestyle

Male gender
Hypercoagulable states
Race (nonwhite)
Excessive alcohol use
C-reactive protein
Asymmetric dimethylarginine (ADMA) plasma
 levels

Clinical manifestations of atherosclerosis include arterial insufficiency, aneurysm formation, and embolism. Usually, manifestations of only one of these conditions are present, but they may coexist.

Arterial insufficiency, or circulatory hypoperfusion, may result from atherosclerotic plaques that have
become large enough to narrow the arterial lumen. In
medium-sized and large arteries, a 50% reduction in arterial diameter on arteriogram correlates roughly with a
75% stenosis of cross-sectional area and enough resistance to decrease flow and downstream pressure.

The hemodynamic circuit consists of the diseased
major artery, a parallel system of collateral vessels, and
the peripheral runoff bed. Collateral vessels are much
smaller, more circuitous, and more numerous than the
major arteries they replace and always have a higher resistance than the original unobstructed artery. The
stimuli for collateral development are the presence of an
abnormal pressure gradient across the collateral system
and increased velocity of flow through intramuscular
channels that connect stem distributing branches with
reentry vessels. In part, this explains the improvement
in collateral circulation that results from a regular exercise program in patients with ischemia of the lower extremities; robust collateral circulation in conjunction
with a muscle training effect contributes to relief of
symptoms of lower extremity ischemia.

When the stenosis approaches total occlusion, the
sharply reduced blood flow eventually leads to thrombosis. The clot propagates in the stagnant column of blood
both proximally and distally to the first major tributaries.
Persistent flow at these sites halts the propagation of clot.
The end result is a totally occluded segment bypassed by
a collateral system (Figure 35–1). Clinical manifestations
of ischemia are related to the effectiveness of the collateral system. The development of additional arterial
stenoses further reduces blood flow; severe chronic ischemia is nearly always due to multiple sites of occlusion
of the major vessels proximal to the affected tissues.

Degenerative aneurysms occur because the vessel
wall is unable to withstand the tensile stress imposed by
the distending pressure of the pulsatile column of
blood. Alterations in the architecture, composition, nutrition, or metabolism of the arterial wall may be the
primary cause of this mechanical failure.

Older literature often refers to atherosclerotic aneurysms. In fact, although patients with arterial aneurysms

Figure 35–1. Development of collateral channels in
response to occlusion of the right common iliac artery
and the aortic bifurcation.

have many of the same risk factors as patients with atherosclerosis and even though atherosclerosis may be
present to varying degrees in aneurysms, atherosclerosis
is probably not causative. Biochemical studies have
shown decreased quantities of both elastin and collagen
in the walls of aneurysms. Excessive protease activity
(elastase or collagenase) or reductions in their naturally
occurring inhibitors (antiproteases) in the arterial wall
have been implicated in aneurysm formation. Elastic
fibers of the media become fatigued, fracture, and disintegrate, and collagen-to-elastin ratios are higher in
aneurysms. A hereditary deficiency of the pyridinoline
cross-linkage in collagen has been found in some patients with aneurysms. Abnormal copper metabolism
and positive family histories have also been found in
patients with aneurysms. There may be as high as a
20% chance that another first-degree family member
may have an aneurysm.

Emboli may arise from the lining of aneurysms or
from debris in necrotic atherosclerotic plaques. They
are composed of aggregated platelets, thrombi, cholesterol crystals, lipids, or other plaque constituents.
Symptoms produced by an embolus depend on its size;
the affected organ and its arterial anatomy; the available
collateral vessels; and the composition of the embolus,
which largely determines its rate of dissolution.

Boger RH et al: Biochemical evidence for impaired nitric oxide
 synthesis in patients with peripheral arterial occlusive disease.
 Circulation 1997;95:2068.

Chengpei X, Zarins CK, Glagov S: Aneurysmal and occlusive atherosclerosis of the human abdominal aorta. J Vasc Surg 2001;
  33:91

Dormandy J, Heeck L, Vig S: Peripheral arterial occlusive disease.
  Clinical data for decision making. Semin Vasc Surg 1999;
  12:93.

Kadar A, Glasz T: Development of atherosclerosis and plaque biology. Cardiovasc Surg 2001;9:109.

McMillan WD, Pearce WH: Increased plasma levels of metallopro-
  teinase-9 are associated with abdominal aortic aneurysms.
  J Vasc Surg 1999;29:122.

Muluk SC et al: Outcome events in patients with claudication: a
  15-year study in 2777 patients. J Vasc Surg 2001;33:251.

Rosenfeld ME et al: Chlamydia, inflammation, and atherogenesis.
  J Infect Dis 2000;181(Suppl 3):5492.

Taylor LM Jr et al: Prospective blinded study of the relationship
  between plasma homocysteine and progression of symptomatic peripheral arterial disease. J Vasc Surg 1999;29:8.

Tegos TJ et al: The genesis of atherosclerosis and risk factors: a review. Angiology 2001;52:89.

PERIPHERAL ARTERIAL INSUFFICIENCY

ESSENTIALS OF DIAGNOSIS

- *Intermittent claudication.*
- *Ischemic rest pain.*
- *Decreased pulses.*
- *Nonhealing of wounds.*
- *Pallor of foot on elevation, rubor on dependency.*
- *Necrosis and atrophy.*
- *Low ankle-brachial index.*

General Considerations

Peripheral arterial insufficiency is predominantly a disease of the lower extremities. In the arms, arterial lesions are confined mostly to the subclavian and axillary
arteries. Stenoses of the radial and ulnar arteries occur
primarily in patients with long-standing diabetes mellitus. Because collateral pathways are so abundant, upper
extremity atherosclerosis rarely produces symptoms. In
the lower extremities, obstructive lesions are distributed
widely (Figure 35–2), and symptoms are related to the
location and number of obstructions. Involvement of
the femoropopliteal system is more common than aortoiliac disease. Tandem lesions are often present, increasing the degree of ischemia.

   Peripheral arterial disease affects at least 20% of individuals older than 70 years. Although most patients
with this disorder do not develop gangrene or require

Figure 35–2. Common sites of stenosis and occlusion
of the visceral and peripheral arterial systems.

amputations, adverse outcomes of systemic atherosclerosis, including death, are common. Even after adjustment for known risk factors, individuals with peripheral arterial disease exhibit a higher mortality rate than
the healthy population. A low ankle-brachial index is
one of the strongest risk factors for all-cause mortality
(Figure 35–3). One of the most important things to remember about peripheral arterial disease is that it is a
marker for early death more so than an indicator of imminent limb loss; thus, recognition and treatment of associated atherosclerotic risk factors are essentials for
treatment.

Clinical Findings

A. SYMPTOMS

1. Intermittent claudication—Intermittent claudication is pain or fatigue in muscles of the lower extremity
caused by walking and relieved by rest. Claudication is
derived from the Latin word for "limping, lame";
strictly speaking, the term should be used only for
symptoms in the lower extremities. The pain is a deep-
seated ache gradually progressing to a degree that forces
the patient to stop walking. Patients occasionally describe "cramping" or "tiredness" in the muscle. Typi-

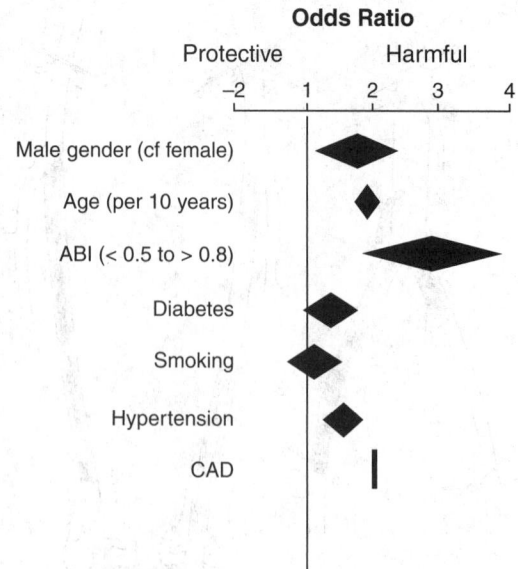

Figure 35–3. Odds ratios for risk factors for all-cause mortality. ABI, ankle-brachial index; CAD, coronary artery disease. (Reproduced, with permission, from TASC Working Group: Management of peripheral arterial disease: epidemiology, natural history, risk factors. J Vasc Surg 2000; 31[1 Suppl]:S22.)

cally, symptoms are completely relieved after 2–5 minutes of inactivity. Claudication is distinguished from other pains in the extremities in that some exertion is always required before it appears; it is reproducible; it does not occur at rest; and it is relieved by cessation of walking. Relief of symptoms is not dependent upon sitting or other positional change. The distance a patient can walk varies with the rate of walking, the level of incline, the degree of arterial obstruction, the development of collateral circulation, and systemic factors (eg, congestive heart failure). The average patient with obstruction of a single arterial segment can walk 90–180 meters on a level terrain at a moderate pace before pain appears. Degree of claudication is traditionally expressed in terms of city blocks, a poorly defined and variable unit. On average, a block is approximately 160 meters. The presence of additional lesions may reduce the walking tolerance to a few meters.

Claudication most commonly occurs in the calf muscles, regardless of which arterial segment is involved, because the calf muscles are most important in normal walking. Occlusions proximal to the origin of the profunda femoris can extend the pain to involve the thigh. Gluteal pain is added by lesions in or proximal to the hypogastric arteries; impotence often accompanies these symptoms. Leriche's syndrome occurs in men as a result of aortoiliac disease and includes claudication of the hip, thigh, and buttock muscles, atrophy of the leg muscles, impotence, and diminished or absent femoral pulses. Occasionally, patients describe transient numbness of the extremity accompanying the pain and fatigue of claudication.

The two conditions that most often mimic claudication are osteoarthritis of the hip or knee and neurospinal compression due to congenital or osteophytic narrowing of the lumbar neurospinal canal (spinal stenosis). Osteoarthritis can be differentiated because pain occurs mostly in joints; the amount of exercise required to elicit symptoms varies; symptoms are characteristically worse in the morning; rest does not relieve symptoms promptly; the severity of symptoms changes from day to day (and may be related to changes in the weather); and anti-inflammatory agents relieve the pain. Neurospinal compression symptoms are produced by increasing lumbar lordosis; therefore, standing as well as walking causes symptoms, which are not relieved until the patient straightens the lumbar spine by sitting or lying down.

Other conditions that can occasionally mimic symptoms of arterial claudication are venous congestion (also called venous claudication), chronic compartment syndrome, and other nonatherosclerotic arterial disorders, including: Buerger's disease and other vasculitides, coarctation of the aorta, popliteal artery entrapment, popliteal cysts, persistent sciatic arteries, external iliac dysplasias (in runners and cyclists), and primary vascular tumors.

Important features to establish the correct diagnosis are the location of pain or symptoms, the quality of the pain, the length of time for relief of symptoms, the reproducibility of symptoms, the distance walked before symptoms begin (initial claudication distance), the maximal distance achieved without pain (maximal walking distance), and the type of rest or position required for symptom relief.

2. Ischemic rest pain—Ischemic rest pain—a grave symptom caused by ischemic neuritis and tissue necrosis—indicates far-advanced arterial insufficiency that usually terminates in gangrene and amputation of the extremity if arterial reconstruction cannot be performed. The term is confusing because it is *not* pain in a muscle group at rest but rather a severe burning pain usually confined to the forefoot distal to the metatarsals. It may be localized to the vicinity of an ischemic ulcer or pregangrenous toe. It is aggravated by elevation of the extremity or by bringing the leg to the horizontal position. Thus, it appears at bed rest (hence the nomenclature) and may prevent sleep. When rest pain first appears, the patient typically rubs the painful foot and tries to walk. Pain is relieved somewhat when the patient is standing erect, as gravity aids the delivery of arterial blood. The patient with continuous rest pain hangs the leg over the side of the bed to obtain relief or sleeps sitting in a chair. Because of constant dependency, the leg and foot of a patient with severe rest pain may be swollen, causing some confusion in diagnosis. Extreme pain may be resistant to opioids for relief. Rest pain indicates an advanced stage of ischemia; it is classically preceded by claudication but may occur de novo in patients whose walking is limited by other illness (eg, angina pectoris). The differentiation of ischemic rest pain from neuropathy in patients with long-standing diabetes mellitus may be difficult. Characteristically, patients with ischemic rest pain experience some relief by placing their limbs in a dependent position, whereas patients with neuropathy do not.

3. Nonhealing wounds or ulcers—Patients with severe lower extremity arterial insufficiency often develop ulcers or wounds on the feet even from seemingly trivial trauma. These lesions are most commonly located on the distal foot and toes, but on occasion they can be in the upper foot and ankle. Typically, the wounds are excruciatingly painful, deep, and devoid of any evidence of healing such as contraction or formation of granulation tissue. Frank gangrene eventually affects these ulcerations.

4. Erectile dysfunction—Inability to attain or maintain an erection may be produced by lesions that obstruct blood flow through both hypogastric arteries and is commonly found in association with obstruction of the terminal aorta. Vasculogenic erectile dysfunction is less common than that due to most other causes (see Chapter 41).

5. Sensation—Although the patient may report numbness in the extremity, sensory abnormalities are generally absent on examination. If decreased sensation is found in the foot, peripheral neuropathy should be suspected.

B. Signs

Physical examination is of paramount importance in assessing the presence and severity of vascular disease. The physical findings of peripheral atherosclerosis are related to changes in the peripheral arteries and to tissue ischemia.

1. Arterial palpation—Hardening of the arterial wall is palpable in vessels near the surface of the extremity. Decreased amplitude of the pulse denotes proximal stenosis. It is unusual for collateral flow to be sufficient to produce a pulse distal to an occluded artery. Two grading systems are commonly used. Both methods of grading are acceptable. Clearly, it is important to include a denominator in order to differentiate the systems (eg, 4+/4+ equals 2+/2+).

GRADING OF PULSES			
Traditional		**Basic**	
4+	Normal	2+	Normal
3+	Slightly reduced	1+	Diminished
2+	Markedly reduced	0	Absent
1+	Barely palpable		
0	Absent		

2. Bruits—A bruit is the sound produced by dissipation of energy as blood flows through a stenotic arterial segment. The sound is caused partly by blood turbulence and partly by arterial wall vibrations. It is heard loudest during systole and, with greater stenosis, may extend into diastole. The bruit is transmitted distally along the course of the artery. Thus, when a bruit is heard through a stethoscope placed over a peripheral artery, stenosis is present *at* or *proximal* to that level. The pitch of the bruit rises as the stenosis becomes more marked, until a critical stenosis is reached or the vessel becomes occluded, when the bruit may disappear. Thus, absence of a bruit does not indicate insignificant disease.

3. Pallor—Pallor of the foot on elevation of the extremity indicates advanced ischemia. Lesser degrees of elevation are necessary to produce pallor in patients with advanced lesions. Pallor on elevation does not occur unless advanced ischemia is present.

4. Reactive hyperemia—The ischemia produced by elevation results in maximum cutaneous vasodilation. When the extremity is returned to a dependent position, blood returning to the dilated vascular bed produces an intense red color in the foot, called reactive hyperemia. Reactive hyperemia does not occur in the absence of provocation of ischemia. The rate of return of skin color when the extremities return to a dependent position is proportionate to the efficiency of the collateral circulation; the more delayed the reactive hyperemia, the more severe the impairment in circulation.

5. Rubor—In advanced atherosclerotic disease, the skin of the foot displays a characteristic dark red cyanosis on dependency. Because of reduced inflow, the blood in the capillary network of the foot is relatively stagnant, and oxygen extraction is high. Hemoglobin becomes deoxygenated, and the capillary blood becomes the color of that found in the venous side of the circulation. The concurrent vasodilation due to ischemia causes blood to suffuse the cutaneous plexus, imparting a purple color to the skin. The purple discoloration due to chronic congestion from venous insufficiency does not become pallid on elevation.

6. Response to exercise—Exercise in a normal individual increases the pulse rate without producing arterial bruits or changes in pulse amplitude. In an individual who complains of claudication but who has minimal findings at rest, exercise will sometimes produce an audible bruit and a decrease in pulse strength and distal arterial pressure, unmasking an otherwise inapparent stenosis.

7. Temperature—With chronic ischemia, the temperature of the skin of the foot decreases. Coolness can best be detected by palpation with the back of the examiner's hand against the dorsum of the patient's foot.

8. Ulceration—Ischemic ulcers are usually very painful and accompanied by rest pain in the foot. They occur in toes or at a site where trauma from a shoe or bedding causes additional ischemia or infection. The margin of the ulcer is sharply demarcated or punched-out, and the base is devoid of healthy granulation tissue. The surrounding skin is pale and mottled, and signs of chronic ischemia are invariably present. Scraping or debriding the ulcer results in little bleeding.

9. Necrosis—Tissue necrosis first becomes apparent in the most distal portions of the extremity, often at an ulcer site. Necrosis halts proximally at a line where the blood supply is sufficient to maintain viability and results in dry gangrene. If the part is infected (wet gangrene), necrosis may extend into tissues that would normally remain viable.

10. Atrophy—Moderate to severe degrees of chronic ischemia produce gradual soft tissue and muscle atrophy and loss of strength in the ischemic zone. Joint mobility may be reduced in the forefeet, as atrophy of the muscles of the feet produces increasing prominence of the interosseous spaces. Subsequent changes in foot structure and gait increase the possibility of developing foot ulceration.

11. Integumentary changes—Chronic ischemia commonly produces loss of hair over the dorsum of the toes and foot and may be associated with thickening of the toenails due to slowed keratin turnover. With more advanced ischemia, there is atrophy of the skin and subcutaneous tissue, so that the foot becomes shiny, scaly, and skeletonized. Hence, a quick glance at a foot can identify the presence or absence of serious arterial insufficiency.

C. NONINVASIVE VASCULAR TESTS

Noninvasive vascular testing may aid in the management of patients with symptoms of peripheral vascular disease. In a patient with severe ischemia, rest pain, or tissue loss, in whom arteriography is clearly indicated,

noninvasive tests are not essential but are useful for comparison purposes. Noninvasive assessment is helpful in a patient with claudication and decreased pulses below the femoral artery, because testing can reveal the severity of hypoperfusion and the sites of hemodynamically significant stenoses or occlusions.

A peripheral vascular testing laboratory should be equipped with a Doppler velocity detector, blood pressure cuffs of different sizes, a sphygmomanometer, a plethysmograph for pulse volume recording, and a motorized treadmill. Treadmill testing may be constant (1.5 miles per hour on a 12% incline) or graded (1.5 miles per hour on a gradually increasing slope). A device to measure the partial pressure of oxygen in tissues (transcutaneous [TC] PO_2) is occasionally useful. With these instruments, blood pressure can be measured at rest and during exercise in the arm, ankle, calf, and thigh, and the rate of recovery of an ischemic area after exercise can be determined. A plethysmograph is any instrument that detects and graphically records volume changes, such as mercury-in-Silastic tube strain gauges or impedance strips encircling the limb at selected levels. A pulse volume recording is produced. By comparing the magnitude and contour of each pulse volume recording at various levels, the presence and location of significant occlusive arterial lesions can be determined. The TC PO_2 in potentially ischemic locations correlates with wound healing, but it is a difficult test to perform. Toe blood pressures can also be measured by plethysmography.

A quick screening test—and the cornerstone of diagnosis—consists of measurement of resting systolic blood pressure at the brachial artery and the posterior tibial or dorsalis pedis artery. The **ankle-brachial index (ABI)** is determined by dividing the pressure obtained at the ankle by the brachial arterial pressure. Normally, the ABI is 1.0 or greater; a value below 1.0 indicates occlusive disease proximal to the point of measurement. ABIs correlate roughly with the degree of ischemia; eg, rest pain usually appears when the ratio is 0.3 or lower. An important limitation of the indirect measurement of extremity pressure is in patients with extreme stiffening and calcification of the vessel wall. Since such a vessel cannot be compressed, an elevated pressure is recorded even though the intraluminal pressure may be low. Wall calcification should be suspected whenever the ABI is above 1.2 or when the value is out of proportion to the patient's clinical status. Patients with diabetes mellitus most commonly exhibit this phenomenon.

Additional noninvasive studies—painless, quick, and accurate in most cases—are useful in localizing disease or determining its severity. Segmental limb pressure measurement accurately detects and segmentally localizes hemodynamically significant large vessel occlusive lesions by determining pressures at the high thigh, low high, upper calf, and lower calf levels in addition to ankle pressures. A sphygmomanometer cuff is placed at a given level with a Doppler probe over one of the pedal arteries. The location of the occlusive lesions can be ascertained from pressure gradients between cuffs.

When standard limb pressures are erroneously high (because of arterial calcification), toe pressures are useful; toe pressures are normally about 10 mm Hg less than ankle pressure and are determined using a special small occlusion cuff and a flow sensor (eg, digital plethysmography using a light-emitting diode). Similarly, segmental plethysmographic pulse volume recordings. document pulsatility by determining volume changes in the limb; pulsatility reflects blood flow and can be especially helpful in patients with severe arterial calcification that precludes accurate pressure measurements.

Functional testing may confirm and quantitate the diagnosis of claudication using treadmill walking. The patient walks at a standard speed and grade until claudication pain is experienced or a time limit is reached. With significant arterial occlusive disease there will be a decrease in the ABI from resting to postexercise level, usually measured 1 minute after cessation of walking. A graded treadmill is similar, but it employs a slowly rising walking platform. Both types of treadmill studies (standard and graded) are useful both for establishing the diagnosis of claudication and for assessing the results of therapy.

D. IMAGING STUDIES

Calcification in the walls of atherosclerotic arteries is often visible on standard x-ray films and may occur without narrowing of the arterial lumen; for this reason, it is not an index of the functional status of the artery.

Color duplex imaging is a painless, relatively inexpensive, and (in experienced hands) accurate method for developing anatomic and some functional information (eg, velocity gradients across stenoses) about arterial insufficiency. Although the accuracy of this study is very operator-dependent, it can supply sufficient information to permit performance of revascularization in selected cases.

Arteriography provides anatomic but little functional information about peripheral arterial disease. It should not be performed as a diagnostic test but reserved for patients warranting invasive intervention such as percutaneous transluminal angioplasty (PTA) or vascular surgery. The Seldinger technique, in which catheters are advanced over flexible guidewires inserted directly into accessible (eg, common femoral) arteries, has supplanted direct arterial punctures for arteriograms of almost all arteries. Complications of angiography are related to technique and contrast media. Technical complications include puncture site hema-

toma, arteriovenous fistula, false aneurysm, retroperitoneal hematoma, subintimal dissection, and distal embolization of blood clot or atheromatous plaque (about 1% risk). Contrast agents may precipitate allergic reactions ranging from mild rash to severe anaphylaxis (about 0.1% risk). Because of their high osmolality, standard chemicals cause heat, vasodilation, and pain upon injection. Use of nonionic agents, carbon dioxide instead of contrast, and digital subtraction angiography (see below) lessens symptoms and the risk of adverse outcomes. Both standard and nonionic agents cause a transient decrease in renal blood flow and increased vascular resistance; in a small proportion of patients, angiography induces acute renal insufficiency. Patients with renal failure, proteinuria, diabetes, and dehydration are at increased risk for contrast-induced renal failure. Adequate hydration of patients before and after angiography reduces the incidence of this complication.

Digital subtraction angiography (DSA) electronically digitizes x-ray signals and enhances the images using computer subtraction techniques. Although the images produced by DSA have contrast, the spatial resolution is less than with conventional arteriography. DSA was first used as a means of obtaining intravenous angiography, which produced poor resolution. It is now most commonly used along with arterial injections to decrease the amount of contrast media and to better delineate small vessels in the foot. DSA has replaced standard arteriography in most medical centers.

Magnetic resonance angiography (MRA) can delineate arteries without using contrast agents. The basic principle of MRA is that the vector of the proton spin becomes aligned with the brief application of a magnetic field. The MRA signal is generated as the protons return to a nonexcited or random alignment. MRA is potentially able to define the components of atherosclerotic plaque, which vary in water and lipid composition, and to differentiate plaque from thrombus. However, current techniques do not distinguish well between tight stenoses and complete occlusions.

Treatment & Prognosis

The objectives of treatment are relief of symptoms and prevention of limb loss. In the lower extremity, the goal is to maintain bipedal gait. In the upper extremity, symptoms are rarely severe enough to require arterial operation, although revascularization is occasionally required for severe symptoms precipitated by exercise of the arm. Viability of fingers or of the hand is rarely jeopardized by arterial disease, unless repeated emboli occur. Upper extremity symptoms of pain and fatigue with exercise are termed "effort fatigue."

The operative risk must be assessed for each patient. Recognition of coexistent cardiac and respiratory systems is particularly relevant, because most patients with peripheral vascular disease also have ischemic heart disease or chronic obstructive pulmonary disease due to prolonged tobacco use. Most patients with peripheral vascular disease have significant concomitant coronary artery obstructions. If the patient is apt to remain incapacitated by angina or dyspnea, there is little to be gained by operation for mild or moderate claudication. The overriding issues in management of patients with intermittent claudication is that they are at significant risk of developing severe and often fatal cardiovascular complications; their most serious problem is not the limitation of walking even though that may be their presenting symptom. Patients with claudication are at a two to four times greater risk of dying from complications of generalized atherosclerosis than people without claudication. (See Figure 35–4.)

In general, patients with peripheral vascular disease have shortened life expectancies. Nondiabetic patients with ischemic disease of the lower extremity have a 5-year survival rate of 70% (Figure 35–3). The survival rate is 60% in patients with associated ischemic heart disease or cerebrovascular insufficiency. Patients with peripheral vascular disease and renal failure have a 2-year survival rate of less than 50%. Most deaths are due to my myocardial infarctions and strokes. Only 20% of deaths are due to nonatherosclerotic causes.

A. MEDICAL TREATMENT

Medical treatment consists of (1) reducing risk factors, (2) exercise rehabilitation, (3) foot care, and (4) pharmacotherapy.

1. Reduction of risk factors—Cigarette smoking is the single most important risk factor for the progression

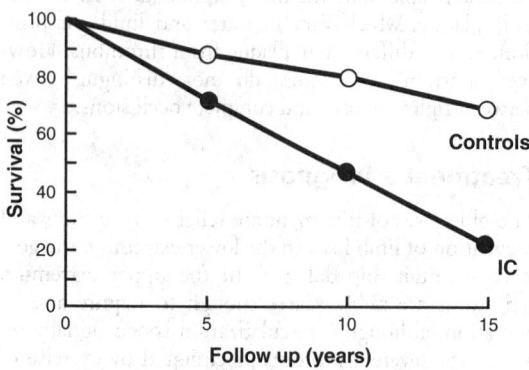

Figure 35–4. Survival of patients with intermittent claudication (IC) and matched controls. (Reproduced, with permission, from TASC Working Group: Management of peripheral arterial disease: epidemiology, natural history, risk factors. J Vasc Surg 2000; 31[1 Suppl]:S19.)

of atherosclerosis, and all patients must stop smoking. Hypertension should be controlled, although the effects of its treatment on the natural history of peripheral arterial disease have not been evaluated. There is no good evidence that beta-blockers adversely affect mild to moderate claudication. In peripheral arterial disease, the major lipid risk factors are elevated LDL cholesterol and triglyceride levels and low HDL cholesterol levels. Lipoprotein(a) is an independent risk factor for peripheral arterial disease, but there are no specific management options to decrease lipoprotein(a) levels except to treat abnormalities in other lipid fractions. Lipid modification is associated with stabilization or regression of arterial plaques. Dietary restrictions should be instituted first. The most effective drugs to treat hyperlipidemia are a group of medications known informally as statins that inhibit hydroxymethylglutaryl coenzyme A (HMG-CoA) reductase. The goals of therapy should be to reduce the LDL cholesterol level to less than 100 mg/dL (2.6 mmol/L). Statins have become the first-line medications for treatment of hyperlipidemia, but other antilipid medications, including bile acid-binding resins (cholestyramine, colestipol), niacin, and fibrates (gemfibrozil) may also be useful. Both type 1 and type 2 diabetes increase the prevalence and severity of cardiovascular disease. Intensive glycemic control reduces the incidence of nephropathy, neuropathy, and retinopathy in diabetes, but it does not correlate with the severity or progression of peripheral arterial disease. In order to reduce microvascular end points and all-cause mortality, however, it is recommended that fasting blood sugars should range from 80 to 120 mg/dL and that postprandial sugars should be < 180 mg/dL; hemoglobin A_{1c} should be less than 7%.

2. Exercise rehabilitation—Exercise, ranging from unsupervised walking in the community to formal supervised exercise on a treadmill, significantly improves walking ability. A 21-study meta-analysis of exercise programs showed an average 180% increase in initial claudication distance and a 120% increase in maximal walking distance achieved through exercise. The precise mechanism behind this improvement is not firmly established. Collateral development seems unlikely because ankle pressures and limb flow do not increase substantially. Possible explanations include improved metabolic capacity in muscles, altered gait using more proximal nonischemic muscles, and favorable modifications in other risk factors (improvement in glucose metabolism, reduction in LDL cholesterol and triglyceride concentrations, increase in HDL cholesterol concentration, decreased obesity, and smoking cessation).

3. Foot care—The feet should be inspected and washed daily and kept dry. Clean cotton socks should be worn beneath dress socks, and shoes must fit properly. Mechanical and thermal trauma to the feet should be avoided. Toenails should be trimmed carefully, and corns and calluses should be attended to promptly. Because even minor foot infections may produce complications that will result in amputation (especially in patients with diabetes mellitus), foot infections or injuries should be treated immediately. Educating the patient to understand peripheral vascular insufficiency and the importance of foot care is a central aspect of treatment.

4. Pharmacotherapy—The Antiplatelet Trialists Collaboration reviewed 189 controlled studies involving secondary prevention of cardiovascular events in over 100,000 patients and found an overall 25% decrease in fatal and nonfatal myocardial infarctions, strokes, and vascular deaths in those treated with antiplatelet agents. Aspirin at dosages ranging from 75 to 350 mg/d is the first-line antiplatelet agent generally recommended, though clopidogrel, which blocks the activation of platelets by ADP is useful in aspirin-intolerant patients or those with large atherosclerotic burdens (ie, coronary artery disease, cerebrovascular disease, and peripheral arterial disease). All patients with peripheral arterial disease, whether symptomatic or asymptomatic, should be considered for antiplatelet therapy to reduce the risk of cardiovascular morbidity and mortality. Only two drugs have been approved by the FDA specifically for treatment of symptoms of intermittent claudication. **Pentoxifylline** improves red cell deformability, lowers fibrinogen levels, and decreases platelet aggregation; it produces a small improvement in both initial claudication distance (about 20%) and absolute claudication distance (about 10%). Cilostazol is a phosphodiesterase III inhibitor with vasodilator, antiplatelet, and antilipid activity. Randomized, placebo-controlled, blinded trials have shown an increase of about 50% in absolute claudication distance in cilostazol-treated patients compared with 10% improvement in controls. Quality-of-life assessments also improved significantly. Other agents are in various stages of development, including carnitine, prostaglandins, vascular endothelial growth factor (VEGF), and L-arginine. Gene therapy for cardiovascular disease is also being investigated, but conclusions regarding safety and efficacy are premature.

B. ENDOVASCULAR THERAPY

Numerous techniques are available for treating atherosclerosis using devices within blood vessels. Percutaneous transluminal angioplasty (PTA) consists of dilation of a stenotic arterial segment using an inflatable balloon catheter that can be inflated to extremely high pressures without deforming the balloon. The deeper layers of the plaque are cracked and sheared circumferentially away from the media. As the balloon expands, it permanently overstretches the media and adventitia,

fracturing atheromatous plaques and expanding the artery to widen the lumen. Because energy losses associated with a stenosis are inversely proportionate to the fourth power of the radius at that point, small increases in radius can result in substantial increases in blood flow.

Percutaneous transluminal angioplasty may be used as primary therapy or as an adjunct to surgery. As noted above, the success rate for percutaneous transluminal angioplasty is highest in the treatment of short stenoses of large proximal arteries. The 1-year success rate is 85% in common iliac disease, 70% in external iliac disease, and only 50% in femoral and popliteal artery disease. Use of percutaneous transluminal angioplasty for calf vessels is limited. The success rate is inversely related to the length of stenosis, and stenoses longer than 10 cm have little chance of remaining patent. In large arteries, the success rate in treating stenoses is about the same as for complete occlusions, but in small vessels the results with stenoses are better.

The initial failure rate of percutaneous transluminal angioplasty is 10–20%. Other complications include disruption of the artery, false aneurysm formation, dissection of an atherosclerotic plaque, and distal embolization. Local thrombosis with acute ischemia of the extremity is unusual. Since disease can be expected to recur in about one-third or more of cases, the patient should be closely followed using noninvasive tests. Repeat percutaneous transluminal angioplasty may be indicated for recurrent disease. The apparent cost savings afforded by percutaneous transluminal angioplasty instead of operative treatment of arterial disease are offset by the need for multiple repeat procedures.

In the past decade, placement of endovascular stents in conjunction with PTA has become increasingly popular. Two basic varieties of stents are currently available: balloon-expandable (Palmaz type) and self-expanding (Wallstent type). Stainless steel, nitinol, and various alloys are used for construction of stents. Most authorities agree on the following indications for placement of intra-arterial stents: post-PTA arterial dissection, inadequate PTA due to elastic recoil, chronic occlusions, restenoses after previous PTAs, and arterial stenoses with ulcerations producing emboli.

Stents have been most successful when placed in the aorta or common iliac arteries, but placement in other arteries, including the mesenteric, renal, external iliac, and femorodistal arteries, is acceptable in certain clinical settings. Use of stents for treatment of carotid occlusive disease is more controversial.

Atherectomy is an endovascular procedure in which plaque is removed piecemeal by a cutting or rotating catheter, leaving a portion of the media and arterial wall behind. In theory, removing the plaque should be more effective than angioplasty in treating stenosis, and it does not produce thermal injury as does laser angioplasty. Varieties of atherectomy catheters each have unique characteristics, but all debulk lesions with an intraluminal cutting device. The short-term results of atherectomy are satisfactory, but restenosis is a major problem.

C. SURGICAL TREATMENT

Arterial reconstruction is performed both for limb salvage and for incapacitating claudication. This latter indication requires prudent surgical judgment, because most patients with claudication alone should be treated nonoperatively. For patients with more advanced disease (eg, rest pain, impending gangrene), operation is mandatory. The choice of operative procedure depends upon the location and distribution of arterial lesions and the presence of associated heart, pulmonary, or other disease.

Direct revascularization operations are applicable for patients with obstructive lesions located anywhere from the abdominal aorta to the arteries of the calf, providing there is demonstrable patency of the arteries distal to the segment to be revascularized. All patients undergoing vascular surgery should have preoperative risk assessments (see Chapter 2). Beta-blocker administration is appropriate for most patients perioperatively to reduce cardiac morbidity.

1. Aortoiliofemoral interventions—Interventional radiologic percutaneous techniques have replaced operative intervention for many lesions involving the aorta and common iliac artery. When stenoses or even occlusions are relatively short and localized, PTA with or without placement of permanent intraluminal stents (Figure 35–5) is the treatment of choice, for patency

rates of such "less invasive" procedures approach the results of operative treatment; moreover, if disease recurs, repeat interventions are possible. The total costs of multiple interventions, however, quickly approach those of surgery. PTA and stenting of the external iliac artery or the common femoral artery generally produce inferior long-term patency rates compared with operation. When operation is required for aortoiliofemoral occlusive disease, an inverted Y-shaped prosthesis is interposed between the infrarenal abdominal aorta and the femoral arteries. On occasion, the lesion is confined to the aorta and common iliac arteries, and endarterectomy is preferable (Figure 35–6). The goal of operation is restoration of blood flow to the common femoral artery or, when occlusive disease of the superficial femoral artery is present, to the profunda femoris artery.

The clinical results of aortoiliofemoral reconstruction are excellent. The operative death rate is 5%; early patency rate, 95%; and late patency rate (5–10 years postoperatively), about 80%. Complications associated with aortoiliac reconstruction include infection, aortointestinal fistula formation, anastomotic aneurysm formation, occlusion of a limb of the graft, bowel infarction, peripheral embolization with limb loss, renal failure, and erectile dysfunction.

Although the risks of aortoiliac reconstruction are acceptably low in the average patient, simpler procedures may be preferable in high-risk patients. If the clinically important lesions are confined to one side, a femorofemoral or iliofemoral bypass graft can be used. A long graft from the axillary to the femoral artery (ie, axillofemoral graft) is used for treating patients with infected abdominal aortic Dacron grafts or aortoenteric fistulas. These "extra-anatomic" methods of arterial re-

Figure 35–5. Percutaneous treatment of iliac artery stenosis: ***A:*** Preoperative arteriogram showing focal iliac artery stenosis. ***B:*** Percutaneous transluminal dilation of lesion. ***C:*** Widely patent arterial segment with stent in place.

Figure 35–6. *Left:* Aortogram showing atherosclerotic occlusive disease of the infrarenal aorta and iliac arteries. *Right:* Postoperative aortogram showing wide patency after aortoiliac endarterectomy.

construction, however, are more prone to late occlusion and infection than are direct reconstructions.

2. Femoropopliteal reconstruction—When disease affects both the aortoiliac and femoropopliteal segments of the arterial tree, aortofemoral bypass (with profundaplasty if indicated) is generally adequate. When disease is confined to the femoropopliteal segment, femoropopliteal bypass is used. The principal indication for these operations is limb salvage. In patients with claudication alone, the indications for femoropopliteal bypass are more difficult to define but must include substantial disability resulting from the claudication symptoms.

A femoropopliteal bypass graft is performed to provide pulsatile blood flow to the popliteal artery (Figure 35–7). The best graft for this purpose is autologous great saphenous vein. The saphenous vein may be left in situ or removed and reversed for use as an arterial conduit. In the former instance, the vein is left in its normal position, special instruments are used to render the valves incompetent, and the venous tributaries are ligated. Expanded polytetrafluoroethylene (PTFE) may also be used as a conduit, particularly when bypassing to the supragenicular popliteal artery. Below the knee PTFE conduits produce much lower patency rates than saphenous veins. Operative death rates are low (2%), and 5-year patency rates range from 60% to 80%. Limb salvage rates are higher than graft patency rates. Patients undergoing femoropopliteal bypass for limb salvage have a survival rate of only about 50% within 5 years. Myocardial infarctions and strokes cause most deaths.

Figure 35–7. *Left:* Femoral arteriogram showing occlusion of the superficial femoral and proximal popliteal arteries. *Right:* Femoral arteriogram showing patency of the femoral and popliteal arteries after endarterectomy.

When profundaplasty alone is performed for limb salvage, the goal is improvement of flow to the profunda femoris artery and thereby through collaterals to the popliteal or tibial arteries. The operative death rate is only 1%, but the 5-year survival rate is 50%. Limb salvage in patients undergoing profundaplasty is 80% when the popliteal artery is patent and 40–50% when the popliteal artery is occluded. Isolated profundaplasty is rarely helpful for treating claudication.

Percutaneous transluminal angioplasty with or without stent placement is occasionally performed for patients with infrainguinal occlusive arterial disease, especially if they are at high risk for surgical complications. However, most patients with limb-threatening ischemia have disease that is too extensive for such percutaneous interventions, and long-term patency rates are low for these procedures.

3. Distal arterial reconstruction—Reconstruction of distal arteries (ie, bypass to the tibial, peroneal, or pedal vessels) is performed only for limb salvage. Autogenous saphenous vein is the best graft material, and either in situ or reversed technique may be used. If the greater saphenous vein is unavailable, a composite graft of lesser saphenous or arm veins is the next best choice. Prosthetic conduits have high failure rates. The operative death rate is about 5%, and the graft failure rate during the first 30 days is 15–35%. Five years after operation, about half of the grafts at risk are still functioning. The survival rate of patients undergoing distal arterial reconstruction is lower than for those undergoing operation for femoropopliteal disease.

Successful revascularization results in lower costs than primary amputation or failed reconstruction. Improvements in patient selection and in vascular reconstructive techniques reduce the high cost of caring for such patients. Occasionally, primary amputation is preferable to revascularization if the likelihood of successful bypass is low, extensive foot infection is present, or patients are nonambulatory.

4. Lumbar sympathectomy—Lumbar sympathectomy is seldom indicated as the only treatment for patients with occlusion of major arteries in the lower extremities. Sympathectomy is ineffective in the management of gangrene of the toes or foot and does not lower the required level for amputation or delay the requirement for amputation. At present, reflex sympathetic dystrophy (causalgia) is the principal indication for sympathectomy.

5. Amputation—If intermittent claudication is the only symptom, amputation of the limb will be necessary in only 5% of patients within 5 years and 10% in 10 years. However, patients with multiple risk factors for atherosclerosis and short-distance claudication are at increased risk for eventual limb loss. Amputation is more likely if patients continue to smoke cigarettes. Of patients who present with ischemic rest pain, however, about 5% require amputation as initial therapy, and most require amputation or revascularization within 5 years.

Ballard JL et al: Aortoiliac stent deployment versus surgical reconstruction: analysis of outcome and cost. J Vasc Surg 1998; 28:1.

Beebe HG et al: A new pharmacological treatment for intermittent claudication: results of a randomized, multicenter trial. Arch Intern Med 1999;159:2041.

Byrne J et al: Infrainguinal arterial reconstruction for claudication: is it worth the risk? An analysis of 409 procedures. J Vasc Surg 1999;29:259.

Chew DK et al: Autogenous composite vein bypass graft for infrainguinal arterial reconstruction. J Vasc Surg 2001;33:259.

Conti CR: Current status of medical therapy of peripheral arterial disease. Clin Cardiol 1999;22:331.

Cronenwett JL, Birkmeyer JD (editors): *The Dartmouth Atlas of Vascular Health Care.* AHA Press, 2000.

de Virgilio C et al: Dipyridamole-thalhum/sestamibi before vascular surgery: a prospective blinded study in moderate-risk patients. J Vasc Surg 2000;32:77.

Donnelly R et al: ABC of arterial and venous disease: vascular complications of diabetes. BMJ 2000;320:1062.

Dormandy J et al: The fate of patients with critical leg ischemia. Semin Vasc Surg 1999;12:142.

Feinglass J et al: Measures of success and health-related quality of life in lower-extremity vascular surgery. Annu Rev Med 2000; 41:101.

Golledge J et al: Outcome of femoropopliteal angioplasty. Ann Surg 1999;229:146.

Gordon IL et al: Three-year outcome of endovascular treatment of superficial femoral artery occlusion. Arch Surg 2001;136:221.

Hill SL, Holtzman G: Vascular surgeons—do they make a difference in peripheral vascular disease? Surgery 2001;129:136.

Jarvis B et al: Clopidogrel: a review of its use in the prevention of atherothrombosis. Drugs 2000;60:347.

Johnson WC et al: A comparative evaluation of polytetrafluoroethylene, umbilical vein, and saphenous vein bypass grafts for femoral-popliteal above-knee revascularization: a prospective randomized Department of Veterans Affairs cooperative study. J Vasc Surg 2000;32:268.

Krupski WC et al: Negative impact of cardiac evaluation before vascular surgery. Vasc Med 2000;5:3.

McDermott MM: Ankle brachial index as a predictor of outcomes in peripheral arterial disease. J Lab Clin Med 1999;133:33.

Mills JL et al: The natural history of intermediate and critical vein graft stenosis: recommendations for continued surveillance or repair. J Vasc Surg 2001;33:273.

Nelemans PJ et al: Peripheral arterial disease: meta-analysis of the diagnostic performance of MR angiography. Radiology 2000; 217:105.

Oppat WF et al: Natural history of composite sequential bypass: ten years' experience. Arch Surg 1999;134:754.

Poldermans D et al: The effect of bisoprolol on perioperative mortality and myocardial infarction in high-risk patients undergoing vascular surgery. N Engl J Med 1999;341:1789.

Powell RJ et al: The durability of endovascular treatment of multisegment iliac occlusive disease. J Vasc Surg 2001;31:1178.

Quinn SF et al: Aortic and lower-extremity arterial disease: evaluation with MR angiography versus conventional angiography. Radiology 1998;206:693.

Rutherford RB et al: Recommended standards for reports dealing with lower extremity ischemia: revised version. J Vasc Surg 1997;26:517.

Savander SJ et al: The Legs for Life screening for peripheral vascular disease. J Vasc Interv Radiol 2001;12:33.

Strandness DE Jr et al: Peripheral vascular disease. Circulation 2000;102(Suppl 4):46.

Tan KH et al: Exercise training and peripheral vascular disease. Br J Surg 2000;87:553.

TASC Working Group: Management of peripheral arterial disease (PAD). J Vasc Surg 2000;31:S1.

Taylor LM et al: The incidence of perioperative myocardial infarction in general vascular surgery. J Vasc Surg 1992;15:52.

Tetterroo E et al: Randomised comparison of primary stent placement versus primary angioplasty followed by selective stent placement in patients with iliac artery occlusive disease. Dutch Iliac Stent Trial Study Group. Lancet 1998;351:1153.

Veith FJ et al: Six-year prospective multicenter randomized comparison of autologous saphenous vein and expanded polytetrafluoroethylene grafts in infrainguinal arterial reconstructions. J Vasc Surg 1986;3:104.

Wain RA et al: Can duplex scan arterial mapping replace contrast arteriography as the test of choice before infrainguinal revascularization? J Vasc Surg 1999;29:100.

ACUTE ARTERIAL OCCLUSION

Sudden occlusion of a previously patent artery supplying an extremity is a dramatic event characterized by the abrupt onset of severe distal ischemia, with pain, coldness, numbness, motor weakness, and absent pulses. Tissue viability depends on the extent to which flow is maintained by collateral circuits or surgical intervention. The clinical manifestations are those of ischemia of nerves, muscle, and skin. When ischemia persists, motor and sensory paralysis, muscle infarction, and cutaneous gangrene become irreversible in a matter of hours. A line of demarcation develops between viable and nonviable tissue. Flow in the distal arteries is reduced progressively by propagating intraluminal thrombus, and surgical restoration of blood flow to the ischemic portion of the extremity eventually becomes impossible.

Acute major arterial occlusion may be caused by an embolus, thrombosis, trauma, or dissection. Embolic occlusion usually results from dislodgment of a blood clot into the bloodstream. The heart is the source of embolus in 80–90% of episodes. The clot most frequently originates from the left atrium in patients with arterial fibrillation or from ventricular mural thrombus in patients with recent myocardial infarction. Prosthetic heart valves may be the source of emboli, although this is uncommon with chronic systemic anticoagulation or use of tissue valves. Septic emboli may emanate from infective endocarditis. Emboli may arise from clots within aneurysms anywhere in the aortofemoral system; popliteal aneurysms that cause emboli have a particularly poor prognosis. Ulceration in atherosclerotic plaques can lead to dislodgment of platelets, thrombus, or debris. Miscellaneous infrequent sources of emboli include cardiac tumors (including cardiac myxoma), and paradoxic emboli (venous thrombi migrating through a patent foramen ovale). Up to 5–10% of spontaneous emboli originate from a source that remains unidentified despite thorough diagnostic interrogation. These have been called **cryptogenic emboli.** In some cases, confusion arises in differentiating in situ thrombosis from peripheral embolism. Hypercoagula-ble states have been implicated, especially in younger patients without evidence of atherosclerosis or in patients with malignancy.

Sudden thrombosis of an atherosclerotic peripheral artery may be difficult to differentiate clinically from embolic occlusion. The usual mechanism is hemorrhagic dissection beneath an atherosclerotic plaque. These patients have preexisting atherosclerotic stenosis and low blood flow, which predisposes to stagnation and thrombosis. Differentiation between embolic and thrombotic occlusions is based on the clinical setting and a history of long-standing symptoms.

Traumatic occlusion may be due to numerous causes, eg, contusion or laceration by a bone after a fracture or dislocation, penetrating injuries, and—more commonly in recent years—as a complication of arterial catheterization or PTA. Intra-arterial injection of drugs of abuse is an increasingly frequent cause of acute arterial occlusion.

Acute arterial dissection may occur in any artery but most commonly occurs in the thoracic aorta (see Chapter 19). This disorder is characterized by separation of the arterial wall by extraluminal blood that enters the wall through an intimal tear. Classically, aortic dissection causes sudden and intense chest and interscapular pain as the dissection occurs; as the dissection progresses, it causes a wide variety of symptoms, leading to the epithet, "the great masquerader." For example, severe abdominal pain may result from mesenteric artery involvement, whereas limb ischemia may occur from involvement of the iliofemoral arteries.

Clinical Findings

Acute arterial occlusion is characterized by the five *P*s: pain, pallor, pulselessness, paresthesias, and paralysis. Severe sudden pain is present in 80% of patients, and its onset usually indicates the time of vessel occlusion. Pain is absent in some patients because of prompt onset of anesthesia and paralysis.

Pallor appears first but is replaced by mottled cyanosis as deoxygenated blood gradually suffuses the extremity. Cutaneous hypesthesia slowly progresses to anesthesia. It is important to separate perception of light touch from that of pressure, pain, and temperature, because the larger fibers serving these latter functions are relatively less susceptible to hypoxia. The onset of motor paralysis heralds impending gangrene. If changes persist beyond 12 hours, limb salvage is unlikely. Tense swelling with acute tenderness of a muscle belly—a common occurrence in the gastrocnemius following superficial femoral artery occlusion—generally denotes irreversible muscle infarction. Skin and subcutaneous tissues have greater resistance to hypoxia than nerves and muscles, which demonstrate irreversible histologic changes after 4–6 hours of ischemia.

The level of demarcation of ischemic changes suggests the site of arterial occlusion. Since collaterals always supply the tissues just beyond the occlusion, the demarcation is as follows:

Site of Occlusion	Line of Demarcation
Infrarenal aorta	Mid abdomen
Aortic bifurcation and common iliac arteries	Groin
External iliacs	Proximal thigh
Common femoral	Lower third of thigh
Superficial femoral	Upper third of calf
Politeal	lower third of calf

If collateral flow increases, it becomes evident by return of warmth and normal color of the skin and a lessening of the sensory deficit. When reversible ischemia has been severe and protracted at the onset, normal sensory function may not return. When collateral flow has reached its maximum, the signs and symptoms are those of chronic occlusion of the involved artery.

Treatment & Prognosis

A. Embolism and Thrombosis

Immediate anticoagulation by intravenous heparin slows the propagation of thrombus and allows time for assessment of adequacy of collateral flow and preparation for operation if indicated. When embolus cannot be differentiated from thrombosis, arteriography should be performed if it can be done without delaying therapy. Diagnosis of acute embolic occlusion is based upon an abrupt block of the artery with little accompanying arterial disease; conversely, acute in situ thrombosis is associated with extensive atherosclerosis and a well-established collateral network.

The operative treatment of the average embolus differs from that of preexisting atherosclerosis. Although some surgeons recommend nonoperative management with anticoagulation as the sole therapy for acute arterial ischemia, this approach is not widely favored. Nonoperative management is best reserved for some emboli to major arteries in the upper extremities, where collateral circulation is outstanding, and for some in the lower extremities when skin color improves or neural function returns quickly after occlusion. If the initial ischemia recedes, the decision for removal of the embolus is based upon an estimate of the disability that will be produced by chronic occlusion of the involved artery. Chronic occlusion of the axillary or brachial arteries is usually well tolerated, whereas chronic occlusion of lower extremity vessels causes claudication at best.

If advanced ischemia persists or is profound, the embolus must be removed. Therapeutic options include catheter-directed thrombolysis, percutaneous mechanical thrombectomy, ultrasound-accelerated thrombolysis, and surgical embolectomy. For patients with severe acute ischemia, operative therapy is preferable because it is usually associated with the least delay in reestablishing perfusion. Surgical embolectomy may be performed through an arteriotomy at the site of the embolus or, most commonly, by extraction with a balloon (Fogarty) catheter inserted through a proximal arteriotomy. Successful embolectomy requires removal of the embolus and the "tail" of thrombus that extends distally or proximally from it. If operation is not performed within the first few hours, the ramifications of this thrombus into arterial branches usually cannot be extracted and revascularization is impossible. Intraoperative infusion of thrombolytic agents is an adjunct to embolectomy when thrombus has propagated. Late thrombectomy (after 12 hours) is successful only when propagation of thrombus has been arrested by collateral blood flow reentering the vessel distal to the embolus. Fasciotomy is normally required after prolonged acute ischemia to treat compartment syndrome. Renal insufficiency—the so-called myonephrotic syndrome—should be anticipated after reperfusion of ischemic muscle. Treatment consists of vigorous hydration and alkalinization of the urine. Administration of free radical scavengers may be helpful in this disorder.

Moribund patients with embolic disease should not be treated surgically. Patients with clearly irreversible limb ischemia should undergo amputation without an attempt at revascularization, because revascularization subjects the patient to the serious hazards of the reperfusion syndrome caused by recirculation of acidotic hyperkalemic venous blood.

Many patients present late with subacute ischemia when it is difficult to ascertain the cause of occlusion. Initial therapy should consist of anticoagulation. The arterial anatomy should be defined by arteriography. Treatment options include continuation of anticoagulants, thrombolytic therapy with streptokinase or urokinase, arterial embolectomy, or arterial reconstruction. Intravenous thrombolytic therapy is ineffective and is associated with a high rate of complications. A safer, more effective regimen involves selective intra-arterial infusion of lower doses of thrombolytic agent (eg, alteplase) directly into the clot. This activates thrombus plasminogen more efficiently, protects the drug from circulating antibodies and inhibitors, and lowers complication rates.

B. Traumatic Arterial Occlusion

Traumatic arterial occlusion must be corrected within a few hours to avoid development of gangrene. Repair of arterial injury is usually performed in conjunction with repair of other injuries. The general principles are described in Chapter 14.

Campbell WB, Ridler BM, Szymanska TH: Current management of acute leg ischaemia: results of an audit by the Vascular Surgical Society of Great Britain and Ireland. Br J Surg 1998; 85:1498.

Greenberg R et al: The role of thrombolytic therapy in the management of acute and chronic lower extremity ischemia. J Endovasc Ther 2000;7:72.

Ouriel K et al: Acute lower limb ischemia: determinants of outcome. Surgery 1998;124:336.

Suggs WD et al: When is urokinase treatment an effective sole or adjunctive treatment for acute limb ischemia secondary to native artery occlusion? Am J Surg 1999;178:103.

Swischuk JL et al: Transcatheter intraarterial infusion of rt-PA for acute lower limb ischemia: Results and complications. J Vasc Interv Radiol 2001;12:423.

EXTREMITY PERIPHERAL MICROEMBOLI

Recurrent microemboli to the small arteries in the extremities can arise from sources already described as well as from ulcerated atheromas. The peripheral aneurysms most commonly implicated are in the popliteal and subclavian arteries. The mural thrombus in the wall of popliteal aneurysms is particularly susceptible to fragmentation with flexion of the knee joint. Subclavian aneurysms are almost always associated with an anomalous cervical rib that compresses the artery, and they develop as extensions of the poststenotic dilation. The source of atheromatous microembolization is almost always a lesion in the aorta-iliac-femoral portions of the arterial tree.

When a microembolus occludes a digital artery, the patient experiences sudden pain, cyanosis, and coldness or numbness in the affected digit. These changes characteristically improve over several days, only to reappear perhaps in a different area of the hand or foot. This clinical entity has been called **blue toe syndrome,** or **trash foot.** The sudden onset of pain and purple discoloration of a toe in the presence of palpable pulses is recognized as a potentially limb-threatening arterial problem. With each succeeding episode, recovery is slower and less complete.

Suddenness of onset differentiates peripheral atheroembolism from other causes of blue toes, such as vasculitis, thromboangiitis obliterans, trauma, or chronic ischemia. It is important to remember that a patent proximal artery to serve as a conduit for the embolus is required for occurrence of this syndrome. Three things are required for the blue toe syndrome: a source of emboli, a conduit, and a target. With embolic occlusion of distal arteries, a normal blood supply is present in adjacent tissue segments. Unless this difference is recog-

nized and the lesion of origin corrected, survival of the foot or hand may be in peril from recurrent microemboli that progressively occlude additional arteries.

Once discovered, the source of microemboli must be removed by appropriate valvular or arterial reconstruction. Catheter-directed thrombolytic therapy may be used to dissolve distal emboli in selected cases. Acute anticoagulation is nearly always indicated and chronic anticoagulation may be necessary, particularly with valvular disease.

Farooq MM et al: Penetrating ulceration of the infrarenal aorta: case reports of an embolic and an asymptomatic lesion. Ann Vasc Surg 2001;15:255.

Matchett WJ et al: Blue toe syndrome: treatment with intraarterial stents and review of therapies. J Vasc Interv Radiol 2000; 11:585.

Sharma PV et al: Changing patterns of atheroembolism. Cardiovasc Surg 1996;4:573.

SMALL ARTERY OCCLUSIVE DISEASE

Obstructing lesions may occur in arteries less than 3 mm in diameter (eg, the radial, ulnar, tibial, or peroneal arteries), most commonly in patients with diabetes mellitus, recurrent microembolization (see above), vasculitis, or thromboangiitis obliterans (Buerger's disease). Hand, foot, or digital ischemia can result from these conditions, and amputation is sometimes required.

Differentiation of occluded arterial segments from vasoconstrictive disorders can best be accomplished in the upper extremity by the **Allen test.** This is done by having the patient make a tight fist while the examiner occludes the radial and ulnar arteries at the wrist and asks the patient to open and close the hand rapidly. With the hand in a relaxed position, patency of the radial artery can be determined by releasing the radial artery and noting the return of color. This maneuver is then repeated for the ulnar artery. The extremity is made ischemic by compressing the proximal artery while the hand is exercised. When the extremity has become pale, the artery is released and the pattern of return color is observed. In a person with normal arteries and normal sympathetic tone, a vivid flush appears almost simultaneously in all areas of the hand. Patients with excess sympathetic tone will have a diffusely delayed but unevenly distributed return of color. When small artery occlusion is present, there will be a prolonged delay in or absence of reperfusion of the cutaneous area supplied by the occluded arteries.

DIABETIC VASCULAR DISEASE

Atherosclerotic arterial disease in patients with diabetes mellitus is more diffuse and more severe than in nondiabetics. Advanced disease often affects both large and medium-sized arteries, and even the smaller arteries (especially those in the calf) may be involved. In nondiabetic patients, atherosclerosis at the bifurcation of the popliteal artery and tibioperoneal trunk usually extends into the tibial vessels for only a short distance. In diabetic patients, however, the tibioperoneal vessels frequently contain irregular atherosclerotic changes as far down as the ankle, and the vessels may be heavily calcified. Hence, the degree of ischemia is often severe and extensive, whereas noninvasive tests may be falsely normal. In addition to extensive femorotibial macrovascular atherosclerotic disease, all diabetics have thickened capillary basement membranes at the microcirculatory level. Treatment of diabetics with angiotensin-converting enzyme (ACE) inhibitors may worsen microvascular circulation.

Diabetic patients also have a high incidence of neuropathy and are therefore more apt to injure themselves. Neuropathy is also responsible for loss of tone of intrinsic foot muscles that leads to subluxation of the metatarsal phalangeal joints, resulting in a "rocker-bottom" foot and ultimately producing complete joint destruction termed a "Charcot foot." Thus, ulceration is prone to occur because of altered foot architecture and diminished sensation. Neurotrophic ulcers over the first metatarsophalangeal joint are termed "malperforans ulcers." Such wounds are particularly susceptible to infection because of white blood cell dysfunction in diabetics. Additionally, inflammatory cells and some bacteria elaborate substances that act as procoagulants.

Akbari CM et al: Diabetes and peripheral vascular disease. J Vasc Surg 1999;30;373.

Bouton AJ et al: The diabetic foot: the scope of the problem. J Fam Pract 2000;49:S3.

Effects of rampiril on cardiovascular and microvascular outcomes in people with diabetes mellitus: results of the HOPE Study and MICROHOPE Substudy. Heart Outcomes Prevention Evaluation (HOPE) Study Investigators. Lancet 2000; 355:253.

Nehler MR et al: Intermediate-term outcome of primary digit amputations in patients with diabetes mellitus who have forefoot sepsis requiring hospitalization and presumed adequate circulatory status. J Vasc Surg 1999;30;509.

NONATHEROSCLEROTIC DISORDERS CAUSING LOWER LIMB ISCHEMIA

Thromboangiitis Obliterans

Thromboangiitis obliterans (**Buerger's disease**) is characterized by multiple segmental occlusions of small arteries in the extremities distal to the brachial and popliteal arteries. In contrast to atherosclerosis, which involves the intima and inner media, thromboangiitis obliterans is manifested by infiltration of round cells in all three layers of the arterial wall. Healing of the arter-

ial wall lesion is associated with fibrous obliteration of the lumen in segmental fashion. Migratory phlebitis is frequently present. The disease occurs almost exclusively in young cigarette-smoking men; commonly, both upper and lower extremities are affected.

Many patients with Buerger's disease have specific cellular immunity against arterial antigens, specific humoral antiarterial antibodies, and elevated circulatory immune complexes. HLA typing can differentiate such patients from patients with atherosclerosis and from normal individuals. The role of cigarette smoking is unclear; it is probably facilitative rather than causative. Symptoms consist of slowly developing digital pain, cyanosis, and coldness, progressing eventually to necrosis and gangrene. Claudication in the muscles of the foot may be the first symptom.

Examination shows an irregular pattern of digital ischemia. The Allen test (see above) demonstrates delayed filling of affected digital arteries and rapid filling in adjacent vessels.

A precise diagnosis can only be made by microscopic examination showing the typical segmental vasculitis with infiltration of lymphocytes into all layers of the vessel wall. Arteriographic findings are distinctive but not pathognomonic. The artery proximal to the occlusions characteristically is tapered, and the arterial wall is smooth and devoid of irregular atherosclerotic plaques; multiple wispy collateral vessels are present. The configuration resembles a dunce cap.

It is essential that the patient stop smoking to avoid progression of the disease. Sympathectomy decreases arterial spasm and is useful in some patients. Amputation is indicated for persistent pain or gangrene and can be performed adjacent to the line of demarcation with satisfactory primary healing.

The disease may become dormant if the patient can stop smoking, but this is unfortunately difficult to achieve in many who ultimately develop gangrene of additional digits.

Popliteal Artery Entrapment Syndrome

A rare cause of popliteal artery stenosis or occlusion occurs as a result of an anomalous course of the popliteal artery. The popliteal artery normally passes between the two heads of the gastrocnemius muscle as it enters the lower leg. In the entrapment syndrome, the artery passes medial to the medial head of the gastrocnemius, causing compression of the popliteal artery when the knee is extended. There are five anatomic mechanisms for popliteal artery entrapment, but all produce similar clinical effects. Fibrous thickening of the intima occurs at the site of compression and gradually progresses to total occlusion. Poststenotic dilation of the artery may occur with mural thrombus and distal embolization.

Symptoms vary from simple calf claudication to those of more severe ischemia depending upon the adequacy of collateral channels and the extent of distal or proximal clot propagation. Popliteal artery entrapment should be considered when a young, otherwise healthy patient presents with calf claudication. Until the artery becomes occluded, the only finding is a decrease in strength of the pedal pulses, most evident using provocative maneuvers of foot dorsiflexion and plantar flexion. MRI studies are most useful confirmation of the diagnosis. Atherosclerotic changes are notably absent. Treatment consists of division of the medial head of the gastrocnemius muscle and resection and graft replacement of the diseased arterial segment. Lumbar sympathectomy is often performed as well.

Cystic Degeneration of the Popliteal Artery

Arterial stenosis is produced by a mucoid cyst in the adventitia, usually located in the middle third of the artery. Calf claudication is the most common symptom, and the only finding is decrease in the strength of the peripheral pulses. Rarely, a mass can be palpated. Arteriography shows a sharply localized zone of popliteal stenosis with a smooth concentric tapering having an hourglass appearance. Ultrasound or CT scans can be used to demonstrate the cyst within the vessel wall. The stenosis may be missed on conventional anteroposterior films and may appear only on lateral exposures. Evacuation of the cyst may relieve the stenosis, but because of the possibility of recurrence, local arterial excision and graft replacement may be required occasionally.

Abdominal Aortic Coarctation

Constriction of the thoracic or abdominal aorta may be congenital and developmental or may result from an inflammatory aortopathy such as Kawasaki's disease or Takayasu's disease. These are rare disorders that may produce symptoms of lower extremity, mesenteric, or renal ischemia depending on the location of the constriction. The congenital variant of this condition is best managed surgically when it is recognized; autogenous repair may be preferable to use of prosthetic grafts. The inflammatory aortopathies are thought to be a variant of autoimmune disease and at least initially are managed medically with anti-inflammatory agents and immunosuppressive agents. In "burned-out" inflammatory aortopathy, however, standard surgical operations appear to work satisfactorily in these patients.

Blank M et al: Monoclonal anti-endothelial cell antibodies from a patient with Takayasu Arteritis activate endothelial cells from large vessels. Arthritis Rheum 1999;42:1421.

Eichorn J et al: Antiendothelial cell antibodies in thromboangiitis obliterans. Am J Med 1998;315:17.

Levien LJ et al: Adventitial cystic disease: a unifying hypothesis. J Vasc Surg 1998;28:193.

Levien LJ et al: Popliteal artery entrapment syndrome; more common than previously recognized. J Vasc Surg 1999;30:587.

Mickley V et al: Coarctations of descending and abdominal aorta: long-term results of surgical therapy. J Vasc Surg 1998:28: 206.

O'Hara N et al: Surgical treatment for popliteal artery entrapment syndrome. Cardiovasc Surg 2001;9:141.

Ring DH Jr et al: Popliteal artery entrapment syndrome: arteriographic findings and thrombolytic therapy. J Vasc Interv Radiol 1999:10:713.

Teoh MK: Takayasu's arteritis with renovascular hypertension: results of surgical treatment. Cardiovasc Surg 1999;7:626.

Tsolakis IA et al: Cystic adventitial disease of the popliteal artery: diagnosis and treatment. Eur J Vasc Endovasc Surg 1998; 15:188.

■ ARTERIAL ANEURYSMS

An aneurysm is a permanent localized dilation of an artery to one and one-half or more times is normal diameter. Arterial aneurysms may be classified according to etiology (eg, degenerative, inflammatory, mechanical, congenital, dissecting); shape (eg, saccular, fusiform); location (eg, central, peripheral, splanchnic, renal, cerebral); or structure (eg, true, false). A **true aneurysm** involves all vessel wall layers (intima, media, and adventitia). Atherosclerosis is coexistent with rather than causative of most true aneurysms; thus, they are best termed degenerative rather than atherosclerotic. Dilation is associated with elongation of the artery. A **false aneurysm** or **pseudoaneurysm** is a pulsatile hematoma not contained by the vessel wall layers but confined by a fibrous capsule. False aneurysms are caused by disruption of the vessel wall or the anastomotic site between graft and vessel, with containment of blood by surrounding tissue.

Degenerative aneurysms are found, in descending order of frequency, in the distal abdominal aorta, the iliac arteries, the popliteal artery (Figure 35–8), the common femoral artery, the arch and descending portions of the thoracic aorta, the carotid arteries, and other peripheral arteries. As the aneurysm enlarges, mural thrombus is deposited on its interior surface because of eddy currents and stagnant flow. The functional lumen of the artery may remain unchanged and may appear relatively normal on arteriograms—a factor that limits the usefulness of angiography in diagnosis.

Numerous mechanisms have been proposed for the cause of abdominal aortic aneurysms. Casting doubt on atherosclerosis as the major cause is the observation that

Figure 35–8. Arteriogram showing aneurysm of the popliteal artery (arrow).

only 20–25% of aortic aneurysms are associated with aortoiliac occlusive disease. Decreased elastin and collagen are present in the walls of aneurysms. Whereas collagen makes up about 25% of the wall of an atherosclerotic aorta, it comprises only 18% of aneurysmal aortic wall. Fragmentation and weakening of the elastic lamellae (elastin) produces insufficient retractive force and allows increases in the length and diameter of the aorta.

An inflammatory process primarily involving activated tissue macrophages have been implicated in abdominal aortic aneurysm formation. This may contribute to increased proteinase activity (collagenase, elastase) or deductions in their naturally occurring inhibitors (antiprotease) in the aortic wall. Structural abnormalities also contribute; reductions in the number of elastic lamellae and virtual absence of vasa vasorum (blood vessels that nourish the arterial wall) in the media of the distal abdominal aorta (compared with the thoracic aorta) may also favor aneurysmal degeneration of this arterial segment. These structural abnormalities combine with hemodynamic factors that place the infrarenal aorta at risk for aneurysm owing to large pulsatile stresses because of its tapering geometry, increased stiffness, and reflected pressure waves from branch vessels.

Genetically linked enzyme differences have been associated with aneurysms in experimental animals. Lysyl oxidase, a copper-containing enzyme that helps regulate collagen cross-linking, is deficient in a strain of mice that develop abdominal aortic aneurysms. This sex chromosome-linked enzyme defect has been found in several large families in which almost every male has an abdominal aortic aneurysm, suggesting the possibility of genetic susceptibility. There is a 19% incidence in first-degree relatives of patients with aortic aneurysms.

Rare causes of true aneurysms of the abdominal aorta include Marfan's syndrome, Ehlers-Danlos syndrome, Behçet's disease, cystic medial necrosis, syphilis, and long-term sequelae of aoartic dissection.

INFRARENAL ABDOMINAL AORTIC ANEURYSMS

Most aneurysms of the abdominal aorta involve the segment of the aorta between the takeoff of the renal arteries and the aortic bifurcation but may include variable portions of the common iliac artery. Abdominal aortic aneurysms are present in 2% of the elderly population, and the incidence is increasing. The abdominal aorta is the most common site of atherosclerotic aneurysms and also the most dangerous site; aneurysms here are much more likely to rupture than are aneurysms of smaller peripheral arteries.

The recently completed ADAM (Aneurysm Detection and Management) study screened 73,451 veterans 50–79 years of age using abdominal ultrasound; an abdominal aortic aneurysm 4 cm or larger was detected in 1031 participants (1.4%). Men are affected more often than women by a ration of 4:1. The incidence of abdominal aortic aneurysm varies with the population studied and is lowest in unselected groups (like the ADAM cohort) and highest in patients with other atherosclerotic lesions. In contrast to the ADAM findings, abdominal aortic aneurysms are found in 5% of patients with coronary artery disease and in as many as 50% of patients with femoral or popliteal aneurysms.

Cigarette smoking is the systemic risk factor for the presence of abdominal aortic aneurysms with an 8:1 preponderance of abdominal aortic aneurysms in smokers compared with nonsmokers. The excess prevalence associated with smoking accounted for 78% of all abdominal aortic aneurysms that were 4 cm or larger in the ADAM study sample. Hypertension is present in 40% of patients with abdominal aortic aneurysms. Surprisingly, diabetes appears to exert a protective effect against abdominal aortic aneurysm formation.

Enlargement of abdominal aortic aneurysms is governed by the law of Laplace, in which wall tension (T) is equal to intraluminal pressure (P) times the radius (R) [T = PR] of a cylinder. Thus, it is predictable that expansion rates correlate directly with aneurysm size and degree of systemic hypertension. Tripling the aortic radius from 2 cm to 6 cm results in a 12-fold increase in wall tension.

Rupture with exsanguination is the major complication of abdominal aortic aneurysms. Ruptured abdominal aortic aneurysm is the thirteenth leading cause of death in the United States, resulting in 15,000 deaths per year. In Great Britain, 1:70 men between the age of 60 and 84 years die of a ruptured abdominal aortic aneurysm. Despite increased recognition and treatment of these lesions, the number of deaths due to ruptured abdominal aortic aneurysms and the perioperative mortality rate after ruptured abdominal aortic aneurysm repair have not significantly changed in the past 20 years.

Clinical Findings

A. SYMPTOMS AND SIGNS

An intact abdominal aneurysm rarely produces more than minimal symptoms, although the patient may be aware of a painless, throbbing mass. Rarely, intact abdominal aortic aneurysms produce back pain due to pressure on nerves or erosion into vertebral bodies. However, most back pain is musculoskeletal in origin and the vast majority of unruptured aneurysms are asymptomatic. Severe pain in the absence of rupture characterizes the rare inflammatory aneurysm that is surrounded by 2–4 cm of perianeurysmal inflammatory reaction.

Heart failure may occur owing to aortocaval fistulas; gastrointestinal hemorrhage or obstruction may result from duodenal erosion or stretching by expanding aneurysms; or pyelonephritis may develop because of ureteral obstruction by an aneurysm.

Usually, the sole physical finding is a palpable fusiform or globular pulsatile abdominal mass. With smaller aneurysms, this mass is centered in the upper abdomen just above the umbilicus, the normal location of the infrarenal portion of the abdominal aorta. Larger aneurysms bulge distally into the abdomen below the umbilicus and proximally into the space behind the rib cage. In obese patients or older individuals in whom aortas become tortuous, physical examination is not reliable. The aneurysm may be slightly tender to palpation. Severe tenderness is found in inflammatory aneurysms, after rupture has occurred, or if the aneurysm has recently expanded. In practice, many if not most abdominal aortic aneurysms are based on routine abdominal examination.

B. IMAGING STUDIES

Plain films of the abdomen in anteroposterior, lateral, and oblique projections reveal calcification in the outer layers of about 20% of degenerative abdominal aneurysms; thus, plain films are not good screening studies and provide minimal anatomic information. CT scans provide valuable information about aneurysm architecture and have been used to predict aneurysm expansion rates. In addition, CT scans show important adjacent structures that impact on abdominal aortic aneurysm repair, such as colonic or pancreatic masses, horseshoe kidneys or other renal abnormalities, and venous anomalies, including retroaortic renal veins, circumaortic renal veins, and left-sided or duplicated vena cavas. Aortograms are not needed preoperatively in all cases but should be obtained for the following indications: (1) suspected suprarenal involvement; (2) symptoms of visceral angina suggesting mesenteric arterial insufficiency; (3) evidence on ultrasound scans of a horseshoe or pelvic kidney; (4) suspected renovascular disease; (5) unexplained impairment of renal function; and (6) clinical evidence of coexistent occlusive disease (which, surprisingly, occurs in less than one of five cases).

Ultrasound is the most useful and least expensive method for accurately measuring the size and position of aneurysms of the infrarenal aorta. Repeated ultrasound examinations are cost-effective for observational management of small abdominal aortic aneurysms. In all cases of groin false aneurysms after Dacron graft placement, ultrasound evaluation of the abdominal aorta and graft should be done to assess the proximal anastomosis. Ultrasound does not reliably detect perigraft collections of blood or fluid, so it should not be relied on to diagnose ruptured abdominal aortic aneurysms. CT scan and MRI are not as cost-effective as repeated ultrasound examination to assess expansion of abdominal aortic aneurysms.

Natural History

The expansion rate of aneurysms of the abdominal aorta is variable and unpredictable in individual patients. Most aneurysms continue to enlarge and will eventually rupture if left untreated. Average expansion rates for abdominal aortic aneurysms are 0.4 cm per year. Rate of expansion and risk of rupture correlate with diastolic blood pressure, initial aneurysm diameter, and degree of obstructive pulmonary disease. The size of the aneurysm correlates best with the risk of rupture. About 40% of aneurysms 5.5–6 cm or more in diameter will rupture within 5 years if untreated, and the average survival of an untreated patient is 17 months. In contrast, the ADAM study found an 0.5% per year rupture rate in small-diameter abdominal aortic aneurysms (4–5.4 cm), an overall rate remarkably similar to a comparable trial in the United Kingdom. Thus, surgery is recommended for nearly all aneurysms 6 cm or more in size, but small aortic aneurysms can be safely observed using serial ultrasound examination to assess expansion. Repair is mandatory for an aneurysm—regardless of size—that is asymptomatic, tender, or enlarging rapidly (> 0.5–1 cm/yr) on sequential ultrasound examinations.

Treatment

When indications exist for abdominal aortic aneurysm repair, two major choices are available. Conventional operative repair, introduced in 1951, is a well-established and successful intervention but entails a major surgical procedure with substantial morbidity and mortality. Endovascular repair, introduced in 1991, is gaining rapid popularity because the stent-graft device is introduced through a small femoral arteriotomy; while it reduces ICU and hospital stay and (possibly) procedure-related morbidity and mortality, it is associated with higher failure rates and device-related expense.

Conventional operative abdominal aortic aneurysm repair consists of replacing the aneurysmal segment with a synthetic fabric graft. Tubular or bifurcation grafts of Dacron or polytetrafluoroethylene (PTFE) are preferred. The proximal anastomosis is usually made to the aorta above the aneurysm—the so-called neck—

Figure 35–9. Exposure of an infrarenal abdominal aortic aneurysm. Arterial clamps are placed at the neck of the aneurysm below the left renal vein and on the common iliac arteries.

and directly below the origin of the renal arteries. The site of the distal anastomosis is determined by the extent of aneurysmal involvement of the iliac arteries. When a tube graft is contraindicated, the iliac arms of a bifurcated graft are anastomosed to the distal ends of the transected common iliac arteries (Figures 35–9 and 35–10). Traditionally, a transperitoneal approach via midline laparotomy has been used for abdominal aortic aneurysm repair, but retroperitoneal operations via flank incision may decrease perioperative pulmonary and gastrointestinal complications.

Abdominal aortic aneurysms in high-risk patients may be treated by thrombosis of the aneurysm induced by outflow obstruction while limb perfusion is maintained by axillofemoral bypass. Adequacy of thrombosis is assessed by CT scan. While this approach would seem to combine a minimal operation with elimination of the risk of rupture, the operative mortality rate is 10%, and rupture may still occur despite adequate thrombosis. This method is rarely used.

Elective infrarenal abdominal aneurysmectomy has a 2–4% operative death rate and a 5–10% rate of com-

Figure 35–10. Replacement of an aortic aneurysm with a synthetic bifurcation graft. The laminated clot within the aneurysm has been removed and the outer wall is closed over the graft.

plications, such as bleeding, renal failure, myocardial infarction, graft infection, limb loss, bowel ischemia, and erectile dysfunction. A very rare complication is paraplegia due to sacrifice of an abnormally distally situated accessory spinal artery (which usually arises from the aorta at the T8–L2 vertebral levels). Malignant tumors are encountered unexpectedly in about 4% of cases. The long-term results of aneurysmectomy are excellent: the graft failure rate is low, and false aneurysm formation at the anastomoses is rare. The long-term survival of these patients is determined principally by the presence or absence of disease in other vascular beds, which may lead to myocardial infarction and stroke—the principal causes of late deaths.

Endovascular Repair

Multicenter, prospective, but nonrandomized trials led the FDA to approve for general use two different devices for endovascular repair of abdominal aortic aneurysms in 1999. Both devices are introduced through femoral arteriotomies using a system of guidewires, introducer-catheters, and delivery systems. Tube and bifurcated systems are available. One device (Ancure) consists of unsupported lightweight crimped woven polyester fixed to the aortic iliac wall by self-expanding attachment frames at the proximal and distal ends of the graft that incorporate hooks placed at intervals around their circumference (Figure 35–11). The other device (AneuRx) is a modular, bifurcated, thin-walled, noncrimped woven polyester graft joined to a nickel-titanium (nitinol) exoskeleton by numerous individual polyester sutures; the self-expanding nitinol stent rings provide both radial and columnar structural support along the length of the graft, but there is no hook fixation in this device (Figure 35–12). Numerous other manufacturers have pulled their devices from the market or have them in various stages of clinical evaluation. In most reports, endovascular patients have less operative blood loss, shorter hospital stays, and a trend toward reduced operative morbidity. Surprisingly, perioperative mortality rates are similar to conventional repair, probably because of higher-risk patients selected for endovascular repair.

Failure of initial placement of endografts averages 5–10% and numerous technical problems can occur, including iliac and aortic rupture from the deployment device. The most important intermediate or long-term adverse outcome is persistent perfusion of the aneurysm ("endoleak"), caused by ineffective proximal or distal sealing, persistent retrograde flow through lumbar or inferior mesenteric arteries, or graft material erosion or modular separation in the device itself. Graft limb oc-

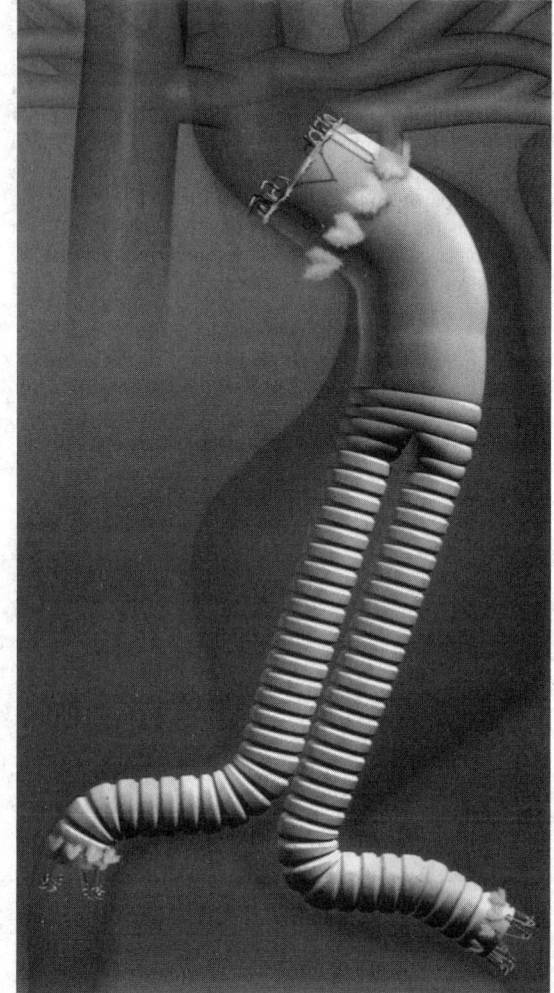

Figure 35–11. Ancure (Guidant Inc) endograft with fixating hooks at both ends

clusions due to kinking and other problems may also occur.

Many endoleaks can be treated using endovascular techniques, and not all endoleaks lead to abdominal aortic aneurysm rupture. Nevertheless, rupture does occur after endograft abdominal aortic aneurysm repair, some of which have been fatal. The rate of late ruptures is uncertain but probably low. Newer iterations of endografts with smaller delivery systems may eventually permit percutaneous insertion while minimizing complications. At present, however, the need for reintervention and the significance of endoleaks are major questions concerning the durability of endovascular abdominal aortic aneurysm re-

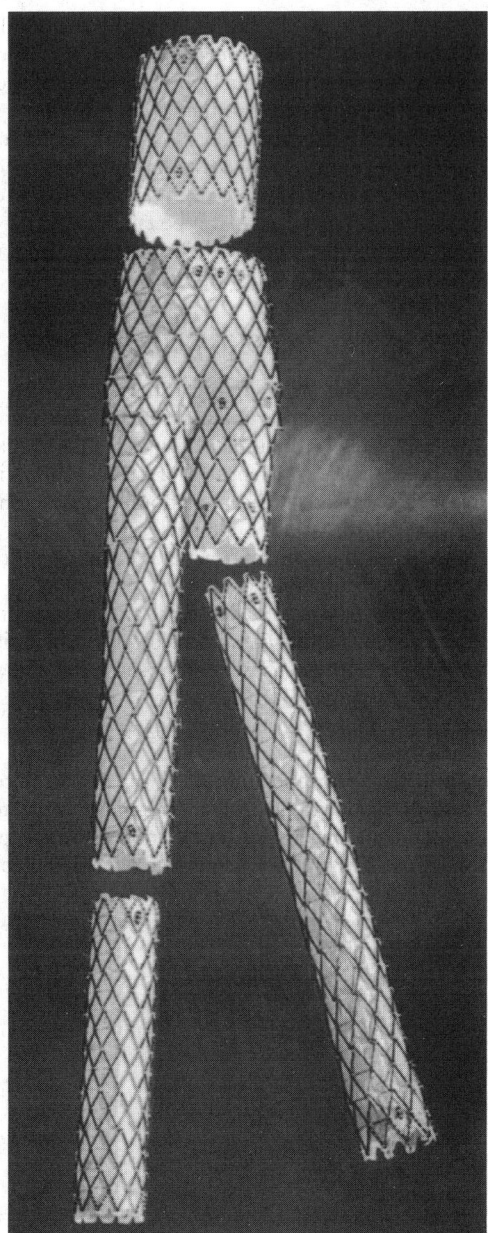

Figure 35–12. AneuRx (Medtronic Inc) endograft with nitinol exoskeleton (modular).

pair. Because these devices are expensive (over 10,000 each) and because lifelong follow-up with regularly scheduled CT scans to exclude late-appearing endoleaks is required, the cost-benefit advantage of shorter hospital stays is offset by the overall expense of endograft repair.

ILIAC ANEURYSMS

Iliac artery aneurysms occur in conjunction with abdominal aortic aneurysms in about 20% of cases. Isolated iliac aneurysms are rare. There is great variability in the estimated prevalence of isolated iliac aneurysms in both autopsy and clinical studies, but in general they occur in less than 1% of the population over 50. About 70% of solitary iliac artery aneurysms occur in the common iliac artery. Solitary aneurysms occur in the internal iliac artery in about 20% of cases, with the remainder in the external iliac. Most patients have two or more involved vessels.

The clinical manifestations of iliac aneurysms depend upon the etiology, size, location, and coexisting disorders (eg, connective tissue disease, intravenous drug abuse). Over half of patients complain of symptoms related to their aneurysms. Symptoms of compression or erosion of surrounding structures and rupture are the most frequent presentations. Sepsis from ureteral obstruction and subsequent pyelonephritis often occurs, and erosion or rupture into the ureter or bladder can cause microscopic or massive hematuria. Compression of femoral, obturator, or sciatic nerves may produce neurologic symptoms. An unusual but dramatic mode of presentation is massive leg swelling and acute congestive heart failure produced by spontaneous rupture of an iliac artery aneurysm into the adjacent vein resulting in a large arteriovenous fistula.

Physical examination can suggest the diagnosis of iliac artery aneurysms if the physician is alert to that possibility. Most symptomatic iliac aneurysms can be palpated as pulsatile masses on abdominal or rectal examinations. Although iliac aneurysms are unusual in women, gynecologic examination may occasionally disclose them. Perianal ecchymosis caused by dissection of blood through the retroperitoneal space and decreased sphincter tone have been reported after rupture of iliac aneurysms. Bruits, thrills, and shock are not specific for aneurysms involving the iliac arteries.

The diagnosis of isolated iliac aneurysms may be confirmed by ultrasonography, CT scans, MRI, and arteriography. Although ultrasound is much less expensive than the other modalities, it is operator-dependent and often inaccurate because of the depth of the arteries in the pelvis or the presence of overlying intestinal gas. Transanal ultrasound may be of use for diagnosing hypogastric artery aneurysms. CT and MRI are equally accurate for diagnosing iliac aneurysms, but MRI is more expensive. Arteriography may miss iliac artery aneurysms because thrombotic debris may fill the aneurysmal sac. However, there is general agreement that arteriography is essential for planning elective repair of iliac aneurysms to assess the pelvic circulation.

There is no large prospective series describing the natural history of isolated iliac aneurysms. Although the natural history of isolated iliac artery aneurysms is largely unknown, rupture occurs frequently. In general, perioperative death occurs in one-half of patients with ruptured aneurysms. The limited number of cases reported, all of which are either anecdotal or retrospective analyses, makes any recommendation for treatment largely empirical. Rupture has been reported in aneurysms as small as 2 cm, but the measurements in these patients were made in the presence of hypotension and may be inaccurate. It is very unusual for an iliac aneurysm under 3 cm to rupture. Similar to aortic aneurysms, iliac aneurysms tend to enlarge unpredictably.

Like aortic aneurysms, size seems to be the most important determinant for rupture of iliac aneurysms. Most authorities recommend that patients with isolated iliac artery aneurysms larger than 3 cm in diameter who otherwise are good operative risks should undergo elective repair. Operative strategy depends on which arteries are involved and the presence or absence of multiple aneurysms, particularly when they are bilateral. Solitary common iliac artery aneurysms (Figure 35–13) are best treated by retroperitoneal exposure and replacement by interposition prosthetic grafts. If the contralateral internal iliac artery is normal, the ipsilateral internal iliac can be safely ligated. If the ipsilateral hypogastric artery is also aneurysmal, it is advisable to open the sac and ligate the branches of the artery from within the aneurysm rather than risk injury to the many adherent veins surrounding the external surface of the aneurysm. Bilateral common iliac artery aneurysms are usually best managed by exclusion using a bifurcated prosthetic interposition graft originating from the abdominal aorta by means of a transperitoneal approach. At least one distal anastomosis should incorporate the lumen of the hypogastric artery. Alternatively; a "jump" graft can be taken to one of the internal iliac arteries. Currently, there is also enthusiasm for treating iliac aneurysms using endografts as well.

SUPRARENAL AORTIC ANEURYSMS

Aneurysms of the segment of aorta between the diaphragm and the renal arteries are uncommon and are usually associated with similar changes in the thoracic and infrarenal aorta. The entire thoracic and abdominal aorta becomes dilated (thoracoabdominal aneurysms). The risk of rupture of the suprarenal segment is not appreciable until the diameter exceeds 7 cm. Symptoms are rare unless rupture occurs.

Aneurysms proximal to the renal arteries cannot be palpated. They should be suspected when chest films show dilation of the descending thoracic aorta. The size and extent of suprarenal aneurysms are best assessed using CT scan with contrast medium.

Resection and graft replacement of the upper abdominal aorta is an operation of far greater magnitude and risk than operations on the infrarenal aorta. A thoracoabdominal approach is usually necessary, and provisions must be made for reimplantation of the celiac

Figure 35–13. Arteriogram of isolated iliac artery aneurysm

axis and the superior mesenteric and renal arteries. At this time, the risks of operation for asymptomatic aneurysms less than 7 cm in diameter at this level are probably greater than the risk of rupture. Paraplegia, renal failure, and bowel ischemia are much more common after repair of these aneurysms than after repair of infrarenal aortic aneurysms.

RUPTURED AORTIC ANEURYSMS

With increasing size, lateral pressure within the aneurysm may eventually lead to spontaneous rupture of the aneurysmal wall. Although immediate exsanguination may ensue, there is usually an interval of several hours between the first episode of bleeding, a self-limited extravasation into the subadventitia or periaortic tissue, and later retroperitoneal. This phenomenon is termed "contained rupture." When periaortic tissue can no longer contain the expanding hematoma, "free rupture" occurs with exsanguination into the free peritoneal cavity. Curiously, ruptured aneurysms are more likely to occur in the autumn and winter.

Clinical Findings

Most aortic aneurysms are asymptomatic until rupture begins. The patient presents with sudden severe abdominal pain that usually radiates into the back and occasionally into the inguinal region. Faintness or syncope results from blood loss. Pain may lessen or faintness may disappear after the first hemorrhage, only to reappear and progress to shock if bleeding continues.

When bleeding remains contained in the periaortic tissue, a discrete, pulsatile abdominal mass can be felt. In contrast with an intact aneurysm, the ruptured aneurysm at this stage is usually tender. As bleeding continues—usually into the retroperitoneum—the discrete mass is replaced by a poorly defined midabdominal fullness, often extending toward the left flank. Shock becomes profound, manifested by peripheral vasoconstriction, hypotension, and anuria. The classic triad of pain, a pulsatile abdominal mass, and hypotension associated with a ruptured abdominal aortic aneurysm is present in less than two-thirds of patients with this disorder.

Emergency abdominal ultrasound examination performed in the emergency room will confirm the presence of an aortic aneurysm but will not disclose hemorrhage. CT scans reliably confirm hemorrhage from an aneurysm, but the delay in obtaining them usually precludes their use in unstable patients.

Treatment & Prognosis

Laparotomy must be performed as soon as intravenous fluids have been started and blood has been sent for cross-matching. There is no time for x-rays, ECGs, scans, blood tests, or other examinations with the exception of the rapid abdominal ultrasound examination to confirm the presence of an aneurysm, if ultrasound is readily available. Control of the aorta proximal to the aneurysm must be obtained immediately. A successful outcome of the operation is related to the patient's condition on arrival, the promptness of diagnosis, and the speed of operative control of bleeding and blood replacement. The operative death rate is about 60–80% and rates average at least 60%. Because many patients with ruptured aneurysms die before reaching the hospital, the overall death rate approaches 90%. Major factors responsible for improved survival are *immediate* operation with rapid proximal aortic control, avoidance of a left thoracotomy for clamping the aorta above the diaphragm, avoidance of technical errors, and expeditious completion of the operation. Without operation, the outcome is uniformly fatal.

INFLAMMATORY ANEURYSMS

Inflammatory aneurysms are true atherosclerotic aneurysms that elicit a unique inflammatory response adjacent to the external calcified layer of the aneurysmal wall. Inflammatory abdominal aortic aneurysms arise from the same or similar antigenic stimuli that are responsible for noninflammatory ones. In contrast to retroperitoneal fibrosis, the inflammation is usually confined to the anterior aorta and iliac arteries. The patient complains of abdominal pain and tenderness over the aneurysm. One-fourth of patients have some degree of ureteral obstruction. CT scanning reliably demonstrates the characteristic thick wall and confirms the diagnosis. Characteristic pathologic changes include infiltration of the aortic wall by lymphocytes, plasma cells, and occasional multinucleated giant cells and lymphoid follicles with germinal centers. The inflammatory reaction tends to be prominent around the vasa vasorum.

Inflammatory aneurysms are easily recognized at operation by the dense shiny white fibrotic reaction that envelopes the adjacent viscera, especially the duodenum, left renal vein, and inferior vena cava, making these structures especially vulnerable to operative injury. Ideally, inflammatory aneurysms should be repaired using a retroperitoneal approach. The transperitoneal approach should be modified as follows: (1) the aorta should be clamped at the diaphragm; (2) the duodenum should not be dissected away from the aneurysm; and (3) the operation should be performed within the lumen after proximal and distal control has been achieved. A retroperitoneal approach to the aneurysm avoids some of the inflammation encountered with transperitoneal exposure.

INFECTED ANEURYSMS

An infected aneurysm develops after bacterial contamination of a preexisting aneurysm, usually from a hematogenous source. This differs from microbial aortitis, in which virulent bacteria (often *Salmonella*) colonize the aorta and cause false aneurysm formation and rupture. In addition, bacterial cultures of mural thrombus in noninfected degenerative abdominal aortic aneurysms are positive in 10–40% of patients. The significance of these positive cultures is unknown, but most have been coagulase-negative staphylococcal species—an organism often found in prosthetic graft infections. The confusing term "mycotic aneurysm" is commonly used to denote infected aneurysms in general, not just fungal infections. The term was coined by Osler at the time when the distinction between bacteria and fungi was unclear.

Contamination may result from septic emboli caused by bacterial endocarditis, hematogenous seeding during episodes of bacteremia, direct extension from a contiguous area of infection, or direct trauma. Streptococci (including *Streptococcus pneumoniae*), haemophilus, staphylococcus, *Escherichia coli*, other gram-negative organisms, and fungi have all been implicated. The chances of rupture are far greater with gram-negative than gram-positive infections. The survival rate of patients with gram-positive infections is about 70%—in contrast to only 25% in patients with gram-negative organisms.

Infectious organisms may involve practically every major artery, but aortic involvement is most common. The typical case presents with a rapidly enlarging, tender pulsatile mass that may feel warm. Fever is invariably present, and half of patients have positive blood cultures. Angiography of these patients may show a *saccular* false aneurysm in which the infection has caused excessive wall necrosis that is likely to rupture.

Treatment consists of excision and extra-anatomic bypass grafting. A prolonged course of antibiotics should be given.

Becquemin J et al: Mid-term results of endovascular versus open repair for abdominal aortic aneurysm in patients anatomically suitable for endovascular repair. Eur J Vasc Endovasc Surg 2000;19:656.

Beebe HG et al: Results of an aortic endograft trial: impact of device failure beyond 12 months. J Vasc Surg 2001;33 (2 Suppl):S55.

Coselli JS et al: Mortality and paraplegia after thoracoabdominal aortic aneurysm repair: a risk factor analysis. Ann Thorac Surg 2000;69:409.

Curci JA et al: Preoperative treatment with doxycycline reduces aortic wall expression and activation of matrix metalloproteinases in patients with abdominal aortic aneurysms. J Vasc Surg 2000;31:342.

Dardik A et al: Surgical repair of ruptured abdominal aortic aneurysms in the state of Maryland: factors influencing outcome among 527 recent cases. J Vasc Surg 1998;28:413.

Dardik A et al: Results of elective abdominal aortic aneurysm repair in the 1990s: a population-based analysis of 2335 cases. J Vasc Surg 1999;30:985.

DiMarzo L et al: Inflammatory aneurysm of the abdominal aorta. A prospective clinical study. J Cardiovasc Surg 1999;40:407.

Holzenbein T et al: Midterm durability of abdominal aortic aneurysm endograft repair: a word of caution. J Vasc Surg 2001;33(2 Suppl):S46.

Johansen K et al: Ruptured abdominal aortic aneurysm: the Harborview experience. J Vasc Surg 1991;13:240.

Johnston KW: Multicenter prospective study of nonruptured abdominal aortic aneurysm: part II. Variables predicting morbidity and mortality. J Vasc Surg 1989;9:437.

Kanazawa S et al: Management of isolated iliac artery aneurysms. J Cardiovasc Surg 2000;41:513.

Lederle FA et al: Prevalence and associations of abdominal aortic aneurysm detected through screening. Ann Intern Med 1997;126:441.

Lederle FA et al: Yield of repeated screening for abdominal aortic aneurysm after a 4-year interval. Aneurysm Detection and Management Veterans Cooperative Study Investigators. Arch Intern Med 2000;160:1117.

Moneta GL et al: Surgical treatment of infected aortic aneurysm. Am J Surg 1998;175:396.

Moore WS et al: Abdominal aortic aneurysm: a 6-year comparison of endovascular versus transabdominal repair. Ann Surg 1999;230:298.

Mortality results for randomized controlled trial of early elective surgery or ultrasonic surveillance for small abdominal aortic aneurysms. The UK Small Aneurysm Trial Participants. Lancet 1998;352:1649.

Parsons RE et al: Midterm results of endovascular stented grafts for the treatment of isolated iliac artery aneurysms. J Vasc Surg 1999;30:915.

Rasmussen TE et al: Inflammatory aortic aneurysms. A clinical review with new perspectives in pathogenesis. Ann Surg 1997;225:155.

Robicsek F et al: Management of inflammatory aneurysm of the infrarenal aorta using retroperitoneal exposure, open aneurysmorrhaphy and descending aorta-to-femoral artery bypass. J Cardiovasc Surg 2000;41:457.

Safi HJ et al: Progress in the management of type I thoracoabdominal and descending thoracic aortic aneurysms. Ann Vasc Surg 1999;13:457.

Sahgal A et al: Diameter changes in isolated iliac artery aneurysms 1 to 6 years after endovascular graft repair. J Vasc Surg 2001;33:289.

Scheinert D et al: Treatment of iliac artery aneurysms by percutaneous implantation of stent grafts. Circulation 2000;102(19 Suppl 3):III253.

Smoking, lung function, and the prognosis of abdominal aortic aneurysm. The UK Small Aneurysm Trial Participants. Eur J Vasc Endovasc Surg 2000;19:636.

Sternbergh WC 3rd et al: Hospital cost of endovascular versus open repair of abdominal aortic aneurysms. J Vasc Surg 2000;31:237.

Sultan S et al: Fifteen-year experience of transperitoneal management of inflammatory abdominal aortic aneurysms. Eur J Vasc Endovasc Surg 1999;18:510.

Zarins CK et al: The AneuRx stent graft: four-year results and worldwide experience 2000. J Vasc Surg 2001;33:5129.

FEMORAL, POPLITEAL, & PERSISTENT SCIATIC ARTERY ANEURYSMS

The popliteal artery is the site of degenerative peripheral arterial aneurysms in 70% of cases. The next most common site is the femoral artery, but this is unusual. However, pseudoaneurysms of the femoral artery following arterial punctures occur with an incidence ranging from 0.05% to 6%. Thrombosis, peripheral embolization, and claudication are the presenting manifestations. Unlike aortic aneurysms, rupture is rare. Occlusion results from fragmentation of the mural thrombus lining the aneurysmal sac, an event that may be due partly to the mobility of the adjacent hip or knee. Thrombus may occlude the lumen of the aneurysm or embolize downstream into smaller arteries in the leg or foot.

These same complications can occur in a rare but very interesting anomaly, **persistence of the sciatic artery.** In the complete form of this syndrome, the large embryonic sciatic artery (originating from the internal iliac system) communicates directly with the popliteal artery, with or without an intact femoropopliteal vessel. The diagnosis of a persistent sciatic artery is suggested by absence of a femoral pulse with intact popliteal and pedal pulses. The prevalence is 0.25:1000 patients studied by angiography. Persistent sciatic arteries have a particular propensity for aneurysmal degeneration, presenting as painful, pulsatile buttock masses.

Clinical Findings

A. SYMPTOMS AND SIGNS

Until progressive stenosis or thrombosis occurs, symptoms are usually minimal or absent. The patient is aware of a throbbing mass when the aneurysm is in the groin, but popliteal aneurysms are usually undetected by the patient. In most patients, the first symptom is produced by the ischemia of acute arterial occlusion. The pathologic findings range from rapidly developing gangrene to only moderate ischemia that slowly lessens as collateral circulation develops. Symptoms from recurrent embolization to the leg are often transient; sudden ischemia may appear in a toe or part of the foot, followed by slow resolution, and the true diagnosis may be elusive. Recurrent ischemic episodes due to occlusion of small arteries in the leg in patients over age 50 are almost always embolic in origin. Rarely, popliteal

aneurysms will produce symptoms by compressing the popliteal vein or tibial nerve.

Palpation of local arterial enlargement suggests the diagnosis. Because popliteal pulses are somewhat difficult to palpate even in normal individuals, a particularly prominent or easily felt pulse is suggestive of aneurysmal dilation. Since popliteal aneurysms are bilateral in 50% of cases, the diagnosis of thrombosis of a popliteal aneurysm is often aided by the palpation of a pulsatile aneurysm in the contralateral popliteal space. One-third of patients with bilateral popliteal aneurysms have abdominal aortic aneurysms.

B. IMAGING STUDIES

Arteriography may not demonstrate the aneurysm accurately, because mural thrombus reduces the apparent diameter of the lumen. Nevertheless, arteriography is advised—especially when operation is considered—to define the status of the arteries distal to the aneurysm.

Duplex color ultrasound is the most efficient investigation to confirm the diagnosis of peripheral aneurysm, to measure its size and configuration, and to demonstrate mural thrombus.

Treatment

Immediate operation or urgent operation after intra-arterial thrombolytic therapy is indicated when acute thrombosis has caused pregangrenous ischemia. Early operation is indicated for recurrent peripheral embolization. The evidence is unclear regarding the advisability of routine operation in the absence of symptoms, but operation is usually recommended if the external diameter of the aneurysm exceeds three times the normal arterial diameter at that site or if a large amount of thrombus is present within the aneurysm. Acute pseudoaneurysms of the femoral artery due to arterial punctures can almost always be successfully treated using ultrasound-guided compression as a noninvasive method of repair.

The standard surgical treatment for both femoral and popliteal degenerative or atherosclerotic aneurysms has been resection with graft replacement. Recently, however, popliteal aneurysms have been satisfactorily managed by exclusion and bypass graft with saphenous vein. If exclusion rather than resection is performed, the geniculate "feeder" arteries within the aneurysm must be ligated or progressive enlargement can still occur. Endovascular graft repair has also been reported. Persistent sciatic artery aneurysms are treated by exclusion of the aneurysm by surgical or interventional radiologic techniques with a femorodistal bypass as required for the resultant ischemia.

Prognosis

The long-term patency of bypass grafts for femoral and popliteal aneurysms depends on the adequacy of the outflow tract. Late graft occlusion is less common than in similar operations for occlusive disease.

Diwan A et al: Incidence of femoral and popliteal aneurysms in patients with abdominal aortic aneurysms J Vasc Surg 2000; 31:863.

Duffy ST et al: Popliteal aneurysms: a 10-year experience. Eur J Vasc Endovasc Surg 1998;16:218.

Henry M et al: Percutaneous endovascular treatment of peripheral aneurysms. J Cardiovasc Surg 2000;41:871.

Levi N et al: Arteriosclerotic femoral artery aneurysms: a short review. J Cardiovasc 1997;38:335.

Steinmetz E et al: Preoperative intraarterial thrombolysis before surgical revascularization for popliteal artery anerurysm with acute ischemia. Ann Vasc Surg 2000;14:360.

EXTRACRANIAL CAROTID ARTERY ANEURYSMS

Aneurysms of the extracranial carotid arteries are rare but may occur at any point along the course of the vessels. True aneurysms of the carotid are usually the result of atherosclerosis but occasionally may be caused by cystic medial necrosis, Marfan's syndrome, or fibromuscular dysplasia. False aneurysms may occur rarely after carotid endarterectomy or as a result of trauma or infection. Pharyngeal abscess was a frequent cause of false aneurysms of the carotid artery in the preantibiotic era.

Clinical Findings

A. SYMPTOMS AND SIGNS

Most patients present with a pulsatile neck mass. A coiled or redundant carotid or subclavian artery is the commonest cause of this type of mass and must be differentiated from aneurysm. On occasion, a carotid aneurysm protrudes into the oropharynx, where it produces symptoms of dysphagia. Pain from the aneurysm may radiate to the angle of the jaw. About 30% of patients will have had a transient neurologic event before presentation. Rupture, which is common with false aneurysms but rare with true aneurysms, may occur into the oropharynx, ear canal, or soft tissues of the neck.

B. IMAGING STUDIES

Duplex ultrasound can differentiate redundant and coiled arteries from aneurysms and should be used as the initial test in patients who present electively. The spectral analysis component of duplex Doppler is useful in demonstrating coexistent occlusive disease. In the assessment of false aneurysms, it is useful to delineate the extent of the lesion, which may not be apparent from arteriography. Arteriography is necessary to plan the operation. Two types of atherosclerotic aneurysms are seen: fusiform and saccular. False aneurysms assume bizarre shapes, depending on location and containment by neck tissues. Size, extent, and the presence of laminar thrombus can be determined using ultrasound.

Treatment

Most accessible true aneurysms should be resected and replaced with a graft of autogenous tissue, although some authorities prefer prosthetic grants to avoid kinking. Endovascular stenting for repair of carotid aneurysms has been described. All false aneurysms should be repaired. Some extensive aneurysms require carotid ligation, which is safe if carotid back pressures is greater than 65 mm Hg. An oculopneumoplethysmography test should be performed preoperatively for such patients. Alternatively, temporary carotid artery balloon occlusion can be used to assess potential neurologic consequences during awake arteriography. If the value is low or the patient experiences neurologic symptoms during provocative temporary occlusion, a superficial temporal-to-middle cerebral bypass may be required at the time of internal carotid ligation.

El-Sabrout R et al: Extracranial carotid artery aneurysms: Texas Heart Institute experience. J Vasc Surg 2000;31:702.

May J et al. Endoluminal repair of internal carotid artery aneurysm: a feasible but hazardous procedure. J Vasc Surg 1997; 26:1055.

Rosset E et al: Surgical treatment of extracranial internal carotid artery aneurysms. J Vasc Surg 2000;31:713.

Carotid Body Tumors

The normal carotid body is a 3- to 6-mm nest of chemoreceptor cells of neuroectodermal origin located on the posterior medial side of the carotid bifurcation. It responds to a decrease in oxygen tension, an increase in blood acidity, and an increase in CO_2 tension or an increase in blood temperature by causing an increase in blood pressure, cardiac rate, and the depth and rate of respiration. Thus, the carotid body serves to correct hypoxia and its effects. In comparison, the carotid sinus is a baroreceptor; stimulation (by surgical manipulation or hypertension) causes reflex bradycardia and hypotension.

Tumors of the carotid body have been called cervical chemodectomas, paragangliomas, glomus tumors, and nonchromaffin paragangliomas. Histologically, the tumors resemble the normal carotid body. While the tumor is capable of metastatic behavior, this only occurs in about 10% of cases. Extension into local structures is the most common complication.

Almost all cases present as slow enlargement of an asymptomatic cervical mass. Rarely, the tumor causes hypertension by secreting catecholamines. A history of slow enlargement is frequently elicited. There is no predilection for either sex. Bilaterality is common when the tumor is familial. The incidence of carotid body tumors may be increased in oxygen-deprived individuals (eg, cyanotic heart disease; chronic hypoxia of high altitude).

A solitary midlateral pulsatile neck mass that is firm and rubbery should always suggest carotid body tumor. Because it is attached to the underlying artery, the mass is more mobile in the horizontal than the vertical plane. Bruits are present over the mass in about half of cases. Rarely, cranial nerve dysfunction occurs from tumor extension.

Angiography shows a characteristic tumor blush at the carotid bifurcation, with wide separation of the internal and external carotid arteries (Figure 35–14). Noninvasive color duplex scanning is also often diag-

nostic. Percutaneous needle biopsy or incisional biopsy is inaccurate and dangerous because of the risk of serious hemorrhage.

Complete excision—the preferred treatment—occasionally requires arterial reconstruction when the lesion is large and complex. Radiation therapy and chemotherapy have no value. Preoperative angiographic embolization of large tumors decreases vascularity but carries a risk of stroke; it is rarely employed. The incidence of cranial nerve injury from operative removal of carotid body tumors is about 40% and is higher with larger masses and prior attempts at resection.

Kohn JS et al: Familial carotid body tumors: a closer look. J Vasc Surg 1999;29:649.

Westerband A et al: Current trends in the detection and management of carotid body tumors. J Vasc Surg 1998;28:84.

VISCERAL ARTERY ANEURYSMS

Splenic Artery Aneurysms

Splenic artery aneurysms are second in frequency to aneurysms of the aortoiliac system among intra-abdominal aneurysms. Aneurysms of the splenic artery account for more than 60% of splanchnic artery aneurysms. Women are affected four times more commonly than men and often during childbearing years. Arterial fibrodysplasia and portal hypertension also predispose to formation of splenic artery aneurysms. Rupture, the major complication, has been reported in less than 2% of splenic aneurysms; rupture rarely occurs with lesions smaller than 2–3 cm in diameter. Rupture during pregnancy tends to occur in the third trimester and is associated with 75% maternal death rate and 90% fetal death rate. Diagnosis is most often made from plain x-ray films of the abdomen, showing concentric calcification in the upper left quadrant.

Operation is indicated for patients with symptomatic aneurysms, pregnant women with splenic artery aneurysms, and patients who are good operative risks and whose aneurysm is greater than 3 cm in diameter. Operative procedures include aneurysm exclusion or excision with or without splenectomy depending on the location of the aneurysm. Laparoscopic ligation is also feasible.

Hepatic Artery Aneurysms

Hepatic artery aneurysms account for 20% of splanchnic artery aneurysms. There is a 2:1 male:female ratio, and the frequency of reported rupture is about 20%. Aneurysm rupture is associated with a 35% mortality rate. Patients usually present with rupture into the peritoneal cavity, biliary tree, or a nearby viscus. Rupture into the biliary tree producing hemobilia is as frequent

Figure 35–14. Carotid body tumor.

as intraperitoneal rupture. The symptomatic triad of intermittent abdominal pain, gastrointestinal bleeding, and jaundice strongly suggests the diagnosis and is present in about one-third of patients. Surgery is usually required for control of bleeding. If the common hepatic artery is involved, the artery may be safely ligated. Aneurysms in other portions of the artery usually require vascular reconstruction.

Superior Mesenteric Artery Aneurysms

Aneurysms of the proximal superior mesenteric artery account for 5% of all splanchnic artery aneurysms. Sixty percent of superior mesenteric artery aneurysms are mycotic, and most of the rest are atherosclerotic. The aneurysm may involve the origin or branches of the artery. The presenting findings include nonspecific abdominal pain and a mobile pulsatile abdominal mass. Rupture is one cause of "abdominal apoplexy." Radiologic evaluation, except for arteriography, is unrewarding, since the lesion is rarely calcified.

Operative therapy includes ligation, endoaneurysmorrhaphy, or replacement with a segment of autogenous vessel. For branch aneurysms, bowel resection is often the best choice.

RENAL ARTERY ANEURYSMS

This uncommon aneurysm occurs in less than 0.1% of the population and is often associated with hypertension. The aneurysm is usually saccular and located at a primary or secondary bifurcation of the renal arteries. Women are affected slightly more frequently than men. There are four principal categories: (1) true renal artery aneurysms, (2) dissecting renal artery aneurysms, (3) aneurysms associated with medial fibrodysplastic disease, and (4) arteritis-related microaneurysms.

Most aneurysms are asymptomatic and are discovered on plain abdominal films or during investigation of hypertension. Renovascular hypertension, which occurs in 30% of patients, may be due to turbulent flow within an aneurysm, associated arterial stenosis, dissection, arteriovenous fistula formation, thromboembolism, or compression of adjacent arterial branches. Spontaneous rupture of renal artery aneurysms is rare except during pregnancy, and although a kidney may be lost, death is uncommon. The rate of rupture is about 3%. Emboli from the aneurysm to the distal renal vessels occur rarely.

Most small renal artery aneurysms should be managed nonoperatively. Blood pressure should be controlled, and CT scans or digital subtraction angiography should be performed every 2 years. Operation is indicated in women of childbearing age, patients with associated renal artery disease, and patients with large aneurysms (although the statistical validity of rupture occurring in larger aneurysms has not been clearly proved in the literature). Most renal artery aneurysms can be repaired in situ, but ex vivo repair is occasionally required. Nephrectomy is usually required for managing ruptured aneurysms.

Area MJ et al: Splenic artery aneurysms: methods of laparoscopic repair. J Vasc Surg 1999;30:184.

Carr SC et al: Visceral artery aneurysm rupture. J Vasc Surg 2001; 33:806.

Dave SP et al: Splenic artery aneurysm in the 1990s. Ann Vasc Surg 2000;14:223.

Messina LM et al: Visceral artery aneurysms. Surg Clin North Am 1997;77:425.

UPPER EXTREMITY ANEURYSMS

Subclavian Artery Aneurysms

Subclavian artery aneurysms are rare; most supraclavicular pulsatile masses represent tortuous vessels. Pseudoaneurysms due to injections by drug addicts are being reported with increasing frequency. A rare congenital variant is an aberrant subclavian artery arising from the proximal portion of the descending thoracic aorta that becomes aneurysmal; this condition has been termed Kommerell's diverticulum, and it can give rise to difficulty in swallowing (called dysphagia lusoria).

A true subclavian artery aneurysm is usually due to exaggerated poststenotic dilation in a patient with cervical rib syndrome or thoracic outlet syndrome. The most common manifestations result from emboli to the fingers. Treatment consists of resection of the first rib or a cervical rib (if present) and division of the scalenus anterior muscle. The aneurysm should be resected and replaced by an autogenous or prosthetic graft. Cervical sympathectomy is occasionally performed for distal ischemia.

Radial Artery False Aneurysms

The incidence of radial artery false aneurysms has increased as a result of increasing use of radial artery catheters. Occasionally, the aneurysm is infected. If the Allen test is normal, treatment consists of excision and ligation. If the ulnar collaterals are insufficient to preserve viability of the hand, excision, mobilization of the vessel, and arterial reconstruction should be performed.

Cina CS et al: Kommerell's diverticulum and aneurysmal right-sided aortic arch: a case report and review of the literature. J Vasc Surg 2000;32;1208.

Gray RJ et al: Management of true aneurysms distal to the axillary artery. J Vasc Surg 1998;28:606.

Witz M et al: Subclavian artery aneurysms. A report of 2 cases and a review of the literature. J Cardiovasc Surg 1998;39:429.

■ VASOCONSTRICTIVE DISORDERS

Vasoconstrictive disorders are characterized by abnormal lability of the sympathetic nervous system that affects the arterial and venous side of the capillary bed to reduce cutaneous blood flow. Sluggish flow of deoxygenated blood causes cutaneous cyanosis, coldness, numbness, and pain.

Raynaud's syndrome can be precipitated by exposure to cold or emotional stress. It consists of sequential pallor, cyanosis, and rubor after exposure to cold and is the visible manifestation of vasoconstriction, sluggish flow, and reflex vasodilation producing characteristic white-blue-red color changes. Raynaud's syndrome may follow a virulent or benign course and may be associated with many conditions such as immunologic and connective tissue disorders (eg, scleroderma, systemic lupus erythematosus, polymyositis, drug-induced vasculitis); non-immune obstructive arterial disease (eg, diabetes mellitus, thromboangiitis obliterans); occupation trauma (eg, vibration injury, cold injury); and other disorders (eg, cold agglutinins, chronic renal failure, neoplasia). An association with *Helicobacter pylori* infections has been reported.

The classic differentiation of Raynaud's syndrome into a benign "disease" and a virulent "phenomenon" is confusing. It is more appropriate to distinguish an occlusive lesion from the purely vasoconstrictive variety. If the underlying cause is an unrelenting disorder (eg, collagen vascular disease), cervical sympathectomy has no lasting effect. If the cause is transient or manageable (eg, emboli), sympathectomy may occasionally be of value. All patients with Raynaud's syndrome should avoid cold exposure, tobacco, oral contraceptives, beta-adrenergic blocking agents, and ergotamine preparations. Calcium channel blockers and transdermal prostaglandins may also help. However, calcium channel blockers frequently produce adverse side effects (mostly related to hypotension) in individuals most likely to present with Raynaud's syndrome (young women). A double-blind placebo-controlled study showed that ketanserin lessened symptoms of Raynaud's syndrome. Cilastazol has also been used with relief of symptoms in some patients.

Acrocyanosis is a common chronic, benign vasoconstrictive disorder related to Raynaud's syndrome that is largely restricted to young females. It is characterized by persistent cyanosis of the hands and feet. Numbness and pain accompany its more severe form. The changes disappear with exposure to a warm environment. Examination in a cool room shows diffuse symmetric cyanosis, coldness, and occasionally hyperhidrosis of hands and feet. Cyanosis of the skin of the calf, thigh, or forearm usually displays a reticulated pattern and has been called **livedo reticularis** and **cutis marmorata**. The peripheral pulses may diminish in the cold but return to normal with rewarming. The Allen test may show a normal response, but in patients with particularly intense vasoconstriction, color return will be slow but even (as compared to the uneven return in patients with scleroderma and thromboangiitis obliterans).

SCLERODERMA

Scleroderma is a connective tissue disease characterized pathologically by fibrosis due to increase and swelling of collagenous tissue, fragmentation and swelling of the elastic fibers in the cutis, and arterial intimal thickening. It may present as a multisystem disease with changes in the lung, kidney, gastrointestinal tract, muscle, and central nervous system. It occurs more frequently in women, and its first manifestations usually appear between ages 25 and 50.

Its most common form involves first the skin and vasculature of the fingers, hands, and forearms. The skin becomes thickened and taut. Flexion of the fingers is limited by the tightness of the overlying skin. The muscles in the forearm develop woody induration.

Symptoms in the early stages consist of progressive coldness and occasional numbness of the fingers. Intermittent episodic blanching of one or more fingers is frequent. With increasing ischemia, one or more of the terminal phalanges become painful and tender. Atrophy and ulceration of the fingertips, with exquisite tenderness, follow. At this stage, cutaneous fibrosis of the hands and fingers is usually far advanced. Gangrene of the ends of the fingers is the terminal ischemic event.

Vascular examination in the early phases may show only chronic cyanosis and coldness of the hands and fingers. Coincident with the development of skin changes, pallor and atrophy of the fingertips appear. Attempts at finger flexion cause blanching of the knuckles. The Allen test shows slow return of color starting in the proximal hand and progressing in an uneven fashion into the fingers.

Treatment is palliative at best, since there is no way to halt the progression of pathologic change. Sympathectomy is rarely of value. Systemic corticosteroid therapy occasionally slows progression. Finger amputation is necessary once gangrene has developed.

Gasbanini A et al: *Helicobacter pylori* eradication ameliorates primary Raynaud's phenomenon. Dig Dis Sci 1998;43:1641.

Knapid-Kordecka M et al: Clinical spectrum of Raynaud's phenomenon in patients referred to a vascular clinic. Cardiovasc Surg 2000;8:457.

Maricq HR et al: An objective method to estimate the severity of Raynaud phenomenon: digital blood pressure response to cooling. Vasc Med 1998;3:109.

McLafferty RB et al: Raynaud's syndrome in workers who use vibrating pneumatic air knives. J Vasc Surg 1999;30:1.

Melone CP Jr et al: Surgical management of the hand in scleroderma. Curr Opin Rheumatol 1999;11:514.

REFLEX SYMPATHETIC DYSTROPHY

The pathophysiology of posttraumatic pain syndromes remains poorly understood. A number of terms are used to refer to the same condition, including causalgia, posttraumatic sympathetic dystrophy, Sudeck's atrophy, shoulder-hand syndrome, traumatic neuralgia, and Mitchell's causalgia. Reflex sympathetic dystrophy occurs with equal frequency in the upper and lower extremities and in men and women. The initial injury may be a missile wound, fracture, crush injury, or laceration.

The most distinctive and dramatic feature of the syndrome is the almost unendurable pain that occurs. It is a burning pain involving the entire hand or foot. The slightest stimuli can produce sudden increase in the severity of pain (eg, a breeze from an open window, the touch of clothing, or a step on the stair).

Increased sympathetic nervous system activity characterizes this syndrome. Vasomotor changes in the foot or hand are marked, and vasoconstriction is a prominent feature. The extremity becomes cold, cyanotic, and moist. After several years, the illness is characterized by increasing pain, dystrophy, and atrophy. The bones may undergo cystic and subchondral erosion as well as diffuse osteoporosis, which is seen on bone scans or x-rays.

Initial management consists of diagnostic sympathetic block with local anesthetic agents. This is successful in relieving pain in the majority of cases. If the patient has long-lasting relief after the block, blocking should be repeated, as this alone will result in permanent cure in about one-third of patients. Surgical sympathectomy is indicated for patients who have only short-lived pain relief after sympathetic blockade. Spinal cord stimulation and intrathecal baclofen may also provide temporary (sometimes permanent) pain relief.

Ciccone DS et al: Psychological dysfunction in patients with reflex sympathetic dystrophy. Pain 1997;71:323.

Kemler MA et al: Spinal cord stimulation in patients with chronic reflex sympathetic dystrophy. N Engl J Med 2000;343:618.

Schwartzman RJ: New treatments for reflex sympathetic dystrophy. N Engl J Med 2000;343:654.

van Hilten BJ et al: Intrathecal baclofen for the treatment of dystonia in patients with reflex sympathetic dystrophy. N Engl J Med 2000;343;6256.

■ THORACIC OUTLET SYNDROME

The term thoracic outlet syndrome refers to the variety of disorders caused by abnormal compression of arterial, venous, or neural structures in the base of the neck. Numerous mechanisms for compression have been described, including cervical rib, anomalous ligaments, hypertrophy of the scalenus anticus muscle, and positional changes that alter the normal relation of the first rib to the structures which pass over it. Patients often describe a history of cervical trauma.

Symptoms rarely develop until adulthood. For this reason, it has been assumed that an alteration of normal structural relationships which occurs with advancing years is the primary factor. Even anomalous cervical ribs seem well tolerated during childhood and adolescence.

Inclusion of these syndromes in discussions of vascular disease originates from a former view that many of the symptoms were the result of intermittent compression of the subclavian or axillary arteries. This assumption was reinforced by the frequent finding that certain postural manipulations could produce depression of the radial pulse. The present view holds that whereas transient circulatory changes may indeed occur, the primary cause of symptoms in most patients is intermittent compression of one or more trunks of the brachial plexus. Thus, neurologic symptoms predominate over those of ischemia or venous compression. However, compression of the subclavian artery and vein in the thoracic outlet can produce even more severe sequelae than neurologic symptoms, which are usually more annoying than debilitating. Compression of the subclavian artery can produce stenosis and reflex poststenotic dilation of the artery, leading to arterial occlusion or emboli. Compression of the vein can produce thrombosis, which can result in severe upper extremity pain and swelling. This process is termed effort thrombosis (also called Paget-Schroetter syndrome).

Clinical Findings

A. SYMPTOMS AND SIGNS

Symptoms consist of pain, paresthesias, or numbness in the distribution of one or more trunks of the brachial plexus (usually in the ulnar distribution). Most patients associate their symptoms with certain positions of the shoulder girdle. These may occur from prolonged hyperabduction, as in house painters, hairdressers, and truck drivers. Others may relate their symptoms to the downward traction of the shoulder girdle produced by carrying heavy objects. Numbness of the hands often wakes the patient from sleep. On physical examination, motor deficits are rare and usually indicate severe compression of long duration. Muscular atrophy may be present in the hand. The radial pulse can be weakened by abduction of the arm with the head rotated to the opposite side (**Adson's test**), though pulse reduction by this maneuver often occurs in completely asymptomatic persons. Light percussion over the brachial plexus in the supraclavicular fossa produces peripheral sensations (**Tinel's test**) and reproduces the symptoms in patients with chronic neurologic impingement. A bruit is commonly heard over the subclavian artery above the center of the clavicle with abduction of the arm. Occlusion of the subclavian vein with upper extremity edema is a frequent complication of thoracic outlet syndrome.

B. DIAGNOSIS

Thoracic outlet compression must be differentiated from other disorders that mimic this condition (eg, carpal tunnel syndrome and cervical disk disease). While cervical x-rays and peripheral nerve conduction studies do not confirm the diagnosis of thoracic outlet syndrome, they are valuable to elucidate other possibilities. Arteriograms may demonstrate subclavian or axillary artery stenosis when the arm is in abduction. This finding can occur in normal individuals and is not diagnostic, but poststenotic dilation of the artery is distinctly abnormal and indicates a definite lesion. Unfortunately, there is no recognized objective study to confirm unequivocally the diagnosis of neurogenic thoracic outlet syndrome.

Treatment

Most patients benefit from postural correction and a physical therapy program directed toward restoring the normal relation and strength of the structures in the shoulder girdle. Surgical techniques for decompression of the thoracic outlet are reserved for patients who have not responded after 3–6 months of conservative treatment. Some surgeons prefer transaxillary first rib section, while others prefer a supraclavicular approach. With either operation, the anterior scalene muscle and any associated fibrous bands should be excised.

When the process produces arterial and venous pathology, operation is almost always required. Symptomatic arterial stenosis and aneurysms require decompression of the thoracic outlet in combination with arterial reconstruction, generally involving reversed vein graft interposition for the diseased subclavian artery. Effort thrombosis of the subclavian vein is usually best treated by catheter-directed thrombolysis of the venous occlusion followed by thoracic outlet decompression with or without operative venous reconstruction or intraluminal stent placement. Insertion of intraluminal venous stents without rib resection is ineffective because the stents themselves are compressed and narrowed by the underlying anatomy.

Angle N et al: Safety and efficacy of early surgical decompression of the thoracic outlet for Paget-Schroetter syndrome. Ann Vasc Surg 2001;15:37.

Kreienberg PB et al: Long-term results in patients treated with thrombolysis, thoracic inlet decompression, and subclavian vein stenting for Paget- Schroetter syndrome. J Vasc Surg 2001;33:5100.

Sharp WJ et al: Long-term follow-up and patient satisfaction after surgery for thoracic outlet syndrome. Ann Vasc Surg 2001; 15:32.

Wilbourn AJ: Thoracic outlet syndromes. Neurol Clin 1999;17: 477.

■ ARTERIOVENOUS FISTULAS

Arteriovenous fistulas, often called "malformations," may be congenital or acquired. Abnormal communications between arteries and veins occur in many diseases and may affect vessels of all sizes and in many locations, including the brain, lungs, bowel, skin, muscle, and elsewhere. Their effects depend upon their size and location—for example, some malformations are composed mostly of veins (venous malformations) that may produce compressive or cosmetic symptoms but rarely bleed or produce heart failure. In congenital fistulas, the systemic effect is often not great, because the degree of communication, though diffuse, is small. Larger acquired fistulas enlarge rapidly. Cardiac dilation and failure result when shunting is excessive, prolonged, or untreated.

Congenital fistulas or malformations are often noted in infancy or childhood. When a limb is involved, muscle mass or bone length may be increased. Arteriovenous malformations frequently involve the brain, visceral organs, or lungs. Gastrointestinal hemorrhage may occur. Osler-Weber-Rendu disease or syndrome (also termed hereditary hemorrhagic telangiectasia) is an autosomal dominant disorder characterized by hemorrhages in the form of epistaxis or gastrointestinal bleeding associated with large arteriovenous anomalies in the lungs and gastrointestinal tract. Pulmonary lesions cause polycythemia, clubbing, and cyanosis.

Acquired fistulas result from injuries that produce artificial connections between adjacent arteries and veins and may be the result of trauma or disease. Penetrating injuries are the most common cause, but fistulas are sometimes seen after blunt trauma. Iatrogenic arteriovenous fistulas after arteriography are becoming increasingly common. Connective tissue disorders (eg, Ehlers-Danlos syndrome), erosion of an atherosclerotic or mycotic arterial aneurysm into adjacent veins, communication with an arterial prosthetic graft, and neoplastic invasion are other causes. A rare but dramatic cause of traumatic arteriovenous fistula is combined injury to the aorta and inferior vena cava or to the iliac arteries and veins during surgical excision of a herniated disk by the dorsal approach.

Clinical Findings

A. SYMPTOMS AND SIGNS

The time of onset and the presence or absence of associated disease should be determined. A typical continuous machinery murmur can be heard over most fistulas and is often associated with a palpable thrill and locally increased skin temperature. Proximally, the arteries and veins dilate and the pulse distal to the lesion diminishes. There may be signs of venous insufficiency and coolness distal to the communication on the involved extremity. Tachycardia occurs in some patients as a feature of increased cardiac output. When the fistula is occluded by compression, the pulse rate slows **(Branham's sign).**

In contrast, venous malformations rarely produce hemodynamic effects. In this disorder, the presence of a mass, which may or may not be tender, is the principal finding. Because flow rates are low, bruits and thrills are absent.

B. IMAGING STUDIES

MRI has become the imaging study of choice for the evaluation and follow-up of peripheral arteriovenous malformations. Precise delineation of arteriovenous fistulas can only be done with appropriate arteriograms. Selective catheter injection techniques have permitted most accurate radiologic diagnosis.

Treatment

Not all arteriovenous connections require treatment. Most venous malformations should be treated conservatively with compression garments when possible. In addition, small peripheral fistulas may be observed and frequently will never cause difficulties. Some are surgically inaccessible.

The indications for intervention include hemorrhage, expanding false aneurysm, severe venous or arterial insufficiency, cosmetic deformity, and heart failure.

Most fistulas are now managed by embolization under radiographic control. The embolic material used includes blood clot, glass beads, Gelfoam, and muscle. A number of centers have reported good results with arteriovenous malformations in various parts of the body. Arteriovenous malformations of the head and neck and of the pelvis appear particularly well suited for this form of therapy. Direct injection of sclerosant compounds into venous malformations under fluoroscopic control is also successful.

Surgical options include ligation of all feeding vessels, amputation of the extremity, en bloc resection of the fistula, and repair of the fistula by reconstruction of the involved arteries and veins. Oversewing the defects in the artery and vein is curative for postarteriography fistulas. Surgery should be avoided in most cases of congenital arteriovenous malformations.

Congenital arteriovenous fistulas are amenable to surgical management only when en bloc resection of all tissue involved in the fistula can be accomplished. When the fistulous connections involve substantial portions of an extremity, local arterial ligation is invariably followed by recurrence, and only temporary palliation can be expected. Moreover, ligation of major feeder vessels obviates embolotherapy by interventional radiology techniques. Amputation may be a last resort to control unmanageable peripheral fistulas.

Prognosis

The results of therapy vary according to the extent, location, and type of fistula. In general, traumatic fistulas have the most favorable prognosis. Congenital fistulas are more difficult to eradicate, because of the numerous arteriovenous connections usually present. These fistulas have a high propensity for recurrence, and most surgeons are reluctant to operate unless the surgical indications are urgent.

Hisamatsu K et al: Peripheral arterial coil embolization for hepatic arteriovenous malformation in Osler-Weber-Rendu disease. Intern Med 1999;38:962.

Iqbal M et al: Pulmonary arteriovenous malformations: a clinical review. Postgrad Med J 2000;76:390.

Jacobowitz GR et al: Transcatheter embolization of complex pelvic vascular malformations: results and long-term follow-up. J Vasc Surg 2001;33:51.

Mattle HP et al: Dilemmas in the management of patients with arteriovenous malformations. J Neurol 2000;247:917.

Mulliken JB et al: Vascular anomalies. Curr Probl Surg 2000;37:517.

White RI Jr et al: Long-term outcome of embolotherapy and surgery for high-flow extremity arteriovenous malformations. J Vasc Interv Radiol 2000;11:1285.

■ CEREBROVASCULAR DISEASE

ESSENTIALS OF DIAGNOSIS

• *Episodic motor and visual dysfunction; stroke; aphasia, ataxia, and sensory dysfunction.*

- *Cervical arterial bruits or pulse deficits, or blood pressure differences in the arms.*
- *Duplex ultrasound confirmation of carotid stenosis.*
- *Selective arteriograms.*

General Considerations

Symptoms of cerebrovascular disease are most often the result of emboli and less often the result of hypoperfusion. About 80% of patients with occlusive cerebrovascular disease have an atherosclerotic lesion in a surgically accessible artery in the neck or mediastinum (Figures 35–15, 35–16, and 35–17) that is the cause of symptoms. Less commonly, symptoms may be due to arterial emboli originating in the heart, fibromuscular disease, arterial dissection, or Takayasu's (giant cell) arteritis.

Cerebral infarction occurs when the blood supply is decreased below a critical level; this causes cellular death within minutes. This event is manifested by a

Figure 35–16. Diagram showing common sites of stenosis and occlusion of the extracranial cerebral vasculature.

fixed or advancing neurologic deficit. It can result from local arterial thrombosis, cerebral embolization, or hemorrhage.

Embolization is the most common mechanism of cerebral infarction from carotid lesions. The atherosclerotic plaque ulcerates, and atheromatous debris or blood clot will dislodge to produce infarction when it reaches the brain. Most lesions of this sort occur at the origin of the internal carotid, but the innominate artery and ascending aorta are implicated occasionally.

Characteristically, lesions of atherosclerosis occur along the outer wall of the carotid bulb. Preferential location of advanced disease has been demonstrated in postmortem anatomic specimens, on angiograms of patients with severe carotid stenosis, and in specimens removed during carotid endarterectomy. Low wall shear stress, flow separation, and loss of unidirectional flow allow for greater interaction of atherogenic particles and vessel walls at this area of the artery.

Neurologic dysfunction without infarction may be produced in two ways: (1) cerebral embolization by small (microembolic) fragments that only temporarily impede arterial flow; and (2) transient reduction in cerebral perfusion short of that required to give irreversible ischemia.

Since most microemboli originate from a lesion in the internal carotid artery, neurologic dysfunction is confined to the carotid territory and appears as "short-lived" paresis or numbness of the contralateral arm or leg. This is called a **transient ischemic attack (TIA).**

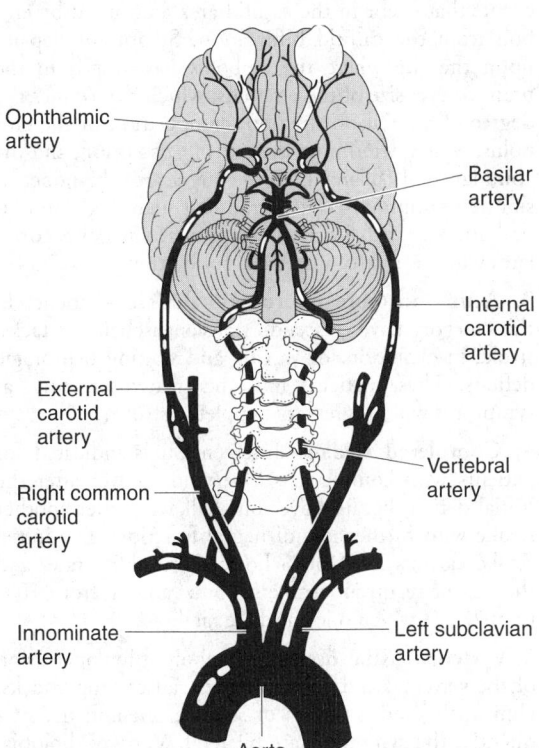

Ophthalmic artery

Basilar artery

Internal carotid artery

External carotid artery

Vertebral artery

Right common carotid artery

Innominate artery

Left subclavian artery

Aorta

Figure 35–15. Diagram of arterial blood supply to the eyes and brain.

Figure 35–17. *Left:* Preoperative carotid arteriogram showing stenosis of the proximal internal carotid artery. *Right:* Postoperative carotid arteriogram showing restoration of normal luminal size following endarterectomy.

The onset is swift, and most TIAs are brief (minutes). By convention, 24 hours is the arbitrary limit of a TIA. A microembolus to the ophthalmic artery, the first branch of the internal carotid artery, produces a temporary monocular loss of vision called **amaurosis fugax.** Emboli may be visible as small bright flecks (**Hollenhorst plaques**) lodged in arterial bifurcations in the retina. Without treatment, one-third of patients with TIAs will eventually develop permanent neurologic impairment either from dislodgment of a macroembolus or thrombotic occlusion of the internal carotid artery, while 20% of patients with amaurosis fugax will suffer strokes. Antiplatelet therapy decreases these stroke rates by about 5%.

Clinical Findings

Patients with cerebrovascular disease may present initially to an internist, family practitioner, neurologist, neurosurgeon, ophthalmologist, or vascular surgeon. Satisfactory management of these patients depends on recognition of disease and appropriate referral for further treatment.

A. SYMPTOMS

Patients with cerebrovascular disease can be grouped into five categories based on symptoms at presentation.

1. Asymptomatic disease—An audible bruit heard in the neck may be the only manifestation of cerebrovascular disease. Severe carotid stenosis may also occur in the absence of a bruit with markedly reduced blood flow.

2. Transient neurologic or visual episodes—Most events that occur in the carotid area are caused by emboli from the carotid bifurcation. Symptoms depend upon the site where the embolus has lodged in the brain or eye; size of the embolus, which determines the degree of arterial obstruction; composition of the embolus, which determines the rate of dissolution; and the abundance of collaterals to the target area. Hypoperfusion less commonly causes transient neurologic and visual attacks. Stroke risk in symptomatic patients correlates with severity of internal carotid artery stenosis.

3. Acute unstable neurologic deficit—Patients in this category have crescendo transient ischemic attacks, stroke in evolution, or waxing and waning neurologic deficits. These patients must be treated urgently, as symptoms will progress to completed stroke.

4. Completed stroke—Intervention is indicated for patients with completed stroke who recover after the initial deficit, because over one-half will suffer another stroke with further loss of neural function. The initial stroke carriers a 20–30% hospital mortality rate, and the risk of recurrent stroke is high, ranging from 10% to 50%t, of which one-third are fatal.

5. Vertebrobasilar disease—Emboli or hypoperfusion of the vertebral and basilar arteries causes drop attacks, clumsiness, and a variety of sensory phenomena. Frequently, the symptoms are bilateral. Vertigo, diplopia, dysphagia, or dysequilibrium occurring *individually* is rarely due to vertebrobasilar disease, but when these symptoms occur in combination the diagnosis becomes more likely. It is unusual for dizziness alone to be due to cerebrovascular disease.

B. SIGNS

Auscultation of the carotid and subclavian arteries usually suggests the diagnosis of major vessel stenosis and may delineate the sites of hemodynamically significant disease. Pulse deficits are unusual in the neck but common in the arms. The following lesions may exist *without* clinical signs: (1) occlusion of the internal carotid artery, (2) high-grade (> 90%) stenosis, (3) occlusion and stenosis of the vertebral arteries, and (4) ulceration without significant hemodynamic stenosis of any vessel.

1. Palpation—In the neck, only the pulse of the common carotid artery can be felt directly. Thus, the internal carotid may be completely occluded in the presence of a normal palpable neck pulse. The status of pulses of the superficial temporal artery and the axillary artery reflects the patency of the external carotid artery and the subclavian artery, respectively.

2. Bruits—A bruit localized to one artery indicates a stenosis at or proximal to the point where it can be heard. A bruit with maximal intensity high in the neck indicates stenosis at the common carotid bifurcation. Bruits caused by stenosis at the origin of the vertebral artery are most prominent over the lower portion of the trapezius muscle at the back of the neck. Bruits due to proximal subclavian stenosis are most audible above the midpoint of the clavicle and are transmitted into the axilla. Innominate artery stenosis produces a bruit heard along the full length of the right common carotid and right subclavian arteries. Cardiac murmurs are loudest over the precordium and radiate along the subclavian and proximal common carotid arteries.

3. Brachial blood pressures—A discrepancy between the blood pressures in the two arms indicates arterial stenosis or occlusion proximal to the brachial artery on the side of reduced pressure. Most commonly, the origin of the left subclavian artery is stenosed.

C. NONINVASIVE TESTS

The most useful noninvasive test for the diagnosis of extracranial carotid artery disease is duplex ultrasound analysis, which combines high resolution B-mode imaging and range-gated Doppler spectral flow analysis. Imaging demonstrates plaque morphology, whereas Doppler spectral velocity analysis determines the degree of stenosis rapidly and accurately. New color-flow duplex devices have further improved the utility of this technology.

Determination of degree of luminal narrowing is based mostly on velocity criteria. As the stenosis increasingly obliterates the lumen of the vessel, the velocity of blood increases in the area of the stenosis so that

the total volume of flow remains constant. Normally, the velocity of the internal carotid artery is low with a large amount of diastolic blood flow because of autoregulation in the cerebral vessels. With increasing degrees of stenosis, the systolic and diastolic flow velocities progressively increase. Although the performance and interpretation of a carotid duplex scan require experience and skill, many clinicians now perform carotid endarterectomy without preoperative arteriography, based solely on color-duplex scanning.

D. IMAGING STUDIES

Cerebral arteriography is still performed in many patients with symptomatic and asymptomatic cerebrovascular disease who are candidates for surgery. Surgery is indicated if the lesion is surgically accessible and meets criteria determined by randomized prospective studies. The two most important such studies in this regard are the NASCET (North American Symptomatic Carotid Endarterectomy Trial) and the ACAS (Asymptomatic Carotid Atherosclerosis Study), which prospectively compared surgical and medical therapy for symptomatic and asymptomatic patients with carotid artery stenoses, respectively (see below). Arteriograms should provide extracranial and intracranial views of the carotid and vertebrobasilar systems. Intravenous digital subtraction angiography (DSA) does not reliably demonstrate cerebrovascular anatomy, but intra-arterial DSA has permitted use of minimal amounts of contrast and small catheters so that outpatient arteriography is now routinely performed.

Treatment

The objective of treatment for cerebrovascular disease is to prevent strokes and TIAs. This is accomplished by improving blood flow or removing a source of microemboli. The NASCET study was reported in two major parts. In the first report, 659 patients with carotid stenoses measuring 70–99% were randomized to carotid endarterectomy plus aspirin versus aspirin therapy alone. The cumulative risks of any ipsilateral stroke at 2 years were 26% in the 331 medical patients and 9% in the 328 surgical patients—an absolute risk reduction of 17%. In the second report, in patients with moderate carotid stenosis (50–69%), the results also favored surgery but less dramatically; the 5-year risk of ipsilateral stroke was 15.7% among patients treated surgically (n = 1108) and 22.2% among those treated medically (n = 1118; P = .045). Patients with stenoses of less than 50% did not benefit from surgery. In the ACAS trial, 1662 patients with asymptomatic carotid artery stenosis of 60% or greater were randomized to medical therapy or carotid endarterectomy. After a median follow-up of 2.7 years, the aggregate risk over 5 years for ipsilateral stroke or death was estimated to be 5.1 % for surgical patients and 11% for patients treated medically (aggregate risk reduction of 53%).

Medical therapy consists of antiplatelet drugs and reduction of atherosclerotic risk factors by smoking cessation, treatment of hypertension, lowering of LDL cholesterol, etc. Oral anticoagulants only variably reduce the incidence of TIAs, do not reduce the risk of completed strokes, and are associated with serious bleeding complications. There have been four large cooperative prospective studies of the efficacy of antiplatelet agents for preventing strokes conducted in the USA, Canada, and France. Of these, only the French study concluded that aspirin prevented strokes, although the others found that when the end-points of stroke, TIA, and death are combined, aspirin was beneficial. Intolerance of aspirin, mostly because of gastrointestinal side effects, is surprisingly common; there is no consensus regarding the optimal dose. A randomized trial comparing another antiplatelet agent, ticlopidine hydrochloride, with aspirin for the prevention of stroke in high-risk patients showed

that ticlopidine was slightly more effective than aspirin, but the risks of serious side effects were greater. Clopidogrel is an antiplatelet thienopyridine that, like ticlopidine, is an ADP-receptor platelet inhibitor. In the CAPRIE (Clopidogrel versus Aspirin in Patients at Risk of Ischaemic Events) trial, long-term administration of clopidogrel to patients with atherosclerotic vascular disease (n = 19,185) was more effective than aspirin in reducing the combined risk of ischemic stroke, myocardial infarction, or vascular death. Based on these results, many neurologists recommend clopidogrel for medical therapy of cerebrovascular disease.

Endarterectomy is the preferred technique for the removal of atherosclerotic lesions at the common carotid bifurcation, in the orifices of the right vertebral and subclavian arteries, and in the innominate artery (Figure 35–18). The left vertebral artery is difficult to approach through the neck, and obstruction at its orifice is more easily managed by transplanting the vertebral artery to the side of the adjacent left common carotid artery. Obstruction at the origin of the left com-

Figure 35–18. Technique of carotid endarterectomy. The common, internal, and external carotid arteries are occluded **(A)**, and a longitudinal arteriotomy is created **(B)**. Plaque is removed **(C–F)** with careful attention to achieve a smooth end point **(G)**. The arteriotomy is closed, using continuous suture technique **(H)**.

mon carotid artery would require an open thoracotomy for endarterectomy. However, thoracotomy and its risks can be avoided by dividing the common carotid low in the neck and transplanting it to the left subclavian artery. Alternatively, a prosthetic graft can be placed from the subclavian to the common carotid artery beyond the stenosis (subclavian-carotid bypass).

Surgery is not performed for recent completed cerebral infarction, because restoration of normal blood flow and arterial pressures to an infarcted area may cause hemorrhage into the infarct or increase edema. In addition, endarterectomy cannot be performed when the internal carotid artery is completely occluded, because thrombosis propagates to the intracranial portion of the artery at the ophthalmic or middle cerebral artery. If patients recover significant neurologic function after strokes, carotid endarterectomy is indicated after the acute infarction has healed.

The **subclavian steal syndrome** is characterized by the development of neurologic symptoms upon exercise of the upper extremity. Anatomically, there is a proximal subclavian stenosis or occlusion, with reversal of flow through the vertebral artery (ie, the vertebral artery serves as a collateral to supply blood to the arm). While this *anatomic* arrangement is often demonstrated on angiograms, the clinical syndrome is very rare. Symptoms of effort fatigue in the involved extremity are far more common than neurologic complaints. Management consists of bypass grafting from the common carotid to the subclavian artery distal to the lesion (Figure 35–19) or transposition of the subclavian artery beyond the lesion to the side of the nearby common carotid artery.

There continues to be considerable debate about the correct approach to management of patients with coexistent **coronary and carotid atherosclerosis.** The priorities appear clear in two groups. The patient with symptomatic carotid stenosis whose coronary artery disease is less symptomatic should undergo carotid operation. Similarly, if the patient has an asymptomatic bruit from noncritical carotid stenosis and symptomatic heart disease, the coronary arteries should take precedence. It is the group of patients with symptoms in both vascular distributions for whom the answer is still not clear. Satisfactory results have been achieved with combined simultaneous carotid and coronary procedures in some centers. There is increasing evidence that the simultaneous procedure is associated with an increased death rate and increased cerebral and cardiac complications over staged procedures, and it is recommended that closely spaced staged procedures be performed whenever possible.

Percutaneous carotid artery angioplasty and stenting in place of operative carotid endarterectomy has gained some acceptance in recent years, but its indications remain controversial. There have been no randomized studies of this procedure, though several are in planning stages. In one recent review of periprocedural complication rates in 528 consecutive patients undergoing carotid stenting, there was an overall 30-day stroke and death

Figure 35–19. *Left:* Arteriogram showing selective injection of the left subclavian artery. There is antegrade flow in the ipsilateral vertebral artery and retrograde flow in the contralateral vertebral artery. *Right:* A later film in this sequence shows filling of the right subclavian artery by retrograde flow in the right vertebral artery. There is proximal occlusion of the right subclavian artery causing the subclavian steal syndrome.

rate of 7.4%, which is higher than most reports describing the results of carotid endarterectomy. High restenosis rates after carotid stenting have also been described.

Other Causes of Cerebrovascular Symptoms

Primary disease of the extracranial arteries other than atherosclerosis is rare.

A. TAKAYASU'S (GIANT CELL) ARTERITIS

Takayasu's arteritis is an obliterative arteriopathy principally involving the aortic arch vessels that often affects young women. High-dose corticosteroids and cyclophosphamide have been shown to arrest and in some cases reverse the progress of the disease. The pararenal abdominal aorta and pulmonary arteries may also be affected. Operative treatment of nonspecific arteritis should be avoided unless arteritis is active, but it may be successful in burned-out disease.

B. DISSECTING ANEURYSMS OF THE AORTA

Dissecting aneurysms of the aorta may extend into the arch branches, producing obstruction and cerebral symptoms. These are discussed in Chapter 20, Part I.

C. INTERNAL CAROTID DISSECTION

Dissection originating in the internal carotid artery and localized to its extracranial segment occurs as an acute event that may narrow or obliterate the internal carotid lumen. The primary lesion is an intimal tear at the distal end of the carotid bulb. It may follow various types of neck trauma or, more commonly, severe hypertension. Dissection may also develop spontaneously, most frequently in young adults.

Cerebral symptoms are the result of ischemia in the ipsilateral hemisphere. Acute neck pain in association with localized cervical tenderness adjacent to the angle of the mandible is a frequent finding.

Arteriography shows a characteristic pattern of tapered narrowing at or just beyond the distal portion of the carotid bulb. The lumen beyond this point may be obliterated or may persist as a barely visible narrow shadow. This gives rise to a faint "string" of contrast visible above the top of the cap. If the lumen persists, it resumes a normal caliber beyond the bony foramen.

Anticoagulation is the treatment of choice for this disorder. Operation is indicated only for patients with recurrent TIAs. In most patients, the intramural clot will be resorbed, restoring a normal lumen. In the rare case in which the dissection is confined to the surgically accessible proximal third, this segment may be resected and replaced with a graft. If the involvement is longer and the TIAs are believed to result from embolization and if the carotid back pressure exceeds 65 mm Hg, proximal ligation can be performed. Extracranial to intracranial bypass can also be performed in this setting.

D. FIBROMUSCULAR DYSPLASIA

Fibromuscular dysplasia is a nonatherosclerotic angiopathy of unknown cause that affects specific arteries, chiefly in young women. Symptoms of cerebrovascular disease can occur when the carotid artery is affected. It is usually bilateral and involves primarily the middle third of the extracranial portions of the internal carotid artery. Several pathologic variants of the disease have been described, but in most of them the primary lesion is overgrowth of the media in a segmental distribution, producing irregular zones of arterial narrowing. The most common result is a series of concentric rings, producing the radiologic appearance of a *string of beads* in a long internal carotid artery. A bruit high in the neck may be the only physical finding on vascular examination, although about one-third of patients are hypertensive because of renal artery involvement.

The prevalence of fibromuscular dysplasia and the portion of patients who develop symptoms are not known. Once symptoms develop, transient neurologic events are the most common manifestation. However, more than 20% of patients have had a stroke by the time of presentation.

Because of the high incidence of neurologic disability, the lesion should be corrected surgically when patients develop symptoms. Treatment of asymptomatic disease is controversial. Use of intraoperative graduated dilators or balloon dilation has given excellent results. Percutaneous transluminal angioplasty has been employed, but the risk of causing embolization appears high.

Surgical Results

Late restenosis or occlusion is uncommon after carotid endarterectomy; many authorities advocate liberal or routine use of the vein or prosthetic patch for closure of the arteriotomy to reduce complications. The main complication of cerebrovascular operations is stroke, which occurs in 1–4% of patients depending on the operative indications and cerebrovascular anatomy. Higher stroke rates occur in the setting of symptomatic stenosis or contralateral carotid occlusion. The operative death rate for all extracranial cerebrovascular operations is less than 1%. Transient cranial nerve injury, which occurs in about 20% of operations, may cause tongue weakness, hoarseness, mouth asymmetry, earlobe numbness, and dysphagia. Less than 5% of peripheral nerve deficits are permanent.

Abou-Zamzam AM Jr et al: Is a single preoperative duplex scan sufficient for planning bilateral carotid endarterectomy? J Vasc Surg 2000;31:282.

Baker WH et al: Effect of contralateral occlusion on long-term efficacy of endarterectomy in the asymptomatic carotid atherosclerosis study (ACAS). ACAS Investigators. Stroke 2000; 31;2330.

Barnett HJJM et al: Benefit of carotid endarterectomy in patients with symptomatic moderate or severe stenosis. N Engl J Med 1998;339:1415.

Beneficial effect of carotid endarterectomy in symptomatic patients with high-grade stenosis. North American Symptomatic Carotid Endarterectomy Trial Collaborators. N Engl J Med 1991;325:445.

Darling RC 3rd et al: Analysis of the effect of asymptomatic carotid atherosclerosis study on the outcome and volume of carotid endarterectomy. Cardiovasc Surg 2000;8:436.

Endarterectomy for asymptomatic carotid artery stenosis. Executive Committee for the Asymptomatic Carotid Atherosclerosis Study (ACAS). JAMA 1995;273;1421.

Ferguson GG et al: The North American Symptomatic Carotid Endarterectomy Trial: surgical results in 1415 patients. Stroke 1999;30:1751.

Golledge J et al: Systematic comparison of the early outcome of angioplasty and endarterectomy for symptomatic carotid artery disease. Stroke 2000;31:1439.

Hobson RW: Carotid angioplasty-stent: clinical experience and role for clinical trials. J Vasc Surg 2001;33:5117.

Kresowik TF et al: Improving the outcomes of carotid endarterectomy: results of a statewide quality improvement project. J Vasc Surg 2000;31:918.

Moore WS et al: Indications, surgical technique, and results for repair of extracranial occlusive lesions. In: *Vascular Surgery,* 5th ed. Rutherford RB (editor): Saunders, 2000.

A randomised, blinded, trial of clopidogrel versus aspirin in patients at risk of ischaemic events (CAPRIE). CAPRIE Steering Committee: Lancet 1996;348:1329.

Rothwell PM et al: Interrelation between plaque surface morphology and degree of stenosis on carotid angiograms and the risk of ischemic stroke in patients with symptomatic carotid stenosis. On behalf of the European Carotid Surgery Trialists' Collaborative Group. Stroke 2000;342:1693.

Roubin GS et al: Immediate and late clinical outcomes of carotid artery stenting in patients with symptomatic and asymptomatic carotid artery stenosis: a 5-year prospective analysis. Circulation 2001;103:532.

Schievink WI: Spontaneous dissection of the carotid and vertebral arteries. N Engl J Med 2001;344:898.

Veith FJ et al: Current status of carotid bifurcation angioplasty and stenting based on a consensus of opinion leaders. J Vasc Surg 2001;33:5111.

■ RENOVASCULAR HYPERTENSION

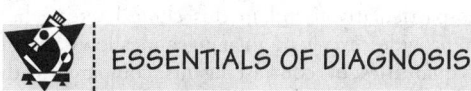

ESSENTIALS OF DIAGNOSIS

- *Severe hypertension.*

- *Declining renal function.*
- *Suspicion of renal artery involvement.*

General Considerations

More than 23 million people in the USA have hypertension, and renovascular disease is the cause in 2–7% of cases. Atherosclerosis of the aorta and renal artery is present in two-thirds of patients with renovascular disease, and fibromuscular dysplasia is present in most of the rest. Less common causes of hypertension include renal artery emboli, renal artery aneurysms, renal artery dissection, hypoplasia of the renal arteries, and stenosis of the suprarenal aorta.

Atherosclerosis characteristically produces stenosis at the orifice of the main renal artery. The lesion usually consists of an atheroma that originates in the aorta and extends into the renal artery. Less commonly, the atheroma arises in the renal artery itself. Renal artery stenosis is more common in males over age 45 years and is bilateral in about 95% of cases.

Fibromuscular dysplasia usually involves the middle and distal thirds of the main renal artery and may extend into the branches (Figure 35–20). Medial fibroplasia is the most common variety of fibroglandular dysplasia, accounting for 85% of these lesions. It is bilateral in 50% of cases. The arterial stenoses are caused by concentric rings of hyperplasia that project into the arterial lumen. Renal artery aneurysms frequently coexist. Fibromuscular dysplasia occurs mainly in women, with onset of hypertension usually occurring before age 45 years. It is the causative disorder in 10% of children with hypertension. Developmental renal artery hypoplasia, coarctation of the aorta, and Takayasu's aortitis are the vascular causes of hypertension in childhood.

Hypertension due to renal artery stenosis results from kidney response to hypoperfusion. Cells of the juxtaglomerular complex secrete renin, which acts on

Figure 35–20. Renal arteriogram showing bilateral fibromuscular hyperplasia of the renal arteries (arrows).

circulating angiotensinogen to form angiotensin I, which is rapidly converted to angiotensin II by angiotensin-converting enzyme (ACE). This octapeptide constricts arterioles, increases aldosterone secretion, and promotes sodium retention. Blood pressure increases in an attempt to overcome renal hypoperfusion. As renovascular hypertension becomes established, pathologic changes occur in the kidneys and other organs, and hypertension becomes volume-dependent.

Clinical Findings

A. SYMPTOMS AND SIGNS

Most patients are asymptomatic, but irritability, headache, and emotional depression are seen in a few. Persistent elevation of the diastolic pressure is usually the only abnormal physical finding. A bruit is frequently audible to one or both sides of the midline in the upper abdomen. Other signs of atherosclerosis may be present when this is the cause of the renal artery disease.

Other clues to the presence of renovascular hypertension include absence of a family history of hypertension; early onset of hypertension (particularly during childhood or, in women, during early adulthood); marked acceleration of the degree of hypertension; resistance to control with antihypertensive drugs; and rapid deterioration of renal function. Patients are more likely to have renovascular hypertension if initial diastolic pressure is greater than 115 mm Hg or if renal function deteriorates while they are being given ACE inhibitors.

B. DIAGNOSTIC STUDIES

Divided urinary excretion studies, which were used to indicate which of the two kidneys was the cause of hypertension, have largely been discarded, because of the frequency of false-negative results when both renal arteries are diseased.

Selective renin determinations from renal vein blood samples are suggestive of the diagnosis if the ratio of the renin from the involved kidney to that of the uninvolved one exceeds 1.5. This is called the renal vein renin ratio (RVRR).

Like urinary excretion tests, selective renal vein renin determinations are difficult to reproduce. All antihypertensive medications must be discontinued at least 1 week before the study, and sodium intake should be diminished (to maximize renin output and exaggerate differences between the kidneys).

When bilateral renal artery disease exists, however, this value may be misleading, because both kidneys produce renin. Systemic serum renin determinations are of little value, because the retention of sodium and water produces a dilutional effect. Only in malignant hypertension are systemic renin concentrations uniformly elevated.

Captopril and enalapril inhibit ACE and cause a precipitous drop in blood pressure in patients with renin-dependent hypertension. Renal function may also deteriorate. The combination of provocative testing with a converting enzyme inhibitor and RVRR determinations increases the accuracy of diagnosis of surgically correctable renovascular hypertension. Captopril renal scintigraphy has emerged as the preferred study to establish the diagnosis.

Duplex ultrasound scanning may also be useful in the diagnosis of renovascular disease. In experienced hands, the overall agreement of duplex findings and angiography is over 90%. Renal artery stenosis is characterized by peak systolic velocities in the range of 180–200 cm/s, and the ratio of these velocities to those in the aorta approaches 3.5. Magnetic resonance angiography (MRA), especially with gadolinium enhancement, may provide high-resolution images of diseased renal arteries. Its lack of nephrotoxicity and noninvasiveness make it an attractive diagnostic test.

C. IMAGING STUDIES

Intravenous urography with rapid injection and rapid sequence exposure is a common screening test that also depends upon comparison of the two kidneys. The ischemic kidney has delayed appearance of dye in the calices and hyperconcentration in the later films as water is extracted by the tubules. The nephrogram phase may show a small kidney on the affected side. Sensitivity of urography is poor, however.

Conventional renal arteriography is the most precise method for delineating the obstructive lesion. Since atherosclerotic disease most often involves the origins of the renal arteries, a midstream aortogram should be obtained in addition to selective renal artery catheterization. Renal arteriography should be performed if the diastolic blood pressure exceeds 110 mm Hg, other clinical criteria are consistent with renovascular hypertension, and long life is otherwise expected. Deteriorating renal function is another indication for arteriography. Oblique and multiple-plane arteriograms improve identification of renal artery stenoses. The presence of collateral vessels circumventing a renal artery stenosis suggests a hemodynamically significant renal artery lesion; a pressure gradient of 10 mm Hg is required for collateral vessel development, and the same amount of pressure difference is associated with activation of the renin system. Intra-arterial digital subtraction arteriography is particularly useful in this clinical setting because it provides excellent imaging and allows use of smaller quantities of contrast agents compared with conventional arteriography, which decreases the potential for contrast-induced nephrotoxicity.

Treatment

A. SURGICAL TREATMENT

Primary surgical treatment consists of revascularization of the renal artery. The indications for arterial reconstruction are influenced by the extent of disease in the renal arteries, the degree of associated arterial disease, the response to medical control of hypertension, the patient's life expectancy, and the anticipated morbidity associated with operation. Nephrectomy should be considered when arterial repair is impossible or especially hazardous and the disease is unilateral.

Endarterectomy is effective in the management of atherosclerotic lesions and is most easily accomplished through an incision into the adjacent aorta. When there is extensive intimal degeneration in the aorta (eg, associated aneurysmal disease in the aorta), a fabric bypass graft may be used as a side arm from the aortic prosthesis.

Arterial replacement is the preferred method of treatment in patients with fibromuscular dysplasia of the renal artery. Autogenous grafts using a segment of saphenous vein or hypogastric artery are advised (Figure 35–21). Nonanatomic bypass procedures are also useful in many patients with renovascular hypertension. The hepatic artery or the iliac arteries may be sites for bypass grafts to the renal artery, especially when originating a graft from the aorta would entail high operative risks. Splenorenal bypasses for left-sided lesions are another type of nonanatomic approach, but the celiac and splenic arteries often have coexistent occlusive atherosclerotic disease that mandates preoperative arteriographic assessment of these vessels. Operative arterial dilation, alone or in conjunction with a bypass procedure, may be necessary for treatment of fibrous intraparenchymal stenotic disease.

Obstructive lesions in the secondary branches of the renal artery due to fibromuscular dysplasia were originally considered to be inoperable. Extracorporeal techniques have recently been developed that in most instances can overcome the technical difficulties. These require removal of the kidney from the abdomen (ex vivo arterial reconstruction), continuous cold perfusion of its vascular tree, and microvascular techniques for arterial replacement. The kidney is then either returned to a site near its original position or transplanted to the ipsilateral iliac fossa.

B. PERCUTANEOUS TRANSLUMINAL ANGIOPLASTY

Percutaneous transluminal angioplasty has a 90% immediate success rate in patients with fibromuscular dysplasia, and 1 year later about 60% of patients remain cured. Results are not as long-lasting in renal atherosclerosis, however, as restenosis occurs in more than half of treated patients. If lesions occur at some distance from the aorta, results are superior to those achieved with angioplasty of primarily aortic lesions. The adjunctive use of stents after renal percutaneous transluminal angioplasty has improved success and durability of this procedure. Renal percutaneous transluminal angioplasty and stenting in properly selected patients must be considered alternative therapy for managing renovascular hypertension.

Prognosis

Operations for revascularization of the renal artery are successful in lowering blood pressure in over 90% of patients with fibromuscular hyperplasia. Operation for atherosclerotic stenosis results in improvement or cure of hypertension in about 60%. Salvage of renal function is even better. Results are better in patients with focal renal artery disease whose only clinical manifestation of atherosclerosis is secondary hypertension than in those with clinically overt extrarenal atherosclerosis affecting the coronary artery, carotid artery, aorta, or extremity vessels. The operative mortality rate of renovascular surgery in children is almost nil, whereas it increases to 2–8% in adults with diffuse atherosclerosis.

Ballard JJ: Renal artery endarterectomy for treatment of renovascular hypertension combined with infrarenal aortic reconstruction: analysis of surgical results. Ann Vasc Surg 2001;15:260.

Cambria RP et al: Surgical renal artery reconstruction without contrast arteriography: the role of clinical profiling and magnetic resonance angiography. J Vasc Surg 1999;29;1012.

Darling RC 3rd et al: Outcome of renal artery reconstruction; analysis of 687 procedures. Ann Surg 1999;230:524.

Figure 35–21. *Top:* Preoperative renal arteriogram of a patient with stenosis of the mid portion of the right renal artery (arrow). *Bottom:* Postoperative renal arteriogram after renal artery bypass with an autograft of the hypogastric artery.

Giroux MF et al: Percutaneous revascularization of the renal arteries: predictors of outcome. J Vasc Interv Radiol 2000;11:713.

Hansen KJ et al: Management of ischemic nephropathy: dialysis-free survival after surgical repair. J Vasc Surg 2000;32:472.

Helin KH et al: Predicting the outcome of invasive treatment of renal artery disease. J Intern Med 2000;247:105.

Hua HT et al: The use of colorflow duplex scanning to detect significant renal artery stneosis. Ann Vasc Surg 20000;14:118.

Iglesias JI et al: The natural history of incidental renal artery stenosis in patients with aortoiliac vascular disease. Am J Med 2000;109:642.

Safian RD et al: Renal-artery stenosis. N Engl J Med 2001; 344:431.

Textor SC et al: Renal artery stenosis: a common, treatable cause of renal failure? Annu Rev Med 2001;52:421.

Teoh MK: Takayasu's arteritis with renovascular hypertension: results of surgical treatment. Cardiovasc Surg 1999;7:626.

Travis JA et al: Aneurysmal degeneration and late rupture of an aortorenal vein graft: case report, review of the literature, and implications for conduit selection. J Vasc Surg 2000;32:612.

van Jaarsveld BC et al: The effect of balloon angioplasty on hypertension in atherosclerotic reinal -artery stenosis. Dutch Renal Artery Stenosis Intervention Cooperative Study Group. N Engl J Med 20001342:1007.

van Rooden CJ et al: Long-term outcome of surgical revascularization in ischemic nephropathy: normalization of average decline in renal function. J Vasc Surg 1999;29:1037.

Woolfson RG: Renal failure in atheroscolerotic renovascular disease: pathogenesis, diagnosis, and intervention. Postgrad Med J 2001;77:68.

Wong JM et al: Surgery after failed percutaneous renal artery angioplasty. J Vasc Surg 1999;30:468.

■ GASTROINTESTINAL ISCHEMIA SYNDROMES

 ESSENTIALS OF DIAGNOSIS

- *Postprandial pain.*
- *Fear of eating.*
- *Weight loss.*
- *Epigastric bruit.*
- *Pain out of proportion to physical findings.*

General Considerations

The celiac axis, the superior and inferior mesenteric arteries, and the two internal iliac arteries are the principal sources of blood supply to the stomach and intestines. The anatomic collateral interconnections between these arteries are numerous and may become quite large. Single or even multiple occlusions are generally well tolerated, because collateral flow is readily available (Figure 35–22).

Chronic stenosis or occlusion of the celiac or superior mesenteric arteries is caused by atherosclerosis in the vast majority of cases. Vasculitis (eg, lupus erythematosus, Takayasu's disease) is the second most common cause. When atherosclerosis is the cause, the usual lesion is a collar or thickened intima that begins in the aorta itself and extends into the orifice of the visceral artery. Associated atherosclerosis in the aorta and its other branches is frequent.

Visceral ischemia due to external compression of the celiac artery, or **median arcuate ligament syndrome,** has been diagnosed most often in women aged 25–50. The existence of this syndrome is controversial.

Acute mesenteric ischemia is a complex and serious disorder. The cause is either embolic or thrombotic. The diagnosis can be difficult and its recognition is often delayed, resulting in irreversible bowel ischemia that requires extensive bowel resection. Patients classically present with excruciating diffuse abdominal pain with a surprising absence of physical findings such as abdominal tenderness or distention—unless actual bowel perforation produces a surgical abdomen. The

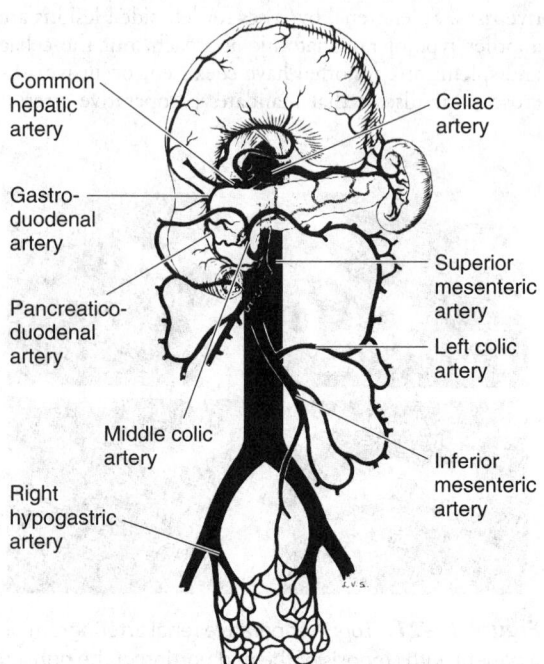

Figure 35–22. Visceral arterial circulation and interconnections.

mortality rate from acute mesenteric ischemia remains high, and patients who require massive bowel resection rarely survive or, if they survive, they develop incapacitating short-gut syndrome. The prognosis improves dramatically if the diagnosis is made expeditiously and if revascularization can be achieved prior to intestinal infarction. Early diagnosis is required for such a successful outcome.

Clinical Findings

The principal complaint is postprandial abdominal pain, which has been labeled abdominal or visceral angina. Pain characteristically appears 15–30 minutes after the beginning of a meal and lasts for an hour or longer. Pain is occasionally so severe and prolonged that opiates are required for relief. Pain occurs as a deep-seated steady ache in the epigastrium, occasionally radiating to the right or left upper quadrant. Weight loss results from reluctance to eat, although mild degrees of malabsorption occur. Thus, gastrointestinal absorption studies are not helpful. Diarrhea and vomiting have been described. An upper abdominal bruit may be heard in over 80% of patients.

Arteriography in the anteroposterior and especially the lateral projections demonstrates both the arterial lesion and the patterns of collateral blood flow (Figure 35–23). Patients should be well hydrated before angiography, because this procedure can precipitate hypercoagulability and osmotic diuresis with dehydration, vascular occlusion, and bowel infarction. Duplex scan-

ning and MRA are used with increasing frequency as less invasive methods of screening.

Treatment

When the obstruction is atherosclerotic, surgical revascularization of the superior mesenteric and celiac axes may be performed by either endarterectomy or graft replacement (Figure 35–23). During endarterectomy, a sleeve of aortic intima and the orifice lesions in the celiac or superior mesenteric arteries are removed. The operation is performed by a retroperitoneal approach to the aorta through a left thoracoabdominal incision. Alternatively, a Dacron graft may be brought from the lower thoracic aorta to the celiac axis or superior mesenteric artery—an operation that is performed from within the abdomen. External compression of the celiac artery by the median arcuate ligament may be relieved by simple division of the ligament in 50% of cases, but simultaneous arterial reconstruction produces the best results. Operation should be avoided in patients with acute vasculitis as the underlying cause of mesenteric ischemia; high-dose steroids and immunosuppressive agents are indicated instead.

In addition, PTA and stenting has gained acceptance as an alternative form of therapy for both chronic and acute mesenteric ischemia. Results are best for focal, nonorificial stenoses.

Prognosis

Surgery for atherosclerotic visceral artery insufficiency almost always results in relief of symptoms if a technically adequate operation is accomplished. If operation is not performed, death will occur from inanition or massive bowel infarction.

Patients with median arcuate ligament compression respond favorably to operation in the majority of instances; however, some of these patients are not improved even though a technically adequate operation is performed.

Figure 35–23. *Left:* Preoperative visceral arteriogram showing severe stenosis of the celiac and superior mesenteric arteries. *Right:* The postoperative visceral arteriogram shows wide patency of the celiac and superior mesenteric arteries after transaortic endarterectomy. The inset shows the atherosclerotic stenotic lesions removed by endarterectomy

Farber MA et al: Distal thoracic aorta as inflow for the treatment of chronic mesenteric ischemia. J Vasc Surg 2001;33:281.

Foley MI et al: Revascularization of the superior mesenteric artery alone for treatment of intestinal ischemia. J Vasc Surg 2000;32:37.

Geelkerken RH et al: Duplex ultrasound examination of splanchnic vessels in the assessment of splanchnic ishaemic symptoms. Eur J Vasc Endovasc Surg 1999;18:371.

Kazmers A: Operative management of chronic mesenteric ischemia. Ann Vasc Surg 1998;12:299.

Leduc FJ et al: Acute mesenteric ischaemia: minimal invasive management by combined laparoscopy and percutaneous transluminal angioplasty. Eur J Surg 2000;166:345.

Mateo RB et al: Elective surgical treatment of symptomatic chronic mesenteric occlusive disease: early results and late outcomes. J Vasc Surg 1999;29:821.

Meaney JF: Non-invasive evaluation of the visceral arteries with magnetic resonance angiography. Eur Radiol 1999;9:1267.

Schulte KM et al: Coral reef aorta: a long-term study of 21 patients. Ann Vasc Surg 2000;14:626.

Vicente DC et al: Acute mesenteric ischemia. Cuff Opin Cardiol 1999;14:453.

■ INTRA-ARTERIAL INJECTIONS & IATROGENIC ARTERIAL TRAUMA

Intra-arterial injections are seen frequently among intravenous drug abusers. Brachial and femoral injections are most frequent. The patient experiences severe burning pain in the affected arterial distribution, followed by intense vasoconstriction and in many cases thrombosis with gangrene of digits or of the entire extremity. In lesser insults, after the period of vasospasm, the extremity becomes swollen and discolored. When intra-arterial injection is recognized, if the needle is still in place, the artery should be copiously irrigated with heparinized saline. Intra-arterial vasodilators (eg, nitroglycerin, papaverine, tolazoline) may be useful to alleviate vasospasm. The patient usually presents late. Infection, pseudoaneurysm formation, and chemical endarteritis are late complications. Various regimens have been advocated—anticoagulants, sympathectomy, dextran, corticosteroids—with mixed results. At present, heparinization is the recommended immediate management. Late complications such as infected pseudoaneurysm formation are often best treated by excision and ligation—in many cases without extra-anatomic revascularization—but with reliance on collateral blood flow to maintain tissue viability.

The marked increase in performance of percutaneous catheter-based vascular interventions combined with anticoagulation regimens has resulted in a greater frequency of peripheral arterial pseudoaneurysms and arteriovenous fistulas. Most of these iatrogenic injuries are self-limited and will resolve spontaneously over time, especially after systemic anticoagulation is discontinued. Emergent operation is rarely indicated unless the iatrogenic arterial trauma results in distal ischemia, severe infection, continuing major hemorrhage, or local integumentary or neurologic compromise. Observation is usually the best treatment for iatrogenic pseudoaneurysms or arteriovenous fistulas. Ultrasound-guided compression and percutaneous duplex-guided thrombin injection are occasionally successful, but their precise roles remain to be determined. A particularly challenging iatrogenic vascular injury is related to technical problems engendered by the use of percutaneous vascular suturing devices employed after percutaneous arterial procedures.

Hye RJ: Compression therapy for acute iatrogenic femoral pseudoaneurysms. Semin Vasc Surg 2000;13:58

Nehler MR et al: Iatrogenic vascular injuries from percutaneous vascular suturing devices. J Vasc Surg 2001;33:943.

Nehler MR et al: Iatrogenic vascular trauma. Semin Vasc Surg 1998;11:283.

O'Sullivan GJ et al: A review of alternative approaches in the management of iatrogenic femoral pseudoaneurysms. Ann R Coll Surg Engl 1999;81:226.

Reddy DJ et al: Infected femoral artery false aneurysms in drug addicts: evolution of selective vascular reconstruction. J Vasc Surg 1986;3:718.

Ting AC et al: Femoral pseudoaneurysms in drug addicts. World J Surg 1997;21:783.

Vermeulen EG et al: Percutaneous duplex-guided thrombin injection for treatment of iatrogenic femoral artery pseudoaneurysms. Eur J Vasc Endovasc Surg 2000;20:302.

Amputation

William C. Krupski, MD, & Mark R. Nehler, MD

Amputations are sometimes necessary as part of surgical care for disorders involving the upper and lower extremities. Amputation may have several goals depending on the indications for operation and the condition or functional status of the patient. These goals have variable success rates and priorities—again contingent on the indication for surgery and the patient population. Amputations have four aims: (1) The removal of all diseased tissue—but this is not always achieved with the initial amputation, particularly when performed for ischemic or infectious disease. (2) The relief of pain is critical—but this may not be achieved because of healing failures and chronic pain syndromes (eg, phantom limb pain and reflex sympathetic dystrophy). (3) Primary healing of the amputation wound is desirable but may not be accomplished because of infection or efforts to maintain limb length. (4) Construction of a stump that will permit the most useful function with or without prosthetic fitting is most consequential in functional patients. Many minimally functional elderly patients develop breakdown and pressure necrosis of their distal lower extremities primarily from inactivity in combination with ischemia. Amputations in these patients are often performed more proximally to ensure healing.

Toe amputations and major leg amputations (transtibial and transfemoral) are common surgical procedures. In contrast, more proximal leg amputations (hip disarticulations, hemipelvectomy) and upper extremity amputations are uncommon. Toe amputations are performed by surgeons of varied specialties, including podiatrists, orthopedic surgeons, and vascular surgeons. Transtibial and transfemoral amputations are usually performed by vascular or orthopedic surgeons. Orthopedic or plastic reconstructive surgeons customarily perform more proximal lower extremity amputations and major upper extremity amputations.

As the average age of the population has risen, the incidence of peripheral arterial disease and diabetes mellitus has increased. More than 90% of the 110,000 amputations performed in the USA each year are for ischemic or infective gangrene. More than half of lower extremity amputations are performed for vascular and infectious complications of diabetes mellitus, and 15–50% of diabetic amputees will lose a second leg within 5 years. This risk is about two times higher for men than for women. Other indications for amputations are nondiabetic infection with ischemia (15–25%), ischemia without infection (5–10%), osteomyelitis (3–5%), trauma (2–5%), and frostbite, tumors, neuromas, and other miscellaneous causes (5–10%).

Many patients facing amputation are near the end of life because of systemic cardiovascular disease. Approximately 20–30% of patients undergoing major amputation (below-knee or above-knee) will be dead within 2 years. The prevalence of many comorbidities in this population is also reflected in the perioperative mortality rates for major amputation, ranging from 5% to 10% for below-knee amputations to 10% or higher for above-knee amputations. In addition, failure of primary below-knee amputation healing ranges from 30% to 90%. Although major amputations do not receive the notoriety of higher-profile operations, they are difficult procedures with higher morbidity and mortality rates than many of the other commonplace major operations.

Level of Amputation

The level of amputation is determined by assessing the likelihood of healing of the limb in association with the functional potential of the patient. Extensive myocutaneous free flap grafting to maintain a below-knee amputation and preserve the use of the knee joint may be appropriate in a young patient with limb loss related to extensive trauma. Conversely, a demented elderly nursing home patient with mild ischemia and heel pressure necrosis may be better treated with a primary above knee amputation to avoid a knee flexion contracture despite adequate blood supply for healing of a below knee-amputation. In general, the knee joint should be preserved if possible in patients who can be rehabilitated. The clinical conundrum in patients with limb ischemia is twofold: (1) determining which limbs have adequate blood supply to heal at the below-knee level and (2) determining which patients with vascular disease have reasonable rehabilitation potential. There is no way of answering either question with confidence.

Technical decisions regarding amputation level are based on adequacy of blood flow, extent of tissue necrosis, and location of tumor. In the upper extremities, circulatory impairment is rare. In the lower extremities, in which impairment is more likely to occur, the circulatory status at different levels may be determined by measurement of the peripheral pulses and the capillary refill time and by noting the presence of rubor, the condition of the skin, and the presence of ischemic atrophy. At present, no single measurement of blood flow can reliably predict the best level of healing. Extremely low or absent blood flow predicts nonhealing, and normal flow predicts healing. However, in most cases the prediction falls in between. The best predictions are based on clinical assessment by an experienced surgeon, assisted by one of the several techniques for determining amputation level. In patients with distinct lines of demarcation (eg, with gangrene) and in those with tumors, the amount of tissue that must be removed is usually more obvious.

For most patients with ambulatory potential, as long a limb as possible should be preserved in order to maintain nearly normal walking with the least expenditure of energy. Compared with normal walking, energy expenditure is increased 10–40% with a transtibial prosthesis, 50–70% with a transfemoral prosthesis, and 60% with crutches. One obvious way to reduce energy cost is to reduce the velocity. The average speed of ambulation for a normal adult is 4.8 km/h, compared with 3.2–4 km/h for a transtibial amputee and 2.4 km/h for a transfemoral amputee.

Determination of Amputation Level

A. CLINICAL EXAMINATION

The presence of palpable pedal pulses in a warm, pink limb is a reliable indicator that arterial flow is adequate to support healing of a below-knee amputation. Conversely, an absent ipsilateral femoral pulse is associated with an 80% chance of failure of a primary below-transtibial amputation. In general, the presence of a palpable pulse in the major artery immediately above the amputation site (eg, femoral pulse for above-knee, popliteal pulse for below-knee) indicates a high probability of amputation primary healing, and absence of a palpable pulse in these locations significantly reduces the likelihood of amputation healing.

B. MEASUREMENT OF BLOOD PRESSURE

In addition to clinical assessment, measurement of blood pressure in the thigh and ankle with a doppler ultrasound device and pneumatic cuffs is a useful technique for determining the level of amputation. Readings are not accurate enough, however, to be the sole basis for decision making. Segmental blood pressures are fallible, and blood pressure in the ankle is an unreliable guide to healing in the foot if the tibial vessels are calcified and cannot be compressed by the cuff, a condition reported in at least

20–25% of diabetics. In addition, significant lower extremity edema hinders accurate measurements. The notion that above-knee amputation is mandatory if the blood pressure in the ankle is below 60 mm Hg is unwarranted. This technique does not adequately demonstrate collateral circulation, and healing is common even when ankle pressures are extremely low or undetectable. Absence of an arterial flow signal in the popliteal space, however, reliably predicts that transtibial amputation will fail to heal.

C. OXYGEN TENSION MEASUREMENTS

Transcutaneous measurement of oxygen tension (using a modified Clark-type oxygen electrode) is another guide to healing. A transcutaneous PaO_2 of zero indicates a high probability that healing will be unsatisfactory at that site, whereas a PaO_2 above 40 mm Hg indicates that good healing is likely. Intermediate values do not correlate closely with the degree of healing. Transcutaneous PaO_2 measurement is noninvasive and very reproducible. Disadvantages of the technique are the expense of the equipment and the time required for examination (about 30 minutes per site). It is important to heat the skin to 44 °C, which causes a temperature-dependent microstructural change in the lipid phase of the stratum corneum from solid to liquid.

D. OTHER MEASURES OF SKIN PERFUSION

Multiple techniques are available to assess the skin perfusion for determination of the optimal amputation level. Most of these methods have not gained widespread use in clinical practice. Problems with these techniques include impracticality, expense, and technical difficulty—and inconsistent confirmatory studies.

1. Xenon Xe 133 studies—Clearance of Xe 133 injected intradermally predicts successful below-knee amputation in 97% of patients when rates of > 2.6 mL/min/100 g of tissue are present and in < 50% of patients when flow rates are < 2 mL/min/100 g of tissue. Because the technique is complex and invasive, it has remained a research tool only. Moreover, pharmaceutical-grade sterile xenon is not commercially available.

2. Laser doppler studies—Laser doppler is a noninvasive technique to determine the velocity of blood flow in the skin microcirculation. This method is popular in Europe but has not been extensively used in North America. Absence of flow reliably predicts nonhealing, but specific flow velocities have not been differentiated.

3. Skin fluorescence—Intravenous injection of fluorescein dye followed by measurements of skin fluorescence with a fluorometer have been reported to predict healing with 80% accuracy. Fluorometers are commercially available, but this technique has not gained widespread application.

4. Skin perfusion pressure—Photoelectric measurement of skin perfusion pressure involves positioning a blood pressure cuff over a photoelectric detector that is connected to a plethysmograph. The external pressure required to prevent skin hyperemia after blanching is recorded. A skin perfusion pressure of 20 mm Hg or higher predicts healing with 80% accuracy.

5. Skin temperature—Infrared thermography has been correlated with skin blood flow. A single report demonstrated a 94% positive predictive value but only an 11% negative predictive value.

E. ARTERIOGRAPHY

Arteriography provides anatomic, not physiologic information. It assesses feasibility of vascular reconstructions but is of little value in selecting the amputation site because findings do not correlate with circulation to the skin. Arteriography provides anatomic information, not physiologic data.

Preparation for Amputation

No pharmacologic treatment can forestall amputation; however, patients must be adequately prepared for operation. Diabetes mellitus, heart failure, and infection should be controlled. Material from sites of potential infection should be cultured and appropriate antibiotics administered preoperatively. In the presence of infection or a necrotic tumor, the first step should be a debriding (guillotine-type) amputation and continued antibiotics. A definitive amputation with primary closure of the wound can be performed 5–7 days later.

Malnutrition adversely affects the healing of amputation sites, and serum albumin levels and total lymphocyte counts correlate with success rates. Assuming that the amputation level is appropriate, healing occurs in 80% of patients when serum albumin is at least 3.5 g/mL and total lymphocyte count is at least 1500 cells/μL, but in less than 30% of patients when values are lower.

When patients are so critically ill that they cannot tolerate a general or regional anesthetic, a "medical amputation" can be used as a temporary measure. This involves placing a tourniquet at the level of amputation and packing the distal extremity in ice, thereby diminishing the systemic metabolic effects of profound ischemia.

Urgent or Emergency Amputation

A. ACUTE ARTERIAL OCCLUSION

Arterial flow can be restored surgically in most patients with acute arterial occlusion, but when flow cannot be restored or when the patient's presentation or the diagnosis is delayed beyond viability, urgent or emergency amputation is required. The most reliable sign of nonliability on physical examination is rigor of the involved muscle bed. The degree of urgency is determined by the extent of ischemia, the mass of ischemic muscle, the amount of pain, and the presence of systemic toxicity and infection. If there is little ischemic or necrotic tissue, amputation may be deferred until demarcation between viable and nonviable tissue becomes evident; this usually takes a day or two. This allows for maximum development of collateral circulation and increases the chances that a limited amputation will heal. When circulatory improvement stops or if toxicity develops, amputation should be performed promptly. The more extensive the tissue destruction, the greater the risk of serious toxicity when amputation is delayed. Myoglobinuria and renal dysfunction are early signs of toxicity. Mental confusion, sepsis, and deterioration of vital signs are late findings. All should mandate emergency amputation, usually above or through the knee.

B. INJURY

In patients with massively injured or crushed extremities, early amputation may greatly shorten the time required for successful rehabilitation. There are several scoring systems for determining the advisability of immediate amputation after major extremity trauma. The most popular is designated MESS (Mangled Extremity Severity Score). In brief, severe major nerve injury in conjunction with bone, soft tissue, and vascular injury warrants consideration of primary amputation, because a neurologically useless extremity is not worth salvaging. In addition, the incidence of postamputation chronic phantom pain syndrome increases the longer a chronically painful posttraumatic limb goes without proper treatment. Whereas plantar sensation is the minimum degree of neural function required for the lower extremity to function, a compromised upper extremity can frequently function better than currently available prostheses. Although severity scores are helpful, the decision to amputate in marginal cases can be postponed until the extremity is clearly nonviable or insensate.

■ SPECIFIC TYPES OF AMPUTATIONS

LOWER EXTREMITY AMPUTATIONS

Obviously, all patients and physicians wish to avoid limb loss. However, with modern prosthetic equipment, improvements in the functional usefulness of wheelchairs, and legislation (Americans With Disabilities Act) mandating wheelchair access to most public facilities, an amputee can be more mobile after than before the procedure. The goals of amputation vary depending on the functional status of the patient.

Lower extremity amputations are done most commonly at one of the following levels: toe (called digit amputations, which may be extended to include resection of the metatarsal and called ray amputations), transmetatarsal, below-knee, and above-knee. Amputations at other levels (Syme's amputation, Chopart's amputation, knee disarticulation, and hip disarticulation) are infrequently performed, usually to treat conditions other than vascular disease.

1. Toe & Ray Amputations

Toes are the most frequently amputated parts of the body. Over two-thirds of amputations in diabetics involve the toes and forefoot. The indications include gangrene, infection, neuropathic ulceration, frostbite, and osteomyelitis limited to the middle or distal phalanx. Good blood flow is required.

Contraindications to digit amputation include indistinct demarcation, infection at the metatarsal level, dependent rubor, and ischemia of the forefoot. Important principles pertaining to digit and ray amputations include the following:

(1) The first metatarsal head is important for patient balance and should be preserved if possible.

(2) Amputation that leaves only one or two remaining digits (unless the first) does not facilitate normal foot function but complicates functional footwear. Patients often develop pressure lesions of the remaining digits due to neuropathy.

(3) Resection of metatarsal heads in diabetic patients with malperforans ulcers often transfers the pressure point responsible for the initial lesion to the adjacent metatarsal head. Therefore, without adequate protection with orthotic shoes or inserts (along with patient compliance), recurrence of these lesions is the rule rather than the exception. This is particularly likely in obese diabetic patients. Several clinical series of toe amputations in diabetic patients have demonstrated the necessity of another toe amputation in up to two-thirds of cases, and below-knee amputation was eventually required in 15–20% of patients.

(4) Digit and ray amputations should be carried out through the shafts of bones because joint cartilage will secrete fluid into the wound and retard healing.

(5) Tendons are avascular structures and should be divided as proximally as possible.

For dry, uninfected gangrene of one or more toes, **autoamputation** may be allowed to occur. During this process, epithelialization occurs beneath the eschar, and the toe spontaneously detaches, leaving a clean residual limb at the most distal site. Although preferable in many patients (and especially frostbit patients), autoamputation sometimes requires months to complete.

Ray or wedge amputation includes removal of the toe and metatarsal head; occasionally, two adjacent toes may be amputated by this method. As with toe amputation, there is modest cosmetic deformity and a prosthesis is not required. Ray amputation of the great toe leads to unstable weight bearing and some difficulty with ambulation resulting from loss of the first metatarsal head.

The extents of toe and ray amputations are shown in Figure 36–1. For distal resections, a circular incision is made at the midpoint of the proximal phalanx, and the phalanx is resected at about its midpoint. If it is necessary to remove the entire phalanx or to excise the distal portion of the metatarsal, the incision is extended proximally over the metatarsal, and the bone is divided behind the metatarsal head. Not uncommonly, the incision must be left open to heal by second intention owing to the presence of local infection.

Complications that may require amputation at higher levels include infection, osteomyelitis of remaining bone, and nonhealing of the incision. These complications have been reported in up to one-third of diabetic patients.

Figure 36–1. Toe and ray amputation.

2. Transmetatarsal Amputation

Transmetatarsal forefoot amputations preserve normal weight bearing. The principal indication is gangrene of several toes or the great toe, with or without soft tissue infection or osteomyelitis. The gangrene should have spread beyond a level that could be treated by a two-ray amputation; there must be no evidence of spreading infection within the foot; and the plantar skin must be healthy. Patients who do not meet these criteria require a higher amputation.

The incision creates a generous plantar flap (Figure 36–2). There is no dorsal flap. On the plantar surface, the incision is continued medially to laterally just proximal to the metatarsophalangeal crease. The metatarsal bones are divided with the medial and lateral shafts cut shorter than those in the middle to preserve the normal architecture of the foot and assist with orthotic fitting postoperatively, and the tendons are pulled down and transected as high as possible.

Transmetatarsal amputation produces an excellent functional result. Walking requires no increase in energy expenditure, and the gait is usually smooth. A prosthesis is not mandatory, but to achieve optimal gait, the shoes must be modified. Lamb's wool or custom-molded foam can be used to fill the toe portion of the shoe. A spring steel shank in the sole of the shoe approximates the action of the longitudinal foot arch during the toe-off phase of walking.

Open transmetatarsal amputations are occasionally necessary in the presence of infection. After the wound has contracted, a split-thickness skin graft may be used for skin coverage. The prosthetic fitting and rehabilitation of these patients are delayed and more difficult, because preservation of the skin graft becomes a primary concern. An ankle-foot orthosis may be necessary.

Chopart's amputation (transtarsal amputation of the forefoot through the talonavicular-calcaneo-cuboid joint), **Lisfranc's amputation** (through the tarsometatarsal joint), and **Piroff's amputation** (removal of the talus and rotation of the calcaneus) are unpopular procedures because they produce an imbalance in the remaining muscles of the foot. This results in equinovarus deformity of the foot, with a tender scar and unsatisfactory weight bearing. The Achilles tendon can be transected in an attempt to improve the situation. Ambulation in these patients is somewhat limited. However, limb salvage may be greater when unconventional foot amputations are used.

3. Syme's Amputation

Syme's amputation is a modification of disarticulation through the ankle joint. Trauma of the forefoot with good vascularity of the heel and ankle are the chief indications for this procedure. It is rarely performed except in young trauma patients. Spreading infection in the spaces of the foot, gangrene involving the heel pad, advanced ischemia of the foot, and a neurotropic foot with absence of heel sensation are contraindications to Syme's amputation.

Syme's amputation is the most technically demanding lower extremity amputation, and strict attention to surgical detail is crucial for success. The incision is shown in Figure 36–3. During the operation, particular

Figure 36–2. Transmetatarsal amputation.

Figure 36–3. Syme's amputation.

attention must be paid to preserving the posterior tibial vessels, which supply the heel pad and inferior margins of the wound. The calcaneus must be dissected from the heel pad with great care in order to avoid injury to the soft tissues of the heel flap. The malleoli are resected flush with the joint surface, and the bones are trimmed so there are no pressure points. These last steps may be delayed for 6–8 weeks and performed as a second-stage procedure.

Syme's amputation produces an end-bearing residual limb and leaves a lower extremity only several inches shorter than normal, thus allowing the patient to walk short distances on safe surfaces without a prosthesis. A prosthesis is not essential, and the patient can wear a cup slipper around the house. A cosmetic prosthesis employs a lightweight foot with a plastic shell into which the amputated limb fits. It is more difficult to fit than a conventional transtibial prosthesis and therefore requires an experienced prosthetist for ultimate success. Walking speed is decreased, but energy consumption is increased very little.

4. Major Leg Amputation

Despite efforts to preserve limb length for rehabilitation purposes, the ratio of above-knee to below-knee amputations is roughly 1.0 and has not changed in several decades. Preservation of the knee joint reduces the oxygen consumption required to ambulate from 60% above baseline levels to 40%. Although young trauma patients undergoing an above-knee amputation may eventually be able to walk, an elderly patient after transfemoral amputation rarely does so. An attempt at performing a below-knee amputation is warranted in almost any patient who appears to be a potential candidate for rehabilitation.

The morbidity and mortality for major limb amputation is substantial, primarily due to the systemic disease burden of the patient population. Mortality rates range from 5% to 30% and are generally highest in patients undergoing above-knee amputations since these patients are the least functional and most ill. Perioperative myocardial infarction is the most common cause of death. Deep venous thrombosis occurs in 10–15% of patients and may be present prior to amputation because of the sedentary state of these patients both preoperatively and postoperatively.

Difficulty in accurately predicting healing has led to a discrepancy in reported healing rates—ranging from 30% to 90%—for below-knee amputations. One-third of patients having below-knee amputations require reamputation. Approximately half of the below-knee amputations that do not heal will require conversion to the above-knee level. Patients undergoing amputation for acute severe infections have wound infections or breakdown of the amputation stump in up to two-thirds of cases. These patients should have primary guillotine amputation as a preliminary step to clear the infectious process before a definitive below-knee stump is created.

Absolute indications for primary above-knee amputation include contracture at the knee joint (observed in debilitated patients with long-standing extremity pain who have been in a prolonged withdrawal posture with the knee flexed) and nonviable calf muscle or skin for creation of the below-knee flap. Primary above-knee amputation is relatively contraindicated in patients who are not candidates for rehabilitation. The frequent failure of healing of below-knee amputation, the higher perioperative morbidity and mortality in this population (making secondary operations more dangerous), and the modest functional benefit of preserving the knee joint in a nonambulatory patient are the major arguments in favor of primary above-knee procedures in such cases.

Amputations can be performed using proximal tourniquets. This offers the advantage of minimizing blood loss, particularly in an infected hyperemic limb. Regional anesthesia is frequently used, but there is scant evidence that this decreases perioperative mortality compared with general anesthesia. Blood transfusions are rarely required since the potential for significant hemorrhage is modest.

Guillotine amputations are simple circular incisions usually just above the ankle (which can be more proximal if necessary) that are carried through sharply to divide all structures at that level (hence the name). Absolute indications for guillotine amputation include severe foot infections that preclude limb salvage. Necrotizing diabetic foot infections with or without gross purulence are the most frequent indication. Removing the grossly infected foot allows the lymphatics to be cleared of infection and reduces the risk of below-knee stump infection. Most surgeons do not perform guillotine amputations prior to an above-knee amputation because the distance from the infection source is felt to be relatively protective. The calf muscles should be compressed to reveal purulence that may have tracked proximally, most commonly in the anterior compartment. The major tibial vessels are oversewn at the end of the stump, and the wound is dressed. Controlling the tibial vasculature can be difficult, particularly in young diabetic patients with normal circulation. The wound is then examined in 48 hours to determine if the infectious process has been controlled. If that is so, a formal below-knee amputation is then performed.

The most common procedure for below-knee amputation is the Burgess technique, which utilizes a long posterior flap.

The blood supply to a posterior flap is generally better than the supply to an anterior flap or to sagittal flaps, because the sural arteries (which supply the gastrocnemius and soleus muscles) arise high on the popliteal artery, an area not often diseased, whereas the more distal popliteal artery or tibial arteries are often diseased, especially in diabetics.

The use of rigid dressings and immediate postoperative prostheses has proved advantageous. Application of a rigid cast bandage has several potential advantages: (1) It controls postoperative edema, which may reduce pain; (2) it protects the stump from trauma, particularly when a patient falls during attempts at mobilization; and (3) it allows the patient to be ambulatory with a temporary prosthesis much sooner. The disadvantages include cost and personnel time to apply the rigid bandages and lack of patient compliance. A single randomized trial in vascular patients did not demonstrate a difference in wound complications with rigid dressings compared with standard bandages.

Use of immediate postoperative prostheses provides two advantages: (1) a rigid dressing and (2) early ambulation. The rigid dressing controls edema, improves healing, prevents joint contractures, and protects from trauma. Early ambulation decreases hospital stay, increases rates of rehabilitation, decreases complications of prolonged bed rest (eg, decubitus ulcers, pneumonia, pulmonary emboli), and improves the patient's psychologic outlook.

The skin flaps are shown in Figure 36–4. The anterior incision is made approximately 7–10 cm below the tibial tuberosity and carried to the midpoint of the leg both medially and laterally. After the muscles of the anterior compartment have been transected, the fibula and tibia are divided, and the tibia is beveled to avoid a sharp projection beneath the skin. The posterior flap is wedge-shaped and contains soleus muscle, gastrocnemius muscle, and skin; it is fashioned to avoid tension when the wound is closed and to provide a generous pad over the distal residual limb. Drains are generally not required for amputations performed for vascular disease, because bleeding is minimal, but they are often necessary for amputations performed for trauma or tumor.

Above-knee amputation may be performed at several levels, including knee disarticulation; the patient is left without a functional knee. Knee disarticulation amputation is technically more demanding than transfemoral amputation at a higher level. When fashioning an above-knee stump, one should preserve as long a lever arm as possible; amputation in the lower thigh is preferable to amputation in the mid or upper thigh.

The technique is straightforward. Short anterior and posterior flaps, sagittal flaps, or a circular incision may

Figure 36–4. Below-knee amputation.

be used. The bone is divided slightly higher than the skin and soft tissue to avoid tension when the wound is closed. A simple dressing is then applied.

5. Hip Disarticulation

Most dysvascular patients requiring high amputations can be successfully treated with transfemoral amputation. Hip disarticulation is reserved for the few dysvascular patients in whom transfemoral amputation fails or who have tumors of the thigh or lower femur. Life-threatening infection that cannot be controlled by hip disarticulation is almost uniformly fatal.

An anterior racket-shaped incision or a long posterior flap can be developed to cover the large defect created by a hip disarticulation. In the presence of vascular insufficiency, the flaps may have to be modified to achieve a closure that heals primarily. The muscles, nerves, and capsule of the hip joint are incised, and the disarticulation is completed by division of the ligamentum teres.

Most of these patients cannot be rehabilitated, but vigorous efforts should be made to rehabilitate selected well-motivated individuals, especially young patients who have undergone operation for tumor.

6. Hemipelvectomy

Hemipelvectomy (hindquarter amputation) is reserved for patients with malignant tumors of the lower extremity or pelvis that cannot be removed by lesser procedures. The classic operation involves removal of the entire lower extremity and varying amounts of the innominate bone (Figure 36–5). If the iliac bone is removed completely, the procedure is termed radical; in conservative hemipelvectomy, part of the iliac bone attached to the sacrum is left in place. Internal hemipelvectomy is the procedure in which the innominate bone and surrounding musculature are removed and the lower extremity is preserved.

The incision for hemipelvectomy is determined by the site of the tumor. For posteriorly placed tumors, an anterior flap of skin, subcutaneous tissue, and fascia lata based on the femoral vessels is appropriate. Alternatively, quadriceps muscle can be used for a myocutaneous flap. Rectus abdominis island flaps and thigh flaps based on the femoral vessels have also been used to close the defect after a hindquarter amputation. In some cases, a combination of Marlex mesh and skin graft may be applied over such defects.

Figure 36–5. Hemipelvectomy.

The operative mortality rate for hindquarter amputation is about 3%, but complications occur in about 50% of cases. Five-year survival rates depend on the kind of tumor and stage of disease at the time of operation. The 5-year survival rate is 75% after hemipelvectomy for fibrosarcomas and chondrosarcomas; few patients with malignant melanoma are alive after 5 years.

UPPER EXTREMITY AMPUTATIONS

The indications for amputation of upper extremities are much different from those of lower extremities because advanced atherosclerosis is unusual in the upper extremity. Upper extremity amputations are most often performed for severe trauma or malignant tumors. Conditions causing arterial ischemia in upper extremities that may require amputation include thromboangitis obliterans, connective tissue disorders, accidental intra-arterial injection of drugs, and diabetic patients with long-standing end-stage renal disease.

Microsurgical techniques now allow previously hopeless cases of traumatic amputation to be treated by **replantation.** Function following replantation of the thumb and other digits is good; after replantation of the palm, wrist, or forearm, function is less satisfactory, but an attempt at limb salvage is warranted in selected cases, especially in children. The advantages and disadvantages of amputation and replantation must be weighed: with amputation, there is a cosmetic defect but a relatively short period of rehabilitation; with replantation, there is normal appearance but a long, costly rehabilitation period.

It is advisable to preserve as much length as possible when performing amputations in the upper extremity. Good skin coverage must be obtained, but length should not be sacrificed for the sake of skin closure; split-thickness skin grafts, musculocutaneous flaps, and skin traction can all help in complex situations. In the hand, maintenance of length should be based on functional considerations (Figure 36–6).

Usefulness of the upper extremity prosthesis is limited by diminished sensory and proprioceptive feedback; thus, auditory and visual control of the prosthesis is required. Limited "gadget tolerance" and high costs due to low demand reduce the availability of electric-powered prostheses. Prostheses with elbow joints and terminal devices activated by body power are generally more acceptable to amputees.

Traumatic amputations do not have to be treated definitively at the initial debridement. Expectant management will permit questionably viable tissues to demarcate and thereby allow maximal preservation of length. When deciding whether to amputate an injured extremity, the physician should assess the status of five structures: skin, tendons, nerves, bones, and joints. If

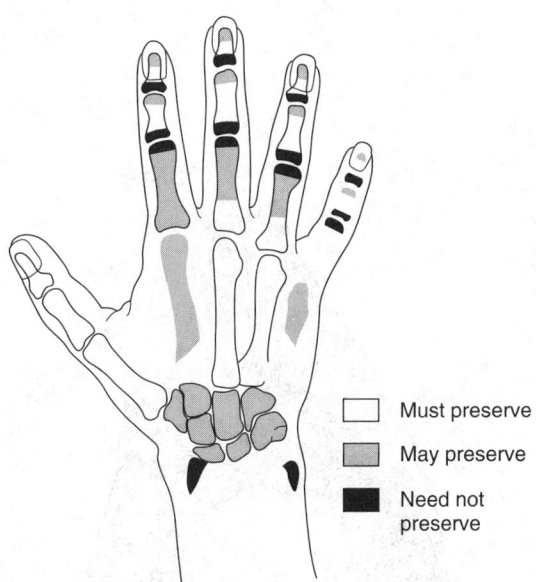

□ Must preserve

▨ May preserve

■ Need not preserve

Figure 36–6. Amputation in the hand.

three or more are compromised, amputation is usually favored over attempts at preserving the part.

1. Wrist Disarticulation

After amputation below the elbow, only about 50% of the ability to perform pronation and supination can be transmitted to a prosthesis, because of the bulk of the proximal forearm and the length of the remaining radius and ulna. The more proximal the amputation, the less pronation and supination is possible. Amputations through the wrist permit the most pronation and supination and provide for better prosthetic control than higher amputations do.

2. Forearm Amputation

Even if only a short residual limb can be achieved, forearm amputation is preferable to above-elbow amputation. As much muscle function as possible should be preserved to maximize control of a prosthesis. Several innovative reconstructive procedures are available that allow upper arm muscles to assist in controlling a prosthesis when a very short residual limb precludes pronation and supination by forearm muscles.

3. Transhumeral Amputation

Every effort should be made to preserve length. Even if a very high amputation is necessary, the head of the humerus should be spared, since it serves as a support for a prosthesis and maintains shoulder width.

4. Forequarter Amputation

Malignant tumor is the usual indication for forequarter amputation. The operation is easiest if done from a posterior approach, but the location and size of the mass may require an anterior approach (Figure 36–7). A thoracotomy or partial neck dissection may be necessary to resect the tumor completely. After the wound has healed, a Silastic foam shoulder cap held in place with straps provides a cosmetically acceptable shoulder.

■ SPECIAL PROBLEMS OF AMPUTEES

Thromboembolism

The amputee is at great risk for deep venous thrombosis (15%) and pulmonary embolism (2%) postoperatively because (1) amputation often follows prolonged immobilization during treatment of the primary disease and (2) the operation involves ligation of large veins, causing stagnation of blood, a situation that predisposes to thrombosis. If immediate-fit prosthetic techniques are not employed, an additional period of inactivity follows the operation, further increasing the risk of thromboembolism.

Pain & Flexion Contracture

Flexion contractures of the knee or hip occur rapidly in the painful limb because of the natural tendency to assume a flexed posture. Measures to prevent contracture are indicated preoperatively, and application of a rigid dressing postoperatively decreases the incidence of this complication.

Persistent pain in a residual limb and phantom limb pain are common. If the cause of pain is residual limb ischemia, higher amputation is the treatment. A neuroma in a residual limb can be treated by injection of a local anesthetic or excision of the neuroma. Causalgia may respond to sympathectomy. Continuous nerve sheath block using catheters placed adjacent to the transected nerve trunks at the time of surgery may reduce early postoperative pain and late phantom pain. However, introduction of infection by the catheters is a concern.

Phantom limb pain is the sensation that a painful limb is present after amputation. Most amputees experience this phenomenon to some degree. Hypotheses concerning etiology include the gate theory (loss of sen-

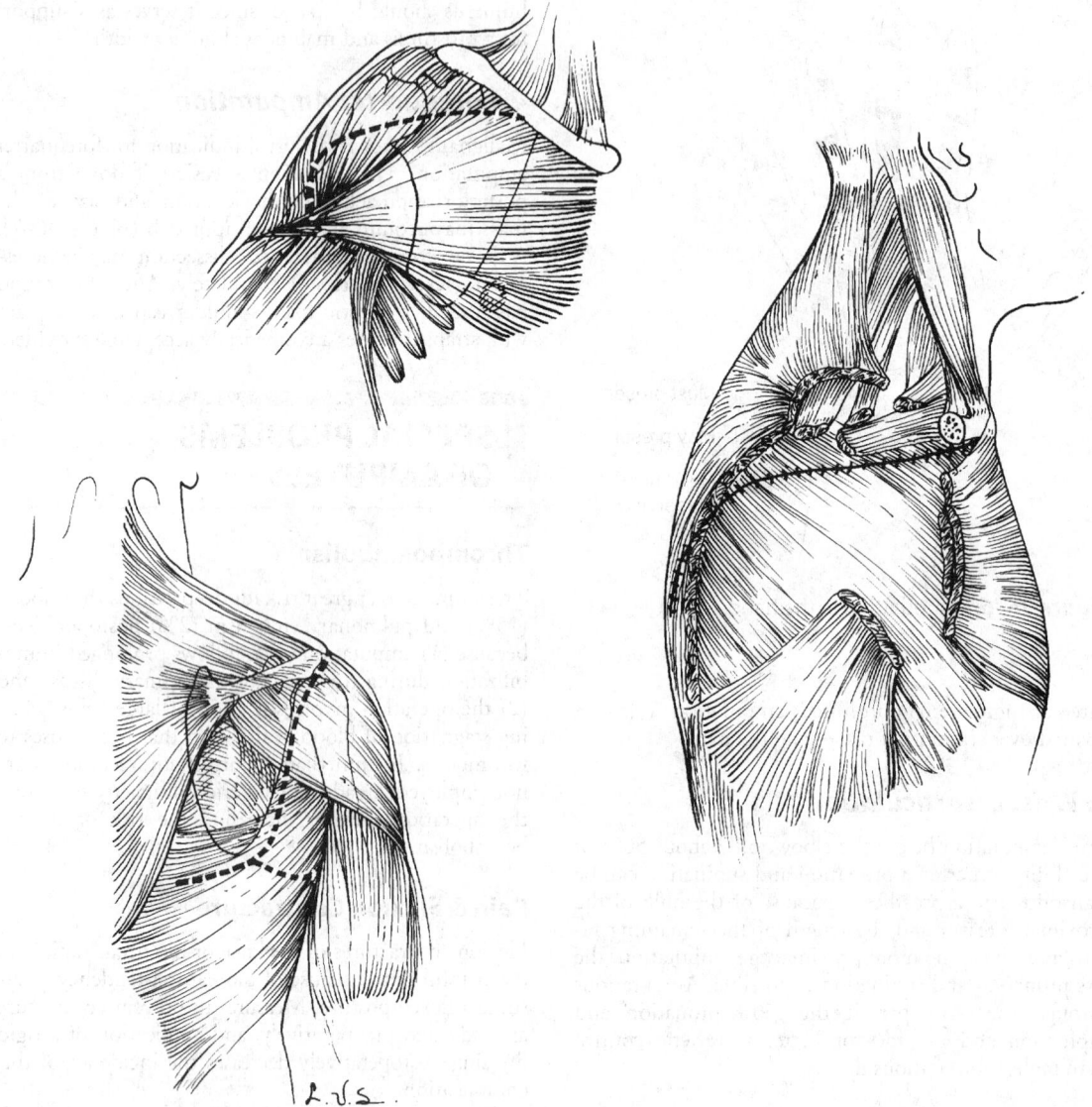

Figure 36–7. Forequarter amputation

sory input decreases self-sustaining neural activity of the gate, causing pain), the peripheral theory (nerve endings in the residual limb represent parts originally innervated by the severed nerve), and the psychologic theory (hostility, guilt, and denial are interpreted as pain). Treatment is difficult; improvement has been reported using tricyclic antidepressants, transcutaneous electrical nerve stimulation (TENS), and calcitonin. The incidence and severity of phantom limb pain are increased if there has been prolonged ischemia before amputation and decreased if postoperative rehabilitation has been rapid.

Increased Mortality Rate

Five-year survival for all lower extremity amputees is less than 50%, compared with 85% for an age-matched population. Diabetic amputees have only a 40% 5-year survival. Two-thirds of all deaths are due to cardiovascular disease.

Trauma to the Residual Limb

Because their gait is relatively unstable, amputees are at increased risk for falls that may lead to fractures or other injury to the residual limb. Disruption of the wound or skin should usually be allowed to heal by secondary intent. About 3–5% of amputees experience fractures at some time, principally of the distal femur and hip. The diagnosis of fracture is overlooked or delayed in 25% of cases. Although most fractures can be successfully treated, one-half of amputees who were ambulatory before injury become wheelchair-bound afterward.

Ischemia in Residual Limbs

Progressive vascular disease results in ischemia of about 8% of transfemoral amputations and 1% of transtibial amputations. Operations are often required to improve arterial flow when gangrene develops in a residual limb. The mortality rate of this condition is high.

■ REHABILITATION FOLLOWING AMPUTATION

The rehabilitation goals following amputation are highly variable. Younger patients universally want to regain ambulatory status and frequently return to work. Elderly patients with significant comorbid conditions may remain wheelchair-bound, and much of their rehabilitation is focused on providing wheelchair access in their living situations and working on independent transfers. It is important to understand that amputation in an elderly patient is frequently an event that occurs near the end of life. For these people, relief of pain and provision for modest function may be the most appropriate outcome in the limited amount of time they have left.

The rehabilitation strategy for a young lower extremity amputee is aggressive and straightforward. Eventual ambulation is the rule rather than the exception. The use of rigid dressings and immediate postoperative prostheses has reduced the interval from operation to the beginning of ambulation to 1 month. Patients are instructed in the use of a compressive garment (stump shrinker) to control edema and are taught massage techniques to soften the scar and decrease its sensitivity. A temporary prosthesis allows gait training.

The rehabilitation strategy for older amputees is much different. Only half of elderly patients undergoing amputation are considered rehabilitation candidates. Because of delays in wound healing, the mean time from amputation to prosthetic fitting averages 9 months. Although up to 80% of patients considered candidates for rehabilitation are fitted with a prosthesis, only one-third are ambulatory outside the home. At 2 years, only two-thirds of the ambulatory patients who initially walk remain ambulatory (primarily as a result of contralateral limb disease or cardiopulmonary restrictions). Therefore, independent ambulation after major limb amputation in an elderly vascular patient is the exception rather than the rule.

The rehabilitation of a major upper extremity amputee is more complicated. Most of these patients are young, since trauma is the most common reason for upper extremity amputation. Loss of an upper extremity has greater functional impact on the patient. In addition, the psychologic effects are frequently more severe. For example, the highest suicide rate for amputees in the Vietnam War was reported in those with major upper extremity loss. The variety of functions performed in daily activities using the upper extremity is far greater than for the lower extremity. Effective prostheses for upper extremity amputees utilizing neuromuscular feedback are currently available. However, owing to cost and cosmesis, up to one-third of upper extremity amputees do not wear the prosthesis at all and a larger number wear their prostheses only intermittently. Finally, because of the traumatic etiology for most major upper extremity amputations, the incidence of postamputation pain syndromes is greater than in patients with major lower limb loss.

The length of the residual limb correlates well with regaining the ability to walk. Cardiopulmonary disease and physical weakness make walking an overwhelming effort for some patients; this emphasizes the importance of preserving as long a residual limb as possible, so that walking will require the least possible amount of energy.

■ PROSTHESES

The patellar tendon-bearing prosthesis is used for 90% of lower extremity amputees. It provides total contact with the residual limb, avoiding excessive pressure in any one area. A cuff suspension strap above the knee maintains close contact between the limb and prosthesis. The solid ankle cushion heel (SACH) prosthesis, the most frequently prescribed foot used for transfemoral and transtibial prostheses, is rugged and adequately simulates ankle motion at heel-strike and toe-off. It is a good initial foot even for the younger, more athletic individual who may go on to a newer, dynamic energy-storing foot after becoming accustomed to the SACH foot.

The most commonly prescribed transfemoral prosthesis is the total-contact suction socket. For older, dysvascular amputees, a single-axis constant friction knee or single-axis "stabilizing" (friction lock) knee is best because it is lightweight. Younger, more athletic transfemoral amputees can tolerate heavier prostheses with hydraulic or pneumatic knees, which permit changes in cadence.

More efficient prostheses requiring less energy are constantly being developed. Components fashioned from new types of plastics, fiberglass casting tapes, and carbon fiber polymers allow construction of ultra-lightweight strong and durable prostheses. They are useful both in elderly amputees (who have less energy reserve) and in young amputees who want to participate in sports.

Gait Analysis

The gait of both transfemoral and transtibial amputees is markedly different from normal gait. The forward velocity of walking is significantly lower in amputees and is lower in transfemoral than transtibial amputees. The time-distance parameters of velocity, cadence, strike length, and gait cycle are 1 SD below normal in transtibial amputees and 2 SD below normal in transfemoral amputees. The normal symmetry of walking is not present, as has been documented by measurements of single-limb support time and motion analyses of the lower extremities, head, arms, and trunk. This asymmetry of motion increases the excursion of the center of mass during each gait cycle and thereby increases the amount of energy used in ambulation.

■ LONG-TERM CARE FOLLOWING AMPUTATION

Patients who have undergone amputation require periodic checks of the prosthesis and residual limb, physical therapy, and in many cases psychologic support for life. Shrinkage of the residual limb requires replacement of the initial prosthesis after about 6 months and again 1 year after amputation. Thereafter, well-made transtibial prostheses should have a useful life of approximately 2 years. Patients must be educated to care for the residual limb, with utmost attention to cleanliness, and shown how to protect areas of pressure, trauma, or insensitivity.

After amputation for vascular disease or complications of diabetes mellitus, symptoms in the opposite leg should be anticipated and reported promptly, and ulcers or other changes in the residual limb should be brought to the attention of the physician as early as possible.

REFERENCES

Adunsky A et al: Non-traumatic lower limb older amputees: a database survey from a geriatric center. Disabil Rehabil 2001; 20:80.

Cutson TM, Borgiorni DR: Rehabilitation of the older lower limb amputee: a brief review. J Am Geriatr Soc 1996;44:1388.

Dirschl DR, Dahners LE: The mangled extremity: when should it be amputated? J Am Acad Orthop Surg 1996;4:182.

Fletcher DD et al: Rehabilitation of the geriatric vascular amputee patient: a population-based study. Arch Phys Med Rehabil 2001;82:776.

Huang ME, Levy CE, Webster JB: Acquired limb deficiencies. 3. Prosthetic components, prescriptions, and indications. Arch Phys Med Rehabil 2001;82:S17.

Kent R, Fyfe N: Effectiveness of rehabilitation following amputation. Clin Rehabil 1999;13(Suppl I):43.

Levy CE et al: Acquired limb deficiencies. 4. Troubleshooting. Arch Phys Med Rehabil 2001;82:S25.

Manord JD et al: Management of severe proximal vascular and neural injury of the upper extremity. J Vasc Surg 1998;27:43.

Mayfield JA et al: Trends in lower limb amputations in the Veterans Health Administration, 1989–1998. J Rehabil Res Dev 2000;37:22.

Nehler MR et al: Intermediate term outcome of primary digit amputations in diabetic patients with forefoot sepsis and adequate circulatory status. J Vasc Surg 1999;30:509.

Pohjolainen T, Alarnta H: Ten-year survival of Finnish lower limb amputees. Prosthet Orthot Int 1998;22:10.

Sewell P et al: Developments in the trans-tibial prosthetic socket fitting process: a review of past and present research. Prosthet Orthot Int 2000;24:97.

Trautner C et al: Incidence of lower limb amputations and diabetes. Diabetes Care 1996;19:1006.

White SA et al: Lower limb amputation and grade of surgeon. Br J Surg 1997;84:509.

Veins & Lymphatics

37

Laura K. Pak, MD, Louis M. Messina, MD, & Thomas W. Wakefield, MD

■ I. THE VEINS

VENOUS ANATOMY

Veins of the lower extremity (Figure 37–1) consist of superficial and deep systems joined by venous perforators. The greater and lesser saphenous veins are superficial veins—the name "saphenous" aptly derived from the Greek word for "manifest, clear," ie, "visible." They contain many valves and show considerable variation in their location and branching points. In up to 10% of patients, the greater saphenous vein may be duplicated. Typically, it originates from the superficial arch of the foot and is found anterior to the medial malleolus at the ankle. As it ascends in the calf just beneath the superficial fascia, it is joined by two major tributaries: an anterior vein, which crosses the tibia; and a posterior arch vein, which arises posterior to the medial malleolus beside the posterior tibial artery. The greater saphenous then enters the fossa ovalis to empty into the deep femoral vein.

The saphenofemoral junction is marked by four or five prominent branches of the greater saphenous vein: the superficial circumflex iliac vein, the external pudendal vein, the superficial epigastric vein, and the medial and lateral accessory saphenous veins. Another important anatomic landmark is the relationship of the greater saphenous vein to the saphenous branch of the femoral nerve; as it emerges from the popliteal space, the nerve follows a course parallel to the vein. Injury during saphenous vein stripping or saphenous vein harvest for bypass produces neuropathic pain or numbness along the medial calf and foot. The lesser saphenous vein arises from the superficial dorsal venous arch behind the lateral malleolus at the ankle and curves toward the midline of the posterior calf, ascending to join the popliteal vein behind the knee.

Deep veins of the leg parallel the courses of the arteries. Two or three venae comitantes accompany each tibial artery. At the knee, these paired high-capacitance veins merge to form the popliteal vein, which continues proximally as the superficial femoral vein. At the inguinal ligament, the superficial and deep (profunda) femoral veins join medial to the femoral artery to form

the common femoral vein. In the pelvis, external and internal iliac veins join to form common iliac veins that empty into the inferior vena cava. The right common iliac vein ascends almost vertically to the inferior vena cava while the left common iliac vein takes a more transverse course. For this reason, the left common iliac vein may be compressed between the right common iliac artery and lumbosacral spine, a condition known as May-Thurner syndrome.

Muscular sinusoids represent another component of the deep veins of the leg. These thin-walled, nonvalved venous lakes run longitudinally within soleus muscle bellies and then coalesce to join the posterior tibial and peroneal veins. Blood empties from these sinusoids during muscle contraction; inactivity leads to stasis and deep venous thrombosis.

Blood flow is directed from superficial to deep veins of the leg via valved perforating (communicating) veins. Perforators are located below the medial malleolus (inframalleolar perforator), in the medial calf (Cockett perforators), at the level of the adductor canal (hunterian perforator), and just above (Dodd's perforator) and below (Boyd's perforator) the knee.

Delicate bicuspid venous valves prevent reflux and direct the flow of blood from the foot and leg toward the heart. Valves are more numerous in the distal part of the extremity, decrease in number proximally, and are virtually absent in the inferior vena cava itself.

The inferior vena cava ascends in the abdomen and ends at the right atrium. It lies to the right of the midline, lateral to the aorta, and receives a number of lumbar veins that connect with the vertebral and paravertebral venous plexuses. The inferior vena cava and its tributaries are derived in the fifth to eighth week of life from the fusion and obliteration of several paired embryonic veins: the anterior and posterior cardinal veins, the subcardinal veins, the supracardinal veins, and the sacrocardinal veins. Because of this complex embryonic development, anomalies in the venous system are not uncommon. The most common abnormality is a circumaortic left renal vein (7% incidence), followed by a retroaortic left renal vein (2–3% incidence), duplication of the inferior vena cava (0.2–3% incidence), and left sided inferior vena cava (0.2–0.5% incidence). An unsuspected retroaortic or circumaortic renal vein can be inadvertently injured during aortic cross-clamping.

Figure 37–1. Anatomy of the superficial and perforating veins of the lower extremity. (Reproduced, with permission, from Rutherford RB, Cronenwett JL, Gloviczki P: *Vascular Surgery.* Philadelphia: Saunders, 2000.)

Veins of the upper extremity are also divided into superficial and deep groups, though direction of flow from superficial to deep is not as distinct as in the lower extremity. Dorsal veins of the hand empty into the cephalic vein ("intern vein") on the radial aspect and into the basilic vein on the ulnar aspect of the forearm. The cephalic vein ascends lateral to the biceps muscle into the deltopectoral groove, where it passes through the clavipectoral fascia to join the axillary vein. The cephalic vein is useful for arteriovenous fistulas because it is superficial and lateral in the arm, allowing easy access for hemodialysis needles. The basilic vein, which runs medially in the arm to become the axillary vein, is deeper and thicker-walled than the cephalic vein. Its many branches make it tedious to harvest, but it can be used for bypass conduit or for a laterally tunneled upper arm dialysis fistula (basilic vein transposition). The median cubital vein links the cephalic and basilic veins in the antecubital space.

Paired brachial veins comprise the deep system of veins. They accompany the brachial artery and join the basilic vein as it becomes the axillary vein. The axillary vein continues medially as the subclavian vein, which passes through a tight space anterior to the first rib and anterior scalene muscle and posterior to the clavicle. The subclavian vein and the internal jugular vein join behind the clavicular head to form the brachiocephalic vein, which empties into the superior vena cava.

Giordano JM et al: Anomalies of the vena cava. J Vasc Surg 1986; 3:924.

Scultetus AH et al: Facts and fiction surrounding the discovery of venous valves. J Vasc Surg 2001;33:435.

VENOUS PHYSIOLOGY

Knowledge of lower extremity venous anatomy is essential to understanding the physiology of venous flow. The volume of blood in the lower extremities may increase by one-half liter when an individual moves from a reclining to an erect position (Figure 37–2). Increased blood volume is accommodated by increased venous capacitance, which is regulated by smooth muscle contractility in the vein walls. Erect posture creates a vertical column of blood, exerting a hydrostatic pressure equal to the distance from the toes to the right atrium (about 100–120 mm Hg). The hydrostatic pressure

Figure 37–2. Pedal venous pressure measurements with exercise. The normal drop in pressure associated with ambulation is impaired by deep vein incompetence and proximal venous obstruction. (Reproduced, with permission, from DeWeese JA: Venous and lymphatic disease. In: *Principles of Surgery*, 4th ed. Schwarz S [editor]. McGraw-Hill, 1983.)

must be overcome to avoid pooling of blood in the legs and to provide venous return to the heart. Several aspects of the venous system make it possible to move blood against the force of gravity. Because the circulation is a closed system, venous return is affected by arterial inflow and by the negative intrathoracic pressure created during inspiration. Valves assure unidirectional movement of blood from superficial to deep systems and from the foot back to the heart. Hydrostatic pressure is dissipated by lack of simultaneous opening of the valves. Soleal venous sinusoids are another central component to the system. When the muscle contracts during exercise, blood empties from the sinusoid into the deep veins of the calf and leg. This high-velocity flow siphons blood from deep veins of the foot upward into the calf—analogous to smoke being drawn up a smokestack by wind blowing past the chimney (Venturi effect).

DISEASES OF THE VENOUS SYSTEM

VARICOSE VEINS

ESSENTIALS OF DIAGNOSIS

- *Dilated, tortuous superficial veins in the lower extremities, usually bilateral.*
- *May be asymptomatic or may be associated with bleeding, localized pain, nocturnal cramps, or aching discomfort and "heaviness" with prolonged standing.*
- *Pigmentation, ulceration, and edema suggest concomitant venous stasis disease.*
- *Increased frequency after pregnancy.*

General Considerations

Varicose veins are very common, afflicting 10–20% of the world's population. Abnormally dilated veins occur in several locations in the body: the spermatic chord (varicocele), esophagus (esophageal varices), and the anorectum (hemorrhoids). Varicosities of the legs were described as early as 1550 BC, and in the 1600s AD were correlated with trauma, childbearing, and "standing too much before kings." Modern studies identify female sex, pregnancy, family history, prolonged standing, and a history of phlebitis as risk factors for varicose veins. In the Framingham Study, the highest incidence was found in women between 40 and 49 years of age.

Varicose veins are classified as either primary or secondary. Primary varicose veins are thought to be due to genetic or developmental defects in the vein wall that cause diminished elasticity and valvular incompetence. Most cases of isolated superficial venous insufficiency are primary varicose veins. Secondary varicose veins arise from destruction or dysfunction of valves caused by trauma, deep venous thrombosis, arteriovenous fistula, or nontraumatic proximal venous obstruction (pregnancy, pelvic tumor). When valves of the deep and perforating veins are disrupted, chronic venous stasis changes may accompany superficial varicosities. It is important to recognize that untreated, long-standing venous dysfunction from either primary or secondary varicose veins may cause chronic skin changes that lead to infection, nonhealing venous ulceration, and chronic disability. To define the optimal method of treatment, the etiologic factors and distribution of disease must be clearly identified.

Clinical Findings

The clinical presentation of patients with varicose veins can be quite variable. Most varicose veins are asymptomatic and come to medical attention because of aesthetic concerns. If symptomatic, varicose veins may be associated with localized pain, a diffuse ache or "heaviness" in the calf—particularly with prolonged standing—or phlebitis. Mild ankle edema may occur. Symptoms generally improve with leg elevation.

The varicosities appear as dilated, tortuous, elongated veins predominantly on the medial aspect of the lower extremity along the course of the greater saphenous vein. Overlying skin changes may be absent even in the presence of extensive large varicosities. Smaller, flat, blue-green reticular veins, telangiectasias, and spider veins may accompany varicose veins and are further evidence of venous dysfunction. A cluster of telangiectasias below the inframalleolar perforator is termed a corona phlebectatica paraplantaris. Secondary varicose veins can cause symptoms characteristic of chronic venous insufficiency, including edema, hyperpigmentation, scaling dermatitis, and venous ulcerations.

Physical examination begins with inspection of all extremities to determine the distribution and severity of the varicosities. Bimanual circumferential palpation of the thighs and calves is helpful. Palpation of a thrill or auscultation of a bruit indicates the presence of an arteriovenous fistula as a possible etiologic factor. The **Brodie-Trendelenburg test** is a useful maneuver for identifying sites of valvular incompetence. With the patient lying supine, the leg is elevated until all varicosities collapse. A tourniquet is placed at the mid thigh to exclude reflux secondary to incompetence at the saphenofemoral junction. With the tourniquet in place, the patient is instructed to stand. If the varicosities stay collapsed, this implies valvular insufficiency at the saphenofemoral junction. If the varicosities rapidly refill, perforator vein incompetence is implicated. The tourniquet can then be moved more distally to identify the location of the incompetent perforator. Today, tourniquet tests have been virtually replaced by venous duplex ultrasound imaging.

Differential Diagnosis

Ulceration, brawny induration, and hyperpigmentation indicate chronic deep venous insufficiency. This is important to recognize because the changes generally do not resolve with saphenous vein stripping, and wound healing following surgery may be jeopardized by failure to treat the venous stasis disease.

If extensive varicose veins are encountered in a young patient—especially if unilateral and in an atypical distribution (lateral leg)—Klippel-Trenaunay syndrome must be considered. The classic triad is varicose veins, limb hypertrophy, and a cutaneous birthmark (port wine stain or venous malformation). Because the deep veins are often anomalous or absent, saphenous vein stripping can be hazardous. Standard treatment for patients with Klippel-Trenaunay syndrome is graduated support stockings, surgery for correction of leg length discrepancy, and limited stab avulsion of symptomatic varices after thorough duplex ultrasound vein mapping.

Treatment

A. NONSURGICAL TREATMENT

Treatment for both primary and secondary varicose veins initially involves a program directed at management of venous insufficiency, including elastic stocking support, periodic leg elevation, and regular exercise. Prolonged sitting and standing are discouraged. For most patients, knee-high or thigh-high gradient compression stockings of 20–30 mm Hg are sufficient. The compression stockings are worn all day to diminish venous distention during standing and are removed at night.

B. SURGICAL TREATMENT

Indications for surgical treatment (Figure 37–3) include persistent or disabling pain, recurrent superficial thrombophlebitis, erosion of the overlying skin with bleeding, and manifestations of chronic venous insufficiency (particularly ulceration).

The operative plan is dependent on determination of the competency of the deep and perforating veins and the location of sites of venous reflux. Surgery can then be tailored to the pattern of disease. High ligation and strip-

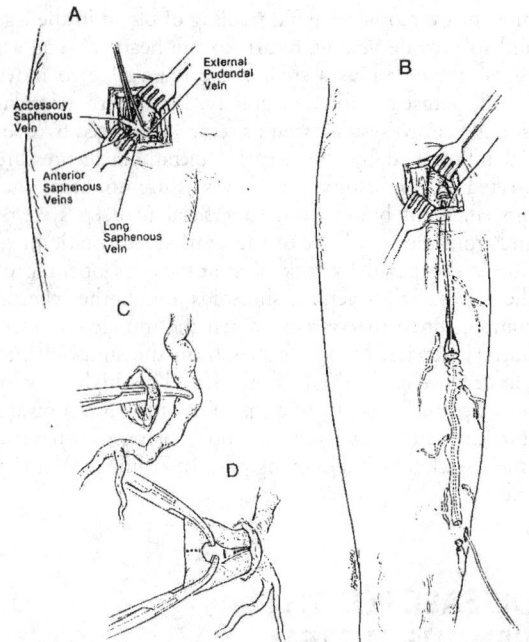

Figure 37–3. Technique of varicose vein stripping. (Reproduced, with permission, from Bergan JJ, Kistner RL: *Atlas of Venous Surgery.* Saunders, 1992.)

ping of the entire saphenous system is reserved for patients with an incompetent valve at the saphenofemoral junction and varicosities throughout the length of the greater saphenous vein. This is performed by ligating the saphenofemoral junction and the major proximal saphenous vein branches through a small incision in the groin, isolating the greater saphenous vein at the medial malleolus, passing a flexible plastic stripper through the vein from bottom to top and securing it proximally to the ligated vein, and then removing the entire vein by withdrawing the stripper.

Alternatively, selective removal of isolated clusters of varicose veins can be accomplished by the stab-avulsion technique. Stab incisions 1.5–2 mm long are made along premarked varicosities and specially designed vein hooks are then used to loop the vein and deliver it through the incision; using forceps, a 4–5 cm length of vein can be extracted.

The combined techniques of high ligation and stab-avulsion are often employed. Some argue that the saphenous vein should be removed from the groin down to the first stab for the best long-term results. With careful patient selection and properly selected operative techniques, the recurrence rate should be approximately 10%. Complications include hematoma formation, infection, and saphenous nerve irritation.

C. COMPRESSION SCLEROTHERAPY

Compression sclerotherapy is usually applied to telangiectasias, spider veins, and small varicosities that persist after vein stripping. With the patient supine, a small volume of sclerosing solution (0.2–3% sodium tetradecyl sulfate) is injected into a varix isolated by proximal and distal digital venous occlusion. Direct pressure with compression stockings is maintained for 1 week afterward. The goal is to obliterate the abnormal vein by inducing localized endothelial destruction and fibrosis. More than one treatment is often required. Complications, including allergic reactions, thrombophlebitis, neoangiogenesis, and skin necrosis or hyperpigmentation, are rare.

Belcaro G et al: Endovascular sclerotherapy, surgery, and surgery plus sclerotherapy in superficial venous incompetence: a randomized, 10 year follow-up trial—final results. Angiology 2000;51:529.

Bradbury A et al: The relationship between lower limb symptoms and superficial and deep venous reflux on duplex ultrasonography: the Edinburgh Vein Study. J Vasc Surg 2000;32:921.

Dwerryhouse S: Stripping the long saphenous vein reduces the rate of reoperation for recurrent varicose veins: five year results of a randomized trial. J Vasc Surg 1999;29:589.

DEEP VEIN THROMBOSIS

ESSENTIALS OF DIAGNOSIS

- *Pain in the thigh or calf sometimes accompanied by edema. Half of patients are asymptomatic.*
- *History of recent surgery, trauma, cancer, prolonged immobilization, or oral contraceptive use.*
- *Homans' sign is accurate in 50% of cases.*
- *Venous duplex ultrasound is the diagnostic modality of choice*

General Considerations

Deep venous thrombosis affects more than 500,000 people per year in the USA and is associated with a mortality of up to 21% in the elderly. Treatment is estimated to cost $1–2.5 billion a year—not including expenditures associated with long-term sequelae of this disease.

Virchow's triad (stasis, vascular injury, and hypercoagulability) should be the cornerstone for assessment of risk factors for deep venous thrombosis. In the majority of cases, the cause is multifactorial.

Stasis can occur with venous insufficiency, severe heart failure, or prolonged bed rest or immobility of an extremity following coma, prolonged ventilatory support, pelvic or limb fracture, paralysis, extended airplane travel, or lengthy operation. Radiolabeled fibrinogen scanning has shown that half of perioperative cases develop in the operating room.

Endothelial injury can result from direct trauma (severed vein, venous cannulation, or transvenous pacing) or local irritation secondary to infusion of chemotherapy, previous deep venous thrombosis, or phlebitis. Damaged endothelium leads to platelet aggregation, degranulation, and formation of thrombus as well as vasoconstriction and activation of the coagulation cascade. Thrombin activation from release of tissue factor and diminished fibrinolysis mediated by plasminogen activator inhibitor are intraoperative events that may be related to endothelial disruption.

Hypercoagulable state can be inherited or acquired. Twenty to 30 percent of patients with new deep venous thromboses have an underlying occult or known malignancy. One-fourth of these are lung cancer, though hypercoagulability may also be seen in patients with cancer of the pancreas, prostate, breast, and ovary. Most of these malignancies are associated with increased fibrinogen or thrombocytosis. Deficiency in antithrombin 3 and proteins C and S may be inherited or may result from nephrotic syndrome, disseminated intravascular coagulation, or liver failure. Increased homocysteine, factor V Leiden mutation, prothrombin gene variant, and paroxysmal nocturnal hemoglobinuria are also associated with venous thrombosis.

Other commonly sited risk factors for deep venous thrombosis include advanced age, type A blood group, obesity, a history of previous deep venous thromboses, multiparity, use of oral contraceptives, inflammatory bowel disease, and systemic lupus erythematosus.

Deep venous thrombosis occurs most frequently in the calf veins, though it may arise in the femoral or iliac veins. Thrombi originate in soleal sinusoids or in valve sinuses, where there are flow eddies. Treatment of isolated calf vein thromboses is controversial, as they are associated with a low risk of pulmonary embolism. However, if untreated, 25% progress to proximal deep veins of the leg, where the incidence of chronic venous insufficiency is 25% and that of fatal pulmonary embolism is 10%. These observations and the improved safety profile of low-molecular-weight heparin are compelling more practitioners to treat isolated calf deep venous thromboses.

Clinical Findings

A. SYMPTOMS AND SIGNS

The diagnosis of deep venous thrombosis cannot be made solely on the basis of presenting symptoms and signs, as up to half of patients with acute thromboses have no abnormality detectable in the involved extremity. Homans' sign (pain on passive dorsiflexion of the ankle) is positive in only half of cases. Some patients present with acute pulmonary embolism unaccompanied by leg edema or pain.

Symptomatic patients most often complain of a dull ache or pain in the calf or leg associated with mild edema. With extensive proximal deep venous thrombosis, there can be massive edema, cyanosis, and dilated superficial collateral veins. Low-grade fever and tachycardia occasionally occur. Iliofemoral venous thrombosis can result in phlegmasia cerulea dolens, characterized by cyanosis of the limb due to venous outflow obstruction. In phlegmasia alba dolens, the leg is pulseless, pale, and cool due to concomitant arterial spasm. These are potentially limb-threatening conditions.

B. IMAGING STUDIES

Because deep venous thrombosis is difficult to diagnose on the basis of physical signs or symptoms, some objective diagnostic study is required before treatment is started. Historically, the standard for diagnosis was ascending phlebography, accomplished by fluoroscopic imaging during contrast injection into an intravenous line on the dorsum of the foot. The patient stands but is non-weight-bearing on the extremity studied. An abrupt cutoff of the contrast column indicates deep venous thrombosis. The complications of this procedure include risk of contrast allergy, contrast-induced nephropathy, and phlebitis.

Duplex ultrasound has now become the test of choice. It is a noninvasive examination, does not expose the patient to radiation, is easily reproducible, and has specificity and sensitivity of greater than 95%. It is also useful to detect other potential pathologic processes such as Baker's cyst. The examination includes both a B-mode image and Doppler flow analysis. Each venous segment is assessed for the presence of thrombosis, indicated by venous dilation and incompressibility during light probe pressure. Doppler findings suggestive of acute deep venous thrombosis are absence of spontaneous flow, loss of flow variation with respiration, and failure to increase flow velocity after distal augmentation. The criteria for the presence of chronic venous thrombosis are less well established. The chronically occluded vein is often narrowed, and there are prominent nearby collaterals. Chronic thrombi are highly echogenic, while acute thrombi are anechoic (and, therefore, not visible) on the B-mode image. Duplex ultrasound is less accurate in detection of calf thromboses and is highly operator-dependent.

Magnetic resonance venography shows promise as a diagnostic study for this disorder. The sensitivity and specificity of magnetic resonance venography are 100% and 96%, respectively. The injection of gadolinium is useful for determining the age of the thrombus.

Measurement of D-dimer levels is too nonspecific and scanning with radiolabeled fibrinogen too time-consuming for use in the acute clinical setting. Older tests such as impedance plethysmography and venous pressure measurements do not achieve the same accuracy as duplex ultrasound and have been largely abandoned.

Differential Diagnosis

Localized muscle strain or contusion or Achilles tendon rupture can often mimic the symptoms of deep venous thrombosis. Cellulitis may cause edema, localized pain, and erythema. Unilateral leg swelling can also result from lymphedema, obstruction of the popliteal vein by Baker's cyst, or obstruction of the iliac vein by retroperitoneal mass or idiopathic fibrosis. Bilateral leg edema suggests heart, liver, or kidney failure or inferior vena cava obstruction by tumor or pregnancy.

Treatment

Treatment is aimed at reducing the incidence of complications associated with deep venous thrombosis, which include varicose veins, chronic venous insufficiency or postphlebitic syndrome, recurrent deep venous thrombosis, or pulmonary thromboembolism. The primary treatment of deep venous thrombosis is systemic anticoagulation. This reduces the risk of pulmonary embolism and extension of venous thrombosis and also decreases the rate of recurrent deep venous thrombosis by 80%. Systemic anticoagulation does not directly lyse thrombi but stops propagation and allows natural fibrinolysis to occur. Heparin is initiated immediately and dosed to a goal PTT of 1.5–2 times normal. Achieving therapeutic heparinization within the first 24 hours after diagnosis is shown to reduce the rate of recurrent deep venous thrombosis.

Warfarin is started after therapeutic heparinization. The two therapies should overlap to diminish the possibility of a hypercoagulable state, which can occur during the first few days of warfarin administration, because warfarin also inhibits the synthesis of natural anticoagulant proteins C and S. The recommended treatment for a first episode of uncomplicated deep venous thrombosis is 3–6 months of warfarin, maintained at a goal international normalized ratio (INR) of 2.0–3.0. After a second episode of deep venous thrombosis, the usual recommendation is lifelong warfarin. The risk for recurrent venous thrombosis is increased markedly in the presence of factor V Leiden mutations, antiphospholipid antibody, and antithrombin III and protein C or protein S deficiencies, so lifelong anticoagulation is usually recommended for these conditions, as well.

Low-molecular-weight heparin (LMWH) has been shown to be as safe and effective as warfarin in the treatment of deep venous thrombosis. It is administered twice daily by subcutaneous injection. LMWH does not require monitoring of its anticoagulant effect because of its predictable dose-response relationship, and this feature of the drug has made feasible the outpatient treatment of deep venous thrombosis. Standard unfractionated heparin inhibits thrombin because it is large enough to make a three-way complex between thrombin, antithrombin, and itself. LMWHs are much smaller than standard heparin molecules and do not inhibit thrombin; their main therapeutic effect comes from inhibition of factor Xa activity. The advantages of LMWHs over standard heparin preparations include a lower risk of bleeding complications and thrombocytopenia, less interference with proteins C and S, less complement activation, and a lower risk of osteoporosis. Moreover, recent randomized trials have shown regression of thrombus with LMWH.

Current research efforts are directed toward development of an oral thrombin inhibitor. This is expected to have a more favorable dose-response curve and side-effect profile than warfarin.

Many studies have evaluated the efficacy of fibrinolytic agents in the treatment of deep venous thrombosis. Recombinant tissue plasminogen activator (rt-PA; alteplase) has generally superseded urokinase and streptokinase in clinical use. Although faster clot lysis and increased venous patency are observed with alteplase versus heparin, this has not translated to a decreased incidence of long-term sequelae such as chronic venous insufficiency. The risk of bleeding complications is higher with alteplase and does not appear to be reduced by selective catheterization for local administration. To be effective, alteplase should be instituted within 1 week after clot formation, before extensive fibrin cross-linking can occur. There has been no demonstrable benefit to selective administration of alteplase, but theoretically this technique may allow medication dose reduction. One possible application for alteplase is acute iliofemoral venous thrombosis complicated by massive extremity edema, cyanosis, or calf compartment syndrome. Iliofemoral thrombectomy achieves a clinical success rate of 40–90% for this disorder, with most treatment failures being due to residual distal thrombosis, stenosis or obliteration of the proximal vein, or recurrent thrombosis.

Prevention

Surgery increases the risk of deep venous thrombosis 21-fold. This disorder is a reported complication for 20% of patients admitted for a general surgical procedure, 24% of those undergoing an elective neurosurgical procedure, and 50–60% of those undergoing hip or knee arthroplasty. These statistics emphasize the need for routine deep venous thrombosis prophylaxis in the surgical patient. The most commonly used measures are elastic stockings with sequential compression devices and low-dose unfractionated heparin, 5000 units given by subcutaneous injection twice daily, or LMWH given at a prophylactic dose of 30 mg subcutaneously twice daily.

Low-dose heparin and LMWH have both been shown to significantly reduce the incidence of postoperative deep venous thromboses and pulmonary embolisms. LMWH appears to be more effective in the orthopedic population and is associated also with a lower risk of bleeding complications (1–5% versus 2–12% with unfractionated heparin). Use of heparin products is contraindicated in patients with history of recent craniotomy, intracranial bleeding, or severe gastrointestinal bleeding. Many practitioners also avoid the use of subcutaneous heparin or LMWH in patients with epidural or spinal anesthesia because of the possibility of spinal hematoma. In any patient receiving subcutaneous heparin or LMWH, the platelet count must be monitored for early detection of heparin-induced thrombocytopenia, which occurs with a peak incidence at 5–10 days of treatment.

Graduated compression stockings and sequential compression devices are beneficial in reducing the risk of calf vein thrombosis but have not been shown to decrease the incidence of pulmonary thromboembolism. They function by increasing venous flow, decreasing venous stasis, and increasing the release of endothelial fibrinolytic factors. They are safe for use on almost all patients.

Guidelines for venous thromboembolism prophylaxis are based on a patient's specific risk factors. For certain low-risk patients, no specific prophylaxis is indicated other than early ambulation. In higher-risk patients, appropriate prophylaxis includes the use of low-dose unfractionated heparin or LMWH with or without intermittent pneumatic compression. In minimally ambulatory patients, treatment continuing beyond hospital discharge may be indicated. Patients with hypercoagulable state or paralysis may benefit from lifetime anticoagulation with low-dose warfarin or prophylactic inferior vena cava filter placement.

Breddin HK et al: Effects of a low-molecular-weight heparin on thrombus regression and recurrent thromboembolism in patients with deep-vein thrombosis. N Engl J Med 2001; 344:626.

Clagett GP: Prevention of venous thromboembolism. Chest 1998; 114:531

Ferrari E et al: Travel as a risk factor for venous thromboembolic disease: a case-control study. Chest 1999;115:440.

Forster A et al: Tissue plasminogen activator for the treatment of deep venous thrombosis of the lower extremity: a systematic review. Chest 2001;119:572.

Heit JA et al: Risk factors for deep vein thrombosis and pulmonary embolism: a population-based case-control study. Arch Intern Med 2000;160:809.

Hirsh J et al: Clinical trials that have influenced the treatment of venous thromboembolism: a historical perspective. Ann Intern Med 2001;134:409.

Ruehm SG et al: Direct contrast-enhanced 3D MR venography. Eur Radiol 2001;11:102.

AXILLARY-SUBCLAVIAN VENOUS THROMBOSIS

 ESSENTIALS OF DIAGNOSIS

- *History of strenuous, repetitive upper extremity activity or recent venous cannulation.*
- *Aching pain, cyanosis, and edema of the anterior chest wall, axilla, shoulder, arm, and hand.*
- *Prominent distended venous collaterals.*
- *Subclavian vein obstruction at the thoracic outlet.*

General Considerations

Thrombosis of the axillary or subclavian vein is a relatively uncommon event, accounting for less than 5% of all cases of deep vein thrombosis. Only 12% result in pulmonary thromboembolism, but local symptoms of upper extremity thrombosis can cause significant disability.

There are two major etiologies. Primary axillary-subclavian thrombosis, also known as Paget-Schrotter syndrome or "effort thrombosis," occurs as a result of intermittent transient obstruction of the vein in the costoclavicular space during repetitive or strenuous activities involving the upper extremity (Figure 37–4). This condition was first described in independent reports by Paget and von Schroetter in the late 19th century. During strenuous repetitive movements of the upper extremity, the subclavian vein is compressed between the first rib and the anterior scalene muscle posteriorly and the clavicle—with underlying subclavius muscle and fibrous costocoracoid ligament—anteriorly. Primary subclavian vein thrombosis can also occur in patients with hypercoagulable states such as antiphospholipid antibody syndrome or factor V Leiden mutation. Secondary subclavian vein thrombosis results from

A

B

C

Figure 37–4. ***A:*** Effort thrombosis in a 13-year-old wrestler. Arrow marks subclavian vein thrombosis refractory to rt-PA thrombolysis. ***B:*** Arm in abduction. Note disappearance of prominent venous collaterals. ***C:*** Immediate postoperative venogram following scalenectomy, first rib resection, and thrombectomy.

venous injury by indwelling central venous catheters, external trauma, or pacemaker wires.

Clinical Findings

A. SYMPTOMS AND SIGNS

Primary axillary-subclavian vein thrombosis usually occurs in healthy young athletes and people who perform heavy manual labor. Men outnumber women 4:1. Most often patients give a history of repetitive arm activity, but sometimes a single strenuous exercise, such as wrestling, can precipitate thrombosis. Most patients present with an aching pain most severe in the axilla, accompanied by edema and cyanosis of the upper extremity. Significant superficial venous distention is usually apparent in the arm, forearm, shoulder, and anterior chest wall. Symptoms may abate somewhat with the arm elevated.

Paget-Schroetter syndrome may also be accompanied by symptoms of neurogenic thoracic outlet syndrome: tingling, numbness, and pain in the hand and anterior chest wall caused by compression of the brachial plexus between hypertrophied or anomalous anterior and middle scalene muscles. Some patients may have a positive Adson test, signifying impingement of the subclavian artery in the thoracic outlet. This test is positive if diminishment of the radial pulse is noted on abducting and externally rotating the arm while turning the head away from the arm examined. Arterial thoracic outlet syndrome is manifested by effort fatigue of the arm and hand, coolness, and digital embolization.

B. IMAGING STUDIES

Upper extremity venous duplex ultrasound is a good screening modality for patients with suspected axillary-subclavian vein thrombosis. If this study is positive, upper extremity venography and thrombolysis should be considered. It is important that the patient undergo positional venography, abducting the arm 120 degrees to confirm extrinsic compression of the subclavian vein at the thoracic outlet. Venous compromise is further evidenced by prominent collateral veins.

Chest x-ray should be obtained on all patients to exclude the presence of cervical rib, which can also cause compression of the subclavian vein.

Treatment

Any indwelling central venous lines or pacemaker wires in the thrombosed vein should be removed if possible. Arm elevation, pain control, and intravenous fluid resuscitation should be instituted.

Distinguishing these types of thoracic outlet syndrome is important in selecting the appropriate mode of therapy. A new standard of care for patients with acute axillary-subclavian vein thrombosis is emerging. Selective catheterization with rt-PA infusion is performed at diagnosis. rt-PA is infused over 12–24 hours through a multi-sideholed catheter centered in the thrombosed vein. Positional venography is repeated after lysis of the clot is achieved. If short-segment stenoses resulting from venous catheterization are identified, these can be corrected by angioplasty. Compression of the vein with the appearance of large venous collaterals when the arm is abducted suggests venous thoracic outlet syndrome, which is best treated with early surgery. A 35–65% risk of rethrombosis and chronic venous stasis is expected without surgery. Delaying surgery to allow epithelial remodeling while on anticoagulation has not been proved to enhance outcome.

Because the etiology of venous thoracic outlet syndrome is compression of the vein between the first rib-anterior scalene muscle origin and the clavicle, surgery consists of anterior scalenectomy, first rib resection, and venolysis (release of the vein from constricting scar). This operative plan may be modified if there is residual thrombus in the vein (thrombectomy with primary closure or patch angioplasty, interposition graft, internal jugular turndown, or jugular-subclavian bypass), or concomitant neurogenic thoracic outlet syndrome (anterior and middle scalenectomy with neurolysis) or arterial thoracic outlet syndrome (anterior and middle scalenectomy with resection of subclavian aneurysm). Positional venography is performed postoperatively, with angioplasty and stenting reserved for tight residual venous stenoses. Warfarin is continued for 1–3 months, and aspirin is then continued indefinitely afterward.

It is the general practice at our institution to evaluate patients for hypercoagulable state, including plasma levels of antithrombin 3, factor V Leiden, cardiolipin antibody, and proteins C and S. As many as 56% of patients presenting with acute axillary-subclavian vein thrombosis are found to be in a hypercoagulable state, the most common of which are mutations in coagulation factor V and antithrombin 3. Because of a 40–60% rate of recurrent thrombosis, these patients are maintained indefinitely on warfarin.

Prognosis

The prognosis after axillary-subclavian vein thrombosis is dependent upon the cause of the condition. Most patients experience fairly rapid resolution of their initial presenting symptoms. For patients with secondary forms of this disease, the outcome is dependent upon resolution of the underlying condition. For patients with Paget-Schroetter syndrome who undergo thoracic outlet decompression, excellent outcomes in terms of continued venous patency and avoidance of symptoms of chronic venous insufficiency can be expected. In contrast, chronic axillary-subclavian vein thrombosis with symptoms persisting for over 3 months does not often respond to rt-PA, mechanical thrombolysis, or prolonged anticoagulation and may cause significant long-term disability.

Angle N et al: Safety and efficacy of early surgical decompression of the thoracic outlet for Paget-Schroetter syndrome. Ann Vasc Surg 2001;15:37.

Hingorani A et al: Upper extremity deep venous thrombosis: an under-recognized manifestation of a hypercoagulable state. Ann Vasc Surg 2000;14:421.

Schneider DB et al: Management of vascular thoracic outlet syndrome. Chest Surg Clin N Am 1999;9:781.

Urschel HC et al: Paget-Schroetter syndrome: what is the best management? Ann Thorac Surg 2000;69:1663.

PULMONARY THROMBOEMBOLISM

 ESSENTIALS OF DIAGNOSIS

- *Acute onset of dyspnea, chest pain, and hemoptysis.*
- *Tachypnea and a widened arterial-alveolar oxygen difference.*
- *Abnormal findings on a ventilation-perfusion lung scan, spiral CT scan, or magnetic resonance angiogram.*

General Considerations

Pulmonary thromboembolism is responsible for up to 50,000 deaths each year in the United States. It is the third leading cause of death among hospitalized patients, yet only 30–40% of those with pulmonary thromboembolism have suspected deep venous thrombosis. Efforts directed at reduction in the mortality rate of pulmonary thromboembolism demand an aggressive approach to diagnosis of this problem in patients identified to be at high risk.

Pulmonary thromboembolisms arise from a number of sources. Air embolism can occur during the placement or removal of central venous catheters. Amniotic fluid emboli may occur during active labor. Fat emboli from long bone fractures cause a syndrome characterized by respiratory insufficiency, coagulopathy, encephalopathy, and an upper body petechial rash. Other less common causes of pulmonary emboli include septic emboli, tumor emboli from atrial myxoma or infe-

rior vena cava extension of renal cell carcinoma, and parasitic emboli. However, deep venous thrombosis remains the most common source of pulmonary thromboemboli. Sixty percent of patients with untreated proximal lower extremity deep vein thrombosis will develop pulmonary thromboembolism.

Fewer than 10% of pulmonary thromboemboli will produce pulmonary infarction. The pathophysiology of pulmonary embolism depends on the size and frequency of the emboli as well as the condition of the underlying lung. Obstruction of large pulmonary arteries results in increases in pulmonary artery pressure and acute right ventricular failure, but many of the clinical manifestations of pulmonary thromboembolism result from release of vasoactive amines that cause severe pulmonary vasoconstriction. Vasoconstriction leads to increased physiologic dead space and systemic hypoxia from a right-to-left shunt. Reflex bronchial vasoconstriction is also common.

Clinical Findings

A. SYMPTOMS AND SIGNS

Dyspnea and chest pain are present in up to 75% of patients with pulmonary thromboembolism. However, these symptoms are nonspecific, especially in patients who may have underlying cardiopulmonary disease. Tachycardia, tachypnea, and altered mental status are highly suggestive findings in an at-risk population. The classic triad of dyspnea, chest pain, and hemoptysis is present in only 15% of patients with pulmonary thromboembolism. Pleural friction rub and the S1Q3T3 morphology on electrocardiography are even less common findings.

B. IMAGING AND OTHER DIAGNOSTIC STUDIES

Chest x-ray is most often normal but may show a pleural cap. Electrocardiography may reveal new-onset atrial fibrillation or ischemic changes, but in most cases only acute sinus tachycardia and nonspecific ST and T wave changes are identified. Arterial blood gas determination shows hypoxia and often a respiratory alkalosis or increased arterial-alveolar oxygen gradient. Plasma D-dimer levels are elevated in the presence of both pulmonary thromboembolism and acute deep venous thrombosis, but this test lacks sufficient specificity to be of diagnostic value.

Until recently, the most common studies used to diagnose pulmonary embolism were ventilation-perfusion (VQ) scan and pulmonary angiogram (Figure 37–5). Ventilation-perfusion scans have sensitivity and specificity that approach 90% if results of the scan correlate with clinical risk factor assessment. For example, treatment can be started in a patient with a high-probability scan and a highly suggestive examination. Unfortu-

Figure 37–5. Pulmonary embolism. ***A:*** Pulmonary angiogram. Arrow marks location of left lower lobe emboli. ***B:*** Spiral CT. Arrow marks location of large embolus in left main pulmonary artery.

nately, two-thirds of studies are inconclusive. Pulmonary angiography remains the most reliable test for diagnosis, but it is invasive, time-consuming, and expensive.

Two newer modalities have improved the accuracy and safety of the diagnosis of pulmonary thromboembolism. Spiral CT scan has virtually replaced VQ scan in the diagnosis of pulmonary thromboembolism. Accuracy supersedes that of VQ scan and does not require clinical correlation. Magnetic resonance angiography has also demonstrated excellent sensitivity and specificity and is now being used widely in many institutions.

Treatment

A. ANTICOAGULATION

Heparin or LMWH anticoagulation is started as soon as the diagnosis is made after initial stabilization with ventilatory support and pressors. Recombinant tissue plasminogen activator (rt-PA; alteplase) thrombolysis is considered for large clot burden, severe respiratory compromise, or hemodynamic instability. When compared with heparin alone, thrombolytic therapy speeds the resolution of pulmonary emboli in the first 24 hours. The disadvantages of lytic therapy are its greater cost and higher risk of significant bleeding complications.

B. INFERIOR VENA CAVA INTERRUPTION

Inferior vena cava interruption is considered in patients who have extension of venous thrombus on adequate heparin therapy or patients in whom heparin anticoagulation is contraindicated or who have had a complication of anticoagulation. More recently, temporary or permanent inferior vena cava filters have been placed prophylactically in high-risk patients such as those with unresectable cancer or major trauma.

Historically, inferior vena cava interruption was performed as an open surgical procedure, involving ligation or plication of the infrarenal vena cava or placement of a serrated clip to "strain" blood returning to the right atrium. The Greenfield filter developed in 1973 was initially deployed by venous cutdown. (Figure 37–6.) Multiple devices are now available for fluoroscopically guided percutaneous placement through a 12F sheath introduced into the common femoral vein or, in cases of femoral thrombus, into the internal jugular vein. The presence of a duplicated inferior vena cava must be excluded by venography at the time of filter placement because lower extremity deep venous thrombosis might still serve as a source of emboli.

C. SURGICAL TREATMENT

Hemodynamically unstable patients in whom thrombolytic therapy has failed or cannot be instituted re-

Figure 37–6. Inferior vena caval filters in a patient with deep venous thrombosis and duplicated inferior vena cava.

quire percutaneous or open surgical extraction of the thrombus. Open surgical pulmonary embolectomy is reserved for patients who develop intractable hypotension, those who fail transcatheter pulmonary embolectomy, and those who have tumor or foreign body emboli. Catheter techniques involve mechanical thrombolysis or removal of intact pulmonary emboli using a suction cup. Initial reports indicate that suction catheter pulmonary embolectomy is successful in approximately 75% of the cases in which it has been used.

Prognosis

Pulmonary embolism is one of the most frequent causes of preventable hospital death. Prevention by use of deep venous thrombosis prophylaxis and early diagnosis by selective testing of high-risk patients are essential steps to reducing the morbidity of this disease.

Anderson FA et al: A population-based perspective of the hospital incidence and case-fatality rates of deep vein thrombosis and pulmonary embolism: the Worcester DVT Study. Arch Intern Med 1991;151:933.

Cross JJ et al: A randomized trial of spiral CT and ventilation perfusion scintigraphy for the diagnosis of pulmonary embolism. Clin Radiol 1998;53:177.

Dalen JD et al: Thrombolytic therapy for pulmonary embolism. Is it effective? Is it safe? When is it indicated? Arch Intern Med 1997;157:2550.

Hull RD: Low-molecular-weight heparin vs. heparin in the treatment of patients with pulmonary embolism: American-Canadian Thrombosis Study Group. Arch Intern Med 2000; 160:229.

Meaney JF: Diagnosis of pulmonary embolism with magnetic resonance angiography. N Engl J Med 1997;336:1422.

Mohan CR et al: Comparative efficacy and complications of vena caval filters. J Vasc Surg 1995;21:235.

Value of the ventilation/perfusion scan in acute pulmonary embolism: results of the prospective investigation of pulmonary embolism diagnosis (PIOPED). The PIOPED Investigators. JAMA 1990;263:2753.

SUPERFICIAL THROMBOPHLEBITIS

ESSENTIALS OF DIAGNOSIS

- *Erythema, induration, and tenderness along the superficial vein.*
- *Usually spontaneous but can follow venous cannulation.*

General Considerations

Superficial thrombophlebitis may appear spontaneously in patients with varicose veins, in pregnant or postpartum women, or in patients with thromboangiitis obliterans or Behçet's disease. It may also occur after intravenous therapy or in an area of localized trauma. The presence of superficial phlebitis—particularly if it occurs in a migratory manner—suggests the presence of an abdominal cancer such as carcinoma of the pancreas (Trousseau's thrombophlebitis). The most common vein affected is the greater saphenous vein and its branches. In up to 20% of cases, a simultaneous deep venous thrombosis exists. Pulmonary emboli are rare unless extension into the deep venous system occurs.

Clinical Findings

The patient usually presents complaining of localized extremity pain and redness. Areas of induration, erythema, and tenderness correspond to dilated and often thrombosed superficial veins. Over time, a firm cord may develop. Generalized edema is absent unless the deep veins are involved. The presence of fever and shaking chills suggests septic or suppurative phlebitis, which occurs most commonly as a complication of intravenous cannulation.

Differential Diagnosis

Superficial thrombophlebitis must be distinguished from ascending lymphangitis, cellulitis, erythema nodosum, erythema induratum, and panniculitis. Unlike these other disorders, superficial phlebitis tends to be well localized over a superficial vein.

Treatment

The primary treatment of superficial venous thrombophlebitis is the administration of nonsteroidal anti-inflammatory drugs, local heat, elevation, and support stockings or ACE wrap. Ambulation is encouraged. In most cases, symptoms will resolve within 7–10 days. Excision of the involved vein is recommended for symptoms that persist over 2 weeks despite treatment or for recurrent phlebitis in the same vein segment. If there is progressive proximal extension with involvement of the saphenofemoral junction or cephalic-subclavian junction, ligation and resection of the vein at the junction should be performed. Alternatively, full-dose anticoagulation can be attempted and followed with monthly venous duplex scans.

Septic thrombophlebitis requires treatment with broad-spectrum intravenous antibiotics. If rapid resolution of the cellulitis occurs, no treatment beyond a short course of antibiotics is required. However, if the patient becomes septic, immediate excision of the infected vein is required. With positive blood cultures, an extended course of antibiotics specific for the identified organism is indicated.

Prognosis

Most episodes of uncomplicated superficial thrombophlebitis respond to conservative management. Cases in which extension into the deep venous system occurs can be associated with thromboembolism.

Belcaro G et al: Superficial thrombophlebitis of the legs: a randomized, controlled, follow-up study. Angiology 1999;50:523.

Lucia MA et al: Images in clinical medicine: superficial thrombophlebitis. N Engl J Med 2001;344:1214.

CHRONIC VENOUS INSUFFICIENCY

The basic physiologic abnormality in patients with chronic venous insufficiency is chronic elevation of venous pressure. The normal venous capacitance can accommodate large-volume changes that occur during exercise with only minimal changes in venous pressure. However, with calf muscle pump dysfunction and valvular reflux, blood pools in the lower extremities and venous hypertension occurs, leading to what Cockett termed "ankle blowout syndrome." Outflow obstruction from proximal obstruction can also produce venous hypertension, resulting in "venous claudication" as the deep venous system fills with blood during exercise. The leg becomes painful, swollen, and heavy, mimicking arterial insufficiency.

Valvular incompetence of the deep veins can be congenital or result from damage following phlebitis, varicose veins, or deep venous thrombosis. Venous reflux is demonstrable in 17% of extremities 1 week after thrombosis but in 66% after 12 months.

Chronic venous stasis changes are centered in the "gaiter areas" around the ankles. This is the location of the commonly affected perforator veins and is a region with sparse soft tissue support to withstand elevated venous pressures. Brawny edema is produced by extravasation of plasma fluid, red blood cells, and plasma proteins. Lysis of red blood cells results in deposition of hemosiderin, which creates a brownish discoloration. Leukocytes become sequestered in the microcirculation, leading to capillary occlusion and release of superoxide radicals, proteolytic enzymes, and growth factors. Macrophages and T lymphocytes are primary mediators of this inflammatory response which results in fibroblast activation and scarring and fibrosis of the subcutaneous tissues. Ultimately, this fibrosis results in compromised skin perfusion and ulceration.

Clinical Findings

A. SYMPTOMS AND SIGNS

Both isolated saphenous vein incompetence and deep venous insufficiency can lead to chronic venous stasis changes. The first symptom to develop is usually ankle and calf edema. Involvement of the foot and toes suggests lymphedema. Typically, the edema is worst at the end of the day and improves with leg elevation. Long-standing disease is characterized by stasis dermatitis, hyperpigmentation, brawny induration, and ulceration. Venous stasis ulcers are large, painless, and irregular in outline. They have a shallow, moist granulation bed, occur in the gaiter area on the medial or lateral aspects of the ankle, and are often accompanied by stasis dermatitis and stasis pigmentation.

B. IMAGING AND OTHER DIAGNOSTIC STUDIES

Duplex ultrasound can identify the presence and location of incompetent perforating veins and has been used to evaluate the function of individual venous valves. However, it does not easily assess calf muscle pump function or the presence of proximal obstruction. These concerns are addressed with use of air plethysmography, which gives a quantitative assessment of venous reflux (by the venous filling index), calf muscle pump function (by the ejection fraction), and overall venous function (by residual volume function). These measurements help to stratify patients into treatment groups. Abnormal residual volume function may indicate poor calf muscle pump function or valvular reflux, but patients with increased venous filling indices and normal ejection fractions would be good candidates for antireflux surgery, while those with normal venous filling indices and decreased ejection fractions would not. Air plethysmography can be utilized during exercise, it is easily and readily repeatable, and it can be used to differentiate superficial from deep venous insufficiency.

Determination of functional outflow obstruction requires venography with or without pressure measurement. In normal limbs, the arm-foot venous pressure differential is less than 4 mm Hg at rest and less then 6 mm Hg with reactive hyperemia. Descending phlebography involves injection of contrast into the common femoral vein to test the valves during normal breathing and with a forced Valsalva maneuver. Using this technique, pathologic reflux can be identified in patients with postthrombotic damage in approximately 30% of cases.

Differential Diagnosis

Congestive heart failure and chronic liver and kidney disease must be considered in the differential diagnosis of bilateral lower extremity edema. Lymphedema is characterized by nonpitting edema of the dorsum of the foot and toes as well as the calf and generally is not associated with ulceration. Severe arterial insufficiency produces ulcers that are painful, well circumscribed, and located over pressure points on the distal end of the extremity and foot. Ulcers due to autoimmune diseases, erythema nodosum, and fungal infections are distinguished by appearance and distribution.

Treatment

Venous insufficiency is an incurable but manageable problem. Most patients respond well to a conservative treatment program composed of intermittent leg elevation, regular exercise, and the use of surgical elastic graduated compression stockings. Although the mechanism by which elastic compression improves the symptoms of chronic venous insufficiency has not been clearly established, recent work suggests that external compression may restore competency of dilated valve cusps and affect venoarterial reflex. Most venous ulceration will improve with leg elevation, external compression, and local wound care. Compression can be achieved with either an inelastic bandage such as a Unna's boot or with an occlu-

sive wound dressing covered by Ace bandage wrapping or surgical support stockings.

Surgery is indicated for a small percentage of patients with nonhealing ulcers or disabling symptoms refractory to conservative management. The two main categories of procedures are antireflux procedures and bypass operations for obstruction. The pathology must be accurately characterized so that an appropriate operative strategy can be developed. The most common abnormality in patients with chronic venous insufficiency is incompetence of the popliteal or tibial veins; 50–60% of patients have incompetent perforators.

Perforating vein ligation is used in patients with recurrent or recalcitrant venous ulcers with demonstrated incompetence of perforating veins under the area of ulceration. It is performed to reverse the local wound complication of venous ulceration and does nothing to change the underlying deep venous hemodynamics of the leg. Therefore, patients must understand that for maximal effectiveness after perforator ligation, standard treatment for chronic venous insufficiency must be continued. Patients who have proximal venous obstruction should have this problem corrected prior to perforator interruption. The incidence of ulcer recurrence after perforator ligation is 15–20%, but the wound complication rate secondary to impaired incisional healing with severe stasis disease ranges from 12% to 55%. Wound complications have been reduced to 5% with the introduction of subfascial endoscopic perforator surgery, which achieves an ulcer recurrence rate of 12–28% at 2 years, equal to the rate following open surgery.

Direct venous reconstructive surgery is indicated for (1) venous reflux not amenable to a conservative treatment regimen, (2) failure to relieve symptoms after vein stripping or perforator ligation, or (3) intractable disabling venous claudication associated with venous outflow obstruction. Procedures for reflux include valvuloplasty, venous segment transposition, and valvular transplantation. The best results with valvuloplasty are achieved when combined with perforator ligation. The reported success rate is 77% in one recent study of 155 extremities with a 1- to 13-year follow-up. Valvuloplasty can be performed by placement of external cuffs or bands, vein wall plication, angioscopic repair, or open valve repair. Venous segment transfer involves replacing a refluxing segment of vein with a healthy segment of autologous axillary vein. Alternatively, a competent segment of profunda vein can be used to replace an incompetent segment of superficial femoral or greater saphenous vein in a vein transposition. Although initial results of these procedures are good, the effect is not long-lasting. Transplantation of individual valves at the level of the popliteal vein is a new technique with reported good clinical results in 60–70% of cases and an improvement in venous hemodynamics by air plethysmography.

Bypasses and angiographic procedures can be performed for venous obstruction. The Palma procedure is a cross-femoral bypass first described in 1958 for iliac vein obstruction. In this procedure, the proximal saphenous vein from the contralateral leg is tunneled suprapubically to the femoral vein on the side of the iliac obstruction. This allows for venous flow to bypass across the pelvis and empty through the patent contralateral iliac vein. Prosthetic material has been used with equivalent clinical outcomes. Overall 5-year graft patency averages 75–80%. Historically, distal femoral arteriovenous fistulas were constructed to improve iliofemoral vein graft patency, but more current experience does not support their continued use in most cases. Patients with short-segment iliac vein obstruction from May-Thurner syndrome have also been successfully treated by angioplasty and stenting.

Saphenopopliteal bypass (May-Husni procedure) can be considered for patients with occlusion of the superficial femoral vein. In this procedure, calf blood flow is shunted around the obstructed superficial femoral vein through the patent saphenous vein. Approximately 75% of patients are reported to show clinical improvement postoperatively.

Criado E et al: The role of air plethysmography in the diagnosis of chronic venous insufficiency. J Vasc Surg 1998;27:660.

DePalma RG et al: Target selection for surgical intervention in severe chronic venous insufficiency: comparison of duplex scanning and phlebography. J Vasc Surg 2000;32:913.

Gruss JD, Heimer W: Bypass procedures for venous obstruction. In: *Surgical Management of Venous Disease.* Raju S, Villavicencio JL (editors). Williams & Wilkins, 1997.

Mohr DN et al: The venous stasis syndrome after deep venous thrombosis or pulmonary embolism: a population-based study. Mayo Clin Proc 2000;75:1249.

Raju : Technical options in venous valve reconstruction. Am J Surg 1997;173:301.

■ II. THE LYMPHATICS

LYMPHEDEMA

ESSENTIALS OF DIAGNOSIS

- *Can be developmental or acquired.*
- *Painless edema of one or both lower extremities, usually involving the ankle, the dorsum of the foot, and the toes.*
- *Edema is usually pitting at first and then becomes firm, rubbery, and nonpitting due to fibrosis.*
- *Frequent episodes of lymphangitis and cellulitis may occur.*

General Considerations

Much less is known about the fluid dynamics of the lymphatic system than of the venous or arterial system. Most energy for lymph propulsion arises from the intrinsic lymphatic smooth muscle contractions that occur rhythmically. Lymphatic luminal pressures are usually 30–50 mm Hg and can exceed arterial pressure under special circumstances. The lymphatic system carries interstitial fluid and macromolecular proteins lost from the capillaries—as well as infectious agents and foreign material—back into the central circulation. Two to 4 liters a day of lymph drain into the subclavian vein.

The fundamental mechanism responsible for lymphedema formation is impairment of lymph flow out of the extremity. Primary lymphedema is caused by abnormal lymphatic development—most often hypoplasia resulting in severe reduction in the number of lymphatics and the lymphatic diameters. It is classified by age at onset of the disease. Congenital lymphedema develops before 1 year of age, is usually bilateral, and affects males more than females; if familial, it is known as Milroy's disease. More often, lymphedema develops during adolescence (lymphedema praecox) and is unilateral; there is a 3.5:1 female predominance. Lymphedema occurring after age 35 is referred to as lymphedema tarda.

Secondary lymphedema results from a wide variety of disease processes that cause obstruction to the lymphatic system. The most common of these is surgical excision and radiation to the axillary or inguinal lymph nodes as part of the treatment of breast cancer, cervical cancer, prostate cancer, melanoma, and soft tissue tumors. Less common causes of secondary lymphedema are bacterial and fungal infections, trauma, and lymphoproliferative diseases. In many developing countries, lymphatic obstruction due to filariasis is caused by three different parasites: *Wuchereria bancrofti, Brugia malayi,* and *Brugia timori.*

Clinical Manifestations

A. SYMPTOMS AND SIGNS

The history of the disease process will usually define the cause of the lymphedema. Development of painless edema in an adolescent girl with a family history of lymphedema would indicate primary lymphedema as a diagnosis. A history of lymph node dissection, irradiation, or the presence of a parasitic infection suggests secondary lymphedema.

Figure 37–7. Acquired lymphedema. Edema is centered at the ankle and involves the foot and toes

Lymphedema development is usually slowly progressive and painless. In the early stages the edema is pitting, but as the disease progresses, chronic fibrosis occurs and the edema becomes nonpitting. The distribution of edema is also characteristic. It is usually centered around the ankle (Figure 37–7) and is most pronounced on the dorsum of the foot, producing a buffalo hump appearance. Unlike edema of venous stasis disease, lymphedema also often involves the toes. In the early stages the skin is normal, but skin thickening and hyperkeratosis occurs with long-standing disease. A chronic eczematous dermatitis may ensue.

Rarely, lymphangiosarcoma or angiosarcoma may develop as a complication of chronic lymphedema. This neoplastic transformation of blood vessels and lymphatics is called Stewart-Treves syndrome.

B. IMAGING STUDIES

Venous duplex scans are performed to rule out venous insufficiency. Lymphangiography is rarely used now, as it can further damage the lymphatics and is unnecessary to establish the diagnosis. Lymphoscintigraphy is a specialized test used for the detection of lymph node metastasis and does not play a significant role in the diagnosis of lymphedema though it may confirm the diagnosis in ambiguous cases. CT and MRI are useful tests in patients with suspected secondary lymphedema from unknown malignancy.

Differential Diagnosis

A variety of diseases can result in bilateral lower extremity edema. These include congestive heart failure, chronic renal or hepatic insufficiency, and hypoproteinemia. In patients with unilateral leg edema, differential diagnosis includes congenital vascular malformations, chronic venous insufficiency, and reflex sympathetic dystrophy.

Treatment

Lymphedema is a chronic disease for which there is no complete cure. However, a variety of conservative measures can substantially reduce the risk of further complications and disability.

No drug therapy is effective. Use of benzopyrones (coumarins) and steroid injections to increase lymphatic transport has not shown consistent benefit. Diuretics can be useful for acute exacerbation of edema secondary to infection or for coexisting venous stasis disease, but these agents are not recommended for long-term use in lymphedema.

The mainstay of treatment is external compression and meticulous skin care. Mechanical reduction of lymphedema can best be achieved with a program of frequent leg elevation, manual lymphatic drainage massage, low-stretch wrapping techniques, and intermittent pneumatic compression. Sequential pneumatic compression devices are traditionally the first line of treatment. Many different devices are available for use on the leg, and Reid sleeves can be custom fit for patients with postmastectomy arm lymphedema. Graduated compression stockings maintain the limb after reduction by pneumatic compression.

Good skin care is imperative in order to prevent infection. Moisturizing lotions should be applied regularly, especially after showering or bathing. Drying and cracking of the skin can create portals of entry for bacteria. Infection is difficult to eradicate because of disordered lymphatic drainage and can be limb-threatening.

The psychologic impact of chronic lymphedema cannot be underestimated. However, with appropriate patient education that results in the prevention of chronic infection or massive edema, this problem can be manageable.

Operation may be considered in rare cases of severe functional impairment and recurrent lymphangitis. The primary goals of these operations are to reduce limb bulk, either by ablative techniques (excision of excess tissue) or physiologic techniques (lymphatic reconstruction). The Charles procedure involves excision of all skin and subcutaneous tissue from the tibial tuberosity to the lateral head of the fibula and wound coverage by a split-thickness skin graft. This has been largely replaced by the Sistrunk procedure, which is a staged subcutaneous tissue excision. Wide skin flaps are raised for excision of subcutaneous tissues in the medial leg and then 3 months later in the lateral leg. Ablative techniques have been less successful in the upper extremity than in the lower extremity.

The Thompson procedure is an indirect lymphatic reconstruction. A flap of dermis is buried in the muscle compartment to promote formation of communications between subdermal and deep lymphatics, Omental free flaps are similarly designed to encourage new lympholymphatic channels. Direct lymphatic reconstruction by creation of lymphovenous anastomoses or lymphatic interposition grafting is achievable by microsurgical techniques and has had limited success in some centers. Long-term efficacy is not yet known.

Ko DS et al: Effective treatment of lymphedema of the extremities. Arch Surg 1998;133:452.

Pain SJ et al: Lymphoedema following surgery for breast cancer. Br J Surg 2000;87:1128.

LYMPHANGITIS

 ESSENTIALS OF DIAGNOSIS

- *Red streaks traveling longitudinally up an extremity towards regional lymph nodes*
- *Shaking chills, fever, and malaise.*

General Considerations

Lymphangitis is usually caused by a hemolytic streptococcal or staphylococcal infection that arises in an area of cellulitis near an open wound. Multiple long red streaks can be seen coursing toward the regional lymph nodes. Severe systemic manifestations include tachycardia, fever, chills, and malaise which untreated can lead to sepsis and death.

Clinical Findings

A. SYMPTOMS AND SIGNS

Pain at the site of the initial wound is present. High fevers develop rapidly. The streaks may be faint in appearance initially, especially in dark-skinned patients. Regional lymph nodes are often enlarged and tender.

B. LABORATORY FINDINGS

An elevated white blood cell count associated with a left shift is almost universally present. Blood and wound cultures should be obtained routinely.

Differential Diagnosis

Lymphangitis should be distinguished from superficial thrombophlebitis, which is usually localized to a single venous segment often with a palpable cord. Patients usually do not appear toxic, as do patients with lymphangitis. Cat-scratch fever should always be considered when lymphadenitis is present. It is also important to differentiate cellulitis and severe soft tissue infections from lymphangitis. In general, lymphangitis is characterized by its superficial location and the linear pattern of erythema.

Treatment

The extremity should be elevated and warm compresses applied. Analgesics and intravenous antibiotics should be instituted immediately. Examination of the wound should be made to determine the need for debridement or incision and drainage of an abscess.

Prognosis

Delayed or inadequate therapy can lead to overwhelming sepsis and death. Aggressive institution of appropriate antibiotic therapy and wound care will usually control the infection within 48–72 hours.

Neurosurgery & Surgery of the Pituitary

38

Mitchel S. Berger, MD

■ DIAGNOSIS & MANAGEMENT OF DEPRESSED STATES OF CONSCIOUSNESS

Cornelia S. von Koch, MD, PhD, & Julian T. Hoff, MD

Definitions

The clinical definition of consciousness ranges from alert wakefulness to deep coma. An **alert**, awake patient responds immediately and appropriately to all stimuli. A **stuporous** patient responds only when aroused by vigorous stimulation. **Coma** implies failure to respond to stimulation. Most cases of depressed states of consciousness lie between these extremes and are best categorized by accurate descriptions of their responses to specific stimuli—eg, auditory, visual, and tactile (touch or pain).

The Neurologic Examination

The most reliable index for assessing the level of consciousness at any moment is the patient's response to external stimuli. (How quick and how accurate are the patient's responses to questions, to touch, to pain, etc?) Brain stem reflexes also allow an accurate estimate of the level of consciousness—pupillary responses to light, corneal reflexes, oculocephalic and caloric responses, cough and gag reflexes, pattern of breathing, etc. Motor activity of the extremities, either spontaneous or induced by the examiner's stimulus, provides assessment of the entire neuraxis. Does the patient move the extremities purposefully, equally, and briskly, or is there failure to move at all? Which extremities do not move? Nonpurposeful or reflex movement of the arms and legs may also establish the level of neuraxis function, though less reliably (eg, decorticate or decerebrate posturing).

Depressed consciousness may occur abruptly (eg, cerebral concussion) or gradually (eg, barbiturate overdose), often with fluctuations in the level of consciousness (eg, waxing-waning consciousness associated with subdural hematoma). Accurate and repeated examina-

tions will establish not only the level of consciousness but also its changing course. The urgency of diagnosis depends largely upon the rate of change in the patient's course as determined by repeated examinations.

Diagnostic Possibilities

Depressed states of consciousness may be due to many causes. Trauma is usually obvious, both from the history and upon examination of the patient. **Metabolic disorders** (eg, diabetes mellitus, uremia, poisoning, electrolyte imbalance, hypoxia) may similarly alter the state of consciousness. In addition to an accurate history and physical examination, laboratory investigations are required to establish a diagnosis of metabolic coma.

Patients with **intracranial neoplasms** may be alert, comatose, or at any level of consciousness in between. A progressive, unrelenting history is a valuable criterion of this initial diagnosis. **Central nervous system infections** (eg, encephalitis, meningitis) are usually accompanied by systemic signs of infection and a progressively worsening course. Cerebral abscess, on the other hand, behaves more like an expanding neoplasm than a fulminating infection.

Vascular occlusions (emboli, thrombosis) usually cause abrupt neurologic deficits without grossly impaired consciousness, whereas cerebral hemorrhage typically causes abrupt coma with profound neurologic deficits. Conversely, subarachnoid hemorrhage may occur without any alteration of wakefulness. **Degenerative diseases** are usually slowly progressive, dementing illnesses that dull consciousness but characteristically do not produce coma.

Diagnostic Tools

Laboratory and radiographic tests help to establish the clinical diagnosis. Routine examinations should include a complete blood count, urinalysis, plasma glucose, blood urea nitrogen, and serum electrolytes.

Urine and blood for toxicologic study are essential if poisoning is a possibility. Skull and cervical spine films and chest x-ray are obvious aids after trauma. Cerebrospinal fluid analysis is an essential step toward diagnosis of meningitis or subarachnoid hemorrhage. Lumbar puncture is rarely helpful in the assessment of head trauma and probably is contraindicated during the initial workup after injury.

Although most patients are unconscious for a single reason, some may have combined or additive reasons. A severe head injury may have been caused by abrupt coma induced by cerebral hemorrhage in a hypertensive patient, or a diabetic patient with glioblastoma multiforme may be in coma from an insulin overdose and not from the expanding neoplasm. The physician must be aware of these possible—though uncommon—complexities.

The administration of intravenous hypertonic glucose (50%, 50 mL) is occasionally diagnostic but should be done only after blood has been taken for glucose measurement and before an intravenous glucose drip has been started.

Most patients with depressed consciousness should undergo CT scanning or MRI to establish the presence or absence of an intracranial mass lesion. Appropriate therapy depends on the early recognition of the specific intracranial problem.

Management

Protection of the airway and control of shock are fundamental principles of management of patients with depressed consciousness. Most complications of coma can be attributed to failure to follow these basic rules. Responsive patients with good cough reflexes can often protect their own airways. Other patients, usually stuporous or comatose, require endotracheal intubation or tracheostomy in order to (1) reduce the likelihood of aspiration of gastric contents and (2) ensure unrestricted gas exchange (PO_2, PCO_2).

Adequate tracheal suctioning, frequent changes in position, pulmonary physiotherapy, and intermittent positive pressure breathing help maintain good pulmonary function once the airway is secure.

Shock must be controlled. If it is due to hypovolemia, blood and fluids must be given intravenously. In the absence of trauma, other causes of hypotension must be sought and treated specifically (eg, gram-negative sepsis).

A nasogastric tube (to sample ingested drugs, to remove gastric contents that might be aspirated into the lungs, etc), intravenous cannulas to administer drugs and fluids, and an indwelling bladder catheter to assess fluid balance are necessary steps in the early management of comatose patients.

ELEVATED INTRACRANIAL PRESSURE

The skull contains brain, cerebrospinal fluid, and blood (Figure 38–1). At normal intracranial pressures of 10–15 mm Hg (120–180 mm H_2O), these three components maintain volumetric equilibrium. Increased volume of one component will elevate intracranial pressure unless the volume of the other two components decreases proportionally (Monro-Kellie doctrine). Because compensatory volumetric changes have physical and physiologic limits, the ability of the skull's contents to maintain normal pressure can be exceeded by a change of volume that is either too fast or too great.

The compensatory properties of the intracranial contents follow a pressure-volume exponential curve (Figure 38–2). Increased volume of any of the three components can be accommodated to a certain point without change in intracranial pressure. Once that critical volume is reached, however, additional volume increase produces an increase in intracranial pressure.

Increased intracranial pressure exerts its deleterious effect (1) by distorting and shifting the brain as pressure gradients develop, and (2) by reducing the effective perfusion pressure of the brain (cerebral perfusion pressure [CPP] = mean arterial pressure [MAP] minus intracranial pressure [ICP]). Common examples of a significant volumetric change in one or more of the three normal intracranial components are cerebral edema (brain), hydrocephalus (cerebrospinal fluid), and cerebral venous occlusion (blood).

An intracranial mass (eg, tumor, hematoma) represents a fourth component, and its presence initiates compensatory adjustments of the other three: (1) Intracranial vessels are compressed, reducing the amount of intracranial blood; (2) cerebrospinal fluid volume is reduced by increased absorption or reduced production (at high intracranial pressure); and (3) intracranial bulk is reduced by brain creeping out of adjacent foramina (eg, transtentorial herniation, tonsillar herniation). Children with expandable skulls due to unfused sutures have an additional compensatory mechanism to accommodate expanding intracranial volume and are thereby partially protected from extreme rises of intracranial pressure.

Clinical Findings

Most brain insults, whether from trauma, ischemia, poisoning, or other sources, are accompanied by raised intracranial pressure. Following head trauma, intracranial pressure may rise quickly to very high levels as a result of vascular congestion, extravasation, and cerebral edema. Intracranial pressure may also rise substantially when a neoplasm occupies the intracranial cavity. Intracranial hypertension may occur after cerebrovascular occlusions (stroke), during central nervous system infections, and following cerebral hypoxia. Intracranial pressure by itself is rarely a clinical problem when coma is the result of a metabolic disorder (eg, uremia, hepatic coma).

Figure 38–1. Intracranial compartments and circulation of cerebrospinal fluid.

1. Internal carotid artery
2. Cortical and deep cerebral arteries
3. Capillary network
4. Cortical and deep cerebral veins
5. Superior sagittal sinus
6. Transverse sinus
7. Internal jugular vein
8. Choroid plexus
9. Lateral ventricles
10. Third ventricle
11. Cerebral aqueduct
12. Fourth ventricle
13. Central canal of spinal cord
14. Foramina of Magendie and Luschka
15. Subarachnoid space
16. Arachnoid granulations

A. SPECIFIC SIGNS OF RAISED INTRACRANIAL PRESSURE

While any of the following clinical signs may result from causes other than raised intracranial pressure, most will appear during raised intracranial pressure if the elevation is severe or prolonged.

1. Cardiovascular—Blood pressure elevation accompanied by bradycardia and respiratory slowing classically results from raised intracranial pressure. This "Cushing response," however, usually appears only when intracranial hypertension is severe.

2. Gastrointestinal—Hemorrhage from gastric ulcerations (Cushing's ulcer) may accompany raised intracranial pressure.

3. Pulmonary—Hemorrhagic pulmonary edema may result from severe elevation of intracranial pressure as

well as from other brain insults. The lung lesion is the end product of a pathophysiologic sequence mediated by the sympathetic nervous system. Few patients survive this hemodynamic storm of neurogenic origin unless intracranial pressure is reduced.

4. Neurologic—Papilledema, abducens nerve paresis (unilateral occasionally; bilateral often), and depressed consciousness are the most common signs associated with generalized intracranial pressure elevations. Loss of visual acuity may occur as a late consequence of optic nerve atrophy. In children, decreased upward gaze is common.

B. SPECIFIC SYNDROMES

Specific syndromes may appear when intracranial pressure is raised by the presence of an intracranial mass.

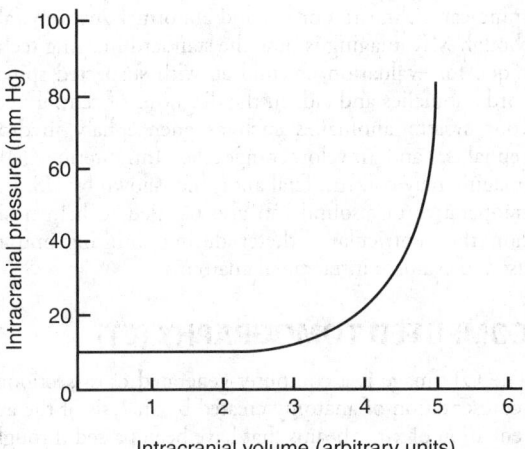

Figure 38–2. Change in intracranial pressure with changes in intracranial compartment volume. The figures along the abscissa represent units of volume.

Table 38–1. Clinical manifestations of transtentorial herniation.

Compressed Structure	Clinical Manifestations
Cranial nerve III	Ipsilateral mydriasis
Midbrain physiologic functional transection	Decerebrate rigidity
Reticular formation	Coma
Ipsilateral cerebral peduncle	Contralateral hemiparesis
Contralateral cerebral peduncle	Ipsilateral hemiparesis (false localizing sign)
Cerebral aqueduct (of Sylvius)	Headache and vomiting due to acute hydrocephalus
Posterior cerebral artery	Contralateral hemianopsia (false localizing (sign)[1]

[1]This sign is a consequence of herniation and does not indicate the localization of the primary process; in this sense, the sign falsely localizes the primary lesion.

1. Transtentorial herniation—A laterally placed supratentorial mass may push the uncus and hippocampus medially into the tentorial incisure. The oculomotor nerves, the cerebral peduncles, the cerebral aqueduct, and the midbrain (containing the reticular formation) are vulnerable to compression from the displaced temporal lobe. Transtentorial herniation may then appear clinically (Table 38–1).

2. Tonsillar herniation—Herniation of the cerebellar tonsils into the foramen magnum causes compression of the medulla. The hallmark of medullary compression is respiratory failure: slow and irregular breathing followed by apnea. Earlier signs of herniation are nuchal rigidity, intermittent opisthotonos, and depressed gag and cough reflexes. Consciousness may be retained until the patient becomes severely hypoxic.

Although raised intracranial pressure usually becomes obvious clinically, it may go undetected for months. Patients with benign intracranial hypertension (pseudotumor cerebri) often have no symptoms despite severe papilledema and intracranial hypertension. Similarly, patients with obstruction of cerebrospinal fluid pathways may tolerate intracranial pressure elevation for weeks or months without developing overt clinical signs. Failing mentation may provide the only clue to progressive hydrocephalus in the latter circumstance.

Treatment

A. SPECIFIC TREATMENT

Management of specific causes of raised intracranial pressure is effective treatment. Removal of intracranial masses, shunting of obstructed cerebrospinal fluid, and removal of toxins (eg, lead, in lead encephalopathy) are examples of specific forms of treatment.

B. NONSPECIFIC TREATMENT

When raised intracranial pressure as such must also be managed, the following nonspecific measures are useful:

1. Control of respiration—Accumulation of CO_2 ($PaCO_2$ > 40 mm Hg) will increase cerebral blood flow and raise intracranial pressure. A therapeutic goal is maintenance of $PaCO_2$ in the range of 30–40 mm Hg.

2. Control of body temperature—Hypothermia reduces cerebral metabolism and lowers intracranial pressure. Hyperthermia increases intracranial pressure. Thus, fever must be controlled.

3. Osmotic diuretics—Mannitol, urea, or glycerin can reduce intracranial pressure by cerebral dehydration.

4. Cerebrospinal fluid drainage—Reduction of cerebrospinal fluid volume by repeated spinal taps or by shunting may control raised intracranial pressure from pseudotumor. Ventricular drainage of cerebrospinal fluid reduces intracranial pressure transiently in severe head injury and in patients with obstructive hydrocephalus.

5. Bony decompression—This nonspecific method of reducing intracranial pressure may be employed when other measures fail.

King BS et al: The early assessment and intensive care unit management of patients with severe traumatic brain and spinal cord injuries. Surg Clin North Am 2000;80:855.

Luerssen TG: Intracranial pressure: current status in monitoring and management. Semin Pediatr Neurol 1997;4:146.

Marshall LF: Head injury: recent past, present, and future. Neurosurgery 2000;47:546.

Wilkins RH, Rengachary SS (editors): *Neurosurgery,* 2nd ed. McGraw-Hill, 1996.

Youmans J: *Neurological Surgery,* 4th ed. Saunders, 1996.

■ NEURODIAGNOSTIC PROCEDURES

William P. Dillon, MD

Magnetic resonance (MR) imaging is the study of choice for the evaluation of most lesions affecting the brain and spine. It has gradually replaced computed tomography (CT) for many indications and has also reduced the need for invasive neuroimaging techniques such as myelography and angiography. CT is more sensitive than MR imaging in visualizing fine osseous detail such as temporal bone anatomy fractures. Recent developments such as helical CT, CT angiography (CTA), MR angiography (MRA), and interventional neuroradiologic procedures have continued to advance the diagnosis and guide the therapy of neurologic disorders.

PLAIN FILM RADIOGRAPHY

CT and MR have largely replaced plain films, especially in cases with neurologic deficits. Plain films of the skull and spine are useful in the initial assessment of spinal trauma and in suspected infection but are rarely indicated otherwise. Plain films are also no longer indicated in the setting of head trauma, as CT or MR reveals more critical information regarding the intracranial contents.

ULTRASOUND

High-resolution ultrasound (US) may image intracranial and spinal anatomy when an acoustic window (bony defect) is present. It is noninvasive, does not involve x-rays, and can be performed with portable equipment. Ultrasound has found wide application in the evaluation of intracranial anatomy in infants with open fontanelles. In the neonatal intensive care unit, ultrasound is the standard technique for evaluating the premature infant for intraventricular hemorrhage and hydrocephalus. Ultrasound examination of the infant spine can delineate normal and abnormal anatomy, although MR imaging is now the standard imaging technique for evaluation of children with suspected spinal cord anomalies and aids in the diagnosis of central nervous system anomalies such as anencephaly, hydrocephalus, and myelomeningocele. Intrauterine MR imaging may confirm fetal anomalies shown by US. Intraoperative ultrasound can also be used to help position the ventricular catheter during shunting and is used to evaluate intracranial anatomy.

COMPUTED TOMOGRAPHY (CT)

The CT image is a computer-generated cross-sectional representation of anatomy created by analysis of the attenuation of x-ray beams that have been passed through various points around a section of the body or brain. The x-ray source is collimated to the desired slice thickness. Sensitive x-ray detectors are aligned 180 degrees from the x-ray source and detect x-rays that are not attenuated by the patient's anatomy. A computer calculates a "back projection" image from the attenuation profile. Greater x-ray attenuation, as caused by bone, results in areas of high "density," while soft tissue structures, which attenuate x-rays less, appear lower in density. The resolution of an image depends on the radiation dose, the collimation (slice thickness), the field of view, and the matrix size of the display. Recent developments in slip ring helical scanners have increased the speed of CT acquisition to as short as 0.5–1 second per scan, or 1–2 minutes for a typical head CT. In the helical scan mode, the table moves continuously through the rotating x-ray beam, generating a "helix" of information that can be reformatted into various slice thicknesses. Advantages of helical CT include shorter scan times, reduced patient and organ motion, and the ability to acquire dynamic CT images during the infusion of intravenous contrast. Dynamic contrast images can be used to construct CT angiograms (CTAs) of vascular structures as well as physiologic maps of vascular perfusion. CTA has proved useful in assessment of the intracranial and extracranial carotid arteries, especially in acute stroke victims. (Figure 38–3). "Multidetector" CT scanners acquire multiple sections with each revolution of the gantry, further decreasing the time per examination and improving the spatial and temporal assessment of vascular anatomy and physiology.

CT is safe and reliable. Radiation exposure is between 3 cGy and 5 cGy per examination. The most frequent complications are associated with use of intravenous contrast agents. Two broad categories of contrast media—ionic and nonionic—are in use. Nonionic agents are preferred; ionic agents are less expensive but are associated with a higher incidence of toxicity and allergic reactions than nonionic agents.

A

B

Figure 38–3. ***A:*** A 50-year-old patient presents with acute left hemiparesis. Noncontrast CT scan demonstrates the "insular string sign"—low density involving the insular cortex—a finding consistent with acute middle cerebral arterial infarction (arrows). ***B:*** Partition from a contrast-enhanced CT angiogram. Note the normally enhancing left internal carotid artery (thin arrow) and nonfilling of the thrombosed right internal carotid artery (thick arrows).

The indications for CT have narrowed since the development of MR imaging. CT is useful in imaging osseous structures of the spine, skull base, and temporal bones. CT is also more sensitive and specific than MR for acute subarachnoid hemorrhage. In the spine, CT is often useful in the evaluation of patients with traumatic spinal injury, osseous spinal stenosis, and spondylosis, but MR is preferred for patients with neurologic deficits. CT obtained following instillation of intrathecal contrast (CT myelography) is useful to evaluate the intracranial cisterns for cerebrospinal fluid fistula, as well as the spinal subarachnoid space in patients with ambiguous MR results. Conditions that are identified with a high degree of accuracy by CT include intracerebral, subdural, and epidural hematomas, cerebral atrophy, and hydrocephalus. Patients with suspected cerebral infarction are also candidates for CT scan, though MR is more sensitive to early infarction. Lesions situated near the calvarium or skull base are more difficult to delineate with CT because of beam-hardening artifacts from adjacent bone. Use of thin sections orthogonal to the area can minimize these artifacts. MR is, however, ideal for detecting and delineating lesions adjacent to the calvarium, as bone artifacts are minimized. Intravenous administration of iodinated contrast media may improve the sensitivity of CT by enhancing the density of lesions with an increased blood pool (eg, meningioma, arteriovenous malformations) or a deficient blood-brain barrier (eg, metastatic tumor and inflammatory lesions).

MAGNETIC RESONANCE IMAGING

The phenomenon of magnetic resonance (MR) is a complex interaction between protons in biologic tissues, static and alternating magnetic field (the magnet), and energy in the form of radiofrequency (Rf) waves of a specific frequency, introduced by coils placed next to the body part of interest. The images that are created reflect the density of hydrogen protons as well as their relaxation rates. The relaxation rate of protons is different for different normal and pathologic tissues. T1- and T2-weighted images can be obtained in order to highlight certain aspects of disease processes. The surrounding molecular environment and atomic neighbors influence the relaxation rates of a hydrogen proton in a tissue. MR images can be generated in sagittal, coronal, axial, and oblique planes without changing the patient's position. Each plane obtained requires a separate sequence lasting 2–10 minutes. Unlike CT, movement of the patient during a sequence will distort all of the images; therefore, patient cooperation is important. Approximately 5% of the population experience claustrophobia in the MR environment, but this can be reduced by mild sedation. MR may be obtained in 2D or 3D modes. Three-dimensional volumetric imaging results in a volume of data that can be reformatted in any plane and manipulated in a real-time fashion to highlight certain disease processes. Fluid-attenuated inversion recovery (FLAIR) is a pulse sequence that produces T2-weighted images in which the cerebrospinal fluid signal is suppressed. FLAIR images are more sensitive than standard spin echo images for cortical lesions and meningeal processes. (Figure 38–4) Echoplanar imaging (EPI) techniques permit rapid MR imaging on the order of milliseconds. EPI is the basis for diffusion imaging, which is the most sensitive technique for identifying acute infarction. and perfusion imaging (Figure 38–5).

The heavy-metal element gadolinium forms the basis of all current intravenous MR contrast agents. Gadolinium is a paramagnetic substance, which reduces the T1 and T2 relaxation times of nearby water protons, resulting in a high signal on T1-weighted images. Gadolinium contrast does not cross a normal blood-brain barrier and thus causes enhancement of brain tissue only at sites of abnormalities in the barrier or lesions with slow vascular flow. Allergic reactions and renal dysfunction are extremely rare side effects of gadolinium agents. These agents can be administered safely to children as well as adults and are often use to increase the sensitivity of MR to various disease states that disrupt the blood-brain barrier.

MR is particularly useful—compared with CT—for identifying lesions in the posterior fossa and the spinal cord. MR imaging has replaced myelography and CT as the initial diagnostic procedure for most conditions of the spine and spinal cord.

Magnetic resonance angiography (MRA) delineates the major extracranial and intracranial vessels without the need for contrast agents, though recent fast scan techniques during a bolus of contrast material have improved the detection of vascular disorders (Figure 38–6). It is important to understand that MRA is a **vascular flow map** and not an anatomic map as revealed by conventional angiography. Two MRA techniques—time-of-flight (TOF) and phase-contrast—are currently in use. TOF, currently the technique used most frequently, relies on the suppression of nonmoving tissue to provide a background for the high signal intensity of flowing blood. A typical TOF angiography sequence results in a series of contiguous thin MR sections (0.9 mm thick) that can be viewed as a maximum intensity projection (MIP) which can be reformatted or viewed in various planes and angles to reveal vascular relationships. Either arterial or venous structures can be obtained (Figures 38–7 and 38–8) The ability to delineate intracranial vascular lesions noninvasively is useful in screening for aneurysms and vascular occlusive disease. MRA has supplanted routine diagnostic

A

B

Figure 38–4. FLAIR MR imaging. Two examples of the utility of FLAIR imaging. **A:** Coronal T2-weighted FLAIR image in a patient with intractable epilepsy demonstrates high signal intensity of the hippocampus consistent with mesial temporal sclerosis (arrow). Note the normal low signal intensity of cerebrospinal fluid in the cisterns and ventricles. **B:** Coronal FLAIR in a patient with subarachnoid hemorrhage. High signal blood replaces the normal low signal blood in the cisterns and in the left hemispheric subdural hematoma.

A

B

Figure 38–5. Diffusion imaging in acute stroke. ***A:*** FLAIR image demonstrates a nonspecific mass of high signal intensity. The differential diagnosis is stroke and tumor. ***B:*** Diffusion-weighted image shows the lesion with high intensity, or restricted, diffusion signal consistent with acute cerebral infarction.

Figure 38–6. Contrast-enhanced MR angiography. Coronal view of contrast-enhanced MRA of the cervical vasculature acquired in 30 seconds during infusion of intravenous gadolinium contrast material. The patient suffered from subclavian artery occlusion and steal syndrome (arrows).

angiography for many purposes, with the exception of patients suspected of vasculitis or other small vessel diseases.

MYELOGRAPHY

Myelography is a radiographic study that outlines the spinal canal and its contents. Water-soluble nonionic contrast material is injected into the subarachnoid space via a lumbar or cervical puncture. The hyperbaric contrast material mixes with cerebrospinal fluid and is manipulated within the spinal canal by tilting the patient into various positions. The flow of contrast material is monitored by fluoroscopy, and radiographs are taken in desired projections to record and preserve with more detail the areas of interest. The agent is excreted by the renal system. CT scanning following subarachnoid instillation of contrast material—"CT myelography"—increases the amount of information obtained com-

Figure 38–7. MRA of aneurysm. 3D time of flight MRA of the circle of Willis demonstrates a small carotido-ophthalmic artery aneurysm (arrow).

pared with routine plain film myelography. Low-dose CT myelography has replaced conventional myelography in most instances; however, CT myelography is still necessary in patients with metallic spinal prostheses or other conditions where MR imaging is contraindicated. Myelography is also useful in detecting cerebrospinal fluid fistula.

DIGITAL SUBTRACTION ANGIOGRAPHY

Radiographic visualization of the arterial and venous systems of the neck, brain, and spinal cord is accomplished by intra-arterial injection of a water-soluble iodinated contrast agent. Injections are made via a long catheter placed into the femoral artery and positioned into the artery of interest. Extremely small catheters have allowed supraselective catheterization of cerebral arteries, permitting endovascular therapies with various devices. Endovascular placement of electrolytically detachable coils has become a standard therapy for certain cerebral aneurysms and assists in the preoperative management of arteriovenous malformations. Digital subtraction angiography is the best procedure for characterizing aneurysms and arteriovenous malformations; however, MRA and CTA have improved in recent years, making possible noninvasive assessment of many of these vascular disorders. Conventional angiography is reserved for cases in which small-vessel detail is essential for diagnosis. Digital subtraction angiography (DSA) permits the use of smaller amounts of contrast material and decreases radiation exposure to the patient. Newer contrast materials and careful attention to technique have reduced the rate of side effects to less than 1%.

A

B

Figure 38–8. MR venography. **A:** Normal lateral view of MRV demonstrates the normal sagittal sinus (arrows). **B:** A patient with acute headaches demonstrates thrombosis of the sagittal sinus (arrows).

RADIONUCLIDE IMAGING

Short half-life gamma-emitting isotopes such as technetium Tc 99m pertechnetate or indium In 113m diethylenetriamine pentaacetic acid (DTPA) are excluded by the intact blood-brain barrier. The isotopes will cross defects in the blood-brain barrier such as those caused by neoplasms or vascular accidents, which appear as an area of increased activity. Intravenous injection of the isotope as a bolus followed by rapid-sequence imaging can give qualitative information about extracranial carotid artery and supratentorial cerebral blood flow.

Isotope cisternography can give qualitative information about cerebrospinal fluid flow and absorption characteristics. An isotope such as indium In 113m DTPA is injected into the subarachnoid space, followed by scanning at intervals of up to 48 hours. This technique is useful for the evaluation of hydrocephalus, cerebrospinal fluid shunt function, and cerebrospinal fluid fistulas (leaks).

Xenon CT is a technique that quantifies regional cerebral blood flow. Inhalation of xenon gas (25–28%) during CT scanning increases the density proportionate to blood flow. This technique may be combined with the administration of acetazolamide, which normally increases cerebral blood flow, to assess circulatory reserve.

Positron emission tomography (PET) relies on the detection of positrons emitted during the decay of a radionuclide that has been injected into a patient. The most frequently used moiety is 2-[^{18}F]fluoro-2-deoxy-D-glucose (FDG), which is an analog of glucose and is taken up by cells competitively with 2-deoxyglucose. Multiple images of glucose uptake activity are formed after 45–60 minutes. Images reveal differences in regional glucose activity among normal and pathologic brain structures. FDG PET scanning has been used to assist in differentiating radiation necrosis from active neoplasm following therapy, in localizing temporal lobe epileptic foci, and in detecting metastatic disease and determining cardiac viability. A lower activity of FDG in the parietal lobes has been associated with Alzheimer's disease.

MAGNETOENCEPHALOGRAPHY (MEG)

Magnetoencephalography (MEG) is a technique that detects the magnetic dipoles intrinsic to the brain during task activation such as sensory stimulation, language tasks, or auditory stimuli. The foci of activity may be mapped onto MRI scans to reveal anatomic localization of somatosensory function.

■ INTRAOPERATIVE NEUROPHYSIOLOGIC MONITORING

Charles D. Yingling, PhD

The last decade has seen a rapid growth in the development of techniques for intraoperative neurophysiologic monitoring. Examples include monitoring cranial nerves during skull base surgery, assessing cerebral perfusion during aneurysm clipping or carotid endarterectomy, monitoring both ascending and descending pathways during spinal surgery, and mapping sensory, motor, and language regions of the cerebral cortex. Most major medical centers now have personnel and equipment dedicated to intraoperative monitoring, and there are many private groups offering monitoring services on a contract basis to smaller hospitals nationwide. Neural monitoring specialists now have national certification offered by the American Board of Neurophysiological Monitoring (supervisory level) and the American Board of Registered Electrodiagnostic Technologists (technologist level). Neurophysiologic monitoring has become an integral part of many neurosurgical procedures as well as of a wide range of orthopedic, otolaryngologic, vascular, pediatric, and neurointerventional radiology procedures.

SKULL BASE SURGERY

One of the first applications of intraoperative neurophysiology was monitoring facial nerve function during acoustic neuroma resection, a technique actually pioneered in the late 19th century which came into widespread use during the 1980s. Small needle electrodes are placed within facial muscles to record electromyographic potentials, and electrical stimulation is used to map the nerve in relation to the tumor by eliciting electromyographic responses when the nerve is contacted. The threshold and amplitude of the responses can be used to quantify facial nerve function and predict postoperative outcome. Electromyographic responses may also be elicited by surgical events such as traction on the nerve and can alert the surgeon to the location of the nerve in the surgical field, which can then be confirmed with stimulation. Conversely, the absence of a response to suprathreshold stimulation indicates an area in which resection can proceed safely. This technique has been shown to dramatically lower the incidence of facial nerve palsy following acoustic neuroma resection, and its routine use has been recommended in an NIH Consensus Conference report.

Similar techniques can be used to monitor other cranial motor nerves by appropriate placement of recording electrodes. For anterior skull base surgery, such as removal of prepontine or cavernous sinus region tumors, the nerves to the extraocular muscles can be monitored by placing fine hookwire electrodes into the inferior rectus, superior oblique, and lateral rectus muscles. The motor component of the trigeminal nerve can be monitored with electrodes in the temporalis or masseter muscles. Lower cranial nerves can be identified with electrodes in the trapezius and genioglossus for tumors of the jugular foramen or foramen magnum region. By intubating with a special electromyographic endotracheal tube (Xomed-Treace), electromyography can be recorded from the vocalis muscles, innervated by the recurrent laryngeal component of the tenth cranial nerve. In all of these cases, electromyographic reactions to surgical manipulations may alert the surgeon to the location of a specific nerve, and electrical stimulation can be used for confirmation.

Development of techniques for monitoring sensory nerves has been more difficult. Visual evoked potentials (VEP), which have long been used in the diagnostic clinic and which are an obvious means of monitoring optic nerve function, are notoriously unstable under anesthesia. Despite repeated efforts with different anesthetic agents, this problem has remained intractable, and optic nerve function is for that reason rarely monitored. Excessive stimulus artifact due to short response latencies has limited the applicability of somatosensory evoked potentials (SEPs) for monitoring trigeminal sensory function. The only sensory cranial nerve that is routinely monitored is the cochlear nerve, which can readily be assessed with only slight modifications of the auditory brain stem response (ABR) technique routinely used in the audiology clinic. However, the small amplitude of this response limits its utility, since signal averaging over 1 or 2 minutes is often necessary to obtain a repeatable response—too slow to be of much use in the surgical context. Direct recordings from the cochlear nerve are much faster but require an invasive electrode which can be difficult to place so that it is stable and not in the way. Digital signal processing techniques show promise for speeding ABR collection times but have yet to come into widespread use. Despite these limitations, ABR monitoring has a place in management of smaller acoustic tumors with good residual hearing. It is also useful in detecting excessive stretching of the cochlear nerve during cerebellar retraction for microvascular decompression or other posterior fossa procedures.

Anesthetic requirements for cranial nerve monitoring are straightforward: No muscle relaxants should be used except for intubation, since electromyographic responses must be unaffected. Otherwise, any desired technique can be used, since the ABR is almost unaffected by normal concentrations of commonly used agents such as N_2O, halogenated vapors, opioids, barbiturates, or propofol.

SPINAL CORD SURGERY

One of the earliest applications of intraoperative neurophysiologic monitoring was the use of somatosensory evoked potentials (SEPs) during scoliosis correction. SEPs are recorded with methods similar to those used in the diagnostic clinic: Appropriate peripheral nerves (usually the median, ulnar, common peroneal, or posterior tibial) are electrically stimulated and averaged responses are obtained from scalp electrodes near somatosensory cortical regions as well as from more peripheral sites. However, since SEPs are mediated primarily by the dorsal columns, it is possible for isolated anterior spine injury or ischemia to remain undetected. There has thus been great interest in development of techniques for monitoring spinal motor pathways as well. An early technique involved stimulation of the cord itself via percutaneous needles placed adjacent to the spinal lamina rostrad to the incision and recording from electrodes placed over peripheral motor nerves. This so-called "neurogenic motor evoked potential" (nMEP) had the advantage that the patient could be maintained on neuromuscular blocking agents to prevent movement in response to stimulation.

Unfortunately, subsequent studies demonstrated that the nMEP response is primarily mediated by antidromic conduction in the dorsal columns, so it is not a true motor evoked potential. The technique now preferred is transcranial electrical stimulation with electrodes placed over the primary motor cortex. A series of brief high-voltage pulses (typically 300–500 volts, four to seven pulses at intervals of 2–3 ms) is delivered through scalp electrodes, and responses are recorded from upper and lower extremity muscles such as abductor pollicis brevis, tibialis anterior, and gastrocnemius. Since antidromic activity cannot cross the somatosensory synapses in the thalamus and dorsal column nuclei, the response is thought to be mediated by corticospinal tracts. Multiple pulses are necessary to elicit the response under general anesthesia, which affects the synapse to the motor nerve in the anterior horn of the spinal cord. The responses are large in amplitude and can thus be seen in single trials without the need for signal averaging. Owing to the predominance of upper extremity representation in the cortical motor areas, lower extremity transcranial MEPs typically have higher thresholds and lower amplitudes than responses in upper extremity muscles. This transcranial motor evoked potential (tcMEP) is quite sensitive to changes in spinal cord perfusion and has been successfully employed not only in scoliosis surgery but also in many other procedures where the spinal cord or its vascular supply is at risk. Spinal tumors, decompressive procedures (both anterior and posterior), and thoracoabdominal aortic aneurysms have all benefited from tcMEP monitoring, which is usually done in conjunction with SEP recording so as to monitor both ascending and descending pathways.

The anesthetic requirements for spinal cord monitoring are much more constraining than for cranial nerve monitoring. The tcMEP technique requires that no muscle relaxants be used, since EMG activity is being recorded. The stimulus causes contractions in scalp muscles which are activated directly, so a bite block must be used to prevent tongue injuries. Some patient movement may be seen in the surgical field, but this is usually minimal; since the responses can be seen in single trials, the surgeon only need pause for a few seconds to allow the pathways to be checked. Both tcMEPs and SEPs are greatly diminished or abolished by high concentrations of commonly used agents such as nitrous oxide or halogenated vapors. The most marked responses are usually obtained with a total intravenous technique based on propofol and narcotics, which can usually be supplemented by low doses of desflurane or similar agents.

Surgery in the lumbar and sacral levels (eg, for tethered cord, myelomeningocele, or lumbosacral tumors) requires a different approach than for cervical or thoracic level surgery. Since the spinal cord terminates at approximately T12 in adults, issues of cord compression, distraction, or perfusion are less relevant than the status of sensory and motor roots in the cauda equina. While it is desirable to preserve innervation of the legs, the most devastating complications of surgery in this region are loss of bowel and bladder control by interruption of lower sacral roots. Motor roots in the cauda equina can be easily monitored using procedures very similar to those developed for cranial motor nerves; the electrodes are simply placed in different muscles. Depending on the level of interest, quadriceps, tibialis anterior, hamstring, gastrocnemius, or intrinsic foot muscles can be easily recorded, as can the external anal sphincter. The urethral sphincter can also be monitored by means of a special ring electrode placed over a standard Foley catheter. The course of roots in relation to lumbosacral tumors can be easily mapped in the same way the facial nerve is mapped in acoustic neuroma. For tethered cord, the filum terminale is identified and stimulated before being transected to ensure that no roots are adherent to its ventral surface, which is a common finding. After all roots are dissected free, stimulation of the filum will produce no responses at intensities from 10 times to 100 times those necessary to activate motor roots. For lumbosacral root monitoring,

anesthetic management is simplified since the only constraint is that no muscle relaxants can be employed.

ANEURYSM SURGERY

Treatment of cerebral aneurysms carries risks of ischemia to structures downstream from the aneurysm. Aneurysm clips may occlude parent vessels or perforators arising from them, and temporary occlusion of a major vessel is often necessary. The risk is particularly high for aneurysm of the posterior communicating or basilar arteries because of the large number of perforators supplying critical brain stem and thalamic structures. Thus, a means of monitoring perfusion in these territories is desirable.

In principle, electroencephalographic recordings could be used to detect cortical ischemia since hypoperfusion causes electroencephalographic slowing, which can be detected readily with digital electroencephalographic techniques. However, because of the risk of ischemia, many vascular neurosurgeons prefer to administer barbiturates prior to clipping or occlusion for cerebral protection. By lowering the cerebral metabolic rate of oxygen consumption ($CMRO_2$), the risk of damage due to cerebral hypoperfusion is reduced; however, since barbiturates produce significant effects on the EEG, such recordings can no longer be used to detect hypoperfusion or ischemia. Fortunately, SEP recordings are also sensitive to decreased cerebral blood flow and can still be recorded even when the EEG is rendered isoelectric by barbiturate administration.

In practice, EEGs and SEPs can be recorded from the same scalp electrodes by directing the signals to separate amplifiers with appropriate filter settings. Electrodes are placed over midline and bilateral parietal and frontal sites. The exact electrode position may have to be altered from standard clinical placements in order to avoid the craniotomy site; since intraoperative changes are assessed rather than comparisons to normative data, this generally does not pose a problem. Baseline recordings under standard anesthesia are obtained first in order to confirm system function and avoid any problems due to positioning; baseline problems are often detected if there is concurrent cervical stenosis and should be corrected by adjusting patient position before proceeding with the craniotomy.

Barbiturates should be administered a few minutes before clipping or occlusion since a new SEP baseline will be necessary. Thiopental sodium is typically administered in a dose comparable to that which would be used for anesthetic induction. The EEG is used to titrate the level of barbiturate to obtain a burst-suppression pattern, in which periods of isoelectricity alternate with higher-amplitude bursts. A burst/suppression ratio of about 20% burst activity is adequate; more than this provides no further cerebral protective effect and will make it more difficult to extubate the patient after the procedure. A new SEP baseline is then obtained; it will typically exhibit prolonged latency and decreased amplitude but will still have a high enough signal/noise ratio to effectively assess intraoperative changes.

For middle cerebral artery aneurysms, either ulnar or median nerve SEPs can be employed. For anterior cerebral or anterior communicating artery aneurysms, posterior tibial nerve SEPs should be used since the lower extremity somatosensory area is in the distal anterior cerebral artery territory. For posterior communicating or basilar artery aneurysms, both upper and lower extremity SEPs should be recorded since occlusion of perforating arteries into the brain stem or thalamus can affect either or both of these pathways. Unilateral changes in SEP amplitude can usually be detected within 2–4 minutes after inadvertent occlusion and are a signal for repositioning clips as necessary to restore baseline values. Such changes are relatively rare in treatment of uncomplicated middle or anterior cerebral artery aneurysms but are encountered more frequently in treatment of posterior circulation aneurysms. This is presumably due to the higher number of small perforating arteries, which are more difficult to visualize with the longer reach from a standard pterional or orbitozygomatic craniotomy.

MAPPING MOTOR PATHWAYS

Surgery for tumors near the central sulcus or internal capsule poses risks of compromised motor function. However, patient survival is enhanced if the most complete resection possible is obtained. In order to locate both cortical and subcortical motor regions, electrical stimulation mapping is employed. For dominant hemisphere tumors resected under local anesthesia, verbal reports from the patient can be used to determine any sensory or motor responses accompanying stimulation. Areas critical for language or memory function can similarly be mapped using appropriate behavioral testing during stimulation. However, when surgery is performed under general anesthesia, this is not possible. If light surgical anesthesia is maintained without the use of muscle relaxants, gross movement of the contralateral body can often be observed in response to direct stimulation of the exposed cortex. However, the sensitivity of this method can be greatly enhanced by simultaneous recording of electromyographic activity from multiple muscles. Consistent electromyographic responses are often observed without any overt motion being detected. This technique is particularly valuable when resecting tumors near subcortical motor pathways, since there is no obvious topography to indicate where a response is likely to be observed. It is much easier to scan multiple electromyographic channels at a slow sweep

speed than to simultaneously observe the entire contralateral body. Since mapping takes little time, it can be repeatedly employed as tumor resection proceeds until responses are obtained. Use of such mapping techniques allows maximal tumor resection to be obtained without compromising motor function.

■ CRANIOCEREBRAL TRAUMA

Martin C. Holland, MD

Trauma is the leading cause of death among persons under 45 years of age, with craniocerebral trauma accounting for a large portion of the deaths. Craniocerebral trauma is second only to stroke as a cause of death from injury to the central nervous system. Though precise numbers are difficult to obtain, it is estimated that the incidence of traumatic brain injury falls between 132 cases and 367 cases per 100,000 population. The 1985–1987 National Health Interview Survey estimated that 1.975 million Americans annually sought medical attention for head injuries. Of these, 373,000 were admitted to hospitals for the injury and 75,000 died.

Traumatic brain injury affects mostly young men, with the male:female ratio falling between 2:1 and 2.8:1. Motor vehicle accidents are the most common cause of serious injury, accounting for approximately 30–55% of admissions. Falls account for 15–35% of cases, assaults and gunshot wounds for 2–25%, and sports-related injuries for 5–20%. As individuals become older, the risk of developing a traumatic brain injury increases—specifically, the incidence of falls and pedestrians-hit-by-automobiles rises after the seventh decade of life.

Craniocerebral trauma can involve injury to the scalp, skull, meninges or brain. Most injuries are not life-threatening, though lifelong sequelae are not uncommon. Fifty to 90 percent of traumatic brain injury-related hospital admissions are for mild injuries, while 10–30% are for moderate injuries and 5–25% for severe ones. These numbers must be interpreted with caution, however, as the definition of "mild" varies considerably. Nevertheless, it is important to note that a minority of hospital admissions following traumatic brain injuries are for severe injuries.

Pathogenesis

Traumatic brain injury can be classified on the basis of mechanism of injury as follows.

A. ACCELERATION-DECELERATION INJURY

Typically seen following high-speed motor vehicle accidents, this type of injury is due to sudden acceleration or deceleration of the brain. The skull and brain usually accelerate differentially, causing the brain to slosh back and forth within the skull. As it does, the brain impacts against intracranial bony irregularities such as the floor of the frontal fossa, the sphenoid wing, or the petrous ridge, leading to the development of superficial cortical contusions. A further consequence of this differential movement between skull and brain is the stretching of cortical draining veins as they cross the subdural space before penetrating the dural sinuses. If stretched enough, these veins tear and bleed into the subdural space, thus forming subdural hematomas. The ultimate consequence of acceleration-deceleration is the transmission of kinetic forces to the brain that cause shear injury to neurons (axons particularly) and blood vessels. This leads to diffuse axonal injury and the development of subcortical, pericentral, and posterolateral mesencephalic hematomas.

B. IMPACT INJURIES

Impact injury is often seen following assaults with blunt objects such as bats or pipes. In such cases, the skull absorbs much of the object's kinetic force, though the brain often absorbs enough to cause a concussion. Skull fractures are common in this type of injury, and dural injury often follows. This also results in the development of epidural hematomas because the meningeal vessels under the fracture tear. Since the skull absorbs much of the impact, the severity of brain injury per se is less severe than that following acceleration-deceleration injuries. Thus, the classic clinical picture is that of initial loss of consciousness at the time of impact followed by a lucid period as the patient recovers from the concussion. In some cases, a second period of decreased mentation develops after the lucid period, as the epidural hematoma expands to compress the brain stem or other vital brain areas. The portion of the skull most vulnerable to fracture is the thin temporal squamosa. Thus, the underlying middle meningeal artery is the blood vessel most vulnerable to injury and a temporal epidural hematoma the most likely result.

C. PENETRATING INJURIES

Penetrating brain injuries can be divided into high-velocity and low-velocity types. The cutoff is somewhat arbitrary but is generally defined as missile velocity of 300 feet per second at impact. Since the energy (E) transmitted to the brain equals one-half the missile mass (M) times its velocity (V) squared (E = ½ × M × V²), the higher the velocity or the greater the missile mass, the greater the energy transmitted to the brain. Since energy varies with the square of the velocity, V has greater impact than M in determining the energy absorbed by the brain. Since low-velocity missiles often cannot penetrate the thick cranial vault, most low-velocity injuries occur though the relatively thin skull base—particularly the orbitocranial window—causing damage to structures along the path of entry, the cerebral vasculature being particularly vulnerable. A multitude of low-velocity missiles have been described, including pens, pencils, chopsticks, branches, arrows, darts, and needlefish.

High-velocity injuries are of a different nature. Though structures along the path of entry are certainly injured, much of the damage occurs away from the missile tract. This is because the missile's kinetic energy is absorbed by the skull and brain as it slows. The resulting transfer of energy to the brain precipitates a diffuse injury similar to that imparted to the brain following acceleration-deceleration injuries. As such, the morbidity and mortality of high-velocity injuries is significantly higher than that of low-velocity injuries. The increased use of military-style assault weapons in United States urban centers has increased the lethality of gunshot wounds, as these are designed to fire with much higher muzzle velocities than conventional firearms.

Pathobiology

Regardless of mechanism, all injuries to the brain share some common physiologic characteristics. The initial impact leads to a number of biochemical alterations, many of which are thought to involve the unregulated release of neurotransmitters due to traumatic depolarization of cerebral neurons. Though many neurotransmitters are released simultaneously, the excitatory neurotransmitter glutamate is released in the greatest quantity. It is thought to initiate a biochemical cytotoxic cascade mediated through N-methyl-D-aspartate (NMDA)/glutamate receptors. This cascade leads to alterations in cellular energy metabolism, cerebral blood flow, transmembrane ion concentration gradients, free radical production, and cytokine release.

In concert with these cellular changes are gross changes such as the development of intracranial hematomas, cerebral edema, and hydrocephalus, all of which can contribute to intracranial hypertension. Systemic problems such as hypotension, seizures, infections, and hypoxia can develop as well, increasing the risk of further neurologic injury.

Clinical Findings

A. SYMPTOMS AND SIGNS

The range of clinical findings and neurologic deficits following craniocerebral trauma is wide and varied, depending on the location, mechanism, and severity of injury. Confounding factors such as spinal cord injury, shock, and the influence of drugs or alcohol can also mask neurologic deficits, making accurate assessment difficult. Finally, the neurologic examination can change drastically—especially in the acute setting—a situation that calls for frequent and careful neurologic assessments.

1. Initial examination—The initial general trauma assessment should focus on the ABCs (airway, breathing, and circulation), and steps should be taken to stabilize the patient hemodynamically. Next, an initial trauma neurologic examination is done, focusing on the patient's mental status, cranial nerve reflexes, and motor function (ABCD, where D is for disability). In this way a quick assessment of the brain, brain stem, and spinal cord can be achieved.

2. Glasgow Coma Scale—Mental status is best assessed using the Glasgow Coma Scale. It is the most widely used neurotrauma scale, is easy to use, and has excellent interexaminer concordance. Based on a scale from 3 to 15, three clinical parameters (eye opening, verbal response, and motor response) are assessed to determine the patient's level of consciousness. All three components are added to give a composite score. Coma is technically considered at a grade of 8 or less—this is also considered a severe injury. Moderate injuries are generally considered at a score of 9–12 and mild ones from 13 to 15.

a. Eye-opening—Graded from 1 to 4, this component assesses the level of stimulus required for a patient to open his or her eyes. Eye-opening to ambient stimulus is graded as a 4; eye-opening to directed verbal stimulus a 3; eye-opening to pain a 2; and no eye-opening at all is graded as a 1.

b. Verbal response—This parameter grades the level or complexity of spontaneous verbal output on a scale of 1–5. Normal speech with normal content is graded a 5; normal speech with inappropriate content receives a 4; words without sentence structure is graded a 3; sound without word structure is a 2; and absence of verbal output is graded as a 1.

c. Motor response—The most sensitive indicator of neurologic dysfunction and the best predictor of outcome, motor response is graded on a scale from 1 to 6. The highest grade (6) is given to patients who follow verbal commands. All other grades are scored in response to a painful stimulus. Patients who localize pain receive a 5; those who withdraw from it are graded as a 4; flexor posturing (also called decorticate posturing) grades as a 3; and extensor posturing (decerebrate posturing) as a 2. No response to painful stimulus receives a 1.

3. Cranial nerve and reflex assessments—The detail and extent of cranial nerve examination depends on the patient's level of consciousness. Patients who are awake and cooperative presumably follow commands allowing full examination of cranial nerve function. Comatose patients, however, can only elicit cranial nerve reflexes. The most simple and directed cranial nerve examina-

tion focuses on three reflexes—the pupillary reflex, the corneal reflex, and the gag reflex. The first assesses pupillary response to light, carrying afferent information via cranial nerve II (optic nerve) and efferent information via nerve III (oculomotor). The corneal reflex carries afferent information via cranial nerve V (ophthalmic portion of the trigeminal nerve) and efferent information via cranial nerve VII (facial). Finally, the gag reflex afferent and efferent signals are carried via the glossopharyngeal (IX) and vagus (X) nerves, respectively. With these three reflexes, the entire brain stem can be quickly assessed as the pupillary reflex is localized in the midbrain, the corneal reflex in the pons, and the gag reflex in the medulla. The presence of a unilaterally dilated or fixed pupil in the comatose patient is of considerable concern as it often indicates transtentorial herniation of the ipsilateral temporal uncus due to supratentorial intracranial hypertension. The loss of the corneal or gag reflex is of much more concern as it indicates severe brain stem injury.

Other cranial reflexes include the oculovestibular reflex (caloric reflex) and oculocephalic reflex (doll's eye), though these are not usually assessed in the trauma bay as they are impractical in the case of the former and unsafe in the latter (due to the potential presence of a cervical injury).

4. Assessment of motor function—The initial motor examination should be limited to a qualitative assessment of movement of all four extremities. It is often impossible to formally examine motor strength because of interference by resuscitation efforts and the presence of pelvic or long bone fractures. As such, it is enough to establish the presence of a paresis or plegia and note which limbs are affected. More detailed examination can wait until initial resuscitation efforts have stabilized the patient. The awake, cooperative, hemodynamically stable patient can be examined more formally and at leisure. A rectal examination assessing sphincter tone is mandatory in the acute period.

Assessment of sensation, deep tendon reflexes, and coordination is completely useless in the comatose patient and can generally be performed along with the more formal motor examination in the awake, cooperative patient.

5. Vital signs—In addition to assessing the patient's neurologic function, it is imperative to closely monitor the vital signs. Hypotension in the presence of tachycardia most frequently indicates hypovolemia, though this picture can also be due to a high to midthoracic spinal cord injury. Hypotension with a normal or low pulse can indicate a cervical injury or primary cardiac pathology such as sick sinus syndrome or junctional rhythm. Hypertension and bradycardia (Cushing's reflex) in the comatose patient usually indicates the presence of intracranial hypertension. This can be manifested in subtle ways. Even trends toward hypertension and bradycardia can be harbingers of intracranial hypertension. As such, the neurosurgeon must be alert to gradually increasing blood pressure with downward drifts in heart rate—even if the patient remains nominally normotensive and tachycardiac.

B. IMAGING STUDIES

Since the advent of computed tomography (CT) in the mid 1970s, the radiographic evaluation of craniocerebral trauma has changed dramatically. No longer are plain skull films, pneumoencephalography, or cerebral angiography mainstays of trauma evaluation—head CT has for all practical purposes supplanted them. It is fast, easy, readily available in any trauma center, and exceedingly sensitive to intracranial blood or air and bony (skull) injury. Most modern CT scanners can obtain a complete head CT with 5 mm thick sections in less than 2 minutes, and the images are of excellent quality and resolution.

Cerebral angiography is still used occasionally if vascular injury is suspected. An example is the patient presenting with massive epistaxis whose head CT indicates a basilar skull fracture involving the carotid canal. This situation calls for emergent angiographic assessment of the petrous carotid with possible endovascular occlusion of the injured vessel.

If the patient is stable, magnetic resonance imaging (MRI) can be used to establish the severity of any intracranial pathologic process not clearly visualized on CT. This is often the case in the posterior fossa, where bone can cause significant artifact on CT images, potentially obscuring cerebellar or brain stem pathology. Magnetic resonance angiography (MRA) is an alternative to conventional angiography in the hemodynamically and neurologically stable patient. The biggest disadvantages of MRI and MRA is that studies take considerably longer than CT scans and cannot be performed in patients with implanted metallic objects such as cardiac pacers, some intracranial pressure monitors, and some older aneurysm clips.

Medical Treatment

The heterogeneous and dynamic nature of craniocerebral trauma makes it impossible to address treatment options as a strict algorithm. However, we can address the two major issues that, if left untreated, can lead to severe disability or death—hemodynamic instability and neurologic instability.

A. HEMODYNAMIC INSTABILITY AND AIRWAY MANAGEMENT

Signs of hemodynamic instability should be treated with rapid and aggressive volume resuscitation. Crystal-loid solutions such as 0.9% sodium chloride or lactated Ringer's solution are the fluids of choice. The author prefers the former to keep the patient mildly hypernatremic (serum sodium 146–148 mmol/L). This both raises the seizure threshold and helps control intracranial hypertension. Packed red blood cells (O-negative or type-specific) and whole blood infusions should be given if the patient has suffered significant blood loss. At least four units of blood products should be ready and available for immediate use during the initial resuscitation period. Trauma patients also commonly develop coagulopathies such as diffuse intravascular coagulopathy, which must be treated aggressively with fresh frozen plasma. Pressor agents such as phenylephrine, dopamine, or norepinephrine must be used judiciously and never before the patient's intravascular volume has been repleted.

In addition to hemodynamic support, the patient's airway ventilation and oxygenation must be rapidly assessed and secured. In some cases, this involves endotracheal intubation or, if necessary, placement of a transcutaneous tracheal airway (via cricothyrotomy or tracheotomy). In any case, in order to minimize risk of injury (or further injury) to the spinal cord, the cervical spine should be manipulated as little as possible. The term "in-line traction" is often used to describe the maneuver used to maintain cervical stability during intubation. This is somewhat of a misnomer, since the spine per se is rarely placed in traction. All that is needed is to maintain normal cervical alignment during intubation.

B. NEUROLOGIC INSTABILITY

Neurologic instability is almost always the result of intracranial hypertension, and in the acute setting is most likely due to an intracranial mass lesion. Seizures, drugs, and systemic hypotension can also present as neurologic instability and must be considered in the differential diagnosis.

1. Seizures—Patients with craniocerebral trauma are at risk for developing seizures. Some patients present actively seizing and should be treated with anticonvulsant medications—phenytoin (or fosphenytoin), 15–20 mg/kg intravenously followed by 300–400 mg/d in adults for 7 days. The advantage of fosphenytoin is that it can be infused more quickly than phenytoin without the risk of inducing hypotension—it is, however, considerably more expensive. Status epilepticus should be treated with benzodiazepines such as lorazepam or diazepam, though barbiturates or even general anesthesia is occasionally needed to control the seizures. Patients with intracranial pathology such as intraparenchymal contusions, subdural hematomas, or large epidural hematomas should also be given anticonvulsants, as they are at risk for developing posttraumatic seizures. If the seizures stop, anticonvulsants can be discontinued at 7 days. This approach decreases the incidence of early posttraumatic seizures yet minimizes the patient's exposure to anticonvulsants. If the patient develops seizures after anticonvulsants are stopped, they should be reinstituted for at least 6 months. Patients who are chronic alcoholics are also at risk for developing alcohol withdrawal seizures and should be treated primarily with benzodiazepines such as chlordiazepoxide (if they are taking oral medications) or diazepam (if nothing by mouth) until they have completed their withdrawal, usually in 5–7 days.

2. Intracranial hypertension—Normal intracranial contents include brain parenchyma, cerebrospinal fluid, and intracranial blood. Since intracranial volume is fixed, volume changes in of any of the three components affect intracranial pressure. The pressure-volume curve described by Langfitt and coworkers demonstrates a curvilinear relationship between intracranial volume and changes in intracranial pressure. As intracranial volume increases, so does intracranial pressure. Initially, the rise in pressure is barely noticeable and the slope of the curve approximates zero. As intracranial volume accumulates, the curve becomes increasingly steeper, eventually approaching vertical. Thus, intracranial pressure varies exponentially with intracranial cerebrospinal fluid, brain, or blood volume. The treatment of intracranial hypertension relies essentially on this relationship and aims at lowering intracranial cerebrospinal fluid, brain, and blood volume. It follows that intracranial pressure management mandates the use of intracranial pressure monitors.

Two basic types of intracranial pressure monitors are currently available: drainage and nondrainage types. The former can be placed in the ventricle, subarachnoid, or subdural space. The latter is usually placed within the brain parenchyma, though it can be placed in virtually any intracranial compartment. Because of its potential therapeutic role, the external ventricular drain is the intracranial pressure monitor of choice at our institution. Not only does it provide information on intracranial pressure—it also allows the physician to drain ventricular cerebrospinal fluid, thus reducing intracranial pressure. If the ventricular catheter cannot be placed, then a nondraining monitor is used. We use fiberoptic monitors because of their ease of placement.

The major risks associated with these monitors are infection and hemorrhage. The infection rates for external ventricular drains versus fiberoptic catheters are 0–27% (average 8%) and 0–1.7%, respectively. The risk of hemorrhage with either type is similar (0–1%). The incidence of malfunction, on the other hand, is considerably higher with fiberoptic technology. Mal-

function or obstruction rates for intraventricular, subdural, and subarachnoid drains are 2.5%, 2.7% and 16%, respectively. The risk of malfunction with the fiberoptic catheter, on the other hand, is 10–30%. In addition, the cost difference between fiberoptic and drainage catheters is enormous, with nondraining monitors costing an order of magnitude more than external ventricular drains. All things considered, the accuracy, reliability, therapeutic value, and cost make the external ventricular drain the most useful intracranial pressure monitor available.

Though the risk of placing either hydrostatic or fiberoptic monitors is small, it is clear that not all traumatic brain injury patients require invasive monitoring. Generally speaking, patients who have a Glasgow score from 9 to 15 are at low risk for developing intracranial hypertension while those with a score of 8 or less are at higher risk. Patients with scores of 8 or less with abnormalities on head CT have been shown to have a 53–63% chance of developing intracranial hypertension compared with a 13% risk in patients with a normal CT. Interestingly, patients with normal CTs but with at least two of the following clinical features—systolic blood pressure < 90 mm Hg; extensor or flexor posturing, or age over 40 years—run a risk of developing intracranial hypertension equal to that of patients with abnormal head CTs.

Intracranial hypertension is treated by decreasing intracranial cerebrospinal fluid, brain, or blood volume. Both surgical and nonsurgical approaches are available, though not all are useful in the acute setting.

a. Cerebrospinal fluid volume—Cerebrospinal fluid volume is generally lowered by use of a ventriculostomy. This can be done in one of two ways—either by keeping the drain constantly open or by monitoring the pressure continuously, draining only if the pressure reaches a set threshold. For most trauma situations, the author finds it most useful to keep the drain for monitoring and intermittent drainage because this permits close monitoring of intracranial pressure spikes that otherwise might not be captured by leaving the drain constantly open. When no amount of drainage controls intracranial pressure, then other pressure-lowering modalities should be started. Medical management of cerebrospinal fluid volume is impractical in the trauma setting because medications such as steroids or acetazolamide are slow-acting and have significant side effects that make their use undesirable.

b. Brain volume—The surgical approach to decreasing brain volume is crude and generally unsatisfactory, as it requires performance of a lobectomy. This is sometimes necessary in order to buy some extra space into which the remaining brain can swell, but lobectomies are generally bloody affairs to be avoided if possible. Medical management of brain volume is more satisfying as it essentially means giving mannitol intravenously and keeping serum sodium at or slightly above the high end of normal. Mannitol does not cross the blood-brain barrier and so establishes an osmotic gradient across the barrier, drawing interstitial water out of the brain and into the vasculature. There are two practical limitations to mannitol: hypotension and serum osmolality. Mannitol not only draws water across the blood-brain barrier, it also is a powerful osmotic diuretic that can reduce a patient's blood pressure substantially. Hypotension, therefore, is a contraindication to mannitol infusion. As for serum osmolality—as it increases, so does viscosity. At levels above 320 mosm/kg, its deleterious effects on blood viscosity overwhelm the benefits of giving mannitol to lower intracranial pressure.

Hypernatremia helps control cerebral edema by normalizing the Na^+ gradient across cellular membranes. As noted earlier, glutamate initiates a series of biochemical changes thought to be mediated through NMDA receptors. One of these changes involves intracellular Na^+ accumulation, which leads to cellular swelling. Increasing serum Na^+ presumably decreases cerebral (cytotoxic) edema by ameliorating intracellular water accumulation. The main issues of concern associated with hypernatremia are two: hyperchloremia and diabetes insipidus. The former results from infusion of large volumes or 0.9% NaCl solution. High serum chloride facilitates renal excretion of serum bicarbonate, which then leads to metabolic acidosis. This can be reversed somewhat by changing from sodium chloride to sodium bicarbonate solution.

c. Blood volume—Of the three components, intracranial blood volume is the most interesting and challenging to manage. The surgical approach is fairly straightforward—its aim is to evacuate intracranial blood clots. The exact approach depends on the type and location of the hematoma and will be described in detail below. Nonsurgical management focuses on the intravascular compartment. This is composed of arterial, capillary, and venous volumes, which we will deal with individually.

Capillary volume—This compartment is passive and cannot be manipulated to any significant degree.

Venous volume—Though also passive, intracranial venous volume can be altered in a number of ways. The main goal is to lower intracranial pressure by decreasing venous volume. This can be accomplished simply by elevating the head of the bed. This facilitates intracranial venous drainage by increasing the pressure differential between intracranial venous pressure and central venous pressure. Another approach is simply to prevent increased intrathoracic pressure, as this would

inhibit intracranial venous outflow and increase intracranial pressure. Causes of increased intrathoracic pressure include Valsalva maneuvers (eg, seizures, coughing, agitation, vomiting, straining) and primary pulmonary disorders (eg, ARDS, pneumonia). By treating the underlying cause of each, we can sometimes control intracranial pressure. Sedatives, paralytic agents, anticonvulsants, stool softeners—all decrease Valsalva maneuvers; optimizing ventilator settings and treating pneumonias can also help control intracranial pressure.

Arterial volume—This compartment is essentially manipulated by taking advantage of cerebral autoregulatory mechanisms. These couple cerebral blood flow to cerebral metabolic demands. First, metabolic autoregulation alters local cerebral blood flow to match changes in local cerebral metabolism. Second, pressure autoregulation is designed to maintain a constant cerebral blood flow over a wide range of blood pressures. Third, osmotic autoregulation maintains blood flow constant with changes in blood viscosity—all other things being equal. They all essentially work through tissue pH as a means of detecting ischemia. As tissue pH drops, autoregulatory mechanisms interpret this as the tissue becoming ischemic and respond by vasodilating upstream arterioles in order to increase local blood flow. Though vasodilation increases local tissue perfusion, it also increases arterial blood volume—which increases intracranial pressure. Conversely, increasing tissue pH leads to vasoconstriction and, consequently, lower intracranial pressure.

The most common way of inducing cerebral vasoconstriction is to decrease serum PCO_2 by means of mechanical hyperventilation. Serum PCO_2 and pH are closely interrelated—decreasing PCO_2 increases serum pH—and by hyperventilating, the cerebral vasculature is "fooled" into believing that the local cerebral blood flow is too high, thus causing vasoconstriction and decreased intracranial pressure. It is easy to see that this approach has the theoretical disadvantage of being capable of causing cerebral ischemia–a notion supported by data suggesting that hyperventilation below a PCO_2 of 30 mm Hg leads to a worse neurologic outcome.

As long as autoregulation remains intact, we can also decrease intracranial pressure through induced systemic hypertension. This maneuver transiently increases cerebral blood flow and causes the brain to respond by inducing cerebral vasoconstriction. This, then, leads to a lowering of intracranial pressure.

Finally, we can decrease cerebral metabolism through medications such as barbiturates and propofol. As the cerebral metabolic rate falls, so does metabolic demand. In response, the cerebral vasculature naturally constricts, thus lowering intracranial pressure. The biggest problem with the last approach is that both barbiturates and, to a lesser degree, propofol can lower blood pressure and decrease cardiac function. Therefore, these medications need to be used with caution.

Surgical Treatment

The surgical treatment of trauma is fairly straightforward. The most difficult aspect is knowing when to operate and when not to. The actual surgical approach depends on the location and effects of the problem. As such we will discuss in sequence the treatment of epidural hematomas, subdural hematomas, intraparenchymal contusions, open skull fractures, and scalp lacerations.

All trauma patients undergo a complete head shave at our institution prior to incision and if time permits (and skull integrity permits) are put in three-point fixation.

A. EPIDURAL HEMATOMA

Epidural hematomas almost always underlie a skull fracture (Figure 38–9). The most common location is the temporal fossa since the temporal squamosa is the thinnest part of the cranial vault, the most likely to fracture, and can easily lacerate the underlying middle meningeal artery. Other less common locations include the frontal and parietal convexity as well as the occipital and infratentorial compartments. Occasionally, a skull fracture will cross a venous sinus—the superior sagittal sinus and transverse sinuses being the most susceptible—causing formation of a venous epidural hematoma.

Dura

Epidural hematoma

Figure 38–9. Epidural hemorrhage. (Reprinted from *Hosp Med* [Oct] 1965;1:9, by permission of the authors and Wallace Laboratories.)

The general approach is to make a curvilinear scalp incision to expose the entire skull overlying the hematoma (or as much of it as possible). One usually encounters a skull fracture on turning the skin flap. If the temporalis muscle is overlying the site, this should also be reflected inferiorly, leaving a thin rim of temporalis fascia attached to the superior temporal line (if possible) to which the muscle can be attached at the end of surgery. Once the bone is exposed, a single burr hole is made with a cutting burr somewhere near the edge of the underlying hematoma. The cranial flap can then be turned using the drill's footplate attachment. The hematoma is then evacuated, any dural bleeding is stopped, and the dura is secured to the craniotomy edge using 4-0 braided nylon sutures. The author usually makes a small dural incision to inspect the subdural space to rule out the presence of a coincident subdural hematoma. Once hemostasis is ensured, the bone flap is re-attached using three "dog bone" titanium plates at the edge of the craniectomy. The musculocutaneous flap is then closed using 00 Vicryl sutures for the galeal layer and staples for the skin. An intracranial pressure monitor is frequently placed at this time before transport to the ICU.

A special note about venous epidural hematoma should be offered: These injuries can cause massive exsanguination in a very short period of time. What makes them so difficult is the state of the underlying venous dural sinus, which is usually criss-crossed by multiple comminuted skull fractures making it hard to localize the dural sinus tear. Massive blood loss occurring at the time of opening makes exposure even harder. The answer is to run the craniotomy parallel and just lateral to the sinus (and, if possible, on both sides of the sinus) and place multiple dural tack-up stitches along its edge. Trying to expose the entire sinus is usually futile and fatal.

B. SUBDURAL HEMATOMA

The approach to subdural hematoma is really no different from that for epidural hematoma except that the craniotomy is usually much larger and the dura is opened (Figure 38–10). The scalp incision is usually a very large curvilinear incision beginning at the hairline in the midline and continuing along the midline to approximately lambda. From here, the incision continues parallel to the lambdoid suture to the level of the asterion and then continues anteriorly just above the ear and curves anterior to the ear to end 1 cm inferior to the root of the zygoma. The temporalis muscle is removed as above, but no time is wasted in preserving the fascial attachment to the superior temporal line. This distinction is in contrast to the approach to epidural hematoma since the author often does not replace the bone flap following evacuation of the hematoma because the brain is much more likely to swell significantly, causing

Subdural hematoma

Dura

Figure 38–10. Subdural hemorrhage. (Reprinted from *Hosp Med* [Oct] 1965;1:9, by permission of the authors and Wallace Laboratories.)

intracranial pressure management problems. In any case, the skull is removed as described above but hugging the periphery of the skin incision and extending the craniotomy down to the frontal floor and pole and the temporal floor and pterion. Though this seems like a lot of surgery, it rarely takes more than 5 minutes to complete the craniotomy from the time of the first skin incision. Once the skull is off, the dura is rapidly and widely opened using tenotomy scissors. At this point, the hematoma is evacuated.

Subdural hematomas resulting from tearing of cortical draining veins typically drain into six areas: the superior sagittal sinus at (1) the frontal pole, (2) along the frontoparietal junction and (3) the occipital pole; (4) the sphenoparietal sinus at the temporal pole, (5) the transverse sigmoid junction and (6) along the superior petrosal sinus. These areas should be inspected to make certain that any active bleeding has stopped. Once hemostasis is ensured, a ventriculostomy is passed through the exposed frontal lobe into the lateral ventricle. A subdural drain is placed, and both catheters are tunneled through the skin outside the musculocutaneous flap. The brain is then covered with Gelfoam and the skin flap closed with 00 absorbable suture and staples. If the bone is replaced, it is done so as described above.

C. INTRAPARENCHYMAL CONTUSION

The approach to intraparenchymal contusion depends on the presence of an overlying subdural hematoma and the degree of cerebral swelling. In the absence of sub-

dural hematoma and significant global cerebral swelling, an approach akin to that employed for epidural hematoma is used. If not, the subdural hematoma approach is used. Once the brain is exposed, a small cortical incision is made where the contusion is closest to the surface of the brain—avoiding eloquent areas such as the primary motor cortex. Once the contusion is encountered, it usually delivers itself with minimal effort. Hemostasis is ensured and the wound closed as above.

D. OPEN SKULL FRACTURES AND SCALP LACERATIONS

These can be discussed together as the surgical approach is similar for both. The main surgical objective is to clean the area to minimize the risk of infection and facilitate wound closure. In the case of skull fractures, attention must be paid to the possibility of underlying dural lacerations or hematomas. If either is present, a more extensive exploration may be necessary. Much emphasis has been placed on the need for meticulous dural repair. In the author's opinion, this is not necessary as long as the area has been cleaned and debrided well. Experience from treatment of penetrating injuries has shown that even these do not require aggressive surgical debridement and dural repair. Scalp wounds require mainly that devitalized tissue be removed, wound edges cleaned, and the galea be closed as completely as possible.

Prognosis

There are many outcome scales used for the long-term assessment of traumatic brain injury. Some measure cognitive function, others physical disability, and still others emotional, neuropsychologic, psychosocial, or behavioral function. There are no outcome scales that fully cover the spectrum of neurologic dysfunction that follows traumatic brain injury. Some of the more common ones are the Galveston Orientation and Amnesia Test (GOAT), which assesses orientation and degree of amnesia; the Paced Auditory Serial Addition Test (PASAT), which assesses attention; and the Trail Making Test B for assessing mental processing. Three others are the Disability Rating Scale, the Rancho Los Amigos Cognitive Functioning Scale, and the Glasgow Outcome Scale (GOS)—all of which assess the patient's disability and handicap. To some degree, the choice of test depends on the patient's disability. Moderately and severely injured patients are most often assessed with the Glasgow Outcome Score, usually administered at 3, 6, and 12 months after injury. This scale places patients into one of five categories: Death, Persistent Vegetative State, Severe Disability (conscious but disabled), Moderate Disability (disabled but independent), and Good Recovery.

As is true of any functional scoring system, those that are most comprehensive are the most difficult to use and those that are the easiest to administer are the least comprehensive. For example, the Halstead-Reitan Neuropsychological Battery (a common standardized neuropsychologic battery) consists of 12 individual tests and can take up to 9 hours to administer. Similarly, the Luria-Nebraska Neuropsychological Battery consists of 248 individual items that can take up to 6 hours to administer. The Glasgow Outcome Score, on the other hand, is reliable, easily used, and takes minutes to score but is relatively insensitive to neurocognitive and behavioral deficits.

The outcome following traumatic brain injury primarily depends on the initial severity of injury and correlates fairly well with the postresuscitation Glasgow Coma Score. Other factors that influence outcome are patient age and the presence of physiologic alterations that can cause secondary brain injury.

A. OUTCOME FOLLOWING MILD TRAUMATIC BRAIN INJURY

Patients who present with a Glasgow Coma Score between 13 and 15 generally do well in the long-run. The most significant sequelae are designated postconcussive symptoms and include headache, fatigue, dizziness, nausea, blurred vision, diplopia, memory difficulties, tinnitus, irritability, and difficulty concentrating (among others). Approximately 50% of patients complain of at least one of these 6 weeks after injury, while 14% still complain of symptoms at 1 year. Generally speaking, persistent symptoms become less severe and less frequent with time. The presence of more symptoms at 1 year compared with at 6 weeks is associated with a higher incidence of pending litigation.

B. OUTCOME FOLLOWING MODERATE TRAUMATIC BRAIN INJURY

Of patients with a Glasgow Coma Score of 9–12, only 60% make a good recovery, while 26% remain moderately disabled, 7% severely disabled, and 7% are either vegetative or dead. Factors that influence outcome within this group are Glasgow Coma Score, patient age greater than 40, abnormality on admission CT scan, and progressive changes on CT scan.

C. OUTCOME FOLLOWING SEVERE TRAUMATIC BRAIN INJURY

Outcome following severe injury is very difficult to predict, especially early in the patient's hospital course. Patients in this group are often hemodynamically and neurologically unstable and can suffer significant secondary injury. Factors contributing to bad outcome are many, but—as is true also of moderate injury—the postresuscitation Glasgow Coma Score (particularly motor score) and age are the most significant. Other significant predictive factors presenting in the acute

postinjury period include pupillary response, pupillary size, midline shift, and intracranial pressure. Some data have shown that early, aggressive intensive care management with focus on hemodynamic and intracranial pressure monitoring, control of ventilation and oxygenation, and prevention of causes of secondary injury has some effect on the Glaucoma Outcome Score following severe traumatic brain injury.

Summary

Traumatic brain injuries are a heterogeneous group of injuries that require early, aggressive treatment, intensive and constant hemodynamic and intracranial monitoring, and frequent critical reassessment of all physiologic and clinical parameters. As we learn more about the physiology of the injury responses, monitoring parameters and treatment options are bound to change. What is dogma today will be anathema tomorrow. As long as we keep this in mind and are willing to change our preconceptions, we are in a great position to advance the treatment of traumatic brain injury.

Bailes JE, Cantu RC: Head injury in athletes. Neurosurgery 2001; 48:26.

Grant IS, Andrews PJ: ABC of intensive care: neurological support. BMJ 1999;319:110.

Haydel MJ et al: Indications for computed tomography in patients with minor head injury. N Engl J Med 2000;343:100.

Rosner S, Rosner M, Johnson A: Cerebral perfusion pressure: management protocol and clinical results. J Neurosurg 1995; 83:949.

Schutzman SA et al: Evaluation and management of children younger than 2 years old with apparently minor head trauma: proposed guidelines. Pediatrics 2001;107:983.

Stiell IG et al: The Canadian C-spine rule for radiography in alert and stable patients. JAMA 2001;286:1781.

■ SPINAL CORD INJURY

Geoffrey T. Manley, MD, PhD, Alexander M. Papanastasio, MD, & Russ P. Nockels, MD

 ESSENTIALS OF DIAGNOSIS

- *Neck or back pain following injury.*
- *Numbness or tingling in the trunk or extremities.*
- *Weakness or paralysis.*
- *Loss of bowel or bladder function.*
- *Imaging studies.*

General Considerations

Spinal cord injury remains one of the most devastating of all survivable traumatic injuries. Each year, more than 11,000 new spinal cord injuries occur in the United States as a result of motor vehicle accidents, falls, sports injuries, and various other types of accidents. Today, more than 200,000 Americans are living with spinal cord injury. Most of the injured are between 16 and 30 years of age at the time of injury, and males are much more likely than females to be injured. While most victims are employed at the time of injury, only 30–40% will be able to return to work. From the time of injury to death, the average cost of care of one patient exceeds $500,000, and the annual cost for acute and chronic care of spinal cord-injured patients is estimated to be $4 billion.

In the past, management of acute spinal cord injury focused on conservative care. The finding that pharmacologic treatment with intravenous methylprednisolone resulted in modest improvements in the National Acute Spinal Cord Injury Studies (NASCIS-1, 2, and 3) has provided new hope that future pharmacologic therapies may further diminish neurologic deficits. Recently, significant advances have also been made in the safety and efficacy of surgical decompression, stabilization, and fixation of the spine, paving the way for perhaps repairing the damage resulting from spinal injury. It is likely that future treatments will combine pharmacologic and surgical approaches to improve the outcome of this devastating injury.

Pathogenesis

In general, injury to the spinal cord follows compression or severe angulation of the vertebral spine. In rare instances, severe hypotension will lead to cord infarction or axial distraction of elements of the vertebral column will result in stretch injury of the cord. Most cord injuries follow subluxation with or without rotation of adjacent vertebral bodies that compress the cord between dislocated bone. Less often, axial compression of the spine will crush or wedge a vertebral body, and either bone or intervertebral disk fragments can be extruded into the spinal canal and compress the spinal cord or the anterior spinal artery. Another injury, seen usually in older patients with degenerative arthritis and stenosis of the cervical spine, involves neck hyperextension with infolding of the ligamentum flavum located in the spinal canal posterior to the cord. The spinal cord is trapped between arthritic bony spurs anteriorly and the ligamentum flavum posteriorly, producing a characteristic injury known as the central cord syndrome.

Early after spinal cord injury, there is a temporary loss of function with little or no demonstrable pathologic change. However, the initial trauma initiates a cascade of downstream injury mechanisms that includes accumulation of excitatory amino acids, neurotransmitters, vasoactive eicosanoids, oxygen free radicals, and by-products of lipid peroxidation and activation of programmed cell death pathways. Loss of the "blood-cord barrier" causes edema and increased tissue pressure that, along with cord hemorrhage, limit the blood supply, with the result that cell ischemia may further damage the cord. The distribution of cord edema, hemorrhage, and infarction dictates the neurologic symptoms and signs elicited at the time of evaluation.

Clinical Findings

A. SYMPTOMS, SIGNS, AND SYNDROMES

In complete spinal cord injuries, there is no voluntary nervous function below the injury site. There is an initial phase of spinal shock, a loss of all reflexes below the injured segment—including the bulbocavernosus and cremasteric reflexes and anal contraction to perianal stimulation—and deep tendon reflexes. This phenomenon may be temporary because of ionic and blood flow changes at the injury site. In incomplete spinal cord injuries, some function is present below the injury site, accounting for a much more favorable overall prognosis. Cord function may improve rapidly as spinal shock clears, or function may improve slowly in the months or years after injury.

The sites of damage within the cord and nerve root will determine what function is lost and what remains:

1. Anterior cord syndrome—This disorder results from damage to spinothalamic tracts and corticospinal tracts with relatively intact dorsal columns and preservation of touch and position sense, often related to injury to the spinal artery.

2. Brown-Séquard's syndrome—A lesion involving the spinal cord extensively on one side of the midline results in ipsilateral motor weakness and loss of proprioception and contralateral loss of pain perception below the level of injury.

3. Central cord syndrome—Hemorrhagic necrosis of the central portions of the cervical spinal cord often follows a brief concussive injury. Because distal leg and sacral motor and sensory fibers are located most peripherally in the cervical cord, the perianal sensation and some lower extremity movement and sensation may be preserved.

4. Nerve root injury—This can occur at the level of vertebral body dislocation. Direct root compression may be relieved by reduction of the dislocation or by removal of fractured bone or disrupted disk.

5. Conus medullaris compression—Injuries at the thoracolumbar region may cause injury to nerve cells of the tip of the spinal cord, descending corticospinal fibers, and lumbosacral nerve roots with a mixed upper motor neuron and lower motor neuron dysfunction.

6. Cauda equina syndrome—This syndrome may arise from bony dislocation or disk extrusions in the lumbar or sacral regions, with compression of lumbosacral nerve roots below the conus medullaris. Bowel and bladder dysfunction as well as leg numbness and weakness occur commonly in this syndrome.

B. PHYSICAL EXAMINATION

Evaluation and initial treatment must be started at the scene of the injury. Early recognition of a spine or spinal cord injury will mandate preventive measures to preserve remaining neurologic function. Patients suspected of having spinal cord injuries must be immobilized with rigid cervical collars and backboards. At the receiving medical facility, care must be taken to treat hypoventilation, hypoxia, and hypercapnia (found with high cervical cord injuries), shock, and hypothermia (secondary to loss of sympathetic nerve function with cervical injuries), paralytic ileus with abdominal sequestration of fluid, and bladder distention.

Even though the combination of head and spinal cord injury is uncommon, until x-rays show otherwise, the examiner must assume that any comatose patient has an unstable spine fracture. Concern about combined injury must not delay resuscitation of hypotension and hypoventilation. If the patient is awake, a history should be taken as soon as possible, including information about the specific nature of the injury and what pain or neurologic symptoms followed. Complaints of numbness and weakness should be noted carefully. Severe headache, particularly occipital pain, is common with odontoid fracture or hangman's fracture (bilateral fracture of the C2 pedicles). To assess weakness, the patient is asked to move hands and feet spontaneously and against resistance. Sensory testing of the extremities, anterior trunk, neck, and face should then be done. Palpation of the spine by sliding the hands under the patient with minimal spine movement can reveal focal bone tenderness or deformity. Deep tendon reflexes must be evaluated in arms and legs; depression or absence of these reflexes will help localize the level of injury (Figure 38–11). Absence of abdominal reflex contraction to skin stimulation of the lower abdomen will localize a lesion in the T9–11 region. Absence of the cremasteric reflex (contraction of scrotal musculature in response to pinching of the medial thigh) indicates a lesion in the T12–L1 region of the cord. An intact bulbocavernosus reflex (anal sphincter contraction to penile or clitoral compression or downward pressure on the bladder trigone by a Foley catheter

balloon when the catheter is gently pulled) indicates that sacral motor and sensory pathways are intact; absence of the bulbocavernosus reflex is consistent with spinal shock or with sacral spinal cord or nerve root injury.

When the patient must be transferred to an x-ray table or bed, the transfer should be done with a fireman's carry, with at least three people *on each side* of the patient and with a seventh person, who directs the move, keeping the head in a neutral position by gentle axial traction (4–7 kg) applied with one hand on the chin and the other on the occiput.

C. IMAGING STUDIES

Along with the physical examination, x-rays are essential for the evaluation of spine injuries. The lateral film is the most informative and should be examined for alignment of the anterior and posterior aspects of adjacent vertebral bodies and for angulation of the spinal canal at any level. Paravertebral or prevertebral soft tissue masses usually indicate hemorrhage into these areas from fractures or ligamentous disruption. Anteroposterior spine films of the thoracic region and other levels permit assessment of lateral displacement of the vertebral bodies or widening or disruption of the pedicles. Oblique views in the cervical and lumbar regions will demonstrate facet fractures or dislocations. Frontal and lateral tomography can further identify bony abnormalities, but this procedure requires movement of the patient onto special tables for study.

MRI gives excellent views of the spine, disks, and spinal cord and is the diagnostic procedure of choice in patients with spinal cord injuries. CT scanning provides superior imaging of the bony spine and extraspinal soft tissue and provides additional insights into the management of spinal injury. Instillation of intrathecal metrizamide can outline the spinal cord and demonstrate cord compression.

Differential diagnosis

A detailed neurologic examination of motor and sensory function allows for classification of a spinal cord injury and differentiation from other pathologic entities. The principal diagnostic obstacle in the setting of trauma is often the inability to assess a patient due to altered mental status from associated brain injury or intoxication. Initial assessment can also be complicated by a period of areflexia, called spinal shock, that resolves over a variable period of time. Other complicating factors in the differential diagnosis include peripheral nerve injuries secondary to fractures of the extremities. Here again, a detailed neurologic examination and an understanding of the anatomy of the peripheral nervous system is essential for making the correct diagnosis. The possibility of factitious symptoms

SENSORY LEVELS

Hearing, equilibrium
Taste
Pharynx, esophagus
Larynx, trachea
Occipital region (C1, 2)
Neck region (C2, 3, 4)
Shoulder (C4, 5)

Arm
{ Axillary (C5, 6)
Radial (C6, 7, 8)
Median (C6, 7, 8)
Ulnar (C8, T1)

Thorax
{ Spine of scapula (T3)
Inferior angle of scapula (T7)

Epigastrium

Abdomen
{ Umbilicus (T10)

Gluteal region (T12, L1)
Inguinal region (L1, 2)

Femoral region (L1, 2, 3)
{ Anterior
Median
Lateral
Posterior

Crural region (L4, 5)
{ Median
Lateral

Scrotum, penis
Labia
Perineum (S1, 2)
Bladder (S3, 4)
Rectum (S4, 5)
Anus (S5, C1)

Spinous processes
Spinal nerves
First rib
Filum terminale

Medulla oblongata
Cervical plexus
Brachial plexus
Intercostal and thoracic muscles
Abdominal muscles
Lumbar muscles
Lumbar plexus
Sacral plexus
Sacro-coccygeal plexus

MOTOR LEVELS

Facial muscles VII
Pharyngeal, palatine muscles X
Laryngeal muscles XI
Tongue muscles XII
Esophagus X
Sternocleidomastoid XI (C1, 2, 3)
Neck muscles (C1, 2, 3)
Trapezius (C3, 4)
Rhomboids (C4, 5)
Diaphragm (C3, 4, 5)
Supra-, infraspinatus (C4, 5, 6)

Arm
{ Deltoid, brachioradialis, and biceps (C5, 6)
Serratus anterior (C5, 6, 7)
Pectoralis major (C5, 6, 7, 8)
Teres minor (C4, 5)
Pronators (C6, 7, 8, T1)
Triceps (C6, 7, 8)

Forearm
{ Long extensors of carpi and digits (C6, 7, 8)
Latissimus dorsi, teres major (C5, 6, 7, 8)
Long flexors (C7, 8, T1)
Thumb extensors (C7, 8)

Hand
{ Interossei, lumbricales, thenar, hypothenar (C8, T1)

Iliopsoas (L1, 2, 3)
Sartorius (L2, 3)
Quadriceps femoris (L2, 3, 4)
Gluteal muscles (L4, 5, S1)
Tensor fasciae latae (L4, 5)
Adductors of femur (L2, 3, 4)
Abductors of femur (L4, 5, S1)
Tibialis anterior (L5)
Gastrocnemius, soleus (L5, S1, 2)
Biceps, semitendinosus, semimembranosus (L4, 5, S1)
Obturator, piriformis, quadratus femoris (L4, 5, S1)
Flexors of the foot, extensors of toes (L5, S1)
Peronei (L5, S1)
Flexors of toes (L5, S1, 2)
Interossei (S1, 2)
Perineal muscles (S3, 4)
Vesicular muscles (S4, 5)
Rectal muscles (S4, 5, C1)

Figure 38–11. Motor and sensory levels of the spinal cord. (Reproduced, with permission, from Waxman SG: *Correlative Neuroanatomy*, 24th ed. Originally published by Appleton & Lange. Copyright © 2000 by The McGraw-Hill Companies, Inc.)

should also be considered, especially when there is a question of psychiatric illness or secondary gain. This diagnosis can be addressed by detailed serial neurologic exams. The potential for other related traumatic injuries must be considered, as nearly 60% of patients with spinal cord injury have other organ system injuries and 10% have additional spinal fractures.

Treatment

Injuries of bony and neural elements of the spine often coexist, and the treatment of both should be coordinated to ensure the best possible outcome. Transection of the spinal cord almost never accompanies spinal cord injury in humans. Thus, strict adherence to the following principles is therefore imperative to protect surviving spinal tissue: First, the injury must be recognized. Second, care must be exercised to prevent further damage ("secondary" injury) and to detect deteriorating neurologic function so that corrective measures can be taken. Third, the patient must be maintained in optimal condition to allow the greatest possible nervous system repair and recovery. Fourth, evaluation and rehabilitation of the patient must be actively pursued to maximize the function of surviving but dysfunctional nervous tissue. These principles must be followed in order to diminish the economic, social, and emotional cost of spinal cord injury.

Emergency resuscitation of the spinal cord-injured patient parallels that of any major trauma, with the modification that spine alignment must be scrupulously maintained. Based on the NASCIS-2 and NASCIS-3 studies, the current recommendation is for all adult patients with acute nonpenetrating spinal cord injury to receive methylprednisolone immediately after recognition of spinal cord injury. Patients should be given 30 mg/kg of methylprednisolone intravenously within 8 hours, and preferably within 3 hours after injury, followed by a continuous infusion of 5.4 mg/kg/h. Those patients that received the initial bolus of methylprednisolone between 3 and 8 hours after injury should receive a 48-hour infusion instead of the standard 24-hour regimen used for patients treated within 3 hours. Adequate blood pressure and ventilation are critical. Patients with cervical cord injuries maintain ventilation only with diaphragmatic activity; if paralytic ileus with abdominal distention occurs—or if the patient tires—initial adequate ventilation may deteriorate, and the patient will become hypoxic and require intubation and mechanical ventilation. After loss of spinal cord sympathetic pathways, blood pressure may be lower than normal. If urinary output is inadequate after catheterization, patients with mild hypotension will respond to low doses of pressor agents, but these should be used only after unsuspected sources of hemorrhage in the chest or abdomen have been excluded.

Unstable cervical fractures should be managed initially with external immobilization. Skeletal fixation with Gardner-Wells tongs or halo traction can be achieved in most emergency rooms, or halter traction can be used temporarily. Thoracic and lumbar fractures are managed by keeping the patient in a neutral position, "logrolling" as necessary for skin care or pulmonary management. Oscillating beds also improve skin and pulmonary care.

Operative management of spinal cord injury must take into account two major considerations: **decompression** and **stability.** Realignment of the spinal canal can be achieved by proper application of traction, postural adjustment, and spine manipulation done by experienced physicians. Surgical exploration for bony realignment may be necessary in some patients. Surgery may also be indicated if bone or a foreign body is in the spinal canal or if the injury is followed by a progressive neurologic deficit that may be the result of a spinal epidural or subdural hematoma. Management of spine instability may include spinal fusion with metal plates, rods, and screws in combination with bone fusion.

Complications

The primary causes of death after spinal cord injury are potentially avoidable. Renal failure following repeated urinary tract infections is best prevented by carefully performed intermittent bladder catheterization, which often can be done by the patient. Decubitus ulcers form easily over bony prominences in anesthetic areas and can be prevented with intermittent turning of patients and rotatory beds.

Prognosis

The neurologic examination and the age of the patient are the most critical prognostic factors for short-term and long-term recovery. In the acute trauma setting, spinal cord injury mortality is 20%. Long-term, patients with complete motor and sensory loss at 72 hours are unlikely to recover function beyond one root level below the level of the injury, but up to 90% of patients with incomplete lesions can ambulate 1 year after injury. Recovery is more likely with limited lesions and in younger patients. Of the incomplete cord syndromes, the central cord syndrome and the Brown-Séquard syndrome have relatively good prognoses, while patients with anterior cord syndrome do less well. Excluding the first 18 months, patients' 25-year survival rate is 70–80%. The most frequent causes of death include respiratory and cardiac disease, and there is a tenfold increased risk of suicide.

The team approach provided by centers that specialize in spinal cord injury has been very successful and has shown that hospital stays can be shortened, complications can be reduced, and costs lowered. Rehabilitation also requires emotional support and patient education for activities of daily living and job retraining. Exciting new insights into molecular mechanisms involved in spinal cord injury hold great promise for improved pharmacologic treatments. Emerging surgical procedures that incorporate advances in bioengineering and functional neurosurgery suggest that restorative neurosurgery will also have an increasing role in improving the functional abilities of patients with spinal cord injuries. It is likely that the evolving multidisciplinary approach will lead to improved treatment, recovery, and outcome for patients with spinal cord injuries.

Belanger E et al: The acute and chronic management of spinal cord injury. J Am Coll Surg 2000;190:603.

Bracken MB et al: Administration of methylprednisolone for 24 or 48 hours or tirilazad mesylate for 48 hours in the treatment of acute spinal cord injury. Results of the Third National Acute Spinal Cord Injury Randomized Controlled Trial. National Acute Spinal Cord Injury Study. JAMA 1997;277:1597.

Chen TY et al: The role of decompression for acute incomplete cervical spinal cord injury in cervical spondylosis. Spine 1998; 23:2398.

DeVivo MJ: Causes and cost of spinal cord injury in the United States. Spinal Cord 1997;35:809.

Kirshblum SC et al: Predicting neurologic recovery in traumatic cervical spinal cord injury. Arch Phys Med Rehabil 1998; 79:1456.

Nesathurai S: Steroids and spinal cord injury: revisiting the NASCIS 2 and NASCIS 3 trials. J Trauma 1998;45:1088.

Vale FL et al: Combined medical and surgical treatment after acute spinal cord injury: results of a prospective pilot study to assess the merits of aggressive medical resuscitation and blood pressure management. J Neurosurg 1997;87:239.

■ TRAUMATIC PERIPHERAL NERVE LESIONS

Nicholas M. Barbaro, MD

 ESSENTIALS OF DIAGNOSIS

- *History of trauma (blunt, laceration, or surgical) followed by neurologic deficit.*
- *Neurologic findings may consist of partial or complete loss of function in one or more nerves.*
- *Electrodiagnostic studies are helpful only after 2–3 weeks.*

General Considerations

Peripheral nerves contain sensory or motor axons (or both), most of which are myelinated. Each axon is surrounded by fine collagen fibers, the endoneurium. Groups of axons called fasciculi are bound together by the perineurium, which consists of Schwann cells and fine collagen fibrils. The epineurium, made of thicker collagen fibrils, surrounds the fasciculi. This layer is thought to elaborate the fibroblastic reaction that is the primary cause of fibrosis subsequent to nerve injury.

The four major causes of nerve injury are laceration, contusion, stretch, and compression. Less commonly, nerves may be injured inadvertently when an injection is given. Irrespective of cause, localized injuries fall into one of three categories: neurotmesis, axonotmesis, and neurapraxia. In **neurotmesis** (eg, nerve laceration), axons and endoneurial tubes are disrupted. The proximal nerve end first swells and then, to a variable degree, undergoes retrograde degeneration. Subsequently, a neuroma develops, composed of connective tissue and a tangle of regenerating axons. The axons in the distal end die (wallerian degeneration), the endoneurial tubes shrink, collagen is deposited, and an end-bulb glioma forms. In **axonotmesis,** there is wallerian degeneration, but because the endoneurial tubes are retained, effective axonal regeneration can occur unless it is impeded by a connective tissue fibroblastic reaction (neuroma in continuity). In **neurapraxia,** there is temporary failure of conduction without loss of axonal continuity.

Clinical Findings

Following nerve injury, the history suggests the type of pathology while the neurologic examination localizes the lesion. A standard neuroanatomy textbook should be available for review of specific motor and sensory innervation and possible anatomic variations. A complete neurologic examination must be done, with emphasis on the nerves involved. Motor, sensory, and reflex deficits must be correlated to determine severity and distribution of involvement. The sensory findings are the least reliable because of overlap from adjacent uninjured nerves. Electromyography and nerve conduction studies establish a baseline for monitoring subsequent recovery but are not helpful until 2–3 weeks after an acute injury.

Differential Diagnosis

An accurate history and a meticulous examination are the key elements. The history will help differentiate traumatic neuropathies from those of infectious origin (diphtheria, mumps, influenza, malaria, syphilis, typhoid, typhus, dysentery, tuberculosis, gonorrhea) or toxic or metabolic origin (diabetes, rheumatic fever, gout, leukemia, vitamin deficiency, polyarteritis nodosa, drug reaction, heavy metals, carbon monoxide).

Complications

Pain resulting from nerve injury (neuropathic pain) can be caused by neuroma formation, by involvement of the sympathetic nervous system (complex regional pain syndrome; CRPS), or by alterations in peripheral and central processing of sensory information. Painful neuromas produce pain when pressure is applied locally. Pain associated with CRPS (formerly known as causalgia or sympathetically maintained pain is burning and dysesthetic and is associated with hyperpathia and trophic skin and joint changes. Early aggressive treatment of CRPS is essential to avoid permanent disability. Local anesthetic blocks of the peripheral and sympathetic nerves may be helpful in diagnosing and treating these problems. Medical management includes tricyclic antidepressants, anticonvulsants (carbamazepine or gabapentin), mexiletine, or sympathetic blocking agents. Surgical treatment includes neurolysis, resection of the neuroma away from sites of mechanical trigger, sympathectomy, or electrical stimulation of the proximal nerve or the spinal cord.

Treatment & Prognosis

The choice of treatment depends on the nature of the nerve injury. Early exploration and repair should be used for clean lacerations. When associated injuries are present (major arterial laceration, shock) or when there is gross contamination, it is better to tag the nerve endings with nonabsorbable suture to prevent excessive retraction and to facilitate subsequent repair. Such injuries should be approached within 10 days if the patient's condition warrants. Patients with nerves injured by stretch or contusion should be followed for clinical signs of recovery. If no recovery is seen within 3 months, exploration is indicated. Intraoperative electrical studies help distinguish between axonotmetic injuries in the process of recovery (compound nerve action potential present) and those with no evidence of recovery. Recovering nerves should be left intact, but in those with no evidence of function, the damaged segment should be resected. Although this approach sometimes results in exploration when the nerves would have recovered spontaneously, initiation of early repair is important in nerve that will not recover. Because nerve regeneration is relatively slow (1 inch per month) and because intraneural fibrosis eventually prevents axonal growth (approximately 18 months), waiting too long may eliminate the chance for recovery.

The techniques of nerve anastomosis depend on whether the primary nerve endings are in close proximity; if so, epineurial repair should be performed with microscopic magnification and fine (8-0 or finer) suture. Nerve repair must be done without tension. If the gap between endings is too long for primary repair, nerve grafts (usually sural) should be used in an interfascicular repair.

Some lesions resulting from contusion or compression are improved by neurolysis. The same is true of some injection neuropathies (depending upon the substance injected).

Prompt institution of physical therapy for improvement of muscle function and maintenance of joint range of motion is indicated. The denervated portion of the limb is subject to muscle atrophy and fibrosis, joint stiffness, motor end-plate atrophy, and trophic skin changes. The longer the denervation persists, the less likely it is that a good functional result will ultimately be achieved.

Only careful grading of sensorimotor function following injury will allow accurate evaluation of recovery, especially after surgical repair. Intraoperative factors such as axial orientation of fasciculi, proper coaptation, suture material, hemostasis, and especially suture line tension determine the outcome. In axonotmetic and neurotmetic injuries, regeneration occurs at a rate of 1 inch per month. Thus, improvement may not be noted for many months, and the patient must be psychologically prepared. Recovery of function should proceed smoothly from proximal to distal; maximum recovery may take 1–2 years. Factors that adversely affect the return of function are the type of nerve injured (mixed), the age of the patient, proximal nerve injury, large nerve defect, and associated tissue injury.

Patients must understand that their role in treatment is an active one, and their motivation must be maintained. Early rehabilitation is important to maintain full joint range of motion while awaiting functional return. Later, physical therapy will help maximize the return of useful function. Neurologic recovery is often incomplete, and the use of tendon transfers may be helpful as a means of improving the functional outcome.

Carter GT et al: Electrodiagnostic evaluation of traumatic nerve injuries. Hand Clin 2000;16:1.

Noble J et al: Analysis of upper and lower extremity peripheral nerve injuries in a population of patients with multiple injuries. J Trauma 1998;45:116.

Penkert G et al: Diagnosis and surgery of brachial plexus injuries. J Reconstr Microsurg 1999;15:3.

Spinner RJ; Kline DG: Surgery for peripheral nerve and brachial plexus injuries or other nerve lesions. Muscle Nerve 2000; 23:680.

■ BRAIN TUMORS

Michael W. McDermott, MD, Sandeep Kunwar, MD, & Mitchel S. Berger, MD

 ESSENTIALS OF DIAGNOSIS

- Headache.
- Seizures.
- Progressive neurologic deficit.
- Change in personality or behavior.

General Considerations

Tumors of the central nervous system are considered either primary or metastatic (secondary). Among primary brain tumors a useful surgical classification is into intra-axial and extra-axial lesions. Intra-axial tumors are those that are within the brain parenchyma, and extra-axial ones are those arising outside the parenchyma, usually attached to leptomeninges or involving the skull or skull base. Primary malignant brain tumors are among the most difficult malignancies to eradicate with treatment. Even low-grade astrocytomas of the cerebral hemispheres or brain stem are generally considered to behave in a "malignant" manner because of their infiltrating and progressive nature and because they lead to death if not treated. There are a few well localized primary brain tumors such as cerebellar astrocytomas, juvenile pilocytic astrocytomas, and gangliogliomas, and dysembryoplastic neuroepithelial (primitive neuroectodermal) tumors (PNETs) that can be removed surgically with long-term control rates without adjunctive therapy (Figures 38–12 and 38–13).

The intracranial compartment is a fixed space, and for that reason growing brain tumors produce nonspecific symptoms as they increase the intracranial pressure. The most common symptom is generalized headache, usually worse in the morning and sometimes relieved by vomiting. Papilledema is a clinical sign that confirms the presence of long-standing increased intracranial pressure. Specific localizing signs are created by invasion or compression of functioning neural tissue such as the speech and language cortices, the motor or primary sensory cortices, or the visual cortex. Given that most primary brain tumors of the astrocytic series arise within the frontal lobe, it is not surprising that one of the most common presenting symptoms is change in personality or behav-

Figure 38–12. Distribution of intracranial tumors in children. (Reproduced, with permission, from Burger PC, Vogel FS: *Surgical Pathology of the Nervous System and Its Coverings*. Wiley, 1976.)

Cerebral hemisphere:
  Astrocytoma, anaplastic astrocytoma
  Glioblastoma multiforme
  Meningioma
  Metastatic carcinoma
  Vascular malformation
  Oligodendroglioma
  Ependymoma
  Sarcoma

Pineal region:
  Germ cell neoplasm

Cerebellum:
  Hemangioblastoma
  Metastatic carcinoma
  Astrocytoma
  Medulloblastoma

Fourth ventricle:
  Ependymoma
  Choroid plexus papilloma
  Meningioma

Region of the foramen magnum:
  Meningioma
  Schwannoma
  Neurofibroma

Cerebellopontine angle:
  Acoustic schwannoma
  Meningioma
  Epidermoid cyst
  Choroid plexus papilloma
  Glomus jugulare tumor

Corpus callosum:
  Astrocytoma, anaplastic astrocytoma
  Glioblastoma multiforme
  Oligodendroglioma
  Lipoma

Region about the third ventricle:
  Astrocytoma, anaplastic astrocytoma
  Glioblastoma multiforme
  Oligodendroglioma
  Ependymoma
  Pilocytic astrocytoma

Lateral ventricle:
  Ependymoma
  Meningioma
  Subependymoma
  Choroid plexus papilloma

Third ventricle:
  Colloid cyst
  Ependymoma

Optic chiasm and nerve:
  Meningioma
  Astrocytoma

Pituitary region:
  Pituitary adenoma
  Craniopharyngioma
  Meningioma
  Germ cell neoplasm

Brain stem:
  Astrocytoma, anaplastic astrocytoma
  Glioblastoma multiforme

Figure 38–13. Distribution of intracranial tumors in adults. (Reproduced, with permission, from Burger PC, Vogel FS: *Surgical Pathology of the Nervous System and Its Coverings.* Wiley, 1976.)

ior. Irritation of cortical tissue or its deafferentation may produce focal or secondarily generalized seizures.

The most recent data from the Central Brain Tumor Registry of the United States indicates that the overall incidence of primary and central nervous system tumors is 12.7 per 100,000 person years. (See Tables 38–2, 38–3, and 38–4.) For the period of data collection between 1992 and 1997, among 38,848 tumors reported, 35.9% occurred in the supratentorial compartment, 6.5% primarily within the infratentorial compartment, and in 17.6% there was an overlap between the two. By histology, neuroepithelial tumors were the most common, accounting for 36% of all primary brain tumors, followed by meningiomas (26%), nerve sheath tumors (7%), and pituitary adenomas (6%). The mean age at diagnosis for all tumors in this study was 54 years. The incidence rates for most primary tumors were higher in males or similar to the rates in females with the exception of meningiomas, which was twice as common in women. Overall, the incidence for brain tumors was highest among per-

Table 38–2. Distribution of all primary brain and central nervous system tumors by site.[1]

Site	Percentage of Total[2]
Supratentorial	35.9%
Infratentorial	6.5%
Intraventricular	1.3%
Pituitary	7.2%
Pineal region	0.5%
Overlapping and not otherwise specified	17.6%
Other central nervous system tumors	31.0%

[1]Central Brain Tumor Registry of the United States, 1992–1997.
[2]Total number of cases = 38,848.

Table 38–3. Distribution of all primary brain and central nervous system tumors by histology.[1]

Histology	Percentage of Total[2]
Glioblastoma	23%
Astrocytomas	13%
Meningioma	26%
Schwannoma	7%
Pituitary adenoma	6%
All others[3]	25%

[1]Central Brain Tumor Registry of the United States, 1992–1997.
[2]Total number of cases = 38,848.
[3]Includes lymphoma, germ cell tumors, hemangioblastoma, craniopharyngioma, epidermoid and dermoid cysts, hemangioma, and chordoma

sons aged 75–84 years. In children, brain tumors are the second most common cause of cancer related deaths; in adolescents and young adults between the ages of 15 and 34, brain tumors are the third leading cause of cancer-related deaths. In the pediatric age group from birth to 19 years, astrocytomas, medulloblastomas, and ependymomas are the most common diagnosis.

In adults, it is generally considered that 70% of primary brain tumors arise in the supratentorial compartment, with the remainder in the infratentorial compartment. In children the distribution is reversed, with 70% of tumors within the posterior fossa. The Central Brain Tumor Registry data show that 61% of primary tumors are located within the brain (intra-axial) and 31% within the leptomeninges (extra-axial).

Table 38–4. Distribution of pediatric primary brain and central nervous system tumors.[1]

Histology	Percentage of Total[2]
Embryonal[3]	15.9%
Pilocytic astrocytoma	15.5%
Astrocytomas	21.7%
Ependymoma	6.3%
Malignant glioma not otherwise specified	8.5%
All others	32%

[1]Central Brain Tumor Registry of the United States, 1992–1997.
[2]Total number of cases = 38,848.
[3]Includes medulloblastoma.

In recent years, advances in molecular biology have identified specific oncogenes or, more commonly, loss of tumor suppressor genes that may be associated with development of a primary brain tumor. Advances in surgical instrumentation and technique and the use of surgical navigation systems for intracranial operations have led to improvements in safety and outcomes. These aspects will be considered further under the specific diagnostic groups.

TUMORS OF NEUROGLIAL CELLS

Neuroglial cell tumors arise from cells derived from the primitive neuroepithelium and account for 50% of all intracranial primary brain tumors. In the past these tumors were collectively known as gliomas, a category which now includes several histologic tumor types. Many classifications for neuroglial tumors have been proposed, and most are based on the identification of reasonably precise etiologic features linking neoplastic elements to normal cell types found both in the mature and in the developing central nervous system. In the widely used World Health Organization (WHO-2) grading system, the main histologic subtypes are graded from one to four. Astrocytomas and oligodendrogliomas—the most common gliomas—are widely distributed throughout the brain, brain stem, and spinal cord. Ependymomas arise from ependymal cells that line the ventricle walls and central canal, which is where they are most commonly located. Medulloblastomas (primitive neuroectodermal tumors of the cerebellum) presumably originate from fetal cells residing in the cerebellum and occur primarily in children. Gliomas represent a very complex set of tumors in classification as well as in treatment. The cardinal property of gliomas is their propensity to undergo anaplastic change to a more malignant lesion, ie, to increase in histologic grade over time. Most of the gliomas are known for their ability to infiltrate into normal tissue, and for that reason patients commonly present with seizures, focal neurologic deficits, or increased intercranial pressure.

1. Astrocytomas & Oligodendrogliomas

There are two categories of low-grade astrocytomas. Pilocytic astrocytomas are most commonly found in children. These lesions are most commonly found in the cerebellum and less commonly in the hypothalamus, then the optic nerve and chiasm, and at times in the brain stem and spinal cord. Pilocytic astrocytomas are well-circumscribed and often cystic neoplasms composed of varying compact and loose-textured astrocytes associated with Rosenthal fibers.

The second type of low-grade astrocytoma is the low-grade fibrillary astrocytoma, or WHO-2 astrocytoma. Fibrillary astrocytomas favor the cerebral hemispheres of young to middle-aged adults and the brain stems of children.

Among patients with low-grade astrocytomas, seizures are more common than functional deficits owing to the absence of cortical destruction, which is more commonly seen with higher-grade lesions. These slow growing neoplasms occur predominantly in the third and fourth decades. Grade II astrocytomas over time can progress to grade III or grade IV tumors.

Anaplastic Astrocytomas

This group of fibrillary astrocytic tumors is intermediate in differentiation between the better-differentiated astrocytoma and the poorly differentiated glioblastoma. Anaplastic astrocytomas are considered WHO-II grade III tumors and occur primarily within the cerebral hemispheres. They most frequently occur a decade later than the grade II astrocytomas, peaking in the fifth and sixth decades. These tumors can also appear in the pons, typically in children (diffuse pontine hypertrophy). Unlike differentiated astrocytomas, anaplastic astrocytomas tend to be more infiltrative and diffuse lesions. A particular variant results in gliomatosis cerebri, a condition in which the tumor infiltrates most of one or both hemispheres.

Glioblastoma Multiforme

The most common glioma, accounting for 23% of primary brain tumors, is biologically and histologically the most malignant of the fibrillary astrocytomas. Histologically, these tumors show pseudopalisading necrosis, endothelial proliferation, and multiple mitotic figures. Some tumors are so poorly differentiated that they provide no histologic evidence of an astrocytic precursor lesion, and most have histologic heterogeneity within different regions of the tumor. More recently, glioblastomas have been classified as primary or secondary glioblastomas. In general, glioblastomas that contain distinct large areas of differentiated astrocytic tumor or have been documented previously as low-grade lesions are classified as secondary glioblastomas and are due to malignant transformation of lower-grade lesions. Primary glioblastomas are believed to arise de novo as malignant tumors. Studies using biologic markers support the notion that primary and secondary glioblastomas are cytogenetically different. By the WHO-2 grading system this is a grade 4 tumor and is extremely infiltrative. Biopsies of adjacent normal tissue up to 2 cm beyond the radiographic boundaries of the tumor show evidence on neoplastic cells intermixed with normal parenchyma. Because of the rapid growth and the degree of adjacent cerebral edema, patients commonly present with symptoms of increased intracranial pressure or focal neurologic deficits.

Oligodendrogliomas

Oligodendrogliomas are infiltrative gliomas composed of oligodendrocytes, which occur primarily in the cerebral hemispheres, especially the frontal lobes. These tumors usually present in adulthood and are often associated with a long history of seizures—sometimes a decade or more. Many of these lesions have mineralization, which is visible on a CT scan. On histologic examination these tumors have perinuclear halos, giving them a "fried egg" appearance. Oligodendrogliomas vary in aggressiveness from low-grade (WHO-2 grade II) to anaplastic oligodendrogliomas (WHO-2 grade III). Tumors can also have a mixed component of oligodendroglial as well as astrocytic components, which are graded separately.

2. Ependymomas

Most ependymomas are slow-growing, well-circumscribed neoplasms arising throughout the neuraxis in intimate relationship with the ependyma or its remnants. Intracranial lesions most often occur in children and adolescents, though adults are also affected. The primary site of ependymomas is heavily age-dependent. The fourth ventricle is the most common site and accounts for up to 60% of these tumors. Among adults, the location in intracranial ependymomas appears to be evenly divided between infratentorial and supratentorial locations. In contrast, the vast majority of spinal ependymomas occur in adults and comprise the main glioma of the spinal cord and phylum terminale (over 60%). Although most ependymomas are slow-growing lesions, because of their location they can produce clinical and radiographic signs of increased intracranial pressure or obstruction of the cerebrospinal fluid pathways. The prognosis of these tumors is markedly improved if total resection can be accomplished. Tumors arising from the floor of the fourth ventricle (dorsal surface of the brain stem) constitute a poor operative risk for gross total resection, resulting in incomplete resections and an increased likelihood of recurrence. Because of the location of these tumors, they may descend along the cerebrospinal fluid pathways.

3. Medulloblastomas

Medulloblastoma is a small-cell neuroectodermal tumor of the cerebellum and is the most common brain tumor of childhood. Over 50% occur in the second half of the first decade, and one-third occur in adolescence and early adulthood. Symptoms may be a reflection of cerebellar dysfunction, increased intracranial pressure, or craniospinal dissemination. The genesis of medulloblastoma is controversial, but it is believed that these cells are bipotential (neuronal and glial) and may arise from immature cells residing in the external granular layer or cells in the posterior medullary velum. Histologically, these tumors are highly malignant, with populations of dense small cells lacking apparent stroma or distinctive architectural features. Medulloblastomas have a propensity to seed throughout the cerebrospinal fluid pathways. These tumors are highly radiosensitive and, depending on tumor stage, 10-year survival rates of 40–50% have been achieved by aggressive resection and radiotherapy.

Choroid Plexus Papilloma & Carcinoma

These tumors are papillary neoplasms derived from choroid plexus epithelium. Choroid plexus neoplasms in children usually arise within the lateral ventricles and most frequently the third ventricles. Plexus tumors in adults are nearly all papillomas, many of which arise within the fourth ventricle or its lateral recess. These tumors can cause hydrocephalus secondary either to obstruction of cerebrospinal fluid flow or to overproduction of cerebrospinal fluid. Malignant variants (choroid plexus carcinomas) occur and carry a very poor prognosis. Most carcinomas are frankly infiltrative and are likely to recur or result in craniospinal dissemination.

NON-GLIAL CELL TUMORS

These tumors arise from a variety of tissues, including the skull base, leptomeninges, pituitary gland, and pineal region. Nerve sheath tumors—most commonly schwannomas—are also included in this group. For the most part, these tumors are benign and produce symptoms by compression of brain rather than invasion as well as by elevation of intracranial pressure.

1. Meningiomas

Meningiomas account for 26% of all primary brain tumors and arise from arachnoid cap cells. At operation they are usually attached to the dura although they do not arise from it. Many are globular in shape, and 85% are histologically benign. They most commonly occur along the faux (falx, parasagittal), sphenoid wing, and convexity dura. In 10% of patients the tumors are multiple, and this may be associated with neurofibromatosis type 2. In children there is a tendency for meningiomas to be histologically and clinically more aggressive. Hyperostosis of bone may occur either in the skull base or in the convexity and usually relates to stimulation of bony activity by invading meningioma. A characteristic clinical picture is of a middle-aged woman with unilateral painless proptosis that usually is seen with a hyperostotic sphenoid wing meningioma.

Meningiomas are known to be induced by radiation therapy with latent intervals of 10–40 years between radiation exposure and tumor appearance. Radiation-induced meningiomas are commonly more atypical or aggressive on histology and have a more aggressive clinical behavior. A possible role of sex steroid hormones has been investigated in an attempt to explain the female preponderance of meningiomas, but no causal relationship has been established. Multiple meningiomas are the hallmark of neurofibromatosis type 2, which develops in response to loss of the tumor suppresser gene on chromosome 22. The most common karyotypic abnormality in meningiomas is monosomy of 22 or loss of the long arm of 22. Other allelic losses on chromosome arms 1-p, 6-q, 9-q, 10-q, 14-q, 17-p, and 18-q may well be important in development and progression of these tumors.

The World Health Organization has classified meningiomas on the basis of the likelihood of recurrence and grade. Brain invasion alone is no longer sufficient for the diagnosis of malignant meningioma (Table 38–5).

2. Nerve Sheath Neoplasms

These benign tumors originate from Schwann cells and have a predilection for the eighth, fifth, and tenth nerves. Clinically, the most common intracranial schwannoma is the vestibular schwannoma, or acoustic

Table 38–5. Classification of meningiomas.[1]

Grade I: Low risk of recurrence
Meningothelial
Fibrous
Transitional
Psammomatous
Angiomatous
Microcystic
Secretory
Lymphoplasmacyte-rich
Metaplastic
Grade II: Intermediate risk of recurrence
Atypical
Clear cell
Choroid
Grade III: High risk of recurrence
Rhabdoid
Papillary
Anaplastic

[1]World Health Organization, 2000.

neuroma, which arises from the superior or inferior portion of the vestibular nerve in the internal auditory canal. As the tumor enlarges, it expands the bony canal and extends into the cerebellopontine angle. Patients who present with unilateral hearing loss confirmed by audiogram more commonly are imaged with magnetic resonance studies, and the diagnosis of these tumors is being made earlier. The presence of bilateral vestibular schwannomas is diagnostic of neurofibromatosis type 2. All age groups are affected, but there is a peak incidence in the fourth to sixth decades. Pathologically, the tumors are composed of spindle-shaped neoplastic Schwann cells with alternating areas of compact stroma with loose, less cellular areas. Most schwannomas are sporadic tumors, and almost all have a mutation of a tumor suppresser *NF2* gene, which encodes for the protein merlin. By Western blotting or immunohistochemistry, almost all tumors appear to have loss of merlin expression. This may be an essential step in schwannoma tumorigenesis.

3. Cranial Meningiomas

These benign tumors of epithelial origin are found in the region of the sella or suprasellar cistern. They account for 1.2–4% of adult intracranial tumors and 6–10% of pediatric brain tumors. The sex incidence is equal. Cranial meningiomas are thought to originate from epithelial rests found within the infundibular stalk or pituitary. During the fourth week of gestation, Rathke's pouch forms as a diverticulum and migrates to meet the infundibulum, which is a downgrowth from the floor of the diencephalon. Two pathologic types are identified: the adamantinomatous craniopharyngioma and papillary craniopharyngioma. The tumors are confined to the sella in only 5% of cases, while the majority involve both the sella and the suprasellar regions. Clinically, patients most often present with visual pathway disturbances, followed in frequency by endocrinopathy or hydrocephalus. The tumors can be solid or cystic (or both). On CT imaging, the adamantinomatous form may show intratumoral calcification. In adult patients, this calcification can be the most prominent imaging characteristic of the tumor. Cystic portions of the tumor may displace the third ventricle and cause obstructive hydrocephalus. While the goal of treatment is complete surgical resection, tumor location around the vital structures makes this goal difficult to achieve.

4. Congenital Tumors

Epidermoid Tumors

Epidermoid tumors were formerly called "pearly tumors" because of the findings at surgery of a smooth, glistening mother-of-pearl appearance related to the accumulation of desquamated epithelium. Epidermoid cysts occur along the basal cisterns, most commonly in the suprasellar or parasellar regions as well as in the cerebellopontine angle. The capsule of these tumors is frequently adherent to adjacent cranial nerves and vascular structures. The aim of surgery is evacuation of the central portion of the cyst in order to eliminate surrounding mass effect. Epidermoid cysts in the sellar region usually present with visual or endocrine disturbances or hydrocephalus. Patients with these cysts have repeated attacks of aseptic meningitis, presumably related to leakage of cyst contents into the cerebrospinal fluid pathways. MRI studies are extremely useful, particularly in the noncontrast T1, proton density, and FLAIR sequences. As compared with arachnoid cysts, epidermoid tumors typically have increased signal intensity In the FLAIR images.

Dermoid Tumors

Dermoid tumors are less common than epidermoid cysts, but they generally grow more quickly and thus present at a younger age than epidermoids. While epidermoid cysts are generally found laterally in basal cistern compartments, dermoid cysts tend to be located in the midline. One-third occur in the region of the fourth ventricle. Obstruction of cerebrospinal fluid pathways and a presentation with hydrocephalus is more common. Dermoid tumors contain adnexal elements as hair, hair follicles, or sebaceous glands. They may be associated with a dermal sinus tract, which may present anywhere on the occipital scalp along the midline. Repeated bouts of bacterial meningitis associated with dermoid tumors should arouse suspicion of such a tract. On imaging studies there is a much higher incidence of calcification in dermoids than in epidermoid tumors. Treatment consists of excision.

Central Nervous System Germ Cell Tumors

This histologically heterogeneous group of tumors is derived from all three germ layers. They tend to occur in the midline, most commonly in the region of the third ventricle or the pineal gland. They constitute less than 1% of all primary intracranial neoplasms and only 3% of those encountered in childhood or adolescence. Their incidence is much higher in East Asian countries for some reason. Approximately 90% of patients with germ cell tumors are under age 20. Because of their location in the pineal or third ventricular regions, they obstruct cerebrospinal fluid pathways and cause hydrocephalus with intracranial hypertension. Positioned within the pineal region along the posterior of the midbrain, they can compress the tectal plate and cause characteristic paralysis of upward gaze and impaired conversions with absence of pupillary light reflex (Parinaud's syndrome). Involvement of the hypothalamic region and pituitary stalk produces diabetes insipidus. Many of these tumors have a propensity for spread within the cerebrospinal fluid, which must be examined in the workup prior to treatment. Oncoproteins are also secreted by some of these tumors, and the most useful markers are alpha-fetoprotein, human chorionic gonadotropin, and placental alkaline phosphatase. Elevation of any of these markers constitutes presumptive evidence that the tumor is a germ cell tumor.

5. Pituitary Tumors

The incidence of pituitary adenomas in autopsy studies is greater than 20%. Most are benign adenomas. They are classified as endocrine-active or endocrine-inactive (nonfunctioning) depending on whether the adenoma secretes a hormone resulting in a hypersecretory syndrome. Of the endocrine-active tumors, those that secrete growth hormone (somatotropic adenomas) result in acromegaly (or gigantism in children), excess secretion of adrenocorticotropic hormone (corticotropic adenomas) results in Cushing's disease, excess secretion of thyroid-secreting hormone (thyrotropic adenomas) results in hyperthyroidism, and hyperprolactinemia results in galactorrhea-amenorrhea in women. Hyperprolactinemia is related to prolactin secretion from the adenoma or to loss of the dopaminergic suppression by the hypothalamus of prolactin from the normal gland, the latter occurring when the pituitary stalk is distorted. Gonadotropic adenomas (secreting FSH or LH) present in a fashion similar to that of endocrine-inactive adenomas.

Pituitary tumors are also divided by size into microadenomas (< 1 cm) or macroadenomas (> 1 cm). Secretory tumors commonly present as microadenomas, whereas endocrine-inactive tumors and prolactinomas in men present as macroadenomas. Macroadenomas result in pituitary dysfunction, with the initial loss of growth hormone and gonadotropin release resulting in diminished libido. Although these tumors are benign, they result in progressive pituitary dysfunction and can compress the optic chiasm, resulting in a bitemporal visual field cut (tunnel vision).

Treatment of pituitary adenomas is excision with the exception of prolactinomas, which can be treated with dopamine agonists to prevent tumor growth and cause shrinkage. Surgery entails either a transsphenoidal approach by a sublabial or transseptal incision or a purely endonasal approach. Postoperative hospitalization is usually 1–2 days, with relatively rapid recovery. Complete resection is curative, but the likelihood of complete resection depends on the size of the tumor and whether there has been invasion of adjacent cavernous sinus or bone. The treatment of prolactinomas by surgery or medical therapy depends on the size and extent of the tumor, the serum prolactin level, and the patient's desires. Radiotherapy for pituitary adenomas is reserved for tumor recurrence or for tumors incurable by surgery alone.

6. Tumors Within the Skull Base

Primary skull neoplasms include both benign and malignant variants. These tumors generally produce symptoms by direct compression of brain tissue or cranial nerves. Benign tumors are often found incidentally in the course of investigation for other processes. These include osteoma, hemangioma, and aneurysmal bone cyst. Malignant primary skull tumors commonly include chordoma and chondrosarcoma. Chordomas are thought to arise from notochordal remnants and usually occur along the clivus. They are slowly growing and histologically benign, though clinically they have a very high rate of recurrence in spite of complete surgical removal. Their location within the skull base surrounding basal blood vessels and cranial nerves makes complete removal difficult. Chondrosarcomas have a more benign course and usually present in men in the fourth decade. They frequently arise in the upper third of the clivus or parasellar region and present with local compressive cranial neuropathy. Treatment both of these tumors is excision plus radiotherapy to reduce the rate of recurrence.

7. Metastatic Tumors

Autopsy studies have revealed the presence of intracranial metastases in one-fourth of cancer patients. Tumors of the lungs, breast, and skin account for over 90% of brain metastases. Choriocarcinoma, renal cell carcinoma, and metastatic melanoma are the most common hemorrhagic metastases. Eighty percent of brain metastases are located within the vascular distribution of the middle cerebral artery. They typically occur near the junction of the gray and white matter and can also occur within the pituitary, the pineal gland, or the choroid plexus. Involvement of the leptomeninges is common and is universally fatal. Approximately 30% of brain metastases are solid at the time of presentation, and a characteristic of these lesions is the abundant vasogenic edema they produce in surrounding brain. Metastases affecting the spinal cord occur in the epidural space, in the leptomeninges, or within the spinal cord. Epidural metastases are the most common clinical pattern of presentation.

Clinical Findings

Symptoms produced by brain tumors are largely related to their site, size, and rate of growth. The clinical manifestations may be divided into two broad categories: those related to elevated intracranial pressure and those related to tumor location.

A. GENERALIZED SYMPTOMS AND SIGNS

Symptoms and signs may be due to elevation of intracranial pressure related to tumor growth, associated cerebral edema, obstruction of cerebrospinal fluid pathways with development of hydrocephalus, obstruction of cerebrospinal fluid absorption mechanisms, or intratumoral hemorrhage. The most common symptom of increased intracranial pressure is headache, which is typically generalized and relatively constant but worse in the morning. Morning headache may be relieved by vomiting. Exacerbation of headache in the early hours of the day may be related to increased venous pressure in the supine position. Any change in the pattern of a preexisting headache syndrome or new onset of severe headache or persistent syndrome should arouse suspicion of brain tumor.

Personality change, easy fatigability, listlessness, mental slowing, and problems with attention and concentration are commonly noted by patients or family when there is a rapidly growing tumor. Without intervention or diagnosis, continued elevation of intracranial pressure leads to deterioration to unconsciousness and ultimately to coma and death.

Signs of increased intracranial pressure may be subtle or marked. In its most obvious form, disturbed level of attentiveness, alertness, or frank coma may be observed. Elevated intracranial pressure that has been present for days, weeks, or months may lead to the development of papilledema. In severe cases this is associated with frank hemorrhages in the nerve fiber layer. Long-standing untreated papilledema eventually leads to loss of nerve fibers with the development of optic atrophy and blindness. A nonlocalizing sign of elevated intracranial pressure is the development of a sixth nerve palsy, resulting in paralysis of the lateral rectus muscle of the eye and inturning of the involved eye. Patients complain of double vision, most marked on looking toward the side of the affected nerve. This is thought to be related in part to the long intradural course of the sixth nerve after it exits the pons to enter a dural fold in the upper third of the clivus. Following treatment of the underlying associated problem, this nerve palsy resolves over weeks to months and in the interim can be corrected with prism glasses.

Seizures, while not a direct manifestation of increased intracranial pressure, are a nonspecific presenting symptom in adults with brain tumors. Tumors of the frontal, temporal, and parietal lobes are more likely to present with seizures than those involving the basal ganglia, brain stem, or cerebellum. Tumors within the occipital lobe may present with irritative phenomena such as nonformed visual hallucinations or a visual field defect.

It should be noted that in children, before closure of the cranial sutures, progressive enlargement of the head and bulging of the anterior fontanelle is a sign of elevated intracranial pressure. This may be due to a number of intracranial conditions including, but not limited to, brain tumor.

B. FOCAL SYMPTOMS AND SIGNS

Intra-axial tumors involving the cerebral hemispheres, basal ganglia, brain stem, or cerebellum may present with specific clinical constellations of symptoms and signs. Extra-axial nonglial neoplasm may also present with focal neurologic symptoms. Focal symptoms and signs are usually due to interference with function of a specific local area of brain. Clinical localization may be assisted by knowledge of the function localized to any of these areas. Some general comments can be made.

1. Cerebral hemispheres—Tumors of the frontal lobe commonly present with alterations in personality, behavior, motivation, mood, and memory. Within the dominant hemisphere, laterally located (usually left) frontal tumors may produce expressive language difficulties. Posterior frontal tumors bordering the primary motor cortex may produce irritative phenomena such as focal simple seizures with motor phenomena or secondary generalization. Direct invasion by glial neoplasms or compression by extra-axial tumors may produce frank loss of function. Initially this will begin in the contralateral extremity and progress in both severity and degree. Face, hand, and arm motor cortices are represented over the lateral frontal cortex, while trunk and legs are represented mesially.

2. Parietal lobe—Within the dominant hemisphere, anterior inferior parietal tumors produce receptive language difficulties. Patients have difficulty with left-right orientation and comprehension of the spoken or written word. Difficulties may also be present with naming, calculating, and reading. It is uncommon for patients with parietal tumors to complain of focal sensory deficits, but they will say that an entire side of the body is numb. Specific to the nondominant parietal lobe are functions related to three-dimensional constructional abilities as well as common daily activities such as dressing. Disturbances in these areas may be indicative of tumor location. There may also be contralateral inattention to both the visual and tactile stimulation.

3. Temporal lobe—In the dominant hemisphere, posterior temporal lobe tumors may produce difficulties with naming, calculation, and reading. Anterior and mid temporal lobe tumors may produce a contralateral quadrant visual sphere defect. Seizures not uncommonly are the presenting manifestation of temporal lobe tumors.

4. Occipital lobe—Occipital lobe tumors usually present with a visual field defect manifested by bumping into objects on the contralateral side of extrapersonal space. They may have irritative visual phenomena with nonformed visual hallucinations as simple as scintillating scotomas. Generalized seizure is not a common presentation of occipital lobe tumors.

5. Sellar and parasellar regions—Tumors in and about the optic nerve chiasm, tract, hypothalamus, and cavernous sinus may produce either visual or endocrine disturbances. Lesions of the optic nerve produce unilateral visual loss while those of the chiasm produce a bitemporal field defect. Disturbance of hypothalamic function results in autonomic disturbances and endocrinopathy. Extension of any process into the third ventricle may produce noncommunicating hydrocephalus. Involvement in structures coursing through the cavernous sinus—ie, cranial nerves III, IV, V, and VI—may produce double vision and facial numbness. Trigeminal neuralgia may be a feature of cerebellopontine angle or skull base extra-axial tumors.

6. Pineal region—Tumors of the pineal region produce symptoms related to elevated intracranial pressure from hydrocephalus and disturbance of coordinated eye movements. Hydrocephalus is usually noncommunicating, related to obstruction or compression of the cerebral aqueduct with enlargement of the third and lateral ventricles. Compression of the midbrain tectum produces problems with upward gaze and convergence. Typically, there is an absence of the pupillary light reflex.

7. Posterior fossa—Tumors of the brain stem typically cause multiple cranial nerve palsies—usually cranial nerves V, VI, and VII—followed by ataxia and long tract sensory and motor signs. Tumors of the midline cerebellum may produce a midline truncal ataxia or ipsilateral limb ataxia or incoordination when involved in the cerebral hemispheres. In many cases there is associated noncommunicating hydrocephalus.

8. Cerebellopontine angle—Vestibular and trigeminal schwannomas as well as petroclival meningiomas are the most common tumors in this location. These tumors produce a combination of specific cranial nerve dysfunction plus cerebellar disturbances and, later, hydrocephalus related to kinking of the cerebral aqueduct.

SPECIAL INVESTIGATIONS FOR SUSPECTED BRAIN TUMORS

Most patients with primary brain tumors do not have specific laboratory findings on routine blood work. However, for germ cell tumors, serum levels of alpha-fetoprotein, human chorionic gonadotropin, and carcinoembryonic antigen, and placental alkaline phosphatase may be elevated. Patients with malignant primitive neuroectodermal tumors require examination of cerebrospinal fluid for central nervous system axis staging that may direct further treatment. For patients with metastatic tumors, evaluation of the primary organ system with appropriate imaging studies is necessary in order to adequately stage the primary tumor locally.

Most patients with intracranial brain neoplasms are imaged using MRI as the standard. The addition of intravenous paramagnetic contrast agents preoperatively helps predetermine the possible grade and the site for the most definitive biopsy. Anatomic detail derived from MRI is superior to that of CT scanning. Functional localization of eloquent areas of brain and their relationship to the associated tumor is also possible with functional MRI techniques using blood oxygen level-dependent (BOLD) contrast imaging. In addition, magnetic resonance spectroscopy can also help define the metabolism of volumes of tumor that are independent from static imaging features. MR imaging of the spinal axis is another important feature for staging those malignant tumors with a propensity for leptomeningeal spread, such as medulloblastoma and germinoma.

Following tumor tissue biopsy or removal, standard histologic and immunohistochemical techniques are used for distinguishing different tumor cell types. The proliferative potential for tumors can be derived by MIB-1 (evaluating Ki-67 expression) or proliferating cell nuclear antigen (PCNE) labeling studies. Molecular markers such as *P53* status and loss of heterozygosity of genes on portions of chromosomes (-1p, -19q for oligodendrogliomas) may have important therapeutic implications.

DIFFERENTIAL DIAGNOSIS OF BRAIN TUMORS

Because brain tumors can cause focal neurologic signs and increased intracranial pressure, many conditions may be simulated by brain tumor. In infants and adolescents, unexplained seizures usually herald the onset of idiopathic epilepsy. In adults, the onset of seizures is usually the first manifestation of a brain tumor. Vascular malformations, degenerative diseases, subdural hematoma, brain abscess, encephalitis, meningitis, and toxic states may mimic a tumor. Parasitic infections with a combination of solid and cystic components may mimic a benign brain tumor. Opportunistic infections in immunocompromised patients may present as mass lesions. Multiple small ring-enhancing lesions, seen with some forms of pyogenic brain abscess, may mimic intracranial metastases from a systemic primary. Even with the advent of modern imaging techniques that now are able to evaluate the metabolic "fingerprint" of a tumor, the final diagnosis still rests with tissue examination of the imaged lesion.

MEDICAL TREATMENT OF BRAIN TUMORS

The medical treatment of patients with brain tumors involves correction of metabolic abnormalities such as hyponatremia, administration of steroids to reduce vasogenic edema, and possibly administration of antiepileptic drugs in patients who present with seizures, to reduce the likelihood of further events.

In patients with elevated intracranial pressure, the syndrome of inappropriate antidiuretic hormone (SIADH) secretion may lead to the development of hyponatremia. Patients should be cautioned against drinking excessive amounts of water in order to flush out metabolic tumor toxins. We generally limit patients who have intra-axial neoplasms with surrounding edema to 1800 mL of fluid per day. No specific dietary restrictions are recommended, though patients scheduled for biopsy or open craniotomy are asked to stop aspirin-containing compounds 10 days prior to the procedure. Other anti-inflammatory agents are stopped 3 days before the procedure.

No agent is more effective than dexamethasone at reversing vasogenic edema related to intracranial tumor. Standard doses for symptomatic patients with elevations of intracranial pressure are 4 mg orally four times daily. This is tapered over time as the clinical condition allows. Patients are cautioned to observe for side effects, which include tremors, sleeplessness, excessive appetite, weight gain, and exacerbation of underlying glucose intolerance. Steroid medications can generally be reduced 1–2 weeks after operation for an intracranial tumor. In this way, long-term complications of excessive steroid use are avoided.

A variety of new antiepileptic drugs are currently available for the treatment of patients who present with epilepsy. As yet there is no good information that prophylaxis prior to surgery is warranted for patients with intra-axial brain neoplasms who did not present with a seizure. Standard agents to be used are carbamazepine, phenytoin, and valproic acid. Serum levels of any antiepileptic drug should be monitored after intravenous or oral loading and after waiting five half-lives

of the drug before a steady state is reached. Modification of drug dosages is necessary in order to achieve a therapeutic serum concentration so that further seizures can be avoided.

SURGICAL TREATMENT OF BRAIN TUMORS

Prior to any operative treatment, the options of simple observation, stereotactic biopsy, or attempt at gross total tumor removal with open craniotomy should be presented to the patient. Realistic steps should be discussed with appropriate risks. The major objectives of surgical treatment are (1) to confirm the pathologic diagnosis in order to recommend appropriate further therapy; (2) to remove as much tumor as possible without increasing neurologic deficits or compromising quality of life; (3) to remove tumor for relief of symptoms of increased intracranial pressure; and (4) to remove tumor for relief of focal neurologic symptoms related to compression about the cortex by adjacent tumor.

For intra-axial glial neoplasms of the cerebral hemispheres, apart from pilocytic astrocytomas, total tumor removal is not always possible. Significant debulking of the tumor can now be accomplished safely through increased use of surgical navigation systems and intraoperative neurophysiologic monitoring and testing. Some data exist supporting the role of cytoreductive surgery for both low-grade and high-grade glial neoplasms. However, some patients live better—though perhaps not longer—after debulking surgery that reduces intracranial pressure and reduces focal mass effect, allowing for improved neurologic function.

For some posterior fossa tumors, complete tumor excision is the goal. For primitive neuroectodermal tumors, the residual volume of the tumor influences the patient's prognosis. Complete removal of lower-grade neoplasms such as ependymoma and choroid plexus papilloma obviates the need for further therapies and allows for simple imaging follow-up.

For extra-axial nonglial tumors such as meningiomas, complete surgical removal of the tumor is the goal. For convexity meningiomas, the excision of a tough normal dura surrounding the globular mass may reduce the chance for a later marginal occurrence. However, marginal excisions of dura cannot be accomplished safely in the region of the falx, major renal sinuses, the skull base, or the parasellar and posterior fossa regions. In these cases, subtotal removal of tumor may be followed by radiotherapy techniques. Fractionated external beam radiotherapy and radiosurgery offer the patient a good chance of extended tumor control not requiring further treatment.

Benign nerve sheath neoplasms of the fifth and eighth cranial nerves are best treated by surgical excision. Depending on their size, fifth nerve schwannomas can either be removed via a lateral subtemporal, anterolateral, or orbitozygomatic craniotomy or a posterolateral combined supra- or infratentorial approach. Vestibular schwannoma, when small and when functional hearing is still present, can be removed by a middle fossa approach. Larger tumors with preserved hearing and without a significant internal auditory canal component can be removed via a suboccipital approach. Large tumors in patients with no useful hearing are usually best managed via a translabyrinthine approach. Radiosurgery remains an option for vestibular schwannomas smaller than 2.5 cm in diameter. We have generally reserved this for the older patient population, but younger patients are now also being treated in this way. This treatment involves the application of a stereotactic head frame for imaging and treatment in a single session. Fractionated stereotactic radiotherapy techniques are also being employed with the hope of reducing facial neuropathy and increasing the chance of preserving useful hearing.

Craniopharyngiomas present a special surgical challenge because of their proximity to the optic apparatus, infundibulum, and hypothalamus. When tumors are almost completely intrasellar, a transsphenoidal approach can be used. However, when there is a significant suprasellar component, a supratentorial approach is usually required through a pterional, unilateral, frontal, or midline subfrontal approach. Residual tumors are best controlled through fractionated external beam radiotherapy.

Benign tumors of the basal cisterns such as epidermoid cysts are approached with standard neurosurgical techniques. In the case of epidermoid tumors, while it is possible to remove the desquamated epithelium from the center of the tumor, removal of the cyst capsule is usually not possible. For dermoid tumors, excision of any associated sinus tract is mandatory, accompanied by repair of the involved dura. These cyst walls may also be adherent to the cranial nerves, arteries, or adjacent brain surface. For pineal region tumors, open surgical approaches are preferred to stereotactic biopsy techniques because of the confluence of deep veins in this region. Supracerebellar infratentorial, occipital transtentorial, and interhemispheric transventricular approaches are used depending on the size, shape, and distribution of tumor.

Bone tumors of the skull base such as chordoma and chondrosarcoma are approached with multiple surgical disciplines, usually involving neurosurgery, neuro-otology, ophthalmology, and plastic surgery. These complicated and prolonged procedures require that the surgeons be skilled in a variety of aspects of neurosurgical care, including vascular neurosurgery.

Postoperative Complications

Surgical risks include those related to general anesthesia and those specific to the procedure. Anesthetic risks include bronchial pneumonia, urinary tract infection, venous thrombosis, skin pressure sores, air embolization, compression neuropraxia of peripheral nerves, and other benign reversible conditions. The risks of intraoperative cardiac death are exceedingly low, usually less than 1%. Risks specific to intracranial operation include the risks of infection of cerebrospinal fluid, brain, or the bone flap. Postoperative intracerebral, subdural, or epidural hematomas are uncommon, occurring in only 2–4% of patients postoperatively. Risks of increased neurologic deficit are related to a number of factors, most importantly tumor location and proximity to major arteries, veins, and venous sinuses. The risks of neurologic deficit when operating close to functional cortex may be reduced by intraoperative neurophysiologic monitoring and testing. Wound complications are more common in patients who have been on long-term steroids, those who have had prior operations or radiotherapy, or those who have a persistent cerebrospinal fluid leak after surgery.

RADIATION THERAPY FOR BRAIN TUMORS

Fractionated external beam radiotherapy is usually administered to patients with malignant primary brain tumors even after the total excision. For low-grade tumors, it remains an option after biopsy or subtotal excision. Techniques from malignant tumors usually include once-a-day treatment, 5 days per week, 180–200 Gy per day to a total of 6000 Gy. Craniospinal axis treatment for primitive neuroectodermal tumors usually requires a dose of 2500–3500 Gy to the entire head and spinal access with a boost to the primary tumor site. Malignant primary brain tumors that receive fractionated radiation therapy as part of a standard treatment protocol include glioblastoma, anaplastic astrocytoma, anaplastic oligodendroglioma, malignant ependymoma, choroid plexus carcinoma, medulloblastoma, malignant meningioma, malignant germ cell tumors, and metastatic tumors. With respect to metastatic brain tumors, persuasive data exist supporting the use of external beam radiation therapy of the entire brain after excision of the lesion. The survival of patients is improved with this combination when compared with whole brain radiation therapy alone.

Radiosurgery is a technique defined by the use of stereotactic methods for target localization and delivery of treatment and involves a single treatment session. Radiosurgery can be delivered with a variety of systems. including linear accelerator, gamma knife, and proton beam units. A great deal of clinical work with radio-surgery has centered around treatment of benign conditions such as vascular malformations and intracranial schwannomas and meningiomas. Control rates of the benign tumors appear to be excellent—above 90% at 5–8 years posttreatment. Further follow-up is required to determine the long-term results of this treatment.

CHEMOTHERAPY FOR BRAIN TUMORS

The therapeutic efficacy of antineoplastic agents against primary or metastatic brain tumors has been disappointing. This is due to several factors, including the presence of a blood-brain barrier that inhibits the transport of chemotherapeutic drugs to the interstitium of the brain. In addition, the endothelial cells within the brain have a high concentration of P-glycoprotein, which actively transports many chemotherapeutic agents out of the brain. Despite these difficulties, there are a few chemotherapeutic agents that have made it to general clinical practice for the treatment of glial neoplasms. These drugs are able to achieve reasonable concentrations within the brain because of their lipophilic nature. The most widely used antineoplastic agent for the treatment of grade III and grade IV astrocytomas are nitrosourea-based compounds. More recently, temozolomide has been shown to have some activity against grade III astrocytomas. Most chemotherapeutic trials have shown the greatest effects in younger patients. In order to overcome the difficulties of drug delivery, several systems have been developed including the use of biodegradable polymers locally implanted into the tumor cavity, hyperosmotic blood-brain barrier disruption, and direct interstitial microinfusion for convection-enhanced delivery. Since conventional chemotherapy agents yield only marginal improvement in survival for glioma patients when compared with radiation therapy alone, new therapeutic strategies are being developed, including monoclonal antibodies, recombinant toxins, and gene transfer therapy.

PROGNOSIS

1. Glial Neoplasms

The prognosis for glia-based neoplasms is strongly dependent on the histology. Among astrocytomas, histologic grade, age, Karnofsky status, and in certain cases the extent of resection influence overall survival. For grade II astrocytomas, median survival varies from 7 years to 10 years. For grade III anaplastic astrocytomas, the median survival ranges from 3 years to 5 years, and for glioblastoma multiforme the median survival is approximately 12–18 months. Longer survival is most often noted in younger patients, and the outlook is especially poor in el-

derly patients with glioblastoma. Tumors with oligodendroglial components tend to have better survival rates. In general, these tumors are more radiation-sensitive as well as chemotherapy-sensitive. Among anaplastic oligodendrogliomas, there is a clear association between chemosensitivity and loss of chromosome-1p are correlated. Long-term survival has been seen in patients with low-grade oligodendroglioma. Medulloblastomas treated by gross total resection and radiation therapy can be associated with 10-year survivals of 40–50%. Significant residual disease postresection or dissemination carries a worse prognosis. Ependymomas, when completely resected, have long-term survival rates, with some patients being cured. Choroid plexus papillomas are cured following complete resection.

2. Nonglial Tumors

Meningiomas

The prognosis of patients treated for intracranial meningioma depends upon the pathologic type and whether the tumor is benign or malignant. The degree of surgical resection also has a significant influence on the probability of recurrence. The recurrence rate ranges from 9% for excision of all tumor and adjacent dura to 39% for partial tumor removal without excision of the dural attachment or involved bone. Recurrence of tumor usually requires consideration of reoperation or external beam radiation therapy. For benign meningiomas recurrent after subtotal resection, the control rates with fractionated external beam radiation therapy are excellent—nearly 90% at 5 years and 80% 10 years after treatment. For malignant meningiomas, the prognosis is poor even with combined treatment, with median survivals of approximately 30% at 3 years posttreatment.

Trigeminal & Vestibular Schwannomas

The prognosis for these patients depends primarily on whether or not their complications are associated with surgical treatment. These tumors are slowly growing, and recurrences can be treated with reoperation or radiosurgery. Unlike meningiomas, subtotal resections are often followed by a prolonged period of no tumor growth and the enhancing mass seen on the scans remain dormant for many years. Recurrence rates after microsurgical resection vary in the literature but are less than 5%. Recurrence rates after radiosurgery are 10–12% at 5–10 years.

Craniopharyngioma

Most of the tumors that can be totally removed are reported to have 80–90% 10-year survivals. Significant endocrine or hypothalamic complications after surgery reduce these numbers. After subtotal removal and radiation therapy, survival figures are similar to those of completely removed tumors, though controversy exists as to which approach gives the best outcome.

Chordoma & Chondrosarcoma

It is rare to accomplish complete surgical excision of these tumors of the skull base. After particle beam radiation therapy, tumor control rates at 5 years are 63% and 78% for chordoma and chondrosarcoma, respectively.

Germ Cell Tumors

Radiotherapy responses for germinoma are excellent, with 5-year survivals of over 90%. With malignant neoplasms such as embryonal cell carcinoma, yolk sac tumor, and choriocarcinoma, 5-year survivals are much worse—on the order of 20–40%.

3. Metastatic Tumors

Survival of patients with metastatic brain tumors depends also to a great extent on the status of their systemic disease and whether or not it is progressive or controlled. Studies of patients with progressive systemic disease within 3 months of diagnosis of their brain metastases have found no benefit for combined surgical and radiotherapy treatment over whole brain radiation therapy alone. Most patients survive somewhere between 8 and 12 months after the original diagnosis, but survival can be very long with some tumors such as renal cell carcinoma that have an indolent course and are responsive to radiosurgical techniques.

Brandes AA, Pasetto LM, Monfardini S: The treatment of cranial germ cell tumours. Cancer Treat Rev 2000;26:233.

Cho BK et al: Pineal tumors: experience with 48 cases over 10 years. Childs Nerv Syst 1998;14:53.

Chung WY et al: Gamma knife radiosurgery for craniopharyngiomas. J Neurosurg 2000;93(Suppl 3):47.

Habrand JL et al: The role of radiation therapy in the management of craniopharyngioma: a 25-year experience and review of the literature. Int J Radiat Oncol Biol Phys 1999;44:255.

Hader WJ et al: Intratumoral therapy with bleomycin for cystic craniopharyngiomas in children. Pediatr Neurosurg 2000; 33:211.

Mainprize TG, Taylor MD, Rutka JR: Pediatric brain tumors: a contemporary prospectus. Clin Neurosurg 2000;47:259.

Maira G et al: Craniopharyngiomas of the third ventricle: trans-lamina terminalis approach. Neurosurgery 2000;47:857.

McDermott MW: Current treatment of meningiomas. Curr Opin Neurol 1996;9:409.

McElveen JR et al: A review of facial nerve outcome in 100 consecutive cases of acoustic tumor surgery. Laryngoscope 2000; 110:1667.

Prasad D, Steiner M, Steiner L: Gamma surgery for vestibular schwannoma. J Neurosurg 2000;92:745.

Rosenberg SI: Natural history of acoustic neuromas. Laryngoscope 2000;110:497.

■ TUMORS OF THE SPINAL CORD

Philip R. Weinstein, MD & Harold Rosegay, MD, PhD

The clinical diagnosis of spinal cord tumor should be considered when signs and symptoms localize an intraspinal lesion. These may consist of pain or numbness in a nerve root distribution, bilateral arm or leg weakness and numbness, Brown-Séquard's syndrome, a sensory level on the torso, or weakness and muscle atrophy with loss of the appropriate deep tendon reflexes at the level of the lesion. In cases in which long tract findings such as spasticity, hyperreflexia, and loss of proprioception predominate, a search for signs of segmental anterior or posterior horn cell loss may indicate the upper level of involvement. Horner's syndrome, when present in conjunction with other signs or symptoms of cord involvement, is helpful in localization. If, in addition, the history is one of progression, and if bladder or bowel function has been impaired, the suspicion of a mass lesion takes precedence over other possibilities. However, valuable time is lost if one expects and waits for the full picture, since decompensation of function begun by compression will accelerate because of the added effect of spinal cord ischemia. Intramedullary tumors may grow to large size while producing only mild sensory loss with sacral sparing, or localized weakness with mild long tract signs.

Certain spinal cord tumors occur in clinical settings that should increase the suspicion of their presence. For example, signs and symptoms of thoracic cord involvement in a middle-aged woman should raise the probability of meningioma. If there is a history of Recklinghausen's disease, one must consider neurofibroma, schwannoma, meningioma, ependymoma, and multiple tumors as likely possibilities. A mass in the posterior mediastinum seen on chest x-ray may have an intraspinal dumbbell extension of a neurofibroma. A patient with lymphoma or Hodgkin's disease who develops impairment of bladder function may have an otherwise asymptomatic extradural tumor implant at the level of the thoracic cord or conus. Cervico-occipital pain with weakness progressing downward on one side of the body and then upward on the other, with nystagmus and atrophy of the intrinsic muscles of the hands, suggests meningioma of the foramen magnum. Subarachnoid hemorrhage for which no intracranial cause can be found may be due to spinal cord tumor or arteriovenous malformation. The rare patient with papilledema or communicating hydrocephalus and elevated cerebrospinal fluid protein levels will have a thoracolumbar neoplasm. Kyphoscoliosis, pain, and weakness occurring in infancy and childhood should suggest the possibility of glioma or neuroblastoma. If the child is known to have an intracranial medulloblastoma or an ependymoblastoma, meningeal seeding may have taken place. A hairy mole or fat pad may be associated with a dermoid or lipomeningocele. Metastatic disease of the spine must always be kept in mind. Intercostal neuralgia may be the first sign of myeloma that has invaded the bone marrow and destroyed the pedicle adjacent to the affected root.

Imaging Studies

On plain x-rays of the spine, one may see the following changes consistent with tumor: destruction of bone or erosion and widening of the pedicles, scalloping of the posterior surfaces of the vertebral bodies, or enlargement of the intervertebral foramina. Calcification is sometimes seen with meningiomas. In general, destructive bony changes are due to metastatic tumor, whereas the more localized erosions are seen with neurofibroma, epidermoid tumor, and ependymoma. Neurofibroma has a predilection for the C1–2 interlaminar space and is shown by marked thinning of the posterior arches. If a thoracic neurofibroma is suspected, one should check for deviation of the mediastinal pleural reflection at the involved level, which is indicative of a dumbbell tumor. CT scans or MRI of the spine may differentiate between extramedullary tumors, syrinx, hemangioblastoma, and lipoma but not between astrocytoma or ependymoma. Myelography was once the definitive test, but MRI with gadolinium enhancement has superseded it as the examination of choice. Occasionally, angiography may provide information of diagnostic value (eg, in hemangioblastoma).

Tumors are distributed along the spinal axis as follows (in order of decreasing frequency): thoracic, lumbar, cervical, and sacral. About two-thirds of primary tumors are extramedullary-intradural and are benign (meningioma, neurofibroma, epidermoid), a fact that makes early diagnosis imperative in order to prevent irreversible loss of function. The common intramedullary tumors, for which treatment is less satisfactory, are astrocytoma, ependymoma, hemangioblastoma, and lipoma.

Treatment

An attempt should be made to completely excise all neurofibromas, schwannomas, and meningiomas with their respective attachments to spinal roots or dura; however, because some extend extradurally and beyond the spinal canal, this attempt may require facetectomy and extraspinal exposure by thoracotomy or a retroperitoneal abdominal approach. A dumbbell tumor protruding discretely through a thoracic intervertebral foramen into the posterior mediastinum should be removed through a curved paraspinal incision that will allow both laminectomy and costotransversectomy to be done. Intramedullary ependymomas and hemangioblastomas that can be demarcated from the surrounding spinal cord after myelotomy may be removed with microsurgical and microbipolar techniques. Infiltrating gliomas may be radically but subtotally resected and then treated with radiation therapy. Recurrence is to be expected and progression of paralysis is inevitable when the tumor is malignant. Laser microsurgery and ultrasonic aspiration are used in excision of intramedullary tumors such as ependymomas with excellent results. Intraoperative ultrasonography is very useful for localization of tumor and cyst. Syringo-pleural shunts are used when necessary to drain persistent syringomyelia caused by intramedullary tumors.

Metastatic tumors not associated with pathologic fracture causing cord compression by bone fragments may be treated with x-ray therapy, which is to be administered on an emergency basis if there is beginning loss of function and a pathologic diagnosis has previously been made. The indications for operation are as follows: (1) rapid progressive loss of function; (2) radioresistant tumors; (3) undiagnosed masses with the possibility of another diagnosis, such as abscess; and (4) recurrence or progression following radiation therapy. Radiation therapy may be used in conjunction with operative decompression. Radiation therapy alone should be used to relieve pain when spinal cord function is intact and there is no bony compression. Lesion-directed surgical approaches have improved the outcome of operation for metastatic disease. Thus, when a metastatic tumor lies anterior to the spinal cord and involves the vertebral body, it is to be approached by anterior vertebrectomy or wide posterolateral laminectomy to allow transpedicular removal of any anterior tumor. Not only compression but also vertebral column stabilization, in some cases with both anterior and posterior instrumentation extending over multiple levels, must also be done. Chemotherapy may be a useful adjunct to radiotherapy in the treatment of myeloma or lymphoma, including Hodgkin's disease.

Coleman RE: Skeletal complications of malignancy. Cancer 199780(8 Suppl):1588.

Houten JK et al: Intramedullary ependymomas: clinical presentation, surgical treatment strategies and prognosis. J Neuro-Oncol 200047:211.

Janjan NA: Radiotherapeutic management of spinal metastases. J Pain Symptom Manage 1996;11:47.

Koeller KK et al: Neoplasms of the spinal cord and filum terminale: radiologic-pathologic correlation. Radiographics 2000;20: 1721.

Newton HB et al: Spinal cord tumors: review of etiology, diagnosis, and multidisciplinary approach to treatment. Cancer Practice 1995;3:207.

■ TUMORS OF PERIPHERAL NERVES

Nicholas M. Barbaro, MD & Charles B. Wilson, MD, DSc, MSHA

 ESSENTIALS OF DIAGNOSIS

- *A mass along the course of a peripheral nerve.*
- *Evidence of motor or sensory dysfunction confined to a single peripheral nerve.*
- *Pain distributed along a single peripheral nerve.*
- *Magnetic resonance imaging (MRI) showing gadolinium-enhancing mass within a peripheral nerve.*

General Considerations

Peripheral nerve tumors may be removable or diffusely invasive. The most common of the former type is the nerve sheath tumor, variously called perineurial fibroblastoma, neurilemmoma, or schwannoma. These tumors may displace a major portion of the nerve to one side and often can be totally or almost totally excised. They are found in patients with neurofibromatosis more often than in the general population. Rarely, these tumors may become malignant, metastasizing to other portions of the body and invading surrounding tissues.

Schwannomas are typically benign tumors that arise from the supporting cells within a nerve. They usually arise from a single fascicle within a nerve, displacing the other fascicles. Symptoms occur when the tumor gets big enough to be felt through the skin or when pressure within the nerve causes pain, numbness, or weakness in the distribution of the parent nerve.

Neurofibromas are characterized by general neoplastic activity within the nerve sheath. A wide spectrum of connective tissue and endoneurial cells intermixed with axons is seen histologically. These diffuse growths usually cannot be excised without resecting a segment of the involved nerve; at times they may spread in a plexiform fashion along all of a nerve's branches. Neurofibromas are most often found in patients with neurofibromatosis.

Nerve sheath tumors tend to be less than 1 mm in diameter but may become quite large—eg, to involve as the entire sciatic nerve in the thigh. They may be excruciatingly painful even early in development or may become gigantic before being noted—especially, for example, when deep within an extremity or the abdomen. Growth activity is often associated with puberty.

Clinical Findings

The symptoms and signs are those of peripheral nerve dysfunction, irritative or paralytic. The nature and distribution of this dysfunction show that it is related to a specific nerve rather than tracts in the spinal cord or brain. Sensory disturbances or muscular atrophy may be noted. Nerve conduction tests and precise electromyography may be of assistance. MRI with gadolinium will image the lesions.

DIFFERENTIAL DIAGNOSIS

Peripheral neuropathies, including those that are the result of pressure (entrapment), may mimic peripheral nerve tumors, but a tumor that produces symptoms is usually large enough to be felt. Nerve tumors may occur anywhere along the course of the nerve, whereas entrapment occurs at characteristic locations. Generalized sensitivity along a nerve is more characteristic of neuritis than dysfunction caused by a primary nerve tumor.

Treatment & Prognosis

The operative approach to peripheral nerve tumors depends on the type of lesion. Schwannomas can almost always be removed with little permanent increase in the preoperative neurologic deficit. Typically, an operating microscope is used, and the lesion is separated from surrounding normal nerve fascicles. Complete resection is curative in these benign lesions. Amputation of the extremity may be necessary for an invasive malignant schwannoma unless it is so advanced that long-term survival is unlikely. Neurofibromas cannot usually be resected without loss of function in the parent nerve. For this reason, true neurofibromas should only be biopsied to ensure that they are not malignant and should be left in place unless the parent nerve can be sacrificed without producing significant neurologic deficit.

In patients with neurofibromatosis, the growths are often multiple, so only the tumors that cause clinical signs and symptoms (eg, pain or sensorimotor loss) should be removed. In this disease, tumors not causing dysfunction should be left alone unless cosmetic deformity is substantial or they are subject to repeated trauma or irritation.

Because most peripheral nerve tumors can be completely removed or are slowly growing lesions confined to a single nerve, the overall prognosis is good. However, moderate disability can be produced by unresectable lesions of major nerves. In addition, patients with neurofibromatosis may have multiple lesions, including those in the craniospinal axis, which can produce progressive and severe neurologic deficits. Malignant peripheral nerve tumors can be fatal if not treated aggressively in their early stages.

Artico M: Benign neural sheath tumours of major nerves: characteristics in 119 surgical cases. Acta Neurochir (Wien) 1997; 139:1108.

Hems TE; Burge PD; Wilson DJ: The role of magnetic resonance imaging in the management of peripheral nerve tumours. J Hand Surg (Br) 1997;22:57.

Vauthey JN; Woodruff JM; Brennan MF: Extremity malignant peripheral nerve sheath tumors (neurogenic sarcomas): a 10-year experience. Ann Surg Oncol 1995;2:126.

Wong WW et al: Malignant peripheral nerve sheath tumor: analysis of treatment outcome. Int J Radiat Oncol Biol Phys 1998; 42:351.

■ PITUITARY TUMORS

Charles B. Wilson, MD, DSc, MSHA

 ESSENTIALS OF DIAGNOSIS

- *Hypopituitarism, ie, hyposecretion of one or more pituitary tropic hormones.*
- *Syndrome of pituitary hypersecretion: acromegaly and gigantism.*
- *Cushing's disease, amenorrhea-galactorrhea.*
- *Visual impairment; typically, bitemporal hemianopia.*
- *Suprasellar expansion detected by MRI.*

General Considerations

In the past, pituitary adenomas were classified according to staining patterns seen with light microscopy. The three types—chromophobe, eosinophilic, and basophilic—did not correspond very closely with the clinical syndromes of pituitary hypersecretion. For example, chromophobe adenomas could produce hypopituitarism, Cushing's disease, acromegaly, and amenorrhea-galactorrhea. Subsequently, electronmicroscopic identification of typical secretory granules and immunocytologic demonstration of the specific hormones contained within secretory granules have been correlated with elevations of specific hormones in blood as determined by radioimmunoassay. Consequently, the term "chromophobe" is meaningless and has been dropped, and pituitary tumors should be classified as endocrine-active or endocrine-inactive.

Pituitary adenomas are classified by size: microadenomas are tumors with a diameter of less than 1 cm, whereas all larger tumors are macroadenomas.

Clinical Findings

Endocrine-active adenomas are the characteristic syndromes, and the larger tumors, by compressing the normal anterior pituitary, may cause a mixed endocrine picture of oversecretion accompanied by hypopituitarism. Microadenomas are discovered in patients with one of the pituitary hypersecretory syndromes; because secretion may not be proportionate to size, endocrine-active adenoma is diagnosed by endocrine testing and confirmed radiographically, primarily with MRI. The endocrinopathy of endocrine-inactive adenomas is pituitary hypofunction—GH, FSH, and LH secretion being affected early and TSH and ACTH late. Diabetes insipidus, a result of direct hypothalamic involvement, is rarely caused by pituitary tumors. Although pituitary adenomas may extend out of the sella to produce huge intracranial masses before affecting the function of suprasellar structures, typically the initial clinical manifestation of macroadenomas is visual impairment caused by the upward extension of the tumor (suprasellar extension) that compresses the optic nerves and chiasm. In 90% of patients with visual involvement, the pattern is some variation of bitemporal hemianopia.

Acromegaly and gigantism are readily recognized. Cushing's *syndrome* is caused by adrenal hypercortisolism; Cushing's *disease* is that form of hypercortisolism produced by an ACTH-secreting pituitary adenoma. Following bilateral adrenalectomy, the same pituitary adenoma produces Nelson's syndrome of unopposed ACTH hypersecretion.

Hyperprolactinemia is the most frequent cause of amenorrhea and galactorrhea, and most young women with this clinical presentation harbor a prolactin-secreting microadenoma. The tumor is less common in men but causes impotence and decreased libido when present.

Differential Diagnosis

For endocrine-active adenomas, the diagnosis is established by laboratory tests of pituitary function, including assessment of target organ responsiveness to available hypothalamic releasing factors. With the exception of some patients with Cushing's disease, MRI of the sella will confirm the diagnosis of an intrasellar mass.

Current MR imaging with coronal and sagittal views will identify all but the smallest (< 2 mm) intrasellar tumors and any extrasellar extensions of tumor. Other masses—eg, craniopharyngioma and giant aneurysms—can mimic endocrine-inactive pituitary adenomas, but MRI should differentiate these conditions from pituitary adenoma.

Cushing's syndrome (adrenal hypercortisolism) has several causes that can be established by appropriate studies. Hyperprolactinemia can result from administration of certain drugs (eg,, phenothiazines), and it may accompany other endocrine disorders such as hypothyroidism.

Treatment

Prolactin-secreting macroadenomas can be treated by transsphenoidal microsurgical removal; rarely, massive tumors require craniotomy. For microadenomas, microsurgical transsphenoidal removal achieves excellent results in patients desiring pregnancy. Nonsurgical therapy involves long-term administration of medication that in the majority of patients reduces or restores prolactin values to normal levels with variable reduction in volume of tumor. Medication-enabled pregnancy in patients with large tumors may be complicated by rapid tumor growth.

Acromegaly and Cushing's disease are treated initially by operation (transsphenoidal), with radiation therapy being used for tumors that cannot be removed completely. For patients not cured by surgery, acromegaly can be treated with somatostatin analogs and Cushing's disease by bilateral laparoscopic adrenalectomy. Nonsecreting (endocrine-inactive) tumors are treated by operation followed in many cases by radiation therapy to prevent regrowth.

Abosch A, et al: Transsphenoidal microsurgery for growth hormone-secreting pituitary adenomas: initial outcome and long-term results. J Clin Endocrinol Metab 1998;83:3411.

Freda PU et al: Long-term treatment of prolactin-secreting macroadenomas with pergolide. J Clin Endocrinol Metab 2000;85:8.

Kovacs K, Horvath E: *Atlas of Tumor Pathology,* Second Series, Fascicle 21. Armed Forces Institute of Pathology, 1986.

Littley MD et al: Hypopituitarism following external radiotherapy for pituitary tumours in adults. Q J Med 1989;70:145.

Mampalam TJ, Tyrrell JB, Wilson CB: Transsphenoidal microsurgery for Cushing's disease: a report of 216 cases. Ann Intern Med 1988;109:487.

Munari C et al: Long term results of stereotactic endocavitary beta irradiation of craniopharyngioma cysts. J Neurosurg Sci 1989;33:99.

Peck WW et al: High-resolution MR imaging of pituitary microadenomas at 1.5 T: experience with Cushing's disease. AJR Am J Roentgenol 1989;152:145.

Peillon F et al: Receptors and neurohormones in human pituitary adenomas. Horm Res 1989;31:13.

Pinzone JJ et al: Primary medical therapy of micro- and macroprolactinomas in men. J Clin Endocrinol Metab 2000;85:3053.

Rush SC, Newall J: Pituitary adenoma: the efficacy of radiotherapy as the sole treatment. Int J Radiat Oncol Biol Phys 1989; 17:165.

Samaan NA et al: Multiple endocrine syndrome type I. Clinical, laboratory findings, and management in five families. Cancer 1989;64:741.

Semple PL et al: Transsphenoidal surgery for Cushing's disease: outcome in patients with a normal magnetic resonance imaging scan. Neurosurgery 2000;46:553.

Tyrrell JB, et al: Transsphenoidal microsurgical therapy of prolactinomas: initial outcomes and long-term results. Neurosurgery 1999;44:254.

Wass JA et al: The treatment of acromegaly. Clin Endocrinol Metab 1986;15:683.

Wilson CB: Endocrine-inactive pituitary adenomas. Clin Neurosurg 1992;38:10.

Wilson CB: Role of surgery in the management of pituitary tumors. Neurosurg Clin North Am 1990;1:139.

■ PEDIATRIC NEUROSURGERY

Nalin Gupta, MD, PhD, & Warwick J. Peacock, MD

Most neurosurgical problems in infancy and childhood are due to one of four causes: congenital malformations, neoplasms, infections, and trauma. They represent a distinct group of disorders that require management tailored to the needs of the developing nervous system. Trauma and infections are discussed elsewhere in this chapter and will be discussed only briefly in reference to specific pediatric problems. Functional disorders such as spastic cerebral palsy and intractable epilepsy are also amenable to surgical treatment.

CONGENITAL MALFORMATIONS

Congenital malformations occur frequently in the nervous system and are exceeded only by prematurity as a cause of death in infants. In most cases, no specific cause can be demonstrated, though a number of teratogenic factors have been recognized: (1) maternal infections, eg, rubella, toxoplasmosis, cytomegalic inclusion disease, and syphilis; (2) drugs ingested by the mother during gestation, eg, thalidomide, LSD, methotrexate; (3) ionizing radiation; (4) maternal anesthesia; and (5) systemic disease, electrolyte imbalance, and dietary deficiencies. Although specific genes responsible for some congenital defects have been identified, it is reasonable to assume that the final phenotype results from a complex interplay of genetic predisposition and various intrauterine factors.

1. Malformations of the Skull or Vertebral Column

A spectrum of anomalies can result from either improper ossification of bony elements, or failed segmentation during early development. Children may be asymptomatic or profoundly disabled.

Craniosynostosis is defined as the premature closure or absence of one or more of the sutures that normally separate the individual bones of the skull (Table 38–6). The majority of these cases involve a single suture and are isolated. The incidence is 4:10,000 births. Sutural closure prevents radial and symmetric growth of the head and is manifest as a deformation of head shape with compensatory growth occurring parallel to the plane of the fused suture. Single-suture synostosis is rarely associated with abnormal neurologic function. When the process involves two or more sutures, growth and development of the brain can be affected, particularly during the first year of life when the brain triples its weight. Primary craniosynostosis must be differentiated from the secondary approximation and fusion of sutures in microcephaly and that which sometimes follows operative procedures on the skull or shunting for hydrocephalus. Premature closure of a specific suture results in a characteristic visual appearance.

Treatment consists of excision of the fused suture and sometimes reconstruction of the skull. Most procedures are performed between 3 months and 6 months of age, when the growing brain is still able to mold the relatively thin cranial vault into a "normal" shape.

Craniofacial syndromes such as Crouzon's and Apert's syndromes involve closure of several sutures, resulting in cranial vault and mid face abnormalities such as hyper- or hypotelorism, maxillary hypoplasia, and proptosis. Treatment may require multiple osteoplastic techniques at the skull base to achieve an acceptable result.

Chiari malformations are related by the presence of abnormalities of the posterior fossa and cerebellum. Chiari type 1 is characterized by a small posterior fossa and caudal displacement of the cerebellar tonsils through the foramen magnum and may be associated with hydrocephalus or syringomyelia (a central cavity in the spinal cord). Chiari type 2 is usually seen in patients with myelomeningocele. In addition to cerebellar herniation, there are other abnormalities such as kinking of the cervicomedullary junction, cortical malformations, and agenesis of the corpus callosum. Types 3 and 4 are rare.

Diastematomyelia is a bony spicule projecting through the middle of the spinal canal to divide the meninges and spinal cord into two compartments. It is usually accompanied by other skeletal anomalies and varying degrees of spinal cord dysfunction.

Basilar impression is the upward displacement of the cervical spine into the base of the skull. It results in reduced capacity of the posterior fossa and stenosis of the foramen magnum, leading to compression of the brain stem and spinal cord.

2. Incomplete Formation of the Neural Tube

Failure of the neuroectoderm to fuse in the midline during the third and fourth weeks of fetal life leads to secondary failure of formation of overlying mesoderm and ectoderm. These defects may be small and concealed or they may be exposed and involve large areas of the spinal cord, meninges, vertebral column, overlying muscles, and skin. The most frequently involved anatomic level is the lumbosacral area; the least frequently involved is the thoracic area (cervical myelomeningoceles are very rare).

Spina bifida occulta is a defect in the fusion of the spinous processes and lamina that is present in many children. It is asymptomatic and does not necessarily

Table 38–6. Types of craniosynostosis.

Suture	Cranial abnormality	Features	Frequency
Sagittal	Scaphocephaly	AP elongation, reduced biparietal distance	40–60%
Unilateral coronal	Anterior plagiocephaly	Recession of the forehead, elevation of the ipsilateral eye	20–30%
Bilateral coronal	Brachycephaly	"Tower-like" pointed head, reduced overall size, flattened forehead	10%
Metopic	Trigonocephaly	Pointed frontal bone, hypotelorism	5–10%
Lambdoid	Posterior plagiocephaly	Flattening of the occipital area, prominence of the contralateral frontal area	1–3%

require treatment. Cases that involve multiple levels and those associated with skin abnormalities (eg, hemangioma, patches of hair, dermal sinus, or subcutaneous lipoma) may produce neurologic dysfunction by tethering of the spinal cord. The clinical picture includes progressive weakness, scoliosis, gait instability, urinary or bowel difficulties, and sometimes pain. MRI is the diagnostic procedure of choice. In newborn infants, spinal ultrasound can assist in determining the position of the conus medullaris and associated spinal cord anomalies. Surgical correction of the tethered cord halts progression of symptoms in most patients and may improve neurologic and urologic function in up to 25% of patients.

Myelomeningocele (spina bifida aperta) (see Figure 38–14) is protrusion of nerve roots or cord elements along with the meninges. It occurs at least ten times more often than simple meningocele and always causes some degree of neurologic deficit. Findings range from mild weakness and slight sphincteric disturbance

to complete sensory and motor paralysis below the lesion and incontinence. Hydrocephalus is associated with at least 80% of lumbosacral myelomeningoceles; Chiari malformation type 2 is always present and may cause brain stem dysfunction.

Meningocele consists of herniation of the meninges through a spina bifida without abnormality of the spinal cord or nerve roots. Neurologic function is usually preserved in these patients.

Encephalocele with cranium bifidum is a much less common midline protrusion of the meninges through the skull. It is usually occipital or at the base of the nose. The extent of brain tissue within the encephalocele often determines the functional outcome.

Treatment

For all open spina bifida lesions, the fundamental surgical principle is reconstitution of the neural tube by layered closure of the dura, skin, and sometimes fascia, usu-

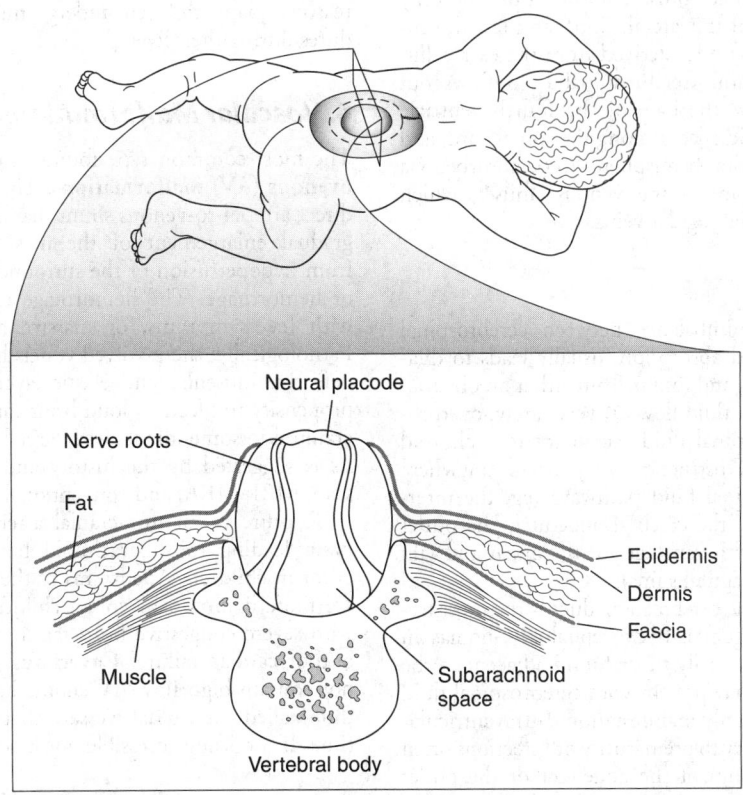

Figure 38–14. Diagrammatic representation of a myelomeningocele. The neural placode is superficial and not covered by any ectodermal or mesodermal elements. Laterally, the dermis fuses with the dura, which is then continuous with the thin lateral edge of the placode. The actual neural placode is usually easily visualized as the most central portion of the defect.

ally within a few days after birth. The goals of early repair are prevention of meningitis, preservation of neurologic function, and facilitation of nursing care. For lesions that are covered by normal skin, repair can be delayed for several months unless symptoms develop. Early recognition and treatment of hydrocephalus is essential.

A team approach is required to manage a broad range of orthopedic (spasticity, club feet, scoliosis), urologic (urinary reflux, neurogenic bladder, hydronephrosis), and rehabilitation (orthoses, therapy, special schooling) concerns. Entry into a normal school, completion of education, and physical independence are the ultimate goals. Urosepsis and shunt malfunction remain the primary causes of long-term morbidity and mortality. Repair of myelomeningoceles is being performed in utero, but the long-term benefits of this approach are unknown.

3. Disturbances of Cerebrospinal Fluid Circulation & Absorption

At least 50% of total cerebrospinal fluid is produced by the choroid plexus of the lateral, third, and fourth ventricles, with the remainder derived from the extracellular fluid of the brain. Cerebrospinal fluid flows out through foramina at the base of the fourth ventricle into the subarachnoid spaces, along the spinal cord, and finally over the cerebral hemispheres to be absorbed via the arachnoid villi into dural venous sinuses, which drain into the internal jugular veins.

Pathogenesis

Hydrocephalus, an imbalance between cerebrospinal fluid production and absorption, usually leads to dilation of the ventricles and results from either an obstruction to cerebrospinal fluid flow or, very rarely, overproduction of cerebrospinal fluid secondary to a choroid plexus papilloma. Obstruction may occur anywhere along the cerebrospinal fluid pathways (eg, the interventricular foramen, the cerebral aqueduct, the outlet foramina of the fourth ventricle, or the arachnoid villi associated with the sagittal sinus).

Obstruction of the cerebral aqueduct is the most frequent cause of congenital hydrocephalus. Gliomas in critical locations, especially those found adjacent to the cerebral aqueduct, may present with cerebrospinal fluid obstruction as their only manifestation. Intraventricular hemorrhage secondary to prematurity or infections often causes gliosis (scarring) of the aqueduct or the outlet foramina of the fourth ventricle, with similar results. Scarring (arachnoiditis) in the basal cisterns or over the cerebral convexities may result from meningitis, intracranial hemorrhage, meningeal carcinomatosis, or, rarely, tumors blocking the foramen magnum or basal cisterns.

Treatment

CT scans and other tests (eg, MRI flow studies, cerebrospinal fluid drainage, nuclear isotope studies, intracranial pressure monitoring) are used to determine the cause of hydrocephalus by identifying the site of cerebrospinal fluid flow obstruction. Although endoscopic third ventriculocisternostomy is successful in treating a subset of patients, thereby avoiding shunt insertion, most cases of hydrocephalus are treated by diverting cerebrospinal fluid to an alternative site. In the vast majority of cases, shunts are placed into the peritoneal cavity (VP shunt), right atrium (VA shunt), or pleural space (VPl shunt).

Within 3 years of insertion, about 40% of shunts will fail for a variety of reasons (eg, obstruction, infection, disconnection, perforation of a viscus). Eighty percent of shunt-related infections occur within 6 months after insertion, with the majority caused by staphylococcal species. A shunt infection requires removal of the shunt, treatment with antibiotics, and replacement with a sterile shunt system. For these reasons, many children undergo multiple shunt procedures during their lives.

4. Vascular Malformations

The most common type found in children are **arteriovenous (AV) malformations.** These lesions contain a direct arterial-to-venous shunt that causes symptoms by gradual enlargement of the mass, cerebral ischemia from hypoperfusion of the surrounding brain, seizures, or hemorrhage. The hemorrhage can be either small, with few symptoms, or massive and at times fatal. Pathologically, the involved vessels have thin walls with defective muscular and elastic layers and thus have a propensity to bleed. A loud bruit can be heard over the cranium in some infants with large lesions. The diagnosis is suggested by the history and confirmed by CT scan, MRI, MRA, and conventional angiography.

Rupture of an intracranial arterial **saccular aneurysm** leading to subarachnoid hemorrhage is a rare event in children. Aneurysms of the great cerebral vein are more common in young children and can present with severe congestive heart failure as a result of high-output cardiac failure. **Cavernous malformations** do not contain high flow AV shunts but are composed of thin-walled sinusoidal vessels that can rebleed over time. If surgically accessible, most are removed.

Treatment

Treatment of AV malformations varies depending on the symptoms, the age and condition of the patient, and the size and location of the malformation. Interventional neuroradiologic procedures can be used to reduce the size of AV malformations and thus allow safer excision. Total excision is preferred but should not be attempted if a severe neurologic deficit is likely. Deep or residual lesions can be treated using tightly collimated radiation (gamma knife or LINAC), which usually results in obliteration of the lesion over months.

NEOPLASMS

Neoplasms of the central nervous system are the most common solid tumors of childhood (3.3:100,000), exceeded in frequency only by lymphoma and leukemia. They differ from those found in adults by their sites of origin and histologic type. Twenty percent of pediatric nervous system tumors are located in the spinal cord and 80% in the brain. Of the latter, 50% arise in the posterior fossa and 50% in the supratentorial compartment (Table 38–7). Meningiomas, pituitary tumors, and metastatic tumors—among the more common adult tumors—are rare in children.

1. Brain Tumors

Brain tumors produce symptoms by increasing intracranial pressure (through occupying space or obstructing cerebrospinal fluid pathways) or by directly invading or compressing neural tissues. In infants and children, the symptoms and signs of increased intracranial pressure are vomiting, headache, papilledema, mental dysfunction, personality changes, and cranial nerve palsy. Symptoms and signs of direct brain involvement are ataxia, incoordination, nystagmus, weakness of extremities, seizures, and head tilt to the side of the lesion (seen with cerebellar hemisphere lesions).

For most common brain tumors (medulloblastoma, ependymoma, and astrocytoma), the extent of surgical resection is a positive predictive factor for survival. For other less frequently encountered tumors (hemangioblastoma, dermoid cyst, craniopharyngioma, or unilateral optic nerve glioma), gross total removal is curative. Therefore, for most patients a definitive surgical procedure is the initial step. For unresectable tumors, cerebrospinal fluid pathways are reopened or bypassed and radiation therapy or chemotherapy is given. Radiation is avoided in children under 3 years of age due to sequelae such as cognitive decline, visual loss, endocrine dysfunction, and second malignancies. A current trend is the use of intensive chemotherapy to delay radiation treatment as long as possible.

Astrocytomas

Astrocytomas (Figure 38–15) are the most common primary brain tumor in children and fortunately are either benign or low-grade by histology. Astrocytomas arising in the cerebellar hemispheres (about 15% of all brain tumors) are almost always benign and can be cured by gross total resection. Approximately 10% of all tumors are astrocytomas arising from the hypothalamus or optic apparatus. This location prevents radical resection. Patients with neurofibromatosis 1 are predisposed to the development of optic pathway gliomas. Some astrocytomas are malignant, and these tumors—particularly those that arise in the brain stem—are infiltrative by nature and have a very poor prognosis regardless of treatment.

Medulloblastoma

This tumor is composed of small, poorly differentiated cells that are identical to those found with pineoblastoma, Ewing's sarcoma, and other primitive tumors. Some pathologists group these tumors together as **primitive neuroectodermal tumors (PNETs).** Medulloblastomas are tumors of children and young adults,

Table 38–7. Types of central nervous system tumors in children and their location.

Cell Type	Incidence	Supratentorial	Infratentorial
Astrocytoma	40%	Common, especially suprasellar	Cerebellar hemisphere
Primitive neuroectodermal tumor	20%	Rare	Midline cerebellum (medulloblastoma)
Ependymoma	10%	Rare	Fourth ventricle
Craniopharyngioma	5%	Suprasellar	Rare
Brain stem glioma	5%	N/A	Pons
Neuronal tumors	3%	Cause seizures	Rare
Dermoid tumors	3%	Rare	Rare
Other	10%		

Figure 38–15. A 2-year-old child presented with headaches and vomiting. Post-gadolinium MR images demonstrate a large hypothalamic astrocytoma filling the third ventricle (sagittal plane on left) and leading to obstruction of cerebrospinal fluid flow and marked enlargement of the lateral ventricles (axial plane on right).

with the majority arising in the posterior fossa. Gross total excision followed by radiation carries the best long-term prognosis. High-risk patients include those whose have residual tumor after surgery, central nervous system spread at diagnosis, and age less than 3 years. For patients without these features, the 5-year survival rate is 60–70%.

Craniopharyngiomas

These histologically benign tumors arise in the suprasellar area and are composed of epithelial tissue with a central cystic area containing desquamated material. Their proximity to vital structures in the suprasellar area makes their management a formidable challenge. Visual, endocrine, and neurologic complications are commonly encountered following either surgery or adjunctive treatment.

2. Spinal Cord Tumors

Spinal cord tumors are uncommon. The clinical presentation is insidious, with gradual progression of symptoms such as back pain, leg weakness, gait instability, torticollis, or bowel and bladder dysfunction. Tumors are classified according to the site of origin. Intramedullary tumors include gliomas such as astrocytomas and ependymomas and undifferentiated tu-

mors such as medulloblastomas. The congenital group (eg, dermoids, teratomas, and neurofibromas) are usually intradural but not within the spinal cord. Extradural tumors are generally metastatic (ie, neuroblastomas and lymphosarcoma) and cause spinal cord compression.

Diagnostic evaluation in the current era requires a detailed contrast MRI study of the spine. Other studies are of limited value. Depending upon the nature of the lesion, the surgical goal is total removal, though in certain cases only a biopsy is possible. For these tumors, radiation therapy or chemotherapy (or both) is the treatment of choice.

TRAUMA

1. Head Injuries

Head injury is the commonest cause of death and disability in children. In general, management follows the same principles as are applicable in adult trauma patients. A few injuries are seen more commonly in children. **Nonaccidental trauma** has a number of synonyms (eg, shaken baby syndrome) and represents a spectrum of injuries including intracranial hemorrhage or contusion, retinal hemorrhage, and extremity fractures. Often there is no relevant history or at best a vague history. Most jurisdictions have legal requirements for reporting these injuries, if suspected, to the appropriate authorities. **Greenstick skull** fractures occur in infants when the skull is pushed inward without fragmenting. These fractures can usually be elevated by leverage through a small burr hole.

2. Spine Injuries

A child's spine develops the biomechanical features of the adult spine by the early teen years. Prior to this, the relatively large size of the head with respect to the body, the immaturity of ligamentous structures, and the orientation of the facet joints predisposes children to cervical spine injures and to C1–C2 injuries in particular. **Spinal cord injury without radiologic abnormality** is the syndrome of a neurologically apparent spinal cord injury in the absence of a detectable vertebral column injury. These injuries are often delayed in onset and are presumed to be caused by hypermobility of the spine or a delayed ischemic event.

FUNCTIONAL DISORDERS

1. Spastic Cerebral Palsy

Extreme prematurity is often the prelude to the later development of spastic cerebral palsy. Spasticity is due to loss of descending inhibition on the spinal reflex arc. Selective posterior rhizotomy has proved to be a safe and effective method of reducing the muscular hypertonicity that interferes with the acquisition of motor skills in the developing child. By dividing selected posterior spinal rootlets, excitatory influence on the anterior horn cells is reduced, leading to improved muscle tone and motor function and normalization of gait patterns. More recently, implantation of a constant infusion baclofen pump has been found to be helpful in some children with spastic cerebral palsy.

2. Surgery for Intractable Seizures in Childhood

Whereas epilepsy surgery in adults is mainly limited to temporal lobectomy, a variety of procedures are extremely helpful in controlling intractable seizures in children. The pathologic basis of seizures and the seizure types found in children differ from those in adults. Resective procedures such as hemispherectomy, lobectomy, and focal resection are often helpful, but when resection is not feasible disconnective surgery is an option. Division of the corpus callosum may eliminate drop attacks, and multiple subpial resections can be used in a seizure focus which is also the site of some important cortical function such as speech or movement. In children with intractable seizures where nei-

ther resection nor disconnection is possible, implantation of a vagus nerve stimulator is useful in significantly reducing seizure frequency.

Botto LD et al: Neural-tube defects. N Engl J Med 1999;341: 1509.

Bruner JP et al: Survival rates in patients with primary malignant brain tumors stratified by patient age and tumor histologic type: an analysis based on Surveillance, Epidemiology, and End Results (SEER) data, 1973–1991. J Neurosurg 1998; 88:10.

Lowe LH, Reed GW: Fetal surgery for myelomeningocele and the incidence of shunt-dependent hydrocephalus. JAMA 1999; 282:1819.

Pollack IF: Pediatric brain tumors. Semin Surg Oncol 1999;16:73.

Rankin J et al: The changing prevalence of neural tube defects: a population-based study in the north of England, 1984–96. Paediatr Perinat Epidemiol 2000;14:104.

■ INTRACRANIAL ANEURYSMS

Philip V. Theodosopolous, MD, &
Michael T. Lawton, MD

 ESSENTIALS OF DIAGNOSIS

- *Clinical symptoms or signs of aneurysm rupture: sudden, severe headache with associated stiff neck, nausea and vomiting, impaired consciousness, seizures, or coma.*

- *Clinical symptoms or signs of an expanding intracranial mass: progressive oculomotor nerve palsy, visual field cut, lower cranial nerve dysfunction, brain stem deficits, or hydrocephalus.*

- *Radiographic evidence of subarachnoid hemorrhage on CT scan (ruptured aneurysms) or the aneurysm itself on CT scan or MRI (unruptured aneurysms). In either case, four-vessel cerebral angiography is needed to confirm the diagnosis and elucidate aneurysm anatomy.*

General Considerations

An aneurysm is a saccular dilation of an artery that typically occurs at a branch point or curve in the artery's course and generally points in the direction of blood flow. Usual aneurysm morphology consists of a neck (where the aneurysm originates from the parent artery), the body or fundus, and the dome. Small perforating branches that supply adjacent brain arise from the neck at some aneurysm sites (anterior communicating artery, internal carotid artery [ICA] bifurcation, and basilar apex). Aneurysms enlarge and rupture at the dome, where walls are thinnest and there is frequently a daughter sac or lobe. Saccular aneurysms are thought to be acquired degenerative defects that develop in response to relentless hemodynamic stress. However, defects in the media or internal elastic lamina may be genetically or congenitally influenced.

Aneurysms are named by their associated branch artery or, when not associated with a discrete branch, by their anatomic location. Aneurysms in the anterior circulation—in order from proximal to distal—include petrous ICA, cavernous ICA, clinoidal ICA, ophthalmic artery (OphA), superior hypophysial artery (SHA), Posterior communicating artery (PCoA), anterior choroidal artery (AChA), ICA bifurcation, anterior communicating artery (ACoA), pericallosal artery, and middle cerebral artery (MCA) aneurysms. Aneurysms in the posterior circulation, in anatomic order from proximal to distal, include vertebral artery (VA), posterior inferior cerebellar artery (PICA), vertebrobasilar junction (VBJ), anterior inferior cerebellar artery (AICA), superior cerebellar artery (SCA), basilar tip, and posterior cerebral artery (PCA) aneurysms. The most common aneurysms are ACoA, PCoA, MCA, and basilar tip aneurysms.

The prevalence rate of intracranial saccular aneurysms is between 0.1% and 9%, with rates around 0.5–1% in angiographic series and around 1–6% in autopsy studies. Approximately 25% of patients have multiple aneurysms. Intracranial arteries lie in the subarachnoid space between the pia and arachnoid layers, a space filled with cerebrospinal fluid and compartmentalized into interconnecting cisterns. Consequently, aneurysms also lie in the subarachnoid space (except for petrous, cavernous, and clinoidal ICA aneurysms), and ruptured aneurysms produce subarachnoid hemorrhage (SAH). In the USA, the annual incidence of SAH is 11 per 100,000, with an estimated 30,000 new cases each year. It accounts for 5–10% of all strokes, afflicts women more than men, and blacks more than whites. SAH occurs most commonly in patients between the ages of 40 and 60 years. Aneurysm rupture is a potentially devastating event. The 30-day mortality rate for SAH is around 45%. Half of these patients die before arriving at a hospital from the effects of the initial hemorrhage, and many of the remainder die later from rebleeding or the effects of vasospasm. Survivors experience neurologic deficits in about 30% of cases.

While saccular aneurysms are the most common type, other nonsaccular aneurysms include fusiform (atherosclerotic), dissecting, traumatic, infectious, and neoplastic aneurysms. Fusiform aneurysms are tortuous, elongated, dilated arteries with separate inflow and outflow, most commonly seen in elderly patients with generalized atherosclerosis. Traumatic aneurysms are the result of direct arterial injury, with rupture of all three arterial layers (intima, media, and adventitia) and fibrous organization of the surrounding hematoma. In contrast, dissecting aneurysms result from tears through—but no deeper than—intima and internal elastic lamina. Infectious and neoplastic aneurysms develop from circulation of infectious material or tumor cells, often from a focus within the heart (eg, bacterial endocarditis or atrial myxoma). Infectious emboli lodge in small distal cerebral arteries and occlude flow, after which intense inflammation in the adventitia and media destroys the integrity of the wall and weakens it. Neoplastic aneurysms have a similar pathogenesis except that arterial invasion is directly from tumor cells. The resulting aneurysms are typically fusiform, eccentric, and at distal sites.

Clinical Findings

A. Symptoms and Signs

Most aneurysms present with rupture. The classic presentation is a sudden, unusually severe headache that may be associated with nausea, vomiting, painful nuchal rigidity, and photophobia. The critical features that distinguish this headache from other headaches are its instantaneous onset and its severity. When asked to evaluate severity on a scale from 1 to 10, patients typically respond with a number off the scale. They describe their headaches as "the worst headache of my life" and can remember vivid details of events surrounding its onset. These symptoms are characteristic of a "sentinel hemorrhage," a small contained leak from the aneurysm without frank rupture. Misdiagnosis of a sentinel hemorrhage can be catastrophic because patients have the highest risk of rehemorrhage in the following 24 hours. An estimated 60% of SAH patients who seek medical attention are misdiagnosed and for that reason have worse outcomes than those who are properly diagnosed.

More severe hemorrhages produce seizures, neurologic deficits, impaired consciousness, and death. These more devastating presentations are often due to intraparenchymal or intraventricular extension of the hemorrhage or sustained elevation of intracranial pressure (ICP). Several grading scales are used to evaluate the severity of hemorrhage, providing a "shorthand" description of a patient's clinical condition and also some guidance in treatment decisions and prognosis. The Hunt-Hess Scale is the most common one (Table 38–8), but others include the Glasgow Coma Scale (GCS) and the World Federation of Neurological Surgeons (WFNS) Scale.

Table 38–8. Classification scales for subarachnoid hemorrhage.

A. Hunt-Hess Scale[1]

Grade	Criteria
I	Asymptomatic, or minimal headache, nuchal rigidity
II	Moderate to severe headache, no neurologic deficit except for cranial nerve palsy
III	Drowsiness, confusion, mild focal deficit
IV	Stupor, moderate to severe hemiparesis, early decerebrate posturing
V	Deep coma, decerebrate posturing, moribund

B. Glasgow Coma Scale

Points	Eye Opening	Verbal	Motor
6			Obeys commands
5		Oriented	Localizes pain
4	Spontaneous	Confused	Withdraws to pain
3	To voice	Inappropriate	Flexes (decorticate)
2	To pain	Incomprehensible	Extends (decerebrate)
1	None	None	None

C. World Federation of Neurological Surgeons Scale

Grade	Glasgow Coma Scale	Motor Deficit
I	15	None
II	13–14	None
III	13–14	Present
IV	7–12	Any
V	3–6	Any

D. Fisher Scale

Grade	Subarachnoid Blood
I	No blood detected
II	Diffuse, < 1 mm thick
III	Localized clot or thick layer, > 1 mm thick
IV	Diffuse or none, with intracerebral or intraventricular blood

[1] Reproduced, with permission, from Hunt WE, Hess RM: Surgical repair as related to time of intervention in the repair of intracranial aneurysms. J Neurosurg 1968;28:14.

Unruptured aneurysms are typically diagnosed incidentally during the evaluation of unrelated problems such as headaches or other neurologic symptoms. Still, unruptured aneurysms can present with symptoms related to mass effect or cerebral ischemia. The cranial nerve most frequently involved is the oculomotor nerve, which runs parallel to the posterior communicating artery and can be compressed by PCoA and basilar apex aneurysms. A patient presenting with a new oculomotor palsy (unilateral dilated pupil with deviation of the eye downward and laterally) should be considered to have an aneurysm until proved otherwise. With PCoA aneurysms, the dilated pupil usually precedes the diplopia because of the greater sensitivity and peripheral location of the parasympathetic fibers within the nerve. Cavernous ICA aneurysms may also present with oculomotor palsy but in addition may involve the trochlear, abducens, and trigeminal nerves. These patients have an immobile eye, retro-orbital pain, and facial numbness or dysesthesias. AChA aneurysms rarely cause oculomotor deficits but can impinge on the mesial temporal lobe to produce epilepsy or can compress the optic tract. ICA bifurcation aneurysms can also compress the optic tract and, when giant, the internal capsule to produce a contralateral hemiparesis.

Ophthalmic artery aneurysms lie under the optic nerve, and their growth to giant sizes (≥ 25 mm) causes progressive visual field loss, initially a unilateral inferior nasal field defect that may enlarge to involve the entire ipsilateral nasal field and the superior temporal loss in the contralateral eye (junctional scotoma). SHA aneurysms project medially towards the sella and produce bitemporal hemianopsias similar to those associated with pituitary tumors.

Large or giant basilar aneurysms can cause pressure on the midbrain, causing a contralateral hemiparesis from compression of the cerebral peduncle or hydrocephalus from occlusion of the cerebral aqueduct. The oculomotor deficits from basilar aneurysms tend to spare the pupil and cause ipsilateral ptosis and weakness of upgaze. Large basilar trunk, vertebrobasilar, and vertebral artery aneurysms can compress lower cranial nerves or nuclei with corresponding dysphasia, dysarthria, hoarseness, gait instability, and incoordination.

Giant aneurysms with intraluminal thrombus can present with ischemic symptoms if clot from the aneurysm embolizes downstream. This is particularly true with ICA and MCA aneurysms, manifesting with symptoms of aphasia and contralateral motor and sensory deficits. Ischemic symptoms account for 5–25% of symptoms from unruptured aneurysms.

B. IMAGING STUDIES

The diagnosis of SAH requires the confirmation of blood in the subarachnoid space, which can be accomplished best with CT scan. Blood is easily seen on noncontrast CT scan, with a sensitivity of greater than 95%. In addition, the location of blood provides clues to the aneurysm location and identifies associated intracerebral and intraventricular hemorrhage. Hydrocephalus is a common finding in these patients because subarachnoid blood interferes with the normal circulation and reabsorption of cerebrospinal fluid. Often this associated hydrocephalus is more responsible for a patient's depressed level of consciousness than the hemorrhage itself and is reversible with ventriculostomy.

Ultimately, the diagnosis of an intracranial aneurysm depends on its identification with catheter angiography. A complete angiogram includes injections of all four major intracranial arteries (both ICAs and both VAs), filmed in two orthogonal views (anteroposterior and lateral). Additional views of the aneurysm are often needed to fully visualize its anatomy. Pre- and postinjection images are digitally subtracted to visualize just the vascular structures, removing shadows cast by the skull, skull base, and overlying opacities. These digital subtraction angiograms provide detailed information about the aneurysm location, anatomy, hemodynamics, other aneurysms, and collateral circulation. It should be remembered that angiographic images show the internal anatomy of an aneurysm, which may be much smaller than the external diameter of the aneurysm if it is filled with thrombus or coil material or thickened with calcium or atherosclerotic changes.

Catheter angiography has its disadvantages, namely, it is invasive, time-consuming, costly, and associated with increased risks (dissection, embolization, aneurysm rupture, and groin hematomas). Still, it is the most definitive test for the diagnosis of aneurysms. Angiograms generated with MR or CT data (MRA and CTA, respectively) are newer imaging modalities that currently do not provide all the information that catheter angiography does. Both CTA and MRA are noninvasive and easier to obtain. CTA results are available quickly and may play a role in unstable patients with ruptured aneurysms that need to get to the operating room right away. MRA is slower and lacks the resolution of CTA or conventional angiography, missing small aneurysms less than 3 mm in diameter. However, MRI or MRA is becoming a common method of detecting unruptured aneurysms in patients with other neurologic issues that have to be dealt with.

C. LABORATORY FINDINGS

Lumbar puncture is the only laboratory study that needs to be considered in the evaluation of an aneurysm patient. It is used in those cases where the patient's history is strongly suggestive of subarachnoid hemorrhage but the CT scan is normal. There are two ex-

planations for this inconsistency. The first explanation is a sentinel hemorrhage that has leaked so little blood that it is not radiographically apparent. In this case, cerebrospinal fluid may be blood-tinged and will not clear in successive tubes. The second explanation is a delayed CT scan performed days after the subarachnoid hemorrhage. A delay in seeking medical attention or in ordering the CT scan allows subarachnoid blood to disperse, making it difficult to detect on the imaging study. In this case, cerebrospinal fluid will be xanthochromic, indicating that blood has been present for days and is being metabolized. If the fluid from a lumbar puncture is positive for new or old blood, further evaluation with an angiogram is indicated. It should be noted that so-called "traumatic taps" yield fluid that initially is bloody but clears in successive tubes. This finding should not be mistaken for true SAH.

Treatment

A. RATIONALE

Once an aneurysm has been diagnosed, a decision needs to be made about treatment. The primary cause of death and disability from aneurysms is the brain injury produced by the initial hemorrhage, and there is no treatment that can reverse it. Existing treatments are aimed instead at preventing the initial rupture or rerupture and reversing the effects of SAH, eg, vasospasm. There is little controversy about the need to treat ruptured aneurysms because of their high risk of rerupture (4% in the first 24 hours and 20% by the first 2 weeks after the initial hemorrhage). Furthermore, the mortality rate associated with rebleeding is 40%. Therefore, treatment is undertaken quickly after diagnosis, usually within 72 hours of the initial bleed. The only treatment controversy arises in poor-grade patients (Hunt-Hess grades IV and V), since these patients have a poor prognosis to begin with and aggressive management will yield good outcomes in only 25–40%. Patients with minimal neurologic function, uncontrollable ICP, or who are moribund are managed expectantly. Still, it is difficult to predict outcome, and an aggressive treatment policy is generally more prudent. In addition to protecting against rerupture, early treatment of ruptured aneurysms enables aggressive postoperative management of delayed vasospasm with induced hypertension.

The treatment of unruptured aneurysms is more controversial because of the difficulty of accurately determining the risks of rupture and the risks of treatment. The annual risk of aneurysm rupture is between 0.05% and 2%. Factors that contribute to rupture risk are the size and location, the presence of another aneurysm that has ruptured, and possibly hypertension and smoking. While there is no critical size or cutoff value, there are prospective data showing increased rupture risk in aneurysms 10 mm or more in diameter. The cumulative natural history risk of an aneurysm is determined by estimating their life expectancy in years and extrapolating the annual rupture risk over this interval. Therefore, a patient's age and general health impact the treatment decision. In making a choice between treating an aneurysm or observing it, one must compare this natural history risk with the treatment risk. Morbidity and mortality rates associated with surgery for unruptured aneurysms vary from 4–15% and 0–4%, respectively. Many factors influence surgical outcome, including aneurysm size, location, and morphology; patient age, symptoms, and medical condition; and the experience of the surgical team and hospital staff. Weighing these factors together, treatment is generally recommended for patients with large or symptomatic aneurysms or another previously ruptured aneurysm. Treatment is favored in young patients with long life expectancies, a family history of aneurysm rupture, multiple aneurysms, or documented growth. Conservative management is favored in older patients, those with small aneurysms and short life expectancies, or severe comorbid medical conditions. Ultimately, patient preferences will determine the final decision with unruptured aneurysms.

B. INITIAL MANAGEMENT OF SAH

After a ruptured aneurysm is diagnosed, the aneurysm is secured as quickly as possible. In the meantime, efforts are made to stabilize the patient and minimize the risk of rerupture. Most important is blood pressure control. Rebleeding is caused by absolute elevations in blood pressure and also rapid variations. Blood pressure should be carefully monitored with invasive arterial lines in an ICU setting where intravenous agents or drips can be administered. Hydrocephalus is present in approximately one-fourth of SAH patients and resolves with the insertion of a ventriculostomy. External ventricular drainage can improve the clinical status of patients dramatically and is recommended in all obtunded or comatose patients. In addition, ventriculostomy allows ICP to be transduced and can guide preoperative management of increased pressures. In poor-grade patients, intubation and mechanical ventilation is usually needed to protect the airway and sometimes to hyperventilate the patient for ICP management. Other comfort measures such as bed rest, sedation, and analgesics help minimize agitation that might precipitate rerupture. Seizures can precipitate rerupture, and anticonvulsants are given in the immediate post-SAH period.

C. SURGICAL MANAGEMENT

Clipping of the aneurysm neck effectively closes the aneurysm and keeps blood from flowing into it. The clip application is done under direct visualization under an operating microscope, allowing preservation of flow in the parent and perforating arteries around its base. Once clipped, an aneurysm can be deflated or opened to removed blood and thrombus that might be compressing neural structures. Blood in the subarachnoid spaces can also be removed directly or diluted with irrigation, which may have some beneficial effects on subsequent vasospasm. Microsurgical clipping provides an immediate, durable cure for aneurysms. The recurrence rate after clipping is less than 1%, and after an immediate postoperative angiogram no follow-up imaging is required.

Surgical clipping requires exposure of the aneurysm. There are many surgical approaches for aneurysms, but the most common is the pterional or frontotemporal craniotomy. It provides direct exposure of the internal carotid artery from its entry into the subarachnoid space to its terminus, working in the space between the frontal and temporal lobes. Extensive removal of bone from the skull base (pterion, sphenoid ridge, and orbital roof) as well as opening the lateral cerebral sulcus to further separate the frontal and temporal lobes, creates ample room to access all ICA, ACoA, MCA, and basilar apex aneurysms. Additional exposure can be gained by removing the orbital rim with the orbitozygomatic approach, commonly used for giant anterior circulation aneurysms and basilar apex aneurysms. Posterior circulation aneurysms are accessed through the far-lateral approach (PICA aneurysms), one of the transpetrosal approaches (VBJ, AICA, and midbasilar artery aneurysms), or a combined transpetrosal-subtemporal approach that communicates the regions above and below the tentorium in front of the sigmoid sinus.

The vast majority of aneurysms (> 95%) can be treated with direct surgical clipping. However, aneurysms that are giant in size, fusiform in shape, or lacking a defined neck may require alternative techniques such as trapping or proximal occlusion. These techniques can be performed safely if trial arterial occlusion with a balloon-tipped catheter is tolerated by the patient without ischemic deficits. Hypotensive challenge or cerebral blood flow studies increase the accuracy of balloon test occlusion (BTO). Bypass procedures are indicated in those patients who do not tolerate their BTO, and a variety of bypasses are available to meet the flow demands of the involved vascular territory. The superficial temporal artery (STA) is a commonly used donor artery that can revascularize the middle cerebral artery territory. Saphenous vein grafts can also be used to bypass aneurysms along the ICA as it travels through the skull base and cavernous sinus, providing flows equal to the native ICA. Intracranial arteries such as the distal MCA, ACA, or PICA can be used as donor arteries to revascularize adjacent arteries with proximal aneurysms. Wrapping an aneurysm with cotton is another surgical alternative used as a last resort, externally reinforcing the walls with a material that elicits an inflammatory reaction to promote scarring and thickening of the aneurysm.

D. Endovascular Management

Endosaccular occlusion of intracranial aneurysms has become an acceptable alternative to microsurgical clipping during the past decade. This technique is performed using electrolytically detachable Guglielmi coils (GDC) deployed through transfemoral intra-aneurysmal catheters and angiographic visualization. In general, aneurysm coiling appears to have lower morbidity and mortality rates than surgery but higher rates of incomplete obliteration and higher rates of recurrence, making its long-term efficacy still unproved. Complications from endovascular coiling are different from those associated with surgery and include arterial dissection, intraoperative aneurysm rupture, parent artery occlusion, distal embolization, and groin hematomas. Although overall complication rates are around 8%, permanent neurologic morbidity is observed in around 4%. Mortality rates are up to 2%. The rates of complete aneurysm occlusion vary according to aneurysm size and morphology and range between 35% and 80%. Consequently, incompletely coiled aneurysms may not be protected from rehemorrhage risk, and new hemorrhages in patients treated with coils have been reported to be around 3–4%. Furthermore, endosaccular coils remain exposed to hemodynamic forces that can shift or compact the coils or promote growth of the aneurysm around the coils. Aneurysm recurrence after coiling has been reported in 5–45% of cases. Therefore, surveillance angiography is required and recurrences can pose complicated treatment issues.

Currently in North America, endovascular coils are used as a primary treatment for elderly patients, those considered to have high surgical risk, and those who are medically unsuitable for surgery. The minimally invasive appeal of this treatment is increasing patient interest and demand. In addition, new deployment techniques that use balloons to protect the parent artery from coil herniation and new devices such as three-dimensional coils and stents make aneurysms with unfavorable anatomy treatable with endovascular methods. For example, stent-supported coil embolization lays a stent across a wide aneurysm neck and deploys coils through the interstices of the stent. Endovascular techniques have become an integral part of multi-

modality therapy for aneurysms and will be increasingly utilized in the future.

E. Vasospasm

Vasospasm is the narrowing of cerebral arteries from smooth muscle cell contraction in the vessel walls, leading to diminished cerebral perfusion, ischemia, and infarction. Vasospasm typically occurs during a time period 4–14 days after SAH and resolves spontaneously thereafter. The pathogenesis is unclear but is related to the amount and distribution of blood in the subarachnoid space. The Fisher Grading Scale is a useful predictor of a patient's likelihood of developing vasospasm. Approximately 70% of patients experience some degree of vasospasm, with 20–30% developing ischemic symptoms. The mortality from vasospasm alone has been estimated between to be 5% and 15%, and the neurologic morbidity has been estimated at around 6%.

Patients at risk of developing vasospasm are monitored closely in an ICU. All patients are given nimodipine, a calcium channel blocker that inhibits vascular smooth muscle cell contraction and platelet aggregation. It is started within 4 days of SAH and continued for 21 days, regardless of admission grade, at a dose of 60 mg every 4 hours. Vasospasm is detected with angiography, transcranial Doppler ultrasonography (TCD), or changes in the neurologic examination. Angiography is the optimal diagnostic study but is limited by its invasiveness. TCD measures velocity of blood flow in cerebral arteries, which increases as arteries narrow with vasospasm. Therefore, measuring TCD velocities indirectly monitors vasospasm. TCD is noninvasive and can be done repeatedly to detect trends. Rising TCD velocities guide the timing of more aggressive measures, like hypertensive therapy and angioplasty.

The mainstay of medical management is hypervolemia, hypertension, and hemodilution (HHH therapy). Volume expansion is achieved with packed red blood cells, albumin solution, or hypertonic saline solution. Invasive monitoring with either a central venous pressure line or a pulmonary artery catheter is required to guide fluid management. Volume expansion to central venous pressures greater than 8 mm Hg or diastolic pulmonary artery pressures of greater than 14 mm Hg is usually enough to dilute the hematocrit to under 35%. In addition, volume expansion may increase systolic blood pressure to desired end points. As the patient's clinical condition demands, the blood pressure is elevated further with pressor agents to systolic values between 180 mm Hg and 220 mm Hg.

Endovascular therapies for vasospasm are becoming increasingly utilized when aggressive medical management fails, when TCD velocities rise, or when there are multiple risk factors for severe vasospasm. Transluminal balloon angioplasty (TBA) mechanically dilates segments of large cerebral arteries that are in spasm, usually restoring the normal caliber of the lumen. This intervention immediately improves blood flow to ischemic brain and typically results in clinical improvement. Furthermore, the effects of angioplasty appear to last up to a week, which corresponds to the duration of vasospasm. The success of this intervention has largely to do with timing. Early angioplasty before or immediately after neurologic deterioration enhances its efficacy.

TBA is limited to large cerebral arteries such as ICA, MCA, and ACA. Transluminal balloon angioplasty is limited to large vessels such as the internal, middle, and anterior cerebral arteries. Smaller distal arteries are not amenable to angioplasty and instead can be treated with intra-arterial papaverine infusion. Superselective infusion of papaverine, a potent vasodilator, can improve the caliber of vasospastic arteries but the effects are short-lived (< 12 hours). Repeated treatments may be needed for severe distal vasospasm, which limits its utility.

Prognosis

Outcome depends on the extent of damage done by the initial aneurysm hemorrhage or subsequent rehemorrhage, complications resulting from treatment, and complications resulting from vasospasm. Of these factors, the initial injury is most important. The patient's preoperative status as assessed by the Hunt-Hess Scale is perhaps the best predictor of outcome. Good recovery, as defined by Glasgow Outcome Scores, can be expected in 97% of grade I patients, 88% of grade II patients, and 81% of grade III patients. In these low-grade patients, 55% resumed in their normal living conditions, 67% returned to full-time work, and 23% reported physical disabilities. In contrast, poor-grade patients (Hunt-Hess grade IV and grade V) have less favorable outcomes. Left untreated, more than 90% of grade V patients will die or be severely disabled. When treated aggressively, between one-fourth and one-third of poor-grade patients will have a favorable outcome.

Brilstra EH et al: Treatment of intracranial aneurysms by embolization with coils: a systematic review. Stroke 1999;30:470.

Chyatte D, Porterfield R: Nuances of middle cerebral artery aneurysm microsurgery. Neurosurgery 2001;48:339.

Dovey Z et al: Guglielmi detachable coiling for intracranial aneurysms: the story so far. Arch Neurol 2001;58:559.

Hacein-Bey L et al: Complex intracranial aneurysms: combined operative and endovascular approaches. Neurosurgery 1998; 43:1304.

Thornton J et al: What percentage of surgically clipped intracranial aneurysms have residual necks? Neurosurgery 2000;46:1294.

Tregiarie-Venzi MM, Suter PM, Romand JA: Review of medical prevention of vasospasm after aneurysmal subarachnoid hemorrhage: a problem of neurointensive care. Neurosurgery 200; 48):249.

■ ARTERIOVENOUS MALFORMATIONS

G. Edward Vates, MD, PhD, &
Michael T. Lawton, MD

 ESSENTIALS OF DIAGNOSIS

- Arteriovenous malformations (AVMs) present with seizures, spontaneous subarachnoid or intracerebral hemorrhage, or progressive neurologic deficit.
- AVMs can present at any age but more commonly become symptomatic during the second or third decades of life.
- CT and MRI often suggest the diagnosis and can provide important information about the location of the lesion in relation to critical brain structures; cerebral angiography is diagnostic and essential for planning therapy.

General Considerations

Arteriovenous malformations (AVMs) occur within the central nervous system as congenital anomalies that allow blood to be shunted directly from arteries to veins without an interposed capillary network. Afferent and efferent vessels are dilated, and they lead to and from a tangle of malformed channels (the nidus) containing arterial blood. Because these abnormal vessels receive blood at arterial pressure, bleeding can result. AVMs can also grow over time through a combination of vessel enlargement and recruitment of new vessels, perhaps involving mechanisms of angiogenesis. Congestion of draining veins with arterial blood flow can also lead to neurologic symptoms by causing venous hypertension and reduced perfusion in adjacent brain areas. Excision of the malformation will restore normal perfusion to the uninvolved brain.

AVMs can be small, with only a single feeding artery, or they can encompass several lobes of the brain and have arterial feeders from multiple sources. They can occur in virtually any portion of the nervous system but are most common in the cerebral hemispheres (90% of AVMs). Cerebral AVMs are usually conical, with the apex near the ventricles and a broad base at the cortical surface; large cortical AVMs commonly present with seizures caused by irritation of adjacent cortical tissue. Small AVMs are more likely to present with spontaneous hemorrhage, causing headache, neurologic deficits, coma, or even death. AVMs can be associated with flow-related aneurysms on feeding arteries or can have aneurysms on vessels within the nidus of the AVM itself. If aneurysms are present, they are usually the source of hemorrhage. AVMs can occur in the cerebellum or brain stem but are much less common. Rarely, AVMs occur within the spinal cord, or they may involve only the dura (intracranial or intraspinal).

Patients with AVMs usually develop symptoms before age 40 (but usually not during childhood). The most common presentation is hemorrhage (50–65%), followed by seizures (15–35%). Mortality and morbidity with each hemorrhage are 10–30% and 15–50%, respectively. For the first year after a hemorrhage, the risk of another hemorrhage is 6%, but for all subsequent years the annual risk drops to 2%, which is the risk of hemorrhage in an unruptured AVM that presents with other signs or symptoms.

Clinical Findings

A. SYMPTOMS AND SIGNS

Hemorrhage may cause symptoms ranging from headaches to focal neurologic deficits to coma, or the defect can be clinically silent. The site of the hemorrhage will determine the neurologic deficit but the size of a hemorrhage is often irrelevant, as small hematomas in eloquent areas cause more impairment than large ones in silent areas of the brain. Hemorrhage into the ventricles of the brain can cause hydrocephalus that must be managed with ventricular drainage. Hemorrhage into the subarachnoid space can cause headache and nuchal rigidity, much like subarachnoid hemorrhage from an aneurysmal hemorrhage. However, the subsequent risk of vasospasm is usually much less after AVM-related subarachnoid hemorrhage than after aneurysmal subarachnoid hemorrhage; this is probably due to differences in the amount and distribution of subarachnoid blood found after AVM versus aneurysmal rupture (AVMs leak less blood that is distributed over the convexities, while aneurysms leak more blood into the basilar cisterns, adjacent to the origins of the major brain arteries as they emerge from the skull base).

Seizures can be focal or general and may cause temporary postictal neurologic deficits. The clinical importance of AVM presentation with seizures is that it may allow for treatment of an AVM prior to symptomatic hemorrhage. There are insufficient data in the literature to predict either the seizure frequency or the prognosis of seizure control based on the size or location of an AVM, though frontal or temporal lobe AVMs are more commonly associated with seizures.

Headaches are common in patients with AVMs, but headache is one of the most common neurologic complaints. It is difficult to show a precise relationship between headache and AVMs, and the literature is inconclusive on the subject of which (if any) headache syndromes reliably predict an underlying AVM.

Focal neurologic deficits can occur in the absence of hemorrhage or seizure in patients with AVMs. These symptoms were once thought to be due to "steal" of arterial blood from adjacent areas of functional brain by the high-flow arteriovenous shunt of an AVM. However, recent studies using measurements of intra-arterial and intravenous pressure and blood flow in AVMs and adjacent cortical territories in patients suggest that focal neurologic symptoms may be produced by venous congestion leading to venous hypertension and ischemia in adjacent cortical territories.

It is worth noting one uncommon but well-known complication of large AVMs in infants and children: arteriovenous shunting leading to left ventricular dysfunction and high-output cardiac failure. Frequently, these children will have an audible cranial bruit and can present with noncommunicating hydrocephalus due to obstruction of the cerebral aqueduct by enlarged basal veins surrounding the midbrain.

B. LABORATORY FINDINGS

If a patient presents with sudden onset headache or neurologic deficits, a CT scan is usually all that is required for diagnosis of an intracranial or subarachnoid hemorrhage (see below). However, if this is not diagnostic, lumbar puncture may be required to establish the presence of subarachnoid blood that would prompt rigorous search for a cause.

C. IMAGING STUDIES

Any young adult presenting with new-onset severe headache, neurologic deficits, coma, or seizures should first be studied by noncontrast CT scan, which will routinely demonstrate intracerebral or subarachnoid blood if a hemorrhage has occurred and, in the absence of bleeding, may suggest a mass lesion without contrast. CT scans also help to guide immediate management decisions such as the need for emergency hematoma evacuation or ventriculostomy for hydrocephalus and intraventricular hemorrhage. MR imaging with intravenous gadolinium contrast defines the relationships of the AVM to surrounding brain structures and can be critical in assessing the surgical risks and choosing the appropriate surgical approach.

Four-vessel cerebral arteriography (both carotid arteries and both vertebral arteries) is the standard test used to define the vascular anatomy of AVMs. This procedure identifies all feeding arteries, all compartments of the nidus, and all draining veins. In addition, angiography can identify associated aneurysms within the nidus or those on feeding arteries far removed from the nidus. Selective external carotid artery injections should be performed on the side of large lesions because many will have feeding artery contributions from the dura or from external-to-internal carotid anastomoses that can be embolized easily. If surgical resection is planned, angiography with endovascular embolization of large feeding arteries can significantly reduce arterial supply to an AVM prior to surgery and thereby make resection much less difficult.

It should be noted that any or all of the studies described above can fail to detect an AVM nidus immediately after acute hemorrhage because the intraparenchymal clot can compress the nidus and close it off, making it radiographically "silent." Therefore, in any patient suspected of having an AVM-related hemorrhage but in whom MRI and angiography are not diagnostic, these studies should be repeated 1–3 months after the hemorrhage. By this time, the hematoma will have been absorbed and any underlying vascular pathology should be evident. On occasion, bleeding may be due to a cavernous malformation, another kind of vascular malformation whose characteristic appearance on MRI is described below.

Differential Diagnosis

Hemorrhage—intracerebral or subarachnoid—can be caused by hypertension, amyloid angiopathy, diabetes mellitus, or hemorrhagic conversion of an ischemic stroke, but these diseases are unlikely in the age group usually affected by AVM-related hemorrhage. Therefore, in the absence of blood dyscrasia, spontaneous intracranial hemorrhage in a child or young adult is the hallmark of an AVM. Other diagnostic considerations include an intracranial aneurysm or a primary brain neoplasm or secondary metastatic lesion within the brain that has bled spontaneously. Each of these has a characteristic appearance on MRI or angiography and can be easily differentiated from an AVM. Cavernous malformations ("cryptic" vascular malformations) are the second most frequently seen cerebrovascular malformation but are nonetheless much less common than AVMs. They are composed of small-caliber venous sinusoidal vascular channels that are commonly thrombosed, and because of their slow flow they are usually angiographically "silent." Their low flow also makes them less likely to bleed (annual risk of 0.7%) and less likely to cause neurologic deficits when they do. These defects have a characteristic "mulberry" appearance on MRI and are usually surrounded by a ring of T2-weighted susceptibility that makes them easy to distinguish from AVMs. They typically present with seizures unless they are located in the brain stem, where even a small venous hemorrhage can cause a profound and sudden neurologic deterioration. These are treated with surgical removal.

A wide range of structural and biochemical disorders can cause seizures although, as noted before, they usually give rise to a radiographic evaluation that can suggest or prove the presence of an AVM.

Treatment

A. MEDICAL TREATMENT

Medical treatment is only effective for relieving symptoms or for reducing posthemorrhagic sequelae. Anticonvulsants can control AVM-incited seizures, and blood pressure control is important after a hemorrhage, especially if the hemorrhage is due to an AVM-related aneurysm.

B. SURGICAL TREATMENT

The ideal treatment of an AVM is excision and removal of any associated hematoma. However, treatment must be guided by two basic principles: (1) The AVM should be removed completely, because any residual nidus can still bleed; and (2) neurologic function should be preserved. Some malformations cannot be removed with reasonable risk, and some of these can be treated by endovascular embolization or focused irradiation (stereotactic radiosurgery; see below).

In an attempt to determine which patients should or should not be offered surgery, a number of grading systems have been developed. AVM grading systems are important for estimating the risk of operation compared with the risks associated with the natural history of the lesion, and for these reasons they should be simple but comprehensive enough to grade all AVMs, address all factors that influence treatment risk, and predict these treatment risks. Most grading systems are based on radiographic features of the lesion. The most widely accepted grading system is the Spetzler-Martin system, which attempts to predict the risk of surgical resection based on three variables: AVM size, pattern of venous drainage, and location in relation to eloquent brain (Table 38–9). Size is scored by measuring the greatest diameter of the AVM on angiography, MRI, or CT and relates to the number of feeding arteries and the degree of flow. Venous drainage is scored by determining whether the AVM empties into the superficial cortical venous system or into the deep venous system (internal cerebral veins, basal veins of Rosenthal, or vein of Galen); this relates to the depth of the AVM and surgical accessibility. Eloquence is scored by the proximity of the AVM nidus to areas of brain that have easily identifiable neurologic function and, when injured, produce disabling neurologic deficits (motor and sensory cortex, deep gray matter, corticospinal tracts, or brain stem). A numerical AVM grade is then assigned by adding the scores for size, venous drainage, and eloquence. AVMs can then be stratified into five grades, with grade 1 lesions being

Table 38–9. Spetzler-Martin grading system for AVMs.

Factor	Point Weight
Factor 1: AVM size	
Small (< 3 cm)	1
Medium (3–6 cm)	2
Large (> 6 cm)	3
Factor 2: Functional eloquence of location	
Noneloquent	0
Eloquent	1
Factor 3: Pattern of venous drainage	
Surface cortical only	0
Deep drainage component	1

Total grade = sum of all three factors (grades 1–5)

small, superficial, and in noneloquent brain and grade 5 lesions being large and deep in eloquent brain.

Prospective analysis of AVM grade and surgical results in 120 patients showed minimal risk associated with surgical resection of AVMs in patients with grade 1 or grade 2 lesions, with no new neurologic deficits after surgery. We therefore recommend aggressive surgical excision of these lesions. In contrast, surgical resection of grade 4 and grade 5 AVMs resulted in 15–20% incidence of new deficits. Patients with grade 4 and grade 5 AVMs are recommended for surgical treatment only when they suffer repeated hemorrhages or are experiencing a rapid and progressive neurologic decline. Grade 3 lesions remain ambiguous in that some studies suggest these lesions can be resected with low surgical morbidity while others report an unacceptable surgical risk. This may be due to the variability in the nature of these lesions as prescribed by the Spetzler-Martin grading system, and patients with grade 3 malformation should therefore be evaluated on an individual basis. Patients whose neurologic condition is deteriorating are typically ready to accept surgical risks, whereas patients who are neurologically intact may prefer to postpone treatment until absolute indications are present and the surgical risks become more acceptable relative to the natural history of the AVM. Because the risk of hemorrhage accrues annually, young patients are exposed to substantial cumulative risk during their lifetimes and may be more amenable to a strategy of surgical excision.

Endovascular embolization as sole treatment of AVMs is usually unacceptable because complete occlusion rates are low and the long-term occlusion rates are unknown. Therefore, embolization should be used as part of a multimodality approach to either devascularize a large lesion before surgery or reduce its size before radiosurgery. In this context, embolization can significantly simplify surgical resection or can convert a large AVM into a much smaller one that can be more effectively treated with radiosurgery.

Stereotactic radiosurgery is rapidly gaining attention as an alternative treatment for AVMs and has been shown to work well for small defects. However, radiosurgical obliteration is inversely related to AVM size, with larger lesions showing a lower rate of occlusion after delivery of radiation. In addition, there is a lag-time in the onset of effectiveness; generally, radiosurgery takes up to 2 years to achieve full effect, and during that time studies suggest that the risk of hemorrhage from an irradiated AVM may actually increase compared with an untreated AVM. Therefore, we do not currently recommend stereotactic radiosurgery for small AVMs, as these lesions can be surgically resected with no morbidity and with immediate elimination of the risk of hemorrhage. Instead, stereotactic radiation can be used as part of a multimodal treatment plan for deep AVMs located in critical brain structures where there is no easy surgical access. Such an AVM can be reduced in size, either by endovascular embolization or partial surgical resection, and then obliterated with stereotactic radiation therapy applied to the much smaller residual nidus.

Postoperative Complications

The complication rates associated with resection of AVMs of different grades are reviewed above. The most important postoperative complication relates to a phenomenon called "normal perfusion pressure breakthrough." Once an AVM has been resected, the shunting of blood through the nidus is gone, thus restoring normal perfusion and normal arterial pressure within vessels of adjacent brain. Because shunting through the AVM has altered the autoregulation of these vessels, these arteries are ill-suited for accommodation of the new influx of arterial blood and can hemorrhage. The actual risk of normal perfusion pressure hemorrhage is unknown, but because of the theoretical risk, blood pressure control is critical during the first 24–48 hours after surgery while arteries adjacent to the AVM nidus reestablish their normal autoregulation.

Postoperative hemorrhage should also sound the alarm for a possible residual AVM nidus. Nothing short of complete AVM resection will protect the patient from further hemorrhage, and all patients should therefore undergo postoperative angiography to verify complete obliteration of the AVM nidus. Intraoperative angiography should be considered in selected cases of either large or deep AVMs where it can be difficult to determine if resection is complete. In addition, any patient treated with stereotactic radiation should undergo follow-up angiography 2–3 years after treatment; if there is residual nidus, this may need to be treated with further stereotactic radiotherapy (staged radiosurgery) or with conventional microsurgical removal.

Prognosis

The annual risk of hemorrhage from an unruptured AVM is approximately 2%. This risk doubles during the first year after a hemorrhage but then drops back to the prehemorrhage annual rate for all subsequent years. The morbidity associated with each hemorrhage is 15–50%, and the mortality is 10–30%. Because the lesion is present at birth, there is a lifelong risk of serious complications from bleeding and neurologic deficits. In contrast, the overall morbidity from AVM treatment is less than 10%, and the overall mortality is less than 5%, though this varies widely depending on the grade of AVM, as described above. The patient's preoperative neurologic condition is also important. Patients who present with devastating hemorrhage may not deteriorate with treatment but will be left with disabling deficits that require prolonged rehabilitation. Age is also an important factor because young patients are much more resilient after treatment than elderly ones. However, with adequate time, full recovery is usually possible; studies have demonstrated that most early neurologic deficits after surgery will resolve.

Drake CG: Cerebral arteriovenous malformations: considerations for and experience with surgical treatment in 166 cases. Clin Neurosurg 1979;26:145.

Hamilton MG, Spetzler RF: The prospective application of a grading system for arteriovenous malformations. Neurosurgery 1994;34:2.

Heros RC, Morcos J, Korosue K: Arteriovenous malformations of the brain. Surgical management. Clin Neurosurg 1993;40:139.

Lawton MT, Hamilton MG, Spetzler RF: Multimodality treatment of deep arteriovenous malformations: thalamus, basal ganglia, and brain stem. Neurosurgery 1995;37:29.

Lunsford LD et al: Stereotactic radiosurgery for arteriovenous malformations of the brain [see comments]. J Neurosurg 1991; 75:512.

Steiner L et al: Microsurgery and radiosurgery in brain arteriovenous malformations [editorial] [see comments]. J Neurosurg 1993;79:647.

■ MOVEMENT DISORDERS RESPONSIVE TO SURGERY

Philip Starr, MD

Recently there has been a resurgence of interest in subcortical brain surgery for movement disorders. Movement disorders amenable to surgical treatment include Parkinson's disease, essential tremor, and generalized dystonia.

PARKINSON'S DISEASE

 ESSENTIALS OF DIAGNOSIS

- *Idiopathic Parkinson's disease is diagnosed clinically since there is no laboratory test short of brain examination at autopsy by which it can be diagnosed with certainty. The criteria for diagnosis are as follows:*
- *At least two of the following four cardinal clinical signs: rigidity, bradykinesia, tremor, and postural instability.*
- *Symptomatic improvement in response to oral administration of levodopa.*
- *Exclusion—by MRI and clinical history—of atypical parkinsonism.*

General Considerations

Surgery for Parkinson's disease has a long history. Beginning in the 1950s, thalamotomy (lesioning of the motor thalamus) and pallidotomy (lesioning of the globus pallidus) were performed before a solid scientific basis for these procedures was established. When treatment of Parkinson's disease with oral levodopa became widespread in the 1960s, surgical treatment was used less often. In the 1990s, several factors combined to produce a resurgence of interest in surgery for this disease: (1) improved surgical techniques, including MRI and CT-guided stereotaxy; (2) recognition of the limitations of long-term medical therapy as the disease advances; (3) understanding of the theoretical basis for basal ganglia surgery in Parkinson's disease; and (4) the development of chronic deep brain stimulation as a reversible, adjustable alternative to lesioning surgery.

Pathogenesis

Parkinson's disease is an idiopathic, progressive neurodegenerative disorder involving loss of dopaminergic cells in the substantia nigra pars compacta (SNc). Loss of dopaminergic neurons of the SNc results in excessive and abnormally patterned activity in the subthalamic nucleus (STN) and in its major target nuclei, the internal segment of the globus pallidus (GPI) and the substantia nigra, pars reticulata (SNr). Since GPi and SNr have inhibitory projections to motor regions of the thalamus, thalamocortical activity is suppressed. This is thought to be the basis for many of the motor abnormalities in Parkinson's disease. As predicted by this model, inactivation of brain tissue in STN or GPi—effectively decreasing the inhibitory influence on the motor thalamus and, thus, "normalizing" thalamocortical activity—was found to be effective in treating parkinsonism in animal models. This provided the theoretical basis for pallidal and subthalamic surgery for Parkinson's disease in humans.

Differential Diagnosis

Idiopathic Parkinson's disease must be distinguished from a variety of atypical parkinsonian symptoms, which include multisystem atrophy and progressive supranuclear palsy. While the symptoms may be similar, atypical parkinsonism should be suspected if the symptoms have never responded robustly to oral dopamine replacement. The distinction is important to neurosurgeons since atypical parkinsonism is unresponsive to basal ganglia surgery.

Treatment

A. MEDICAL TREATMENT

A variety of pharmacologic treatments are initially effective in reducing the symptoms of Parkinson's disease. Treatment with levodopa in combination with carbidopa (Sinemet) is the mainstay of pharmacotherapy. Sinemet is usually supplemented with dopamine agonists such as pergolide or pramipexole. The activity of levodopa may be prolonged by inhibitors of catechol-*O*-methyltransferase (COMT) such as entacapone. After 5–15 years of treatment, Sinemet still produces a beneficial response, but its utility is compromised by peak-dose dyskinesias and a shorter, less predictable duration of action. When patients develop these complications of medical therapy, they are considered for surgery.

B. SURGICAL TREATMENT

Three types of surgery for Parkinson's disease are in current practice or under clinical investigation: lesioning surgery, deep brain stimulation, and intrastriatal transplantation of dopamine-secreting cells. Lesioning and deep brain stimulation procedures attempt to compensate for (rather than correct) the brain defect in Parkinson's disease by interruption of abnormal basal ganglia output. Deep brain stimulation has effects on motor function similar to those of lesioning but has several advantages: It is reversible in the event of an un-

wanted stimulation-induced effect, it can be adjusted as symptoms change, and it is safer for bilateral use.

In contrast, cell transplantation strategies attempt to correct the biochemical defect of Parkinson's disease by replacing lost dopaminergic brain cells. In the future, such "restorative" biologic therapies may emerge as effective and possibly curative interventions for Parkinson's disease. Although theoretically very attractive, much more laboratory work must be done in order to make cell transplantation therapies practical and effective. Human fetal substantia nigra allografts can survive in the human brain without long-term immunosuppression. Porcine xenograft tissue has also been used, but graft survival is less than is true for allograft.

Outcomes of surgery are measured by changes in the Unified Parkinson's Disease Rating Scale (UPDRS), a quantitative rating scale of overall function in Parkinson's disease. At this time, bilateral deep brain stimulation of the globus pallidus or subthalamic nucleus appears to offer the greatest symptomatic relief, producing 40–60% improvements in the motor subscore of the UPDRS in the off-medication state . The best results of intrastriatal human allograft transplantation produce only a 20–30% improvement.

C. SURGICAL TECHNIQUES

Because the basal ganglia are deep structures, they are approached through small skull openings without direct visualization of the target structures rather than by open craniotomy. Target localization is performed by the method of stereotaxis. In stereotactic neurosurgery, a stereotactic frame is fixed to the patient's head to provide both an external coordinate system and a mechanical platform on which to mount instruments and direct them to known coordinates in the patient's brain. A brain image, such as CT or MR, is then obtained to visualize both the frame and the target within the patient's brain. The coordinates of the brain target—in the coordinate system defined by the frame—are calculated. In the operating room, instruments are mounted on the frame and directed toward the image-defined stereotactic target. Correct identification of the target is confirmed by intraoperative physiologic studies such as neuronal recording with microelectrodes. The neurologic status of the patient (such as strength, vision, and improvement of motor function) must be monitored frequently during the procedure.

Postoperative Complications

Hemorrhagic stroke occurs in 1–5% of patients undergoing stereotactic neurosurgery for movement disorders. Transient postoperative confusion is common in elderly patients or following bilateral surgery. For deep brain stimulation implants, perioperative infection of the device occurs in 3–5% of cases.

Prognosis

Idiopathic Parkinson's disease is progressive, with slow worsening of all motor symptoms and, in the late-stages, cognitive decline. It is currently unknown whether any of the surgical treatments alters the course of Parkinson's disease. It is hypothesized that subthalamic nucleus stimulation may prevent progression of Parkinson's disease by suppression of ongoing excitotoxic insult to the SNc that may result from chronic subthalamic nucleus overactivity.

ESSENTIAL TREMOR

Essential tremor is characterized by tremor of the arms, head, or voice, without other neurologic signs. The arm tremor is more prominent with outstretched postures and action than at rest. In about 50% of cases, there is a clear family history. Essential tremor is not a degenerative disease, as the brain MRI and pathologic examination of the brain are normal.

Three classes of drugs can be used to treat essential tremor: beta-blockers such as propranolol, barbiturate derivatives such as primidone, and benzodiazepines such as clonazepam. Surgery should be considered if the tremor interferes with activities of daily living and fails to respond to these medications. Lesioning or deep brain stimulation of the ventralis intermedius nucleus of the motor thalamus are both effective for essential tremor, though in a randomized study thalamic stimulation was associated with a slightly lower complication rate.

DYSTONIA

Dystonia is a movement disorder defined as a syndrome of sustained muscle contractions—frequently causing twisting and repetitive movements—and abnormal postures. Electromyographic studies show abnormal cocontraction of agonist and antagonist muscles, prolongation of the electromyographic bursts, and overflow of electromyographic activity into muscle groups outside the area of intended movement. Reciprocal inhibition in spinal and brain stem reflexes is diminished. Dystonia may be classified according to body part (focal, segmental, or generalized), age at onset, or according to presumed etiology. Four etiologic subcategories of dystonia are now recognized: primary dystonia, dystonia-plus syndromes, secondary dystonia, and heredodegenerative dystonias.

Medical therapy with anticholinergic drugs such as trihexyphenidine or injection of botulinum toxin into the affected muscles should be the initial treatment. Lesioning or deep brain stimulation of the globus pallidus have been shown to be effective for primary generalized dystonia, particularly in cases associated with a mutation in the *DYT1* gene. The efficacy of pallidal surgery for secondary dystonias—such as those due to stroke or cerebral palsy—is not well documented. Surgical techniques and complications are similar to those described above for Parkinson's disease.

Benabid AL et al: Chronic electrical stimulation of the ventralis intermedius nucleus of the thalamus as a treatment of movement disorders. J Neurosurg 1996;84:203.

Coubes P et al: Treatment of DYT1-generalized dystonia by stimulation of the internal globus pallidus. Lancet 2000;355:2220.

Fahn S, Bresman SB, Marsden CD: Classification of dystonia. Adv Neurol 1998;78:1.

Freeman TB et al: Bilateral fetal nigral transplantation into the postcommissural putamen in Parkinson's disease. Ann Neurol 1995;38:379.

Ghika J et al: Efficiency and safety of bilateral contemporaneous pallidal stimulation (deep brain stimulation) in levodopa-responsive patients with Parkinson's disease with severe motor fluctuations: a 2 year follow-up review. J Neurosurg 1998;89:713.

Guridi J, Lozano AM: A brief history of pallidotomy. Neurosurgery 1997;41:1169.

Koller WC, Pahwa R, Busenbark KL: High frequency unilateral thalamic stimulation in the treatment of essential and parkinsonian tremor. Ann Neurol 1997;42:292.

Krauss JK et al: Bilateral stimulation of the globus pallidus internus for treatment of cervical dystonia. Lancet 1999;354:837.

Limousin P et al: Electrical stimulation of the subthalamic nucleus in advanced Parkinson's disease. N Engl J Med 1998;339:1105.

Limousin P, Speelman JD, Gielen F: Multicentre European study of thalamic stimulation in parkinsonian and essential tremor. J Neurol Neurosurg Psychiatry 1999;66:289.

Lindvall O: Update on fetal transplantation: the Swedish experience. Mov Disord 1998;13:83.

Lozano AM et al: Globus pallidus internus pallidotomy for generalized dystonia. Mov Disord 1997;12: 865.

Ondo WG et al: Pallidotomy for generalized dystonia. Mov Disord 1998;13:693.

Rodriguez MC, Obeso JA, Olanow CW: Subthalamic nucleus-mediated excitotoxicity in Parkinson's disease: a target for neuroprotection. Ann Neurol 1998;44(Suppl 1):S175.

Shuurman PR et al: Comparison of continuous thalamic stimulation and thalamotomy for suppression of severe tremor. N Engl J Med 2000;342:461.

Starr PA, Vitek JL, Bakay RA: Ablative surgery and deep brain stimulation for Parkinson's disease. Neurosurgery 1998;43:989.

Tronnier VM, Fogel W: Pallidal stimulation for generalized dystonia. J Neurosurg 2000;92:453.

Vitek JL et al: GPi pallidotomy for dystonia: clinical outcome and neuronal activity. Adv Neurol 1998.78:211.

■ PAIN

Nicholas M. Barbaro, MD

Pain has been defined as "an unpleasant sensory and emotional experience associated with actual or potential tissue damage, or described in terms of such damage." This definition takes into account that pain is a well-recognized signal of damage and, as such, an important symptom of numerous diseases. Pain resulting from injury to the nervous system (neuropathic pain) may not indicate tissue damage and thus may not be a useful sensory phenomenon; rather, it may constitute a pathologic process in itself. The above definition of pain also takes into account the emotional aspects of pain, which can be all-consuming for a patient, and suggests the importance of psychologic factors in evaluation and treatment.

Patients with pain can be divided into two groups: those with diseases that limit life expectancy, such as malignant tumors (malignant or cancer pain); and those with normal life expectancy (chronic benign pain). For practical purposes, patients expected to live 2 years or less are put into the malignant pain group. The medical and surgical management of these two groups is very different.

In general, the approach to treating pain begins with an attempt to diagnose the cause. The natural history of the underlying problem must also be considered. For example, pain in a recently operated region is expected to resolve with wound healing. When possible, the source of the pain should be treated directly (eg, removal of a herniated disk, treatment of a primary tumor). If the pain cannot be treated directly or if the source of the pain is unknown, efforts are made to treat the pain as such.

MALIGNANT PAIN

The main goal in treating patients with malignant pain is to reduce suffering during a terminal illness. Therapies that might be inappropriate in patients with normal life expectancies can be considered. Opioids, for example, can be used in high doses unless excessive sedation, respiratory depression, severe constipation, or other significant adverse effects occur. Any dose that relieves pain and maximizes useful function can be used. Other medications, such as tricyclic antidepressants, anticonvulsants, and nonsteroidal anti-inflammatory agents, may provide additional relief. When medical

management fails to reduce the pain sufficiently, surgical treatment is indicated. Surgical management of malignant pain involves two approaches: (1) epidural or intrathecally administered morphine and (2) ablation to interrupt pain transmission.

The spinal cord contains opioid receptors which, when activated by locally administered morphine, produce rather profound pain relief. Temporary percutaneous catheters can be used to test this therapy; if significant pain relief is demonstrated, prolonged spinal administration of morphine is indicated. This can be accomplished by implanting a subcutaneous reservoir attached to an epidural or intrathecal catheter; morphine can be injected into the reservoir by the patient or caregiver. Although this technique provides useful pain relief, it is impractical because repeated skin punctures are required and there is a risk of infection. If the patient's life expectancy is more than a few months, implantation of an infusion pump is recommended. Spinal morphine is most effective for midline and multifocal pain problems, such as sacral pain associated with prostate tumors, pelvic pain from carcinoma of the cervix, and multifocal bone pain from widely metastatic disease. Other drugs such as bupivacaine and clonidine may relieve pain related to nerve invasion.

Cancer pain that is unilateral and focal may be treated with cordotomy, creating a lesion in the spinothalamic tract designed to interrupt pain transmission. An open cordotomy, which requires laminectomy, produces excellent analgesia and can be done in the thoracic region for leg pain. Percutaneous cordotomy using a radiofrequency needle is done at the C1–2 level. This is less traumatic for the patient and may produce analgesia in both the arm and the leg. Bilateral high cervical cordotomy is not recommended because of the risk of respiratory depression.

Other ablative techniques for treating cancer pain are used relatively rarely. These include midline myelotomies, rhizotomies (open or percutaneous), and neurectomies.

POSTOPERATIVE PAIN

Some pain is experienced by nearly every patient after invasive surgical procedures. The amount and duration of pain varies with the type of procedure, with the individual patient, and with many other factors, including the rapidity of healing and associated complications such as infection. The fact that pain is expected after surgical procedures does not mean it should not be treated aggressively. Reducing postoperative pain not only lessens the most unpleasant aspect of the procedure for the patient, it also reduces the incidence of other types of morbidity, such as pneumonia and deep vein thrombosis. For these reasons, appropriate doses of opioids and other pain-reducing drugs such as anti-inflammatory agents are an essential part of postoperative care.

The treatment of postoperative pain has improved substantially in recent years. These improvements include the use of epidural or intrathecal opioids and the use of long-acting nerve blocks at the end of a procedure. In addition, new delivery techniques such as patient-controlled analgesia, in which the patient self-administers small incremental doses of opioid analgesic, reduce overall postoperative pain and actually decrease the amount of analgesic required during the postoperative period.

CHRONIC BENIGN PAIN

Patients with a life expectancy longer than 2 years who have pain that cannot be eliminated by treating the underlying cause are considered to have chronic benign pain. Such patients should be evaluated by a team of individuals experienced in pain treatment (pain clinic), including specialists in anesthesiology, psychology, psychiatry and neurology or neurosurgery, physical therapy, and pharmacology. This multidisciplinary approach takes into account the multifactorial cause of long-standing pain.

The medical management of such patients is beyond the scope of this chapter. In general, drugs with little or no potential for addiction or significant dependence should be used. When opioids are used, long-acting drugs on a time-contingent rather than pain-contingent schedule are preferred, and short-acting opioids should be avoided. Anticonvulsant and tricyclic antidepressant drugs may be effective and are best administered by physicians with experience in their use.

When medical management fails to reduce pain adequately, surgical treatment can be considered. Ablative techniques such as rhizotomy (cutting of nerve roots), neurectomy, and cordotomy are inappropriate in these cases except as noted below. Techniques of neuromodulation that do not cause neural injury should be used instead.

Neuromodulation techniques take advantage of the capacity of the nervous system to reduce the access of painful stimuli to higher central nervous system centers. Transcutaneous electrical nerve stimulation, the least invasive of these techniques, uses skin electrodes to activate the large fibers in peripheral nerves. This selective activation reduces the ability of nociceptive fibers (A δ and C) to activate spinal neurons, which transmit pain signals to higher centers. This technique is limited by the inability to stimulate large painful areas and by the inconvenience of wearing electrodes for long periods.

A more invasive approach to neuromodulation involves direct or percutaneous implantation of electrodes into the spinal canal to electrically stimulate the dorsal columns. Spinal cord stimulation is most effective for pain in the extremities, such as pain after nerve injury, peripheral neuropathies, and complex regional pain syndromes. In patients with ischemic pain, spinal cord stimulation not only reduces the pain but may also improve blood flow in the involved extremities as well.

SPECIFIC PAIN SYNDROMES

1. Trigeminal Neuralgia

Trigeminal neuralgia is an episodic lancinating facial pain that conforms to one—or perhaps two—divisions of the trigeminal nerve. It is more common in elderly patients except when seen as a manifestation of multiple sclerosis, and is slightly more common in women. The mainstay of treatment is the anticonvulsant drug carbamazepine and, more recently, gabapentin. Patients who do not respond to medical management may be treated with a percutaneous, open, or radiosurgical procedure. Percutaneous approaches involve placing a needle through the foramen ovale at the skull base. The trigeminal nerve is then partially damaged with glycerol, a mildly toxic alcohol, a radiofrequency-induced heat lesion, or by balloon compression of the trigeminal ganglion. The percutaneous approaches are minimally invasive and require very short hospitalization, but the recurrence rate is higher than with an open approach, and patients are left with some loss of facial sensation, perhaps including protective corneal sensation.

Many cases of trigeminal neuralgia are caused by irritation of the trigeminal nerve at the brain stem by blood vessels, such as the superior cerebellar and anterior inferior cerebellar arteries. This syndrome can often be cured by moving the offending vessel away from the nerve. When the trigeminal nerve is exposed and such a neurovascular relationship cannot be demonstrated, partial rhizotomy (nerve sectioning) can provide excellent pain relief. A recent addition to the surgical treatment of trigeminal neuralgia is radiosurgery, a stereotaxic technique used to deliver high levels of radiation to precise brain regions. Typically, a single dose of radiation (70–80 Gy) is delivered to the trigeminal nerve between its entrance in the pons and the gasserian ganglion behind the cavernous sinus. Such treatment is very effective in reducing or eliminating the pain of trigeminal neuralgia, but longer follow-up is required to determine whether it will become the treatment of choice for this condition.

2. Pain After Amputation

A variety of pain syndromes may follow limb amputation. Most patients experience sensory phenomena in the amputated limb. In a minority of cases, these so-called phantom sensations are painful. Phantom limb pain is described as a continuous pain, as if fingernails were digging into the palm or the limb were being twisted into painful postures. Some patients have painful neuromas at the cut ends of peripheral nerves; the pain is usually electrical and occurs each time the stump is pressed. Injury to the cutaneous nerves may cause painful skin sensitivity in the stump. Medications such as tricyclic antidepressants and anticonvulsants may be effective in these cases, but opioids usually are not. Surgical options include revision and burying of painful neuromas and, in refractory cases, spinal cord or brain stimulation.

3. Spinal Nerve Root Avulsion Pain

Injuries that radically displace the head and shoulder can avulse the spinal nerves from the spinal cord. This commonly occurs after motorcycle accidents in which the head and shoulder are rapidly and severely distracted. This type of brachial plexus injury is not surgically reparable and usually is not painful. In some cases, however, the pain is severe; typically, it is a burning pain and may include a phantom-like pain sensation. When such pain is refractory to medical management, it can be alleviated in 80% of cases by a dorsal root entry zone lesion. In this procedure, the spinal cord is exposed, and the region where dorsal roots formerly entered the spinal cord is identified. Lesions are made either with small needles (radiofrequency) or with a laser. Care must be taken to avoid damaging nearby spinal tracts.

4. Spinal Cord Injury Pain

Most patients with severe spinal cord injury experience some pain. In some cases, it is severe and requires specific medical treatment. Pain after spinal cord injury may occur at the border zone between normal and abnormal sensation or may affect large areas of the body with little or no sensory function. The former may be treated with the dorsal root entry zone procedure described above; lesions are created at the region immediately above and below the spinal cord injury. More diffuse spinal cord injury pain is very difficult to treat and does not respond well to any surgical procedures. Such patients should be referred to multidisciplinary pain clinics.

Barker FG 2nd et al: The long-term outcome of microvascular decompression for trigeminal neuralgia. N Engl J Med 1996; 334:1077.

Dickenson AH: Central acute pain mechanisms. Ann Med 1995; 27:223.

Kondziolka D et al: Gamma knife radiosurgery for trigeminal neuralgia: results and expectations. Arch Neurol 1998;55:1524.

North RB, Roark GL: Spinal cord stimulation for chronic pain. Neurosurg Clin North Am 1995;6:145.

Stanton-Hicks M, Salamon J: Stimulation of the central and peripheral nervous system for the control of pain. J Clin Neurophysiol 1997;14:46.

Taha JM, Tew JM Jr: Comparison of surgical treatments for trigeminal neuralgia: reevaluation of radiofrequency rhizotomy. Neurosurgery 1996;38:865.

Wasner G, Backonja MM, Baron R: Traumatic neuralgias: complex regional pain syndromes (reflex sympathetic dystrophy and causalgia): clinical characteristics, pathophysiological mechanisms and therapy. Neurol Clin 1998;16:851.

■ INTERVERTEBRAL DISK DISEASE

Philip R. Weinstein, MD, & Julian T. Hoff, MD

Anatomic Considerations

A. THE INTERVERTEBRAL DISK

The intervertebral disk has three parts: the circumferential annulus, which consists of dense fibrous tissue and is very strong; the central nucleus, which consists of fibrocartilage and has little tensile strength but great elasticity; and the vertebral body end-plates, which are cartilaginous and form the interface between bone and disk above and below each joint. Fibrocartilage may be fragmented acutely or may degenerate gradually with time. It heals poorly because of limited blood supply. Nutrient arteries atrophy with age beginning in the second decade. The nucleus contains approximately 80% water at birth; it gradually dehydrates and loses its elasticity with age. The annulus, however, has more capacity to heal and is buttressed by thick anterior and posterior longitudinal ligaments that add strength.

Intervertebral disk disease may occur at any level from C2 to L5. The midcervical and lower lumbar areas are affected most often. Thoracic disk disease is uncommon.

B. THE SPINAL CORD AND NERVE ROOTS

Knowledge of the anatomic and physiologic relationships of the spinal cord, nerve roots, vertebrae, and neural foramina is useful for understanding the principles for diagnosis of intervertebral disk disease.

The cervical spinal cord occupies about half of the cross-sectional area of the normal spinal canal, is centrally placed, and moves rostrally and caudally a few millimeters during flexion and extension of the neck.

Anteroposterior and lateral motion is restricted by the tethering effect of the intradural dentate ligaments.

The spinal cord terminates as the conus medullaris at L1–2. Posterior and anterior nerve roots emerge from the conus separately, passing within the lumbar sac to their respective intervertebral foramina, where they exit from the spinal canal. The roots join to form a peripheral nerve within the neural foramen, which also contains the dorsal root ganglion. Sacral nerve roots are medial and central within the lumbar sac, adjacent to the filum terminale, the meningeal structure that attaches the conus to the caudal end of the spinal canal.

In the neck, the C1 root emerges from the spinal canal above the C1 vertebra; the C2 root emerges below C1. Thus, the nerve root that emerges from the spine between the C5 and C6 vertebrae is the C6 root. C8 emerges between C7 and T1, and the T1 root emerges below the pedicle of the T1 vertebra crossing through the T1–T2 foramen.

Sensation around the deltoid area is basically related to the C5 root; sensation in the thumb and possibly in the index finger is a C6 root function. Sensation in the third and fourth fingers is a C7 root function, whereas the fifth finger is supplied by C8. Biceps muscle strength and the biceps tendon reflex require an intact C6 root; triceps reflex and strength are dependent upon the C7 root. Intrinsic muscles of the hand allowing abduction and adduction of the fingers are innervated by C8 and T1.

Lumbosacral nerve roots carry on the same relationships to the vertebrae determined by emergence of the T1 nerve root below the T1 vertebra. That is, the L4 nerve root emerges below the L4 pedicle, and the S1 root emerges below S1.

Each root (eg, L4) passes laterally toward the neural foramen as it descends within the spinal canal. It crosses the adjacent intervertebral disk (eg, L4–5) at the extreme lateral edge of the disk after exiting the spinal canal below the pedicle of the L4 vertebra inferolaterally. The nerve root (eg, L5) that descends to the next lowest foramen passes across the same intervertebral disk (eg, L4–5) more medially, in a location that is more vulnerable to diseases involving intraspinal displacement of the disk.

The sensory distribution of L5 is on the medial aspect of the foot and the great toe. S1 sensation is experienced over the lateral aspect of the foot, the fifth toe, and the lateral sole of the foot. Pain or sensory deficit in those dermatomal areas implies involvement of either L5 or S1 fibers. Plantar flexion is primarily an S1 motor function; dorsiflexion of the foot is an L5 function. Knee extension by the quadriceps muscle group is subserved primarily by the L3 and L4 motor roots. The ankle jerk is primarily dependent upon the S1 root, whereas the knee jerk depends upon L3 and L4. The L5

fibers may contribute to both reflexes or to neither one. The L5 nerve root selectively supplies the great toe extensor muscle (extensor hallucis longus).

The sensory distribution of the remaining sacral roots S2–5 is in the "saddle" area over the buttocks and on the soles of the feet. Voluntary motor control of the urinary bladder and anal sphincters is subserved by the S2–4 nerve roots. Thus, the cauda equina syndrome, a rare complication of massive extrusion of a lumbar disk, is associated with sensory loss over the perineal area and buttocks and with urinary and fecal incontinence.

CERVICAL DISK SYNDROME

ESSENTIALS OF DIAGNOSIS

Subjective:

- *Pain in the suboccipital, cervical, interscapular, thoracic, and shoulder areas radiating into the upper extremities.*
- *Discomfort aggravated by neck movement.*
- *Pain, paresthesias, and dysesthesias radiating into the cervical dermatomes.*

Objective:

- *Straightening of cervical lordosis, limitation of cervical movements, and paraspinous muscle spasm.*
- *Weakness, fasciculations, muscle atrophy, depression of deep tendon reflexes, and dermatome sensory change in the upper extremities.*
- *Spasticity, weakness, and extensor plantar sign in the lower extremities.*
- *Spastic bladder dysfunction.*
- *Radiologic evidence of narrowed disk spaces, formation of osteophytes, and spinal stenosis.*
- *Myelographic, CT, or MRI evidence of extradural cervical cord or root displacement or compression, often at multiple levels.*

General Considerations

If the cervical intervertebral disk ruptures and extrudes through the annulus and posterior longitudinal ligament, adjacent neural structures may be compressed. Compression of the spinal cord may result in paraplegia or quadriplegia, depending on the segment involved. Compression of a spinal root may cause weakness and sensory loss in structures of the upper extremity innervated by it. The severity of the clinical syndrome depends upon the site and severity of compression by the displaced disk fragment. Often, intrinsic disruption of the disk occurs, but the adjacent ligaments hold, preventing complete extrusion of the fragmented disk. The annulus may separate from its attachment to the vertebral body margin or tear sufficiently to allow the disk to bulge into the spinal canal or foramina. Thus, neural structures also may be compressed by protrusion of an injured or degenerated disk.

After trauma or spontaneously, the annulus may rupture and the nucleus may herniate into the spinal canal or neural foramen acutely. Often, however, the nucleus does not extrude but simply becomes desiccated and progressively degenerates, losing its biomechanical function and elasticity. The disk space gradually narrows, the joint becomes looser, and the cartilaginous end-plates of the adjacent vertebra touch, stimulating reactive osteogenesis. Bony spurs develop at the joint in reaction to the increased mobility and stress. If a bony spur (osteophyte) forms in the neural foramen, the nerve root passing through may be chronically irritated and compressed. If the osteophyte forms within the spinal canal, spinal cord compression may result in the development of myelopathy with signs and symptoms of impaired cord function. Formation of osteophytes around the joints of vertebrae is termed **spondylosis.**

Cervical spondylosis is common and may even be "normal" in aging persons. Radiographic evidence of cervical spondylosis exists in 85% of people over 65 years of age. It may not be associated with symptoms of cord or root compression, however, unless the neural canal or foramina are narrowed. Developmental reduction of canal dimensions, resulting in spinal stenosis, may contribute to the appearance of symptoms that are the result of entrapment of neural elements.

Clinical Findings

A. SYMPTOMS AND SIGNS

The onset of symptoms and signs of an extruded disk fragment may be acute or insidious. Acute symptoms may follow trauma or be unrelated to injury. Neck and radicular pain radiating down the arm occur simultaneously, but spinal cord symptoms are rare. There is usually limitation of neck motion, tenderness over the brachial nerves, and straightening of the normal cervical lordosis. Decrease in a deep tendon reflex (biceps or triceps jerk) is common with or without weakness in the muscles supplied by the compressed root. With foraminal osteophytes, episodes of cervical discomfort may recur over many months or years before radicular symptoms occur. Interscapular aching and suboccipital head-

aches are common associated complaints that may be explained as episodes of sequential radiation of referred skeletal pain. The signs and symptoms of cervical spondylosis are those of progressive cervical radiculopathy and, in advanced cases, spastic paraparesis with mild to moderate sensory deficit on the torso and in the lower extremities as well as in a cervical dermatome pattern. Neck and arm pain may or may not be present along with some limitation of cervical spine movement.

B. IMAGING STUDIES

Plain x-rays may be normal except for straightening of the cervical lordosis. The lateral view may demonstrate narrowing of one or more disk spaces. X-rays may show osteophyte formation at the appropriate neural foramen in association with disk narrowing. This is usually best seen on oblique views. In cervical spondylosis, there is usually x-ray evidence of osteophytes and disk narrowing at several levels, and in most cases with neurologic symptoms and signs, the sagittal diameter of the cervical spinal canal is also congenitally narrowed. When the diameter of the canal is 10 mm or less, clinically significant spinal cord compression can be expected to occur.

MRI is now being used with increasing success as the initial diagnostic study for patients with cervical radiculomyelopathy. Subarachnoid cerebrospinal fluid spaces, spinal cord, nerve roots, and vertebral structures can be visualized without injection of contrast material, but resolution of osseous anatomic details may not always be as clear as is obtained with CT scanning, especially for visualization of vertebral fractures.

CT scans of the spine are useful for evaluating the diameter of the canal and the foramina in patients with cervical spine stenosis. Osteophytes and posttraumatic deformities of the vertebral bodies and facet joints can be identified; soft tissue lesions such as displaced disk or hypertrophied ligaments and joint capsules that may cause compression of neural elements in patients with spondylosis are less well visualized in the cervical and thoracic areas.

Following acute disk herniation, MRI may show a small ventral extradural defect obliterating the nerve root cuff. In cervical spondylosis, the sagittal image shows bar-like ventral defects at the disk space, usually at several levels and sometimes associated with apparent widening of the cord shadow on the axial projection if the spinal diameter is narrowed. CT scanning in conjunction with myelography also provides images of the relationship between vertebral and neural elements in the axial plane or in the sagittal and oblique planes using reformatted views. With contrast material demonstrating the size and configuration of the subarachnoid space, compression or atrophy of the cervical cord and nerve roots can be clearly visualized and the lesions identified.

Differential Diagnosis

Cervical disk disease must be differentiated from traumatic and inflammatory disease affecting the soft tissues and joints of the neck and pectoral girdle, such as subdeltoid or subacromial bursitis and cervical and shoulder sprains. Nerve entrapment syndromes in the upper extremities such as cervical rib and scalenus anticus syndrome, carpal tunnel syndrome, and tardy ulnar palsy may also cause neck and arm pain, weakness, and numbness. Other conditions that must be considered include coronary insufficiency and angina pectoris; neoplasms of the pulmonary apex (eg, Pancoast tumors), primary peripheral or central nervous system tumor of the brachial plexus, cervical cord, or cervicomedullary junction; fractures, dislocations, or subluxations of the cervical spine; and inflammatory disease of the cervical theca such as arachnoiditis, sarcoidosis, and Pott's disease. The condition that is most difficult to distinguish from cervical radiculopathy is brachial neuritis, an idiopathic inflammatory disease that affects the brachial plexus.

The disorder that most frequently mimics cervical disk disease is invasion of the cervical spine by metastatic tumor. Biopsy and surgical decompression or radiation therapy are indicated as emergency procedures, especially when a pathologic fracture or epidural mass lesion threatens spinal cord function.

Complications

Permanent damage to the nerve roots and spinal cord may occur, with loss of motor and sensory function. This is particularly true in cervical stenosis and spondylosis, in which both direct pressure on the spinal cord and compression of its vascular supply may produce a severe, progressive irreversible myelopathy with spastic paraplegia or quadriplegia that does not respond to surgical decompression. Such patients are also vulnerable to acute onset of paraparesis or quadriparesis initiated by relatively mild cervical hyperextension injuries sustained during a fall or motor vehicle accident.

Treatment

A. MEDICAL MEASURES

Initially, cervical disk disease should be treated medically unless there is evidence of spinal cord compression or radicular motor loss in an extremity from severe neural compression. Medical therapy for patients suffering from radiculitis includes immobilization of the neck with a cervical collar. Physical therapy to pain sites, including mild traction with the cervical spine in a neutral position, may be helpful. Analgesics, anti-inflammatory agents, muscle relaxants, and local heat are frequently used in combination with physical therapy.

B. SURGICAL TREATMENT

There are two methods of treating cervical disk disease surgically: (1) posterior decompression of the nerve roots, spinal cord, or both, with or without fusion; and (2) anterior decompression of nerve roots spinal cord or both, with or without fusion. The choice is based on consideration of a particular patient's anatomic lesions as demonstrated with MRI, CT, or myelography. It may be necessary to use both an anterior and a posterior approach in separate stages if satisfactory recovery is not observed within 3–6 months after the initial operation.

Prognosis

Seventy-five percent of patients will recover following an adequate trial (10–14 days) of medical therapy, even though some continue to have cervical or interscapular discomfort or mild paresthesias. In some patients, radicular or myelopathic symptoms recur upon return to full activity. Although many patients with cervical disk disease can be managed symptomatically for years with intervals of physical therapy and a cervical collar, others eventually require surgical therapy. For the 25% who do not respond to conservative therapy, operation is required. Even after surgery, symptoms may reappear, perhaps because of residual or recurrent disease at the same or adjacent disk levels. In some instances, reevaluation for additional surgery is indicated.

Improvement follows operative treatment of a cervical disk in approximately 80% of patients. Surgical treatment of cervical spondylosis with myelopathy results in improvement in 70% of cases and arrest of progression in many of the remainder.

THORACIC DISK DISEASE

Although the disorder is rare, knowledge of thoracic disk disease is essential, because it is associated with significant deficit when it does occur. Occasionally, the nucleus of a thoracic disk extrudes into the spinal canal as a result of forceful trauma. Because the thoracic canal is small in relation to the spinal cord within it, severe cord compression often results from disk rupture. The onset of paraplegia is often abrupt, and paralysis may be permanent. More often, however, osteophyte formation due to a degenerated thoracic disk accounts for spinal canal narrowing. The occurrence of cord compression is then more gradual and progressive.

Treatment for ruptured thoracic disk associated with intractable pain or disabling neurologic deficit is primarily surgical and consists of removal of the offending disk or spur by the anterior thoracotomy, lateral extracavitary costo-transversectomy, or posterolateral transpedicular approach. Posterior decompression by laminectomy is the least effective approach in the thoracic area and has the highest risk of complications.

LUMBAR DISK SYNDROME

 ESSENTIALS OF DIAGNOSIS

- *History of back injury or stress or a discrete episode of spontaneous onset.*
- *Low back pain.*
- *Pain aggravated by activity and relieved by bed rest.*
- *Signs of root compression, associated with the onset of radicular radiation to the legs, eg, sciatica.*
- *Abnormal straight leg-raising test.*
- *Neurologic findings variable; usually mild.*

General Considerations

If the nucleus of a lumbar intervertebral disk extrudes through the annulus and elevates or tears the posterior longitudinal ligament, lumbosacral nerve roots may be displaced or compressed. Sensory loss, dermatomal pain, motor loss in the myotomes innervated by those roots, and loss of the knee and ankle tendon jerks may result. The severity of the syndrome produced depends upon the site and severity of nerve root compression. Occasionally, the entire cauda equina may be compressed, resulting in paraplegia and loss of motor and sensory function below the lesion, including bowel and bladder sphincter control. Disk rupture may occur in the midline, compressing centrally placed sacral nerve roots preferentially, without involvement of laterally placed lumbar roots at the level of herniation.

Disruption of a lumbar disk may occur without extrusion of the nucleus. In that event, elasticity of the joint is reduced and mobility is increased. The annulus may bulge without tearing. As time passes, osteophytes form around the degenerated disk and may encroach upon the spinal canal and foramina. Lumbar spondylosis, a condition common in the elderly, is the end result. Stenosis of the lumbar canal and foramen may also present as a developmental defect, aggravating the compressive effects of degenerative disk disease and spondylosis.

Clinical Findings

Over 90% of problems arise from the L4–5 and L5–S1 intervertebral areas, with most of the remainder occurring at L3–4. Lumbar disk disease rarely involves higher levels.

A. SYMPTOMS AND SIGNS

Although pain is usually acute when associated with frank herniation, it may also be chronic. There may be back pain, leg pain, or both. The radiation of low back pain into the buttock, posterior thigh, and calf is usually the same with disease at the L4–5 or L5–S1 interspaces. This radiating pain may be aggravated by coughing, sneezing, or the Valsalva maneuver. Bending or sitting accentuates the discomfort, whereas lying down characteristically relieves it. Most commonly, the back pain is described as deep, aching, and constant (lumbago) with a sharp shooting element traveling from the buttock down the leg posteriorly to the foot or toes (sciatica). Sometimes pain and paresthesias radiate to the groin (L3), medial thigh (L4), big toe (L5), or little toe (S1).

Palpation of the paravertebral area and the buttock (less frequently, over the vertebral spinous processes) reveals tenderness at the affected disk level or over the sciatic notch. Palpation of the sciatic nerve in the popliteal fossa may also elicit tenderness or referred pain. The paravertebral musculature may be in spasm, and reactive scoliosis may be present. Straight leg raising produces back or leg pain that may be accentuated with further stretching of the sciatic nerve (by ankle dorsiflexion). Pain produced when the leg opposite the affected side is raised is highly suggestive of disk extrusion.

Weakness of the anterior calf musculature (with the extensor hallucis longus being the first affected) is a common finding, especially with L4–5 disk herniation and L5 radiculopathy. Foot drop can occur in advanced cases. Weakness of the gastrocnemius suggests L5–S1 disease. Weakness of the quadriceps may occur with L3–4 herniation. Atrophy may be present in cases of long-standing radiculopathy. Comparison of knee and ankle reflexes is important. Depression of the ankle jerk is common with L5–S1 disease but is also present in a significant number of cases of L4–5 disease. The knee jerk may be depressed in L3–4 disease.

Sensory patterns are variable. Numbness or paresthesias in the legs are present in fewer than one-third of patients. Rarely, bowel and bladder sphincter dysfunction is reported. Hypesthesia on the dorsum of the foot is common; sensory deficit on the little toe and the lateral surface of the foot is more frequent with L5–S1 disease, and deficit on the big toe and medial aspect of the foot is more frequent with L4–5 disease.

B. IMAGING STUDIES

Plain films of the lumbosacral spine should be taken to identify congenital or acquired skeletal abnormalities.

Narrowing of the disk spaces occurs with equal frequency in symptomatic and asymptomatic patients and therefore has no diagnostic value.

MRI scans are useful to image the thecal sac, disks, and vertebral elements. Thoracolumbar tumors can be excluded and, in some instances, peridural scar tissue can be distinguished from recurrent disk herniation in postoperative patients by administration of a paramagnetic contrast agent that enhances signal intensity in scar or granulation tissue but not disk. When certain imaging parameters are selected, the cerebrospinal fluid can be demonstrated, and the need to inject contrast material into the lumbar or cervical subarachnoid space is eliminated. Lumbar puncture is not necessary. MRI of the lumbar spine is rapidly replacing both myelography and CT as the initial diagnostic procedure of choice.

CT scanning of the lumbar spine usually provides adequate diagnostic information if disk protrusion or rupture has occurred. Because the neural canal is larger in the lumbar area, soft tissue lesions such as tumors or cysts as well as spinal canal stenosis may be identified. Sagittal and coronal section reformatting of axial scans provides images showing the longitudinal configuration of the lumbar thecal sac. In patients with an appropriate history of disk rupture and a neurologic deficit that correlates anatomically with the level of abnormality shown on the CT scan, myelography may not be necessary. However, if more than one level is involved or if previous disk disease has been treated surgically, CT scanning without myelography will not provide sufficient diagnostic information.

MRI is diagnostic in 80–90% of cases and is important in localizing the disease and ruling out intraspinal tumors. The scan must include the lower thoracic cord and conus in order to eliminate the possibility of more rostral compression of the lumbosacral nerve roots by tumor or disk. False-positive and false-negative results may occur.

C. SPECIAL EXAMINATIONS

Electromyography may demonstrate denervation of the muscles in the appropriate nerve root distribution and can be used as an adjunct to neurologic examination when diagnosis is difficult. Electromyography alone is not diagnostic of disk rupture.

Although rarely indicated in current practice, discography may demonstrate an abnormal disk. Radiopaque contrast material is injected under fluoroscopic control into the disk space and a CT scan is obtained. Degenerated and extruded disks may be identified. Internal disruption or degeneration of the annulus without dislocation of the nucleus into the neural canal can be demonstrated by discography. Such information can often be obtained with MRI without injection of contrast material. Report by the patient of concordant pain typical of the predominant symptoms at one level that is also anatomically abnormal and not during injection of adjacent levels may localize the site of incapacitating discogenic back pain.

Differential Diagnosis

Back pain with radiation to the leg has many causes: (1) bony abnormalities such as spondylolisthesis, spondylosis, spinal stenosis, or Paget's disease; (2) primary and metastatic tumors of the cauda equina or the pelvic region; (3) inflammatory disorders, including abscess in the epidural space or retroperitoneal lumbosacral plexus, postinfectious or posttraumatic arachnoiditis, and rheumatoid spondylitis; (4) degenerative lesions of the spinal cord and peripheral neuropathies; and (5) peripheral vascular occlusive disease.

Treatment

A. MEDICAL MEASURES

A trial of medical treatment is indicated in all patients who do not demonstrate progressive weakness or sphincter dysfunction. This consists initially of bed rest with application of hot packs to the pain site, anti-inflammatory medications, analgesics, and skeletal muscle relaxants. Pelvic traction that partially immobilizes the patient may help relieve muscle spasm. Physical therapy and graded exercise are indicated in chronic cases or after an acute episode subsides. A corset or back brace provides external support and allows patients to return to activity earlier. A body cast or plastic jacket may be required in cases where chronic pain is relieved by immobilization.

B. SURGICAL TREATMENT

Surgical treatment is indicated in patients with progressive neurologic deficits and chronic disabling pain. Acute onset of symptoms associated with muscle weakness or sphincteric disturbance must be treated with urgent decompression.

A simple laminotomy and foraminotomy is made posteriorly at the appropriate interspace, with care to protect the nerve root and dura. Microsurgical technique allows adequate exposure through a smaller incision that reduces muscle dissection. Endoscopic instrumentation is also available and in use. If disk extrusion has occurred, the surgeon attempts to remove this piece and diligently searches for other detectable portions of the disk. When herniation without extrusion has occurred, the surgeon makes a window in the posterior longitudinal ligament and annulus and removes all accessible degenerated material from the intervertebral space. Some surgeons recommend that a fusion be done primarily or as a secondary procedure in chronic back pain cases where preoperative immobilization has relieved symptoms of joint instability. Total diskectomy through bilateral posterior laminotomies or an anterior lumbar transperitoneal approach by laparotomy can be followed by interbody fusion that replaces the disk with iliac crest bone grafts and titanium or bone dowel cages for relief of intractable discogenic pain syndromes and stabilization of the intervertebral joint. Posterior pedicle screw fixation may also be added for circumferential arthrodesis of the motion segment.

Transcutaneous injection of enzymes (eg, chymopapain, collagenase) into lumbar disks has been used in the past to dissolve fibrocartilage or collagen material to relieve pain and radiculopathy without surgery. Needle placement is guided by fluoroscopy. Although satisfactory results were reported in 60% of patients, complications related to nerve root injury, transverse myelitis, and systemic anaphylaxis occurred. Patients with fragments of disk material that detach and extrude into the spinal canal are unlikely to benefit from such treatments. Percutaneous coagulation or aspiration of degenerated disk material has been attempted through an ultrasonic nucleotome cannula, a radiofrequency electrode, or a laser probe inserted into the intervertebral space as a safer method for relieving painful in situ disk protrusions. Fragmentation and excision of pieces of degenerated fibrocartilage can also be accomplished through a fiberoptic arthroscopic cannula using microsurgical instruments under fluoroscopic or fiberoptic videoscope control. Further studies are in progress to evaluate long-term results with these techniques.

Prognosis

With medical treatment, most patients improve sufficiently to return to full activity. Lumbar disk syndrome may recur intermittently with stress or exertion. Recurrent herniation may again be treated surgically, often successfully.

About 10–20% of cases require surgical management. The best results are obtained in patients with extrusion of disk material and acute radiculopathy. Those with chronic poorly localized discogenic pain and no neurologic deficit are less likely to benefit from diskectomy. If joint instability is demonstrated at one or two levels, spinal fusion with or without discectomy may be indicated.

Thus, if the syndrome has resulted from an extruded disk fragment and is accompanied by an unequivocally positive radiographic study that correlates with clinical findings, 85% of patients will recover completely after surgical treatment. If the syndrome is not associated with a ruptured disk and a positive scan or myelogram, intensive physiotherapy for postural correction and strengthening of spinal and abdominal support musculature is indicated. Emotional and economic factors, in-

cluding litigation and compensation for injury, play an important role in outcome regardless of whether treatment is medical or surgical.

Joanes V: Cervical disc herniation presenting with acute myelopathy. Surg Neurol 2000;54:198.

Leufven C, Nordwakk A: Management of chronic disabling low back pain with 360 degrees fusion. Results from pain provocation test and concurrent posterior lumber interbody fusion, posterolateral fusion, and pedicle screw instrumentation in patients with chronic disabling low back pain. Spine 1999;24:2042.

Levi N, Gjerris F, Dons K: Thoracic disc herniation. Unilateral transpedicular approach in 35 consecutive patients. J Neurosurg Sci 1999;43:37.

Modic MT: Degenerative disc disease and back pain. Magn Reson Imaging Clin N Am 1999;7:481.

Wang JC et al: The outcome of lumbar discectomy in elite athletes. Spine 1999;24:570.

Witzmann A, Hejazi N, Krasznai L: Posterior cervical foraminotomy. A follow-up study of 67 surgically treated patients with compressive radiculopathy. Neurosurg Rev 2000;23:213.

■ SURGICAL INFECTIONS OF THE CENTRAL NERVOUS SYSTEM

Cornelia S. von Koch, MD, PhD, &
Mark L. Rosenblum, MD

BRAIN ABSCESS

 ESSENTIALS OF DIAGNOSIS

- *History of predisposing factors such as sinusitis, dental abscess, otitis, systemic infection (especially pulmonary infection or endocarditis), congenital cyanotic heart disease, or brain damage from trauma or surgery.*
- *Headache, localized neurologic signs, seizures, fever.*
- *Positive CT or MRI brain scan.*
- *Acute or subacute course (days to weeks).*
- *Immune status.*

General Considerations

Brain abscess is a relatively rare disease; large medical centers see only four to six cases each year. In patients with normal immune systems, brain abscesses usually occur secondary to intracranial extension of infections of the paranasal sinuses, middle ear, lungs, heart, and teeth. Congenital cyanotic heart disease resulting in right-to-left shunting and open cranial wounds from trauma or surgical procedures are predisposing factors for abscess formation; however, in 10–60% of patients, no cause can be identified. The organisms most commonly responsible for infections are streptococcus, staphylococcus, and enteric gram-negative rods. However, brain abscess in neonates and infants is caused exclusively by proteus and citrobacter species. Anaerobic organisms are found in 50%, with bacteroides and fusobacterium being the most common, and multiple microbes in up to 69% of cultures from abscesses; 3–50% are sterile.

Abscesses arising from frontal and ethmoid sinusitis usually occur in the frontal lobes, whereas those arising from middle ear disease occur in the posterior temporal lobe. Hematogenous abscesses commonly involve the middle cerebral artery distribution.

Immunosuppressed patients and patients with AIDS are predisposed to brain abscesses caused by fungi and protozoal infections. AIDS patients are especially vulnerable to toxoplasma, cryptococcus, nocardia, and mycobacteria.

Clinical Findings

A. SYMPTOMS AND SIGNS

The usual presenting symptoms depend on the location of the abscess and the immune status of the patient and include low-grade fever (40–70%), headache (60–90%), focal neurologic deficits (50–75%), seizures (10–50%), and an altered level of consciousness due to increased intracranial pressure (10–70%).

B. LABORATORY FINDINGS

Blood studies may show mild polymorphonuclear leukocytosis and an elevated sedimentation rate. *Lumbar puncture should not be performed with suspected abscess unless CT scan or MRI shows only a small mass or no mass.* Cerebrospinal fluid analysis is rarely helpful and often normal, with negative cultures or nonspecific results.

C. IMAGING STUDIES

The diagnosis of brain abscess is made on CT or MRI scans, which show a discrete mass with a smooth, symmetric contrast-enhancing ring, low-density center, and variable surrounding edema. Magnetic resonance spectroscopy has recently been used to better distinguish brain abscesses from ring-enhancing brain tumors.

Differential Diagnosis

Brain abscess must be differentiated from brain tumor, cerebral infarction, resolving intracranial hemorrhage, subdural empyema, extradural abscess, and encephalitis.

Complications

The major complications of brain abscess are rupture into the ventricles or subarachnoid space, obstruction of cerebrospinal fluid pathways, and transtentorial herniation, because of the mass effect of the abscess and the reactive brain swelling.

Treatment

A. MEDICAL TREATMENT

Before starting antibiotic therapy, obtain cultures of blood, nasopharyngeal secretions, sputum, urine, or draining material from paranasal sinuses or wounds, as may be indicated by the suspected source of infection. Culture of the cerebrospinal fluid should only be performed when no mass effect is seen on imaging and symptoms of meningitis are present. Whenever possible, antibiotics should not be started prior to abscess aspiration, since doing so preoperatively results in cultures that frequently do not grow out organisms.

Vancomycin, a third-generation cephalosporin, and metronidazole are started when the diagnosis is made. As soon as the organism is identified, specific antibiotics that are cytotoxic and can cross the blood-brain barrier are instituted. The duration of administration of parenteral antibiotics is largely empiric and can range from 4 weeks to 8 weeks. Infectious disease consultation is strongly advised. Toxoplasma abscesses will usually respond to treatment with pyrimethamine and sulfadiazine. Treatment of fungal abscesses relies on the use of agents such as amphotericin B, but the results have been discouraging.

Since new antibiotics with improved activity and ability to cross the blood-brain barrier are being developed every year, the reader is referred to the infectious disease literature for the most recent updates.

If there is an extracerebral focus of infection (sinus, mastoid, wound, etc), it should be drained surgically.

B. SURGICAL TREATMENT

Surgical treatment consists of excision of the abscess or aspiration through a burr hole. CT-guided stereotaxic aspiration, performed under local anesthesia, is the procedure of choice for most abscesses, especially small, deep abscesses or diseases found in patients who are poor candidates for surgery. Solitary abscesses larger than 1.5 cm in diameter and multiple abscesses larger than 3 cm in diameter should be aspirated without delay. Medical treatment is justified only if the patient has a known predisposing factor, a CT scan that suggests the presence of an abscess, is alert and either clinically stable or improving with antibiotic therapy, if the abscess is small (less than 1.5 cm in diameter), and if there is little associated mass effect or if the patient has a bleeding diathesis. Aspiration of the abscess may be necessary if the organism is not otherwise identifiable and is essential if the patient deteriorates or if CT or MRI shows an increase in abscess size. After the organism is identified, antibiotics are adjusted appropriately. Corticosteroids are given only when there is significant mass effect from the abscess and surrounding edema, both of which may put the patient at significant risk. Anticonvulsants should be used. An abscess will occasionally resolve with antibiotic treatment alone, as shown by serial CT or MRI scans. In patients with multiple abscesses, small lesions can be followed with antibiotics after the organism has been identified by aspiration of the largest lesion. The decision to treat with antibiotics alone requires frequent follow-up visits, with CT or MRI scans and treatment planning by a neurosurgeon who is ready to operate whenever the patient's condition deteriorates or serial imaging demonstrates an increase in abscess size or no change after 4 weeks of antibiotic therapy.

Postoperative CT or MRI scans are done for early detection and management of complications such as hemorrhage and recurrent abscess. Monitoring for 1 year is indicated to make certain that no recurrence develops.

LESS COMMON PYOGENIC INFECTIONS

Epidural Abscess

Epidural abscess in the cranial or spinal epidural space produces focal neurologic deficit by pressure on the underlying neural tissues. In the cranium, it is usually secondary to adjacent osteomyelitis or head trauma or to cranial operations. In the spine, epidural abscesses are usually metastatic from a remote infection in the pelvis or lower extremities, or from bacteremia usually caused by urinary tract infection or illicit intravenous drug use.

Treatment consists of immediate drainage of the pus and appropriate treatment of the primary infection with antibiotics. Operations should also be performed on the primary focal sites of infection.

Subdural Abscess

Subdural abscess or empyema, a serious complication of sinus and ear infections and of meningitis in infants, progresses rapidly and has a high death rate. Immediate

MRI scan followed by surgical drainage and antibiotic therapy are indicated.

Cerebral Thrombophlebitis

Cerebral thrombophlebitis is a rare complication of meningitis, epidural and subdural abscesses, and thrombophlebitis of facial veins. The lateral, cavernous, and superior sagittal sinuses are most commonly involved, producing neurologic deficit by venous infarction. Treatment is with specific antibiotics and surgical drainage of the original site of infection. If marked cerebral edema is associated, treatment with glucocorticoids, diuretics, and mannitol should be considered.

CLOSED DISK SPACE INFECTIONS FOLLOWING REMOVAL OF LUMBAR INTERVERTEBRAL DISK

Closed disk space infection is seen in approximately 1–3% of patients following lumbar diskectomy and is thought to be due to pyogenic infection confined to the disk space. The most common organism is *Staphylococcus aureus*. Symptoms usually occur 1–3 weeks or longer after operation. Preoperative sciatica has usually resolved when the patient complains of severe pain localized in the back and thighs, aggravated by any motion. The patient may run a low-grade fever or be afebrile; the white count may be normal or slightly elevated. The erythrocyte sedimentation rate and C-reactive protein are elevated. Starting at about 4 weeks, plain films reveal destruction of the vertebral end-plates and narrowing and eventual bony fusion of the disk space. MRI shows characteristic changes in disk spaces and vertebral bodies as early as 3–5 days after onset of symptoms.

Treatment consists of immobilization with a brace and analgesics. A needle biopsy of the interspace should be performed before antibiotic therapy is planned; antibiotics should be given for 6–8 weeks. Surgery consisting of disk space debridement and fusion is indicated if conservative treatment fails.

TUBERCULOSIS OF THE SPINE (Pott's Disease)

Tuberculous infections of the spine have recently become more prevalent in the United States due to the emergence of multidrug-resistant strains. The thoracic cord is most commonly involved, followed by the cervical cord and the lumbar cord segments. Radiographically, there is usually destruction of one or more intervertebral disks, apposition of the adjacent vertebral bodies, and destruction of one or more vertebral bodies. Soft tissue swelling is usually evident around the affected area, and a soft tissue mass of varying size is commonly present.

Treatment consists of isoniazid, rifampin, and pyrazinamide with or without ethambutol depending on the susceptibility of the organism. Continuation of antibiotic treatment for up to 12 months may be indicated. For advanced disease and unstable spines, surgical drainage and anterior or posterior fusion is necessary. The affected area must be immobilized.

Bockova J et al: Intracranial empyema. Pediatr Infect Dis J 2000; 19:735.

Calfee DP et al: Brain abscess. Semin Neurol 2000;20:353.

Heilpern KL et al: Focal intracranial infections. Infect Dis Clin North Am 1996;10:879.

Khan IA et al: Management of vertebral diskitis and osteomyelitis. Orthopedics 1999;22:758.

Luk KD: Tuberculosis of the spine in the new millennium. Eur Spine J 1999;8:338.

Moon MS: Tuberculosis of the spine: controversies and a new challenge. Spine 1997;22:1791.

Sampath P et al: Spinal epidural abscess: a review of epidemiology, diagnosis, and treatment. J Spinal Disord 1999;12:89.

Vidyasagar C, Muethy HKRS: Management of tuberculosis of the spine with neurological complications. Ann R Coll Surg Engl 1994;76:80.

Otolaryngology— Head & Neck Surgery

39

Lee D. Rowe, MD

Otolaryngology is a regional surgical specialty devoted to diseases of the head and neck. An understanding of head and neck anatomy, physiology, and pathology is necessary to manage diverse disorders of head and neck structures, ranging from hearing and communication impairments to disorders calling for facial plastic and reconstructive surgery.

■ EAR

Sound waves travel as alternating compressions and rarefactions of the elastic medium through which they are transmitted (sound travels at about 1100 ft/s [346 m/s]). Sound waves exhibit several physical characteristics, including amplitude and frequency, that are related to the subjective psychoacoustic attributes of loudness and pitch. The intensity range of human hearing is great—the most intense tone that can be perceived as sound is several million times louder than the faintest detectable one.

The auricle serves to localize sound in space and to amplify sound waves impinging on the tympanic membrane through the resonance capabilities of the external auditory canal. Sound waves strike the tympanic membrane and produce in-and-out vibrations that transmit sound energy to the ossicular chain. The tympanic membrane protects the round window from simultaneous sound exposure by interposing an air-filled middle ear space. With large perforation of the tympanic membrane, sound simultaneously strikes the round window and the tympanic membrane, decreasing the energy transmitted to the oval window.

Acoustic energy at the tympanic membrane is transformed by the malleus, incus, and stapes into energy within the oval window perilymph. Sound is amplified by the lever mechanism of the ossicular chain and also as a function of the large ratio of the tympanic membrane area to the area of the small stapes footplate. Therefore, the middle ear and ossicular system act as an efficient device for transferring acoustic energy from one elastic medium (air) to another medium of different impedance (fluid).

Movement of the stapes footplate produces a traveling wave in the scala vestibuli perilymph that is propagated along the basilar membrane of the cochlea from the base to the apex and down the scala tympani to the round window. Vibration of the basement membrane produces a shearing movement between the tectorial membrane and the hairs of the hair cells, generating electrical activity within the cochlea and auditory nerves. The point of maximal displacement of the basilar membrane is dependent upon the frequency (or pitch) of the wave. High-frequency tones cause maximal displacement near the base of the cochlea, and low-frequency tones cause maximal stimulation near the apex.

Cochlear frequency encoding involves depolarization of afferent neurons that synapse in the cochlear nuclei in the brain stem. The attendant perception of loudness and pitch depends upon the total number of neurons activated and their frequency specificities. The central auditory pathway is a complex system with many crossovers and relay stations to the auditory cortex.

CLINICAL AUDIOLOGY

Audiology is the study of hearing and disorders in sound recognition. Sound carried by air to the ear and perceived in the normal way represents hearing by **air conduction.** Tests of hearing by air conduction provide information about the patency of the external auditory canal, the efficiency of sound transmission by the tympanic membrane and the ossicular chain, and the integrity of the cochlea, acoustic nerve, and central auditory pathway. A defect in the auditory system from the external auditory canal to but not including the cochlea causes conductive hearing loss and raises the intensity threshold for perception of sound. The conductive hearing loss applies only to air conduction. Otitis media with effusion is the most common cause of conductive hearing loss in children. Other causes include ceruminous impactions in the external auditory canal, large tympanic membrane perforations, ossicular chain discontinuities from trauma or infection, otosclerosis, and temporal bone neoplasms involving the external auditory canal or middle ear.

If the sound source is placed on the skull or teeth, the vibration will directly stimulate the cochlear periplymph and bypass the external and middle ear. **Bone conduction** hearing tests thus examine the integrity of the cochlea, the eighth nerve, and the central auditory pathway. Bone conduction hearing losses are secondary to lesions of the sensory (cochlea) and neural (acoustic nerve) components of the auditory system and are designated **sensorineural** hearing losses. The most common cause of sensorineural hearing loss is aging (presbycusis), which is associated with progressive loss of outer hair cells within the organ of Corti and neural degeneration. However, noise exposure (especially industrial noise), ototoxic drugs including neomycin and other aminoglycosides, temporal bone fractures, labyrinthine infections, and arterial insufficiency may also produce sensorineural hearing disorders. Composite or mixed losses have both conductive and sensorineural elements.

Hearing is clinically evaluated by a careful history and physical examination that includes tuning fork testing, whispered voice assessment, and audiometric analysis. Because of the importance of hearing in speech acquisition and intellectual maturation, it is critical to diagnose disorders early. By noting the verbal responses to spondaic words or phrases (eg, "football," "hot dog," "childhood," "heartbreak"—taking care to sustain the accent on both syllables), the examiner can grossly establish the level of hearing loss in each ear. The degree of loss may be estimated from Table 39–1 by determining the voice level at which the words are no longer perceived.

It is important to provide masking (noise) by rubbing the tragus or hair in front of the ear not being tested when the loud whispered level is reached. Otherwise, sound or speech may cross over to the nontested ear, yielding a false result.

Table 39–1. Estimation of hearing loss by voice level.[1]

Examiner's Voice Level	Decibel Equivalent	Degree of Loss
Soft whispered voice (inaudible to examiner)	25 dB	None
Moderate whispered voice (just audible to examiner)	25–40 dB	Mild
Loud whispered voice	40–55 dB	Moderate
Moderately loud spoken voice	70–90 dB	Moderately severe
Loud spoken voice	90–120 dB	Profound

[1]The degree of hearing loss may be estimated by determining the voice level at which the patient understands the examiner's voice. If the patient hears the examiner's whispered voice distinctly, hearing is probably normal.

Further characterization of the type of hearing loss requires the use of tuning forks to differentiate a conductive from a sensorineural defect. In the **Weber test,** placement of a 512-Hz tuning fork on the skull in the midline or on the teeth stimulates both cochleae simultaneously. If the patient has a conductive hearing loss in one ear, the sound will be perceived loudest in the affected ear (ie, it will lateralize). When a unilateral sensorineural hearing loss is present, the tone is heard in the unaffected ear. The **Rinne test** compares air conduction (AC) with bone conduction (ie, AC > BC) in one ear, and commonly utilizes the 256-Hz and 512- Hz tuning forks. Sound stimulation by air in front of the pinna is normally perceived twice as long as sound placed on the mastoid tip (ie, AC > BC). With conductive hearing loss, the duration of air conduction is less than bone conduction (ie, BC > AC; negative Rinne test). In the case of sensorineural hearing loss, the duration of both air conduction and bone conduction are reduced; however, the 2:1 ratio remains the same (ie, AC > BC; positive Rinne test). The results of these two tuning fork tests are assessed to determine the type of hearing loss.

Further quantification of the type and degree of hearing loss and the ability to hear and understand speech requires pure tone audiometry, speech reception threshold testing, and speech discrimination analysis. An audiometer is an electronic device capable of delivering pure sound frequencies by both air and bone conduction from 125 Hz to 8000 Hz at intensities ranging from 0 to 110 decibels (dB) in 5-dB steps. The decibel is a logarithmic ratio of two sound pressure levels or intensities that are related to a reference intensity, measured in dynes per square centimeter. The threshold intensity of sound perception in a normal individual is 0–25 dB within the speech frequencies (300–4000 Hz). The ear has the greatest sensitivities between these frequencies, because the tympanic membrane and ossicular chain transmit sound most efficiently in this range. Pure tone audiometry will demonstrate normal thresholds at all frequencies for both air and bone conduction (Figure 39–1). A conductive hearing loss raises the threshold for sound perception in air. With air conduction hearing loss of 60 dB, for example, the threshold is 10,000-fold greater than normal (Figure 39–2). Sensorineural hearing losses result in equal increases in the threshold for air conduction and bone conduction and produce a characteristic audiogram (Figure 39–3).

Speech perception can be evaluated by presenting the patient with a list of spondaic words at an intensity corresponding to 50% comprehension. The resulting speech reception threshold should approximate the average hearing levels for the speech frequencies of 500 Hz, 1000Hz, and 2000 Hz. These frequencies are extremely important for understanding conversation in English and fall within the 300-Hz to 3000-Hz transmission range of the telephone. The ability to discrimi-

Air conduction

O	Right ear (red)
X	Left ear (blue)
△	Right ear with _____ dB masking in left
□	Left ear with _____ dB masking in right

Bone conduction

>	Right ear (red)
<	Left ear (blue)
▶	Right ear with _____ dB masking in left
◀	Left ear with _____ dB masking in right
↓	No response at maximum limits of audiometer

SPEECH DISCRIMINATION SCORES

X   LEFT EAR: 100%
O   RIGHT EAR: 100%

To convert the above readings based on the 1964 ISO reference thresholds to readings based on the 1951 ASA reference thresholds, subtract the following (rounded) difference in dB:

125	250	500	1000	2000	4000	8000
10	15	15	10	10	5	10

Figure 39–1. Normal hearing.

nate speech is ascertained by presenting a list of 50 phonetically balanced monosyllabic words 30–40 dB above the speech reception threshold. The percentage of words the patient repeats correctly is called the **discrimination score** and should normally be between 90% and 100%. In conductive hearing loss, the discrimination score is normal; in sensorineural hearing losses, the discrimination score decreases with progressive cochlear and neuronal impairment.

Because the tests described above require a voluntary response, they are of little use if age or illness prevents the patient from performing the required tasks.

Figure 39–2. Bilateral severe conductive hearing loss due to otosclerosis.

Figure 39–3. Bilateral high-frequency sensorineural hearing loss.

For example, infants with a high risk of hearing loss (eg, congenital rubella) are unable to give voluntary responses; therefore, an objective method of determining auditory thresholds is necessary to fully evaluate a suspected hearing loss. **Evoked response** or **brain stem audiometry** measures electrical responses to sound stimuli (clicks) from the acoustic nerve, cochlear nuclei, and inferior colliculi from the surface of the scalp and the mastoid prominence or ear lobe of the test ear. These techniques are particularly useful in evaluating patients with suspected sensorineural hearing losses secondary to acoustic neuroma, cerebellopontine angle tumor, or a brain stem lesion. **Brain stem evoked response audiometry (BSERA)** is especially important in newborn nurseries for identifying infants at risk of hearing impairment. These include low-birth-weight infants (< 1500 g), infants with low Apgar scores, infants with hyperbilirubinemia (> 20 mg/dL) or neonatal meningitis, or infants with the TORCH (toxoplasmosis, rubella, chlamydia) complex (Table 39–2). Accordingly, a protocol for audiologic screening of at-risk newborn infants (Table 39–3) is indicated using BSERA. If hearing loss is identified, habilitation should begin by age 6 months. BSERA is also used for evaluating potential candidates for pediatric cochlear implantation.

Gelfand SA et al: Apparent auditory deprivation in children: implications of monaural versus binaural amplification. J Am Acad Audiol 1993;4:313.

CONDUCTIVE HEARING LOSS

1. Otitis Media With Effusion

Otitis media with effusion is the leading cause of hearing loss in childhood. More than 30% of all children have had three or more episodes of otitis media by their second birthday. Although otitis media with effusion

Table 39–2. High-risk criteria for hearing loss.[1]

1. Family history of childhood hearing impairment
2. Congenital perinatal infection, eg, cytomegalovirus, rubella, herpes, toxoplasmosis, syphilis, TORCH
3. Anatomic malformation of the head or neck
4. Birthweight < 1500 g
5. Hyperbilirubinemia at level exceeding indications for exchange transfusion
6. Bacterial meningitis, especially *Haemophilus influenzae*
7. Severe asphyxia, including infants with Apgar scores of 0–3 who fail to start spontaneous respiration by 10 minutes and those with hypotonia persisting to 2 hours of age

[1]Joint Committee on Infant Hearing, 1982.

Table 39–3. Protocol for screening infants at risk for hearing loss.

1. Newborn infants with no risk factors are not screened unless the parent is concerned about auditory behavior or speech and language development. Parents of infants not at risk are to be given information and education.
2. Infants at risk are screened by BSERA prior to discharge. Parents of at-risk infants are to be given information and education.
   a. Infants who passed the screening procedure are provided with follow-up as needed for medical and developmental consideration.
   b. Infants who pass the screening procedure but are at risk for progressive hearing impairment are monitored audiologically and managed as needed.
   c. Infants who fail the screening procedure are evaluated, given follow-up, and provided with a management system.

occurs in all age groups, it is most common from the newborn period to age 7. The term **nonsuppurative otitis media** denotes a broad range of middle ear effusions characterized by an inflammatory exudate and various amounts of mucus. Several distinct types are recognized: (1) serous otitis media—a sterile, pale, low-viscosity transudate; (2) secretory otitis media—a chronic **glue ear** with infiltration of lymphocytes, histiocytes, plasma cells, leukocytes, and markedly increased glandular production of mucus; and (3) aerotitis media secondary to barotrauma or direct temporal bone injury. Chronic otitis media with effusion is unsterile in 50% of cases; *Haemophilus influenzae, Streptococcus pneumoniae, Moraxella catarrhalis,* and *Streptococcus pyogenes* are the organisms most often found. Although many factors may be implicated, including rhinoviruses, upper respiratory bacteria, passive smoking, and inflammatory mediators of arachidonic acid metabolism, the common denominator appears to be auditory tube (eustachian tube) dysfunction. The physiologic role of the auditory tube is to protect the middle ear from nasopharyngeal secretions, clear middle ear secretions into the nasopharynx, and, more importantly, ventilate the middle ear space. Auditory tube dysfunction develops from barotrauma when the nasopharyngeal pressure exceeds middle ear pressure during rapid descent in an airplane or from adenoidal hypertrophy that produces lymphatic or mechanical obstruction of the auditory tube. In addition, over half of children with cleft palate deformities manifest auditory tube dysfunction secondary to malfunction of the tensor veli palatini muscle, resulting in inefficient opening of the auditory tube.

If auditory tube function is compromised—as it frequently is in young children—early diagnosis and treatment are critical to prevent impairment of speech development. On physical examination, the tympanic membrane is retracted, the short process of the malleus is extremely prominent, and the light reflex is frequently lost. Pneumatic otoscopy discloses marked reduction of tympanic membrane mobility, and a characteristic yellow or amber color is often seen in the middle ear space. Middle ear effusions can be confirmed by the presence of an air-fluid level in the middle ear.

Unfortunately, otoscopy is not a reliable method of assessing middle ear effusions. Impedance audiometry (tympanometry) is a more accurate means of diagnosing otitis media with effusion. The overall compliance of the tympanic membrane and middle ear system, which varies inversely with its impedance, is measured by delivering to the tympanic membrane a continuous 220-Hz tone signal via a sealed probe tip and recording the amount of energy reflected from the surface. The pressure in the external auditory canal is varied from +400 mm H_2O to −400 mm H_2O, and the reflected energy is recorded. The resulting tympanogram correlates well with the presence or absence of effusion. A normal type A tympanogram is characterized by peak compliance at 0 mm H_2O pressure; the absence of a peak of maximal compliance is commonly encountered in middle ear effusion (type B tympanogram). By contrast, type C tympanograms exhibits a peak of maximal compliance of less than −100 mm of H_2O and are chiefly associated with a retracted tympanic membrane with or without effusion.

Initial management of otitis media with effusion consists of identifying the cause. In adults, a malignant neoplasm of the nasopharynx such as carcinoma or lymphoma should be carefully excluded. Unilateral hearing loss secondary to otitis media with effusion is a common manifestation of obstruction of the auditory tube by tumor. Allergy and enlargement of the adenoids may play a causative role in children. Group day care settings are associated with a high risk of otitis media with effusion. Conservative treatment with sympathomimetic amines and antihistamines is often attempted first, though there is no evidence that they alter the clinical course. Nonoperative therapy also includes antibiotics, autoinflation (Valsalva's maneuver), and control of etiologic factors (nasal infections, sinusitis, allergy, etc). Many consultants would start with a course of amoxicillin in doses twice the current recommendations of 40 mg/kg/d in three divided doses. Some patients may respond to a 3- to 4-week course of antibiotics. Failure of medical treatment necessitates myringotomy and insertion of ventilating tubes (Figure

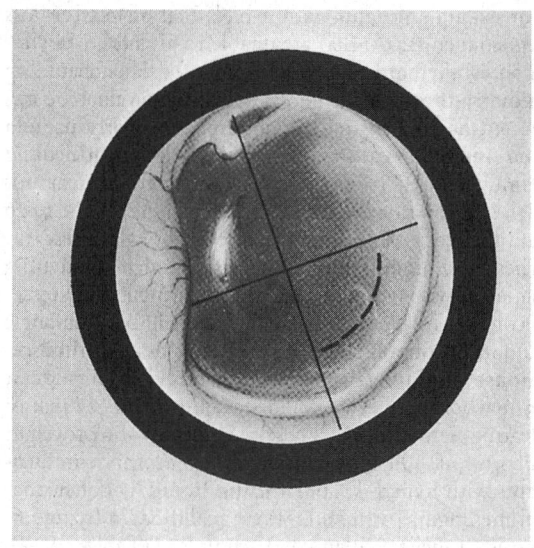

Figure 39–4. Site of myringotomy.

39–4). Usually this is defined as 3 months of chemoprophylaxis with amoxicillin-clavulanate potassium, amoxicillin, or sulfisoxazole. Current indications for sustained middle ear ventilation with tubes include (1) significant conductive hearing loss; (2) persistent tympanic membrane atelectasis and negative middle ear pressure of less than 150 mm H_2O; (3) cleft palate; and (4) impending cholesteatoma. Approximately 80% of intubated patients respond after one insertion and require no further treatment. Surgical treatment immediately corrects the conductive hearing loss, reduces the incidence of recurrent infections, and improves the child's learning capacity. Adenoidectomy, which is recommended for children requiring more than one set of myringotomy tubes, reduces recurrent middle ear infections, since chronically infected adenoids obstruct the auditory tube and serve as a persistent source of infection in the middle ear. Otitis media-prone children carry nontypable *H influenzae* at an unusually high rate.

Bluestone CD et al: "Appropriateness" of tympanostomy tubes: setting the record straight. Arch Otolaryngol Head Neck Surg 1994;120:1051.

Grundfast KM: Management of otitis media and the New Agency for Health Care Policy and Research Guideline. Arch Otolaryngol Head Neck Surg 1994;120:797.

Managing otitis media with effusion in young children. Arch Otolaryngol Head Neck Surg 1994;120:793.

Rosenfeld RM: Comprehensive management of otitis media with effusion. Otolaryngol Clin North Am 1994;27:443.

2. Chronic Otitis Media

The long-term sequela of chronic auditory tube dysfunction is chronic otitis media, which involves chronic perforation of the tympanic membrane that may or may not be associated with recurrent acute suppuration, destruction of the ossicular chain, or both. The perforation of the tympanic membrane may take two forms: (1) a central (or safe) perforation, in which a remnant of the tympanic membrane is interposed between the rim of the perforation and the annulus of the tympanic membrane (Figure 39–5); and (2) marginal (or dangerous) perforation, in which the annulus of the tympanic membrane has been destroyed, primarily in the posterosuperior quadrant. In the former case, the middle ear is usually dry; in the latter, suppuration commonly occurs. The pars flaccida is frequently involved in marginal perforations, and central perforations are restricted to the pars tensa. However, suppuration may develop in either situation as a result of the introduction of staphylococci or gram-negative rods (commonly *Pseudomonas aeruginosa,* klebsiellae, and Enterobacteriaceae) via the auditory tube or external auditory canal. Foul-smelling otorrhea characteristic of anaerobic streptococcal infection should be treated by vacuum drainage of the external auditory canal and instillation of neomycin plus polymyxin otic drops with or without an oral fluoroquinolone such as ciprofloxacin, norfloxacin, grepafloxacin, or ofloxacin. These are avoided, however, in children aged 16 and younger and in infants. Alternative therapy may be instituted with gentamicin drops plus clindamycin orally, or tobramycin with hydrocortisone topically. Some clinicians add metronidazole to this regimen. In recalcitrant cases, parenteral azlocillin, ticarcillin, or ceftazidime may prove beneficial if no cholesteatoma is present. Intravenous ciprofloxacin or grepafloxacin may also be considered in adults.

Complications of chronic otitis media such as seventh nerve paralysis, labyrinthitis, lateral semicircular canal fistula, petrositis (Gradenigo's syndrome), or intracranial suppuration are less frequently associated with central perforations than with marginal ones. If squamous epithelium migrates into the middle ear or mastoid, a keratinizing aural cholesteatoma develops. The desquamating epithelium produces bone-destroying collagenase and tends to remain infected. The associated middle ear inflammation interferes with the tenuous blood supply to the stapes and the long process of the incus, resulting in ossicular destruction with a conductive hearing loss of 50–60 dB. White amorphous debris is often observed in the pars flaccida. If untreated, a cholesteatoma may progressively destroy the ossicular chain and erode into the inner ear, producing profound hearing loss. Computed tomography is essential in the management of chronic otitis media in determining the extent of the disease, the presence of any associated complications, and the degree of pneumatization of the mastoid. For example, the finding of a large radiolucent defect secondary to bone destruction may imply an aggressive cholesteatoma.

Bacterial invasion of the cranium from an infected cholesteatoma may occur as a result of osteitis, thrombophlebitis, bony erosion, or along a preformed pathway such as the oval or round windows, perilymphatic duct, or endolymphatic duct. In the preantibiotic era, the onset of severe temporoparietal headache and nuchal rigidity in a patient with chronic otitis media was an ominous sign. The most common intracranial complication of chronic otitis media is meningitis secondary to pneumococcal or other streptococcal infection. Additional potential problems include epidural abscesses, temporal lobe abscess, cerebellar abscess, lateral sinus thrombosis, subdural empyema, and otitic hydrocephalus. Fortunately, these complications are now rare and can be prevented by early surgical treatment of chronic otitis media and cholesteatoma. Intracranial complications of chronic otitis media are best evaluated by MRI with or without CT. Management includes drainage, mastoidectomy, and penicillin or clindamycin (for anaerobic bacteria) and ceftazidime (for pseudomonas, staphylococcus, and most gram-negative species) as initial agents. An alternative antibiotic choice is tobramycin and ticarcillin/clavulanate.

Figure 39–5. Perforation of eardrum.

Simple central tympanic membrane perforations are repaired by grafting the tympanic membrane with temporalis fascia or canal wall skin. In the absence of cholesteatoma, associated ossicular discontinuity is repaired with an autogenous homograft or alloplastic materials to reestablish the sound-transforming capability of the middle ear. With advanced middle ear and mastoid disease and associated cholesteatoma, more radical surgery is required. In a radical mastoidectomy, the remnants of the tympanic membrane, ossicles, and cholesteatoma are removed and the mastoid air cells, antrum, and middle ear are converted into an open cavity that is periodically inspected and cleaned. If the cholesteatoma lies above and superficial to the tympanic membrane and middle ear ossicles, either a canal wall-up mastoidectomy or canal wall-down mastoidectomy is performed depending on the location of the cholesteatoma. The primary goal of each is to eradicate infection and provide a temporal bone free of cholesteatoma.

Merfield DO et al: Therapeutic management of chronic suppurative otitis media with otic drops. Otolaryngol Head Neck Surg 1993;109:77.

Naguib MB et al: Surgical management of epitympanic cholesteatoma with intact ossicular chain: the modified Bondy Technique. Otolaryngol Head Neck Surg 1994;111: 545.

3. Otosclerosis

In otosclerosis, a unique localized disease of the otic capsule, new spongy bone replaces normal bone, producing ankylosis or fixation of the stapes footplate. The resulting primarily conductive hearing loss starts insidiously in the third and fourth decades of life and progressively involves both ears in 80% of individuals. Otosclerosis is an inherited disease, more common in whites, with an incidence of approximately 12% in temporal bone series. Bilateral otosclerosis is present more commonly in women by a ratio of 2:1. In adults with normal-appearing tympanic membranes, it is the most common cause of progressive conductive hearing loss. Evaluation of the hearing loss requires tuning fork and audiometric testing, including air conduction, bone conduction, and speech audiometry. The patient with a significant hearing loss secondary to otosclerosis has several options. If the hearing loss is unilateral, no treatment may be necessary. Hearing aids or surgery can be offered to improve hearing. The complete-in-the-canal hearing aid, which fits close to the tympanic membrane of the ear canal, is extremely effective for patients with otosclerosis. The hearing loss may be treated in selected cases by microsurgical removal of the stapes and reconstruction with a metallic prosthesis (3.7–4.5 mm in length) crimped over the long process of the incus. The medial end of the prosthesis is placed over vein or fascia inserted in the oval window. Alternatively, a small hole is created in the footplate of the stapes with a pick or microdrill (stapedotomy) and a Teflon wire or platinum ribbon prosthesis (4.25–0.5 mm) inserted. Argon, KTP (potassium titonyl phosphate), and CO_2 lasers can be used for small-fenestra stapedotomy. Stapedectomy or stapedotomy corrects the conductive hearing loss in most patients and may cause partial or total sensorineural hearing loss in fewer than 1% of patients. Revision stapedectomy may be necessary because of recurrent conductive hearing loss or because of a suspected oval window fistula associated with vertigo, fluctuating hearing loss, or tinnitus.

Emmett JR: Physical examination and clinical evaluation of the patient with otosclerosis. Otolaryngol Clin North Am 1993; 26:353.

Glasscock M et al: Twenty-five years of experience with stapedectomy. Laryngoscope 1995;105:899.

Vartiainen E et al: Hearing levels of patients with otosclerosis 10 years after stapedectomy. Otolaryngol Head Neck Surg 1993; 108:251.

SENSORINEURAL HEARING LOSS

Disorders affecting the cochlea and auditory neurons distort the perception of sound, producing sensorineural hearing loss. The deficit is generally greater in the higher frequencies and is associated with decreased speech discrimination scores (ie, ability to understand complex speech is impaired). It is estimated that one out of a thousand individuals have significant hearing impairment at birth. Children born with bilateral profound hearing loss or who acquire profound hearing loss before speech acquisition (2 years of age) are termed prelingually deafened. Those children and adults deafened after language development are termed postlingually deafened.

The most common cause of sensorineural hearing loss is presbycusis, a gradual deterioration that starts after 20 years of age in the highest frequencies and often involves all speech frequencies by the sixth and seventh decades. The impaired hearing stems from degenerative changes in the hair cells, auditory neurons, and cochlear nuclei. Tinnitus (ringing in the ear) is a common complaint. Hearing rehabilitation includes physician counseling and formal aural rehabilitation, encompassing the range from assisted listening devices, in-the-canal aids, in-the-ear aids, behind-the-ear aids, body aids, and bone conduction aids up to cochlear implants. Profound bilateral sensorineural hearing loss in adults who are postlingually deaf and unresponsive to conventional amplification may benefit from cochlear implants. A cochlear implant provides sound awareness, permits identification of environmental sounds, and improves ability to communicate through auditory clues such as prosody, rhythm, and intensity. A cochlear implant has two components: an external component, consisting of a small microphone to pick up auditory information, a speech processor that changes the mechanical acoustical sound energy into an electrical transmitter coil to send the information via radiofrequency through the skin; and an internal component, consisting of one or more electrodes implanted directly into the cochlea as well as a signal receiver and stimulator that interprets the electrical signal sent by the processor.

Injury to the inner ear or acoustic trauma from a sudden very loud noise (ie, painful, > 140 dB) may produce a permanent sensorineural hearing loss. More importantly, prolonged exposure (8 hours daily or more) to intense nonpainful sound such as industrial noise above 90 dB may result in destruction of the outer hair cells of the organ of Corti and a sensorineural hearing loss that characteristically initially affects perception at 4000 Hz. These patients may also experience tinnitus. Up to 10 million Americans are routinely exposed to potentially hazardous noise levels. Further noise exposure should be prevented with ear protectors (earmuffs or earplugs) and a hearing conservation program initiated at work.

Additional causes of sudden sensorineural hearing loss include diabetes mellitus, hypothyroidism, cochlear artery insufficiency, aminoglycosides, ototoxic diuretics (eg, ethacrynic acid), antimetabolites such as cisplatin and mechlorethamine, tumors of the vestibular nerve (vestibular schwannoma) or cerebellopontine angle, perilymph fistulas, trauma, autoimmune inner ear disorders such as Cogan's syndrome, Wegener's granulomatosis and systemic lupus erythematosus, congenital inner ear malformations, multiple sclerosis, and AIDS. Rubella in the first trimester of pregnancy, Rh incompatibility, birth trauma, hyperbilirubinemia, prematurity, congenital syphilis, meningitis, treatment of postnatal infection with ototoxic drugs such as kanamycin, gentamicin, tobramycin, and streptomycin, and congenital anomalies are often associated with profound bilateral prelingual deafness, and infants at risk should be tested immediately with brain stem evoked response audiometry (BSERA). Unfortunately, over 90% of infants with congenital sensorineural hearing loss have no known risk factors. Genetic causes for sensorineural hearing loss in children resulting in pre- and postlingual deafness represent approximately 50% of the cases. The remainder are divided equally among environmental and idiopathic causes. Profoundly impaired children with puretone averages at 500, 1000, and 2000 Hz greater than 90 dB who are unable to detect speech at 60 dB or greater with an appropriately fitted hearing aid should be considered for cochlear implantation.

Children must be at least 2 years of age at most centers to be considered for implantation.

In cases of sudden sensorineural hearing loss when no cause can be identified, viruses such as mumps, measles, influenza, and adenoviruses are the most likely cause. Laboratory testing, which is essential to determine the cause, may include a complete blood count, erythrocyte sedimentation rate, determination of rheumatoid arthritis factor and antinuclear antibody levels, quantitative serum immunoglobulin levels, FTA-ABS, fasting blood glucose, serum cholesterol and triglycerides, and thyroid functions tests. In addition, MRI with gadolinium testing should be done. Prednisone (60 mg daily for 9 days and then tapering over 5 days) may be beneficial in preventing permanent hearing loss.

Callanan V et al: Cochlear implantation for children and adults. Lancet 1996;347:412.

Dodds A et al: Cochlear implantation after bacterial meningitis: the dangers of delay. Arch Dis Child 1997;76:139.

Langman AW et al: Cochlear implants in children. Pediatr Clin North Am 1996;43:1217.

OTALGIA

Ear pain may be caused by a primary disorder of the ear or may be referred from structures with a common sensory innervation. Inflammation of tissues innervated by the fifth cranial nerve—including the nose, paranasal sinuses, nasopharynx, mandible, and salivary glands—may produce otalgia. Inflammatory lesions of the oropharynx, the larynx, and the base of the tongue are commonly associated with otalgia. Unfortunately, however, neoplastic lesions do not produce otalgia until they are significantly advanced.

Inflammation of the external auditory canal (otitis externa) is commonly caused by bacteria (*Proteus mirabilis, Pseudomonas aeruginosa,* staphylococci) and occasionally by otomycoses (*Aspergillus niger, Candida albicans*). Predisposing causes are water immersion, high humidity, instrumentation in the external auditory canal, and ceruminous impaction. Patients complain of otalgia, pruritus, otorrhea, and decreased hearing and intermittent blockage of the canal. Pain on traction of the pinna or tragus differentiates otitis externa from acute otitis media. Hyperemia, edema, and otorrhea are seen on inspection of the external auditory canal. Treatment consists of early precise debridement, topical broad-spectrum antibiotics (eg, polymyxin B, bacitracin, neomycin), and hydrocortisone to reduce canal wall inflammation. In neomycin-sensitive individuals, topical 2% aqueous acetic acid is effective. Contact with water should be avoided, and dry heat hastens resolution. Diabetics are particularly at risk of developing pseudomonas invasive otitis externa. If untreated, invasive otitis externa can progressively involve the underlying skin, cartilage, or bone, leading eventually to osteomyelitis of the skull, multiple cranial nerve palsies, and death. Patients with invasive otitis externa are treated with immediate debridement and an intravenous semisynthetic penicillin such as ticarcillin with clavulanate, mezlocillin, piperacillin, or azlocillin, and an aminoglycoside (tobramycin or amikacin) for 4–6 weeks. Some clinicians would choose imipenem or meropenem as the primary choice. Monotherapy with ceftazidime has proved effective in some cases. Two fluoroquinolones, ciprofloxacin (available for intravenous use) and ofloxacin, administered orally may be effective for invasive pseudomonas otitis externa. Most clinicians would switch to oral antibiotics only when pain, drainage, and granulation tissue are substantially decreased. At 4 weeks of therapy a gallium scan (which identifies collections of granulocytes) is obtained. If the patient is symptom-free and the scan is negative, antibiotics are discontinued and the patient is followed clinically. If symptoms persist and the scan remains positive, treatment for an additional 2–3 weeks is continued. A repeat scan is obtained. Late to advanced malignant external otitis requires more than 6 weeks of intravenous antibiotics, reserving surgery for a walled-up abscess or dead bone that serves as a nidus of infection.

Inflammation that progresses to involve the auricular appendage may result in **perichondritis** and then **chondritis** with cartilaginous necrosis. Perichondritis or chondritis of the pinna may also follow auricular trauma and hematoma, frostbite, or surgical drainage of a furuncle of the external auditory canal. It is manifested by edema, erythema, and tenderness of the pinna. Treatment consists of a systemic antistaphylococcal penicillin or, as an alternative, cephalothin or clindamycin and incision and drainage of any hematoma or abscess. Cotton soaked in an antiseptic solution (eg, povidone iodine) is placed within the recesses of the auricle, and a mastoid dressing is applied. Failure to adequately drain an auricular hematoma or abscess will result in a **cauliflower ear** deformity secondary to cartilaginous destruction and fibrosis.

Paradise JL: Managing otitis media: a time for change. Pediatrics 1995;96:712.

Poole MD: Otitis media complications and treatment failures: implications of pneumococcal resistance. Pediatr Infect Dis J 1995;14(4 Suppl):S23.

ACUTE OTITIS MEDIA

Acute suppurative otitis media is a very common problem in pediatric and family practice, with otalgia the most common ear complaint in childhood. Twenty per-

cent of children under 8 years of age experience at least one episode. The peak prevalence is between 6 and 11 months of age. Recurrence is common, especially if the initial episode occurs during the first 12 months of life. Viruses may cause otitis media, but suppuration is predominantly caused by bacteria, especially *S pneumoniae*. *H influenzae*, *M catarrhalis*, *S pyogenes* (group A) or *S aureus*, and anaerobes are also seen. *H influenzae* (non-type B) infection occurs more commonly in the age group under 5 years. In the newborn, gram-negative infections with *Escherichia coli*, *Klebsiella pneumoniae*, enterobacter species, *P aeruginosa*, and *P mirabilis* predominate.

The presenting clinical signs and symptoms are variable: In adults, otalgia and a conductive hearing loss are most common; infants may exhibit only fever, lethargy, or irritability. The tympanic membrane is commonly red, bulging, and extremely painful. Spontaneous perforation of the tympanic membrane with purulent otorrhea and hemorrhage is often present in infants when first seen by a physician. Prompt antibiotic therapy hastens resolution of the disease and prevents the development of temporal bone and intracranial complications. Topical vasoconstrictors such as phenylephrine should be instilled into the nasal cavities, and systemic vasoconstrictors, including ephedrine, pseudoephedrine, or phenylpropanolamine, may be prescribed to improve auditory tube function. In nonallergic low-risk patients over 6 weeks of age, amoxicillin may be recommended, and erythromycin and sulfisoxazole may be used in penicillin-allergic individuals. Patients who fail to respond may have an infection caused by β-lactamase-producing *H influenzae* type B and should be given cefpodoxime, cefprozil, loracarbef, cefuroxime, or cefixime. In infants under 1 month of age, therapy must also be directed against gram-negative enteric organisms.

Emerging *S pneumoniae* resistance to penicillin secondary to alterations of penicillin-binding proteins may require limiting choices to amoxicillin or amoxicillin and clavulanate at doses of 80–100 mg/d in divided doses, based upon the amoxicillin component. When penicillin-resistant pneumococci cause bacteremia or other more serious infections, vancomycin with or without ceftriaxone is the treatment of choice. In infants with impending otologic or intracranial complications such as meningitis, labyrinthitis, or lateral sinus thrombosis, ceftriaxone is recommended. In children over 4–6 weeks of age, *H influenzae* type B is the most common cause of meningitis. Because of this organism's high resistance to ampicillin and rare resistance to chloramphenicol, ceftazidime or ceftriaxone is recommended. Early administration of dexamethasone in children with meningitis in a dosage of 0.15 mg/kg four times a day for 4 days may lower the incidence of severe hearing loss. Myringotomy is indicated to relieve severe pain unresponsive to opioids or to identify antibiotic-resistant organisms. The development of sudden facial paralysis is an indication for emergency myringotomy. The incision should be made in the posteroinferior quadrant, midway between the umbo and the annulus. When repeated episodes of acute otitis media occur, it is important to rule out associated infection such as chronic adenoiditis or chronic sinusitis. Occasionally it is necessary to do serum IgG subclass testing to identify immune system immaturity. Children who continue to have episodes of otitis media in spite of adequate chemoprophylaxis and who do not clear their middle ear effusions between episodes should undergo tympanostomy tube placement.

Alho OP et al: Which children are being operated on for recurrent acute otitis media? Arch Otolaryngol Head Neck Surg 1994;120:807.

Haddad J: Treatment of acute otitis media and its complications. Otolaryngol Clin North Am 1994;27:431.

ACUTE MASTOIDITIS

Acute mastoiditis is a complication of acute otitis media and develops as a result of pus retention in the mastoid. It is most likely caused by *S pneumoniae; H influenzae* and *S aureus* are also commonly identified. The destruction of bony septa results in a coalescence of mastoid air cells and subsequent erosion of the cortices of the mastoid process of the temporal bone. Otalgia, aural discharge, and fever are characteristically observed 2–3 weeks after an episode of acute suppurative otitis media. Examination reveals severe mastoid tenderness, lateral displacement of the pinna, or postauricular mastoid swelling secondary to subperiosteal abscess. Ceftriaxone with or without metronidazole is given, and if a subperiosteal abscess develops, the mastoid and its air cells must be surgically drained. Alternative antibiotic choices include imipenem or chloramphenicol plus vancomycin or nafcillin. A complete mastoidectomy through a postauricular incision includes exenteration of the infected bone and pus and inspection of the dura of the posterior and middle cranial fossae to exclude epidural abscess.

FOREIGN BODIES IN THE EAR

Foreign bodies of the external auditory canal frequently traumatize the epithelium and may also perforate the tympanic membrane or disrupt the ossicular chain, producing a conductive hearing loss. Oval or round window injury may cause a concomitant sensorineural hearing loss. All kinds of objects are inserted into the external canal, especially by children. In addition, insects such as cockroaches may enter the canal, attaching their pincers to the tympanic membrane. Most foreign bodies can be removed with a right-angled hook or forceps if they are not lodged significantly medial to the isthmus of the external auditory canal. Gentle expulsion of nonvegetable matter with a soft rubber syringe (similar to the removal of cerumen) is effective. In young children or adults with firmly embedded objects, a general anesthetic is necessary to avoid injuring the tympanic membrane or ossicular chain. Insects may be suffocated by instilling mineral oil or lidocaine into the external auditory canal.

Bressler K et al: Ear foreign body removal: a review of 98 consecutive cases. Laryngoscope 1993;103:367.

TINNITUS

Tinnitus is the subjective sensation of noise in the ear or head not of psychogenic origin. Tinnitus is extremely common, affecting an estimated 10 million Americans. It is reported by patients as a constant or intermittent buzzing, ringing, or humming sound. Tinnitus originates from the inner ear when localized loss of outer hair cells occurs while the inner hair cells are still functional. An accompanying decrease of neuronal signals coming from the outer hair cell system leads to compensatory mechanisms within the auditory pathways which enhance tinnitus-related neuronal activity. The presence of depression and anxiety increases the perception of tinnitus. It has been estimated that up to 50% of tinnitus sufferers are depressed. Tinnitus is experienced by patients with presbycusis, noise-induced hearing loss, ceruminous impaction, otosclerosis, temporomandibular joint disorders, and otitis media (acute and chronic). Exposure to ototoxic drugs, closed head trauma, endolymphatic hydrops (Meniere's disease), and vestibular schwannoma (acoustic neuroma) are other causes. Highly vascular lesions of the temporal bone less commonly may elicit pulsatile tinnitus; examples are glomus jugulare or tympanicum tumors (non-chromaffin-producing neoplasms of paraganglionic cell origin). Aneurysms or arteriovenous malformations are rare causes of true tinnitus. In fact, pulsatile tinnitus can emanate from any arterial or venous structure within the cranial cavity, head and neck region, and thoracic cavity. The venous type can originate from jugular bulb anomalies but also occurs in young morbidly obese women suffering from benign intracranial hypertension.

Comprehensive management includes assessment of hypertension, blood lipids, thyroid function, and allergies and informing patients of factors that aggravate tinnitus, including stress, caffeine, nicotine, and aspirin. Treatment is determined by the primary disease, but since most cases are caused by presbycusis, effective therapy is often unavailable. Attempts at symptomatic relief have included diuretics, antihistamines (eg, dexchlorpheniramine maleate), anticonvulsants (eg, clonazepam), anxiolytics such as alprazolam and diazepam, and antidepressants (eg, nortriptyline, amitriptyline). Masking of tinnitus with frequency-specific hearing aids or extraneous noise such as a radio or stereo—especially before sleep—may be helpful in motivated patients. Biofeedback therapy has been used successfully in anxious patients. Cochlear nerve section may be offered when hearing acuity is severely diminished, and in rare circumstances microvascular decompression of the intracranial portion of the auditory nerve may provide relief from incapacitating tinnitus. Recent success has been reported with an electrical radiofrequency transmitter transmitting audio frequencies across the skin. Other modalities, including acupuncture, psychotherapy, and hypnotherapy, have given inconsistent results and are not recommended. Currently, habituation training aimed at habituating the reactions induced by tinnitus and blocking out the perception of tinnitus is being studied.

Brooke GB: Vascular decompression surgery for severe tinnitus. Am J Otol 1996 17:569.

Jastreboff PJ et al: Neurophysiological approach to tinnitus patients. Am J Otol 1996;17:236.

Nodar RH: Tinnitus reclassified: new oil in an old lamp. Otolaryngol Head Neck Surg 1996;114:582.

TEMPORAL BONE FRACTURES

Fractures of the skull base from blunt trauma commonly involve the temporal bone. Hemorrhagic otorrhea, ecchymosis of the postauricular area (Battle's sign), and disturbances in cochlear or vestibular function may be encountered. Eighty percent of fractures of the temporal bone are longitudinal to the petrous ridge; the remainder are transverse or perpendicular. Longitudinal fractures are chiefly secondary to parietal blows with the fracture line extending across the floor of the middle cranial fossa and through the roof of the external auditory canal, rupturing the tympanic membrane. The incudostapedial joint is frequently disrupted and requires ossiculoplastic reconstruction. The labyrinth is often spared, and only 35% of patients develop a sensorineural hearing loss. Twenty percent of patients develop delayed seventh nerve paralysis caused by ischemia and compression rather than neural disruption.

Transverse fractures, on the other hand, are caused by a blow to the occiput and are associated with a higher death rate. The fracture may involve the foramen magnum, pass through or near the jugular foramen, and cross the internal auditory canal to reach the foramen lacerum or foramen spinosum. Often the fracture line will splinter to reach the medial wall of the inner ear. The tympanic membrane remains intact, with a blue-black hemotympanum, and cerebrospinal fluid rhinorrhea is not uncommon. In one-third to one-half of cases, the seventh nerve is lacerated or transected, typically in the labyrinthine or mastoid segment, resulting in immediate facial paralysis. In addition, disruption of the membranous labyrinth leads to complete loss of cochlear-vestibular function and subsequent sensorineural hearing loss and vertigo.

If there is a cerebrospinal fluid leak, it is treated with head elevation, fluid restriction, and diuretics. In 85% of cases, the leak stops by 7 days and no repair is necessary. If the leak continues beyond several weeks, surgical repair is indicated. The development of progressive facial paralysis and loss of greater than 90% electrical stimulability of the facial nerve within 2 weeks requires immediate neuronal decompression of the facial canal. If the nerve has been anatomically disrupted, debridement and end-to-end anastomosis or nerve grafting will be necessary.

NEOPLASMS OF THE SKULL BASE

Squamous cell and **basal cell carcinomas** are the most common malignant tumors of the pinna, occurring in sun-exposed individuals. Small lesions may be removed by V-wedge excision while those complex morpheaform neoplasms require MOHS (microscopically oriented histologic surgical) technique for primary control. Adjunctive radiation therapy is considered for recurrent or deeply invasive tumors. Tumors invading the cartilage require wide surgical excision. Melanoma of the pinna is a dangerous neoplasm which can spread to the cervical lymph node chain as well as distantly. Most melanomas can be removed with wedge resection while some require partial or total auriculectomy. A functional elective neck dissection is considered for lesions over 1.5 mm thick. Squamous cell or basal cell carcinomas arising in the external auditory canal require wide excision for the best chance of cure. MRI is important to define surgical limits, as it better visualizes infiltration of the infratemporal fossa, parotid, dura, and temporomandibular joint than CT scanning. En bloc resection of the external auditory canal is possible for lesions not involving the middle ear or mastoid, whereas more invasive tumors require parotidectomy, partial or total temporal bone resection, and, for tumors extending beyond the temporal bone, skull base surgery. Squamous cell carcinomas arising in the middle ear should be treated by resection of the temporal bone combined with full-course radiation therapy (6000–7000 cGy).

Glomus jugulare and **glomus tympanicum** tumors are vascular neoplasms that usually arise from the jugular bulb and tympanic plexus, respectively. Both tumors spread cephalically and posteriorly into the middle ear and mastoid. Both are non-chromaffin-producing paragangliomas and are histologically the same as carotid body tumors, the most common chemodectomas of the neck. In addition, a **glomus vagale** neoplasm arising in the skull base and neck may extend superiorly into the cranial vault. The natural history of these tumors is one of slow, progressive growth and gradual invasion of the jugular foramen and its nerves (cranial nerves IX, X, XI) as well as cranial nerves VII, XII, and VIII. The overall incidence of central nervous system invasion is less than 20%.

The principal manifestation of a tumor of the middle ear is conductive hearing loss and a violaceous retrotympanic mass; pulsatile tinnitus is often present if the tumor is highly vascular. **Brown's sign** may be present (pulsation of the tympanic membrane that is inhibited by positive pressure applied to the tympanic membrane by a pneumatic otoscope). Thin-section, high-resolution CT scanning in combination with gadolinium-enhanced MRI is used to delineate the extent of tumor. Angiography is used for preoperative assessment of tumors requiring embolization. The treatment of choice is lateral cranial base surgical removal if the lesion does not involve the carotid siphon and has not spread by distant metastases. Small glomus tympanicum tumors may be cured by total surgical removal. When intracranial extension is present, a neurosurgical approach is required in addition to the neuro-otologist's lateral skull-based surgery. Radiotherapy causes tumor shrinkage but not eradication and is best combined with surgical excision of the tumor.

Benign facial nerve schwannoma is another skull base and temporal bone neoplasm. This fusiform lesion typically is elongated to involve more than one segment of the nerve. MRI with gadolinium is the current standard screening procedure for suspected tumors because of the high false-negative rate associated with BSERA testing. Microsurgical excision is the procedure of choice via either a translabyrinthine, middle fossa, or retrosigmoid approach depending on the tumor size and level of hearing. Observation is the best choice for management of patients with smaller tumors who have limited life expectancy.

Jackson CG et al: Hearing conservation in surgery for glomus jugulare tumors. Am J Otol 1996;17:425.

Prasad S et al: Efficacy of surgical treatments for squamous cell carcinoma of the temporal bone: a literature review. Otolaryngol Head Neck Surg 1994;110:270.

Thomas SS et al: Squamous cell carcinoma of the pinna: a six year study. Br J Plast Surg 1994;47:81.

CONGENITAL DEFORMITIES OF THE EAR

Lop-ear, the most common congenital deformity of the auricle, is the result of failure of development of the antihelical fold or excessive protrusion of the conchal cartilage. Treatment consists of otoplasty, the surgical creation of an antihelical fold or reduction of conchal cartilage projection (or both). Treatment before 5 or 6 years of age, when the auricle is three-fourths adult size, avoids ridicule of the child by its peers.

Preauricular cysts and sinus tracts are common unilateral or bilateral congenital defects found anterior to the upper helix or tragus. They develop following incomplete fusion of the auricular hillocks. Many subsequently become infected, requiring complete excision, which may be hazardous because of ramification of the sinus tracts near facial nerve branches. Congenital aural atresia varies widely in severity from mild narrowing of the external auditory canal—with or without dysplasia of the tympanic membrane and middle ear space—to entire absence of the middle ear cleft and auricle and bony atresia of the external auditory canal. Complete congenital aural atresia is rare, occurring in one in 10,000 births, with males affected more commonly than females. In the presence of complete bony atresia, anomalies of the middle ear cavity and structures are more common. Congenital aural atresia can occur in isolation or in association with microtia and other craniofacial dysplasias such as Treacher Collins', Crouzon's, Goldenhar's, Möbius', and Pierre Robin syndromes. Additional congenital anomalies include colobomas, heart defects, atresia of the choana, retarded growth or development, and genital hypoplasia, which have been observed in a unique group of patients afflicted with the so-called CHARGE association. Facial nerve palsies and laryngotracheal abnormalities are also common in this group. Initial treatment requires first establishing the presence of adequate hearing in the opposite ear. If hearing in the opposite ear is normal, surgical repair is not recommended, because the potential risk to the seventh nerve, which takes an anomalous course through the temporal bone, is too great. However, the use of a nerve monitoring unit during external ear canal and middle ear reconstruction will help reduce the risk of injury to the seventh nerve. If there is a profound conductive hearing loss on both sides, however, surgical reconstruction of the middle ear is indicated if feasible; if not, bilateral bone conduction hearing aids should be used. Auricular reconstruction for severe microtia or complete atresia is a challenging cosmetic surgical problem, often requiring soft tissue flaps and autogenous cartilaginous grafts, and should be done prior to middle ear reconstruction typically at 6 years of age when rib length is large enough to allow an adequate cartilage block for auricular sculpting. Four stages are required, beginning with the autogenous cartilage framework and construction of a cutaneous pocket, leading to transposition of lobular remnants, elevation of the auricular framework, and tragal reconstruction with conchal bowl definition.

Briggs RJS et al: Correction of conductive hearing loss in children. Otolaryngol Clin North Am 1994;27:607.

Cressman WR et al: Surgical aspects of congenital aural atresia. Otolaryngol Clin North Am 1994;27:621.

Hayes D: Hearing loss in infants with craniofacial anomalies. Otolaryngol Head Neck Surg 1994;110:39.

Nagata S: Secondary reconstruction for unfavorable microtia results utilizing temporoparietal and innominate fascia flaps. Plast Reconstr Surg 1994;254.

SYSTEMIC DISORDERS AFFECTING THE EAR

A variety of systemic illnesses are associated with hearing loss, including diabetes mellitus, hypothyroidism, renal disease, Paget's disease of the bone, and others. It is now well recognized that the human immunodeficiency virus (HIV) can cause hearing loss and vestibular complaints. Indeed, 50% of HIV-positive patients have abnormal auditory and vestibular testing. Patients with AIDS are subject to reactivation of otosyphilis and sudden sensorineural hearing loss secondary to cryptococcal meningitis and *Pneumocystic carinii* infection.

Immune-mediated inner ear disease can cause progressive hearing loss with or without vestibular symptoms secondary to the production of autoantibodies directed toward inner ear structures. Although many patients do not exhibit signs of autoimmune disease, some may have other evidence of autoimmune illnesses such as systemic lupus erythematosus, Sjögren's syndrome, rheumatoid arthritis, Wegener's syndrome, and Cogan's syndrome. Treatment is with steroids and occasionally antimetabolites.

Osteogenesis imperfecta, an autosomal dominant inherited disorder, may appear with ossicular abnormalities, including otosclerosis with stapes fixation. Four different types (I–IV) are recognized and are associated with varying degrees of systemic skeletal involvement, multiple fractures, and growth retardation. Conductive hearing loss and sensorineural hearing loss can occur in osteogenesis imperfecta, and the stapes abnormality does not respond as well to stapedectomy as in otosclerosis.

Chen AY et al: Otolaryngologic disease progression in children with human immunodeficiency virus infection. Arch Otolaryngol Head Neck Surg 1996;122:1360.

■ VESTIBULAR SYSTEM

The vestibular system serves to maintain balance, posture, and spatial orientation in concert with vision and peripheral proprioception. Loss of two of these three sensory modalities is severely incapacitating. The vestibular end organs are dynamic structures that respond to linear acceleration (saccule and utricle) and to angular acceleration (semicircular canals). Angular acceleration of the head displaces endolymph and deflects hair cell cupulae in the cristae. Hair cell deflection results in either an increase or a decrease in neuronal impulses to the vestibular nuclei. Because the six semicircular canals are arranged in three pairs with one member of a pair (right) lying in a plane parallel to the plane of the other member (left), differences in acceleration between the right and left sides of the body are monitored in the vestibular nuclei. Normally, when a person is resting or moving at a constant rate, sensory input from the paired horizontal semicircular canals and two pairs of posterior and superior semicircular canals is balanced. Angular acceleration with subsequent hair cell deflection results in unilateral increased vestibular output and increased muscle tone in the extraocular and skeletal muscles, maintaining balance, posture, and spatial orientation. Failure of the vestibular apparatus to sustain the organism's balance produces vertigo, nystagmus, falling, and past-pointing. Sudden unilateral diminution of function in the vestibular system, in Meniere's disease, perilymph fistula, acute labyrinthitis, or temporal bone fracture, causes an imbalance of neuronal information arriving in the temporal lobe cortex. The cortical interpretation is constant motion or vertigo aggravated by head movement. Similarly, neuronal imbalance arriving at the extraocular motor nuclei and reticular formation produces rapid nystagmus, nausea and vomiting, and parasympathetic discharge. In response to overwhelming vestibular dysequilibrium, the cerebellum inhibits vestibular nuclei, but only incompletely. Ultimately, restoration of balance will require (1) functional repair of the diseased end organ, requiring hours or days; (2) central nervous system suppression of the normally functioning side, requiring months; or (3) generation of new neuronal output in the hypofunctioning labyrinth.

Clinical Assessment of the Dizzy Patient

Nowhere in medicine and surgery is a carefully taken history more important than in evaluating patients with dizziness. Nonvertiginous or extravestibular dizziness is far more common than otogenic or true vertiginous imbalance. The sensation of lightheadedness or syncope points to nonvestibular causes of dizziness such as cardiac arrhythmias, vasovagal episodes, orthostatic hypotension, or hyperventilation, which are not associated with the perception of the room spinning around. The clinical evaluation of the vestibular system includes examination of cerebellar function (gait, Romberg, two-step Fukuda, finger-to-nose, dysdiadochokinesis, and dysmetria testing) and the cranial nerves and observation of spontaneous positional nystagmus. The vestibular ocular reflex can be evaluated qualitatively at the bedside with doll's-eye, dynamic visual acuity, and ice water caloric tests. Because visual fixation with the eyes open may suppress nystagmus, it is important to record eye movements with electronystagmography. This is a technique for recording changes in the corneoretinal potential with skin electrodes and an electronic apparatus. Spontaneous, positional, and positioning nystagmus may be recorded to determine whether the vertigo is peripheral or central in origin.

Additional information is obtained with the Hallpike caloric stimulation test. Caloric stimulation of the labyrinth via the tympanic membrane induces convection currents within the horizontal semicircular canal, producing cupular deflection in one direction with 30 °C water and in the opposite direction with 44 °C water. With the patient supine and the head elevated 30 degrees, irrigation of the external auditory canal with cold water (30 °C) produces the rapid component of nystagmus to the opposite side; warm water (44 °C) produces nystagmus to the same side. The mnemonic device is COWS ("cold to the opposite" and "warm to the same"). Decreased vestibular response to caloric stimulation (canal paresis) indicates a vestibular end organ, vestibular nerve, or brain stem lesion.

Baloh RW: Approach to the evaluation of the dizzy patient. Otolaryngol Head Neck Surg 1995;112:3.

Honrubia V: Contemporary vestibular function testing: accomplishments in future prospective. Otolaryngol Head Neck Surg 1995;112:64.

Lindstrom CJ: Office management of the dizzy patient. Otolaryngol Clin North Am 1992;25:745.

MENIERE'S DISEASE (Endolymphatic Hydrops)

Meniere's disease is characterized by a tetrad of symptoms of unknown cause: episodic vertigo, fluctuating sensorineural hearing loss, a sensation of aural fullness, and tinnitus. The tinnitus is usually low-pitched and roaring. The hearing loss is more severe in the lower frequencies, in many cases progresses over several years, and remains confined to one ear in most patients. The attacks are associated with nausea, vomiting, and prostration. Pathologically, there is generalized dilation of the membranous labyrinth that includes the scala media and endolymphatic sac and is associated with occasional membrane breaks and intermingling of endolymph and perilymph. Circulating immune complexes may be involved in the pathogenesis of Meniere's disease.

Patients with severe hydrops should be treated with diuretics, salt restriction, a low-caffeine diet, avoidance of nicotine, and labyrinthine sedatives such as diazepam, 5 mg three times daily, to prevent recurrent attacks. Antihistamines such as meclizine, dimenhydrinate, and cyclizine are used to reduce the severity of vertigo. Associated vertigo, nausea, and vomiting are controlled without antiemetics by combining the synergistic effects of a cholinergic antagonist (scopolamine) and an adrenergic agonist (dextroamphetamine).

Surgical treatment is currently reserved for patients with severe incapacitating vertigo or tinnitus or to prevent further deterioration of hearing. In patients with useful hearing, decompression of the endolymphatic sac and insertion of a shunt between the membranous labyrinth and subarachnoid space improves symptoms in over half of cases. Vestibular neurectomy through either a middle cranial fossa or retrolabyrinthine approach may conserve hearing. With severe loss of hearing and speech discrimination, a total transmastoid labyrinthectomy is used, which relieves vertigo in over 90% of patients. Unilateral chemical ablation of vestibular function has been accomplished with the intratympanic installation of gentamicin once or twice weekly for 2 or 3 weeks. The main complication has been sensorineural hearing loss, which occurs in 5–25% of patients depending upon the protocol used.

Cohen H et al: Disability in Meniere's disease. Arch Otolaryngol Head Neck Surg 1995;121:29.

Goycooleh MV et al: Overall view and rationale for surgical alternatives for incapacitating peripheral vertigo. Otolaryngol Clin North Am 1994;27:283.

Hirsh BE et al: Intratympanic gentamicin therapy for Meniere's disease. Am J Otol 1997;18:44.

Santos PM: Diuretic and diet effect on Meniere's disease evaluated by the 1993 committee on hearing and equilibrium guidelines. Otolaryngol Head Neck Surg 1993;109:680.

Telischi FF et al: Long-term efficacy of endolymphatic sac surgery for vertigo in Meniere's disease. Otolaryngol Head Neck Surg 1993;109:83.

Wackym PA: Histopathologic findings in Meniere's disease. Otolaryngol Head Neck Surg 1995;112:90.

VESTIBULAR SCHWANNOMA

Vestibular schwannomas account for about 8% of intracranial tumors and arise twice as often from the vestibular division of the eighth nerve as from the auditory division. They develop in one per 100,000 individuals yearly. Growth varies according to the patient's age. Although vestibular schwannomas account for about 80% of all cerebellopontine angle neoplasms, other lesions in the cerebellopontine angle may produce a nearly identical clinical picture. These include meningiomas, primary cholesteatomas, metastatic tumors, and aneurysms. Vestibular schwannomas, which are derived from Schwann cells, initially produce a high-frequency sensorineural hearing loss. Tinnitus is less common, and true vertigo is unusual. However, unsteadiness or balance disorders may develop as the tumor enlarges. Hallpike caloric testing commonly reveals canal paresis on the affected side. MRI with gadolinium is the current standard for screening for suspected vestibular schwannomas because of the high false-negative rate associated with BSERA.

Management of acoustic neuromas depends on the tumor's size and growth rate, the patient's age, and the state and prognosis of bilateral hearing. For patients under 65, small intracanalicular tumors (within the internal auditory canal) may be surgically removed through the transmastoid labyrinthine route if no useful hearing remains; a middle cranial fossa or retrosigmoid approach is utilized to preserve serviceable hearing for tumors 1.5 cm or less if the puretone average is less than 30 dB and the discrimination score is greater than 70%. Both routes maintain the integrity of the facial nerve. Larger tumors (> 3 cm) are associated with an increased incidence of hearing loss, dysequilibrium, headache, facial numbness, and diplopia and are removed via a suboccipital craniotomy; huge ones can only be removed via a combined suboccipital and translabyrinthine approach if the facial nerve is to be preserved. For patients over age 65 with slowly growing tumors, observation is the preferred treatment.

Dornhoffer JL et al: Presentation and diagnosis of small acoustic tumors. Otolaryngol Head Neck Surg 1994;111:232.

Grey PL et al: Audio vestibular results after surgery for cerebellopontine angle meningiomas. Am J Otol 1996;17:634.

Kartush JM et al: Acoustic neuroma update. Otolaryngol Clin North Am 1996;29:377.

Sekhar LN et al: The best treatment for vestibular schwannoma (acoustic neuroma): microsurgery or radiosurgery? Am J Otol 1996;17:676.

LABYRINTHITIS

In the preantibiotic era, acute suppurative labyrinthitis developing as a complication of acute otitis media or meningitis was not rare. More common today, however, is viral inflammation of the labyrinth or inner ear, causing vestibular neuritis or labyrinthitis. The clinical picture is a sudden onset of vertigo lasting days to a week, with gradual resolution of unsteadiness over weeks or months. Unilateral hearing loss can occur, and an electronystagmogram will often show reduced caloric response in one ear. Initial treatment with vestibular suppressants such as meclizine or diazepam are helpful. These should be removed as soon as possible and a vestibular rehabilitation program started to facilitate central cerebellar compensation.

BENIGN PAROXYSMAL POSITIONAL VERTIGO

Benign paroxysmal positional vertigo is associated with brief (< 30 seconds) episodes of sudden onset of intense vertigo precipitated by head or body movement. Hallpike positional testing often reveals horizontal rotatory nystagmus toward the involved undermost ear in the lateral decubitus position. The disorder is believed to result from degenerative otoconia from the utricular macula in the posterior semicircular canal. These particles may float free and, because they have a higher specific gravity than endolymph, produce abnormal cupular deflection in the semicircular canal with certain head movements.

Vestibular rehabilitation exercise programs have been prescribed for this problem. The particle repositioning maneuver developed by Epley appears to be the most effective form of therapy and is designed to disperse the otoconia back into the utricle, where they cannot cause cupular deflection.

GERIATRIC DYSEQUILIBRIUM

There are many vestibular disorders in the elderly, including vascular disease with ischemia (vertebral basilar insufficiency) or infarction (lacunar, brain stem, or cerebellar), endolymphatic hydrops, and benign paroxysmal positional vertigo (see above). Vertebral basilar insufficiency usually results from atherosclerosis involving the subclavian, vestibular, or basilar arteries and is associated with visual changes, weakness, paresthesias, and drop attacks. In addition, degenerative changes and loss of otoconia, vestibular epithelium, vestibular nerves, Scarpa's ganglion, and cerebellum occur with aging. The resulting dizziness and falls that are common among persons over age 65 are usually caused by central discoordination, but positional vertigo not uncommonly plays a central role. Because these peripheral vestibular aging changes are compensated by visual input, more dysequilibrium occurs at night. Gait abnormalities and a positive Romberg test, especially with the eyes closed, predominate. The vestibular rehabilitation exercises are most helpful. The morbidity and mortality associated with falls in the elderly are substantial and increase with age.

Blakley BW: Randomized controlled assessment of the canalith repositioning maneuver. Otolaryngol Head Neck Surg 1994;110:391.

Herdman SJ et al: Single treatment approaches for BPPV. Arch Otolaryngol Head Neck Surg 1993;119:450.

FACIAL NERVE PARALYSIS

Paralysis of the seventh nerve immobilizes the muscles of facial expression: The eye fails to close, the forehead does not wrinkle (as opposed to central or supranuclear facial paralysis with forehead sparing), and the angle of the mouth droops, so the patient drools. Peripheral seventh nerve paralysis suggests serious disease, such as tumor of the cerebellopontine angle, acoustic neuroma, facial nerve neuroma, neoplasm of the middle ear, or parotid gland neoplasm. Acute otitis media, temporal bone fracture, and chronic otitis media with or without cholesteatoma may produce facial paralysis. Other causes include surgical trauma, Guillain-Barré syndrome, Lyme disease, AIDS, and herpes zoster oticus (Ramsay Hunt's syndrome). When the cause is unknown, the condition is known as Bell's palsy. Although Bell's palsy is the commonest cause of peripheral seventh nerve paralysis, the pathogenesis is mysterious. Current theories implicate vascular ischemia and compressive edema within the facial canal as the cause of neurapraxia and cessation of axoplasmic flow. There is evidence that Bell's palsy is part of a viral cranial polyneuropathy that usually resolves in 6–12 weeks. Recent herpes simplex viral DNA has been clearly demonstrated in the geniculate ganglion of a patient with Bell's palsy.

All patients with facial paralysis should have a thorough history and physical examination. In addition, a high-resolution CT scan of the temporal bones and gadolinium-enhanced MRI should be obtained. The latter frequently demonstrates better soft tissue visualization and gadolinium enhancement in Bell's palsy, herpes zoster oticus, facial neuromas and vestibular schwannomas. MRI is indicated in patients experiencing weakness lasting more than 2 months or with progressive or recurrent palsies. The following special diagnostic tests should be performed: puretone audiometry, speech reception thresholds and speech discrimination; glucose tolerance tests to rule out diabetes mellitus; and Lyme titers; supramaximal electroneurography nerve excitability testing over the peripheral branches and main trunk of the seventh nerve is often used to predict the need for surgical decompression. With electroneurography, a supramaximal stimulus is delivered to the seventh nerve trunk and a compound action potential is recorded using surface electrodes. In patients with a greater than 90% loss of compound action potential prior to day 14 after the onset of paralysis, middle cranial fossa decompression is indicated.

The initial medical management of Bell's palsy is controversial. However, routine eye care with petroleum-based ocular lubricants (eg, Lacrilube) at night and artificial tears every 2–3 hours during the day is not. Approximately 70% of patients recover completely, but the prognosis for complete recovery falls to 10% in the presence of dry eye. Early treatment with corticosteroids (eg, 60–80 mg of prednisone daily with gradual tapering over 7–10 days) is felt by some experts to hasten resolution of edema and improve the outcome (ie, prevent permanent paralysis or synkinesis). Acyclovir, 800 mg orally five times a day, or valacyclovir, 500 mg orally twice daily, is recommended. In patients with herpes zoster oticus, intravenous acyclovir with prednisone is helpful. Nonpregnant adults with facial paralysis secondary to Lyme disease are best treated with doxycycline; amoxicillin, erythromycin, ceftriaxone, and cefuroxime may be used as substitutes.

Rehabilitation of the paralyzed face exhibiting no recovery is a challenging problem. Unilateral facial paralysis is unlikely to recover if a year has passed since the injury and no voluntary motion is noted. If paralysis persists, placement of a gold weight eyelid implant will be necessary to provide adequate ocular closure and thus prevent exposure keratitis. Nerve crossover procedures using a hypoglossal to seventh nerve anastomosis are recommended for restoring resting facial tone in cases of complete paralysis where a proximal facial nerve stump is not available for grafting or repair. For traumatic lesions, immediate neural repair or interposition grafting of the damaged segment with a greater auricular or sural nerve graft may be efficacious. Occasionally, decompression of the facial nerve combined with rerouting through the temporal bone is sufficient. Finally, neuromuscular transfer techniques utilizing either temporalis or masseter muscle pedicles or microvascular free muscle transfer are effective for facial reanimation in patients who are not candidates for cable nerve grafts or hypoglossal nerve transposition.

Adour KK: Bell's palsy treatment with acyclovir and prednisone compared with prednisone alone. Ann Otol Rhinol Laryngol 1996;105:371.

Burgess RC et al: Polymerase chain reaction of herpes simplex viral DNA from the geniculate ganglion of a patient with Bell's palsy. Ann Otol Rhinol Laryngol 1994;103:775.

Seiff SR et al: Management of ophthalmic complications of facial nerve palsy. Otolaryngol Clin North Am 1992;25:669.

NOSE & PARANASAL SINUSES

NASAL FOREIGN BODIES

Nasal foreign bodies are common in children, who frequently place pebbles, beads, seeds, buttons, or paper into the nares. A severe inflammatory reaction ensues, especially with organic matter, and this is associated with a foul-smelling unilateral nasal discharge. Chronic foreign bodies may encrust with calcium and magnesium to form rhinoliths. Removal of foreign body requires topical vasoconstrictors such as phenylephrine and topical anesthesia with lidocaine or cocaine. General anesthesia may be needed in uncooperative children.

NASAL VESTIBULITIS

Inflammation of the nasal vestibule may assume two forms: a localized acute furunculitis or a chronic diffuse dermatitis. Acute staphylococcal furunculitis of the pilosebaceous follicles in the vestibule may develop into a spreading cellulitis of the tip of the nose. Treatment includes hot soaks and oral cephalexin. Incision and drainage of a localized abscess is rarely necessary, since the majority of cases drain spontaneously. Diffuse nasal vestibulitis is treated with antibiotic ointments containing polymyxin B, bacitracin, and neomycin. Early treatment of all acute infections of the nose, paranasal sinuses, and face is important to prevent the occurrence of retrograde thrombophlebitis and cavernous sinus thrombosis, as well as facial cellulitis. If these complications occur, intravenously therapy with a broad-spectrum agent such as ampicillin-sulbactam or ceftriaxone plus clindamycin is essential.

ACUTE RHINITIS
(Coryza, Common Cold)

Acute rhinitis is often secondary to infection with respiratory viruses, including rhinoviruses, coronaviruses, and papillomaviruses. It is associated with sneezing, watery rhinorrhea, tearing, malaise, and headache. The incidence of colds increases during the fall, remains elevated during the winter, and generally declines during the spring. Examination of the nasal mucous membrane reveals hyperemia, edema, and watery mucosal discharge. Later, the secretions may become thick and yellow-green in color. Tenderness to palpation over the paranasal sinuses may be found. Nonnarcotic analgesics such as aspirin, decongestants, and antihistamines as well as fluids and rest will alleviate symptoms. Topical vasoconstrictors such as oxymetazoline and phenylephrine provide symptomatic relief. Antibiotic therapy is not necessary unless secondary bacterial invasion occurs. The condition usually resolves within 5–10 days.

ALLERGIC RHINITIS

Antigens inhaled and deposited on the mucous membranes of the nasal cavities of hypersensitive individuals elicit an IgE-mediated rhinitis. This perennial or seasonal disorder is often associated with other respiratory allergies such as asthma, chronic laryngitis, or tracheobronchitis. Allergens such as animal danders, molds, dust, and pollens are commonly implicated, and sensitivity to them may be confirmed by skin end point titration, skin prick testing, or in vitro radioallergosorbent testing (RAST). Allergic rhinitis is characterized by sneezing, watery rhinorrhea, tearing, dysosmia, and nasal obstruction. The mucous membrane appears edematous and pale, with a thin discharge. Individuals with chronic allergic rhinitis commonly develop nasal polyps and acute or chronic sinusitis. Polyps may arise from the middle meatal region at the sinus ostia and appear as pale gray, glistening edematous masses within the nasal cavity. Occasionally, a large antrochoanal polyp arises from the maxillary sinus ostia in conjunction with chronic maxillary sinusitis and presents as a long pedunculated mass in the nasopharynx. Treatment requires removal of the polyp and drainage of the maxillary sinus.

Treatment for mild allergic rhinitis is started with an antihistamine (Table 39–4) and avoidance of the allergen if possible. Topical nasal steroids in the form of beclomethasone dipropionate, triamcinolone acetonide, budesonide, fluticasone, mometasone, or flunisolide or the use of topical cromolyn sodium delivered intranasally is effective in reducing or eliminating moderate symptoms in some patients. These nasal sprays are given in concert with saline nasal rinses. For severe conditions, oral glucocorticoids or intramuscular steroids are em-

Table 39–4. Oral antihistamines for allergic rhinitis.

Drug	Usual Adult Dose
Alkylamines	
Brompheniramine maleate	4 mg every 4–6 hours
Chlorpheniramine maleate	4 mg every 4–6 hours
Ethanolamines	
Clemastine fumarate	1.34–2.68 mg every 12 hours
Diphenhydramine hydrochloride	20–50 mg every 4–6 hours
Others	
Fexofenadine	60 mg every 12 hours, or 180 mg daily
Azatadine maleate	1–2 mg every 12 hours
Cyproheptadine hydrochloride	4 mg every 6–8 hours
Pheniramine tartrate	25 mg every 4–6 hours
Terfenadine	60 mg every 12 hours
Astemizole	10 mg daily
Loratadine	10 mg daily
Cetirizine	5–10 mg daily

ployed in addition to antihistamines, nasal steroids, and oral decongestants. Desensitization immunotherapy should be considered if pharmacotherapy insufficiently controls symptoms or produces undesirable side effects; if there are positive skin tests or serum specific IgE that correlates with rhinitis symptoms; if there is a history of allergic rhinitis for at least two seasons or 6 months (perennial); or if appropriate measures to avoid indoor allergens fail to control symptoms. Finally, surgical removal of nasal polyps associated with allergic rhinitis combined with endoscopic surgical drainage of obstructed maxillary and ethmoid sinuses is performed for severe nasal obstruction and chronic sinusitis unresponsive to medical therapy.

Baraniuk JN: Pathogenesis of allergic rhinitis. J Allergy Clin Immunol 1997;99:S763.

Durham SR et al: Changes in allergic inflammation associated with successful immunotherapy. Int Arch Allergy Immunol 1995;107:282.

Ferguson BJ: Allergic rhinitis. Options for pharmacotherapy and immunotherapy. Postgrad Med 1997;101:117.

Fornadley JA et al: Allergic rhinitis: clinical practice guidelines. Otolaryngol Head Neck Surgery 1996;115:115.

Nightingale CH: Treating allergic rhinitis with second-generation antihistamines. Pharmacotherapy 1996;16:905.

RHINITIS MEDICAMENTOSA

Misuse or abuse of intranasal vasoconstrictors (eg, phenylephrine, cocaine) may lead to mucosal edema, hyperemia, and watery rhinorrhea. The resulting nasal obstruction is severe, prompting the individual to increase the use of topical decongestants and thus perpetuate the cycle. Successful treatment requires complete cessation of intranasal medications for 2–3 weeks, and an oral decongestant such as pseudoephedrine must be used. A short course of systemic corticosteroid therapy or the gradual substitution of topical steroids for topical decongestant therapy seems to assist the withdrawal process. Unfortunately, the new complex of nasal septal perforation, palatal retraction, pharyngeal wall ulceration, and nasal collapse secondary to cocaine abuse that mimics midline granuloma does not respond to this management. Invariably, these lesions are colonized with *S aureus* and require intravenous antistaphylococcal penicillin and, in rare cases, external beam radiation therapy.

VASOMOTOR RHINITIS

Vasomotor rhinitis results from hyperreactivity of parasympathetic control of the nasal vasculature and glands. The vasomotor reaction is characterized by vascular engorgement mediated by the release of acetylcholine (a powerful vasodilator) at parasympathetic nerve endings. This commonly occurs in response to changes in external temperature and humidity and is not caused by allergens. Exposure to inhalant irritants such as tobacco smoke, perfume, and industrial pollutants may provoke parasympathetic activity. There is often a history of trauma. The patient complains of nasal obstruction, sneezing, and watery rhinorrhea. Systemic decongestants such as pseudoephedrine and phenylpropanolamine give some relief. Antihistamines help combat the problem through their anticholinergic action. Corticosteroid nasal spray is occasionally effective, while the use of intranasal cromolyn sodium may benefit the patient by preventing the release of mediators from mast cells. A recent option for control of vasomotor rhinitis is the application of nasal ipratropium bromide at either 0.03% or 0.06% concentration (two puffs three times a day) for control of congestion and rhinorrhea. Septoplasty to correct traumatic nasal septal obstruction with or without bilateral partial inferior turbinectomy is successful in relieving nasal airway obstruction.

PARANASAL SINUSITIS

Inflammation of the paranasal sinuses is commonly precipitated by an acute upper respiratory tract infection of viral origin. Edema of the nasal mucosa produces obstruction of the sinus ostia, resulting in secondary bacterial invasion and localized pain and tenderness. Headache that is exacerbated by changes in position and barometric pressure is very common. Other common symptoms are auditory tube dysfunction with otalgia, rhinorrhea, nasal congestion, postnasal discharge, and sometimes anosmia in adults. Acute sinusitis is defined by persistence of upper respiratory tract symptoms beyond the usual 7-day course of the predisposing viral illness. Microorganisms responsible for acute sinusitis are most often *S pneumoniae, M catarrhalis,* and *H influenzae.* Because β-lactamase production is common among strains of *H influenzae* and particularly *M catarrhalis,* therapy with amoxicillin-clavulanic acid, cefuroxime, or erythromycin and trimethoprim-sulfamethoxazole for 2–3 weeks is preferred initial management of acute sinusitis. In persons allergic to penicillin, erythromycin plus a sulfonamide is recommended. Therapy also includes oral decongestants, antihistamines for patients who have a substantial component of allergic rhinitis, immunotherapy with IgE desensitization, and corticosteroids in the form of topical nasal sprays, systemic agents, or both. Chronic sinusitis in adults is defined as 12 weeks of persistent signs and symptoms or four episodes per year of recurrent acute sinusitis. If there is no improvement with previous antibiotic treatment, anaerobic and *S aureus* coverage should be included with either amoxicillin-clavulanate and metronidazole or cefuroxime plus metronidazole. In HIV-infected patients who develop pseudomonas infections, ciprofloxacin plus clindamycin or an aminoglycoside has proved effective. For chronic sinusitis, first-line antibiotics include amoxicillin-clavulanate, second-generation cephalosporins, and the newer macrolides and fluoroquinolones. Cefixime is an excellent choice when resistant *H influenzae* and moraxella are implicated but fails in managing *S pneumoniae* infection. Treatment is continued for 3 weeks.

Endoscopic sinus surgery is indicated for patients with persistent facial pain, headache, or nasal congestion and those who fail to respond to aggressive medical management. CT scans should be obtained in the axial and coronal planes to evaluate the persistence of chronic sinusitis and the presence of sinus abnormalities such as nasal septal deformity, pneumatization of the middle turbinates (concha bullosa), inferior turbinate hypertrophy, or substantial obstruction of the osteomeatal complex. Because the flow of mucus in the sinuses is toward the natural ostium, relief of obstruction of the osteomeatal complex (hiatus semilunaris and ethmoid infundibulum) is indicated to restore drainage from the sinuses and prevent persistent symptoms. Reestablishment of ethmoid and maxillary sinus ventilation and elimination of foci of ethmoid disease are necessary for success. The introduction of the nasal endoscopy combined with articulating video cameras and video imaging allows removal of just enough mucosa to restore drainage. The commonest site of infection in chronic sinusitis is the anterior ethmoid air cells. Endoscopic sinus surgery is most effective in controlling localized disease, recurrent acute sinusitis, and sinusitis secondary to anatomic obstruction, particularly in patients with no previous sinus surgery or in those who have a maxillary sinus mycetoma. The prognosis is unfavorable in patients with immunodeficiencies, immotile cilia syndrome, severe allergy, triad asthma with nasal polyposis and aspirin sensitivity, sarcoidosis, multiple prior operations, diffuse severe polypoid disease, or polyposis with diffuse extramucosal fungal infection.

Patients undergoing successful endoscopic sinus surgery show the greatest improvement with respect to resolution of facial pain. Frequently, simultaneous septoplasty and partial inferior turbinectomies is necessary for adequate exposure and endoscopic drainage of the sinuses. Patients with opacification of the sphenoid sinus have a poorer outcome, whereas those who have no purulent drainage or reformation of polypoid mucosa postoperatively have a dramatic resolution of facial pain, nasal obstruction, postnasal discharge, rhinorrhea, and improvement in their history of recurrent asthma. If maxillary sinus disease remains after this approach, a Caldwell-Luc procedure through an incision in the gingival labial sulcus may be necessary. For patients who have persistent ethmoid disease, external ethmoidectomy is indicated via a Lynch incision midway between the dorsum of the nose and the medial canthal ligament of the eye.

Complications of acute sinusitis are rare in infancy and childhood. Acute maxillary sinusitis and, more commonly, ethmoiditis may be complicated by orbital cellulitis and abscess formation. The progressive development of chemosis, scleral erythema, proptosis, and ophthalmoplegia points to orbital infection and potential intracranial invasion. A CT scan with contrast enhancement will detect an orbital abscess and evaluate other causes of unilateral proptosis. Treatment consists of intravenous ceftriaxone and clindamycin or ampicillin-sulbactam. In patients developing an orbital abscess, drainage through a Lynch incision must be performed early to avoid serious intracranial complications such as meningitis, epidural abscess, subdural abscess, cerebral abscess, and cavernous sinus thrombosis. Several factors in pediatric sinusitis are critical: (1) Chronic purulent rhinosinusitis in children has an immunologic (IgG subclass deficiencies) or anatomic origin. (2) Children under age 7 with nasal polyposis and chronic sinusitis must be considered to have cystic fibrosis or ciliary abnormalities causing poor mucus transport until proved otherwise. (3) Sinusitis exacerbates asthma. (4) Atopic children are more likely to develop sinusitis. (5) Allergy must be suspected in the age group from 3 years to 5 years, particularly when the symptoms include eczema, colic, and a family history of allergy.

Acute frontal sinusitis is more common in adults and frequently occurs following nasal trauma involving the nasal frontal duct. In the adolescent, it is the major source of orbital infection. In cases refractory to medical management, treatment consists of trephination of the anterior floor of the frontal sinus in the medial portion of the eyebrow. Chronic frontal sinusitis unresponsive to medical treatment and development of a mucocele are additional indications for operation. Endoscopic removal of frontal sinus mucoceles is now possible. A mucocele results from mucosal membrane duplication and obstruction of the sinus ostium secondary to chronic infection or trauma. It gradually enlarges to destroy the frontal bone and encroach upon the orbit or anterior cranial fossa. In large mucoceles of the frontal sinus that cannot be approached endoscopically, a bicoronal incision with an osteoplastic flap is used to excise and obliterate the sinus with fat or muscle. Finally, if patients have persistent postendoscopic drainage with facial pain, headache, or recurrent asthma, a repeat CT scan is indicated.

Gungor A et al: Pediatric sinusitis: a literature review with emphasis on the role of allergy. Otolaryngol Head Neck Surg 1997; 116:4.

Kennedy DW et al: Functional endoscopic sinus surgery: theory and diagnosis. Arch Otolaryngol 1995;11:576.

Kuhn FA et al: Postoperative care following functional endoscopic sinus surgery. Otolaryngol Clin North Am 1997;30:479.

EPISTAXIS

The nasal cavity is a common site of spontaneous hemorrhage. The blood supply to the nose is derived both from the external and the internal carotid artery systems. In 90% of cases, the epistaxis originates in the anterior nasal septum in the rich vascular plexus (Kiesselbach's plexus) in Little's area. The terminal septal branches of the anterior and posterior ethmoidal arteries arising from the internal carotid artery (via the ophthalmic artery) anastomose in this area along with branches from the superior labial artery (via the external facial) and the sphenopalatine artery (via the internal maxillary artery). Both originate from the external carotid artery system. Because of their location, vessels on the anterior septal mucosa are readily susceptible to trauma from nasal picking, drying, crusting, and infection. Severe caudal septal deformities may lead to mucosal drying over the point of deflection, causing spontaneous hemorrhage. In addition, the concomitant use of alcohol, aspirin, or other NSAIDs interferes with platelet function, increasing the risk of epistaxis.

Mild epistaxis from the anterior septum is readily controlled with digital pressure for 5–10 minutes. Persistent hemorrhage requires topical cocainization and cauterization with a silver nitrate applicator or electrocautery. If hemorrhage is still not controlled, ¼-inch gauze packing impregnated with petrolatum should be placed atraumatically in the nasal cavity. Bleeding associated with leukemia, uremia, hepatic failure, coagulopathies, or hereditary hemorrhagic telangiectasia (Rendu-Osler-Weber syndrome) should be treated with absorbable gelatin sponge (Gelfoam) soaked in topical thrombin, oxidized regenerated cellulose (Surgicel), microfibrillar collagen hemostat (Avitene Hemostat), or a compressed Merocel sponge inserted into the nasal cavity for 4–5 days. All packing should be coated or saturated with an antibiotic to prevent toxic shock, which is caused when the pack is colonized by S aureus strains that express TSS toxin-1, enterotoxin B, or enterotoxin C. Treatment of underlying coagulopathy, leukemia, uremia, or liver disorder is obviously important. Moderate long-term success in hemorrhagic hereditary telangiectasia has been achieved with estrogen derivatives and septal dermoplasty. Septal dermoplasty involves removing the diseased mucosa together with subepithelial telangiectasias and replacing it through a lateral rhinotomy with a skin graft. The YAG laser is currently used in recalcitrant cases for photocoagulation of nasal hemorrhagic telangiectasias.

Posterior epistaxis from the terminal branches of the sphenopalatine and internal maxillary arteries is more serious and is frequently associated with hypertension, diabetes, or major systemic vascular disorders. It arises from a plexus of vessels located in the posterior 1 cm of the nasal floor, inferior meatus, inferior turbinate, and middle turbinate. Successful treatment requires the use of both anterior and posterior packing, inserted with topical 4% cocaine anesthesia. The posterior pack is made by tying folded 4 × 4 gauze squares to the end of a catheter that has been passed transnasally and brought out through the mouth. Two strings are tied to the pharyngeal end of the catheter and brought out through the nares. They are then tied over an anterior nasal pack and bolster (Figure 39–6). The remaining third string is brought out through the mouth and taped to the cheek, where it can be grasped and removed in 4–5 days. These techniques are extremely uncomfortable, lower arterial oxygen saturation, and may induce dysrhythmias or an acute myocardial infarction in patients with severe cardiovascular disease. Because toxic shock syndrome has been reported with the use of nasal packs, patients are started on intravenous cephalothin. Packing is left in place for 3–5 days. If bleeding fails to respond to posterior packing or posterior endoscopic cauterization under general anesthesia, transantral ligation of the internal maxillary artery through a Caldwell-Luc approach with or without anterior ethmoid artery ligation or angiographic embolization will be required. Currently, both ligation and embolization are specifically indicated for epistaxis secondary to vascular anomalies, bleeding disorders, trauma, or tumor. This practice has the advantage that it can be conducted under local anesthesia with conscious sedation. Its most frequently reported complication is facial paralysis. Transantral internal maxillary ligation, on the other hand, is associated with risk of dental injury, oral antral fistula, facial pain and paresthesias, postoperative sinusitis, and intraoperative bleeding. Unlike embolization, internal maxillary ligation requires a general anesthetic, which may place a patient at significant cardiovascular risk.

Elahi MN et al: Therapeutic embolization in the treatment of intractable epistaxis. Arch Otolaryngol Head Neck Surg 1995;121:65.

Elden L et al: Angiographic embolization for the treatment of epistaxis: review of 108 cases. Otolaryngol Head Neck Surg 1994;111:44.

Hartley C et al: The Foley catheter in epistaxis management—a scientific appraisal. J Laryngol Otol 1994;108:399.

McGarry GW et al: Idiopathic epistaxis, hemostasis and alcohol. Clin Otolaryngol 1995;20:174.

Strong EB et al: Intractable epistaxis: transantral ligation versus embolization: efficacy review and cost analysis. Otolaryngol Head Neck Surg 1995;113:674.

Figure 39–6. Packing to control bleeding from the posterior nose. **A:** Catheter inserted and pack attached. **B:** Pack drawn into position as catheter is removed. **C:** Strip tied over a bolster to hold pack in place with anterior pack installed "accordion pleating" style. **D:** Alternative method using balloon catheter instead of a gauze pack.

Winstead W: Sphenopalatine artery ligation: An alternative to internal maxillary artery ligation for intractable posterior epistaxis. Laryngoscope 1996;106:667.

NASAL TRAUMA

Nasal bone fractures are the most common fractures of the maxillofacial skeleton and frequently are associated with septal fractures and epistaxis. Clinical findings commonly include periorbital edema and ecchymosis, displacement of the bony dorsum to the right with depression of the left nasal bone (secondary to a "right hook" fisticuffs injury), crepitus, and, occasionally, laceration of the dorsum. In severe facial trauma, because the other facial bones are often broken, the entire facial skeleton should be assessed by x-ray.

Early reduction under local anesthesia before significant swelling appears produces an excellent result. Elevation with a periosteal elevator— combined with laterally applied digital pressure—is usually effective. An external plaster of Paris splint or commercially available splint is applied and removed in 1 week. It may be necessary to reduce severely impacted nasal bones with a Walsham forceps, one blade placed intranasally and the other extranasally. If the nasal fracture is encountered after severe edema has developed, it is better to postpone reduction for several days to allow resolution of edema. In children, the facial skeleton heals so fast that fracture must be reduced within 4–5 days to avoid malunion. Malunion in adults is treated by rhinoplasty and often concomitant septoplasty to repair the deviated nasal septum.

Complications of nasal trauma include septal hematoma and abscess formation, septal perforation, septal deviation, and cerebrospinal fluid rhinorrhea secondary to fracture of the cribriform plate, the roof of the ethmoid sinus, the posterior table of the frontal sinus, or the sphenoid sinus.

A septal hematoma is a collection of blood underneath the mucoperichondrium or mucoperiosteum of the septum. Physical examination discloses a bulging red septum, and nasal obstruction is usually complete and bilateral. Unless the hematoma is immediately incised and drained, a staphylococcal abscess may develop that results in cartilaginous necrosis and saddle nose deformity. Intravenous nafcillin, oxacillin, cefazolin, or clindamycin should be given to prevent cavernous sinus thrombosis and meningitis.

A septal deviation, especially along the nasal floor, produces varying degrees of nasal obstruction depending upon the severity of deflection into the nasal cavity. The caudal end of the septum may be deflected into the nasal vestibule, causing obstruction or external deformity. Nasal septoplasty through a caudal submucoperichondrial incision is used to reconstruct and straighten the septum.

Septal perforations are repaired only if complicated by persistent epistaxis, crusting with nasal obstruction, or, rarely, whistling. The repair involves an open transcolumellar rhinoplastic approach, using a temporalis fascial or perichondrial graft and advancement of two bipedicled mucoperichondrial flaps to cover the defect. Alternatively, an alloplastic septal button can be created to close the perforation.

Fractures of the nasal bones, nasoethmoidal region, and frontal region may occur in association with a dural defect and cerebrospinal fluid rhinorrhea. This provides a potential route for ascending infection and meningitis. The dural defect may communicate with the nasal cavity via the ethmoidal, frontal, or sphenoidal sinuses or the cribriform plate. A basilar skull fracture with an intact tympanic membrane may also present with cerebrospinal fluid rhinorrhea.

The diagnosis should be suspected upon finding watery rhinorrhea with an increased glucose content and may be confirmed by thin-section coronal CT following subarachnoid instillation of metrizamide by intrathecal injection. Fluid should be sent for β_2-transferrin determination, which is found only in cerebrospinal fluid and aqueous humour. The source of cerebrospinal fluid leak may be demonstrated in many cases by placing fluorescein dye (0.5 mL of 5% solution) in the lumbar subarachnoid space. Thirty minutes later, the nose can be endoscopically examined to determine the fistula site—front sinus, sphenoid sinus, roof of the ethmoid (fovea ethmoidalis), cribriform plate, or middle ear (via the auditory tube). Cerebrospinal fluid appears as a yellowish-green fluid using a xenon light source, and Wood's lamp is not necessary.

Acute posttraumatic cerebrospinal fluid rhinorrhea is treated conservatively with bed rest in the semisitting position, fluid restriction, lumbar drainage, and diuretics for 5–7 days. The patient should avoid straining, blowing the nose, sneezing, or vigorous coughing. Indications for surgery are persistent cerebrospinal fluid leakage of more than 6 weeks' duration, recurrent meningitis, pneumoencephalos, or intermittent leakage. In sinusitis or osteitis, intravenous ceftriaxone is indicated.

Small defects of the cribriform plate, fovea ethmoidalis, and sphenoid sinus have been successfully repaired through an external ethmoidectomy incision using a variety of septal or middle turbinate mucoperiosteal flaps. However, an endoscopic approach using free grafts of fascia, nasal mucoperichondrium, muscle, fascia lata, or fibrin glue is preferred. Fibrin glue, composed of 10% calcium chloride and topical thrombin, added to cryoprecipitate in separate syringes, becomes gelatinous when combined and effectively seals the leak. The fibrin glue will last about 7–10 days and then dissolve. In all cases, the graft and glue are held in position by an absorbable packing such as Gelfoam, Surgicel, or Oxycel. Alternatively, Avitene paste may be used. Small defects of the posterior table of the frontal sinus are best managed by a bicoronal incision, osteoplastic flap approach, and obliteration of the frontal sinus with abdominal fat. Large defects will necessitate anterior fossa craniotomy and repair. Bone fragments are stabilized with low-contour titanium plates and screws.

Other soft tissue facial injuries and fractures of the zygoma, maxilla, orbit, and mandibles are discussed in Chapter 44.

Dodson EE et al: Transnasal endoscopic repair of cerebral spinal fluid rhinorrhea and skull base defects: a review of 29 cases. Otolaryngol Head Neck Surg 1994;111:600.

El Jamel MS et al: Localization of inactive cerebral spinal fluid fistulas. J Neurosurg 1995;83:795.

El Jamel MS: Fractures of the middle third of the face and cerebral spinal fluid rhinorrhea. Br J Neurosurg 1994;8:289.

Teichgradber JF et al: The management of septal perforations. Plast Reconstr Surg 1993;91:229.

CONGENITAL NASAL MALFORMATIONS

Congenital malformations of the nose and central face are unusual. Facial clefts, such as cleft lip and palate or a bifid nose, commonly result from genetic or teratogenic factors operating in the second month of fetal life. Although atresia and stenosis of the anterior nares are rare, they should be suspected in any infant who has difficulty breathing. Bilateral bony posterior choanal atresia is more commonly the cause of congenital neonatal respiratory impairment. Because they are obligatory nasal breathers during the first several weeks of life, newborns develop apnea and cyanosis when crying stops and the mouth is closed. The definitive diagnosis is confirmed by inability to pass a catheter transnasally.

Initial treatment includes either an oral endotracheal tube or McGovern nipple (which allows mouth breathing), followed by early transnasal or transpalatal correction of the atresia. The atretic plate can be successfully removed endoscopically with diamond burrs, powered oscillating blades, or the CO_2 laser. The surgically created posterior choana is kept patent with a 16F or 18F polyvinylchloride (Portex) endotracheal tube that is removed in 6–8 weeks. Unilateral choanal atresia, on the other hand, is usually not diagnosed until later in childhood or early adulthood and is associated with unilateral nasal obstruction or rhinorrhea. Repair is best performed when the nasal cavities and hard palate have reached adult size.

Other congenital lesions that may produce nasal obstruction include nasal gliomas, encephaloceles, meningoceles, and teratomas (dermoids, teratoids, true teratomas, and epignathi). Nasal gliomas are composed of neural and glial elements. Similarly, meningoceles and encephaloceles that have intracranial connections through the cribriform plate, fovea ethmoidalis, or sphenoid bone may present as a nasal mass that may be mistaken for a nasal polyp. Not infrequently, these heterotopic brain elements are seen as a mass on the nasal dorsum that is frequently confused with a midline dermoid cyst. CT scans or MRI of the anterior cranial fossa and cribriform plate must be obtained to rule out intracranial connections. Treatment of heterotopic brain elements with an intracranial connection requires a combined craniotomy and transfacial approach. If the diagnosis remains in doubt, frontal craniotomy is performed before transfacial excision to avoid development of cerebrospinal fluid rhinorrhea and meningitis. Other surgical approaches for complete excision of congenital nasal masses include open rhinoplasty and transnasal, endoscopic, or combined transcranial-endoscopic techniques.

Koltai PJ: The external rhinoplasty for the correction of unilateral choanal atresia in young children. Ear Nose Throat J 1991; 70:450.

ORAL CAVITY

WHITE LESIONS OF THE ORAL CAVITY

The mucous membrane of the oropharynx resembles the skin in that individual cells arise from the germinal layer and mature, but they do not keratinize. Mechanical, thermal, and chemical trauma (eg, alcohol; nicotine, including smokeless tobacco products) may lead to thickening of the germinal layer and later development of a nonnucleated keratinized layer that appears as gray-white nonulcerated plaques on the oral cavity mucosa (leukoplakia). Because the histologic appearance varies considerably and up to one-half of these lesions may exhibit malignant transformation, biopsy is indicated to rule out early carcinoma. The treatment is surgical excision of small lesions with a knife or with a CO_2 or KTP laser and avoidance of further exposure to irritants. Laser excision has a lower recurrence rate plus the advantages of better precision, bloodless field, excellent tissue healing, and less pain and discomfort.

Lichen planus, though primarily a dermatologic disorder affecting up to 2% of the population, may involve any mucous membrane exposed to trauma or chronic irritation such as tobacco—eg, the buccal mucosa frequently develops white papules or striae from repetitive biting. Hyperkeratosis, acanthosis, and subepithelial edema complete the histologic picture. Because of the clinical similarities between lichen planus and discoid lupus erythematosus and lichenoid stomatitis—and because of its relationship to liver disease and oral cancer—biopsy of representative lesions is indicated to confirm the diagnosis and rule out other disorders. Topical triamcinolone is often useful for associated submucosal inflammation. In some cases, this may undergo malignant degeneration into squamous cell carcinoma.

Finally, ill-fitting dentures may elicit raised folds of white tissue in the gingivolabial sulcus that histologically consist of fibrous tissues proliferation and overlying epithelial hyperplasia. An inflammatory papillary hyperplasia on the hard palate may occur as a result of improperly fitting dentures. These polypoid lesions are hyperemic, soft, and mobile. Surgical removal is often necessary, followed by denture readjustment.

Bagan JV et al: Oral lichens planus and chronic liver disease: a clinical and morphometric study of the oral lesions in relationship to transaminase elevation. Oral Surg Oral Med Oral Pathol 1994;78:337.

Banard NA et al: Oral cancer development in patients with oral lichen planus. J Oral Pathol Med 1993;22:421.

INFLAMMATORY DISEASES OF THE GINGIVA

Inflammation of the gums (gingivitis) frequently develops as a result of poor oral hygiene, heavy smoking, and lowered resistance. **Acute necrotizing ulcerative gingivitis** (Vincent's gingivitis) is due to an overgrowth of the normal oral bacterial symbionts. Clinically, it is characterized by painful hemorrhagic gums, ulceration, fever, lymphadenopathy, and a yellow-gray gingival pseudomembrane. Treatment consists of topical hydrogen peroxide, proper oral hygiene with removal of plaque and tartar at the tooth margins, and oral penicillin. Clindamycin is an acceptable antibiotic alternative, especially for penicillin-resistant anaerobic infections.

Although not limited to the gingivae, recurrent **aphthous stomatitis** (canker sores) frequently presents on the gingivae as round or ovoid, discrete, erythematous macules 2–30 mm in diameter that rapidly indurate and ulcerate but do not vesiculate (as do herpetic lesions). They are the most commonly reported oral ulcers, occurring in approximately one-fourth of the population. They may elicit enough pain to interfere with mastication and speaking. Tetracycline solution, 250 mg held in the mouth for 20 minutes four to six times a day and the analgesic dyclonine 0.5%, plus diphenhydramine elixir are effective treatment. Alternative therapy includes an emollient paste such as 0.1% triamcinolone acetonide in sodium carboxymethylcellulose or an aqueous 0.1% or 0.2% suspension alone or combined with initial bursts of prednisone (40–60 mg). The application of silver nitrate to the ulceration base is also useful. The cause is uncertain, but evidence suggests that aphthous stomatitis is a noninfectious inflammatory mucosal disease that may have multiple causes, including stress and gastroesophageal reflux. Severe recurrent aphthous stomatitis may also respond to oral colchicine and dapsone.

Trauma to the tooth may provoke inflammation of the periodontal membrane **(acute periodontitis),** rendering it tender to touch. If the traumatic stimulus is removed, the inflammation resolves. Recurrent gingivitis coupled with poor dental hygiene may cause chronic periodontitis, pyorrhea, and regression of the periodontal ligament from the neck of the tooth. The gingival sulcus deepens, pockets form between the roots of the teeth and the surrounding gingivae, and debris and tartar accumulate. Mild periodontitis is characterized by gingival erythema, edema, tenderness, and hemorrhage. Severe periodontitis is associated with gingival necrosis, halitosis, and loss of unstable teeth. Unless the cycle is broken, periapical abscess formation and tooth devitalization will continue. Frequent flossing and regular professional dental care are recommended.

HERPETIC STOMATITIS

Herpetic lesions of the oral cavity are divided into primary gingivostomatitis, herpes labialis, and intraoral herpes—all caused by human herpes virus type 1 (HHV-1) and presenting as small vesicles that rupture, yielding a yellow-white superficial ulcer surrounded by a red halo. They are usually located on the labial and buccal mucosa, gingivae, and tongue. In contrast to recurrent aphthous ulcers, recurrent HHV-1 lesions are limited to the attached gingiva and hard palate. In severe cases, the gingivae are edematous and bleed readily. The primary form is accompanied by fever, pain,

malaise and cervical lymphadenopathy. Although the primary disease is self-limiting, virus may be reactivated by physical trauma and endogenous stress. Treatment is supportive, including topical anesthetics in solution or troche form. If herpetic stomatitis occurs as part of a disseminated infection or in an immunocompromised patient, systemic acyclovir (200 mg five times daily) is prescribed. Newer antiviral agents—valacyclovir and famciclovir—have been used successfully. Topical acyclovir has limited usefulness in treating herpes labialis but can be effective if prescribed early in the prodromal stage. Penciclovir cream has also been reported to be effective in reducing the clinical signs and symptoms of recurrent herpes labialis.

Spruance SL et al: Penciclovir cream for the treatment of herpes simplex labialis. A randomized, multicenter, double-blind, placebo-controlled trial. JAMA 1997;277:1374.

ORAL CANDIDIASIS

Oral candidiasis (thrush) is caused by the yeast-like fungus *C albicans* and characterized by a white pseudomembranous lesion closely adherent to the mucous membrane, which bleeds and ulcerates when it sloughs. It also occurs in a hyperplastic form, characterized by superficial fungal invasion of the epithelium and leukoplakia; in an erythematous or atrophic form; and as angular cheilitis. Candida is normally a part of the oral biota but may become pathogenic after prolonged administration of antibiotics; radiation therapy to the cavity or pharynx; immunotherapy for carcinoma, leukemia, or lymphoma; or immune deficiency associated with corticosteroid therapy, diabetes, hepatic disease, etc. In addition, candidiasis along with oral hairy leukoplakia (nontender, caused by Epstein-Barr virus) is identified in patients with AIDS. Other local causative factors include xerostomia, smoking, smokeless tobacco, and mechanical changes in the oral environment such as dentures or poor oral hygiene. Oral nystatin, clotrimazole, or miconazole is effective treatment. For immunocompromised hosts who develop systemic candidal infections, amphotericin B is recommended. Ketoconazole administered orally is the drug of choice for chronic mucocutaneous candidiasis. The treatment of chronic mucocutaneous candidiasis may also include immunologic therapy with thymic transplants and infusion of lymphocytes from immunocompetent donors. Severely immunocompromised patients may benefit from the protracted use of prophylactic fluconazole. Chlorhexidine rinses have proved useful in treating oral candidiasis in children with leukemia.

Como JA et al: Oral azole drugs as systemic antifungal therapy. N Engl J Med 1994;330:263.

Lynch DP: Oral candidiasis: history, classification and clinical presentation. Oral Surg Oral Med Oral Pathol 1994;78:189.

Scully C et al: Candida and oral candidosis: a review. Crit Rev Oral Biol Med 1994;5:125.

CONGENITAL ORAL CAVITY MALFORMATIONS

Torus Palatinus & Torus Mandibularis

Torus palatinus, a common developmental abnormality of the oral cavity, consists of a bony exostosis of varying size and shape in the midline of the palate. Clinically, it may interfere with proper fitting of dentures and require surgical removal. It must be distinguished from tumors of the minor salivary glands and fissural cysts of the palate.

Torus mandibularis, like its palatal counterpart, is a bony exostosis usually situated on the lingual surface of the mandible adjacent to the cuspid and first bicuspid teeth. It is asymptomatic until an attempt is made at fitting a denture.

Macroglossia

Isolated macroglossia is rare and may be seen in cretinism, Down's syndrome, and acromegaly. It may also be caused by lymphangiomatous invasion of the tongue. Relative macroglossia is encountered in Pierre Robin syndrome (micrognathia and cleft palate). The relatively large tongue may obstruct the upper airway, necessitating insertion of an oral airway or tongue-lip adhesion. The tongue base is sutured over an anterior neck button to assist in anterior displacement of the tongue. These measures are only necessary until the oral cavity enlarges enough to accommodate the tongue. Tracheostomy is rarely necessary.

Ankyloglossia

Tongue-tie or partial ankyloglossia is manifested by an abnormally short and thick lingual frenulum. Various degrees of ankyloglossia occur, ranging from mild restriction with only a mucous membrane band to those in which both the frenulum and the underlying fibers of the genioglossus muscle are markedly fibrosed. Rarely, complete ankyloglossia with fusion of the tongue to the floor of the mouth may be encountered. Limitation of movement of the tongue tip results in malocclusion with an anterior "open bite" deformity, early prognathism, and swallowing and speech difficulties. Children with severe ankyloglossia meeting any of these criteria require frenulectomy, genioglossus myotomy, and mucous membrane closure with multiple Z-plasties.

Ranula

A ranula is a transparent retention cyst in the floor of the mouth arising from the sublingual salivary glands. The cyst enlarges gradually, penetrating the deep structures of the floor of the mouth above the mylohyoid muscle. It should be excised if it is small; marsupialization is necessary for large cysts, owing to the multiple ramifications.

■ SALIVARY GLANDS

There are three pairs of major salivary glands (parotid, submandibular, and sublingual) responsible for the secretion of saliva and stimulated by swallowing. Hundreds of minor salivary glands maintain resting levels of saliva necessary for moisturizing, lubrication, cleansing, digestion, and immunologic protection of the mouth.

ACUTE BACTERIAL SIALADENITIS

Acute bacterial sialadenitis may develop secondary to obstruction, stasis of saliva, or decreased secretion. There is diffuse painful enlargement of the gland, often with erythema and tenderness. Typically this occurs in the older patient who is taking diuretics or is dehydrated. The most common organism responsible, especially in acute parotitis, is *S aureus.* Other organisms include streptococci, *E coli,* and anaerobes. Antibiotic therapy is with a first-generation cephalosporin (cephalothin or cephalexin) or dicloxacillin. Alternatives are clindamycin, amoxicillin-clavulanate, or ampicillin-sulbactam.

VIRAL SIALADENITIS

Mumps is the most common viral cause of acute salivary inflammation. Young children 4–10 years of age are most commonly affected, developing bilateral swelling of the parotid glands 2–3 weeks after exposure. Symptoms last 7–10 days. Cytomegalovirus (CMV) is the second most common cause of acute viral sialadenitis and may mimic infectious mononucleosis clinically and hematologically.

CHRONIC SIALADENITIS

Chronic or recurrent bacterial sialadenitis or submandibular sialadenitis may develop as a result of antecedent acute suppuration or viral inflammation. More commonly, however, there is a history of ductal obstruction. Recurrent bacterial invasion of the parotid gland or submandibular gland leads to destruction and fibrosis of acini with ductal ectasia. The subsequent decrease in salivary flow creates a cycle of ascending sialadenitis, ductal ectasia, acinar atrophy, and obstructive fibrosis. Clinically, the patient complains of recurrent parotid pain and swelling, typically while eating. Initial treatment should be conservative, utilizing sialagogues (lemon balls or chewing gum), adequate oral hydration to stimulate salivary flow, and amoxicillin-clavulanate or cephalexin. In patients with recalcitrant disease, an extended course of clindamycin, cefoxitin, nafcillin, or vancomycin plus metronidazole may be necessary if methicillin-resistant *S aureus* and penicillin-resistant streptococci are considered. Superficial parotidectomy is recommended if prolonged conservative management fails.

White AK: Salivary gland diseases in infancy and childhood: nonmalignant lesions. J Otolaryngol 1992;21:422.

SIALOLITHIASIS

Salivary gland stones are both a cause and a consequence of chronic sialadenitis. In addition, they may produce acute suppurative sialadenitis. The stones are composed of inorganic calcium and sodium phosphate salts that are deposited in the duct on an organic nidus of mucus or cellular debris. Eighty to ninety percent of salivary calculi occur in the submandibular gland and may lead to complete acute obstruction of the gland, with most stones occurring in the ducts rather than the gland itself. The patient complains of painful swelling, especially with meals, and may report extrusion of gravel from the duct.

The diagnosis is confirmed by palpation of a stone or by demonstration of decreased salivary flow from the duct. Soft tissue films may reveal a radiodense stone, and CT may show sialoliths, though 20–40% of calculi are radiolucent on plain films. Treatment consists of intraoral removal of stones that are close to the duct orifice by ductal dilation and massage. Stones in the hilum of the submandibular gland necessitate excision of the gland if associated with chronic pain and swelling. Parotid sialoliths are managed in a similar fashion.

SALIVARY GLAND TRAUMA

Injuries to the salivary glands may be intraoral or extraoral, blunt or lacerating. The parotid gland is most commonly injured along with associated structures, including the facial nerve, Stensen's duct, soft tissues, mandible, or zygoma. Laceration of the parotid duct may occur with a facial laceration posterior to the anterior edge of the masseter muscle and results in simultaneous injury to the buccal branch of the facial nerve. The severed duct is repaired over a small polyethylene

catheter using fine interrupted sutures. The associated seventh nerve injury is repaired by anastomosing the cut ends with 10-0 monofilament suture. All lacerations in the parotid gland region must be examined for seventh nerve injury. Injury may occur either to the main trunk proximal to the pes anserinus or to one of the branches within the parotid gland. Facial injuries anterior to a vertical line from the lateral canthus of the eye generally do not require exploration, and the nerve will regenerate spontaneously. However, some surgeons advocate microscopic repair to offer a better chance of complete recovery without development of synkinesis (mass movement of the face). If injury to the nerve is suspected, each of the five major branches is assessed by observing voluntary movements and responses to nerve excitability testing. If transection of the facial nerve is likely, exploration and precise repair through a parotidectomy incision with the operating microscope is crucial. The greater auricular or sural nerve may be used as a cable graft for avulsed segments of the facial nerve. An exception to this approach would be an extensively contaminated wound such as a shotgun injury. In this situation, it is better to explore and debride the wound, tag the proximal and distal branches of the injured nerve with metal clips, and delay nerve repair until wound healing is more complete. This should be performed within 30 days after injury to achieve the best results.

May M et al: Managing segmental facial nerve injuries by surgical repair. Laryngoscope 1990;100:1062.

■ PHARYNX

PHARYNGITIS

Acute pharyngitis is usually caused by viruses (especially the adenoviruses and rhinoviruses) or group A beta-hemolytic streptococci. Clinically, erythema, edema, and occasional membrane formation are present, and the patient complains of pain on swallowing. In bacterial pharyngitis, the white count and fever are higher and cervical adenopathy is more marked. Pneumococci, *H influenzae, M catarrhalis, Neisseria gonorrhoeae,* and coagulase-positive staphylococci are the primary pathogens. Pharyngeal cultures are obtained. Antibiotic treatment is primarily directed toward group A beta-hemolytic streptococcus with penicillin or erythromycin, even in the face of a negative rapid strep test because of the potential sequelae of rheumatic fever and glomerulonephritis. The goal of antibiotic therapy is to eliminate infections, avoid suppurative complications, hasten recovery, and prevent rheumatic fever. Other bacterial agents, including *Mycoplasma pneumoniae* and chlamydia species, may account for a third of bacterial pharyngitis in adults. Treatment is with a macrolide (erythromycin, clarithromycin, or azithromycin). Gonococcal pharyngitis occurs in 1–2% of the sexually active population and is treated with a single dose of intramuscular ceftriaxone or oral cefixime. Concurrent treatment for chlamydia is required.

One must differentiate acute bacterial pharyngitis from diphtheritic pharyngitis and infectious mononucleosis. *Corynebacterium diphtheriae* is a potentially lethal bacterium in a nonimmunized host. Characteristic features are odynophagia, fever, and the development of a gray pseudomembrane on the oropharynx associated with a fetid odor. The membrane bleeds easily when removed and may gradually involve the larynx, producing acute upper airway obstruction. Infectious mononucleosis may mimic diphtheria, exhibiting faucial arch edema, a pharyngeal pseudomembrane, and laryngeal edema. A positive heterophil agglutination or Monospot test, absolute lymphocytosis, generalized lymphadenopathy, and hepatosplenomegaly differentiate this disease from diphtheria. Tonsilloadenoidal hyperplasia may be so marked as to obstruct the upper airway, necessitating intubation and tonsilloadenoidectomy.

Acute tonsillitis secondary to group A betahemolytic streptococcal infection commonly occurs in children under 10-years of age and may occasionally present in epidemic form. Clinically, pyrexia, odynophagia, referred otalgia, and malaise predominate. The usual signs of viral upper respiratory tract infection—cough, coryza, and conjunctivitis—are absent. The tonsils appear hyperemic and edematous with or without a purulent exudate filling the tonsillar crypts that coalesces to form a yellow-white pseudomembrane. A 7- to 10-day course of penicillin or cephalexin is adequate therapy, but amoxicillin is frequently substituted because of its dosing schedule. An alternative choice is erythromycin in patients allergic to penicillin. Clindamycin, amoxicillin-clavulanate, or dicloxacillin is indicated for those who do not respond to these drugs. With emerging worldwide *S pneumoniae* resistance to penicillin, clinicians must consider culturing in order to guide treatment when treatment failures occur. The mechanism of streptococcal resistance primarily involves alterations in penicillin-binding proteins responsible for binding β-lactam antibiotics in general rather than the production of β-lactamase enzymes. Amoxicillin, 80–100 mg/kg/d in divided doses, plus amoxicillin-clavulanate may be necessary.

Chronic tonsillitis may follow acute or subacute episodes of tonsillitis, especially in older children, and is associated with recurrent odynophagia, cough, and findings of tonsillar enlargement, debris in tonsillar crypts, and cervical lymphadenitis. There is increasing evidence that *H influenzae* plays a major role in this disorder as well as in the pathogenesis of tonsillar hypertrophy. In addition, *S aureus* has become a more prominent offender, along with actinomycetes. In view of the high incidence of β-lactamase-producing organisms, amoxicillin-clavulanate, clindamycin, or an antistaphylococcal penicillin is recommended. Tonsillectomy is indicated if there are four to six documented episodes of acute tonsillitis per year, three to four episodes in each of the preceding 2 years or three episodes in each of the preceding 3 years.

Acute tonsillitis may in some instances extend beyond the tonsillar tissue into the space between the anterior and posterior tonsillar pillars into the soft palate, producing a **peritonsillar abscess,** or quinsy, which is frequently associated with *S pyogenes* infection. Physical examination reveals an edematous, bulging, anterior tonsillar pillar with medial displacement of the soft palate and uvula. Immediate therapy includes incision and drainage of the abscess through the anterior tonsillar pillar or needle aspiration, intravenous penicillin or clindamycin, hydration, and antipyretics followed by either immediate tonsillectomy or an interval tonsillectomy in 6 weeks. The advantages of immediate tonsillectomy in carefully selected patients include complete abscess drainage without recurrence, rapid relief of symptoms, greater technical simplicity with less hemorrhage, less severe illness, and shorter hospitalization.

Pulmonary hypertension, cor pulmonale, and congestive heart failure (Noonan's syndrome) secondary to chronic hypoxia have been reported in young children with hyperplasia of Waldeyer's ring. More recently, chronic hypersomnolence and periodic apnea have been recognized in children with upper airway obstruction secondary to tonsilloadenoidal hyperplasia. During sleep, these patients experience episodes of hypopnea and periods of cessation of nasal-oral air flow of longer than 10 seconds, persistent chest wall movement, and subsequent hypoxia and hypercapnia. The obstructive sleep apnea syndrome is characterized by frequent arousals during sleep and more subtle clinical findings such as weight loss, behavioral disturbances, learning disabilities, daytime somnolence, and enuresis. Tonsillectomy and adenoidectomy are indicated to relieve upper respiratory tract obstruction.

Isolated adenoidal hypertrophy secondary to physiologic enlargement of the adenoids or chronic viral nasopharyngitis may produce nasal airway obstruction. These children exhibit chronic rhinorrhea, mouth breathing, dental abnormalities, an elongated face, and snoring during sleep. Adenoidectomy is curative.

The obstructive sleep apnea syndrome in adults (Pickwickian syndrome) is commonly seen in obese middle-aged men and spans a wide range of severity. It is defined as daytime sleepiness with altered cardiopulmonary function associated with frequent obstructive apneas or hypopneas during sleep. It is characterized by loud, stertorous snoring. Snoring is caused by high-frequency oscillation of the soft palate, resulting in intermittent narrowing of the pharyngeal airway. An estimated 25% of the adult male population snores every night. The degree of severity of airway obstruction is ascertained by obtaining a polysomnogram that measures the number, frequency, and duration of apneic episodes, the degree of arterial oxygenation saturation, the presence of cardiac arrhythmias associated with apnea, and the degree of daytime impairment. There are many forms of treatment, including behavioral, surgical, medical, and mechanical, some of which can be used in combination. In mild sleep apnea, behavioral treatment—particularly weight reduction—is sufficient. Alcohol consumption should be reduced in the evening hours, and sedative medications that can worsen sleep apnea should be avoided. Mechanical treatment is the best choice for many patients. Nasal continuous positive airway pressure (CPAP) is given by a silicone mask over the nose that is attached by tubing to an air pump. It acts as a pneumatic splint to maintain the patency of the airway. Alternative systems include the use of bi-level pressure (BiPAP). If this is not tolerated, the upper airway obstruction can be corrected with nasal septoplasty and turbinectomy to reduce nasal resistance plus a uvulopalatal pharyngoplasty (UPPP) and tonsillectomy for patients with collapse at either the retropalatal or the velopharyngeal level.

April MM et al: The effect of intravenous dexamethasone in pediatric adenotonsillectomy. Arch Otolaryngol Head Neck Surg 1996;122:117.

Deutsch ES: Tonsillectomy and adenoidectomy. Changing indications. Pediatr Clin North Am 1996;43:1319.

Doern GV et al: Antimicrobial resistance of Streptococcus pneumonia recovered from out patients in the United States during the winter months of 1994 to 1995: results of a 30-center national surveillance study. Antimicrob Agents Chemother 1996;40:1208.

Kiselica D: Group A beta-hemolytic streptococcal pharyngitis: current clinical concepts. Am Fam Physician 1994;49:1147.

Riley RW et al: Obstructive sleep apnea in the hyoid: a reviewed surgical procedure. Otolaryngol Head Neck Surg 1994; 111:717.

Sherae et al: The efficacy of surgical modifications of the upper airway in adults with obstructive sleep apnea syndrome. Sleep 1996;19:156.

Strollo PJ et al: Obstructive sleep apnea. N Engl J Med 1996; 334:99.

Wood AJ: Antimicrobial drug resistance. N Engl J Med 1996; 335:1415.

BENIGN NEOPLASMS OF THE PHARYNX

The most common benign tumor of the nasopharynx is the juvenile angiofibroma, a highly vascular, nonencapsulated, invasive neoplasm with a propensity to occur in adolescent males. The hormone-dependent tumor is stimulated by testosterone and in vitro its growth rate is reduced by antiandrogens such as cyproterone and flutamide.

Onset of clinical signs and symptoms may be at any time from 7 years to 21 years of age. Epistaxis occurs in 75% of cases in addition to nasal obstruction and rhinorrhea. Anosmia is common. Preoperative digital subtraction angiography and CT scanning should be performed to evaluate the blood supply and the anatomic extent of the tumor. The major blood supply is from the internal maxillary artery. Preoperative embolization of the tumor and estrogen therapy markedly decrease blood loss at surgical resection. For lesions confined to the nasopharynx, a transpalatal approach is satisfactory. Larger tumors with involvement of the nasal cavity, the maxillary sinus, the ethmoid sinus, or the sphenoid sinus require a lateral rhinotomy and transpalatal or Caldwell-Luc approach (or both) for complete excision. Although these neoplasms are only moderately responsive to radiation therapy, such therapy is often the treatment of choice for orbital or intracranial invasion.

Hagen R et al: Juvenile nasopharyngeal fibroma: androgen receptors and their significance for tumor growth. Laryngoscope 1994;104:1125.

PHARYNGEAL FOREIGN BODIES

Irregular foreign bodies entering the pharynx are likely to lodge in the lingual or palatine tonsils, valleculae, or piriform sinuses. Smooth round or ovoid objects commonly lodge at the opening to the esophagus or the cricopharyngeus muscle, especially in children. Dysphagia, odynophagia, or aphagia may result. In a young child or infant, drooling is a characteristic sign. Dyspnea, wheezing, or persistent cough may develop secondary to compression of the larynx or trachea. If the esophagus is penetrated by a sharp object such as a pin or fish bone, subcutaneous emphysema can be palpated in the neck. Foreign bodies lodging more distally in the esophagus such as at the level of the aortic arch, left main bronchus, or gastroesophageal junction generally do not produce early symptoms.

Chest x-ray, anteroposterior and lateral neck films, and occasionally a barium swallow are necessary to delineate the site of a foreign body. Foreign bodies of the palatine and lingual tonsils are removed directly with a curved hemostat: objects located in the hypopharynx or esophagus require direct laryngoscopy or esophagoscopy under general anesthesia.

■ LARYNX

The larynx has four functions: (1) protection of the lower airway, (2) phonation, (3) respiration, and (4) fixation of the chest. Laryngeal dysfunction can therefore lead to abnormalities such as aspiration, weak cry, hoarseness, stridor, and poor cough. These problems point to laryngeal dysfunction and should prompt an inspection of the larynx with a laryngeal mirror (indirect laryngoscopy) or fiberoptic nasopharyngolaryngoscopy during phonation, swallowing, and deep inspiration. Cinefluoroscopy with barium sulfate allows assessment of the competency of the larynx during swallowing. Neoplasms and traumatic lesions of the larynx are effectively evaluated by CT scan or MRI. In any individual with hoarseness of more than 2–3 weeks' duration, the larynx should be inspected as described above. If the larynx cannot be inspected in this way, transnasal fiberoptic laryngoscopy or direct laryngoscopy under general anesthesia is required. A specimen of larynx is obtained at direct laryngoscopy for biopsy examination for suspected neoplasms.

FOREIGN BODIES OF THE LARYNX & TRACHEOBRONCHIAL TREE

For children, a variety of objects, including seeds, beans, pins, and tiny toys, may be aspirated into the tracheobronchial tree. In adults, meat is the most common cause of obstruction and is associated with a number of factors: (1) large, poorly chewed pieces of food, (2) elevated blood alcohol, and (3) upper and lower dentures. The development of a **café coronary** is frequently confused with a myocardial infarction.

Foreign bodies entering the tracheobronchial tree must pass (1) the epiglottis, (2) the upper laryngeal inlet, (3) the false cords (ventricular bands), (4) the true vocal cords, and (5) the cough reflex. If a foreign body lodges in the larynx, there is immediate pain and laryngospasm, dyspnea, and inspiratory stridor proportionate to the degree of upper airway obstruction. The voice may be hoarse or aphonic.

If partial airway obstruction is present and the victim can exchange air and cough, no attempt should be made to move the foreign body at that time. If the victim is aphonic, unable to cough or exchange air, and is clutching his or her neck, complete airway obstruction is present. If equipment is not at hand for emergency tracheotomy or cricothyrotomy, the Heimlich maneuver is recommended for relieving foreign body airway obstruction: a series of four manual thrusts are administered to the upper abdomen, exerting downward pressure on the diaphragm and compressing the lung. Finally, if the foreign body remains in the larynx or pharynx after these maneuvers, manual removal with the finger probe may be successful.

In the conscious adult patient with adequate air exchange, indirect laryngoscopy supplemented with anteroposterior and lateral x-rays of the neck and chest will confirm the position of the foreign body. Removal of a laryngeal foreign body necessitates general anesthesia and a laryngoscope and alligator forceps. Foreign bodies in the tracheobronchial tree also require general anesthesia and open bronchoscopy with forceps removal.

The reaction of the tracheobronchial tree to a foreign body depends upon the degree of obstruction and the physical nature of the foreign body. For example, a bean acts as a ball valve, rising with expiration and occluding the distal airway on inspiration. Vegetable matter produces a violent bronchitis that may be associated with chronic suppurative pneumonitis; and nonobstructive metallic objects may remain within the tracheobronchial tree for an extended period causing little tissue damage.

Tracheal foreign bodies produce inspiratory and expiratory wheezing. With distally located objects, three different patterns may occur: (1) partial (bypass valve) bronchial obstruction, in which the foreign body permits the passage of air during both inspiration and expiration; (2) expiratory check valve obstruction, where ingress of air is minimally impaired but egress is checked, resulting in obstructive emphysema; and (3) stop valve obstruction, in which no air enters the subjacent lung, resulting in atelectasis. Radiographic evaluation is invaluable. The recommended protocol includes anteroposterior and lateral neck and chest films, inspiratory and expiratory films, and, in selected cases, fluoroscopy and decubitus films. Currently, open (rigid) bronchoscopy is the standard way to remove foreign bodies of the tracheobronchial tree and will result in fewer complications and missed foreign bodies. Flexible fiberoptic bronchoscopy is reserved for removing peripheral foreign bodies in patients being maintained on mechanical ventilators or in patients with cervical or maxillofacial trauma.

Hayashi AH et al: Management of foreign body bronchial obstruction using endoscopic laser therapy. J Pediatr Surg 1990; 25:1174.

Inglis AF et al: Lower complication rates associated with bronchial foreign bodies over the last 20 years. Ann Otol Rhinol Laryngol 1992;101:61.

Limper AH et al: Tracheobronchial foreign bodies in adults. Ann Intern Med 1990;112:604.

Mu L et al: The causes and complications of late diagnosis of foreign body aspiration in children. Report of 210 cases. Arch Otolaryngol Head Neck Surg 1991;117:876.

Sataloff RT: Office evaluation of dysphonia. Otolaryngol Clin North Am 1992;25:843.

LARYNGEAL TRAUMA

Trauma to the larynx and trachea may occur from iatrogenic causes (prolonged endotracheal intubation or inappropriate tracheotomy, laryngotomy, or cricothyrotomy) or extrinsic injuries (automobile accidents, neck blows, strangulation, etc). The passenger in the front seat of an automobile is particularly vulnerable to hyperextension injury of the neck. This results in compression of the larynx, hyoid bone, and upper trachea between the dashboard and the cervical spine. Injuries of the larynx are less common in children because of the higher position of the larynx in the neck and the resulting protection provided by the mandible. Severe laryngotracheal injury may occur, however, in children riding bicycles, motor bikes, snowmobiles, etc, who strike a horizontal cable or fall against the handlebars.

The most common injury to the larynx is vertical fracture of the thyroid cartilage with or without fracture of the cricoid cartilage. Because the cricoid cartilage is the only complete cartilaginous ring in the respiratory tract, its functional integrity is critical in maintaining a patent airway. An unreduced fracture of the cricoid may result in subglottic stenosis. Associated injuries of the pharynx, trachea, esophagus, soft tissues, and neurovascular structures of the neck are common. Escape of air into the mediastinum may produce tension pneumothorax.

Clinical findings in laryngotracheal trauma include (1) subcutaneous emphysema or crepitus, (2) dysphonia, (3) loss of the laryngeal prominence (Adam's apple), (4) dysphagia, (5) odynophagia, (6) stridor, (7) hemoptysis, and (8) cough.

Conservative treatment with cool mist, intravenous fluids, cefazolin, and parenteral corticosteroids will suffice for laryngeal soft tissue edema without significant airway obstruction or impaired vocal cord mobility. CT scanning is done to evaluate the laryngeal skeleton for fracture and determine the subsequent course of treatment. It is not performed in patients with an obvious penetrating wound who will require immediate tracheotomy and exploration. More severe laryngotracheal injury requires endotracheal intubation or tracheotomy. In an emergency, an endotracheal tube may be introduced through an open laryngotracheal wound. Ideally, tracheotomy should be performed after the airway is controlled by intubation or open bronchoscopy. However, this may not be possible in cases of complete laryngotracheal separation. If a high tracheotomy or a cricothyro-

tomy has been performed, it should be revised as soon as possible to the third or fourth tracheal ring to prevent vocal cord paralysis and subglottic stenosis. Open reduction and stabilization of all cartilaginous, mucosal, and soft tissue defects with internal fixation and a soft stent is done immediately if the patient's general condition permits. This is recommended within 24 hours. Late laryngeal stenosis may be successfully treated in some patients with the CO_2 laser. Ultimately, the following factors affect wound healing within the larynx and trachea and determine the success or failure of therapy: (1) mechanical loss of lumen-supporting structures, (2) loss of blood supply to cartilaginous structures, (3) presence of chondritis, and (4) degree of progressive fibrosis and stenosis.

Bent JP et al: Acute laryngeal trauma: a review of 77 patients. Otolaryngol Head Neck Surg 1993;109:441.

Schaefer SD: The acute management of external laryngeal trauma. A 27-year experience. Arch Otolaryngol Head Neck Surg 1992;118:598.

Weymuller EA et al: Problems associated with prolonged intubation in the geriatric patient. Otolaryngol Clin North Am 1990;23:1057.

PEDIATRIC AIRWAY OBSTRUCTION

Airway obstruction at birth or in the first several months of life is commonly secondary to congenital and neoplastic disorders. At birth, immediate differentiation must be made between respiratory depression, with cyanosis and shallow, slow respirations; and respiratory tract obstruction, producing tachypnea, stridor, and suprasternal and subcostal retractions.

Stridor (noisy breathing) is the most prominent symptom and is an expression of partial respiratory tract obstruction secondary to external compression or partial occlusion within the airway. The character and intensity of stridor depend upon the site and degree of obstruction and the airflow velocity and pressure gradient across the point of obstruction. Obstruction at the level of the true vocal cords produces high-pitched inspiratory stridor. By contrast, stridor that occurs chiefly during expiration and is lower in pitch is commonly associated with tracheal obstruction. The quality of the cry remains normal in most infants with airway obstruction who do not have a laryngeal lesion. A weak or absent cry at birth suggests neurogenic vocal cord impairment. In addition to evaluating the cry and breathing patterns, the physician should also assess swallowing function in all infants with stridor. Mediastinal tumors and vascular rings producing extrinsic esophageal and tracheal compression cause feeding difficulties and failure to thrive. The presence of recurrent pneumonitis and aspiration suggests a laryngeal lesion or tracheoesophageal fistula. All infants with stridor should have an anteroposterior and lateral chest film and barium swallow followed by endoscopy.

Newborns & Small Infants

The most common cause of infantile stridor is **laryngomalacia,** or **congenital flaccid larynx.** During inspiration, there is extreme infolding of the omega-shaped epiglottis and aryepiglottic folds owing to inadequate cartilaginous support. The presence of staccato stridor with expiration helps identify laryngomalacia. The supine position or head flexion aggravates the stridor, whereas patency of the airway is improved by the prone position and head extension. The stridor gradually resolves in most infants within 2–3 months. Endoscopic inspection is necessary in infants with persistent or progressive stridor.

Congenital subglottic stenosis is the second most frequently encountered laryngeal lesion and may become evident several weeks or more after birth, following an upper respiratory tract infection. Because the subglottic region is the narrowest point in the upper respiratory tract (4.5–5.5 mm at full term, 3.5 mm when premature), a small amount of edema will critically narrow this conduit. Subglottic stenosis is present when the subglottic airway measures less than 4 mm in a full-term infant or 3 mm in a preterm infant. Isolated congenital subglottic stenosis may involve soft tissue stenosis or cartilaginous stenosis of the cricoid cartilage (or both). **Pediatric laryngotracheal stenosis** may be more commonly caused by neonatal intubation as well as external trauma, high tracheotomy, infections, inflammation or burns. It may be isolated to the subglottic space or may occur in combination with supraglottic, glottic, or subglottic stenosis. It often extends into the upper trachea. The subglottis is almost universally involved. A grading system from grade 1, which represents no obstruction, to grade 4, when no detectable lumen can be found, can be used to plan therapy. For grade 1 and 2 stenosis, which ranges from less than 50% obstruction to 70% obstruction, endoscopic CO_2 laser techniques may be the primary therapy for isolated supraglottic, glottic, or subglottic pathology, while anterior laryngotracheal split with either costal or auricular cartilage may be necessary for grade 2 lesions. In grades 3 and 4, where the obstruction ranges from 71% to 100%, anterior and posterior laryngotracheal splits or cricotracheal resection with thyrotracheal anastomosis are required. In most cases, concomitant tracheotomy or stenting of the airway will be necessary until an adequate airway with vocal cord movement is confirmed by microlaryngoscopy and bronchoscopy.

Progressive laryngeal stridor and a croup-like illness in the first several months of life suggest a lesion simulating subglottic stenosis, ie, the **subglottic hemangioma.** The neoplasm is a soft, compressible, bluish tumor below the level of the true vocal cords that is frequently poorly delineated from surrounding tissue. There is a 2:1 female to male preponderance, and 50% of the lesions are associated with cutaneous hemangiomas. The lateral neck film confirms the presence of a localized subglottic soft tissue mass.

Mechanical airway obstruction is treated with tracheotomy; however, early therapy with systemic corticosteroids may decrease the need for tracheotomy. Hemangiomas producing severe airway obstruction that do not respond to corticosteroids or regress spontaneously should be surgically removed. Because they are so vascular, these lesions are best excised with the neodymium:YAG or CO_2 laser in a staged manner.

Larger Infants & Children

Supraglottitis is an acute inflammatory disorder of the larynx secondary to infection with *H influenzae type B*

Table 39–5. Laryngotracheobronchitis and supraglottitis.

Laryngotracheobronchitis	Supraglottitis
Onset and history Relatively slow in onset as the terminal event of a 4- or 5-day respiratory tract infection	Rapid in onset and progressive, advancing to severe airway obstruction within 6–8 hours. Usually no antecedent respiratory infection.
Etiology Usually viral but may be bacterial	Usually bacterial (*Haemophilus influenzae*) but may be viral
Symptoms Stridor, barking cough, sometimes horseness	Stridor preceded by severe sore throat and dysphagia (drooling)
X-ray findings Narrowing of the subglottic airway ("steeple sign")	Enlarged epiglottis on soft tissue lateral to the pharynx and larynx (thumbprint sign)
Treatment Early: Moist oxygen, corticosteroids, antibiotics, and nebulized epinephrine Late: Endoscopic intubation with or without tracheostomy	Immediate moist oxygen and early establishment of an airway by endoscopic intubation. This is followed by administration of intravenous antibiotics.

that affects the epiglottis, aryepiglottic folds, arytenoids, and ventricular bands (Table 39–5). There is usually no prodromal phase, and dysphagia, odynophagia, and shortness of breath rapidly progress to drooling, inspiratory stridor, and a muffled but clear voice. The disease affects principally children 2–6 years of age. Most children are extremely toxic, with fever, tachycardia, and tachypnea. The child sits erect, anxious and increasingly exhausted, drooling, and hungry for air. Lateral neck films confirm the diagnosis and reveal massive edema of the epiglottis (Figure 39–7). However, an x-ray is not essential for the diagnosis. It should not delay immediate treatment.

Immediate control of the airway is mandatory and lifesaving. Children are given 100% humidified oxygen and taken immediately to the operating room, where rapid halothane and oxygen anesthetic induction is followed by atraumatic peroral endotracheal intubation. Pharyngeal and epiglottic blood cultures are obtained, and an intravenous line is started. A course of parenteral

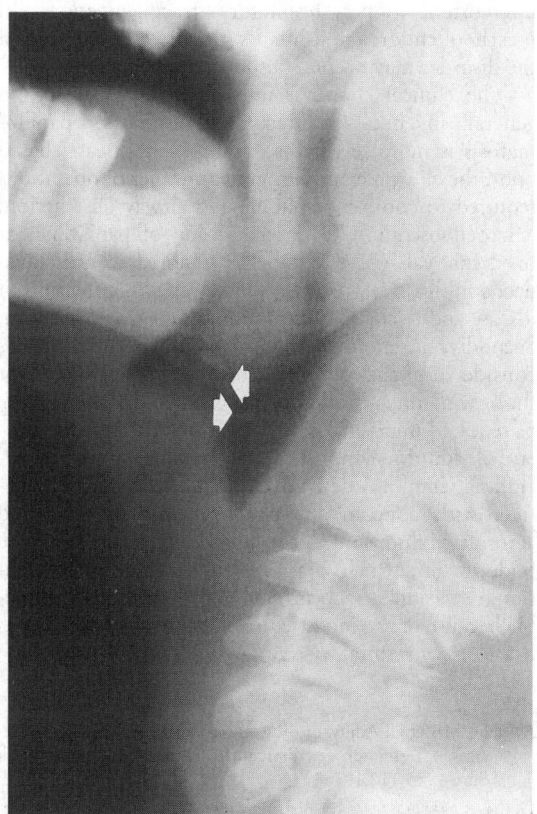

Figure 39–7. Lateral neck film in child with acute supraglottitis. Note the enlarged epiglottis (arrows).

antibiotics consisting of ceftriaxone, cefotaxime, or cefuroxime is initiated pending culture and sensitivity reports. Many consultants today prefer ceftriaxone. If a history of penicillin allergies is obtained, aztreonam or chloramphenicol alone is begun. Direct laryngoscopy is performed to rule out other potential causes of acute laryngeal obstruction. Direct inspection of the larynx reveals a cherry-red swollen epiglottis. At this time, the endotracheal tube is changed to a nasotracheal tube (one or two sizes smaller than normal). A tracheotomy set should be available in case the nasal tracheal tube cannot be properly positioned. Within 72 hours, the infant is generally afebrile and coughing around the tube during suctioning and may be successfully extubated. Of interest is a shifting trend in supraglottitis toward the older pediatric patient and adult. Since the introduction of the Hib vaccine in 1985, a marked decrease in pediatric supraglottitis has occurred. As a result, a relative increase in adult supraglottitis has developed, with two to nine cases per 100,000 in adults and only one per 100,000 in children. Unlike children, adults with supraglottitis have a more gradual onset of symptoms of 36–48 hours, with odynophagia, dysphagia, fever, and leukocytosis—and fewer requiring intubation. Nevertheless, patients should be admitted to an ICU for airway monitoring, intravenous hydration, and intravenous antibiotics aimed at *H influenzae* with equipment available for rapid intubation if necessary.

By contrast, **acute laryngotracheobronchitis** is a viral illness which is far more common than acute supraglottitis (Table 39–5). This illness occurs chiefly in late autumn and winter, with parainfluenza virus the most common cause and adenovirus, rhinovirus, and respiratory syncytial virus also responsible. The principal lesion is subglottic edema, with a variable component of tracheobronchial inflammation. Infants 3 months to 2 years of age are principally affected, exhibiting a 2:1 male:female ratio. The symptoms of a seal-like barking cough, hoarseness, inspiratory and expiratory stridor, and substernal retractions are frequently preceded by an insidious upper respiratory tract illness lasting 1–7 days. In contrast to children with supraglottitis, the infant appears sick but not toxic. Anteroposterior neck films confirm the clinical impression of marked subglottic narrowing (steeple sign) and assist in excluding aerodigestive tract foreign bodies, mediastinal tumors, laryngotracheal neoplasms, and vascular compression of the trachea (Figure 39–8). Initial treatment in the emergency room includes high humidification, oxygenation, hydration, and parenteral corticosteroids (dexamethasone, 0.5–1 mg/kg). Racemic epinephrine is administered by nebulizer with or without intermittent positive pressure, decreasing airway obstruction within 10–30 minutes after administration with the effect waning after 2 hours. The L-isomer is

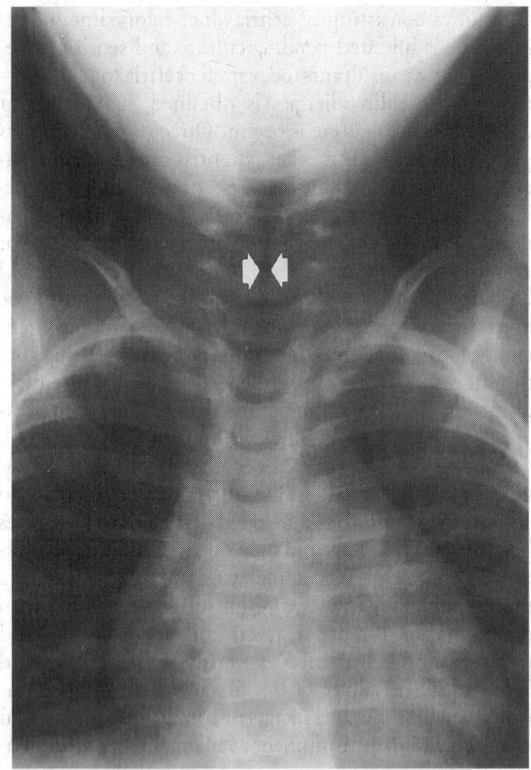

Figure 39–8. Anteroposterior chest film in infant with laryngotracheobronchitis. Marked narrowing of the subglottic space is seen (arrows).

more effective, and the recommended dosage is 0.25 mL of 1:1000 epinephrine if the patient is less than 6 months of age and 0.5 mL of 1:1000 epinephrine if the patient is older. Patients with progressive hypoxia, cyanosis, hypercapnia, and increasing tachypnea and tachycardia who do not respond to medical management should be intubated. The choice of tracheotomy versus oral or nasal intubation is controversial. The rationale against intubation is that in 5% of patients who are intubated subglottic stenosis occurs. This may, however, be reduced by the use of an endotracheal tube that is at least 0.5 mm smaller than the predicted size.

Barrow HN et al: Adult supraglottitis. Otolaryngol Head Neck Surg 1993;109:474.

Carey MJ: Epiglottitis in adults. Am J Emerg Med 1996;14:421.

Frantz TD et al: Acute epiglottitis: changing epidemiologic patterns. Otolaryngol Head Neck Surg 1993;109:457.

Senior BA et al: Changing patterns in pediatric supraglottitis: a multi-institutional review, 1980–1992. Laryngoscope 1994; 104:1314.

RECURRENT RESPIRATORY PAPILLOMATOSIS

The most common benign laryngeal neoplasm is the papilloma. The term juvenile laryngeal papillomatosis was at one time used to describe this condition, but currently the term recurrent respiratory papillomatosis is preferred because it reflects the involvement of the entire upper respiratory tract and its tendency to recur. Caused by human papillomavirus types 6 and 11, one-half of the cases are of juvenile onset, occurring from early infancy through 12 years of age. Adult-onset disease has a peak incidence during the third and fourth decades of life. A history of maternal condylomas is found in up to one-half of patients with juvenile-onset disease. Adult-onset recurrent respiratory papillomatosis is presumed to occur on the basis of sexual contact— primarily oral and genital exposure.

Clinically, because the vocal fold is the first and predominant site of a papilloma lesion, hoarseness is the primary symptom in both juvenile-onset and adult-onset cases. Upper airway obstruction of varying degrees of severity may worsen or initially occur during an intercurrent upper respiratory tract infection. In preschool children and infants, the first presentation of the disorder may occur as a sudden airway crisis.

The clinical course is unpredictable. However, in general, juvenile-onset recurrent respiratory papillomatosis is more severe than adult-onset disease, based upon the clinical extent or on the number of operations required to control dysphonia and airway obstruction. Microendoscopic CO_2 laser excision of papillomas at fixed intervals (2, 4, 6 months) tailored to individual needs fulfills the two main objectives of elimination of disease and maximal preservation of normal epithelium. Secondly, interferon alfacon-1 adjunctive therapy is considered in patients with moderately severe disease or those with uncontrolled or progressive disease in spite of repeated microendoscopic excision. Of the wide variety of additional nonsurgical adjuvants available, including vitamin A derivatives, hematoporphyrin derivatives with concomitant photodynamic therapy, and aerosolized fluorouracil, the most effective appears to be podophyllin, which is applied at the time of conventional excision. Tracheotomy is to be avoided if possible because of the increased risk of spread of papillomas in the lower respiratory tract.

Avidano MA et al: Adjuvant drug strategies in the treatment of recurrent respiratory papillomatosis. Otolaryngol Head Neck Surg 1995;112:197.

Derkay CS: Task force on recurrent respiratory papillomas: a preliminary report. Arch Otolaryngol Head Neck Surg 1995; 121:1386.

Doyle DJ et al: Recurrent respiratory papillomatosis: juvenile versus adult forms. Laryngoscope 1994;104:523.

Eicher SA: Isotretinoin therapy for recurrent respiratory papillomatosis. Arch Otolaryngol Head Neck Surg 1994;120:405.

Hartley C et al: Recurrent respiratory papillomatosis—the Manchester experience, 1974–1992. J Laryngol Otol 1994;108:226-9.

Kashima H et al: Sites of predilection in recurrent respiratory papillomatosis. Ann Otol Rhinol Laryngol 1993;102(8 Part 1):580.

Kashima HK et al: Recurrent respiratory papillomatosis. Obstet Gynecol Clin North Am 1996;23:699.

LARYNGITIS

Acute laryngitis often occurs in association with a general viral upper respiratory tract infection caused mainly by rhinoviruses, respiratory syncytial virus, and adenoviruses. However, if hoarseness persists for more than several days, the possibility of secondary bacterial invasion by *M catarrhalis, H influenzae,* or *S pneumoniae* must be considered. Hoarseness, cough, and odynophagia are often marked, with minimal edema or erythema of the true vocal folds. Treatment includes voice rest, hydration, humidification, and oral cefuroxime, amoxicillin-clavulanate, or a macrolide (clarithromycin, azithromycin).

Chronic laryngitis culminating in polypoid chorditis, on the other hand, is related to many factors, including voice misuse, inhalation of irritants, gastroesophageal reflux, and chronic allergies. Pathologically, fluid accumulates in the subepithelial space of the vocal cords (Reinke's space) on the superior surface of the musculomembranous fold. In some individuals, large sessile polyps may develop and occupy the entire vocal cord or a portion thereof. The voice is severely affected, having a hoarse and breathy character with an abnormally low pitch. Females present with these complaints more frequently than males. In adults, polyps and chronic laryngitis are managed by voice rest, cessation of smoking, avoidance of chronic irritants, and speech therapy. Microdirect laryngoscopy and surgical excision with microforceps or the CO_2 laser are necessary for polyps not responding to conservative management. In patients with gastroesophageal reflux disease, nocturnal heartburn, chronic throat pain, dysphonia, wheezing, and cough are common complaints. The origin is multifactorial: smoking, large meals; drugs such as theophylline, diazepam, and calcium channel blockers; and dietary factors, including caffeine, alcohol, chocolate, fats, and mints contribute to the problem. The resulting chronic posterior laryngitis is related to reflux of acid into the pharynx and may occur without the classic symptoms of gastroesophageal reflux disease. The diagnostic evaluation of GERD-induced posterior laryngitis includes flexible endoscopic examination of the larynx and barium esophagography. Medical therapy includes dietary and lifestyle changes with total acid suppression. Two classes of drugs which are effective are histamine H_2 receptor antagonists (cimetidine, ranitidine, famotidine, nizatidine) and the proton pump inhibitors (omeprazole, lansoprazole). Many clinicians would concomitantly consider esophagogastroduodenoscopy to establish a diagnosis of GERD and stage reflux esophagitis to exclude other esophageal diseases. This permits biopsy of the distal esophagus if columnar metaplasia (Barrett's esophagus), dysphagia, or carcinoma is suspected. As an alternative diagnostic test, 24 hour double-probe pH monitoring and pressure manometry may be appropriate if the patient fails to improve with symptomatic treatment. Omeprazole or lansoprazole for over 6 months may be effective in recalcitrant cases.

Hanson DJ et al: Outcomes of antireflux therapy for the treatment of chronic laryngitis. Ann Otol Rhinol Laryngol 1995;104:550.

Kahrilas PJ: Gastroesophageal reflux disease. JAMA 1996;276:983.

Shaker R et al: Esophagopharyngeal distribution of reflux gastric acid in patients with reflux laryngitis. Gastroenterology 1995;109:1575.

Thompson AR: Pharmacological agents with effects on voice. Am J Otolaryngol 1995;16:1218.

VOCAL NODULES

Misuse of the voice, particularly shouting or roaring in a very high or very low tone of voice, will result in condensation of hyaline connective tissue at the junction of the anterior and middle thirds of the true vocal cords. Vocal nodules occur in both children and adults and produce a hoarse and breathy voice. In children, most nodules regress with voice therapy, and surgical removal is unnecessary. In both children and adults, however, voice therapy must be instituted for persistent nodules before they are endoscopically removed with the laser or microforceps.

VOCAL CORD PARALYSIS

The recurrent laryngeal nerves of the vagus nerves are the primary innervators of the abductors and adductors of the vocal folds. Isolated injury of the recurrent laryngeal nerve results in paralysis of the vocal cord in the paramedian position on one side 2–3 mm lateral to the laryngeal midline. Combined injury of the recurrent and superior laryngeal nerves paralyzes the vocal cord in the intermediate position several millimeters lateral to the paramedial position.

Vocal cord paralysis may be unilateral or bilateral, central or peripheral. Unilateral left vocal cord paralysis is most common. Fewer than 20% of cases are bilateral. Thyroidectomy is by far the most common cause of bilateral vocal cord paralysis. Central causes include brain stem and supranuclear lesions and account for only 5% of all cases. Supranuclear or cortical causes of vocal cord paralysis are exceedingly rare, owing to the bilateral crossed neural innervation to the brain stem medullary centers in the nucleus ambiguus. The most frequent central cause is vascular insufficiency or a stroke affecting the brain stem. Cortical lesions usually do not produce spastic or flaccid paralysis. The patients present with aphonia or speech apraxia. Brain stem lesions, on the other hand, cause flaccid paralysis of the vocal muscles, producing severe dysfunction with weakness of the larynx, pharynx, or tongue and accompanying sensory deficits. Congenital central lesions are usually secondary to Arnold-Chiari malformation or brain stem dysgenesis and are often associated with additional cranial neuropathies.

Most cases of peripheral vocal cord paralysis are secondary to thyroidectomy or nonlaryngeal neoplasms, including bronchogenic, esophageal, and thyroid carcinoma. Other less common lesions causing paralysis of a vocal cord include tumors of the deep lobe of the parotid gland, carotid body tumors, glomus jugulare vagale tumors, and neurogenic neoplasms of the tenth nerve and jugular foramen. External penetrating wounds to the neck or prolonged endotracheal intubation may also traumatize the recurrent laryngeal nerve, producing vocal cord paralysis. Finally, toxic neuropathy and idiopathic causes account for the remaining cases. Idiopathic vocal cord paralysis is a diagnosis of exclusion and is considered to be a viral mononeuropathy. In the majority of these cases, spontaneous recovery occurs within 4–6 months.

In adults, unilateral recurrent laryngeal nerve paralysis generally produces hoarseness and a weak, breathy voice with varying amounts of aspiration of liquids, vocal fatigue, and dysphagia. The normal vocal cord may cross the midline to approximate the paralyzed vocal cord in the paramedian position. In children, varying degrees of inspiratory stridor may also be present. Bilateral vocal cord paralysis is commonly associated with inspiratory stridor, shortness of breath, and dyspnea on exertion.

Diagnostic assessment of vocal cord paralysis includes flexible fiberoptic examination of the larynx and vocal cord movement, examination of the head and neck for neoplasms, chest x-ray, CT scan of the base of the skull to the carina, and perhaps endoscopic evaluation of the aerodigestive tract. Stroboscopic examination of the vocal fold vibratory pattern as well as laryngeal electromyography may be helpful to assess recurrent laryngeal nerve function, determine prognosis for recovery, and evaluate treatment outcomes. In cases of laryngeal trauma, thin-cut (2 mm) CT scanning of the larynx should be obtained to look for arytenoid dislocation or laryngeal fracture.

Management of unilateral vocal cord paralysis due to lesions of the recurrent laryngeal nerve includes observation, speech therapy, and surgery. Compensation by the opposite cord over the first 3–6 months may be sufficient in many patients to preclude the necessity for operation. The options for surgical management are medialization and reinnervation of the paralyzed cord. Medialization options include injection into the paralyzed vocal cord of Teflon paste or Gelfoam under local anesthesia, mobilizing it medially. Medialization is valuable in the therapy of aspiration and results in dramatic improvement in voice quality. Other injection options for glottic insufficiency include bovine collagen, and autologous medialization of the paralyzed cord may also be accomplished externally via a thyroidotomy and placement of a Silastic wedge implant inside the thyroid cartilage in a small pocket deep to the paralyzed vocal cord. An additional external medialization approach—arytenoid adduction through the posterior border of the thyroid lamina—is ideal for correction of a glottic gap involving the posterior and mid portion of the vocal cord. In the past, bilateral paramedian vocal cord paralysis was commonly managed by permanent tracheotomy. Medial arytenoidectomy through an endolaryngeal approach using the CO_2 laser is performed leaving the phonatory glottis intact. This procedure may be complicated by loss of adequate voice production and exacerbation of aspiration. Attempts to treat bilateral abductor vocal cord paralysis with nerve-muscle transposition of the ansa hypoglossi nerve and the omohyoid muscle to the posterior cricoarytenoid muscle have met with qualified success. This reinnervation technique attempts to provide inspiratory neuronal input to the sole abductor of the vocal cord, the posterior cricoarytenoid muscle. Direct anastomosis of the ansa cervicalis to the recurrent laryngeal nerve may reinnervate the larynx and allow the tracheostomy tube to be removed.

Berninger MS: Evaluation and treatment of the unilateral paralyzed vocal cord. Otolaryngol Head Neck Surg 1994;111:497.

Crumley RL: Endoscopic laser medial arytenoidectomy for airway management in bilateral laryngeal paralysis. Ann Otol Rhinol Laryngol 1993;102:81.

McCaffrey TV: Transcutaneous Teflon injection for vocal cord paralysis. Otol Laryngol Head Neck Surg 1993;109:54.

Netterville JL et al: Silastic medialization and arytenoid adduction: the Vanderbilt experience. A review of 116 phonosurgical procedures. Ann Otol Rhinol Laryngol 1993;102:413.

Shindo ML et al: Autologous fat injection for unilateral vocal cord paralysis. Ann Otol Rhinol Laryngol 1996;105:602.

■ INFLAMMATORY NECK MASSES

Acute suppurative lymphadenitis usually occurs in infants and children with viral upper respiratory tract infections. In adults with AIDS or who are immunocompromised for any reason, it may initially present with painful lymphadenopathy in the neck. Bacterial lymphadenitis commonly develops secondary to infection with group A streptococci, *S aureus, S pneumoniae,* or mouth anaerobes and may evolve into a deep neck abscess forming a lateral neck mass. These abscesses are most commonly mixed infections, with anaerobic organisms predominating. Mixed infections are synergistic, and β-lactamase production is common. High fever, neck stiffness, odynophagia, trismus, and leukocytosis characterize this complication. Material obtained from a deep neck infection should be routinely submitted to the laboratory for Gram stain, culture, and sensitivity testing. Deep neck abscesses may develop in the prevertebral, sublingual, submandibular, submental, or retropharyngeal spaces as well as in the lateral neck region. Abscesses of the neck are compartmentalized by two of the three envelopes of the deep cervical fascia—the superficial, middle, and deep layers. Infections may spread from one space to another or extend downward into the mediastinum. In addition, cellulitis or abscess formation in the retropharyngeal space or sublingual space (Ludwig's angina) can obstruct the airway. Infection around the carotid sheath may also produce serious hemorrhage by necrosis of the great vessels and their branches. Necrotizing cervical fasciitis is a particularly virulent form of deep neck infection and is invariably polymicrobial and of dental origin with a significant role played by anaerobes.

Patients with deep neck infections should be hospitalized immediately. Broad-spectrum antibiotic therapy directed against β-lactamase-resistant organisms and anaerobic bacteria is started. Treatment includes ampicillin-sulbactam or clindamycin or cefuroxime plus metronidazole. Methicillin-resistant *S aureus* is often found in patients with deep neck infections secondary to drug abuse. Vancomycin should be considered in these cases. Preoperative localization of the abscess is performed with CT scanning. MRI may be superior to CT in some cases. The presence of free gas in the neck should warn of a possible necrotizing fasciitis. The airway should be controlled with an endotracheal tube or tracheostomy before the abscess is incised and drained. The surgical approach to a deep neck abscess depends on the space involved. Proximal control of the carotid artery should be obtained. The lateral pharyngeal space is approached through an incision parallel to the anterior border of the sternocleidomastoid muscle. Most well-localized retropharyngeal abscesses are drained intraorally. A more conservative approach is transcervical. Submandibular abscesses are approached through an incision 2 cm below the inferior border of the mandible.

Chronic granulomatous infections, which may involve the cervical lymph nodes, include tuberculosis, cat-scratch disease, infections with atypical mycobacteria, and occasionally actinomycosis. Tuberculous adenitis commonly develops following pulmonary tuberculosis and usually responds to triple-drug chemotherapy. Persistently enlarged or suppurative nodes should be excised. Atypical mycobacterial adenitis, on the other hand, is seldom associated with pulmonary disease, and routine tuberculin skin tests are either negative or weakly positive. In contrast to tuberculous adenitis, these atypical infections do not respond well to chemotherapy alone and frequently must be excised or curettaged. Neck masses may result from intravenous cervical drug abuse. *S aureus* is the most common pathogen, and treatment with incision and drainage and intravenous nafcillin or cephalothin is recommended.

Finally, actinomycosis may present as an abscess with multiple draining sinuses near the angle of the mandible, discharging pus with characteristic sulfur granules. Often there is underlying dental disease or osteomyelitis of the adjacent bone. Long-term (3–4 weeks) intravenous penicillin in high doses is necessary; surgical excision should be reserved for persistent disease.

Armstrong M Jr et al: Radiographic imaging of sinusitis and HIV infection. Otolaryngol Head Neck Surg 1993;108:36.

Beitler JJ et al: Low-dose radiotherapy for multicystic benign lymphoepithelial lesions of the parotid gland in HIV-positive patients: long-term results. Head Neck 1995;17:31.

Bielamowicz SA et al: Spaces and triangles of the head and neck. Head Neck 1994;16:383.

Brook I et al: Clinical and microbiological features of necrotizing fasciitis. J Clin Microbiol 1995;33:2382.

Carbone A et al: Head and neck lymphomas associated with human immunodeficiency virus infection. Arch Otolaryngol Head Neck Surg 1995;121:210.

Friedman M et al: Treatment of aphthous ulcer in AIDS patients. Laryngoscope 1994;104:566.

Kennedy TL: Curettage of nontuberculous mycobacterial cervical lymphadenitis. Arch Otolaryngol Head Neck Surg 1992;118:759.

Lazor JB et al: Comparison of computed tomography and surgical findings in deep neck infections. Otolaryngol Head Neck Surg 1994;111:746.

Lee KC et al: Contemporary management of cervical tuberculosis. Laryngoscope 1992;102:60.

Singh B et al: Kaposi's sarcoma of the head and neck in patients with acquired immunodeficiency syndrome. Otolaryngol Head Neck Surg 1994;111.

Stuart MG et al: Nontuberculous mycobacterial infection of the head and neck. Arch Otolaryngol Head Neck Surg 1994; 120:873.

■ AIDS IN OTOLARYNGOLOGY

Because of AIDS, the otolaryngologist is encountering previously rare diseases more often. Examples include cranial and cervical herpes zoster, oral hairy leukoplakia, and oral candidiasis. There are many similarities between AIDS and primary immunodeficiency disorders, including ataxia-telangiectasia, common variable immunodeficiency disease, Wiscott-Aldrich syndrome, and severe combined immunodeficiency disease. As immunosuppressed patients survive longer, they are beginning to manifest cancers such as lymphomas and squamous cell carcinomas in addition to Kaposi's sarcoma.

The most common manifestations of AIDS in the head and neck region are sinusitis and postnasal discharge. Maxillary sinusitis is more common and more severe in AIDS patients than in the general population. In the mouth, Kaposi's sarcoma may occur, primarily on the hard palate, but is also now seen in the larynx. Overall, 15% of AIDS patients present with Kaposi's sarcoma of the head and neck. Lymphoma and oral candidiasis are also common. Oral candidiasis is treated with nystatin or clotrimazole. Oral ketoconazole and fluconazole are alternative agents. Hairy leukoplakia, a nontender lesion caused by the Epstein-Barr virus, is frequently seen with major aphthous ulcers. These ulcers are treated with intralesional injection of triamcinolone acetonide (20–40 mg/mL) depending upon the size of the ulcers. Ulcers are reinjected biweekly as needed. An oral mixture of diphenhydramine, dexamethasone, nystatin, and tetracycline may also prove beneficial. In the cervical region, Kaposi's sarcoma, lymphoma, and *Mycobacterium avium-intracellulare* infections are also encountered.

The otologic manifestations of AIDS are primarily hearing loss, otalgia, otorrhea, vertigo, and tinnitus. Sensorineural hearing loss is the most common finding, with the loss greater in high frequencies. Most commonly, Kaposi's sarcoma presents as a flat lesion involving the auricle. Kaposi's sarcoma of the ear canal is easily managed with the argon laser. *Pneumocystis carinii* granuloma of the ear canal is treated by resection and trimethoprim-sulfamethoxazole. There is no evidence of increased external ear canal fungal infection in AIDS. However, serous otitis media due to auditory tube dysfunction secondary to benign lymphoid hyperplasia is frequent.

Herpes zoster oticus syndrome (Ramsay Hunt's syndrome) is associated with facial paralysis, vertigo, and hearing loss and is best treated with either acyclovir or famciclovir for acyclovir-resistant varicella-zoster virus. Ototoxic drugs used in the treatment of AIDS include acyclovir (which produces vertigo), trimethoprim-sulfamethoxazole (which produces vertigo and tinnitus), and zidovudine (which causes vertigo and hearing loss). HIV infection may alter the natural course of latent syphilis, and patients may present with otosyphilis that is difficult to treat because of the poor vascularity of the otic capsule and its isolation from cerebrospinal fluid. Early treatment with zidovudine (AZT) may help control progression of the disease. Alternatively, didanosine (ddI) or zalcitabine (ddC) may be used for patients unresponsive to AZT or for concurrent use with AZT in advanced cases. Treatment for Kaposi's sarcoma and non-Hodgkin's lymphoma is combination chemotherapy or chemotherapy plus erythropoietic support drugs. Multicystic benign lymphoepithelial lesions of the parotid gland are increasingly seen in patients with HIV and can produce considerable physical discomfort as well as cosmetic deformity. Low-dose radiation therapy provides reliable and temporary palliation for these large lesions.

Armstrong M Jr et al: Radiographic imaging of sinusitis in HIV infection. Otolaryngol Head Neck Surg 1993;108:36.

Beitler JJ et al: Low-dose radiotherapy for multicystic benign lymphoepithelial lesions of the parotid gland in HIV-positive patients: long-term results. Head Neck 1995;17:31.

Carbone A et al: Head and neck lymphomas associated with human immunodeficiency virus infection. Arch Otolaryngol Head Neck Surg 1995;121:210.

Weber PC, Adkins WY Jr: The differential diagnosis of Meniere's disease. Otolaryngol Clin North Am 1997;30:977.

The Eye & Ocular Adnexa

40

Stephen A. Kamenetzky, MD, Linda M. Tsai, MD, & Khalid F. Tabbara, MD

EXAMINATION OF THE EYE

Evaluation of the eye and its adnexa requires a good history, physical examination of the eyes, and assessment of visual function. The history should include general information about the patient's age, occupation, and health status as well as ocular complaints. Occasionally, special examinations may be required to identify specific ocular disorders or to establish the presence of associated systemic disease.

The basic office equipment required for a routine eye examination by a nonophthalmologist includes the following: (1) a hand-held flashlight, (2) a binocular magnifying loupe, (3) an ophthalmoscope, (4) a visual acuity chart, and (5) a tonometer.

The basic medications required for an eye examination are (1) a local anesthetic such as proparacaine 0.5% or tetracaine 0.5%; (2) fluorescein strips; and (3) dilating drops, such as phenylephrine 2.5% or tropicamide 0.5–1%.

Visual Acuity Testing

Central visual acuity should be part of the routine examination of the eye in all patients. The Snellen chart is most commonly used. The patient faces the test chart at a distance of 6 meters (20 feet). The patient is tested by occluding one eye at a time and reading the chart with the unoccluded eye. Visual acuity corresponds to the smallest line the patient can read and is recorded as 20/20, 20/30, 20/40, 20/50, etc. The patient who is unable to read the large letters at the top of the chart should be moved progressively closer until the characters can be read, whereupon the distance between the patient and the chart should be recorded as the numerator. If the patient wears eyeglasses for distance, the visual acuity should be repeated with the glasses on and the results recorded as uncorrected vision and corrected vision. Preschool children or illiterates should be properly instructed and then tested with the illiterate E chart.

Visual Field Testing

Confrontation visual fields can be used to grossly detect visual field defects such as quandrantanopia, hemianopia, or severe visual field constriction. With one eye occluded, the patient is asked to fixate on the examiner's face and detect finger count or hand motion in each quadrant. Formal visual field testing (perimetry) is used to more carefully examine the central and peripheral visual fields. The technique is performed separately for each eye. It is used to measure the function of the retina, the optic nerve and intracranial visual pathway. Because perimetry relies on subjective patient responses, the results will depend on the patient's alertness and cooperation. Several methods are used to assess visual field functions, including the tangent screen, Goldmann perimetry, and computerized automated perimetry.

Tonometry

Tonometry measures intraocular pressure. The most common instruments used are the Schiotz tonometer and the applanation tonometer. Tonometers measure the amount of corneal indentation produced by a preset amount of weight or force. The softer the eye, the less force required to indent the cornea. The normal intraocular pressure varies between 10 mm Hg and 20 mm Hg.

Inspection of Anterior Segment & Adnexa

Inspection of the external ocular structures—lids, conjunctiva, cornea, sclera, and lacrimal apparatus—should include everting the upper eyelids for inspection of the conjunctival surface with the patient looking down. The exposed surfaces are inspected for anatomic defects, foreign bodies, lacerations, inflammation, discharge, tearing, dryness, or other abnormalities. In patients who are unconscious or in coma, the degree of lid closure and the presence of Bell's phenomenon—upward position of the cornea during sleep—are significant findings. Corneal sensation and reflexes in each eye should be noted before any anesthetic drops are used. With the aid of a hand-held flashlight and magnifying loupe or with a biomicroscope (slit lamp), the eye and adnexa can be inspected.

A direct ophthalmoscope focused on the ocular surface may provide some magnification. In addition, considerable detail of the ocular surface can be observed using a +20 diopter lens and a hand-held flashlight.

The depth of the anterior chamber should be noted by shining a light across the eye.

Assessment of Pupillary Functions

Examination of the pupils should be performed before any dilating drops are instilled. Both direct and consensual light reflexes of the pupils should be assessed. The reaction of the pupils with accommodation should be noted. The size of the pupil should be noted, and any differences between the size of the right and left pupil should be recorded and described. In hospitalized patients and those with neurologic disorders, pupils should be dilated with discretion and only with short-acting mydriatics.

Eye Movements

Ocular motility should be assessed in different directions of gaze. In examining eye movements, one should note random movements, the position of the eyes in primary gaze, latent nystagmus, the convergence of the eyes, and ductions in the cardinal positions of gaze. The oculocephalic reflex (doll's head) may be tested, and the response to forced eyelid closure (Bell's phenomenon) should be noted. The light reflection ("reflex") on the cornea from a penlight is at the same point in each eye when the eyes are straight.

Ophthalmoscopy

Ophthalmoscopy is important for the diagnosis of both ocular and systemic conditions. It can be critical in neurologic and neurosurgical contexts. In most instances, the optic nerve head can be clearly seen without dilating the pupils. In hospitalized patients with neurologic and neurosurgical disorders, dilation of the pupils should be avoided unless absolutely necessary. In exceptional cases, short-acting mydriatics such as tropicamide 0.5% should be used to dilate the pupils.

SYMPTOMS & SIGNS OF OCULAR DISORDERS

Visual disturbances or decrease in visual acuity may be due to a number of ocular and systemic diseases.

Decrease in Visual Acuity

Decrease in visual acuity may be unilateral or bilateral, painful or painless, and persistent or transient. The duration of the decrease in visual acuity is important. Was the change noted recently? Was it gradual or sudden? Was it binocular or monocular? Was it discovered accidentally? Unilateral acute painful loss of vision may be due to angle-closure glaucoma, endophthalmitis, or uveitis. Painless unilateral loss of vision may be due to ischemic optic neuropathy, optic neuritis, central retinal artery or vein occlusion, retinal detachment, vitreous hemorrhage, or retinal hemorrhages. Transient painless acute loss of vision in one eye may be due to migraine or amaurosis fugax. Bilateral acute loss of vision may be due to pituitary abnormality, ophthalmic migraine, conversion reaction, or intracranial occipital vascular occlusion.

Disturbances in Vision

Disturbances in vision may consist of image distortion, photophobia, color change, spots before the eyes, visual field defects, night blindness, momentary loss of vision, or halos around lights. Distortion of normal shape is most often due to astigmatism or macular lesions. Photophobia is commonly due to corneal inflammation, iritis, ocular albinism, or aniridia. Changes in color (chromatopsia) such as yellow vision are due to retinal lesions or the use of systemic medications such as digoxin. Spots before the eyes are reported by patients with vitreous opacities or in association with intraocular inflammation. Visual field defects may be due to lid edema, retinal and optic nerve lesions, lesions in the visual pathway, or cortical abnormalities. Night blindness may be genetic, as in patients with retinitis pigmentosa, or acquired—eg, as a result of vitamin A deficiency, glaucoma, optic atrophy, cataract, or retinal degeneration. Transient loss of vision may imply impending cerebrovascular accident or partial occlusion of the internal carotid artery. Colored halos around lights or bright objects are associated with acute angle-closure glaucoma. Incipient cataract may also cause halos (colorless) around point light sources.

Double Vision

Double vision (diplopia) can be constant or intermittent and may occur suddenly in certain positions of gaze or only at certain distances. It is important to differentiate between horizontal diplopia and vertical diplopia, because the nerve pathways are different. Monocular diplopia occurs with refractive error, lenticular changes, macular lesions, malingering, or conversion reactions. Binocular double vision is most often due to misalignment of the eyes from extraocular muscle dysfunction or neurologic abnormalities.

Ocular & Orbital Pain

Ocular pain may result from corneal lesions, inflammation, sudden increase in intraocular pressure, anterior uveitis, cyclitis, scleritis, or optic neuritis. Other causes of pain include inflammation of the orbital contents or tumors in the orbit. Dacryocystitis may also cause severe pain. Eyelid pain may arise from infections of the meibomian glands and the glands of Zeis and Moll.

Redness of the Eye

Acute redness (injection) of the eye not associated with trauma may be due to conjunctivitis, acute anterior uveitis, acute angle-closure glaucoma, corneal infection, or corneal abrasion (Table 40–1). Subconjunctival hemorrhage may also present as a red eye, but this is usually painless and otherwise asymptomatic. Conjunctivitis is the most frequent cause of red eye and can be due to bacterial, chlamydial, viral, or allergic causes. Nonspecific irritation by exogenous agents or a foreign body may also cause redness of the eye. Physical (thermal and irradiation), chemical, and mechanical injury to the eye may lead to redness of the eye and swelling of the periocular and adnexal structures. "Dry eye" or ocular surface anomalies will cause redness, a foreign body sensation, and variable degrees of decreased vision.

Discharge

Ocular discharge may be noted as watery, mucopurulent, purulent, or chronic crusting of the lid margins. When the discharge is watery and not associated with redness or pain, it may be due to excessive tear formation or obstruction of the lacrimal passages. Watery discharge with photophobia, pain, or irritation may be due to keratitis or keratoconjunctivitis. Purulent discharge is a sign of bacterial infection, severe inflammation of the conjunctival surface, or bacterial infection of the lacrimal sac or canaliculus. Mucopurulent discharge may be due to infections with bacterial organisms (eg, pseudomonas or haemophilus species). When the discharge forms mucoid strings, it is characteristic of allergic disorders involving the conjunctiva or dry eye syndrome.

Swelling of the Eyelids

Swelling of the eyelids may be unilateral or bilateral. In unilateral swelling, the patient may suffer from infection of the glands of Meibom, Zeis, or Moll; bilateral swelling may indicate blepharitis or allergic dermatitis. Systemic diseases associated with water retention, hyperthyroidism, or hypothyroidism may also be associated with swelling or puffiness of the eyelids.

Displacement of the Eyes

Forward displacement of the eyes (exophthalmos, proptosis) may be due to abnormalities of the thyroid gland or to tumors of the orbit.

Strabismus

Strabismus results from misalignment of the eyes due to muscle imbalance and may be in the form of tropia

Table 40–1. Differential diagnosis of common causes of inflamed eye.

	Acute Conjunctivitis	Acute Iritis[1]	Acute Glaucoma[2]	Corneal Trauma or Infection
Incidence	Extremely common	Common	Uncommon	Common
Discharge	Moderate to copious	None	None	Watery or purulent
Vision	No effect on vision	Slightly blurred	Markedly blurred	Usually blurred
Pain	None	Moderate	Severe	Moderate to severe
Conjunctival injection	Diffuse; more toward fornices	Mainly circumcorneal	Diffuse	Diffuse
Cornea	Clear	Usually clear	Steamy	Change in clarity related to cause
Pupil size	Normal	Small	Moderately dilated and fixed	Normal
Pupillary light response	Normal	Poor	None	Normal
Intraocular pressure	Normal	Normal	Elevated	Normal
Smear	Causative organisms	No organisms	No organisms	Organisms found only in corneal ulcers due to infection

[1]Acute anterior uveitis.
[2]Angle-closure glaucoma.

(manifest deviation) or phoria (latent deviation). Ocular deviations may be lateral (exotropia) or medial (esotropia) and upward (hypertropia) or downward (hypotropia).

Leukocoria

A white pupil in a child indicates a serious eye disorder. The most frequent cause of leukocoria is congenital cataract, which requires urgent management to prevent amblyopia. Other causes include retinoblastoma, retrolental fibroplasia (retinopathy of prematurity), toxocariasis, persistent hyperplastic primary vitreous, vitreous hemorrhage, retinal detachment, retinal dysplasia, incontinentia pigmenti, Coats's disease, and Norrie's disease.

Other Symptoms

Patients may present with other symptoms such as burning, itching, gritty and foreign body sensations, or a "sandy" feeling. These symptoms in elderly patients are suggestive of dry eye syndrome. Itching is frequently associated with allergic disorders.

■ DISEASES OF THE EYE & ADNEXA

ACUTE HORDEOLUM

Acute hordeolum (sty) is a common infection of the glands of the eyelids involving the glands of Zeis or Moll (external hordeolum). The meibomian glands may be infected, leading to internal hordeolum. The usual causative agent is *Staphylococcus aureus.*

Acute hordeolum is characterized by pain, swelling, and redness of the eyelid. A large hordeolum is infrequently associated with a preauricular lymph node but may lead to an abscess in the eyelid.

If pus is localized and pointing out to the skin or conjunctiva, treatment consists of making a local horizontal (skin) or vertical (conjunctiva) incision. If there is no evidence of abscess formation, the patient can be treated with warm compresses three times daily and topical antibiotic drops such as tobramycin or sulfacetamide 10% three or four times daily for 5–7 days. Ophthalmic ointments such as erythromycin or bacitracin may alternatively be used twice daily for 5–7 days. Oral antibiotics, especially tetracycline derivatives, may be required as an adjunct in patients with acne rosacea.

CONJUNCTIVITIS

Acute conjunctivitis is the most frequent cause of red eye. Infectious causes include bacterial, viral, chlamydial, fungal, and parasitic agents. Less common causes of conjunctivitis include chemical irritation, allergy, hypersensitivity to topical medications, vitamin A deficiency, dry eye syndrome, and injury.

Clinical Findings

A. SYMPTOMS AND SIGNS

Patients with conjunctivitis complain of redness, irritation, a foreign body sensation, and conjunctival discharge. One or both eyes may be affected. In patients with bacterial conjunctivitis, the eyelids may be stuck together in the morning. Examination reveals conjunctival hyperemia with purulent or mucopurulent discharge and variable degrees of lid swelling.

B. LABORATORY FINDINGS

If bacterial conjunctivitis is suspected, conjunctival swabs and scrapings should be taken for culture on blood agar and chocolate agar and for staining with Gram and Giemsa stains.

Treatment

In patients with suspected bacterial conjunctivitis and until laboratory reports are received, topical broad-spectrum antibacterial agents can be prescribed, eg, sulfacetamide 10% eye drops or ciprofloxacin 0.3% eye drops four times daily during the day plus erythromycin or bacitracin ophthalmic ointment at bedtime.

Viral conjunctivitis does not need to be treated and is self-limited. However, if the diagnosis is unclear, topical antibiotics are often used. Contact precautions are useful in all situations of bacterial and viral conjunctivitis since spread of disease is through contact with tears, either directly or through fomites.

Treatment of patients with allergic conjunctivitis consists of topical decongestants (naphazoline 0.1%), and H_1 receptor blocker (livocabastine), or a mast cell stabilizer (cromolyn). Combination mast cell and antihistamine drops such as olopatadine are also available. In severe cases of allergic conjunctivitis, topical corticosteroids may be used with the assistance of an ophthalmologist.

CORNEAL ULCERS

Corneal infections leading to ulceration may be due to bacteria (including chlamydiae), viruses, fungi, or protozoa. The most serious infection of the cornea is caused by pseudomonas species.

Clinical Findings

A. SYMPTOMS AND SIGNS

Patients with corneal ulcers complain of pain, photophobia, and blurring of vision. Patients develop conjunctival hyperemia and chemosis, with ulceration of the cornea and whitish or yellowish infiltrate. Hypopyon (pus in the anterior chamber) may be present in cases due to bacterial or fungal infections.

B. LABORATORY FINDINGS

Laboratory studies include culture and cytologic inspection of corneal scrapings.

Treatment

Corneal ulceration is a serious condition that should be managed carefully and followed closely. The most severe and devastating infection of the cornea is caused by *Pseudomonas aeruginosa*. Topical and subconjunctival antibiotics should be given on an empirical basis until the results of culture and sensitivity tests are obtained. Organism-specific antimicrobial treatment should then be given. Central corneal ulcers may leave corneal scars, causing loss of vision. Patients so affected may require penetrating keratoplasty (corneal transplant).

Patients wearing contact lenses should be advised to stop wearing them. Patients using topical corticosteroids should stop using them.

DACRYOCYSTITIS

Dacryocystitis is a common infection of the lacrimal sac. It may be acute or chronic and occurs most often in infants and in persons over age 40 years. It is usually unilateral and always secondary to obstruction of the nasolacrimal duct. In rare instances, the nasolacrimal duct may be obstructed by a tumor.

Normally, the nasolacrimal duct opens spontaneously during the first month of life. Failure of canalization leads to obstruction of the sac and secondary dacryocystitis.

The cause of acquired nasolacrimal duct obstruction is usually unknown, but trauma to the nose or infection may be responsible. In infants, dacryocystitis leading to obstruction may be due to *Haemophilus influenzae*, staphylococci, or streptococci. In patients with trachoma, nasolacrimal and canalicular obstruction is common. The cause of acute dacryocystitis in adults is usually *Staphylococcus aureus* or beta-hemolytic streptococci. In chronic dacryocystitis, *Streptococcus pneumoniae* is a common pathogen.

Clinical Findings

A. SYMPTOMS AND SIGNS

Acute dacryocystitis is characterized by pain, swelling, tenderness, and redness in the tear sac area; pus may be expressed. In chronic dacryocystitis, tearing and discharge are the principal signs. Mucus or pus may be expressed from the tear sac.

B. LABORATORY FINDINGS

Pus can be expressed from the upper or lower puncta and should be examined by Gram stain and culture and sensitivity testing.

Treatment

A. ADULTS

Acute dacryocystitis responds well to systemic antibiotic therapy, but recurrences are common if the obstruction is not surgically relieved.

B. INFANTS

When ductal obstruction is due to failure of canaliculization in the first month of life, daily forceful massage of the tear sac is indicated, and topical antibiotics should be instilled in the conjunctival sac four or five times daily. If this is not successful, probing of the nasolacrimal duct is indicated. Most ophthalmologists postpone probing until the age of 6 months since in most cases the ducts that will open spontaneously have opened by that time. The probe should be passed through both the upper and the lower canaliculi.

ORBITAL CELLULITIS

Orbital cellulitis is manifested by an abrupt onset of swelling and redness of the lids, accompanied by proptosis, decreased vision, diplopia, and fever. It is usually caused by staphylococci or streptococci. Immediate treatment with intravenous antibiotics is indicated to prevent abscess formation and rapid increase in the orbital pressure, which may interfere with the blood supply to the eye. The response to antibiotics is excellent, but surgical drainage may be required if an abscess forms. CT is indicated to rule out abscess formation. Preseptal cellulitis is limited to the area anterior to the orbital septum and may be treated with oral antibiotics while monitoring closely for progression to orbital infection.

PTERYGIUM

Pterygium is a fleshy, triangular encroachment of the conjunctiva onto the nasal side of the cornea and is usually associated with excessive exposure to wind, sun, sand, and dust. Pterygium may be either unilateral or bilateral. There may be a genetic predisposition, but no hereditary pattern has been described. Excision is indicated if the growth threatens vision by approaching the visual axis, though recurrence is common.

Treatment is by superficial excision. After excising large or recurrent pterygia, autologous conjunctival tissue transplantation is indicated. A thin layer of conjunctiva is obtained from the upper bulbar conjunctiva and sutured to the area where the pterygium was removed. This leads to rapid restoration of anatomic integrity of the epithelial surface and may prevent further recurrences. Patients should be advised to wear sunglasses out of doors. Topical mitomycin eye drops have been used to prevent recurrences of the disease, but serious complications such as scleral thinning and keratitis have been reported.

CATARACT

Cataract is an opacity in the lens that may lead to decrease in vision when it occupies the visual axis. Cataract is the leading cause of curable blindness in the world.

There are three types: (1) congenital cataract, (2) cataract associated with other disorders, and (3) age-related (senile) cataract. Some cataracts are rapidly progressive, while others may show slow progression.

1. Congenital Cataract

Congenital cataract may be genetically determined or may be caused by intrauterine factors that interfere with normal development of the lens. Intrauterine viral infections (the most common is rubella), for example, can lead to congenital cataract.

Congenital cataract may be unilateral or bilateral and complete or incomplete. Dense cataract present at birth is an indication for urgent operative management to prevent amblyopia. Phacoemulsification or simple aspiration with central posterior capsulotomy and limited anterior vitrectomy is recommended for congenital cataract. Preservation of the peripheral posterior capsule and zonules is important for future implantation of intraocular lenses. If the cataract is aspirated, leaving the posterior capsule intact, the posterior capsule becomes opaque, requiring capsulotomy at a later stage. Correction with soft contact lenses can be started immediately after surgery. Posterior chamber intraocular lenses may be implanted when the child is older. Restoration of true binocular vision in very young children is seldom achieved after removal of unilateral congenital cataracts.

2. Cataracts Associated With Other Disorders

Many systemic conditions may be associated with cataracts, including diabetes mellitus, galactosemia, hypocalcemia, myotonic dystrophy, Down's syndrome, and cutaneous disorders such as atopic dermatitis. Certain systemic medications and eye drops containing corticosteroids can also cause cataracts. Other disorders of the eye such as retinal detachment or chronic uveitis may also be associated with cataracts. Physical, mechanical, and thermal injury or ionizing radiation may also lead to cataract.

The treatment of such cataracts is similar to that of senile cataract.

3. Senile Cataract (Age-Related Cataract)

Senile cataract—due to aging of the lens—is the most common type. The rate of progression is variable. Diagnosis is by slit lamp examination. In advanced cataract, a white opacity may be seen in the pupillary area upon gross inspection.

Treatment

Once the cataract leads to visual impairment, treatment is by surgical removal of the lens. Clinical trials of agents that may delay or prevent the formation of cataracts are under way, but no pharmacologic means of prevention is available at present.

Cataract surgery can be done in three different ways. All three methods give excellent results, with complete restoration of visual acuity. In rare cases where intraocular lenses are contraindicated, such as certain forms of uveitis, optical correction can be achieved with eyeglasses or contact lenses.

A. Intracapsular Lens Extraction

Intracapsular extraction, rarely used today, removes the lens entirely with its capsule either by forceps or a cryoprobe. This procedure cannot be performed on children or young adults because of the adhesion between the lens and the vitreous.

B. Extracapsular Extraction

With standard extracapsular cataract extraction (Figure 40–1), the anterior capsule of the lens is removed, the nucleus of the cataract is expressed, and the residual cortical material is aspirated from the eye through a 9–11 mm incision. The posterior capsule is left intact

Figure 40–1. Extracapsular cataract extraction. **A:** Performing a circular anterior capsulotomy. **B:** Removal of the excised anterior capsule of the cataract. **C:** Expression of the nucleus of the cataract. **D:** Removal of the remaining cortical material by irrigation and aspiration.

and an intraocular lens which restores vision is placed in the capsular bag. The incision is then sutured with 10-0 nylon. In 25–35% of patients undergoing extracapsular cataract extraction, the posterior capsule may become opacified. This is treated by Nd:YAG laser capsulotomy. If such a laser is not available, surgical incision of the opaque posterior capsule is required.

C. PHACOEMULSIFICATION

Phacoemulsification, now the most common form of extracapsular cataract extraction, involves fragmenting the nucleus of the lens with a high-frequency ultrasonic probe and simultaneously aspirating the nuclear fragments from the eye. The advantage of phacoemulsification is that the incision size can be reduced and the patient more quickly rehabilitated. The cortical material is removed by irrigation and aspiration. The use of foldable lenses allows placement of the lens implant through the small incision, and in many cases no suture is required.

ANGLE-CLOSURE GLAUCOMA (Acute Glaucoma)

About 1% of people over age 35 have anatomically narrow anterior chamber angles. In such patients, if the pupil dilates spontaneously or is dilated with a mydriatic or cycloplegic agent, the angle may close and an attack of acute glaucoma may be precipitated. For this

reason, it is a wise precaution to estimate the depth of the anterior chamber angle before instilling these drugs.

Acute angle-closure glaucoma is manifested by an acute onset of pain, headache, and blurring of vision. Some patients develop nausea and vomiting. The eye is red, the cornea is hazy, and the pupil is mid-dilated and does not react to light. Intraocular pressure is elevated.

The attack is aborted by use of topical pilocarpine, beta-blockers, apraclonidine and latanoprost drops, systemic acetazolamide, and, if necessary, an intravenous hyperosmotic agent such as mannitol. Definitive treatment consists of peripheral iridotomy, which establishes a communication between the posterior and anterior chambers. This is usually done with an argon or Nd:YAG laser. Rarely, surgical peripheral iridectomy is required.

OPEN-ANGLE GLAUCOMA (Chronic Simple Glaucoma)

In open-angle glaucoma, the intraocular pressure is usually consistently elevated. Over a period of months or years, this results in optic atrophy, with loss of vision varying from slight constriction of the upper nasal peripheral visual fields to complete blindness. The cause of the decreased rate of aqueous outflow in open-angle glaucoma has not been clearly demonstrated. The disease is bilateral but can be asymmetric and is probably genetically influenced. Blacks are particularly at risk.

Clinical Findings

Patients with open-angle glaucoma have no symptoms initially. On examination, there may be slight cupping of the optic disk. The visual fields gradually constrict, but central vision remains good until late in the disease. Tonometry, ophthalmoscopic visualization of the optic nerve, and visual field testing are the three principal tests used for the diagnosis and continued clinical evaluation of glaucoma.

The normal intraocular pressure is about 10–20 mm Hg. The diagnosis is never made on the basis of a single tonometric measurement. Transient elevations of intraocular pressure do not constitute glaucoma for the same reason that periodic or intermittent elevations of blood pressure do not constitute hypertensive disease. All persons over age 20 should have tonometric and ophthalmoscopic examinations every 3–5 years. The examination may be performed by the general physician, internist, or ophthalmologist. If there is a family history of glaucoma or other risk factors, annual examination is indicated. Low tension glaucoma is an uncommon condition characterized by visual field changes and optic nerve cupping in the presence of normal ocular pressure.

Treatment

Most patients can be controlled with topical beta-blockers (eg, timolol maleate 0.25-0.5%, 1 drop twice daily), topical alpha-adrenergic agonists (eg, brimonidine 0.2%, 1 drop twice daily), topical carbonic anhydrase inhibitors (eg, dorzolamide 2%, 1 drop twice daily), or topical prostaglandins (eg, latanoprost 0.005%, 1 drop once daily). Oral carbonic anhydrase inhibitors (eg, acetazolamide) are used in patients with persistently uncontrolled high intraocular pressures. Miotics (eg, pilocarpine 1–4%, 1 drop four times daily) and epinephrine eye drops (0.5–2.0%, 1 drop twice daily) are less commonly used. (*Caution:* Epinephrine is contraindicated if the anterior chamber angle is narrow.)

Argon laser trabeculoplasty can be helpful in decreasing the intraocular pressure in some patients. In those with persistent pressure elevation, surgery is indicated. The most common filtering procedure is trabeculectomy. The success of this procedure has been improved by the use of intraoperative application of mitomycin to inhibit the fibrosis and closure of the filtering channels. In certain types of glaucoma such as neovascular glaucoma or aphakic glaucoma with failed filtering procedures, valves can be used.

RETINAL DETACHMENT

Detachment of the retina is usually spontaneous but may be secondary to trauma. Spontaneous detachment occurs most frequently in persons over 50 years of age.

Retinal tears or holes are the most important predisposing factors. Increased risk of retinal detachment is also associated with cataract surgery and high myopia.

In the presence of a retinal tear or hole, fluid from the vitreous cavity enters the defect and transudation from choroidal vessels—combined with abnormal vitreous traction on the retina and the force of gravity—leads to detachment of the retina from the pigment epithelium. The superior temporal area is the most common site of detachment. The area of detachment rapidly increases, causing progressive visual loss. Central vision remains intact until the macula becomes detached.

On ophthalmoscopic examination, the retina is seen as an elevated gray membrane. One or more retinal tears may be seen.

Treatment

All cases of retinal detachment should be referred immediately to an ophthalmologist. If the patient must be transported a long distance, the head should be positioned so that the detached portion of the retina will recede with the aid of gravity. For example, a patient with a superior temporal retinal detachment in the right eye should lie supine with the head turned to the right. Position is less important for a short trip.

Retinal detachment is a true emergency if the macula is threatened. If the macula is detached, permanent loss of central vision may occur even though the retina is eventually successfully reattached by surgery. Treatment consists of closure of retinal tears by cryosurgery, laser, or scleral buckling. This produces an inflammatory reaction that causes the retina to adhere to the choroid. The laser is of value in a limited number of cases of minimal detachment. The laser creates an inflammatory adhesion between the choroid and the retina. Its main use is in the prevention of detachment by sealing small retinal tears before detachment occurs.

In uncomplicated retinal detachment with a superior retinal tear and healthy vitreous, pneumoretinopexy may be performed. The procedure consists of injection of air or certain gases into the vitreous cavity through the pars plana, and positioning the patient to augment sealing of the retinal hole and permit spontaneous reabsorption of the subretinal fluid.

About 85% of uncomplicated cases can be cured with one operation; an additional 10% will need repeated operations; and the remainder never reattach. The prognosis is worse if the macula is detached, if there are many vitreous strands, or if the detachment is of long duration.

Without treatment, retinal detachment almost always becomes total in 1–6 months. Spontaneous detachments are ultimately bilateral in 20–25% of cases.

STRABISMUS

Any child under age 7 (especially infants and young children) with strabismus should be seen without delay to prevent amblyopia and to treat it at an early stage. In adults, the sudden onset of strabismus usually follows head trauma, microvascular infarct, intracranial hemorrhage, or brain tumor. About 3% of children are born with or develop strabismus. In descending order of frequency, the eyes may deviate inward (esotropia), outward (exotropia), upward (hypertropia), or downward (hypotropia).

Clinical Findings

Children with frank strabismus first develop diplopia. They soon learn to suppress the image from the deviating eye, and the vision in that eye therefore fails to develop. This is the first stage of amblyopia. Most cases of strabismus are obvious, but if the angle of deviation is small or if the strabismus is intermittent, the diagnosis may be missed.

Amblyopia due to strabismus can be detected by routine visual acuity examination of all preschool children. Visual acuity testing with an illiterate E card can be used by those who cannot be tested with a standard eye chart.

Treatment

The objectives in treatment of strabismus (Figure 40–2) are to achieve good visual acuity in each eye; straight eyes, for cosmetic purposes; and coordinate function of both eyes (fusion). The best time to initiate treatment is at about age 6 months. If treatment is delayed beyond this time, the child will favor the straight eye and suppress the image in the other eye. This results in failure of visual development (amblyopia) in the deviating eye.

If the child is under age 6 years and has an amblyopic eye, vision may be improved by occluding the good eye. At age 1 year, patching may be successful within 1 week; at 6 years, it may take a year to achieve the same result, ie, to equalize the visual acuity in both eyes. Surgery to align the eye is usually performed after the visual acuity has been equalized. The prevention of blindness by these simple diagnostic and treatment procedures is one of the most rewarding experience in medical practice.

Surgery for correction of strabismus consists of weakening or strengthening the extraocular muscles. For correction of exotropia, the lateral rectus muscles in each eye are weakened by recession. The muscle is detached at its insertion and then resutured posteriorly to the sclera at a distance not to exceed 8 mm from the original insertion. Alternatively, a lateral rectus muscle may be recessed and the medial rectus muscle in the same eye cut at its insertion and a part of the muscle not to exceed 6 mm resected. The muscle is then resutured to its original insertion. The amount of recession and resection and the number of extraocular muscles resected or recessed is determined by the degree of ocular deviation. In patients with esotropia, both medial recti are recessed or a single medial rectus is recessed in combination with resection of the lateral rectus in the same eye. For vertical deviation, the vertical muscles are recessed, resected, tucked, or weakened by myectomy (usually the inferior oblique).

■ OCULAR BURNS

CHEMICAL BURNS

Apart from the history, the diagnosis of chemical eye burns is usually based on the presence of swelling of the eyelids and marked conjunctival hyperemia and chemosis. The limbus may show blanched patchy areas and conjunctival sloughing, especially in the interpalpebral area. There is usually corneal stromal haze and diffuse edema, with wide areas of epithelial cell loss and corneal ulcerations. Defects in the cornea can be better visualized with the instillation of fluorescein.

Alkali burns of the eye are serious because the agents tend to rapidly penetrate intraocularly and damage the tissue. Retained particles in the conjunctival fornices may cause progressive damage and must be promptly removed. Patients are managed by instilling a

Figure 40–2. **A:** Exposure of an extraocular muscle in surgery for strabismus. **B:** Recession of the muscle behind its original insertion followed by suturing to the sclera with absorbable suture.

topical anesthetic agent and then promptly irrigating copiously with isotonic saline solution. Double eversion of the upper eyelid should be performed to look for and remove material lodged in the superior fornix. This can be easily done by using a forceps or moist cotton applicator. A lid speculum is placed after the instillation of tetracaine 0.5% eye drops, and the eye is irrigated with saline. Topical dilating drops such as atropine 1% or homatropine 5% are instilled, and a topical antibiotic ointment such as ophthalmic erythromycin and bacitracin should be applied.

Acid burns cause rapid damage but are in general less serious than alkali burns. Management consists of immediate irrigation with sterile isotonic saline solution, water, or whatever safe liquid is available. A topical anesthetic agent is instilled to minimize pain during irrigation. The patient is then given an analgesic and the eye is patched. Topical antibiotic ointment may also be used.

THERMAL BURNS

The treatment of thermal burns of the eyes is similar to the treatment of burns elsewhere on the body. Systemic analgesia should be provided. A topical anesthetic agent such as proparacaine 0.5% or tetracaine 0.5% is used to minimize pain during manipulation. In cases of burns involving the cornea, topical dilating drops such as atropine 1% or homatropine 5% are instilled. Antibiotic drops are often prescribed for 3–5 days.

BURNS DUE TO ULTRAVIOLET RADIATION

Injuries to the corneal epithelium by ultraviolet rays may be mild or severe. This is referred to as actinic keratitis, snow blindness, welder's arc burn, or flash burn, depending on the source of ultraviolet radiation. Patients present with severe pain and photophobia. The examination reveals diffuse punctate staining of the cornea, best seen with fluorescein staining, proper magnification, and a cobalt blue light.

A topical antibiotic such as ophthalmic erythromycin or bacitracin ointment is instilled. Topical nonsteroidal drops such as diclofenac or ketorolac tromethamine may be used for pain.

■ OCULAR TRAUMA

Ocular trauma may be classified as penetrating or nonpenetrating. Trauma can lead to permanent reduction or loss of vision. Eye injuries are common in spite of the protection afforded by the bony orbit. The use of safety goggles at work helps prevent most serious occupational injuries to the eye.

Clinical Evaluation

A careful history of the injury should be obtained from the patient or someone who knows what happened. Visual acuity should be measured with and without glasses. The eyelids, conjunctiva, cornea, anterior chamber, iris, lens, vitreous, and fundus should be inspected for lacerations, breaks, or hemorrhage. Detection of corneal damage (such as abrasions) can be performed by instilling fluorescein dye and examining the eye using a cobalt blue light under magnification. X-ray examination is helpful in looking for fractures of the orbital bones and trying to rule out radiopaque foreign bodies. CT scan is performed when available. Patients with severe injuries should have immediate ophthalmic consultation. Further damage can be caused by manipulation, which for that reason should be avoided.

PENETRATING OR PERFORATING INJURIES

Penetrating or perforating ocular injuries require immediate careful attention and prompt surgical repair to prevent functional loss.

Many facial injuries—especially those occurring in automobile accidents—are associated with penetrating ocular trauma. Some injuries may be undetected and inapparent because of eyelid swelling or because the patient's other injuries have demanded the attention of the emergency room staff. Such injuries, if not promptly attended to or adequately managed by an ophthalmologist, may lead to loss of vision. Accurate records and a description of how the injury occurred should be obtained. The eye and ocular adnexa should be examined, including vision testing and testing of ocular motility. *Do not apply pressure on the globe.* X-ray examination and CT scan are performed to rule out fractures of orbital bones or the presence of intraocular foreign bodies.

Careful repair and approximation of corneal and scleral lacerations should be performed in the operating room. Metallic intraocular foreign bodies can often be removed with a magnet at the time of suturing of the corneal or scleral lacerations. The major objectives in management of ocular penetrating or perforating injuries are to relieve pain, preserve or restore vision, and achieve good cosmetic results. Pain relief may be achieved by the administration of morphine, 2–4 mg intravenously or subcutaneously, or meperidine, 50–75 mg intramuscularly as needed. Sedatives such as diazepam, 5 mg, may be given orally as required.

The injured eye should be covered gently with sterile gauze or an eye pad and a protective Fox shield, but no pressure should be applied. Parenteral broad-spectrum antibiotics such as cefazolin or gentamicin should be given. Antiemetics—ondansetron, 4 mg intravenously—should be given to patients who are vomiting to prevent further injury.

LACERATIONS OF THE OCULAR ADNEXA

Lacerations of the eyelids and the periorbital skin should be carefully evaluated and inspected. Superficial laceration of the skin can be sutured by approximation. In cases of deep eyelid lacerations, intraocular or orbital damage should be ruled out. The skin of the eyelids has good elasticity, is loosely attached to underlying tissue, and in adults is frequently present in surplus quantities. This facilitates the development of flaps and grafts. Small linear skin lacerations may be easily sutured and the wound secured with interrupted 6-0 nylon suture. Because of the good blood supply, the sutures may be removed in 3–5 days. In deep lacerations of the eyelids, if the wound divides the orbicularis muscle parallel to its fibers, only skin sutures are generally required. When the muscle fibers are transversely divided they should be approximated with absorbable sutures using 6-0 Vicryl or Dexon sutures. The skin can be approximated with fine silk or nylon sutures. In patients with lacerations resulting in round or oval losses of skin, the skin is undermined and the laceration approximated. In larger defects, reconstruction with flaps may be required. Flaps used in reconstruction of the eyelids are advancement flaps, rotational flaps, transposition flaps, island flaps, and Z-plasty flaps.

In large defects, when flaps cannot be used, free skin grafts may be obtained from behind the ear or from the skin of the inner upper arm.

The main problem that complicates suturing of the lower eyelid is retraction or eversion from vertical tension, which for that reason should be avoided.

BLUNT TRAUMA TO THE OCULAR ADNEXA & ORBIT

See Table 40–2.

Contusions of the eyeball and ocular adnexa may result from blunt trauma. The outcome of such an injury cannot always be determined, and the extent of damage may not be obvious upon superficial examination. Careful eye examination is needed, along with x-ray or CT scan.

Table 40–2. Types of ocular injury associated with blunt trauma.

Eyelids	Ecchymosis, swelling, laceration, abrasions, conjunctival or subconjunctival hemorrhages.
Cornea	Edema, lacerations.
Anterior chamber	Hyphema, recession of angle, secondary glaucoma.
Iris	Iridodialysis, iridoplegia, rupture of iris sphincter.
Ciliary body	Hyposecretion of aqueous humor.
Lens	Cataract, dislocation.
Vitreous	Vitreous hemorrhage.
Ciliary muscle	Paralysis.
Retina	Commotio retinae, retinal edema, choroidal breaks in Bruch's membrane, choroidal hemorrhage.

BLOWOUT FRACTURE OF THE FLOOR OF THE ORBIT

Blowout fracture of the floor of the orbit can be associated with enophthalmos, double vision in primary position or in upper gaze, limitation of ocular movement in upper gaze, hypotropia, and decreased or absent sensation over the maxillary area. CT scan of the orbit shows orbital floor displacement.

The management of patients with blowout fractures of the orbital floor should be carefully assessed by both an ophthalmologist and an otolaryngologist because of potential associated fractures of the maxilla or zygoma. The patients is usually treated with a systemic antibiotic (cephalothin or amoxicillin/potassium clavulanate), told not to blow his nose, and reassessed within 1 week by an ophthalmologist. Operative management is recommended if there is significant enophthalmos, continued diplopia in primary gaze, or significant instability of the orbital floor.

CORNEAL & CONJUNCTIVAL FOREIGN BODIES

Patients may give a history of working with high-speed tempered steel tools, or drilling, or hammering against a hard object. There may be no history of trauma to the eye, and the patient may not be aware of a foreign body. In most cases, however, the patient complains of foreign body sensation in the eye or under the eyelid, pain, tearing, and photophobia.

Malignant Tumors of the Eyelids

Squamous cell carcinoma has a tendency to grow slowly and painlessly. It begins as a small lesion covered by a layer of keratin. The lesion may erode, causing an ulcer with hyperemic edges. It may enlarge to form a fungating mass and may invade the orbital cavity. Early excision may result in cure. If early treatment is not provided, squamous cell carcinoma may spread via the lymphatic system to the preauricular and submandibular lymph nodes.

Basal cell carcinoma begins as a slowly growing, locally invasive tumor forming the so-called rodent ulcer with raised nodular borders. Inner canthal basal cell carcinoma may invade locally and extend into the orbit. Treatment should include complete excision to prevent recurrence.

Malignant melanomas of the eyelids are similar to malignant melanomas of the skin elsewhere on the body.

CONJUNCTIVAL TUMORS

Benign tumors of the conjunctiva include melanocytic nevi (pigmented or nonpigmented), papillomas, granulomas, dermoid tumors, and lymphoid hyperplasia. Malignant tumors of the conjunctiva include carcinoma, malignant melanoma, and, rarely, lymphoma. Carcinoma of the conjunctiva arises frequently at the limbus or the inner canthus in the exposed area of the bulbar conjunctiva. Early in the course of the disease, the lesion may resemble a pterygium. The tumor is slightly elevated, with a gelatinous surface, and may spread over the corneal surface. The growth of this lesion is slow. Treatment is by excisional biopsy.

INTRAOCULAR TUMORS

Benign Intraocular Tumors

Melanocytic nevi of the iris, ciliary body, or choroid are common. No treatment is required for these lesions. Retinal angioma may be seen in patients with phacomatoses (eg, Bourneville's disease). Choroidal hemangioma is another less frequently encountered benign intraocular tumor.

Malignant Intraocular Tumors

Malignant intraocular tumors include malignant melanoma of the uvea, retinoblastoma, and a rare tumor of the ciliary body known as diktyoma or medulloepithelioma.

Malignant melanoma of the uvea is most common primary intraocular tumor in adults. It typically occurs in the fifth or sixth decade and is almost always unilateral. The most frequent site is the choroid, but malignant melanoma may occur also in the ciliary body or iris. Malignant melanomas of the choroid may cause decrease in vision and may undergo necrosis, leading to intraocular inflammation. Histopathologic examination shows spindle-shaped cells with or without prominent nuclei and large epithelioid tumor cells. Intraocular malignant melanomas may spread directly through the sclera by local invasion or directly into the central nervous system via optic nerve extension.

Malignant melanomas can be detected by ophthalmoscopy after pupillary dilation.

Treatment of malignant melanoma consists of enucleation or radiotherapy, using radioactive plaques or charged particles. Extension outside the eye may require exenteration of the orbit. Patients with small melanomas—less than 10 mm in diameter—can be observed by serial photography of the fundus. Similarly, small melanomas of the iris that have not invaded the iris root can be safely followed and observed until growth is documented. If there is growth of the iris tumor, treatment is by local iridectomy. If the iris malignant melanoma invades the root and ciliary body, it can be removed surgically by iridocyclectomy.

Retinoblastoma is a rare but life-threatening condition in childhood. It is the most frequent intraocular malignant tumor in children arising from embryonic cone cells of the photoreceptor layer. Most patients with retinoblastoma present in the first or second year of life. Patients may present with leukocoria or strabismus. Retinoblastoma may be multifocal, and both sporadic and inherited forms occur. It may grow slowly to fill the intraocular space and undergo necrosis, leading to calcific deposits. Tumor cells may seed on the iris and in the anterior chamber, causing fluffy whitish exudates.

Spontaneous remission of retinoblastoma has been reported. Treatment oiptions include radiotherapy, cryotherapy, chemotherapy, and enucleation.

ORBITAL TUMORS

Orbital tumors may be of two types: those arising from orbital tissues (primary orbital tumors) and those invading the orbit from adjacent structures (secondary orbital tumors). Primary orbital tumors include benign tumors such as dermoid cysts, hemangiomas, lipomas, fibromas, osteomas, chondromas, neurofibromas, and lacrimal gland tumors. Malignant tumors of the orbit include rhabdomyosarcoma, adenocarcinoma of the lacrimal gland, and lymphomas. Invading tumors include malignant melanoma and retinoblastoma from the intraocular structures and malignant melanomas and carcinomas from the skin of the eyelids and conjunctiva. Metastatic lesions may reach the orbit from the lung or breast. Neuroblastoma may also metastasize to the orbit in children. Meningiomas of the cranial nerves may invade the orbit through the optic canal.

Treatment and prognosis in all cases depend on the type of tumor.

■ LASER TREATMENTS FOR OCULAR DISEASE

The laser has many useful applications in ophthalmology. Using various gases, a single-wavelength beam can be produced that can be absorbed by selective tissues in they eye.

DIABETIC MACULAR EDEMA

Macular edema occurs in the preproliferative stage of diabetic retinopathy and is characterized by retinal thickening with or without exudates within the central macular area. This procedure is performed with a slit-lamp delivery system with a contact lens and is aided by fluorescein angiography. Improvement may take up to 3 months to occur. Long-term studies by the National Institutes of Health have shown that treatment with an argon laser may improve visual outcome by up to 50%.

PANRETINAL PHOTOCOAGULATION

Panretinal photocoagulation is indicated for treatment of proliferative diabetic retinopathy. Using a contact lens and a slitlamp delivery system, extensive destruction of peripheral retina is undertaken to decrease production of vasoproliferative factors and increase retinal oxygenation, thus causing regression of abnormal blood vessels that lead to hemorrhage, scarring, and retinal detachment.

LASIK SURGERY FOR CORRECTION OF REFRACTIVE ERROR

Laser in-situ keratomileusis (LASIK) is a lamellar refractive surgical procedure which involves creation of a partial-thickness corneal flap under high suction. The flap is then lifted and an ArF (argon-fluoride) excimer beam is used to ablate stromal tissue with minimal damaging thermal effect. The flap is then replaced and allowed to heal. The combination of accuracy, precision, minimal postoperative discomfort, and quick visual recovery has made this the most popular refractive technique.

PHOTODYNAMIC THERAPY

Photodynamic therapy is a laser procedure that allows selective treatment for wet exudative age-related macular degeneration in patients who have subfoveal choroidal neovascularization. The choroidal lesion must be predominantly classic in nature, which means more than half of it must be evident on fluorescein angiography. The procedure involves intravenous infusion of a photosensitizer, verteporfin, which collects onlyin abnormal tissue and is then photoactivated by a non-thermal laser light applied through a slitlamp delivery system. The theory is that photoactivation leads to cellular damage and subsequent vessel occlusion and regression of abnormal blood vessels without damage to surrounding normal tissue.

Urology

Richard D. Williams, MD, Christopher S. Cooper, MD, & James F. Donovan, Jr., MD

EMBRYOLOGY OF THE GENITOURINARY TRACT

A basic understanding of genitourinary embryology facilitates the learning of many aspects of urology. Embryologically, the genital and urinary systems are intimately related. Associated anomalies of the two systems are commonly encountered.

The Kidneys

The kidneys pass through three embryonic phases (Figure 41–1): (1) The **pronephros** is a vestigial structure without function in human embryos that, except for its primary duct, disappears completely by the fourth week. (2) The pronephric duct gains connection to the **mesonephric tubules** and becomes the mesonephric duct. While most of the mesonephric tubules degenerate, the mesonephric duct persists bilaterally; from where it bends to open into the cloaca, the ureteral bud grows cranially to interact with the metanephric blastema. (3) This forms the **metanephros,** which is the final phase. The metanephros develops into the kidney. During cephalad migration and rotation, the metanephric tissue progressively enlarges, with rapid internal differentiation into the nephron and the uriniferous tubules. Simultaneously, the cephalad end of the ureteral bud expands and divides within the metanephros to form the renal pelvis, calices, and collecting tubules.

The Bladder & Urethra

Subdivision of the cloaca (the blind end of the hindgut) into a ventral (urogenital sinus) and a dorsal (rectum) segment is completed during the seventh week and initiates early differentiation of the urinary bladder and urethra. The urogenital sinus receives the mesonephric duct and absorbs its caudal end, so that by the end of the seventh week the ureteral bud and mesonephric duct have independent openings. The ureteral orifice migrates upward and laterally. The mesonephric duct orifice moves downward and medially, and the structure in between (the trigone) is formed by the absorbed mesodermal tissue, which maintains direct continuity between the two tubes (Figure 41–2).

The fused müllerian ducts also meet the urogenital sinus at Müller's tubercle. The urogenital sinus above Müller's tubercle differentiates to form the bladder and the part of the prostatic urethra proximal to the seminal colliculus in the male or the bladder and the entire urethra in the female (Figure 41–3). Below Müller's tubercle, the urogenital sinus differentiates into the distal part of the prostatic urethra and the membranous urethra in the male or the distal vagina and vaginal vestibule in the female. The rest of the male urethra is formed by fusion of the urethral folds on the ventral surface of the genital tubercle. In the female, the genital folds remain separate and form the labia minora.

The prostate develops at the end of the 11th week as several groups of outgrowths of urethral epithelium both above and below the entrance of the ejaculatory duct (distal vas deferens). The developing glandular element (seminal colliculus) incorporates the differentiating mesenchymal cells surrounding it to form the muscular stroma and capsule of the prostate. The seminal vesicles form as duplicate buds from the distal end of the mesonephric duct (vas deferens).

The Gonads

The potential to differentiate along male or female lines is present in every embryo initially. The development of one set of sex primordia and the gradual involution of the other are determined by the genetic sex of the embryo and differential secretion of numerous hormones. The *SRY* gene—or testis-determining factor—on the Y chromosome drives the gonad to differentiate into a testicle. Gonadal differentiation begins during the seventh week (Figure 41–3). If the gonad develops into a testis, the germinal epithelium progressively grows into radially arranged, cord-like seminiferous tubules. The production of müllerian inhibiting factor (MIF) by the testicle causes regression of the müllerian duct and acts in a local (paracrine) fashion so that only the ipsilateral müllerian duct is affected. The subsequent production of testosterone by the testicle leads to masculinization of the mesonephric (wolffian) duct structures (ie, epididymides, vas deferens, seminal vesicles, and ejaculatory duct). If the gonad develops into an ovary, it becomes differentiated into a cortex and a medulla; the cortex later differentiates into ovarian follicles containing ova. The lack of testosterone leads to the disappearance of the mesonephric duct.

Figure 41–1. Schematic representation of the development of the nephric system. Only a few of the tubules of the pronephros are seen early in the fourth week, while the mesonephric tissue differentiates into mesonephric tubules that progressively join the mesonephric duct. The first sign of the ureteral bud from the mesonephric duct is seen. At 6 weeks, the pronephros has completely degenerated and the mesonephric tubules start to do so. The ureteral bud grows dorsocranially and has met the metanephric blastema. At the eighth week, there is cranial migration of the differentiating metanephros. The cranial end of the ureteral bud expands and starts to show multiple successive outgrowths (renal calices).

The testes remain in the abdomen until the seventh month and then pass through the inguinal canal to the scrotum, following the path of the gubernaculum. The mechanism of descent remains uncertain. Lack of complete testicular descent is known as cryptorchidism; descent to an abnormal site beyond the external inguinal ring known as testicular ectopia.

The ovary, which is attached to ligaments, undergoes internal descent to enter the pelvis.

In the female, the genital duct system develops from the müllerian ducts, which fuse at their caudal ends and differentiate into the uterine tubes, the uterus, and the proximal two-thirds of the vagina.

The external genitalia start to differentiate by the eighth week. The genital tubercle and genital swellings develop into the penis and scrotum in the male and the clitoris and labia majora in the female. The external genitalia are masculinized by dihydrotestosterone (DHT), which is created from testosterone under the influence of 5α-reductase.

With the breakdown of the urogenital membrane in the seventh week, the urogenital sinus achieves a separate opening on the undersurface of the genital tubercle. The expansion of the infratubercular part of the urogenital sinus will form the vaginal vestibule and the distal third of the vagina. The two folds on the undersurface of the genital tubercle unite in the male to form

the penile urethra; in the female, they remain separate to form the labia minora.

Patten RM et al: The fetal genitourinary tract. Radiol Clin North Am 1990;28:115.

ANATOMY OF THE GENITOURINARY TRACT: GROSS & MICROSCOPIC

The Kidneys

The kidneys lie retroperitoneally in the posterior abdomen and are separated from the surrounding renal fascia (Gerota's fascia) by perinephric fat. The renal vascular pedicle enters the renal sinus; the vein is anterior to the artery, and both are anterior to the renal pelvis. The renal artery divides just outside the renal sinus into anterior and posterior branches that undergo further subdivisions with variable extents of distribution. They are end arteries and thus result in segmental infarction when occluded. The venous tributaries anastomose freely and usually drain into one renal vein.

The Renal Parenchyma

The renal parenchyma consists of more than 1 million functioning units (nephrons) and is divided into a pe-

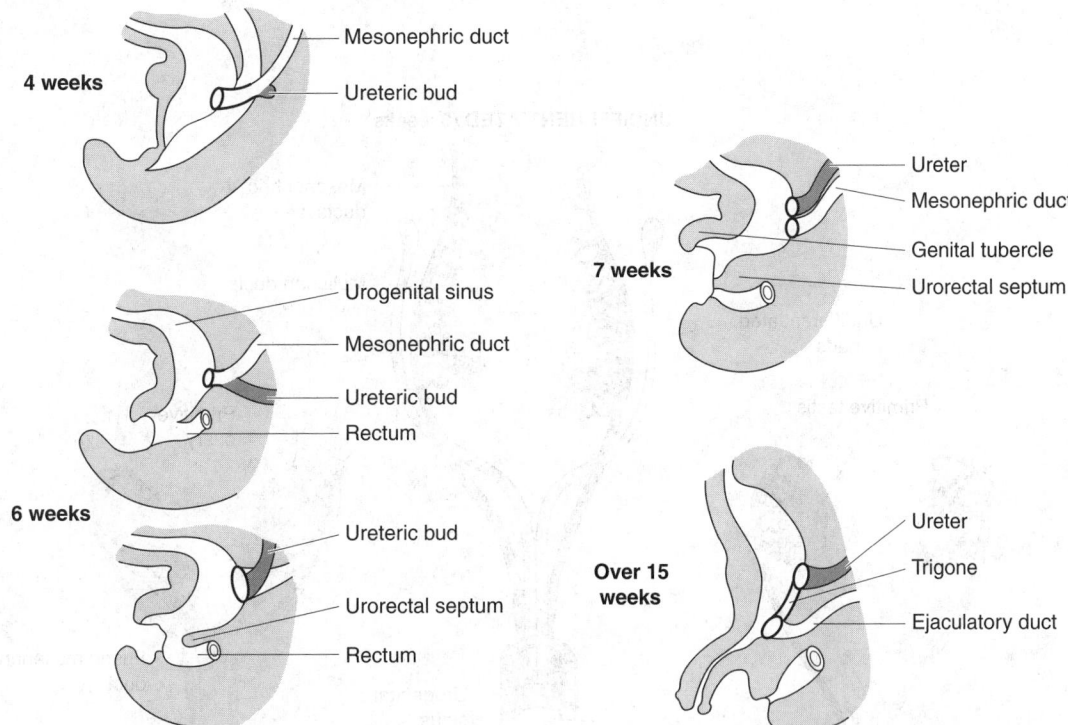

Figure 41–2. The development of the ureteral bud from the mesonephric duct and their relationship to the urogenital sinus. The ureteral bud appears at the fourth week. The mesonephric duct distal to this ureteral bud will be gradually absorbed into the urogenital sinus, resulting in separate endings for the ureter and the mesonephric duct. The mesonephric tissue that is incorporated into the urogenital sinus will expand and form the trigonal tissue. The mesonephric duct will form the vas deferens in the male and Gartner's duct (if present) in the female.

ripheral cortex containing secretory elements and a central medulla containing excretory elements. The nephron starts as Bowman's capsule, which surrounds the glomerulus and leads to elongated proximal and distal convoluted tubules with the loop of Henle in between, ending in a collecting duct that opens into a minor calix at the tip of a papilla.

The Renal Pelvis & Calices

The renal pelvis and calices are within the renal sinus and function as the main collecting reservoir. The pelvis, which is partly extrarenal and partly intrarenal (but occasionally is totally extra- or intrarenal), branches into three major calices that in turn branch into several minor calices. These calices are directly related to the tips of the medullary pyramids (the papillae) and act as a receiving cup to the collecting tubules. The pelvicaliceal system is a highly muscular structure; the fibers run in many directions and are directly con-

tinuous from the calices to the pelvis, allowing synchronization of contractile activity.

The Ureter

The ureter connects the renal pelvis to the urinary bladder. It is a muscularized tube; its muscle fibers lie in an irregular helical arrangement and function primarily in peristaltic activity. Ureteral muscle fibers are directly continuous from the renal pelvis cranially to the vesical trigone distally.

The blood supply to the renal pelvis and ureters is segmental, arising from multiple sources, including the renal, gonadal, and vesical arteries—with rich subadventitial anastomoses.

The Bladder

The bladder is primarily a reservoir with a meshwork of muscle bundles that not only change from one plane to

Figure 41–3. Transformation of the undifferentiated genital system into the definitive male and female systems.

another but also branch and join each other to constitute a synchronized organ. Its musculature is directly continuous with the urethral musculature and thus functions as an internal urethral sphincteric mechanism in spite of the lack of a true circular sphincter.

The ureters enter the bladder posteroinferiorly through the ureteral hiatus; after a short intravesical submucosal course, they open into the bladder and become continuous with the trigone, which is superimposed on the bladder base though deeply connected to it.

The Urethra

The adult female urethra is about 4 cm long and is muscular in its proximal four-fifths. This musculature is arranged in an inner longitudinal coat that is continuous with the inner longitudinal fibers of the bladder and an outer circular coat that is continuous with the outer longitudinal coat of the bladder. These outer circular fibers comprise the sphincteric mechanism. The striated external sphincter surrounds the middle third of the urethra.

In the male, the prostatic urethra is heavily muscular and sphincteric. The membranous urethra is within the urogenital diaphragm and is surrounded by the striated external sphincter. The penile urethra is poorly muscularized and traverses the corpus spongiosum to open at the tip of the glans.

The Prostate

The prostate surrounds the proximal portion of the male urethra; it is a fibromuscular, cone-shaped gland about 2.5 cm long and normally weighing about 20 g in the adult. It is traversed from base to apex by the urethra and is pierced posterolaterally by the ejaculatory ducts from the seminal vesicles and vas deferens that converge to open at the verumontanum (seminal colliculus) on the floor of the urethra.

The prostatic glandular elements drain through about 12 paired excretory ducts that open into the floor of the urethra above the verumontanum. The prostate is surrounded by a thin capsule, derived from its stroma, which is rich in musculature, and part of the urethral musculature and the sphincteric mechanism. A rich venous plexus surrounds the prostate, especially anteriorly and laterally. Its lymphatic drainage is into the hypogastric, sacral, obturator, and external iliac lymph nodes.

The Testis, Epididymis, & Vas

The testis is a paired organ surrounded by the tunica albuginea and subdivided into numerous lobules by fibrous septa. The extremely convoluted seminiferous tubules gather to open into the rete testis, where they join the efferent duct and drain into the epididymis. The epididymis drains into the vas deferens, which courses through the inguinal canal into the pelvis and is joined by the duct from the seminal vesicle to form the ejaculatory duct, which opens before opening into the prostatic urethra on either side of the verumontanum.

Arterial supply is via the spermatic, vas deferential, and external cremasteric arteries. Venous drainage is through the pampiniform plexus, which drains into the internal spermatic veins; the right spermatic vein joins the vena cava and the left joins the renal vein.

Testicular lymphatics drain into the retroperitoneal lymph nodes; the right primarily into the interaortocaval area, the left into the para-aortic area, both just below the renal vessels.

de Groat WC: Anatomy and physiology of the lower urinary tract. Urol Clin North Am 1993;20:383.

Preuss HG: Basics of renal anatomy and physiology. Clin Lab Med 1993;13:1.

PHYSIOLOGY OF THE GENITOURINARY TRACT

The Kidneys

The kidneys maintain and regulate homeostasis of body fluids by the following mechanisms:

A. GLOMERULAR FILTRATION

This is dependent on glomerular capillary arterial pressure minus plasma colloid osmotic pressure plus Bowman's capsular resistance. The resultant glomerular filtration pressure (about 8–12 mm Hg) forces protein-free plasma through the capillary filtering surface into Bowman's capsule. Normally, about 130 mL of plasma is filtered every minute through the renal circulation; the entire volume of plasma recirculates through the kidney and is subjected to the filtration process once every 27 minutes.

B. TUBULAR REABSORPTION

About 99% of the filtered volume will be reabsorbed through the tubules, together with all the valuable constituents of the filtrate (chlorides, glucose, sodium, potassium, calcium, and amino acids). Urea, uric acid, phosphates, and sulfates are also reabsorbed to varying degrees. The process of reabsorption is a combination of active and passive transport mechanisms. Reabsorption of water and electrolytes is under the control of adrenal, pituitary, and parathyroid hormones.

C. TUBULAR SECRETION

This helps (1) to eliminate certain substances and thus maintain their plasma levels and (2) to exchange valuable ions from the filtrate for less desirable ions in the plasma (eg, a sodium ion from the urine for a hydrogen ion in the plasma). Failure of adequate secretory function leads to the acidosis commonly encountered in chronic renal disease.

The Ureteropelvicaliceal System

This system is one continuous tubular structure with a syncytial type of smooth musculature that is imperceptibly in motion from one segment to the other. Waves of peristaltic contractions start from the calices and are propagated along the smooth muscle cells to the renal pelvis. At normal urine flow rates, many of these contractions waves are terminated at the ureteropelvic junction; however, some are transmitted to the ureter and down toward the urinary bladder. These peristaltic waves occur at a rate of about 5–8/min, involve a 2- to 3-cm segment at a time, and usually proceed at the velocity of 3 cm/s. Frequency, amplitude, and velocity are influenced by urine output and flow rate. In a state of diuresis, there may be a 1:1 relationship between caliceal contractions and ureteral contractions. Ureteral filling is primarily passive and occurs by reception of a bolus of urine from a renal pelvis contraction. The ureteropelvic junction closes after passing a bolus of urine, preventing back pressure and back flow of urine unto the renal pelvis secondary to the elevated ureteral contraction pressure. A contraction ring forms in the proximal ureter, and as it migrates down the ureter it pushes the bolus of urine antegrade. In states of diuresis, the size of the bolus increases and the pressure in the bolus may be greater than the pressure in the contraction ring ahead of it. In this case, the ureteral walls cannot coapt, and urine is transported as an uninterrupted column of fluid.

The Ureterovesical Junction

The ureterovesical junction allows flow of urine from the ureter to the bladder and at the same time prevents retrograde flow. The continuity and the specific muscular arrangement of the intravesical ureter and the trigone provide a muscularly active valvular mechanism that can efficiently adapt itself to the variable phases of bladder activity during filling and voiding.

The normal resting pressure of the ureterovesical junction (10–15 cm H_2O) is greater than the more cephalad ureteral resting pressure (0–5 cm H_2O). Progressive bladder filling leads to firm occlusion of the intravesical ureter against retrograde urine flow and to increased resistance to antegrade flow resulting from trigonal stretching. During voiding, trigonal contraction completely seals the intravesical ureter against any antegrade or retrograde flow of urine.

The Urinary Bladder

The urinary bladder functions primarily as a reservoir that can accommodate variable volumes without increasing its intraluminal pressure. When the bladder reaches full capacity, the detrusor muscle voluntarily contracts following relaxation of the external sphincter and maintains its contraction until the bladder is completely empty. Funneling of the bladder outlet with progressive downward movement of the dome ensures complete emptying.

The vesical sphincteric mechanism is primarily a smooth muscle sphincter in the bladder neck and male prostatic urethra and in the proximal four-fifths of the female urethra. There is no purely circular sphincteric entity, but there are abundant circularly oriented smooth muscle fibers that are directly continuous with the outer coat of the detrusor muscles. The sphincter has an abundance of alpha receptors that respond to sympathetic neural input from the pelvic nerve to maintain urethral closure. Parasympathetic input from the pelvic nerve facilitates bladder contracture and voiding.

There is a voluntary striated muscle sphincter that is part of the urogenital diaphragm and surrounds the mid urethra in the female and the membranous urethra in the male. It responds to somatic neural input from the pudendal nerve. It is essential for continence when the internal sphincter is nonfunctional. Its pathologic irritability or spasticity can lead to obstructive manifestations.

Benigni A et al: Functional implications of decreased renal cortical atrial natriuretic peptide binding in experimental diabetes. Circ Res 1990;66:1453.

Diamond JR: Effects of dietary interventions on glomerular pathophysiology. Am J Physiol 1990;258:F1.

■ DEVELOPMENTAL ANOMALIES OF THE GENITOURINARY TRACT

Genitourinary tract anomalies constitute about one-third of all congenital abnormalities and occur in over 10% of the population. The severity varies from lesions incompatible with life to insignificant findings detected during diagnostic studies for unrelated reasons. The anatomic abnormalities are often not intrinsically harmful, yet they may predispose to infection, stone formation, or chronic renal failure.

RENAL ANOMALIES

Bilateral absence of the kidneys is rare and is associated with oligohydramnios, Potter facies, and pulmonary hypoplasia. It occurs more often in males and results in death shortly after birth. Unilateral renal agenesis is seen more often but is not usually associated with illness. **Renal agenesis** is thought to be due to both lack of a ureteral bud and lack of subsequent development of the metanephric blastema. The trigone is absent on the affected side. Because adrenal gland development is unrelated to kidney development, both adrenals are usually present in the normal position. Rarely, more than two kidneys are seen, a condition clearly dissimilar to ureteral duplication, as described later.

Abnormal ascent of the metanephros leads to an **ectopic kidney,** which may be unilateral or bilateral. Lumbar, pelvic, and the less common thoracic and crossed ectopic varieties are seen. Ectopic kidneys are associated with genital anomalies in 10–20% of cases. Fusion abnormalities are also associated with failure of normal ascent and include fused pelvic kidneys and **horseshoe kidneys** (the most common), which are typically fused at the lower poles. Intravenous urography typically establishes the diagnosis. The relationship of the kidneys to the psoas muscles is abnormal: instead of an oblique orientation with the medial border of the kidney parallel to the psoas muscle, the kidneys are vertical and the medial border intersects and crosses the

psoas muscle (Figure 41–4). Horseshoe kidneys have a high incidence of vesicoureteral reflux and are at increased risk of ureteropelvic junction obstruction. The latter may be related to a high ureteral insertion in the renal pelvis, crossing of the ureter over the isthmus, or compression by one of many anomalous arteries. Failure of rotation during ascent results in "malrotated" kidneys and is rarely significant.

Polycystic Kidneys

Parenchymal anomalies include a variety of cystic and dysplastic lesions. Polycystic kidney disease is hereditary and bilateral. The infantile form is a rare autosomal recessive disease that leads to progressive renal failure and a short life expectancy without dialysis or transplantation. The cause is cystic dilation of the cortical tubules without apparent connection to the collecting system. It is also associated with biliary dysgenesis and congenital hepatic periportal fibrosis.

The adult form is autosomal dominant and related to the *PKD1* gene, located on chromosome 6. It occurs in 1:1000 to 1:500 individuals and is a major cause of end-stage renal disease in adults. Large kidneys are seen, with cysts of varying sizes throughout the renal parenchyma. Cysts may also be present in the liver, pancreas, and spleen, and cerebral arterial aneurysms may occur. Renal cystic enlargement exerts pressure on

A

B

Figure 41–4. **A:** Excretory urogram showing horseshoe kidney with expansion of left side of isthmus and compression of lower left caliceal system. **B:** Gross pathology of horseshoe kidney.

normal parenchyma, leading to its gradual destruction and glomerulosclerosis.

The diagnosis is often made during a workup for hypertension or uremia discovered in the third to sixth decades. Hematuria with or without flank pain is a common finding. An intravenous urogram will reveal the enlarged kidneys, with marked elongation of the calices, which are compressed by large cysts (Figure 41–5). Ultrasonography or CT scan will readily make the diagnosis.

Surgery is rarely warranted. Therapy is medical and ultimately includes dialysis. Renal transplantation is often indicated, though potential family donors must be carefully screened to determine whether they have the same disorder.

Medullary Sponge Kidney

Medullary sponge kidney results from collecting tubular ectasia (see Polycystic Kidneys) and is associated with recurrent urolithiasis and an increased incidence of infection in 50% of patients. The lesion is often bilateral and may involve all of the calices. Intravenous urograms reveal dilated collecting tubules as a "blush" in the renal papilla. Microscopic hematuria is common. Specific antibiotics should be given for documented infections, and prophylactic therapy for renal stones should be recommended, based on the results of metabolic stone evaluation.

Simple Renal Cysts

Simple renal cysts are common (approximately 50% after age 50) and are thought to arise from tubular dilation. They may be solitary or bilateral and multiple. They rarely have pathologic significance except in the

Figure 41–5. Polycystic kidneys. Excretory urogram in a child, showing elongation, broadening, and bending of the calices around cysts. Renal function was normal.

differentiation from solid renal masses. (See Renal Adenocarcinoma, below.)

Multicystic Dysplastic Kidney

Multicystic dysplastic kidney is a congenital abnormality consisting of macroscopic cysts of variable sizes compressing dysplastic renal parenchyma. It is usually associated with an atretic proximal ureter. The disorder occurs in about 1:2400 live births and is frequently noted on prenatal ultrasound. Rarely, it may occur bilaterally and associated with oligohydramnios and renal failure. It may be distinguished from other causes of hydronephrosis by the absence of any renal function on renal scan. There is an increased incidence of contralateral ureteropelvic junction obstruction (5–10%) and reflux (18–43%).

The chance of developing a malignancy in multicystic dysplastic kidney appears to be no greater than 1:2000. There may also be an increased incidence of hypertension. These two factors constitute a rationale for treatment by nephrectomy. However, conservative management with routine ultrasound examinations at intervals of 6–12 months is reasonable practice, since about half involute within 5 years.

Renal Vascular Abnormalities

Multiple renal arteries occur in 15–20% of patients and are significant only when they cause ureteropelvic junction obstruction. Congenital **renal artery aneurysms** are infrequent; they are differentiated from acquired lesions by their location at the bifurcation of the main renal artery or at a distal branch point. The lesions are usually asymptomatic, but they can cause hypertension. They require surgical treatment only if hypertension is uncontrolled, if they are incompletely calcified, or if they have a diameter of more than 2.5 cm. **Congenital arteriovenous fistulas** are rare but may result in hematuria, hypertension, or cardiac failure necessitating operative treatment.

Renal Pelvis Anomalies

Ureteropelvic junction obstruction is one of the more common causes of hydronephrosis in childhood. The condition may be associated with compression by anomalous renal arteries or intrinsic stenosis of the junction. The diagnosis is not uncommonly made when gross hematuria follows minor trauma. Renal ultrasound provides a safe screening technique in patients suspected of ureteropelvic junction obstruction. Intravenous urography will suggest the diagnosis, and diuretic renal scan or retrograde pyelography, or both, will confirm it and suggest functional significance. Bilaterality is not uncommon, and the condition will require surgical repair if symptomatic or severe. Percutaneous incision of the obstruction with short-term stenting has been successful. Symptoms include flank pain, particularly with orally induced diuresis.

Bulas D: Unilateral renal agenesis may result from in utero regression of multicystic renal dysplasia. J Urol 1993;150:793.

Gabow PA: Autosomal dominant polycystic kidney disease. N Engl J Med 1993;329:332.

Mesrobian HG, Rushton HG, Bulas D: Unilateral renal agenesis may result from in utero regression of multicystic renal dysplasia. J Urol 1993;15:793.

URETERAL ANOMALIES

Congenital Obstruction of the Ureter

Congenital obstruction of the ureter may be due to ureterovesical and ureteropelvic junction obstruction or to neurologic deficits such as sacral agenesis or myelomeningocele. Functional ureteral obstruction—also known as **primary obstructive megaureter**—is not uncommon (Figure 41–6). Symptoms are renal pain during oral diuresis or those resulting from pyelonephritis. Excretory urograms depict dilation above the obstruction. Vesicoureteral reflux is uncommonly associated with megaureter. Milder forms without symptoms or significant hydronephrosis are the

Figure 41–6. Excretory urogram showing bilateral megaureter.

rule and do not require treatment if renal function is normal. When treatment is necessary, it consists of division of the ureter proximal to the obstruction and reimplantation of the ureter into the bladder.

Duplication of Ureters

Bifurcation of the ureteral bud before it interacts with the metanephric blastema results in incomplete ureteral duplication, commonly in the mid or upper ureter. A second ureteral bud from the metanephric duct leads to complete ureteral duplication (Figure 41–7A; right kidney) draining one kidney. This represents the most common ureteral anomaly, occurring in 1:125 people. It occurs twice as often in females. The presence of more than two ureters on each side is not common, but bilaterality of ureteral duplication occurs 40% of the time. Usually, all of the duplicated ureters enter the bladder; the ureter draining the upper pole of the kidney enters closest to the bladder neck (due to its later reabsorption into the bladder). Because of this relationship, the ureter draining the lower pole often has a short intramural tunnel and an inadequate surrounding musculature and is thus prone to vesicoureteral reflux. The ureter draining the upper pole may be ectopic (again because of its late absorption) and thus empty into the bladder neck, urethra, or genital structures (vagina or vestibule in the female and seminal vesicle or vas deferens in the male [Figure 41–7A; left kidney]). The ureter draining the upper pole is prone to obstruction and may be associated with a ureterocele, which is a common cause of obstruction. Duplication becomes significant when hydronephrosis or pyelonephritis occurs. The diagnosis is made by intravenous urography (Figure 41–7). Ureteral reimplantation to prevent recurrent infection is necessary in some cases. An anastomosis between the upper pole renal pelvis and the lower pole ureter or a low ureteroureterostomy are alternatives in selected cases. The upper pole of the kidney and its ureter may require removal if obstruction is severe and renal function of that segment is poor.

Ectopic Ureteral Orifice

Ureteral ectopia can occur in the absence of duplication and drain into any of the abnormal positions mentioned above. If the orifice lies proximal to the external urinary sphincter, no incontinence ensues, but vesicoureteral reflux is common. In contradistinction to the female, the ectopic orifice in the male never lies distal to the external sphincter, making incontinence an extremely rare presentation. Should it drain into the vagina or at the vestibule, there may be continuous leakage of urine apart from voiding. Most ectopic orifices involve the ureter draining the upper pole of a duplicated system, and most are observed in females. Hy-

A   B

Figure 41–7. **A:** Duplication of ureters and ectopic ureteral orifice. Complete duplication with obstruction to one ureter with ectopic orifice on left. The ureter with the ectopic opening always drains the upper pole of the kidney. **B:** Excretory urogram showing left complete ureteral duplication.

droureteronephrosis of the involved segment frequently occurs due to ureteral obstruction as it traverses the muscle of the bladder neck.

An ectopic orifice may be seen beside the urethral orifice or in the roof of the vagina on endoscopy. Renal ultrasound or intravenous urograms will often demonstrate hydroureteronephrosis of the upper renal segment. Cystography may show reflux into the ectopic orifice but may require cyclic voiding first to decompress the obstructed segment with bladder neck relaxation and subsequently to permit reflux. In the rare case when there is significant upper pole renal function, the ureter can be divided and reimplanted into the bladder or lower pole ureter. Usually, however, heminephroureterectomy is necessary.

Ureterocele

A ureterocele is a ballooning of the distal submucosal ureter into the bladder. This structure commonly has a pinpoint orifice and therefore leads to hydroureteronephrosis. If large enough, it may obstruct the vesical neck or the contralateral ureter. It is most common in

females with ureteral duplication and always involves the ureter draining the upper renal pole.

Most ureteroceles are now detected by prenatal ultrasound. Symptoms are usually those of pyelonephritis or obstruction. Intravenous urograms may show a negative shadow in the bladder cast by the ureterocele (Figure 41–8). The ureter and renal calices may be normal or may reveal marked dilation or no excretory function at all. A cystogram may show reflux into the ipsilateral lower pole ureter.

Treatment of ureteroceles depends upon multiple factors, including the presence or absence of reflux in any or all of the ureters as well as whether or not the ureterocele is completely contained within the bladder (orthotopic) or if a portion is at the bladder neck or urethra (ectopic). A simple method of establishing drainage involves cystoscopy and puncture of the ureterocele. Associated reflux, if present, can be managed with prophylactic antibiotics until the child has grown larger, at which time a technically easier ureteral reimplant may be performed with a decompressed ureter. In the relatively uncommon situation when there is no associated reflux, an upper pole heminephrectomy is con-

Figure 41–8. Ureterocele. Excretory urogram showing bilateral space-occupying lesions in the bladder caused by ureteroceles (arrows).

sidered. Minimally obstructive ureteroceles within the bladder in adults do not require treatment.

Cooper CS et al: Long-term follow-up of endoscopic incision of ureteroceles: intravesical versus extravesical. J Urol 2000; 164:1097.

VESICOURETERAL REFLUX

The main function of the ureterovesical junction is to permit free drainage of the ureter and simultaneously prevent urine from refluxing back from the bladder. Anatomically, the ureterovesical junction is well equipped for this function, because the ureteral musculature continues uninterrupted into the base of the bladder to form the superficial trigone. Additionally, the terminal 4–5 cm of ureter are surrounded by a musculofascial sheath (Waldeyer's sheath) that follows the ureter through the ureteral hiatus and continues in the base of the bladder as the deep trigone (Figure 41–9).

Direct continuity between the ureter and the trigone offers an efficient, muscularly active, valvular function. Any stretch of the trigone (with bladder filling) or any trigonal contraction (with voiding) leads to firm occlusion of the intravesical ureter, thus increasing resistance to flow from above downward and sealing the intravesical ureter against retrograde flow (Figure 41–10).

Etiology & Classification

Vesicoureteral reflux may be classified as primary reflux due to developmental ureterotrigonal weakness or associated with ureteral anomalies such as ectopic orifice or ureterocele, and secondary reflux due to bladder outlet or urethral obstruction, neuropathic dysfunction, iatro-

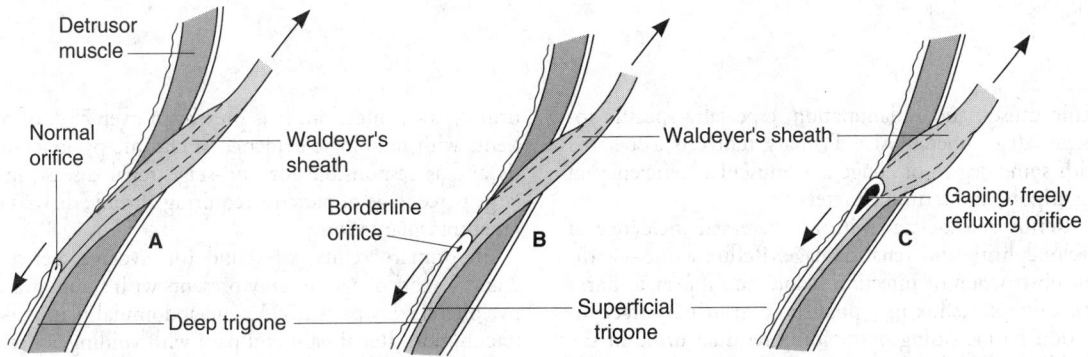

Figure 41–9. Vesicoureteral reflux. The length and fixation of the intravesical ureter and the appearance of the ureteral orifice depend upon the muscular development and efficiency of the lower ureter and its trigone. **A:** Normal structures. **B:** Moderate muscular deficiency. **C:** Marked deficiency results in a golf hole distortion of the submucosal ureter.

Waldeyer's sheath

Ureter

Superficial trigone
(white zone)

Deep trigone

Waldeyer's sheath

Ureter

Superficial trigone

Deep trigone

The ureteral muscle extends
downward and becomes the
superficial trigone

Waldeyer's sheath extends
downward and becomes the
deep trigone

Bladder neck

Figure 41–10. Normal ureterotrigonal complex. ***A:*** Side view of ureterovesical junction. Waldeyer's muscular sheath invests the juxtavesical ureter and continues downward as the deep trigone, which extends to the bladder neck. The ureteral musculature becomes the superficial trigone, which extends to the verumontanum in the male and stops just short of the external meatus in the female. ***B:*** Waldeyer's sheath is connected by a few fibers to the detrusor muscle in the ureteral hiatus. This muscular sheath, inferior to the ureteral orifices, becomes the deep trigone. The musculature of the ureters continues downward as the superficial trigone. (Adapted from Tanagho EA, Pugh RCB: Br J Urol 1963;35;151.)

genic causes, and inflammation, especially specific infection (eg, tuberculosis). Primary reflux is associated with some degree of congenital muscular deficiency in the trigone and terminal ureter.

Reflux is associated with an increased incidence of pyelonephritis and renal damage. Reflux alone—without obstruction or infection—does not appear to harm the kidneys. Reflux may predispose to urinary tract infection by increasing postvoiding residual urine in the bladder, enhancing bacterial growth from the stasis of urine. It also allows bacteria free access from the bladder to the kidney.

Reflux is the most common cause of pyelonephritis and is found in 30–50% of children presenting with

urinary tract infection. It is present in over 75% of patients with radiologic evidence of chronic pyelonephritis and is responsible for end-stage renal disease in a large percentage of patients requiring chronic dialysis or renal transplantation.

In primary reflux, the child (on average, between 2 and 3 years of age) usually presents with symptoms of pyelonephritis or cystitis. Vague abdominal pain is not uncommon. Renal pain and pain with voiding are relatively uncommon. On rare occasions, the patient may present with advanced renal failure with bilateral renal parenchymal damage. Significant reflux and its sequelae are more common in females and are usually detected earlier. About one-third of the siblings of a child with reflux will also have reflux, and one-half of the children of a mother with reflux will also have reflux.

In secondary reflux, manifestations of the primary disease (neuropathic, obstructive, etc.) are usually the presenting symptoms.

Clinical Findings

A. SYMPTOMS AND SIGNS

With acute pyelonephritis, fever, chills, and costovertebral angle tenderness may be present. Children usually do not have renal pain but may complain of vague abdominal pain. Occasionally, daytime frequency, incontinence, or enuresis may be caused by infection associated with reflux. In cases of obstruction or neuropathic deficit, a palpable hydronephrotic kidney or a distended bladder may be found. The diagnosis may be elusive in infants who present with ill-defined symptoms.

B. LABORATORY FINDINGS

Urinalysis will usually reveal evidence of infection (pyuria and bacteriuria). Urine cultures are mandatory when infection is suspected. Renal function tests may be abnormal if reflux and infection have caused renal scarring.

C. IMAGING STUDIES

The most useful study for conclusive diagnosis of reflux continues to be voiding cystourethrography (Figure 41–11). This study demonstrates the grade of reflux as well as the urethral anatomy. Radionuclide voiding studies are extremely sensitive at detecting reflux but do not demonstrate the anatomic detail seen with a voiding cystourethrogram. Radionuclide voiding studies are often performed as follow-up after an initial voiding cystourethrogram since they offer the advantage of decreased radiation exposure.

Radioisotopic renal scanning provides accurate differential renal function data and detection of renal scars. Ultrasound can provide accurate measurement of renal size and may demonstrate the presence of renal scarring and ureteral or caliceal dilation. In many cases, there may be no abnormality visible in the upper urinary tract, or only mild distal ureteral dilatation may be seen.

D. URODYNAMIC CONSIDERATIONS

A significant number of children with dysfunctional voiding present with urinary tract infections and are subsequently found to have reflux. These children contract the bladder against a closed external sphincter. Elevated voiding pressures associated with dysfunctional voiding may increase renal damage with an associated urinary tract infection and may also lessen the chance for either spontaneous or surgical resolution of reflux.

Figure 41–11. Voiding cystourethrogram showing total left vesicoureteral reflux.

When the history suggests the possibility of voiding dysfunction (incontinence, frequency, urgency), urodynamic studies are conducted to evaluate the voiding dynamics. Treatment of voiding dysfunction may result in resolution of the reflux.

Treatment

Although some children with reflux may not require antibiotics, the current standard of care requires that any child with reflux be maintained on prophylactic antibiotics. Prompt treatment of pyelonephritis prevents renal scar formation. Factors causing secondary reflux—such as dysfunctional voiding or obstruction—should be corrected.

In many children, reflux will resolve with time and growth. Reflux is graded as seen on voiding cystourethrography as follows:

Grade I: Contrast enters ureter

Grade II: Contrast enters the renal collecting system

Grade III: Slight dilation of the calices or ureter

Grades IV and V: Progressively increased amounts of caliceal dilation and ureteral dilation or tortuosity

Reflux most likely to resolve is of lower grade or detected at a younger age. Over 70% of children with grades I, II, or unilateral grade III reflux will have resolution within 5 years. Resolution in children with grade V or bilateral grade IV reflux can be anticipated in less than 10% of cases.

In obstructive secondary reflux (eg, posterior urethral valves), release of obstruction may cure reflux. Occasionally, surgical reimplantation is still required. In neuropathic reflux, intermittent catheterization for control of infection may allow return of valvular competence. However, many cases will require bladder augmentation for a noncompliant bladder and ureteral reimplantation. In reflux associated with ectopic orifices, duplication with ureterocele, and other congenital malformations, reimplantation is generally required.

The aim of surgery is to correct the reflux. This is accomplished by the creation of a longer submucosal tunnel for the ureter. With bladder filling and increased pressure, the ureter is compressed between the mucosa and underlying detrusor muscle. This flap valve prevents reflux of urine. The necessary length of the tunnel to stop reflux depends upon the diameter of the ureter, with a 5:1 length to diameter ratio being ideal. One of three methods is used in most cases: (1) In suprahiatal repair (Politano-Leadbetter procedure), a new ureteral hiatus is developed about 2.5 cm above the original one and the ureter—after passing through a submucosal tunnel—is sutured to the cut edge of the trigone at the level of the original orifice. (2) In the cross-trigonal repair (Cohen procedure), the original hiatus is maintained, and the ureter is advanced through a submucosal tunnel, extending across the trigone to the contralateral bladder wall. (3) A totally extravesical ureteral advancement procedure (extravesical ureteroplasty) achieves results similar to those achieved with the intravesical methods described above, with a shorter hospital stay and shorter convalescence.

Teflon paste or collagen gel injections have also been used to increase submucosal support of the ureter. With proper placement beneath the ureteral orifice under endoscopic vision, these injections act to bolster the deficient antireflux mechanism. Concern regarding late sequelae of Teflon injections (eg, particle migration) has prevented use of this approach in the United States. Collagen injections are still available but have a lower long-term success rate than Teflon injections or open surgical correction.

Prognosis

The long-term prognosis is excellent for patients with mild to moderate reflux successfully treated with antibiotic prophylaxis. There are few instances of recurrent infection or renal insufficiency. Patients with more significant reflux or persistent urinary tract infections will benefit from collagen injection or surgical reimplanta-

tion; the success rate is approximately 95% (cessation of reflux, clearance of renal infection, and absence of obstruction). Unfortunately, for patients with advanced disease (irreversible ureteral decompensation and chronic pyelonephritis, which is now thought to be a self-perpetuating immune complex process), the prognosis is less favorable. These patients account for a significant proportion of patients with end-stage renal disease who ultimately require chronic dialysis, renal transplantation, or both.

Bjorgvinsson E et al: Diagnosis of acute pyelonephritis in children: comparison of sonography and ^{99}Tc-DMSA scintigraphy. AJR Am J Roentgenol 1991;157:539.

Cooper CS et al: The outcome of stopping prophylactic antibiotics in older children with vesicoureteral reflux. J Urol 2000; 163:269.

Elder JS et al: Pediatric Vesicoureteral Reflux Guidelines Panel summary report on the management of primary vesicoureteral reflux in children. J Urol 1997;157:1846.

Frey P et al: Prevention of vesicoureteral reflux by endoscopic injection. Br J Urol 1992;69:1.

Jodal U et al: Infection pattern in children with vesicoureteral reflux randomly allocated to operation or long-term antibacterial prophylaxis: the international reflux study in children. J Urol 1992;148:1650.

Koff SA: Relationship of dysfunctional voiding and reflux. J Urol 1983;130:1138.

Leonard MP et al: Endoscopic injection of glutaraldehyde cross-linked bovine dermal collagen for correction of vesicoureteral reflux. J Urol 1991;145:115.

Noordzij JW et al: A view on the anatomy of the ureterovesical junction. Scand J Urol Nephrol 1993;27:371.

BLADDER ANOMALIES

Anomalies of the bladder are infrequent and include the following: (1) **agenesis,** or complete absence, which results in a persistent cloaca; (2) bladder **duplication,** which may be complete, with separate ureteral openings drained by duplicated urethras, or incomplete, with a septum or hourglass deformity; and (3) **urachal anomalies,** which in the most severe forms appear as a patent opening at the umbilicus and are usually associated with some form of bladder outlet obstruction. In less severe forms, a **urachal diverticulum** may be present at the dome of the bladder or a **urachal cyst** along the course of the partially obliterated urachus. These latter conditions may cause abdominal pain and umbilical or bladder infection requiring surgical treatment. Occasionally, adenocarcinoma develops in a urachal remnant (see section on Tumors of the Bladder, below).

Failure of cloacal division results in a persistent cloaca. Incomplete division is more frequent (though still rare) and results in a rectovesical, rectourethral, or rectovestibular fistula (usually with imperforate anus or anal atresia).

Exstrophy of the Bladder

Exstrophy of the bladder is the most severe bladder anomaly—the result of a complete ventral defect of the urogenital sinus and the overlying inferior abdominal wall musculature and integument (Figure 41–12A). The lower central portion is devoid of skin and muscle. The anterior bladder wall is absent, and the posterior wall is contiguous with surrounding skin. Urine drains onto the abdominal wall, the rami of the pubic bones are widely separated (Figure 41–12B), and the open pelvic ring may affect gait. In males, the penis is shortened and the urethra is epispadiac. The exposed bladder mucosa tends to be chronically inflamed.

Currently, the favored treatment is bladder salvage, which includes closure of the bladder in the newborn period. Urethral closure and penile reconstruction have also been advocated at the time of the initial bladder closure. Ureteral obstruction or vesicoureteral reflux may develop and require ureteral reimplantation. The closed bladder may have a small capacity, and incontinence is often a complication. Patients frequently require multiple operations, including bladder augmentation and bladder neck reconstruction. Good results have been observed in more than half of all patients

Figure 41–12B. Roentgenogram of pelvis with widely separated pubes (arrows) in patient with exstrophy.

treated, with preservation of renal function and continence.

Cooper CS et al: Pediatric reconstructive surgery. Curr Opin Urol 2000;10:195.

Prune Belly Syndrome

Prune belly syndrome consists of a triad of abnormalities: deficient abdominal wall musculature, bilateral cryptorchidism, and variable amounts of dilation of the urogenital tract. The cause is not known. Almost all children with prune belly syndrome have reflux. The incidence of eventual renal failure is 25–30%. Risk factors for renal failure include bilateral abnormal kidneys on ultrasound or renal scan, a serum creatinine that never falls below 0.7 mg/dL, and clinical pyelonephritis. These children are managed with prophylactic antibiotics and frequent urine cultures, followed by prompt treatment of any urinary tract infections. Abdominoplasty may be performed to help correct the abdominal wall defect.

Noh PH et al: Prognostic factors of renal failure in children with prune belly syndrome. J Urol 1999;162:1399.

Congenital Neurovesical Dysfunction

Congenital neurovesical dysfunction frequently accompanies a posterior myelomeningocele and sacral agenesis, with associated spinal abnormalities. Both conditions may result in incontinence and recurrent urinary infection with late sequelae (ureteral reflux, pyelonephritis, and renal failure). These children require frequent evaluation of their kidneys and kidney function

Figure 41–12A. Photograph of male patient with bladder exstrophy.

since high bladder storage pressures may harm the kidneys.

PENILE & URETHRAL ANOMALIES

Hypospadias

Hypospadias rates in the United States have doubled over the past 30 years. It results from failure of fusion of the urethral folds on the undersurface of the genital tubercle. The urethral meatus is ventrally displaced on the glans on the shaft of the penis or more proximal at the level of the scrotum or perineum. With more proximal displacement, chordee (ventral curvature of the penile shaft) frequently occurs and requires treatment or it will preclude straight erections and normal intercourse (Figure 41–13). The midscrotal hypospadiac penis may resemble female external genitalia with an enlarged clitoris and labia. Sexual assignment in these latter infants requires hormonal and chromosomal analysis.

In hypospadias with the meatus positioned proximal to the corona, the prepuce is abnormal—not forming a complete cylinder due to a ventral defect. Circumcision should not be done in these patients, as the prepuce can be used later in surgical repair.

The degree of hypospadias dictates the need for repair. If the opening is glandular or coronal (85% of pa-

Figure 41–13. Hypospadias, penoscrotal type. Redundant dorsal foreskin that is deficient ventrally; ventral chordee.

tients), the penis is usually functional both for micturition and procreation, and repair is done primarily for cosmetic reasons. Openings that are more proximal on the shaft require correction to allow voiding while standing, normal erection, and proper sperm deposition during intercourse. Surgical plastic repair of hypospadias is currently accomplished by a variety of highly successful one-stage operations and is routinely performed between 6 and 19 months of age. The most common complications of hypospadias surgery include meatal stenosis and fistula formation; however, improved techniques have decreased the incidence of these complications.

Epispadias

Epispadias is a rare congenital anomaly that is commonly associated with bladder exstrophy. When it occurs alone, it is considered a milder degree of the exstrophy complex.

The urethra opens on the dorsum of the penis, with deficient corpus spongiosum and loosely attached corpora cavernosa. If the defect is extensive, it may extend to the bladder neck, causing incontinence. The pubic bones are separated, as in exstrophy. Marked dorsiflexion of the penis is usually present.

Treatment consists of correction of penile curvature, reconstruction of the urethra, and reconstruction of the bladder neck in incontinent patients.

Urethral Strictures

Congenital urethral strictures are rare but when present are most common in the fossa navicularis (just proximal to the meatus) and in the bulbomembranous urethra. Commonly, these strictures are thin diaphragms that may respond to simple dilation or to direct vision internal urethrotomy. Rarely is open surgical repair necessary. Congenital urethral strictures in girls and meatal stenosis in boys are very uncommon. When the latter does occur, it appears to be acquired, as it is seen only in circumcised boys.

Urethral Diverticulum

In males, urethral diverticula are nearly always in the pendulous or bulbous urethra. They are often associated with an obstructive flap of the urethral mucosa (anterior urethral valve)—thought to represent incomplete closure of the urethral folds. Treatment by endoscopic unroofing is usually successful, though most diverticula are small and require no therapy. In females they occur in adult life and are usually manifested by irritative symptoms and recurrent infection. The cause is unknown, but the disorder is most likely congenital. Treatment is usually by transvaginal excision. Diverticula may occasionally harbor stones or tumors.

Posterior Urethral Valves

Posterior urethral valves are the most common obstructive urethral lesion in newborn and infant males. They consist of obstructive folds of mucosa, seen only in males, which originate at—or are attached at some point to—the verumontanum in the prostatic urethra. The embryologic derivation is indefinite. They are partially obstructive and thus lead to variable degrees of back pressure damage to the urinary bladder and upper urinary tract. Progressive renal damage may occur as a result of early obstruction at the ureterovesical junction because of trigonal hypertrophy and later development of reflux. Dilation and obstruction of the prostatic urethra are always present. Spontaneous urinary ascites from the kidneys is often seen in neonates. This clears when the obstruction is relieved.

About one-third of children with posterior urethral valves are now diagnosed by prenatal ultrasound. Another one-third are diagnosed in the first year of life, with the remaining third presenting later. Clinical manifestations consist of difficult voiding, a weak urinary stream, and a midline lower abdominal mass that represents a distended bladder. In some cases, the kidneys are palpable. Urinary incontinence and urinary tract infection may occur. Laboratory findings include elevated serum urea nitrogen and creatinine and evidence of urinary infection. Ultrasound shows evidence of bladder thickening and trabeculation, hydroureter, and hydronephrosis. Demonstration of urethral valves on a voiding cystourethrogram establishes the diagnosis, as does endoscopic identification of valves.

Posterior urethral valves must be differentiated from neuropathic dysfunction, tumors, and meatal stenosis. If meatal stenosis and phimosis are excluded, any lower urinary tract obstructive disorder in a newborn or young boy should be considered posterior urethral valves until proved otherwise.

Treatment consists of destruction of the valves by endoscopic incision. In a premature infant with a small urethra prohibiting transurethral resection, a temporary cutaneous vesicostomy may be required to provide drainage and improve impaired kidney function.

The prognosis depends upon the original degree of kidney damage and the success of efforts to prevent or treat infection. In cases seen early, the prognosis is quite favorable. Many of these children have delayed development of urinary continence due to bladder changes and impaired urinary concentration.

Cooper CS et al: Preservation of urethral plate spongiosum: technique to reduce hypospadias fistulas. Urology 2001;57:351.

Hulbert WC et al: The predictive value of ultrasonography in evaluation of infants with posterior urethral valves. J Urol 1992; 148:122.

Kirsch AJ et al: Laser tissue soldering for hypospadias repair: results of a controlled, prospective clinical trial. J Urol 2001; 165:574.

Paulozzi LJ et al: Hypospadias trends in two U.S. surveillance systems. Pediatrics 1997;100:831.

SCROTAL & TESTICULAR ANOMALIES*

Testicular Torsion

Neonatal testicular torsion (extravaginal torsion) is an extremely rare condition. The entire testicle and the tunica vaginalis are twisted. No trigger mechanism associated with the torsion has been identified. Though the vast majority are necrotic and nonsalvageable, several studies have reported salvage of testicular tissue when torsion is detected immediately following birth. Any scrotal swelling in the neonate requires close follow-up. Intravaginal testicular torsion in adolescents is described later in this chapter.

Cooper CS et al: Bilateral neonatal testicular torsion. Clin Pediatr 1997;36:653.

Scrotal Lesions

Congenital scrotal lesions include hypoplasia of the scrotum (unilateral or bilateral) in association with cryptorchidism (see below) and bifid scrotum with extensive hypospadias.

Berkowitz GS et al: Prevalence and natural history of cryptorchidism. Pediatrics 1993;92:44.

Burks DD et al: Suspected testicular torsion and ischemia: evaluation with color Doppler sonography. Radiology 1990; 175:815.

Das S, Singer A: Controversies of perinatal torsion of the spermatic cord: A review survey and recommendations. J Urol 1990; 143:231.

■ ACQUIRED LESIONS OF THE GENITOURINARY TRACT

OBSTRUCTIVE UROPATHY

Obstruction is one of the most important abnormalities of the urinary tract, since it eventually leads to decompensation of the muscular conduits and reservoirs, back pressure, and atrophy of renal parenchyma. It also invites infection and stone formation, which cause addi-

---

* Undescended testicles (cryptorchidism) and hydroceles in infants are discussed in Chapter 46.

tional damage and can ultimately end in complete uni-lateral or bilateral destruction of the kidneys.

Both the level and the degree of obstruction are important to an understanding of the pathologic consequences. Any obstruction at or distal to the bladder neck may lead to back pressure affecting both kidneys. Obstruction at or proximal to the ureteral orifice leads to unilateral damage unless the lesion involves both ureters simultaneously. Complete obstruction leads to rapid decompensation of the system proximal to the site of obstruction. Partial obstruction leads to gradual progressive muscular hypertrophy followed by dilation, decompensation, and hydronephrotic changes.

Etiology

Acquired urinary tract obstruction may be due to inflammatory or traumatic urethral strictures, bladder outlet obstruction (benign prostatic hyperplasia or cancer of the prostate), vesical tumors, neuropathic bladder, extrinsic ureteral compression (tumor, retroperitoneal fibrosis, or enlarged lymph nodes), ureteral or pelvic stones, ureteral strictures, or ureteral or pelvic tumors.

Pathogenesis

Regardless of its cause, acquired obstruction leads to similar changes in the urinary tract, which vary depending on the severity and duration of obstruction.

A. URETHRAL CHANGES

Proximal to the obstruction, the urethra dilates and balloons. A urethral diverticulum may develop, and dilation and gaping of the prostatic urethra and ejaculatory ducts may occur.

B. VESICAL CHANGES

Early, detrusor and trigonal thickening and hypertrophy compensate for the outlet obstruction, allowing complete bladder emptying. This change leads to progressive development of bladder trabeculation, cellules, saccules, and, finally, diverticula. Subsequently, bladder decompensation occurs and is characterized by the above changes plus incomplete bladder emptying (ie, postvoid residual urine). Trigonal hypertrophy leads to secondary ureteral obstruction owing to increased resistance to flow through the intravesical ureter. With detrusor decompensation and residual urine accumulation, there is stretching of the hypertrophied trigone, which appreciably increases ureteral obstruction. This is the mechanism of back pressure on the kidney in the presence of vesical outlet obstruction (while the ureterovesical junction maintains its competence).

Catheter drainage of the bladder relieves trigonal stretch and improves drainage from the upper tract.

A very late change with persistent obstruction (more frequently encountered with neuropathic dysfunction) is decompensation of the ureterovesical junction, leading to reflux. Reflux aggravates the back pressure effect on the upper tract by transmitting abnormally high intravesical pressures and favors the onset or persistence of urinary tract infection.

C. URETERAL CHANGES

The first change noted is a gradual increase in ureteral distention. This increases ureteral caliber and stimulates hyperactive ureteral contraction and ureteral muscular hypertrophy. Because the ureteral musculature runs in an irregular helical pattern, stretching of its muscular elements leads to lengthening as well as widening, causing the dilated ureter to assume a tortuous, serpiginous course, weaving back and forth across the relatively straight course of the ureteral vessels, which are unaffected by the ureteral obstruction. This is the start of ureteral decompensation, where tortuosity and dilation become apparent. These changes progress until the ureter becomes atonic, with infrequent, ineffective, or completely absent peristalsis.

D. PELVICALICEAL CHANGES

The renal pelvis and calices, subjected to increased volumes of retained urine, distend. First, the pelvis shows evidence of hyperactivity and hypertrophy, and then progressive dilation and atony. The calices show similar changes to a variable degree, depending on whether the renal pelvis is intrarenal or extrarenal. In the latter, caliceal dilation may be minimal in spite of marked pelvic dilation. In the intrarenal pelvis, caliceal dilation and renal parenchymal damage are maximal. The successive phases seen with obstruction are rounding of the fornices, followed by flattening of the papillae and finally clubbing of the minor calices.

E. RENAL PARENCHYMAL CHANGES

With continued pelvicaliceal distention, there is parenchymal compression against the renal capsule and, more importantly, compression of the arcuate vessels results in a marked drop in renal blood flow leading to parenchymal ischemic atrophy. With increased intrapelvic pressure, there is progressive dilation of the collecting and distal tubules, with compression and atrophy of tubular cells.

Clinical Findings

A. SYMPTOMS AND SIGNS

The findings vary according to the site of obstruction.

1. Infravesical obstruction—Infravesical obstruction (eg, due to urethral stricture, benign prostatic hypertrophy, bladder neck contracture) leads to difficulty in initiation of voiding, a weak stream, and a diminished flow rate with terminal dribbling. Burning and frequency are common associated symptoms. A distended or thickened bladder wall may be palpable. Urethral induration due to stricture, benign prostatic hypertrophy, or cancer of the prostate may be noted on rectal examination. Meatal stenosis and impacted urethral stones are readily diagnosed by physical examination.

2. Supravesical obstruction—Renal pain or renal colic and gastrointestinal symptoms are commonly associated. Supravesical obstruction (eg, due to ureteral stone, ureteropelvic junction obstruction) may be completely asymptomatic when it develops gradually over a period of months. An enlarged kidney may be palpable. Costovertebral angle tenderness may be present.

B. LABORATORY FINDINGS

Evidence of urinary tract infection, hematuria, or crystalluria may be seen. Impaired renal function may be noted in cases of bilateral obstruction. Postrenal azotemia (serum changes reflecting impaired renal function due primarily to obstruction) is suggested by elevation of serum urea nitrogen and serum creatinine with a ratio greater than 10:1.

C. IMAGING STUDIES

Radiologic examination is usually diagnostic in cases of stasis, tumors, and strictures. Dilation and anatomic changes occur above the level of obstruction whereas distal to the obstruction, the configuration is usually normal. This helps in localizing the site of obstruction. Combined antegrade imaging by intravenous urograms and retrograde imaging by ureterograms or urethrograms is sometimes needed to demonstrate the obstructed segment. In supravesical obstruction, demonstration of stasis and delayed drainage is essential to establish and quantitate the severity of obstruction.

1. Antegrade urography—Antegrade urography via percutaneous needle or tube nephrostomy is valuable when the obstructed kidney fails to excrete the radiopaque material on excretory urography. The Whitaker test requires percutaneous catheter access to the collecting system above the site of suspected obstruction. This permits fluid introduction into the renal pelvis and simultaneous measurement of urine flow rate and pressures in the bladder and renal pelvis, thus providing a quantitative assessment of the degree and severity of obstruction. The fluid transport can be measured and the degree of obstruction estimated by the use of a pressure monitor.

2. Ultrasonography—This will reveal the degree of dilation of the renal pelvis and calices and allows for diagnosis of hydronephrosis even in the prenatal period. Color Doppler ultrasound can reveal blood flow and restrictive indices to help determine functional impairment.

3. Isotope studies—A technetium Tc 99m DMSA scan portrays the degree of hydronephrosis as well as renal function. Use of diuretics during the scan can provide specific data on the significance of the obstruction and the need for treatment. Multiple studies can reveal ongoing functional changes.

4. CT scan—This is of particular value in revealing the degree and site of obstruction as well as the cause in many cases. The use of contrast agents will allow estimation of residual renal function.

Complications

The most important complication of urinary tract obstruction is renal parenchymal atrophy as a result of back pressure. Obstruction also predisposes to infection and stone formation, and infection occurring with obstruction leads to rapid kidney destruction.

Treatment

The first goal of therapy is relief of the obstruction (eg, catheterization for relief of acute urinary retention). Definitive therapy often requires surgery, but minimally invasive techniques are becoming utilized more often. Simple urethral stricture may be managed by dilation or internal urethrotomy (incision of the stricture under direct vision through the resectoscope). However, urethroplasty (open surgical graft or flap of skin or bladder or buccal mucosa to replace urethral diameter) may be required and is usually more successful. Benign prostatic hyperplasia and obstructing bladder tumors classically require excision, but thermal and laser techniques are providing satisfactory outcomes with less morbidity. Impacted ureteral stones may either be removed or bypassed by a catheter unless it is thought that they may pass spontaneously.

Ureteral or ureteropelvic junction obstruction requires surgical repair; however, endoscopic approaches within the ureter or by laparoscopy may be equal to open repair. Renal stones may be removed instrumentally via percutaneous nephrostomy or by irrigation through a tube placed directly into the kidney.

Preliminary drainage above the obstruction is sometimes needed to improve kidney function. Occasionally, intestinal urinary diversion or permanent nephrostomy is required. If damage is advanced, nephrectomy may be indicated.

Prognosis

The prognosis depends on the cause, site, duration, and degree of kidney damage and renal decompensation. In general, relief of obstruction leads to improvement in kidney function except in seriously damaged kidneys, especially those destroyed by inflammatory scarring.

Bauer SB, Joseph DB: Management of the obstructed urinary tract associated with neurogenic bladder dysfunction. Urol Clin North Am 1990;17:395.

Cockett AT et al: Indications for treatment of BPH: the AUA Study Cancer 1992;70(Suppl 1):280.

Rink RC, Mitchell ME: Physiology of lower urinary tract obstruction. Urol Clin North Am 1990;17:329.

Staskin DR: Hydroureteronephrosis after spinal cord injury: effects of lower urinary tract dysfunction on upper tract anatomy. Urol Clin North Am 1991;18:309.

URETEROPELVIC JUNCTION OBSTRUCTION

Stenosis of the renal pelvis outlet is commonly due to congenital narrowing of the junction or compression by anomalous vessels. However, the lesion may be acquired. Presentation is similar in either case, with abrupt onset of flank pain usually following ingestion of large amounts of fluids.

The diagnosis is made by intravenous urography, which reveals hydronephrosis with a dilated renal pelvis and thin renal cortex. Occasionally, patients present with intermittent hydronephrosis and normal urograms except during attacks of pain when x-rays show typical obstruction. These patients generally have normal renal parenchyma. Retrograde ureteropyelography is usually needed in patients with chronic moderate to severe obstruction to determine the extent of the lesion and to provide assurance that the distal ureter is normal (Figure 41–14). Marked obstruction may make it difficult to determine whether kidney function is surgically salvageable. In these cases, it may be necessary to perform either (1) differential radioisotope renography with use of a diuretic during the study or (2) percutaneous nephrostomy with flow measurement through the pelvic junction (Whitaker test) and differential creatinine clearance collection.

Severe obstruction with minimal remaining renal function is best treated by unilateral nephrectomy. If renal function is adequate (> 10% of total renal function or > 10 mL/min creatinine clearance), surgical repair of the stenosis, either by creation of a renal pelvis flap or by resection of the stenotic area and reanastomosis, is warranted. The use of percutaneous ureteroscopy or nephroscopy with endopyelotomy, incising the strictured ureteropelvic junction, offers an alternative method of therapy. Laparoscopic repair has proponents as well. The surgical results of these methods are excellent in terms of

Figure 41–14. Retrograde ureteropyelogram showing right ureteropelvic junction obstruction.

functional preservation, improvement of urine flow, and relief of symptoms, but dilation of the calices may persist.

Ben Slama MR et al: Extraperitoneal laparoscopic repair of ureteropelvic junction obstruction: initial experience in 15 cases. Urology 2000;56:45.

Van Cangh PJ et al: Endopyelotomy. Prognostic factors and patient selection. Urol Clin North Am 1998;25:281.

URETERAL STENOSIS

Acquired ureteral stenosis is less common than the congenital types. Causes include (1) ureteral injury (surgical, traumatic, radiation therapy), (2) compression of the ureter by lymph nodes harboring cancer, (3) prolonged compression by an anomalous blood vessel, (4) tuberculous or bilharzial ureteritis, (5) retroperitoneal fibrosis, (6) aneurysm of the aorta following aortofemoral bypass grafts, (7) ureteropelvic junction obstruction secondary to reflux, (8) occlusion of the ureterovesical junction by infiltrating cancer of the bladder or cervix, and (9) functional obstruction of the ureterovesical junction secondary to hypertrophy of the trigone developing from obstruction distal to the bladder neck.

Symptoms are usually those of obstruction to urine flow from the kidney, though many cases are asymptomatic. An unsuspected lesion is often discovered on excretory urography.

Therapy consists of treatment of the cause, eg, resection of the stenosed segment with end-to-end anastomosis. Endoscopy-guided ureteral dilation or incision may be curative. Ureteral stents may be beneficial for postoperative ureteral stricture or following injury due to radiation therapy.

RETROPERITONEAL FIBROSIS

See also Chapter 23.

One or both ureters may be compressed by a chronic inflammatory process, usually of unknown cause, which involves the retroperitoneal tissues of the lumbosacral area. Patients treated for migraine with methysergide may develop this fibrosis. Sclerosing Hodgkin's disease and fibrosis from metastatic cancer have also been implicated. Symptoms include renal pain, low backache, and those associated with uremia. Some patients present with complete anuria. Urinary infection is unusual. If both ureters are obstructed, the serum creatinine is elevated.

Excretory urograms show hydronephrosis and a dilated ureter down to the point of obstruction. The ureters are displaced medially in the lumbar area. Retrograde ureterograms show a long segment of ureteral stenosis, though a catheter passes easily through the ureter. Sonograms and CT scans may demonstrate fibrous plaques with proximal hydroureteronephrosis. If the patient is anuric, indwelling ureteral catheters or percutaneous nephrostomy should be done. When the patient's condition has improved, definitive therapy can be accomplished. If methysergide is suspected to be the causative agent, fibrosis may subside when the drug is discontinued. These patients may benefit from administration of corticosteroids. Chronic indwelling ureteral stents have also been used successfully. If these methods fail, ureterolysis must be performed to free the ureter from the fibrous plaque. The involved ureter should be dissected from the plaque, moved to a lateral position, and wrapped with omentum to prevent recurrent entrapment.

BENIGN PROSTATIC HYPERPLASIA

 ESSENTIALS OF DIAGNOSIS

- *Prostatism: nocturia, hesitancy, slow stream, terminal dribbling, frequency.*
- *Residual urine.*
- *Acute urinary retention.*

- *Uremia in advanced cases.*

General Considerations

The cause of benign prostatic enlargement is not known but is probably related to hormonal factors. By upsetting the mechanism for opening and funneling the vesical neck at the time of voiding, hyperplasia of the prostate causes increased outflow resistance. Consequently, a higher intravesical pressure is required to accomplish voiding, causing hypertrophy of the vesical and trigonal muscles. This may lead to the development of bladder diverticula—outpocketings of vesical mucosa between the detrusor muscle bundles. Hypertrophy of the trigone causes excessive stress on the intravesical ureter, producing functional obstruction and resulting in hydroureteronephrosis in late cases. Stagnation of urine can lead to infection; the onset of cystitis will exacerbate the obstructive symptoms. The periurethral and subtrigonal prostate enlargement produces the most significant obstruction.

The prostate in young men has an anatomic capsule like an apple peel. In men with prostatic enlargement, there is a thick "surgical" capsule similar to an orange peel, composed of peripherally compressed true prostatic tissue. This permits intracapsular enucleation of the enlarged periurethral glands (Figure 41–15).

Clinical Findings

A. SYMPTOMS AND SIGNS

Typically, the patient notices hesitancy and loss of force and caliber of the stream. He may also be awakened by the urge to void several times at night (nocturia). Postvoid dribbling ("terminal dribbling") is particularly disturbing. The complication of infection increases the degree of obstructive symptoms and is often associated with burning on urination. Acute urinary retention may supervene. This is associated with severe urgency, suprapubic pain, and a distended, palpable bladder.

The size of the prostate rectally is not of primary diagnostic importance, since there is a poor correlation between the size of the gland and the degree of symptoms and amount of residual urine.

B. LABORATORY FINDINGS

Urinalysis may reveal evidence of infection. Residual urine is commonly increased, and a timed urinary flow rate will be decreased. The serum creatinine may be elevated in cases with prolonged severe obstruction.

C. IMAGING STUDIES

Excretory urograms are often normal and are thus not required. In late-stage cases, the study may show hy-

Anatomic capsule

Hypertrophied
periurethral tissue
(transition zone)

Surgical
capsule

True prostate (peripheral zone)

Figure 41–15. Benign prostatic hyperplasia. The enlarged periurethral glands are enclosed by the surgical capsule. The true prostate has been compressed.

droureteronephrosis if severe obstruction is present. This almost always resolves after prostatectomy. The enlarged gland may cause an indentation in the inferior surface of the bladder, which may result in a "J-hook" deformity of the distal ureter. The postvoiding film may reveal varying amounts of residual urine. Renal ultrasound examination may obviate the need for urograms; however, imaging is not required to make the diagnosis nor to determine the need for or method of treatment. Pelvic ultrasound can also accurately predict the amount of residual urine.

D. Endoscopic Examination

The presence of residual urine may be documented if the patient is catheterized immediately after voiding. Endoscopy will reveal secondary vesical changes (eg, trabeculation) and enlargement of the periurethral prostatic glands. Endoscopy is not required to make the diagnosis, however.

E. Urodynamic Studies

Simultaneous physiologic monitoring of bladder filling and emptying, urethral sphincter activity, abdominal

pressure, and pelvic floor muscle (electromyography) can be extremely useful in documenting whether bladder outlet obstruction, poor bladder function, or other causes are responsible for lower urinary tract symptoms. While urodynamic studies are not required for diagnosis in all cases, they are helpful in equivocal cases to help determine management.

Differential Diagnosis

Neuropathic bladder may produce a similar syndrome. A history suggesting a neuropathic difficulty may be obtained. Neurologic deficit involving S2–4 is particularly significant.

Cancer of the prostate also causes symptoms of vesical neck obstruction. Symptoms and signs of osseous metastases may also be present. Typically, the cancerous gland is stony hard. Serum prostate-specific antigen may be slightly elevated in patients with benign prostatic hypertrophy, but if it is over 10 ng/mL, cancer should be suspected (normal is < 4 ng/mL). Serum alkaline phosphatase is usually increased if the tumor has spread to bone.

Acute prostatitis may cause symptoms of obstruction, but the patient is septic and has infected urine. The prostate is exquisitely tender.

Urethral stricture diminishes the caliber of the urinary stream. There is usually a history of gonorrhea or local trauma. A retrograde urethrogram will show the stenotic area. A stricture blocks the passage of an instrument or catheter.

Complications

Obstruction and residual urine lead to vesical and prostatic infection and occasionally pyelonephritis; these may be difficult to eradicate.

The obstruction may lead to the development of bladder diverticula. Infected residual urine may contribute to the formation of calculi.

Functional obstruction of the intravesical ureter, caused by the hypertrophic trigone, may lead to hydroureteronephrosis.

Treatment

The indications for operative management are impairment of or threat to renal function and bothersome symptoms. Because the degree of obstruction progresses slowly in most patients, conservative treatment (watchful waiting) may be adequate. Drugs that relax the prostatic capsule and internal sphincter (α-adrenergic blocking agents) or decrease the volume of the prostate (5α-reductase inhibitors or antiandrogens) have been tried with considerable success.

A. CONSERVATIVE MEASURES

Treatment of chronic prostatitis may reduce symptoms. The resolution of a complicating cystitis will usually afford some relief. In order to protect vesical tone, the patient should be cautioned to void as soon as the urge develops. Forcing fluids over a short time causes rapid vesical filling, decreasing vesical tone; this is a common cause of sudden acute urinary retention and thus should be avoided. These conservative measures are of only temporary help—if any—in patients with prostatic hyperplasia.

Controversy surrounds choices in the treatment of benign prostatic hyperplasia. No treatment may be appropriate in patients who complain of mild to moderate symptoms. Interest has focused on nonoperative medical therapy. Alpha-adrenergic blocking agents relax the internal (bladder neck) sphincter and prostatic capsule. Selective agents that are long-acting and preferentially work for this purpose include doxazosin and tamsulosin. 5α-Reductase inhibitors block conversion of testosterone to dihydrotestosterone (the androgen active in promoting prostate growth) and are particularly useful for large glands and in combination with an alpha-blocker.

Catheterization is mandatory for acute urinary retention. Spontaneous voiding may return, but a catheter should be left indwelling for 3 days while detrusor tone returns. If this fails, treatment is indicated.

B. SURGICAL MEASURES

There are four classic approaches used in prostatectomy: transurethral, retropubic, suprapubic, and perineal. The transurethral route is preferred in patients with glands weighing under 50 g because morbidity rates are lower and the hospital stay is shorter. Larger glands may require open surgery, depending on the preference of the urologist. The death rate is low in each procedure (1–2%). Potency is at greatest risk when the transperineal exposure is used, but impotence occasionally results following transurethral resection of the prostate.

An alternative approach to the treatment of benign prostatic hyperplasia is transurethral incision of the prostate (TUIP). This procedure consists of incision of the prostate at the bladder neck up to the verumontanum, allowing expansion of the entire prostatic urethra. It is especially effective when the primary point of obstruction is caused by a "median bar" or high posterior lip of the bladder neck.

Prognosis

Most patients with marked symptoms receive considerable relief and substantial improvement in urine flow following surgical treatment; however, those with milder forms may benefit from drug therapy.

URETHRAL STRICTURE

Acquired urethral strictures in males may be due to external trauma or to prior instrumentation (most common). Strictures may be inflammatory, due to gonorrhea, tuberculous urethritis, or schistosomiasis, or may rarely be a complication of cancer. The common presenting symptoms are dysuria, weak stream, splaying of the urinary stream, urinary retention, and urinary tract infection. Evidence of scarring due to trauma or induration and perineal fistula may be seen. Urethroscopy reveals the degree of narrowing. A retrograde urethrogram will delineate the site and degree of stricture.

Urethral stricture must be differentiated from bladder outlet obstruction due to prostatism, impacted urethral stones, urethral foreign bodies, and tumors.

Initial treatment consists of transurethral direct vision internal urethrotomy (incision of the stricture). Successful results are obtained in 75% of patients. For long dense strictures or those failing to respond to internal urethrotomy, open surgical repair is indicated. This is probably best achieved by the transpubic or perineal route if the lesion involves the membranous urethra. If the mid urethra is involved, the perineal approach is indicated; if the distal urethra is involved, the penile approach is appropriate. End-to-end anastomosis is satisfactory, but a one-stage inlay patch graft, tube, or pedicle flap of preputial skin is currently favored for most strictures.

Andrich DE et al: Urethral strictures and their surgical treatment. BJU Int 2000;86:571.

Barry MJ et al: The American Urological Association symptom index for benign prostatic hyperplasia. J Urol 1992;148:1549.

Ekman P: Finasteride in the treatment of benign prostatic hypertrophy: an update. New indications for finasteride therapy. Scand J Urol Nephrol 1999;203(Suppl):15.

Garraway WM et al: Benign prostatic hyperplasia: effects on quality of life and impact on treatment decisions. Urology 1994;44:629.

Gerber GS et al: Endopyelotomy: Patient selection, results and complications. Urology 1994;43:2.

Kavoussi LR et al: Laparoscopic pyeloplasty. J Urol 1993;150: 1891.

Lepor H et al: A dose titration study evaluating terazosin, a selective, once-a-day α-blocker for the treatment of symptomatic benign prostatic hyperplasia. J Urol 1990; 144:1393.

McAninch JW: Reconstruction of external urethral strictures: circular fasciocutaneous penile flap. J Urol 1993;149:488.

Moul JW: BPH: New concepts in the 1990's. Postgrad Med 1993; 94:141.

Wessels H et al: Current controversies in anterior urethral stricture repair: free-graft versus pedicled skin-flap reconstruction. World J Urol 1998;16:175.

■ URINARY TRACT INFECTIONS

Urinary tract infection is the second most common type of infection in humans and is frequently encountered by primary care physicians as well as urologists.

These infections are caused by a variety of pyogenic bacteria which typically produce a nonspecific tissue response. The most common organisms are gram-negative bacteria, particularly *Escherichia coli*. Less common are *Enterobacter aerogenes, Proteus vulgaris, Proteus mirabilis, Pseudomonas aeruginosa,* and *Enterococcus faecalis.*

Owing to the short length of the female urethra and bacterial colonization of the introitus, ascending infection is a common occurrence in young girls and in sexually active women. In males, ascending infection is usually a consequence of urethral instrumentation.

Though relatively uncommon, descending or hematogenous urinary tract infection is usually associated with local urinary tract disorders—most commonly, obstruction and stasis; less commonly, trauma, foreign bodies, or tumors.

Lymphatic spread occasionally occurs from the large bowel or from the cervix and adnexa in the female through the perivesical and periureteral lymphatics.

Direct extension to the urinary bladder of nearby inflammatory processes—eg, appendiceal abscess, enterovesical fistula, or pelvic abscess—may occur.

Predisposing Factors

Infection is usually initiated or sustained by predisposing factors. Predisposing systemic factors include diabetes mellitus, immunosuppression, and malnutrition; these disorders probably favor urinary tract infection by interfering with normal bladder and body defense mechanisms. Predisposing local factors include organic or functional obstruction, stasis (residual urine), foreign bodies (especially catheters and stones), tumors or necrotic tissue, and trauma (especially to the kidneys). Vesicoureteral reflux facilitates transport of bacteria from the bladder to the kidney, and this subsequently predisposes to pyelonephritis.

Classification of Urinary Tract Infection

Urinary tract infection is classified as (1) upper urinary tract infection (most commonly, acute or chronic pyelonephritis or infection due to renal abscess); (2) lower urinary tract infection (cystitis or urethritis); or

(3) genital infection (prostatitis, epididymitis, seminal vesiculitis, or orchitis).

Urologic Instrumentation or Surgery & Urinary Tract Infection

In the absence of urinary tract infection, surgery of the upper urinary tract rarely requires prophylactic antibacterial therapy. In the presence of infection, one attempts to sterilize the system before operation. If stenting or tube drainage is required and there are no symptoms of infection, colonization by urea-splitting organisms such as *P mirabilis* or *Klebsiella pneumoniae* does not call for antibacterial therapy until the stent or tube is to be removed. Urine culture is obtained approximately 24 hours before removal, and specific antibacterial therapy is started at that time.

With lower urinary tract surgery, the situation is different. Even when the urine is sterile, antibacterial therapy is advised before operations involving the urethra and the bladder, especially for women in whom contamination from vaginal organisms is likely. Men undergoing prostatectomy for obstructive prostatism often have urinary tract infection, particularly when catheter drainage is used preoperatively. In these cases, antimicrobial therapy is necessary before and after surgery to prevent bacteremia.

In the presence of urinary tract infection, any urethral instrumentation poses a threat of bacteremia—more apt to occur in males than in females. Appropriate antibacterial coverage should be instituted before manipulation.

When the urinary tract cannot be sterilized, effective serum levels of antibiotic (eg, aminoglycoside plus ampicillin) should be achieved before instrumentation.

A. PRINCIPLES OF CATHETERIZATION

After a short-term single catheterization, the rate of infection is 1–5%. However, in certain patients—pregnant women, elderly or debilitated patients—and in the presence of urologic disease, the risk is much higher. An indwelling catheter often leads to colonization, especially in women. The incidence is proportionate to the duration of catheterization and reaches approximately 95% after 5 days.

Strict aseptic technique is of critical importance in catheterization. Proper cleansing of the genitalia is essential. Iodophor preparations may be used for cleaning the vaginal introitus or the glans penis. Many common urinary tract pathogens are present in normal colonic flora, and these organisms often gain access to the urinary tract of catheterized patients. Cross-contamination of urinary catheters (passive transmission of bacteria from patient to patient on the hands of hospital personnel) is a frequent mode of transfer of resistant organisms. Measures directed to the prevention of catheter cross-contamination are essential. Closed catheter drainage is probably the best way to reduce cross-contamination.

With sterile technique during catheterization and a closed drainage system, most catheters can be kept sterile for 48–72 hours. In a closed drainage system, an added airlock or one-way valve preventing reflux of urine from the collecting bag to the draining tubes also helps prevent infection. The general principles are as follows: (1) Indwelling catheters should be used only when absolutely necessary. (2) Catheters should be inserted with strict aseptic technique. (3) A closed drainage system, preferably with a one-way valve, is advisable. (4) Nonobstructed dependent drainage is essential. (5) Unnecessary irrigation of the system should be avoided. (6) If the catheter is needed for a prolonged period, it should be changed every 2–3 weeks to minimize encrustation and stone formation. (7) The urine of catheterized patients should be cultured before manipulation. (8) Catheterized patients with asymptomatic catheter colonization should be given antibiotics just before the catheter is removed—not during the period of catheterization unless symptomatic infection occurs.

B. ANTIBACTERIAL THERAPY

The choice of antibiotics depends on the type of organism and its sensitivity, as determined by urine cultures. For uncomplicated infection, adequate urine concentrations of the antibiotic determine efficacy, but in cases of bacteremia and septic shock, serum concentrations are crucial. Commonly used oral medications are sulfonamides, nitrofurantoin, ampicillin, trimethoprim-sulfamethoxazole, fluoroquinolones, and oxytetracycline. For parenteral therapy, aminoglycosides and cephalosporins are effective against the most common organisms, ie, *P mirabilis, E aerogenes,* and *P aeruginosa.*

ACUTE PYELONEPHRITIS

ESSENTIALS OF DIAGNOSIS

- Chills, fever, and flank pain.
- Frequency and urgency of urination; dysuria.
- Pyuria and bacteriuria.
- Bacterial growth on urine cultures.

General Considerations

Except in the presence of stasis, foreign bodies, trauma, or instrumentation, pyelonephritis is an ascending type of infection. Pathogenic organisms usually reach the kidney from the bladder, often via an incompetent ureterovesical junction.

Clinical Findings

A. SYMPTOMS AND SIGNS

In acute attacks, pain is present in one or both flanks. Young children commonly present with poorly localized abdominal pain; irritative lower urinary tract symptoms may be present. Chills and fever are common. Severe infection may produce hypotension, peripheral vasoconstriction, and acute renal failure. Gross hematuria is not common.

B. LABORATORY FINDINGS

Pyuria and bacteriuria are consistent findings. Leukocytosis with a shift to the left is common. Urine culture identifies the organism.

C. IMAGING STUDIES

In acute attacks, only minimal changes such as delayed visualization and poor concentrating ability are noted on intravenous urography. CT scans may demonstrate zones of decreased enhancement in the renal parenchyma as well as perinephric fat stranding. Renal or ureteral calculi may be seen on plain abdominal x-rays or nonenhanced CT scans. Chest x-ray may show a small ipsilateral pleural effusion.

Differential Diagnosis

Pneumonia, acute cholecystitis, or splenic infarction can be confused with pyelonephritis. Acute appendicitis will sometimes cause pyuria and microhematuria. Any acute abdominal illness such as pancreatitis, diverticulitis, or intestinal angina can simulate pyelonephritis. Appropriate chest x-rays and urinalysis will usually make the distinction.

Complications

If the diagnosis is missed in the acute stage, the infection may become chronic. Both acute and chronic pyelonephritis lead to progressive renal damage.

Treatment

Specific antibiotic therapy should be given for at least 4 days to eradicate the infecting organism after proper identification and sensitivity determination. Symptomatic treatment is indicated for pain and irritative voiding symptoms. Adequate fluid intake to assure optimum urinary output is required. Failure to simultaneously identify and treat predisposing factors (eg, obstruction) is the principal cause of failure to respond to therapy, leading to chronic pyelonephritis.

Prognosis

The prognosis is good with adequate treatment of both the infection and its predisposing cause, depending on the degree of preexisting renal parenchymal damage.

EMPHYSEMATOUS PYELONEPHRITIS

Emphysematous pyelonephritis is a form of acute pyelonephritis secondary to a gas-producing bacteria (most often *E coli*). It is commonly seen in diabetic patients with upper urinary tract obstruction. The diagnosis is made by the usual signs of acute pyelonephritis and by the presence of gas in the renal collecting system and parenchyma seen on plain films, ultrasound, or CT. The condition is life-threatening, with a mortality rate of 60–80% with intravenous antibiotics alone. Operative treatment, including nephrectomy and drainage along with antibiotics, decreases the mortality rate to less than 20%.

CHRONIC PYELONEPHRITIS

Chronic pyelonephritis is the result of inadequately treated or recurrent acute pyelonephritis. The diagnosis is primarily made by x-ray, since patients rarely have signs or symptoms until late in the course, when they develop chronic flank pain, hypertension, anemia, or renal failure. Pyuria is not a consistent finding. Because chronic pyelonephritis may be a progressive localized immune response initiated by bacteria long since eradicated, urine cultures are usually sterile. Early cases may have no findings on intravenous urography, whereas in late cases it may reveal small kidneys with typical caliceal deformities (clubbing), with evidence of peripheral scarring and a thin cortex. Voiding cystourethrography may document vesicoureteral reflux as the cause. Complications include hypertension, stone formation, and chronic renal failure.

Antibiotic treatment is not helpful in these patients unless ongoing infection can be documented. The prognosis depends on the status of renal function but is generally not good, particularly when the disease is contracted in childhood. Progressive deterioration of renal function usually occurs.

Xanthogranulomatous pyelonephritis is a form of chronic pyelonephritis seen most frequently in middle-aged diabetic women and rarely in children. The disease is usually unilateral and is associated with prolonged obstructing nephrolithiasis. Patients often have nonspecific symptoms similar to those of acute pyelonephritis but have an enlarged kidney with calculi and a mass often indistinguishable from tumor. Proteus species are common causative agents. Nephrectomy is usually the treatment of choice, though a partial nephrectomy may be performed for focal disease. Histologic examination confirms the diagnosis following nephrectomy by the demonstration of foamy lipid-laden macrophages.

PAPILLARY NECROSIS

This disorder consists of ischemic necrosis of the renal papillae or of the entire pyramid. Excessive ingestion of analgesics, sickle cell trait, diabetes, obstruction with infection, and vesicoureteral reflux with infection are common predisposing factors.

The symptoms are usually those of chronic cystitis with recurring exacerbations of pyelonephritis. Renal pain or renal colic may be present. Azotemic manifestations may be the presenting symptoms. In acute attacks, localized flank tenderness and generalized toxemia may occur. Laboratory findings consist of pyuria, occasionally glycosuria, and acidosis. Impaired kidney function is shown by elevated serum creatinine and urea nitrogen. Intravenous urography usually shows impaired function and poor visualization in advanced cases. Evidence of ulceration, cavitation, or linear breaks in the base of the papillae and radiolucent defects due to sloughed papillae may be seen; the latter may become calcified. Retrograde urograms may be needed for proper imaging if kidney function is markedly impaired.

Preventive measures consist of proper management of diabetic patients with recurrent infections and avoidance of chronic use of analgesic compounds containing phenacetin and aspirin.

Intensive antibacterial therapy may be needed, though it is commonly unsuccessful in eradicating infection. Little can be done surgically except to remove obstructing papillae and correct predisposing factors (eg, reflux, obstruction) if identified.

In severe cases, the prognosis is poor. Renal transplantation may be required.

RENAL ABSCESS

While renal abscess is occasionally due to hematogenous spread of a distant staphylococcal infection, most abscesses are secondary to chronic nonspecific infection of the kidney, often complicated by stone formation. The onset may be acute, with high fever, but occasionally low-grade fever and general malaise are the presenting symptoms. Localized costovertebral angle tenderness and a palpable flank mass may be present. A mass may be evident on intravenous urograms, DTPA scans, sonograms, CT scans, or renal angiograms. If the abscess is due to hematogenous spread, the urine will not contain bacteria unless the abscess has broken into the pelvicaliceal system. More frequently, gram-negative organisms are found, as would be expected in light of the preponderance of ascending infection.

If organism sensitivity can be established by appropriate tests (blood and urine cultures and sensitivity tests), treatment with the proper antibiotic is indicated. Many infections have responded to percutaneous drainage and irrigation with antibiotic solutions, especially in cases of unilocular abscess cavity seen on either ultrasound or CT examination. In multilocular abscess or persistent bacteremia despite percutaneous drainage, surgical drainage or even heminephrectomy may be necessary.

When the abscess is found to be secondary to chronic renal infection, nephrectomy is usually indicated because of advanced destruction of the kidney.

PERINEPHRIC ABSCESS

Abscess between the renal capsule and the perirenal fascia most often results from rupture of an intrarenal abscess into the perinephric space. *E coli* is the most common causative organism. The pathogenesis usually begins with severe pyonephrosis secondary to obstruction, as with renal or ureteral calculi. Clinical findings are similar to those of renal abscess. A pleural effusion on the affected side and signs of psoas muscle irritation are common. Abdominal plain films may show obliteration of the psoas muscle shadow, and an intravenous urogram may show poor concentration of contrast medium and hydronephrosis. CT scan is the current study of choice for diagnosis.

Treatment involves prompt drainage of the abscess and use of appropriate systemic antibiotics, including coverage of anaerobes. Percutaneous drainage is often successful; however, open surgical drainage is necessary if percutaneous drainage is incomplete. Mortality ranges between 20% and 50% with antibiotics and drainage, whereas treatment with antibiotics alone increases this rate to 75–100%.

CYSTITIS

Cystitis is more common in females and is usually an ascending infection. In males, it usually occurs in association with urethral or prostatic obstruction, prostatitis, foreign bodies, or tumors. The urinary bladder is normally capable of clearing bacterial inoculation unless an underlying pathologic process interferes with its defensive mechanisms.

In the acute phase, the principal symptoms of cystitis are dysuria, frequency, urgency, and hematuria; low-grade fever and suprapubic, perineal, and low back pain may be present. In chronic cystitis, irritative symptoms are usually milder.

Evidence of prostatitis, urethritis, or vaginitis may be present. Laboratory findings, in addition to hematuria, consist of bacteriuria and pyuria. Leukocytosis is not common. Urine culture identifies the organism. Cystoscopy is not advisable in the acute phase. In chronic cystitis, evidence of mucosal irritation may be present.

In any documented recurrent lower urinary tract infection (particularly in males), a complete urologic workup is indicated. Instrumentation is contraindicated in the acute phase, but cystoscopy is essential to identify the predisposing factor in chronic or recurrent bacterial cystitis.

Specific antibacterial therapy is given according to sensitivity testing of recovered organisms (*E coli* in > 80% of cases). Sterilization of urine should usually be followed by a variable period of continuous antibiotic therapy (depending upon the predisposing factor or the chronicity and recurrence of the disease). Prolonged suppressive medication is usually indicated in cases associated with voiding dysfunction.

In women with recurrent postcoital cystitis, premedication (eg, sulfonamides, nitrofurantoin) on the night of intercourse and the following day in addition to immediate postcoital voiding decreases recurrences.

PROSTATITIS

Acute Bacterial Prostatitis

Acute bacterial prostatitis is a severe acute febrile illness caused by ascending coliform bacteria which frequently colonize the male urethra. Symptoms include high fever; chills; low back and perineal pain; and urinary frequency and urgency, with diminished stream or retention. On examination, the prostate is extremely tender, swollen, and warm to the touch. A fluctuant abscess may be palpable. The prostate must be examined cautiously, because vigorous palpation may cause acute septicemia. Laboratory findings include pyuria, bacteriuria, and leukocytosis.

Transurethral manipulation by catheter or cystoscopy should be avoided; urinary retention should be treated by introducing a percutaneous suprapubic tube. Treatment with systemic antibiotics (fluoroquinolones or aminoglycosides and ampicillin-cephalosporin) should be started immediately and should be adjusted later when results of culture and sensitivity tests are known. *E coli* is found in 80% of cases. Treatment with oral antibiotics for several weeks after the initial phase has subsided is necessary to eradicate the bacteria completely. A prostatic abscess usually requires open perineal drainage or transurethral unroofing. The prognosis is good if treatment is thorough and prompt.

Chronic Prostatitis

Chronic prostatitis is a common and complex problem. With differential diagnosis including urethritis, bacterial and nonbacterial prostatitis, prostatodynia, and seminal vesiculitis, assigning the correct diagnosis may challenge even the expert. The symptoms are varied and include suprapubic pain, low back pain, orchialgia, dysuria at the tip of the penis, and urinary frequency and urgency. The urinalysis may be normal. There may be a clear white urethral discharge. Prostate examination may reveal a soft, boggy prostate.

Expressed prostatic secretions may contain numerous leukocytes (> 10 per high-power field) in clumps as well as macrophages. Cultures of urine are usually sterile, but cultures of expressed prostatic secretions and urine obtained after prostatic massage are usually positive in bacterial prostatitis. Chlamydia or ureaplasma may be an offending organism, particularly in males under age 35. Determination of the site of infection may require differential cultures. The first part of the voided urine stream is collected as VB_1 and the midstream specimen as VB_2. The prostate is then massaged to obtain expressed prostatic secretions (EPS), and the postmassage urine is collected as VB_3. The differential leukocyte and bacterial counts from each of these specimens can help localize the site of infection. If VB_1 has high levels of leukocytes and bacteria relative to the other specimens, urethritis is likely; if VB_2 has high levels, a site above the bladder neck is likely; and if the EPS, VB_3, or both, have high counts, prostatitis is likely.

Treatment depends on culture results, but if there is no bacterial growth on culture, tetracycline, 250–500 mg four times a day for 14 days, may be curative. For chronic bacterial prostatitis, at least a 6-week course of a fluoroquinolone or trimethoprim-sulfamethoxazole is often given. Surgical treatment for prostatitis is rarely indicated or helpful. Some patients improve following discontinuation of caffeine and alcohol, and a few respond to repeated prostatic massage. Patients with no evidence of bacterial infection or obstructive findings and those who have recurrent pelvic pain in association with voiding dysfunction (eg, intermittent or weak urinary stream) may be treated with α-adrenergic blocking agents or biofeedback to decrease the internal and external sphincter tone.

ACUTE EPIDIDYMITIS

Acute epididymitis is most commonly a disease of young males, caused by bacterial infection ascending from the urethra or prostate. The disease is less common in older males, but when it does occur, it is most often due to infection secondary to urinary tract obstruction or instrumentation.

The symptoms are sudden pain in the scrotum, rapid unilateral scrotal enlargement, and marked tenderness that extends to the spermatic cord in the groin and may be relieved by scrotal elevation (**Prehn's sign**). Fever is present. An acute hydrocele may result, and secondary orchitis with a swollen, painful testicle may occur. Laboratory studies reveal pyuria, bacteriuria, and marked leukocytosis.

Epididymitis must be differentiated from torsion of the testis, testicular tumor, and tuberculous epididymitis. A technetium Tc 99m pertechnetate scan reveals increased uptake with epididymitis but decreased uptake with torsion. Scrotal ultrasound will distinguish between the solid mass of a testicular tumor and an enlarged, inflamed epididymis and can also identify epididymal or testicular abscess, which will require operative treatment. Increased blood flow on Doppler ultrasound also helps distinguish epididymitis from torsion, though it is not completely reliable.

Cultured aspirates from inflamed epididymides of men under age 35 tend to show gonococci and chlamydiae; in men older than 35, *E coli* is most common. Epididymal aspiration for culture is not required routinely, however. Pyuria with a negative urine culture suggests the presence of chlamydial infection in both prostate and epididymis. (See also Tuberculosis, below.)

Treatment consists of antibiotics, usually ceftriaxone and doxycycline in men under age 35 and fluoroquinolones in those over age 35. In some patients, pain is relieved by scrotal hypothermia, and consideration should be given to infiltration of the spermatic cord by 1% bupivacaine. Some clinicians recommend giving nonsteroidal anti-inflammatory drugs such as ibuprofen or indomethacin to aid in pain relief. In most instances, prompt treatment will result in rapid resolution of pain, fever, and swelling. Patients must refrain from exertion for 1–3 weeks.

Exacerbations can be controlled by treating the predisposing factor. Chronic epididymitis rarely resolves completely; it has no consequences except, occasionally in bilateral cases, sterility due to scarring and obstruction of the delicate epididymal tubule. Rarely, epididymectomy is necessary.

TUBERCULOSIS

Tuberculosis is a commonly missed genitourinary infection that should be considered in any case of pyuria without bacteriuria or in any case of urinary tract infection that does not respond to treatment.

Genitourinary tuberculosis is always secondary to pulmonary infection, though in many cases, the primary focus has healed or is quiescent. Infection occurs via the hematogenous route. The kidneys and (less commonly) the prostate are the principal sites of urinary tract involvement, though any part of the genitourinary system can be affected.

Pathology

Renal tuberculosis usually starts as a tuberculoma that gradually enlarges, caseates, and finally ulcerates, breaking into the pelvicaliceal system. Caseation and scarring are the principal pathologic features of renal tuberculosis. In the ureter, tuberculosis usually leads to distal strictures, periureteritis, and mural fibrosis.

In the bladder, the infection is characterized by areas of hyperemia and a coalescent group of tubercles, followed by ulcerations. Bladder wall fibrosis and contraction are the end results.

Urethral involvement in the male is uncommon but when present leads to urethral stricture, usually in the bulbous portion. Periurethral abscess and fistula are possible complications.

Genital tuberculosis may involve the prostate, seminal vesicles, and epididymides, either separately or in association with renal involvement. Tubercle formation with later caseation and fibrosis is the basic pathologic feature. The prostate becomes enlarged, with palpable nodules and an irregular consistency. The affected seminal vesicle is fibrotic and distended. Induration and thickening of the epididymis and beading of the vas deferens are characteristic findings. The testicles are rarely involved.

Clinical Findings

A. SYMPTOMS AND SIGNS

The patient commonly presents with lower urinary tract irritation, usually with pyuria. Less common manifestations are hematuria, renal pain, and renal colic.

B. LABORATORY FINDINGS

"Sterile" pyuria is the rule, but 15% of cases have secondary bacterial infection (eg, *E coli*). *Mycobacterium tuberculosis* can be identified on an acid-fast stain of the centrifuged sediment of a 24-hour urine specimen or by culture of the first morning urine collected on 3 successive days (positive in 90% of cases).

C. IMAGING STUDIES

Radiologic findings that suggest genitourinary tuberculosis include moth-eaten, caseous cavities or bizarre, irregular calices. Strictures in straight, rigid, moderately dilated ureters and a contracted bladder with vesicoureteral reflux are all suggestive evidence.

Treatment

A. MEDICAL TREATMENT

Tuberculosis must be treated as a systemic disease. Once the diagnosis is established, medical treatment is indicated regardless of the need for surgery. Whenever possible, medical treatment should be continued for at least 3 months before operation.

Active medications against tuberculosis include rifampin, isoniazid, pyrazinamide, ethambutol, and streptomycin. Standard initial treatment is with rifampin, isoniazid, and pyrazinamide for 8 weeks. Pyridoxine, 100 mg/d, is given in divided doses to counteract the vitamin B_6 depletion effect of isoniazid. In patients with more severe infections, ethambutol or streptomycin may be added to the initial treatment. Following the initial 8 weeks of therapy, rifampin and isoniazid are continued in combination three times per week for another 8 weeks. Liver function tests must be followed in view of the hepatotoxicity of rifampin, isoniazid, and pyrazinamide.

B. SURGICAL MEASURES

If medical therapy fails to cure a unilateral lesion, nephrectomy may be necessary. However, this is rare. In bilateral disease that has seriously damaged one kidney and is in an early stage in the other, unilateral nephrectomy may be considered; in localized polar lesions, partial nephrectomy may be done.

In unilateral epididymal involvement, epididymectomy plus contralateral vasectomy is indicated to prevent descent of the infection to the prostate; bilateral epididymectomy should be done if both sides are involved.

For a severely contracted bladder, augmentation enterocystoplasty will increase vesical capacity following eradication of the infection.

Prognosis

In a high percentage of cases, cure is obtained by medical means. Unilateral renal lesions have the best prognosis.

Cooper CS et al: The outcome of stopping prophylactic antibiotics in older children with vesicoureteral reflux. J Urol 2000; 163:269.

Eastham J et al: Xanthogranulomatous pyelonephritis: clinical findings and surgical considerations. Urology 1994;43:295.

Jones BF et al: Acute renal failure due to acute pyelonephritis. Am J Nephrol 1991;11:257.

Lang EK: Renal, perirenal, and pararenal abscesses: percutaneous drainage. Radiology 1990;174:109.

Loughlin KR: Management of urologic problems during pregnancy. Urology 1994;44:159.

Lucas MJ et al: Urinary infection in pregnancy. Clin Obstet Gynecol 1993;36:855.

Mokrzycki MH: Renal malacoplakia with papillary necrosis and renal failure. Am J Kidney Dis 1992;19:587.

Petersen L et al: Male genitourinary tuberculosis: report of 12 cases and review of the literature. Scand J Urol Nephrol 1993; 27:425.

Saw KC et al: Tuberculosis prostatitis: nodularity may simulate malignancy. Br J Urol 1993;72:249.

Stapleton A et al: Postcoital antimicrobial prophylaxis for recurrent urinary tract infection: a randomized, double-blind, placebo-controlled trial. JAMA 1990;264:703.

Talner LB et al: Acute pyelonephritis: can we agree on terminology? Radiology 1994;192:297.

■ CALCULI

RENAL STONE

ESSENTIALS OF DIAGNOSIS

- *Flank pain, hematuria, pyelonephritis, previous stone passage.*
- *Costovertebral tenderness.*
- *Red cells in urine.*
- *Stone visualized on urography, ultrasonography, or CT scan.*

General Considerations

Most stones are composed of calcium salts (oxalate, phosphate) or magnesium-ammonium phosphate—the latter secondary to urea-splitting organisms. Most calcium stones are idiopathic (ie, idiopathic hypercalciuria). In patients with hyperparathyroidism or those who ingest large amounts of calcium or vitamin D or in patients who are dehydrated or immobilized, hypercalciuria promotes stone formation.

The less common metabolic stones, cystine and uric acid, usually form secondary to hypersecretion of these substances or to a defect in urinary acidification. Owing to the radiodensity of sulfur, cystine stones are radiopaque (albeit less so than calcium stones), whereas uric acid stones are radiolucent. Stones that obstruct the ureteropelvic junction or ureter lead to hydronephrosis and infection.

Clinical Findings

A. SYMPTOMS AND SIGNS

If the stone acutely obstructs the ureteropelvic junction or a calix, moderate to severe renal pain will be noted, often accompanied by nausea, vomiting, and ileus.

Hematuria is common. Symptoms of infection, if present, will be exacerbated. Nonobstructing calculi are usually painless. This includes staghorn calculi, which may form a cast of all calices and the pelvis. In the symptomatic patient, there may be costovertebral angle tenderness and a quiet abdomen. Infection secondary to obstruction may lead to high fever and a rigid abdomen.

B. LABORATORY FINDINGS

With acute infection, leukocytosis is to be expected. Urinalysis may reveal red and white blood cells and bacteria. A pH of 7.6 or higher implies the presence of urea-splitting organisms. A pH consistently below 5.5 is compatible with the formation of uric acid or cystine stones. If the pH is fixed between 6.0 and 7.0, renal tubular acidosis should be considered as a cause of nephrocalcinosis. Crystals of uric acid or cystine in the urine are suggestive. A 24-hour urine collection for calcium may reveal hypercalciuria, which occurs with hyperparathyroidism and idiopathic hypercalciuria.

Increases in urine calcium and phosphate plus hypercalcemia (and hypophosphatemia) suggest the presence of hyperparathyroidism. Measurement of serum intact parathyroid hormone is helpful in patients suspected of having hyperparathyroidism. Excessive urinary uric acid is compatible with uric acid stone formation.

A qualitative test for urinary cystine should be part of the routine evaluation. If levels are elevated, a 24-hour quantitative measurement should be made. Hyperchloremic acidosis suggests renal tubular acidosis with secondary renal calcifications. Total renal function will be impaired only if the stones are bilateral, and particularly if chronic infection complicates the clinical presentation.

C. IMAGING STUDIES

About 90% of calculi are radiopaque (calcium, cystine). Excretory urography is necessary to verify their location within the urinary tract and also affords a qualitative measure of renal function (Figure 41–16). An acutely obstructed kidney may show only increasing density of the renal shadow without significant radiopaque material in the calices. A nonopaque stone (uric acid) will be seen as a radiolucent defect in the opaque contrast media. Calculi larger than 1 cm cast a specific acoustic shadow on ultrasonography. Spiral CT has become the study of choice in emergent situations, as the entire urinary tract can be scanned rapidly and without contrast injection. Calculi can be readily identified and distinguished from clot or tumor. Plain x-ray of the skeletal system may identify Paget's disease, sarcoidosis, or osteoporosis due to prolonged immobilization responsible for hypercalciuria.

Figure 41–16. Bilateral staghorn calculi and left upper ureteral stone. *Left:* Plain film. Arrow points to ureteral stone. *Right:* Excretory urogram showing bilateral impaired function.

D. STONE ANALYSIS

If a stone has previously been passed or if one is recovered, its chemical composition should be analyzed. Such information may be useful when planning a preventive program.

Differential Diagnosis

Acute pyelonephritis may begin with acute renal pain mimicking that of renal stone. Urinalysis reveals pyuria, and urograms or CT fails to reveal a calculus.

Renal adenocarcinoma may bleed into the tumor, causing acute pain mimicking that of an obstructing stone. Imaging can make the differentiation.

Transitional cell tumors of the renal pelvis or calices will mimic uric acid stone; both are radiolucent. CT scan without contrast or ultrasound will reveal the stone by virtue of increased density compared with adjacent soft tissues.

Renal tuberculosis is complicated by stone formation in 10% of cases. Pyuria without bacteriuria is suggestive. Urography reveals the moth-eaten calices typical of tuberculosis.

Papillary necrosis may cause renal colic if a sloughed papilla obstructs the ureteropelvic junction. Imaging (particularly CT) will settle the issue.

Renal infarction may cause renal pain and hematuria. Evidence of a cardiac lesion, nonfunction of the kidney on urography, and exclusion of a calculus help in differentiation. Infarction is confirmed by angiography, radioisotopic renography, or color Doppler ultrasound.

Complications

Acting as a foreign body, a stone increases the probability of infection. However, primary infection may incite stone formation. A stone lodged in the ureteropelvic junction leads to progressive hydronephrosis. A staghorn calculus, as it grows, may destroy renal tissue by pressure, and the infection that is usually present also contributes to renal damage.

Prevention

An effective preventive regimen depends upon stone analysis and chemical studies of the serum and urine.

A. GENERAL MEASURES

Ensure a high fluid intake (3–4 L/d) to keep solutes well diluted. This measure alone may decrease stone-forming potential by 50%. Combat infection, relieve stasis or obstruction, and advise the patient to avoid prolonged immobilization. For calcium stone formers, stop vitamin D supplements and foods and medications containing calcium salts.

B. SPECIFIC MEASURES

1. Calcium stones—Remove the parathyroid tumor, if present. Reduce dairy products (milk, cheese) in the diet. Calcium in the diet should be less than 400 mg/d. Dietary sodium may promote calcium absorption, and restriction to 100 meq/d may be helpful. Limitation of proteins and carbohydrates may also reduce hypercalciuria.

Oral orthophosphates are effective in reducing the stone-forming potential of urine by decreasing urine calcium and increasing inhibitor activity. Thiazide diuretics such as hydrochlorothiazide, 50 mg twice daily, decrease the calcium content in urine by 50%. If hyperuricosuria is coincident with calcium urolithiasis, then allopurinol and urinary alkalinization can reduce the formation of urate crystals, which may act as a nidus for calcium crystallization.

For a patient with primary absorptive hypercalciuria, cellulose sodium phosphate can be given. This substance will combine with calcium in the gut to prevent absorption.

2. Oxalate stones (calcium oxalate)—Prescribe phosphate or a thiazide diuretic (see above) and limit calcium intake. Elimination of excessive oxalate in coffee, tea, colas, leafy green vegetables, and chocolate may also be helpful. Vitamin C in excess of 1 g can be metabolized in some individuals to oxalate and thus should be avoided.

3. Magnesium-ammonium-phosphate stones—These stones are usually secondary to urinary tract infection due to bacteria that produce urease (primarily proteus species). Eradication of the infection will prevent further stone formation but is impossible when stones are present. After all calculi have been removed, prevention of stone growth is best accomplished by urinary acidification, long-term use of antibiotics, and, perhaps, use of acetohydroxamic acid, a urease inhibitor that maintains an acid urinary pH and may potentiate antibiotic action.

4. Metabolic stones (uric acid, cystine)—These substances are most soluble at a pH of 7.0 or higher. Give sodium-potassium citrate solution, 4–8 mL four times daily orally ; monitor the urine pH with a paper indicator. For uric acid stone formers, limit purines in the diet and give allopurinol. Patients with mild cystinuria may need only urinary alkalinization, as described above. For severe cystinuria, giving penicillamine, 30 mg/kg/d orally, will reduce urinary cystine to safe levels. Penicillamine should be supplemented with pyridoxine, 50 mg/d orally. Propionyl glycine preparations have been used with similar results and fewer side effects.

Treatment

A. CONSERVATIVE MEASURES

Intervention is not required for small nonobstructive, asymptomatic caliceal stones. Hydration and dietary management may be sufficient to prevent growth of existing or new calcium stones in patients without metabolic abnormalities. Those with identifiable metabolic disorders may benefit from the specific measures described previously. Patients with primary renal tubular acidosis and secondary stones can be treated with hydration and urinary alkalinization.

B. PERCUTANEOUS INTERVENTION (ENDOUROLOGY)

In selected patients with symptomatic or large pelvic stones, percutaneous stone removal may be successful.

A percutaneous tract enters the renal collecting system through an appropriate calix (**percutaneous nephrostomy**). The tract is subsequently dilated, and endoscopic extraction of the stones (**percutaneous nephroscopy and percutaneous nephrolithotomy**). Pulverization by means of ultrasonic, electrohydraulic, or laser probes passed through the nephrostomy tract may also be useful. Residual infection stones may be dissolved by percutaneous irrigation with hemiacidrin. For cystine and uric acid stones, alkaline or other irrigants that increase the specific crystal solubility may be used (eg, N-acetyl-L-lysine or propionyl glycine for cystine stones). Specific antibiotic treatment for infection must be given before irrigation to prevent sepsis.

Success with these endourologic methods approaches 100%. The advantages over surgical procedures include no incision, use of local anesthesia in many cases, and rapid recovery and return to employment. Disadvantages include the occasional need for multiple treatments to completely remove the calculi and the uncommon occurrence of significant hemorrhage.

C. EXTRACORPOREAL SHOCK WAVE LITHOTRIPSY (ESWL)

With this technique, patients are positioned in the path of shock waves focused on the renal calculi with the aid of fluoroscopy or ultrasound. General or regional anesthesia is required in selected patients, but sedation is sufficient in most cases. The shock waves (more than 1500 are usually given) pulverize the stones, and the small particles pass spontaneously over 2–5 days. Results to date have been excellent. Calcium stones and magnesium-ammonium-phosphate stones have been treated successfully. Because of the physical properties of the crystal lattice, ESWL is not as effective in fragmenting cystine stones. Radiolucent uric acid stones, which can be "visualized" using contrast via intravenous pyelography or retrograde ureteropyelography, are amenable to ESWL treatment. Staghorn calculi are amenable to a combined approach: percutaneous nephrolithotomy to remove the major bulk of the stone followed by ESWL to pulverize any inaccessible fragments. Fewer than 10% of patients treated with ESWL have required subsequent endourologic or surgical treatment.

A variety of devices now effectively pulverize stones using less energy and thus can be used with only intravenous sedation; an increased number of pulses are required to obtain the same results as with previous higher-energy devices. Some newer instruments use ultrasound instead of x-ray for stone localization.

D. OPEN SURGICAL REMOVAL OF STONES

Endourologic intervention and ESWL have markedly decreased the indications for open surgery. Rarely, both percutaneous nephrolithotomy and ESWL will be contraindicated, and open nephrolithotomy will be necessary. The goal of any approach is to remove all stone fragments, and the approach chosen must allow for intraoperative localization by radiography or ultrasonography. Incisions into the renal pelvis (pyelolithotomy) or the renal parenchyma (radial nephrotomy or anatrophic nephrolithotomy) may be required for complete stone removal. Instillation of a mixture of thrombin and calcium into the kidney causes the fragments to become trapped in a dense clot which is removed through a pyelotomy incision (coagulum pyelolithotomy). Operative nephroscopy allows a full view of all the calices and removal of all fragments. "Bench" surgery with autotransplantation of the kidney may be required in some instances. Rarely, poorly functioning kidneys containing symptomatic stones require nephrectomy.

Prognosis

The recurrence rate of renal stone is high unless sufficient attention is paid to measures for prevention of stone formation. The danger of recurrent stone is progressive renal damage due to obstruction and infection.

URETERAL STONE

ESSENTIALS OF DIAGNOSIS

- Severe ureterorenal colic.
- Hematuria.
- Nausea, vomiting, and ileus.
- Stone visible on excretory urography.

General Considerations

Ureteral stones originate in the kidney. When symptoms occur, ureteral obstruction is implicit and renal function endangered. Complicating infection may occur. Most ureteral stones pass spontaneously.

Clinical Findings

A. SYMPTOMS AND SIGNS

The onset of pain is usually abrupt. Pain is felt in the costovertebral angle and radiates to the ipsilateral lower abdominal quadrant. Nausea, vomiting, abdominal distention, and gross hematuria are common. When the stone approaches the bladder, symptoms mimic cystitis. If the kidney is infected, acute ureteral obstruction exacerbates the infection.

The patient is usually in such agony that only parenteral opioids will give relief. Costovertebral angle tenderness and guarding may be evident. Absence of bowel sounds and abdominal distention signify ileus. Fever may occur as a result of complicating renal infection.

B. LABORATORY FINDINGS

Laboratory findings are the same as for renal stone.

C. IMAGING STUDIES

Excretory urograms or spiral CT is essential. Plain films may reveal an opacity in the region of the ureter. Confirmation of ureteral location requires demonstration of confluence of stone and ureteral contrast (Figure 41–17). Excretory urograms with oblique films are diagnostic. This procedure depicts the degree of obstruction and the size and position of the stone, information that permits selection of appropriate treatment. A radiolucent stone will appear as a filling defect within a proximally dilated ureter—indistinguishable from a ureteral tumor or blood clot by intravenous urography. CT scan will discriminate between stone and tumor or clot density. Cystoscopy, ureteral catheterization, retrograde urography, and ureteroscopy may also be helpful.

Figure 41–17. Excretory urogram showing right ureteral stone causing hydronephrosis. Large irregular filling defect from unsuspected vesical neoplasm.

Differential Diagnosis

A tumor of the kidney or renal pelvis may bleed, and passage of a blood clot may cause ureteral colic. Urograms may reveal a radiolucent area in the ureter surrounded by the radiopaque urine. A CT scan without contrast agents will reveal no radiopacity.

A primary tumor of the ureter may cause obstructing pain and hematuria. The urogram will reveal the ureteral filling defect, often with secondary obstruction. A CT scan will differentiate a stone from tumor. Urinary cytologic study may reveal malignant transitional cells.

Acute pyelonephritis may cause pain as severe as that seen with stone. Pyuria and bacteriuria are found but do not rule out stone. Stone is absent on urography.

A sloughed papilla traversing the ureter may cause colic and will produce a urogram compatible with uric acid stone. Papillary sloughs should be evident, however.

Complications

If obstruction from the ureteral stone is prolonged, progressive renal damage may ensue. Bilateral stones may cause anuria, requiring immediate drainage of the proximal collecting system with indwelling ureteral catheters or percutaneous nephrostomy.

Infection may supervene, but many renal infections are iatrogenic, ie, introduced at the time of stone manipulation.

Prevention

See Renal Stone.

Treatment

A. GENERAL MEASURES

Most ureteral stones pass spontaneously—particularly those less than 0.5 cm in diameter. Once the diagnosis has been established, analgesics should be given and the patient hydrated. Periodic plain films should be taken to follow the progress of the stone and interval renal ultrasound studies obtained to assess the degree of hydronephrosis. The urine should be strained until the stone passes in order to recover the calculus for analysis. With larger stones, acute obstruction can be temporarily relieved by inserting an indwelling ureteral stent.

B. SPECIFIC MEASURES

If the stone causes intractable pain, progressive hydronephrosis, or acute infection, it should be removed. Obstructing stones in the upper two-thirds of the ureter can often be successfully treated by simultaneous ureteral catheterization and manipulation of the stone

back to the renal pelvis followed by ESWL or percutaneous nephrolithotomy as described above. Ureteroscopy permits ultrasonic or laser fragmentation or stone basket retrieval under direct vision. Retrograde basket extraction under fluoroscopic control may be used to remove small distal ureteral stones. Open surgical removal (ureterolithotomy) is only very rarely required for ureteral stones. ESWL has been applied to ureteral stones in the proximal ureter but is more problematic in the distal ureter owing to bone interference by surrounding pelvis, which interferes with imaging and attenuates shock wave force.

Prognosis

About 80% of ureteral stones pass spontaneously. Periodic plain films of the abdomen or excretory urograms will portray progress of the stone and warn of ensuing renal damage that would prompt operative intervention.

VESICAL STONE

Primary vesical calculi are rare in the USA but are common in Southeast Asia and the Middle East. The cause is probably dietary. Secondary stones usually complicate vesical outlet obstruction with residual urine and infection; 90% of those affected are men. Other causes of bladder stasis such as neurogenic bladder and bladder diverticula also promote vesical stone formation. They are common in vesical schistosomiasis or in association with radiation cystitis. Foreign bodies in the bladder may act as a nidus for the precipitation of urinary salts. Most stones contain calcium; some are composed of uric acid.

Clinical Findings

A. SYMPTOMS AND SIGNS

Symptoms of bladder neck obstruction are elicited. There may be sudden interruption of the stream and urethral pain if a stone occludes the bladder neck during voiding. Hematuria is common. Vesical distention may be noted; evidence of urethral stricture or an enlarged prostate is usually found.

B. LABORATORY FINDINGS

Pyuria and hematuria are almost always present.

C. IMAGING STUDIES

Vesical calculi are usually radiopaque. Excretory urograms will reveal that the stones are intravesical; residual urine is usually depicted on the postvoiding film. If nonopaque areas are noted, CT scan or ultrasound will differentiate between stones and vesical tumors or blood clots, but direct vision endoscopically is preferred.

D. Instrumental Examination

Inability to pass a catheter or sound into the bladder signifies urethral stricture. Catheterization may demonstrate residual urine. Cystoscopy will visualize the stones and may reveal an obstructing prostate.

Differential Diagnosis

A pedunculated vesical tumor may suddenly occlude the vesical neck during voiding. Excretory urograms, pelvic ultrasound CT scan, ultrasound, or cystoscopy leads to definitive diagnosis.

Extravesical opacifications may simulate stones on a plain film. Excretory urograms, CT scan, or cystoscopy will make the differentiation.

Complications

Acting as foreign bodies, bladder stones exacerbate urine infection and foil antibiotic therapy given for the purpose of sterilizing the urine. Stones obstructing the urethra must be removed.

Prevention

Prevention requires relief of the primary obstruction, removal of the stones, and sterilization of the urine.

Treatment

A. General Measures

Analgesics should be given for pain and antimicrobials for control of infection until the stones can be removed.

B. Specific Measure

Small stones can be removed or crushed transurethrally **(cystolitholapaxy).** Larger stones are often disintegrated by transurethral electrohydraulic lithotripsy (shock wave generating probe), or may require suprapubic transvesical removal (vesicolithotomy). The obstructive lesion must also be corrected.

Prognosis

Recurrent vesical stone is uncommon if the obstruction and infection are treated.

NEPHROCALCINOSIS

Nephrocalcinosis is a precipitation of calcium in the tubules, parenchyma, and, occasionally, the glomeruli. It always causes renal functional impairment, often severe. Stones may be found in the calices and pelvis. The common causes are primary hyperparathyroidism, excessive milk-alkali or vitamin D intake, and hyperparathyroidism secondary to severe renal damage associated with hyperchloremic acidosis, renal tubular acidosis, or sarcoidosis. Calcifications may also be seen in the skin, lungs, stomach, spleen, and corneas or around the joints.

Clinical Findings

A. Symptoms and Signs

There are no specific symptoms. In childhood, the patient may merely fail to thrive. Stones or sand may be passed. The complaints are usually those of the primary disease. Physical examination may reveal an enlarged parathyroid gland, corneal calcifications, and pseudorickets.

B. Laboratory Findings

The urine may be infected. In renal tubular acidosis, the pH is fixed between 6.0 and 7.0. Urinary calcium is high in hyperparathyroidism, both primary and secondary. Tests of renal function are depressed; uremia is common. Hypercalcemia and hypophosphatemia are seen with primary hyperparathyroidism; secondary hyperparathyroidism may be associated with a low serum calcium and an elevated serum phosphate. Hyperchloremic acidosis and hypokalemia accompany renal tubular acidosis.

C. Imaging Studies

A plain x-ray will reveal punctate calcifications in the papillae of the kidneys. Caliceal or pelvic stones may also be noted. The pattern of calcification may have to be differentiated from renal tuberculosis and medullary sponge kidney.

Complications

Complications include renal damage caused by the calcifications and renal and ureteral calculi. Chronic renal infection may complicate the primary disease.

Treatment & Prognosis

The primary cause should be treated, if possible (eg, parathyroidectomy). Discontinue vitamin D, give a low-calcium diet, and force fluids. With hyperchloremic acidosis, alkalinize the urine with potassium citrate. Osteomalacia requires administration of vitamin D and calcium even though nephrocalcinosis is present.

If nephrocalcinosis is secondary to primary renal disease, the outlook is poor. If the cause is correctable and renal function is fairly good, the prognosis is more favorable.

Pak CYC: Southwestern Internal Medicine Conference: medical management of nephrolithiasis—a new, simplified approach for general practice. Am J Med Sci 1997;313:215.

Preminger GM: Is there a need for medical evaluation and treatment of nephrolithiasis in the "age of lithotripsy"? Semin Urol 1995;12:51.

Ramakumar S et al: Renal calculi: percutaneous management. Urol Clin North Am 2000;27:617.

Sarica K et al: 371 bladder calculi in a benign prostatic hyperplasia patient. Int Urol Nephrol 1994;26:23.

Segura JW et al: Nephrolithiasis Clinical Guidelines Panel summary report on the management of staghorn calculi. The American Urological Association Nephrolithiasis Clinical Guidelines Panel. J Urol 1994;151:1648.

Shokeir M: Transurethral cystolitholapaxy in children. J Endourol 1994;8:157.

Spencer BA et al: Helical CT and ureteral colic. Urol Clin North Am 2000;27:231.

Stanley KE, Winfield HN: Management of staghorn calculi: percutaneous nephrolithotripsy versus extracorporeal shock wave lithotripsy. Semin Urol 1994;12:15.

Vieweg J et al: Unenhanced helical computerized tomography for the evaluation of patients wit acute flank pain. J Urol 1998;160:679.

■ GENITOURINARY TRACT TRAUMA

INJURIES TO THE KIDNEY

 ESSENTIALS OF DIAGNOSIS

- *History or evidence of trauma, usually local.*
- *Hematuria.*
- *Flank mass.*
- *Failure to opacify the kidney or extravasation of urine on excretory urography.*

General Considerations

Renal injury is uncommon but potentially serious and often accompanied by multisystem trauma. The most common causes are athletic, industrial, or automobile accidents. The degree of injury may range from contusion to laceration of the parenchyma or disruption of the renal pedicle.

Clinical Findings

A. SYMPTOMS AND SIGNS

Gross hematuria following trauma means injury to the urinary tract. Pain and tenderness over the renal area may be significant but could be due to musculoskeletal injury. Hemorrhagic shock may result from renal laceration and lead to oliguria. Nausea, vomiting, and abdominal distention (ileus) are the rule. Physical examination may reveal ecchymosis or penetrating injury in the costovertebral angle or flank. Extravasation of blood or urine may produce a palpable flank mass. Other injuries should be sought.

B. LABORATORY FINDINGS

Serial hematocrit determinations will give clues to persistent bleeding. Hematuria is to be expected, but the absence of hematuria does not exclude renal injury (as in renal vascular injury).

C. IMAGING STUDIES

A plain film may reveal obliteration of the psoas shadow; this suggests the presence of a retroperitoneal hematoma or urinary extravasation. Bowel gas may be displaced from the area. Evidence of transverse vertebral process fractures or rib fracture may be noted. Excretory urograms may show a normal kidney if it is mildly contused or may show extravasation of contrast if the kidney is lacerated. Nonfunction suggests injury to the vascular pedicle. The excretory urogram should demonstrate that the contralateral kidney is normal. Retrograde urograms are seldom necessary. CT scan is frequently helpful in assessing the extent of renal injury and may be used in place of excretory urography. CT scans may miss urinary extravasation if performed too rapidly following intravenous contrast administration—before the contrast is excreted into the collecting system and ureter. If renal vascular damage is suspected and the patient's condition is stable, preoperative renal angiography should be performed to facilitate planning of renovascular reconstruction. In special circumstances, selective renal artery embolization may control bleeding. Renal imaging is indicated in any adult with gross hematuria or microscopic hematuria with shock. Imaging is also required with deceleration injuries and is indicated in children with any grade of hematuria.

Differential Diagnosis

Bony fractures or contusion of soft tissues in the region of the kidney may cause confusion. Hematuria might be secondary to vesical injury. The absence of a perirenal mass (ie, hematoma or urinoma) or contrast extravasation on urograms or CT scan would rule out significant trauma.

Complications

A. EARLY

The most serious complication is continued perirenal hemorrhage, which may be fatal. Serial hematocrit, blood pressure, and pulse determinations are essential. Serial CT scans may also be useful. Evidence of an enlarging flank mass implies persistent bleeding. In most cases, bleeding stops spontaneously, probably as a result of tamponade by the perirenal fascia. Delayed bleeding 1 or 2 weeks later is rare. Infection of the perirenal hematoma may occur.

B. LATE

Ultrasound should be obtained 1–3 months after surgery to look for progressive hydronephrosis from ureteral obstruction. The blood pressure should be checked at regular intervals, because hypertension may be a late sequela.

Treatment

Treat shock and hemorrhage with fluids and transfusion. Most patients with blunt renal trauma stop bleeding and heal spontaneously. Bed rest is indicated until hematuria resolves. If bleeding persists, laparotomy is indicated.

Penetrating renal trauma requires exploration. Lacerations may be sutured, the collecting system closed, and urinary extravasation drained. Nephrectomy or partial nephrectomy may be necessary to remove devitalized tissue and secure the collecting system.

Late complications may occur. Perinephric abscess should be drained. Hypertension due to renal ischemia requires vascular reconstruction or nephrectomy.

Prognosis

Most injured kidneys heal spontaneously, though the patient must be examined at intervals for the onset of hypertension due to renal ischemia or progressive hydronephrosis due to secondary ureteral stricture. Many patients with genitourinary trauma have associated injuries. In most cases, death is due to associated injury rather than renal injury.

INJURIES TO THE URETER

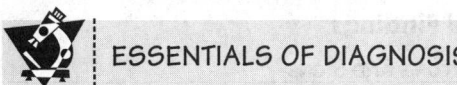

ESSENTIALS OF DIAGNOSIS

- Anuria or oliguria; prolonged ileus or flank pain following pelvic operation.
- Onset of urinary drainage through wound or vagina.
- Demonstration of urinary extravasation or ureteral obstruction by urography.

General Considerations

Most ureteral injuries are iatrogenic in the course of pelvic surgery. Ureteral injury may occur during transurethral bladder or prostate resection or ureteral manipulation for stone or tumor. Ureteral injury is rarely a consequence of penetrating trauma. Unintentional ureteral ligation during operation on adjacent organs may be asymptomatic, though hydronephrosis and loss of renal function will result. Ureteral division leads to extravasation and ureterocutaneous fistula.

Clinical Findings

A. SYMPTOMS

If the ureteral injury is not recognized at surgery, the patient may complain of flank and lower abdominal pain on the injured side. Ileus and pyelonephritis may develop. Later, urine may drain through the wound (or through the vagina following transvaginal surgery). Wound drainage may be evaluated by comparing creatinine levels found in the drainage fluid with serum levels: urine exhibits very high creatinine levels when compared with serum. Intravenous administration of 5 mL of indigo carmine will cause the urine to appear blue-green; therefore, drainage from a ureterocutaneous fistula becomes blue, while serous drainage remains yellow. Anuria following pelvic surgery not responding to intravenous fluids means bilateral ureteral ligation until proved otherwise. Peritoneal signs may occur if urine leaks into the peritoneal cavity.

B. LABORATORY FINDINGS

Microscopic hematuria is usually found but may be absent. Tests of renal function may be normal unless both ureters are occluded.

C. IMAGING STUDIES

Excretory urograms may show evidence of ureteral occlusion. Extravasation of radiopaque fluid may be seen in the region of the ureter. Retrograde ureterography will depict the site and nature (occlusion or division) of the injury.

Ultrasonography will reveal hydroureter and hydronephrosis or a fluid mass representing urinary extravasation. Radionuclide scanning will show delayed excretion, with an accumulation of counts in the pelvis and renal parenchyma resulting from ureteral obstruction; although urinary extravasation is detected, anatomic specificity for site of injury is not clearly defined.

Differential Diagnosis

Ureteral injury may mimic peritonitis if urine leaks into the peritoneal cavity. Excretory urography will reveal the ureteral involvement.

Oliguria may be due to dehydration, transfusion reaction, or bilateral incomplete ureteral injury. A survey of fluid and electrolyte intake and output, including serial body weights, should prove definitive. Total anuria implies bilateral ureteral injury and indicates the need for immediate urologic investigation.

Vesicovaginal and ureterovaginal fistulas may be confused. Methylene blue solution instilled into the bladder will stain the drainage of a vesicovaginal fistula. Cystoscopy may show the vesical defect. Retrograde ureterography should reveal a ureteral fistula.

Complications

These include urinary fistula, ureteral obstruction or stenosis with hydronephrosis, renal infection, peritonitis, and uremia (with bilateral injury).

Prevention

Before operation for large pelvic masses, which may cause displacement of the ureters, catheters should be placed in the ureters to facilitate their identification at surgery.

Treatment

A. Injury Recognized at Surgery

1. Ureteral division—Repair of a ureter inadvertently cut during surgery consists of anastomosis of the ends over an indwelling stent (**ureteroureterostomy),** reimplanting the ureter into the bladder if the injury is juxtavesical (**neoureterocystostomy),** or anastomosing the proximal segment of divided ureter to the side of the contralateral ureter (**transureteroureterostomy).** The anastomosis must be tension-free and the area of repair must be drained.

2. Ureteral resection—Repair of a ureter from which a segment has been removed requires interposition of a ureteral substitute or mobilization of the proximal and distal ureter and urothelium to provide a tension-free anastomosis. With loss of the distal ureter, the bladder may be hitched cephalad to the psoas muscle or a bladder flap may be created to facilitate a ureteral implant. In extreme cases, autotransplant of the kidney to the pelvis may be necessary.

B. Injury Discovered After Surgery

Early reoperation is recommended. Depending on the findings, the following procedures may be utilized: ureteroureterostomy, neoureterocystostomy, and trans-

ureteroureterostomy. A psoas hitch (as noted above) or a Boari flap may be used when the proximal ureter is short. If a long segment of ureter is not viable, an intestinal ureter may be constructed. If hydronephrosis is advanced or if sepsis develops, percutaneous nephrostomy should precede repair. When the patient's condition is stable, definitive repair can be accomplished. Nephrectomy may be indicated if the contralateral kidney is normal and there is a contraindication to transureteroureterostomy (such as calculi or upper tract transitional cell carcinoma).

Prognosis

In cases of iatrogenic injury, the results are best if the injury is recognized at the time of surgery. Late repair, if severe periureteral fibrosis has developed, is less likely to afford a good outcome.

INJURIES TO THE BLADDER

 ESSENTIALS OF DIAGNOSIS

- *History of trauma (including surgical or endoscopic).*
- *Fracture of the pelvis.*
- *Suprapubic pain and abdominal muscle rigidity.*
- *Hematuria.*
- *Extravasation shown on cystogram.*

General Considerations

The most common cause of vesical injury is an external blow over a full bladder. Rupture of the organ is seen in 15% of patients with pelvic fracture. The bladder may be inadvertently opened during pelvic surgery or injured by cystoscopic maneuvers, eg, transurethral resection of bladder tumor. If the injury is intraperitoneal, blood and urine will extravasate into the peritoneal cavity, producing signs of peritonitis. If it is extraperitoneal, a mass will develop in the pelvis.

Clinical Findings

A. Symptoms and Signs

There is usually a history of hypogastric or pelvic trauma. Hematuria and suprapubic pain are expected. Associated injury may cause hemorrhagic shock. There is suprapubic tenderness and guarding. Intraperitoneal extravasation causes peritoneal signs, while extraperitoneal extravasation results in formation of a pelvic uri-noma.

B. LABORATORY FINDINGS

A falling hematocrit reflects continued bleeding. Hematuria is expected in patients who are able to void. A patient who cannot void should be catheterized unless pelvic fracture (and urethral injury) is suspected or blood is noted at the urethral meatus.

C. IMAGING STUDIES

A plain film may reveal fracture of the pelvis. An extraperitoneal collection of blood and urine may displace the bowel gas laterally or out of the pelvis. If bladder trauma is suspected, cystography should precede excretory urography. Extravasation is most reliably demonstrated by a postdrainage cystogram film. If one suspects urethral trauma, a retrograde urethrogram should precede catheter insertion. The excretory urogram may suggest the diagnosis of bladder perforation but by itself is insufficient to exclude bladder injury. As in the case of renal injury, CT scan may provide necessary information and obviate the need for cystography.

Differential Diagnosis

Renal injury is also associated with trauma and usually presents with hematuria. Excretory urograms show changes compatible with renal trauma; the cystogram is negative.

Injury to the membranous urethra can mimic extraperitoneal rupture of the bladder. A urethrogram will reveal the site of injury. Urethral disruption is a contraindication to urethral catheterization.

Complications

Extraperitoneal extravasation may lead to pelvic abscess. Intraperitoneal extravasation will cause delayed peritonitis, oliguria, and azotemia.

Treatment

Treat shock, hemorrhage, and other life-threatening injuries. Marked extraperitoneal extravasation should be drained, the bladder decompressed by either a suprapubic or urethral catheter, and appropriate antibiotics administered. Small extraperitoneal extravasations are treated nonoperatively by urethral catheter.

Intraperitoneal extravasation of bladder urine requires exploratory laparotomy, bladder closure, and bladder catheter drainage. Penetrating injuries (ie, gunshot, stabbing) require exploration and closure of the bladder. The ureters should also be evaluated in all cases of bladder injury by preoperative imaging or intraoperative assessment, which may be done by inject-

ing indigo carmine and looking for ureteral extravasation or retrograde passage of 5F feeding tubes through the ureteral orifice.

Prognosis

Early diagnosis minimizes morbidity and mortality rates. The prognosis depends chiefly upon the severity of associated injuries.

INJURIES TO THE URETHRA
Membranous Urethra

Injury to the membranous urethra is usually a consequence of pelvic fracture and thus is associated with hemorrhage and multi-organ injury. The mechanism of injury is blunt trauma and deceleration resulting in shearing forces applied to the prostate and urogenital diaphragm. Penetrating injuries result from external missiles or laceration by bone fragments acting as secondary projectiles.

If the urethral disruption is incomplete, the patient may be able to void, and hematuria would be inevitable. Urethral injury is suspected if blood is expressed from the urethral meatus. In cases of complete avulsion, extravasation causes a suprapubic mass. Rectal examination may reveal a nonpalpable or upwardly displaced prostate.

X-ray reveals a fractured pelvis; urethrography delineates any extravasation, and cystography identifies an associated bladder injury (Figure 41–18). An immediate excretory urogram or CT scan should be obtained in all cases to assess kidney and ureteral function.

Treatment must be coordinated with care of associated injury. Once a membranous urethral injury with urinary extravasation has been identified, suprapubic cystostomy should be performed either at the time of laparotomy or percutaneously before placement of external pelvic fixation. Definitive urethral repair may be delayed until the patient has recovered from the acute injury and pelvic fractures have healed. Occasionally, when urethral disruption is incomplete, late repair is unnecessary. Primary repair may be indicated in cases of severe prostatomembranous dislocation, major bladder neck laceration, or concomitant pelvic vascular or rectal injury.

Late sequelae are urethral stricture, impotence, and incontinence. Urethral stricture must be identified by retrograde urethrography and may be treated by transurethral incision of the stricture or urethroplasty. Impotence due to injury of nerves to the corpora cavernosa that course adjacent to the membranous urethra may resolve without treatment during the year following injury. Vascular injury of the hypogastric or pudendal ar-

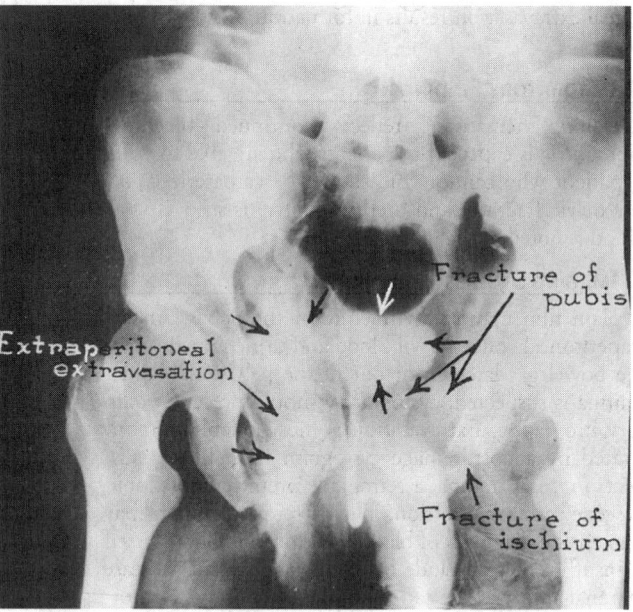

Figure 41–18. Vesical injuries. *Left:* Retrograde cystogram showing intraperitoneal extravasation. Note radiopaque material in both lumbar gutters. *Right:* Retrograde cystogram showing extraperitoneal rupture of the bladder secondary to fracture of the pelvis.

teries may cause impotence following trauma. Cavernosometry and arteriography will confirm the diagnosis; appropriate treatment may include vascular reconstruction. Incontinence depends upon the neurologic status of the patient. Medical or surgical therapy is utilized to increase bladder capacity and bladder outlet resistance.

Bulbous Urethra

The bulbous urethra may be injured as a result of instrumentation or, more commonly, falling astride an object (straddle injury). Urethral contusion may cause a perineal hematoma without injury to the urethral wall. Laceration will lead to urinary extravasation.

Perineal pain and some urethral bleeding are to be expected. Sudden swelling in the perineum may develop following attempted urination. Examination reveals a perineal mass; swelling due to extravasation of blood and urine involves the penis and scrotum and may spread onto the abdominal wall.

If the patient can void well and the perineal hematoma is small, no treatment is necessary. If urethrography reveals significant extravasation, suprapubic cystostomy should be performed. Minor injury without extravasation (contusion, compression by hematoma) may be managed by careful insertion of a urethral catheter (Figure 41–19).

The only serious complication is stricture, which requires internal urethrotomy or surgical repair.

Pendulous Urethra

External injury to this portion of the urethra is not common, since the penis is so mobile. The erect organ, however, is vulnerable. Most trauma to this area is secondary to instrumentation or sex play. As a rule, these injuries are mild, although a few may be complicated by stricture.

Urethral bleeding and penile swelling are to be expected. A urethrogram will reveal the site and severity of injury.

If voiding is normal, no treatment is required. A large hematoma may require drainage. If significant injury is present, a suprapubic tube should be inserted and delayed surgical repair performed after swelling and inflammation have resolved.

INJURIES TO THE PENIS

Mechanisms of penile injury include penetration, blunt trauma to the erect penis during sexual activity (eg, fracture of corpora cavernosa), avulsion of skin (also known as "power takeoff injury"), and amputation. Pendulous urethral injury is rare (discussed above).

Figure 41–19. Injury to the membranous urethra. *Left:* Retrograde cystogram showing periprostatic extravasation; laceration of membranous urethra with fracture of pelvis. *Right:* Oblique urethrogram showing extravasation in region of bulbous urethra. Pressure injection caused radiopaque solution to enter venous system. (This is the mechanism for emboli if oily lubricants are injected into the urethra.)

Tourniquet injury is also uncommon; the circumferential compression may be due to a rubber band, a steel ring, string, or a hair and may be exacerbated by subsequent erection. The tourniquet may have been applied unintentionally, but child abuse cases have been reported in which the penis has been ligated as punishment for enuresis.

Treatment includes assessment and care of urethral injuries if present. Removal of tourniquet, split-thickness skin grafting of avulsion injuries, and primary closure of corporal lacerations are principles of therapy. The penis may be acutely reimplanted up to 16 hours following amputation using microsurgical techniques.

INJURIES TO THE SCROTUM & TESTIS

Avulsion of the scrotal skin may require a meshed split-thickness skin graft. If the avulsion is severe, involving the skin and dartos muscle, then the testes may be implanted in the subcutaneous tissue of the thigh or left out and dressed with 0.25% acetic acid-soaked gauze. Scrotal reconstruction is performed at a later time, frequently by using skin grafts, as noted above.

Penetrating trauma rarely injures the mobile testes. Lacerations should be explored, debrided, and closed primarily. If hemorrhage into the tunica vaginalis is noted, drainage is indicated.

Blunt trauma to the testes may cause contusion or rupture. Rupture of the tunica albuginea may be demonstrated by ultrasonography as abnormal echotexture of the parenchyma. In cases of rupture, scrotal exploration allows debridement and closure of the tunica albuginea. The testes may ultimately undergo atrophy despite these efforts.

Brubaker LT, Wilbanks GD: Urinary tract injuries in pelvic surgery. Surg Clin North Am 1991;71:963.

Colodny AH: Acute urologic conditions. Pediatr Ann 1994;23:207.

Gay SB, Sistrom CL: Computed tomographic evaluation of blunt abdominal trauma. Radiol Clin North Am 1992;30:367.

Husmann DA, Morris JS: Attempted nonoperative management of blunt renal lacerations extending through the corticomedullary junction: the short-term and long-term sequelae. J Urol 1990;143:682.

Levine E: Acute renal and urinary tract disease. Radiol Clin North Am 1994;32:989.

McAleer IM et al: Genitourinary trauma in the pediatric patient. Urology 1993;42:563.

Morey AF et al: Reconstruction of posterior urethral disruption injuries: outcome analysis in 82 patients. J Urol 1997;157;506.

Wessels H et al: Criteria for nonoperative treatment of significant penetrating renal lacerations. J Urol 1997;157:24.

■ TUMORS OF THE GENITOURINARY TRACT*

Tumors of the genitourinary tract are among the most common neoplastic diseases found in adults. Prostate cancer, for example, is the most common cancer in males (36%); renal and bladder cancer account for nearly 10% of all malignant tumors in adults. Even though excellent diagnostic methods are available, nearly half of all genitourinary tumors are not found until regional or distant spread has occurred. Advances in diagnosis and treatment of genitourinary tract tumors have occurred in recent years, and the prognosis has improved in conditions such as Wilms' tumor, testicular cancer, and bladder cancer. The mainstay of diagnosis continues to be physical examination, complete urinalysis, intravenous urography, and cystoscopy whenever indicated. Curative treatment of these tumors continues to be surgical in most instances.

RENAL ADENOCARCINOMA (Renal Cell Carcinoma)

ESSENTIALS OF DIAGNOSIS

- *Painless gross or microscopic total hematuria.*
- *Solid renal parenchymal mass on intravenous urography with nephrotomograms, renal ultrasound, or abdominal CT scan.*
- *Paraneoplastic syndromes common.*

General Considerations

Malignant tumors of the kidney account for approximately 6% of all tumors in adults. Often the diagnosis is suspected because of microscopic hematuria or manifestations of metastases such as pathologic fractures or superficial skin nodules. The cause is unknown, though a hormonal influence is suspected, as the disease occurs in males three times more commonly than in females. Tobacco use is also implicated. A suppressor gene on chromosome 3p has been shown to be present in von Hippel-

Lindau renal cancers as well as in most sporadic renal adenocarcinomas. The cell of origin is in the proximal convoluted tubule, as determined by morphologic and cell surface antigen homology; thus, 90% of these tumors are adenocarcinomas. The tumor metastasizes commonly to the lungs (30%), adjacent renal hilar lymph nodes (25%), ipsilateral adrenal (12%), opposite kidney (2%), and bones (lytic lesions in mainly long bones).

There are numerous conditions that predispose to renal cell cancer, including adult polycystic kidney disease, von Hippel-Lindau syndrome (cerebellar hemangioblastomas, retinal angiomatosis, and bilateral renal cell carcinoma), and acquired renal cystic disease developing in patients with end-stage renal disease. Paraneoplastic syndromes are common in renal cell carcinoma and are often what suggests the diagnosis, yet they rarely have prognostic significance. These syndromes include hypercalcemia, erythrocytosis (but not polycythemia), hypertension, fever of unknown origin, anemia, and hepatopathy **(Stauffer's syndrome)**. Renal cell carcinoma has a predilection for producing occlusive tumor thrombi in the renal vein and the inferior vena cava (particularly from the right), manifested by signs of lower extremity edema and acute scrotal varicocele when occluding the left renal vein. This phenomenon of inferior vena cava thrombus occurs in approximately 12% of patients. Occasionally, the tumor thrombus reaches up through the inferior vena cava to the right atrium.

Clinical Findings

A. SYMPTOMS AND SIGNS

Painless gross or microscopic hematuria throughout the urinary stream ("total hematuria") occurs in 60% of patients. The degree of hematuria is not necessarily related to the size or stage of the tumor. Although a triad of hematuria, flank pain, and a palpable flank mass suggests renal cell carcinoma, fewer than 10% of patients will so present. Both pain and a palpable mass are late events occurring only with tumors that are very large or invade surrounding structures or when hemorrhage into the tumor has occurred. Symptoms due to metastases may be the initial complaint (eg, bone pain, respiratory distress).

B. LABORATORY FINDINGS

Microscopic urinalysis will reveal hematuria in most patients. The erythrocyte sedimentation rate may be elevated but is nonspecific. Elevation of the hematocrit, prothrombin time, and levels of serum calcium, alkaline phosphatase, and aminotransferases occur in less than 10% of patients. These findings nearly always resolve with curative nephrectomy and thus are not usually signs of metastases. Anemia unrelated to blood loss

---

* Wilms' tumor is discussed in Chapter 46.

occurs in 10–15% of patients, particularly those with advanced disease.

C. IMAGING STUDIES

The diagnosis of renal cell carcinoma is often made by intravenous urography performed as an initial step in the workup of hematuria, an enigmatic metastatic lesion, or suspicious laboratory findings (Figure 41–20). Ultrasonography and CT scan often reveal incidental renal masses which now account for 40% of the initial diagnoses of renal cancer in patients without manifestations of renal disease. Plain abdominal x-rays may reveal a calcified renal mass, but only 20% of renal masses contain demonstrable calcification. (Twenty percent of masses with peripheral calcification are malignant; over 80% with central calcification are malignant.) The initial technique for workup of hematuria is intravenous urography with nephrotomography; intravenous urography alone will define only 75% of renal mass lesions. Differentiation of the most common renal mass (ie, a simple benign cyst) can be made by the finding of a radiolucent center with a thin wall and a sharp interface between the mass and the renal cortex (the typical "beak sign" of a cortical cyst).

1. Ultrasonography—Further definition of all renal masses seen on intravenous urography is required. Abdominal ultrasonography can define the mass as a benign simple cyst or a solid mass in 90–95% of cases (Figure 41–21D). Previously, cytologic study of aspirated fluid was considered necessary to confirm the presence of simple cysts, but ultrasound techniques are accurate enough in all but a few equivocal cases to obviate such studies. Abdominal ultrasound can also identify a vena caval tumor thrombus and its cephalad extent in the cava.

2. Isotope scanning—Occasionally, a renal mass will be suspected on intravenous urography but is equivocal or not seen on ultrasound. In these cases, a renal cortical isotope scanning agent such as technetium Tc 99m DMSA will be helpful. Isotope scans of a renal tumor or cyst will show an area of decreased uptake, whereas an area of increased uptake indicates a renal "pseudotumor" or a hypertrophied column of Bertin.

3. CT scan—CT scan is the diagnostic procedure of choice when a solid renal mass is noted on ultrasound. CT scan accurately delineates renal cell carcinoma in over 95% of cases. Over 80% of tumors are enhanced by iodinated contrast medium, reflecting their high vascularity (Figures 41–21A and 21B). Because of the high accuracy of CT scan, renal angiography is rarely indicated and only when CT scan is equivocal (Figure 41–22). The accuracy of angiography is lower (80%) and the morbidity rates and cost higher than those of CT scan. CT scan is usually not required for diagnosis of renal cysts; these lesions do not concentrate contrast agents.

CT scan is also helpful in local staging and can reveal tumor penetration of perinephric fat; enlargement of local hilar lymph nodes, indicating metastases; or tumor thrombi in the renal vein or inferior vena cava.

4. Magnetic resonance imaging (MRI)—MRI (Figure 41–21C). It is not preferred at present since it is not more accurate than CT and is much more expensive. It is the most accurate noninvasive means of detecting renal vein or vena caval thrombi. With the further refinement of pulse sequencing and the use of paramagnetic contrast agents, MRI has become one of the primary techniques for staging solid renal masses. Magnetic resonance angiography (MRA) has become particularly useful for mapping the blood supply and the relationship to adjacent structures in candidates for partial nephrectomy.

D. OTHER DIAGNOSTIC OR STAGING TECHNIQUES

Isotopic bone scanning, chest x-ray, and CT scan of the chest can be used to examine the most common sites of metastases and are necessary before determining treatment. There are no useful tumor markers for renal cell carcinoma. Occasionally, aspiration cytology of the mass can be useful in an enigmatic case. Previously, such procedures were discouraged because of fear of disseminating the tumor along the needle tract, but this has proved to be rare, and the technique is safe. The diagnosis is most often made by noninvasive means, and needle aspiration is required only in indeterminate cases (< 10%).

Figure 41–20. Adenocarcinoma of the kidney. Intravenous urogram. Distortion of the pelvis and the middle and lower calices of the right kidney. The left kidney is normal.

Figure 41–21. A: Nonenhanced CT scan showing renal cell carcinoma in the right kidney. The mass, which is difficult to identify, is lateral to the lower pole of the kidney. **B:** Contrast-enhanced CT scan in the same patient clearly shows heterogeneous enhancement of the tumor. **C:** T1-weighted magnetic resonance image (MRI) delineates an obvious mass in the same patient without contrast injection. **D:** Renal ultrasound shows a solid mass within the renal parenchyma of the left kidney in another patient.

Differential Diagnosis

A variety of lesions in the retroperitoneum and kidney other than renal cysts may simulate renal cancer. These include lesions due to hydronephrosis, adult polycystic kidney disease, tuberculosis, xanthogranulomatous pyelonephritis, angiomyolipoma or other benign renal tumors, or adrenal cancer and retroperitoneal lipomas, sarcomas, or abscesses. In general, the radiographic and ultrasonographic techniques described above should make the differentiation. Hematuria may be caused by renal, ureteral, or bladder calculi; renal pelvis, ureteral,

or bladder tumors; or many other benign conditions usually delineated by the studies described. Cystoscopy is obligatory in hematuric patients with a normal intravenous urogram to rule out disease of the bladder and to determine the source of the hematuria.

Complications

Occasionally, patients may present with acute flank pain secondary to hemorrhage within a tumor or colic secondary to obstructing ureteral clots. Tumor in the renal vein or vena cava may cause a varicocele or lower

Figure 41–22. Adenocarcinoma of the kidney. Selective renal angiogram showing marked vascularity of mass in lower portion of right kidney typical of malignant tumor.

extremity edema associated with proteinuria. Pathologic fractures due to osteolytic metastases in long bones are common, as are symptomatic brain metastases.

Treatment

Staging is the key to designing the treatment plan (Table 41–1). Patients with disease confined within the renal fascia (Gerota's fascia) or limited to nonadherent renal vein or vena caval tumor thrombi (stages I, II, and IIIA) are best treated by open radical nephrectomy. This involves en bloc removal of the kidney and surrounding Gerota's fascia (including the ipsilateral adrenal), the renal hilar lymph nodes, and the proximal half of the ureter. Para-aortic node dissection has not been beneficial and is not recommended. In patients with large tumors and normal contralateral kidneys, open radical nephrectomy is recommended. Patients with tumors in solitary kidneys, those with diabetes mellitus or renal insufficiency, and those with tumors under 4 cm (even with a normal opposite kidney) should be considered for partial nephrectomy because the prognosis in such cases (if negative surgical margins are obtained) is the same as that of radical nephrectomy. Laparoscopic radical or partial nephrectomy has been advocated as a method equal to the open approach with the advantages of less blood loss, shorter hospitalization, and earlier return to normal function. Laparo-

scopic cryoablation of renal cancer has also shown considerable promise.

Nephrectomy has not been associated with improved survival rates in patients with multiple distant metastases (stage IV), and the procedure is not recommended unless patients are symptomatic or a promising therapeutic protocol is being studied. Southwestern Oncology Group data have shown, however, that up to a 6-month improvement in survival can be achieved with nephrectomy—even with metastasis—in selected patients. Patients with solitary pulmonary metastases have benefited from joint surgical removal of both the primary lesion and the metastatic lesion. Preoperative arterial embolization in patients with or without metastases does not improve survival rates, though it may be helpful as a single treatment measure in patients with symptomatic but nonresectable primary lesions. Radiation therapy is of little benefit except as treatment for symptomatic bone metastases. Medroxyprogesterone for metastatic renal cell carcinoma has given an equivocal 5–10% response rate of short duration. Vinblastine has also had a response rate of approximately 20%, again of minimal duration. There are no other cytotoxic chemotherapeutic agents of benefit.

Immunotherapy with interferon alfa has had a 15–20% response rate. Other interferons, alone (interferon beta, interferon gamma) or in combination with chemotherapeutic agents, have been less effective than interferon alfa. Adoptive immunotherapy—using lymphocytes (lymphokine-activated killer [LAK] cells) from exposure of the patient's own peripheral blood lymphocytes to interleukin-2 (IL-2) in vitro followed by reinfusion into the patient along with systemic IL-2 infusion—has shown up to 33% objective response rates. High-dose intravenous IL-2 causes a profound capillary leak syndrome and substantial toxicity. Subsequent studies have shown only a 16% response rate. Studies using lymphocytes isolated from the patient's own tumor (tumor-infiltrative lymphocytes [TIL]) expanded in IL-2 in vitro followed by reinfusion of the selected CD8 TIL and systemic IL-2 have shown limited response rates. Finally, clinical trials of combined IL-2 and interferon alfa show a 30% response rate with extended survival, and this is currently the best conventional method available.

Prognosis

Patients with localized renal cancer (stages I, II, and IIIA) treated surgically have 5-year survival rates of approximately 70–80%, whereas rates for those with local nodal extension or distant metastases are 30% and less than 10%, respectively. Most patients who present with multiple distant metastases succumb to disease within 15 months (Table 41–1).

Table 41–1. TNM staging classification and prognosis of renal cell cancer.

Stage	T	N	M	Five-Year Survival (%)
I. Tumor confined by renal capsule	T1 (< 7.5 cm tumor with minimal caliceal distortion) T2 (> 7.5 cm tumor with caliceal deformity)	N0 (nodes negative)	M0 (lack of distant metastases)	60–70
II. Tumor extension to perirenal fat or ipsilateral adrenal but confined by Gerota's fascia	T3a	N0	M0	50–65
IIIa. Renal vein or inferior vena cava involvement	T3b (renal vein involvement) T3c (renal vein and caval involvement below the diaphragm) T4b (caval involvement above the diaphragm)	N0	M0	50–60 (renal vein) 25–35 (vena cava)
IIIb. Lymphatic involvement	T1–3	N1 (single homo-lateral regional node involved) N2 (multiple regional, contralateral, or bilateral nodes involved) N3 (fixed regional nodes) N4 (juxtaregional nodes involved)	M0	15–35
IIIc. Combination of IIIa and IIIb	T3–4	N1–4	M0	15–35
IVa. Spread to contiguous organs except ipsilateral adrenal	T4a	N3–4	M0	0–5
IVb. Distant metastases	T1–4	N0–4	M1	0–5

RENAL SARCOMA

Renal sarcomas include rhabdomyosarcoma, liposarcoma, fibrosarcoma, and leiomyosarcoma; the latter is the most common, though all are very uncommon. Sarcomas are highly malignant and are usually detected at a late stage and thus have a poor prognosis. The diagnostic approach is similar to that of renal cell carcinoma. The histology of the lesion is rarely suspected preoperatively. These tumors have a tendency to surround the renal vasculature and do not exhibit neovascularity on arteriography.

Treatment is surgical, with wide local excision; however, local recurrence and subsequent distant metastases are the rule. There is no therapy of proved benefit for metastatic disease.

SECONDARY MALIGNANT RENAL TUMORS

Metastases to the kidney often develop from primary tumors of distant sites, most commonly the lung, stomach, and breast. It is rare for the diagnosis to be made before autopsy; this suggests that renal metastasis is a late event. There are usually no symptoms, though microscopic hematuria occurs in 10–20% of cases. Intravenous urograms may be normal, since the tumors are located peripherally in the parenchyma. Contiguous spread of a tumor adjacent to the kidney is not infrequent (eg, tumors of the adrenal, colon, and pancreas and retroperitoneal sarcomas). Tumors such as lymphoma, leukemia, and multiple myeloma may also infiltrate the kidney. Routine radiologic, hematologic, and chemical examinations should demonstrate the primary tumor in most cases.

BENIGN RENAL TUMORS

Renal Adenoma

Renal adenoma is the most common benign solid parenchymal lesion. Tumors less than 3 cm in diameter have been considered benign and those larger than 3 cm malignant; however, small lesions are not histologically distinguishable from renal adenocarcinomas, and the biology cannot be predicted preoperatively. These tumors should be considered malignant and should be treated by total excision.

Renal Oncocytoma

Renal oncocytoma is a subtype of adenoma. The tumors are generally asymptomatic, unassociated with the paraneoplastic syndromes often encountered in patients with renal adenocarcinoma. There commonly is a central stellate scar, and these tumors produce a typical spoke-wheel pattern on angiography. However, because neither this nor any other diagnostic finding is specific enough to exclude malignancy preoperatively, total removal is most often performed for these lesions.

Mesoblastic Nephroma

Mesoblastic nephroma is a benign congenital renal tumor seen in early childhood, which must be distinguished from the highly malignant nephroblastoma, or Wilms' tumor (see Chapter 46). Unlike Wilms' tumor, mesoblastic nephroma is commonly diagnosed within the first few months of life. Histologically, it is distinguished from Wilms' tumor by cells resembling fibroblasts or smooth muscle cells and by the lack of epithelial elements. The prognosis is excellent; complete surgical resection is curative, and neither chemotherapy nor radiotherapy is required.

Angiomyolipoma

Angiomyolipoma is a benign hamartoma seen most often in adults with tuberous sclerosis (which also includes adenoma sebaceum, epilepsy, and mental retardation). The tumor is also common in middle-aged women, but only unilaterally. It is often detected following spontaneous retroperitoneal hemorrhage. The tumors may be quite large and are commonly multiple and bilateral. CT scan defines these tumors; a negative CT number is seen in areas of fat within the mass. Occasionally, an angiomyolipoma will elude diagnosis preoperatively and will require nephrectomy. Asymptomatic patients with

small (< 5 cm) tumors and typical findings on CT scan of fat within the tumor do not require surgery, as the prognosis is excellent without treatment. Those presenting with a retroperitoneal hemorrhage or a size greater than 5 cm should be surgically removed.

Other Benign Renal Tumors

Other benign renal tumors include the following: (1) **fibroma,** a renal parenchymal capsular or perinephric fibrous mass; (2) **lipoma,** an adipose deposit within or around the kidney, often perihilar or within the renal sinus; (3) **leiomyoma,** a common retroperitoneal tumor that may arise from the renal capsule or renal vascular walls; and (4) **hemangioma,** which is occasionally found to be the elusive cause of hematuria. Hemangiomas are generally quite small, and the diagnosis is confirmed by angiography or direct vision of the lesion in the renal collecting system. Because these and other benign tumors are infrequent, the final diagnosis is generally made by the pathologist after the kidney is removed.

TUMORS OF THE RENAL PELVIS & CALICES

ESSENTIALS OF DIAGNOSIS

- *Gross or microscopic hematuria.*
- *Radiolucent filling defect in the renal pelvis or the calices on intravenous urography.*
- *Malignant cells on urine cytologic study.*

General Considerations

In over 90% of cases, tumors involving the collecting system of the kidney are urothelial transitional cell carcinomas. Less than 5% of tumors in this location are squamous carcinomas (often in association with chronic inflammation and stone formation) or adenocarcinomas. The cause of transitional cell carcinoma of the upper urinary tract is similar to that of epithelial tumors in the ureter or bladder; there is a strong association with cigarette smoking and exposure to industrial chemicals. Excessive use of phenacetin-containing analgesics and the presence of Balkan nephritis are also predisposing factors.

Clinical Findings

A. SYMPTOMS AND SIGNS

Gross or microscopic painless hematuria occurs in over 70% of patients. The lesions are usually asymptomatic unless bleeding causes acute flank pain secondary to obstructing clots. Presenting symptoms are often due to metastases to bone, the liver, or the lungs. Physical examination is not usually helpful.

B. Laboratory Findings

Microscopic hematuria on urinalysis is the rule. Pyuria is not seen. Cytologic examination of voided urine specimens may be diagnostic in high-grade tumors. Urine obtained from the ureter by retrograde catheterization or by brushing with specialized ureteral instruments can improve the diagnostic accuracy of cytologic examinations. Direct biopsy during ureteroscopy is the most accurate. There are no commonly associated paraneoplastic syndromes or diagnostic serum tumor markers in transitional cell carcinoma. A large number of urine markers are currently being studied, but none can be recommended.

C. Imaging Studies

The diagnosis is commonly made on intravenous urography and confirmed by retrograde pyelography, which reveals a radiolucent filling defect in the renal pelvis or calices (Figure 41–23). Renal ultrasound or CT scan can be used to rule out calculus. CT scan is also useful in local staging of the tumor. Transitional cell carcinoma is usually avascular on arteriography, and for that reason the study is not diagnostically useful. The tumors metastasize to the lungs, liver, and bone, so chest films, CT scan of the lungs and liver, and a bone scan are useful to determine the presence of metastases. Transitional cell carcinoma tends to be multifocal in the urinary tract, involving the opposite kidney (1–2%), ipsilateral ureter, or bladder (40–50%). Surveillance of these potential sites is important.

Figure 41–23. Retrograde pyelogram showing transitional cell carcinoma of left upper pole collecting system.

D. Endoscopic Findings

Cystoscopy is necessary when gross hematuria is present to determine the location of the bleeding. Retrograde pyelography and ureteral cytologic studies or brushing as described above can be useful, though mildly abnormal cytologic findings may occur in patients with upper tract inflammation or calculi. Rigid or flexible ureteroscopes can be used to view the upper ureter and renal pelvis directly. Biopsy of upper tract lesions is possible through these instruments. Although percutaneous approaches to the renal collecting system have been perfected, their use for diagnosis or treatment of suspected transitional cell carcinoma in routine cases is not recommended, because of the possibility of spreading tumor cells outside the kidney.

Differential Diagnosis

A variety of conditions may mimic transitional cell carcinoma of the renal pelvis, including calculi, sloughed renal papillae, tuberculosis, and renal cell carcinoma with pelvic extension of the tumor. These can usually be ruled out by the diagnostic studies described above.

Complications

Occasionally, bleeding may be severe enough to require immediate nephrectomy. Infection may develop, particularly when there is obstruction and hydronephrosis, requiring prompt use of systemic antibiotics.

Treatment

Renal transitional cell carcinoma is treated by nephroureterectomy (perifascial nephrectomy and removal of the entire ureter, down to and including the ureteral orifice within the bladder). Transureteral or percutaneous endoscopic techniques for resection of selected low-grade lesions have been described. High recurrence rates and the potential for local tumor spread would argue against this approach except in unusual circumstances (renal insufficiency or solitary kidney). Laparoscopic nephroureterectomy has been reported as well. Para-aortic lymphadenectomy has not been shown to improve survival rates and is not recommended. Because 50% of these patients will develop transitional cell carcinoma of the bladder, cystourethroscopy must be performed postoperatively; it is usually done quarterly during the first year, twice the second year, and then annually.

Prognosis

Because most of these tumors are low-grade and noninvasive, the 5-year tumor-free survival rate is higher than 90% for lesions treated with complete removal of the ipsilateral upper urinary tract. Survival rates are much lower for lesions that invade the renal parenchyma or are of histologic grade III or higher. A poor prognosis is associated with tumors having histologic features of squamous carcinoma or adenocarcinoma. These tumors are mildly radiosensitive, but pre- or postoperative radiotherapy has not been particularly helpful. Metastatic lesions are particularly problematic, and survivors are rare. Chemotherapy combinations, which have shown benefit in transitional cell carcinoma of the bladder (methotrexate, cisplatin, and vinblastine [CMV] or, with the addition of doxorubicin [Adriamycin], M-VAC) are also efficacious in transitional cell carcinoma of the upper urinary tract. Both VIG (vinblastine, ifosfamide, and gallium) and paclitaxel alone have achieved substantial responses as well.

TUMORS OF THE URETER

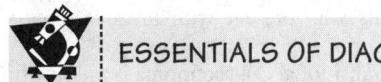

ESSENTIALS OF DIAGNOSIS

- *Gross or microscopic hematuria.*
- *Radiolucent filling defect in the ureter on intravenous urography or retrograde pyelography.*
- *Malignant cells on urine cytologic study.*

General Considerations

Ureteral tumors are rarely benign, but benign fibroepithelial polyps do occasionally occur within the ureter. More than 90% of ureteral tumors are transitional cell carcinomas. The cause is unknown, but tobacco smoking and exposure to industrial chemicals are known to be associated. Ureteral transitional cell carcinoma is often found in association with renal pelvis transitional cell carcinoma and slightly less often with bladder transitional cell carcinoma. The lesions develop in persons age 60–70 and are twice as common in men as in women. More than 60% of these tumors occur in the lower ureter.

Clinical Findings

A. SYMPTOMS AND SIGNS

Gross or microscopic hematuria is the rule (80% of cases). Because ureteral tumors grow slowly, they may not cause symptoms even though they completely obstruct the kidney. Occasionally, gross hematuria may cause acute obstruction because of clots. The initial presentation may be due to symptomatic metastases to bone, lungs, or liver. Extensive mid and lower ureteral tumors may be palpable.

B. LABORATORY FINDINGS

Urinalysis commonly reveals hematuria. There are no biochemical markers specific to the diagnosis, though patients with metastases may have abnormal liver function tests or anemia. Serum creatinine levels may be elevated with complete unilateral obstruction in elderly patients. Cytologic studies of voided urine or ureteral urine or brush studies may be diagnostic.

C. IMAGING STUDIES

The diagnosis may be made on intravenous urography, though the tumor often obstructs the ureter completely, so that cystoscopy and retrograde pyelography are required for definition of the lesion. These studies often reveal a filling defect in the ureter (classically described as a "goblet sign") (Figure 41–24). The ureter is dilated proximal to the lesion. CT scan is useful in ruling out nonopaque calculi and in abdominal tumor staging. Arteriography is of little value. Chest x-ray, CT scans, and bone scans are helpful in determining the presence of metastases.

Figure 41–24. Retrograde ureterogram showing "negative" shadow caused by transitional cell carcinoma of the obstructed lower right ureter and the typical "goblet sign."

D. ENDOSCOPIC FINDINGS

Cystoscopy is necessary when gross hematuria is present to determine the site of bleeding. Retrograde pyelography may then be necessary. Ureteroscopy may provide a direct view of the tumor and access for biopsy.

Differential Diagnosis

Nonopaque calculi, sloughed renal papillae, blood clots, or extrinsic compression by retroperitoneal masses or nodes may all produce signs, symptoms, and x-ray findings similar to those with ureteral tumors. The radiographic, cytologic, and endourologic studies listed above should make the distinction, but surgical exploration will be required occasionally.

Treatment

Most ureteral transitional cell carcinomas are not associated with metastases and can be definitively treated with nephroureterectomy. Selected patients with noninvasive low-grade lesions may be treated by segmental ureteral resection with end-to-end anastomosis (ureteroureterostomy). In selected patients with low-grade tumors and renal insufficiency or solitary kidney, an endoscopic transureteral resection can be considered. Para-aortic lymphadenectomy has not been helpful. Pre- or postoperative radiation therapy appears to be of no benefit. As with renal pelvis and bladder transitional cell carcinoma, cystoscopy should be performed periodically postoperatively. Patients with metastases are rarely helped by removal of the primary tumor. These tumors are responsive to chemotherapy. A small series of metastatic ureteral cancer patients treated with CMV (cisplatin, methotrexate, and vinblastine) showed a 60% response rate; however, there are no reports of durable remissions or long-term survivors.

Prognosis

The 5-year survival rate for patients with low-grade noninvasive lesions treated surgically approaches 100%. Those with high-grade or invasive lesions have a poorer prognosis, and those with metastases have a 5-year survival rate of less than 10%.

TUMORS OF THE BLADDER

 ESSENTIALS OF DIAGNOSIS

- *Gross or microscopic hematuria.*
- *Malignant cells on urine cytologic study.*

- *Cystoscopic visualization of the tumor.*
- *Histologic confirmation of the lesions.*

General Considerations

Vesical neoplasms account for nearly 2% of all cancers and are the second most common cancer of the genitourinary tract. Males are affected twice as often as females. More than 90% of tumors are transitional cell carcinomas, while a few are squamous cell carcinomas (associated with chronic inflammation, as in bilharziasis) or adenocarcinomas (often seen at the dome of the bladder in patients with a urachal remnant).

Most transitional cell carcinomas are superficial (not invasive into the bladder wall) when recognized, and over 80% remain so even when they recur. Twenty percent of recurrent tumors will become invasive. Eighty percent of patients who present with invasive disease will not have had prior superficial tumors.

The cause of transitional cell carcinoma is unknown; there is a strong association with chronic cigarette smoking and exposure to chemicals prevalent in dye, rubber, leather, paint, and other chemical industries. Common use of artificial sweeteners such as cyclamates and saccharin was thought to be related to bladder tumor development, but evidence to substantiate this claim has not been forthcoming.

The treatment and prognosis depend entirely on the degree of anaplasia (grade) and the depth of penetration of the bladder wall or beyond (Table 41–2). Most of these tumors develop on the trigone and the adjacent posterolateral wall; thus, ureteral involvement with obstruction is common. Tumors tend to be multifocal within the bladder. Approximately 5% of patients develop upper urinary tract transitional cell carcinoma as well.

Clinical Findings

A. SYMPTOMS AND SIGNS

Gross hematuria is a common finding, though microscopic hematuria often leads to the diagnosis. Patients with diffuse superficial tumors, particularly carcinoma in situ, may have urinary frequency and urgency. Occasionally, large necrotic tumors become secondarily infected, and patients exhibit symptoms of cystitis. Pain secondary to clot retention, tumor extension into the bony pelvis, or ureteral obstruction may occur but are not frequent presenting complaints. When both ureters are obstructed, azotemia with attendant secondary symptoms may be the finding that requires diagnostic studies.

Table 41–2. Treatment and prognosis of bladder tumors related to stage of disease.

Conventional Stage	TNM Stage	Tumor Involvement	Treatment	Five-Year Survival (%)
O	Ta	Mucosa only	Transurethral resection	85–90
A	T1	Submucosal invasion (lamina propria)	Transurethral resection and intravesical chemotherapy	60–80
B1	T2a	Superficial muscle invasion	Total cystectomy and pelvic lymphadenectomy	50–55
B2	T2b	Deep muscle invasion		30–50
C	T3	Perivesical fat invasion		30–40
D1	T3–4 N+	Regional lymph node invasion	Systemic chemotherapy	6–35
D2	T3–4 M1	Distant metastases		0–10

External physical examination is not generally revealing, though occasionally a suprapubic mass may be palpable. Rectal examination may reveal large tumors, particularly when they have invaded the pelvic side walls. Thus, bimanual examination is a necessary part of staging evaluation.

B. LABORATORY FINDINGS

Microscopic hematuria is the only consistent diagnostic finding. Patients with bilateral ureteral obstruction may have azotemia and anemia. Liver metastases may cause elevation of serum transaminases and alkaline phosphatase. There are no paraneoplastic syndromes or tumor markers consistently present in patients with transitional cell carcinoma. Urinary markers currently being studied are various tumor-associated antigens, growth factors, and nuclear matrix proteins, but none are proved to be accurate enough to obviate cystoscopy for diagnosis.

C. IMAGING STUDIES

Small bladder tumors will not be seen on intravenous urography, but larger tumors will usually produce filling defects in the bladder (Figure 41–25). Ureteral obstruction with hydroureteronephrosis may be seen as well. Invasion of the bladder wall may be predicted in patients with asymmetry or marked irregularity of the bladder wall. Noninvasive lesions seen on intravenous urography tend to be exophytic within the bladder, without evidence of bladder wall distortion.

Ultrasonography by external, transrectal, or transurethral routes can accurately define moderate-sized bladder tumors and can often depict deep invasion. Vesical angiography is of little benefit in the diagnosis or staging of bladder neoplasms.

CT scan can be useful for staging, but the depth of bladder wall penetration and delineation of tumor deposits in adjacent nonenlarged lymph nodes are not accurately defined. In patients with nodal metastases suspected on CT scans, fine-needle aspiration and cytologic studies may confirm the diagnosis and eliminate the need for surgical exploration. MRI is helpful in the pelvis, where motion artifacts are minor and the scant pelvic fat is just enough to provide organ differentiation. However, the information is not superior to that obtained with CT.

Figure 41–25. Excretory urogram showing space-occupying lesion (transitional cell carcinoma) on the left side of the bladder. The upper tracts are normal.

D. Urinary Cytologic Studies

Transitional cell tumors shed neoplastic cells into the urine in large numbers. Low-grade tumor cells may not appear abnormal on cytologic examination, but higher-grade tumor cells can be detected by cytologic study. These studies are most useful in checking for recurrence of transitional cell carcinoma. Flow cytometry (differential staining of DNA and RNA within urine cells to measure the amount of nuclear protein and thus the relative number of aneuploid [abnormal] cells) has been used to screen patients with some success. This technique may be useful for early diagnosis of recurrence.

E. Endoscopic Findings

Cystoscopy is mandatory in any adult patient with unexplained hematuria and a normal intravenous urogram. Many transitional cell carcinomas will not be seen on intravenous urography. Cystoscopic examination should detect nearly all tumors in the bladder (Figure 41–26). Only a few patients will have carcinoma in situ (superficial high-grade tumor) that is not visible. Any tumor seen should be biopsied. Superficial-appearing tumors can be diagnosed and removed transurethrally at the same time. The entire bladder, including the bladder neck, should be routinely scrutinized in all patients with microscopic hematuria. In patients without visible tumor and no other causes of hematuria, random biopsies may be diagnostic of carcinoma in situ. A bimanual examination should be done during cystoscopy in all patients with transitional cell carcinoma to be certain that the bladder is not fixed, signifying extensive extravesical extension.

Figure 41–26. Transitional cell (papillary) carcinoma of the bladder with minimal invasion of the bladder wall.

F. Staging

Therapy depends on the stage of the tumor as seen on histologic sections and examinations for metastases. Table 41–2 sets forth the stage, treatment, and prognosis of patients with transitional cell carcinoma of the bladder. The histologic grade of the tumor is also important in determining treatment and prognosis, but in general, low- and high-grade histologic characteristics tend to occur in low- and high-stage tumors, respectively.

As previously discussed, CT scan, MRI, or both may be helpful in predicting the stage of the tumor. Isotope bone scanning, chest x-ray, and chest CT scan will eliminate the possibility of bone or pulmonary metastases and should be done before determining therapy in patients with invasive lesions.

Treatment

A. Transurethral Resection, Fulguration, and Laser Therapy

Endoscopic transurethral resection of superficial and submucosally invasive low-grade tumors can be curative. Nevertheless, because the tumor recurs in more than 50% of patients, cystoscopy should be performed periodically. Quarterly examinations are recommended during the first year following tumor resection, every 6 months during the second year, and annually thereafter. Periodic urinary cytologic examinations can be helpful as well. Intravenous urography is recommended yearly for the first 3–5 years but is not mandatory. Recurrent small tumors without obvious invasion may be treated by fulguration only, though biopsy is recommended to document the stage and grade.

Neodymium:YAG lasers have been used for desiccation of low-grade, low-stage tumors. There is as yet no proven advantage to this approach except that patients can be treated under local anesthesia as outpatients and perhaps that tumor cells are rendered nonviable and thus incapable of reimplantation elsewhere in the bladder or urethra. Biopsies for diagnosis and staging are still required, however. An alternative approach involves using photosensitizing agents that are preferentially taken up by tumors when given systemically. Selective wavelengths of laser light (630 nm) directed to the bladder transurethrally in patients previously given a photosensitizer can selectively destroy tumor cells and perhaps adjacent premalignant cells as well.

B. Intravesical Chemotherapy

A variety of chemotherapeutic agents have been used in patients with recurrent low-grade, low-stage (O–A) tumors. Thiotepa is instilled into the bladder by catheter (30–60 mg in 60 mL of water) and left indwelling for 2 hours. Patients are treated once a week for 1 month and then monthly for up to 2 years. Treatment results in decreased frequency of recurrence or no recurrence in nearly 50% of patients. Other agents include mitomycin and doxorubicin. Immunotherapeutic drugs, which include BCG, are effective in prophylaxis (60%) of recurrent papillary tumors and curative (70%) in carcinoma in situ, a highly malignant lesion less responsive to the cytotoxic agents described above. Side effects of BCG include vesical irritability (90%) and systemic BCG-osis (1%). Although the mechanism of action of BCG is not entirely known, it is suspected to induce T cell recruitment and subsequent cytokine release locally at the tumor site. It is the most effective agent currently used. Interferon alfa has also been studied and is effective (nearly 50% of cases) for carcinoma in situ, with less toxicity than BCG; however, its durability as a single agent is poor. The combination of BCG and interferon alfa has shown improved results over either agent used alone.

C. Radiation Therapy

Definitive radiation therapy should be reserved for patients who have inoperable muscle-invasive bladder cancer localized to the pelvis or who refuse surgical treatment, as the 5-year survival rate is only 30%. In some patients with recurrence after radiation therapy, "salvage cystectomy" can be curative (in at least 30% of cases), though surgical morbidity rates are high.

Much controversy surrounds the use of radiation therapy preoperatively. Some workers have claimed a down-staging effect with 2000 cGy given over 1 week or 4000 cGy given over 3–4 weeks. The studies were poorly controlled, however, and subsequent reports have not confirmed these findings. Currently, urologic oncologists rarely use preoperative radiation therapy.

D. Surgical Therapy

Occasional patients are seen with invasive lesions (B_1, B_2) localized to an area in the bladder well away from the bladder base or orifices and without tumor in other sites of the bladder (proved by multiple biopsies) or beyond. Partial cystectomy (removal of the tumor and a 3-cm surrounding margin of normal bladder) is appropriate in these patients. Such tumors are rare, and patients must be selected carefully for partial cystectomy. Administration of one dose of 1000 cGy preoperatively to prevent tumor wound seeding may be considered. All other patients with high-grade or invasive (B_1, B_2, and C) lesions without distant spread or a fixed pelvis on bimanual examination are best treated by cystectomy and pelvic lymph node dissection. This includes removal of the bladder and the prostate in males. Removal of the entire urethra may be necessary in selected patients with tumors at the bladder neck or in the prostate or in those with diffuse carcinoma in situ in the bladder. In females, the uterus,

the urethra, and the anterior vaginal wall are usually removed. Urinary diversion is required and is commonly accomplished by creation of an ileal diversion. Continent cutaneous urinary diversions (orthotopic) requiring intermittent cutaneous catheterization rather than cutaneous bag drainage became popular in the late 1980s. The basic principles are large-volume reservoirs with detubularization of bowel to maintain low intrapouch pressures and construction of an intussuscepted or plicated ileal segment to provide cutaneous continence. Orthotopic reservoirs have been devised using bowel configurations similar to those described above to connect directly to the membranous urethra, permitting the patient to void normally. These procedures are appropriate in both men and women and have been shown to be safe, with minimal increase in morbidity over cutaneous diversions.

E. Systemic Chemotherapy

Chemotherapy in the form of CMV (cisplatin, methotrexate, vinblastine) or M-VAC (CMV plus doxorubicin [Adriamycin]) has been used precystectomy (neoadjuvant) or postcystectomy (adjuvant) for muscle-invasive tumors or as treatment of metastatic urothelial cancer. The neoadjuvant series all show an approximate 60% downstaging from clinical to pathologic stage and a 30% rate of complete tumor eradication. As with the prior preoperative radiation studies, however, there is no evidence as yet that these results will eventuate in a higher long-term survival rate. An intergroup randomized trial of cystectomy alone versus neoadjuvant chemotherapy and cystectomy is now in progress in the USA to answer this important question. Adjuvant chemotherapy may be useful, but few patients have been studied and no definitive prospective randomized trials comparing adjuvant versus no adjuvant treatment have been reported. Several reports of efficacy with either CMV or M-VAC for treatment of metastatic disease have shown a 60% overall objective response rate with a 30% complete response rate. A few long-term survivors with apparent cure have been reported (10–15%), and either of these regimens thus appears to be a definite advance in the treatment of urothelial cancer. Newer approaches include paclitaxel, carboplatin, and gemcitabine in various regimens that appear to have similar efficacy with less toxicity, but no phase III studies have been reported. These results have caused a few investigators to study chemotherapy alone or in combination with radiation to attempt bladder salvage in patients with invasive bladder cancer. To date, these studies are incomplete.

Prognosis

Approximately half of the low-grade superficial tumors will be controlled by transurethral surgery or intracavitary use of chemotherapeutic agents (Table 41–2). Following radical cystectomy, the 5-year survival rate varies with the extent, stage, and grade of the tumor but averages about 30–55%. The complications of urinary diversion (ureteral obstruction with hydronephrosis, pyelonephritis, and nephrolithiasis) also influence the outcome.

CARCINOMA OF THE PROSTATE

ESSENTIALS OF DIAGNOSIS

- *Palpable rock-hard nodule in the prostate on rectal examination.*
- *Serum PSA elevation.*
- *Histologic confirmation on needle biopsy.*
- *Osteoblastic bone metastases and elevated serum acid phosphatase in advanced cases.*

General Considerations

In adult males, prostate cancer is the most common neoplasm (after skin cancer) and the second most common cause of death due to cancer. The tumor is more prevalent in black males than in any other group in the USA. The tumor rarely occurs before age 50, and the incidence increases with age such that in the eighth decade, more than 60% of men have prostate cancer (at autopsy). In most of these older men, however, the disease is not clinically apparent; only 10% of men over age 65 develop clinical evidence of the disease. Ninety-five percent of tumors are adenocarcinomas. The tumor arises primarily in the peripheral zone (70%), an area that differs in embryologic derivation from the periurethral (transition) zone, which is the site of formation of benign prostatic hyperplasia. Thus, the causes of the two diseases are considered to be different; they may occur simultaneously but are not related. The cause of prostate cancer is unknown, but many factors appear to be involved, including genetic, hormonal, dietary (particular high-fat diets), and perhaps environmental carcinogenic influences.

Screening

Advances in transrectal ultrasound (TRUS) and prostate-specific antigen (PSA) monitoring have allowed for enhanced detection of nonpalpable tumors. Much controversy currently exists over whether men over age 50 should be encouraged to undergo screening. While available data show a decrease in the mortality rate of prostate cancer, there is as yet little evidence that screening has been the cause of this change. Even so, the realities of clinical practice are that the combination of digital rectal examination and serum PSA monitoring is the most effective screening protocol.

Clinical Findings

A. SYMPTOMS AND SIGNS

Incidental or stage A (T1) carcinoma of the prostate presents no physical signs (it is nonpalpable) and is only diagnosed by the pathologist when prostate tissue is removed as treatment for symptomatic bladder outlet obstruction presumed to be caused by benign prostatic hyperplasia or is found by an elevated PSA. Patients with stage B (T2) or higher disease have a hard nodule on the prostate that can be felt during rectal examination (Table 41–3). In over 60% of these men, the cancer causes obstructive symptoms, urinary retention, or urinary infection (Figure 41–27). Previously, 50% of patients presented with evidence of metastases, including weight loss, anemia, bone pain (commonly in the lumbosacral area), or acute neurologic deficit in the lower limbs. Today, however, fewer than 20% of patients present in this way because earlier diagnosis is the rule.

B. LABORATORY FINDINGS

Patients with extensive metastases may have anemia due to bone marrow replacement by tumor. Those with bilateral ureteral obstruction secondary to trigonal compression by tumor may exhibit azotemia and uremia. Serum alkaline phosphatase is often elevated in patients with bone metastases but not in those with localized disease.

Prostate-specific antigen is elevated in the serum of approximately 60% of men with prostate cancer. Levels above 4 ng/mL are abnormal and can be falsely elevated due to cystoscopy, prostate biopsy, or urethral catheterization but *not* by normal digital rectal examination. Methods for enhancing PSA specificity include the following: age-specific PSA (younger men [under age 55 years] normal < 2.5 ng/mL; older men [over age 65 years] normal > 6.5 ng/mL); PSA density (PSA divided by prostate volume), where < 0.15 ng/mL suggests cancer; percent-free PSA (total PSA minus complexed PSA), where when < 10%, the risk of prostate cancer is 60% (only useful with total PSA 2–10 ng/mL); and complexed PSA (similar specificity to percent-free PSA). While total PSA is useful for staging, it is not absolute.

Methods for enhancing PSA specificity include the following: age-specific PSA (younger men [under age 55 years] normal > 2.5 ng/mL; older men [over age 65 years] normal > 6.5 ng/mL); PSA density (PSA divided by prostate volume), where > 0.15 ng/mL suggests cancer; percent-free PSA (total PSA minus complexed PSA), where when < 10%, the risk of prostate cancer is

Table 41–3. Treatment and prognosis of prostate cancer related to tumor stage.

Conventional Stage	TNM Stage	Clinical Findings	Treatment	Fifteen-Year Survival (%)
A1	T1a	Nonpalpable tumor; incidental finding at prostatectomy (low-grade cancer seen in < 5% of prostate).	Observation	Normal
A2	T1b	Same as above except tumor is high-grade, or > 5% of prostate is involved, or both.	Total prostatectomy with pelvic lymph-adenectomy	30–45
B1	T2a	Localized nodule 1–1.5 cm in diameter in one lobe.		50–60
B2	T2b	Tumor is ≥ 1.5 cm in diameter or in more than one lobe.		35–45
C	T3, T4	Periprostatic extension.	Radiation with or without pelvic lymphadenectomy	20–30
D	N+ or M+	Pelvic lymph node involvement or distant metastases.	Hormonal therapy (orchiectomy or LHRH/antiandrogen) when symptomatic. Irradiation for isolated bone pain.	0–10

60% (only useful with total PSA 2–10 ng/mL); and complexed PSA (similar specificity to percent-free PSA).

While total PSA is useful for staging, it is not absolute. PSA appears to be most helpful in following patients after treatment, as levels fall to almost nil with complete response and rise early (as much as 6 months before serum acid phosphatase) when tumor recurs.

Figure 41–27. Advanced carcinoma of prostate; trabeculation of bladder wall.

Extensive carcinoma involving capsule, anterior portion, and seminal vesicles

Note that neither acid phosphatase nor PSA alone can be used for screening. Newer methods for measuring unbound (free) PSA have substantial promise for differentiating benign from malignant disease.

C. IMAGING STUDIES

Transrectal ultrasound (TRUS) has become very useful for evaluating tumor volume and guiding biopsy needles into the peripheral zone and other specific areas, such as the base, the apex and the transition zone of the prostate. The study can also reveal typical hypoechoic peripheral zone lesions in 70% of patients with palpable lesions (Figure 41–28). Because many prostate cancers are not hypoechoic and not all hypoechoic lesions are cancer, TRUS alone for screening for prostate cancer is not recommended. An intravenous urogram may reveal urinary retention or distal ureteral obstruction. Extensive lesions may exhibit a ragged-edged filling defect in the bladder base. A chest x-ray may help in identifying the uncommon lung metastases but more often shows typical osteoblastic metastases in the thoracic spine or ribs. An abdominal x-ray may reveal metastases in the lumbosacral spine or ilium. A CT scan of the pelvis may show an enlarged prostate and large pelvic or para-aortic lymph nodes; however, the study is rarely accurate for staging and is not routinely recommended unless the PSA is > 20 ng/mL or the Gleason sum of the tumor is ≥ 7, or the tumor is palpably outside of the prostate (stage C/T3). Fine-needle aspiration and cytologic studies of abnormal nodes may provide important staging data and perhaps obviate staging laparotomy.

A **B**

Figure 41–28. Transrectal ultrasound of the prostate. **A:** Transaxial plane. Transition zone is shown at short arrows and hypoechoic prostate cancer in the peripheral zone at long arrows. **B:** Sagittal plane, showing large hypoechoic prostate cancer at arrows. (B = bladder.)

MRI appears to be more helpful in pelvic staging of prostate cancer than is CT scan, but like CT it is incapable of accurately differentiating intraprostatic lesions (Figure 41–29). A monoclonal antibody, Cyt-356 (which identifies prostate-specific membrane antigen), has been coupled with a radioisotope for diagnosis of soft tissue metastases. Results show that the Prostascint scan is 60% accurate but that it has a false-positive rate which limits its usefulness.

D. BIOPSY

The diagnosis is established by TRUS-guided transrectal biopsies in most instances. Because the great major-

ity of patients have biopsies due to an elevated serum PSA (stage T1a) and no abnormal findings on TRUS, symptomatic biopsies of the base, middle, and apex of the prostate—concentrating on the peripheral zone with three to six biopsies per side of the prostate—are required for accurate diagnosis.

Differentiation of the tumor is graded by the pathologist using the Gleason scale, which assigns a grade of 1–5 for both the primary and secondary forms of the tumor. The two numbers are added, and the cancer can thus be Gleason sum 2–10, with 10 being the most poorly differentiated cancer. The likelihood of metastasis can be inferred from the Gleason sum, as 7 or more is an aggressive cancer.

E. STAGING

Rectal examination can provide initial staging in patients with palpable tumors (Table 41–3). Needle biopsy is confirmatory, and histologic grading can fairly accurately predict the metastatic potential of the tumor. A normal isotopic (technetium Tc 99m) bone scan will rule out bone metastases. A pelvic CT scan may be useful to define pelvic lymphadenopathy in patients with high-grade lesions. The laparoscopic approach to pelvic lymph node dissection has provided the same prognostic information as an open surgical procedure with less morbidity and a markedly reduced hospital stay. This approach is useful in patients with high-grade or high-stage lesions, those considered for radical perineal prostatectomy. Cystoscopy is not required except in large lesions suspected to involve the bladder neck and trigone.

Figure 41–29. T2-weighted MRI in the transaxial plane showing transition zone at short arrows and peripheral zone at long arrows, with hypointense area in right posterior zone of prostate cancer.

Differential Diagnosis

Nodules caused by benign prostatic hyperplasia may be difficult to distinguish from cancer; benign nodules are usually rubbery, whereas cancerous nodules have a much harder consistency. Fibrosis following a prior prostatectomy or secondary to chronic prostatitis may be associated with lesions indistinguishable from cancerous nodules and require biopsy for definition. Occasionally, phleboliths or prostatic calculi on the surface of the prostate may be confusing; however, TRUS can be helpful in the differentiation and for biopsy guidance.

Treatment

See also Table 41–3.

A. CURATIVE THERAPY

Patients with low-grade, low-stage incidental lesions (stage A1; T1a) have a prognosis similar to that of patients without cancer of the prostate and require observation only. Patients with clinical stage A2 (T2b), B0, B1 (T2a), or B2 (T2b) lesions are candidates for curative therapy. The pendulum has recently swung from external-beam radiation therapy back toward prostatectomy as the procedure of choice in these patients. Recently, the use of radioactive seed placement trasnperitoneally into the prostate has been gaining popularity. Complete staging, including pelvic lymph node dissection, is important, so that appropriate candidates will be selected. Patients with grossly positive pelvic lymph nodes are not candidates for total prostatectomy. Recent advances in surgical technique have led to a low incidence of incontinence (1–4%) and preservation of potency in up to 70% of patients. Alternative procedures include external-beam pelvic irradiation plus interstitial radiation (with ^{125}I, ^{103}Pd, and ^{192}Ir). The 15-year results of radiotherapy are nearly as good as those of total prostatectomy in patients with localized disease.

Patients with stage C cancer are best treated with neoadjuvant androgen deprivation and external-beam radiation therapy, but when the lesion is large, palliation only is expected.

B. PALLIATIVE THERAPY

Patients with metastatic disease cannot be cured, but significant palliation can be offered. Androgen deprivation therapy in the form of oral estrogen (diethylstilbestrol, 3 mg/d) or bilateral orchiectomy is effective in 70–80% of symptomatic patients. Choice of therapy depends on patient preference (many patients find castration unacceptable) or coexistent disease (eg, estrogens have numerous side effects—about 25%—including congestive heart failure, thrombophlebitis, and myocardial infarction, and thus should not be used except in selected patients). These hormonal treatments are not additive, and use of both treatments simultaneously has no advantages over use of either alone. Luteinizing hormone-releasing hormone (LHRH) agonists have shown efficacy comparable to that of estrogen or orchiectomy, with reduced side effects. The drug must be given by injection every three to four months and is expensive. Studies have also shown that if an LHRH agonist is used, concomitant administration of an antiandrogen (flutamide or bicalutamide) improves survival. Studies to determine if orchiectomy plus an antiandrogen is more effective than orchiectomy alone have not shown an advantage to the combination.

Controversy continues concerning whether to treat asymptomatic patients at the time of diagnosis or to wait until symptoms develop. Because either approach is palliative only and there are no definitive studies showing survival advantages with early treatment, is recommended that treatment be withheld until symptoms occur except in patients who cannot accept a no-treatment philosophy.

Patients in whom hormonal therapy has failed can be treated by aminoglutethimide or ketoconazole (both of which inhibit adrenal androgen production) or oral corticosteroids for short-term relief of bone pain. Radiation therapy for symptomatic bone lesions can be helpful, as can local irradiation for an obstructing or bleeding prostate tumor. A bone-seeking radioisotope (strontium) appears to have some efficacy in therapy of bone metastases. On occasion, transurethral prostatectomy will be required to relieve bladder outlet obstruction. Chemotherapy has not shown dramatic results, though cyclophosphamide, doxorubicin, and cisplatin have all produced minor objective responses in some patients. Mitoxantrone and prednisone have been approved by the FDA for symptomatic bone metastasis, but there is no evidence that survival is prolonged.

Prognosis

Radical prostatectomy cures 70–80% of the patients suitable for that operation, but its use should be limited to those with a reasonable life expectancy (Table 41–3). Currently, about 50% of patients with prostatic cancer are amenable to curative therapy when their disease is discovered. Careful annual rectal examination to check for suspicious areas of induration and serum PSA monitoring should be performed in all men over age 50—and over age 40 if there is a positive family history in a first-degree relative (father, brother) or in blacks—if this cure rate is to be improved.

SARCOMA OF THE PROSTATE

Sarcoma of the prostate is rare. Half of all cases occur in boys under age 5. The tumor is highly malignant and metastasizes to the pelvic and lumbar lymph nodes, lungs, liver, and bone. Symptoms of urinary tract obstruction are present. The prostate is enlarged. Cystography or excretory urography may show superior displacement of the bladder or encroachment of the tumor into the bladder. Endoscopy will reveal the mass and allow biopsy.

Total prostatocystectomy, postoperative radiotherapy, and chemotherapy have cured a few cases in adults. In children, combination chemotherapy with surgery for residual tumor has shown increasing success. The tumor is relatively radioresistant.

TUMORS OF THE URETHRA

Malignant tumors of the urethra are rare. The disease is more common in females than in males. Squamous cell types are seen most often in both sexes.

In females, urethral bleeding is the most common symptom. Distal urethral lesions of low grade and without extension can be treated by radiotherapy or wide local excision. Extensive or proximal lesions are best treated by preoperative irradiation and anterior exenteration (removal of the bladder, uterus, adnexa, and urethra with the anterior vaginal wall), including pelvic lymphadenectomy and urinary diversion. The prognosis is excellent for distal lesions without extension, but 5-year survival rates are less than 50% for those with proximal lesions.

In males, the lesion is most commonly in the bulbomembranous urethra and is associated with a history of chronic urethral strictures, often secondary to gonorrheal infection. Patients present with urethral bleeding, a weak urinary stream, and a perineal mass. The diagnosis is made by urethroscopy and biopsy. Distal penile lesions can be treated by partial or total penectomy. Lesions in the bulbous urethra or more proximal lesions require extensive surgical resection, including en bloc removal of the penis, urethra, prostate, bladder with overlying pubis, and pelvic lymph nodes and urinary diversion. Preoperative radiation therapy (2000–4000 cGy) is recommended, although too few patients have been treated to determine the benefit. In both males and females with distal lesions, groin lymphatics may be involved, but node dissection is required only when gross disease is palpable. Prophylactic node dissection is controversial. Five-year survival rates are 60% for distal urethral tumors but less than 40% for the more common proximal lesions.

Primary irradiation—other than to distal lesions in the female—is rarely helpful. Patients with metastatic disease may respond to methotrexate or cisplatin alone or in combination, but objective remissions are usually of short duration.

TUMORS OF THE TESTIS

ESSENTIALS OF DIAGNOSIS

- *Painless, firm mass within the testicle in a man aged 18–40.*
- *Elevated serum levels of the beta subunit of human chorionic gonadotropin (β-hCG), alphafetoprotein (AFP), lactic dehydrogenase (LDH), or all three.*
- *Enlarged retroperitoneal nodes on abdominal CT scan.*
- *Palpable abdominal mass in advanced cases.*

General Considerations

Most testicular tumors are malignant germ cell tumors. Non-germ cell tumors such as Sertoli cell tumors and Leydig cell tumors are rare and usually benign. Germ cell tumors are categorized as either seminomatous (35%) or nonseminomatous (embryonal, 20%; teratocarcinoma, 38%; teratoma, 5%; choriocarcinoma, 2%). Cryptorchidism predisposes to testicular cancer, with the incidence increasing inversely with the level of testicular descent (ie, testicles remaining in the abdomen have a much higher incidence of cancer). Metastases first develop in the retroperitoneal nodes; right-sided tumors metastasize primarily to the interaortocaval region just below the renal vessels, and left-sided tumors primarily to the left para-aortic area at the same level. Distant spread is to supraclavicular areas (left, primarily) and the lungs. Just under 50% of patients have metastases when first seen.

Clinical Findings

A. SYMPTOMS AND SIGNS

Testicular tumors present as a painless firm mass within the testicular substance. They often have been present for several months before the patient seeks consultation. Occasionally (10%), a hydrocele will be present, obscuring palpation of the mass. A few patients have spontaneous bleeding into the mass, causing pain. Patients with high serum levels of hCG may have gynecomastia. Patients with extensive abdominal metastases may present with abdominal pain, anorexia, and weight loss. Examination may reveal palpable retroperitoneal nodes when spread is extensive, or palpable supraclavicular nodes, particularly on the left side.

B. LABORATORY FINDINGS

In general, testicular tumors do not alter the usual laboratory parameters, but serum tumor markers are diagnostically helpful. Patients with extensive retroperitoneal metastases may have bilateral ureteral obstruction that causes azotemia and anemia.

Serum lactic dehydrogenase (LDH), particularly isoenzyme I, is elevated in approximately 60% of patients. β-hCG, a particularly sensitive marker, is a glycoprotein produced by 65% of nonseminomatous testicular tumors but only 10% of seminomas. The alpha subunit of the molecule is identical to luteotropic hormone (LH), but the beta subunit is unique to testicular tumors in adult males. There is cross-reactivity in some assays between the alpha and beta subunits; treated patients who develop modest elevations should have simultaneous assay of LH to be certain the marker detected is β-hCG}. Urinary βhCG studies have been even more sensitive than serum levels but are useful only in selected patients with suspected early recurrences.

Alpha-fetoprotein (AFP) is elevated in 70% of patients with nonseminomatous testicular cancer but is not elevated in patients with seminoma. Patients in whom histologic study has shown seminoma but in whom serum AFP is elevated should be suspected of having nonseminomatous elements in the primary specimen or metastatic lesions.

Approximately 85% of patients demonstrate elevation of one of these markers at presentation. Serum levels decrease when the tumor is completely removed or regresses. Markers are used mainly to follow tumor regression or predict recrudescence, as even minute amounts of tumor may cause serum elevations; however, tumor may be present without elevation of serum markers.

C. IMAGING STUDIES

An intravenous urogram, though not essential, may reveal deviated or obstructed ureters secondary to retroperitoneal metastases. Abdominal CT scan will define enlarged lymph nodes in approximately 90% of cases when they are present. Chest x-ray and CT scan will detect most pulmonary metastases.

Scrotal ultrasound is useful for identifying the typical hypoechoic lesion in the testicle when there are equivocal physical findings. Regardless of the findings on ultrasound, however, a young man with an intratesticular mass on palpation requires surgical definition of the mass.

Differential Diagnosis

Testicular masses in men age 18–40 are almost always malignant and should be treated accordingly. Confusion can occur with scrotal hydroceles, cord hydroceles, epididymal masses or cysts, or epididymitis. Most of these can be differentiated from masses within the testicle by palpation, but if not, transillumination or scrotal ultrasound (or both) is usually helpful. Hydrocele aspiration with a fine needle may be helpful, but care must be exercised not to puncture the mass and thus spread tumor cells.

Treatment

See also Table 41–4.

Inguinal orchiectomy with high ligation of the cord at the internal ring is proper initial treatment for all kinds of testicular cancer. Rarely is incisional biopsy of the testicle advisable. Recommendations for further therapy (retroperitoneal dissection, chemotherapy, radiation therapy) are then based on the pathologic findings. A staging workup, including measurement of serum markers, chest x-ray and chest CT scan, and abdominal CT scan, is conducted to determine the extent of disease.

A. NONSEMINOMATOUS TUMORS

Following orchiectomy, retroperitoneal lymph node dissection is recommended for all patients with non-

Table 41–4. Treatment and prognosis of testicular cancer related to tumor stage.

Conventional Stage	TNM Stage	Clinical Findings	Treatment	Five-Year Survival (%)
I	T1	Confined to testicle	Inguinal orchiectomy; retroperitoneal lymphadenectomy (irradiation for seminoma)	>95
IIA	N1–N2a	< 6 microscopic nodes		> 90
IIB	N2b	> 6 microscopic nodes		> 85
IIC	N3	Bulky abdominal nodes	Orchiectomy and chemotherapy followed by resection of residual disease	~70
III	M+	Distant metastases		

seminomatous testicular cancer except in the presence of bulky abdominal or distant metastases. Patients with pure choriocarcinoma are an exception and do not usually retroperitoneal surgery, because the disease in such cases is invariably systemic and requires multiagent chemotherapy. The extent of lymphadenectomy depends on the testicle involved but in general includes para-aortic and paracaval nodes from the renal vessels down to the aortic bifurcation and along the external iliac artery to the internal inguinal ring on the involved side. Seminal emission can be preserved; loss of this function was previously a complication of retroperitoneal lymph node dissection because of interruption of autonomic nerves crossing the aorta and near the aortic bifurcation.

Because of the associated morbidity, some have proposed that retroperitoneal lymph node dissection be withheld after orchiectomy in patients with normal serum markers and no evidence of retroperitoneal nodal disease on abdominal CT scan and lymphangiography and who have no findings of distant metastases on chest x-ray and CT scan. The rationale was that only 20% of these patients will develop recurrent disease, which could then be treated when it appeared. This approach should be discussed at length with the patient to ensure his reliable compliance with a program for frequent follow-up.

Patients with any nonseminomatous cell type who have extensive retroperitoneal or chest metastases are best treated after orchiectomy by multiagent chemotherapy followed by excision of persistent masses. Combination chemotherapy with bleomycin, etoposide, and cisplatin achieves over a 90% cure rate in stage I and stage II patients and a 70% cure rate in stage III patients. Patients who do not respond may be treated with ifosfamide, doxorubicin, or both, with some expectation of success.

B. SEMINOMA

In the absence of extensive distant spread, patients with pure seminoma should be treated with external-beam radiation therapy (2500 cGy) to the abdomen following orchiectomy. In the presence of bulky abdominal disease or more distant metastases, survival rates are better with multiagent chemotherapy (described above) given initially in lieu of radiation therapy. Patients with substantial residual tumor (> 3 cm) after chemotherapy may benefit from surgical removal of the remaining tumor.

Prognosis

The prognosis for the various stages of testicular cancer is outlined in Table 41–4. Even in the presence of metastases, many of these patients can be cured. The only exception is patients with choriocarcinoma, who still have a poor survival rate (35% at 5 years) despite extensive chemotherapy.

TUMORS OF THE PENIS

Cancer of the penis is a rare disease occurring in the fifth to sixth decades. The cause is uncertain. The disease is rarely seen in circumcised men. The lesion commonly is on the glans penis or foreskin. Early cases may exhibit a painless red, velvety lesion, but most often the lesion is an exophytic nodular or wart-like growth with secondary infection. The initial diagnosis is made by a generous incisional biopsy of the lesion, which reveals squamous cell carcinoma in over 95% of cases. The tumors tend to metastasize to superficial or deep inguinal nodes, though the attendant infection may cause enlarged, tender nodes, which may be difficult to differentiate from metastatic cancer.

The differential diagnosis includes syphilitic chancre, soft chancre due to haemophilus infection, and simple or giant condyloma. Biopsy will usually differentiate between these conditions.

Small noninfiltrating lesions can be treated with fluorouracil cream, external-beam radiation, or laser therapy. However, close follow-up is mandatory in patients so treated. Larger lesions not involving deep structures are treated by partial penile amputation at least 2 cm proximal to the lesion, leaving enough of the penis for adequate direction of the urinary stream. Deeply infiltrating lesions require total penectomy, with formation of a perineal urethrostomy.

Palpable inguinal nodes should be treated by antibiotics for 6 weeks following treatment of the primary lesion to eliminate infection. Persistently palpable nodes will require bilateral ilioinguinal lymphadenectomy. Prophylactic node dissection has not been associated with increased survival rates in patients without palpable nodal involvement. Even those who undergo delayed node dissection when the nodes become palpable can be cured. Radiation therapy for palpable nodes or as prophylaxis for nonpalpable nodes has been effective.

Patients with distant metastases (to the lungs or bone) have a poor prognosis, though cisplatin and methotrexate have shown objective but not durable responses. Five-year survival rates for patients with noninvasive lesions localized to the penis are 80%; for those with inguinal node involvement, 50%; and for those with distant metastases, nil.

Atkins MB et al: Randomized phase 11 trial of high-dose interleukin-2 either alone or in combination with interferon alfa-2b in advanced renal cell carcinoma. J Clin Oncol 1993; 11:661.

Baselli EC et al: Intravesical therapy for superficial bladder cancer. Oncology 2000;14;719.

Carter BS et al: Hereditary prostate cancer: epidemiological and clinical features. J Urol 1993;150:797.

Chodak GK et al: Results of conservative management of clinically localized cancer. N Engl J Med 1994;330:242.

Cookson MS et al: Management of stage T_1 bladder cancer with intravesical bacillus Calmette-Guérin therapy. J Urol 1992; 148:797.

Einhorn LH et al: Vinblastine, ifosfamide and gallium (VIG) combination chemotherapy in urothelial carcinoma. J Clin Oncol 1994;12:2271.

Epstein JI: PSA and PAP as immunohistochemical markers in prostate cancer. Urol Clin North Am 1993;20:757.

Fleischmann J, Goldberg G: Management of superficial transitional cell carcinoma of the bladder. Semin Urol 1993;11:193.

Fleming C et al: A decision analysis of alternative treatment strategies for clinically localized prostate cancer. JAMA 1993; 269:2650.

Foster RS et al: Testicular cancer: what's new in staging, prognosis, and therapy. Oncology 1999;13:1689.

Garnick MB: Prostate cancer: screening, diagnosis and management. Ann Intern Med 1993;118:804.

Gill IS et al: Laparoscopic renal cryoablation: initial clinical series. Urology 1998;52:543.

Gill IS: Laparoscopic radical nephrectomy for cancer. Urol Clin North Am 2000;27:707.

Gschwend JE et al: Radical cystectomy for invasive bladder cancer: contemporary results and remaining controversies. Eur Urol 2000;38:121.

Heidenreich A et al: Quality-of-life issues in the treatment of testicular cancer. World J Urol 1999;17:230.

Jarrett TW et al: Endourologic management of upper tract transitional cell carcinoma. World J Urol 2000;18:243.

Kahn D et al: Radioimmunoscintigraphy with ^{111}In-labeled monoclonal antibody 7E11-C5 (CYT 356) in subjects with occult recurrent prostate cancer. J Urol 1994;152:1490.

Kamat AM et al: Intravesical therapy for bladder cancer. Urology 2000;55:161.

Kaufman DS et al: Selective bladder preservation by combination treatment of invasive bladder cancer. N Engl J Med 1993; 329:1377.

Lamm DL: Complications of bacillus Calmette-Guérin immunotherapy. Urol Clin North Am 1992;19:565.

Litwin MS, deKernion J: Perspectives on the problem of prostate cancer. J Urol 1994;152:1680.

Pentyala SN et al: Prostate cancer: a comprehensive review. Med Oncol 2000;17:85.

Rassweiler JJ et al: Laparoscopic partial nephrectomy: the European experience. Urol Clin North Am 2000;27:721.

Steele GS et al: Management of low-stage nonseminomatous germ cell tumors of the testis. Compr Ther 2000;26:210.

Stockle M et al: Advanced bladder cancer (stages pT3b, pT4a, pN1 and pN2): Improved survival after radical cystectomy and 3 adjuvant cycles of chemotherapy: Results of a controlled prospective trial. J Urol 1992;148:302.

Taneja SS et al: Management of disseminated kidney cancer. Urol Clin North Am 1994;21:625.

Tierney AC et al: Laparoscopic radical and partial nephrectomy. World J Urol 2000;18:249.

van den Ouden D et al: Management of locally advanced prostate cancer. 1. Staging, natural history, and results of radical surgery. World J Urol 2000;18:194.

Vasey PA: Immunotherapy for renal carcinoma: theoretical basis and current standard of care. Br J Clin Pharmacol 2000; 50:521.

Walther PJ: Contemporary chemotherapeutic approaches for the treatment of hormone-refractory prostate carcinoma. World J Urol 2000;18:216.

Whitmore WF Jr: Localized prostate cancer: management and detection issues. Lancet 1994;343:1263.

■ NEUROPATHIC (NEUROGENIC) BLADDER

A neuropathic bladder has abnormal activity secondary to a neurologic condition. To understand the variety of neuropathic bladder conditions, a basic understanding of the normal innervation and myoneurophysiology is required.

Myoneural Anatomy

The urinary bladder and its involuntary sphincter develop and differentiate from the tubular urogenital sinus. The differentiation of the encasing mesenchymal cells forms the musculature of the detrusor and urethral sphincter.

Innervation

The innervation of the bladder and its involuntary sphincter is via the autonomic nervous system. The parasympathetic supply to the bladder and the sphincter is via the pelvic nerves, which arise from S2–4. These fibers also carry the stretch sensory receptors to the same spinal cord center (S2–4).

The sensory supply for pain, touch, and temperature is carried via the sympathetic fibers arising from the thoracolumbar segments (T11–L2).

Motor and sensory supply of the trigone is via the thoracolumbar sympathetic fibers.

The striated external sphincter, as well as the entire urogenital diaphragm, receives its motor and sensory innervation from the somatic fibers arising from S2–4 (via the pudendal nerve).

It is clear that the S2–4 segment is the origin of the motor supply to the bladder musculature, to the involuntary sphincter, and to the striated external sphincter. The trigone is the only structure that is partly independent in its innervation. This is why segment S2–4 is called the spinal cord center for micturition. It is located at the level of the T12 and L1 vertebral bodies. There are connections between the spinal reflex center and the midbrain and cerebral cortex. Through these connections, inhibition and control of the spinal cord reflexes can be maintained. The micturition reflex is coordinated in the pontine micturition center.

Myoneurophysiology

The primary functions of the urinary bladder are to store and empty urine at a safe pressure and in a continent fashion. Intact myoneural elements are essential for these functions. The primary reservoir function is possible because of the specialized detrusor muscle arrangement and because of the bladder compliance phenomenon. The normal bladder can accommodate volumes up to 400 mL without increasing intravesical pressure. Bladder fullness is perceived through increases in stretching of bladder mechanoreceptors.

Distention and stretch initiate detrusor activity that can be controlled and inhibited by the high cortical centers or can be allowed to progress to active detrusor contraction and voiding. Normally during voiding, detrusor contraction continues until the bladder is completely empty unless voiding is voluntarily interrupted or inhibited.

Before voiding begins, the pelvic floor and the striated external sphincter relax, the bladder base descends, and the bladder outlet assumes a funnel shape. As a result, urethral resistance decreases. This is followed by detrusor muscle contraction and a rise in intravesical pressure to 20–40 cm of water, which results in a urine flow of about 15–30 mL/s. When the bladder is completely empty, the pelvic floor and striated external sphincter contract, elevating the bladder base, increasing urethral pressure, and ending voiding. Intact nerve pathways are essential for these synchronized activities to occur.

Cystometry

Cystometry is a simple method for testing the bladder's storage function and gives the following information: bladder capacity, extent of accommodation or compliance, the ability to sense bladder filling and temperature, and the presence of an appropriate detrusor muscle contraction. In addition, postvoid residual urine can be measured at the same time. A normal cystometrogram is shown in Figure 41–30.

Uroflowmetry

Uroflowmetry is the measurement of urine flow rate. If detrusor contraction is properly coordinated with

Figure 41–30. Cystometrograms. *A:* Normal cystometrogram. *B:* Cystometrogram in a patient with hyperreflexic bladder caused by transection of the spinal cord above S2. *C:* Cystometrogram in a patient with an areflexic flaccid neuropathic bladder caused by a myelomeninogocele.

sphincter relaxation, then the outlet resistance will fall as the bladder pressure increases, and the flow rate will be adequate. Normally, the flow rate changes with age but is > mL/s in males under 60 and > 25 mL/s in females under 50 years of age. is 20–25 mL/s in males and 25–30 mL/s in females. Any flow rate below 15 mL/s suggests obstruction or detrusor dysfunction. A flow rate under 10 mL/s strongly suggests underlying pathology.

Urodynamics

Urodynamic studies require measurement of bladder pressure during micturition. The pressure measured within the bladder (intravesical pressure) is a combination of the intra-abdominal pressure and the pressure generated by the detrusor. To determine the detrusor pressure, the intra-abdominal pressure is measured with a rectal catheter and this pressure is subtracted from the total intravesical pressure (measured by the bladder catheter). The urine flow rates may then be assessed in light of the detrusor pressure. No consensus exists on a critical value for pressure and flow that is diagnostic of obstruction. Nomograms have been developed for evaluating the pressure-flow relationship and thus to categorize these values as obstructed, equivocal, or unobstructed.

Electromyographic Recording

Needle or patch electrodes may be employed to record the activity of the external sphincter. This information is useful when obtained during micturition. Increased activity in the sphincter after voiding begins suggests detrusor-sphincter dyssynergia.

Classification & Clinical Findings

Several classification systems exist that describe the variety of pathologic bladder conditions which develop secondary to neuropathies. Many bladder conditions are predictable based on the neurologic lesion. A lesion above the brain stem (ie, stroke) affecting micturition frequently results in involuntary bladder contractions (detrusor hyperreflexia) with coordinated (synergistic) sphincter relaxation. These patients will have urge incontinence.

A complete lesion of the spinal cord (ie, trauma) above the T12 vertebral body may leave the spinal reflex center intact. This often leads to what has been categorized as an upper motor neuron lesion. These patients have detrusor hyperreflexia and uncoordinated sphincter activity (detrusor-sphincter dyssynergia). Although detrusor contractions can generate abnormally high intravesical pressure, they are not effective in producing adequate urine flow because of the spastic external sphincter and are not sustained. Thus, there is always residual urine. Bladder capacity is reduced. Detrusor contraction and mass reflexes can be initiated from certain trigger areas.

Figure 41–30B is a typical cystometrogram of a hyperreflexic bladder.

An injury to the spinal reflex center or below often leads to what has been categorized as a lower motor neuron lesion. These patients often develop detrusor areflexia. Trauma is the most common cause, but tumors, ruptured intervertebral disks, and meningomyelocele may also cause this type of neuropathic bladder. Both motor and sensory fibers are usually affected, and there is loss of sense of fullness (Figure 41–30C). These contractions are usually weak and unsustained, and bladder emptying is incomplete, resulting in large amounts of residual urine.

The bladder dynamics in a person with a neuropathic bladder often change over time. This may occur secondary to changes in innervation (ie, tethering of spinal cord, multiple sclerosis, recovery from spinal shock) or changes in the bladder. For example, a patient with a hyperreflexic bladder and dyssynergic sphincter often develops a trabeculated, noncompliant bladder over time. These changes require periodic reevaluation of all patients with neuropathic bladders regardless of the initial classification.

Differential Diagnosis

Cystitis, interstitial cystitis, and organic obstruction are occasionally confused with neuropathic bladder, but associated neurologic lesions usually make the diagnosis of neuropathic bladder easy. Psychosomatic disturbances can cause spasm of the external sphincter, incomplete voiding, retention, or incontinence.

Complications

Common complications include urinary tract infection, stone formation, and incontinence. The most serious consequences of these lesions are the hydrodynamic back pressure on the kidneys, hydronephrosis, infection, decompensation of the ureterovesical junction, and loss of renal function.

Treatment

Immediately following spinal cord injury, there is a shock phase that may last a few weeks to 2–3 years. The average time is 2–3 months. The bladder is completely dissociated from nervous control and thus has no sensation and is areflexic.

Treatment is aimed at avoiding the aforementioned complications in the hope of partial or complete recovery. During the shock phase, continuous closed drainage or, preferably, clean intermittent (every 4–6 hours) catheterization should be instituted until bladder activity is restored.

A. HYPERREFLEXIC BLADDER

In the hyperreflexic bladder, attaining a functional bladder depends upon mobilizing residual urine and increasing the bladder capacity. Residual urine volume can be decreased by reducing urethral resistance by several methods: transurethral prostatectomy, division of the external sphincter, pudendal nerve manipulation (ablation or electrical stimulation), or alpha-blocker pharmacologic therapy.

Functional capacity can be increased by decreasing detrusor instability with an anticholinergic-parasympatholytic drug (oxybutynin), or by operative augmentation. This is often performed with small or large intestine (enterocystoplasty).

Conversion to a flaccid areflexic bladder can be achieved by cord rhizotomy. The storage function of the bladder is preserved, and the patient can be managed by clean intermittent catheterization.

Supravesical urinary diversion may be called for in patients with upper tract deterioration due to elevated storage pressures or female incontinence. Male incontinence may be controlled by a condom catheter.

B. AREFLEXIC BLADDER

Function of the flaccid bladder can be improved by measures that facilitate complete emptying; these include voiding by Credé's maneuver (suprapubic pressure), transurethral resection of the bladder neck to reduce outlet resistance, and timed voiding or timed clean intermittent catheterization. An indwelling urethral catheter or suprapubic cystostomy is required in a few cases, but chronic intubation should be avoided if possible.

Suprapubic urinary diversion (ileal or colon conduit, etc) can circumvent decompensation of the ureterovesical junction if deterioration of upper tracts occurs. The quality of detrusor contraction has been improved by means of electrodes implanted in the sacral roots. Implantable prosthetic sphincters, periurethral collagen injections, or urethral slings may also improve urinary control.

Prognosis

Renal injury from elevated bladder pressure and infection are the most serious consequences of neuropathic bladder. When diversion or bladder augmentation is required, proper timing of the operation is essential for preservation of kidney function. Patients with a neuropathic bladder require close follow-up of their kidneys with renal ultrasound and serum creatinine determinations.

Appell RA: Collagen injection therapy for urinary incontinence. Urol Clin North Am 1994;21:177.

Cooper CS et al: Pediatric reconstructive surgery. Curr Opin Urol 2000;10:195.

Hollander JB et al: Urinary diversion and reconstruction in the patient with spinal cord injury. Urol Clin North Am 1993; 20:465.

Jensen JK et al: The role of patient history in the diagnosis of urinary incontinence. Obstet Gynecol 1994;83(5 Part 2):904.

Peggs JF: Urinary incontinence in the elderly: pharmacologic therapies. Am Fam Physician 1992;46:1763.

Perkash I: Long-term urologic management of the patient with spinal cord injury. Urol Clin North Am 1993;20:423.

Rousseau P et al: Urinary incontinence in the aged. Part 1: patient evaluation. Geriatrics 1992;47:22.

Rousseau P et al: Urinary incontinence in the aged. Part 2: management strategies. Geriatrics 1992;47:37. (Published erratum appears in Geriatrics 1992;47:87.)

Webster GD et al: Voiding dysfunction following cystourethropexy: its evaluation and management. J Urol 1990; 144:670.

■ OTHER DISEASES & DISORDERS OF THE GENITOURINARY TRACT

SIMPLE RENAL CYST

A simple renal cyst is usually unilateral and solitary but may be multiple and bilateral. The cause of this disorder is unclear. The cyst can compress and destroy adjacent parenchyma. Cysts contain fluid that resembles (but is not) urine. Most are diagnosed in patients after the fourth decade. Occasionally, what appears to be a simple cyst may in fact be a papillary cystadenocarcinoma—an uncommon form of renal cancer with both solid and cystic components. In those cases, however, ultrasound will usually demonstrate a complex mass with both cystic and solid components.

Flank pain may be a presenting symptom, though most renal cysts are found incidentally on urography done for other purposes. A mass may be felt in the flank or upper quadrant and must be distinguished from tumor. Urinalysis and tests of renal function are normal. Excretory urograms reveal a mass that distorts adjacent calices. Nephrotomography shows a radiolucent mass (in contradistinction to tumor). If the CT scan or ultrasound reveals an equivocal cystic mass, cyst aspiration may be performed, the fluid submitted for cytologic examination, and the cyst filled with contrast material to delineate its wall. A simple cyst must be distinguished from adenocarcinoma of the kidney; ultrasonography or CT scan usually makes that distinction.

Complications are rare, but bleeding into or infection of a cyst may occur.

If the diagnosis of cyst is established, surgery is not necessary unless the lesion causes pain or endangers renal function. Simple percutaneous aspiration with instillation of 95% ethanol may suffice. If sclerosis fails, operative excision may be performed.

RENAL ARTERY ANEURYSM

Aneurysm of the renal artery is relatively rare. It results from weakening of the artery wall by arteriosclerosis, poststenotic dilation, intimal or perimedial fibroplasia, or trauma. If the aneurysm causes stenosis of the artery, hypertension may ensue secondary to ischemia and activation of the renin-angiotensin system. A plain abdominal x-ray may reveal a ring-like calcification in the wall (Figure 41–31). Angiography or CT scan is diagnostic.

Surgery is indicated in the following situations: (1) secondary renal ischemia and hypertension, (2) dissecting aneurysm, (3) aneurysm associated with pain or

Figure 41–31. Intrarenal aneurysm of renal artery. Plain film showing calcified structure over the right renal shadow.

hematuria, (4) anticipation of pregnancy, (5) aneurysm coincident with significant stenosis, (6) radiographic evidence of incomplete calcification or increase in size on serial films, and (7) aneurysm containing thrombus with evidence of distal embolization. If the aneurysm ruptures, emergency nephrectomy may be necessary.

RENAL INFARCTION

The common causes of renal artery occlusion include emboli due to subacute infective endocarditis, atrial or ventricular thrombi, arteriosclerosis, polyarteritis nodosa, trauma, and, in the neonate, umbilical artery catheterization. Multiple emboli are common and lead to patchy renal ischemia. Occlusion of a main renal artery will cause renal infarction.

The patient may suffer from flank pain, or the lesion may be silent. Hematuria is common. Excretory urograms may reveal no excretion of radiopaque material or may only opacify a portion of the kidney. With complete acute occlusion of the main renal artery, a ureteral catheter will drain no urine, yet the retrograde urogram will reveal normal anatomy. Renal angiography, color Doppler ultrasound, or magnetic resonance angiography makes the diagnosis by revealing occlusion of the artery or arterioles; a renal scan will show similar findings. CT scan after the intravenous injection of ra-

diopaque medium will show no concentration in the ischemic area. Ureteral stone may mimic renal infarction, but urograms, CT scan, or angiograms will distinguish one from the other. Following renal infarction, hypertension may develop secondary to renal ischemia; it may later resolve spontaneously.

If the diagnosis is made promptly (within 5–8 hours), thrombectomy or endarterectomy should be considered. Otherwise, anticoagulation therapy should be instituted (eg, heparin). Thrombolytic therapy (eg, streptokinase) may be used to lyse the clot. If permanent hypertension develops, definitive treatment of the arterial occlusion or nephrectomy (preferably laparoscopic) should be performed.

RENAL VEIN THROMBOSIS

Thrombosis of the renal vein affects both infants and adults and can be either acute or chronic. In children, thrombosis may be caused by severe dehydration (eg, due to ileocolitis and diarrhea or the nephrotic syndrome). In adults, it may be secondary to renal infection, ascending thrombosis of the vena cava, or caval occlusion due to tumor thrombus. There is usually flank pain and a palpable distended kidney. If renal vein thrombosis is secondary to infection, the patient is septic and urinalysis reveals pus cells and bacteria. In noninfectious cases, the urine may reveal microhematuria and mild proteinuria. The patient with bilateral involvement is azotemic. Nephrotic syndrome may develop. Excretory urograms show delayed opacification in an enlarged kidney. The calices are elongated. Later, the kidney may become atrophic. Renal angiography reveals stretching and bowing of arterioles. Selective renal venography will demonstrate the thrombus, as will renal ultrasound (Figure 41–32).

Treatment should attempt to eliminate the underlying cause whenever possible. If the diagnosis of unilateral infected renal vein thrombosis can be established, nephrectomy should be performed. In bilateral disease, anticoagulant or thrombolytic therapy (or both) is required.

VESICAL FISTULAS

Vesical fistulas may be congenital or acquired. Congenital fistulas usually involve the urachus. Acquired fistulas may be iatrogenic or due to trauma, tumor, or inflammation.

The most common types of vesical fistulas are vesicovaginal, vesicointestinal, and vesicocutaneous. Vesicovaginal fistulas are commonly secondary to gynecologic or birth trauma; rarely, they occur as a complication of infiltrating cervical carcinoma. Vesicointestinal fistulas are most often due to inflammatory bowel disease: Crohn's disease, diverticulitis, and appendicitis. Cystostomy in

Figure 41–32. Thrombosis of renal vein. Selective left renal venogram showing almost complete occlusion of vein. Veins to lower pole failed to fill. Note large size of kidney.

the presence of bladder outlet obstruction, bladder cancer, or foreign body may result in vesicocutaneous fistula.

Diagnostic maneuvers include cystoscopy, conventional cystography, barium enema or barium swallow, and CT scan with contrast infusion. Oral charcoal may be useful for detecting a urinary intestinal fistula, as the granules can be seen in spun urine under the microscope.

Therapy for vesicovaginal fistula requires surgical closure, with placement of an omental flap between the bladder and the vagina. For vesicointestinal fistula, the primary intestinal lesion must be resected and the bladder closed. An indwelling urethral catheter is necessary during the healing period.

INTERSTITIAL CYSTITIS

This lesion is most commonly found in middle-aged women. Urinary frequency both day and night is most often accompanied by suprapubic pain with bladder distention. The cause is uncertain, though some suggest an autoimmune collagen disease while others have documented the presence of mast cells and mast cell mediators (histamine and prostaglandin) in bladder biopsy specimens of affected patients.

The diagnosis is based on the history and the results of cystoscopy under general anesthesia. Cystoscopy re-

veals a small-capacity bladder and punctate hemorrhage following forceful distention. (Studies suggest this is a nonspecific finding.) Biopsy may reveal lymphocytic infiltration, mast cell infiltration, and submucosal fibrosis. In patients suspected of having interstitial cystitis, one must rule out carcinoma in situ; urine cytologic study precedes cystoscopy and random bladder biopsy.

Treatment of established cases of interstitial cystitis often fails. Response has been obtained with hydraulic bladder overdistention, intravesical treatment with 50% DMSO, 0.4% oxychlorosene sodium, or sodium pentosanpolysulfate. Systemic corticosteroids have their proponents as well, and BCG has been tried with some success. Some patients require operative augmentation of bladder capacity by enterocystoplasty or, rarely, cystourethrectomy and permanent urinary diversion.

URINARY STRESS INCONTINENCE

Involuntary loss of urine during stress (coughing, sneezing, or physical strain) is a common complaint of postmenopausal women. The cause is related to pelvic relaxation with age, resulting in descent of the trigone and proximal urethra. There is obliteration, of the urethrovesical angle, which normally provides resistance at the bladder outlet. The diagnosis is made by the history and physical examination and urodynamic evaluation. When the bladder is full, the patient should be asked to cough while in both the supine and upright positions, producing incontinence. Digital pressure applied to the paraurethral tissues in an anterior direction through the vagina will reestablish the urethrovesical angle and prevent stress incontinence (Marshall's test).

Treatment in patients with normal bladder function and low residual urine is initiated with behavioral therapy and perineal exercises; if unsuccessful, pharmacologic methods include oxybutynin and ephedrine. Definitive management is surgical. This can be accomplished by retropubic urethrovesical resuspension either using the Marshall-Marchetti-Krantz procedure or the Stamey modification of the Pereyra procedure. Currently, the most effective surgical approach is a sling procedure with a piece of autologous or synthetic fascia attached to the rectus muscle or os pubis and surrounding the urethra at the bladder neck. Newer approaches include the use of collagen injection into the periurethral tissues, resulting in increased urethral outflow resistance.

FEMALE URETHRITIS & PERIURETHRITIS

Urethritis in the female may be acute or chronic. Acute urethritis can be gonorrheal in origin. Chemical urethritis is occasionally acquired from exposure to soap or bath oils. Chronic urethritis is a common problem in females, since the female urethra is exposed to pathogenic bacteria because of its anatomic location. Urethral trauma, instrumentation, and increase in the number of pathogenic organisms lead to infection and overt urethritis. Urethritis usually precedes cystitis.

Hormonal changes associated with menopause cause vaginal and urethral mucosal changes, leading to irritative symptoms and increased susceptibility to inflammation.

Urethritis usually causes irritative voiding symptoms similar to those of cystitis and, occasionally, functional obstructive symptoms. Examination may reveal urethral discharge, marked tenderness, or congested everted mucosa at the external meatus. Induration of the urethra may be associated with vaginitis and cervicitis. Endoscopy may reveal obstruction, mucosal congestion, and inflammatory polyps. Urethral calibration rarely reveals obstruction. Spasm of the external sphincter may be noted.

Treatment is directed to the underlying cause. Estrogen cream is indicated for senile vaginitis. Surgical treatment consists of urethral dilation and opening and draining infected periurethral ducts. Alpha-blockers given orally may also help decrease urethral resistance. Correction of vaginitis, cervicitis, and cervical erosions helps in ameliorating symptoms.

FEMALE URETHRAL CARUNCLE

Urethral caruncle, commonly seen after menopause, represents granulomatous overgrowth of the posterior lip of the external meatus. The caruncle is tender and causes pain with intercourse and urination. The primary concern is exclusion of urethral cancer. Treatment is complete excision.

FEMALE URETHRAL DIVERTICULUM

Urethral diverticulum in the female commonly presents as recurrent lower urinary tract infection. It should be suspected whenever urinary infection fails to resolve with treatment. Symptoms are urinary dribbling and cystic swelling in the anterior vaginal wall during voiding. If diverticulum is suspected, it can usually be identified during panendoscopy and opacified by contrast on a voiding cystourethrogram while occluding the external meatus. These lesions occasionally contain stones or tumors.

Treatment consists of transvaginal diverticulectomy.

SPERMATOCELE

Spermatocele is a retention cyst of a tubule of the rete testis or the head of the epididymis. The cyst is distended with a milky fluid that contains sperm. Located at the superior pole of the testis and caput epididymidis, the spermatocele is soft and fluctuant and can be transilluminated.

No treatment is needed unless the spermatocele is painful, in which case surgical excision may be performed.

VARICOCELE

Varicocele is due to incompetent valves in the testicular vein, permitting transmission of hydrostatic venous pressure; distention and tortuosity of the pampiniform plexus results. Varicocele is on the left side in 98% of cases, presumably because of venous drainage of the left testes to the left renal vein, causing increased retrograde venous pressure. The varicocele is bilateral in up to 50% of cases.

Mild varicoceles are commonly asymptomatic, but a dragging scrotal sensation may be noted. Varicocele may lead to infertility in some men (see Male Infertility).

Asymptomatic varicocele is best untreated unless it is a suspected factor in male infertility. Treatment then consists of operative ligation of the spermatic vein at or above the internal inguinal ring. In recurrent varicocele, transfemoral catheterization and occlusion or ablation of the spermatic vein may be performed with a detachable balloon or sclerosing agents. The technical success rate is high.

TORSION OF THE SPERMATIC CORD

Torsion of the spermatic cord (intravaginal torsion) is most common in adolescent boys. A twist in the spermatic cord interferes with testicular blood supply. If torsion is complete, testicular infarction may occur within 4–6 hours. The cause is unknown, but an underlying anatomic abnormality (spacious tunica vaginalis, loose epididymotesticular connection, undescended testis) is usually present.

Clinical findings consist of precipitous onset of lower abdominal and scrotal pain and scrotal swelling. There may be a history of previous attacks in young adolescents. The testis is swollen, tender, and retracted. The pain is not relieved by testicular support. The cord above the swelling is normal. The cremasteric reflex is absent on the affected side.

Torsion must be differentiated from orchitis, epididymitis, and pain due to testicular trauma. Technetium Tc 99m pertechnetate scan *may* differentiate orchitis-epididymitis from testicular torsion if performed early in the course of symptoms: the former will demonstrate increased blood flow, in contrast to the ischemic pattern of torsion. Color Doppler ultrasound is more definitive and less time-consuming and can delineate the lack of testicular blood flow. If the diagnosis cannot be established by examination, history, and imaging, exploration is required.

Torsion of the spermatic cord is a surgical emergency! Contralateral orchiopexy is always necessary because of frequent bilateral involvement—ie, the "bell clapper" deformity (lack of fixation of the cord structures by the testicular mediastinum)—and the high incidence of recurrent torsion and infertility in bilateral cases.

TORSION OF TESTICULAR APPENDAGES

The epididymis and the testicle often have a vestigial remnant of embryologic ducts known as an appendix testis or appendix epididymidis. These structures can undergo spontaneous infarction usually in young boys, causing acute testicular pain and swelling that may be difficult to differentiate from testicular torsion. Occasionally, the infarcted appendage can be seen through the scrotal wall as a "blue dot" sign on the scrotum. This sign is only visible early in the course, prior to hydrocele formation and onset of scrotal edema. Scrotal ultrasound occasionally delineates the enlarged appendage and a normal testicle, establishing the diagnosis. In most cases—and certainly in equivocal ones—immediate scrotal exploration and removal of the infarcted appendage is required to rule out testicular torsion. Although the appendages often occur bilaterally, appendiceal torsion does not; thus, removal of the opposite appendage is not indicated.

MALE INFERTILITY*

Male infertility accounts for 30–50% of infertile couples (10–15% of marriages). Both partners should be evaluated for causes of infertility.

The causes of male infertility include the following: congenital anomalies (genetic, such as Klinefelter's syndrome; or developmental, such as absent vas deferens), trauma (both testicular, resulting in atrophy; and neurologic, resulting in erectile or ejaculatory dysfunction), infections (either systemic or reproductive organ specific), endocrine disorders (pituitary insufficiency, androgen deficiency), acquired anatomic abnormalities (varicocele, vasectomy), drug side effects (nitrofurantoin, estrogens, antineoplastic agents).

DIAGNOSIS

The most important aspect of infertility evaluation is the history, which uncovers the cause in many patients. The physical examination is no less important and may

reveal small testicles, a varicocele, or absence of the vas deferens.

A. Semen Analysis

Semen analysis is essential in evaluation of male factor infertility. At least three samples should be analyzed, since values may vary over time and with the method of collection. The specimen is produced by masturbation after 3 days of ejaculatory abstinence and collected in a clean wide-mouth container and examined within 2 hours. Determination of the volume, pH, liquefaction, sperm count, viability, abnormal forms, and motility constitutes a complete analysis. Normal values include volume of more than 1.5 mL, 20 million sperm per milliliter, 60% motile sperm, and 60% normal oval sperm heads.

B. Hormone Studies

Patients with no sperm in the ejaculate (azoospermia) or very low counts (oligospermia) should have serum FSH, LH, prolactin, and testosterone levels measured. Patients with elevated prolactin levels should be investigated for pituitary tumor; those with markedly elevated FSH levels have primary testicular abnormalities which are not amenable to therapy.

C. Testicular Biopsy

Testicular biopsies are indicated in azoospermic patients to distinguish obstructive versus parenchymal disease. Testicular biopsy should be performed in patients with unexplained oligospermia to establish a histologic diagnosis, to assess prognosis, and to direct treatment. If the serum FSH is more than two times normal, one may presume the presence of severe and irreversible testicular damage without confirmatory testis biopsy.

Vasography requires injection of contrast material into the vas. The purpose of this study is to delineate obstruction of the vas, epididymis, seminal vesicle, or ejaculatory duct. Vasography is used in patients who are azoospermic and have no evidence of retrograde ejaculation while demonstrating normal spermatogenesis on testicular biopsy. Seminal fructose levels should be obtained before operative exposure of the vas. Absence of fructose would indicate obstruction of the ejaculatory duct, and if this diagnosis is confirmed by vasography, the obstructing tissue may be resected by transurethral methods.

D. Other Diagnostic Studies

The **sperm penetration assay,** performed by incubation of sperm with hamster eggs whose zona pellucida has been enzymatically removed, offers an objective method of determining the ability of sperm to penetrate the ovum. The **cervical mucus penetration test** compares sperm motility in cervical mucus with a

---

* Female infertility is discussed in Chapter 42.

known standard. Although these two important parameters of sperm function can be evaluated, neither test alone can establish the cause of male factor infertility.

Antisperm antibodies can be measured in the serum of either the male or female partner, or in the seminal fluid. This assessment is indicated when spontaneous sperm agglutination or decreased sperm motility is noted on semen analysis. If antisperm antibodies are found, immunosuppressive therapy in the form of steroids may be effective in reducing agglutination (clumping) and increasing motility. Another method of treating autosperm antibodies is in vitro sperm washing with immunobeads coated by anti-human antibody. The sperm not bound by antibody remain in the supernatant and can be used for intrauterine insemination.

Studies to detect a nonpalpable varicocele include **venous Doppler, scrotal thermography, venography,** and **ultrasound with color Doppler.** Physical examination is the most effective method of detecting clinically significant varices. Venography is reserved for patients with recurrent varices, since identification of collateral venous channels would direct choice of therapy.

Transrectal ultrasound is used to support the diagnosis of ejaculatory duct obstruction in the azoospermic patient. Absence of the seminal vesicles or distention due to distal obstruction can be identified. This study should be preceded by measurement of fructose in the ejaculate (lack of fructose suggests obstruction of the ejaculatory duct) and examination of postejaculate urine (to determine the presence of sperm, suggesting retrograde ejaculation).

Treatment

A. Nonoperative Treatment

Primary male infertility may be caused by hypogonadotropic hypogonadism, diagnosed by demonstrating low serum levels of FSH, LH, and testosterone. Spermatogenesis may be stimulated by administration of hCG followed by FSH. Isolated absence of either FSH or LH is rare; the LH deficiency is overcome by administration of testosterone, and lack of FSH is treated by administration of menotropins. Hyperprolactinemia may contribute to male infertility and would be treated with bromocriptine.

Infection of the reproductive organs should be treated when found during evaluation of male infertility. Infection may cause infertility immediately by several mechanisms: decreased spermatogenesis due to hyperthermia, immune interaction with sperm causing agglutination and decreased motility, as well as later sequelae such as obstruction of the ejaculatory tract. Pyospermia suggests the diagnosis, and treatment should

be designed to eliminate the common pathogens: *Neisseria gonorrhoeae, Chlamydia trachomatis,* and *Ureaplasma urealyticum* (all are sensitive to tetracycline).

If antisperm antibodies are found in either partner, steroids may be used to suppress the immune system. One must use steroids with caution and after thoroughly discussion of possible side effects with the patient; acne, hypertension, gastrointestinal bleeding, and avascular necrosis of the hip have been reported with steroid administration. Response to treatment is assessed by repeat semen analysis and measurement of antisperm antibodies in the patient's serum. Sperm washing in an attempt to remove cytotoxic antibodies may improve motility and decrease clumping; washed semen may then be instilled into the uterus (artificial insemination of the husband's semen; AIH) or used in conjunction with in vitro fertilization techniques.

Retrograde ejaculation or lack of seminal emission—usually due to spinal cord injury or sympathetic nerve injury during retroperitoneal surgery leading to bladder neck (ie, internal sphincter) incompetence—can be treated with α-adrenergic drugs or antihistamines to reestablish internal sphincter function and antegrade ejaculation. Alternatively, alkalinized postejaculate urine can be collected and centrifuged and the concentrated sperm instilled into the female partner's uterus.

Other medications under investigation include clomiphene and tamoxifen. Currently, these drugs have not been objectively shown to be effective.

B. Operative Therapy

Ligation of varicocele will yield pregnancy in 30–50% of patients. Several approaches are available, including inguinal and retroperitoneal. Transvenous occlusion of the spermatic vein by balloon is useful especially in cases of recurrent varicocele.

Obstruction of the epididymis-vas system may be amenable to vasovasostomy or vasoepididymostomy. Currently, these procedures are performed with the aid of the operating microscope, and patency is established in 50–90%.

Obstruction of the ejaculatory ducts is rare. When this diagnosis is made, transurethral resection of the ducts may establish patency.

C. Assisted Reproductive Techniques

These include the following: artificial insemination with husband's sperm (AIH), gamete intrafallopian transfer (GIFT), and in vitro fertilization (IVF) using intracytoplasmic sperm injection (ICSI) after retrieving eggs by transvaginal ultrasound guidance and sperm by testicular aspiration in selected partners. In cases of male factor infertility not amenable to treatment, artificial insemination by donor sperm is also available.

PRIAPISM

Priapism is a rare disorder in which prolonged, painful erection occurs, usually not associated with sexual stimulation. The blood in the corpora cavernosa becomes hyperviscous but not clotted. About 25% of cases are associated with leukemia, metastatic carcinoma, sickle cell anemia, or trauma. In most cases, the cause is uncertain.

If the erection does not subside, needle aspiration of the sludged blood of the corpora followed by lavage with alpha-adrenergic agents such as phenylephrine should be performed. Delayed or unsuccessful treatment may result in impotence. Unsuccessful treatment calls for the Winter procedure, in which a biopsy needle is passed through the glans into one of the corpora. A piece of tunica albuginea is removed, creating a fistula between corpora cavernosa and corpus spongiosum. This simple procedure is highly successful, and potency is usually maintained. Other procedures include cavernosal-glandular shunt, cavernosal-spongiosum shunt, and saphenous vein-cavernous shunt. If priapism persists, impotence results.

In sickle cell anemia, hydration and hypertransfusion often give relief and should constitute initial therapy.

PEYRONIE'S DISEASE (Plastic Induration of the Penis)

Fibrosis of the dorsal covering sheaths of the corpora cavernosa occasionally occurs without known cause in men over age 45. The fibrosis will not permit the involved surface to lengthen with erection, thus leading to dorsal chordee. The disorder may be due to vasculitis in the connective tissues. Palpation of the penile shaft reveals a raised, firm plaque dorsally. There is an association with Dupuytren's contracture.

Controversy exists regarding treatment. Expectant therapy or medical treatment, including vitamin E and aminobenzoic acid, may limit or cure the disease in half of patients. Operative therapy is necessary for patients who do not respond or for impotent patients. In the potent patient, a Nesbit procedure—excision of an ellipse of tunica albuginea from the ventral convex aspect of the shaft and suture closure—or plaque excision and dermal grafting has been used successfully. If the patient is impotent, insertion of a penile prosthesis is the procedure of choice.

PHIMOSIS & PARAPHIMOSIS

Phimosis—inability to retract the foreskin to expose the glans—may be congenital but is more often acquired. At birth, the foreskin cannot be easily retracted, but by age 3, the prepuce becomes pliant and the glans can be exposed and cleansed. If the foreskin is then retractable, circumcision is not necessary. Acquired phimosis is usually a result of chronic and recurrent bacterial balanitis (infection of the prepuce), common in patients with diabetes or balanitis xerotica obliterans. These patients are best treated by circumcision.

Paraphimosis is the inability to reduce a previously retracted foreskin. The prepuce becomes fixed in the retracted position proximal to the corona. With prolonged retraction, lymphedema of the prepuce exacerbates the condition and increases the circumferential pressure of the shaft proximal to the glans. Manual reduction can usually be accomplished using the index fingers to pull the prepuce distally while pushing the glans into the prepuce. If this measure fails, the preputial cicatrix may be incised (dorsal slit) and the foreskin reduced with relative ease. Circumcision may be performed as an elective procedure once the edema has subsided.

CONDYLOMATA ACUMINATA

Condylomata acuminata are wart-like lesions that occur on the penis, scrotum, urethra, and perineum in men and the vagina, cervix, and perineum in women. They are caused by human papillomavirus and are usually transmitted by sexual contact. Pain and bleeding are common presenting complaints. Warts outside the urethra can be treated with excision, application of podophyllum resin, liquid nitrogen, or CO_2 laser. Urethroscopy is needed to determine the proximal extent of lesions in the urethra. Intraurethral fulguration, CO_2 laser treatment, injection of fluorouracil solution, or IFN-α can be curative.

IMPOTENCE

Impotence is the inability to obtain and sustain an erection satisfactory for sexual intercourse.

Causes of Impotence

Causes can be grouped into the following categories: neurologic, vascular, endocrine, systemic, pharmacologic, and psychologic. Treatment is directed accordingly.

A. NEUROLOGIC

Reflex erections are mediated by the afferent fibers of the pudendal nerve and efferent fibers of the parasympathetic outflow (S2–S4). Psychogenic erections are initiated via cerebral centers. Specific neurologic diseases that may cause impotence may be congenital (spina bifida), acquired (cerebrovascular accident,

Alzheimer's disease, multiple sclerosis), iatrogenic (electroshock therapy), neoplastic (pituitary or hypothalamic tumors), traumatic (cord compression), infectious (tabes dorsalis), and nutritional (vitamin deficiency).

B. Vascular

Vascular causes of impotence may be cardiac (anginal syndromes, congestive failure), aortoiliac disease (Leriche's syndrome, atherosclerosis, other embolic phenomena), microangiopathy (diabetes, radiation injury), and abnormal venous drainage.

C. Endocrine

The accepted endocrine causes of impotence are hypogonadism, hyperprolactinemia, pituitary tumors, hypothyroidism, Addison's disease, Cushing's syndrome, acromegaly, and testicular feminizing syndrome.

D. Pharmacologic

Impotence is a common and often unsuspected complication of many therapeutic and illicit drugs. Major groups that may cause sexual dysfunction are the following: tranquilizers, antidepressants, antianxiety agents, anticholinergic drugs, antihypertensives, and many drugs with abuse potential. One should recognize that virtually all antihypertensives (including diuretics) can be associated with impotence or ejaculatory dysfunction. Drugs with abuse potential include alcohol (both as a direct affect and secondary to cirrhosis) and cocaine.

E. Psychogenic

Up to 50% of cases of impotence are related to psychogenic factors. Establishing an organic cause of impotence is important in choosing appropriate therapy. Factors that indicate a psychogenic cause are the following: selective erectile dysfunction (episodic, normal nocturnal erections, normal erections with masturbation), sudden onset, associated anxiety or external stress, affect disturbances (anger, anxiety, guilt, fear), and patient convinced of an organic cause.

Diagnosis

The history and physical examination suggest the cause in most cases. Confirmatory tests are necessary to ensure an appropriate choice of therapy.

In investigating a possible neurologic cause of impotence, the neurologic examination should include review of systems with respect to bladder and bowel function. More invasive studies would include a cystometrogram with bethanechol supersensitivity testing, electromyography of the external urethral sphincter, and bulbosphincteric reflex latency.

Vascular impotence is suggested by signs of peripheral vascular disease as well as a history of atherosclerotic heart disease. Noninvasive diagnostic testing is performed by Doppler penile-brachial index. A penile blood pressure to brachial blood pressure ratio less than 0.6 suggests a vascular cause. Venous leak requires cavernosography and cavernosometry. Arteriography is rarely required but may be indicated in patients with a history of pelvic trauma.

Endocrine evaluation mandates measurement of serum testosterone and prolactin; many investigators would include assessment of follicle-stimulating and luteinizing hormones. Routine automated chemical screening may suggest other hormonal abnormalities that require additional testing. These studies should also detect systemic disease capable of causing impotence: cirrhosis, renal failure, scleroderma, and diabetes.

Psychogenic impotence may be established by nocturnal penile tumescence monitoring or outpatient snap-gauge cuffs. Additional testing includes one of the following: Minnesota Multiphasic Personality Inventory, DeRogatis Sexual Function Inventory, and Walker Sex Form.

Treatment

A. Nonoperative Treatment

In patients without arterial-vascular causes of impotence, intracorporal injections of papaverine, phentolamine, or prostaglandin E_1 (or all three) offer a nonoperative means of restoring sexual function. Intractable psychogenic impotence may also respond to this treatment. Intraurethral pellets of alprostadil (prostaglandin E_1) can also be used; however, they often cause pain and are not favored by most patients. Sildenafil, a phosphodiesterase inhibitor, is the first successful oral agent for erectile dysfunction. It works in patients who have normal blood flow and neurologic innervation, but it is expensive and is contraindicated in men with heart disease. Finally, a vacuum erection device can be used to sustain erection.

Endocrine disturbances responsible for impotence include hypotestosteronemia and hyperprolactinemia. Testosterone deficiency is treated by replacement therapy using a depot testosterone intramuscular injection every 2–3 weeks. Hyperprolactinemia is currently treated by bromocriptine therapy; the patient should be evaluated to assess the presence of a pituitary tumor.

Pharmacologic causes of impotence require altering medical treatment to ameliorate or eliminate secondary impotence. The ability to change medications depends upon the severity of the underlying disease.

Psychogenic impotence is treated by a trained sex therapist, and response may be anticipated in a majority of cases. The importance of eliminating organic causes of impotence before embarking upon psychologic therapy is obvious: the best psychologic methods applied to organic impotence will not resolve the dysfunction but will serve to frustrate both the therapist and patient.

B. OPERATIVE TREATMENT

Penile prosthesis insertion is currently the most common operative method for treatment of impotence. Two categories of prosthesis are in use: semirigid and inflatable. The semirigid prostheses are composed of a rigid shaft and a flexible hinge at the penile-pubic junction or a malleable soft metal case within the prosthesis; the erection is constant and is satisfactory to effect vaginal penetration, but the penile circumference is not equal to that of a natural erection.

Inflatable prostheses offer erections more similar in size to those experienced by the patient prior to the onset of impotence when compared to those achieved by semirigid prostheses. Two types of inflatable prostheses are available: the standard inflatable prosthesis consists of two corporal inflatable rods, a reservoir situated in the retropubic space, and a pump placed in the scrotum; the new inflatable rods combine the simplicity of two corporal rods with the sophistication of a self-contained pump and reservoir system (FlexiFlate and Hydroflex), permitting the convenience of inflation and deflation without tubing and multiple components.

Satisfactory results are achieved in 85% of patients. Complications common to both types of prostheses are infection and erosion of skin or urethra. The inflatable prostheses are also at risk for mechanical failure of the pump, tubing or reservoir leak, and aneurysm or rupture of the corporal cylinders.

Arterial revascularization of the penile arteries has met with limited success. Aortoiliac reconstruction improves erectile function in only 30% of cases. Microsurgical revascularization of the penile arteries (dorsal artery of the penis or deep corporal arteries) is successful in 60% of patients. While these methods avoid the risks of prosthetic infection and offer the advantage of reestablishing the natural physiologic mechanisms or erection, the mediocre success rate (when compared with the results of prosthetic insertion) would suggest that microsurgical penile revascularization be reserved for carefully selected cases.

Carrier S et al: Pathophysiology of erectile dysfunction. Urology 1993;42:468.

Chuang AT et al: Male infertility: evaluation and nonsurgical therapy. Urol Clin North Am 1998;25:703.

Donovan JF et al: Laparoscopic varix ligation. J Urol 1992;147:77.

Erickson DR et al: Interstitial cystitis. Int Urogynecol J 1998; 9:174.

Hansen SW et al: Long-term fertility and Leydig cell function in patients treated for germ cell cancer with cisplatin, vinblastine and bleomycin versus surveillance. J Clin Oncol 1990; 8:1695.

Howards SS: Treatment of male infertility. N Engl J Med 1995; 332:312.

Kamischke A et al: Analysis of medical treatment of male infertility. Hum Reprod 1999;14:1.

Lamb DJ et al: Male infertility: recent advances and a look towards the future. Curr Opin Urol 2000;10:359.

Martin-du Pan RC, Campana A: Physiopathology of spermatogenic arrest. Fertil Steril 1993;60:937.

Sant GR et al: Insterstitial cystitis. Curr Opin Urol 1999;9:297.

Schlesinger MH et al: Treatment outcome after varicocelectomy: a critical analysis. Urol Clin North Am 1994;21:517.

Sigman M: Assisted reproductive techniques and male infertility. Urol Clin North Am 1994;21:505.

Simon LJ et al: The Interstitial Cystitis Data Base Study: concepts and preliminary baseline descriptive statistics. Urology 1997;49(Suppl 5A):64.

Gynecology

42

Edward C. Hill, MD, & Elena A. Gates, MD

■ CONGENITAL ANOMALIES OF THE FEMALE REPRODUCTIVE SYSTEM

Edward C. Hill, MD, & Elena A. Gates, MD

Congenital defects of the female reproductive system arise as a result of abnormal embryonic development of the müllerian ducts and urogenital sinus. The most common defects are imperforate hymen, septate or double vagina, transverse septum of the vagina, congenital absence of the vagina, and duplication defects of the uterus. Although most such defects are idiopathic, some result from in utero exposure to teratogenic agents such as diethylstilbestrol or androgenic progestins during the first 4½ months of fetal development.

An adequate physical examination will detect or at least arouse suspicion of defective development. Careful examination of the genitalia of the newborn is especially important; errors have been made in gender assignment because of casual examinations. Imaging with ultrasound (or, preferably, MRI), pelvic examination under anesthesia, and laparoscopic or hysteroscopic examination can provide additional information. The urinary tract should be imaged as well because one-third to one-half of cases are associated with anomalies of the urinary tract such as absent kidney, horseshoe kidney, and duplication of the collecting system. Injury to the urinary tract can result from failure to recognize associated urinary tract anomalies during corrective surgery.

VAGINAL ANOMALIES

Imperforate Hymen

Imperforate hymen is often not recognized until puberty, when, despite the appearance of menstrual symptoms such as cramping, no bleeding is seen. Examination at this time will reveal the bulging imperforate hymen. Rectal examination may demonstrate a large cystic pelvic mass representing a distended vagina

(hematocolpos) and even a cystically enlarged uterus (hematometra). Urinary obstruction has been reported as a result of a large hematocolpos from accumulation of menstrual fluid behind an imperforate hymen.

Imperforate hymen is treated by cruciate incisions (hymenotomy) or laser excision of the mucous membrane, releasing the trapped menstrual fluid and correcting the hematocolpos and hematometra. Antibiotics should be given when there is significant hematocolpos and hematometra in order to prevent secondary infection.

Duplication of the Vagina

Duplication of the vagina may occur with or without duplication of the uterine corpus. The duplication may be only partial and may take the form of a longitudinal septum, in which case excision may be required if soft tissue dystocia occurs in labor or if coitus is obstructed. Complete duplication of the vagina usually requires no treatment.

Occasionally, the duplication takes the form of a hemivagina, a rudimentary vagina that fails to communicate with the second vagina or the introitus. This may result in formation of hematocolpos at menarche, with an apparent paravaginal cystic mass as a presenting sign. Renal agenesis may occur ipsilateral to the hemivagina. Marsupialization of the rudimentary vagina with the primary vagina is the usual method of management.

Transverse Septum of the Vagina

A transverse vaginal septum usually is incomplete. If imperforate, it may be mistaken for congenital absence of the vagina. Transverse vaginal septa are treated by excision.

Absence of the Vagina

Absence of the vagina usually is associated with absence of the uterus as well. Often there is a very small lower vagina representing the portion that develops from the urogenital sinus. The condition is commonly not recognized until the physician is consulted because of primary amenorrhea in a teenager. Treatment is frequently desired in an attempt to achieve more satisfactory sexual function.

Congenital absence of the vagina is managed by creation of an artificial vagina. This should be deferred until the patient has a desire and a need for a functioning vagina. In a well-motivated patient, congenital absence of the vagina may be corrected by nonoperative dilation and elongation of the vulvar vestibule. Success has been reported with vaginal dilators, vaginal molds, and with intercourse alone. Should a conservative approach fail or seem inappropriate to the management of an individual patient, the condition can be managed by surgical construction of an artificial vagina. A variety of techniques have been described and typically involve segments of small or large bowel, skin graft, or vulvoperineal skin flaps placed in an artificially created channel between the bladder and the rectum.

DUPLICATION DEFECTS OF THE UTERUS

Duplication defects of the uterus are often detected in the course of investigation for habitual abortion or for repeated premature labor. While many women with uterine anomalies have normal pregnancy outcomes, these anomalies are associated with increased rates of first- and second-trimester loss, cervical incompetence, preterm labor, and malpresentation of the fetus. Conception rates do not appear to be affected. Anomalies may vary from a simple midline septum in a single uterus (septate uterus) to duplication of the uterine horns (bicornuate uterus) to complete duplication of the corpus and cervix (uterus didelphys). These types of uterine anomalies may be suspected after physical examination, especially during pregnancy. Diagnosis can be confirmed using MRI or hysterosalpingography. The latter should be combined with ultrasonography or laparoscopy to distinguish a large septum from a bicornuate state. A combined laparoscopic-hysteroscopic evaluation is also useful, particularly if operation is planned.

The principal indication for surgical correction of uterine anomalies is recurrent pregnancy loss. It is important to select surgical candidates carefully, as cervical incompetence can be associated with uterine anomalies and is best treated by cerclage. The septate uterus is most often treated by hysteroscopic metroplasty with transcervical incision or resection of the septum. If the septum cannot be successfully resected hysteroscopically, abdominal metroplasty may be warranted. Pregnancies occurring after abdominal metroplasty should be delivered by cesarean section as the risk of uterine rupture is increased. When uterine anomalies are responsible for a poor obstetric history with high fetal wastage, one can expect significant improvement following surgical correction.

Grimbizis G et al: Hysteroscopic septum resection in patients with recurrent abortions or infertility. Human Reproduction 1998;13:1188.

Heinonen PK: Reproductive performance of women with uterine anomalies after abdominal or hysteroscopic metroplasty or no surgical treatment. J Am Assoc Gynecol Laparosc 1997; 4:311.

Hensle TW et al: Vaginal reconstruction. Urol Clin North Am 1999;26:39.

Li S et al: Association of renal agenesis and müllerian duct anomalies. J Comput Assist Tomogr 2000;24:829.

■ CORRECTION OF INFERTILITY DUE TO TUBAL ABNORMALITIES

Marcelle Cedars, MD

A couple may be considered infertile if a pregnancy does not occur after 1 year of normal coital activity (12 ovulatory exposed cycles) without contraceptives. About 15% of couples are infertile, and in approximately 40% of these there is a significant male factor (low sperm count, impaired motility, or anomalous forms). One-third of infertile couples have more than one problem. Anatomic abnormalities of the pelvic organs are the single most common cause of infertility in women. The list may include chronic salpingitis, endometriosis, and peritubal adhesions from previous appendicitis (with rupture). The bacteria involved with an inflamed appendix may be quite "toxic" to the female tube. Desire to reverse previous tubal sterilization may also be a reason for tubal surgery.

History

Specific questions should elicit information regarding any history of sexually transmitted disease, pelvic inflammatory disease, and any abdominal surgery. Patients should also be asked about worsening dysmenorrhea or deep dyspareunia that might suggest endometriosis.

Clinical Findings

Pelvic examination should always be performed. The size and mobility of the uterus should be assessed and the presence of adnexal masses excluded. Rectovaginal examination is required to evaluate the uterosacral ligaments for nodularity and tenderness (suggesting endometriosis). Ultrasound is often helpful. The ovaries can be evaluated for the presence of iso-echoic masses that might suggest endometriosis (endometriomas). A large hydrosalpinx may be easily seen on ultrasound and may modify treatment recommendations.

Even if the examination is normal, a hysterosalpingogram may reveal an obstruction at the cornu, a hydrosalpinx, partial fimbrial occlusion, or tubo-ovarian adhesions. For safety reasons, the procedure should always be performed first with a water-based dye; if the tubes are patent and there is no extravasation of the dye, an oil contrast medium may then be used. Data suggest that this procedure improves pregnancy rates in patients with unexplained infertility and minimal to mild endometriosis.

Laparoscopy with direct visualization of the pelvic organs may be warranted if the above findings are inconclusive. Evaluation of the pelvic organs, as well as therapeutic (corrective) measures, can be performed at the same time with this procedure. This treatment might involve lysis of adhesions or fulguration of endometrial implants. If the hysterosalpingogram is entirely normal, there is about a 30% chance that an abnormality will be found on laparoscopy. Almost 80% of these abnormalities will be minimal or mild (peritoneal) endometriosis. Only about 6% of patients will have adhesive disease not suspected on the hysterosalpingogram.

Treatment

Transvaginal tubal catheterization (much like an angioplasty) may be performed either by radiologic guidance (by the interventional radiologist) or by hysteroscopy (by the gynecologist) to relieve proximal tubal obstruction. This may avoid the need for more elaborate procedures such as tubal reimplantation.

Tuboplasty operations are designed to reestablish tubal patency or return pelvic anatomy to normal by lysis of adhesions. These surgical procedures are more successful if the damage is localized and there is little intrinsic damage to the tube (eg, with fimbrial adhesions or previous tubal ligation). Reestablishment and maintenance of tubal patency have been more successful with the development of microsurgical techniques that require gentle tissue handling. Salpingolysis, reimplantation of the tube into the uterus, end-to-end anastomosis, and fimbrial salpingostomy may be performed. The use of laparoscopy (avoiding exposure of the bowel and peritoneal surfaces to air and handling) decreases the chances for new adhesion formation. Minimizing manipulation to the tissues and minimizing bleeding and necrosis limit the re-formation of adhesions. Newer agents that act as barriers to separate tissues and prevent adhesion re-formation are under investigation.

Evaluation of the extent of tubal damage (damage to the fimbria and internal tubal structures) and of peritubal adhesive disease is critical to the estimation of expected success with any tubal repair. Tubal surgery statistics are generally quoted as the cumulative pregnancy rate over a 2-year period of time. Therefore, other infertility factors must be evaluated and will influence the likelihood of success following surgery. The female partner's age and the presence of other infertility factors (eg, ovulatory dysfunction, male factor) might make tubal surgery a less attractive option even when the anatomy would suggest the likelihood for a good anatomic repair.

In vitro fertilization is an alternative when tubal obstruction cannot be remedied or when multiple infertility factors exist. If a hydrosalpinx is visible on ultrasound, consideration should be given to its removal (or obstruction) prior to proceeding to in vitro fertilization as implantation rates are lower and miscarriage rates higher in their presence.

Prognosis

When the female partner is young (under 35) and only mild disease exists, pregnancy rates may reach 70%. With the most severe disease, this rate drops to < 15%. Ectopic (tubal pregnancy) rates are approximately 10%, and all tubal surgery patients should be followed closely until an intrauterine pregnancy is documented. Tubal reanastomosis rates may be as high as 80–90% for an isthmic-isthmic anastomosis. All rates for tubal surgery must be compared with the success of the local in vitro fertilization program to determine the best option for an individual patient.

Benadiva CA et al: In vitro fertilization versus tubal surgery: is pelvic reconstructive surgery obsolete? Fertil Steril 1995; 64:1051.

Spielvogel K et al: Surgical management of adhesions, endometriosis, and tubal pathology in the woman with infertility. Clin Obstet Gynecol 2000;43:916.

Watson A et al: Techniques for pelvic surgery in subfertility. Cochrane Database Syst Rev 2000;(2):CD000221.

Watson A et al: Liquid and fluid agents for preventing adhesions after surgery for subfertility. Cochrane Database Syst Rev 2000;(2):CD001298.

■ ABNORMAL UTERINE BLEEDING

Abner Korn, MD

Abnormal uterine bleeding may occur at any age. In the newborn, it is frequently related to removal of the infant at birth from the influence of maternal estrogen, which has produced endometrial proliferation in the baby's uterus. During the reproductive years, it may occur as **hypermenorrhea** (or **menorrhagia**), excessive or prolonged bleeding at the normal time of menstruation; **polymenorrhea,** bleeding that occurs more frequently than every 3 weeks; or **intermenstrual bleeding** (or **metrorrhagia**), which occurs during the interval between normal menstrual periods.

Hypermenorrhea may be due to such organic conditions as uterine leiomyoma, endometrial polyps, and blood dyscrasias or it may be related to a functional disturbance such as irregular shedding of the endometrium, presumably resulting from faulty regression of the corpus luteum of the ovary. Polymenorrhea may be related to early ovulation with a shortened proliferative phase, which frequently is secondary to hypothyroidism. One of the most frequently encountered problems is the completely acyclic and sometimes heavy and prolonged bleeding of the anovulatory patient, leading to so-called **dysfunctional uterine bleeding.** This condition is seen most often in adolescents and in perimenopausal women and is due to a failure in regular ovulatory function. The endometrium is proliferative in type at a time in the menstrual cycle when it would show secretory changes if ovulation had occurred. In many instances there is, after a period of time, the development of endometrial hyperplasia owing to the prolonged stimulus of estrogen on the endometrium without the modifying influence of progesterone. Intermenstrual bleeding may be due to the slight drop in estrogen titer associated with ovulation, in which event it occurs quite regularly at about mid cycle. Other causes of intermenstrual bleeding that occurs at any time are polyps, submucous leiomyomas, blood dyscrasias, genital tuberculosis, and cancer of the cervix, uterine corpus, or uterine tube. Complications of pregnancy should not be overlooked as a cause of abnormal bleeding in women of reproductive age.

Postmenopausal bleeding—vaginal bleeding occurring a year or more after menopause—is of concern because it may be indicative of endometrial cancer. The exogenous administration of estrogenic substances, including their use in cosmetic preparations and herbal supplements, is also an important cause. Atrophic changes, polyps, trauma, blood dyscrasias, hypertensive cardiovascular disease, and estrogen-producing tumors of the ovary are less frequent causes. The bleeding may be represented by a scant brownish vaginal discharge, or it may be frank, profuse, bright red bleeding. Because it looms so large in the etiology of postmenopausal bleeding, cancer should be considered the cause until proved otherwise.

Clinical Findings

In the assessment of any type of menstrual disorder, the following points should be considered:

(1) Careful documentation of the menstrual history and a record of the temporal relationship of the abnormal bleeding to the menstrual cycle are necessary. A special menstrual calendar kept by the patient or a basal body temperature graph can be very helpful.

(2) A history of hormonal medication, herbal supplement, or hormone-containing cosmetic use.

(3) A general history and physical examination may lead to the correct diagnosis of hypothyroidism, blood dyscrasia (most commonly in adolescents), anticoagulant use, genital tuberculosis, etc.

(4) A carefully performed pelvic examination will often reveal vaginal, cervical, uterine, or adnexal disease.

(5) Cervical cytologic examination is essential in all patients, and the specimen should be collected prior to the introduction of lubricating jelly into the vagina.

(6) A complete blood count and measurement of red cell indices will reflect the degree of iron deficiency secondary to acute or chronic blood loss. Additional blood studies may be necessary when endocrine disorders or blood dyscrasias are suspected.

(7) Endometrial biopsy is often required to establish the cause of abnormal menstrual bleeding. Biopsy should be done at an appropriate time in the menstrual cycle—eg, after the 16th day of the cycle if anovulatory bleeding is suspected—but can be done at any time to evaluate for hyperplasia or carcinoma. Endometrial sampling with a disposable suction-device (Pipelle, Vabra, etc) can be accomplished in an office setting.

(8) Hysteroscopy may help establish the cause of bleeding and offers the opportunity for simultaneous treatment. Hysteroscopy can be accomplished in an office or outpatient surgical setting and is recommended when bleeding is recurrent or resistant to therapy or when structural abnormalities of the endometrium (eg, myomas) are suspected.

(9) Transvaginal ultrasound can show endometrial thickness and structural abnormalities of the uterus (such as polyps or myomas), especially when saline is introduced into the endometrial cavity (sonohysterogram). Using an endometrial thickness threshold of 5 mm, 96% of cancers are detected with a specificity of 92% when hormone replacement therapy is not being used and 77% when hormone replacement is used.

Treatment

Dilation and curettage is a most effective short-term method of controlling uterine bleeding. Longer-term treatment will generally be directed toward the cause of the abnormal uterine bleeding.

In chronic blood loss due to hypermenorrhea produced by leiomyomas, reduction in bleeding can be achieved by the administration of progestins. A gonadotropin-releasing hormone agonist will result in menstrual suppression and amenorrhea. Bleeding due to leiomyomas can be lessened by removal of the fibroid tumors (myomectomy) or cured by hysterectomy.

Dysfunctional bleeding due to chronic anovulation is treated with cyclic progestin therapy (medroxyprogesterone acetate, 10 mg/d for 10 days every 4 weeks), with oral contraceptive pills, or, for women who desire to become pregnant, with clomiphene for ovulation induction. Control of acute heavy bleeding may be achieved through the use of higher dose combination oral contraceptives (one pill four times a day for 3 or 4 days to control bleeding, then tapered to one pill a day over the ensuing week). An antiemetic is often needed when using high-estrogen therapy. A low-dose oral contraceptive is started and continued for 3 months or longer, if the patient desires. Intravenous conjugated estrogen, 25 mg every 4 hours, has been used also to control acute bleeding. Such a regimen must be followed by administration of a progestin to stabilize the endometrium. This can then be followed by daily use of an oral contraceptive pill for longer-term control. Termination of hormonal treatment will result in withdrawal bleeding. A 5-year intrauterine device (IUD) containing levonorgestrel produces amenorrhea in about 25% of women and light bleeding in the remainder.

Severe and intractable bleeding of a dysfunctional nature may rarely require hysterectomy. In the absence of other causes, hypermenorrhea associated with ovulatory cycles can be ameliorated with nonsteroidal anti-inflammatory drugs. Hysteroscopic endometrial ablation by Nd:YAG laser or electrosurgery may avoid hysterectomy in the premenopausal patient with intractable bleeding. These operations generally require a normal uterine cavity. About 20% of women have amenorrhea following endometrial ablation, but up to 35% will require hysterectomy within 5 years. Alternative methods of endometrial ablation developed recently (eg, thermal balloons) seem to have efficacy equal to hysteroscopic ablation but are technically simpler to perform. The levonorgestrel IUD has been shown in recent randomized, controlled trials to be nearly as effective as hysteroscopic ablation operations.

Postmenopausal bleeding of nonneoplastic origin may require estrogen therapy if it is due to atrophic changes. More commonly, it is seen as a side effect of hormone replacement therapy (HRT) and can be treated by discontinuing HRT or choosing an alternative regimen. Curettage is curative if the bleeding is due to endometrial polyps. Endometrial carcinoma is a contraindication to estrogen therapy and is treated by total abdominal hysterectomy and bilateral salpingo-oophorectomy with or without preoperative radiation therapy. Well-differentiated endometrial adenocarcinoma in young women who desire to maintain fertility

has been successfully treated using high-dose progestins in about three-fourths of cases.

Randall, TC: Progestin treatment of atypical hyperplasia and well-differentiated carcinoma of the endometrium in women under age 40. Obstet Gynecol 1997;90:434–40.

A randomised trial of endometrial ablation versus hysterectomy for the treatment of dysfunctional uterine bleeding: outcome at four years. Aberdeen Endometrial Ablation Trials Group. Br J Obstet Gynaecol 1999;106:360.

Smith-Bindman R et al: Endovaginal ultrasound to exclude endometrial cancer and other endometrial abnormalities. JAMA 1998;280:1510.

Stewart, A: The effectiveness of the levonorgestrel-releasing intrauterine system in menorrhagia: a systematic review. Br J Obstet Gynaecol 2001;108:74.

■ CHRONIC PELVIC PAIN

Lee Learman, MD, PhD

Chronic pelvic pain is most often defined as 6–12 months of pain below the umbilicus producing a significant impact on a patient's quality of life. A 1994 Gallup Poll found that one in seven reproductive-age women had experienced chronic pelvic pain and estimated the annual cost of illness to be $882 million in outpatient visits alone. The evaluation and treatment of chronic pelvic pain accounts for 15–40% of all referrals to gynecologists, 40% of all laparoscopies, and 12% of all hysterectomies.

Diagnosis

The differential diagnosis and comorbidity of chronic pelvic pain make it one of the most challenging issues encountered in ambulatory practice. While many patients attribute their pain to a gynecologic cause, the physician must conduct a meticulous patient interview and physical examination to assess a wide range of nongynecologic diagnoses. The most common of these are irritable bowel syndrome and inflammatory bowel disease; nephrolithiasis and interstitial cystitis; abdominal wall hernia, muscle strain, or nerve injury; and depressive disorders or somatization. Patients may also have mood symptoms as a consequence of living with pain and are more likely to have suffered sexual assault as an adult or child.

The gynecologic causes of chronic pelvic pain are grouped into cyclic and continuous symptom patterns. Cyclic causes include primary dysmenorrhea, in which periods are painful but no pelvic pathology can be identified; and secondary dysmenorrhea due to endometriosis, adenomyosis, or perhaps chronic salpingitis. Midcycle ovulatory pain (mittelschmerz) occurs during oocyte release from an ovarian follicle and thus produces lateral pain that migrates from one side to the other from month to month. Gynecologic causes of continuous pain include later stages of endometriosis and adenomyosis, uterovaginal prolapse, and chronic salpingitis or pelvic adhesions. Ovarian remnant syndrome occurs after oophorectomy when residual ovarian tissue is trapped in a retroperitoneal location. Ovarian dystrophy occurs when an ovary undergoes progressive ischemic injury after ligation of the uterine circulation at hysterectomy or tubal surgery.

Clinical Findings

The pelvic examination for chronic pelvic pain proceeds in a slow and methodical fashion in which the patient remains fully informed of each step in the examination and is allowed to interrupt or terminate the examination at any time. The goal is first to determine what the background degree of tenderness is and then to identify focal tender areas that exceed this background level. The patient is instructed before the examination to indicate which maneuvers during the examination reproduce their pain. A rectovaginal examination should be conducted to evaluate cul-de-sac tenderness or mass and to palpate the uterosacral ligaments for evidence of endometriosis. A pelvic mass found on examination is usually further characterized by ultrasound into suspicious versus nonsuspicious for neoplasm, and surveillance, medical treatment, or surgical excision is then planned accordingly. An abnormal pelvic examination has about an 80% predictive value for pelvic abnormalities noted at laparoscopy but only about a 45% sensitivity and a 40% negative predictive value.

Treatment

After ruling out nongynecologic causes by history, physical examination, and appropriate studies and referrals, reproductive-age women are often offered treatment consisting of analgesics and ovulation suppression. A typical regimen would include low-dose combined oral contraceptives (to be used in patients over 35 years old only if they are nonsmokers) and nonsteroidal anti-inflammatory agents. When pain is refractory to medical management or when physical examination findings are abnormal, diagnostic laparoscopy is conducted. This procedure includes a survey of upper abdominal structures and meticulous inspection of the pelvic peritoneum, bladder, uterus, tubes, ovaries, appendix, rectum, and sigmoid colon. Approximately one-third of patients will have evidence of endometriosis, one-third will have adhesions or evidence of chronic salpingitis, and one-third will have a normal pelvis. The presence of abnormalities may not explain the pain,

however. Among pain-free patients undergoing laparoscopy for other indications, about 30% will have abnormal findings.

Although the evidence for success of laparoscopic treatments is not strong, patient preference and clinical experience support correction of focal abnormalities and other procedures that could credibly lessen the patient's pain. These procedures include lysis of adhesions, destruction or removal of endometriotic implants and ovarian endometriomas, and interruption of the autonomic nerve tracts through which pain messages travel from the pelvis to the spinal cord (presacral neurectomy, uterine nerve ablation). The best available data indicate that laparoscopic treatments will produce a short-term improvement in pain in 62–82% of patients. The treatment success data come primarily from case series reports and thus are likely to overestimate real-world success. While the interventions to improve pelvic pain could also be performed via laparotomy, this is avoided out of a concern that laparotomy is more adhesiogenic than laparoscopy because there is greater peritoneal injury.

In nondepressed patients who have completed their childbearing or who wish definitive treatment, hysterectomy is a highly effective therapy with success rates of 75–95% if uterine pathology is present and 50–91% if no pelvic pathology is noted. The success rate plummets to less than 5% if the patient has any neurovegetative signs or symptoms of depression. Patients with endometriosis should also be offered bilateral ovarian removal to prevent stimulation of residual implants. Finally, patients with refractory pain after multiple medical regimens and surgical procedures should be referred to a multidisciplinary clinic where the myriad causes of pelvic pain can be systematically investigated and chronic pain management instituted.

Jamieson DF et al: The prevalence of dysmenorrhea, dyspareunia, pelvic pain, and irritable bowel syndrome in primary care practices. Obstet Gynecol 1996;87:55.

Mathias SD et al: Chronic pelvic pain: prevalence, health-related quality of life, and economic correlates. Obstet Gynecol 1996;87:321.

■ CONTRACEPTION

Philip D. Darney, MD

The majority of the world's people who want to avoid an unintended birth rely on methods of family planning that require some sort of operative procedure, including sterilization operations for men and women, the insertion of contraceptives into the uterine cavity or under the skin, and termination of unwanted pregnancies by therapeutic abortion. These family planning procedures are in fact the world's most commonly performed operations. In the United States, nearly one million sterilization operations and more than a million abortions are performed yearly. Nearly 40% of American women rely on their own tubal sterilization or the male partner's vasectomy for contraception. These common operations are simple, safe, and effective, but specialized equipment, knowledge of methods of pain relief, and training are required. It is beyond the scope of this chapter to provide more than an overview of these procedures. Texts listed in the bibliography provide technical details.

Americans use sterilization for contraception more than the people of most countries because temporary methods such as intrauterine and oral contraceptives have an undeservedly bad reputation in the United States. An increase in both female and male sterilization procedures occurred between 1973 and 1988, a period during which the use of intrauterine contraception declined and the use of oral contraception decreased substantially. Since the late 1980s, oral contraception has regained some of its popularity.

Sterilization by tubectomy was first proposed by James Blundell in lectures at Guy's Hospital in London, but the operation did not become common until the 1930s. Many methods of female sterilization were developed, including the Madelener, Irving, Uchida, and the still popular Pomeroy operations, but these all required laparotomy. Not until laparoscopic tubal occlusion was introduced did female sterilization become more common than the simpler male vasectomy. In laparoscopic procedures, the oviducts are occluded with Filshie titanium clips, Hulka spring-loaded clips, Yoon Silastic bands, or unipolar or bipolar electrocautery. A 10-year follow-up study has shown that long-term failure of all these operations is higher than expected, ranging from 2% to 4%—comparable to the failure rates of copper or hormonal intrauterine contraceptives and subdermal implants. This study did not demonstrate adverse health or menstrual effects of tubal occlusion operations. Because tubal occlusion reversal is difficult and expensive, 2–25% of women express regret at having had the operation. Both mini laparotomy for Pomeroy-type tubal excision and laparoscopic tubal occlusion are commonly performed under local anesthesia with conscious sedation in about 20 minutes.

Modern intrauterine contraceptives carry copper or progestational hormones to the uterine cavity where they inhibit sperm motility and block fertilization. They are packaged with disposable inserters that can usually be passed through the cervical canal without local anesthesia or cervical dilation. Both copper and progestin devices are highly effective and have long durations of action (less than 5% failure at 10 years of use). These modern intrauterine contraceptives do not increase the risk of pelvic infection. On the contrary, the levonorgestrel-containing system, like other hormonal contraceptives, actually decreases the risk of pelvic inflammatory disease. Ectopic pregnancy rates in users of these intrauterine contraceptives are reduced to a tenth of those reported in women not using contraception of any kind.

The principal side effect of intrauterine contraceptives is change in menstrual bleeding: the copper devices increase blood loss and the progestin devices decrease it to about half the normal flow. Because of this action, the levonorgestrel device has been shown to be as effective as uterine surgery for treatment of abnormal uterine bleeding as well as to protect the endometrium from precancerous hyperplasia during estrogen replacement therapy. The copper device is an effective postcoital (emergency) contraceptive, but progestin devices cannot be used in this way.

Despite the safety and efficacy of intrauterine contraceptives, they are much less used in the USA than in the rest of the world. For example, in Germany and Denmark, about 20% of women practicing contraception use intrauterine methods, while in the USA less than 1% do.

Subdermal implant contraception uses low serum concentrations of contraceptive progestins found in birth control pills to thicken cervical mucus and inhibit ovulation. These actions result in failure rates comparable to those reported following sterilization and intrauterine contraception. Their duration of action ranges from 1 year to 7 years depending on the number of implants, the progestin employed, and the delivery system. As with intrauterine contraceptives, the principal side effect is change in menstrual bleeding; the majority of users experience a diminution in blood loss but an increase in number of days of bleeding, sometimes at unpredictable intervals.

Contraceptive implants require subdermal insertion with a disposable trocar under local anesthesia. They are removed under local anesthesia with a scalpel and forceps. These procedures take only a few minutes, and pain and infections are rare. The 7-year system (Norplant) uses six capsules, requiring more time for insertion and removal. Newer single-rod systems (eg, Implanon and Uniplant) are easier to use, have a shorter life, and are associated with somewhat more acceptable bleeding patterns.

Although new contraceptives are safe and highly effective, they are not perfect. Unintended pregnancies result in the need for about one million abortions per year in the USA. In the past, contraceptive failure meant an unwanted birth or recourse to dangerous secret abortion services. Changes in the law and in abortion techniques have meant that in most countries of the world women need not risk their lives to limit family size. Uterine aspiration procedures using manual or electric sources of vacuum have led to safe induced abortions in the first trimester, with mortality rates of less than 1:200,000 procedures. Second-trimester terminations require more complex equipment and greater surgical skill: The principal determinant of the morbidity and mortality of abortion is the duration of gestation, with abortion at 20 weeks being ten times as risky as abortion at 10 weeks.

Medical methods of abortion using prostaglandins with or without progesterone antagonists (eg, mifepristone) are employed at gestations earlier than 9 weeks and beyond 20 weeks, but surgical abortion remains much more common and less expensive in both the first and second trimester. The principal complications are hemorrhage and uterine perforation (primarily with second-trimester operations), but the principal cause of death associated with abortion is anesthesia. Local anesthesia, with or without conscious sedation, is safer than general anesthesia.

Darney P et al: *Protocols for Ambulatory Gynecologic Surgery.* Blackwell Science, 1996.

Speroff L et al: *A Clinical Guide for Contraception,* 3rd ed. Lippincott Williams & Wilkins, 2001.

■ PELVIC ORGAN PROLAPSE & URINARY INCONTINENCE

Sharon Knight, MD, & Elaine Waetjen, MD

An understanding of pelvic floor relaxation requires a thorough knowledge of the anatomic relationship of the pelvic viscera and their supporting tissues. These conditions are thought to result initially from stretching and tearing of the muscles, nerves, and connective tissues of the pelvis during vaginal childbirth. Other factors thought to contribute to loss of support include chronic or repetitive increases in intra-abdominal pressure (eg, chronic cough, constipation, heavy lifting, obesity).

Anatomically, multiple factors play a role in pelvic support. The paired levator ani muscles collectively form the pelvic floor. The collagenous support of the pelvis includes the endopelvic fascia, which is continuous with the cardinal and uterosacral ligaments. The bladder, upper vagina, and rectum all rest horizontally upon and are supported by the levator ani muscles, which actively contract to maintain the position of those structures in the pelvis.

Obstetric injuries to the pelvic floor can involve damage (stretching or breaks) to the investing endopelvic fascia and the supporting ligaments of the uterus as well as muscular and neurologic injury, which may also contribute to loss of levator function and thus

loss of support. Careful repair of lacerations occurring during delivery will avoid these problrems.

Stress incontinence is involuntary loss of urine from the urethra with increases in intra-abdominal pressure (eg, Valsalva maneuver) in the absence of detrusor activity. It can be demonstrated clinically during pelvic examination by asking the patient to cough. Stress incontinence should be distinguished from other common types of urinary incontinence. With **urge incontinence,** the patient experiences the loss of urine with bladder filling and the desire to void. Stress and urge incontinence may occur simultaneously and are referred to as **mixed incontinence. Overflow incontinence** may present with symptoms of any of the other described types of incontinence. It can be ruled out by checking a postvoid residual urine volume during examination. Surgical correction of stress incontinence may produce a temporary urge incontinence that may persist in 10–15 % of patients.

The bladder and urethra are supported by the muscles of the pelvic floor and the endopelvic fascia. There are two primary mechanisms of stress incontinence. In women with normal pelvic support, the proximal urethra is held in a pelvic position and is subjected to the same intra-abdominal pressure changes as those affecting the bladder. Thus, increases in abdominal pressure (eg. during coughing) are distributed equally to the urethra and bladder and in this way the greater "closing pressure" of the urethra is maintained and the patient remains continent. In patients with anterior vaginal wall relaxation, however, increased abdominal pressure causes descent of the proximal urethra and bladder base into the vagina (hypermobile urethra). Thus, pressure is no longer equally distributed (intravesical pressure exceeds intraurethral pressure) and urinary leakage occurs.

The second mechanism of stress urinary incontinence, **intrinsic sphincter deficiency,** involves loss of integrity of the urethral sphincter. Risk factors include previous surgery to treat incontinence, a history of radiation therapy, and age over 50 years. This diagnosis is independent of pelvic support.

In cases of pelvic organ prolapse beyond the hymen, stress incontinence may be unmasked only after correcting the prolapse. This should be evaluated preoperatively with office cytometrics, formal urodynamic testing, or a pessary test.

Clinical Findings

Mild degrees of pelvic organ prolapse are found in many women without significant symptoms. Prolapse is measured in various ways. The Baden and Walker system is the most commonly used clinical method: Grade 0 indicates no prolapse. In grade 1, the leading edge of the prolapse is beyond the midvaginal line but above the vaginal hymen. In grade 2, the prolapse is no more than about 4 cm beyond the hymen. Grade 3 occurs with complete uterine (total procidentia) or vaginal prolapse.

Descent and bulging of the anterior vagina usually indicates the presence of a cystocele or, less commonly, an anterior enterocele. Similarly, an anatomic defect in the posterior vagina signifies that a rectocele or enterocele (or both) exists. All of these conditions can be demonstrated during examination with the patient in the lithotomy or standing position by asking her to bear down or strain.

The symptoms of pelvic organ prolapse may include: pelvic pressure or a sensation of "falling out" of the pelvic organs, a mass protruding from the vagina (which may be a cystocele, rectocele, cervix, or all of these), stress incontinence, fecal incontinence, and other difficulties with defecation.

Differential Diagnosis

There are few entities in the differential diagnosis of pelvic organ prolapse. Urethral diverticula may simulate cystocele and produce a bulge of the anterior vaginal wall. The diverticulum is usually palpable as a discrete mass, and pressure against the mass often expresses purulent material from the urethral meatus. Endoscopic and urethrocystographic examinations confirm the diagnosis.

With regard to urinary incontinence, urodynamic studies are helpful in distinguishing stress incontinence from urge incontinence and are used to rule out intrinsic sphincter deficiency.

Treatment

A. NONOPERATIVE TREATMENT

The postmenopausal woman with mild to moderate anatomic defects may have some improvement of symptoms after the administration of a topical estrogen. Pelvic floor muscle (Kegel) exercises may improve symptoms in up to 60% of patients with stress or urge urinary incontinence. A pessary to support the descending pelvic structures often provides relief of symptoms, including those of urinary incontinence. Pessaries are good options for patients who do not want or cannot have surgery.

B. SURGICAL TREATMENT

There are many different surgeries to correct pelvic organ prolapse. The choice involves consideration of specific anatomic defects as well as the patient's age, health status, previous surgeries, and sexual activity. In cases of uterine prolapse, hysterectomy is often involved. Common procedures done for specific defects

include the following: (1) for cystocele or anterior vaginal prolapse, anterior colporrhaphy and abdominal or vaginal paravaginal repair; (2) for rectocele, posterior colporrhaphy; (3) for vaginal apex or vault prolapse, vaginal procedures such as sacrospinous ligament fixation, uterosacral suspension, and iliococcygeus suspension, or abdominal sacrocolpopexy. In patients for whom sexual activity is not an issue, closure (colpocleisis) or removal (colpectomy) of the vagina is an option. Surgical correction of prolapse has variable results—up to one-third of patients require reoperation for recurrent prolapse. There is some suggestion that the abdominal approach (sacrocolpopexy) may be more durable.

Many surgeries have been described for the treatment of stress urinary incontinence. Retropubic urethropexy and suburethral sling procedures are the most commonly performed and most durable procedures. Success of these two procedures is approximately 85% at 5 years. Sling procedures are the operation of choice in patients with intrinsic sphincter deficiency with a hypermobile urethra. In patients who have intrinsic sphincter deficiency with a nonmobile urethra, transurethral collagen injection is a minimally invasive treatment option. Anterior repairs and transvaginal needle suspensions have much lower success rates and should not be done for urinary incontinence.

Benson JT et al: Vaginal versus abdominal reconstructive surgery for the treatment of pelvic support defects: a prospective randomized study with long-term outcome evaluation. Am J Obstet Gynecol 1996;175:1418.

Black NA et al: The effectiveness of surgery for stress incontinence in women: a systematic review. Br J Urol 1996;78:497.

Bump RC et al: Epidemiology and natural history of pelvic floor dysfunction. Obstet Gynecol Clin North Am 1998;25:723.

Olsen AL et al: Epidemiology of surgically managed pelvic organ prolapse and urinary incontinence. Obstet Gynecol 1997;89:501.

■ FISTULAS

Robert Domush, MD

URINARY TRACT FISTULAS

Urinary tract fistulas to the vagina are of three kinds: vesicovaginal (most common), ureterovaginal, and urethrovaginal. They occur most often as a result of accidental injury to the urinary tract at the time of pelvic surgery or because of ischemic necrosis resulting from an impaired blood supply. The latter can occur either following radiation therapy for carcinoma of the reproductive organs (especially the cervix) or following prolonged impaction of the fetal head during labor. Fistulas may also occur as a result of tumor invasion of the vesicovaginal septum.

Total abdominal hysterectomy is the operation most often complicated by the development of vesicovaginal fistula. Fistulas caused by urinary tract injury can be prevented by skillful surgical technique. The surgeon should be alert for injuries, which should be repaired at the time of operation.

Clinical Findings

A. SYMPTOMS AND SIGNS

Constant urinary leakage is the cardinal symptom. Urine can usually be seen coming through an opening in the vagina. In vesicovaginal and ureterovaginal fistulas, the vaginal ostium is at or near the vault closure (post hysterectomy) whereas the urethrovaginal fistula opens along the anterior wall of the vagina. If the urethrovaginal fistula involves the distal urethra, the patient may remain continent and lose urine into the vagina only at the time of voiding.

A communication between the urinary bladder and the vagina can be demonstrated by instilling sterile milk or a dye (methylene blue or indigo carmine) into the bladder via a catheter and watching it pass through into the vagina on speculum examination. If leakage of urine into the vagina cannot be demonstrated in this fashion, the defect probably is ureteral and can be demonstrated by giving the patient methylene blue tablets by mouth and later finding a blue stain on a cotton pledget placed in the vagina.

B. UROLOGIC EXAMINATION

Cystoscopy and x-ray studies of the urinary tract will localize the urinary tract opening of the fistulous tract. Occasionally, the fistulous tracts are branching or multiple.

Treatment

Urinary tract fistulas rarely close spontaneously. Most must be repaired surgically, but sufficient time should elapse after diagnosis to allow for resolution of edema and inflammatory reactions. Otherwise, attempts at repair are likely to be unsuccessful. The use of cortisone as an anti-inflammatory agent has been challenged, and surgical results are excellent without its use. Urinary tract infections should be treated and skin excoriation and infection resolved before surgical correction is attempted.

Ureterovaginal fistulas are repaired by performing a ureteroureterostomy or by implanting the severed ureter into the bladder (ureteroneocystostomy). Attempts at conservative measures to close vesicovaginal fistulas include prolonged Foley drainage or cauterization with silver nitrate or electrocautery. Surgery via both abdominal (suprapubic) and vaginal approaches are used to repair vesicovaginal fistulas, and a number of techniques are available (layered closure, partial colpocleisis). Regardless of the method used, the principles of repair are the same: meticulous technique, using fine suture material; approximation of broad surfaces without tension; and maintenance of bladder decompression postoperatively until healing can occur. Improvement in surgical outcomes will increase with the use of interpositioning grafts.

Radiation fistulas are more complex because of tissue ischemia. They may require the introduction of a new blood supply provided by bulbocavernosus or gracilis myocutaneous flaps for successful repair.

RECTOVAGINAL & SIGMOIDOVAGINAL FISTULAS

Rectovaginal fistulas can occur as a result of obstetric injury, surgical procedures, cervical cancer, radiation therapy, inflammatory bowel disease, or diverticulitis. The symptoms are those of incontinence of flatus or feces through the vagina. Foul vaginal discharge with or without blood may be the presenting sign. The vaginal ostium usually can be demonstrated by speculum examination, and a probe passed through the fistulous tract can be palpated by the rectal diagnosing finger. A sigmoidovaginal fistula may require colonoscopy or retrograde dye studies.

Low rectovaginal fistulas near the introitus should be repaired after the surrounding inflammatory reaction and edema have subsided. This may require 3–4 months from the time of diagnosis. Those found high in the vagina—particularly fistulas resulting from radiation therapy—are often best managed with an initial diverting colostomy which is then closed 2–3 months after a successful repair. Before surgical repair of a rectovaginal fistula, the bowel should be prepared with a low-residue diet, antibiotics, cleansing enemas, and oral bowel-emptying agents.

Fistulas that are related to inflammatory bowel disease (Crohn's disease) carry a very poor prognosis and usually will not heal when repair is attempted unless the disease is clearly in remission. Ileostomy and abdominoperineal resection are necessary in patients whose symptoms are unacceptable despite medical management. Fistulas that occur as a result of cancer are not amenable to surgical repair. A diverting colostomy may give the patient considerable comfort.

Tancer ML et al: Genital fistulas secondary to diverticular disease of the colon: a review. Obstet Gynec Surv 1996;51:67.

Woo HH et al. The treatment of vesicovaginal fistulae. Eur Urol 1996;29:1.

■ BENIGN TUMORS OF THE VULVA & VAGINA

Elena A. Gates, MD

Hidradenoma

Hidradenomas are small, discrete, firm, mobile structures in the subcutaneous tissues of the labia or perianal region. These sweat gland tumors are benign but may be mistaken for cancer because of an adenomatous microscopic pattern. Treatment consists of local excision.

Sebaceous Cysts

Sebaceous cysts are small, raised, discrete, white cystic structures in the skin of the labia majora or minora that contain white sebaceous material. They may become infected, producing small abscesses. Most sebaceous cysts require no therapy. If they cause discomfort, simple excision is indicated.

Bartholin Cyst

Bartholin cysts—typically cysts of the gland duct—occur secondary to inflammation and occlusion of the duct opening. Located deep to the posterior labium majus, they vary in size from 1 cm to several centimeters in diameter. The larger masses tend to bulge into the vestibule of the vulva and the lower vagina. They may be asymptomatic or may cause local pressure symptoms and dyspareunia. Secondary infection occurs frequently, producing a painful abscess.

Symptomatic cysts and low-grade abscesses can be drained using a small mushroom catheter or word catheter introduced through a stab incision in the fluctuant medial aspect of the mass just cephalad to the hymen. The catheter should remain in place for 2 weeks to allow the tract to epithelialize and act as a new duct opening. In the event of surrounding cellulitis, antibiotic therapy can be added. If drainage fails, the cyst can be marsupialized. Rarely, excision of the gland itself is required.

Solid nodules within a Bartholin cyst should be biopsied to evaluate for malignancy.

Gartner Duct Cysts

These occur as small round or fusiform cystic swellings beneath the mucosa of the anterolateral wall of the vagina. They arise from remnants of the vaginal portion of the mesonephric (wolffian) duct and contain a clear serous fluid. They are usually asymptomatic and are discovered in the course of routine physical examination. Occasionally, they reach 5–6 cm in size. Small asymptomatic cysts require no therapy. Larger masses should be excised.

■ ENDOMETRIOSIS

Marcelle Cedars, MD

Endometriosis is the presence of functioning endometrial tissue in extrauterine sites, most commonly the ovaries, the uterosacral ligaments, and the cul-de-sac peritoneum. Other sites are the uterine tubes, the serosal surface of the uterus, the rectovaginal septum, the sigmoid colon, the pelvic peritoneum, and the small intestine (Figure 42–1). Ectopic endometrium has been found in the umbilicus, in abdominal scars, and (rarely)

Figure 42–1. Endometriosis.

in the breasts, the extremities, the pleural cavity, and the lungs.

Endometriosis is thought to occur by one or more of three mechanisms: (1) retrograde menstruation and implantation; (2) müllerian metaplasia of coelomic epithelium; and (3) lymphatic and venous dissemination. Retrograde menstruation through the uterine tubes is common. What is not known is what favors the growth and development of these tissues in the peritoneal cavity in some women and its regression and resorption in others. In some women, menstrual endometrium implants on the surface of the ovaries and falls by gravity into the cul-de-sac (pouch of Douglas), where it implants and responds to the cyclic hormonal influences of the menstrual cycle, shedding and bleeding at the time of menstruation. Conditions favoring retrograde passage of menstrual flow—eg, cervical stenosis or congenital anomalies such as vaginal atresia or transverse vaginal septum—predispose to endometriosis.

The reported prevalence of endometriosis is generally accepted to be 10–20%. Diagnosis at the time of laparoscopy for infertility may be as high as 20–47% while patients undergoing laparoscopy for tubal sterilization have an incidence of only 1–5%. The incidence of endometriosis appears to increase with several social and environmental factors such as delayed childbearing, a family history of the disease, declining use of oral contraceptive pills, and exposure to some toxins (such as dioxin).

It has been claimed that teenagers do not have endometriosis, but newer information suggests otherwise. Endometriosis may rarely occur following menopause but almost always in response to hormonal replacement therapy.

Carcinoma has been known to develop in areas of endometriosis within the pelvis and usually takes the form of endometrioid adenocarcinoma. Adenoacanthomas and endometrial stromal sarcomas have been reported, but these also are quite rare.

Classification

A staging system for endometriosis has been developed by the American Fertility Society (AFS)—now the American Society of Reproductive Medicine. The Revised AFS classification system now accepted worldwide is useful in that the inspection required for staging requires meticulous evaluation of the entire pelvis. Unfortunately, this staging system is only broadly predictive of outcome with treatment and may not correlate at all with patient pain. A newer system that recognizes the varied presentation of endometriosis (eg, atypical and deep infiltrating implants) and reflects scientifically based scores as a marker for disease activity has been suggested. (See accompanying box.)

STAGING OF ENDOMETRIOSIS

Minimal, mild (stages I and II)
  a. Scattered pelvic implants over the peritoneal surfaces of the pelvis (< 4 cm total).
  b. Rare superficial implants on ovaries.
  c. No significant adhesive disease.

Moderate (stage III)
  a. Multiple implants or small endometriomas (< 3 cm) involving one or both ovaries.
  b. Minimal periovarian or peritubal adhesions.
  c. Scattered implants with scarring on other structures.

Severe (stage IV)
  a. Large ovarian endometriomas (> 3 cm).
  b. Significant periovarian or peritubal adhesions.
  c. Tubal obstruction.
  d. Obliteration of cul-de-sac.
  e. Bowel or bladder adhesions.

Clinical Findings

A. SYMPTOMS AND SIGNS

Endometriosis has various presentations. Some patients with extensive disease—even with large bilateral ovarian endometriomas—may remain asymptomatic. Others with small peritoneal implants may be incapacitated by pain. The disease is typically first manifested as dysmenorrhea developing in the third or fourth decade. This may progress to pain that occurs not only with menstruation but also for several days preceding or following menses. This pain is often accompanied by dyspareunia and tenesmus. Some women complain of low back pain and of painful defecation associated with the menstrual period. This symptom is quite characteristic of cul-de-sac and rectovaginal septum involvement. Patients may also have pain in the buttock or radiating down the leg from involvement in the sciatic nerve.

Bladder involvement may cause a suprapubic pressure-type pain with or without dysuria and hematuria at the time of menstruation. Involvement of the bladder mucosa is quite rare. If an endometriotic implant involves the peritoneum overlying the ureter, the resulting tissue reaction may produce hydroureter and hydronephrosis with flank and lower abdominal pain.

Bowel obstruction may occur when endometrial implantation involves the small or large bowel. Mechanical ileus may result from the numerous dense adhesions that form as a result of the inflammatory reaction in response to cyclic bleeding from peritoneal implants.

Rupture of a large ovarian endometrial cyst occasionally causes symptoms of an acute abdominal emergency. Treatment is important to prevent pelvic adhesions and future infertility.

In some cases the only symptom is infertility. Endometriosis should be considered in all infertile patients.

B. PELVIC EXAMINATION

Bimanual pelvic examination is essential for assessment of the mobility of the uterus and the presence of adnexal masses. Rectovaginal examination is the only way the cul-de-sac, the uterosacral ligaments, and the posterior wall of the uterine corpus can be adequately palpated. The ovaries frequently are prolapsed and adherent to the posterior leaf of the broad ligament lateral to the cul-de-sac and are best felt by the rectal finger. Examination just preceding the menstrual period is the best time for palpation of the characteristic shotty nodules in the pouch of Douglas. Suspicious findings on pelvic examination should be further evaluated by ultrasound. The presence of isoechoic masses within the ovaries is highly suggestive of endometrioma.

C. SPECIAL EXAMINATIONS

Serum concentrations of CA-125 are elevated (> 35 units/mL) in approximately one-third of patients with advanced disease. As a screening test, CA-125 lacks specificity and sensitivity, but in patients with advanced disease it may serve as a marker of recurrence of disease after treatment.

Laparoscopic examination is required to establish the diagnosis. A finding of characteristic raspberry or blueberry implants of ectopic tissue or the powder-burn marks of scarred endometrium is diagnostic. Endometriosis may also appear in "atypical" lesions recognized as red glandular excrescences, petechiae, white nodules (subperitoneal glands) or clear vesicular lesions. These may, in fact, be more active disease than the classic powder-burn bluish-gray lesions. Any questionable lesions should be biopsied and sent for pathologic diagnosis. The diagnosis requires the presence of glands and stroma in the ectopic site. Microscopic disease is sometimes evident as a ground-glass appearance of the peritoneum. Laparotomy is rarely necessary and may involve major resection of the pelvic organs or bowel.

Prevention

The early diagnosis and treatment of menstrual obstruction (dilation of the cervix, hymenotomy, metroplasty, removal of vaginal septum) may help to prevent or delay the development of endometriosis in those pa-

tients with outflow obstruction. Early multiparity appears to prevent the development of endometriosis. There is evidence that long-term contraceptive pill users are less likely to develop endometriosis, particularly if the pill contains a small amount of estrogen in combination with a potent progestin.

Treatment

Treatment should be tailored to fit the circumstances with respect to the age of the patient, her symptoms, her desire for children, and the extent of the disease. Therapy may vary, therefore, from mere observation, reassurance, and analgesia if necessary to complete surgical removal of the uterus, tubes, and ovaries. A conservative approach is recommended for the patient who is symptom-free or only mildly symptomatic and with minimal pelvic findings such as slightly tender cul-de-sac nodules. Regular examinations should be scheduled at intervals of not more than 6 months. Evidence of progression of the disease—in the form of either increasing symptomatology, infertility, or the development of pelvic masses—requires more specific treatment.

A. MEDICAL TREATMENT

All medical treatment induces a remission and not a cure of endometriosis. Recurrence of symptoms is common when treatment is discontinued. Long-term suppression with oral contraceptive pills should be considered in all women, but particularly those who have had a recurrence of symptoms following prior successful treatment. Medical treatment is not indicated for endometriosis associated with infertility.

The induction of amenorrhea has been successful in bringing about regression in a high percentage of patients with endometriosis. This may be accomplished in several ways:

1. Danazol—This synthetic androgen derived from ethisterone has been found to be effective in the medical treatment of endometriosis. It acts by suppressing the secretion of gonadotropins. It is given in doses of 200–800 mg daily and continued without interruption for 6–9 months. Drawbacks are expense and androgenic side effects.

2. Progestins—Norethynodrel, norethindrone acetate, and medroxyprogesterone acetate are the agents most commonly used. Continuous progestins induce amenorrhea (although breakthrough bleeding may occur). Symptomatic improvement is reported in up to 80% of patients. Induction of decidualization and ultimately necrosis in the implants as well as cessation of menses seem to be important in the response. This treatment can be continued for 6–12 months or longer in some patients. Side effects include breakthrough bleeding, fluid retention, and headaches.

3. Oral contraceptive pills—The production of a pseudopregnancy state through hormonal therapy with combined estrogen and progestin is another alternative. Treatment with cyclic or continuous oral contraceptive pills for 6–12 months is effective in about 80% of patients. This treatment can be continued long-term until fertility is desired. The most frequent indication for prolonged use is recurrent endometriosis following a conservative operation or other medical therapies. Side effects are nausea, breast tenderness, fluid retention, and breakthrough bleeding.

4. GnRH analogs—The analogs of gonadotropin-releasing hormone (eg, leuprolide, nafarelin, goserelin) act by down-regulation of the GnRH receptor in the pituitary and elimination of FSH and LH secretion. Without gonadotropin secretion, estradiol levels fall to the castrate range. In the face of this hypoestrogenism, endometrial implants regress and about 80% of patients report symptomatic improvement. Side effects are those of menopause with vasomotor symptoms, vaginal dryness, sleep disturbances and moodiness, and bone loss with long-term treatment. So-called "add-back" therapy with either norethindrone acetate or combined hormone replacement therapy reduces side effects while not interfering with efficacy.

B. Surgical Treatment

The surgical approach to endometriosis may be designed to improve fertility, prevent further progression of the disease with preservation of the ovaries, or eliminate the disease by removal of the uterus and adnexal structures. Surgical treatment is required for large endometriomas (> 4 cm) as these will not respond to medical therapy. Their persistence may increase the risk for destruction of normal ovarian tissue and for premature development of diminished ovarian reserve.

1. Conservative surgery—Preservation of childbearing function by removal or cauterization of implants, freeing up of tubal adhesions, presacral neurectomy for the relief of pain, and perhaps by uterine suspension is indicated for the patient who desires to preserve childbearing capacity and has failed medical therapy. Conservative surgery in which an attempt to preserve a single ovary at the time of hysterectomy and oophorectomy for severe disease carries a 20% risk for a subsequent surgery to remove the remaining ovary. Laparoscopic surgery on an ambulatory basis has all but eliminated the need for laparotomy.

2. Definitive surgery—This requires the removal of the uterus and the tubes and ovaries. Since endometriosis is dependent upon ovarian function for its continued growth and development, total hysterectomy and bilateral salpingo-oophorectomy should be done in patients with extensive disease, particularly those with bowel involvement. It is critically important not to mistake bowel implants for cancer. Unnecessary abdominoperineal resections have been performed in young women for unrecognized endometriosis. Provided there has been a preoperative bowel preparation, bowel implants can be locally resected.

Oral estrogen replacement therapy in the form of conjugated estrogens, 0.625–1.25 mg/d, may be given without danger of exacerbating the endometriotic process. The use of estrogen-progestin combinations is not required. A 6 month course of continuous progestins may reduce vasomotor symptoms, protect the bone, and allow suppression of residual disease. Estrogen replacement therapy may then be instituted.

Henzl MR et al: Administration of nasal nafarelin as compared with oral danazol for endometriosis: a multicenter double-blind comparative clinical trial. N Engl J Med 1988; 318:485.

Hoeger KM et al: An update on the classification of endometriosis. Clin Obstet Gynecol 1999 Sep;42:611.

Hughes E et al: Ovulation suppression for endometriosis. Cochrane Database Syst Rev 2000;CD000155.

Lebovic DI et al: Immunobiology of endometriosis. Fertil Steril 2001;75:1.

Moore J et al: Modern combined oral contraceptives for pain associated with endometriosis. Cochrane Database Syst Rev 2000;CD001019.

Reddy S et al: Treatment of endometriosis. Clin Obstet Gynecol 1998;41:387.

ADENOMYOSIS

Lee Learman, MD, PhD

Adenomyosis occurs when fingers of endometrium extend into the myometrium to a depth greater than two low-power microscopic fields. It may be a focal or a diffuse process and may involve the entire thickness of the myometrium. The pathogenesis is not known, but the theory of direct growth of the basal layer of endometrium into the myometrium is widely accepted. Estrogen has been implicated as a stimulus to the development of adenomyosis, and the symptomatic improvement that occurs with the onset of menopause supports this concept. The disease is seen most often in the decade preceding menopause.

Clinical Findings

The condition is most common in women between ages 35 and 50 and leads to hypermenorrhea, polymenorrhea, or intermenstrual bleeding with dysmenorrhea or dyspareunia. It may be associated with endometriosis. Examination will reveal a slightly to moderately enlarged symmetric, mobile uterus that may be tender to palpation, particularly in the premenstrual phase of the cycle.

The preoperative diagnosis of adenomyosis is very difficult. MRI is somewhat more effective than ultrasonography in suggesting the diagnosis. The use of needle biopsy of the uterus has been reported as a means of diagnosing the condition, though the sensitivity of this approach is only fair. The definitive diagnosis is made by pathologic examination of uterine tissue, generally after hysterectomy.

Differential Diagnosis

Adenomyosis must be distinguished principally from leiomyomas of the uterus. An analogous condition, endolymphatic stromal myosis (stromal endometriosis, low-grade stromal sarcoma), although histologically benign, clinically behaves as a low-grade cancer. Connective tissue cells resembling those of the endometrial stroma infiltrate the lymphatic and venous spaces of the myometrium, and the process may extend into the vessels of the broad ligament, in which event local recurrence is possible following hysterectomy. Metastases to the ovary, peritoneal surfaces, and lung have been reported in rare cases. This disease, usually of the postmenopausal years, is very rare and should not be confused with adenomyosis.

Treatment

Total hysterectomy with or without bilateral salpingo-oophorectomy is curative. Hormonal approaches that are successful in treating endometriosis are also useful. These include continuous progestin therapy administered orally, by depot injection, or as an intrauterine system, and gonadotropin-releasing hormone analogs.

Prognosis

Adenomyosis is a self-limited process that undergoes spontaneous regression, becoming asymptomatic after the menopause.

Fedele L et al: Treatment of adenomyosis-associated menorrhagia with a levonorgestrel-releasing intrauterine device. Fertil Steril 1997;68:426.

Vercellini P et al: Treatment with a gonadotropin releasing hormone agonist before endometrial resection: a multicentre, randomised controlled trial. Br J Obstet Gynaecol 1996; 103:562.

Vercellini P et al: Transvaginal ultrasonography versus uterine needle biopsy in the diagnosis of diffuse adenomyosis. Hum Reprod 1998;13:2884.

■ LEIOMYOMAS OF THE UTERUS

Alison Jacoby, MD

Leiomyomas of the uterus are found in at least 20% of women over age 30. The true prevalence is unknown because most women with myomas have no symptoms. Black women have a threefold to ninefold higher incidence than white women. Myomas arise from proliferation of a single clone of uterine smooth muscle cells under the influence of estrogen, progesterone, and other growth factors. As a result, myomas often have an increased growth rate during pregnancy and a cessation of growth after menopause. They are usually multiple and can be located within the myometrium (intramural), beneath the external surface (subserous), or adjacent to the endometrium (submucous). Other types of myomas are intraligamentous (between the leaves of the broad ligament), parasitic (detached from the uterus and deriving blood supply from other abdominal organs), and cervical. Myomas may vary in size from tiny "seedlings" to massive tumors filling the entire pelvis and abdomen.

On cut section, leiomyomas are well-circumscribed, pearly-gray, solid tumors with a pseudocapsule and a whorled appearance. Microscopically, myomas are composed of fascicles of uniform, spindle-shaped smooth muscle cells. Mitotic figures are rare. Other common features include hyaline, cystic, and carneous degeneration, edema, calcifications, and focal hemorrhage.

Clinical Findings

A. SYMPTOMS AND SIGNS

The clinical presentation depends on the location, number, and size of the myomas. Although myomas are frequently discovered in the course of a routine pelvic examination, the majority of these women have no symptoms. The most common symptoms reported are heavy, prolonged menses, a sensation of pelvic pressure, abdominal distention, and urinary frequency. In addition, women can develop urinary retention, dyspareunia, low back pain, and constipation. When degenerative changes occur, mild symptoms may suddenly become severe and require treatment. Submucous and intracavitary myomas are liable to cause heavy, prolonged and frequent bleeding, at times alarmingly profuse. These myomas may become pedunculated and protrude through the cervix.

Palpation of the uterus reveals an irregular and enlarged structure that may be felt on abdominal examination. It is usually firm and nontender but may become soft and tender following an episode of degeneration.

Hydronephrosis can occur from external compression of the ureters by the enlarged uterus.

B. Laboratory Findings

Anemia may result from acute or chronic blood loss. An endometrial biopsy should be performed in women with abnormal uterine bleeding to rule out endometrial hyperplasia and cancer.

C. Imaging Studies

Pelvic sonography is the most useful radiographic study for diagnosing leiomyomas. When a submucous myoma is suspected clinically, saline sonohysterography and hysteroscopy are useful for visualizing the contour of the uterine cavity. MRI is reserved for evaluation of a radiographically atypical leiomyoma and for the precise localization of myomas prior to myomectomy.

Differential Diagnosis

Before surgery, it can be difficult to distinguish a uterine myoma from a uterine sarcoma (leiomyosarcoma, endometrial stromal sarcoma, and mixed mesodermal tumor). However, the incidence of uterine sarcoma among women operated on for uterine myomas is extremely low (0.23%). Even rapidly growing myomas, defined as an increase by 6 weeks gestational size in 1 year, are unlikely to be malignant. However, a postmenopausal woman with an enlarging uterine mass, especially if accompanied by vaginal bleeding, should be evaluated for sarcoma.

Solid ovarian tumors and pedunculated subserous myomas may be difficult to differentiate on physical examination. Pelvic sonography is useful. MRI or laparoscopy is sometimes necessary to identify the origin of the mass. Enlargement of the uterus by a myoma may mimic a pregnant uterus or vice versa. A pregnancy test should be done in all suspected cases.

Complications

Hemorrhage from a submucous myoma or chronic menorrhagia often results in secondary iron deficiency anemia. Patients with torsion of a pedunculated subserous myoma present with severe pain and evidence of an acute abdomen.

Infertility may occur secondary to myomas, particularly if the uterine cavity is enlarged or distorted by a submucous myoma. Miscarriage, preterm labor, premature rupture of membranes, and postpartum hemorrhage can be caused by myomas. Rarely, a large myoma in the lower uterine segment can obstruct passage of the fetus during labor. The majority of women with myomas have uncomplicated pregnancies and deliveries.

Treatment

Asymptomatic myomas require no therapy. Reexamination is recommended every 6–12 months to assess symptoms and record the rate of growth. Women with heavy, prolonged, or frequent episodes of bleeding can benefit from a trial of cyclic or continuous birth control pills or progestins. GnRH agonists decrease myoma size and stop menstruation prior to surgery. Long-term use of GnRH agonists causes osteoporosis, and myomas regrow soon after the medication is discontinued.

For women with pelvic pressure or bleeding unresponsive to medical management, several surgical and nonsurgical treatment options are available. Women who have not completed childbearing usually undergo a myomectomy, though women who do not desire pregnancy often choose this option as well. Myomectomy can be performed by laparotomy, laparoscopy, or hysteroscopy depending on the location, number, and size of the myomas. Women who have completed childbearing and seek an alternative to hysterectomy may benefit from uterine artery embolization. This nonsurgical procedure involves diminishing blood flow to the uterus. Subsequently, the uterus and myomas decrease in size by 30–50% and symptoms such as heavy bleeding and pelvic pressure improve in 80–90% of women. Hysterectomy is definitive treatment for women with symptomatic myomas. Alternatives to total abdominal hysterectomy include vaginal hysterectomy, supracervical hysterectomy, and laparoscopic hysterectomy.

Prognosis

Myomas are benign neoplasms. There is no evidence that myomas can transform into sarcomas. Myomectomy results in symptom improvement in 80% of women. The risk of recurrence following myomectomy is approximately 25%, but only 10% of these women require a second operation. The outcome following uterine artery embolization appears favorable, but the duration of follow-up in the published literature is 3 years or less. Hysterectomy is definitive therapy for myomas.

Hurst BS et al: Uterine artery embolization for symptomatic uterine myomas. Fertil Steril 2000;74:855.

■ ADNEXAL MASSES

Lisa Everson, MD

Adnexal masses are abnormal structures found in the ovary, uterine tube, or broad ligament. It is often impossible to determine the origin of adnexal masses by physical examination or radiographically.

The differential diagnosis of adnexal masses is broad (see Table 42–1). The majority are benign, though the likelihood of malignancy increases significantly with age. It is estimated that approximately 13% of persistent adnexal masses are malignant in 13% of premenopausal women and in 45% of women who are postmenopausal.

MANAGEMENT OF ADNEXAL MASSES

Functional Cysts

The most common adnexal mass in a premenopausal woman is either a follicular or corpus luteum cyst. While these functional cysts typically measure 3 cm or less, they can reach sizes up to 8–10 cm. Functional cysts are usually self-limited and will regress over time. Follow-up examination with ultrasound after 4–6 weeks will reveal a decrease in size, and nearly all will ultimately resolve without treatment. Oral contraceptives are often initiated at the time of identification of a presumed functional cyst. While this practice may prevent development of a second functional cyst that could ultrasonographically mimic the original cyst—giving the impression that no reduction in size has taken place—the clinical benefit of oral contraceptives in this setting has not been clearly demonstrated.

While the vast majority of functional cysts resolve without incident, they will occasionally rupture or cause torsion of the ovary, resulting in severe acute abdominal pain. Torsion requires prompt surgical inter-

Table 42–1. Differential diagnosis of adnexal masses.

Follicular or corpus luteum cyst
Mature cystic teratoma
Immature teratoma
Cystadenofibroma
Endometrioma
Serous or mucinous cystadenoma
Epithelial ovarian carcinoma
Tumors of low malignant potential
Sertoli-Leydig cell tumor
Theca lutein cyst
Granulosa cell tumor
Fibroma
Thecoma
Endodermal sinus tumor
Choriocarcinoma
Uterine tube carcinoma
Paraovarian or paratubal cyst
Hydrosalpinx
Pedunculated leiomyoma

vention to untwist the vascular infundibulopelvic ligament before significant ischemia and necrosis of the ovary occurs so that the ovary can be preserved. This is frequently accomplished laparoscopically. Cyst rupture can occur spontaneously or at the time of sexual intercourse. Once a diagnosis of cyst rupture is made, the decision for inpatient or outpatient management depends on the degree of pain, the hemodynamic stability of the patient, and the certainty of the diagnosis. Typically, a woman will be observed in a hospital setting for 24 hours, allowing for the administration of intravenous analgesia and serial examinations and blood counts. Recovery is usually rapid. Occasionally, a ruptured functional cyst will demonstrate ongoing bleeding requiring operation to achieve hemostasis. This is usually accomplished by cautery via laparoscopic access. If this is unsuccessful, cystectomy is indicated.

Persistent Adnexal Masses

Adnexal masses that do not decrease in size over time are likely to be neoplasms. Differentiating benign from malignant masses is one of the challenges in women's health care. Benign masses can generally be removed effectively by the general gynecologic surgeon, often endoscopically, while malignancies are more effectively treated by specialists with training in appropriate surgical staging and maximal cytoreduction, which are important in optimizing the outcome.

Transvaginal ultrasonography is an important tool in evaluation of the uterine adnexa. It has been shown to have a sensitivity for identifying malignant neoplasms of about 90%. However, the specificity has been reported at about 60%. In an effort to improve specificity without sacrificing sensitivity, a number of diagnostic models based on combinations of ultrasonographic features, age, serum CA-125 measurements, and menopausal status have been devised. Unfortunately, attempts at prospective external validation of these models have found them to be less accurate than initially reported. MRI appears to have a promising role in the characterization of adnexal masses, but its sensitivity is somewhat less than that of ultrasound, in particular for early stage tumors of low-malignant potential.

Because it is difficult with radiographic and laboratory evaluation to determine conclusively if persistent adnexal masses are benign or malignant, persistent adnexal masses should generally be surgically removed either laparoscopically or via laparotomy. The size of the mass, its sonographic appearance, and one's level of concern about malignancy are all factors in choosing the operative approach. The decision to perform cystectomy or oophorectomy is typically based on the degree of concern for malignancy, as well as the age of the patient. Ovarian conservation is generally attempted in women under 45, as they can expect to have at least 5 more years of ovarian steroidogenesis prior to menopause. Masses with worrisome sonographic features should be removed by oophorectomy. This allows for complete histologic examination of the ovary. In addition, although intraoperative spillage of malignant cyst fluid into the peritoneal cavity has not been conclusively shown to worsen the outcome, it seems prudent to avoid rupture of the cyst during removal. Oophorectomy probably minimizes the risk of intraoperative cyst rupture.

If a menopausal woman with a cystic adnexal mass is not a good candidate for surgery or simply wants to avoid operation, one can cite several series demonstrating that simple unilocular cysts measuring less than 5 cm in women with low serum CA-125 levels have a very small likelihood of being malignant. However, occasional malignancies have been found even when these criteria are met. Carefully following these women and recommending operation if the cyst size or characteristics change considerably is a reasonable option in such cases.

Aslam N et al: Prospective evaluation of three different models for the pre-operative diagnosis of ovarian cancer. Br J Obstet Gynaecol 2000;107:1347.

Dottino PR et al: Laparoscopic management of adnexal masses in premenopausal and postmenopausal women. Obstet Gynecol 1999;93:223.

Gallup DG et al: Management of the adnexal mass in the 1990s. South Med J 1997;90:972.

Kinkel K et al: US characterization of ovarian masses: a meta-analysis. Radiology 2000;217:803.

■ ECTOPIC PREGNANCY

Mindy Goldman, MD

The incidence of ectopic pregnancy has increased with the use of advanced reproductive technologies, occurring in approximately two in every 100 pregnancies. Given that many ectopic pregnancies are now diagnosed and treated in clinicians' offices, the true incidence of ectopic pregnancy is probably underestimated. Death as a result of ectopic pregnancy has decreased because of earlier diagnosis and currently is about 0.3% of ectopic pregnancies. Risk factors for ectopic pregnancy include prior ectopic pregnancy, conditions that lead to tubal scarring such as pelvic inflammatory disease and prior pelvic surgery, a history of infertility, in vitro fertilization, current IUD use, smoking, diethylstilbestrol exposure, and increased age. The largest risk is felt to be due to salpingitis, with about a sevenfold increased risk of an ectopic pregnancy after acute pelvic inflammatory disease. Infertility patients who have undergone in vitro fertilization are at special risk.

Ninety-five percent of ectopic pregnancies occur in the uterine tube, usually in the ampullary portion. Less common locations include interstitial or cornual pregnancies, which can cause significant intraperitoneal bleeding if rupture occurs, and, more rarely, pregnancies in the abdomen, ovary, or cervix. In vitro fertilization has also increased the rate of heterotopic pregnancy, which is the occurrence of an intrauterine pregnancy with an ectopic, but this is rare.

Fertilization normally occurs in the outer third of the uterine tube, and anything that inhibits transport of the fertilized zygote can result in implantation within the wall of the tube. As the fertilized ovum implants within the tube, there is vascular engorgement and trophoblastic invasion that may weaken the wall of the tube. This can lead to rupture with marked blood loss into the peritoneal cavity. Early diagnosis can help prevent rupture and subsequent complications, including shock and death.

Clinical Findings

A. SYMPTOMS AND SIGNS

The clinical signs and symptoms of an ectopic pregnancy can be variable. Fortunately, because of earlier diagnosis, most women do not present with the classic signs of rupture, including severe abdominal pain and hemodynamic instability. Typically, patients present with amenorrhea and some degree of vaginal bleeding with or without pelvic pain. An adnexal mass may be present on pelvic examination, but findings may be as subtle as vaginal spotting without other clinical symptoms. The uterus is usually slightly enlarged because of decidualization of the endometrium resulting from increased estrogen and progesterone levels.

B. LABORATORY FINDINGS AND IMAGING STUDIES

Laboratory evaluation may show a low hematocrit, particularly if there are clinical signs of rupture. Because the clinical presentation can vary considerably, other tests such as transvaginal ultrasound and serum β-hCG are useful in distinguishing an ectopic from a threatened spontaneous abortion and a failed intrauterine pregnancy. In some cases, serum progesterone levels or findings on suction curettage may be helpful in diagnosis.

1. Human chorionic gonadotropin and transvaginal ultrasound—Trophoblastic cells of the chorionic villi produce β-hCG after implantation of the blastocyst. In early pregnancy, β-hCG typically rises in a curvilinear fashion, doubling approximately every 48 hours. For practical purposes, a rise of at least 66% should be observed every 48 hours until levels plateau at a gestational age of 7–8 weeks. In general, ectopic pregnancies have lower values of β-hCG and subnormal increases, but 15% of ectopics may have normal doubling times. An absolute β-hCG does not permit distinction between an ectopic and a nonviable intrauterine pregnancy. Another problem with β-hCG evaluation is the existence of different reference standards for β-hCG assays, so it is important to ensure that serial values are reported from the same standard.

The use of transvaginal ultrasound has allowed intrauterine pregnancies to be diagnosed at an earlier gestational age, usually within 5 weeks of the last menstrual period. In general, transvaginal sonography allows anatomic landmarks to be seen about 1 week earlier than transabdominal sonography. The concept of a "discriminatory β-hCG zone," defined as a threshold value above which an intrauterine gestational sac should be seen by endovaginal sonography, is highly predictive for diagnosing an ectopic pregnancy unless a multiple gestation is present. The discriminatory zone value varies depending on the β-hCG assay, the reference standard, and the quality of ultrasound resolution. For the First and Second International Reference Preparations (IRP), the value is usually between 1000 and 2000 mIU/mL. Institutions should determine their own discriminatory β-hCG level depending on the assay used and skills of the ultrasonographers. Other findings that ultrasound can detect include free fluid in the cul-de-sac and in some cases an adnexal gestational mass.

2. Serum progesterone—Serum progesterone levels increase during pregnancy, and viable intrauterine pregnancies tend to have higher levels than spontaneous abortions and ectopic pregnancies. In most studies, progesterone levels < 5 ng/mL are associated with abnormal pregnancies and levels > 25 ng/mL are consistent with viable pregnancies. Absolute values vary with ectopic pregnancies, and in many laboratories the assay is not immediately available, thus limiting the practical utility of this test.

3. Suction curettage—If the β-hCG value is less than the discriminatory zone and β-hCG titers have plateaued or are rising abnormally, suction curettage may be helpful in distinguishing between a nonviable intrauterine pregnancy and an ectopic gestation. In a woman without signs of spontaneous abortion the absence of chorionic villi on curettage in the presence of an elevated hCG is predictive of an ectopic pregnancy, though in very early gestations products may be missed by curettage.

Treatment

Treatment of ectopic pregnancy has been traditionally surgical, with procedures done to remove the ectopic gestation and preserve as much uterine tube as possible.

Procedures include salpingostomy, where the ectopic pregnancy is removed through an incision in the antimesenteric aspect of the tube, leaving the remainder of the tube intact; and partial salpingectomy, where the involved portion of the tube is removed. In cases of extensive tubal damage, complete salpingectomy is recommended. In the past, laparotomy was required, but the laparoscopic approach is now preferred unless the patient is hemodynamically compromised. If conservative approaches such as salpingostomy are used, β-hCG titers should be followed after the procedure to make certain that no viable trophoblastic tissue remains.

For many patients, medical management with the folic acid antagonist methotrexate is a viable option. Criteria include a hemodynamically stable patient who is compliant and has no medical contraindication to methotrexate. Relative contraindications include an unruptured mass > 3.5 cm, fetal cardiac motion, or a β-hCG level > 15,000 mIU/mL, since these characteristics decrease the likelihood of success. Published success rates average 84% for single-dose therapy. There are algorithms for the use of methotrexate, though no standardized protocol has been defined. β-hCG levels are monitored until they fall to zero, and if levels have not fallen at a specified rate, a second dose may be required. Time to resolution can be quite variable and operation is needed for treatment failures. During methotrexate use, patients should discontinue folic acid supplements and refrain from sexual intercourse. They are instructed about ongoing risks of rupture. Patients who are Rh negative are given $RH_o(D)$ immune globulin whether treated medically or surgically. Other developments in medical management include the use of other agents such as potassium chloride, prostaglandins, and mifepristone, but these have not been studied as well as methotrexate.

As with spontaneous abortions, some patients with ectopic pregnancies may actually have spontaneous resolution. Expectant management of a documented ectopic pregnancy may be an option if β-hCG levels are declining rapidly and the patient is stable. Patients need to be aware of the risks of rupture and hemorrhage, and emergency management must be readily available.

Most studies show similar success rates for methotrexate and conservative surgical therapy (mainly salpingostomy). Future conception rates are felt to be similar, but more studies are needed regarding the impact of methotrexate on future fertility. In general, the approach to ectopic pregnancy today is to achieve earlier diagnosis in the unruptured state to minimize morbidity and mortality as well as allow for more conservative treatment options.

ACOG Practice Bulletin. Medical management of ectopic pregnancy. Number 3, December 1998. In: 2001 Compendium of Selected Publications. American College of Obstetricians and Gynecologists, 1998.

Lehner R et al: Ectopic pregnancy. Arch Gynecol Obstet 2000; 263:87.

Lipscomb GH et al: Nonsurgical treatment of ectopic pregnancy. N Engl J Med 2000;343:1325.

GYNECOLOGIC MALIGNANCIES

Lee-May Chen, MD, & Bethan Powell, MD

CARCINOMA OF THE VULVA

The vast majority (90–95%) of vulvar cancers are squamous cell carcinomas, and these tumors represent about 5% of all cancers of the female reproductive tract. Human papillomavirus (HPV) plays a role in etiology, but a relationship to invasive cancer has not been conclusively established. Vulvar intraepithelial neoplasia is considered precancerous and occurs more commonly in premenopausal women. Other types of vulvar cancer are Bartholin gland adenocarcinoma, Paget's disease of the vulva, basal cell carcinoma, malignant melanoma, and metastatic carcinoma from the cervix, endometrium, ovary, or elsewhere. Rarely, sarcomas are found arising primarily in the vulvar soft tissues.

The area most often involved is the labium majus (about 50% of cases). Approximately 25% of cases occur on the labium minus; the clitoris and Bartholin's gland are less common sites.

Metastasis to the regional lymph nodes (inguinal, femoral, iliac, and obturator) occurs in about 30% of operable lesions. Lymph node status is the most important factor predicting survival. Risk factors for node metastasis are clinical node status, age degree of differentiation, tumor stage, tumor thickness, depth of stromal invasion, and presence of capillary-lymphatic space invasion.

There is a high incidence of second primary cancers in vulvar cancer patients, particularly in the cervix, endometrium, and breast. Cancer of the vulva should be classified and clinically staged according to the recommendations of the Cancer Committee of the International Federation of Gynecology and Obstetrics (Table 42–2).

Clinical Findings

In situ squamous cell carcinoma of the vulva may be seen in women age 25–40 years as small, slightly raised or papillary (resembling condylomas) white, red, or brownish patches on the skin or mucosa. One-third of lesions are solitary, and two-thirds are multiple. The early invasive lesion is a small, elevated, superficial pap-

Table 42–2. FIGO staging for vulvar cancer.

Stage 0	Carcinoma in situ; intraepithelial carcinoma
Stage I	Tumor confined to the vulva or perineum; 2 cm or less in greatest dimension; no nodal metastasis
IA	Stromal invasion ≤ 1 mm
IB	Stromal invasion > 1 mm
Stage II	Tumor confined to the vulva or perineum; no more than 2 cm in greatest dimension; no nodal metastasis
Stage III	Tumor of any size with adjacent spread to the urethra, vagina, or anus or with unilateral regional lymph node metastasis
Stage IVA	Tumor invades upper urethra, bladder mucosa, rectal mucosa, pelvic bone; or bilateral regional node metastases
Stage IVB	Any distant metastasis, including pelvic lymph nodes

illary or ulcerated lesion with underlying subcutaneous induration. Late cancers present either as large, fungating, infected tumors or as shallow ulcers with indurated margins. The larger the primary lesion, the greater the chance of lymph node involvement; but palpatory evidence is misleading, as regional node enlargement may be related to secondary infection in these tumors. Furthermore, metastatic disease in the lymph nodes may not be palpable. There may be submucosal spread of the tumor cephalad to involve the vagina and urethra—or there may be involvement of the posterior vulva with invasion of the anus and rectum. All suspicious lesions should be examined frequently by biopsy.

Differential Diagnosis

Chronic hypertrophic and atrophic skin conditions may or may not be associated with vulvar cancer. Multiple biopsies are necessary to establish the correct diagnosis. Granulomatous venereal lesions of the vulva may be clinically suspicious, and biopsy of the involved area is mandatory. The complement fixation test may be helpful, but it must be remembered that granulomatous disease and cancer of the vulva may occur simultaneously.

Prevention

Treatment of precancerous lesions is thought to reduce the subsequent development of invasive carcinoma. Vulvar intraepithelial neoplasia is diagnosed by colposcopic examination after treatment of the vulva with

3–5% acetic acid. Lesions usually will appear white. Eliminating cigarette smoking may also contribute to the reduction of vulvar cancer.

Treatment

Vulvar intraepithelial neoplasia, if localized, may be treated by wide excision or laser vaporization. Skinning vulvectomy with split-thickness skin grafting, if necessary, is done for diffuse, multifocal disease.

Microinvasive lesions (< 1 mm invasion) are adequately treated by wide local excision with 1 cm margins. All other stage 1 lesions, if well lateralized, can be treated with radical local excision with a 2 cm margin along with an ipsilateral inguinofemoral nodal dissection. Contralateral groin dissection is performed if ipsilateral positive nodes are found. Medial stage 1 lesions and more advanced stages which are operable are treated with radical vulvectomy plus bilateral inguinofemoral lymph node dissection. Radiation therapy with concurrent chemosensitization is required for inoperable lesions and for cases with close margins or positive nodes.

Prognosis

Adequate surgery is effective in a high percentage of patients, even when there is evidence of spread to the inguinal and femoral nodes. When the nodes are not involved, 5-year cure rates of 90% are reported, and a 50% salvage rate is possible in the presence of lymph node involvement.

Creasman WT et al: The National Cancer Data Base report on early stage invasive vulvar carcinoma. The American College of Surgeons Commission on Cancer and the American Cancer Society. Cancer 1997;80:505.

Grendys EC Jr et al: Innovations in the management of vulvar carcinoma. Curr Opin Obstet Gynecol 2000;12:15.

CARCINOMA OF THE VAGINA

Carcinoma in situ of the vagina occurs either as a direct extension of the process from the portio vaginalis of the cervix or as a separate area in a "neoplastic field." It should be suspected whenever carcinoma in situ or invasive carcinoma of the vulva or cervix is present, and it may appear in the vagina many months or years after successful treatment of either of those two conditions. Carcinoma in situ of the vagina is most often diagnosed by cytologic examination, colposcopy, and biopsy of acetic acid-staining or Schiller-positive lesions, ie, those that do not take up the iodine stain after application of Lugol's solution. As in carcinoma of the cervix and vulva, human papillomavirus is an etiologic factor.

Treatment is by local excision of involved areas when they are few and small. Electrocautery, laser ther-

apy, and topical fluorouracil have been used; failure rates are 25–50%. Extensive involvement of the vaginal mucosa may require partial or complete vaginectomy with complete colpocleisis in the elderly, sexually inactive patient or with skin graft construction of an artificial vagina in the patient who wishes to retain coital function.

Invasive squamous cell carcinoma of the vagina, arising primarily from the vagina, is an unusual lesion, most cancers of the vagina being extensions from an epidermoid carcinoma of the cervix. The lesion is most often ulcerative, with a cauliflower configuration being less common. There is firm induration surrounding the ulcerative lesion, which is easily palpated, whereas a small, soft papillary lesion may be missed. The upper third of the vagina is the site in about 75% of patients. In many cases the only symptom is a bloody vaginal discharge, and the diagnosis is made by biopsy.

Treatment is by radiation therapy or radical surgery. Unfortunately, these tumors grow rapidly and insidiously, and in over 50% of patients they have penetrated the vaginal wall at the time of the initial examination. Involvement of the bladder and rectum is common. As a result, the overall 5-year survival figures are in the range of 20–30%.

Adenocarcinoma of the vagina has occurred in teenage girls, apparently arising in areas of vaginal adenosis (probably müllerian duct remnants). There appears to have been a relationship between the appearance of this tumor in these young patients and the administration of diethylstilbestrol to their mothers during the fetal life of the patient.

The classification and staging of carcinoma of the vagina is outlined in Table 42–3.

Table 42–3. FIGO staging for vaginal cancer.

Stage 0	Carcinoma in situ; intraepithelial carcinoma.
Stage I	The carcinoma is limited to the vaginal wall.
Stage II	The carcinoma has involved the subvaginal tissue but has not extended to the pelvic wall.
Stage III	The carcinoma has extended to the pelvic wall.
Stage IV	The carcinoma has extended beyond the true pelvis or has involved the mucosa of the bladder or rectum. Bullous edema as such does not permit a case to be alloted to stage IV.
IVA	Spread of the growth to adjacent organs or direct extension beyond the true pelvis.
IVB	Spread to distant organs.

Metastatic carcinoma of the vagina is much more common than primary vaginal carcinoma, the most frequent sources being the cervix, vulva, bladder, urethra, rectum, endometrium, and ovary.

Rare primary tumors of the vagina are sarcoma (mixed mesodermal tumors, including sarcoma botryoides of infants, fibrosarcoma, leiomyosarcoma, and hemangiosarcoma), adenocarcinoma arising from mesonephric (Gartner's) duct or müllerian duct remnants, embryonal carcinoma, and malignant melanoma. Radical surgical removal offers the best hope of cure for the majority of these neoplasms.

Fine BA et al: The curative potential of radiation therapy in the treatment of primary vaginal carcinoma. Am J Clin Oncol 1996;19:39.

Manetta A et al: Primary invasive carcinoma of the vagina. Obstet Gynecol 1990;76:639.

CARCINOMA OF THE CERVIX

Carcinoma of the cervix is now the second most common invasive cancer of the female reproductive tract. Early sexual activity, multiple partners, multiparity, and chronic inflammation are associated factors. Herpesvirus hominis type 2 and human papillomavirus (HPV) have been found to be frequently associated with cervical cancer, and there is increasing evidence that HPV infections, particularly types 16, 18 and 31, are the most important risk factor for high-grade squamous intraepithelial lesions of the cervix and cervical cancer. The precancerous potential of low-grade squamous intraepithelial neoplasia has not been established.

The majority of cervical cancers are squamous cell (85%); the remainder consist of adenocarcinomas, mixed carcinomas (adenosquamous), and rare sarcomas (mixed mesodermal tumors, lymphosarcomas).

The earliest squamous cell carcinoma is confined to the epithelial layers (carcinoma in situ, intraepithelial carcinoma, preinvasive carcinoma), and it is thought that the disease remains confined to the mucous membrane for several years before invading the subjacent stroma. Carcinoma in situ occurs most frequently in the fourth decade, whereas invasive carcinoma is encountered most often in women between age 40 and age 50.

Following penetration of the basement membrane and involvement of the cervical stroma, the disease spreads by direct contiguity to the vagina and the adjacent parametrium and via the lymphatic channels (which are abundant in this area) to the regional lymph nodes of the pelvis (iliac and obturator) and to the periaortic lymph nodes. Estimating the extent of the malignant process is extremely important in determining the mode of therapy and in estimating the prognosis. This is judged clinically as shown in Table 42–4.

It is known from an examination of surgical specimens that the probability of lymph node metastasis increases according to the local extent of the disease, being approximately 15% in stage I, 30% in stage II,

Table 42–4. FIGO staging for cervical cancer.

Stage 0	Carcinoma in situ
Stage I	Cervical carcinoma confined to uterus (extension to corpus should be disregarded)
IA	Invasive carcinoma, diagnosed only by microscopy. All macroscopically visible lesions—even with superficial invasion—are TIB/TIBI. Stromal invasion with a maximum depth of 5 mm measured from the base of the epithelium and horizontal spread of 7 mm or less. Vascular space involvement, venous or lymphatic, does not affect classification
IAI	Measured stromal invasion 3 mm or less and 7 mm or less in horizontal spread
IA2	Measured stromal invasion more than 3 mm and not more than 5 mm with a horizontal spread of 7 mm or less
IB	Clearly visible lesion confined to the cervix or microscopic lesion greater than TIA2
IBI	Clearly visible lesion 4 cm or less in greatest dimension
IB2	Clearly visible lesion more than 4 cm in greatest dimension
Stage II	Cervical carcinoma invades beyond uterus but not to pelvic wall or to the lower third of vagina
IIA	Tumor without parametrial invasion
IIB	Tumor with parametrial invasion
Stage III	Cervical carinoma extends to the pelvic wall and/or involves lower third of vagina or causes hydronephrosis or nonfunctioning kidney
IIIA	Tumor involves lower third of the vagina, no extension to pelvic wall
IIIB	Tumor extends to pelvic wall or causes hydronephoris or nonfunctioning kidney
Stage IV	Cervical carcinoma involving the mucosa of adjacent organs, or distant metastases
IVA	Tumor invades mucosa of bladder or rectum and/or extends beyond true pelvis
IVB	Distant metastasis

and 45% in stage III. About 80% of patients with stage IV cancer have lymph node involvement.

Clinical Findings

A. CARCINOMA IN SITU

High-grade squamous intraepithelial lesions and carcinoma in situ do not cause symptoms. Fifteen to 20 percent of patients with carcinoma in situ have no visible lesion. Cytologic examination (Papanicolaou) of a representative specimen collected from the squamocolumnar junction (transformation zone) of the cervix will demonstrate severely dysplastic or frankly malignant cells in 95% of women with this stage of disease.

The Schiller test, using Lugol's solution, is often helpful in demonstrating areas of abnormal epithelium—even in a cervix that appears normal on gross inspection—because the lack of glycogen in these cells makes them unable to take up the stain. The test is not specific for neoplasm, since areas of ectopy, cervicitis, atrophy, and dysplasia are also iodine-negative. A sharply demarcated border of nonstaining is more suggestive of epithelial neoplasia.

Colposcopic examination of the cervix may define areas of dysplasia and carcinoma in situ and should be done in all women who have abnormal (dysplastic or malignant) epithelial cells unrelated to an inflammatory condition. This method is based primarily upon changes that occur in the capillary vascular pattern of the cervix associated with epithelial proliferation.

Punch biopsy is required in all cases in which there is a visible area of redness, an iodine-negative area, or an area of colposcopic abnormality. A cone biopsy and curettage should be done when cytologic examination reveals moderate or severe dysplasia, carcinoma in situ, or perhaps invasive carcinoma and (1) if colposcopy is not available and there is no visible lesion and no iodine-nonstaining area; (2) when colposcopy reveals no abnormalities of the exocervix or when an abnormal transformation zone is seen that extends into the endocervical canal; (3) when a colposcopically directed punch biopsy reveals microinvasive carcinoma; or (4) when colposcopically directed biopsies fail to explain the abnormal cytologic findings.

B. INVASIVE CARCINOMA

With the exception of early stromal involvement, invasive carcinoma of the cervix usually produces symptoms. Intermenstrual or postcoital bleeding is often the first symptom. A watery vaginal discharge, occasionally blood-streaked, may be the only symptom. Pain is a manifestation of far-advanced disease. In most patients with invasive cancer, inspection of the cervix reveals an ulcerated or papillary lesion of the cervix that bleeds on contact. The cytologic examination almost always demonstrates exfoliated malignant cells, though it should be remembered that false-negative Papanicolaou smears are more frequent in the face of invasive carcinoma than in intraepithelial neoplasia. Biopsy usually reveals the invasive nature of the lesion. An occasional endocervical endophytic lesion will produce enlargement of the cervix without becoming evident on the portio vaginalis.

Differential Diagnosis

Chronic cervicitis can be distinguished from cancer of the cervix only by multiple negative cytologic and biopsy examinations. Polyps of the cervix should be examined by a pathologist to exclude malignant change.

Complications

The complications are those caused by spread of the disease or occurring secondary to treatment. Obstruction of the ureter, resulting in hydroureter, hydronephrosis, and uremia, occurs with advancing disease. Bilateral obstruction of the ureters leads to failure of kidney function and death. Involvement of the iliac and obturator lymph nodes may lead to lymphatic obstruction, with lymphedema of the lower extremity. The lumbosacral plexus may become infiltrated by tumor, causing pain in the low back, hip, and leg.

Vesicovaginal and rectovaginal fistulas occur as a result of tumor involvement of these structures or as complications of radiation therapy. A cloaca may result from massive slough of necrotic tumor tissue. Widespread metastases to lung, liver, brain, and bone may occur.

Complications of radiation therapy such as cystitis, colitis, and proctitis are not uncommon but are usually only transitory problems in modern treatment centers. Ovarian failure is an unavoidable complication of radiation therapy. Severe radiation damage to the bladder and rectum may result in hemorrhage, fistulas, and strictures. Radiation necrosis of the cervix and diffuse radiation pelvic fibrosis are rare complications.

The complications of surgery are hemorrhage, infection, thromboembolism, and fistula formation (ureterovaginal, vesicovaginal, and rectovaginal).

Prevention

Invasive cancer of the cervix can be prevented by detecting and properly treating chronic cervicitis, cervical dysplasia, and carcinoma in situ of the cervix. Regular pelvic examinations, with cervical cytologic examination every 1–3 years, have proved to be effective in the prevention of this disease. Cigarette smoking also contributes to the incidence of cervical cancer.

Treatment

The proper treatment of cervical cancer requires individualization of therapy for each patients according to the clinical circumstances. Cervical epithelial dysplasia is destroyed by cauterization or cryosurgery or by laser therapy.

A. CARCINOMA IN SITU

Carcinoma in situ and lesser degrees of cervical intraepithelial neoplasia are best treated by eradication of the entire transformation zone. This can be accomplished by cauterization, cryotherapy, laser vaporization, cone biopsy, electrosurgical loop excision, or cervicectomy. Hysterectomy may be done if there is another indication for removing the uterus. Regardless of the procedure, close follow-up is necessary in order to ensure that treatment has indeed been adequate.

B. INVASIVE CARCINOMA

Stage 1A1 cases can be managed conservatively with cone excision (with negative margins) or hysterectomy. Radical hysterectomy with bilateral pelvic lymph node dissection is a treatment option in cases of small (stage 1A2, IB, IIA) disease in young women or invasive carcinoma complicating pregnancy. These women also have the option of radiation therapy with equal cure rates. More advanced invasive carcinomas are best treated by irradiation under the cooperative management of a radiotherapist and a gynecologist experienced in the treatment of cancer. Both internal sources (radium or cesium) and external sources (x-ray, ^{60}Co, betatron, linear accelerator) should be employed. Several randomized phase III trials have shown an overall survival advantage for cisplatin-based therapy given concurrently with radiation therapy. The risk of death from cervical cancer was decreased by 30–50% by concurrent chemoradiation. This is now recommended in most cases. Recurrent or persistent cancer following radiation therapy may require pelvic exenteration.

Prognosis

The earlier the disease is treated, the better the prognosis. Carcinoma in situ is almost 100% curable. The prevalence of invasive carcinoma of the cervix is decreasing, partly as a result of detection and treatment in the intraepithelial stage of the disease. The best results in stage I cancer of the cervix approach a 90% 5-year survival rate. For stage II, the figure drops to 60%; for stage III, to 30%; and for stage IV, to less than 10%.

Hricak H et al: Role of imaging in cancer of the cervix. American College of Radiology. ACR Appropriateness Criteria. Radiology 2000;215(Suppl):925.

Morris M et al: Pelvic radiation with concurrent chemotherapy compared with pelvic and para-aortic radiation for high-risk cervical cancer. N Engl J Med 1999;340:1137.

Rose PG et al: Concurrent cisplatin-based radiotherapy and chemotherapy for locally advance cervical cancer. N Engl J Med 1999;340:1144.

Sawaya GF et al: Current approaches to cervical-cancer screening. N Engl J Med 2001;344:1603.

ENDOMETRIAL CARCINOMA

Endometrial carcinoma is primarily a disease of postmenopausal women, with a peak incidence in the decade from 55 to 65 years of age. It also occurs in premenopausal women, particularly those with prolonged anovulation. Evidence suggests that prolonged unopposed (by progesterone) estrogen stimulation of the endometrium may be a predisposing factor in the development of endometrial carcinoma. The prolonged use of exogenous estrogens (and tamoxifen) in postmenopausal women multiplies the risk of endometrial cancer about seven times. There is also an association of obesity, hypertension, and diabetes with endometrial cancer.

Complex hyperplasia with atypia is a precursor of endometrial cancer. Well-differentiated (grade 1) tumors tend to be superficial, whereas higher-grade (2, 3) cancers are associated with deep myometrial invasion. Fortunately, deep myometrial penetration, extension beyond the corpus of the uterus, lymph node involvement, and distant metastases occur relatively late in the disease, so that most lesions are detected early. Anaplastic or high-grade tumors and the papillary serous, clear cell, and squamous cell variants behave more aggressively. Adverse prognostic factors include grade, histology, depth of myometrial invasion, cervical extension, tumor size, and extension beyond the uterus.

Endometrial cancer is now staged surgically as shown in Table 42–5.

Clinical Findings

Postmenopausal bleeding is the primary symptom and should be considered to be caused by cancer until proved otherwise. About 40% of women with vaginal bleeding following the menopause will have reproductive tract cancer, and in the vast majority of these cases the cancer is endometrial. Cervical stenosis with pyometra or hematometra is highly suggestive of endometrial carcinoma. Pain is not a common symptom but there may be mild uterine cramping, particularly if there is any degree of stenosis of the cervix. Vaginal cytology is positive in 40–80% of cases. Endometrial biopsy will almost always detect an endometrial carcinoma, as will cytologic sampling of the endometrial cavity. Curettage, first of the endocervix and then of the endometrial cavity, with careful

Table 42–5. FIGO staging for endometrial cancer.

Stage IA	Tumor limited to endometrium
Stage IB	Invasion to less than half the myometrium
Stage IC	Invasion to more than half the myometrium
Stage IIA	Endocervical glandular involvement only
Stage IIB	Cervical stromal invasion
Stage IIIA	Tumor invades serosa and/or adnexa and/or positive cytologic findings
Stage IIIB	Vaginal metastases
Stage IIIC	Metastases to pelvic and/or para-aortic lymph nodes
Stage IVA	Tumor invasion of bladder and/or bowel mucosa
Stage IVB	Distant metastases, including intra-abdominal and/or inguinal lymph nodes

examination under anesthesia is considered the most definitive method of diagnosing and clinically staging the disease. Myometrial involvement is suspected if the corpus is enlarged. MRI may be helpful in defining myometrial penetration.

Endometrial carcinoma that is histologically poorly differentiated, or high-grade, may disseminate relatively early in the course of the disease. Metastatic spread may occur to the vagina, regional pelvic and para-aortic lymph nodes, ovaries, lungs, brain, and bone. The most frequent site of recurrence following treatment for endometrial carcinoma is the vaginal vault.

Prevention

There is presumptive evidence that progesterone therapy will reduce the possibility of endometrial carcinoma in the anovulatory patient as well as in postmenopausal women receiving estrogen replacement therapy. Detection and adequate therapy of the precursors of the disease (hyperplasia with atypia and carcinoma in situ of the endometrium) will prevent the subsequent development of endometrial carcinoma.

Treatment

Total abdominal hysterectomy and bilateral salpingo-oophorectomy is definitive therapy for endometrial carcinoma. Washings of the peritoneal cavity for cytologic examination should be obtained at the time. Pelvic and para-aortic lymph node sampling should be done in most patients with endometrial cancer, with the exception of those with low-risk lesions, small grade 1 cancers without myometrial invasion.

If the cervix is grossly involved, patients should receive preoperative radiation followed by hysterectomy and node sampling or, if they are young, should undergo a radical hysterectomy with pelvic and para-aortic node sampling.

Adjuvant radiation therapy is administered to those with nodal disease, high-grade or deep myometrial involvement, and those with extension beyond the uterus. Radiation alone can be used in patients who are considered poor surgical risks. Poor-risk surgical patients with grade 1 tumors can also be treated with progestin therapy.

Disseminated endometrial carcinoma is treated with large-dose progestin therapy (hydroxyprogesterone caproate, medroxyprogesterone, or megestrol), which produces satisfactory remission of the metastatic disease in about 35% of cases, particularly in patients with tumors that are positive for progesterone receptors. Subjective improvement is noted in the majority of patients so treated. Cisplatin or carboplatin, doxorubicin, or paclitaxel is given to those with high grades, absent receptors, and disseminated disease.

Prognosis

Five-year survival rates of 70–90% are recorded in stage I disease. This drops to 60% in stage II. Histologic undifferentiation, deep myometrial penetration, and absence of estrogen and progesterone receptors all worsen the prognosis.

Kinkel K et al: Radiologic staging in patients with endometrial cancer: a meta-analysis. Radiology 1999;212:711.

Rose PG: Endometrial carcinoma. N Engl J Med 1996;335:640.

SARCOMAS OF THE UTERUS

Uterine sarcomas are relatively rare. They may arise from the myometrium itself, from the endometrial stroma, or, rarely, in preexisting leiomyomas. Mixed tumors (carcinosarcoma, mixed mesodermal tumors) containing both epithelial and connective tissue malignant cells are also encountered. Sarcomas of the uterus metastasize via the bloodstream and lymphatics and spread by contiguity. The lungs are a frequent site of metastatic disease.

In patients in whom the tumor is confined to the pelvic organs, treatment consists of total hysterectomy and bilateral salpingo-oophorectomy, with individualized postoperative radiation or chemotherapy (or both) for those with deep myometrial invasion.

The outlook for patients with uterine sarcoma is variable. Leiomyosarcomas with more than ten mitoses per ten high-power fields carry a poor prognosis, with recurrence within 5 years in about two-thirds of patients. About 40% of patients with malignant mixed müllerian tumors survive.

Doxorubicin has been reported to be effective in the treatment of some leiomyosarcomas. High-dose progestin therapy will bring about complete resolution of metastatic low-grade endometrial sarcoma in some patients. Unresectable or recurrent malignant mixed mesodermal tumors may respond to cisplatin and ifosfamide.

Gonzalez-Bosquet E et al: Uterine sarcoma: a clinicopathological study of 93 cases. Eur J Gynaecol Oncol 1997;18:192.

Levenback CF et al: Uterine sarcoma. Obstet Gynecol Clin North Am 1996;23:457.

TUMORS OF THE UTERINE TUBE (Adenocarcinoma)

Benign tumors of the uterine (fallopian) tubes are very rare. Primary carcinoma of the tube is the most common malignant lesion, but it is rarely encountered, constituting less than 1% of female reproductive tract cancers. Women with *BRCA1/2* mutations are at risk for uterine tube cancer as well as the more common breast and ovarian cancers.

Postmenopausal vaginal bleeding is the usual presenting complaint. There may be a history of intermittent and profuse, serous, yellow, or bloody vaginal discharge (hydrops tubae profluens). An adnexal mass may or may not be palpable.

The diagnosis of primary carcinoma of the uterine tube is rarely made preoperatively. Total abdominal hysterectomy and bilateral salpingo-oophorectomy constitute the treatment of choice in operable lesions. Tumors that are inoperable yet are confined to the pelvic structures should receive radiation therapy, followed by operation if there is a favorable response as judged by increased mobility and diminution in tumor size. Radical hysterectomy and bilateral pelvic lymph node dissection have been advocated as possibly a more curative procedure than simple hysterectomy and bilateral salpingo-oophorectomy.

If the disease is confined to the tube, the prognosis is quite good. Unfortunately, most of these tumors are advanced at the time of discovery, and the overall 5-year cure rate is in the range of 10–20%.

Early use of the laparoscope or the CT scanner may be of aid in the earlier diagnosis of this disease and should be considered in any postmenopausal woman with a vague adnexal mass, particularly if it is accompanied by a watery discharge or postmenopausal bleeding.

Uterine tube cancers are staged and treated as ovarian cancers.

Nikrui N et al: Fallopian tube carcinoma. Surg Oncol Clin N Am 1998;7:363.

OVARIAN CANCER

Ovarian malignancies may develop in the form of epithelial tumors, germ cell tumors, sex cord-stromal tumors, and various mixtures of these groups. Epithelial carcinomas arise from the coelomic epithelium and account for 85–90% of malignant ovarian neoplasms. The peak incidence of epithelial ovarian carcinoma is in the fifth and sixth decades of life, while malignant germ cell tumors are more likely to occur under the age of 30. Stromal tumors seem to be more evenly distributed among the age groups.

The common epithelial histologies are serous, mucinous, endometrioid, clear cell, transitional cell, and undifferentiated adenocarcinoma. Spread of disease is primarily by exfoliation of cells that implant in the peritoneal cavity, but lymphatic channels and hematogenous spread are also common. Serous histology is the most common, comprising approximately 40% of ovarian carcinomas. Mucinous tumors in particular may become very large and distend the entire abdomen. Endometrioid carcinomas are the second most frequent variety (24% of ovarian cancers) and sometimes are associated with endometriosis. Clear cell tumors are also associated with endometriosis but have a significantly more aggressive histologic appearance. Borderline tumors or atypical epithelial proliferation of low malignant potential are considered less aggressive histologic subtypes yet are still considered malignancies because of their risk for recurrence and metastasis.

Tumors of germ cell origin include dysgerminomas (the homolog of testicular seminomas), immature teratomas, endodermal sinus tumor, and choriocarcinoma. While benign cystic teratomas are among the most common benign ovarian tumors, malignant change occurs in rare instances; such tumors are usually squamous cell carcinomas and not immature teratomas.

Less common are the hormone-producing neoplasms. The granulosa-theca cell tumors are the most frequent of the hormonally active tumors, constituting about 4–6% of ovarian cancers. About two-thirds are benign in their clinical behavior. Sertoli-Leydig cell tumors are rare and usually manifest themselves first by producing defeminization (amenorrhea, atrophy of the breast) and then masculinization (deepening of the voice, hirsutism, clitoral hypertrophy). Like granulosa-theca cell tumors, the majority are benign, the reported incidence of cancer being about 20%. Metastatic carcinoma from the gastrointestinal tract (Krukenberg tumor), breast, pancreas, and kidney must always be considered as a possible diagnosis whenever there is bilateral malignant disease of the ovaries.

Although only 10–15% of ovarian cancers are thought to be hereditary, family history is one of the strongest risk factors for epithelial ovarian cancer. Genetic inheritance of a mutation in the *BRCA1* or *BRCA2* gene imposes a 20–40% lifetime risk of developing ovarian cancer along with a 60–80% lifetime risk of developing breast cancer. An increased risk has also been observed in women from families with a background of colorectal and endometrial cancer. Other reproductive factors associated with an increased risk include infertility, probably independent of the use of ovulation induction agents.

Clinical Findings

Despite the common belief that early-stage ovarian cancer is without symptoms, most women with ovarian cancer have vague symptoms such as lower abdominal pressure. The most important sign is the presence of a pelvic mass on physical examination. Any enlargement of the ovary in women of menopausal or post-menopausal age should be regarded as malignant until proved otherwise. A solid, irregular, fixed pelvic mass is highly suggestive of an ovarian malignancy, particularly in combination with an upper abdominal mass or ascites. The CA-125 tumor is helpful to differentiate between a benign or malignant process, though the marker may be negative in half of early-stage ovarian cancers. Although ultrasonography or CT scanning may be helpful, it is often impossible to determine the benign or malignant nature of an ovarian tumor until laparotomy. If an ovarian malignancy is suspected preoperatively, it is appropriate to refer the patient for surgical exploration, staging, and cytoreduction by a gynecologic oncologist.

On occasion, an ovarian malignancy is not detected until it is discovered at operation for another intra-abdominal disorders. Papillations of the external surface, adherence to surrounding structures, and peritoneal implants are signs of cancer. The tumor should be removed without spilling its contents into the peritoneal cavity and should be submitted to a pathologist in the operating room for gross examination and frozen-section microscopic analysis of any suspicious areas. These cystic enlargements may represent simple cysts, serous or mucinous cystadenomas, adenofibromas, or cystadenocarcinomas. Solid enlargements of the ovary may be benign fibromas or thecomas. If a malignancy is identified or suspected, a gynecologic or surgical oncologist should be consulted for thorough surgical staging.

Differential Diagnosis

Ovarian neoplasms may be benign, borderline, or malignant. Pelvic masses may arise from the uterus, adnexa, bowel, or occasionally the genitourinary tract. In most instances the correct diagnosis can be made if an accurate medical history is obtained, a careful physical examination performed, and judicious use made of ancillary diagnostic procedures such as ultrasound, CT scanning, and serum tumor markers. Surgery is often required in order to establish the definitive diagnosis of an ovarian mass and, if the mass is malignant, to accurately assess the extent of disease.

Prevention

Bilateral salpingo-oophorectomy at the time of hysterectomy for benign uterine disease in women over age 40—and after childbearing function has been completed in younger women with strong family histories—is advocated by many to prevent the development of ovarian cancer. To date, no effective screening test for ovarian cancer is applicable to the general population, though women with a strong family history should be considered for genetic counseling and close clinical surveillance. Known protective factors for ovarian cancer include childbearing and use of oral contraceptive pills. Even 6 months of pill use seems to decrease the relative risk for ovarian cancer, and the effects appear to remain protective for up to 10 years. For patients with genetic mutations predisposing them to increased risk, prophylactic oophorectomy may be performed with or without prophylactic mastectomy as well.

Treatment

Accurate pathologic evaluation and thorough surgical staging (Table 42–6) are essential to the management of early stage disease. When a complex adnexal mass is removed in the operating room, washings should be obtained first, and the mass should be removed intact. Laparoscopy may be considered for some lesions, but puncturing the ovarian mass in a bag before removal still risks the possibility of intraperitoneal spill and spread. Solid or papillary projections are particular areas of suspicion. A frozen section should be obtained to exclude malignancy. If an ovarian malignancy is confirmed or suspected, surgical staging includes removal of the uterus, the contralateral ovary, pelvic and para-aortic lymph nodes, and omentum. Peritoneal and bowel surfaces should be carefully inspected and suspicious areas biopsied. Even in ovarian malignancies clinically confined to the ovary, there can be occult metastatic disease in the lymph nodes or omentum. In women without any evidence of extra-ovarian disease who want to maintain future childbearing capacity, the uterus and contralateral ovary may be preserved, with consideration of later removal on completion of childbearing. Complete surgical staging gives the most accurate prognosis of disease, and if early-stage disease is confirmed it may obviate the need for additional chemotherapy. Patients with stage IA grade 1 or grade 2

Table 42–6. FIGO staging for ovarian cancer.

Stage I	Tumor limited to the ovaries
IA	Limited to one ovary, no tumor on external surface, capsule intact; negative peritoneal cytology
IB	Limited to both ovaries, no tumor on external surface, capsule intact; negative peritoneal cytology
IC	IA or IB tumor, but with surface tumor, ruptured capsule, or positive ascites or peritoneal cytology
Stage II	Tumor extending to the pelvis
IIA	Metastasis to the uterus or tubes
IIB	Metastatasis to other pelvic tissues
IIC	IIA or IIB tumor, both with surface tumor, ruptured capsule, or positive ascites or peritoneal cytology
Stage III	Tumor extending outside the pelvis and/or retroperitoneal or inguinal nodes. Extension to small bowel, omentum, or superficial liver are considered Stage III lesions
IIIA	Histologically confirmed microscopic disease of abdominal peritoneal surfaces; lymph nodes are negative
IIIB	Implants of abdominal or peritoneal surfaces not exceeding 2 cm in diameter; lymph nodes are negative
IIIC	Implants of abdominal or peritoneal surfaces greater than 2 cm in diameter, or positive retroperitoneal or inguinal lymph nodes
Stage IV	Tumor metastatic to distant sites including pleural effusions or liver parenchyma

tumors have a very good prognosis and usually are not treated with additional chemotherapy.

When the disease extends beyond the ovaries into the pelvis or abdomen, cytoreduction of all bulky disease contributes to an advantage in chemotherapy response and survival. Even in stage IV disease, tumor debulking improves survival if the intraperitoneal disease can be resected to minimal residual. A hysterectomy and bilateral salpingo-oophorectomy should be performed along with removal of the omentum. Intestinal resection, diaphragm resection, splenectomy, and other upper abdominal procedures may also be indicated if the patient can be left with minimal residual disease. In one series of patients resected to less than 0.5 cm disease, median survival was 40 months, compared with a median survival of 18 months for patients whose disease was only less than 1.5 cm. Successful cytoreductive surgery may be successful in over 70% of patients when performed by gyneco-

logic oncologists, subspecialists trained in ovarian cancer surgery. The CA-125 tumor antigen is a poor marker for ovarian cancer screening but is elevated in over 75% of ovarian carcinomas and can serve as a marker in assessing the effectiveness of therapy.

Chemotherapy is very effective in ovarian cancer as adjuvant therapy and in achieving clinical remission. The current standard regimen for advanced epithelial ovarian carcinoma in the United States is a combination of a taxane and platinum agent for at least six cycles, usually using paclitaxel and carboplatin. Patients who are not surgical candidates may be considered for primary chemotherapy with these agents as well, and many will have a significant tumor response. The current standard regimen for malignant germ cell tumors is cisplatin, etoposide, and bleomycin.

Prognosis

The prognosis for epithelial ovarian carcinoma is related primarily to stage and histologic grade. Because most ovarian cancers are of advanced stage at the time of initial diagnosis, the overall cure rate for ovarian cancer is approximately 50%. Five-year survival rates for patients with stage III or stage IV disease are around 20–35%. Nevertheless, significant disease-free remission can be achieved by combining accurate surgical staging and thorough surgical cytoreduction with chemotherapy. For stage I disease, 5-year survival rates can be over 80–85%, emphasizing the need for improved early detection.

Bomalaski JJ: The treatment of recurrent ovarian carcinoma: balancing patient desires, therapeutic benefit, cost containment and quality of life. Curr Opin Obstet Gynecol 1999;11:11.

Lynch HT et al: Genetics and ovarian carcinoma. Semin Oncol. 1998;25:265.

Marsden DE et al: Current management of epithelial ovarian carcinoma: a review. Semin Surg Oncol 2000;19:11.

Scully RE et al: *Tumors of the Ovary, Maldeveloped Gonads, Fallopian Tube, and Broad Ligament.* Armed Forces Institute of Pathology, 1998.

GESTATIONAL TROPHOBLASTIC DISEASE

Gestational trophoblastic neoplasms are chorionic tumors arising from placental tissue. Hydatidiform moles are related to the swelling of the villi in the absence of a fetal circulation and are accompanied by varying degrees of trophoblastic proliferation. There is a tendency for myometrial penetration that may progress to frank deep invasion of the uterine wall (chorioadenoma destruens, or invasive mole), and a small percentage (about 2–3%) of hydatidiform moles are followed by development of the highly malignant choriocarcinoma.

Hydatidiform moles can be classified as either complete or partial, based on cytogenetics and histopathology. Most complete moles have a 46,XX karyotype, with chromosomes entirely of paternal origin. Most partial moles have a triploid karyotype (69,XXY or 69,XYY), with extra chromosomes again derived from the father. Complete moles have a higher incidence of persistent gestational trophoblastic disease.

Staging of gestational trophoblastic tumors is outlined in Table 42–7.

The frequency of hydatidiform mole is about 1:2000–1:1500 pregnancies in the USA and about 1:650–1:240 pregnancies in the Far East and Mexico. Hydatidiform mole is also more common in women over 40 years of age.

Trophoblastic disease should be assessed for risk of persistent disease to determine optimal treatment and follow-up. (See Table 42–8.)

Clinical Findings

The usual picture is one of a nonviable gestation or presumed threatened abortion. Often there is vaginal bleeding. This may go on for several weeks with little or no abdominal pain. Examination reveals a disproportionately large uterus for the duration of the pregnancy in about 50% of cases. There may be bilateral cystic enlargement of the ovaries (theca lutein cysts). Preeclampsia may develop in women with large moles, and molar pregnancy should be suspected in any patient who develops hypertension, edema, and proteinuria in the first half of pregnancy. Anemia is common.

Serum and urinary β-hCG levels are unusually high and persist at high levels beyond the 12th week, when in normal pregnancy there is usually a significant drop. Ultrasound is quite accurate in the diagnosis of molar pregnancy, with a characteristic appearance of multiple small sonolucencies due to the presence of hydropic villi. Correlating sonographic findings with hCG levels may differentiate the finding of a molar pregnancy from a missed abortion.

In many cases, the diagnosis is not made until the patient spontaneously aborts the molar pregnancy. Any products of conception in which hydropic change is suggested on gross examination should be formally examined by a pathologist. Care must be taken by the pathologist in distinguishing degenerating products of conception from hydropic villi with trophoblastic proliferation. Placental site trophoblastic tumor is a rare form of trophoblastic disease that can arise from any type of pregnancy. β-hCG is a less reliable tumor marker in this disease, and it is relatively insensitive to chemotherapy compared with other chorionic tumors.

Differential Diagnosis

A diagnosis of threatened abortion or missed abortion is often entertained in the presence of a mole. Multiple pregnancy must be considered because it may produce unusually high levels of chorionic gonadotropin. Ultrasound diagnosis is quite reliable in complete hydatidiform mole. There may be an aneuploid fetus in cases of partial hydatidiform mole; however, the presence of focal cystic spaces in the placenta is often diagnostic. There are rare cases of a normal fetus coexisting with a molar pregnancy.

Complications

About 15% of moles become locally invasive (chorioadenoma destruens) and impose a danger of hemorrhage owing to penetration of the vascular uterine wall or pelvic infection from perforation. About 2–3% of moles are followed by choriocarcinoma, a highly malignant tumor. Although this cancer may occur after normal pregnancy, abortion, or ectopic pregnancy, about half of cases develop from an antecedent hydatidiform mole. Metastases are found in the lungs, liver, central nervous system, bone, vagina, and vulva. Despite the

Table 42–7. FIGO staging of gestational trophoblastic tumors.

Stage I	Disease confined to uterus
A	No risk factors
B	1 risk factor
C	2 risk factors
Stage II	Disease extending outside uterus, limited to genital structures—adnexa, broad ligament, vagina
A	No risk factors
B	1 risk factor
C	2 risk factors
Stage III	Disease extending to lungs, with or without genital tract involvement
A	No risk factors
B	1 risk factor
C	2 risk factors
Stage IV	Disease involving other metastatic sites
A	No risk factors
B	1 risk factor
C	2 risk factors

Table 42–8. WHO scoring system for risk of gestational trophoblastic tumors.

	≤ 4 = low risk 5–7 = intermediate risk > 7 = high risk			
Score → Prognostic Factors	0	1	2	4
Age	≤ 39	> 39		
Prior pregnancy	Mole	Abortion	Term	
Interval (months)	< 4	4–6	> 6	
β-hCG titer	< 1000	1001–10,000	10,000–100,000	> 100,000
ABO group	O, A, or A, O	B, AB		
Largest tumor (cm)	< 3	3–5	> 5	
Metastatic site		Spleen Kidney	Liver GI tract	Brain
Number of metastases		1–3	4–8	> 8
Prior chemotherapy			One drug	Two or more drugs

highly aggressive nature of this tumor, gestational trophoblastic disease is one of the most curable forms of malignancy.

Treatment

Once the diagnosis of a molar pregnancy has been established, the uterus should be emptied. This is done by both suction and sharp dilation and curettage. Larger moles are better evacuated with the simultaneous administration of intravenous oxytocin. All specimens are examined pathologically for evidence of proliferative activity of the trophoblast, which serves as an indication of the probability of malignant change.

Lutein cysts of the ovaries, which occur in about one-third of molar pregnancies, will regress following removal of the mole and should not be surgically excised.

All patients with hydatidiform mole should be followed weekly after evacuation of the uterus for the possible development of persistent gestational trophoblastic disease. Patients should be given effective contraceptive advice and counseled not to become pregnant for at least a year. Weekly serum β-hCG levels should be obtained until the titer is normal for 3 weeks; thereafter, monthly levels are measured until the titer is normal for 6–12 months. It may take as long as 14–16 weeks for hCG to reach normal levels following molar

evacuation. A plateau or rising titer, particularly with the disappearance of the hormone followed by a later reappearance, is strongly suggestive of choriocarcinoma or invasive mole if pregnancy can be ruled out.

Patients with persistent gestational trophoblastic tumors should be evaluated with a metastatic workup and considered for chemotherapy based on their risk factors (Table 42–8). The workup should include a pelvic examination, pelvic ultrasound, chest x-ray, a complete blood count, and renal and liver function tests. If these tests are normal, other sites of metastasis are not likely to be present. If metastatic lesions are suspected, a CT scan of the head, chest, abdomen, and pelvis should be performed.

Single-agent chemotherapy is the preferred treatment for patients with stage I or low-risk disease who wish to maintain reproductive options. If future childbearing is not an issue, patients with invasive mole should be considered for hysterectomy and single-agent adjuvant chemotherapy. Prophylactic chemotherapy should be considered in older women with extremely high gonadotropin titers given their high risk of persistent disease after evacuation. Single-agent management with methotrexate or dactinomycin has resulted in similar response and remission rates for gestational trophoblastic tumors. Methotrexate competes with folic acid in cellular metabolism and is given either by weekly intramuscular injection or as infusions 5 days in a row given every other week. Dactinomycin is a vesicant agent but is also given as five daily infusions given every other week or as a single bolus infusion given every other week. Both of these regimens can be quite cytotoxic and should be administered under the guidance of a gynecologic oncologist or medical oncologist. Intermediate-risk gestational trophoblastic disease can be treated with combination chemotherapy: methotrexate, dactinomycin, and cyclophosphamide or chlorambucil. Even in high-risk patients, a combination regimen of etoposide, methotrexate, dactinomycin, cyclophosphamide, and vincristine is still effective in drug-resistant disease.

Prognosis

The prognosis for cure of gestational trophoblastic tumors is excellent. Before chemotherapeutic agents became available, the outlook for choriocarcinoma was very poor. Five-year remission rates in the range of 80% or better are now being reported even in the presence of metastatic disease. Follow-up of a reliable tumor marker and assessment of risk factors to select an efficacious chemotherapy regimen have made gestational trophoblastic disease one of the success stories in oncology. The risk in subsequent pregnancies for another molar pregnancy is slightly increased (about 1%), and early ultrasound is recommended to confirm normal gestation. The placenta or products of conception should be examined after delivery, and follow-up hCG levels should be obtained to exclude the possibility of persistent trophoblastic disease.

Berkowitz RS et al: Chorionic tumors. N Engl J Med 1990; 335:1740.

Bower M et al: EMA/CO (etoposide, methotrexate, actinomycin-D, cyclophosphamide, vincristine) for high-risk gestational trophoblastic tumous: results from a cohort of 272 patients. J Clin Oncol 1990;15:2636.

Newlands ES et al: Recent advances in gestational trophoblastic disease. Hematol Oncol Clin North Am. 1999;13:225.

Orthopedics

Bobby K-B Tay, MD, William W. Colman, MD, Sigurd Berven, MD, Roger Fontes, Jr., MD, Stephen Gunther, MD, William Holmes, MD, Hubert T. Kim, MD, PhD, Lisa Lattanza, MD, Edward Diao, MD, Serena S. Hu, MD, & David S. Bradford, MD

Orthopedic surgery and orthopedic medicine have evolved substantially over the last decade. Improvements in implant design and materials have been responsible for major breakthroughs in our ability to treat patients with complex orthopedic problems. The limitations on what we can achieve with engineering advances have motivated us to seek greater understanding of the biologic mechanisms that determine the optimal outcomes for our patients.

A Note on Terminology

In general, the use of eponyms to denote fractures or deformities is best avoided by the student and nonorthopedist. Although well-entrenched eponyms are included in this chapter, it is often less confusing to use anatomic terms.

Varus and **valgus** are descriptive terms frequently used in the characterization of angular musculoskeletal deformities. They refer to the direction of the apex of the deformity in relation to the midline of the body. If the apex points away from the midline, the deformity is varus; if toward the midline, the deformity is valgus. Knock-knees are an example of valgus deformity; the entire lower limb is abnormally angulated, with the apex of the deformity (the knee) pointing toward the midline. In bowlegs, the angle of deformity points away from the midline; this condition is called varus knees or genu varum. Similar designations apply to angular deformities of the elbow (cubitus varus or valgus) and the hip (coxa vara or valga).

When a long bone such as the femur or humerus is fractured, the limb may be visibly deformed. The relationship between the main fracture fragments, or the alignment, can be characterized by describing the angular deformity in the sagittal and coronal planes. In this case, the fracture itself constitutes the apex of the deformity and may be designated as varus or valgus. However, in practical use, the angulation of the fracture is more clearly described by noting the apex of the deformity (apex anterior, posterior, lateral, or medial) The fracture is said to be comminuted if the bones are fragmented. The fracture is displaced when the main bony fragments are translated or separated from each other. Fracture displacement is then subcategorized into minimally, moderately, and completely displaced.

If there is a wound overlying the fracture through which the fracture is either exposed or through which it may have communicated with the external environment, the fracture is described as **open.** In this situation, fracture contamination must be promptly addressed by surgically cleaning the wound and the underlying bone to minimize the likelihood of developing osteomyelitis.

Joint dislocations also warrant immediate treatment. The maneuver to restore proper alignment of a joint or fracture is called **reduction.** Vascular structures spanning the joint may be injured at the time of injury or may be compressed by malalignment of bony structures. The arterial pulses distal to the injury should be assessed and documented. Absent pulses are often restored after reduction of the joint. If the vessels are torn, early repair or reconstruction is often required to restore distal circulation to the limb.

Joint or fracture reduction may be performed by **open (surgical)** or **closed (nonsurgical)** techniques. A dislocation or fracture is described as unstable if there is a high likelihood of further deformation. Following reduction, unstable fractures or dislocations may be stabilized by closed or open techniques. Closed techniques involve traction, casts, splints, or braces; open techniques involve exposure of the fracture and reduction of the fracture fragments with maintenance of the reduction with some form of internal or external fixation device. The surgical management of an unstable fracture or dislocation is therefore described as "open reduction and internal or external fixation."

■ FRACTURES & JOINT INJURIES

FRACTURES & DISLOCATIONS OF THE SPINE

Demographics

In a recent survey of 165 trauma centers evaluating a total of 111,219 trauma patients, the incidence of cervical spine injury was 4.3%, with a 1.3% incidence of spinal cord injury. Most studies report an incidence of 3.2–5.3 new spinal-cord injuries per 100,000 persons at risk in the United States. There is a bimodal distribution in the prevalence of spinal column injury, with peaks occurring in people between 15 and 24 years of age and in people 50 years of age and older. The percentage of the population over 50 years of age is constantly increasing as a result of longer life expectancies. The elderly are also more active, and as this subset of the population increases in number the incidence of spinal cord injury in the elderly will certainly increase as well. Improvements in emergency medical care and trauma care have reduced the mortality and morbidity associated with these injuries. The mortality from spinal cord injury also decreased from 20% to 9%. Clearly, the cost savings to society from this improved care is significant.

Most patients with spinal column injury are young men (up to 30% were men in their thirties). The most common causes in this age group are motor vehicle accidents, followed by falls, gunshot injuries, and sports injuries. In the pediatric population, motor vehicle accidents are the most common cause of injury; in the elderly, falls are the most common cause. Disturbingly, the proportion of spinal cord injuries from gunshot wounds is increasing, and controversy continues over optimal management of a patient with a bullet in the spinal canal.

As with internal fixation of extremity fractures, internal fixation of spine fractures has allowed early mobilization and rehabilitation, resulting in improvements in outcome. Internal fixation has also made it easier to achieve decompression of the neural elements.

Anatomy

The spinal column consists of multiple individual motion segments made up of the vertebral bodies and the intervertebral disks. Mobility is greatest in the cervical spine, least in the thoracic spine, and of intermediate range in the lumbar spine. Injuries may occur anywhere along the spinal column depending upon the mechanism of injury. However, most nonpathologic vertebral column fractures occur in the more mobile segments (cervical and lumbar spines) and at the junctions between flexible and less flexible segments (cervicothoracic junction, thoracolumbar junction, and lumbosacral junction).

The bony vertebral column also protects the neural elements from injury. In the cervical and thoracic spine, the spinal canal contains the spinal cord, nerve roots, and spinal nerves as they exit from the neural foramina. The spinal cord is composed of central gray matter (neuronal cell bodies) surrounded by white matter (axons). Within a cross section of the cord, several important anatomic structures can be identified. These include the lateral spinothalamic tracts that are responsible for transmitting pain and temperature sensation; the lateral corticospinal tracts, responsible for motor function at that level; and the posterior columns, which transmit position sense, vibratory sensation, and deep pressure sensation. The spinothalamic tracts cross to the opposite side of the spinal cord within three levels of entering the cord. In contrast, the corticospinal tracts and the posterior columns decussate at the craniocervical levels. The most central portions of the corticospinal tracts control the function of the more proximal areas of the body, and the more peripheral portions control the function of the distal areas.

The spinal roots exit the vertebral column through the intervertebral foramina. In the cervical spine, the C1 root exits above the C1 body; the C2 root exits below the C1 body; and the C8 root exits below the C7 body. In the thoracic and lumbar spine, each root exits under the pedicle with the same number.

During development, the spinal cord does not grow longitudinally as rapidly as the vertebra, so the terminal segment of the spinal cord (conus medullaris) ends near the lower border of the first lumbar vertebra. The dural sac distal to the L1 contains the spinal nerves for all the segments from L2 through S5.

Initial Management & Clinical Assessment of Spinal Injury

Treatment is initiated at the scene of the injury. Without exception, all victims of trauma are suspected of having a spinal column injury until such an injury has been ruled out. Cervical spine injury has been closely linked to the presence of severe head injury (odds ratio 8.5), a high-energy mechanism (odds ratio 11.6), or a focal neurologic deficit (odds ratio 58). Initial stabilization begins with the application of a rigid cervical collar, a spine board, and sandbags.

Careful evaluation and documentation of the patient's neurologic status will allow the physician to determine the appropriate treatment plan and estimate the prognosis for functional recovery. Once at the trauma center, clinical assessment of a suspected spine injury begins with evaluation of the patient's airway, breathing, and circulation. Significant retropharyngeal soft tissue swelling, especially in the upper cervical spine, may lead to upper airway obstruction. High cervical injuries causing diaphragmatic and chest wall muscle paralysis will result in respiratory failure. Neurogenic shock can cause significant hypotension and bradycardia. Sensory deficits caused by either cord or root level injuries can result in the rapid development of decubiti over insensate skin over high-pressure areas of the body (especially heels and ischium). Prompt assessment and removal of the patient from the spine board and onto an appropriate bed may help to prevent decubiti. Airway and breathing are ensured by intubation and mechanical ventilation. Nasotracheal intubation is the safest method of airway control in the acute setting because it causes less cervical spine motion than direct oral intubation. The diastolic pressure should be kept above 70 mm Hg to maximize spinal cord blood flow. In the polytrauma setting, this is initially done with fluid resuscitation. However, once the diagnosis of neurogenic shock is established, the blood pressure should be managed with vasopressors to prevent fluid overload. Methylprednisolone, if given within 8 hours after injury, improves motor function recovery after incomplete spinal cord injury. NASCIS-2 (National Acute Spinal Cord Injury Studies) and NASCIS-3 trials have demonstrated that an initial bolus of 30 mg/kg given over the first 15 minutes followed by 5.4 mg/kg/h over the following 24 hours (if steroids were started within 3 hours after injury) or 48 hours (if steroids were started within 3–8 hours after injury) were beneficial in improving long-term motor recovery.

After the initial resuscitation, the primary survey can be performed to evaluate for any life-threatening injuries. At this time, information from emergency medical personnel about the mechanism of injury and the accident scene may alert the physician to possible associated injuries. After the primary survey is complete, the secondary survey should include inspection and palpation of the entire spine. Ecchymosis, soft tissue swelling, tenderness, crepitation, and gaps between the spinous processes suggest underlying spinal column injury. Noncontiguous spinal injuries occur in 6% of patients, and these can easily be missed if there is associated head injury, upper cervical injury, or cervicothoracic injury.

In addition to spinal trauma, other injuries should be assessed since they may influence the treatment of the spinal lesion and may alter the outcome. Suspicion of associated injuries is dependent on the mechanism of the initial traumatic event that is responsible for the characteristic spinal injury pattern. In cervical spine trauma, much attention has been devoted to the investigation of possible vertebral artery injury. Reports indicate a 20-25% incidence of vertebral artery injury after cervical spine injury; the incidence increases with fractures extending into the transverse foramen. Bilateral or dominant vertebral artery injury can cause fatal ischemic damage to the brain stem and cerebellum. Delayed cortical blindness and recurrent quadriparesis can also occur from occult vertebral artery injury after cervical trauma. Despite the high incidence of vertebral artery injury with cervical trauma as well as the potential morbidity and mortality associated with vertebral artery injury, the great majority of these injuries are clinically silent. Up to 50% of all flexion-distraction injuries (seat-belt injuries) of the thoracolumbar spine are associated with intra-abdominal injuries. Axial loading injury mechanisms that are responsible for the majority of burst fractures in the lumbar spine are also responsible for axial loading injury patterns in the lower lumbar spine and lower extremities. These include fractures of the pars interarticularis of the L5 vertebra, the tibial plafond, and the calcaneus.

Classification of Injury

A. CLASSIFICATION OF BONY INJURY

The spinal column consists of four major components that contribute to its stability: (1) the vertebral bodies; (2) the posterior elements (pedicles, laminae, spinous process, and interlocking paired facets at each level); (3) the intervertebral disk; and (4) the ligamentous and musculoaponeurotic sleeves attached to the bone (interspinous ligaments, facet capsules, ligamentum flavum). In general, an injury disrupting only one of the three components will be relatively stable if protected, whereas if all three components are disrupted the spinal column will be significantly unstable at the level of injury, with risk of reinjury to the spinal canal contents. If injury is present in two of the components, the degree of instability will lie between these extremes. For example, the common mild anterior compression fracture at the thoracolumbar junction of the vertebral body is stable, whereas anterior dislocation of the cervical vertebrae is quite unstable. In the latter injury, there is complete anterior displacement of the facets, disruption of the posterior elements, rupture of the interspinous ligaments and the capsule of the facet joints, and disruption of the entire annulus fibrosus with or without a small fracture of the anterior vertebral body beneath the dislocation.

B. CLASSIFICATION OF NEUROLOGIC INJURY

The motor and sensory examination outlined by the American Spinal Injury Association (ASIA) is the most widely accepted and utilized system to assess the impact on the patient of spinal cord injury. It involves the use of a grading system to evaluate the remaining sensory and motor function. The system allows the patient to be assessed through scales of impairment and functional independence. A thorough neurologic examination should be performed and documented when the patient is initially seen and at frequent intervals thereafter both to ensure that there is no further neurologic deterioration and to document the resolution of spinal shock. Spinal shock is the initial period after spinal cord injury during which metabolic rather than structural derangements in the injured cord (depletion of adenosine triphosphate) result in spinal cord dysfunction characterized by paralysis, hypotonia, and areflexia. Once spinal shock has resolved, the motor and sensory examination allows the patient to be graded on a scale of functional impairment. Return of the bulbocavernosus reflex heralds the end of spinal shock. In most cases, this local reflex arc returns within 48 hours after injury. If a patient has a complete neurologic deficit after spinal shock has resolved, the chance for recovery of neurologic function below the level of injury is practically nonexistent. In contrast, patients with root level injuries (at or below the cauda equina) will recover from functionally complete injuries if they have not been transected and if initial compression by bone fragments, malalignment, disk material, etc, has been relieved.

Determination of Sensory Levels

The sensory level is determined by the patient's ability to perceive pinprick (using a disposable needle or safety pin) and light touch (using a cotton ball). Testing of a key point in each of the 28 dermatomes on the right and left sides of the body as well as evaluation of perianal sensation is required. The variability in sensation for each individual stimulus is graded on a 3-point scale:

0 = Absent
1 = Impaired
2 = Normal
NT = Not testable

In the cervical spine, the C3 and C4 nerve roots supply sensation to the entire upper neck and chest in a cape-like distribution from the tip of the acromion to just above the nipple line. The next adjacent sensory level is the T2 dermatome. The brachial plexus (C5–T1) supplies the upper extremities.

ASIA also recommends testing of pain and deep pressure sensation in the same dermatomes as well as evaluation of proprioception by testing the position sense of the both index fingers and both great toes.

Determination of Motor Levels

The motor level is determined by manual testing of a key muscle in the ten paired myotomes from rostral to caudal. The strength of each muscle is graded on a six-point scale:

0 = Total paralysis
1 = Palpable or visible contraction
2 = Full range of motion of the joint powered by the muscle with gravity eliminated
3 = Full range of motion of the joint powered by the muscle against gravity
4 = Active movement with full range of motion against moderate resistance
5 = Normal strength
NT = Not testable

For myotomes that are not clinically testable by manual muscle evaluation, the motor level is presumed to be the same as the sensory level (C1–4, T2–L1, S2–5).

ASIA also recommends evaluation of diaphragmatic function (via fluoroscopy; C4 level) and the abdominal musculature (via Beevor's sign, ie, upward migration of the umbilicus resulting from upper abdominal contraction in the absence of lower abdominal contraction due to paralysis at the T10 level). Evaluation of medial hamstring and hip adductor strength is also recommended but not required.

ASIA Impairment Scale

Once spinal shock has resolved, motor and sensory examination allows the patient to be graded on a scale of functional impairment. The grading system used is a modification of the Frankel classification system.

ASIA A (complete): No sensory or motor function is preserved below the level of injury, including the sacral segments S4–5.

ASIA B (incomplete): Sensory function is spared but there is no motor function below the level of injury except for the preservation of sacral segments S4–5.

ASIA C (incomplete): Motor function is preserved below the neurologic level, and more than half of the key muscles below the neurologic level have a muscle strength less than grade 3.

ASIA D (incomplete): Motor function is preserved below the neurologic level, and at least half of the muscles below the neurologic level have a muscle strength of at least grade 3.

ASIA E: No neurologic deficit.

Imaging Studies

1. Cervical spine—Plain radiographs are used as the first imaging modality for the cervical spine. The standard series includes an anteroposterior, lateral, and an open-mouth view. Eighty-five percent of all significant injuries to the cervical spine will be detected on the lateral view of the cervical spine. If the standard lateral view does not adequately visualize the C7–T1 junction, further studies such as a swimmer's view, oblique views, or CT of this area are necessary.

2. Thoracolumbar spine—All patients with significant injury and pain in the spinal area require anteroposterior and lateral x-rays of appropriate regions of the thoracic and lumbar spine. Overlying shadows (ribs, transverse processes, visceral soft tissue shadows) can make accurate interpretation of the fracture configuration difficult. CT scanning is useful in assessing the degree of bony injury as well as the amount of bony encroachment into the spinal canal. CT is helpful also for preoperative planning and optimizing the choice of spinal fixation necessary to reduce and stabilize the fracture. MRI is extremely helpful in assessing the degree of neural injury and helps in determining outcome. For example, the presence of intraparenchymal hemorrhage in the spinal cord implies a very poor prognosis for neurologic recovery after incomplete injuries.

Complications

Patients with cervical spine injury may have impaired pulmonary function secondary to intercostal nerve paralysis. Mobilization of secretions by chest physical therapy and frequent suctioning are critical in preventing atelectasis and pulmonary infections. All patients with sensory deficits and paralysis are at high risk of developing decubiti. Padding and suspension of high-risk pressure points (heels), frequent turning, and vigilant nursing care are necessary.

Patients with thoracolumbar spine fractures with or without spinal cord injury may have paralytic ileus secondary to sympathetic chain dysfunction. Oral intake should be limited to clear fluids initially, and gastric suction may be necessary if the degree or duration of ileus is significant.

The stress caused by the injury itself—in combination with systemic corticosteroid therapy—can increase the incidence of gastrointestinal ulceration and bleeding. High-dose corticosteroids can also contribute to the development of pancreatitis and infections.

Venous thromboembolic disease remains a significant problem in the management of patients with spinal injury. Pulmonary embolism is the most common cause of preventable death in hospitalized patients. After major trauma, the incidence of deep venous thrombosis has been estimated to be approximately 58%. The prevalence of deep venous thrombosis in patients with spinal cord injury approaches 100%. Symptomatic and fatal pulmonary embolism occurs in up to

6% of trauma patients despite improvements in trauma care and deep venous thrombosis prophylaxis. Fatal pulmonary embolism occurs in 1–2% of people with spinal cord injury.

Deep venous thrombosis typically occurs within the first 3 weeks after spinal cord injury. However, it can also occur late in the setting of a chronic spinal cord injury, with 83% of the events occurring within the first 6 months. In a recent study, Powell noted that 11.6% of all new spinal cord injury admissions to their rehabilitation unit were diagnosed with a new episode of deep venous thrombosis. Having had a previous deep venous thrombosis increases the risk of developing a subsequent episode by a factor of 2.4.

Optimal prophylaxis against thromboembolic disease in the spinal injury patient has not been determined. Early in the course of management, sequential compression devices and foot pumps are a reasonable alternative to pharmacologic anticoagulation. However, after the first few days of recovery from surgery, pharmacologic prophylaxis has the greatest promise for effective prevention of deep venous thrombosis and pulmonary thromboembolism in spinal cord injury. Low-molecular-weight heparins have shown the greatest promise for efficacy and safety in this population.

Treatment

A. SPINE FRACTURES OR DISLOCATIONS WITHOUT NEUROLOGIC DEFICIT

The goal of treatment is to maintain enough stability to protect the neural elements from further mechanical injury while allowing early mobilization and ameliorating pain.

1. Stable fractures—Fractures with a stable configuration, such as an anterior wedge compression, can be managed by external immobilization in a rigid brace that controls motion and maintains satisfactory alignment at the fracture site. Adult patients with anterior compression greater than 50% of normal vertebral height—especially in the lumbar spine with posterior ligamentous injury—are best treated with open reduction and short-segment posterior fusion and spinal instrumentation. This allows early mobilization and prevents late development of spinal deformity.

2. Unstable fractures or fracture-dislocations—These injuries require external immobilization (cast or brace), skeletal traction, or reduction and internal fixation. In most cervical spine fractures, skeletal traction in the long axis will achieve adequate reduction and restore canal integrity. If used as definitive treatment, 6–12 weeks of traction in recumbency is required, followed by bracing for another 6–12 weeks. Because of this, other forms of immobilization are preferable to extended periods of traction. Halo-vest or halo-cast immobilization may allow adequate control of the fracture with earlier ambulation. External immobilization alone is inadequate for significant ligamentous injuries, as these are less likely than fractures to heal with immobilization. Ligamentous disruptions with spinal instability are best managed with open reduction, internal fixation, and spinal fusion.

Unilateral and bilateral facet subluxations are flexion-distraction injuries that disrupt the posterior ligaments and facet capsules while leaving the intervertebral disk uninjured. A small amount of kyphosis (< 10 degrees) may be seen on lateral radiographs. These subluxations must be differentiated from more severe flexion-distraction injuries that have spontaneously reduced with neck extension.

Bilateral perched facets are at the next level of severity with the flexion-distraction mechanism. The inferior facets slide superiorly and anteriorly over the superior facet until the tips engage on each other. Perching of the facets creates a significant kyphotic deformity of the cervical spine. Disruption of the ligamentum flavum and the posterior annulus of the disk occurs in this injury. Treatment consists of reduction and stabilization with posterior fusion and instrumentation.

Unilateral facet dislocations are caused by adding a rotational force to the flexion-distraction mechanism. This results in attenuation of the interspinous ligament and disruption of the facet capsule and the posterolateral corner of the disk. The overall result of the injury mechanism is a rotational deformity of the spine.

Bilateral facet dislocations are the terminal stage of the flexion distraction injury. On lateral x-rays, there can be 50% anterior translation of the superior vertebra. Up to 60% of cases of bilateral facet dislocations will have associated disk disruption, and disk herniation can be present before reduction of facet dislocations in as many as 55% of cases. This is especially worrisome if the disk fragment is associated with the superior translated vertebra, since reduction of the dislocation is apt to push the herniated disk material into the spinal canal.

Controversy exists over the practicality of imaging the intervertebral disk at the level of the injury prior to reduction in an alert, awake, and neurologically intact patient. This debate is based upon several observations: Despite the alarming frequency of disk herniation associated with these injuries, a large proportion of these disk herniations will be clinically insignificant. In addition, most neurologic deficits have occurred during operative reduction under general anesthesia. Thus, several studies have concluded that immediate traction and reduction of facet dislocations in alert and awake patients can be done safely without the need for preliminary MRI. These studies also noted that immediate re-

duction leads to improved neurologic recovery as compared with delayed reduction. It is important to point out that these patients were treated at either a level I trauma center or a spinal cord injury unit with staff who have developed an expertise in the closed treatment of facet dislocations. Furthermore, the ability to perform a detailed neurologic examination between each incremental increase in cervical traction is a critical step in the technique. Any deterioration in neurologic function can be immediately addressed. Patients who present with severe spinal cord injury (Frankel grades A and B) should undergo immediate closed reduction of the dislocation. Patients who have worsening neurologic status, those who have a spinal cord injury not explained by CT scan, and those with dislocations not reducible with less than 40–60 lb of traction should be evaluated by MRI.

Thoracolumbar fractures may be reduced or maintained in an acceptable position using a rigid orthosis. Open reduction and internal fixation are justified when bracing fails to correct the position (increase in deformity, pain that prevents mobilization, development of a neuralgic deficit). Facet dislocation in the thoracolumbar spine is best treated with open reduction, short-segment instrumentation, and fusion. With the development of improved anterior and posterior spinal fixation systems (such as pedicle screws and rods), reduction and stable fixation can be achieved over fewer spinal segments. This has the advantage of preserving uninjured motion segments and minimizing the development of problems with the adjacent vertebral levels. The injured segment should be fused by placement of an onlay bone graft; the internal fixation device may be removed after the fracture and graft have healed.

B. Spine Fractures or Dislocations With Neurologic Deficit

1. Incomplete neurologic deficit—Patients with stable fractures can be treated in the same way as patients with no neurologic abnormalities if angulation is corrected and if MRI shows no evidence of bone or disk fragments significantly compromising the neural elements. This is with the caveat that the external brace is able to adequately immobilize the injured segment to prevent further neurologic injury. If a significant degree of canal compromise is demonstrated at the spinal cord level or if there is a neurologic deficit, surgical decompression is justified. This can be done either through an anterior approach (followed by strut graft) and internal fixation, a posterior costotransversectomy approach, or a combined anterior and posterior approach. The operative plan is individualized to the particular patient. In general, the anterior or combined approach allows easier decompression of the spinal canal and minimizes the number of levels that need to be included in the fusion. (Figure 43–1.)

Patients with incomplete neurologic deficits and unstable fractures or fracture-dislocations have the same stability requirements as patients without neurologic deficits. They are best managed with open reduction, instrumentation, and spinal fusion. Neural canal com-

promise should be managed as in the preceding paragraph.

2. Complete neurologic deficit—No operative procedure has been devised that will achieve recovery in cases of complete neurologic deficit that has persisted beyond the stage of spinal shock. However, surgical stabilization

Figure 43–1. ***A:*** Anteroposterior radiograph of a 25-year-old woman who was a belted passenger in a motor vehicle accident, sustaining a duodenal injury and a flexion distraction injury at L1–L2. ***B:*** Lateral radiograph showing widening of the posterior elements and injury to the facet joints of L1–L2. ***C:*** CT scan showing subluxation of the inferior facet of L1. ***D:*** and ***E:*** Anteroposterior and lateral radiographs after posterior stabilization with pedicle screws and plates and posterior spinal fusion.

is often necessary (1) because spinal instability may interfere with early mobilization and rehabilitation training and (2) because it may result in loss of function at a higher level by causing mechanical injury on the root or cord segment just above the level of injury.

All stable bony injuries are treated in the same way as those that occur in neurologically intact patients except that any orthosis which extends below the level of sensory loss can cause pressure ulcerations on insensate skin. Patients with unstable injuries of the cervical spine can be managed with continuous traction for 6–12 weeks. Frequent turning—either in an ordinary hospital bed or on a turning frame—and good skin care are necessary to prevent pressure ulceration. However, halo-vest immobilization or internal fixation and spinal fusion is preferable to an extended period of traction.

Relatively early mobilization of patients with cervical spine injuries can be achieved using halo-vest immobilization. Cervical burst fractures with impingement on the spinal cord are best treated with anterior decompression of the spinal cord through removal of the fractured vertebra and anterior spinal fusion using autogenous structural graft, cadaveric strut graft, or a titanium fusion cage. The addition of an anterior cervical plate will allow early mobilization of the patient in a cervical collar.

Thoracolumbar spine injuries with neurologic injury are best treated with internal fixation and short-segment fusion (Figure 43–2).

C. External Support

1. Cervical spine—The halo vest or halo cast is constructed by connecting the halo to either a plaster body cast or a padded plastic vest. The body cast offers better fixation if properly molded over the iliac crests, but it cannot be used if sensory impairment is present.

In stable injuries of the cervical spine, cervical collars or cervical thoracic braces (four-poster) are adequate (Figure 43–3).

2. Thoracolumbar spine—In the thoracolumbar spine, cast or brace immobilization for fractures with potential instability must extend from the sternal notch to the symphysis pubica and should be molded to fit body contours. Thoracic braces are not able to immobilize injuries above the T7 level and must be modified to extend to the cervical spine. As noted above, if brace support is used in patients with sensory deficits, frequent monitoring for potential pressure necrosis of skin requires that the cast or brace be removable to permit inspection of all body surfaces at frequent intervals.

Anderson PA, Bohlman HH: Anterior decompression and arthrodesis of the cervical spine: Long-term motor improvement: part II—Improvement in complete traumatic quadriplegia. J Bone Joint Surg Am 1992;74:683.

Bohlman HH, Anderson PA: Anterior decompression and arthrodesis of the cervical spine: long-term motor improvement: part I—Improvement in incomplete traumatic quadriparesis. J Bone Joint Surg Am 1992;74:671.

Bracken MB et al: Administration of methylprednisolone for 24 or 48 hours or tirilazad mesylate for 48 hours in the treatment of acute spinal cord injury. Results of the Third National Acute Spinal Cord Injury Randomized Controlled Trial. National Acute Spinal Cord Injury Study. JAMA 1997;277:1597.

Carl AL, Tromanhauser SG, Roger DJ: Pedicle screw instrumentation for thoracolumbar burst fractures and fracture-dislocations. Spine 1992;17(8 Suppl):S317.

Cybulski GR et al: Complications in three-column cervical spine injuries requiring anterior-posterior stabilization. Spine 1992;17:253.

Denis F, Burkus JK: Shear fracture-dislocations of the thoracic and lumbar spine associated with forceful hyperextension (lumberjack paraplegia). Spine 1992;17:156.

Ferree BA, Wright AM: Deep venous thrombosis following posterior lumbar spinal surgery. Spine 1993;18:1079.

Garvey TA, Eismont FJ, Roberti LJ: Anterior decompression, structural bone grafting, and Caspar plate stabilization for unstable cervical spine fractures and/or dislocations. Spine 1992;17(10 Suppl):S431.

Gertzbein SD: Scoliosis Research Society: multicenter spine fracture study. Spine 1992;17:528.

Heary RF et al: Acute stabilization of the cervical spine by halo/vest application facilitates evaluation and treatment of multiple trauma patients. J Trauma 1992;33:445.

Jeanneret B, Magerl F: Primary posterior fusion C½ odontoid fractures: indications, technique, and results of transarticular screw fixation. J Spinal Disord 1992;5:464.

Maynard FM Jr et al: International Standards for Neurological and Functional Classification of Spinal Cord Injury. American Spinal Injury Association. Spinal Cord 1997;35:266.

Roy-Camille R et al: Treatment of lower cervical spinal injuries—C3 to C7. Spine 1992;17(10 Suppl):S442.

Vaccaro AR et al: Neurologic outcome of early versus late surgery for cervical spinal cord injury. Spine 1997;22:2609.

FRACTURES & DISLOCATIONS OF THE PELVIS

Pelvic fractures are among the most serious injuries and account for 3% of all fractures. About 60% result from vehicular trauma (eg, automobile, motorcycle, bicycle), 30% from falls, and 10% from crush injuries, athletic injuries, or penetrating trauma. Pelvic fractures are the third most commonly seen injury in fatalities due to motor vehicle accidents.

Life-threatening hemorrhage, deformity, neurologic injury, and genitourinary injury are all potential complications that must be identified and treated early in the setting of a pelvic fracture. The literature shows that the mortality rate varied from 9% to 20% in the 1970s and seemed to decrease in the 1980s to 6–10%. Despite this apparent decrease, pelvic fractures pose a formidable clinical challenge. Hemodynamically unstable

Figure 43–2. A: and **B:** Anteroposterior and lateral radiographs of a severe burst fracture of L1 with canal retropulsion. **C:** Sagittal T2-weighted MRI showing injury to the conus medullaris and intraparenchymal hemorrhage. **D:** and **E:** Anteroposterior and lateral images after L1 vertebrectomy and reconstruction with an anterior titanium cage and short segment posterior fusion.

patients who present to the emergency department with pelvic fracture have a mortality rate of 40–50%.

Anatomy

An understanding of pelvic anatomy is essential for identifying fracture patterns and complications. The pelvis is made up of three bones: two innominate bones and the sacrum. The innominates are further subdivided into the ilium, ischium, and pubis. Stability of the pelvic ring depends entirely on the strong ligamentous connection of the innominate bones and the sacrum. A thick fibrocartilaginous disk joins the anterior aspects of the innominate bones to form the pubic symphysis. This joint acts as a supporting strut for the pelvis because the stability of the ring depends almost entirely upon the sacroiliac joints.

The posterior ligamentous structures can be divided into anterior and posterior complexes. The anterior sacroiliac joint ligaments are broad and flat and connect the iliac wing and the sacral ala. These ligaments primarily resist external rotation and torsional forces. However, posterior ligamentous stability is chiefly imparted by the tension band effect of the posterior

Figure 43–3. Thirty-year-old woman suffering a cervical burst fracture following a motor vehicle accident in which she hit her head on the windshield. ***A–C:*** Lateral radiograph, CT scan, and MRI showing burst fracture of C5. ***D:*** The burst fracture was treated with a vertebrectomy of C5 and fusion from C4 to C6 with a tricortical iliac crest bone graft and plate.

sacroiliac ligament complex. Composed of the interosseous sacroiliac ligaments within the joint and the posterior sacroiliac ligaments spanning the sacrum between the posterior iliac spines, the posterior complex is considered to be the strongest ligament in the human body. The posterior sacroiliac complex resists shear forces between the sacrum and the ilium, clinically preventing displacement of the ilium onto the sacrum.

Finally, the pelvic floor contains two strong ligaments, the sacrospinous and the sacrotuberous ligaments. The sacrospinous ligament exerts strong restraint upon torsional forces while the sacrotuberous ligament resists torsion, shear, and flexion forces on the sacroiliac joint.

Stability

Pelvic stability can be defined as the ability of the pelvic ring to withstand physiologic forces without abnormal deformation. Pathologically, the pelvic ring fails under one or more of three basic modes. External rotation strains the pubic symphysis and the sacrotuberous, sacrospinous, and anterior sacroiliac joint ligaments. After roughly 2.5 cm of diastasis, the pelvic floor liga-

ments and the anterior sacroiliac ligaments begin to fail, giving rise to gross rotatory instability. Because the posterior ligament complex is largely intact, superior or posterior displacement of the involved hemipelvis does not occur. Combined external and shear forces are necessary to completely disrupt pelvic stability. Conversely, internal rotation places the pubic rami under compression and the posterior ligament complexes under tension. The rami often fail in their midportions with transverse fractures and sacral alar impaction. The pelvic floor ligaments remain intact, and gross posterior stability is maintained. Therefore, fractures involving torsional forces on the pelvis often have partial instability in the rotatory plane only, with maintenance of stability to other displacement.

Complete instability, however, disrupts both the anterior and the posterior ligamentous restraints. These injuries often present with widely displaced sacroiliac joints and multiaxial instability of the involved hemipelvis. Such fractures have components of superior and posterior displacement relative to the sacrum in addition to rotational displacement in the sagittal and horizontal planes.

Clinical Findings

Physical examination includes palpation of the pelvic bony landmarks, compression maneuvers to assess stability, and rectovaginal examination looking for bony spikes protruding through the mucosa representing an open fracture. The mortality rate of open pelvic fractures is as high as 50%—compared with 8–15% for closed fractures. Associated injuries should be assessed systematically—lower urinary tract injuries, distal vascular status—and a thorough neurologic examination should be performed.

The anteroposterior radiograph required in all patients with blunt trauma rapidly identifies the major pelvic injury. Inlet and outlet radiographs are often required to supplement the anteroposterior film and better define the position and degree of pelvic instability. Eventually, CT scanning will further delineate fracture stability.

Acute Management

Immediate care of the polytrauma patient with a pelvic fracture must address associated retroperitoneal hemorrhage, pelvic ring instability, and injuries to the genitourinary system and rectum as well as fractures open to the peritoneum. Cessation of blood loss, minimization of septic sequelae, and stabilization of the fracture, allowing early and safe patient mobilization, are the immediate treatment goals. Hemorrhage is the leading cause of death in patients with pelvic fracture, accounting for 60% of the deaths. Most of the blood loss is from the fracture site or injured retroperitoneal veins; only 20% of the deaths are associated with major arterial injury. An average blood replacement of 5.9 units has been reported.

General resuscitative principles are applied to stabilize the patient and provide adequate tissue perfusion. Once other sites of hemorrhage have been ruled out, active bleeding from a pelvic fracture may be controlled by the use of an external fixator device. Major fracture fragments are stabilized, and the pelvic and retroperitoneal space available for fluids is decreased or at least prevented from increasing. If this fails to control hemorrhage, arterial embolization is indicated. Definitive internal fixation is usually required after hemorrhage has been controlled and the patient has been stabilized.

Classification & Treatment

Fractures may be classified as type A (rotationally and vertically stable), type B (rotationally unstable and vertically stable, or type C (rotationally and vertically unstable). Common radiographic signs of pelvic instability include (1) displacement of the posterior sacroiliac complex more than 5 mm in any plane; (2) the presence of a posterior fracture gap rather than an impaction; and (3) the presence of an avulsion fracture of the transverse process of the fifth lumbar vertebra or the sacro-ischial end of the sacrospinous ligaments.

Type A fractures involve the pelvic ring in only one location and are considered stable. Type A1 fractures are avulsion fractures which usually occur at muscle origins such as the anterosuperior iliac spine, anteroinferior iliac spine, and ischial apophysis. These fractures most often occur in adolescents, and conservative treatment is usually sufficient. If displacement is minimal, prompt healing without disability is to be expected. If displacement is marked (ie, > 1 cm), reattachment by open operation is justifiable.

Rarely, symptomatic nonunions develop and are best treated surgically. Type A2 fractures are isolated fractures of the iliac wing without involvement of the hip or sacroiliac joints and are usually a result of direct trauma. Even with significant displacement, bony healing is expected and treatment is therefore symptomatic. Healing may be accompanied by ossification of the hematoma with exuberant new bone formation. Finally, type A3 fractures are isolated fractures of the obturator foramen and usually involve minimal displacement of the pubic or ischial rami. The posterior sacroiliac complex is intact, and the pelvis remains stable. Treatment is symptomatic, with early ambulation and weightbearing as tolerated.

Type B fractures involve breaks in the pelvic ring in two or more sites. This creates a pelvic fracture that is rotationally unstable but vertically stable. Type B1 fractures are open book fractures that occur from anteroposterior compression. Unless the anterior separation of the pubic symphysis is severe (> 6 cm), the posterior sacroiliac complex is usually intact and the pelvis is relatively stable to vertical forces. Significant associated injuries to the perineal and urogenital structures are often present and should always be looked for. For minimally displaced symphysial injuries (< 2.5 cm), only symptomatic treatment is needed. For more displaced fracture-dislocations, reduction is done by lateral compression using the intact posterior sacroiliac complex as the hinge on which the "book is closed." Reduction can be maintained with the use of an external fixator; however, internal fixation is currently favored. "Closing the book" decreases the space available for hemorrhage, increases patient comfort, facilitates nursing care, and allows early mobilization. The use of a sheet in the resuscitative period to tie the thighs together can provide temporary stability and help control hemorrhage.

Type B2 and B3 fractures involve a lateral force applied to the pelvis, causing inward displacement of the hemipelvis through the sacroiliac complex and ipsilateral (B2) or, more often , contralateral (B3) pubic rami fractures. The degree of involvement of the posterior sacroiliac ligament complex will determine the degree of instability. The hemipelvis is infolded, with overlapping of the pubic symphysis. Reduction can be accomplished with external fixation, with internal fixation, or with both. External fixation facilitates nursing care but is not strong enough for ambulation. Definitive care usually is accomplished with internal fixation of both the anterior and posterior aspects of the pelvic ring. Major hemorrhage is associated with these fracture types.

Type C fractures are both rotationally and vertically unstable. They often result from a vertical shear injury such as a fall from a height. Anteriorly, the pubic symphysis or pubic rami may be disrupted. Posteriorly, the sacroiliac joint may be disrupted and dislocated, or there may be a fracture through the sacrum or adjacent iliac wing. The hemipelvis is completely unstable, and there may be associated massive hemorrhage and injury to the lumbosacral pelvis. External fixation is insufficient to maintain reduction, but it may help to control hemorrhage and ease nursing care in the acute stage. Internal fixation is usually required as definitive treatment.

FRACTURES OF THE ACETABULUM

The acetabulum is the portion of the pelvic bone that articulates with the femoral head to form the hip joint. It results from closure of the Y or triradiate cartilage and is covered with hyaline cartilage.

Fractures of the acetabulum (Figure 43–4) occur through direct trauma on the trochanteric region or indirect axial loading through the lower limb. The position of the limb at the time of impact (rotation, flexion, abduction, or adduction) will determine the pattern of injury. Comminution is common.

Classification

Acetabular fractures are classified based on which column is involved. The anterior column comprises the anterior iliac crest, the anterior half of the acetabulum, and the pubic ramus. The posterior column includes the sciatic buttress and the sciatic notch, the posterior half of the acetabulum, and the ischial tuberosity. These two columns unite in an inverted Y pattern whose center articulates with the femoral head. Fractures may involve one or both columns in a simple or complex pattern.

Proper fracture classification requires x-rays of good quality. Two oblique views (Judet views) taken 45 degrees toward and away from the involved side complement the standard anteroposterior view of the pelvis. CT scanning gives further information on the fracture pattern, the presence of free intra-articular fragments, and the status of the femoral head and the rest of the pelvic ring.

Letournel has classified acetabular fractures into ten different types: five simple patterns (one fracture line) and five complex patterns (the association of two or more simple patterns). This is the most widely used classification system as it allows the surgeon to choose the most appropriate surgical approach.

Figure 43–4. Forty-year-old man who fell from a height, sustaining a posterior hip dislocation and an acetabular fracture of the weightbearing dome. ***A:*** Coronal CT reconstructions showing large fragment of the superior dome of the right acetabulum. ***B:*** Oblique radiograph demonstrating concentric reduction of the hip and restoration of the articular surface after open reduction and internal fixation.

Treatment

The goal of treatment is to achieve a spherical congruency between the femoral head and the weightbearing acetabular dome and to maintain it until the bones are healed. As with other pelvic fractures, acetabular fractures are frequently associated with abdominal, urogenital, and neurologic injuries, which should be systematically sought and treated. Significant bleeding is often present and should be stopped as soon as possible.

The stabilized patient should be put in longitudinal skeletal traction through a distal femoral or proximal tibial pin pulling axially in neutral position. A trochanteric screw for lateral traction is contraindicated as it will create a contaminated pin tract and thus preclude possible further surgical treatment. Postreduction x-rays are obtained. In general, a displaced acetabular fracture is rarely reduced adequately by closed methods. If the reduction is judged acceptable, traction is maintained for 6–8 weeks until bone healing is evident. Another 6–8 weeks is necessary before full weightbearing can be attempted. Most authors now feel that any residual displacement after traction is an indication for open reduction and internal fixation as there is a clear correlation between anatomic reduction and prognosis. The choice of approach is of primary importance, and more than one approach will sometimes prove necessary. Acetabular surgery uses extensile approaches and sophisticated reduction and fixation techniques and is best performed by pelvic surgeons. Other surgical indications include free osteochondral fragments, femoral head fractures, irreducible dislocations, or unstable reductions.

Complications

Complications inherent to the injury include posttraumatic degenerative joint disease, heterotopic ossification, femoral head osteonecrosis, deep vein thrombosis, and other complications related to conservative treatment. Surgery is performed to prevent or delay osteoarthritis, but it increases the possibility of complications such as infection, iatrogenic neurovascular injury, and increased heterotopic ossification. When the reduction is stable and fixation is solid, the patient can be mobilized after a few days with nonweightbearing ambulation, and weightbearing may begin as early as 6 weeks. Most pelvic surgeons now routinely use postoperative prophylactic anticoagulation and heterotopic bone formation prophylaxis with irradiation or indomethacin or both.

Lowe MA et al: Risk factors for urethral injuries in men with traumatic pelvic fractures. J Urol 1988;140:506.

McLaren AC, Rorabeck CH, Halpenny J: Long-term pain and disability in relation to residual deformity after displaced pelvic ring fractures. Can J Surg 1990;33:492.

Schafermeyer R: Pediatric trauma. Emerg Med Clin North Am 1993;11:187.

Siegel JH et al: Safety belt restraints and compartment intrusions in frontal and lateral motor vehicle crashes: mechanisms of injuries, complications, and acute care costs. J Trauma 1993; 34:736.

Sinnott R, Rhodes M, Brader A: Open pelvic fracture: an injury for trauma centers. Am J Surg 1992;163:283.

SHOULDER INJURIES

1. Clavicular Fracture

Fractures of the clavicle are commonly associated with a fall on the shoulder or outstretched hand. They may also be associated with a direct blow from high-energy trauma or contact sports. It is vital to evaluate these patients for associated injuries such as brachial plexus palsy, vascular injury, rib fracture, and pneumothorax, which are often more serious than the fracture. These fractures are divided into middle third fractures (most common), lateral third, and medial third fractures. The distal fragment is typically displaced downward by the weight of the arm, and the medial fragment is pulled superiorly by the trapezius and sternocleidomastoid muscles. Open fractures are rare. Anteroposterior and anteroposterior-lordotic x-rays (oblique cephalad projection) should be obtained.

Treatment

All nondisplaced clavicular fractures may be treated in a sling for 4–6 weeks if there is no open wound communicating with the fracture and no tenting of the skin. General indications for surgery are open fractures and fractures with significant displacement (especially if there is tenting of the skin). Neurovascular injuries requiring repair may also require surgical fixation. Fractures of the lateral third of the clavicle may require surgical treatment if they are displaced. Most fractures of the middle third heal with nonoperative treatment unless there is significant overlap of the fracture fragments. Most medial fractures are not significantly displaced and many are missed, since this area overlaps the ribs on x-ray. These are also usually treated with a sling or cuff and collar. Open reduction and internal fixation may be performed with an intramedullary screw or extramedullary plate. Complications of open reduction include infection, migration, or breakage of the fixation device; nonunion; and neurovascular injury (Figure 43–5).

Pyper JB: Non-union of fractures of the clavicle. Injury 1978;9:268.

Zenni FJ, Krieg JK, Rosen MJ: Open reduction and internal fixation of clavicular fractures. J Bone Joint Surg Am 1981; 63:147.

Figure 43–5. Intramedullary screw fixation of a severely displaced middle-third clavicular fracture.

2. Acromioclavicular Dislocation

Dislocation (separation) of the acromioclavicular joint is usually caused by a fall on the tip of the shoulder. The acromion is displaced downward by the weight of the arm, and the clavicle is pulled superiorly by the trapezius. These injuries can be classified by degree of displacement, which correlates with the force of injury. Type I acromioclavicular separation is a strain of the acromioclavicular ligament. Type II injury involves rupture of the acromioclavicular ligament and strain of the coracoclavicular ligament complex. This causes the clavicle to be displaced superiorly. Type III injury involves rupture of both the acromioclavicular and the coracoclavicular ligaments, which causes marked superior migration of the lateral end of the clavicle and a drooping appearance of the shoulder. Occasionally, the clavicle is violently ruptured through the deltotrapezial fascia, locked on the acromion, or displaced under the coracoid process. Anteroposterior x-rays should be taken of both shoulders with the patient standing erect.

Treatment

Most acromioclavicular joint injuries are managed non-operatively with a sling for approximately 4 weeks followed by gradual return to full activity. Most patients do not have significant dysfunction or any need to modify their activities. Surgical reconstruction may be indicated for severe injuries, especially in the population of young athletes.

Bjerneld H, Hovelius L, Thorling J: Acromio-clavicular separations treated conservatively. A 5-year follow-up study. Acta Orthop Scand 1983;54:743.

Galpin RD, Hawkins RJ, Grainger RW: A comparative analysis of operative versus nonoperative treatment of grade III acromioclavicular separations. Clin Orthop 1985;193:150.

Larsen E, Bjerg-Nielsen A, Christensen P: Conservative or surgical treatment of acromioclavicular dislocation: a prospective, controlled, randomized study. J Bone Joint Surg Am 1986; 68:552.

Smith MI, Stewart MJ: Acute acromioclavicular separations: a 20-year study. Am J Sports Med 1979;7:62.

3. Sternoclavicular Joint Dislocation

Dislocation of the sternoclavicular joint is rare. The mechanism of injury is usually a motor vehicle accident or sporting injury. Physical examination and anteroposterior and anteroposterior-cephalic tilt x-rays may demonstrate asymmetry. However, confirmation of the diagnosis with a CT scan is often necessary, especially with retrosternal displacement. It is important to identify the direction of displacement because posterior displacement can cause injury to the esophagus, trachea, great vessels, subclavian artery, carotid artery, and pneumothorax. Dislocations of the sternoclavicular joint in children are often associated with physial fractures.

Treatment

Most injuries to the sternoclavicular joint may be treated with a sling or figure-of-eight harness. Posterior dislocations may require emergent reduction if there is associated vascular compression or injury to the trachea, esophagus, or lungs. Closed reduction of posterior dislocations has been described using shoulder retraction and a towel clip. Rarely, open reduction may be necessary.

Barth E, Hagen R: Surgical treatment of dislocations of the sternoclavicular joint. Acta Orthop Scand 1983;54:746.

Selesnick FH et al: Retrosternal dislocation of the clavicle. J Bone Joint Surg Am 1984;66:287.

4. Scapular Fracture

Scapular fractures are classified by location. Scapular body fractures are often associated with other injuries such as subclavian vessel injury, aortic rupture, pneumothorax, rib fractures, brachial plexus injuries, and other soft tissue injuries associated with high-energy trauma. Fractures of the acromion and coracoid occur rarely. Glenoid fractures must be carefully evaluated for articular surface step-off and associated glenohumeral instability. These fractures may be caused by a blow on the shoulder or by a fall on the outstretched arm. Diagnosis with anteroposterior x-ray in the plane of the scapula and axillary x-ray may be supplemented by an axial view of the scapular body and transscapular Y-view. CT scan may also be helpful if surgery is being considered.

Treatment

Most scapular fractures are treated nonoperatively in a sling for 4–6 weeks. Associated injuries may need to be treated emergently and should not be overlooked. Surgical reconstruction of the scapular body or glenoid is indicated for joint surface malreduction and glenohumeral instability. Comminution of articular surface fragments is common, and surgical reconstruction is technically demanding.

Armstrong CP, Van der Spuy J: The fractured scapula: importance and management based on a series of 62 patients. Injury 1984;15:324.

Froimson AI: Fracture of the coracoid process of the scapula. J Bone Joint Surg Am 1978;60:710.

Wilber MC, Evans EB: Fractures of the scapula: an analysis of forty cases and a review of the literature. J Bone Joint Surg Am 1977;59:358.

5. Proximal Humerus Fracture

Fractures of the proximal humerus occur most commonly in elderly individuals with osteoporosis. The weakened bone and the propensity for falls in this population predispose to hip and shoulder fractures. Initial assessment should seek to determine the cause of any related fall as well as the fracture pattern. Prodromal symptoms related to a syncopal episode, myocardial infarction, stroke, transient ischemic attack, or seizure are not rare. Patients in this population are prone also to associated neurovascular injuries and rotator cuff tears. Careful evaluation is important.

Diagnosis is established by x-rays, occasionally supplemented with CT scan. The radiographic examination should consist of a high-quality anteroposterior x-ray in the plane of the scapula (approximately 30 degrees oblique to the frontal plane of the chest) and axillary x-ray. This may be supplemented with a transscapular Y view, but this x-ray is usually less helpful than the axillary view.

Treatment

Most proximal humerus fractures are nondisplaced and can therefore be treated in a sling or cuff and collar and early gentle range of motion exercises. The most commonly used classification system of proximal humerus fractures defines displacement of more than 1 cm or 45 degrees of the humeral head, humeral shaft, greater tuberosity, or lesser tuberosity. Displaced fractures usually require operative reduction and fixation. Surgical

Figure 43–6. Four-part proximal humerus fracture, impacted on inferior glenoid rim.

reconstruction ranges from closed reduction alone or closed reduction and percutaneous fixation to open reduction and internal fixation or prosthetic arthroplasty (Figures 43–6 and 43–7). Patients do not invariably regain symmetric range of motion, but excellent pain relief and function can be attained. There are many potential complications both from the initial injury and from surgical reconstruction. Avascular necrosis of the humeral head can result from injury to the anterior humeral circumflex artery, and stiffness is common.

Neer CS II: Displaced proximal humeral fractures. 1. Classification and evaluation. 2. Treatment of three-part and four-part displacement. J Bone Joint Surg Am 1970;52:1077, 1090.

Paavolainen P et al: Operative treatment of severe proximal humerus fractures. Acta Orthop Scand 1983;54:374.

Weseley MS, Barenfeld PA, Eisenstein AL: Rush pin intramedullary fixation for fractures of the proximal humerus. J Trauma 1977;17:29.

6. Dislocation of the Shoulder Joint

The shoulder (glenohumeral) joint is the most commonly dislocated joint in the body because it is less constrained than other joints and motion is possible in multiple planes. The constraints that prevent instability include the concavity of the glenoid articular cartilage as it conforms to the humeral head and labrum, negative pressure of the joint, and check-rein glenohumeral ligaments. The rotator cuff also provides dynamic stability by compressing the humeral head against the glenoid. These static and dynamic stabilizers create a delicate balance between motion and stability.

Dislocations are usually related to overhead trauma when the arm is in abduction, extension, and external rotation—eg, when an athlete dislocates a shoulder by

Figure 43–7. Surgical reconstruction with hemi-arthroplasty.

falling on an outstretched hand away from the body. This most common position causes a traumatic anterior dislocation. Most traumatic dislocations are anterior, but posterior dislocations can occur. Shoulder instability is classified by several factors such as traumatic versus atraumatic, initial versus recurrent, acute versus chronic, direction, and voluntary versus involuntary.

Anterior Dislocations of the Shoulder Joint

Anterior dislocations can be diagnosed by history and physical examination. The arm is usually extremely painful and held in a position of slight abduction and external rotation. The anterior shoulder area appears full, and there is a vacant sulcus in the posterior shoulder area. Anteroposterior x-ray in the plane of the scapula and axillary x-ray are necessary to determine the direction of the dislocation and the presence of fracture if any. Humeral head impression fractures and glenoid rim fractures are easily missed if the radiographs are inadequate. Dislocation may also be complicated by injury to the brachial plexus (most commonly the axillary nerve) and rotator cuff tear. The examiner should check particularly over the lateral aspect of the arm for sensory changes due to injury of the axillary nerve.

Posterior Dislocation of the Shoulder Joint

Posterior dislocation is characterized by fullness beneath the spine of the scapula, flattening of the anterior shoulder, prominence of the coracoid, and restriction of motion in external rotation. This injury is frequently missed even by experienced surgeons. The reported incidence of missed diagnosis is as high as 60%. The injury occurs either from direct or indirect force to the anterior shoulder, so that the humeral head is pushed out posteriorly. Common causes of posterior dislocation of the shoulder are indirect forces produced with convulsive seizures or electric shock. Anteroposterior x-rays of the chest may look deceptively normal with posterior dislocation, but an axillary view and an anteroposterior x-ray in the scapular plane will show the true position of the head in relation to the glenoid. This dislocation may also be reduced by longitudinal and gentle transverse traction. The reduction may be held in a sling for 3–6 weeks with some external rotation if necessary.

Multidirectional Instability

Patients with congenital or acquired laxity may develop symptomatic shoulder instability in multiple directions. These patients should be initially treated with 6–9 months of rehabilitation and strengthening monitored by a physical therapist. Most of these patients recover stability with muscular strengthening of the rotator cuff and scapular stabilizing muscles.

Voluntary Dislocators

Patients who voluntarily dislocate their shoulders have a high recurrence rate after surgical procedures. Therefore, surgery is usually avoided in this population.

Treatment

The treatment of shoulder dislocations consists of closed reduction after careful examination and documentation of neurovascular status and high-quality x-rays. Many methods of closed reduction have been described, including gentle traction in the prone position and traction-countertraction with a sheet. All methods of reduction rely on adequate analgesia and relaxation. Forceful reductions should be avoided because they may cause brachial plexus injury, vascular injury, or fracture. Postreduction x-rays document a concentric reduction and rule out any associated fracture. Once reduced, the arm is placed in a sling for 3–4 weeks before protected motion exercises are initiated.

Surgical reconstruction is indicated for anterior traumatic instability that is recurrent. The incidence of recurrent instability approaches 80–90% for active young athletes. Therefore, the indication for surgery depends on age and activity level as well as the number of traumatic dislocations and associated fracture or soft tissue injury. After operative repair, the shoulder is usually immobilized in a shoulder immobilizer for 3–6 weeks before active motion is begun. Open surgical repairs for anterior dislocation are successful in preventing further episodes of dislocation in 90–95% of patients. Arthroscopic repair may also be performed.

Aronen JG, Regan K: Decreasing the incidence of recurrence of first time anterior shoulder dislocations with rehabilitation. Am J Sports Med 1984;12:283.

Cisternino SJ et al: The trough line: a radiographic sign of posterior shoulder dislocation. AJR Am J Roentgenol 1978;130:951.

Engelhardt MB: Posterior dislocation of the shoulder: report of six cases. South Med J 1978;71:425.

Morrey BF, Janes JM: Recurrent anterior dislocation of the shoulder: long-term follow-up of the Putti-Platt and Bankhart procedures. Bone Joint Surg Am 1976;58:252.

Rowe CR: Acute and recurrent anterior dislocations of the shoulder. Orthop Clin North Am 1980;11:253.

Rowe CR, Zarins B: Chronic unreduced dislocations of the shoulder. J Bone Joint Surg Am 1982;64:494.

7. Rotator Cuff Tears

Rotator cuff tears and rotator cuff impingement are common sources of shoulder pain. Four rotator cuff muscles (supraspinatus, infraspinatus, teres minor, and subscapularis) function to move the arm and stabilize the shoulder joint. There is a full spectrum of injury ranging from minor irritation (tendonitis, bursitis, strain) of the rotator cuff to bony impingement and rotator cuff tears. The most severe condition is a massive, chronic rotator cuff tear that subsequently leads to proximal migration of the humeral head, local osteopenia, and arthritic changes of the humeral head. This is rotator cuff arthropathy.

Patients with "rotator cuff syndrome" usually present with pain and weakness related to attempted overhead activities and active movements with the arm away from the body. Physical examination demonstrates impingement pain with certain overhead movements and sometimes significant rotator cuff weakness. Diagnosis is made by history and physical examination. Specific shoulder x-rays can be helpful to evaluate any bony impingement from the acromion, acromioclavicular joint, or coracoacromial ligament. MRI is the most useful test to evaluate rotator cuff tears and associated intra-articular pathology (Figure 43–8).

Treatment

The treatment of shoulder pain related to rotator cuff pathology (inflammation, degeneration, tear) depends on other patient variables such as age, activity level, hand dominance as well as the chronicity and level of

Figure 43–8. T2-weighted MRI showing a massive rotator cuff tear.

pain and dysfunction. Tears may result from single event trauma (a fall on the outstretched hand), repetitive trauma (baseball pitchers), or degeneration of the rotator cuff in older patients.

Most cases of shoulder pain related to the rotator cuff are initially treated nonoperatively. Activity modification, NSAIDs, physical therapy, home exercises—all can be beneficial. Some patients require a subacromial lidocaine with corticosteroid injection to control inflammation and pain. Rotator cuff tears can also be treated with surgical reconstruction if they continue to be painful and disabling despite attempted nonoperative therapy. One exception to this general rule is the acute traumatic massive rotator cuff tear, which should be repaired acutely in order to prevent rotator cuff atrophy and retraction. Acromioplasty and distal clavicle excision are performed at the same time if coracoacromial arch impingement contributes to the rotator cuff tear.

Bassett RW, Cofield RH: Acute tears of the rotator cuff. Clin Orthop 1983;175:18.

Gore DR et al: Shoulder-muscle strength and range of motion following surgical repair of full-thickness rotator-cuff tears. J Bone Joint Surg Am 1986;68:266.

Hawkins RJ, Misamore GW, Hobeika PE: Surgery for full-thickness rotator-cuff tears. J Bone Joint Surg Am 1985;67:1349.

Neer CS, Marberry TA: On the disadvantages of radical acromionectomy. J Bone Joint Surg Am 1981;63:416.

Tibone JE et al: Shoulder impingement syndrome in athletes treated by an anterior acromioplasty. Clin Orthop 1985;(198):134.

8. Glenohumeral Arthritis

Arthritis of the glenohumeral joint may be caused by osteoarthritis, inflammatory disease, previous trauma, previous surgery, or arthritis of recurrent instability. Patients have pain with activities and rainy weather just as in arthritis in other joints. They also complain of stiffness, which is usually progressive over time. Physical examination discloses limited motion and usually crepitus with motion (even with the arm at the side). Examination by proper shoulder x-rays shows the characteristic joint space narrowing, humeral head osteophytes, and eburnation of the subchondral bone.

Before operative treatment is elected, a thorough course of conservative measures is indicated such as physical therapy, analgesics, and nonsteroidal anti-inflammatory drugs. An intra-articular lidocaine-steroid injection can be helpful for nonsurgical candidates with debilitating pain. Surgery becomes an option for patients with significant pain and limitation of activity because of their arthritis. Arthroscopic debridement can be helpful for some patients but may offer only a short term solution. Shoulder arthroplasty (hemiarthroplasty, total shoulder replacement) offers a longer-term solution with an excellent 10-year symptom-free function rate. Pain relief is consistent and function is usually improved. Contraindications to total arthroplasty are active or latent septic arthritis, paralysis of the shoulder musculature, and neuropathic joints. Another option for younger patients with severe bone destruction is surgical arthrodesis.

Cofield RH: Total shoulder arthroplasty with the Neer prosthesis. J Bone Joint Surg Am 1984;66:899.

Cofield RH, Briggs BT: Glenohumeral arthrodesis: operative and long-term functional results. J Bone Joint Surg Am 1979; 61:668.

Rybka V, Raunio P, Vainio K: Arthrodesis of the shoulder in rheumatoid arthritis: a review of forty-one cases. J Bone Joint Surg Br 1979;61:155.

Neer CS, Watson KC, Stanton FJ: Recent experience in total shoulder replacement. J Bone Joint Surg Am 1982;64:319.

Post M, Haskell SS, Jablon M: Total shoulder replacement with a constrained prosthesis. J Bone Joint Surg Am 1980;62:327.

Ranawat CS, Warren R, Inglis AE: Total shoulder replacement arthroplasty, Orthop Clin North Am 1980;11:367.

FRACTURES OF THE SHAFT OF THE HUMERUS

Most fractures of the shaft of the humerus result from direct trauma. X-rays in two planes are necessary to determine the configuration of the fracture and the direction of displacement of the fragments. The shoulder and elbow must be included on the initial x-rays to rule out the possibility of fracture or dislocation involving adjacent joints. Before definitive treatment is initiated, a careful neurologic examination should be performed in order to determine the status of the radial nerve and brachial vessels.

Treatment

Most midshaft humeral fractures can be treated nonoperatively in a cast, splint, or brace. The coaptation splint may be molded to improve reduction of the fracture. Alignment should be verified on anteroposterior and transthoracic x-rays with the patient standing. If stabilization has not taken place after 6–8 weeks, consideration of internal fixation and bone grafting is justified. About 5–10% of humeral fractures demonstrate radial nerve involvement. Fractures of the distal third of the humerus are especially vulnerable because the nerve is fixed to the proximal fragment by the intermuscular septum and is more easily injured at the time of displacement. Most radial nerve injuries are the result of stretching or contusion, and function will return in days or months. Open reduction of closed fractures may be indicated if adequate apposition of major fragments cannot be obtained by closed methods, the fracture communicates with an open wound, or arterial circulation has been interrupted.

Balfour GW, Mooney V, Ashby ME. Diaphyseal fractures of the humerus treated with a ready-made fracture brace. J Bone Joint Surg Am 1982;64:11.

Mast JW et al: Fractures of the humeral shaft: a retrospective study of 240 adult fractures. Clin Orthop 1975;(112):254.

Pollock FH et al: Treatment of radial neuropathy associated with fractures of the humerus. J Bone Joint Surg Am 1981;63:239.

FRACTURES & DISLOCATIONS ABOUT THE ELBOW

Anatomy & Biomechanics

The elbow is a complex hinged joint that consists of three bony articulations: the radiocapitellar joint, the ulnohumeral joint, and the proximal radioulnar joint. The bony architecture lends stability to the elbow, but the soft tissue restraints play an important role as well. On the medial side of the elbow, the anterior band of the medial (ulnar) collateral ligament is the primary stabilizer to valgus stress. The lateral ulnar collateral ligament is the primary stabilizer on the lateral side of the elbow. Disruption of this portion of the lateral collateral ligament complex leads to posterolateral instability.

The normal range of motion of the elbow is up to 150 degrees of flexion. Normal pronation and supination are 75 degrees and 85 degrees, respectively. The carrying angle is the resting point of the elbow in full extension. In males, the carrying angle is generally 10–15 degrees valgus; in females, 15–20 degrees valgus.

When elbow injury is suspected, it is important to perform a thorough physical examination of the entire upper extremity including the shoulder and the wrist, looking for associated injuries. Inspections for swelling and deformity as well as palpation are important. Careful neurovascular examination is also critical prior to implementing treatment. Do not forget to assess components of the forearm and hand.

The type of fracture or dislocation sustained is dependent on the mechanism of the injury. A minimum of three x-ray views of the elbow should be obtained: anteroposterior, lateral, and oblique. If examination or subjective complaints indicate the possibility of an associated wrist or forearm injury, x-rays of these areas should also be obtained.

Probably the most useful classification system for distal humerus fractures is the AO system, based on the concept of column integrity and intra-articular involvement. Type A fractures are extra-articular and are further subdivided into A1–A3 fractures based on degree of comminution. This would include epicondylar, supracondylar, and transcondylar fractures. Type B fractures involve only a portion of the articular surface, as in unicondylar and intercondylar fractures. Type B1 fractures are lateral column fractures only; type B2 fractures are medial column fractures only; and type B3 fractures involve only the distal articular surface without either column. Type C fractures involve the entire distal articular surface and are subclassified as C1–3 based on the amount of metaphysial and articular comminution.

Supracondylar Fractures of the Humerus

A. In Children

Supracondylar fractures are much more common in the pediatric population, generally from a direct blow to the elbow from a fall. There are extension (96%) and flexion type fractures. In the extension type, the fragment is displaced posteriorly; in the much less common flexion type, the distal fragment is displaced anteriorly.

These are extra-articular fractures that occur proximal to the olecranon fossa. They are AO type A fractures. Understating normal radiographic anatomy of the elbow is crucial to diagnosing any elbow fracture, especially in the pediatric patient. They require emergent treatment. In the skeletally immature patient, stable and nondisplaced fractures can be treated in a posterior splint or long arm cast for 3–4 weeks with careful weekly x-ray follow-up.

Displaced A2 fractures with the posterior cortex intact can usually be reduced with gentle manipulation by applying longitudinal traction, an anteriorly directed force on the fragment, and flexing the elbow to 120 degrees under sedation or general anesthetic (Figure 43–9). If reduction can be obtained, this can be treated in a long arm cast or splint. However, close follow-up is imperative. Many surgeons will elect to do a closed reduction and percutaneous pinning with Kirschner wires in order to avoid complications of late loss of reduction and malunion or vascular compromise (Volkmann's ischemic contracture) if it is necessary to keep the elbow flexed > 90 degrees to hold the reduction.

Completely displaced, unstable A3 fractures require fixation. They are often associated with neurovascular injury, and this must always be evaluated. Closed reduction and percutaneous pinning is the first choice if the reduction can be achieved. Some surgeons prefer to make an incision on the medial side to visualize the ulnar nerve and avoid injury during pin placement. If closed reduction is unsuccessful, open reduction and pin placement are required.

Figure 43–9. Reduction of a supracondylar humerus fracture. Reduction of the extension injury is accomplished by longitudinal traction *(A)* and flexion of the elbow *(B).* (Reproduced, with permission, from Charnely J: *Closed Treatment of Common Fractures,* 3rd ed. Churchill Livingstone, 1972.)

If there is any question of vascular injury, angiography or open exploration should be undertaken to avoid vascular compromise. Careful postoperative monitoring is always indicated in these injuries.

Occasionally in the patient with multiple injuries, surgery is not an option. Under these circumstances, unstable fractures can be treated with olecranon pin skeletal traction.

B. IN ADULTS

Supracondylar fractures are uncommon after the physes have closed. The transcondylar fracture is even less common but is more common in the older age group. As in the pediatric patient, there are both extension and flexion types, with the extension type being much more common.

Examination and diagnosis are the same as previously described for the pediatric patient. Treatment consists of closed manipulation with longitudinal traction and manipulation of the distal humeral fragment into position with the thumb. If reduction can be achieved, the patient is then splinted in the degree of flexion necessary to maintain the reduction. However, if extreme flexion is necessary and there are risks of vascular compromise, an alternative method of fixation must be used—closed reduction and percutaneous pinning, open reduction and fixation with screws or plates, or external fixation. Some advocate surgical fixation to prevent vascular compromise and allow earlier range of motion activity.

The rare flexion supracondylar fracture should be converted to an extension type if possible. If that cannot be done, the fracture is reduced by longitudinal traction on the humerus with the elbow flexed 90 degrees. The distal fragment is pushed posteriorly while the humerus is translated anteriorly. The same recommendations concerning immobilization versus surgery are followed as for the extension type.

Epicondylar Fractures of the Humerus

Lateral epicondylar fractures are rare, but medial epicondylar fractures are not uncommon especially in children and adolescents. If displacement is minimal < 2–3 mm), closed treatment is appropriate. However, if the fragment is displaced more than a few millimeters, open reduction and fixation with smooth pins or screws would be the recommended treatment. On the medial side, open treatment is preferred over percutaneous fixation so that the ulnar nerve can be visualized and protected. Occasionally, the fragment remains symptomatic or can cause ulnar nerve irritation after healing. If this occurs, the fragment can be excised.

INTRA-ARTICULAR FRACTURES OF THE HUMERUS

Condylar Fractures

These are uncommon fractures, accounting for only 3–5% of distal humeral fractures. Lateral condylar fractures are more frequent than medial condylar fractures and occur in the sagittal plane by one of two mechanisms. Avulsion fractures occur by indirect force, and the fragment ends up distal to its origin. An axial load causes a shear fracture and displaces the fragment proximally.

The classification system used is that described by Milch (Figure 43–10). A type I lateral condylar fracture involves part or all of the capitellum. A type II lateral condylar fracture extends into part or all of the trochlea. Type I medial condylar fractures do not extend beyond the trochlear groove, and type II fractures extend into the trochlear sulcus. Type II condylar fractures are unstable injuries and are technically fracture-dislocations.

Undisplaced type I fractures can be treated with splint or cast immobilization and close follow-up to check for displacement. Displaced type I fractures can be treated with closed reduction and immobilization if reduction is successful. Type II fractures are inherently unstable and should be treated with open reduction and screw fixation. It is important to obtain joint congruity.

Malunion of type I lateral condylar fractures can lead to tardy ulnar nerve palsy. Malunion of type I lateral and medial condylar fractures can be treated with open wedge osteotomy. Type II malunions are more difficult to deal with secondary to the joint incongruity and subluxation.

LATERAL CONDYLE FRACTURES   MEDIAL CONDYLE FRACTURES

Figure 43–10. Condyle fractures. Milch classification. The type II fracture involves the lateral lip of the trochlea—thus its inherent instability. (Reproduced, with permission, from Milch H: Fractures and fracture dislocation of the humeral condyles. J Trauma, 1964.)

Fractures of the Capitellum

This fracture accounts for less than 1% of all elbow fractures. It is important to distinguish it from the lateral condylar fracture. The most widely accepted classifications system is as follows (Figure 43–11): Type I (most common) involves most or all of the capitellum and sometimes part of the trochlea; type II involves a variable amount of articular surface, usually with very little subchondral bone attached; and type III is a comminuted compression fracture of the articular surface.

The mechanism of injury is usually a fall on the outstretched hand for type I and type III fractures and a shearing indirect force for type II fractures. There is often an associated radial head fracture. Diagnosis requires careful scrutiny of the radiographs and suspicion on physical examination. Tomograms may be necessary to see the fragment.

In general, with large fragments, an attempt should be made for open reduction and internal fixation. Small fragments should be excised.

Intercondylar Fractures

These are commonly described as T or Y condylar fractures and are among the most challenging to treat. The mechanism of injury is a wedge effect of the proximal ulna on the trochlear groove of the humerus causing a splitting of the humerus. Comminution in usually associated with these injuries. Classification systems used are the AO classification described earlier and a more succinct system described by Riseborough and Radin in 1969, as follows (Figure 43–12): Type I, undisplaced

Figure 43–12. Intercondylar fractures. **A:** Type I undisplaced T-condylar fracture of the elbow. **B:** Type II displaced but not rotated T-condylar fracture. **C:** Type III displaced and rotated T-condylar fracture. **D:** Type IV displaced rotated and comminuted T-condylar fracture. (Reproduced, with permission, from Bryan RS: Fractures about the elbow in adults. In: *American Academy of Orthopaedic Surgeons: Instructional Course Lectures,* vol. 30. Mosby, 1981.)

Figure 43–11. Fractures of the capitellum. The type I fracture involves a large portion of bone, often the entire structure. Type II is a shear fracture, often with minimal subchondral bone, and may displace posteriorly **(A).** A type III fracture is a comminuted fracture with varying amounts of displacement of the fracture fragments **(B).** (Reproduced, with permission, from Morrey B: *The Elbow and Its Disorders,* Saunders, 1985.)

fracture between the capitellum and trochlea; type II, separation of the capitellum and trochlea without appreciable rotation of the fragments in the frontal plane; type III, separation of the fragments with rotational deformity; and type IV, severe comminution of the articular surface with wide separation of the humeral condyles.

Traditional treatment consisted of closed reduction and casting or traction. Open reduction and internal fixation is now the treatment of choice for certain types of fractures. Type I fractures can be treated closed with early mobilization when swelling subsides and the fracture has had two weeks or so to consolidate. Most type II and type III fractures should be treated with open reduction and internal fixation with plates and screws. Type IV fractures are the most difficult to treat, especially in the older patient with osteopenia. With diffuse osteopenia in the elderly, type IV fractures are probably best treated with the "bag of bones" technique—in other words, conscientious neglect. This means short-term immobilization and early range of motion exercises without trying to reduce the comminuted fragments. In the younger patient with good quality bone and a type IV fracture, it is reasonable to attempt reconstruction. Bone grafting of defects may be necessary.

It is important to realize that there are two distinct components which require reduction and fixation with intercondylar fractures: the intra-articular intercondylar component and the supracondylar one. Kirschner wires or, preferably, screw fixation can be used to stabilize the intercondylar component. This is the most important part of the reduction, reestablishing joint congruity. It is recommended then that the medial and lateral columns be stabilized with plates. The critical issue is to obtain rigid fixation if open reduction and internal fixation are undertaken. Early mobilization can then begin. Operation without obtaining rigid fixation is the worst option of all, as stiffness and joint ankylosis is accelerated.

FRACTURES OF THE PROXIMAL ULNA

Olecranon Fractures

The olecranon is the most proximal palpable portion of the ulna. It is located subcutaneously without much soft tissue coverage. The triceps has a broad insertion at this level.

Anteriorly, the olecranon forms the greater sigmoid (semilunar) notch of the ulna, which articulates with the trochlea. The most proximal anterior portion of the ulna is the coronoid process, which lends stability to the elbow joint.

Olecranon fractures usually occur with a direct blow or as an avulsion injury with forceful triceps contraction. They have been classified as undisplaced, displaced, transverse, oblique, and comminuted. Fracture type dictates appropriate treatment.

A true lateral radiograph of the elbow is essential to accurately assess fracture type. An anteroposterior view and an oblique view should be obtained as well. The goals of treatment are to restore articular congruity and stability, to preserve triceps function, to prevent stiffness, and to avoid complications.

Undisplaced fractures can be managed in a long arm splint or cast with the arm in mid flexion. Careful follow-up with radiographs should be done at weekly intervals for at least 2 weeks. In general, there is sufficient stability at 3 weeks to allow early motion from full extension to 90 degrees of flexion, with progression of flexion at 6 weeks.

There are two options available for displaced fractures—again, depending on fracture pattern and demands of the patient: open reduction and internal fixation or excision.

The tension band wire technique with either longitudinal Kirschner wires or a 6.5 mm cancellous screw is the preferred method for most fractures with minimal comminution. Segmental fractures or comminuted fractures are often better addressed with plating.

External fixation is also an option for comminuted fractures and those with accompanying soft tissue disruption, as in open fractures.

If there is significant comminution or in the elderly patient with poor bone quality, excision of the fragment with reattachment of the triceps is acceptable treatment. Stability must be considered if excision is to be undertaken. If there is also anterior fracture (coronoid) or soft tissue disruption, simple excision could render the elbow unstable.

The most frequent complication of these fractures is prominent implants that must be removed after healing has occurred. Loss of fixation and elbow stiffness have also been reported.

Coronoid Fractures

The coronoid process is the anterior beak-shaped portion of the ulna, forming the buttress anteriorly of the greater sigmoid notch. The anterior portion of the medial collateral ligament attaches here, as well as a portion of the anterior capsule. It therefore contributes to elbow stability.

Isolated fractures of the coronoid are uncommon and are more frequently associated with elbow dislocations or other fractures about the elbow. The mechanism of injury is usually forced posterior displacement of the proximal ulna as with a dislocation or hyperextension force of the elbow. It is important to obtain oblique radiographic views in assessing these fractures as they are sometimes difficult to see on lateral and anteroposterior views.

These fractures have been classified by Regan and Morrey into three types as follows (Figure 43–13): Type

Figure 43–13. Coronoid fractures. The coronoid fracture has been classified into three types by Regan and Morrey. (Reproduced, with permission, from Browner B et al: *Skeletal Trauma.* Saunders, 1992.)

I, avulsion of the tip of the coronoid; type II, a single or comminuted fragment involving 50% or less of the coronoid process; and type III, a single or comminuted fragment involving over 50% of the coronoid process.

Type I fractures can be treated with immobilization in flexion for 3 weeks (or less if the fragment and elbow are stable). Associated fractures should be treated as appropriate in each case with the goal of fracture stability for early range of motion. Isolated coronoid fractures without elbow instability can be treated in the same way as type I fractures. If there is associated elbow instability from soft tissue damage or other fractures, consideration should be given to open reduction and internal fixation. If there is one large fragment, this can be achieved with a screw, Kirschner wire fixation, or suture technique. With comminution, the best approach may be application of an external fixator. Type III fractures are most often associated with significant elbow instability. They are treated in the same way as unstable type II fractures. Excision of fragments is not recommended as this can lead to permanent elbow instability.

FRACTURES OF THE PROXIMAL RADIUS

Radial Head Fractures

Radial head fractures are caused by an axial load on the pronated forearm. The fracture can be isolated or associated with elbow dislocation. Anteroposterior, lateral, and radial head view radiographs will show the fracture. There is usually a fat pad sign on the lateral x-ray.

The Mason classification system is the one most commonly used to describe these fractures. There are three types (Figure 43–14): Type I, nondisplaced; type II, displaced (often a single fragment); and type III, comminuted. Some also add a type IV, fractures associated with dislocation, as this calls for different treatment and implies a worse prognosis.

Other than amount of displacement and comminution, elbow motion is another important factor in considering appropriate treatment. Motion should be assessed acutely by aspirating the hematoma and injecting local anesthetic into the elbow joint. If full range of motion is present, treatment is based on the radiographic findings. However, if there is an obstacle to full range of motion, that must be considered in planning operative versus nonoperative intervention.

Type I (nondisplaced) fractures are treated with a brief period of immobilization in a sling followed by early motion at about 10–14 days after injury. This generally yields good results, with the most common complication being loss of full extension.

There is controversy and about what is the proper treatment of type II fractures. If displacement is minimal and range of motion is full, some would advocate

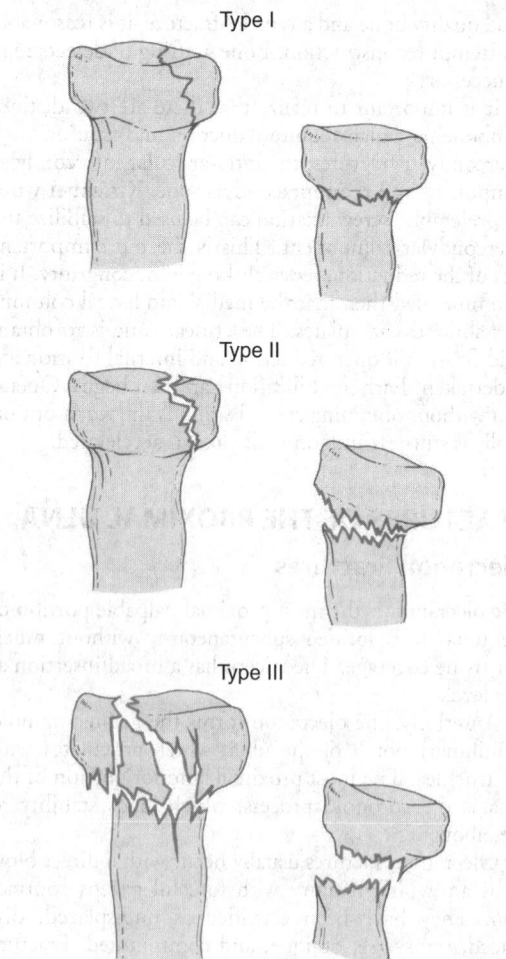

Figure 43–14. Radial head fractures. The modified Mason classification system for radial head fractures. (Reproduced, with permission, from Browner B et al: *Skeletal Trauma.* Saunders, 1992.)

treating with a period of immobilization. If the amount of displacement is unacceptable or there is bony block, operation is necessary. Options include open reduction with internal fixation and excision of part or all of the radial head. If the radial head is excised in its entirety, the decision must be made whether or not to replace it with an implant. If there is instability after removal of the head or if there is concomitant injury to the wrist, a radial head implant should be used. Titanium implants are preferable to Silastic.

Type III fractures are treated by excision of fragments with or without implant replacement, based on the same criteria as set forth above for type II fractures.

Type IV fractures are treated with reduction of the dislocation followed by treatment of the radial head based on its type as described above.

ACUTE INSTABILITY OF THE ELBOW JOINT

The elbow is the second most commonly dislocated joint in the adult (after the shoulder). It occurs when the load placed on the structures about the elbow exceed the intrinsic stability provided by the bony anatomy and ligamentous and muscular constraints. As with any other joint dislocation, the goal of treatment is expeditious reduction.

Dislocations are classified by the direction of displacement of the distal bone. Because there are two bones in the forearm, in addition to the anterior, posterior, medial, and lateral dislocation, one can also have a divergent dislocation when the radius and ulna are forced apart by the distal humerus (Figure 43–15) This is a rare situation. It is also possible to have partial dislocations in which only the radial head or the ulna alone is dislocated. Isolated radial head fractures are rare and are usually accompanied by a fracture of the ulna (Monteggia's fracture).

Standard anteroposterior, lateral, and oblique radiographs of the elbow should be obtained to determine the direction of dislocation as an aid in determining the appropriate reduction maneuver. If fracture about the elbow has occurred with the dislocation, overall treatment is usually dictated by the fracture. The elbow may not be rendered stable until the fractures are fixed. Adequate fracture care will usually cause secondary reduction of the dislocation. Careful neurovascular examination both before and after reduction is critical. Postreduction radiographs should always be obtained—not only to determine the success of the reduction but also to look for any other injury that may have been obscured on the initial x-rays or caused by the reduction maneuver. These patients should be observed for 24 hours to watch for the development of compartment syndrome.

Posterior Elbow Dislocations

This is by far the most common type of elbow dislocation. It results from an axial force being applied to the extended elbow. The extremity may appear to be shortened and the elbow flexed. Both collateral ligaments are disrupted regardless of whether the dislocation is posteromedial or posterolateral.

With adequate anesthesia (conscious sedation, local joint infiltration, or perhaps general anesthesia), traction is applied with the forearm flexed to 90 degrees,

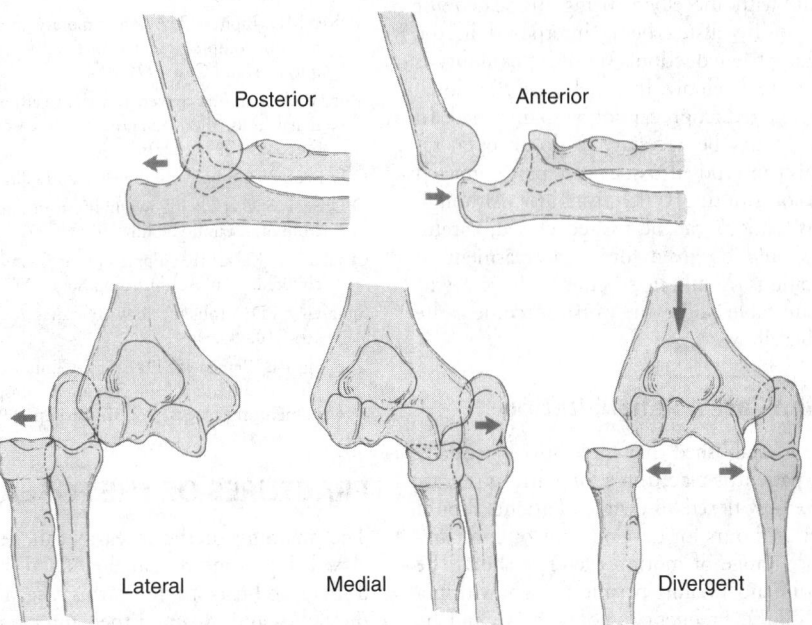

Figure 43–15. Elbow dislocations. An elbow dislocation is defined by the direction of the forearm bones. (Reproduced, with permission, from Browner B et al: *Skeletal Trauma.* Saunders, 1992.)

and the concomitant medial or lateral displacement is then corrected. This should be a gentle maneuver. A "clunk" is usually appreciated as the elbow is reduced back into position. The elbow is then taken through a full range of motion to check for bony block as well as instability. Repeat neurovascular examination and radiographs are obtained.

Anterior Elbow Dislocations

These are relatively rare. Treatment is similar to that of posterior dislocations except that the reduction maneuver is reversed.

Medial & Lateral Elbow Dislocations

With lateral dislocations, some joint motion may be maintained as the ulna may be displaced into the groove between the trochlea and capitellum. The anteroposterior radiograph best shows the direction of dislocation. Again, after adequate anesthesia, the joint is reduced by first applying a distraction force and then a medial or lateral force depending on the direction of dislocation.

Irreducible Dislocations

Very rarely, it is not possible to reduce the elbow by closed reduction techniques. This may be due to delayed treatment, with the elbow being dislocated for days to weeks, or by tissues being interposed in the joint and blocking the reduction. Another possibility is the extremely unstable elbow, in which case the elbow is reducible but the reduction cannot be maintained. In these instances, it may be necessary to do an open reduction to extract interposed tissues or repair damaged tissues that are contributing to the instability. Although most elbow dislocations can be treated closed, careful consideration should be given for open treatment of unstable dislocations. While it is better to have a stiff elbow than an unstable elbow, the worst outcome is the stiff and unstable elbow.

Postreduction Care & Rehabilitation

Once it has been established that the elbow is reduced and stable, the patient is placed in a long arm posterior splint with the elbow flexed 90 degrees. Patients should be observed for 24 hours for development of compartment syndrome. Range of motion exercises should be started when pain and swelling permit, usually within a few days after injury. Frequent radiographs should be taken to confirm that the elbow remains reduced during early rehabilitation. The splint is generally discontinued in 1 or 2 weeks if the elbow is stable.

Complications

Several complications that can occur with this injury, both acutely and chronically. Acute complications are mainly those of nerve and vascular injury. Careful assessment is required both before and after treatment, with early intervention for the development of compartment syndrome. Other complications include continued instability or stiffness with loss of motion. Instability is addressed surgically in most cases. Stiffness can usually be avoided with early range of motion exercises, but if it does occur and is severe it can be addressed with surgical capsulectomies. Heterotopic ossification can also be seen—more commonly in the brain-injured or burn patient. It is generally recommended that areas of heterotopic ossification be excised not earlier than 6 months after injury. In high-risk patients, indomethacin or radiation can be used as prophylaxis.

Davidson PA, Moseley JB Jr, Tullos HS: Radial head fracture: a potentially complex injury. Clin Orthop 1993;(297):224.

Helfet DL, Schmeling GJ: Bicondylar intra-articular fractures of the distal humerus in adults. Clin Orthop 1993;(292):26.

Hotchkiss RN: Displaced Fractures of the Radial Head: internal Fixation or Excision. J Am Acad Orthop Surg 1997;5:1.

Jupiter JB, Mehne DK: Elbow trauma: fractures of the distal humerus. Orthopaedics 1992;15:825.

Kuhn JE, Louis DS, Loder RT: Divergent single-column fractures of the distal part of the humerus. J Bone Joint Surg Am 1995;77:538.

McKee MD, Jupiter JB: A contemporary approach to the management of complex fractures of the distal humerus and their sequelae. Hand Clin 1994;10:479.

Morrey BF: Current concepts in the treatment of fractures of the radial head, the olecranon, and the coronoid. J Bone Joint Surg Am 1995;77:316.

O'Driscoll SW: Elbow instability. Hand Clin 1994;10:405.

O'Driscoll SW et al: Elbow subluxation and dislocation: a spectrum of instability. Clin Orthop 1992;(280):186.

Otsuka NY, Kasser JR: Supracondylar fractures of the humerus in children. J Am Acad Orthop Surg 1997;5:19.

Sponseller PD: Problem elbow fractures in children. Hand Clin 1994;10:495.

Topping RE, Blanco JS, Davis TJ: Clinical evaluation of crossed-pin versus lateral pin fixation in displaced supracondylar humerus fractures. J Pediatr Orthop 1995;15:435.

FRACTURES OF THE FOREARM

The anatomy of the forearm can be thought of as a closed ring, somewhat analogous to the pelvis. It is very difficult to break a ring (in this case, a ring composed of the radius and ulna and their intervening proximal and distal joints) in only one place. Isolated radial or ulnar fractures are therefore uncommon except as a result of a direct blow to that bone.

Fractures of both forearm bones simultaneously or of one bone with a concomitant joint injury to the elbow or wrist joint are more commonly seen than fracture of either bone in isolation.

It is important in evaluating these fractures to obtain anteroposterior, lateral, and oblique radiographs of the forearm that include the elbow and the wrist. In this way, distal radioulnar joint or radial head dislocations can be evaluated. As always, careful neurovascular evaluation and documentation both before and after reduction are critical.

FRACTURES OF THE SHAFT OF THE RADIUS

Isolated Radial Shaft Fractures

An isolated radial shaft fracture should arouse suspicion of a concomitant injury to the wrist or elbow. Closed treatment of this injury is acceptable practice only if very strict criteria are satisfied: There cannot be any displacement of the radius; the normal bow of the radius must be maintained; and there cannot be any concomitant injury to the elbow or wrist. In the adult, essentially no amount of displacement is acceptable as it may limit the return of forearm rotation. If there is displacement, open reduction and internal fixation are recommended.

Galeazzi's Fracture

This is a fracture of the shaft of the radius (most commonly the distal third) in conjunction with a distal radioulnar joint injury. Wrist pain on physical examination arouses suspicion. However, the diagnosis should be confirmed radiographically. The following radiographic findings are suggestive of a distal radioulnar joint disruption when an isolated radial shaft fracture is present: fracture at the base of the ulnar styloid, widening of the distal radioulnar joint space on the anteroposterior radiograph, dislocation of the radius relative to the ulna on a true lateral radiograph, and radial shortening greater than 5 mm relative to the distal ulna.

In adults, these fractures should always be addressed surgically. The recommendation is for open reduction with internal fixation of the radius fracture and then intra-operative evaluation of the stability of the distal radioulnar joint. If after fixing the radius the joint is stable through full pronation and supination, there is no need for immobilization (other than short-term until the incision is healed). If the joint can be reduced but is unstable with rotation, additional treatment is necessary. If there is a repairable ulnar styloid fracture, then open reduction with internal fixation of this piece will often render the distal radioulnar joint stable. If

there is no ulnar styloid fracture but the distal radioulnar joint is reducible but unstable with rotation, then two 0.0625 inch Kirschner wires are used to pin the distal ulna to the radius in a reduced position (usually supination). With both open reduction with internal fixation of the ulnar styloid or the use of transfixing pins, the forearm should be immobilized in full supination in an above-elbow cast or brace for 4–6 weeks. The transfixing pins are removed prior to allowing forearm range of motion. Rarely, the distal radioulnar joint cannot be reduced. In this instance, a dorsal approach to the joint is used to extract interposed tissues blocking reduction. This is most commonly the extensor carpi ulnaris tendon.

Complications of this injury include malunion, nonunion, chronic distal radioulnar joint instability (usually only if this injury is missed and not treated initially) and nerve injury at the time of open reduction with internal fixation.

FRACTURES OF THE SHAFT OF THE ULNA

Isolated Ulnar Shaft Fractures (Nightstick Fractures)

This fairly common injury is caused by a direct blow to the ulna. Radiographic evaluation should include the elbow and wrist to rule out associated injuries. For the nondisplaced isolated fracture, some advocate long arm casting for 6–8 weeks. Functional bracing also gives good results. Some even advocate minimal (Ace bandage) or no bracing with isolated nondisplaced ulnar shaft fractures. In general, it is probably preferable to provide some immobilization until pain subsides. In isolated displaced ulnar shaft fractures, open reduction and internal fixation with plate and screws is the treatment of choice.

Monteggia's Fracture

Monteggia's fracture is fracture of the proximal third of the ulna with dislocation of the radial head. It was first described by Monteggia of Milan in 1814. Bado extended the description to include the entire spectrum of ulnar shaft fractures associated with radial head dislocations. They are classified as follows (Figure 43–16).

Type I: Fracture of the ulnar diaphysis with anterior angulation and anterior dislocation of the radial head (60% of cases).

Type II: Fracture of the ulnar diaphysis with posterior or posterolateral dislocation of the radial head (15% of cases).

Figure 43–16. Monteggia's fractures. The classification of Monteggia lesions by Bado. **A:** Type I: anterior angulation of the ulnar fracture and anterior dislocation of the radial head. **B:** Type II: posterior angulation of the ulnar fracture and anterior dislocation of the radial head. **C:** Type III: fracture of the proximal ulna metaphysis and lateral dislocation of the radial head. **D:** Type IV: anterior dislocation of the radial head and fracture of the radial and ulnar shafts. (Reproduced, with permission, from Browner B et al: *Skeletal Trauma.* Saunders, 1992.)

Type III: Fracture of the ulnar metaphysis with lateral or anterolateral dislocation of the radial head (20% of cases).

Type IV: Fracture of he ulna and radius at the proximal third with anterior dislocation of the radial head (5% of cases).

If an isolated ulnar shaft fracture is noted on x-ray, adequate elbow radiographs must be taken to rule out Monteggia's fracture and careful neurovascular evaluation is required. Injury to both the radial nerve and the posterior interosseous nerve have been described with this injury.

In the child, closed reduction of ulnar shaft fracture usually also reduces the radial head dislocation. In the adult patient, open reduction and internal fixation of the ulnar shaft fracture with compression plating is the treatment of choice. Once the ulnar shaft fracture is anatom-

ically reduced and fixed, the radial head usually reduces. Failure of the radial head to reduce is either secondary to malreduction of the ulna or due to interposed soft tissue, rarely requiring open reduction of the radial head for removal. After reduction, the stability of the radial head should be checked, preferably under fluoroscopy.

Complications include nerve palsy, malunion, nonunion, a stiff elbow, and occasional formation of a radioulnar synostosis. This is seen more often with type IV fractures.

Both-Bone Forearm Fractures

Fractures of both radius and ulna are caused by high-energy injuries such as motor vehicle accidents or falls from a height. The fractures are usually displaced. Careful examination to rule out neurovascular injury and compartment syndrome should be performed. Radiographs of the entire forearm including the elbow and wrist are necessary.

In children with open physes, closed reduction and long arm cast immobilization is usually adequate, since they have the potential to remodel small amounts of deformity. Bayonet apposition with 10–20 degrees of angular deformity and maintained interosseous space is considered acceptable depending on the age of the child. Frequent (weekly) radiographs are necessary to look for displacement. Older children close to skeletal maturity should be treated more like adults.

Treatment for both-bone forearm fractures in adults consists of open reduction and internal fixation with compression plating using 3.5 mm dynamic plates. This affords the best results by restoring normal anatomy and therefore rotation of the forearm. Bone grafting is recommended for comminuted fractures with bone loss. The radius can be approached through an anterior Henry incision regardless of the location of the fracture. Some prefer the dorsal Thompson approach for proximal third radius fractures. The ulna is approached dorsally on its subcutaneous border. To avoid development of a compartment syndrome postoperatively, the fascia is not closed after reduction and plating. Patients are splinted immediately postoperatively for comfort and to allow healing of the skin incisions. With solid fixation, active range of motion of the forearm and elbow can be started at 10–14 days. Open fractures can also be treated successfully with these methods. However, if there is excessive soft tissue damage or wound contamination, the use of an external fixator may be a preferable option.

Complications of this fracture include compartment syndrome, neurovascular injury, malunion, nonunion, synostosis, and loss of motion.

COMPARTMENT SYNDROME

Compartment syndrome is caused by increased pressure in an enclosed space that leads to compromise of circulation and function of tissues in that space. It can be the result of swelling from trauma or postsurgical swelling. It should be differentiated from primary nerve or vascular injury. Careful inspection after trauma or surgery is essential to prevent this devastating complication, especially in the obtunded patient. Pain with passive range of motion of the digits is thought to be the most sensitive early sign of compartment syndrome. Paresthesias and a tense swollen forearm are also signs of compartment syndrome. Pulselessness can occur but is a late sign and does not always occur.

Compartment syndrome is a surgical emergency. If it is suspected, compartment pressures should be mea-sured immediately. If they are elevated, immediate forearm fasciotomy is indicated to avoid permanent damage to muscles, nerves, and vessels.

INJURIES OF THE WRIST REGION

Anatomy

The radius and ulna structurally support the forearm. The distal radius and ulna have specialized articulations with the carpus and with each other. The distal radius has three articular components: the scaphoid fossa, the lunate fossa, and the sigmoid notch. The scaphoid and lunate fossae articulate with their respective carpal bones (the scaphoid and lunate), making up the radiocarpal joint. The sigmoid notch articulates with the distal ulna, forming the distal radioulnar joint. The shafts of the radius and ulna are nearly parallel to one another. The ulnar shaft is fixed in its rotation at the ulnohumeral joint, and it is therefore the radius that rotates around the ulna in pronation and supination. The shaft of the radius and ulna are connected by the interosseous membrane, which is important in transmission of force between the two bones. It also provides muscular attachment for the flexors and extensors of the wrist and digits. The orientation of the distal radius is 5–10 degrees of volar tilt and 22 degrees of radial inclination. These become important parameters in interpreting adequate position of distal radius fractures.

In addition to the bony architecture, there is complex ligamentous and soft tissue anatomy of the wrist. The distal ulna has an ulnar styloid that provides attachment for the triangular fibrocartilage complex, the volar and dorsal ulnar carpal ligaments, and the ulnar collateral ligaments of the wrist. There are also volar and dorsal radiocarpal ligaments that attach to the radius along with the radial collateral ligaments. There are six dorsal compartments of the wrist which contain wrist and digital extensor tendons. On the volar surface, the pronator quadratus lies across the distal radius and ulna. Just anterior to the pronator quadratus are the contents of the carpal canal, containing nine digital flexor tendons and the median nerve. Anterior to the transverse carpal ligament lie the flexor carpi radialis, flexor carpi ulnaris, and palmaris longus muscles. Guyon's canal contains the ulnar nerve and artery. It is bounded by the volar retinacular ligament and flexor retinacular ligament, the hook of the hamate radially, and the pisiform ulnarly.

1. Wrist Sprain

The diagnosis of wrist sprain is made only after ruling out fractures and dislocations of the wrist. Radiographs should be taken at presentation. Careful palpation and examination are necessary to localize the area of injury. If radiographs are negative for fracture or dislocation, the patient should be immobilized in a volar wrist splint for comfort for a period of 2 weeks. If pain and swelling persist, x-rays should be repeated to look for more subtle occult fractures. MRI or an MR arthrogram may be necessary to discern ligamentous injury or damage to the triangular fibrocartilage complex of the wrist. If symptoms improve with a short period of immobilization, range of motion and strengthening exercises should be introduced in a graded fashion.

2. Distal Radius Fracture

Mechanism

Distal radius fractures most commonly occur from a fall on the outstretched hand. They are more common in the middle years and old age and in patients with osteoporosis. High-energy injuries such as motor vehicle accidents and falls from a height can produce this injury in young patients.

Classification of Fractures

In 1814—long before the availability of radiographs—Abraham Colles described the dorsally angulated and displaced distal radius metaphysial fracture. The term Colles fracture is often inappropriately used today to describe any distal radius fracture. Other names for distal radius fractures are Smith's fracture (reverse Colles fracture), an extra-articular metaphysial fracture with volar angulation and displacement; Barton's fracture, a displaced unstable articular fracture-subluxation of the distal radius with volar displacement of the carpus along with the articular fragment; Chauffeur's fracture, intra-articular fracture of the radial styloid; and "die punch" fracture, an intra-articular depression fracture of the lunate fossa. Although these term are commonly used, more complete and descriptive classification systems are now available and preferred.

The Frykman classification system categorizes these fractures based on the presence or absence of ulnar styloid fractures and whether the fracture lines are extra-articular, intra-articular involving the radial carpal joint, intra-articular involving the distal radioulnar joint, or intra-articular involving both the radiocarpal and distal radioulnar joints (Figure 43–17).

The AO/ASIF classification separates distal radius fractures into three groups as shown in the accompanying box. It should be noted that injury to the distal radioulnar joint can occur with any of these fractures.

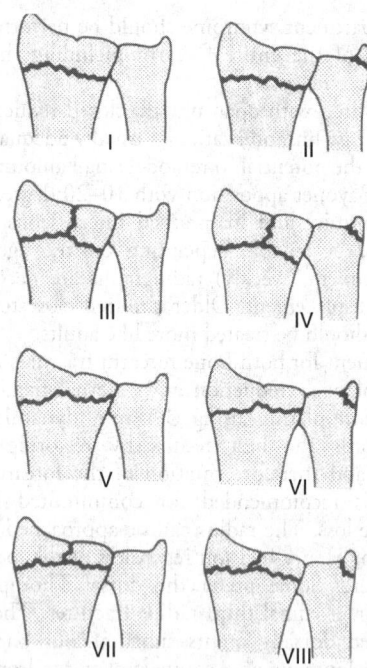

Figure 43–17. Frykman classification of distal radius fractures. Types I, III, V, and VII do not have an associated fracture of the distal ulna. Fractures III–VIII are intra-articular fractures. Higher-classification fractures have worse prognoses. (From Green D, Hotchkiss R, Pederson W: *Green's Operative Hand Surgery.* Churchill Livingstone, 1993.)

AO/ASIF CLASSIFICATION OF DISTAL RADIUS FRACTURES

Type A: Extra-articular fractures
1. Isolated distal ulnar fracture
2. Simple radius fracture
3. Radial fracture with metaphysial impaction

Type B: Intra-articular complex fracture
1. Radial styloid fracture
2. Dorsal rim fracture
3. Volar rim fracture

Type C: Intra-articular complex fracture
1. Metaphysial fracture with radiocarpal congruity preserved
2. Articular displacement
3. Diaphysial-metaphysial involvement

Treatment

Radiographs in the anteroposterior, lateral, and oblique planes should be obtained. If examination shows pain at the forearm or elbow, these radiographs should also be taken. The median nerve can be damaged by fracture fragments or compression from swelling and hematoma and the function of this nerve should be carefully documented both before and after reduction.

Treatment of distal radius fractures depends on many factors, including the amount of displacement and angulation, the degree of comminution, the age of the patient, the quality of the bone, and the functional demands required.

A. Nonoperative Treatment

Nondisplaced, stable fractures can be treated with cast immobilization. Displaced extra-articular fractures that can be reduced and are stable can also be treated in a cast or sugar-tong splint. Because it is often difficult to assess stability, once the fracture is reduced, radiographic evaluation should be done on a weekly basis for the first 2–3 weeks to make sure the alignment is maintained. Volar tilt, radial length, and radial inclination should be restored to acceptable parameters.

B. Indications for Surgical Management

Operation is warranted if reduction cannot be achieved or maintained by closed methods. Very comminuted fractures, even if they are extra-articular, often will shorten and displace in a cast. Fractures with intra-articular stepoff or gap of more than 2 mm require surgical fixation. Volar tilt should be restored to at least neutral in all but the very low demand wrist. Certain types of fractures such as the volar Barton's fracture are known to be unstable and always require volar buttress plating.

C. Techniques of Surgical Management

There are many techniques for surgical management of distal radius fractures. Choice is determined by the pattern of the fracture, the quality of the bone, and the surgeon's preference.

1. Closed reduction and percutaneous pinning— This is an effective method for securing large fragments to help prevent collapse after reduction of unstable fractures. In general, 0.0625 inch Kirschner wires are used in either an interfragmentary or an intrafocal pinning technique. With the interfragmentary technique, wires are passed across the fracture site after the fracture is reduced. With the intrafocal technique, the wire is placed in the fracture site, used there to achieve reduction, and then driven into the bone. These techniques can be used alone or in combination (Figure 43–18). Patients are placed in a cast or splint. The wires are generally left

Figure 43–18. Closed reduction and percutaneous pinning of a distal radius fracture using a combination of intrafocal and interfragmentary techniques.

in place for 6 weeks and then removed in the office after adequate healing has occurred.

2. External fixation—This is a very effective way of treating distal radius fractures. It is especially helpful in treating very comminuted fractures and intra-articular fractures where there are too many small pieces for pins or open reduction. External fixation devices take advantage of ligamentous tension and indirect reduction of the fracture fragments. External fixation is also used for open fractures with soft tissue compromise. It can be used in conjunction with percutaneous pins.

3. Open reduction and internal fixation with plates and screws—This is an effective technique in younger patients with good bone quality and large fragments. It has the added advantage of allowing early range of motion if the fixation is rigid. Many different plating systems are available, including a new Tri-Med system designed for treating intra-articular fractures by obtaining purchase on the intact proximal bone.

Disadvantages of open reduction and internal fixation with plates and screws include a potential for scarring, soft tissue stripping causing devascularization of small fragments, and the possibility of needing to have implants removed in the future.

4. Arthroscopic assisted reduction—The use of wrist arthroscopy to aid in reduction and also assess the quality of reduction is becoming more widely used for intra-articular fractures. It is often somewhat difficult to assess intra-articular fracture reduction with radiographs alone. With the use of wrist arthroscopy, the articular surface can be directly visualized and manipulated. It is also useful for identifying other concomitant pathology such as triangular fibrocartilage complex tear. This technique can be used in conjunction with percutaneous pins, external fixation, or plates and screws.

Complications

The most common complication of distal radius fractures is stiffness of the wrist and digits. Patients should be instructed to begin range of motion exercises for the digits immediately after the fracture is initially treated. Other complications include median nerve injury, unnoticed derangement of the distal radioulnar joint, infection (after operation), malunion, and late rupture of the extensor pollicis longus tendon after nondisplaced fractures. Stiffness of the shoulder and reflex sympathetic dystrophy can also occur.

FRACTURES OF THE ULNAR STYLOID

Fractures of the ulnar styloid are commonly seen in conjunction with distal radius fractures and but can also be seen in isolation. Fractures of the ulnar styloid are often too small to fix. However, large fragments (the entire styloid from its base) that are displaced should be treated by open reduction and internal fixation with small screws, pins, or tension band wires. If these large fragments are not fixed, the patient can go on to have chronic pain in this area as well as instability of the distal radioulnar joint.

DISTAL RADIOULNAR JOINT DISLOCATION

This is discussed earlier in conjunction with the Galeazzi fracture. It should be pointed out that this injury can also occur with a simple distal radius fracture. Careful examination of radiographs and the distal radioulnar joint will keep the clinician from missing this injury in the face of a distal radius fracture.

FRACTURES & DISLOCATIONS OF THE CARPUS

Most carpal bone fractures occur in the proximal carpal row. The scaphoid is the carpal bone most commonly fractured. Carpal bone fractures usually occur in younger people, often from high-energy falls on an outstretched wrist such as may occur while skiing, snowboarding, or rollerblading. Wrist radiographs can be difficult to interpret, and careful scrutiny is necessary so as not to miss these injuries. In addition to the standard anteroposterior, lateral, and oblique views of the wrist, special radiographic views such as a scaphoid view, clenched fist view, or carpal tunnel view can often be helpful.

1. Fracture of the Scaphoid

Treatment of scaphoid fractures can be difficult due in large part to the poor blood supply of this bone, which makes it susceptible to delayed union, nonunion, and avascular necrosis. Blood supply is from branches of the radial artery entering the distal aspect of the bone. Proximal pole blood supply is from retrograde flow. If a fracture occurs at the scaphoid waist or more proximally, the blood supply to this region is interrupted.

The most common area in the scaphoid for fracture is the scaphoid waist. Fractures can also occur in the distal tubercle and proximal pole. Patients present with pain in the radial side of the wrist, more specifically in the "anatomic snuffbox." If a patient has pain in this region, a scaphoid view radiograph of the wrist should be added to the wrist series. Nondisplaced fractures should be treated in a thumb spica cast. Nondisplaced fractures with more unstable oblique patterns should probably be treated in a long arm thumb spica cast for the first 3–4 weeks. Weekly radiographic follow-up for the first 3 weeks is necessary to look for displacement. The average time to healing is 12 weeks. Absence of clinical tenderness and bridging trabeculae on x-ray indicate healing. If no fracture is seen on initial x-ray examination but the patient has pain at the scaphoid, treatment should be as for nondisplaced scaphoid fracture. Scaphoid fractures are often not visible on initial x-ray. Radiographs out of plaster should be repeated in 2–3 weeks. If x-rays show no fracture and the pain has resolved, the cast can be left off. If the x-rays show no fracture and the patient continues to have pain, MRI should be done in a search for occult fracture.

Even with optimal cast treatment, some of these fractures will be complicated by delayed union or nonunion. Treatment in such cases consists of operation with bone grafting and internal fixation, usually with a screw (Figure 43–19). Some surgeons have advocated percutaneous screw fixation even for nondisplaced fractures. The advantages are shorter immobilization time and faster time to union (an average of 7 weeks versus 12 weeks in one study). This is somewhat controversial.

All displaced fractures should be treated with open reduction and internal fixation, either through a dorsal or a volar approach depending on the type of fracture. A bone graft from the distal radius or iliac crest is often used to increase healing potential or correct deformity, especially in the case of delayed union or late presentation. Most surgeons are using screw fixation, though under some circumstances pin fixation may be necessary.

Avascular necrosis of the proximal pole can occur even with adequate treatment but is more common when treatment is delayed. This is a difficult problem to treat. Some surgeons are using vascularized bone grafts to address this problem. In other cases, salvage

Figure 43–19. Scaphoid fracture. *A:* Scaphoid fracture nonunion. *B:* Open reduction and internal fixation of scaphoid nonunion.

procedures are necessary. Patients with long-standing scaphoid nonunions go on to develop early arthritis of the radioscaphoid joint secondary to altered mechanics of the wrist.

2. Fracture of the Lunate

The lunate is the carpal bone most likely to dislocate, but fractures are rare. Small dorsal or volar avulsion fractures can be treated in a splint or cast for 4 weeks. The lunate has a tenuous blood supply and can also develop avascular necrosis, which is known as Kienböck's disease when it occurs in the lunate.

3. Fracture of the Hamate

This fracture generally occurs from a direct blow to the area such as occurs when swinging a baseball bat or golf club that suddenly comes to an abrupt stop as it encounters a firm surface. The fracture can occur through the body or proximal pole but by far the most common place is in the hook of the hamate. Patients present with ulnar-sided hand pain over the hamate hook. Fracture will often not be seen on routine wrist and hand radiographs. A carpal tunnel view should be obtained if this fracture is suspected. If the diagnosis is suspected clinically but the radiographs show no fracture, a CT scan should be obtained. Hook of the hamate fractures are best treated with excision as they do not heal with immobilization and remain painful.

4. Other Carpal Bone Fractures

Fractures can occur in any of the other carpal bones as well, but much less commonly. Triquetral avulsion or

dorsal impaction fractures can occur from falls on the outstretched hand. Isolated fractures of the remaining carpal bones are rare and generally occur with high-energy trauma and other injuries.

5. Traumatic Carpal Instability

Severe injury to the wrist causing damage to the complex ligamentous structures may lead to carpal bone dissociation, carpal dislocations, and fracture dislocations.

Scapholunate dissociation secondary to disruption of the scapholunate ligament leads to altered kinematics of the wrist and early degenerative arthritis. Diagnosis is made by clinical examination and radiography. Patients will have a history usually of falling on an outstretched wrist. There will be tenderness to palpation over the scapholunate interval. If this injury is suspected, a "clenched fist view" should be added to the routine series of wrist radiographs. With a complete tear of the scapholunate ligament, this view will show abnormal gapping between the scaphoid and lunate bones. An increased scapholunate angle will be seen on the lateral projection. With partial tears there may be no radiographic changes. If the diagnosis is made acutely, the ligament can generally be repaired. Chronic scapholunate ligament disruptions do not do well with repair. There are reconstructive options prior to the onset of arthritic changes. However, once arthritis has developed, only salvage options exist.

In cases of severe high-energy trauma, perilunate dislocations, transscaphoid perilunate fracture-dislocations, and lunate dislocations can occur. Perilunate dislocations and lunate dislocations are on a continuum of the same type and mechanism of injury with increasing disruption of the ligamentous structures of the wrist. Patients present with severe wrist pain and swelling after trauma. Good-quality anteroposterior, lateral, and oblique radiographs must be obtained in order to make this diagnosis, which is missed sometimes even by experienced physicians. The relationship of the carpal bones to each other and to the distal radius must be carefully scrutinized. With lunate dislocation, on the lateral radiograph the lunate will be volar to the rest of the carpus and not in alignment with the distal radius. With a perilunate dislocation, the lunate remains in its normal position, articulating with the distal radius, but is angled volar ward, and the rest of the carpus is dislocated. On occasion these injuries occur and then reduce when the splint is applied in the field or when radiographs are taken. In this case, careful attention to the radiographs is necessary to make the diagnosis.

Immediate closed reduction under adequate anesthesia should be attempted. Even if closed reduction is successful, most surgeons feel that open reduction and fixation should be performed to restore the normal relationships of the carpal bones and distal radius. Closed reduction is sometimes not possible, and these patients should be taken emergently to the operating room for open reduction and fixation. If a scaphoid fracture is present with the dislocation, it should be repaired first—rigidly with a screw or pins—and attention then turned to restoring the carpal bone relationships and holding them with pins that will later be removed. Controversy exists as to whether these injuries should be approached volarly, dorsally, or via a combined approach.

Even with the best care, carpal bone and ligament injuries can be devastating, with long-term sequelae of pain, stiffness and early arthritis.

6. Management of Posttraumatic Arthritis of the Wrist

Arthritis of the wrist is treated in most cases only when it becomes painful. Intermittent splinting and anti-inflammatory medication can be helpful for mild cases in the low-demand wrist. There are many salvage options available depending on which joints are affected and how much pain the patient is having. If radioscaphoid arthritis is present and painful but the radiolunate joint is in good condition, a four-corner fusion can be a successful operation. The scaphoid is excised and the lunate, capitate, triquetrum, and hamate are fused. The uninvolved radiolunate joint now bears most of the force across the wrist. In cases of painful arthritis of multiple joints of the wrist, a total wrist arthrodesis provides a stable, pain-free wrist. However, the patient must be willing to accept the loss of motion.

Proximal row carpectomy is a good option in the non-laborer if the capitate is not involved. Total wrist arthroplasty has not gained wide acceptance because of its high reported failure rate over time.

Bond CD et al: Percutaneous screw fixation versus cast immobilization for non-displaced scaphoid fractures. J Bone Joint Surg Am 2001;83:483.

Cassidy C et al: Traumatic wrist disorders—what's in and what's out. AAOS 68th Annual Meeting Instructional Course, 2001.

Jupiter JB et al: Update on the management of traumatic and reconstructive problems of the scaphoid. AAOS 68th Annual Meeting Instructional Course, 2001.

Kozion SH: Peri-lunate injuries: diagnosis and treatment. J Am Acad Orthop Surg 1998;6:114.

Shin AY, Bishop AT, Berger RA: Vascularized pedicled bone grafts for disorders of the carpus. Techniques in Hand and Upper Extremity Surgery 1998;2:94.

Trumble TE et al: Intra-articular fractures of the distal aspect of the radius. AAOS Instructional Course Lecture, Vol 48, 1999.

FRACTURES & DISLOCATIONS ABOUT THE HAND

In evaluating any fracture of the metacarpals and phalanges, certain principles should be kept in mind. For suspected metacarpal fractures, anteroposterior, lateral, and oblique radiographs of the hand should be obtained. When a phalanx fracture of a specific digit is suspected, anteroposterior, lateral and oblique radiographs of just that digit will give better detail. Assessment of neurovascular status of the hand and digits must be done to rule out other injuries, including tendon injury. It is critical to assess rotation and angular deformity of the digit in both extension and flexion. The digit may look fine in extension but when the digits are flexed into a fist there can be rotational malalignment causing overlap of the digits. Fractures of the metacarpals and phalanges should not be immobilized for more than 3 weeks except under unusual circumstances. Fractures of the small bones of the hand heal more rapidly than fractures of larger bones, and prolonged immobilization can cause stiffness and loss of motion that can be difficult or impossible to regain. The safe position for splinting or casting of the hand is with slight wrist extension, the MP joints flexed 60–90 degrees, and the PIP and DIP joints extended.

1. Metacarpal Fractures

Metacarpal Neck Fractures

The most common metacarpal neck fracture is the "boxer's fracture" of the fifth metacarpal, usually caused by the fist striking a stationary object. Metacarpal neck fractures can occur in all of the metacarpals. There is controversy over what is an acceptable amount of angulation. Because there is less compensatory movement at the base of the second, third, and fourth metacarpals, less angulation is accepted in these digits. A general rule is that there should be no more than 10 degrees of dorsal angulation in the index metacarpal, 20 degrees in the middle metacarpal, 30 degrees in the ring metacarpal, and 40 degrees in the small finger metacarpal.

Stable, nondisplaced fractures can be treated in a cast that extends to the PIP joint of the involved digit. Unstable, displaced fractures may require closed reduction and pinning or open reduction with plates and screw. The advantage of open reduction and rigid fixation is that early range of motion exercises can be started almost immediately. The disadvantage is scarring and a possible need for later removal of the implants.

Metacarpal Shaft Fractures

These are described as transverse, oblique, or spiral. Angulations of more than 20 degrees in the ring metacarpal and 30 degrees in the small finger metacarpal should be reduced. Essentially no angulation is acceptable in the index and middle finger metacarpals since in would leave a cosmetically unacceptable prominence on the dorsum of the hand. Rotational deformity should be corrected and held with either percutaneous pins or plates and screws. Multiple metacarpal shaft fractures in the same hand are best treated by means of open reduction with internal fixation to prevent shortening and deformity.

Bennett's Fracture

This is an intra-articular fracture with subluxation at the base of the thumb metacarpal. The volar oblique ligament of the thumb remains attached to the small Bennett fragment (which lies volar and ulnar) and the trapezium. The remainder of the metacarpal slips radially, proximally, and dorsally as a result of the muscular and tendinous attachments. These injuries cannot be adequately treated with casting alone as they tend to slip. The treatment of choice is closed reduction and percutaneous pinning for reducible small fragments that are less than 25% of the joint surface. For larger fragments or those that cannot be reduced by closed means, open reduction and fixation with pins or a screw is preferable.

Fracture-Dislocation of the Small Finger Carpometacarpal Joint

Intra-articular fracture-dislocation of the small finger carpometacarpal joint is an inherently unstable fracture, difficult to assess on x-ray. Some say it is analogous to

Bennett's fracture of the thumb. Most surgeons recommend either closed reduction and percutaneous pinning or open reduction and pinning. For extremely comminuted fractures where articular congruity cannot be restored, some advocate arthrodesis.

2. Phalanx Fractures

Fractures of the proximal and middle phalangeal shafts can be treated closed if they are nondisplaced and stable. Many of these fractures are unstable and require percutaneous pin fixation in order to avoid angular and rotational deformity. Intra-articular fractures with displacement pose a special challenge. Stiffness is always a problem, so that methods of fixation which allow immediate range of motion activity (such as rigid screw fixation, hinged external fixation; Figure 43–20) or traction splinting are recommended.

Distal phalanx tuft fractures do not usually cause much of a problem and require only a short period of splinting for comfort. Nail bed lacerations are often associated with these injuries and should be repaired. Unstable transverse fractures of the distal phalanx may require pin fixation. A special type of distal phalanx fracture is the bony mallet finger, which is avulsion of the terminal insertion of the extensor tendon. These can be treated with a dorsal extension splint of the DIP joint. If the joint is dislocated or if more than 50% of the articular surface is involved, surgical repair may be indicated.

3. Dislocations of the Digits

Dislocations of the PIP and MP joints are the most common dislocations in the digits. Painful swelling and

Figure 43–20. PIP hinged external fixation. Fixation of intra-articular fracture-dislocation of the PIP joint with a hinged external fixation device.

deformity is the presentation, plus limited range of motion. Radiographs will confirm the diagnosis (Figure 43–21). Most often these injuries can be reduced closed by accentuating the deforming force and applying gentle pressure to reduce the joint. Dorsal MP joint dislocations sometimes cannot be reduced closed because of interposed volar plate. Distraction forces applied for reduction actually prevent reduction by causing a "noose effect" around the metacarpal neck. These dorsal MP dislocations require open reduction through either a dorsal or volar approach.

4. Ligamentous Injuries in the Digits

The ulnar collateral ligament of the thumb MP joint is the most commonly injured ligament in the digits. The acute injury is called skier's thumb, whereas chronic injury from repetitive trauma is referred to as gamekeeper's thumb. A sprain without instability can be treated with thumb spica casting or splinting for 4–6 weeks and then range of motion exercises. In the unstable situation, the ligament should be repaired—or reconstructed if adequate tissue is not available for repair.

The collateral ligaments of the other MP joints and the PIP joints can also be injured. In most cases these are treated with splinting or buddy taping to protect

Figure 43–21. MP joint dislocation of the index and middle fingers.

the ligament and early range of motion activity to prevent joint stiffness. In rare circumstances when instability remains, open repair may be in order.

Freeland AE, Benoist LA: Open reduction and internal fixation methods for fractures at the proximal interphalangeal joint. Hand Clin 1994;10:239.

Schuind F et al: Small external fixation devices for the hand and wrist. Clin Orthop 1993;(293):77.

INJURIES OF THE HIP REGION

1. Fracture of the Femoral Neck

Fracture of the femoral neck occurs most commonly in patients over age 50. If displacement has occurred, the extremity is externally rotated and shortened. Motion of the hip causes pain. If the fragments are not displaced and the fracture is stable, pain at the extremes of passive hip motion may be the only significant finding. The fact that the patient can actively move the extremity often interferes with early diagnosis. Before treatment is instituted, anteroposterior and lateral films of excellent quality must be obtained. Gentle traction and internal rotation of the extremity while the anteroposterior film is exposed may provide a more favorable relation of fragments to demonstrate the fracture cleft.

Fractures may be classified as stable or unstable. Stable fractures include stress fractures and impacted fractures. The unstable category includes displaced and comminuted fractures.

Stable Fractures of the Femoral Neck

Patients with stress fractures or impacted fractures may have minimal groin pain and may be able to walk with some pain and a limp. No obvious deformity or shortening is apparent on physical examination, and for that reason the diagnosis may be elusive. If initial x-rays do not reveal the stress fracture, a repeat x-ray, radionuclide study, or MRI may be necessary to confirm the diagnosis. An impacted fracture is usually in valgus position. Impaction must be seen on both anteroposterior and lateral films for diagnosis.

Stress fractures can be treated by crutch ambulation to minimize weightbearing stress. The patient should be instructed not to place the leg in stressful positions or use it for leverage. If the fracture appears to be healing, partial weightbearing may be started at 6 weeks after injury, with progression to full weightbearing when the fracture is healed. Healing usually takes place in 3–6 months.

Impacted fractures may also be treated nonoperatively, but the tendency for displacement is much greater than in stress fractures. Most surgeons prefer to use internal fixation for impacted fractures to allow maintenance of reduction, earlier crutch ambulation, and earlier weightbearing. Multiple screw or pin fixation is in many cases the best treatment and should be secure enough to allow weightbearing immediately. Truly impacted fractures treated with internal fixation without disruption of the fracture have healing rates approaching 100%.

Unstable Fractures of the Femoral Neck

Displaced and comminuted femoral neck fracture can be a life-endangering injury, especially in elderly persons. Treatment is directed toward preservation of life and restoration of function to the hip joint. In most cases, reduction and internal fixation are the treatment of choice. Immobilization of this fracture by means of a plaster spica is unreliable. Definitive treatment by skeletal traction requires prolonged recumbency with constant nursing care and is associated with more numerous complications than early mobilization. Operative treatment usually consists of internal fixation or primary arthroplasty and should be done as soon as the patient is medically prepared for surgery. In general, the younger the patient, the more effort is justified to save the femoral head.

A. Internal Fixation

The goal of internal fixation is to preserve the femoral head fragment by providing a setting for bony healing of the fracture. The objective is to allow the patient as much general physical activity during healing as is compatible with the mechanics of fixation. To permit necessary preoperative evaluation of the patient when internal fixation is elected, initial treatment may be by balanced suspension, skeletal traction, and prompt closed reduction of the fracture. Persistent displacement may cause further compromise of the retinacular blood supply to the articular fragment.

Anatomic or near-anatomic reduction and firm fixation are desirable to provide optimal conditions for bone healing. Comminution at the fracture site, injury to the retinacular blood supply of the capital fragment, excessive stressing of the fracture site, and insecure fixation are some of the factors that lead to failure.

When the fragments are undisplaced or minimally displaced, manipulation is unnecessary. Displacement may be corrected by closed reduction preliminary to fixation or by surgical exposure of the fragment site. Adequate closed reduction is usually obtained by traction and marked internal rotation of the extremity—frequently to 90 degrees. The fixation apparatus may consist of multiple screws applied percutaneously or more elaborate implants that require open operation. After operation, the patient does not require traction and may be mobilized immediately.

Depending upon the relative security of fixation, the extent of early weightbearing must be regulated until bone continuity is restored to the point where displacement of fragments is unlikely. Patients may be ambulatory on crutches or with a walker within a few days after operative treatment.

B. Primary Arthroplasty

In electing primary arthroplasty, the surgeon realizes that the main proximal fragment must be sacrificed because of injury to the blood supply, preexisting disease, or inability to obtain satisfactory reduction of the fracture for internal fixation.

When the acetabulum is undamaged or is not the site of preexisting disease, the commonly accepted technique is hemiarthroplasty using a femoral component (generally of the intramedullary type) that may or may not be stabilized by a grouting substance such as methylmethacrylate. In the rare circumstance when there is concomitant involvement of the acetabulum, total joint replacement may be justified. Primary head and neck resection may be indicated when there is preexisting infection or local tumor.

The most common sequelae of fracture of the femoral neck are redisplacement after reduction and internal fixation, failure of bone healing, and avascular necrosis of the head fragment. Avascular necrosis and associated collapse occur in 15–35% of these patients from interruption of the blood supply to the femoral neck at the time of injury. It is most likely to appear during the 2 years after fracture. Secondary osteoarthritis (posttraumatic arthritis) appears somewhat later and may be complicated by any of the common sequelae mentioned above. The most serious complication of any open operative treatment is infection.

2. Trochanteric Fractures

Fracture of the Lesser Trochanter

Isolated fracture of the lesser trochanter is quite rare but may develop as a result of the avulsion force of the iliopsoas muscle. It occurs commonly as a component of intertrochanteric fracture. Rarely, a symptomatic nonunion may require fragment fixation or excision. Avulsion fractures may also represent a pathologic fracture secondary to metastatic disease.

Fracture of the Greater Trochanter

Isolated fracture of the greater trochanter may be caused by direct injury or may occur indirectly as a result of the activity of the gluteus medius and gluteus minimus muscles. It occurs most commonly as a component of intertrochanteric fracture.

If displacement is less than 1 cm and there is no tendency to further displacement (determined by repeated x-ray examinations), treatment may be by bed rest with the affected extremity in balanced suspension until acute pain subsides. As rapidly as symptoms permit, activity can increase gradually to protracted weightbearing with crutches. Full weightbearing is permitted as soon as healing is apparent, usually in 6–8 weeks. If displacement is greater than 1 cm and increases on adduction of the thigh, extensive tearing of surrounding soft tissues may be assumed, and open reduction and internal fixation are indicated.

Intertrochanteric Fractures

These fractures occur most commonly among elderly persons, usually after a fall. The cleft of an intertrochanteric fracture extends upward and outward from the medial region of the junction of the neck and lesser trochanter toward the summit of the greater trochanter. Peritrochanteric fracture includes both trochanters and is likely to be comminuted (Figure 43–22).

It is important to determine whether comminution has occurred and the magnitude of displacement. These fractures may vary from fissure fracture without significant separation to severe comminution into four major fragments: head-neck, greater trochanter, lesser trochanter, and shaft. Displacement may be marked, with obvious extreme rotation and shortening of the extremity more severe than with femoral neck fractures.

These fractures are extracapsular and occur through cancellous bone that has a good blood supply. Healing occurs in 3–4 months, and lack of healing is uncommon.

Initial treatment of the fracture in the hospital can be by balanced suspension and, when indicated, by the addition of traction. The selection of definitive treatment—closed or operative techniques—depends in part upon the general condition of the patient and the type of fracture. Rates of illness and death are lower when the fracture is internally fixed, allowing for early mobilization. Operative treatment is indicated as soon as the patient is medically able to tolerate surgery.

If the patient is unable to tolerate anesthesia or if the fracture is too severely comminuted to permit internal fixation with good stability, the fracture may be treated by skeletal traction with a Kirschner wire through the proximal tibia. Within 3–4 months, healing is usually sufficient to allow the patient to be out of bed. Long-term traction is associated with many complications, including bedsores, pulmonary complications, deterioration of mental status, and varus position of the fracture.

Figure 43–22. Comminuted intertrochanteric hip fracture. ***A:*** Anteroposterior radiograph. ***B:*** Anteroposterior radiograph after fixation with a compression hip screw and sideplate.

Open reduction may be done electively or may be mandatory for optimal treatment. Reduction of the fracture can be accomplished by closed techniques or it can be an integral part of the open operation. Some surgeons do not prefer to anatomically reduce unstable fractures caused by comminution of the medial femoral cortex. It is argued by some authors that medial displacement of the upper end of the main distal fragment enhances mechanical stability (although it may cause concomitant varus deformity), and this advantageously permits earlier weightbearing and earlier healing. The chief objective of open operation is to provide sufficient fixation of the fragments by a metallic surgical implant so that the patient need not be confined to bed during the healing process.

The fixation most widely used is a sliding screw with a side plate. The screw can slide in the barrel of the side plate, allowing the fracture to impact. A fixed nail and side plate may cause the fracture to be "nailed apart" and contribute to lack of healing. As the fracture impacts, the nail cannot slide and may instead cut through the head of the femur.

Subtrochanteric Fracture

Subtrochanteric fracture due to severe trauma occurs below the level of the lesser trochanter at the junction of cancellous and cortical bone. It is most common in men during the active years of life. Soft tissue damage is extensive. The direction of the fracture cleft may be transverse or oblique. Comminution occurs, and the fracture may extend proximally into the intertrochanteric region or distally into the shaft.

Closed reduction should be attempted by continuous traction to bring the distal fragment into alignment with the proximal fragment. If comminution is not extensive and the lesser trochanter is not detached, the proximal fragment is often drawn into relative flexion, external rotation, and abduction by the predominant activity of the iliopsoas, gluteus medius, and gluteus minimus muscles.

Internal fixation, unless contraindicated, is now the treatment of choice. If conservative treatment is elected, the patient should be placed in distal femoral skeletal traction with the hip and knee flexed 90 degrees to counteract the deforming forces. Traction should be continued for 6–8 weeks in this position until the fracture is "sticky" and then progressively brought to a neutral position for another 6–8 weeks until clinical and radiographic signs of healing are present. Using a hip spica can be an alternative to traction.

Internal fixation is most widely favored. Temporary skeletal traction will maintain femoral length until definitive surgical treatment can be performed. This

Figure 43–23. Subtrochanteric femur fracture with fracture of the distal third of the ipsilateral femoral shaft treated with a reconstruction type intramedullary nail.

should be done early to allow mobilization and prevent malunion.

Closed intramedullary interlocking nails have gained popularity recently (Figure 43–23). Newer devices with intracephalic proximal interlocking allow fixation where conventional nails may be contraindicated. Fixation can also be obtained with nails of the Zickel type, blade plates or lag screws with long sideplates. Retrograde flexible nailing (Ender type) has also been used with less success in providing stability and rotational control.

The activity status after operative treatment depends upon the adequacy of internal fixation. If fixation is secure and the patient is agile and cooperative, ambulation on crutches (nonweightbearing or partial weightbearing) on the affected side may be allowed immediately after the operation. The fracture is usually healed at 3–4 months, but delayed union and nonunion are not uncommon. Hardware failure commonly occurs in these cases, requiring repeat internal fixation and bone grafting.

3. Traumatic Dislocation of the Hip Joint

Traumatic dislocation of the hip joint (Figure 43–24) may occur with or without fracture of the acetabulum or the proximal end of the femur. It is most common during the active years of life and is usually the result of severe trauma unless there is preexisting disease of the femoral head, acetabulum, or neuromuscular system. The head of the femur cannot be completely displaced from the normal acetabulum unless the ligamentum teres is ruptured or deficient from some unrelated cause. Traumatic dislocations can be classified according to the direction of displacement of the femoral head from the acetabulum.

Posterior Hip Dislocation

The head of the femur is usually dislocated posterior to the acetabulum while the thigh is flexed, as may occur in a head-on automobile collision when the driver's or passenger's knee is driven violently against the dashboard.

The significant clinical findings are shortening, adduction, and internal rotation of the extremity. Anteroposterior, transpelvic, and, if fracture of the acetabulum is demonstrated, oblique x-ray projections are required. Common complications are fracture of the acetabulum, injury to the sciatic nerve, and fracture of the head or shaft of the femur. The head of the femur may be displaced through a rent in the posterior hip joint capsule, or the glenoid lip may be avulsed from the acetabulum.

Figure 43–24. Posterior hip dislocation with concomitant fracture of the posterior wall and weightbearing dome of the acetabulum.

The short external rotator muscles of the femur are commonly lacerated. Fracture of the posterior margin of the acetabulum can create instability.

If the acetabulum is not fractured or if the fragment is small, reduction by closed manipulation is indicated. General anesthesia provides maximum muscle relaxation and allows gentle reduction. Reduction should be achieved as soon as possible, preferably within the first few hours after injury as soon as the patient's general status has been adequately assessed. The main feature of reduction is traction in the line of deformity, followed by gentle flexion of the hip to 90 degrees with stabilization of the pelvis by an assistant. While manual traction is continued, the hip is gently rotated into internal and then external rotation to obtain reduction.

The success of reduction is determined immediately by anteroposterior and lateral x-rays. Interposition of capsule substance or bone fragments will be manifested by widening of the joint cleft. If x-rays are difficult to interpret, CT scan can be helpful in assessing concentricity of reduction. If reduction is adequate, the hip will usually be stable, with the extremity in extension and slight external rotation. Stability of the hip should be tested immediately after reduction by motion of the hip in flexion and adduction to assess the maximum limits of stability. A very easy manipulative reduction (eg, the hip "slides in" with very little effort) may suggest major instability and a potential for redislocation even though the hip is maintained in traction.

Postreduction treatment may be by immobilization in traction or balanced suspension or in a plaster spica cast. Since this is primarily a soft tissue injury, sound healing should occur in 4 weeks. Opinion differs on when unsupported weightbearing should be resumed. Some authors believe that disability caused by ischemic osteonecrosis of the femoral head is less likely when complete weightbearing is deferred for 6 months after injury; others believe that early loading is not harmful.

If the posterior or superior acetabulum is fractured, dislocation of the hip must be assumed to have occurred even though displacement is not present at the time of examination. Undisplaced fissure fractures may be treated initially by bed rest and avoidance of full weightbearing for 2 months. Frequent examination is necessary to make certain that the head of the femur has not become displaced from the acetabulum.

Minor fragments of the posterior margin of the acetabulum may be disregarded unless they are in the hip joint cavity. Larger displaced fragments often cannot be reduced adequately by closed methods. If the fragment is large and the hip is unstable following closed manipulation, open operation is indicated. The fragment is then placed in anatomic position and fixed with bone screws or a bone plate and screws.

After the operation, if fixation is tenuous because of severe comminution of the fracture, the patient is placed in bed with the extremity in balanced suspension with 5–8 kg of skeletal traction on the tibial tubercle for about 4–6 weeks until healing of the acetabular fracture is sound. If fixation is stable, the patient may be allowed out of bed in a few days with progression to ambulation on crutches that is nonweightbearing on the injured side. Full weightbearing is not permitted until healing is complete—a process that takes about 3–6 months.

Anterior Hip Dislocation

Anterior dislocation of the hip is much rarer than posterior dislocation. It usually occurs when the hip is extended and externally rotated at the time of impact. Associated fractures of the acetabulum and the femoral neck occur rarely. The femoral head usually remains lateral to the obturator externus muscle but can rarely be found beneath it (obturator dislocation) or under the iliopsoas muscle in contact with the superior pubic ramus (pubic dislocation).

The hip is classically flexed, abducted, and externally rotated. The femoral head is palpable anteriorly below the inguinal flexion crease. Anteroposterior and transpelvic lateral radiographic projections are usually diagnostic.

Closed reduction under general anesthesia is generally successful. Concentric reduction must be obtained. The patient starts mobilization within a few days when pain is tolerable. Active and passive hip motion, excluding external rotation, are encouraged, and the patient is usually fully weightbearing by 4–6 weeks.

Eiskjaer S, Ostgard SE: Survivorship analysis of hemiarthroplasties. Clin Orthop 1993;(286):206.

Daum WJ: Traumatic posterior acetabular defects reconstructed with iliac crest autograft: a report of two cases. Clin Orthop 1993;(291):188.

Desjardins AL et al: Unstable intertrochanteric fracture of the femur: a prospective randomised study comparing anatomical reduction and medial displacement osteotomy. J Bone Joint Surg Br 1993;75:445.

Hinton RY, Smith GS: The association of age, race, and sex with the location of proximal femoral fractures in the elderly. J Bone Joint Surg Am 1993;75:752.

Karachalios T et al: Reconstruction nailing for pathological subtrochanteric fractures with coexisting femoral shaft metastases. J Bone Joint Surg Br 1993;75:119.

Mullaji AB, Thomas TL: Low-energy subtrochanteric fractures in elderly patients: results of fixation with the sliding screw plate. J Trauma 1993;34:56.

Nilsson LT, Johansson A, Stromqvist B: Factors predicting healing complications in femoral neck fractures: 138 patients followed for 2 years. Acta Orthop Scand 1993;3;64:175.

Oransky M, Sanguinetti C: Surgical treatment of displaced acetabular fractures: results of 50 consecutive cases. J Orthop Trauma 1993;7:28.

Parfenchuck TA, Carter LW, Young TR: Ipsilateral fractures of the femoral neck and shaft. Orthop Rev 1993;22:356.

Pitsaer E, Samuel AW: Functional outcome after intertrochanteric fractures of the femur: does the implant matter? A prospective study of 100 consecutive cases. Injury 1993;24:35.

Ragnarsson JI et al: Instability and femoral head vitality in fractures of the femoral neck. Clin Orthop 1993;(287):30.

Roffi RP, Matta JM: Unrecognized posterior dislocation of the hip associated with transverse and T-type fractures of the acetabulum. J Orthop Trauma 1993;7:23.

Schlickewei W et al: Hip dislocation without fracture: traction or mobilization after reduction? Injury 1993;24:27.

Shaw JA, Wilson S: Internal fixation of proximal femur fractures: a biomechanical comparison of the Gamma Locking Nail and the Omega Compression Hip Screw. Orthop Rev 1993;22:61.

Snorrason F, Karrholm J, Holmgren C: Fixation of cemented acetabular prostheses: the influence of preoperative diagnosis. J Arthroplasty 1993;8:83.

Swiontkowski MF: Intracapsular fractures of the hip: current concepts review. J Bone Joint Surg Am 1994;76:129.

Operations for Sequelae of Fractures & Dislocations of the Hip Region

A. Osteotomy

Osteotomy is usually performed in the predominantly cancellous intertrochanteric region, and the bone fragments are generally stabilized by a fixation device. An indication for osteotomy is correction of torsional or varus deformity. Supportive osteotomy is used to minimize displacing stresses at unhealed fracture sites. Abduction, adduction, or rotational osteotomy has been performed for relief of pain associated with ischemic osteonecrosis of the femoral head or secondary osteoarthritis. Although osteotomy preserves joint motion and provides stability, the prognosis for relief of pain is unpredictable.

B. Arthrodesis

Arthrodesis may be intra-articular, extra-articular, or a combination of both. Bone grafting to aid fusion and internal fixation to provide support at the coxofemoral relationship are elective supplemental features. Arthrodesis has been a favored operation as an adjunct in the control of chronic hip joint infection. When arthrodesis is bony—although articular pain is relieved and mechanical stability of the joint is ensured—added stress is placed on the lumber spine and knee joint. Pain from degeneration in those areas is a frequent result. The patient must also accept some disability because of loss of hip joint function.

C. HEAD & NECK RESECTION (GIRDLESTONE ARTHROPLASTY)

The indications for resection of the head and neck of the femur for treatment of fractures, dislocations, and fracture-dislocations have been frequently modified. This operation allows motion but causes significant shortening of the extremity and creates instability that usually requires one or two crutches for ambulation as well as a large shoe lift. Currently, its chief application is in the treatment of chronic hip joint infection. It is useful occasionally in the treatment of pathologic fracture of the proximal femur due to primary or metastatic tumors. Rarely is osteopenia or destruction of bone from causes other than those mentioned above so extensive that resection is preferable to an endoprosthesis

D. TOTAL HIP JOINT REPLACEMENT

Total hip joint replacement (Figure 43–25) has been widely accepted as an excellent operation to relieve the pain and dysfunction caused by arthritis of the hip. This technique implies substitution of at least the articular surfaces of both the acetabulum and the head of the femur by implants made of metal or plastic. The femoral component is usually made of cobalt-chrome alloy, stainless steel, or titanium. The acetabular constituent is usually made of polyethylene of very high molecular weight or a combination of a metal hemispherical shell that supports a liner of polyethylene, ceramic, or metal.

The main indications for any type of hip arthroplasty are relief of incapacitating pain and restoration or improvement of joint function. The presence of joint sepsis is a contraindication to replacement arthroplasty.

Total hip joint replacement requires removal of the entire head of the femur and part of the femoral neck as well as extensive remodeling of the acetabulum. The femoral head and acetabular components are stabilized in bone either by a "press fit" or with polymethylmethacrylate cement. Total hip joint replacement has wider application in the treatment of posttraumatic arthritis resulting from fractures and dislocations of the hip joint in the adult than in their primary treatment. It is useful as a reconstructive procedure in the treatment of failure of the joint without infection. Success rates of over 90% have been reported. Because long-term reliability has not been established, the operation should be reserved for patients over age 50 unless specific factors warrant its use in younger persons.

Failure of total hip joint replacement can be caused by recurrent dislocation within the prosthesis complex, loosening of the components at the interface between the bone and the cementing substance, breakage of the femoral component, sepsis, and undetermined causes of

Figure 43–25. Hybrid total hip replacement with porous coated acetabular shell and cemented femoral stem performed for osteoarthritis.

disabling pain. The long-term effects of wear of the material and the effect of wear debris on the surrounding tissues have not been determined. Infection is the most serious complication; even if it is promptly discovered and vigorously treated, removal of the device complex may be necessary. Removal of the prosthesis leaves the patient with a severely shortened extremity and an unstable hip and necessitates indefinite use of crutch support for ambulation.

Many attempts have been made to develop prostheses that do not require such extensive removal of bone, so that if failure occurs major shortening and instability are less likely to develop. The younger the patient, the longer the time the prosthesis will be subjected to loading and wear. Thus, several revision arthroplasties over the patient's lifetime may be needed. Long-term failure of total hip arthroplasty has been linked to bony resorption around the implant from foreign particle wear debris (usually polyethylene) that causes activation of bone resorbing cells (osteoclasts). Newer formulations of polyethylene as well as alternative bearing surfaces and medical treatment (bisphosphonates) hold great promise to minimize endoprosthetic failure from these mechanisms.

E. HEMIARTHROPLASTY (ENDOPROSTHESIS)

Hemiarthroplasty involves replacement of the femoral head and neck fragment and implies the presence of a normal or nearly normal acetabulum. The procedure is useful when the femoral head is extensively involved with a degenerative process or when treatment is required for unhealed femoral neck fracture. The femoral stem may be stabilized in the femoral canal by a "press fit" or with methylmethacrylate cement. The choice is dependent upon the patient's age and bone quality. Best results are obtained with patients who are motivated to participate in a vigorous rehabilitation program. Functional improvement continues over several years. Causes of failure include motion between the implant and cement or bone, acetabular deterioration secondary to wear, and postoperative infection.

F. BIPOLAR OR UNIVERSAL ENDOPROSTHESIS

These prostheses are intermediate steps between the conventional femoral head prosthesis (endoprosthesis) and the total hip joint prosthesis. The femoral head is removed and replaced with an endoprosthesis with the stem cemented or press-fit in the femoral intramedullary canal. A polyethylene liner is fixed in a metallic cup, and the edges of the liner are so fashioned that the socket "snap fits" on the head. The acetabulum is not altered. Motion occurs between the outer surface of the metallic cup and the articular surface of the acetabulum and between the head of the femoral prosthesis and the polyethylene liner. Theoretic advantages of this prosthesis are that there may be less erosion of the acetabulum than with an endoprosthesis alone, and if revision to the total hip joint is necessary later, only the cup may have to be replaced. One major disadvantage is that dislocation within the prosthetic complex is virtually impossible to reduce by closed manipulation. In addition, the polyethylene liner in a bipolar endoprosthesis may generate more polyethylene wear.

Gebhard JS et al: A comparison of total hip arthroplasty and hemiarthroplasty for treatment of acute fracture of the femoral neck. Clin Orthop 1992;(282):123.

Jalovaara P et al: Treatment of hip fracture in Finland and Sweden: prospective comparison of 788 cases in three hospitals. Acta Orthop Scand 1992;63:531.

Kim YH, Oh JH, Koh YG: Salvage of neglected unstable intertrochanteric fracture with cementless porous-coated hemiarthroplasty. Clin Orthop 1992;(277):182.

Moeckel BH et al: Modular hemiarthroplasty for fractures of the proximal part of the humerus. J Bone Joint Surg Am 1992; 74:884.

Parker MJ: Internal fixation or arthroplasty for displaced subcapital fractures in the elderly? Injury 1992;23:521.

INFECTIONS ASSOCIATED WITH JOINT REPLACEMENTS

Infections that occur following joint replacement arthroplasty may be due to organisms introduced at surgery or may result from late hematogenous contamination. They are generally more serious than infections that follow fractures, since the implanted prosthesis is intended to be a permanent substitute for a failed joint and not a temporary fixation such as is used for fracture healing. Removal of the prosthesis shortens the limb and produces instability unless arthrodesis is achieved, fusing the adjacent bones to prevent motion. Removal of a prosthetic joint without arthrodesis leaves a so-called "excisional arthroplasty," which may offer an acceptable salvage. Arthroplasty following removal of a total hip prosthesis is often called Girdlestone arthroplasty after the surgeon who proposed hip joint excision as primary treatment for certain disorders. While such a salvage procedure may be well tolerated, crutches are usually required and pain is a frequent problem. Furthermore, even removal of all of the implanted material may fail to cure the infection.

It is sometimes possible to control infection and repeat the prosthetic arthroplasty. However, early failure rates tend to be at least 15%, and questions remain about long-term results following revision arthroplasty for infection. Chronic oral antibiotic treatment—to suppress rather than cure infection—may be a reasonable alternative to removal or replacement of the prosthesis for appropriately selected patients.

Treatment of infected joint replacements depends upon the time of occurrence, the virulence of the infecting organism, and the mechanical stability of the prosthesis. Infection must be suspected whenever pain develops following prosthetic arthroplasty. Loosening of the prosthetic components within their bony seats may be due to infection, mechanical failure, or both. Either loosening or infection may cause pain. Relatively avirulent organisms cause infection with a low-grade smoldering course that slowly spreads through the bone adjacent to the prosthesis. Aspiration for culture and sensitivity testing is essential for early diagnosis. Treatment requires surgery and skillful antibiotic management. If the prosthesis is loose, it will require removal, which is necessary for adequate debridement of most chronic infections. All foreign material and infected granulation tissue must be debrided. Viable bone should be preserved. Currently, a hip spacer composed of antibiotic containing methylmethacrylate achieves high local antibiotic concentrations while preserving soft tissue tension around the joint. Wound closure over drains, 4–6 weeks of intravenous antibiotic treatment to achieve adequate serum bactericidal levels (usually 1:8 dilution or more), and adequate mechanical support of the limb are advised. Following removal of a total hip prosthesis, an antibiotic cement spacer, is often placed, and so traction is rarely needed. Decisions must be made about whether or not to replace the removed prosthesis and, if replacement is chosen, whether to proceed immediately or defer reimplantation for weeks or months until the wound is quiescent. Two-stage reimplantation of an infected total hip prosthesis may be more successful than single-stage reimplantation, but this remains controversial. Adding antibiotics to the acrylic cement used to seat prosthetic components is another adjunct that appears to improve the success rate of total hip revision for infection.

Beck-Sague CM et al: Outbreak of surgical wound infections associated with total hip arthroplasty. Infect Control Hosp Epidemiol 1992;13:526.

Fitzgerald RH Jr: Total hip arthroplasty sepsis: Prevention and diagnosis. Orthop Clin North Am 1992;23:259.

Schmalzried TP et al: Etiology of deep sepsis in total hip arthroplasty: the significance of hematogenous and recurrent infections. Clin Orthop 1992;(280):200.

FRACTURE OF THE SHAFT OF THE FEMUR

Fracture of the shaft of the femur (Figure 43–26) usually occurs as a result of severe trauma. Indirect violence, especially torsional stress, is likely to cause spiral fractures that extend proximally or, more commonly, distally into the metaphysial region. Most are closed fractures; open fracture is often the result of compounding from within. Extensive soft tissue injury, bleeding, and shock are commonly present.

The most significant features are severe pain in the thigh and deformity of the lower extremity. Surgical shock is likely to be present, as several units of blood may be lost into the thigh with only moderate swelling becoming apparent. Careful x-ray examination in at least two planes is necessary to determine the exact site and configuration of the fracture cleft. The hip and knee should be examined and x-rays obtained to look for associated injury. A femoral neck fracture may occur

Figure 43–26. Femoral shaft fracture. ***A:*** Anteroposterior x-ray showing fracture of the midshaft of the femur. ***B:*** Anteroposterior x-ray after closed reduction and intramedullary fixation using an antegrade titanium locked nail. ***C:*** Anteroposterior x-ray showing fixation of a midshaft femoral fracture and ipsilateral femoral neck fracture with a retrograde intramedullary nail.

in association with a femur fracture and if overlooked can increase patient morbidity.

Injuries to the sciatic nerve and to the superficial femoral artery and vein are not common but must be recognized promptly. Surgical shock and secondary anemia are the most important early complications. Later complications are those of prolonged recumbency, joint stiffness, malunion, nonunion, leg-length discrepancy, and infection.

Treatment

A. CLOSED TREATMENT

Treatment depends upon the age and medical status of the patient as well as the site and configuration of the fracture. Closed treatment of femoral shaft fractures in adults is rarely indicated. Skeletal traction is generally the most effective form of closed treatment. However, 2–3 months of traction are often required, followed by external plaster or brace support. Acceptable alignment may be difficult to maintain, and joint stiffness is frequent. Other complications of prolonged recumbency like pressure sores and deep vein thrombosis can have disastrous consequences. Fractures of the distal femoral shaft are more suitable for cast-brace treatment. After about 6 weeks in traction, the patient may be placed in a cast-brace (long-leg cast with a hinged knee) to allow early knee motion and progressive weightbearing.

B. OPERATIVE TREATMENT

Most fractures in the middle third of the femur can be internally fixed by an intramedullary rod. Intramedullary fixation of femoral shaft fractures allows immediate mobilization of the patient, more anatomic alignment, improved knee function by decreasing the time spent in traction, and a substantial decrease in the cost of hospitalization.

The procedure may be performed open or "blind." In open nailing, the fracture site is opened and the nail is driven retrograde from the fracture site into the proximal fragment. The fracture is then reduced and the nail driven across the fracture into the distal fragment. This requires a large incision and major manipulation of the fracture fragments, with significant blood loss.

In blind nailing, the fracture is reduced by closed manipulation on the fracture table under fluoroscopic control. An 8 cm to 10 cm incision is made proximal to the greater trochanter, and the nail is inserted through the trochanteric notch down into the intramedullary canal. The fracture site is not opened. Blind nailing decreases the chance of infection and nonunion by decreasing the amount of soft tissue dissection necessary and by leaving the fracture site closed.

If the fracture is comminuted, interlocking nails can be used to maintain length by increased fixation proxi-

mally and distally. These may allow patients early mobilization even with comminuted femoral shaft fractures. If there is extensive soft tissue loss surrounding the fracture, stability of the bone fragments may be achieved with an external fixation device.

Complications of this procedure usually involve technical problems at the time of surgery, resulting in malalignment or shortening from choosing a rod that is too short or too narrow. Infection can occur after any open procedure but is very uncommon in blind nailing. Occasionally, a painful bursa may develop over the proximal end of the nail that causes discomfort when the patient sits or walks. The rod may be removed after healing is complete—usually after 1 year to 1½ years. The healing rate of femoral shaft fractures in general is very high and approaches 100% after blind nailing.

Benirschke SK et al: Closed interlocking nailing of femoral shaft fractures: assessment of technical complications and functional outcomes by comparison of a prospective database with retrospective review. J Orthop Trauma 1993;7:118.

Hajek PD et al: The use of one compared with two distal screws in the treatment of femoral shaft fractures with interlocking intramedullary nailing: a clinical and biomechanical analysis. J Bone Joint Surg Am 1993;75:519.

Parfenchuck TA, Carter LW, Young TR: Ipsilateral fractures of the femoral neck and shaft. Orthop Rev 1993;22:356.

Wu CC et al: Treatment of segmental femoral shaft fractures. Clin Orthop 1993;(287):224.

INJURIES OF THE KNEE REGION

1. Fractures of the Distal Femur

Supracondylar Fracture of the Femur

These fractures involve the distal metaphysis and epiphysis of the femur. It is important to distinguish between extra-articular and intra-articular supracondylar femur fractures (Figure 43–27). The distal fragment is usually rotated into extension from traction by the gastrocnemius muscles. The distal end of the proximal fragment is apt to perforate the overlying quadriceps and may penetrate the suprapatellar pouch.

The distal fragment may impinge on the popliteal neurovascular bundle, and an immediate thorough neurovascular examination is mandatory. Absence or marked decrease of pedal pulses is an indication for immediate reduction. If this fails to restore adequate circulation, an arteriogram should be obtained immediately and the vascular lesion repaired as indicated.

Extra-articular Fractures

For simple fracture patterns, closed reduction under general anesthesia is occasionally successful. Most of these fractures, however, are best treated with internal

Figure 43–27. ***A:*** Anteroposterior radiograph demonstrating a comminuted supracondylar femur fracture with intra-articular extension. ***B:*** Lateral radiograph.

fixation, which allows early mobilization of the patient and of the neighboring joints. Most fractures are treated with internal fixation. Closed interlocked intramedullary nailing is recommended for somewhat more proximal fractures. An interlocked intramedullary device introduced in a retrograde fashion from the intercondylar notch has shown promising results. Most fractures are best treated with open reduction and internal fixation with screws and plates and screwplate devices. Skeletal traction is reserved for patients for whom surgery is contraindicated and is fraught with all the previously mentioned complications that can accompany prolonged recumbency.

Intra-articular Fractures

As for all intra-articular fractures, maximal functional recovery of the knee joint requires anatomic reduction of the articular components. Closed reduction of displaced fractures is almost never successful. Nondisplaced fractures can be treated with a cast brace for about 12 weeks or with percutaneous pinning or open internal fixation, which allows earlier mobilization of the joint.

Intercondylar Fractures

These comminuted fractures of the distal femoral epiphysis are classically described as T or Y fractures according to the configuration of the articular fragments.

Displaced fractures are best treated by open reduction—to restore anatomic alignment of the articular surface—and by internal fixation using lag screws and plates to allow early motion. Even if anatomic alignment is achieved, joint stiffness, pain, and posttraumatic arthritis are not uncommon outcomes.

Condylar Fractures

Isolated fractures of the lateral or medial femoral condyles are rare. They usually result from varus or valgus stress to the knee joint with possible associated ligamentous injuries to the knee. Fractures of the posterior portion of one or the other condyle in the frontal plane can also be seen.

Closed reduction of displaced fragments is very rarely successful. Open reduction with screws is usually indicated. If fixation is solid, postoperative motion is started immediately. Weightbearing is allowed at 3 months when clinical and radiographic healing is present.

2. Fracture of the Patella

Transverse Fracture of the Patella

Transverse fracture of he patella is the result of indirect violence, usually with the knee in semiflexion. Fracture may be due to sudden voluntary contraction of the quadriceps muscles or sudden forced flexion of the leg when these muscles are contracted. The level of fracture is most often in the middle. The extent of tearing of the patellar retinacula depends upon the degree of force of the initiating injury. The activity of the quadriceps muscles causes displacement of the proximal fragment; the magnitude of displacement is dependent upon the extent of the tear of the quadriceps expansion.

Swelling of the anterior knee region is caused by hemarthrosis and hemorrhage into the soft tissues overlying the joint. If displacement is present, the defect in the patella can be palpated, and active extension of the knee is lost.

Open reduction is indicated if the fragments are offset or separated more than 2–3 mm. The fragments must be accurately repositioned to prevent early posttraumatic arthritis of the patellofemoral joint. If the minor fragment is small (no more than 1 cm in length) or severely comminuted, it may be excised and the rectus or patellar tendon (depending upon which pole of the patella is involved) sutured directly to the major fragment. If the fragments are approximately the same size, repair by wire cerclage or figure-of-eight wire is preferred. Accurate reduction of the articular surface must be confirmed by lateral x-rays taken intraoperatively.

Comminuted Fracture of the Patella

Comminuted fracture of the patella is caused only by direct violence. Little or no separation of the fragments occurs because the quadriceps expansion is not extensively torn. Severe injury may cause extensive comminution of the articular cartilages of both the patella and the opposing femur. If comminution is not severe and displacement is insignificant, immobilization for 8 weeks in a plaster cylinder extending from the groin to the supramalleolar region is sufficient.

Severe comminution requires excision of the patella and repair of the defect by imbrication of the quadriceps expansion. Excision of the patella can result in decreased strength, pain in the knee, and general restriction of activity.

Tear of the Quadriceps Tendon

Tear of the quadriceps tendon occurs most often in patients over age 40. Preexisting attritional disease of the tendon is apt to be present, and the causative injury may be minor. The tear commonly results from sudden deceleration, such as stumbling, or slipping on a wet surface. A small flake of bone may be avulsed from the superior pole of the patella, or the tear may occur entirely through tendinous and muscle tissue.

Pain may be noted in the anterior knee region. Swelling is due to hemarthrosis and extravasation of blood into the soft tissues. The patient is unable to ex-

tend the knee completely. X-rays may show avulsion of a bit of bone from the superior patella.

Operative repair is recommended for complete tear. If treatment is delayed until partial healing has occurred, the suture line can be reinforced by transplantation of the iliotibial band from the upper area of the tibia.

Tear of the Patellar Ligament

The same mechanism that causes tears of the quadriceps tendon, transverse fracture of the patella, or avulsion of the tibial tuberosity may also cause tear of the patellar ligament. The characteristic finding is proximal displacement of the patella. A bit of bone may be avulsed from the lower pole of the patella if the tear takes place in the proximal patellar tendon.

Operative treatment is necessary for complete tear. The ligament is resutured to the patella, and any tear in the quadriceps expansion is repaired. The extremity should be immobilized for 8 weeks in a tubular plaster cast extending from the groin to the supramalleolar region. Guarded exercises may then be started.

Dislocation of the Patella

Acute traumatic dislocation of the patella should be differentiated from episodic recurrent dislocation, since the latter condition is likely to be associated with occult organic lesions. When this injury occurs alone, it may be due to direct violence or muscle activity of the quadriceps, and the direction of dislocation of the patella is usually lateral. Spontaneous reduction is apt to occur if the knee joint is extended; if so, the clinical findings may consist merely of hemarthrosis and localized tenderness over the medial patellar retinaculum. Gross instability of the patella, which can be demonstrated by physical examination, indicates that injury to the soft tissues of the medial aspect of the knee has been extensive. Recurrent episodes require operative repair for effective treatment.

Dislocation of the Knee Joint

Traumatic dislocation of the knee joint is uncommon. It is caused by severe trauma. Displacement may be transverse or torsional. Complete dislocation can occur only after extensive tearing of the supporting ligaments and is apt to cause injury to the popliteal vessels or the tibial and peroneal nerves.

Signs of neurovascular injury below the site of dislocation are an absolute indication for prompt reduction, preferably under general anesthesia, since failure of circulation will undoubtedly result in gangrene of the leg and foot. Axial traction is applied to the leg to obtain reduction. If pedal pulses do not return promptly, patency of the popliteal vessels should be investigated immediately by angiography. Even if pulses do return, angiography is usually indicated to rule out an intimal tear of the vessel. Inadequate assessment and treatment of the vascular injuries can lead to an amputation rate of 50%. If a vascular injury is confirmed, repair should be started as soon as the patient's general status allows. Ischemia of more than 4 hours is associated with a poor prognosis for limb salvage. Prophylactic fasciotomy of the leg compartments should be performed at the time of vascular repair to eliminate the compartment syndrome caused by postischemic edema.

Anatomic reduction of uncomplicated dislocation should be attempted. If impinging soft tissue cannot be removed by closed manipulation, arthrotomy is indicated. After reduction, repair of the major ligamentous injuries may be performed, but this should not be done if the time and dissection necessary will further jeopardize survival of the limb. The extremity should be immobilized in a plaster cast extending from the inguinal region to the toes, with the knee in slight flexion. A window should be cut in the plaster over the dorsum of the foot to allow for frequent determination of dorsalis pedis artery pulsation. In anteroposterior dislocations, adequacy of reduction should be assessed at frequent intervals during the first 3–4 weeks to rule out posterior subluxation. If subluxation occurs, the knee joint must be reduced and placed in an external fixation device. After 8 weeks of immobilization, the knee can be protected by a long-leg brace. Intensive quadriceps exercises are necessary to minimize functional loss.

Appel MH, Seigel H: Treatment of transverse fractures of the patella by arthroscopic percutaneous pinning. Arthroscopy 1993;9:119.

Braun W et al: Indications and results of nonoperative treatment of patellar fractures. Clin Orthop 1993;(289):197.

Rasul AT Jr, Fischer DA: Primary repair of quadriceps tendon ruptures: results of treatment. Clin Orthop 1993;(289):205.

Schenck RC Jr, Heckman JD: Injuries of the knee. Clin Symp 1993;45:1.

Shrewing DJ, Meggitt BF: Fractures of the distal femur treated with the AO dynamic condylar screw. J Bone Joint Surg Br 1992;74:122.

Tucker JB, Corsetti J, Gregg JR: Arthroscopically assisted proximal quadricepsplasty for patellar instability. Clin Sports Med 1993;12:81.

INJURIES TO THE LIGAMENTS, MENISCI, & CARTILAGE OF THE KNEE JOINT

Internal derangement of the knee joint mechanism is usually caused by trauma but can also result from overuse. Injuries to the ligaments, cartilage, and meniscus commonly occur as combined lesions.

X-rays are typically the first-line radiographic modality but are often normal in suspected ligament or cartilage injury. Arthroscopy and MRI are valuable adjuncts in diagnosis when the usual methods are inconclusive.

Arthroscopy is a valuable adjunct to the history, physical examination, and x-ray studies for evaluation of the knee joint. The arthroscope introduced into the knee joint through a small stab incision allows examination of most structures inside the knee without major surgical exploration.

Arthroscopy can be helpful in diagnosis of any confusing knee problem, but MRI has largely replaced arthroscopy for the diagnosis of injuries to the menisci and ligaments. MRI also assists with preoperative confirmation of a clinical diagnosis (eg, patients with anterior cruciate tears, meniscal tear, or chondromalacia) and for follow-up evaluation after therapy.

Surgical procedures such as meniscus repair, meniscectomy, synovial biopsy, or removal of loose bodies can be performed through the arthroscope with minimal postoperative morbidity compared with open procedures. However, this is a demanding technique and requires considerable experience for good results.

Injury to the Menisci

Injury to the medial meniscus is the most frequent internal derangement of the knee joint. Clinical findings after acute injury are swelling, pain, and varying degrees of restriction of flexion or extension. True locking (inability to fully extend the knee) is highly suggestive of meniscal tear. A marginal tear permits displacement of the medial fragment into the intercondylar region (bucket handle tear) and prevents either complete extension or complete flexion. Motion may cause pain over the anteromedial or posteromedial joint line. Tenderness can often be elicited at the point of pain. Forcible rotation of the foot with the knee flexed to a right angle may cause pain over the medial joint line. If symptoms have persisted for 2–3 weeks and the patient avoids weightbearing on the knee, weakness and atrophy of the quadriceps femoris may be present. Injury to the lateral meniscus is less common but may also cause mechanical blockage of joint motion. Pain and tenderness may be present over the lateral joint line, and MRI is the imaging modality of choice for diagnosing medial and lateral meniscus tears.

Initial treatment may be conservative. Swelling and pain can be relieved by aspiration, and younger patients usually prefer to be ambulatory on crutches. Isometric quadriceps exercises should be performed frequently throughout the day with the knee in maximum extension, and the emphasis should be placed on restoring range of motion. Physical therapy and nonsteroidal anti-inflammatory drugs are helpful.

Arthroscopy with either meniscectomy or meniscus repair is advisable for recurrent or persistent "locking," recurrent effusion, or pain. Isometric quadriceps exercises and range of motion exercises are started immediately and are gradually increased in frequency. As soon as the patient is able to perform these exercises comfortably, graded resistance maneuvers should be started. Exercises should be continued until motion and strength is equal to the other healthy knee.

Injury to the Ligaments

Ligaments in general prevent displacement or angulation beyond its normal envelope of motion. When the knee is in full extension, the collateral ligaments are taut; in flexion, only the anterior fibers of the tibial collateral ligament are taut.

A. MEDIAL COLLATERAL LIGAMENT

This ligament—often referred to as the tibial collateral ligament—is the primary restraint to valgus. Forced abduction of the leg at the knee causes injury varying from complete rupture to tearing of a few fibers of the ligament. A bit of bone may be avulsed from its femoral or tibial attachment.

A history of a twisting injury at the knee with valgus strain can usually be obtained. Pain is present over the medial aspect of the knee joint. In severe injury, joint effusion may be present. Tenderness can be elicited at the site of the lesion. When only an isolated ligamentous tear is present, x-ray examination may not be helpful unless it is made while valgus stress is applied.

Treatment of an incomplete tear consists of protection from further injury while healing progresses in a brace that allows motion but protects the knee from valgus injury. It may be helpful to bend the brace into varus to take load off of the ligament.

Tear of the medial collateral ligament is frequently associated with other lesions, such as tear of the medial meniscus, rupture of the anterior cruciate ligament, or fracture of the lateral condyle of the tibia. Bony injury is more common in young patients.

B. LATERAL COLLATERAL LIGAMENT

Tear of the lateral collateral ligament is often associated with injury to surrounding structures, eg, the popliteus muscle tendon or the iliotibial band. Avulsion of the apex of the fibular head may occur, and the peroneal nerve may be injured.

Pain and tenderness are present over the lateral aspect of the knee joint, and hemarthrosis may be present. X-rays may show bone avulsion from the fibular head.

The treatment of partial tear is similar to that described for partial tear of the medial collateral ligament. If complete tear is suspected, healing is rare without operative measures, and exploration and reconstruction will probably be required.

C. ANTERIOR CRUCIATE LIGAMENT

The function of the anterior cruciate ligament is prevention of anterior displacement of the tibia. Injury to the anterior cruciate ligament is often associated with injury to the menisci or the medial collateral ligament. The cruciate ligament may be avulsed with part of the tibial tubercle (Figure 43–28), but it usually ruptures within the substance of its fibers.

The characteristic clinical sign of tear of the anterior cruciate ligament is a positive anterior drawer sign: the knee is flexed to 90 degrees and pulled forward, and if excessive anterior excursion of the proximal tibia (in comparison with the opposite normal knee) occurs, tearing of the anterior ligament is suspected. Other tests include the Lachman test (anterior drawer with the knee flexed 20 degrees) and the pivot shift test. MRI is very accurate for the diagnosis of these injuries. Reconstruction is usually required for young active patients who wish to participate in sports that call for sudden cutting or twisting movements. Reconstruction is delayed until full range of motion is obtained.

With avulsion, displaced tibial bone is present, and attachment of the fragment in anatomic position by arthrotomy or arthroscopy is necessary. When the fragment of bone is large, displaced, and not treated until several weeks after injury, excision of the fragment and reinsertion of the ligament may be necessary to eliminate the blocking effect of the bone fragment and permit recovery of function.

Figure 43–28. Lateral T1-weighted MRI image showing an acute rupture of the anterior cruciate ligament (arrow).

D. POSTERIOR CRUCIATE LIGAMENT

Tear of the posterior ligament may occur within its substance or by avulsion of a fragment of bone at its tibial attachment. Tear of the posterior cruciate ligament can be diagnosed by the posterior "drawer" sign: The knee is flexed at a right angle, and the upper tibia is pushed backward; if excessive posterior excursion of the proximal tibia can be noted, tear of the posterior ligament is likely. MRI is very accurate for diagnosis of these injuries.

Treatment is directed primarily at the associated injuries and maintenance of competency of the quadriceps musculature. Primary repair of tears within the fibers is difficult and of dubious value. Open reduction and fixation of a fragment of tibia with the attached ligament is feasible and is apt to restore functional competency of the ligament.

Cartilage Injury

Damage to the cartilage is common with trauma to the knee and should be differentiated from osteoarthritis. Developments in cartilage transplantation, including autograft and allograft tissue, have greatly improved the prognosis for these injuries. Arthroscopy and MRI are required for accurate diagnosis (Figure 43–29). Cartilage is biopsied from the knee, cultured, and then reimplanted at a later date.

Ligamentous Reconstruction of the Knee

Knee joint instability may be (1) single plane (medial, lateral, posterior, or anterior), (2) rotatory, or (3) a

Figure 43–29. Intraoperative photograph showing a full-thickness cartilage injury.

combinations of the two. To speak of repair of ligaments denotes treatment of acute injuries, whereas the term reconstruction is reserved for treatment of ligamentous laxity several months after injury.

Reconstructive procedures to replace the function of the anterior and posterior cruciate ligament include use of a portion of autograft or allograft tendon introduced through drill holes in the proximal tibia and the posterior femur.

Indications for major reconstruction of knee ligaments depend on the patient's age and activity level and the status of the articular cartilage within the knee. Early results of these procedures are often excellent, but the integrity of the repair tends to deteriorate after 2–5 years.

Andriacchi TP, Birac D: Functional testing in the anterior cruciate ligament-deficient knee. Clin Orthop 1993;(288):40.

De Smet AA et al: Diagnosis of meniscal tears of the knee with MR imaging: effect of observer variation and sample size on sensitivity and specificity. AJR Am J Roentgenol 1993;160:555.

DiStefano V: Anterior cruciate ligament reconstruction: autograft or allograft? Clin Sports Med 1993;12:1.

Frank CB, Jackson DW. The science of reconstruction of the anterior cruciate ligament. J Bone Joint Surg Am 1997;79:1556.

Gillquist J: Repair and reconstruction of the ACL: is it good enough? Arthroscopy 1993;9:68.

Halling AH, Howard ME, Cawley PW: Rehabilitation of anterior cruciate ligament injuries. Clin Sports Med 1993;12:329.

Jackson DW et al: Cartilage substitutes: overview of basic science and treatment options. J Am Acad Orthop Surg 2001;9:37.

Newman AP, Daniels AU, Burks RT: Principles and decision making in meniscal surgery. Arthroscopy 1993;9:33.

Woo SL, Livesay GA, Engle C: Biomechanics of the human anterior cruciate ligament: muscle stabilization and ACL reconstruction. Orthop Rev 1992;21(8):935.

FRACTURES OF THE PROXIMAL TIBIA

1. FRACTURES OF THE TIBIAL PLATEAU

Fractures of the tibial plateau (Figure 43–30) account for about 1% of all fractures. As with most orthopedic injuries, they occur primarily in two demographic groups: younger patients sustaining high-energy injuries and elderly patients as a result of minor trauma.

Mechanism of Injury

Fractures of the tibial plateau occur as a result of a combination of axial compression and strong valgus or varus load applied to the knee. A classic example is a pedestrian struck by a car in which the car bumper produces an extreme valgus or varus load on the knee while the leg is axially loaded and fixed by the foot to the

Figure 43–30. Schatzker II tibial plateau fracture. **A:** Anteroposterior radiograph. **B:** Radiograph after fixation with lateral plate and bone grafting.

ground. With this injury mechanism, the femoral condyle exerts both a compressive and shearing force on the corresponding tibial plateau. The fracture pattern may be a pure split, a pure compression, or a combination of both. Older patients with osteoporosis will usually have some component of bony compression.

It must be emphasized that injuries to the soft tissues about the knee are commonly associated with plateau fractures. One report identified injuries of the menisci (20%), medial collateral ligaments (20%), and anterior cruciate ligaments (10%) in 56 patients treated operatively for tibial plateau fractures.

Clinical Findings

A. SYMPTOMS AND SIGNS

Patients will invariably present with a painful and swollen knee. As with all intra-articular fractures, hemarthrosis will be present. Physical examination will show tenderness of the bone and soft tissues. Care should be taken to palpate both collateral ligaments and assess for tenderness. Active and passive range of motion of the joint will be painful and limited. Careful assessment of knee stability should be performed if the patient permits it. Intra-articular injection of lidocaine and aspiration of the hemarthrosis will often give enough pain relief to allow this examination in the emergency room.

B. IMAGING STUDIES

Anteroposterior, lateral, and two oblique views centered on the proximal tibia are usually adequate to make the diagnosis. CT scans can be helpful to assess articular congruence and plan surgical approaches. MRI is increasingly being used because it has been shown to be as effective as CT at demonstrating the bony anatomy but has the added benefit of identifying injuries of the menisci and ligaments.

Treatment

The goal of treatment is to obtain a stable, congruent, mobile, and painless joint. While there are no accurate data on the amount of tibial articular surface depression necessary to produce posttraumatic arthritis, it has been shown that more than 3 mm of depression significantly increases joint reactive forces. This is now generally accepted as the maximum acceptable fracture displacement. However, treatment is determined as much by the characteristics of the patient as by the characteristics of the fracture. For this reason, the patient's age, functional status, and comorbidities along with fracture displacement, comminution, and associated soft tissue injuries must influence treatment options. Closed treatment usually consists of gentle reduction and placement in a locked hinged knee brace. Frequent follow-up radiographs are needed to assess fracture alignment, since malalignment can develop in the brace. Knee motion in the hinged brace is allowed once the fracture has healed sufficiently to avoid fracture displacement. Surgical treatment may consist of a variety of techniques, including open or arthroscopically assisted elevation of depressed joint fragments followed by internal fixation sufficient to allow early range of motion. Strict avoidance of weightbearing is maintained for 12 weeks regardless of the treatment utilized.

2. Fracture of the Tibial Tuberosity

Violent contraction of the quadriceps muscle may cause avulsion of the tibial tuberosity. When avulsion is complete, active extension of the knee is not possible. This injury may also occur in children through the apophysis of the proximal tibia.

If displacement is minimal, treatment is by immobilization in a cylinder cast extending from the inguinal to the supramalleolar region with the knee in full extension. Immobilization is maintained for 8 weeks or until sufficient healing has occurred to allow early protected range of motion activity.

A loose fragment that has been displaced more than 5 mm can be treated either by closed reduction and percutaneous fixation or by open reduction and internal fixation

3. Fracture of the Tibial Eminence

This injury usually occurs in association with a comminuted fracture of the tibial plateau. The medial intercondylar tubercle may be avulsed with adjacent bone attached to the anterior cruciate ligament, and injury to this structure is of greater importance. In addition to avulsion of the anterior cruciate ligament, there may also be injury to the tibial collateral ligament and the medial knee joint capsule. Hemarthrosis is always present.

Isolated, undisplaced fractures with a stable knee may be treated by immobilization of the extremity for 6 weeks in a long-leg plaster cast with the knee in 15–20 degrees of flexion to minimize tension on the anterior cruciate ligament. Displaced eminence fractures or fractures in unstable knees or those associated with other intra-articular injuries require surgical stabilization of the bony fragment if it is large enough or anterior cruciate ligament reconstruction if it is not.

Benirschke SK et al: Immediate internal fixation of open, complex tibial plateau fractures: treatment by a standard protocol. J Orthop Trauma 1992;6:78.

Bennett WF, Browner B: Tibial plateau fractures: a study of associated soft-tissue injuries. J Orthop Trauma 1994;8:183.

Honkonen SE, Jarvinen MJ: Classification of fractures of the tibial condyles. J Bone Joint Surg Br 1992;74:840.

Mallik AR, Covall DJ, Whitelaw GP: Internal versus external fixation of bicondylar tibial plateau fractures. Orthop Rev 1992; 21:1433.

Kode L et al: The evaluation of tibial plateau fractures: efficacy of MR Imaging compared to CT. AJR Am J Roentgenol 1994; 163:141.

O'Dwyer KJ, Bobic VR: Arthroscopic management of tibial plateau fractures. Injury 1992;23:261.

TOTAL KNEE REPLACEMENT

Reconstructive surgery for the arthritic knee (Figure 43–31) has been characterized by the development of total replacement prostheses designed to compensate for varying degrees of cartilage, bone, or ligamentous destruction. Indications for knee replacement include intractable pain (with or without deformity) along with x-ray evidence of arthritis, either rheumatoid, posttraumatic, or degenerative. The many designs of implants available vary in the degree to which they constrain knee motion. The unconstrained implants are mainly resurfacing replacements and require intact collateral and posterior cruciate ligaments. A minimum amount of bone is removed from the articular surfaces of the distal femur and proximal tibia and is replaced by metal on the femoral side and polyethylene (or a metal tray with a polyethylene insert) on the tibial side. The components are cemented in place with polymethylmethacrylate. The largest number of prostheses fall into the semiconstrained category and provide varying amounts of intrinsic stability. Fully constrained prostheses permit motion only in the sagittal plane and are used in joints with severe deformity or major ligamentous laxity. These prostheses require removal of a significant amount of bone to allow room for the device, to correct deformity, and to permit placement of the intramedullary stems.

Enthusiastic early short-term reports of total knee arthroplasty have been qualified by more thoughtful long-term studies, with reoperation rates of 15% and higher. The most common mechanism of failure has been loosening of the prosthetic components, usually on the tibial side. Factors contributing to loosening include inadequate fixation, less than optimal cementing techniques, and restricted rotation of the prosthesis. Obesity, overactivity, and insufficient bone stock are patient factors contributing to failure.

Patients with preoperative varus deformity appear to have a higher incidence of loosening. Other complications include peroneal nerve palsy, problems with wound healing, and deep infection, which frequently requires removal of the prosthesis and arthrodesis of the knee joint.

Pain relief is achieved in 80–90% of patients, and a mild to moderate increase in a range of motion of the knee can be expected. Patients must be motivated to participate in a vigorous rehabilitation program for maximum results.

If osteoarthritis involves one compartment of the joint only, unicompartmental replacement has been successful in elderly patients. In young active patients who have varus deformity of less than 10 degrees, no subluxation, and flexion of 80 degrees or more, high tibial osteotomy to correct varus deformity is advocated.

Figure 43–31. ***A–B:*** Patient with rheumatoid arthritis and severe joint destruction of the right knee. ***C–D:*** Patient was treated with a cemented right total knee replacement.

Cates HE et al: Intramedullary versus extramedullary femoral alignment systems in total knee replacement. Clin Orthop 1993; (286):32.

Edgerton BC, Mariani EM, Morrey BF: Distal femoral varus osteotomy for painful genu valgum: a five-to-11-year follow-up study. Clin Orthop 1993;(288):263.

Skinner HB: Pathokinesiology and total joint arthroplasty. Clin Orthop 1993;(288):78.

Whiteside LA: Correction of ligament and bone defects in total arthroplasty of the severely valgus knee. Clin Orthop 1993; (288):234.

FRACTURE OF THE SHAFTS OF THE TIBIA & FIBULA

Fracture of the shaft of the tibia or fibula (Figure 43–32) may occur at any age but is most common during adolescence and active adulthood. Fractures of the tibial shaft have the highest rate of nonunion of all long bone fractures and, in cases of open tibia fracture, the highest rate of infection. Injury mechanisms range from low-energy rotational injuries to violent, high-energy injuries such as those associated with motorcycle accidents. These are clearly different injuries with different types and incidences of complications, different rates of healing and in many cases very different goals of treatment.

Clinical Findings

A. Symptoms and Signs

Patients present with pain, swelling, and inability to bear full weight on the affected limb. The fracture will be tender to palpation, and crepitation may be present. The injury mechanism should be carefully documented. The condition of the soft tissue envelope surrounding the fibula and especially the almost entirely

Figure 43–32. ***A:*** and ***B:*** Anteroposterior and lateral radiographs of a displaced midshaft tibia fracture.

subcutaneous tibia should be carefully inspected. Any open wounds should be measured, cleaned of any gross contamination, and covered with a sterile saline-soaked gauze dressing. Gross malalignment should be corrected without delay and the limb splinted. As with all long bone fractures, an examination of the joints above and below the fracture (knee and ankle) must be performed.

B. IMAGING STUDIES

X-rays in the anteroposterior and lateral projection of the entire lower leg, including both the knee and ankle joints, are always necessary, and oblique projections are often desirable. The surgeon must know the exact site, configuration, and direction of displacement of the fragments. Inadequate x-ray examination can lead to incomplete diagnosis.

1. Fracture of the Shaft of the Fibula

Isolated fracture of the shaft of the fibula is uncommon though it can occur with a direct blow to the side of the lower leg. Particular attention should be given to clinical and radiographic examination of the ankle and knee to rule out ligamentous or other subtle bony injuries. If no other injury is present, immobilization is for comfort only. Three weeks or a month in a walking cast or

removable cast boot is usually sufficient, and complete healing can be expected.

2. Fracture of the Shaft of the Tibia

Isolated fractures of the shaft of the tibia are not common and tend to be caused by indirect injury such as a torsional movement and can be recognized by the spiral fracture pattern produced. These low-energy injuries tend to be relatively stable because the periosteum around the tibia is typically intact and the fibula provides additional support.

The goal of treatment is to obtain fracture healing with less than 5 degrees of angulation in the coronal plane and 10 degrees of angulation in the sagittal plane. Closed reduction may be needed in cases exceeding these limits. Typically, isolated fractures of the tibia heal well with plaster cast or similar immobilization but may take up to 5 months before clinical and radiographic union is complete. Frequent radiographic follow-up is required during the early stages of fracture consolidation because the intact fibula can cause secondary varus angulation of the tibia. Operation is indicated if acceptable angulation cannot be achieved through closed reduction or if an acceptable reduction is lost during cast treatment.

3. Fracture of the Shafts of Both Bones in Adults

Simultaneous fractures of the shafts of the tibia and fibula are almost always unstable moderate-energy to high-energy injuries that tend to displace despite reduction. Treatment remains controversial though there is increasing support in the orthopedic literature for some form of surgical treatment for all displaced fractures of the tibia and fibula. However, many orthopedists still feel that an attempt at closed reduction and cast or fracture brace treatment should be considered in certain circumstances.

Absolute indications for surgical treatment include open fractures, fractures with associated nerve or vascular injury, and fractures with associated compartment syndrome. Relative indications for surgical treatment include multiply injured patients, head-injured patients, and patients with compromised soft tissue around the fracture site.

Closed treatment can be considered in those patients without the indications for open treatment listed above. The single most important determinant of fracture healing in an acceptable position is the position of the fracture at the time of presentation—ie, the more displaced or angulated a fracture is at presentation, the more likely it is that displacement or angulation will occur in the cast. Other factors increasing risk of displacement in the cast include high-energy injuries, comminuted and segmental fractures, and fracture patterns in which the fractures of the tibia and fibula are at the same level. If an acceptable position can be obtained, casting initially should be with a long-leg cast. Extreme vigilance on the part of the practitioner and the patient for signs of developing compartment syndrome in the cast is critically important for the first 4-5 days. Frequent radiographs are needed to verify that the fracture position remains acceptable in the cast. Six weeks in a long-leg cast is usually sufficient to allow conversion to a short leg cast or fracture brace and at least some protected weightbearing. Some form of external support is typically needed for 4–6 months until fracture healing is complete.

If surgical treatment is indicated—either because closed treatment failed or because indications for acute open treatment are present—treatment can be with intramedullary rodding, external fixation, or open reduction and internal fixation. The majority of tibia fractures are now treated with intramedullary fixation because this form of treatment allows early functional rehabilitation of the knee and ankle, permits early weightbearing, and imposes the lowest risk of infection and soft tissue complications.

Bone LB et al: Displaced isolated tibial shaft fractures treated with either cast or intramedullary nailing. J Bone Joint Surg Am 1997;79:1336.

Brumback RJ: Open tibial fractures: current orthopaedic management. Instr Course Lect 1992;41:101.

Dagher F, Roukoz S: Compound tibial fractures with bone loss treated by the Ilizarov technique. J Bone Joint Surg Br 1991; 73:316.

Garcia-Cimbrelo E et al: Ilizarov technique: results and difficulties. Clin Orthop 1992;(283):116.

Piecioni L, Guanche CA: Clinical experience with unreamed locked nails for open tibial fractures. Orthop Rev 1992;21:1213.

Siebenrock KA, Schillig B, Jakob RP: Treatment of complex tibial shaft fractures: arguments for early secondary intramedullary nailing. Clin Orthop 1993;(290):269.

Wiss DA, Johnson DL, Miao M: Compression plating for nonunion after failed external fixation of open tibial fractures. J Bone Joint Surg Am 1992;74:1279.

ACUTE COMPARTMENT SYNDROME

Compartment syndrome is caused by increased pressure in a closed fascial space, compromising perfusion of nerves and muscles. The fascial compartments of the lower leg and forearm are most commonly involved. The syndrome can be caused by a fracture with subsequent hemorrhage and edema in the compartment, limb compression or crush, vigorous exercise, burns, or any other pathogenic factor that increases intra-compartmental pressures. While a large variety of inciting mechanisms exist, the essential feature of compartment syndrome is increased intracompartmental pressure leading to tissue ischemia. Severe ischemia for 6–8 hours or more leads to muscle and nerve death.

The late signs of arterial insufficiency are pain, pallor, paresthesias, paralysis, and pulselessness. However, these are usually late findings, and if nerve and muscle ischemia has been present long enough to result in paralysis and paresthesias, tissue damage has probably already occurred. Furthermore, compartment syndrome can occur at intracompartmental pressures well below arterial pressure, and compartment syndrome can therefore exist in a pink limb with normal pulses.

Clinical findings include swelling and palpable tenseness over a muscle compartment. Paresthesias, pallor, pulselessness, and paralysis should be sought and documented. However, the two most reliable early indicators of compartment syndrome are pain out of proportion to what is expected for a given injury and pain with passive stretch of the muscles in the compartment suspected of having compartment syndrome. Suspicion is perhaps the physician's best aid in diagnosis of this problem.

If compartment syndrome cannot be diagnosed clinically, intracompartmental pressure must be measured directly. This is performed by inserting a large-bore catheter into the compartment using sterile technique. The catheter is then connected to a pressure monitor via intravenous tubing filled with sterile saline solution. Another option is a self-contained compartment pressure measuring system which is now commercially available. Compartments with pressures above 30–40 mm Hg or within 30 mm Hg of the diastolic pressure should be considered for fasciotomy.

Fasciotomy should be performed with complete release of the skin and fascia of the involved compartments. Compartment pressures are rechecked after fasciotomy to make certain that decompression has been achieved. The wounds are usually left open and covered with sterile dressings and are then treated days later by delayed primary closure or skin grafting.

Cameron SE: Acute compartment syndrome of the triceps: a case report. Acta Orthop Scand 1993;64:107.

Fakhouri AJ, Manoli A 2d: Acute foot compartment syndromes. J Orthop Trauma 1992;6:223.

McQueen MM, Court-Brown CM: Compartment monitoring in tibial fractures: the threshold for decompression. J Bone Joint Surg Br 1996:76: 99.

INJURIES OF THE ANKLE REGION

1. Ankle Sprain

Ankle sprain is most often caused by forced inversion of the foot, as may occur in stumbling on uneven ground. Pain is usually maximal over the anterolateral aspect of the joint; greater tenderness is apt to be found in the region of the anterior talofibular and talocalcaneal ligaments. Eversion sprain is less common; maximal tenderness and swelling are usually found over the deltoid ligament.

Sprain is differentiated from major partial or complete ligamentous tears by anteroposterior, lateral, and 30-degree internal oblique (mortise view) x-ray projections; if the joint cleft between either malleolus and the talus is greater than 4 mm, major ligamentous tear is probable. Occult lesions can be demonstrated by x-ray examination under inversion or eversion stress after infiltration of the area of maximal swelling and tenderness with 5 mL of 1% lidocaine.

If swelling is marked, elevation of the extremity and avoidance of weightbearing for a few days are advisable. The ankle can be supported with Gibney strapping, air cushion splints, or a cast for 2–3 weeks to relieve pain and swelling. Further treatment may be by warm foot baths and elastic bandages. Treatment should be continued until muscle strength and full joint motion are recovered. Tears of major ligaments of the ankle joint are discussed below.

Nyska M et al: Radiological assessment of a modified anterior drawer test of the ankle. Foot Ankle 1992;13:400.

Raatikainen T, Putkonen M, Puranen J: Arthrography, clinical examination, and stress radiograph in the diagnosis of acute injury to the lateral ligaments of the ankle. Am J Sports Med 1992;20:2.

2. Fractures of the Ankle Joint

Ankle trauma accounts for between 3% and 12% of all emergency room visits. The frequency and severity of ankle fractures has been increasing as our population ages yet remains active. In fact, ankle and foot fractures are among the most common fractures among elderly women. Obesity, intoxication, and high-heeled or platform shoes are also risk factors for ankle fracture. Motor vehicle accidents remain a common cause of high-energy injuries despite the development of secondary restraint systems such as airbags, which appear to provide little protection for foot and ankle injuries.

Although most patients who present to the emergency room with ankle pain will have radiographs taken, only 7–36% will have fractures. In an effort to reduce the number of unnecessary radiographs, the Ottawa clinical decision rule was developed to guide physicians in their use of radiographs in ankle and foot injuries. This rule states that radiographs need be obtained only if patients have pain near the malleoli and one of the following: (1) age over 54, (2) inability of bear weight immediately after the injury and for four steps in the emergency room, and (3) bony tenderness at the posterior edge or tip of either malleolus. The rule does not apply for patients with obvious ankle deformities or for patients who are obtunded or have impaired ability to communicate. The overall sensitivity of the Ottawa scale for predicting ankle fracture ranges from 93% to 100%. However, it should not replace sound clinical judgment when considering ordering radiographs.

Clinical examination will reveal swelling and point tenderness over damaged ligaments or fractured bones. The examining physician should palpate both tibia and fibula up to the knee as some ankle fracture patterns propagate the skeletal or soft tissue injury well up the lower leg. The skin should be carefully inspected for wounds which may communicate with the bone. A neurologic examination should also be performed. Radiographic examination should consist of a lateral and mortise view of the ankle. The standard anteroposterior view has been shown to add very little to the diagnostic work up. The mortise view is obtained by obtaining an anteroposterior view of the ankle with the leg internal rotated 20 degrees. This view, when obtained correctly in a non-injured ankle, should show an equal "clear space" between the talar dome and its articulations with the distal tibia, the medial malleolus, and the lateral malleolus.

Fracture of the Medial Malleolus

Fracture of the medial malleolus may occur as an isolated lesion of any part of the malleolus (including the tip) or may be associated with (1) fracture of the lateral malleolus, with medial or lateral dislocation of the talus; and (2) dislocation of the inferior tibiofibular joint, with or without fracture of the fibula. An isolated fracture of the medial malleolus does not usually cause instability of the ankle joint.

Undisplaced isolated fractures of the medial malleolus should be treated by immobilization in a short leg cast with the ankle flexed to a right angle and the foot slightly inverted to decrease tension on the deltoid ligament. Immobilization without weightbearing should be continued for 6–8 weeks or until bone healing is demonstrated bother clinically and radiographically. The rate of nonunion in isolated medial malleolus fractures treated nonoperatively has been reported to be as high as 20%.

Displaced isolated fracture of the medial malleolus can be treated by closed manipulation under general or local anesthesia. The essential maneuver consists of anatomic realignment by digital pressure over the distal fragment followed by immobilization in a plaster cast (as for undisplaced fracture) until bone healing occurs. If anatomic reduction cannot be achieved by closed methods, open reduction and internal fixation with one or two screws is required.

Fracture of the Lateral Malleolus & Combined Injury Patterns

A fracture of the lateral malleolus may occur as an isolated lesion or may be associated with a fracture of the medial malleolus, a tear of the deltoid ligament, or disruption of the syndesmotic ligaments between the distal tibia and fibula. If the structures on the medial side of the ankle (either bony or ligamentous) are injured, lateral subluxation or instability of the talus may be present.

When a lateral malleolus fracture is noted, particular care should be directed toward the physical and radiographic finding on the medial side of the ankle. Medial tenderness without a medial malleolus fracture suggests deltoid ligament injury. Medial clear space widening of more than 4 mm on the mortise view confirms deltoid or syndesmosis ligament disruption. In these cases, anatomic reduction may not be achievable or maintainable with closed manipulation and casting.

Isolated stable fractures of the lateral malleolus can be treated with a short leg cast. Weekly radiographs are obtained in the cast to verify that an acceptable position has been maintained. Casting normally needs to be continued for 4–6 weeks until fracture healing is sufficient to allow some weightbearing in a removable over-the-counter cast boot. Long-term results of this type of treatment have been shown to be quite satisfactory.

The vast majority of fractures that involve both malleoli or that consist of a lateral malleolar injury in conjunction with a deltoid or syndesmotic ligamentous disruption will require open reduction and internal fixation to achieve anatomic reduction. In addition to the benefit afforded by anatomic reduction, open reduction with internal fixation typically allows the patient to begin weightbearing and physical therapy much sooner than is possible with closed reduction and casting.

Fractures of the Distal Tibia

Perhaps no other fracture in orthopedics offers such an astounding variety of injury mechanisms, fracture patterns, and treatment pitfalls as a distal tibia fracture (Figure 43–33). These injuries may consist of everything from very low energy avulsion fractures of the posterior or anterior distal tibial rim to high-energy fractures in which the distal tibia disintegrates within—and often through—the meager envelope of soft tissue surrounding it. Treatment is guided by the mechanism of injury, the fracture configuration, and, most importantly, the condition of the surrounding soft tissues.

Bonar SK, Marsh JL: Unilateral external fixation for severe pilon fractures. Foot Ankle 1993;14:57.

McFerran MA et al: Complications encountered in the treatment of pilon fractures. J Orthop Trauma 1992;6:195.

3. Dislocation of the Ankle Joint

Complete dislocation of the ankle joint is rare because the talus cannot be completely dislocated from the joint unless all ligaments are torn. Major ligamentous injuries in the region of the ankle joint with incomplete dislocations are usually associated with fracture.

Tear of the Deltoid Ligament

Complete tear of the talotibial portion of the deltoid ligament can permit interposition of the posterior tibial tendon between the medial malleolus and the talus. Associated injury is usually present, especially fracture of the lateral malleolus with lateral dislocation of the talus.

Pain, tenderness, swelling, and ecchymosis in the region of the medial malleolus without fracture suggest partial or complete tear of the deltoid ligament. If fracture of the lateral malleolus or dislocation of the distal tibiofibular joint is present, the cleft between the malleolus and the talus is likely to be widened. If significant widening is not apparent, x-ray examination under stress is necessary.

Interposition of the deltoid ligament between the talus and the medial malleolus often cannot be corrected by closed manipulation. If widening persists after closed manipulation, surgical exploration is indicated

Figure 43–33. Axial loading injury to the ankle joint with the foot in dorsiflexion leading to a fracture of the tibial plafond. Anteroposterior **(A)** and lateral **(B)** radiographs.

so that the ligament can be removed and repaired by suture.

Associated fracture of the fibula can be treated by fixation with a plate and screws to ensure maintenance of anatomic reduction.

Tear of the Talofibular Ligament

Isolated tear of the anterior talofibular ligament is caused by forced inversion of the foot. X-ray examination under stress may be necessary, using local or general anesthesia. Both feet are forcibly inverted and internally rotated about 20 degrees while an anteroposterior film is exposed. If the tear is complete, the talus will be seen to be axially displaced from the tibial articular surface (talar tilt). Up to 25 degrees of talar tilt has been reported in normal ankles without a history of injury.

Rupture of the anterior talofibular ligaments may be associated with tear of the calcaneofibular ligament. Tear of both ligaments may be associated with fracture of the medial malleolus and medial dislocation of the talus.

Instability of the ankle joint, characterized by a history of recurrent sprains, may result from unrecognized tears of the anterior talofibular ligament.

Recent isolated tear of the anterior talofibular ligament or combined tear of the calcaneofibular ligament should be treated by immobilization for 4 weeks in a plaster boot. Associated fracture of the medial malleolus

creates an unstable mechanism. Unless anatomic reduction can be achieved and maintained by closed methods, open reduction of the malleolar fragment is indicated—followed by internal fixation of the fracture and repair of the ligamentous injury.

Toohey JS, Worsing RA: A long-term follow-up study of tibiotalar dislocations without associated fractures. Clin Orthop 1989; (239):207.

INJURIES OF THE FOOT

1. The Talus

Dislocation of the Subtalar & Talonavicular Joints

Dislocation of the subtalar and talonavicular joints without fracture occasionally occurs. Displacement of the foot can be by either inversion, in which case the calcaneus dislocates medially, or eversion, in which the calcaneus dislocates laterally. Inversion injuries are classically low-energy injuries and are frequently seen in situations in which a simple ankle sprain was initially suspected. Eversion injuries are classically high-energy injuries. Fortunately, both dislocation patterns are typically easy to reduce in the emergency room though occasionally incarceration of structures—eg, the posterior tibial tendon trapped in the talonavicular joint—can block reduction. After reduction, the extremity should be immobilized in a cast for 3 weeks.

Fracture of the Talus

The talus is composed of the body, neck, and head. More than 60% of the talus is covered by articular cartilage. Three principal arteries that form an anastomotic ring around the neck of the talus provide the blood supply to the entire talus, including the body through retrograde flow. This blood supply, while robust, can be compromised by any fractures of the neck or dislocation of the body. Though rare, fractures of the talus present dual treatment challenges—to restore anatomic alignment in a bone with seven distinct articular surfaces while preserving the tenuous blood supply.

Fracture of the Talar Neck

Talar neck fractures comprise over 50% of talus fractures and are thought to occur by forced dorsiflexion of the forefoot with axial loading. These are usually high-energy injuries, often seen in the brake foot of a driver involved in a high-speed motor vehicle accident. The injury begins as a simple talar neck fracture, but additional energy can propagate the injury to include dislocation of the subtalar, ankle, or talonavicular joints. Surprisingly, neurovascular compromise is rare. Open fractures are common, occurring in up to 25% of talus fractures, and have very high infection rates (38%) despite aggressive management.

An absolutely undisplaced fracture of the neck can be treated adequately with a nonweightbearing cast for 8–12 weeks. Any displacement of the talar neck is an orthopedic emergency and requires immediate operation to restore the alignment and—to the extent possible—minimize any compromise in talar perfusion.

Fractures of the Talar Body & Head

Fractures of the body and head of the talus are rarely isolated injuries and are frequently associated with other injuries of the talus, calcaneus, or subtalar joint. Treatment is directed toward restoring anatomic alignment of articular surfaces. For fractures that are truly nondisplaced, cast immobilization and avoidance of weightbearing is acceptable treatment. Any measurable displacement requires operative treatment. Displaced talar body fractures have a high rate of avascular necrosis despite operative management.

Fractures of the Lateral Process of the Talus

This injury—now called "the snowboarder's fracture" because of its frequent association with that recreational activity—deserves separate mention only because of the frequency with which the diagnosis is initially missed. The mechanism of injury is thought to be forced inversion under axial loading. The physical finding is lateral ankle pain and swelling, often very difficult to differentiate from an ankle sprain. However, careful palpation may show the exact site of maximal tenderness to be slightly more distal and anterior to the tip of the lateral malleolus than a typical ankle sprain. Plain radiographs often miss this fracture. CT scan should be obtained if the diagnosis is uncertain. Early treatment gives the best result, with undisplaced fractures treated with a nonweightbearing cast for 4–6 weeks. Displaced fractures require open reduction.

2. The Calcaneus

Fracture of the Calcaneus

The most common mechanism of injury for calcaneus fracture (Figure 43–34) is a fall from a height. Patients with calcaneus fractures frequently have other associated injuries, including fractures of the spine at the thoracolumbar junction. Comminution and impaction are general characteristics. While various classifications have been advocated, the key distinction that must be made is whether the fracture disrupts the subtalar and calcaneocuboid articulations. In general, fractures asso-

Figure 43–34. Axial CT section showing a fracture of the calcaneus caused by an axial loading mechanism.

ciated with involvement and displacement of the articular surfaces are candidates for some type of surgical reduction. High-energy, comminuted, and open fractures of the calcaneus continue to have high rates of subtalar arthrosis despite more aggressive surgical management.

Fracture of the Calcaneal Tuberosity

Isolated fractures of the tuberosity are not common. They may occur in a horizontal or vertical direction. A horizontal fracture may be limited to the superior portion of the region of the former apophysis and represents an avulsion by the Achilles tendon. When the superior fragment is widely displaced proximally with the tendon, open reduction and fixation may be necessary to obtain the best functional result. Further extension of the fracture cleft toward the subtalar joint in the substance of the tuberosity creates a so-called beak fracture. The fragment may be displaced proximally by the action of the Achilles tendon. If displacement is significant, open reduction is advised.

Vertical fracture occurs near the sagittal plane somewhat medially through the tuberosity. Because the medial fragment normally is not widely displaced, immobilization is not required but will reduce pain.

Fracture of the Anterior Process of the Calcaneus

Fracture of the anterior process of the calcaneus is caused by forced inversion of the foot. It must be differentiated from midtarsal and ankle joint sprains. The firmly attached bifurcated ligament (calcaneonavicular and calcaneocuboid components) avulses its bony attachment on the calcaneus. Maximal tenderness occurs midway between the tip of the lateral malleolus and the base of the fifth metatarsal. The lateral x-ray view projected obliquely demonstrates the fracture cleft. Treatment is with a nonweightbearing cast with the foot in neutral position for 4 weeks.

Fracture of the Body of the Calcaneus

A. NONARTICULAR FRACTURE

Where fracture of the body occurs posterior to the articular surface, the direction of displacement of the tuberosity fragment is proximal. Since the subtalar joint is not disrupted, symptomatic posttraumatic degenerative arthritis is rare though some joint stiffness may persist permanently. Marked displacement can usually be corrected with percutaneous manipulation and pinning.

B. ARTICULAR FRACTURE

The management of intra-articular fractures continues to be controversial. The need for surgery or for closed reduction and the methods used with either approach have all been occasions for debate. The inability to consistently demonstrate superior outcomes after operation reflects this controversy.

Closed treatment continues to be favored by many surgeons. When closed treatment is selected, early range of motion is important to preserve as much ankle, subtalar, and calcaneocuboid motion as possible. A number of studies have shown inferior outcomes in fractures with displaced articular fragments owing to the inability to elevate these fragments with closed techniques.

A better understanding of the biomechanical consequences of articular incongruence is driving an increasing trend for operative management of these fractures. The goals of operation are to restore the calcaneal width and height and restore the articular surface congruence.

Persistent and disabling pain originating in the deranged subtalar joint may require subtalar arthrodesis for adequate relief. Concomitant involvement of the calcaneocuboid joint is an indication for the more extensive triple arthrodesis.

3. The Navicular

Minor avulsion fractures of the tarsal navicular may occur as a feature of severe midtarsal sprain and require neither reduction nor specific treatment. Avulsion fracture of the tuberosity near the insertion of the posterior tibialis muscle is uncommon and must be differentiated from a persistent ununited apophysis and from the supernumerary sesamoid bone, or os tibiale externum.

In general, the fracture occurs either through the middle of the navicular in a horizontal or, less commonly, in a vertical plane. Only noncomminuted fractures with displacement of the dorsal fragment can be satisfactorily reduced. Closed manipulation by strong traction on the forefoot and simultaneous digital pressure over the displaced fragment can restore it to its normal position. If the reduction is not stable, fixation with a percutaneously placed Kirschner wire or interfragmentary screw is needed. Fractures in which acceptable reduction cannot be achieved by closed means should undergo open reduction and fixation. Nonweightbearing immobilization in a plaster cast is required for a minimum of 6 weeks.

4. The Cuneiform & Cuboid

Because of their relatively protected position in the mid tarsus, isolated fractures of the cuboid and cuneiform bones are rarely encountered. Minor avulsion fractures occur as a component of severe midtarsal sprains. Extensive fracture usually occurs in association with other injuries of the foot and often is caused by severe crushing. The most important fracture is the "nutcracker" fracture, which is a compression injury of the lateral column. When more than 2–3 mm of cuboid shortening is present, lateral column lengthening and bone grafting are indicated.

5. Midtarsal Dislocations

Midtarsal dislocation through the cuneonavicular and calcaneocuboid joints or more proximally through the talocalcaneonavicular and calcaneocuboid joints may occur as a result of twisting injury to the forefoot. Fractures of adjacent bones are frequently present as well. When treatment is given soon after the accident, closed reduction by traction on the forefoot and manipulation is generally effective. If reduction is unstable and displacement recurs upon release of traction, stabilization for 4 weeks by percutaneously inserted Kirschner wires is recommended.

6. Fractures & Dislocations of the Metatarsals

Fractures of the metatarsals and tarsometatarsal dislocations are typically caused by a direct crush or indirect twisting injury of the forefoot.

Tarsometatarsal Dislocations

Dislocations of the tarsometatarsal (Lisfranc) joints may present as subtle midfoot sprains or obvious open fracture dislocations. The most common mechanism of injury is axial loading on a hyperplantarflexed midfoot. Midfoot swelling and pain with transverse midfoot compression are hallmarks of these injuries. Anteroposterior, lateral, and oblique radiographs should be obtained, preferably with weightbearing if tolerated by the patient. Careful review of the radiographs will reveal malalignment between the medial border of the second metatarsal and the medial cuneiform and the medial border of the fourth metatarsal and the medial border of the cuboid. CT scan is very sensitive for detecting subtle displacement of this three-dimensional joint.

The goal of treatment is to obtain and maintain anatomic reduction because long-term outcome has been found to correlate best with the quality of the reduction. For widely displaced dislocations, attempted closed reduction should not be deferred. Closed reduction and percutaneous pinning are recommended if perfect reduction can be achieved. The difficulty in achieving anatomic reduction—and particularly in verifying it—have led most authors to recommend open reduction when treating tarsometatarsal fracture-dislocations.

Fracture of the Metatarsal Shafts

Undisplaced fractures of the metatarsal shafts cause no permanent disability unless they fail to heal. Displacement is rarely significant in those fracture patterns in which the middle metatarsals are fractured but the first and fifth are uninjured because the peripheral metatarsals act as in situ splints.

Care should be taken to correct angular malposition in the longitudinal axis of the shaft. Untreated apex dorsal angulation causes plantar prominence of the head of the involved metatarsal, which can cause concentrated local plantar pressure and lead to painful callosities or even full-thickness pressure-induced ulceration. Every effort should be made to correct convex dorsal angulation by distraction of impacted fragments and appropriate manipulation. Closed reduction is best achieved by use of the Chinese fingertrap applied to the toes of the involved metatarsals. If closed reduction is not successful, open reduction with Kirschner wire fixation should be performed. If correction after closed manipulation is acceptable, a plaster cast should be well molded to the plantar aspect of the foot to minimize recurrence of deformity and to support the longitudinal and transverse arches.

Fatigue Fracture of the Metatarsal Shafts

Fatigue fracture of the shafts of the metatarsals has been given various names (eg, march, stress, and insufficiency fracture). Its protean clinical manifestations cause difficulty in precise recognition—even to the point of confusion with osteogenic sarcoma. It commonly occurs in active young adults—such as military recruits—who are unaccustomed to vigorous and excessive walking. A history of a single significant injury is lacking. Incipient pain of varying intensity in the forefoot that is accentuated by walking, swelling, and localized tenderness of the involved metatarsal are cardinal manifestations. Depending upon the stage of development of the injury, x-rays may not demonstrate fracture, and extracortical callus formation may ultimately be the only clue. More striking findings may vary from an incomplete fissure to an evident transverse cleft. Persistent unprotected weightbearing may cause arrest of bone healing and even displacement of the distal fragment. The second and third metatarsals are most frequently involved near the junction of the middle and distal thirds. The lesion can occur more proximally and in other lesser metatarsals. Since weightbearing is likely to prolong and aggravate symptoms, treatment is by protection in either a walking cast or removable cast boot. Weightbearing should be restricted until pain subsides and bone continuity has been restored radiographically.

Fracture of the Tuberosity of the Fifth Metatarsal

Forced adduction of the forefoot may cause avulsion fracture of the tuberosity of the fifth metatarsal. If displacement of the fragment is minimal, adhesive strapping or a stiff-soled shoe is adequate treatment. If displacement is greater than 3–4 mm, treatment should consist of a walking boot until bone healing occurs. Nonunion is rare, but the time to radiographic union can often lag well behind clinical fracture healing.

7. Fractures & Dislocations of the Phalanges of the Toes

Fractures of the phalanges of the toes are caused most commonly by direct injury such as crushing or stubbing.

Comminuted fractures of the proximal phalanx of the great toe, alone or in combination with fracture of the distal phalanx, is the most disabling injury. Since wide displacement of fragments is not likely, correction of angulation and support with an adhesive dressing and splint usually suffices. A weightbearing plaster cast may be useful for relief of symptoms arising from associated soft tissue injury. Spiral or oblique fracture of the proximal phalanges of the lesser toes can be treated adequately by binding the involved toe to an adjacent uninjured toe. Comminuted fracture of the distal phalanx is treated as a soft tissue injury.

Traumatic dislocation of the metatarsophalangeal joints and the uncommon dislocation of the proximal interphalangeal joint usually can be reduced by closed manipulation. These dislocations are rarely isolated and usually occur in combination with other injuries to the forefoot.

8. Fracture of the Sesamoids of the Great Toe

Fracture of the sesamoid bones of the great toe is rare, but it may occur as a result of a crushing injury. It must be differentiated from a bipartite sesamoid. Undisplaced fracture requires no treatment other than a foot support or a metatarsal bar. Displaced fracture may require immobilization in a walking plaster cast, with the toe strapped in flexion.

FRACTURES THAT FAIL TO UNITE

Delayed fracture healing and nonunion are most common in long bone fractures associated with severe soft tissue damage or infection. However, closed fractures with minimal displacement occasionally fail to unite for reasons that remain obscure. The long bone with the

highest risk of nonunion is the tibia. Nonunions of the carpal scaphoid and the femoral neck are not uncommon and are thought to be associated with damage to the blood supply of the fractured area at the time of injury.

Differentiating a slowly healing fracture (delayed union) from a fracture which is never going to heal (nonunion) remains a clinical challenge. Most orthopedic traumatologists reserve the term nonunion for a fracture that is not healed within the average time for a typical fracture in that location to heal and, more importantly, has lost the ability to heal without some type of operative treatment. The treatment of nonunions is based on several factors, including the biology of the fracture, the mechanics of the fracture, the anatomy of the fracture, the patient, and the presence or absence of infection. In general, hypertrophic nonunions that are not infected can be treated successfully with some type of orthopedic construct, whether internal or external, to increase fracture stability. Uninfected atrophic nonunions result from poor healing potential due to absence of necessary biologic factors and require some type of bone grafting procedure to bring new healing potential to the fracture site. Infected nonunions require simultaneous treatment of the fracture and infection because eradication of infection is nearly impossible in the setting of an unstable fracture.

Burdeaux BD Jr: The medical approach for calcaneal fractures. Clin Orthop 1993;(290):96.

Cameron HU et al: Repair of nonunion of tibial osteotomy. Clin Orthop 1993;(287):167.

Marsh JL et al: Major open injuries of the talus. J Orthop Trauma 1995;9:371.

McCrory P et al: "Snowboarder's fracture": fracture of the lateral process of the talus. J Am Board Fam Pract 1994;7:130.

Stephenson JR: Surgical treatment of displaced intraarticular fractures of the calcaneus: a combined lateral and medial approach. Clin Orthop 1993;(290):68.

Swanson TV, Bray TJ, Holmes GB Jr: Fractures of the talar neck: a mechanical study of fixation. J Bone Joint Surg Am 1992; 74:544.

Mody BS et al: Nonunion of fractures of the scaphoid tuberosity. J Bone Joint Surg Br 1993;75:423.

■ PEDIATRIC ORTHOPEDICS

CHILDREN'S FRACTURES & DISLOCATIONS

Children are not "small adults," and their skeletal injuries are different from those of adults in several significant ways. The most striking characteristic of immature bone is its potential for growth. Longitudinal growth occurs at the physis, or cartilaginous growth plate. Bones increase in diameter by appositional growth from the periosteum. Injuries can affect normal growth, usually by impeding it. However, growth may be accelerated, especially by femoral shaft fractures in mid childhood. Growth may help correct deformity of some but not all children's fractures. Such correction is greatest in young children with a lot of growing yet to be achieved. Growth tends to correct angulation in the plane of motion of an adjacent joint but improves varus or valgus deformities only in the very young and does not correct rotational malalignment. Children's bones heal rapidly, and nonunion is exceedingly rare. A child's periosteum is thick and strong. It surrounds a long bone like a sleeve and must be torn to permit displacement of a fracture. Usually the displaced fracture end protrudes through a rent in the periosteum, but the remaining intact portion of the sleeve bridges the fracture area to facilitate reduction and maintenance of alignment.

Any injury in a young child, especially one under 3 years of age, must be considered a sign of possible battered child syndrome (see Chapter 46). State law in all jurisdictions requires that suspected cases be reported to local authorities. Good patient care requires thorough pediatric and social service assessments.

Closed treatment is usually sufficient for children's fractures. Manipulative reduction under general anesthesia may be required for significant displacement. Open fractures, epiphysial fractures with articular surface displacement, and the very rare fracture that cannot be reduced satisfactorily by closed manipulation are the generally accepted indications for open treatment of fractures in children.

Although children's fractures do heal rapidly and pain soon ceases to interfere with function, it is important to recognize that callus bridging a fracture may deform plastically and angulate if the fracture is loaded too early. Immobilization rarely causes joint stiffness in children, so that casts can and should be left on until union is secure.

Because bone in children is mechanically different from that in adults, there are several unique fracture types in this age group. Immature bone is more porous and fails in compression as well as in tension. The result is the so-called buckle or torus fracture that occurs near the metaphysis. The distal forearm provides a typical example. This stable injury should be protected in plaster for 3 weeks to control symptoms and prevent further trauma to the weakened bone.

Immature bone is less brittle than that of adults, and children's bones may therefore bend significantly rather than fracture. Two potential injury patterns result. The first is traumatic bowing, in which the shaft of a bone is bent. Bowing may produce significant deformity—eg, bowing of the ulna may prevent reduction of an associated displaced fracture of the radius. Depending upon the age of the child, some correction of the deformity can occur, but osteotomy may be required for severe traumatic bowing.

Greenstick fracture, the second fracture type related to the plasticity of children's bones, incompletely disrupts a long bone, so that the bone fractures partially on the tension side but maintains continuity of a portion of the opposite cortex. The periosteum also remains intact on the concave side. Depending upon how much it has been bent, the intact cortex promotes persisting angulation. This can be prevented by briskly overcorrecting the deformity, thereby completing the fracture. The remaining periosteum prevents actual reversal of the deformity and facilitates maintenance of reduction. If angulation of a greenstick fracture exceeds 15 degrees, reduction should be carried out as described. Following reduction—or without it if angulation is minimal—the fracture is immobilized in a long plaster cast with three-point molding to keep tension on the intact periosteal hinge during healing.

1. Growth Plate Fractures (Epiphysial Fractures, Epiphysial Separations)

About 15% of children's fractures involve a growth plate—most commonly the distal radius, distal tibia or fibula (or both), and distal humerus.

Classification

Classification of physial injuries helps to distinguish patterns that may disturb growth and also provides some guidance for treatment. However, it should be recognized that even "benign" injuries of the distal femoral and tibial growth plates can have clinically significant consequences. Naturally, injuries to nearly mature physes have little effect on growth no matter what their type or location.

Physial injuries are classified according to the Salter and Harris system (Figure 43–35). A given injury may have different degrees of severity. For example, an apparent Salter-Harris type II fracture may have sustained sufficient compression adjacent to the metaphysial fragment so that a localized area of type V injury is present, with attendant growth abnormality.

A. Type I

Type I injuries have fracture lines that follow the growth plate, separating epiphysis from metaphysis. Unless the periosteum is torn, displacement cannot occur. Without displacement, radiographs appear nor-

Figure 43–35. Salter-Harris classification of physial injuries occurring at the zone of provisional calcification of the growth plate.

mal, and only tenderness localized over the physis instead of an adjacent collateral ligament confirms that a growth plate injury has occurred. Healing occurs rapidly, usually within 2–3 weeks. Complications are rare.

B. TYPE II

In type II injuries, the fracture line separates epiphysis from metaphysis much as in type I injuries but also enters the metaphysis, so that a flake of metaphysial bone is carried with the epiphysis. This finding is known as the Thurston-Holland sign and is diagnostic of a growth plate injury. Type II injuries are the commonest physial fractures. Gentle closed reduction should achieve satisfactory alignment. Healing is rapid, and growth is rarely disturbed. Type II injuries of the distal ends of the femur and the tibia may result in impaired growth that should be watched for.

C. TYPE III

Type III physial injuries are quite uncommon separations of a portion of the epiphysis along the physis, with the fracture line then passing through the epiphysis to the articular surface. This generally occurs when the growth plate is partially fused. Although growth disturbances are therefore rare, displacement of these injuries disturbs the joint surface and therefore may merit open reduction.

D. TYPE IV

Salter-Harris type IV fractures potentially interfere with normal growth. The fracture line crosses the physis, separating a peripheral fragment of bone that includes portions of epiphysis, physis, and metaphysis. Because it involves the articular surface, it may compromise normal joint mobility and long-term function. Anatomic reduction, maintained until healing, is essential to minimize the after-effects of type IV growth plate fractures. If they are displaced, open reduction and internal fixation are advisable. Very gentle technique is essential,

with avoidance of unnecessary periosteal elevation. Fixation is best obtained with fine smooth Kirschner wires that do not cross the physis or do so temporarily through its most central portion, since screw threads and even peripherally placed smooth wires can interfere with physial growth. Unless anatomic reduction is obtained, growth disturbance, nonunion, and joint incongruity are common complications. Even with perfect reduction, growth may be affected, and the prognosis is guarded. The commonest example of type IV injury is fracture of the lateral humeral condyle. If anatomic alignment is not maintained, the fractured lateral condyle fails to unite and makes no further contribution to elongation of the distal humerus. With relative overgrowth of the medial condyle, a progressive cubitus valgus deformity develops. As it becomes stretched around the medial epicondyle, the ulnar nerve develops a "tardy" palsy.

E. TYPE V

Type V growth plate injuries are due to severe axial loading. Some or all of the physis is so severely compressed that growth potential is destroyed. Since initial radiographs may appear normal, the history of a significant fall with swelling and tenderness over the physis should suggest the possibility of such an injury. Subsequent follow-up radiographs confirm it by demonstrating failure to grow, with premature closure of the physis, or progressive angular deformity from tethering of one side of the growth plate. The outlook for these rare injuries is poor. Progressive angulation can be stopped—if a third or less of the physis is involved—by resecting the bridging bone and filling the defect with autogenous fat or a Silastic spacer. This should allow normal growth to resume. An alternative, which stops growth, is to obliterate any remaining physial plate. Osteotomy may be required to correct significant angulation. Any resulting leg length inequality may require treatment.

Imaging Studies

Radiographs are essential but may be difficult to interpret. In addition to the usual anteroposterior and lateral views, oblique projections may be helpful to show displacement or a small Thurston-Holland fragment of metaphysis. Localized soft tissue swelling and signs of hemarthrosis should be heeded. Comparison views of the opposite normal limb may be helpful, especially if exactly symmetric projections are obtained. Epiphysial injuries that are undisplaced may be demonstrated by varus or valgus stress films, which are required for differentiating ligament disruptions from growth plate injuries in skeletally immature children.

Treatment

A. CONSERVATIVE TREATMENT

Most fractures involving the physis may be managed nonoperatively. Undisplaced injuries of any type should be protected in plaster casts until healed. A cast for 3–6 weeks is usually sufficient depending upon the child's age and the site and type of injury. Displaced type I and type II injuries should be treated by gentle closed reduction followed by immobilization as above. Acceptance of some deformity is better than repeated vigorous attempts to correct it, since these efforts involve a risk of additional damage to the physis.

B. OPERATIVE TREATMENT

Displaced type III and type IV injuries usually require open reduction and internal fixation. Type V injuries should be protected in a cast or splint, but the poor outcome of these fortunately rare injuries cannot be improved by any early treatment.

Prognosis

All injuries that involve physes should be followed long enough to confirm that normal growth has not been disrupted. This may require several years, especially if the child is growing slowly or if interference is slight. If the child sustains a type III or type IV injury or any injury of the distal femoral physis, the parents should be warned of the possibility of altered growth. Close follow-up observation is required after growth plate injuries to permit timely diagnosis and treatment of any resulting growth abnormality. Progressive angular deformity may result from an incomplete bony bridge crossing and tethering one side of the physis. Such bridges can be resected, with interposition of a free fat graft, to restore normal growth. A number of techniques are now available to correct limb length inequality due to complete growth arrest. Traditionally, the most frequent has been epiphysiodesis to stop growth of the contralateral limb. Lengthening techniques are being developed that often permit restoration of the short limb to its normal length.

2. Upper Extremity Fractures & Dislocations

Proximal Humeral Fractures

An occasional birth injury causes separation of the unossified proximal humeral epiphysis. The child's failure to use the arm raises the possibility of brachial plexus palsy. Such pseudoparalysis resolves quickly, and radiographs in 10 days demonstrate abundant callus, confirming the nature of the original trauma. Older children usually sustain type II epiphysial fractures. Most are only slightly displaced and can be treated in a sling for 3 weeks. If more displacement is present, manipulation under anesthesia and skin or skeletal traction can improve alignment. There is so much potential for remodeling in the proximal humerus that the best obtainable closed reduction is preferable to open surgery. Deformity, nonunion, and restricted motion are almost never problems for children who sustain proximal humerus fractures.

Supracondylar Fractures of the Humerus

Hyperextension of a child's elbow may cause an undisplaced greenstick supracondylar fracture. There is elbow pain, swelling, and tenderness of both epicondylar ridges. Radiographs confirm swelling and usually show a positive fat pad sign, indicating elbow hemarthrosis. The fracture line is easily missed but may be found where it crosses the olecranon fossa transversely. Careful inspection of a lateral radiograph of the distal humerus shows loss of normal anterior angulation of the capitellum, which may be compared with the other elbow if necessary. Closed reduction is advised if angulation is more than 20 degrees from normal. Whether or not closed reduction is performed, the fracture should be protected for 3 weeks in a long-arm cast or splint, with the elbow flexed above 90 degrees and the arm restrained to the chest with a secure sling or collar and cuff.

Rotation superimposed upon a hyperextended elbow produces a displaced supracondylar fracture of the humerus. A sharp corner of the proximal piece penetrates the periosteum but leaves an intact hinge on the side toward which the distal fragment is displaced. The anteroposterior radiograph shows the direction of displacement and thus the site of the periosteal hinge. Displaced supracondylar fractures of the humerus are serious injuries that threaten the neurovascular status of the involved limb and may result in unsightly deformity if reduction is not accurate. Before radiographs are taken, the elbow should be splinted in moderate extension rather than flexed to a right angle. The wrist pulses and the function of the radial, ulnar, and median (including anterior interosseous) nerves should be checked immediately. Ischemia may be present initially or may develop during early treatment. If left to progress, ischemia causes Volkmann's contracture, with loss of motor and sensory function and necrosis of some of the forearm flexor muscles. The involved muscles contract as they are replaced by scar, so that the wrist develops a flexion contracture and the fingers become clawed. Irreversible muscle necrosis begins after 4–6 hours of ischemia. Effective treatment requires prompt restoration of arterial flow and, if necessary, reduction of elevated compartmental pressure in the forearm. It is mandatory to recognize the signs of ischemia: pain in the forearm (rather than the elbow) and progressive loss of sensory and motor function. Ischemic pain is usually increased when the involved muscles are stretched, so that pain on extension of the fingers is a danger sign. Pulses may be felt at the wrist, and the skin may appear well perfused in spite of elevated compartmental pressure. Alternatively, the pulses may be diminished or absent without dangerously impaired perfusion as long as the forearm is comfortable and the hand warm and pink, with intact sensation and motion. If elevated compartmental pressure is suspected, prompt measurement of tissue pressures is indicated (see Acute Compartment Syndrome, above). Ischemia with supracondylar fractures may be due to (1) vascular injury, which requires surgical repair; (2) vascular entrapment, which usually resolves with reduction; or (3) compression from marked elbow flexion—in which position the elbow may have been placed to preserve fracture alignment—or from tight casts or bandages.

Prompt reduction of deformity is the next step toward restoration of normal perfusion and venous drainage. Acute flexion helps maintain closed reduction but is contraindicated if it impairs perfusion of the forearm. Ischemia that develops during treatment must be corrected by release or removal of any constricting bandages and by extension of the elbow as necessary to reestablish arterial flow. Prompt surgical exploration of the brachial artery and forearm musculature may be required if ischemia is evident. Arteriography usually adds little helpful information, and indirect attempts to restore flow (stellate ganglion blocks, anticoagulants, or vasodilators) waste time and are usually not successful.

Supracondylar humerus fractures can usually be managed without open operation. If displacement and soft tissue damage are mild to moderate, closed reduction is done under general anesthesia by manipulating the distal fragment into position and flexing the elbow

to hold it. A bandage or cast that leaves the antecubital fossa free is applied, and the arm is secured to the chest to prevent rotation. If the fracture is badly displaced or unstable, if soft tissue swelling is marked, or if the amount of flexion required to hold the reduction obliterates the radial pulse, some other means must be chosen. Overhead skeletal traction with an olecranon pin or screw is effective. Dunlop's skin traction with the arm out to the side is less effective. The currently favored approach is to maintain the reduction with pins inserted percutaneously across the fracture with fluoroscopic guidance, following which the elbow can be splinted in sufficient extension to avoid interfering with perfusion.

The "gunstock deformity" of cubitus varus is the commonest late problem after supracondylar fracture. It is caused by inadequate reduction or reduction that is not maintained during healing. Radiographic monitoring is difficult but must be done with care, since correction is much easier and safer before healing has occurred than with a late osteotomy.

Subluxation of the Radial Head (Pulled Elbow, Nursemaid's Elbow)

This common minor injury occurs in children under 4 years of age. It is caused by a sudden pull on the extended pronated arm, usually by an adult tugging on a reluctant toddler. The pronated radial head slips partially under the annular ligament whose proximal portion displaces into the radiocapitellar joint. The distressed child suddenly stops using the arm, which is held flexed and pronated. Tenderness, usually mild, is well localized to the radial head region, and all motions are permitted except supination. After these physical findings are confirmed, the physician performs reduction by firmly supinating the forearm with one hand while the other supports the elbow in 90 degrees of flexion, feeling for a "click" near the radial head just as full supination is achieved. Radiographs, if obtained, show no abnormalities—in fact, positioning for elbow films will often reduce the subluxation. Promptly after reduction, the child becomes less apprehensive and soon resumes use of the limb. A sling may be applied for a few days. Recurrence is an occasional complication that may require more formal immobilization.

Other Elbow Region Fractures & Dislocations

It is essential to remember that "sprains" rarely occur and that swelling, tenderness, and difficulty in moving an injured elbow suggest a serious problem. Radiographic interpretation is difficult because many of the pertinent structures ossify late in childhood. However, precise early diagnosis is necessary to identify several exceptions to the general principle of nonoperative treatment of children's fractures. Surgery is needed for displaced lateral condylar fractures, displaced medial epicondylar fractures, and badly angulated radial neck fractures that resist closed manipulation. Displaced olecranon fractures, if not reduced by elbow extension, will also require internal fixation. Significant distortion of the elbow region by any fracture or dislocation raises the specter of vascular compromise and resulting Volkmann's contracture. Hospitalization for a day or so is advisable if swelling is severe or if the parents cannot be relied on to bring the child in promptly for follow-up visits.

Forearm Fractures

Fractures of the shafts of both the radius and the ulna occur frequently in children. Neurovascular complications, including those due to constricting plasters, are always possible. Initial elevation of the limb and close observation are thus advisable, and children treated as outpatients must be supervised by an observant and informed adult. Forearm fractures in children unite reliably. The commonest problem is malunion with angular or rotational deformity and limited supination-pronation. Closed reduction almost always corrects angulation. Greenstick fractures are reduced as described above. If displacement is complete, general anesthesia is advisable. Direct manipulation or traction can be used to align the fracture. End-on-end reduction is not essential. Side-by-side ("bayonet") apposition is acceptable in a growing child, but angulation must be minimal; the space between radius and ulna must be preserved; and rotational alignment must be correct. Radiographs are repeated weekly for 3 weeks to permit early remanipulation should a potentially unstable fracture displace in plaster. More distal fractures may involve the physis but rarely interfere with growth.

It is important to be aware of the possibility of dislocation of one forearm bone in association with an isolated displaced fracture of the other. With Monteggia's fracture, there is dislocation of the radial head at the elbow, associated with a broken or bent ulnar shaft. Galeazzi's fracture combines dislocation of the distal radioulnar joint with fracture of the radial shaft. Fracture lines attract attention on radiographs, but dislocations are not as obvious. To avoid missing these injuries, check for tenderness, swelling, and deformity at the wrist and elbow in any patient with trauma to the forearm. Look carefully at radiographs of the wrist and the elbow to ascertain whether the normal bony relationships are present. Children with these injuries, unlike adults, can usually be treated successfully with closed reduction of both the fracture and the joint dislocation. Open reduction is required if joint alignment cannot be restored by closed manipulation.

3. Lower Extremity Fractures & Dislocations

Traumatic Hip Dislocation

In children, traumatic dislocation is more common than fracture of the hip and has fewer complications. Prompt closed reduction under general anesthesia with good muscle relaxation is usually successful. Interposed soft tissue or bone fragments may necessitate open reduction. Following reduction, the hip should be protected for 4–6 weeks until soft tissue healing has occurred. Balanced suspension, traction, or a spica cast may be used. With prompt reduction, avascular necrosis is a rare problem.

Fractures of the Proximal Femur

Proximal femur fractures are rare in children. This is fortunate, as displacement and injury to the growth plate and blood supply predispose to frequent complications such as avascular necrosis, nonunion, and deformity that imperil the hip joint. The strength and resiliency of the proximal femur are such that a fracture in this region can only occur with severe trauma—another factor increasing the likelihood of complications.

Birth fractures, now quite unusual, may displace the proximal femoral epiphysis. Pain and swelling suggest septic arthritis, and the deformity raises fears of dislocation. Aspiration or arthrography yields no pus but demonstrates that the femoral head is located in a normal acetabulum and that deformity is at the neck-shaft junction. Splinting in abduction and flexion, a spica cast, or skin traction will maintain alignment during the 2–3 weeks required for healing. Remodeling may occur with any of these injuries, but nonunion, avascular necrosis, and deformity are possible.

In older children, most hip fractures involve the mid and lower portions of the femoral neck. If there is no displacement, spica cast immobilization maintains alignment during healing, but close radiographic monitoring is required for prompt identification and rectification of any displacement. Displaced fractures of the femoral neck should be treated with three or four small pins, preferably placed short of the physis. Postoperatively, a spica cast is advisable until healing is progressing. Satisfactory results are achieved in half or less of cases, with avascular necrosis, varus malunion, epiphysial arrest, nonunion, and postoperative wound infection the principal complications. Intertrochanteric and subtrochanteric fractures can generally be managed by use of traction for 3–4 weeks until early fracture stability is present, at which time a 1½ hip spica is applied for 8–12 weeks. Late problems (eg, angular deformity, unequal limb lengths) are rare but do occur.

Femoral Shaft Fractures

Femoral shaft fractures are fairly common childhood injuries. They often result from significant trauma, so that other injuries may also be present. Radiographs of the hip are required to ensure that fracture or dislocation is not present. The knee should also be x-rayed. Alignment of a femoral shaft fracture is achieved with skin or (for older children) skeletal traction or immediate spica application. Rotational alignment should be corrected. Children 2–10 years of age will usually demonstrate transiently stimulated growth of a fractured femur. It is conventional to align their fractures with about a 1 cm overlap to compensate for this overgrowth. Protection must be continued until mature bony callus has developed, a process that takes roughly as many weeks as the child's age in years. So-called Bryant's skin traction, with both legs suspended vertically, may cause severe ischemia and Volkmann's contracture, even of the uninjured leg. This technique is dangerous for children over the age of 2 years. Femoral fractures in children who are closer to maturity are often most effectively managed with intramedullary nailing, especially if there is head trauma or if multiple injuries have been sustained.

Distal Femoral Growth Plate Fractures

Fractures of the distal femoral growth plate are potentially serious injuries that cause growth abnormalities in up to 45% of patients. They must be suspected whenever a child sustains a knee injury and are suggested by the finding of an intra-articular fat-fluid line on a cross-table lateral radiograph of the knee. Stress radiographs may be required to demonstrate instability. With marked displacement, the popliteal artery or peroneal nerve may be injured. Treatment must be individualized. Gentle anatomic reduction should be accomplished, and reduction should be maintained until healing is secure. A hip spica cast is often required to prevent displacement. If instability is marked, fixation with smooth pins may be required; if open reduction is necessary, such fixation is advisable. The distal femoral epiphysis is responsible for 70% of the growth of the femur and 35% of the growth of the entire lower extremity. Even small disturbances of growth can produce significant limb length inequality if the injured child is young enough. Follow-up of distal femoral growth mechanism injuries should be continued until skeletal maturity is achieved.

Fractures of the Tibia & Fibula

Fractures of the tibia and fibula are not unusual in childhood. An occult undisplaced spiral fracture may be the cause of an acute gait disturbance ("toddler's fracture"). Oblique radiographs may reveal this injury. Most are easy to manage and heal rapidly in a long-leg cast. The spectrum of injuries is quite wide, however, so that each must be evaluated carefully and treated according to its particular attributes. Nerve and vessel damage may be present, especially with displaced fractures of the proximal metaphysis. Nearly undisplaced valgus greenstick fractures of the proximal tibia are pernicious causes of deformity. The initial angulation may not be appreciated, or progressive medial overgrowth may follow apparently satisfactory healing. Fractures in this region with any valgus deformity should be completely reduced and held extended in a long-leg or single-spica cast molded into varus. In some cases, open reduction may be required to remove interposed soft tissues. Another cause of angular deformity is an intact fibula, which may have been bent by the original injury or may encourage collapse into varus by providing relatively more support to the lateral aspect of the leg. One must critically assess the postreduction and early follow-up radiographs following casting to permit timely treatment of angulation. Rotational alignment requires careful visual comparison with the other limb, as it is not obvious on radiographs.

Fractures of the Distal Epiphyses of the Tibia & Fibula

Fractures of the distal epiphyses of the tibia and the fibula occur frequently in children, often from trauma that would produce ligamentous injury in an adult. Suspicion, physical examination that localizes tenderness to a growth plate, and carefully evaluated radiographs will usually suggest the diagnosis. Additional radiographic views, including stress films, will occasionally be required for confirmation. Salter-Harris type I fractures, type II fractures of the fibula, and undisplaced (within 2 mm of anatomic position) type III and type IV fractures have little risk of growth disturbance. Type II fractures of the distal tibial epiphysis are unpredictable, with a higher risk of growth disturbance that does not correlate well with original displacement. Displaced type III and type IV injuries and comminuted epiphysial fractures have a 30% chance of growth disturbance.

If displaced, growth plate injuries of the ankle should be treated by gentle closed reduction, usually under general anesthesia. If this does not correct displacement, type III and type IV injuries should be treated by open reduction and internal fixation, whereas moderate deformity, especially in the sagittal plane, can generally be accepted in type I and type II fractures. Distal fibular growth plate injuries usually have few complications, but those of the distal tibia should be followed until skeletal maturity is achieved.

GAIT DISORDERS & LIMB DEFORMITY

Abnormalities of the lower extremities in children are often a source of parental concern and are frequently noticed when the child is first learning to walk. Rotational alignment—indicated by the orientation of the feet to the line of progression—and angulation at the knees are the two commonest areas of concern.

1. Intoe Gait (Pigeon Toe)

Children normally walk with their feet externally rotated 10 degrees externally from the line of progression. Significant variation occurs from step to step, so that gait must be observed more than just briefly before a reliable conclusion can be made about whether a problem exists. Metatarsus adductus—medial deviation of the forefoot at the tarsometatarsal junction—is a deformity occasionally present at birth. If it persists beyond early childhood, gait appears intoed.

Tibial torsion, the relative rotational alignment of the ankle joint axis compared with that of the knee, increases in an outward direction during childhood. The ankle axis is a line connecting the tips of the medial and lateral malleoli. In a very young child whose leg is hanging freely with the knee flexed 90 degrees and the tibia in neutral rotation, the ankle axis is in the same plane as the knee axis. By adulthood, the transmalleolar axis is externally rotated about 20 degrees. Children 1–3 years of age with intoeing will frequently have relative internal tibial torsion, which almost always corrects spontaneously with growth. Treatment is necessary only if there is significant interference with gait and if spontaneous correction is not occurring. A Denis Browne splint is a metal bar that connects the shoes and holds them in external rotation. It is worn while the child sleeps. This treatment is usually effective. Only rarely—and only in children over 8 years of age—must tibial osteotomy be considered.

Excessive femoral anteversion is a common finding in older children who walk with their feet turned in. Observation reveals that the whole limb is internally rotated, so that the patella—as well as the foot—points medially. Anteversion is the normal anterior inclination of the femoral neck when the distal femur is positioned with the knee axis in a frontal plane. From about 40 degrees in the newborn, femoral anteversion decreases normally to about 15 degrees by adulthood. Excessive femoral anteversion also decreases, often to a normal

range, although significant correction is unlikely to occur after age 8 years. Precise measurement of femoral anteversion requires complicated radiographic techniques, but a good clinical determination can be made by internally rotating the extended hip to produce maximal lateral prominence of the greater trochanter. The required amount of internal rotation is roughly equivalent to the degree of femoral anteversion. Significant anteversion is the usual cause of limited external rotation of the extended hip, with associated increase of the range of internal rotation. The normal newborn's hips have an external rotation contracture, presumably the result of intrauterine posture. This diminishes during the first 3 years of life independently of changes in anteversion of the femoral neck. Femoral anteversion can be corrected only by rotational osteotomy. If the limb can be externally rotated beyond neutral, osteotomy is rarely needed.

2. Angular Deformity of the Lower Extremities (Knock-Knees & Bowlegs)

The angle (varus denotes tibia deviated medially; valgus denotes tibia deviated laterally) between femur and tibia in the frontal plane is age-dependent. Bowlegs (genu varum) are normal in the newborn but progress toward valgus, passing through neutral at about age 18 months. Valgus becomes maximal between ages 2 and 3 years, gradually resolving so that the average leg appears straight by age 6 or 7 years. In young children, angular deformity of the knees requires x-ray evaluation (and perhaps measurement of serum calcium, phosphate, and alkaline phosphatase) if it is not symmetric; if it is associated with abnormally short stature; or if it is severe (more than 10 cm between the knees with the ankles touching in genu varum, or more than 10 cm between the ankles with the knees touching in genu valgum). Operative treatment may be considered in severe cases to improve function and appearance and perhaps to decrease the risk of degenerative joint disease in middle age. Angulation can be corrected by stapling one side of a physis to obtain asymmetric growth or by osteotomy with removal or addition of a wedge of bone.

Pathologic Genu Varum

It is important to distinguish symmetric infantile bowlegs, which should resolve by age 3–5 years, from varus deformity produced by rickets, Blount's disease, or skeletal dysplasias, in which involvement is often bilateral but usually asymmetric. Blount's disease (tibia vara) is a frequently bilateral disorder that has both infantile and adolescent types. Radiologic changes in the medial proximal tibial metaphysis consist of lucency, sclerosis, and fragmentation. Unilateral varus suggests a traumatic origin. In young patients, the metaphysial-diaphysial angle of the tibia helps to differentiate between physiologic bowing and infantile tibia vara prior to development of typical radiologic signs. The angle is formed between the line of the lateral tibial cortex and the line of the prominent medial and lateral metaphysial beaks. A metaphysial-diaphysial angle of greater than 11 degrees strongly suggests Blount's disease. Progressive tibia vara should be treated with corrective osteotomy of the proximal tibia and fibula to achieve physiologic valgus alignment of both knees.

SYSTEMIC DISORDERS AFFECTING BONES & JOINTS IN CHILDREN

1. Juvenile Rheumatoid Arthritis

Rheumatoid arthritis is an autoimmune disorder whose exact cause remains elusive. It is a systemic disease that in its most florid form is characterized by rash, fever, and enlargement of lymph nodes and spleen. There are three basic clinical types of juvenile rheumatoid arthritis. Pauciarticular arthritis generally involves the knee or the ankle but occasionally the hip or an upper extremity (mainly the elbow or the wrist). One joint or only a few joints are affected. Insidious onset of swelling, with effusion, synovial thickening, and often flexion contracture, are noted. Except for possible sedimentation rate elevation, systemic manifestations are absent. A serious complication of juvenile rheumatoid arthritis, most common in the pauciarticular form, is iridocyclitis—inflammation of the iris and ciliary body. This insidious process can lead to glaucoma and blindness if left untreated. Early diagnosis is essential and requires slit lamp examination every 3–6 months in these patients. The outlook for patients with pauciarticular juvenile rheumatoid arthritis is said to be good, but—even though residual involvement may be minimal—few patients remain truly asymptomatic.

Polyarthritis is characterized by multiple joint involvement and minimal evidence of systemic disease. Fingers and toes, the neck, and the temporomandibular joints are more likely to be involved. The course is persistent, with periods of exacerbation.

Polyarthritis with systemic rheumatoid disease (Still's disease) usually presents with multiple (more than five) involved joints, fever, lymphadenopathy, hepatosplenomegaly, rash, subcutaneous nodules, and pericarditis. The course may be remitting or relentless, causing severe permanent disability.

Inflamed joints develop synovial hypertrophy and pannus, which destroy articular cartilage. The associated hyperemia can stimulate the adjacent physes, with resulting overgrowth, or physial arrest may occur. Damage to underlying bone and ligament can produce severe deformity and joint subluxation. In polyarthritis, musculoskeletal involvement is more likely to include the cervical spine, typically with spontaneous fusion of the apophysial joints. C1–2 instability will occasionally occur, as in the adult with rheumatoid arthritis.

When a single joint is inflamed, it is necessary to exclude septic arthritis, foreign body synovitis, and transient synovitis of the hip. Polyarticular juvenile rheumatoid arthritis must be differentiated from rheumatic fever and leukemia. Lyme disease may present as joint inflammation.

Management is initially medical, with anti-inflammatory drugs, rest, splinting, and range of motion exercises, followed by strengthening as synovitis resolves and appropriate bracing to minimize deformity and allow function. Synovial biopsy—percutaneously with a needle, via arthroscopy, or with formal arthrotomy—may be helpful for diagnosis, especially to rule out infection. Synovectomy is controversial but may retard the progression of arthritis if medical measures fail. To be successful, it must be done before joint destruction has progressed too far. Contractures may require soft tissue releasing procedures. Osteotomy may be needed to correct bony deformity, and symptomatic destroyed joints can be treated by arthrodesis or arthroplasty. Extensive orthopedic surgery can often be avoided if the pediatrician and the orthopedist cooperate to provide maximal medical control and appropriate use of bracing and physical therapy.

2. Brachial Plexus Palsy

Brachial plexus palsy due to birth injury has three general patterns of involvement: (1) Erb's palsy, involving C5 and C6 roots; (2) Klumpke's paralysis, involving C8 and T1; and (3) whole arm paralysis, where the extent of involvement of individual roots may vary. Erb's palsy is most common and affects the shoulder, with loss of extension, abduction, and external rotation. Also affected are elbow flexion and forearm supination. Spontaneous improvement will occur and will level off by age 1½ years. Initial treatment is directed at maintaining shoulder motion by positioning and passive stretching to prevent the characteristic contracture in adduction and internal rotation. If muscle imbalance persists at the shoulder, the pectoralis major and subscapularis muscles can be lengthened with posterior transfer of the latissimus dorsi and teres major muscles, so that they become external rotators. Humeral osteotomy may be preferable to tendon transfer when the shoulder joint is unstable. These procedures will position the hand where it can best be used, but a normal limb is not achieved.

SCOLIOSIS & SPINAL DEFORMITY

The spine has an important role in supporting erect posture, stabilizing the limbs relative to the trunk, supporting the abdominal and thoracic cavities, and in protecting neural elements. The spine is in balance when the head is aligned with the pelvis in the coronal and sagittal planes. Scoliosis is spinal curvature of more than 10 degrees in the coronal or frontal plane. An important component of scoliotic deformity is a concurrent rotational asymmetry around the vertical axis of the body. Deformity may also exist in the sagittal plane, with kyphosis, flexion of the spine anteriorly; and lordosis, extension of the spine posteriorly.

Spinal deformity in children may be caused by congenital anomalies, neuromuscular disorders, connective tissue abnormalities, or infection or injury to the developing spine. Most commonly, the cause is unknown, or idiopathic.

Clinical Findings

A. SYMPTOMS AND SIGNS

Spinal deformity may present in the perinatal period or during infancy in children with congenital anomalies of the spine. More commonly, deformity of the spine due to all causes is detected during the preadolescent growth spurt, when the spine is growing most rapidly. The cause of deformity is an important determinant of the natural history, treatment options, and the goals of management. The history should include age at initial presentation, family history, neuromuscular or connective tissue disorders, prior surgery to the spine or trunk, prior trauma or infection, coexisting skeletal, cardiac, renal, or pulmonary abnormalities, and information on growth and the progression of the deformity.

The initial detection of spinal asymmetry is variable between individuals and across communities. Spinal deformity is often detected by family members, friends, or patients with deformity. Routine screening for spinal deformity remains controversial because there is little evidence that routine screening reduces rates of surgery for spinal deformity or in any way improves outcomes of management. The Adams forward bending test is the most common method of screening for scoliosis. An angular measurement of a line connecting the rib prominences relative to horizontal demonstrates axial rotation of the spine, a characteristic of scoliosis. Angular measurements of greater than 7 degrees are associated with coronal deformity greater than 10 degrees and are therefore an indication for radiographic evaluation.

Physical examination of the patient with spinal deformity includes both examination of the spine and a comprehensive examination of the patient. Examina-

tion of the spine may include the location of the curve, curve magnitude, deviation of the trunk from the midline, shoulder asymmetry, pelvic obliquity, and flexibility of the spine. Examination of reflexes (including abdominal reflexes), strength, clonus, hamstring tightness, muscle weakness and contractures, and foot deformity may reveal abnormalities suggestive of intraspinal pathology, including tethering of the cord or a syrinx. Skin examination will include detection of dermal sinuses, hemangiomas, nevi, and hyperelasticity that may be associated with spinal deformity. Chest wall deformity, preauricular skin tags, cleft palate, radial dysplasia, scapular elevation, and thumb duplication or hypoplasia may be found on examination of a patient with congenital deformity of the spine. Scoliosis due to connective tissue pathology may present with joint hypermobility, ocular findings, and cardiac murmurs.

B. IMAGING STUDIES

Spinal deformity occurs in three dimensions, and most imaging studies are limited by providing only a two-dimensional representation. Plain radiographs are useful for the detection of deformity and will provide an accurate quantification of progression of deformity. The Cobb technique is used to accurately measure deformity in the coronal and sagittal planes and is important in demonstrating changes in curve magnitude and pattern. The Cobb technique uses a standing or weightbearing film, and an angular measurement is made between the end-vertebrae that are most tilted from the horizontal at either end of the curve (Figure 43–36) Other plain radiographic measures may include trunk shift relative to the pelvis and overall sagittal and coronal balance of the spine measuring a plumbline between C7 and the sacrum.

MRI examination of the entire spine is an important imaging tool because of the association between intraspinal anomalies with certain types of spinal deformity. Congenital scoliosis may be associated with intraspinal abnormalities, including tethering of the cord, syringomyelia, diastematomyelia, diplomyelia, lipoma, teratoma, and neuroenteric cysts. MRI of the entire spine is indicated for congenital deformity, patients with abnormal neurologic findings on physical examination, and atypical curve patterns including left thoracic curves in females.

1. Idiopathic Scoliosis

Idiopathic scoliosis is the most common cause of spinal deformity in children and adolescents. The prevalence of adolescent idiopathic scoliosis, or deformity in the coronal plane measuring greater than 10 degrees, is 2–3% at age 16. Curves larger than 20 degrees are present in 0.3–0.5% of adolescents. The ratio of affected

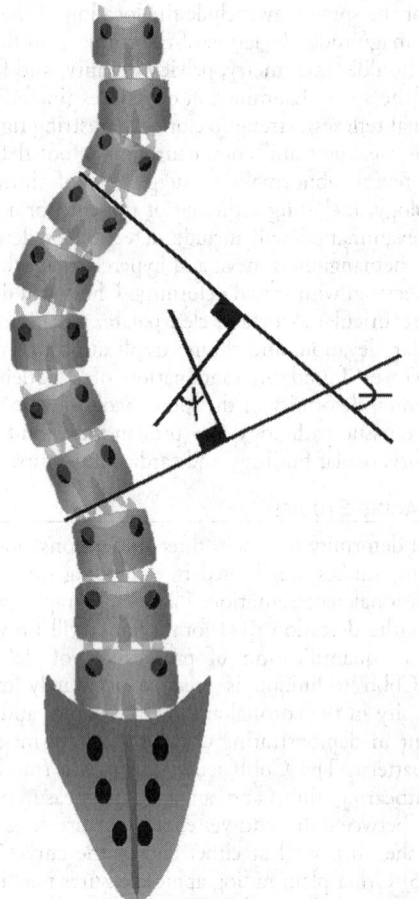

Figure 43–36. Measurement of spinal deformity using the Cobb method.

males to females is equal in curves less than 15 degrees. However, for curves larger than 20 degrees, females are seven times more likely to be affected than males.

Nonoperative management of adolescent idiopathic scoliosis is intended to prevent progression of deformity during the growing years. Bracing is the only nonoperative treatment that has demonstrated efficacy in the management of progressive idiopathic scoliosis. Exercises alone, electrical stimulation, and manipulation of the spine have not demonstrated efficacy relative to the natural history of curve progression. Bracing is recommended for curves of magnitude between 30 and 45 degrees. Curves measuring less than 30 degrees should demonstrate progression before initiation of bracing, while curves measuring greater than 50 degrees may not be managed effectively in a brace.

Treatment

Surgical management of adolescent idiopathic scoliosis is generally indicated to prevent the future consequences of progressive deformity. It is important that the patient, family, and care provider share an accurate understanding of the future consequences of adolescent scoliosis in order to participate in an informed decision regarding surgical care. Future consequences of concern include ongoing progression of deformity, cardiac or pulmonary compromise, neurologic deterioration, unacceptable appearance, and possible development of progressive pain. With information gained from studying the natural history of untreated idiopathic scoliosis, we have useful insight into predicting the future consequences of spinal deformity in general.

2. Neuromuscular Scoliosis

Neuromuscular scoliosis develops secondary to loss of muscular control of the trunk. The term encompasses a multitude of disorders all of which result in some compromise of the patient's ability to control posture and trunk position. The severity of deformity is related to the severity of weakness or spasticity, the patient's age at presentation of neuromuscular pathology, and the rostral or caudal level of involvement within the spinal cord. Spinal deformity may be the reason for initial presentation of a patient with a neuromuscular disorder. Therefore, a detailed history including birth circumstances, family history, and timing of developmental milestones is important in evaluating the child with spinal deformity. Similarly, neurologic examination including documentation of muscle tone, strength, reflex symmetry, and ataxia may reveal a neuromuscular cause of scoliosis. More commonly, a child will have a known neuromuscular disorder and the orthopedic surgeon will monitor the patient for the development of spinal deformity in concert with management of associated deformities, including involvement of the hips, feet, and upper extremities.

Neuromuscular scoliosis may present in patients with disorders involving upper motor neurons, lower motor neurons, or primary myopathies. Upper motor neuron disorders may include cerebral palsy, spinocerebellar degeneration (Friedreich's ataxia, Charcot-Marie-Tooth disease, Roussy-Levy disease), syringomyelia, spinal cord tumor, and spinal cord trauma. Lower motor neuron disorders include poliomyelitis, spinomuscular atrophy, myelodysplasia, dysautonomia, and trauma. Poliomyelitis was the most common cause of neuromuscular scoliosis before the development of vaccination and remains an important cause of neuromuscular deformity in many parts of the world. Primary myopathies that may lead to neuromuscular deformity of the spine include muscular dystrophy, arthrogryposis, and congenital hypotonia.

Neuromuscular scoliosis characteristically presents with long, sweeping patterns, involving more vertebrae than idiopathic curves, with fewer compensatory curves. This may result in imbalance of the trunk relative to the pelvis. Pelvic obliquity is common in neuromuscular scoliosis, resulting in poor sitting balance and skin breakdown. Pulmonary compromise may be an important feature of neuromuscular curves due to the combination of thoracic deformity with intercostal and accessory muscle weakness. Therefore, the child with neuromuscular spinal deformity presents with comorbidities and functional considerations that are distinct from the patient with idiopathic or congenital scoliosis.

Treatment

In the neuromuscular patient who sits and is nonambulatory, goals of surgery include restoration of sitting balance and lumbar lordosis, prevention of sacral and ischial skin breakdown, and improvement of the ability of caregivers to assist with patient transfers and mobility. In the patient with neuromuscular scoliosis that is ambulatory, management includes consideration of maintenance of truncal balance relative to the pelvis, pulmonary function, and functional ability in transfers and gait.

Orthotics—including molded body jackets and thoracolumbar orthoses—may be useful in preserving sitting balance and delaying surgical correction and stabilization. Orthotics do not appear to effectively slow curve progression. Surgical correction and stabilization of the spine is the most effective management. Indications for surgery include curve progression, poor sitting balance, respiratory compromise, and skin compromise. In the patient who is ambulatory, fusion of the spinal column to the pelvis may compromise functional independence.

3. Congenital Scoliosis

Congenital anomalies of the spine are caused by defects in the embryologic formation and segmentation of spinal elements. The formation of the spine begins during the third week of embryonic development with cells from the epiblast layer invaginating into the primitive pit and migrating cephalad to the prochordal plate. These epiblast cells form a notochordal process that separates ectoderm from mesoderm. Proliferation of notochordal cells creates a solid notochord that serves as a midline axis for the axial skeleton. During the fourth week of embryonic development, sclerotomal segments shift to surround the notochord and the

neural tube. The process of formation and resegmentation of sclerotomes is induced by the notochord, and the formation of the posterior arch of the spine is induced by the neural tube. Abnormalities of either the notochord or the neural arch may cause congenital anomalies of the spine. Congenital anomalies may include unilateral failure of formation (hemivertebrae and wedge vertebrae), unilateral or bilateral failure of segmentation, rib fusion, and mixed or complex anomalies. Solitary anomalies of the spine appear sporadic and are not hereditary. Multiple congenital anomalies of the spine may have a heritable basis.

Progression of deformity in congenital scoliosis is related to the type of vertebral anomaly, the position of the vertebral anomaly, and the growth potential for that segment of the spine. Congenital anomalies of the spine have the potential for rapid progression and development of fixed deformity. Therefore, patients with congenital scoliosis warrant early identification and close observation. The patient with a congenital deformity of the spine may have associated intraspinal and systemic abnormalities. Intraspinal disorders associated with congenital scoliosis includes tethering of the cord, syringomyelia, diastematomyelia, diplomyelia, lipoma, teratoma, and neuroenteric cysts. Extraspinal disorders, including tracheoesophageal fistula, esophageal atresia, renal anomalies, bowel malrotation, anal atresia, radial forearm and hand anomalies, and cardiac septal defects, may be detected in the child with congenital deformity of the spine.

Bracing the spine may delay surgery in the young child, and is appropriate for long flexible deformities. Most patients with congenital deformity of the spine detected before 10 years of age will require operative management for control of curve progression. The goal of surgery in young patients is to prevent the development of a severe rigid deformity. Timing of operation requires understanding of curve progression patterns.

SEPTIC ARTHRITIS OF THE HIP

 ESSENTIALS OF DIAGNOSIS

- *Limited hip motion, with local swelling and tenderness.*
- *Variable signs of systemic illness.*
- *Purulent exudate in the hip joint, confirmed by aspiration or arthrotomy.*

Figure 43–37. Septic arthritis of the hip in a 2-year-old boy. ***A:*** Lateral radiograph shows signs of proximal femoral osteomyelitis. ***B:*** T2-weighted MRI showing large effusion in the hip joint and edema of the proximal femur.

General Considerations

See Figure 43–37.

Infection is usually hematogenous and more frequent in infants exposed to invasive measures likely to cause bacteremia. The joint can be primarily involved, or secondary involvement may occur by spread of hematogenous osteomyelitis from the proximal femur. Hip sepsis has also followed penetration of the joint during attempted blood aspiration from the femoral vein.

Staphylococcus aureus and *Streptococcus pyogenes* are the most common causative organisms.

Clinical Findings

A. SYMPTOMS AND SIGNS

Impaired voluntary and reflex motion of the entire involved limb—pseudoparalysis—is the most typical early finding. Fever is unlikely in very young children, but sepsis may be suggested by irritability and failure to thrive. Another focus of infection should increase suspicion. The hip is held flexed in slight abduction and external rotation, with local swelling becoming evident as disease progresses. The area is tender, and attempts to move the hip are resisted and seem especially painful. If pathologic dislocation has occurred, hip asymmetry and instability may be noted.

B. LABORATORY FINDINGS

The sedimentation rate is elevated, but the white blood count may be normal. Leukocytes are abundant in the joint fluid, and Gram-stained smears of fluid show microorganisms as well. Bone scan may initially be negative, especially in children under 6 months of age, but usually shows increased uptake around the involved joint before radiographic changes become evident.

C. IMAGING STUDIES

The early radiographic signs are subtle, with obliteration of soft tissue planes and a suggestion of capsular distention. Lateral subluxation and complete dislocation may occur. Decreasing bone density and periosteal erosion or new bone formation occur later. Ultrasound imaging provides an early indication of joint effusion.

Differential Diagnosis

Alternative diagnoses in the neonate are fractures of the femur occurring during birth and acute hematogenous osteomyelitis of the proximal femur that has not yet spread into the hip. Congenital hip dislocation is not painful and limits motion to a lesser extent. In older children, transient synovitis, rheumatoid arthritis, pelvic osteomyelitis, and acute hemarthrosis from hemophilia must also be considered.

Complications

Structural sequelae include pathologic dislocation; avascular necrosis that may cause total and irreversible destruction of the femoral head and neck; and leg length discrepancy, usually due to undergrowth of the involved femur. Chronic persisting infection may also result.

Treatment

Surgical drainage is required as an emergency procedure. Side effects from negative arthrotomy are so few that exploration is warranted if the diagnosis is uncertain. Gram-stained smears of intra-articular pus guide the initial choice of parenteral antibiotic, which is modified if necessary according to the results of culture and sensitivity tests. Suction-irrigation tube drainage will maintain adequate decompression. Postoperatively, traction or a spica cast is used to rest and align the joint.

Course & Prognosis

If the diagnosis is made and surgical drainage performed within a few days after onset, the long-term results are good. Delay and nonoperative treatment are predictably followed by the complications mentioned above.

TRANSIENT SYNOVITIS OF THE HIP (Irritable Hip Syndrome, Toxic Synovitis, "Observation Hip")

This syndrome of unknown origin is the most common cause of painful hip in young children. A respiratory illness often precedes the complaint of pain, which may be localized in the knee, thigh, or hip. The short duration of symptoms, absence of diagnostic radiographic signs, and nearly normal laboratory studies suggest a benign process. Children of any age may be affected, though the average age is 6 years. Perhaps the most important aspect of transient synovitis is to recognize it appropriately and not confuse it with more serious causes of hip joint inflammation.

Clinical Findings

A. SYMPTOMS AND SIGNS

When first seen, the child has rarely been symptomatic for more than a week. Pain in the lower extremity with activity (or even with rest) is the commonest complaint. Limp and refusal to walk are also common. Localization of pain to the hip region is not reliable, and a specific provocative test of hip motion must always be part of the physical examination of a child with lower extremity complaints. Passive range of motion of the hip must be checked and compared carefully with the opposite side. Normally, the child should be able to relax and motion should be free and easy without "guarding," which is especially noticeable on rotation or at extremes of flexion or extension. Low-grade fever may be present, but the child does not appear ill.

B. LABORATORY FINDINGS

Although the white blood cell count and erythrocyte sedimentation rate may be somewhat elevated, they are usually normal. Bone scan often shows increased activity in the hip joint, without the decreased femoral head uptake suggestive of early avascular necrosis. Hip aspiration, if performed to help clarify a confusing case, reveals clear synovial fluid with a low white cell count, no organisms on Gram-stained smears, and negative cultures for all types of organisms.

C. IMAGING STUDIES

Radiographs are essential to rule out other diagnoses. X-rays are usually normal with transient synovitis of the hip. Shadows adjacent to the femoral neck sometimes suggest "hip effusion," but the significance is questionable, since they can be produced by abduction and external rotation of a normal hip. Occasionally, the joint space will be widened.

Differential Diagnosis

Pyogenic or tuberculous sepsis is the primary concern. Legg-Perthes disease (avascular necrosis), slipped capital femoral epiphysis, and, rarely, other forms of inflammatory joint disease such as rheumatoid arthritis or rheumatic fever must be considered.

Treatment

Hospitalization is often advisable to ensure that an infection is not missed. The hip is placed at rest in 4–5 lb of Buck's or Russell's skin traction. This almost always relieves symptoms promptly and also helps confirm the diagnosis. A few days of rest may be required to regain normal hip motion. A week or so of protection from weightbearing with bed rest at home or with crutches is usually advised. The child should then be reexamined to make certain that normal hip motion and comfort have been achieved. Anteroposterior and lateral x-rays are repeated in 2–3 months to ensure that avascular necrosis has not developed. Occasionally, signs of systemic reaction are more pronounced or the child continues to guard the hip longer than usual. In such cases, needle aspiration confirmed by arthrogram should be performed to rule out infection.

Prognosis

Recurrent symptoms may develop after release from the hospital and resumption of activity but usually resolve with more rest. Permanent (but usually unnoticeable) limitation of motion is present in about 18% of cases. A small number of patients develop other abnormalities and may represent errors in initial diagnosis.

CONGENITAL DYSPLASIA & DISLOCATION OF THE HIP

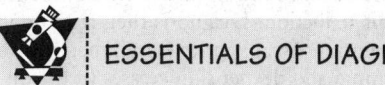 ESSENTIALS OF DIAGNOSIS

- *Mechanical instability of the hip.*
- *Persistent limitation of abduction.*

- Shortening or other asymmetry of the hip if unilateral.
- Widening of buttocks and perineum if bilateral.
- Abnormal gait once walking begins.

General Considerations

Congenital hip dysplasia may be manifested by dislocatability, dislocation, or inadequate joint development that results in early degenerative arthritis of the hip. True dislocation is not necessarily present at birth but develops early in life in some infants with dislocatable hips. The incidence of dislocation is 1 in 1000 infants. Both hips may be involved. Congenital hip dysplasia is more common in females and in patients with other congenital deformities. It is neither painful nor disabling in children but causes significant symptoms in adults if successful atraumatic closed reduction is not achieved in early childhood. If atraumatic reduction is not possible, surgical release of the obstructing or limiting soft tissues should be performed.

Clinical Findings

A. SYMPTOMS AND SIGNS

The physical signs of congenital hip dislocation are the key to diagnosis. They may be subtle, however, and can be missed by the most experienced examiner. This emphasizes the need for repeated evaluation of the hips during routine "well baby" checks.

1. Dislocatable hip—The examiner attempts to displace the infant's femoral head posterolaterally from the acetabulum by means of the subluxation provocation test (Figure 43–38). In a positive test, the femoral head is felt to displace with a jerk, which is repeated as the femur slides back into the acetabulum upon release of the displacing force. Mechanical instability—not a "click"—is the essential finding. Dislocatability is most easily demonstrated shortly after birth and should resolve within a few days.

2. Dislocated hip—Ortolani described the sign of "snapping" produced by relocation of a dislocated femoral head when the examiner abducts the flexed hip and lifts the greater trochanter anteriorly. This test can appear normal in the presence of congenital hip dysplasia if the soft tissues surrounding the joint are not lax enough to permit reduction. Diagnosis then rests upon other signs: limitation of abduction, asymmetry with apparent shortening, and deeper skin creases (if the dislocation is unilateral). As the child begins to walk, an abnormal gait becomes apparent. Trendelenburg's sign is positive, the contralateral side of the pelvis drooping

Figure 43–38. Upper window: Subluxation provocation test. Holding the thighs of the relaxed infant as illustrated, the examiner stabilizes the pelvis with one hand while gently but firmly trying to displace the opposite femoral head posteriorly out of the acetabulum. Adduction of the thigh aids this maneuver. If mechanical instability of the femoral head is present, a "jerk" will be felt, indicating that the hip is subluxable. **Lower window:** In Ortolani's test, abduction and lifting with the fingers produces a corresponding jerk when the dislocated femoral head slides back into the acetabulum.

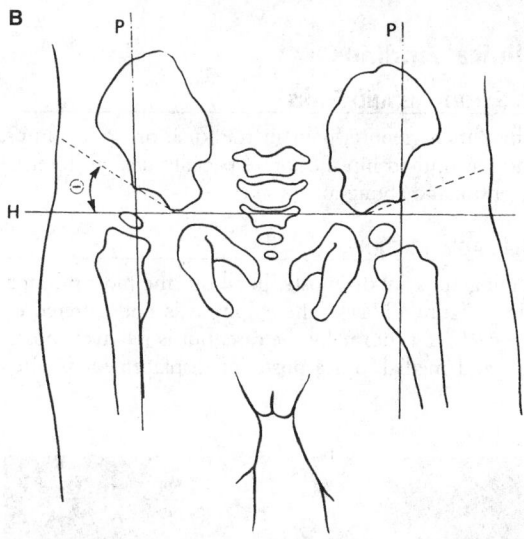

when the child stands on the affected limb. If dislocation is bilateral, the diagnosis is more challenging. The perineum and buttocks are widened, and abduction limitation is bilateral. Gait is "waddling," and lumbar lordosis is prominent.

B. IMAGING STUDIES

Until the cartilaginous acetabulum and femoral head become substantially ossified, x-rays may fail to indicate the true condition of the hip joint. Obvious abnormalities must be considered significant, but apparently normal radiographs do not exclude congenital hip dysplasia until a well-ossified femoral head is adequately contained by the acetabulum. Femoral head ossification is usually present by 6 months of age but is often delayed in dislocated hips. Figure 43–39 shows several of the many radiographic relationships that are important for evaluation of the hip joint in infants. In older children, the femoral head should be adjacent to the radiolucent triradiate cartilage that forms the medial wall of the acetabulum. Displacement of the femoral head confirms dislocation. A shallow acetabulum that poorly covers the femoral head is termed dysplastic. Hip arthrography or CT scans help evaluate reduction of the unossified hip joint. Ultrasonography is gaining popularity as a technique for assessing the infant's hip prior to calcification of the cartilaginous joint structures. Congenital hip disease in the adult is shown in Figure 43–40.

Differential Diagnosis

Congenital abduction contracture of the hip is not unusual in neonates. Proximal femoral focal deficiency and congenital coxa vara are rare conditions that produce shortening or instability in the hip region. Patho-

Figure 43–39. **A:** X-ray of congenital dislocation of the right hip. **B:** Analysis of hip radiographs presupposes adequately exposed films of a properly positioned patient. Hilgenreiner's horizontal line is drawn through both triradiate cartilages (H), and Perkins's vertical line is drawn through the outer margin of each acetabulum (P). If the hip is located, the proximal femoral epiphysis will lie in the inferomedial quadrant formed by the two intersecting lines. Proximal or lateral displacement indicates dislocation. Abnormal acetabular development is suggested by lack of obvious concavity and by an acetabular index (⊖) greater than 30 degrees.

Figure 43–40. Adult with left total hip arthroplasty and persistent dislocation of the right hip caused by bilateral congenital hip dislocations.

logic dislocation can occur rapidly in infected hips; the femoral head is displaced from a radiographically normal acetabulum. Hip dislocation may be caused by muscle imbalance in some children with cerebral palsy or myelomeningocele.

Complications

Complications include inability to gain or maintain a stable reduction, avascular necrosis of the femoral head following operative or nonoperative treatment, and limitation of motion.

Treatment

A. DISLOCATABLE HIP

Neonates with confirmed dislocatable hips should be treated by means of abduction splinting (Pavlik harness, Frejka cushion, etc) until stability and normal radiographic development are confirmed. It is important to flex the hips and abduct them no more than 60 degrees to avoid interfering with the blood supply, so that avascular necrosis does not occur.

B. DISLOCATED HIP

1. Birth to 18 months—In this age group, closed reduction is usually possible. Reduction can be maintained with removable splints as mentioned above if the parents are reliable and careful medical supervision can be continued. A plaster spica cast is often safer. If closed reduction is not possible or cannot be maintained, open reduction is required. X-rays to confirm reduction and its maintenance are essential to any form of treatment.

2. Eighteen months to 4 years—Preliminary traction and open reduction are more likely to be required in this group. If adequate reduction is obtained, more than 90% of patients should have satisfactory results.

3. Older children and adults—Treatment of newly diagnosed congenital hip dysplasia in this age group is difficult. Acetabular remodeling through growth is slight. Mere achievement of a concentric reduction does not ensure a stable pain-free hip. Choices of treatment are operation or no treatment at all. Several osteotomies of the innominate bone have been described for improving acetabular coverage of the femoral head. Pain and limitation of motion will eventually necessitate total hip arthroplasty for many of these individuals.

SLIPPED CAPITAL FEMORAL EPIPHYSIS

During the period of rapid growth in early adolescence, the normal relationship of the femoral head with the femoral neck may become distorted by a shearing displacement through the growth plate—so-called slipped capital femoral epiphysis. The head remains within the acetabulum, while the femoral neck shifts anteriorly and laterally. This displacement may occur rapidly, often in response to minor trauma, or it can be gradual, as indicated by reactive bone formation and remodeling of the femoral neck adjacent to the growth plate. An acute slip may be superimposed upon a gradual "chronic" one. An acute slip is not a traumatic injury to a normal growth plate but is a "pathologic fracture" through a plate that is abnormally weak. Boys are more likely to be affected than girls. Involvement is bilateral in at least 25% of cases. The condition is progressive and can lead to severe deformity and limitation of hip motion if untreated. Marked deformity may cause early degenerative joint disease and is associated with increased risk of avascular necrosis and chondrolysis, though it is difficult to differentiate between the natural history of the disease and the complications of its treatment.

Clinical Findings

A. SYMPTOMS AND SIGNS

The patient reports pain in the knee or groin, limps, and has limited hip motion, especially flexion, internal rotation, and abduction.

B. IMAGING STUDIES

Radiographs are diagnostic in all but the most minimal slips (Figure 43–41). The epiphysis is not centered on the neck, as is normally the case, but is relatively posterior and medial. Since posterior displacement is often

Figure 43–41. Left slipped capital femoral epiphysis. Note that a line extended along the lateral side of the femoral neck misses the capital epiphysis. On the normal right side, this line enters the femoral head, which should overlap the neck on both anteroposterior and lateral views.

more marked, the deformity may not be as evident on the anteroposterior view as on the lateral view. Bony callus, or widening of the metaphysis adjacent to the growth plate, indicates a chronic slip. A significant slip produces a bony prominence on the anterolateral femoral neck, restricting hip motion.

Treatment

Surgical stabilization of the proximal femoral epiphysis is advised. As soon as the diagnosis is made, the patient is hospitalized and placed in skin traction. An internal rotation strap may help reduce an acute slip; this is preferable to forceful manipulation under anesthesia, which increases the risk of avascular necrosis. In situ pinning of the epiphysis is then performed. The surgeon should make sure that pins do not enter the joint space. Gradual mobilization with protected weightbearing follows. The goal of pinning is to prevent further slip and gain closure of the physis. The opposite side must be watched until it closes because of the significant risk of its slipping as well. If severe deformity prevents normal motion, a subtrochanteric osteotomy or excision of the bony hump may be considered. Interference with function rather than abnormality on radiographs is the indication for such procedures.

LEGG-PERTHES DISEASE (Legg-Calve-Perthes Disease; Coxa Plana)

Legg-Perthes disease is an uncommon hip affliction that occurs in about one in 2000 children, generally between the ages of 4 and 10. Boys are affected five times as often as girls, who tend to have more severe involvement. About 10–15% of patients have bilateral disease. The process is self-limited and of unknown cause. Its hallmark is avascular necrosis of the capital femoral epiphysis. When avascular necrosis of the femoral head occurs in adults, little potential exists for reconstitution of dead bone; however, the growing child with Legg-Perthes disease is able to completely replace the necrotic bone with new live bone. Some patients achieve normal hip development. Others acquire permanent deformity of the femoral head, with limited motion and degenerative joint disease becoming symptomatic in middle age.

Determinants of Final Outcome

A. STAGE OF ILLNESS

The earliest signs are an apparent increase in density of the capital epiphysis and thickening of the surrounding cartilage. As revascularization occurs, femoral head density increases, a subchondral crescent-shaped radiolucent fracture appears transiently, and the metaphysis

may widen. The epiphysis itself appears irregular and flattened. Gradually, living bone replaces cartilage and fibrous tissue, so that the femoral head is completely ossified. The ultimate shape will depend upon the molding of the malleable head during replacement of the necrotic epiphysis. A spherical head correlates well with good long-term results.

B. AGE OF PATIENT

Younger patients have a better prognosis. They are lighter in weight, have more rapid healing of necrotic bone, and have more growth time in which remodeling of residual deformity may occur.

C. SEVERITY OF INVOLVEMENT

Catterall has classified patients with Legg-Perthes disease into four groups—according to the extent of involvement of the epiphysis—from group I, with only the anterior part of the epiphysis involved, to group IV, with involvement of the entire head. The extent of involvement is an indicator of the likelihood that the femoral head will deform and thus helps suggest the outcome for a given patient.

D. THE "HEAD AT RISK"

Catterall also proposed certain clinical and radiographic criteria for determining whether the femoral head might deform in the course of the disease. The clinical criteria are (1) obesity, (2) decreasing range of motion of the involved hip, and (3) adduction contracture. The radiographic criteria are (1) lateral subluxation of the femoral head, (2) Gage's sign (widening of the lateral part of the growth plate, so that the superior portion of the femoral neck appears convex), (3) calcification lateral to the epiphysis in the cartilaginous femoral head, (4) diffuse metaphysial reaction, and (5) a horizontal growth plate. Others agree that these signs are helpful indications of which patients are likely to have a poor outcome and might thus benefit from treatment aimed at maintaining a spherical femoral head.

Clinical Findings

A. SYMPTOMS AND SIGNS

Insidious development of limp and sometimes pain in the groin, anterior thigh, or knee eventually bring the patient to a physician. An occasional case presents as acute synovitis. Examination shows antalgic gait, decreased hip motion (especially abduction and internal rotation), and sometimes flexion-adduction contracture. Passive motion is guarded rather than free.

B. LABORATORY FINDINGS

Bone scan may help with early diagnosis and assessment of the extent of head involvement.

C. IMAGING STUDIES

Well-exposed radiographs in both anteroposterior and frog-leg lateral views are essential. If synovitis significantly limits hip motion, a period in traction may be required before adequate positioning can be achieved. Findings will depend upon the stage and severity of disease, as discussed above, but initial films usually show increased density and deformity of the femoral head epiphysis, which may be flattened or fragmented (Figure 43–42).

Differential Diagnosis

The early inflammatory stage of Legg-Perthes disease can be confused with toxic synovitis, septic (including tuberculous) arthritis, and rheumatoid arthritis. The epiphysial abnormalities are similar to those seen in epiphysial dysplasias, hypothyroidism, and avascular necrosis from other causes, notably sickle cell anemia, Gaucher's disease, and chronic use of corticosteroid drugs.

Treatment

Rational treatment requires categorization according to the stage of disease, the extent of head involvement, and the condition of the hip joint at the time of presentation. The mobility of the involved joint must be determined and then followed as an important indicator of prognosis.

A. OBSERVATION

Treatment is unnecessary and contraindicated for the following patients: children with involvement of less than half the femoral head, young children (under 5 years of age) without "at risk" signs, and children who

Figure 43–42. X-ray of Legg-Perthes disease, with significant deformity of right femoral head.

already show radiologic evidence of healing. If significant deformity exists and insufficient growth time remains for remodeling, only symptomatic treatment is appropriate.

B. REST AND TRACTION

If joint motion is limited, bed rest and traction are employed to decrease synovitis and muscle spasm. Muscle releasing procedures may be required if contractures have developed. Once the hip is mobilized, containment of the femoral head within the acetabulum is necessary to maintain its spherical shape. If it is allowed to extrude laterally from the acetabulum, it will become deformed.

C. BRACING

Containment can be achieved with bracing, which should be maintained until reossification is under way; an average of 18 months is required.

D. SURGICAL TREATMENT

An alternative to prolonged bracing is surgery to reorient the acetabulum or the proximal femur to achieve containment. Both innominate osteotomy and varus proximal femoral osteotomy have advocates. Surgical containment properly achieved appears to be as effective as containment by bracing and to be much more expeditious.

Prognosis

Prolonged follow-up is necessary to determine the outcome. Poor results on x-rays do correlate positively with pain, limited motion, and disability. However, the affected hip may not be symptomatic for years. If Legg-Perthes disease of all degrees of severity is untreated, 55% of patients report good results and 45% report fair and poor results. If group I patients are excluded, the figures can be reversed. Following osteotomy of selected patients with more severe disease, two-thirds or more are reported to have a favorable outcome.

FOOT DEFORMITIES IN CHILDREN

Positional deformities of the foot are described with the following specific terms. Equinus refers to plantar flexion. Calcaneus is the opposite position, or dorsiflexion. Varus indicates angulation in the frontal plane, with inversion of the involved part. The forefoot alone may be in varus, or the deformity may be present in the hindfoot as well. Valgus is the opposite of varus and implies eversion of the involved part. Inversion and eversion of the forefoot (metatarsus) describe rotation about the long axis of the foot. Adduction of the forefoot is the term used to distinguish deviation of the metatarsals toward the medial side of the foot without the rotational component suggested by the term varus.

The goal of treatment of foot deformity is a pain-free, flexible, plantigrade foot—ie, a foot whose plantar surface is level with the ground during normal gait.

1. Clubfoot

Talipes equinovarus, or clubfoot, is most commonly an idiopathic congenital condition affecting approximately one in 1000 children. It occurs twice as often in boys and is bilateral half the time. There is a familial tendency, with a 5% chance that a sibling will also be affected.

Clinical Findings

A. Symptoms and Signs

In congenital clubfoot, there is more or less rigid inversion of the hindfoot, adduction of the forefoot, and limited dorsiflexion—an equinovarus deformity. While the cause is not certain, the deformity involves medial subluxation of the navicular and calcaneus on the talus. The joints principally involved are thus the subtalar and talonavicular joints. The adjacent ankle and midtarsal joints are affected to a lesser degree. The overlying soft tissues are contracted, and the longer the subluxation remains, the more deformed become the involved bones, which are composed largely of malleable cartilage. Successful treatment requires early reduction of joint subluxations and maintenance of correction throughout growth.

B. Imaging Studies

X-rays are useful primarily for assessing the adequacy of correction rather than for establishing the diagnosis of clubfoot. At birth, only the ossific nuclei of the calcaneus, talus, and metatarsals are present. Navicular ossification does not begin until about age 4. Therefore, radiographs of the newborn foot provide less information than the clinical examination. A good photograph documents the deformity more adequately. By 2–3 months of age, the ossification centers of the talus and calcaneus have elongated sufficiently to indicate their long axes, so that radiographs can provide helpful data about interosseous relationships. An anteroposterior view of a normal foot shows divergence of the talus and calcaneus, the former directed along the first ray and the latter along the fifth ray. In clubfoot, the talus usually points more laterally and may actually appear superimposed upon the calcaneus. On a lateral radiograph of a normal foot in maximal dorsiflexion, the calcaneus is dorsiflexed, so that its axis crosses that of the navicular, and the anterior ends of their shadows overlap. Clubfoot prevents this dorsiflexion and overlapping. Full

calcaneal dorsiflexion is a valuable radiographic indicator of adequate treatment.

Treatment

Initial treatment is always nonoperative and should be started as soon as possible, preferably the day the infant is born.

A. Manipulation

Gentle manipulation into a corrected position should be done in order to stretch the contracted soft tissues—specifically, to align the calcaneus and navicular relative to the talus. Gentleness is required to avoid tissue trauma and to prevent overcorrection of the forefoot relative to persisting tarsal deformity.

B. Casting

After several minutes of manipulation, a plaster cast is applied and molded to maintain the maximally corrected position. Manipulation and cast application should be repeated weekly.

Casts are advisable for at least 6 months, followed by a Denis Browne bar with attached out-flare shoes. Similar shoes are worn when the child begins to walk, but the Denis Browne bar splinting should be continued at night and during nap times for several more years. During this time, close follow-up is required, with immediate use of a plaster cast if deformity recurs. Correction achieved by age 7 years is usually permanent. Carefully and conscientiously pursued, nonoperative treatment has been sufficient to correct clubfoot deformity in 35–90% of cases in large series. If satisfactory correction has not been achieved by age 3 months, operative management should be considered.

C. Surgical Treatment

Operations for clubfoot are many and varied. The present trend is toward a single combined procedure to release all of the posteromedial contracted tissues and permit open realignment of the talonavicular and talocalcaneal joints. Temporary percutaneous wire fixation is advocated by some surgeons. Postoperative care requires persistent follow-up and prolonged support in a plaster cast, splints, and special shoes. Satisfactory results from posteromedial release are reported in 75–85% of patients. Triple arthrodesis and other surgical procedures provide salvage for symptomatic patients in whom posteromedial release does not provide good results.

2. Metatarsus Adductus

The terms "metatarsus varus" and "metatarsus adductus" are used more or less interchangeably for deformity characterized by medial "hooking" of the forefoot. The adduction is at the tarsometatarsal joint, and the hindfoot is either in neutral position or in valgus. Metatarsus adductus is somewhat commoner than clubfoot and seems to have a stronger familial tendency. The deformity is often quite mobile. If passively correctable, there is an 85% chance of spontaneous correction by age 3 years. No treatment is required if stroking of the lateral border of the foot provokes active correction. Easy passive correction also suggests that treatment is unnecessary. If the forefoot cannot readily be returned to a normal position, restoring a concave lateral border to the foot, treatment is advisable. The surgeon stabilizes the hindfoot with one hand while manipulating the forefoot to correct the deformity with the other hand. A well-molded plaster cast is applied to maintain this position. The cast is changed every 1–2 weeks for 6–8 weeks, followed by night splints for several months. Only a very rare severe deformity will require surgical release or osteotomy and fusion of the tarsometatarsal joints.

Cook DA et al: Observer variability in the radiographic measurement and classification of metatarsus adductus. J Pediatr Orthop 1992;12:86.

3. Flatfoot

The normal newborn foot appears flat because subcutaneous fat fills the longitudinal arch. This fat deposit recedes over the first 4 years of life to reveal the typical adult appearance of a medial arch under the midfoot, which does not touch the floor with weightbearing. An inadequate bony arch, which permits the medial portion of the midfoot to bear weight, is the essential feature of true flatfoot. This deformity is classified as rigid or flexible.

Rigid flatfoot is identified by the absence of normal mobility of the foot. Obvious deformity with convexity of the sole is present in congenital convex pes valgus, where congenital dorsal dislocation of the talonavicular joint is the cause. Early open reduction is advisable. Rigid flatfoot presenting later in childhood is usually due to coalition of the tarsal bones. Associated episodic foot pain and spasm of the peroneal muscles are typical. Depending on the child's age and symptoms and the site of coalition, resection may be advisable or nonoperative treatment may suffice.

In flexible flatfoot, weightbearing obliterates the medial arch and also produces obvious valgus alignment of the calcaneus. Standing on tiptoes or sitting with the feet hanging free will restore the arch and substantially correct heel valgus. Some patients with flexible flatfoot develop foot pain with weightbearing. Pain may range from minimal to severely incapacitating and is not clearly related to the severity of the deformity.

Treatment of asymptomatic flexible flatfoot in children is controversial. Parents distressed by the foot's appearance or by abnormal shoe wear often request treatment, but there is little evidence that treatment prevents future symptoms, and many young children with flexible flatfoot have minimal deformity or symptoms in adulthood.

The child with painful flexible flatfoot deformity deserves treatment. Exercises to stretch tight gastrocsoleus muscle groups or to strengthen intrinsic plantar muscles are usually advised, and external support for the mediolongitudinal arch can be provided if necessary by flexible or rigid arch supports or shoe modifications. If nonoperative treatment fails to control symptoms or if deformity precludes use of normal footwear, surgery may be considered. Many procedures have been proposed. If present, an accessory navicular may be excised, with transposition of an abnormally inserted tibialis posterior tendon. Ligament reconstructions, arthrodeses, and osteotomies may be used separately or in combination to attempt restoration of the arch. A major risk of all such procedures is that a flexible deformity will be exchanged for a potentially more painful rigid one.

Briggs TW, Orr MM, Lightowler CD: Isolated tibial fractures in children. Injury 1992;23:308.

Caine D et al: Stress changes of the distal radial growth plate: a radiographic survey and review of the literature. Am J Sports Med 1992;20:290.

Heath CH, Staheli LT: Normal limits of knee angle in white children: genu varum and genu valgum. J Pediatr Orthop 1993;13:259.

Heinrich SD et al: Stabilization of pediatric diaphyseal femur fractures with flexible intramedullary nails (a technique paper). J Orthop Trauma 1992;6:452.

Henderson RC, Kemp GJ, Campion ER: Residual bone-mineral density and muscle strength after fractures of the tibia or femur in children. J Bone Joint Surg Am 1992;74:211

Hennrikus WL et al: The function of the quadriceps muscle after a fracture of the femur in patients who are less than seventeen years old. J Bone Joint Surg Am 1993;75:508.

Hope PG, Cole WG: Open fractures of the tibia in children. J Bone Joint Surg Br 1992;74:546.

Kling TF Jr et al: Distal tibial physeal injuries in children that may require open reduction. J Bone Joint Surg Am 1984;66:647.

Krueger-Franke M, Siebert CH, Pfoerringer W: Sports-related epiphyseal injuries of the lower extremity: an epidemiologic study. J Sports Med Phys Fitness 1992;32:106.

Krueger-Franke M, Siebert CH, Pfoerringer W: Sports-related epiphyseal injuries of the lower extremity: an epidemiologic study. J Sports Med Phys Fitness 1992;32:106.

Levy J, Ward WT: Pediatric femur fractures: an overview of treatment. Orthopedics 1993;16:183.

Marcinko DE, Azzolini TJ, Mariash SA: Enigma of pediatric vertical talus deformity. J Foot Surg 1990;29:452.

Meyers MC et al: Delayed treatment of a malreduced distal femoral epiphyseal plate fracture. Med Sci Sports Exerc 1992;24:1311.

Oestreich AE, Ahmad BS: The periphysis and its effect on the metaphysis: I: definition and normal radiographic pattern. Skeletal Radiol 1992;21:283.

Salo JM et al: Congenital flat foot: different clinical forms. Acta Orthop Belg 1992;58:406.

Salter RB, Best TN: Pathogenesis of progressive valgus deformity following fractures of the proximal metaphyseal region of the tibia in young children. Instr Course Lect 1992;41:409.

■ PAIN SYNDROMES

PAIN SYNDROMES OF THE SHOULDER

1. Painful Arc Syndrome (Rotator Cuff Tendinitis, Subacromial Bursitis)

 ESSENTIALS OF DIAGNOSIS

- *Pain over the anterior or lateral shoulder, most severe during abduction.*
- *Restriction of joint motion.*

General Considerations

Inflammation within the glenohumeral joint is the most frequent cause of shoulder pain and limitation of motion. The patient is typically middle-aged. Repeated minor trauma from occupational or sports activity is the cause, and the most common site of inflammation at onset is the rotator cuff, particularly the supraspinatus tendon. The location of the supraspinatus tendon between the greater tuberosity of the humeral head and the overhanging acromion process renders it particularly vulnerable to mechanical compression. Rotator cuff inflammation will often spill over into the subacromial bursa, and subdeltoid soreness frequently radiates along the lateral humerus to the deltoid insertion.

Clinical Findings

Active abduction becomes especially painful when the shoulder moves between 60 and 120 degrees because the inflamed rotator cuff and overlying bursa are compressed beneath the acromion. Because of this characteristic feature, the condition is known as painful arc syndrome. The range of active abduction may be extended if the patient is instructed to rotate the arms so that the palms face upward. This rotates the greater tuberosity posteriorly, so that the attached rotator cuff tendons pass behind the acromion, resulting in diminished pain with continued abduction.

Treatment

Treatment of rotator cuff tendinitis and subacromial bursitis is with analgesics such as aspirin or nonsteroidal anti-inflammatory agents (naproxen, ibuprofen), and local application of cold packs. Physical therapy may be useful in preserving full range of motion. Slings and shoulder immobilization should not be used for more than a few days, since capsular adhesions and prolonged stiffness may result. Gentle passive range-of-motion exercises by a therapist or family member should be started as soon as tolerated, followed by active pendulum exercises consisting of circular swinging motions of the dangling arm while leaning forward. Active exercise is gradually increased while passive range of motion is extended with exercises such as pulley-enhanced abduction using a bath towel over a shower curtain rod.

If pain does not respond to oral anti-inflammatory agents, prolonged relief may be obtained by injecting 40 mg of methylprednisolone acetate (or equivalent) and 1–2 mL of lidocaine into the subacromial bursa. The patient should be warned that injection may produce a brief exacerbation of pain before relief is noted and should be provided with analgesic medications. When full function has been recovered, reduction of stressful activities should be advised.

2. CALCIFIC TENDINITIS

 ESSENTIALS OF DIAGNOSIS

- *Excruciating shoulder pain.*
- *Severe restriction of joint motion.*

General Considerations

Calcium deposition in the degenerative rotator cuff may lead to a variant form of tendinitis in the shoulder region. Asymptomatic bilateral calcium deposits in the shoulder tissues are a common finding in persons over age 40. The pathogenesis is unclear. The deposits may enlarge or rupture into the subacromial bursa.

Clinical Findings

A. SYMPTOMS AND SIGNS

The presentation of acute calcific tendinitis or bursitis is dramatic, with excruciating pain and severe restriction of shoulder motion. The patient may refuse even the gentlest examination for fear of motion-induced muscle spasm.

B. IMAGING STUDIES

X-rays reveal either focal calcium deposits within the rotator cuff or a large "cap" of calcium overlying the humeral head, which represents dissemination of calcium into the subacromial bursa.

Treatment

Treatment of acute calcific tendinitis includes immediate injection of a corticosteroid and lidocaine solution into the tendon near the calcium deposit or into the bursa if calcium has entered that structure. Multiple needle punctures into the calcium deposit may break up the deposit and provide dramatic relief. Mobilization of the shoulder should proceed as described in the preceding section.

3. Biceps Tendinitis

ESSENTIALS OF DIAGNOSIS

- *Localized tenderness over the bicipital groove.*
- *Pain during supination of the forearm against resistance.*

General Considerations

A common inflammatory lesion producing shoulder pain involves the biceps tendon in the bicipital groove. Biceps tendon inflammation usually affects individuals whose occupation involves repetitive biceps flexion against resistance or whose recreational activities include forceful throwing of a ball. Pain is prominent over the anterior aspect of the arm and is aggravated by shoulder motion. Symptoms are worse at night and improve with rest. Deltoid muscle spasm may be present and may limit both active and passive motion.

Clinical Findings

Biceps tendinitis can be distinguished from rotator cuff tendinitis by localization of tenderness to the bicipital groove. Forearm supination against resistance with the elbow flexed at the patient's side elicits extreme tenderness in the region of the bicipital groove when the tendon is palpated near the shoulder. Instability of the tendon in the groove is occasionally manifested by a snapping sensation as the arm is abducted and externally rotated. Subluxation of the tendons can be pro-

voked for diagnostic verification by Yergason's maneuver, in which the patient actively flexes the elbow against resistance while the physician rotates the humerus externally. An unstable tendon will "pop" out of the groove.

Treatment

Treatment of bicipital tendinitis includes cessation of offending activities and short-term immobilization of the shoulder in a sling; a trial of aspirin or nonsteroidal anti-inflammatory agents; and, occasionally, local injection of corticosteroids. Repeated corticosteroid injections may result in tendon attrition or rupture and should be avoided. Surgery is occasionally required to stabilize a subluxating tendon.

When discomfort has subsided, progressive mobilization is begun with exercises similar to those described in the section on rotator cuff tendinitis.

4. Adhesive Capsulitis (Frozen Shoulder)

ESSENTIALS OF DIAGNOSIS

- *Diffuse shoulder tenderness.*
- *Restriction of shoulder joint motion.*

General Considerations

A common cause of shoulder pain in middle-aged and elderly patients is adhesive capsulitis, or so-called frozen shoulder. This disorder may complicate other inflammatory shoulder ailments, particularly in individuals immobilized for prolonged periods. It may also occur without any identifiable inciting trauma and has been associated with cardiovascular disease, rheumatoid arthritis, and degenerative cervical spine disease. Though the exact pathogenesis is unknown, the end result is a chronically inflamed, contracted fibrotic capsule densely adherent to the humeral head, the acromion, and the underlying biceps and rotator cuff tendons. Normal bursae are obliterated by scarring.

Clinical Findings

A. SYMPTOMS AND SIGNS

The onset of symptoms is usually gradual and heralded by complaints of diffuse tenderness with disproportionately severe restriction of active and passive motion. Motion is not improved by lidocaine or corticosteroid injection.

B. Imaging Studies

Arthrography reveals a contracted joint capsule and no bursal filling. X-rays may reveal severe osteoporosis of the humeral head.

Treatment

The success of various treatments is difficult to assess, as the natural history of adhesive capsulitis is spontaneous resolution. Subsidence of pain and return of nearly full motion can be anticipated, though the process may persist for 6 months to several years. Efforts to speed return of function have included intensive physical therapy, oral corticosteroids and antiinflammatory agents, and a procedure called infiltration brisement, which consists of pressure injection of the joint with 50 mL of saline and corticosteroid solution in order to break the adhesions binding the capsule to the surrounding structures.

Clearly, the best treatment of this condition is prevention. Prolonged disuse or immobilization of a painful shoulder must be avoided. Early mobilization is stressed, with initiation of gentle range of motion exercises and persistent encouragement and guidance by the physician and the physical therapist.

Ekelund AL, Rydell N: Combination treatment for adhesive capsulitis of the shoulder. Clin Orthop 1992;(282): 105.

PAIN SYNDROMES OF THE ELBOW

1. Tennis Elbow (Humeral Epicondylitis)

ESSENTIALS OF DIAGNOSIS

- *Tenderness over the lateral humeral epicondyle.*
- *Pain at the elbow with flexion or extension of the wrist.*

General Considerations

Though far more common in nonathletes, humeral epicondylitis is commonly termed tennis elbow. This overuse syndrome is uncommon before age 18 years and most frequent in the fourth and fifth decades. Though frequently blamed on faulty backhand motion, tennis elbow is occasionally seen in professional players but is far more common in nonathletes performing activities that require frequent rotary motion of the forearm, such as gardening, use of screwdrivers or wrenches, turning of doorknobs, and even operation of vehicles without power-assisted steering.

Clinical Findings

Tennis elbow is characterized by tenderness and pain at the humeral epicondyle provoked by extension or flexion of the wrist, depending on which epicondyle is involved. The lateral aspect of the elbow is far more often involved, and the origin of the inflamed common extensor muscle is the source of discomfort. Underlying synovitis may accompany the tendinitis. The pain is readily reproduced with traction on the extensor muscles by passive flexion of the fingers and wrist with the elbow extended.

Though the pathogenesis of tennis elbow is unknown, symptoms are usually attributed to inflammation of the origin of the common extensor muscle and, in some cases, to a tear in the origin of the extensor carpi radialis brevis. The tears are thought to be the result of repeated stress on degenerated tendon fibers. Elbow motion remains normal.

Differential Diagnosis

Differential diagnosis includes radial nerve irritation at the elbow, which may often be delineated by electromyography.

Treatment

A. Medical Treatment

Most patients with tennis elbow respond favorably to a brief period of rest and administration of analgesics followed by a program of gradually increasing exercise to strengthen the forearm muscles. Anti-inflammatory drugs or subtendinous injection of soluble corticosteroids with lidocaine may be required in more severe cases. Repeated injections may further weaken tendons and should be avoided.

After the acute symptoms subside, a nonelastic forearm band is prescribed to be worn near the elbow during occupational or recreational activities that aggravate the condition. The band is thought to be effective either because it limits full contraction of the tender muscles or because it slightly alters the position of the extensor tendons. Tennis players are advised to warm up slowly. Changes in the tension of racket strings and racket size or composition may also be of benefit.

B. Surgical Treatment

Some patients with severe or refractory symptoms may require operative treatment. Most surgeons repair the origin of the torn wrist extensor tendon after excision of granulation tissue and any rough subjacent bone.

Lengthening of the short wrist extensor has also been advocated, though loss of strength has been reported with this procedure.

2. Olecranon Bursitis

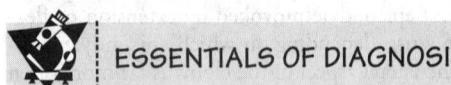

ESSENTIALS OF DIAGNOSIS

- Tenderness and swelling over the olecranon.
- Limitation of elbow flexion.

General Considerations

Olecranon bursitis is a common cause of periarticular elbow pain. Like epicondylitis, this condition is often related to occupational activities, in this case prolonged periods of leaning on the elbow while studying ("student's elbow"), gardening, working on plumbing, or carpentry.

Clinical Findings

A. SYMPTOMS AND SIGNS

The subcutaneous olecranon bursa becomes distended, sometimes to dramatic proportions. The skin of the extensor surface of the forearm may be edematous and pitted. Traumatic bursitis is often only mildly painful despite marked swelling.

B. LABORATORY FINDINGS

Because of the tenderness of the skin over the bursa, elbow motion is limited only in extreme flexion. Fluid obtained by aspiration demonstrates a predominance of mononuclear cells, with fewer than 1000 white cells per microliter. Red cells are numerous, and mucin clot formation is poor. Strict aseptic technique is advised during aspiration of the bursa, as superinfection is common after multiple aspirations. Penetration of the inner wall of the cavity must be avoided; in septic olecranon bursitis, penetration may result in inoculation of bacteria into the underlying triceps tendon, leading to disastrous extension of infection into the posterior aspect of the arm.

Differential Diagnosis

Laboratory findings will differentiate septic olecranon bursitis, in which aspiration fluid demonstrates a predominance of PMNs in far greater numbers. Gout may affect the olecranon bursa, but urate crystals are present.

Treatment

Treatment of idiopathic or traumatic olecranon bursitis consists of protecting the bursa from further pressure or irritation. Aspiration and compression dressings may be necessary if symptoms are prolonged. Recurrence is not uncommon. Water-soluble corticosteroid injection may be helpful once infection has been ruled out as a possible cause. Excision of the bursa may be required for rare persistent cases. The bursa must be totally excised and the overlying skin sutured to the olecranon periosteum to ensure obliteration of the space.

Labelle H et al: Lack of scientific evidence for the treatment of lateral epicondylitis of the elbow: an attempted meta-analysis. J Bone Joint Surg Br 1992;74:646.

Wittenberg RH, Schaal S, Muhr G: Surgical treatment of persistent elbow epicondylitis. Clin Orthop 1992;(278):73.

PAIN SYNDROMES OF THE HIP

1. Bursitis & Tendonitis of the Hip

Bursitis and tendonitis are frequent causes of pain around the hip area. These conditions most commonly affect middle-aged and elderly patients. Patients with a history of prior hip surgery, such as hip replacement or fixation of a hip fracture, may be especially prone to these conditions.

Clinical Findings

A. SYMPTOMS AND SIGNS

A common complaint is the inability to sleep or rest on the affected side. The painful area is localized over the prominence of the greater trochanter, and the pain is reproduced by firm palpation. Hip bursitis may be associated with tendonitis of the hip abductors that insert onto the greater trochanter. Pain due to tendonitis may be reproduced with active hip abduction against resistance.

It is important to differentiate extra-articular sources of hip pain such as bursitis and tendonitis from intra-articular sources such as osteoarthritis. Intra-articular pathology is suggested by pain localized to the groin or buttock, decreased passive internal rotation, and reproduction of the patient's pain at the limits of rotation.

B. IMAGING STUDIES

Plain radiographs are extremely useful in the evaluation of hip joint disorders.

Treatment

Trochanteric bursitis often responds to rest, oral anti-inflammatory medications, and ice. Corticosteroid injection is highly effective in refractory cases. Typically, a mixture of lidocaine and corticosteroid is injected into the areas of maximal tenderness. This often requires a spinal needle to reach the trochanteric bursa that lies just superficial to the trochanter itself. Rapid relief of symptoms confirms injection of the proper area. Treatment of hip abductor tendonitis should include stretching exercises in addition to anti-inflammatory medication and ice. Direct injection of steroid into the tendon should be avoided.

2. The Snapping Hip

The painful snapping hip is most commonly caused by the iliotibial band snapping over the prominence of the greater trochanter. Less commonly, the iliopsoas tendon may be the cause of pain as it snaps over the hip joint capsule.

Snapping due to the iliotibial band can be reproduced with passive flexion of the hip starting from an adducted position. Snapping of the iliopsoas tendon may be reproduced with passive extension and internal rotation of the hip starting from a flexed and externally rotated position. Fluoroscopy after injection of the iliopsoas bursa with contrast can help to confirm this diagnosis.

Treatment usually consists of stretching and strengthening exercises. In rare circumstances, surgical release may be indicated for refractory cases.

3. Avascular Necrosis of the Femoral Head

Avascular necrosis of the femoral head is a disease process that results in focal areas of bone death within the femoral head. Subsequent collapse and flattening of the head may occur. The usual area of involvement is the subchondral bone in the anteromedial portion of the femoral head. The precise cause is not fully understood, but it appears that the final common pathway is disruption of the microcirculation that supplies the cancellous bone within the femoral head.

The most frequent cause of avascular necrosis is prior trauma to the hip. In particular, hip dislocation and fractures of the femoral neck are associated with a high incidence of subsequent avascular necrosis. These types of trauma often result in disruption of the retinacular vessels that are the primary blood supply to the femoral head. Avascular necrosis may also occur in the absence of trauma. In many cases, a predisposing factor or factors can be identified. Known risk factors include the use of systemic steroids (even a single dose), alcohol abuse, blood dyscrasias such as sickle cell disease, Gaucher's disease, and radiation therapy.

Clinical Findings

A. SYMPTOMS AND SIGNS

Patients present with hip or groin pain that typically worsens with activity and weightbearing. On clinical examination, the patient may limp and have increased discomfort with passive internal rotation of the hip. The earliest stage of the disease may be asymptomatic. Because this disease is often bilateral (up to two-thirds of cases), careful evaluation of the opposite hip is essential.

B. IMAGING STUDIES

Plain radiographs serve as the basis for staging the extent of disease and to monitor its progression. MRI is extremely useful in identifying patients with the earliest stages of avascular necrosis, before abnormalities can be detected with plain radiographs.

Treatment

The treatment of avascular necrosis depends on the stage of the disease and the age of the patient. Patients identified with early stage disease, before collapse of the femoral head, may benefit from "core decompression," a procedure in which a reamer is used to create a channel into the affected area of the femoral head. The use of vascularized fibular grafts has also been advocated. However, these procedures are not uniformly successful, and the specific indications remain somewhat controversial.

Patients with more advanced disease, particularly elderly patients, may be good candidates for joint replacement surgery. Replacement may involve either the femoral side alone or both the femoral side and the acetabular side depending on the condition of the acetabular cartilage. Some surgeons prefer to replace both sides in all cases because of more consistent pain relief. Because of the limited durability of prosthetic hip joints, joint replacements in young patients should be reserved for those who have exhausted all conservative measures.

4. Osteoarthritis

 ESSENTIALS OF DIAGNOSIS

- Joint pain and stiffness.
- Pain increases with activity.
- Tenderness along joint line.
- Joint space narrowing and osteophytes on x-ray.

General Considerations

Osteoarthritis is commonly referred to as "wear and tear" arthritis. Patients present with complaints of joint pain and stiffness. Pain due to osteoarthritis constitutes the most common joint complaint for which patients seek medical attention. The onset of symptoms may be insidious or may be associated with mild trauma. It is common for patients to experience a waxing and waning course, but gradual progression is expected. The severity of symptoms, particularly pain, typically increases with activity. As the disease progresses, night pain becomes a more frequent complaint. Osteoarthritis affecting an otherwise normal joint is termed primary osteoarthritis, while disease that is the sequela of a specific event or condition, such as trauma or infection, is termed secondary osteoarthritis.

Osteoarthritis is the most common of all arthropathies. Onset of symptomatic disease is typically in the sixth decade. Most people over the age of 55 have some radiographic evidence of osteoarthritis, though less than half develop joint symptoms. Genetic factors may play a role in the development of osteoarthritis, but only a small fraction of patients have been found to carry genetic markers known to be associated with the disease.

Mechanical factors that result in abnormally high loads across joint surfaces are associated with the development of osteoarthritis. Such predisposing factors include limb malalignment, joint instability, damaged or resected menisci, and malreduced intra-articular fractures. At a cellular level, osteoarthritic chondrocytes exhibit abnormal responses to anabolic and catabolic signaling molecules. They also express increased levels of proteolytic enzymes that lead to extracellular matrix degradation. The matrix of osteoarthritic cartilage is characterized by alterations in the structure and relative abundance of its key structural components, collagen and proteoglycans. These changes make osteoarthritic cartilage a less effective bearing surface and contribute to a vicious cycle of cartilage degeneration and an ineffective repair response.

Clinical Findings

A. Symptoms and Signs

Patients with osteoarthritis complain of a painful joint or joints, particularly with increased levels of activity. The pain is often reproduced with passive motion and loading of the involved joint. Commonly, both active and passive ranges of motion are decreased. Crepitation and mild swelling may also be present. Associated findings include juxta-articular prominences from bone spurs and angular deformities, particularly varus or valgus deformities of the knee. Examination of an arthritic knee often reveals pain along the affected joint line, due either to the arthritis itself or to an associated degenerative meniscal tear.

B. Imaging Studies

Plain radiographs are the primary imaging tool used in the evaluation of osteoarthritis. Weight-bearing films are essential for complete evaluation of weightbearing joints. Special views, such as a bent knee posteroanterior projection, are often requested. Early findings include joint space narrowing, subchondral sclerosis, and early osteophyte formation. Later findings include progressive loss of joint space to the point of bone-on-bone contact, subchondral cyst formation, large osteophytes, joint subluxation, and even severe bone erosion.

Treatment

A. Bracing

Bracing may be effective treatment for a subset of patients with osteoarthritis. The benefits of bracing can be derived from immobilization of a painful joint (such as the use of an molded ankle support) or by decreasing the load across a joint (such as the use of an "unloader brace" for medial compartment arthritis of the knee).

B. Medical Treatment

Nonsteroidal anti-inflammatory drugs remain the mainstay for the pharmacologic treatment of osteoarthritis. The risk of gastrointestinal bleeding is of great concern, particularly with long-term use that is common for these patients. The recent introduction of COX-2 selective agents may decrease this complication. Acetaminophen may also be helpful. The role of nutritional supplements such as glucosamine and chondroitin sulfate remains unclear.

C. Surgical Treatment

Operation is indicated once more conservative measures prove inadequate in providing a level of function acceptable to the patient. Surgical options include joint debridement (either open or arthroscopic), osteotomy, joint fusion, joint reconstruction or resection, and joint replacement.

Joint debridement can be effective in delaying or preventing the need for more aggressive operative management. Joints such as the knee are particularly suitable for arthroscopic debridement, which is associated with minimal morbidity and, in some cases, lasting improvement.

Osteotomies are most commonly performed around the knee to treat isolated medial or lateral compartment degeneration. Osteotomies of the hip are performed to prevent progression of joint degeneration, particularly in patients felt to be too young for joint replacement.

Joint fusion can provide excellent pain relief at the expense of joint motion. Fusion of small joints, such as the interphalangeal joints, is well tolerated whereas fusion of large joints, such as the hip or knee, is often unsatisfactory. Nevertheless, fusion may be the procedure of choice, particularly in the case of active infection.

Some arthritic joints are amenable to reconstructive procedures that can provide effective and durable results. One example is reconstruction of the carpal-metacarpal joint of the thumb using a rerouted tendon and partial or total resection of the trapezium. In other cases, resection of the diseased joint itself may be an effective option, such as removal of the proximal row of carpal bones to treat wrist arthritis.

Prosthetic joint replacement has revolutionized the management of severe and disabling osteoarthritis. Hip, knee, or shoulder arthroplasty provides excellent pain relief and improved function and with current implants and techniques lasts 10 years or more in over 90% of cases. New bearing surfaces hold significant promise in extending the life of these implants even further. Replacements of the elbow, wrist, and ankle are performed less commonly. In general, these surgeries are not as consistently successful as the replacement of larger joints.

5. Rheumatoid Arthritis

ESSENTIALS OF DIAGNOSIS

- *Joint pain and swelling.*
- *Morning stiffness improving with activity.*
- *Elevated rheumatoid factor and ESR.*
- *Periarticular erosions and osteopenia on x-ray.*

General Considerations

Rheumatoid arthritis is a chronic systemic inflammatory, disease characterized by joint pain, swelling, and joint destruction. The incidence is 0.5–3% worldwide, increasing with age with a peak in the fifth decade. Women are affected three times as commonly as men. Rheumatoid arthritis in many cases results in partial or total disability and is associated with a shortened life expectancy.

The cause of rheumatoid arthritis is not known. However, the molecular and cellular basis of the disease is becoming clearer. The fundamental mechanism is characterized by dysregulation of the immune system with activation of inflammatory cells, including T cells, B cells, monocytes, and macrophages. These activated immune cells secrete factors that lead to chronic inflammation, cartilage destruction, and soft-tissue damage.

Clinical Findings

A. SYMPTOMS AND SIGNS

The onset and clinical course of rheumatoid arthritis are variable. A gradual onset with polyarticular involvement is the most common clinical presentation. About 20% of patients have disease that will abate within 2 years, and perhaps 5% will remain in long-term remission. The remainder will have either multiple flares or a progressive course. Major clinical features of active disease include symmetric polyarthritis with joint swelling, tenderness, and morning stiffness lasting an hour or longer. Involvement of the synovium and soft tissues precedes erosion of the cartilage and bone. The hands and feet often are the first sites to be affected with inflammation, joint and tendon subluxation, and, in later stages, joint destruction and tendon rupture. Rheumatoid arthritis affects mainly small and medium-sized joints. The joints most frequently involved are the metacarpophalangeal, proximal interphalangeal, and metatarsophalangeal joints. Less commonly affected joints include the wrist, elbow, shoulder, hip, knee, and mid foot. In addition, the upper cervical spine is frequently involved.

B. LABORATORY FINDINGS

Although no specific laboratory test can be used to make the diagnoses of rheumatoid arthritis, a high titer of rheumatoid factor is present in 80% of patients. The acute-phase reactants, markers, erythrocyte sedimentation rate, and C-reactive protein are also commonly elevated. Antinuclear antibodies are often present in patients with severe rheumatoid arthritis, but their presence is not specific for the disease. Joint aspiration during an acute flare typically reveals 500–25,000 leukocytes/μL.

C. IMAGING STUDIES

The typical radiographic findings in rheumatoid arthritis include periarticular erosions and osteopenia. Joint space narrowing occurs in later stages of the disease. Advanced changes include bone resorption, deformity, dislocation, and fragmentation. In addition, protrusio acetabuli (medial migration of the femoral head into the pelvis) is not uncommonly seen in rheumatoid arthritis as well as in other forms of inflammatory arthritis.

Differential Diagnosis

Rheumatoid arthritis is usually easily distinguished from osteoarthritis based upon presentation, physical examination, and radiographic findings. Other inflammatory arthritides that may mimic rheumatoid arthritis include psoriatic arthritis, Reiter's syndrome, and arthritis associated with systemic lupus erythematosus, hepatitis, and inflammatory bowel disease. The differential diagnosis is more difficult in early stages of rheumatoid arthritis when joint involvement may be monoarticular and relatively mild. Joint aspiration to rule out infectious arthritis and crystal-induced arthritis may be indicated.

Treatment

A. SPLINTING

When acute inflammation is present, rest and splinting of joints can decrease symptoms and limit deformity. In particular, splinting small joints of the hand may prevent the development and progression of finger flexion and hyperextension deformities.

B. MEDICAL TREATMENT

1. Nonsteroidal anti-inflammatory drugs (NSAIDs)—NSAIDs reduce inflammation and pain but rarely eliminate altogether the symptoms of active rheumatoid arthritis. Both nonselective and COX-2 selective agents are utilized. Although COX-2 selective drugs have a more favorable safety profile, their efficacy is not substantially different from that of the nonselective agents. There is no convincing evidence that these drugs affect long-term progression of the disease.

2. Corticosteroids—Corticosteroids are potent suppressors of inflammation and are highly effective in controlling severe polyarticular disease. However, the detrimental effects of systemic corticosteroids are well described and they should be used sparingly. Intraarticular steroid injection can provide temporary relief of joint symptoms without associated systemic effects.

3. Disease-modifying antirheumatic drugs (DMARDs)—DMARDs are a diverse class of agents that target the mechanisms responsible for tissue destruction in rheumatoid arthritis. Their use is associated with reduced morbidity and mortality in patients with rheumatoid arthritis. Combination therapy is often employed for better disease control. The most commonly used agent in the United States is methotrexate. Other DMARDs include hydroxychloroquine, sulfasalazine, cyclosporine, and azathioprine. Some traditional agents, such as penicillamine and gold, are now less frequently used with the advent of more effective agents that have better-understood mechanisms of action.

4. Anticytokine agents—This new class of drugs (infliximab, etanercept) shows great promise in the treatment of rheumatoid arthritis. These agents specifically target cytokines that are key mediators of the inflammatory response.

C. SURGICAL TREATMENT

1. Synovectomy—In early stages of the disease, synovectomy of tendon sheaths can be effective in preventing or delaying some tendon ruptures. Open or arthroscopic synovectomy of affected joints may have a limited role in providing symptomatic relief but does not affect the long-term prognosis.

2. Joint fusion—Joint fusion is effective in providing pain relief and correction of joint deformity at the expense of joint motion. In many cases, joint motion is already severely restricted by the disease. Fusion is commonly performed for joints of the hand and wrist with good long-term results.

3. Joint replacement—Joint replacement for patients with advanced rheumatoid arthritis can provide excellent pain relief and function. Joints that are commonly replaced include the hip, knee, shoulder, elbow, and metacarpophalangeal joints. Because patients with rheumatoid arthritis generally are not as active as patients with osteoarthritis, the question of implant durability in younger patients is less of a concern.

Howie DW, Cornish BL, Vernon-Roberts B: The viability of the femoral head after resurfacing hip arthroplasty in humans. Clin Orthop 1993;(291):171.

Lafforgue P et al: Early-stage avascular necrosis of the femoral head: MR imaging for prognosis in 31 cases with at least 2 years of follow-up. Radiology 1993;187:199.

Sadat-Ali M: Avascular necrosis of the femoral head in sickle cell disease: an integrated classification. Clin Orthop 1993; (290):200.

Swiontkowski MF et al: The effect of fracture on femoral head blood flow: osteonecrosis and revascularization studied in miniature swine. Acta Orthop Scand 1993;64:196.

Takatori Y et al: Avascular necrosis of the femoral head: natural history and magnetic resonance imaging. J Bone Joint Surg Br 1993;75:217.

PAIN SYNDROMES OF THE NECK

1. Cervical Strain

 ESSENTIALS OF DIAGNOSIS

- *Paraspinous neck pain with or without radiation to the shoulder.*
- *Limitation of neck rotation.*

General Considerations

Neck pain is a common complaint in most outpatient clinics. It has been estimated that at any given time in the general population, one of every ten persons is suffering from neck and arm pain. Taking all ages together, 40% of all persons have suffered from neck and arm pain at some time. In most cases, symptoms are mild and self-limited.

Cervical muscle strain is perhaps the most frequent cause. Patients are usually in their forties or fifties. Symptoms typically appear within 24 hours after an episode of overexertion or in response to prolonged tension or poor posture.

Clinical Findings

A. SYMPTOMS AND SIGNS

Pain is most intense in the paraspinous muscles, within the superior trapezius fibers between the spine and the scapula, or at the periosteal site of muscle attachments in the scapula or occiput. Discomfort is characterized as deep aching or a boring sensation, and pain may occasionally radiate to the posterior shoulder or upper arm. This symptom complex is often difficult to differentiate from radicular pain. Discrete "trigger points"—specific points of deep tenderness—may be present. Spasm within the trapezius, levator scapulae, or paraspinous muscles may be palpable as a firm "knot." The neck is held in a guarded position with the head slightly flexed. Active and passive motion of the neck are often limited by voluntary splinting of the painful muscles. Rotation of the head away from the afflicted side is often resisted. The patient may also complain of headache or dizziness. The neurologic examination is always normal.

B. IMAGING STUDIES

X-ray examination may show some straightening of the cervical spine. Mild or severe degenerative changes may be present, including osteophytes of the vertebral bodies or posterior facets. Radiographs are often normal.

Differential Diagnosis

The differential diagnosis includes cervical spondylosis or herniated cervical disk. A patient with a herniated cervical disk will complain of radicular symptoms in a specific dermatomal distribution corresponding to the affected disk level. These patients will often exhibit abnormalities in the neurologic examination such as muscle weakness in the corresponding myotomes, diminished reflexes, and diminished sensation or paresthesias. Pain arising from cervical spondylosis is often indistinguishable from that due to cervical strain. Whatever the precise anatomic source of pain, distinguishing cervical muscle sprain from early degenerative disk symptoms is

of little importance, since both conditions are usually self-limited and are best managed conservatively.

Treatment

Treatment of acute cervical spine pain consists primarily of rest and immobilization. If pain is severe, mild halter traction may help to alleviate some of the pain arising from paraspinous muscle spasm. Halter traction with 2.5–3.5 kg (5–7 lb) may be used conveniently at home by most patients. Hospitalization is rarely required or indicated in the treatment of these patients. Analgesics and muscle relaxants are prescribed as needed to facilitate rest. Limited use of a soft collar to keep the head in a slightly flexed position may be helpful for daily function. To prevent both cervical muscle atrophy and psychologic dependence, the collar should not be used for more than 1–2 weeks. Injection of trigger points with 0.5% lidocaine, acupuncture, or electrical stimulation may help to alleviate spasm. Ice or heating pads may also diminish discomfort.

Severe neck pain from cervical strain often subsides within 1 week. When acute pain has subsided, the patient should begin exercises to strengthen cervical muscles and improve posture. Exercises are isometric and may be performed at home after instruction by the therapist. When all pain has resolved, range of motion exercises are added to improve flexibility.

Prevention of flare-ups also depends upon maintenance of good posture with avoidance of overhead work, long automobile rides, or prolonged cervical flexion and extension posture. Patients are cautioned to avoid sleeping in the prone position, which places the neck in excessive extension. A cylindric pillow (cervical pillow) may help to keep the neck in neutral position during sleep.

Course & Prognosis

The prognosis in cervical pain syndrome not associated with disk degeneration is good if the above measures are undertaken. Symptoms may recur, but early institution of home traction and avoidance of offending activities greatly limit the duration of pain.

2. Whiplash Injury

 ESSENTIALS OF DIAGNOSIS

- *Pain in paraspinous muscles radiating to arms.*
- *Occipital headache.*
- *Limitation of neck rotation.*

General Considerations

A well-known type of soft tissue injury of the neck is the acceleration-deceleration injury called **whiplash.** The most common cause is a rear-end automobile collision during which the trunk of the victim's body is rapidly accelerated by the force of impact and the head is "left behind" because of lack of head contact with the seat. Head acceleration (which is an angular acceleration) is always greater than vehicle acceleration. In experimental models, a 10 mph impact produced 11 g of angular acceleration of the head. Acute hyperextension injures the anterior soft tissue structures of the neck, including the anterior longitudinal ligament, the intervertebral disk, the strap muscles, and the esophagus. The longus colli and sternocleidomastoid muscles are particularly vulnerable. The cervical sympathetic plexus may also be injured. The hyperextension movement also overloads and injures the posterior facet joints. When acceleration of the vehicle stops, the head recoils into flexion, leading to injuries to the facet capsules, posterior ligaments, and paraspinal musculature.

Clinical Findings

A. Symptoms and Signs

The symptom complex following whiplash injury is highly variable. Onset of pain may be delayed as long as 24 hours. Neck pain and stiffness are the most common symptoms. Occipital headaches and retro-ocular pain are also frequently noted. The presence of numbness in the medial hand and forearm has been attributed to scalenus muscle spasm. Visual blurring may result from stretch injury to the cervical sympathetic plexus, and Horner's syndrome may rarely occur. Dysphagia may represent retropharyngeal hematoma or swelling. Vertebral artery spasm occasionally causes tinnitus, dizziness, and vertigo. When the neck is rotated at the time of injury, symptoms are more pronounced on the side toward which the head is turned.

Physical findings are usually attributable to muscle spasm and only rarely to nerve root compression or disk herniation. Spasm is manifested by diminished neck motion and predominant anterior paracervical tenderness to palpation. Posterolateral pain may occur if articular facet joint damage is present. Neurologic examination, including testing of reflexes and muscle strength, is often normal.

B. Imaging Studies

X-rays are usually normal. Care must be taken to avoid overlooking subtle hyperextension injuries such as widening of an anterior disk space, avulsion fractures of the anterior vertebral body, retropharyngeal swelling, or fracture of the posterior facet. Loss of cervical lordosis may imply spasm but may also be artifactual. Reversal of cervical lordosis, resulting in an S-shaped (swan-neck) deformity, signifies damage to the posterior joints. The kyphosis is most often seen at the C4–5 and C5–6 levels.

Treatment

Management of whiplash injuries is as for other soft tissue injuries—analgesics, rest, and immobilization in a soft cervical collar until the pain is controlled, followed by gradual mobilization. Isometric strengthening exercises are initiated when range of motion normalizes. Occasionally, facet injections may be both therapeutic and diagnostic.

Course & Prognosis

Most patients respond well to conservative measures, though anticipated litigation may complicate management. However, up to 45% of patients continue to have symptoms at 2 years even if their litigation has been settled. Degenerative changes in the cervical spine and minor neck discomfort are more common following whiplash injuries, but persistent pain and prolonged disability are unusual.

3. Degenerative Cervical Disc Disease (Cervical Spondylosis)

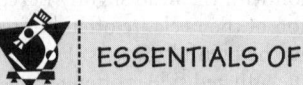 ESSENTIALS OF DIAGNOSIS

- *Neck pain radiating down the arm.*
- *Muscle weakness.*
- *Dermatomal sensory changes.*

General Considerations

The degenerative changes typically associated with aging are collectively termed spondylosis of the cervical spine. Men and women are affected equally. Among persons over age 50, radiologic signs of degeneration of the cervical spine are extremely common. It is estimated that by the seventh decade, 75% of individuals demonstrate such degeneration, though most are asymptomatic. Disk degeneration is therefore considered a natural aging phenomenon.

Cervical spondylosis is characterized initially by tears in the posterior annulus followed by softening and fragmentation of the disk. The weakest area of the annulus is the posterolateral region, which is the commonest site of bulging of the disk. The hydrostatic support provided by the degenerating disk steadily diminishes, and the adjacent vertebral bodies converge. The longitudinal ligaments become lax and are stripped from their bony attachments by the bulging disks. Degenerative calcification of the ligaments produces the familiar bony spurs. The ligamentum flavum also becomes lax and may bulge into the spinal canal. The posterolateral regions of the vertebral bodies become closely approximated and ultimately form an area of friction. These so-called uncovertebral joints of Luschka become increasingly hypertrophic, creating prominent spurs that may encroach onto the neural foramen and spinal canal.

As the vertebral bodies converge because of loss of disk support, the facet joints become subluxated as the superior facet slides posteriorly. Mechanical dysfunction of the joints results in osteoarthritic degeneration and osteophyte formation. Osteophytes about the facets may project into the intervertebral foramina and impinge upon the exiting nerve roots.

Clinical Findings

A. Symptoms and Signs

Clinical symptoms may or may not accompany the degenerative changes of cervical spondylosis. Neurologic compromise may result from nerve root compression (cervical spondylotic radiculopathy) or compression of the cord itself (cervical spondylotic myelopathy). Very rarely, vertebral artery and radicular artery stenosis may occur from osteophyte formation. This may cause vertebrobasilar insufficiency or cervical cord ischemia.

1. Cervical spondylotic radiculopathy—Cervical spondylotic radiculopathy results from pressure on a nerve root as it emerges from the cord to pass peripherally through the intervertebral foramen. A bulging or herniated disk or osteophytes are usually the cause of the compression. The onset of symptoms may be acute or insidious. Patients will usually complain of neck pain with radiation into the infrascapular area.

2. Cervical spondylotic myelopathy—Cervical spondylotic myelopathy is the most common form of spinal cord dysfunction in people over the age of 55. Patients over age 60 are more likely to have multisegmental disease. Spinal cord compression is caused by a combination of factors, including anterior and posterior osteophytes, bulging or herniated intervertebral disks, and a buckled ligamentum flavum. In the Japanese population, ossification of the posterior longitudinal ligament is a common cause of multisegmental cervical compression and myelopathy.

In addition to the mechanical compression of the spinal cord, vascular insufficiency from compression of the anterior spinal artery and the radicular arteries contributes to the neurologic injury. The severity of the myelopathy is dependent upon three factors: (1) the degree of initial compression on the spinal cord, (2) the length of time over which the compression occurs, and (3) the constancy or intermittency of the compressive force. The average space available for the spinal cord in the subaxial cervical spine is between 17 mm and 18 mm. Cervical stenosis is felt to exist if the space available for the spinal cord is less than 13 mm (Figure 43–43). It is important to note that these measurements are taken using the lateral cervical spine radiograph with the neck in neutral position. In the case of multisegmental disease, the actual space available for the cord may be much smaller when the neck is extended.

The symptoms of cervical myelopathy occur and progress very gradually, with functional losses occurring over many years in a "stepladder" type distribution. Radicular pain is often absent, and it may be a long time before the patient seeks medical attention. A few patients demonstrate steadily progressive deterioration leading to spastic paraplegia or quadriplegia.

The patient usually complains of "numbness" in the arms and legs and often of clumsiness and burning in

Figure 43–43. The space available for the spinal cord in the subaxial cervical spine can be measured as the developmental anterior-posterior diameter (DAPD) in patients with developmental spinal stenosis and as the spondylolytic anterior-posterior diameter (SAPD) in patients with cervical spondylosis.

the hands and difficulty in handling small objects. Walking is difficult initially because of balance problems and later due to loss of motor strength. Diffuse, nonlocalized "pins and needles" in the forearm and anterior thigh are also typical. Neck pain may be present or absent, but neck motion is frequently limited.

When myelopathy is precipitated by trauma, symptoms are similar to those described above. Hyperextension injuries in the face of preexisting cervical stenosis causes the classic central cord syndrome with quadriparesis. Limb involvement is usually more symmetric, with more weakness in the arms and hands than in the lower extremities. The acute injury generally subsides, though neurologic deficits frequently persist.

Physical examination of patients with spondylotic myelopathy is characterized by marked motor findings and relatively few sensory changes. Spasticity is present in the upper and lower extremities. Clonus and hyperreflexia are common though often asymmetric. An inverted radial reflex and a scapulohumeral reflex may also be seen. Long tract signs, including positive Babinski and Hoffman signs, may be present. Fine motion of the fingers is often lacking, and intrinsic muscle wasting may be profound. The patient may have an abnormal gait characterized by wide-based, shuffling movements. Generalized muscle wasting and weakness are less common. Sphincter control is generally preserved, though mild difficulty with micturition is common. Erectile dysfunction is a frequent complaint. Vibration sensation in the lower extremities may be diminished.

B. IMAGING STUDIES

The roentgenographic changes in cervical spondylosis include narrowing of the disk space, seen most clearly on a lateral projection (Figure 43–44). Osteophyte formation at the vertebral body margins and in particular at the posterolateral uncovertebral joints is best observed on an anteroposterior projection. Arthritic degeneration of the facet joints with osteophyte formation is best demonstrated in oblique views. The highest incidence of degeneration is observed in segments C5–6 because of the concentration of mechanical forces in this region. C6–7 is the next most common level. In the lateral projection, the size of the spinal canal can be measured to assess the degree of cervical stenosis.

MRI has improved our ability to determine the levels that are affected by the compression. Electromyography may be useful to demonstrate generalized motor impairment resulting from motor neuron involvement.

Differential Diagnosis

A. CERVICAL SPONDYLOTIC RADICULOPATHY

The syndrome is difficult to distinguish from cervical muscle strain unless there are objective radicular signs such as muscle atrophy and sensory changes in a dermatomal distribution.

B. CERVICAL SPONDYLOTIC MYELOPATHY

Differential diagnosis includes tumors and vascular malformations of the spinal cord, syringomyelia, amyotrophic lateral sclerosis, subacute combined degeneration, and multiple sclerosis. In advanced stages, radiculopathy is commonly seen in association with myelopathy. At this point the syndrome is referred to as a myeloradiculopathy. Upper motor neuron involvement producing spasticity in the extremities distinguishes myelopathy with radiculopathy from isolated radiculopathy, in which pain and weakness in the extremity are limited to the specific neural segment involved. Radiculopathy is aggravated by neck motion

Figure 43–44. A: Lateral radiograph of a 50-year-old man with neck pain and myelopathy. ***B:*** Sagittal T2-weighted MRI showing spinal cord compression at C4–5 at the level of the spondylolisthesis.

and is associated with more profound dermatomal sensory loss. Multiple sclerosis tends to occur in younger patients, with a peak onset between ages 20 and 40 years, and seldom appears for the first time after age 50 years. Though many of the motor signs are similar, onset in multiple sclerosis is usually more abrupt. Cranial nerve palsies are common in multiple sclerosis, as is cerebellar dysarthria, giving rise to characteristic "scanning speech" (speech punctuated by long, regularly occurring pauses). Elevated cerebrospinal fluid IgG levels and abnormal visual evoked responses also accompany multiple sclerosis. Remission in multiple sclerosis is frequently more complete than in spondylotic myelopathy.

Neoplasm of the cervical cord is usually more profound and progressive. The segmental level is more discrete with spinal tumor, and cerebrospinal fluid protein is elevated. Loss of sphincter control is rare in spondylotic myelopathy and extremely common with neoplasms. MRI is the diagnostic test most useful for differentiating tumor from a degenerative process.

Treatment

A. CERVICAL SPONDYLOTIC RADICULOPATHY

Most patients with acute onset of cervical spondylotic radiculopathy have regression of symptoms over 4–6 weeks. Progression to myelopathy is rare, and most patients require only rest, analgesics, and immobilization to relieve pain. Paresthesias and slight sensory changes may persist after neck and arm pain have subsided. Chronic symptoms may involve an element of nerve root inflammation that may require vigorous anti-inflammatory drug therapy.

If pain persists longer than expected, MRI of the cervical spine should be performed to accurately localize the site of compression. Only when a discrete herniation is documented is surgical decompression required, either with foraminotomy through a posterior approach or by complete removal of the involved cervical disk and osteophytes through an anterior approach followed by anterior interbody fusion. Patients with significant neck pain, kyphosis, bilateral symptoms, or a central disk herniation should be treated by an anterior approach (Figure 43–45). Young patients with little or no neck pain and pure radiculopathy with unilateral disk herniation can be managed by either approach.

B. CERVICAL SPONDYLOTIC MYELOPATHY

Management of cervical spondylotic myelopathy depends upon the course and severity of symptoms.

1. Medical measures—The management of slowly progressive disease in elderly patients is conservative,

Figure 43–45. Lateral postoperative radiograph of a patient who underwent C4–C5 anterior cervical discectomy and fusion with a titanium plate and tricortical iliac crest bone graft.

and judicious use of a cervical collar for support is generally sufficient. New anti-inflammatory medications that are cyclooxygenase 2 selective hold great promise for symptom relief while minimizing the chance of gastrointestinal ulceration. Cyclooxygenase 2 inhibitors (celecoxib, rofecoxib) are newer NSAIDs with minimal tendency to cause gastrointestinal ulceration with chronic use.

2. Surgical treatment—When symptoms are more severe or progressive despite use of a collar and when they occur in younger patients, operative treatment may be necessary. The choice of treatment depends upon the nature of the compression (disk, vertebral body, posterior osteophytes, hypertrophied ligamentum flavum, ossified posterior longitudinal ligament), the sagittal alignment of the cervical spine (kyphotic, neutral, or lordotic), and the number of levels involved. Compression confined to the intervertebral disks can be relieved by means of single-level or multiple-level anterior discectomies and fusion. When the disease is limited to two vertebral body levels or if there is a preexisting kyphosis greater than 15 degrees, anterior vertebrectomy, foraminotomy, and fusion with a strut graft allows excellent decompression and stabilization of the degenerative segments. When the compression involves more than two vertebral body levels, the morbidity associated with the anterior approach increases significantly. In this case, a posterior decompression via multilevel laminectomy with or without fusion or laminoplasty is preferred (Figure 43–46).

Figure 43–46. *A:* Lateral postoperative radiograph of a patient who had multisegmental cervical stenosis and myelopathy treated with canal expansive cervical laminoplasty from C3 to C7. *B:* Postoperative axial MRI image showing significant canal expansion after the procedure.

Course & Prognosis

A. CERVICAL SPONDYLOTIC RADICULOPATHY

The course is benign. Most cases resolve in 4–6 weeks with conservative management.

B. CERVICAL SPONDYLOTIC MYELOPATHY

In general, the results of surgical management of spondylotic myelopathy are better when symptoms are mild and of relatively shorter duration. However, complete postoperative resolution of symptoms is rare even in these cases. It is noteworthy that the natural evolution of spondylotic myelopathy will often produce at least partial spontaneous remission. Chronic myelopathy and multiple-level involvement are associated with poorer surgical results, particularly in elderly individuals who have lost the ability to ambulate.

Evans RW: Some observations on whiplash injuries. Neurol Clin 1992;10:975.

Poggi JJ et: Cervical spondylolysis. J Spinal Disord 1992;5:349.

Yoshida M et al: Indication and clinical results of laminoplasty for cervical myelopathy caused by disc herniation with developmental canal stenosis. Spine 1998;23:2391.

PAIN SYNDROMES OF THE BACK

1. Low Back Pain

 ESSENTIALS OF DIAGNOSIS

- *Paraspinous low back pain aggravated by exertion.*
- *Radiation of pain into the buttock or thigh.*

General Considerations

In the United States, 400,000 workers are disabled by back pain each year. It has been estimated that 80% of the population suffers low back pain at some time. All physicians are called on at least occasionally to advise patients with this complaint, and a systematic approach is necessary to differentiate the numerous possible causes. Diagnosis and management can be frustrating because the precise cause of most cases of low back pain is uncertain and no cure is known. The first task is to identify the relatively few cases with specific causes that can be treated. The less rewarding and more demanding task is to provide long-term guidance and management for patients for whom specific remedies are unavailable.

Clinical Findings

A. SYMPTOMS AND SIGNS

The most common cause of low back pain is mechanical strain. Patients complain of pain related to overexertion. Pain may immediately follow lifting or other forms of exertion or may have a more insidious onset after prolonged physical activity. Many patients in this group demonstrate generally poor conditioning, with poor abdominal muscle tone and poor posture.

Pain from lumbar strain is exacerbated by bending or lifting and relieved by rest. Pain is often described as a deep-seated ache that is dull and somewhat diffuse. Pain is most severe in the lumbosacral area and may radiate into the buttocks. Palpation reveals tenderness in the paraspinous area, with "trigger points" or "knots" in the erector spinae muscle. Spasm of the paraspinous muscles is a common finding, and the patient may have a slight list toward the nonpainful side. Motion of the lumbar spine is limited by pain.

The neurologic examination is often normal. Deep tendon reflexes are present and symmetric. Motor power and sensation in the lower extremities are normal. Rectal tone is normal. Provocative tests such as straight leg raising and the crossed straight leg raising are negative. The former is performed with the patient supine on the examining table. The examiner then lifts the patient's leg, which is extended at the hip and knee. This maneuver passively stretches the sciatic nerve and results in transmission of tension to the lumbosacral roots that contribute to the nerve. Absence of radicular leg pain associated with straight leg raising reduces the likelihood of spinal nerve compression as the source of symptoms.

B. IMAGING STUDIES

X-ray examination may reveal changes such as lumbar disk space narrowing and osteophytosis or may be entirely normal. Because x-ray signs are nonspecific, many clinicians avoid x-ray studies during the initial evaluation. X-rays should be obtained for persons over age 50, in whom metastatic tumors are more likely to be present, and those under age 20, in whom symptomatic congenital or developmental anomalies may be present. For other patients, x-rays may be obtained during subsequent visits if symptoms do not resolve within several weeks.

Treatment

Management of lumbar strain includes analgesics and rest during the acute phase. A firm board beneath the patient's mattress provides support for tender spinal muscles. Abdominal conditioning and spinal muscle strengthening exercises are prescribed only when the pain subsides. Typical exercises include bent-knee sit-ups and hamstring and spinal muscle stretching. Lumbosacral corsets with steel stays provide mechanical support for the spine by compressing and reinforcing the flaccid abdominal wall. Proper body mechanics should be discussed with the patient, especially the correct manner of lifting objects while bending the legs rather than the spine. Postural exercises may be useful and are most effectively taught by physical therapists.

Course & Prognosis

The usual course of lumbar strain is spontaneous remission with time. Relapses of pain are commonly precipitated by stressful activity, though months may pass without symptoms. Some patients complain of constant pain. Probing inquiry frequently reveals profound depression in these individuals, for whom illness and disability have become dominant elements in their lives. When strain is attributed to working conditions, the clinical course may be complicated by considerations of secondary gain.

Patients who fail to respond to rest and supportive measures must be carefully reexamined to assess for neurologic compression. Those judged to be neurologically normal must be encouraged to return to normal activities as rapidly as possible. Prolonged reliance upon analgesics (especially opioids) must be discouraged.

2. Lumbar Disk Syndrome

 ESSENTIALS OF DIAGNOSIS

- Low back pain radiating into the thigh, leg, and foot.
- Paresthesia in the affected dermatome.

General Considerations

Relapse of low back pain may or may not be associated with leg pain. Patients who present with low back and leg pain frequently recall earlier episodes of postexertional pain limited to the low back. Though specific evidence is lacking, the pattern of leg pain developing secondarily has led many clinicians to attribute the initial episode of localized low back pain to early degeneration of the annulus fibrosus. With annulus degeneration, the nucleus pulposus bulges into the defect, causing further concentration of stress on the damaged fibers. The annulus is richly innervated with pain fibers, and further degeneration tends to be associated with more frequent and episodes of more severe pain. Locking and stiffness characterize the pain-free periods. Degeneration continues with alteration in the collagen structure of both the annulus and the nucleus, culminating in fibrosis and nuclear fragmentation. The shock-absorbing capacity of the nucleus is diminished, and forces are transmitted in a progressively irregular fashion. Fragments of the deteriorating nucleus are pushed outward against or through the weakened annulus, which tends to be weakest at the posterolateral margin of the annulus fibrosus. The protrusion begins as a posterolateral bulge that causes variable compression and irritation of neural structures.

The dural sac below L1 contains only nerve rootlets. Each nerve root emerges below its respective vertebra, hugging the inferomedial border of its respective pedicle, and enters the neural foramen just above the intervertebral disk of that level. A paracentral disk herniation just misses the exiting nerve root at the specific spinal level and compresses the traversing root to the lower adjacent level. Thus, an L4–5 paracentral disk herniation will compress the traversing L5 nerve root. In contrast, a far lateral disk herniation occurs near the exit zone of its respective neural foramen and therefore is most likely to compress the exiting root at that level. The L4–5 and L5–S1 disk levels correspond to the region of maximal mechanical stress in the lumbar spine. Lesions affecting the L5 and S1 nerve roots account for over 90% of disk-mediated nerve root lesions.

Clinical Findings

A. SYMPTOMS AND SIGNS

Sciatica (pain radiating down the posterior leg) is the most common presentation. Prolonged compression results in nerve root inflammation and pain referred in a specific dermatomal distribution. The onset of leg pain is usually insidious, but pain may begin acutely when sudden disk herniation follows injury.

Pain is piercing, burning, or electrical in nature and typically radiates from the thigh into the leg and foot. Activities such as coughing, sneezing, or bearing down during bowel movements increase intra-abdominal pressure, which is directly transmitted to intraspinal structures, provoking or exacerbating pain.

When nerve root compression results from annular bulging, it is often accentuated by prolonged sitting or standing and relieved at least partially by rest. A patient usually prefers to sleep on one side in the fetal position and when sitting prefers a straight-backed chair. When disk extrusion occurs, pain may be less responsive to rest.

Compression of nerve roots often produces objective sensory changes early, with paresthesia and loss of sensation detectable in the affected dermatome. With continued root compression, motor weakness may develop. Motor weakness corresponds to the specific myotomes innervated by the compressed nerve root. With involvement of the L4 root, the patellar tendon reflex may be diminished and slight quadriceps weakness may be observed. Sensation may be diminished over the medial calf. Since the foot dorsiflexors are innervated by L4 and L5, slight weakness of the foot dorsiflexors may also be noticed on side-to-side testing. With involvement of the L5 root, weakness is frequently manifested by loss of strength in great toe dorsiflexion. Pain and numbness are present in the anteromedial leg and foot. First sacral root involvement affects the calf muscles, and the Achilles tendon reflex may be lost on the involved side. Weakness is best demonstrated by the patient's inability to rise on the toes repeatedly. Sensory findings include pain and numbness in the posterolateral leg and foot. Muscle atrophy may accompany sensory and motor changes.

Occasionally, acute posterior midline disk prolapse at the L2–3 level may cause compression of many nerve roots in the cauda equina. This is known as acute cauda equina syndrome. Symptoms include intense leg pain in one or both extremities, with severe muscle weakness or paralysis. Compression of sacral roots results in acute urinary retention. An MRI of the lumbar spine will reveal the site of compression, which is best treated by urgent decompression.

In the presence of severe disk space degeneration and spondylosis, a generalized narrowing of the lumbar spinal canal occurs. Lumbar spinal stenosis occurs as a consequence of the degenerative process of aging. It is a multifactorial narrowing of the spinal canal from facet joint hypertrophy, disk degeneration and loss of disk height, and hypertrophy and buckling of the ligamentum flavum. Spinal stenosis afflicts people in their mid to late fifties and early sixties. There is no clear gender predominance. Early symptoms include generalized backache and stiffness. Narrowing of the lateral recess occurs early in the process, causing unilateral nerve root symptoms. Neurogenic claudication becomes the chief complaint once the central spinal canal becomes narrowed.

B. DIAGNOSTIC TESTS

With less well defined signs of root compression, several tests may help to detect the presence of lumbar disk disease. The straight leg raising test is performed by lifting the extended leg of the supine patient. The test produces tension in the lumbosacral roots and frequently reproduces sciatica in the presence of inflamed or irritated lumbosacral roots.

The straight leg raising test can also be performed on the leg without symptoms. The crossed straight leg raising test is positive if it produces sciatica in the symptomatic leg. Many clinicians believe that a positive test is strong evidence of disk herniation.

Lasègue's test is performed with the patient lying supine. The hip and knee are flexed 90 degrees. The knee is then slowly extended, producing sciatic stretch as in the straight leg raising maneuver.

In patients with spinal stenosis, extension typically exacerbates the symptoms. Flexion of the spine improves the symptoms. Typical physical findings include diminished or asymmetric reflexes in the lower extremities. The extensor hallucis longus is most often found to be weak.

C. IMAGING STUDIES

X-ray examination may reveal degenerative changes, such as disk space narrowing and osteophytosis, or the results may be entirely normal. A myelogram, CT scan, or MRI will confirm the diagnosis.

Differential Diagnosis

Whether nerve root signs are present or not, the main differential concern with back pain is spinal tumor or infection. In addition, palpation of the distal pulses and abdominal aorta is necessary to rule out the presence of aortic aneurysm.

The most common extradural tumors in adults are metastatic, most often from carcinoma of the breast in women and of the prostate in men. Lung, thyroid, and uterine tumors are less common sources of metastases. Multiple myeloma also frequently involves the spine and often causes pain by weakening of bony structures, causing pathologic fractures. Intradural spinal tumors are less common than metastases in adults and include neurofibromas, meningiomas, and ependymomas. Diagnosis of these slow-growing tumors is often quite difficult, as symptoms may mimic discogenic pain and may appear to improve with conservative measures. Metastatic tumors of bone are often detected on routine x-ray studies.

The history may suggest the possibility of spinal tumor. A history of primary tumors elsewhere should immediately arouse this suspicion. A complaint of pain that is more severe at night than during the day is also strongly suggestive of spinal tumor. The reasons for this phenomenon are unclear but may be related to nocturnal increase in cerebrospinal fluid pressure. Persistent bilateral leg pain with no history of back pain also suggests spinal tumor. Both primary and metastatic tumors are easily detected by MRI.

Discitis and vertebral osteomyelitis can cause back pain in the absence of significant neurologic symptoms. Pyogenic vertebral osteomyelitis is due to bacterial infection of the vertebra that can arise from a number of sources, including direct inoculation, contiguous spread from a local infection, and hematogenous seeding. Local spread of bacteria or fungi can occur following intra-abdominal and retroperitoneal abscesses. Direct inoculation results from penetrating injuries and from surgical procedures performed on the intervertebral disk (chemonucleolysis, discography, discectomy). Although local spread from direct inoculation of bacteria into the spine is becoming more prevalent, hematogenous seeding of infection is by far the most common mechanism by which these infections occur. The sources of pathogenic organisms include skin and soft tissue infections, infected vascular access sites, and the urinary tract.

Once the infection is established in the metaphysis, it can then rupture through the end plate into the adjoining disk and infect the adjacent vertebral body. The disk material is relatively avascular and is rapidly destroyed by the bacterial enzymes. Infection in the cervical spine can extend into the mediastinum or into the supraclavicular fossa with disastrous sequelae. In the lumbar spine, abscess formation may occur in the psoas muscle, the buttock (piriformis fossa), the perianal region, the groin, or even the popliteal fossa. Extension of infection into the spinal canal can result in an epidural abscess or bacterial meningitis. Destruction of the vertebral body and intervertebral disk can lead to instability and collapse of the vertebral body. In addition, retropulsion of infected bone and granulation tissue into the spinal canal can cause neural compression or vascular occlusion. If a spinal infection is suspected, the pathogenic organism must be identified before appropriate treatment with antibiotics (with or without surgical debridement) can be instituted. An MRI with gadolinium will clearly delineate the location of the infection as well as the presence of an epidural abscess (Figure 43–47).

Treatment

Management of acute lumbar disk disease is controversial.

A. CONSERVATIVE MANAGEMENT

If symptoms are produced by bulging rather than by extrusion of the herniated disk, conservative measures such as bed rest, analgesics, and anti-inflammatory medications often result in complete resolution of symptoms.

Figure 43–47. Sagittal MRI images of a patient with low back pain due to L5–S1 discitis, vertebral osteomyelitis, and a small anterior epidural abscess. ***A:*** T1-weighted image. ***B:*** T1-weighted image with gadolinium vascular contrast. ***C:*** T2-weighted image.

B. PERCUTANEOUS DISCECTOMY

If pain becomes intractable or if neurologic symptoms progress or fail to respond to conservative measures, laminotomy and removal of the herniated disk may be required. This can be performed via standard microdiscectomy techniques or though a "minimally invasive" endoscopic approach that is done through a paramedian muscle splitting exposure.

C. LAMINECTOMY

If free fragments are present in the spinal canal, laminectomy is clearly indicated if pain or neurologic symptoms fail to respond to conservative measures. However, if the symptoms are tolerable, free fragments have a higher likelihood of spontaneous resorption over time than the classic herniated disk. Complications of laminectomy for disk removal include recurrence of pain due to reherniation of residual disk fragments or scar formation involving the nerve roots; damage of nerve roots, resulting in neurologic deficit; tear of the dura, with resulting dural leak of cerebrospinal fluid; and penetration of the anterior annulus during diskectomy, with damage to the great vessels lying anterior to the spine. Hemorrhage in this situation may be catastrophic owing to difficulties in detection and control.

In the patient with persistent neurogenic claudication that fails to respond to conservative measures, decompressive laminectomy is very effective in relieving symptoms and improving function. If spinal instability (degenerative spondylolisthesis) of deformity is also present, the spine should also be stabilized and fused over the affected levels.

3. Mechanical Back Pain (Facet Syndrome)

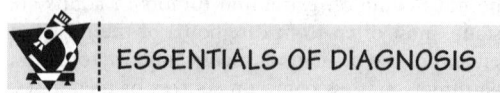

ESSENTIALS OF DIAGNOSIS

- *Pain in the low back.*
- *"Locking" of back during bending.*

General Considerations

People with long-standing lumbar disk disease may develop numerous degenerative changes in the involved segments (facet syndrome). Collapse of the disk results in abnormal motion both anteriorly, between the vertebral bodies; and posteriorly, between the intervertebral facets. Osteophytes form as a result of abnormal stress on the annulus and the joint capsules of the facets.

Clinical Findings

Symptoms may arise from inflammation surrounding the abnormal facets and generally include diffuse aching that may or may not radiate into the buttock or posterior thigh.

The mechanical nature of the pain is reflected by postural discomfort and by locking of the low back during stooping or attempts to straighten the back after forward bending. Abnormal motion is the presumed cause of irritation that leads to reflex muscular inhibition and spinal "locking."

Differential Diagnosis

Experimental injection of hypertonic saline into normal facet joints has been noted to cause low back pain associated with sciatica as well as limitation of straight leg raising. These experimentally induced symptoms are eradicated by injection of the facets with lidocaine. These observations make it clear that sciatica without weakness or sensory deficit is insufficient evidence on which to base a diagnosis of nerve root compression.

Treatment

Patients demonstrating symptoms suggestive of facet syndrome may respond well to systemic anti-inflammatory agents or to fluoroscopically guided injection of the lumbar facets with corticosteroids and lidocaine. Lumbar fusion by anterior or posterior techniques has been advocated to eliminate abnormal motion, but results have been inconsistent.

Fischgrund JS, Montgomery DM: Diagnosis and treatment of discogenic low back pain. Orthop Rev 1993;22:311.

Frank A: Low back pain. Br Med J 1993;306:901.

Frymoyer JW: Predicting disability from low back pain. Clin Orthop 1992;(279):101.

Haldeman S, Rubinstein SM: Cauda equina syndrome in patients undergoing manipulation of the lumbar spine. Spine 1992; 17:1469.

Lang IM et al, MR imaging appearances of cervical epidural abscess. Clin Radiol 1995;50:466.

Omarini LP, Garcia J: CT-guided percutaneous puncture-biopsy of the spine. Review of 104 cases. Schweiz Med Wochenschr 1993;123:2191. (In French.)

PAIN SYNDROMES OF THE FOOT

1. Morton's Neuroma

The interdigital nerve to the third and fourth toes is formed by the third digital branch of the medial plantar nerve and a connecting branch from the lateral plantar nerve. In 1876, Morton described a painful condition of the forefoot that he attributed to neuritis of this digital nerve. The symptoms included pain centered around the fourth metatarsophalangeal joint and in the third intermetatarsal space. Pain is exacerbated by weightbearing, particularly while wearing shoes, and in some cases is steadily progressive. Neuroma pain is distinguishable from simple structural forefoot pain by the fact that it is constant and not relieved by rest. Structural metatarsalgia is experienced almost exclusively during weightbearing and is relieved by rest. The incidence of Morton's neuroma is eight to ten times higher in women than in men.

Interdigital nerve neuroma has been attributed to the course the nerves follow on the way to their destinations in the skin of the toes. Each nerve passes beneath the deep intermetatarsal ligament and then changes its course in a dorsal direction. The more dorsally situated digital branches then enter adjacent toes and provide cutaneous sensation. Dorsiflexion of the toes produces constant friction along the edge of the intermetatarsal ligament. Friction causes fibrosis and enlargement of the nerve sheath, which in turn increase the potential for impingement. The third and fourth interdigital nerves are most commonly involved. This predilection is attributed to the peculiar mobility of the fourth metatarsal, which is least rigidly anchored at its base. The second and third interdigital nerves are sometimes affected, and the first nerve is only rarely involved. The disease very rarely involves two digital nerves simultaneously in the same foot.

Clinical Findings

Diagnosis is based on the history and physical examination. A complaint of unremitting pain in the interspaces of the toes is highly suggestive. Palpation of the space reproduces sharp, stabbing pain, as does compression of the interspaces produced by squeezing the forefoot circumferentially. Simple metatarsalgia should be ruled out by the physical examination. Neuroma pain will rarely respond to orthotics alone.

Treatment

Treatment initially is nonsurgical, emphasizing the need for shoes with a wide toe box and low heel. Some patients respond well to a metatarsal pad. Corticosteroid injections give transient relief in many cases, but long-term relief has not been consistently achieved. Intractable neuroma pain in the intermetatarsal space unresponsive to conservative measures requires operative treatment. Treatment consists of excision of the nerve through a longitudinal incision in the dorsal web space. The neuroma is usually located at the bifurcation into digital branches. The excision must be made well proximal to the intermetatarsal ligament to prevent subsequent adhesion of the cut nerve end and the ligament, with recurrence of pain. Denervation of the digits with sensory loss has proved inconsequential to patients, who usually describe dramatic relief of symptoms immediately after surgery.

2. Metatarsalgia

ESSENTIALS OF DIAGNOSIS

- *Pain beneath the metatarsal heads with weight-bearing.*
- *Plantar callosities.*

General Considerations

Metatarsalgia is a descriptive term denoting a group of disorders causing pain beneath the metatarsophalangeal joints. Mechanical factors are perhaps the chief cause. Laxity of the transverse intermetatarsal ligament permits collapse of the transverse metatarsal arch, resulting in loss of the concavity beneath the central metatarsal heads. The normal concentration of weightbearing by the first and fifth metatarsal heads is dispersed, with relatively greater loads delivered to the second and third metatarsals.

Clinical Findings

Plantar keratoses (callosities) form in areas of excessive stress and are particularly common beneath the second metatarsal head. This is in part due to the prominence of the condyle on the fibular aspect of the central metatarsal heads. Constant irritation of hypertrophic callosities results in inflammation and pain with weightbearing. Symptoms vary from intermittent discomfort to severe and disabling pain.

Collapse of the transverse arch may result from laxity of the intermetatarsal ligament. Ligamentous laxity may exist as a congenital deformity or may result from obesity, prolonged standing, injury, or aging. Intramuscular paralysis may also permit collapse of the arch, and shoes that crowd the toes also create abnormal stress concentration beneath the metatarsal heads.

Differential Diagnosis

Diagnosis is easily made if callosities are evident. Reactive keratoses are occasionally mistaken for plantar warts, but the latter are rarely located beneath metatarsal heads.

Treatment

A. ORTHOTICS

Therapy is directed toward relieving pressure beneath the metatarsal heads by placing felt or rubber pads into the shoe behind the central metatarsal heads. Shoes that comfortably accommodate the padded forefoot are mandatory.

B. SURGICAL TREATMENT

In cases where pain is intractable despite conservative measures, operative treatment is required. Procedures designed to relieve metatarsal pressure include excision of the plantar condylar prominence, osteotomy to shorten the metatarsal, resection of the metatarsal head, and, in particularly resistant cases, excision of the entire offending metatarsal. The latter procedures may cause increased disability and should be undertaken only after failure of less radical procedures, such as condylectomy.

3. Hallux Valgus

ESSENTIALS OF DIAGNOSIS

- *Prominence of the medial first metatarsal.*
- *Lateral deviation of the great toe.*

General Considerations

Hallux valgus is subluxation of the first metatarsophalangeal joint, which results in lateral deviation (valgus) of the great toe and formation of a medial prominence by the first metatarsal head. The cause is a topic of controversy, though a number of factors are involved.

Anatomic factors predisposing to hallux valgus include varus alignment of the first metatarsocuneiform joint. The medially directed first metatarsal widens the angle between the first and second metatarsal beyond the normal 5–8 degrees. This so-called metatarsus varus adds mechanical advantages to the adductor hallucis tendon insertion on the proximal phalanx of the great toe, with resulting lateral deviation of the toe. Ligamentous laxity may also aggravate the imbalance.

The most significant extrinsic causative factor in development of hallux valgus is improper footwear. The predominance of women in all reports of this deformity has been interpreted as a strong indictment of women's shoe styles. Bunching up of the toes in a pointed shoe buckles the first metatarsophalangeal joint by forcing the great toe into a marked valgus deformity. The first metatarsal is levered medialward. With prolonged use of offending footwear, the medial joint capsule becomes attenuated, further lowering the resistance to deformation. The abductor hallucis tendon is pulled plantarward, and its ability to resist great toe adduction is lost. The long flexor and extensor tendons are pulled laterally with the great toe. When the displaced tendons contract, they create a bowstring effect, further exacerbating the deformity.

Clinical Findings

The "bunion" of hallux valgus represents a prominence of the medial first metatarsal head, which results when the great toe becomes progressively laterally subluxated. True exostosis is uncommon, though the ligamentous structures overlying the medial eminence may be thickened, and an adventitial bursa may form over the prominent medial metatarsal head. Pain from irritation of the bursa and the overlying skin occurs as these tissues are compressed between the shoe and underlying bone.

Treatment

A. ORTHOTICS

Conservative measures for treatment of hallux valgus emphasize selection of footwear of proper size and shape to accommodate the deformed forefoot. The pain associated with irritation of the bunion can in many cases be minimized by this simple measure. Night splints have also been recommended, though hallux valgus may progress despite their use. Only when the pain significantly interferes with the patient's lifestyle should surgery be recommended.

B. SURGICAL TREATMENT

Over 50 operations have been advocated for the correction of hallux valgus, which is by way of saying that there is no perfect bunion operation. The main indications for surgery include intractable pain and inability to find comfortable shoes. The elements of surgical correction include excision of the medial prominence of the metatarsal head (bunionectomy), release of the deforming adductor hallucis tendon, excision of the lateral sesamoid bone if it is widely displaced, and reefing of the medial capsular structures to reinforce static resistance to recurrence of the deformity. When the varus deformity of the first metatarsal is excessive, sutures are placed between the capsules of the first and second metatarsal heads or corrective osteotomy of the metatarsal is performed.

Recurrence of the deformity and overcorrection creating hallux varus deformity are the major complications of surgery. Both problems are more apt to occur when correction of severe hallux valgus deformity has been attempted. Some loss of first metatarsophalangeal joint motion can be expected in most cases. Adequate vascularity must be confirmed prior to any correction procedure. The complication rates are low when surgery is performed by experienced surgeons. Ambulation is usually possible shortly after surgery. Careful at-

tention must be paid to postoperative dressings, which should immobilize the great toe and thus reinforce the surgical repair.

Coughlin MJ: Treatment of bunionette deformity with longitudinal diaphyseal osteotomy with distal soft tissue repair. Foot Ankle 1991;11:195.

Schoenhaus HD, Cohen RS: Etiology of the bunion. J Foot Surg 1992;31:25.

■ ORTHOPEDIC INFECTIONS

OSTEOMYELITIS DUE TO EXTENSION OF ADJACENT SOFT TISSUE INFECTION

Infections that develop in the soft tissues of the fingers or toes can extend into and destroy adjacent bone. Septic arthritis from puncture wounds may have a similar result. Prompt treatment of the initial infection will prevent this complication and avoid the need either for amputation or for joint resection and fusion to salvage some function. A more common form of osteomyelitis due to extension from an established infected site is that which occurs beneath trophic ulcers associated with arterial insufficiency, diabetes mellitus, or neuropathy due to other causes. Such chronic soft tissue ulcers inevitably become infected, usually with a mixture of organisms that frequently includes anaerobes. Persisting infection may spread to involve adjacent bone, but usually only its surface unless septic arthritis develops or the infection is of exceptionally long duration. The possibility of osteomyelitis is raised by radiographs of the involved area. Focal demineralization may be present without bone infection. Cortical erosion and periosteal new bone formation are more suggestive, but only the presence of necrotic sequestered bone is convincing evidence of osteomyelitis. MRI has been found to be very sensitive for detecting osteomyelitis.

In fact, persistence of such trophic ulcers rarely results from osteomyelitis but instead from inadequate debridement of soft tissues, continuing mechanical trauma, or inadequate blood supply. Treatment should be directed at these factors. Ray resection or amputation may be necessary to achieve soft tissue healing. Superficially involved bone at the base of an ulcer may require only superficial debridement. Prolonged antibiotic treatment is not necessary in such cases if healing is progressing and will be insufficient if it is not.

Joints adjacent to pressure sores (decubitus ulcers) or neurotrophic or ischemic ulcers may develop septic arthritis that is easily overlooked without synovial fluid aspiration or arthrography. Without adequate joint drainage and debridement, there is little hope for controlling these serious infections it is important to be aware of the marked radiographic abnormalities produced by neuropathic joint destruction in diabetes mellitus as well as other causes of peripheral neuropathy. These can be confused with infection or can coexist with it.

CHRONIC OSTEOMYELITIS

The foregoing discussions should suggest that there is often no clear division between acute and chronic osteomyelitis. From a practical viewpoint, however, the concept of chronic osteomyelitis is valuable because it emphasizes the persisting, recurring nature of infections involving bone and because it is usually associated with more or less easily definable areas of necrotic bone that harbor the causative microorganisms and thus provide a source for recurrences. Chronic osteomyelitis will not be cured without removal of this sequestered and necrotic bone.

Clinical Findings

A. SYMPTOMS AND SIGNS

Chronic osteomyelitis may recur as apparent cellulitis in the region of previously infected bone or as an obvious soft tissue abscess. This may "point" and rupture to produce a sinus tract that persists or drains periodically. Persistent or recurring serous or purulent wound drainage from an area of previous osteomyelitis is highly suggestive, if not diagnostic, of chronic osteomyelitis.

B. LABORATORY FINDINGS

Cultures of a draining sinus usually yield organisms but rarely differentiate the true pathogenic bacteria from bacterial soup colonizing a chronic wound. Tissue biopsy or deep aspiration is necessary for reliable bacteriologic diagnosis, which is the key to appropriate antibacterial therapy. Chronic bone infections may be caused by mycobacteria or fungi, so stains and cultures appropriate for these microorganisms are always required. When tissue is obtained for culture, an adjacent specimen should also be sent for histopathologic study.

C. IMAGING STUDIES

Radiographs demonstrate both destructive and reactive bone changes, with more or less circumscribed areas of lucency, sclerosis, and often periosteal or appositional new bone formation. Involucra and sequestra may be obvious or may require CT scans or MRI for demonstration. A sinogram obtained after gentle injection of iodinated soluble contrast medium will delineate the area of involvement and may indicate the source of recurring infection. Occasionally, a sinus that appears to arise from the pelvis communicates with infection originating in the gastrointestinal tract or genitourinary tract.

Differential Diagnosis

Chronic osteomyelitis must be differentiated from benign and malignant bone tumor, bone dysplasia, and traumatic lesions, including fatigue fracture.

Complications

Failure to eradicate the infection is common. Infection may spread systemically or locally. Pathologic fracture may occur, especially after bone debridement. Bone deformity or shortening, nonunion, malunion, and stiffness or ankylosis of adjacent joints may cause significant loss of function. Amputation may be necessary to control infection or to provide a more functional limb than would remain after prolonged infection and repeated surgery. After years of drainage, malignant degeneration may occur in the sinus tract. This should be suspected if increasing pain or drainage develops with long-standing osteomyelitis.

Treatment

A. CONSERVATIVE TREATMENT

When chronic osteomyelitis is quiescent, no treatment is necessary, and the patient may live an essentially normal life. Dressing changes alone may be sufficient for minor exacerbations with drainage.

B. MEDICAL TREATMENT

If symptoms are more severe, rest with elevation of the involved limb, analgesics as needed, and systemic antibiotics are advisable. The choice of antibiotic may be aided by culture and sensitivity test results from prior symptomatic episodes; by aspiration or biopsy of the involved area; or, least desirably, by a more or less educated guess at the infecting organism and its antibiotic sensitivities. In the early phases of recurrence, without abscess or sinus tract, these measures alone may produce a prompt—though usually temporary—clinical resolution. The optimal duration of antibiotic treatment for chronic osteomyelitis remains unclear. Some authors recommend only brief usage, during acute exacerbations and surgical procedures. Current opinion among infectious disease experts supports a 4- to 6-week course, though the results of this regimen are not well documented. It is clear that antibiotics are adjuncts to adequate debridement and are not in themselves sufficient treatment. Adjunctive oral antibiotic coverage for at least 6 months appears to be beneficial for treatment of chronic staphylococcal osteomyelitis due to susceptible organisms.

C. SURGICAL TREATMENT

Surgical treatment will be necessary if rest and antibiotics do not result in prompt improvement or if significant drainage, bone destruction, or sequestration is evident. Soft tissue abscesses require incision and drainage. The resulting wound may be left open or closed over suction-irrigation tubes. Tubes can be managed in several ways. Continuous flow systems are complicated. Doses of antibiotics delivered by continuous flow may be too large, and toxicity may occur. Scrupulous sterile precautions must be followed with all techniques, and tubes should generally be removed within a few days to minimize the risk of superinfection.

The following regimen has been effective: Periodic irrigation is performed with small volumes of antibiotic solution, followed by prolonged suction to prevent fluid accumulation and minimize soft tissue dead space. As a rule, no more than 10–20 mL of solution (eg, 0.1% gentamicin in normal saline) is injected every 12 hours, allowed to stay in the wound for a few hours, and then withdrawn by suction applied to the tube via a three-way stopcock that also permits irrigation. A single tube is used for small wounds, but double tubes may be needed for larger ones (Figure 43–48). Suction-irrigation tube systems are not a substitute for adequate surgical drainage of pus and adequate debridement of poorly vascularized, chronically infected tissue. Neither do they replace systemic antibiotic treatment with appropriate drugs. They do offer an effective means of ob-

Figure 43–48. Jergesen tube system for periodic suction-irrigation. A tube with several openings near the end is positioned in the area to be drained and brought out obliquely through the soft tissues and skin. The tube is attached to a sterile three-way stopcock and sterile trap bottle. Small volumes of irrigating solution containing antibiotics are injected via the stopcock with sterile technique. The solution is allowed to remain in the wound for a few hours before the stopcock is opened for suction for several more hours. The process is then repeated.

taining early closure of an infected wound that would otherwise require open management.

Removal of bone may be necessary to extract a sequestrum or to unroof an intraosseous abscess. The resulting cavity acts as a "dead space," which fills with hematoma rather than healthy, well-perfused tissue and leaves a potential focus for recurrence of infection. Saucerization and then exteriorization of the cavity may be followed by split-thickness skin grafting or open cancellous bone grafting once the defect is lined with healthy granulation tissue. A better alternative is to fill the defect with a muscle graft, either with its own local blood supply or as a free microvascular transfer. Coverage of adequately debrided chronic osteomyelitis with a well-perfused muscle pedicle appears to be the most effective surgical treatment for significantly symptomatic chronic osteomyelitis. Extensive bone debridement is often required, resulting in a need for bone grafts if function and structural integrity are to be preserved. Free vascularized muscle grafts make adequate debridement and reconstruction possible when the involved area is too large to be managed with locally available tissue resources.

Prognosis

Whatever the initial cause, once an infection involving bone has become well-established, with focally necrotic bone and scar tissue and microabscesses scattered through the involved area, the long-term outlook must remain guarded. Although infection may be controlled with adequate debridement and prolonged treatment with antibiotics, there is always a risk of late recurrence, even after many years of quiescence.

SEPTIC ARTHRITIS

ESSENTIALS OF DIAGNOSIS

- Joint pain.
- Limitation of motion.
- Joint swelling, effusion, warmth, and tenderness.
- Pus and organisms in aspirate of synovial fluid.

General Considerations

Septic arthritis is an inflammatory joint disease caused by bacteria or fungi. Primary infection is caused by direct inoculation of the joint by trauma, including surgery. Secondary infection occurs hematogenously or by extension from adjacent osteomyelitis. Septic arthritis characteristically involves a single joint. This disease must always be considered in the differential diagnosis of monarticular arthritis.

Occasionally, septic arthritis will develop in a joint already involved by another form of arthritis. This possibility must be considered whenever an arthritic joint "flares" or an arthritic patient becomes systemically ill. Septic arthritis is more common in children and debilitated elderly individuals except when gonococci are the cause.

Septic arthritis destroys articular cartilage. The initial reaction to joint infection is acute synovitis, with effusion that develops an increasing concentration of PMNs. The fluid tends to coagulate, producing loculations within the joint cavity. Inflammatory cells infiltrate the synovium, and the overlying tissues become edematous. With continuing infection, the cartilage matrix is destroyed, collagen is lost, and chondrocytes are killed. The damaged cartilage is susceptible to mechanical trauma and is eroded at points of loading. Continued infection may destroy synovial and capsular components as well as cartilage and bone. Spread to adjacent bone produces osteomyelitis. Following successful treatment of early infections, there may be no permanent sequelae, but extensive tissue destruction rarely resolves completely. Fibrous or complete bony ankylosis may result, as well as painful postinfectious degenerative arthritis.

Gonococci are probably the commonest cause of septic arthritis at present, at least in sexually active individuals, and must be considered whenever a seemingly sterile pyarthrosis is encountered. *Staphylococcus aureus* is by far the next most common pathogen. Septic joints in children 6 months to 2 years of age are often due to *Haemophilus influenzae*. Gram-negative bacilli have recently become a more frequent cause of septic joints, especially in adults with chronic debilitating illness. However, almost every bacterial pathogen has been reported to cause septic arthritis, and the clinical presentation is not helpful for determining the causative organism.

Clinical Findings

A. SYMPTOMS AND SIGNS

In acute hematogenous arthritis, the larger joints (knee, hip, elbow, shoulder, and ankle) are more commonly involved. Infections of other organ systems (skin, respiratory tract, genitourinary tract, etc) are possible sources of blood-borne infections. Although infections in adults usually involve only one joint, multiple joint involvement occurs occasionally in children. Any joint may be involved secondarily by spread of a nearby acute or chronic infection. Systemic disease or another serious infection may divert attention from the infected joint. Systemic symptoms usually include fever, chills, and malaise—and, occasionally, misleading migratory polyarthralgia. Pain is progressive and accentuated by joint motion. Local tenderness and warmth are accompanied by soft tissue swelling, and an effusion is palpable if the joint is superficial.

B. LABORATORY FINDINGS

Examination of joint fluid is crucial. By the time infection is clinically apparent, the fluid is usually turbid or purulent. The white cell count is often over $50,000/\mu L$, with more than 90% PMNs. Synovial fluid glucose is decreased, usually to 50 mg/dL below a simultaneously obtained blood glucose level. Gram-stained smears and cultures are essential. The stain will often dictate the choice of first antibiotic pending sensitivity confirmation. Pyarthrosis without visible organisms on a Gram-stained smear is usually gonococcal in origin. Culture specimens for this fastidious organism must be conveyed promptly to the bacteriology laboratory for proper plating on a selective medium and incubation in 5% carbon dioxide. The erythrocyte sedimentation rate is almost always elevated, and the white count may be. Blood cultures are sometimes positive even when organisms are not recovered from joint fluid.

C. IMAGING STUDIES

The appearance of significant x-ray findings depends upon the duration and virulence of infection. X-ray changes lag behind the clinical and pathologic process. During the first 2 weeks, the joint capsule may appear distended, the overlying soft tissues swollen, and fat planes obscured. In infants especially, increased intra-articular pressure from effusion may cause widening of the radiologic "joint space," with possible progression to pathologic dislocation. Comparative x-rays of the opposite normal joint can aid in identification of subtle changes. With persistent hyperemia and disuse, demineralization of subchondral bone occurs and extends proximal and distal to the joint. Trabecular detail is progressively lost, and the compact subchondral bone appears accentuated. Destruction of cartilage is reflected by narrowing of the width of the joint space until subchondral bone is in apposition, a finding accentuated by x-rays taken during weightbearing.

Complications

Complications consist of joint destruction, osteomyelitis, and direct or hematogenous spread to other sites. The risk of complication is increased by delayed diagnosis.

Differential Diagnosis

Acute pyogenic arthritis must be differentiated from other acute arthropathies (reactive arthritis, systemic lupus erythematosus, rheumatoid arthritis, gout, pseudogout, neurogenic arthropathy, etc). Hematogenous osteomyelitis (especially of the proximal femur), rheumatic fever, and epiphysial trauma may mimic acute septic arthritis in childhood. Lyme disease must also be considered.

Acute pyogenic arthritis may complicate almost any type of preexisting joint disease, especially rheumatoid arthritis and neuropathic arthropathy. Concomitant or recent treatment with locally injected or systemic corticosteroids may both predispose to infection and interfere with diagnosis. Polyarthralgia occurs in systemic viral infections and allergic reactions, but the other features of septic arthritis are lacking. Acute infections or inflammations of periarticular structures (eg, septic bursitis and tenosynovitis, osteomyelitis, cellulitis, and acute calcific tendinitis) may be especially difficult to differentiate. Aspiration, examination, and culture of joint fluid are essential to establish or rule out infection of a joint. Occasionally, synovial biopsy is helpful in diagnosing obscure cases of synovitis.

Treatment

A. GENERAL MEASURES

Analgesics and splinting of the involved joint in the position of maximal comfort alleviate pain. Other foci of infection and any coexisting medical conditions must be identified and treated appropriately. Fluid replacement and nutritional support may be required.

B. SPECIFIC MEASURES

Definitive treatment requires drainage of the pyarthrosis and prompt institution of effective antibiotic therapy. The technique of drainage depends upon the joint involved, the stage of infection, and the response of the patient. Although many infected joints can be drained satisfactorily with repeated needle aspiration, the hip—and perhaps other joints that are difficult to aspirate—will require arthrotomy as soon as possible after identification of joint sepsis. Other indications for surgical drainage of septic arthritis are inability to aspirate loculated pus, lack of prompt response to nonoperative management, long-standing infection, and joint infections after surgery or penetrating wounds.

Parenteral antibiotics are indicated for septic arthritis. If organisms are not seen on Gram-stained smears and the patient is a previously healthy adult, gonococcal arthritis is an appropriate working diagnosis, and penicillin should be started as outlined below. Children under 4 years of age have a significant incidence of *H influenzae* arthritis. Preliminary antibiotic treatment in this age group must be effective against this organism, which also may be difficult to see on Gram-stained smears. In adults with negative results on Gram-stained smears and a suspected cause of infection other than gonococci, treatment should be started with a cephalosporin or a beta-lactamase-resistant penicillin and an aminoglycoside.

When organisms are seen, initial antibiotic therapy should be based on that finding. Culture results and clinical response must subsequently be used to ensure an appropriate antibiotic regimen. Parenteral antibiotics are continued at high doses until inflammation resolves significantly. Ten to 14 days of treatment is usually required. An additional 3–4 weeks of oral antibiotic therapy is often advised after parenteral treatment. Briefer treatment usually suffices for gonococcal arthritis. Intravenous penicillin G, 10 million units/24 h, should be continued until significant improvement is achieved. While the response is often prompt, several days of treatment may be required. Once local signs resolve, the antibiotic can be changed to oral ampicillin, 500 mg four times daily, to complete a 7-day course.

Prognosis

Satisfactory results are achieved in 70% or more of patients with septic arthritis if early diagnosis and treatment are provided. Joint destruction—especially of the hip in infants—and joint stiffness in the elderly are the commonest causes of failure. Deaths are rare.

Chaudhuri K et al: Septic arthritis of the shoulder after mastectomy and radiotherapy for breast carcinoma. J Bone Joint Surg Br 1993;75:318.

Dagan R: Management of acute hematogenous osteomyelitis and septic arthritis in the pediatric patient. Pediatr Infect Dis J 1993;12:88.

Ostrum RF: Nocardia septic arthritis of the hip with associated avascular necrosis; a case report. Clin Orthop 1993;(288):282.

Rankin KC, Rycken JM: Bilateral dislocation of the proximal humeral epiphyses in septic arthritis: a case report. J Bone Joint Surg Br 1993;75:329.

■ BONE TUMORS

Primary tumors of bone are relatively uncommon in comparison with secondary or metastatic neoplasms. However, they are of great clinical significance because of the possibility of cancer and because some grow rapidly and metastasize widely. Persistent skeletal pain, localized tenderness, and an enlarging mass with or without limitation of motion of adjacent joints or spontaneous fracture are indications for prompt clinical, radiographic, laboratory, and perhaps biopsy examination. Histologic characteristics generally provide the best information about the nature of the lesion, but they must be correlated with all other related facts. The diagnosis of bone tumors is most precise when made by the clinician, the radiologist, and the pathologist in close consultation.

Operative Technique

There are several surgical approaches to the treatment of bone tumors. With intralesional excision (curettement, debulking), the tumor is entered, but gross as well as microscopic tumor may remain. Excision indicates local removal of a tumor following visualization of the capsule or pseudocapsule to establish the plane of dissection. Tumor cells may be left in the wound even if the capsule is not grossly violated. Wide excision indicates a margin of normal tissue between the capsule or pseudocapsule and the planes of dissection. Radical resection implies removal of the entire anatomic compartment containing the tumor. Amputation may be any of these depending on the margin, but it is usually "wide excision" or "radical resection."

Radiologic Characteristics

A. BENIGN CHARACTERISTICS

1. Cystic expansion of a diaphysis or metaphysis with mature cortex around the area of expansion.
2. The presence of a definable though thin cortical end plate (capsule) around an intraosseous area from which cancellous or cortical bone has been lost, sometimes referred to as a "geographic lesion."
3. No periosteal new bone formation.

B. MALIGNANT CHARACTERISTICS

1. Permeative destruction of either cancellous or cortical bone, manifested by gradual transition from a region of gross destruction with loss of bony continuity to a region of lesser destruction and normal bone. There is no clear line of demarcation between abnormal and normal bone.
2. Gross bone destruction with cortical defects, manifested by loss of large areas of bony substance without encapsulation.
3. Periosteal or bone formation within the tumor or at its margins may be manifested by multiple layers of parallel periosteal reaction (onionskin formation) or sunburst (spiculated, hair-on-end) linear areas of calcification. The latter generally parallel the expansile direction of the tumor as it breaks through bone.
4. A few metastatic tumors (breast, prostate) incite local reactive new bone formation and are classified as osteoblastic rather than osteolytic tumors (the latter are more common in metastatic cancer).

Grading & Staging of Bone Tumors

Some tumor categories can be subclassified into varying degrees of malignancy (grading) according to histologic criteria, radiologic appearance, and clinical course. Grade 0 is benign; grade 1 is low-grade malignancy; and grades 2 and 3 indicate increasingly higher degrees of malignancy. Grading reflects the biologic behavior of the lesion.

The size of the tumor, the presence or absence of local invasion of adjacent compartments or lymph nodes, and the presence or absence of distant metastases can be combined with the surgical grade to establish stage categories that reflect prognosis. When grading and staging are possible, treatment options may be more realistically chosen.

Among musculoskeletal neoplasms, chondrosarcomas lend themselves to grading, though in tumors occurring secondary to osteochondroma, size is of less significance than it is with other sarcomas. Grading and staging of soft tissue sarcomas by histologic criteria, intra- or extracompartmental location, and metastatic spread have prognostic value and aid in planning treatment.

In osteogenic sarcoma and Ewing's sarcoma, the prognosis is not easily determined from the histologic pattern, and grading is therefore not as useful as in soft tissue sarcomas or chondrosarcomas.

Biopsy

The possibility of cancer exists in almost every lesion prior to histologic examination. Therefore, the choice of excision and the extent of exposure for biopsy should be planned to avoid unnecessary contamination of tissue planes with tumor cells, which would complicate subsequent local resection. This consideration takes precedence over more standard surgical approaches used for trauma and reconstruction. In the extremities, biopsy incisions should be longitudinal and placed where minimal dissection is needed to reach the tumor. Frozen section guidance should be obtained. This may permit immediate definitive diagnosis and operation. Even when this is not so, the surgeon can be assured that an adequate and representative sample has been examined and may occasionally be forewarned that the lesion is inflammatory rather than neoplastic. For the latter reason, it is also advisable to take appropriate culture specimens of some of the tissue removed at biopsy even though the clinical picture and x-ray appearance may seem typical of a neoplastic lesion.

Chemotherapy

Adjunctive chemotherapy following appropriate management of the primary lesion delays the appearance and lowers the incidence of metastases and the 2-year death rates for osteogenic sarcoma, Ewing's sarcoma, and primary lymphoma of bone. Alterations in drug combinations, dosage, and frequency continue to be made. For this reason, specific protocols for chemotherapy will not be set forth here. The reader is referred to reports of the appropriate cancer study groups of the National Cancer Institute for current guidelines.

Radiation Therapy

Radiation therapy combined with chemotherapy has become standard treatment for Ewing's sarcoma and primary lymphoma of bone. Radiation therapy used alone sometimes produced dramatic initial control of primary lesions, but 5-year survival rates for these tumors did not improve significantly until chemotherapy was added.

Radiation therapy plus chemotherapy has a less well defined role in the treatment of primary osteogenic sarcoma. Irradiation alone will produce a temporary response manifested largely by brief cessation of the prior rapid rate of growth. However, even when chemotherapy is added, sufficient control of the primary lesion is not achieved.

Radiation therapy of benign lesions of bone is undesirable if the primary can be controlled surgically, since radiation-induced sarcoma of bone occurs with an incidence of 0.2% in normal bone (ie, in radiation fields in patients treated for other lesions). The risk appears to be greater in growing bone than adult bone. Certain benign but locally aggressive tumors of bone with high local recurrence rates necessitate consideration of radiation therapy if the anatomic location makes the risk of morbidity and death associated with surgical removal unacceptable (spine, skull, or facial bones).

METASTATIC BONE TUMORS

The commonest form of cancer affecting the skeleton is metastatic tumor deposits from primary lesions elsewhere in the body. Eighty percent of these metastatic lesions are from primary carcinomas—particularly of the breast, prostate, lung, kidney, thyroid, pancreas, or stomach, in that order of frequency.

The presenting symptom is usually pain. Pathologic fracture may be present and is more common in the lower than the upper extremity.

The presenting radiologic finding is destruction of bone—usually osteolytic but in the case of breast or prostate metastasis either partly or solely osteoblastic. The size of an individual lesion is usually less than what is seen in primary tumors of bone at the time of first diagnosis.

In a patient with a known primary malignant tumor presenting with a painful lytic lesion of bone, a diagnosis of metastatic deposit can be made with some assurance; but there are individuals in whom the primary is not yet recognized at the time the early metastatic lesion becomes painful. Bone scan or skeletal survey will aid the prebiopsy workup since there is a high probability of more than one area of skeletal involvement. The most common primary source of solitary skeletal metastases at the time of first diagnosis is carcinoma of the kidney. Therefore, an excretory urogram should be part of the prebiopsy workup of solitary metastases with no obvious primary. Metastases from carcinoma of the kidney are extremely vascular—an important point to remember when planning biopsy.

The treatment of metastatic cancer has two goals: management of the neoplasm and management of the symptoms produced by the local lesion.

Management of the neoplasm at the metastatic site depends upon the type and prognosis in each case but usually involves radiation therapy, chemotherapy, hormone therapy, or a combination of these treatment methods.

Operative treatment with internal fixation for pathologic fracture is often desirable in metastatic tumors of long bones, particularly in the lower extremities, so that the patient can remain ambulatory and more comfortable during the months or even years of life that remain. Although less commonly indicated because of the nonweightbearing function of the upper extremity, internal fixation may be necessary for pain control or to improve the patient's ability to manage crutches. In addition to the usual techniques for fracture fixation, methylmethacrylate supplementation frequently is necessary to substitute for bone loss and possible lack of healing response.

MYELOMA

In one sense, multiple myeloma is the commonest malignant tumor affecting bone, but since it arises from the hematopoietic marrow, it is not, strictly speaking, a tumor "of bone." Its incidence is about equal to that of all malignant tumors of bone combined. Pain is the principal presenting symptom, and local swelling is uncommon. Pathologic fractures do occur but are not a common initial symptom. The lesions can occur in any bone, but small bone involvement is infrequent. There is a slightly higher incidence in males than females, with peak incidence in the sixth and seventh decades. The bony lesions are manifested radiologically by osteolytic areas of bone destruction, with little or no reactive bone.

As indicated by the term multiple myeloma, there frequently are multiple lesions at the time of initial diagnosis.

The treatment strategy is essentially the same as that outlined above for metastatic tumors.

MALIGNANT BONE TUMORS

1. Osteogenic Sarcoma

Osteogenic sarcoma is the most common primary malignant tumor of bone, with an incidence of 0.25 cases per 100,000 population per year. It usually occurs in the distal femoral metaphysis, proximal tibial metaphysis, proximal humeral metaphysis, pelvis, or proximal femur, in that order of frequency. Most patients are in the adolescent age group, and males predominate in a 3:2 ratio.

The usual presenting manifestations are pain, tenderness, and swelling near a joint. Some limitation of motion may be present.

X-rays show a permeative destructive lesion in the metaphysis that rarely crosses the epiphysial plate and is commonly accompanied by periosteal elevation. Periosteal new bone frequently presents in the form of Codman's triangle at the diaphysial end of the lesion (Figure 43–49). The more central area will show evidence of tumor extension beyond the confines of the cortex and contains sunburst or hair-on-end radially oriented filaments of calcification and bone formation. There is considerable variation in the degree of osteolytic versus osteoblastic activity in these lesions.

The natural history of this tumor is one of relentless growth, early metastasis to the lungs, and death if appropriate treatment is not given. Lymphatic involvement is not common. Treatment by resection (usually amputation) of the primary lesion in past years produced a 5-year survival rate of 15–20%. Most deaths occurred in the first 2 years. With adjunctive chemotherapy following amputation or other local complete resection of the tumor, the appearance of pulmonary metastases has been significantly delayed, and the projected 5-year survival rate currently is about 60%. The apparent ability of adjunctive chemotherapy to destroy microscopic metastases suggests that local resection of primary lesions followed by adjunctive chemotherapy may be substituted for amputation. This is still experimental, however, since at this time 5-year rates for both survival and absence of local recurrence in a suitably functioning limb are not available. Lesions in the pelvis or spine might have boundaries too close to vital structures and hence should be treated with local excision, adjunctive chemotherapy, and perhaps radiation therapy.

Rare variants of osteogenic sarcoma with a less ominous history are parosteal, periosteal, and central sarcomas. These variants may be more amenable to local resection.

Figure 43–49. Osteosarcoma with Codman's triangle.

2. Primary Chondrosarcoma

The incidence of chondrosarcoma is about half that of osteogenic sarcoma. Most of these tumors are located either in the pelvic girdle, ribs, or shoulder girdle, in that order. The peak incidence is in the late fifth and early sixth decades, with a 2:1 male predominance.

The presenting symptom is usually local discomfort. A visible or demonstrable mass is seldom present.

The x-ray appearance is that of a central, slightly expansile, radiolucent lesion containing flocculent areas of calcific density in the lower-grade forms of the tumor. High-grade chondrosarcomas may simulate osteogenic sarcoma on x-rays. The tumor occurs commonly in the metaphysial region when present in long bones but has a predilection for flat bones, as evidenced by the high incidence in the pelvis and ribs and a relatively high incidence in the scapula. The gross pathologic anatomy is that of firm, translucent, usually gritty gray tissue of cartilaginous density with demonstrable fine sediment of calcific density. The natural history is one of continued growth, with a high rate of local recurrence if all tumor is not removed. Metastases to distant sites—particularly the lungs—occur much later than is the case with most other bone sarcomas.

The treatment of chondrosarcoma is individualized in terms of how radical the attempt at surgical removal must be. There is no evidence that x-ray therapy will control the lesion or that chemotherapy will affect the outcome. Complete surgical removal will result in cure at 5 years in almost all grade 1 tumors and a significant percentage of grade 3 tumors. When these tumors are graded, it is important to be certain that all of the tumor has been well sampled, since there may be considerable variation in different geographic areas within the tumor.

3. Ewing's Tumor (Ewing's Sarcoma)

Ewing's sarcoma occurs with an incidence of 0.1 cases per 100,000 population per year. The male:female ratio is 3:2. The tumor occurs most commonly in the second decade. Patients tend to be slightly younger than those with osteogenic sarcoma. Ewing's tumor is most common in the extremities, particularly the lower extremities and pelvic girdle. The symptoms and signs are pain, local swelling, and occasionally fever, with an elevated white blood count.

The x-ray appearance is that of a permeative destructive lesion, usually in the metaphysis but also in the diaphysis more often than osteogenic sarcoma. Periosteal new bone formation is common. The gross pathologic picture is nonspecific, with neoplastic tissue permeating bone and muscle with a consistency varying from firm gray connective tissue to liquefaction necrosis. The latter has at times mimicked purulence secondary to bacterial infection and may be confused with osteomyelitis. These facts reinforce the general wisdom of routinely obtaining material both for culture and for histopathologic examination whether the clinical diagnosis is infection or neoplasm.

The early history is one of progressive local growth, early distant metastases, and death if proper treatment is not given. Metastasis is most commonly to the lung but may occur in other tissues (including bone) more frequently than is the case with osteogenic sarcoma. Radiation therapy to the primary tumor combined with multiple-drug chemotherapy has improved the 5-year survival rate to about 60%.

Treatment of Ewing's sarcoma of the pelvis has a significantly higher failure rate following such combination therapy. Anatomically feasible resection or wide excision following initial tumor response to combined treatment should therefore be considered. If the primary tumor is in an expendable bone, wide excision or resection may be considered after an initial course of combined treatment.

4. Fibrosarcoma

The incidence of fibrosarcoma is about 0.05 cases per 100,000 population per year. Males and females are equally affected. More than half of cases occur in the long bones, and the distal femur and proximal tibia are the commonest sites. The humerus and scapula together have been reported as representing perhaps the second or third most common site. These tumors have been reported in every decade through the ninth but are most common in the third and fourth decades. If fibrosarcoma in Paget's disease or other preexisting disease is included, the mean age at diagnosis is the mid 50s.

The signs and symptoms are those of pain and, at times, local swelling. The incidence of pathologic fracture is relatively high.

X-rays show a destructive lesion of bone, almost universally osteolytic, with little or no calcification within the tumor mass but with periosteal reactions at the margins, which may be horizontal (onionskin) in character or spiculated (hair-on-end). The periosteal reaction is less prominent than in osteogenic sarcoma. The lesions are usually quite large at first presentation. The gross pathologic anatomy is nonspecific, and the tumor itself consists of tissue of connective tissue density and is seldom accompanied by liquefaction necrosis.

The natural history is one of progressive growth, frequent pathologic fracture, and distant metastases usually to the lung, with death if appropriate treatment is not given. Treatment consists of local removal of the primary tumor, which in most situations requires amputation. Neither radiation therapy nor chemotherapy has been helpful. The 5-year survival rate is 30–35%.

5. Malignant Lymphoma (Reticulum Cell Sarcoma of Bone)

This tumor occurs with an estimated incidence of 0.1 case per 100,000 population per year. There is a slight (3:2) male predominance. The tumor is commonest between the third and sixth decades. It is relatively rare in the forearm, hand, and foot.

The usual presenting signs and symptoms are pain, local tenderness, and, occasionally local swelling. The x-ray appearance is usually that of a permeative diffuse, destructive lesion with minimal or absent periosteal reaction, even in the case of rather large lesions. The gross pathologic picture is nonspecific.

If systemic generalized involvement is excluded by appropriate staging, the treatment of choice is radiation, which is associated with a 5-year survival rate of 35–50%. The generalized disease, which may be present with localized symptoms initially, requires combined radiation therapy and chemotherapy and has a reported 5-year survival rate of 23%.

BENIGN BONE TUMORS

1. Osteochondroma

Osteochondromas (bony exostoses) comprise at least 45% of benign bone tumors. These tend to occur at the metaphyses of long bones but may also occur in the spine and ribs. The most common sites are the distal ends of the femur and the proximal ends of the humerus. The patients are usually under 20 years of age at the time of initial excision. Since these are very slow-growing tumors, the time of diagnosis or excision does not coincide with the time of onset.

The x-ray appearance is that of a bony stalk with a cartilaginous cap extending from the metaphysial region near the epiphysial plate and usually inclined away from the joint. These lesions rarely enlarge after childhood. The usual reasons for operation are local mechanical problems related to tumor size or perhaps pressure against musculotendinous structures operating in the vicinity. Sarcomatous degeneration occurs in 1% of cases. Thus, a sudden increase in size or a change in symptomatology warrants exploration and biopsy.

Multiple congenital osteochondromas (exostoses) occur as a heritable autosomal dominant characteristic. There is usually some growth retardation and bowing deformity of the long bones. The incidence of sarcomatous degeneration is variously reported to be 5–15% in this group, but this may simply reflect the larger number of lesions present.

The treatment of symptomatic lesions is by surgical excision, which should include the entire stalk and its base. Secondary chondrosarcoma requires complete removal (resection, with some anatomic areas requiring amputation).

2. Enchondroma (Chondroma)

Enchondroma is most commonly in the hand, including the metacarpals and phalangeals, and next most commonly in the proximal end of the humerus. It is equally distributed between males and females and accounts for about 10% of benign tumors. It may occur from the first decade through the seventh, with the mean age in the mid thirties. The x-ray appearance is that of a cystic, slightly expansile lesion in the shaft of a long bone, with some scalloping of the cortex but without periosteal new bone formation. A speckled, calcific series of shadows within the cystic lesion is characteristic. The gross pathology is that of firm, translucent gray-white granular material.

The natural history is one of slow growth and a low incidence of pathologic fracture. Pain is often present. Except for lesions in the clavicle or small bones of the hand or foot, visible or palpable masses are uncommon.

Treatment consists of curettement and bone grafting.

3. Giant Cell Tumor of Bone

Giant cell tumor (Figure 43–50) is most common around the knee, the sacrum, the distal radius, and the proximal humerus. It occurs with a female:male ratio of 3:2. It is almost never seen before closure of the epiphysial plate. It tends to be centered in the epiphysial area and to extend eccentrically beyond the epiphysial plate boundary. The chief symptom is pain. Pathologic fracture is rare, and the pain usually leads to diagnosis before there is visible or palpable external swelling.

X-rays show a cystic expansion of the involved bone. The area of destruction has a soap bubble appearance,

Figure 43–50. Giant cell tumor of proximal humerus.

with normal trabeculae and little reactive bone at the margins. Grossly, the lesion is filled with an orange and brown soft tumor mass without calcification. Ninety-eight percent of cases are benign and the remainder are malignant, with potential for metastatic spread. The neoplastic portion of the tumor is the mesenchymal stromal cell rather than the giant cell element. Benign giant cell tumor may recur and become malignant.

The natural history without treatment is one of continuous growth resulting in an enormous tumor, pathologic fracture, and in some cases necrosis of overlying skin. Treatment is by operative removal, and complete cure can be expected if the lesion is completely resected. Since it is most common in nonexpendable bones, thorough curettement and grafting is the standard initial treatment. This form of treatment carries a risk of recurrence as high as 40%. If tumor recurs, biopsy should be performed again to verify the absence of malignant change. If malignant change has not taken place, resection followed by allograft, arthrodesis, or prosthetic replacement has the greatest probability of preventing recurrence. But curettement—followed by filling the cavity with methylmethacrylate—is not inappropriate.

In addition to a high recurrence rate, this lesion also carries a higher rate of postoperative wound infection than comparable operations in the same anatomic region.

Radiation therapy is probably not justified because of a risk of later postradiation sarcoma—except in the spine or sacrum, where complete surgical removal is not possible.

4. Aneurysmal Bone Cyst

Aneurysmal bone cyst is most common in the metaphyses of long bones and in the vertebrae, particularly the posterior elements. The peak incidence is in the second decade. The male:female incidence is equal. The most common symptoms and signs are pain and swelling. Pathologic fractures are rare.

The x-ray appearance is that of an eccentric metaphysial lesion containing expansile cysts with septa. A large thin shell portion protrudes beyond the normal confines of the bony anatomy. Grossly, the tumor is a blood-filled cavity with a soft membrane lining the bony margins.

These tumors are locally destructive by expansile growth but do not metastasize.

Treatment consists of operative removal. Radiation therapy is justified only for lesions in areas where local resection (or thorough curettement) is not feasible (eg, the spine). A recurrence rate ranging from 30% to 60% has been reported following curettement. Several factors relating to recurrence are (1) the adequacy of surgical removal; (2) the age of the patient (risk is much greater in patients under age 15); and (3) tumor size (large tumors in young patients have a high recurrence rate). There may also be a correlation between the frequency of mitotic figures and an increased risk of recurrence.

Resection is the treatment of choice where location permits. Some giant cell tumors and some osteogenic sarcomas will have an aneurysmal cystic element, and diagnosis therefore requires a representative sample.

5. Unicameral Bone Cyst

The incidence of unicameral bone cyst in the general population is not clearly defined, since this is a benign lesion with a tendency to be self-limited and possibly self-healing. Most patients are children, usually between the ages of 5 and 15 years, with a slight (3:2) male preponderance. These tumors are usually asymptomatic until pathologic fracture produces pain.

The roentgenographic appearance is that of a multilocular expansile, cystic lesion, principally radiolucent, with its proximal end at or near the epiphysial plate (Figure 43–51). The overlying cortex is attenuated, but no periosteal new bone formation is present. The central portion is rarefied, and undisplaced fracture is the most common initial symptom.

Grossly, the cyst is predominantly a fluid-filled space with a thin capsule. The fluid may vary from serous to sanguineous. The lesions are of varying size, from moderately large to small, and are occasionally seen in x-rays taken for other reasons in asymptomatic patients. At first presentation, however, they classically encompass the entire diameter of the metaphysis. Recognition that these tumors are seen in asymptomatic patients permits the assumption that some are self-healing. Spontaneous regression has been documented following fracture in about 15% of these lesions.

In the past, the usual treatment was curettement and autogenous bone graft to fill the space. The recurrence rate following this treatment varies from 20% to 50% and is reported to be twice as high in patients under age 10 compared with those over age 10. Subtotal resection techniques, with excision of most of the cyst wall including the bony shell, both with or without grafting, have been associated with a recurrence rate of 5–9%, but the number of cases from which these figures are derived is small. If the proximal end of the cyst is in contact with the epiphysial plate, the cyst is classified as "active"; if the cyst is separated from the plate by normal cancellous metaphysial bone, it is classified as "latent." Active cysts carry the greater risk of recurrence following curettement and grafting and also (owing to

Figure 43–51. Unicameral bone cyst with fracture.

the proximity to the epiphysial plate) carry a higher risk of damage to the plate at the time of operation. Intracystic injection of methylprednisolone is a safe alternative to surgical treatment of these lesions. Results of this procedure show a recurrence rate of 5–10% with few complications.

Expectant treatment can be offered until the pathologic fracture is healed, at which time needle biopsy should be done. Although details of classification are sometimes difficult with needle biopsy because of the small sample, this procedure will clearly separate the classic cyst from solid tumor lesions simulating unicameral bone cyst. If the mass is identified as cystic, consideration of operative removal can be postponed (particularly if the patient is under 10 years of age) and the progress of the cyst merely observed. If a second pathologic fracture occurs and the cyst does not show signs of resolution, either curettement with grafting or steroid injection may be tried.

Oppenheim WL, Gallend H: Operative treatment versus steroid injection in the management of unicameral bone cysts. J Pediatr Orthop 1984;4:1.

6. Eosinophilic Granuloma

Eosinophilic granuloma is a solitary lytic lesion of bone that is classified with disorders of the reticuloendothelial system and may not be a true neoplasm. It is relatively rare, and the most common site is the skull. The male:female ratio is 3:2, and the peak incidence is between 7 years and 8 years of age. Most cases occur before age 30.

Pain is the principal presenting complaint. There is almost never any demonstrable tumor mass on physical examination.

The radiologic appearance is that of a lytic defect, which in long bones frequently expands the shaft and may be accompanied by periosteal new bone formation, usually of the horizontal (onionskin) type. In flat bones, the lesion is also lytic but tends to be flattened to conform to the shape of the host bone.

Grossly, the tissue is soft (sometimes semigelatinous) and gray or yellow. Hemorrhagic areas are occasionally seen.

If the systemic variants of histiocytosis X (Hand-Schüller-Christian disease, Letterer-Siwe disease) are excluded, the lesions are probably self-limited and may run through a rapid growth cycle followed by spontaneous healing. There is evidence that they heal following biopsy with or without bone grafting. Low-dose irradiation has been used for treatment, particularly for symptomatic spine lesions, but it is more appropriate to merely observe the patient following biopsy in the hope that spontaneous healing will occur. If pathologic frac-

tures are present, they should be treated by cast or fixation.

7. Chondroblastoma

Chondroblastoma is a relatively rare lesion that characteristically occurs in the epiphysis prior to closure of the epiphysial plate. This location is a rare site of other primary or secondary tumors in growing bone. Ninety percent of cases occur between the ages of 5 and 25 years. The male:female ratio is 2:1. The epiphyses around the knee and the proximal humerus are the common locations. Pain and joint effusion are common, with associated local tenderness and limitation of motion of the adjacent joints.

The x-ray appearance is that of a lytic lesion in the epiphysial body or, if the plate is closed, in its former location. The lesions are usually not expansile and seldom as large as giant cell tumors. They rarely extend significantly across the old epiphysial plate in patients whose physial lines are closed. The lesions tend to be eccentric in the epiphysis and have a mottled appearance compatible with calcification within the tumor. Pathologic fracture and subperiosteal reaction are uncommon. The gross pathologic anatomy is that of granular tissue of cartilaginous density containing foci of calcification. A chondroblastoma grows slowly and lacks malignant characteristics, although a few cases of metastases have been reported.

The commonest treatment is curettement and bone grafting, since the location frequently does not permit resection. The recurrence rate varies from 10% to 40% in different series. If recurrence does occur, recurettement with grafting is still the treatment of choice if the site is one that does not permit resection. There is no evidence that radiation therapy or chemotherapy has any value in these lesions.

Conway WF, Hayes CW: Miscellaneous lesions of bone. Radiol Clin North Am 1993;31:339.

Caso Martinez J et al: En-bloc resection of the distal fibula for aneurysmal bone cyst. Acta Orthop Belg 1993;59:87.

Hudson TM, Stiles RG, Monson DK: Fibrous lesions of bone. Radiol Clin North Am 1993;31:279.

McCarthy CS, Becker JA: Multiple myeloma and contrast media. Radiology 1992;183:519.

Mercuri M et al: The management of malignant bone tumors in children and adolescents. Clin Orthop 1991;(264):156.

Pennington DG, Marsden W, Stephens FO: Fibrosarcoma of metacarpal treated by combined therapy and immediate reconstruction with vascularized bone graft. J Hand Surg Am 1991;16:877.

Simon MA, Finn HA: Diagnostic strategy for bone and soft-tissue tumors. J Bone Joint Surg Am 1993;75:622.

Steiner RM et al: Magnetic resonance imaging of diffuse bone marrow disease. Radiol Clin North Am 1993;31:383.

Plastic & Reconstructive Surgery

44

Luis O. Vasconez, MD, & Henry C. Vasconez, MD

Plastic surgery, although thought of as a technique-oriented specialty, is in fact a problem-solving field. The training of a plastic surgeon allows him or her to see surgical problems in a different light and select from a variety of options to solve surgical problems. Plastic surgeons have received broad training, and most have completed residencies in other fields such as general surgery, ENT surgery, orthopedics, urology, or neurosurgery.

The basic principles of plastic surgery are careful analysis of the surgical problem, careful planning of procedures, precise technique, and atraumatic handling of tissues. Alteration, coverage, and transfer of skin and associated tissues are the most common procedures performed. Plastic surgery may deal with closure of surgical wounds—particularly recalcitrant wounds such as those occurring post radiation or poorly healing wounds in immunocompromised patients—removal of skin tumors, repair of soft tissue injuries or burns, correction of acquired or congenital deformities of the breast, or repair of cosmetic defects. Operations on the head and neck and the hand may require special surgical training.

In the past 2 decades, increased knowledge of anatomy and the development of many new techniques have brought about important changes in plastic surgery. It is now known that in many areas the blood supply of the skin is derived principally from vessels arising from underlying muscles and larger perforating blood vessels rather than solely from vessels of the subcutaneous tissue, as was formerly thought. One-stage transfer of large areas of skin and muscle tissue can be accomplished if the axial pedicle of the underlying muscle is included in the transfer. With the use of microsurgical techniques, musculocutaneous units or combinations of bone, muscle, and skin can be successfully transferred and vessels and nerves less than 1 mm in size can be repaired. These so-called free-flap transplantations are a major advance in the treatment of defects that were previously untreatable or required lengthy or multistaged procedures. More sophisticated knowledge of the blood supply to the skin has introduced a concept of perforator flaps whereby one perforating vessel is identified that may supply a large segment of overlying skin. Similarly, the concept of neurocutaneous arteries and flaps has given rise to the design of additional flap territories such as the so-called sural flap in the lower leg.

The plastic surgeon, as a member of the craniofacial surgical team, is able to dramatically improve the appearance and function of children with severe congenital deformities. Children of normal intelligence who previously had been social outcasts are now able to lead relatively normal lives. Improved understanding of facial growth and abnormal development and diagnostic techniques such as the CT scan, MRI, and three-dimensional computer-assisted imaging enable the reconstructive surgeon to develop a complex strategy for remodeling the deformed craniofacial skeleton. This may involve remodeling or repositioning part or all of the cranial vault, the orbits, the mid face, and the mandible. These complex and at times formidable reconstructions, which were performed by moving both units and adding bone grafts from the ileum, have more recently been somewhat simplified with the introduction of the miniplate method of fixation as well as of bone substitutes that may serve as a scaffold upon which normal bone can regrow.

A recent notable advance in craniofacial surgery has been the introduction of distraction osteogenesis, which borrows from the Ilizarov principle of distraction where one makes a cortical cut in the bone and then applies a distraction apparatus so that in measured amounts (usually 1 mm per day) the bone is transported to bridge a gap. In craniofacial surgery it is more commonly brought to bear to enlarge or cause overgrowth of areas such as an underdeveloped mandible.

Additional areas of involvement for the plastic surgeon entail allotransplantation, particularly with the increasing number of clinical limb allotransplants, which unfortunately at present still require immunosuppression. It is hoped that immunotolerance will some day become a reality, thus allowing transplantation of nonessential organs.

Tissue engineering of bone, cartilage, and nerve is an area of ongoing research for plastic surgeons. Although encouraging experimental results have been reported in anatomic areas difficult to reconstruct such as the external ear, there are as yet no clinical applications.

Fetal surgery—an area pioneered by a number of plastic surgeons—appears to be in a quiescent stage, particularly because of advances in the treatment of cleft lip and cleft palate in the newborn.

Jones JW et al: Successful hand transplantation. One-year follow-up. Louisville Hand Transplant Team. N Engl J Med 2000; 343:468.

■ I. GRAFTS & FLAPS

SKIN GRAFTS

A graft of skin detaches epidermis and varying amounts of dermis from its blood supply in the **donor area** and is placed in a new bed of blood supply from the base of the wound, or **recipient area.** Although the technique is relatively simple to perform and generally reliable, definite considerations about the donor area and adequacy of the recipient area are important. Skin grafting is a quick, effective way to cover a wound if vascularity is adequate, infection is not present, and hemostasis is assured. Color match, contour, durability of the graft, and donor morbidity must be considered.

Types of Skin Grafts

Skin grafts can be either split-thickness or full-thickness grafts (Figure 44–1). Each type has advantages and disadvantages and is indicated or contraindicated for different kinds of wounds (Table 44–1).

A. SPLIT-THICKNESS GRAFTS

Thinner split-thickness grafts (0.01–0.015 inch) become vascularized more rapidly and survive transplantation more reliably. This is important in grafting on less than ideal recipient sites, such as contaminated wounds, burn surfaces, and poorly vascularized surfaces (eg, irradiated sites). A second advantage is that donor sites heal more rapidly and can be reused within a relatively short time (7–10 days) in critical cases such as major burns.

In general, however, the disadvantages of thin split-thickness grafts outweigh the advantages. Thin grafts exhibit the highest degree of postgraft contraction, offer the least amount of resistance to surface trauma, and are least like normal skin in texture, suppleness, pore pattern, hair growth, and other characteristics. Hence, they are usually aesthetically unacceptable.

Thicker split-thickness skin grafts (> 0.015 inch) contract less, are more resistant to surface trauma, and are more similar to normal skin than are thin split-thickness grafts. They are also aesthetically more acceptable but not as acceptable as full-thickness grafts.

The disadvantages of thick split-thickness grafts are relatively few but can be significant. They are less easily vascularized than thin grafts and thus result in fewer successful takes when used on less than ideal surfaces. Their donor sites are slower to heal (requiring 10–18 days) and heal with more scarring than donor sites for thin split-thickness grafts—a factor that may prevent reuse of the area.

Meshed grafts are usually thin or intermediate split-thickness grafts that have been rolled under a special cutting machine to create a mesh pattern. Although grafts with these perforations can be expanded from one and one-half to nine times their original size, expansion to one and one-half times the unmeshed size is the most useful. Meshed grafts are advantageous because they can be placed on an irregular, possibly contaminated wound bed and will usually take. Also, complications of hemostasis are fewer, because blood and serum exude through the mesh pattern. The disadvantage is poor appearance following healing (alligator hide).

Donor sites for split-thickness grafts heal spontaneously by epithelialization. During this process, epithelial cells from the sweat glands, sebaceous glands, or hair follicles proliferate upward and spread across the wound surface. If these three structures are not present, epithelialization will not occur.

B. FULL-THICKNESS GRAFTS

Full-thickness skin grafts include the epidermis and all the dermis. They are the most aesthetically desirable of the free grafts since they include the highest number of skin appendage elements, undergo the least amount of contracture, and have a greater ability to withstand trauma. There are several limiting factors in the use of full-thickness grafts. Since no epidermal elements remain to produce epithelialization in the donor site, it must be closed primarily, and a scar will result. The size and number of available donor sites is therefore limited. Furthermore, conditions at the recipient site must be optimal in order for transplantation to be successful.

Figure 44–1. Depths of full-thickness and split-thickness grafts.

Table 44–1. Advantages and disadvantages of various types of skin grafts.

Type of Graft	Advantages	Disadvantages
Thin split-thickness	Survive transplantation most easily. Donor sites heal most rapidly.	Fewest qualities of normal skin. Maximum contraction. Least resistance to trauma. Sensation poor. Aesthetically poor.
Thick split-thickness	More qualities of normal skin. Less contraction. More resistant to trauma. Sensation fair. Aesthetically more acceptable.	Survive transplantation less well. Donor site heals slowly.
Full thickness	Nearly all qualities of normal skin. Minimal contraction. Very resistant to trauma. Sensation good. Aesthetically good.	Survive transplantation least well. Donor site must be closed surgically. Donor sites are limited.

Areas of thin skin are the best donor sites for full-thickness grafts (eg, the eyelids and the skin of the postauricular, supraclavicular, antecubital, inguinal, and genital areas). Submammary and subgluteal skin is thicker but allows camouflage of donor area scars. In grafts thicker than approximately 0.015 inch, the results of transplantation are often poor except on the face, where vascularity is so good.

C. Composite Grafts

A composite graft is also a free graft that must reestablish its blood supply in the recipient area. It consists of a unit with several tissue planes that may include skin, subcutaneous tissue, cartilage, or other tissue. Dermal fat grafts, hair transplant grafts, and skin and cartilage grafts from the ear fall into this category. Obviously, composite grafts must be small or at least relatively thin and will require recipient sites with excellent vascularity. These grafts are generally used in the face.

D. Cultured Epithelial and Dermal Grafts

Epithelial cells were first to be cultured in vitro and made to coalesce into sheets that could be used to cover full-thickness wounds. Although these culture epithelial sheets were used in the treatment of burns, the result was unsatisfactory because the coverage was very fragile and unsatisfactory. More recently, success has been obtained with artificial dermis which when placed in an appropriate bed will revascularize and can then be covered by a very thin (0.05 cm) split-thickness skin graft. This artificial dermis is increasingly being used in the treatment of burns. Modifications of this concept have also been applied to the care of chronic ulcers, particularly in the leg. The artificial dermis is made out of a collagen matrix and has very low or no antigenicity.

Obtaining Skin Grafts

Instruments used for obtaining skin grafts include razor blades, skin grafting knives (Blair, Ferris Smith, Humby, Goulian), manual drum dermatomes (Padgett, Reese), and electric or air-powered dermatomes (Brown, Padgett, Hall). The electric and air-powered dermatomes are the most widely used because of their reliability and ease of operation. A surgeon, even with only limited experience, can successfully obtain sheets of split-thickness skin grafts, using the electric dermatomes.

The Skin Graft Recipient Area

To ensure survival of the graft, there must be (1) adequate vascularity of the recipient bed, (2) complete contact between the graft and the bed, (3) adequate immobilization of the graft-bed unit, and (4) relatively few bacteria in the recipient area.

Since survival of the graft is dependent upon growth of capillary buds into the raw undersurface of the graft, vascularity of the recipient area is of prime importance. Avascular surfaces that will not generally accept free grafts are tissues with severe radiation damage, chronically scarred ulcer beds, bone or cartilage denuded of periosteum or perichondrium, and tendon or nerve without their paratenon or perineurium, respectively. For these surfaces, a bed capable of producing capillary buds must be provided; in some cases, excision of the deficient bed down to healthy tissue is possible. All unhealthy granulation tissue must be removed, since bacterial counts in granulation tissue are often very high. If bone is exposed, it can be decorticated down to healthy cancellous bone with the use of a chisel or power-driven burr, and a meshed split-thickness skin graft can be applied. If an adequate vascular bed cannot be provided or if the presence of essential structures such as tendons or nerves precludes further debridement, skin or muscle flaps are generally indicated for coverage.

Inadequate contact between the graft and the recipient bed can be caused by collection of blood, serum, or lymph fluid in the bed; formation of pus between the graft and the bed; or movement of the graft on the bed.

After the graft has been applied directly to the prepared recipient surface, it may or may not be sutured in place and may or may not be dressed. Whenever the maximum aesthetic result is desired, the graft should be cut exactly to fit the recipient area and precisely sutured into position without any overlapping of edges. Very large or thick split-thickness grafts and full-thickness grafts will usually not survive without a pressure dressing. In areas such as the forehead, scalp and extremities, adequate immobilization and pressure can be provided by circular dressings. Tie-over pressure stent dressings are advisable for areas of the face, where constant pressure cannot be provided by simple wraparound dressings, or areas where movement cannot be avoided, such as the anterior neck, where swallowing causes constant motion; and areas of irregular contour, such as the axilla. The ends of the fixation sutures are left long and tied over a bolus of gauze fluffs, cotton, a sponge, or other suitable material (Figure 44–2).

Grafts applied to freshly prepared or relatively clean surfaces are generally sutured or stapled into place and dressed with pressure. A single layer of damp or other nonadherent fine-mesh gauze is applied directly over the graft. Immediately over this are placed several thicknesses of flat gauze cut in the exact pattern of the graft.

Figure 44–2. Tie-over stent dressing.

On top of these is placed a bulky dry dressing of gauze fluffs, cotton, a sponge, or other material. Pressure is then applied by wraparound dressings, adhesive tape, or a tie-over pressure stent dressing.

In many cases, it is permissible—and sometimes even preferable—to leave a skin graft site open with no dressing. This is particularly true in slightly infected wounds, where the grafts tend to float off in the purulent discharge produced by the wound. These wounds are best treated with meshed grafts, so that liquid forming between the graft and the wound bed can exude and be removed without disturbing the graft. This treatment can also be used for noninfected wounds that produce an unusual amount of serous or lymphatic drainage, as occurs following radical groin dissections.

In severely ill patients, such as those with major burns, where time under anesthesia must be kept to a minimum, large sheets of meshed split-thickness skin grafts are rapidly applied but not sutured. Skin staples may be used to fix the graft rapidly. Grafts need not be dressed if the area is small, but if the area is large or circumferential, a dressing should be applied. Meshed grafts should generally be covered for 24–48 hours to prevent dryness, since their dermal barrier has been partly disrupted.

Various biologic adhesives, in particular autologous fibrin glue, is being used to immobilize skin grafts. This is especially useful in the face or hands, or areas where bandaging is difficult or cumbersome.

Skin graft dressings may be left undisturbed for 5–7 days after grafting if the grafted wound was free of infection, if complete hemostasis was obtained, if fluid collection is not expected, and if immobilization is adequate. If any one of these conditions is not met, the dressing should be changed within 24–48 hours and the graft inspected. If blood, serum, or purulent fluid collection is present, the collection should be evacuated—usually by making a small incision through the graft with a scalpel blade and applying pressure with cotton-tipped applicators. The pressure dressing is then reapplied and changed daily so that the graft can be examined and fluid expressed as it collects.

The Skin Graft Donor Area

The ideal donor site would provide a graft identical to the skin surrounding the area to be grafted. Since skin varies greatly from one area to another as far as color, thickness, hair-bearing qualities, and texture are concerned, the ideal donor site (such as upper eyelid skin to replace skin loss from the opposite upper eyelid) is usually not found. However, there are definite principles that should be followed in choosing the donor area.

A. COLOR MATCH

In general, the best possible color match is obtained when the donor area is located close to the recipient area. Color and texture match in facial grafts will be much better if the grafts are obtained from above the region of the clavicles. However, the amount of skin obtainable from the supraclavicular areas is limited. If larger grafts for the face are required, the immediate subclavicular regions of the thorax will provide a better color match than areas on the lower trunk or the buttocks and thighs. When these more distant regions are used, the grafts will usually be lighter in color than the facial skin in whites. In people with dark skin, hyperpigmentation occurs, producing a graft that is much darker than the surrounding facial skin.

B. THICKNESS OF THE GRAFT AND DONOR SITE HEALING

Donor sites of split-thickness grafts heal by epithelialization from the epithelial elements remaining in the donor bed. The ability of the donor area to heal and the speed with which it does depends upon the number of these elements present. Donor areas for very thin grafts will heal in 7–10 days, whereas donor areas for intermediate-thickness grafts may require 10–18 days and those for thick grafts 18–21 days or longer.

Since there is a normal anatomic variation in the thickness of skin, donor sites for thicker grafts must be chosen with the potential for healing in mind and should be limited to regions on the body where the skin is thick. Infants, debilitated adults, and elderly people have thinner skin than healthy younger adults. Grafts that would be split-thickness in the normal adult may be full-thickness in these patients, resulting in a donor site that has been deprived of the epithelial elements necessary for healing.

C. MANAGEMENT OF THE DONOR SITE

The donor site itself can be considered a clean open wound that will heal spontaneously. After initial hemostasis, the wound will continue to ooze serum for 1–4 days, depending on the thickness of the skin taken. The serum should be collected and the wound kept clean so that healing can proceed at a maximal rate. The wound should be cared for as described above for clean open wounds in either of two ways.

The more common method is the open (dry) technique. The donor site is dressed with porous sterile fine-mesh or nonadherent gauze. After 24 hours, the dry gauze is changed but the nonadherent gauze is left on the wound and exposed to the air, a heat lamp, or a blow dryer. A scab will form on the gauze and will peel off from the edges as epithelialization is completed underneath. This method has the advantage of simple maintenance once the wound is dry.

The second method is the closed (moist) technique. Studies have demonstrated that the rate of epithelialization is enhanced in a moist environment. In contrast to the dry technique, pain can be reduced or virtually eliminated. Moist-to-moist gauze dressings that require frequent wetting have been replaced by newer synthetic materials. A gas-permeable membrane (OpSite) that sticks to the surrounding skin provides an artificial blister over the wound. Occasionally there is a break in the protective seal covering leakage of serum collected under the membrane. This increases the risk of infection, especially in a contaminated zone. Newer hygroscopic dressings actually absorb and retain many times their weight in water. They are permeable to oxygen yet impervious to bacteria. Infection is still a concern, however, because of occasional exposure of the wound during healing.

Kishi K, Nakajima H, Tajima S: Differential responses of collagen and glycosaminoglycan syntheses and cell proliferation to exogenous transforming growth factor beta 1 in the developing mouse skin fibroblasts in culture. Br J Plastic Surg 1999; 52:579.

van Zuijlen PP et al: Graft survival and effectiveness of dermal substitution in burns and reconstructive surgery in a one-stage grafting model. Plast Reconstr Surg 2000;106:615.

Wang JC, To EW: Application of dermal substitute (Integra) to donor site defect of forehead flap. Br J Plastic Surg 2000; 53:70.

FLAPS

The term "flap" refers to any tissue used for reconstruction or wound closure that retains part or all of its original blood supply after the tissue has been raised and moved to a new location. That part still connected through which the blood supply enters and exits is referred to as the base of the flap. With local skin flaps, a section of skin and subcutaneous tissue is raised from one site and moved to a nearby area, with the base remaining attached at its original location.

Flaps can be classified according to the pattern of blood supply to the skin into random or axial pattern. Flaps can further be classified according to their tissue content into muscle, musculocutaneous, fasciocutaneous, and others.

Random Pattern Flaps

Random pattern flaps consist of skin and subcutaneous tissue cut from any area of the body in any orientation, with no distinct pattern or particular relation to the blood supply of the skin of the flap. Such flaps receive their blood supply from vessels in the subdermal tissue. Although commonly used, this is the least reliable type of flap, and except when cut from facial and scalp skin the ratio of length to width cannot safely exceed 1.5:1. Its use should be minimized. Presently, in any reconstructive effort, one should use a flap with known reliability and a predictable blood supply.

Axial Pattern Flaps

The axial pattern flap has a well-defined arteriovenous system running along its long axis. Because of good vascular supply, it can be made comparatively long in relation to width. Foremost among the axial flaps are the deltopectoral and the forehead flaps, which are based on perforating branches of the internal mammary artery and supraorbital and supratrochlear or superficial temporal vessels, respectively. Other axial flaps are the groin flap, based on the superficial circumflex iliac artery; the dorsalis pedis flap, based on the artery of the same name; the radial forearm flap; the scapular flap; the lateral upper arm flap; and various scalp flaps.

Muscle & Musculocutaneous Flaps

Musculocutaneous flaps consist of skin and underlying muscle, which provide reliable coverage with usually one operation. The use of musculocutaneous units has developed as surgeons have gained more knowledge of the way in which blood is supplied to the skin. The technique has revolutionized reconstructive surgery.

The subdermal plexus of vessels from which skin flaps derive their blood supply is augmented or directly supplied in many areas by sizable perforating vessels arising from underlying muscles. Many muscles receive their blood supply from a single axial vessel, with only minor contributions from other sources (Figure 44–3).

The skin over these muscles can be completely circumscribed and elevated in continuity with the underlying muscle up to its major vascular pedicle. If the vessels in the pedicle are preserved, the unit can be moved in wide arcs to distant areas of the body while normal or near normal blood flow is continued to the skin island as well as to the muscle. The donor sites of such flaps can often be closed primarily.

Knowledge of the anatomy of muscles and their nerve and blood supply is necessary for the successful design of musculocutaneous flaps. Although almost any skeletal muscle can be used, muscles with a dominant arterial pedicle and reliable perforating vessels to the skin are most useful.

In addition to their reliability, musculocutaneous flaps clean up recipient sites that are heavily contaminated with bacteria better than skin flaps do. This is why muscle-containing flaps are the best choice for coverage of wounds caused by radiation or osteomyelitis or those that have a high probability of infection.

The most commonly used muscles and musculocutaneous flaps are the latissimus dorsi, pectoralis major, tensor fasciae latae, rectus femoris, rectus abdominis, trapezius, temporalis, serratus anterior, gluteus maximus, gracilis, and gastrocnemius muscles.

A. LATISSIMUS DORSI

The latissimus dorsi musculocutaneous unit is supplied by the thoracodorsal vessels. Use of this unit has been widely applied in the one-stage reconstruction of the breast following radical or modified radical mastectomy (see rectus abdominis muscle below). The entire latissimus dorsi muscle can be detached from its origin and transposed to the anterior chest. An island of skin can

Figure 44–3. Arterial supply to skin from main artery supplying muscles, as occurs in musculocutaneous flaps.

also be included in the center of the muscle to restore the skin lost on the anterior chest wall. Refinements in technique utilize only enough muscle to carry the skin island, thus leaving intact a good portion of innervated, functional muscle. This unit is also useful for coverage of defects on the anterior chest, shoulder, head and neck, and axilla and even for restoration of flexion of the elbow. It is a popular muscle for free tissue transfer due to its long and relatively large and reliable vascular pedicle.

B. Pectoralis Major

The pectoralis major musculocutaneous unit obtains its vascular supply from the thoracoacromial axis of the subclavian artery just medial to the medial border of the pectoralis minor. It derives a dual blood supply from medial intercostal perforators branching from the internal mammary artery. The entire unit may be transposed medially, especially after disinsertion from the humerus, to cover defects of the sternum, neck, and lower face. Also, an island of skin can be outlined low on the chest and made to reach intraoral defects following cancer excision.

C. Trapezius

The trapezius musculocutaneous unit, based on the descending branch of the transverse cervical artery, is useful for covering defects in the neck, face, and scalp. When skeletonized as an island, the flap will reach the top of the head. When it is used in conjunction with a neck dissection, the transverse cervical artery must be preserved. Functional preservation of shoulder elevation may be accomplished by selectively sparing the transverse, superior fibers of the muscle.

D. Temporalis

The temporalis muscle extends from the temporal fossa to the coronoid process of the mandible. It is supplied by the deep and superficial temporal systems. It is commonly used to fill orbital defects. However, it can cover neighboring cranial, maxillary, palatal and pharyngeal regions.

E. Tensor Fasciae Latae

The tensor fasciae latae musculofascial unit is supplied by the lateral femoral circumflex artery, a branch of the profunda femoris. It has a wide arc of rotation anteriorly and posteriorly. It is elevated with the fascia lata and thus can be used to reconstruct the lower abdominal wall. It has been used to cover defects following excision of osteoradionecrotic ulcers of the pubis or groin. It is also the method of choice for coverage of greater trochanteric pressure ulcers.

F. Rectus Femoris

The rectus femoris, a more robust flap than the tensor fasciae latae with a shorter arc of rotation, has sup-

planted the latter for reconstruction of the lower abdominal wall and for coverage to postradiation ulcers in the pubis and groin. It has a dual blood supply: a muscular branch from the profunda femoris and an axial branch from the superficial femoral artery to the overlying skin and fascia.

G. Rectus Abdominis

The rectus abdominis is supplied by the deep superior and inferior epigastric vessels that run in the undersurface of the muscle and anastomose with the segmentally arranged intercostal vessels to form the epigastric arcade. These vessels send perforating branches throughout the length of the muscle, perforating the anterior rectus sheath and supplying the overlying skin. The flap, when based on the superior epigastric vessel and including the infraumbilical skin, has become the method of choice for autologous tissue breast reconstruction. In situations of marked deformity such as a radical mastectomy associated with radiation therapy or previous abdominal surgery, reconstruction of the breast can be accomplished reliably with infraumbilical skin and adipose tissue based on both rectus muscles. This superiorly based rectus abdominis musculocutaneous flap involves an abdominoplasty as well as reconstruction of the breast. It is a technically demanding operation but gives a very satisfying result. When based on the deep inferior epigastric vessel and using the supraumbilical skin (the "flag" flap), the flap can cover defects of the abdominal wall, flank and thigh.

H. Gluteus Maximus

The gluteus maximus is useful as a muscle or musculocutaneous unit for covering pressure sores or traumatic defects over the sacrum and ischium. The muscle has a double blood supply from the superior and inferior gluteal arteries to the respective halves of the muscle. In ambulatory patients, it is advisable to perform a function-preserving operation by advancing the muscle medially and preserving its insertion laterally.

I. Gracilis

The gracilis muscle receives its dominant blood supply proximally from the medial femoral circumflex artery. Its arc of rotation makes it an excellent source of coverage for ischial pressure sores and vaginal reconstruction. Other recent uses have included transportation of the muscle alone for repair of a persistent perineal sinus following abdominal-perineal resection.

J. Gastrocnemius

The gastrocnemius musculocutaneous unit is based on either the medial or lateral head of the muscle. Each head is supplied by a sural artery, a branch of the popliteal artery that enters the muscle at its most proximal third near its origin. The flap is most useful to cover defects of the knee and proximal anterior tibia. Coverage of exposed bone in the middle and lower leg, where this unit cannot reach, can be accomplished by use of local muscle flaps such as the soleus. Complex bone and soft tissue injuries of the middle and lower leg are best handled with free muscle flaps.

Perforator Flaps

A sophisticated variation on the use of the musculocutaneous principle has been the development of perforator flaps. This usually entails taking a large branch from the major vascular pedicle that may perforate the muscle to arborize and form a subcutaneous vascular plexus that will supply a considerable amount of overlying skin. This is best exemplified by the transverse rectus abdominis muscle perforator flap method of breast reconstruction, where one can isolate the perforating vessels, avoid sacrifice of the rectus abdominis muscle and still maintain the same skin territory. This has also been applied to territories of skin over the perforator segments of the latissimus dorsi myocutaneous units and others.

Fasciocutaneous Flaps

A plexus of vessels is located on top of the muscular fascia and is supplied from vessels that run within the intermuscular septa. These vessels tend to run axially along the fascia, sending perforators to the skin at intervals. Flaps can be designed that are safer than random flaps and that need not contain an entire muscle unit for their transfer. Furthermore, it is possible to make fasciocutaneous or septocutaneous flaps that safely exceed the traditional limits of a 1:1 ratio between length and width. Examples of fasciocutaneous flaps are those overlying the gastrocnemius, quadriceps, and rectus abdominis muscles. Other commonly used flaps are the radial forearm, lateral arm, scapular, and deltopectoral flaps.

Neurocutaneous Flaps

Anatomic studies have confirmed the presence of an arterial pedicle accompanying a sensory nerve such as the sural nerve. Consequently, one may be able to outline a skin territory over the trajectory of a sensory nerve with good viability of the overlying skin.

Free Flaps

Free flaps involve tissue transplantation using microvascular surgery. The term is actually incorrect, since the blood supply from the main axial pedicle of the flap is completely detached and then reattached at a distance to recipient vessels near the wound area.

An operating microscope with two viewing binocular lenses, specialized instruments, and swaged-on needles of 60–80 μm are required for microsurgery; 8-0, 9-0, and 10-0 suture is used to anastomose vessels as small as 0.5 mm in diameter.

Examples of free flaps in current use are axial pattern skin flaps, such as groin and scapular flaps, which are used when only skin is needed, and musculocutaneous flaps, such as latissimus dorsi, gracilis, and rectus abdominis flaps, which are used when the bulk and vascularity of muscle are needed. Composite free flaps such as the fibular flap with its overlying skin are most helpful free flaps for reconstruction of the mandible as well as the floor of the mouth following head and neck tumor extirpations.

The vascular pedicle areas of some flaps contain functional nerves, which can also be reattached with microscopic guidance. Examples are inferior gluteal, thigh, and tensor fasciae latae flaps, which contain sensory nerves. Attempts using **sensory flaps** to provide protective sensation in critical areas such as the feet or the ischium in paraplegic patients have so far been clinically unsuccessful. More encouraging is the work being done to provide sensibility to the floor of the mouth with a sensory innervated radial forearm flap. **Motor flaps** can restore functions such as forearm flexion or facial expression.

Bone and functional joints can be transplanted as free flaps. Flaps from the ribs, fibula, and iliac crest have all been successfully transferred to areas such as the mandible and tibia. The toe-to-thumb transfer is an example of a complex transplantation, that includes bone with a functional joint, tendons and nerves as well as skin.

Blondeel N et al: The donor site morbidity of free DIEP flaps and free TRAM flaps for breast reconstruction. Br J Plast Surg 1997;50:322.

Coskunfirat OK et al: Reverse neurofasciocutaneous flaps for soft-tissue coverage of the lower leg. Ann Plast Surg 1999;43:14.

de Almeida OM et al: Distally based fasciocutaneous flap of the calf for cutaneous coverage of the lower leg and dorsum of the foot. Ann Plast Surg 2000;44:367.

Imanishi N et al: Venous drainage of the distally based lesser saphenous-sural veno-neuroadipofascial pedicled fasciocutaneous flap: a radiographic perfusion study. Plast Reconstr Surg 1999;103:494.

■ II. PRINCIPLES OF WOUND CARE

There are many types of wounds and many factors to consider when choice of coverage procedure is made. Skin type and color, glandular association, and hair-bearing characteristics must be considered. Avascular wound beds, such as exposed bone, cartilage, or tendon, will not accept skin grafts unless viable periosteum, perichondrium, or paratenon (respectively) is present. Other areas with poor vascularity are joint capsules, radiation-damaged tissue, and heavily scarred tissue. Exposed or implanted alloplastic material cannot be used as a graft bed. Such areas must be covered with tissue that is attached to its own blood supply. Skin flaps can be used but are sometimes inadequate because their blood supply is tenuous and the layer of subcutaneous fat is even less reliably vascular and may not attach to the underlying avascular surface. Muscle or musculocutaneous flaps are generally required for avascular areas.

The coverage tissue may need to have more bulk than the original tissue. Areas such as bony surfaces and prominences, weight-bearing surfaces, densely scarred areas, and areas of potential pressure breakdown may require thick, durable covering. Again, skin grafts or skin flaps may not be of adequate thickness even though they may survive and cover the wound. Musculocutaneous flaps are more successful. Bulkiness may be undesirable in areas such as the scalp, face, neck, or hand. Defects in these areas that for other reasons require a musculocutaneous flap for coverage may need to be debulked in a secondary procedure. Axial skin flaps or free axial pattern flaps may be a better choice than musculocutaneous flaps in some areas.

Contraction begins during the proliferative phase of healing and continues to a large degree in wounds covered only by split-thickness skin grafts. The grafted area may shrink to 50% of its original size, and both the graft and surrounding tissue may become distorted. Splinting of the area for 10 days or longer may favorably alter contraction. Full-thickness skin grafts rich in dermis, attached to a fresh wound bed will considerably reduce contraction and skin flaps will eliminate it altogether. In an orifice or tubular passageway, such as the nasal airway, pharynx, esophagus, or vagina, absence of contraction is critical.

The effects of atrophy and gravity should also be considered when technique of coverage is chosen. A denervated muscle will atrophy up to 60% of its regular size. The muscle tissue in a musculocutaneous flap will atrophy even when the nerve to the muscle is preserved in the pedicle, because the muscle's functional tension is generally not restored. Gravity will cause sagging of any tissue that does not have enough plasticity or muscle dynamics to counteract gravitational pull. Reconstructions in the face often tend to sag.

Wounds at risk for or known to have bacterial contamination also require certain types of coverage (eg, pressure sores, lower extremity defects, and wounds resulting from incision and drainage of abscesses). If the area can be skin grafted, meshed split-thickness grafts are most effective, since bacterial exudate will not collect under these grafts. Musculocutaneous flaps are associated with fewer residual bacteria over time than are random pattern skin flaps. This is probably due to the vastly superior vascularity of musculocutaneous flaps.

Contaminated wounds or wounds that are exuding a considerable amount of fluid can be treated by negative-pressure wound dressings. This entails the application of a sponge-like material connected to a suction device which keeps the wound dry as it suctions the exudate and may speed up the process of wound contracture.

Wounds associated with nearby injuries that will probably require further surgery (eg, injuries to tendons or nerves) should be covered with flaps, because the flaps can be incised or undermined to allow for additional surgery. Skin grafts do not have sufficient vascularity to allow for these procedures.

Choice of Coverage

Table 44–2 shows some of the indications for choice of coverage in various types of wounds.

Once a given type of flap is chosen, there are still at least two major considerations in the selection of the exact flap to be used. The most significant consideration is the degree of injury that will occur in the donor area. There is always a trade-off when tissue is taken from one area and used in another. This trade-off is minimal when a well-designed, well-placed skin flap leaves a donor defect that can be closed primarily, but the trade-off is great when the donor defect is as severe as the original wound (eg, skin graft donor sites that become infected or musculocutaneous donor sites that fail to heal).

The patient can often participate in the choice of donor locations and should certainly be made aware of potential donor site scars and complications. The tendency has been to use muscle flaps instead of musculocutaneous flaps to permit easy primary closure of the donor site. The muscle can then be resurfaced with a split-thickness skin graft during the same procedure to give a satisfactory result. This provides for an acceptable donor site scar rather than risking disruption of a tight closure or an otherwise ugly donor site.

The second consideration in selection of a flap is that some or all of the graft or flap may be lost. In general, if the patient's overall condition is poor or the loss of a flap would result in a devastating defect, a very reliable type of flap should be chosen. For example, a microvascular anastomosis can be performed on a leg with one remaining arteriosclerotic vessel to the foot, but if the anastomosis fails, the vessel may thrombose and the leg may be lost. In this case, a flap that is safer, al-

Table 44–2. Indications for various types of tissue coverage.

Type of Wound	Type of Coverage	Reason for Choice
Mildly ($< 10^5$) infected wounds (including burns)	Thin split-thickness or meshed	Difficulty in obtaining successful take of thicker grafts. Donor sites may be reused sooner.
Significantly ($> 10^5$) infected wounds (osteomyelitis)	Thin split-thickness or meshed skin grafts or muscle or musculocutaneous flaps	Rich muscle vascular supply can sterilize an infected wound.
Wounds with poorly vascularized surfaces	Thin split-thickness skin grafts or flaps	Difficulty in obtaining successful take of thicker grafts. Flap with intrinsic blood supply may be required.
Small facial defects	Full-thickness skin graft or local flap	Produces best aesthetic result.
Large facial defects	Thick split-thickness skin grafts or flaps	Cannot use full-thickness graft, because of limited size of donor sites.
Full-thickness eyelid loss	Local flap or composite graft	Repair requires more than one tissue element.
Deep loss of nasal tip	Local flap or composite graft	Repair requires thicker tissue than present in split- or full-thickness grafts.
Avulsive wounds with exposed tendons and nerves	Flap	Requires thick protective coverage without graft adherence to tendons and nerves.
Exposed cortical bone or cartilage	Skin or muscle flap	Free grafts will not survive on avascular recipient site.
Wounds resulting from radiation burns	Muscle or musculocutaneous flap	Free grafts will not survive on avascular recipient site. Damaged tissue extends deeper than may be apparent.

though more time-consuming to place, may be chosen, such as a cross-leg flap.

Elevation & Transposition of Flaps

Additional considerations in reconstructive surgery involve the technique of elevating and transposing flaps. For random skin flaps, these considerations include proper length-to-width ratio, careful planning to allow for transposition with minimal tension and adjustments at the recipient site, accurate dissection in the subcutaneous plane to avoid injury to the subdermal plexus, and avoidance of folding or kinking of the flap. Surgical technique must be atraumatic, and hemostasis must be achieved. With axial pattern flaps, the surgeon must have knowledge of the important underlying blood vessels as well.

Closure Technique

Closure technique is as important as elevation and transposition technique. Flaps should not be allowed to dry out. The wound bed should be irrigated. Closed-

system, nonreactive suction drains are routinely used in both the wound bed and the donor defect for most flaps of any significant size. Suction evacuates blood or serum that may accumulate and keeps the flap firmly pressed against the wound bed. External pressure is both ineffective and detrimental for these purposes. Sutures should accurately and completely appose skin edges without strangulating the epithelium, particularly on the flap side. Buried half-mattress (flap) sutures are recommended (Figure 44–4). Dressings over flaps should be minimal and should not cause pressure or constriction. Emollient dressings, such as petrolatum gauze, antibiotic ointment, or silver sulfadiazine cream, have been shown to aid in preventing desiccation and subsequent necrosis of areas of marginal vascularity.

After a flap is at least temporarily tacked into its final position, adequacy of vascularity can be determined by intravenous injection of fluorescein dye, 10–15 mg/kg, and examination under ultraviolet light (Wood's light). Areas that fluoresce within 10 minutes following dye injection can be expected to survive. Areas that do not fluoresce usually lack arterial inflow, which may be due to temporary arterial spasm but is often due to insuffi-

- Epidermis
- Dermis
- Subcutaneous fat
- Fascia

A. The strength of the closure lies in the dermis. Occasionally, the subcutaneous fat is incorporated to obliterate dead space.

B. The suture is placed so that the knot will lie in the deepest part of the wound. Take care to avoid incorporating the epidermis with this suture, since epithelial cysts will form and result in suture extrusion.

C. The dermal suture is tied just tightly enough to approximate the wound margins. Synthetic absorbable sutures are most commonly used for closure of the dermis.

D. After the dermis is approximated, a fine "epidermal" suture is placed to align the wound edges. This suture adds little to the tensile strength of the wound closure.

E. The epidermal suture is tied just tightly enough to approximate the epidermal edges of the wound. Since the strength of this closure lies in the dermis, the epidermal suture can be removed after 2–3 days. Skin tapes are often used to support the wound for an additional 7–10 days.

Figure 44–4. Layered cutaneous closure (buried half-mattress [flap] sutures). (Reproduced, with permission, from Ho MT, Saunders CE [editors]: *Current Emergency Diagnosis & Treatment*, 4th ed. Originally published by Appleton & Lange. Copyright © 1992 by The McGraw-Hill Companies, Inc.)

cient perfusion that will result in necrosis. A good clinical evaluation of the flap on the operating table is usually sufficient. Any sign of mottling or cyanosis or flap congestion that indicates a degree of venous obstruction warrants serious consideration of reexploration.

Excision & Primary Closure

The ideal type of wound closure is primary approximation of the skin and subcutaneous tissues immediately adjacent to the wound defect, producing a fine-line scar and the optimal aesthetic result in skin texture, thickness, and color match.

All excisions and wound closures should be planned with this ideal in mind. Obviously, large lesions cannot be excised and closed primarily. With invasive cancers, such as sarcomas, the primary goal is performance of adequate en bloc resection, with the type of wound closure being of secondary importance. Nevertheless, even larger excisions, such as mastectomies, can be planned with definite consideration for closure and subsequent reconstruction.

In most cases, minimal scars can be achieved only if the line or lines of incision are placed in, or parallel to, the skin lines of minimal tension. These lines lie perpendicular to the underlying muscles. On the face, they are obvious as wrinkles or lines of facial expression that become more pronounced with age, since they are secondary to repeated muscle contraction (Figure 44–5). On the neck, trunk, and extremities, the lines of mini-

mal tension are most noticeable as horizontal lines of skin relaxation on the anterior and posterior aspects of areas of flexion and extension.

So-called Langer's lines, which were determined by cadaver study, probably show the direction of fibrous tissue bundles in the skin and are no longer considered accurate guides for placing skin incisions.

If the lines of expression cannot be followed, the line of incision should (if possible) be placed at the junction of unlike tissues such as the hairline of the scalp and the forehead, the eyebrow and the forehead, the mucosal and skin junction of the lips, or the areolar and skin margins of the breast. Scars will be partially hidden if incisions are placed in inconspicuous areas such as the crease of the nasal ala and cheek, the auricular-mastoid sulcus, or the submandibular-neck junction. Lines of incision should never purposely cross flexor surfaces such as the neck, axilla, antecubital fossa, or popliteal space or the palmar skin creases of the fingers and hand, because of the risk of contracture formation. A transverse oblique or S incision should be incorporated when crossing these sites.

If a lesion is to be excised, an elliptic incision placed parallel to the skin lines of minimal tension will give the best result if the amount of tissue to be excised does not preclude primary closure.

If the ellipse is too broad or short, a protrusion of skin, commonly called a "dog-ear," will occur at each pole of the wound closure (Figure 44–6). This is most easily corrected by excising the dog-ear as a small ellipse.

A dog-ear may also be present if one side of the ellipse is longer than the other (Figure 44–7). In this case, it may be easier to excise a small triangle of skin and subcutaneous tissue from the longer side.

A. Z-PLASTY

One of the most useful and commonly used techniques in primary wound closure is the Z-plasty. The procedure is illustrated in Figure 44–8. The angles formed by the Z-shaped incision are transposed as shown, in order (1) to gain length in the direction of the central limb of

Figure 44–5. Sites of elliptic incisions corresponding to wrinkle lines on the face.

Figure 44–6. Correction of dog-ear.

Figure 44-7. Alternative method of correction of dog-ear.

the Z or (2) to change the line of direction of the central limb of the Z. Ninety-degree angles would provide the greatest gain in length of the central limb, but smaller angles, such as 60-degree angles, are usually used, because the incision is easier to close and significant gain in length is still achieved. The Z-plasty is used for scar revision and reorientation of small wound incisions so that the main incision will be in a more ideal location. The lengthening function is used for the release or breakup of scar contractures across flexion creases. Frequently, many small Z-plasties in series rather than one large one are done. Occasionally, incisions will be placed under excessive vertical tension after the release of an underlying contracture, such as Dupuytren's contracture in the hand.

B. Suture Technique

Suture technique in primary closure is important but will not compensate for poorly planned flaps, excessive tension across the incision, traumatized skin edges, bleeding, or other problems. Sometimes even a skillfully executed closure may result in an unsightly scar because of healing problems beyond the control of the surgeon.

The goal of closure is level apposition of dermal and epithelial edges with minimal or no tension across the incision and no strangulation of tissue between sutures. This is usually accomplished by placement of a layer of interrupted or running absorbable sutures in the subcuticular level at the base of the dermis. A running monofilament permanent suture can also be used and pulled out after healing has progressed. This suture prevents tension from forming in the upper dermis and epithelium and also causes the surface planes to be level. The epithelial edges can then be opposed with interrupted or running monofilament sutures, which can be removed within a week (within 3–4 days in the face), so the suture tracks can be avoided. Sterile adhesive tape (Steri-Strips) placed across the incision will also prevent surface marks and can be used either primarily or after surface sutures have been removed. Taping will not correct errors in suturing that have resulted in uneven edges or tension across the incision. Tape burns may occur if there is excessive tension or swelling around the incision.

The size and even the type of suture material are less important than careful suture placement and observance of previously mentioned factors. Almost any suture properly placed and removed early enough will provide closure without leaving suture marks. The use of monofilament nylon or polypropylene suture material is advised, however, since these types of sutures cause the fewest reactions of currently available suture materials, excluding stainless steel. Running subcuticular, pullout type monofilament sutures may be left in for up to 3 weeks without causing reactions. Even buried nylon sutures are well tolerated and generally cause fewer problems than braided or absorbable sutures.

Sutures should be removed as soon as possible, depending on the healing characteristics of the skin involved and tension created locally by movement of shearing. The incision should be free of crusts, debris, and bacteria.

Avery C et al: Clinical experience with the negative pressure wound dressing. Br J Oral Maxillofac Surg 2000;38:343.

(a) Incisions outlined. (b) Incisions made and flaps undermined. (c) Flaps transposed. (d) Completed closure.

Figure 44-8. Z-plasty

Machens HG et al: Postoperative blood flow monitoring after free-tissue transfer by means of the hydrogen clearance technique. Plast Reconstr Surg 1997;99:493.

■ III. SPECIFIC DISORDERS TREATED BY PLASTIC SURGERY

DISORDERS OF SCARRING

HYPERTROPHIC SCARS & KELOIDS

In response to any injury severe enough to break the continuity of the skin or produce necrosis, the skin heals with scar formation. Under ideal circumstances a fine, flat hairline scar will result. The details of wound healing are presented in Chapter 7.

However, hypertrophy may occur, causing the scar to become raised and thickened, or a keloid may form. A keloid is a true tumor arising from the connective tissue elements of the dermis. By definition, keloids grow beyond the margins of the original injury or scar; in some instances, they may grow to enormous size.

The tendency should be resisted to regard all thickened scars as keloids and to label as keloid formers all patients with unattractive scars. Hypertrophic scars and keloids are distinct entities, and the clinical course and prognosis are quite different in each case. The overreactive process that results in thickening of the hypertrophic scar ceases within a few weeks—before it extends beyond the limits of the original scar—and in most cases, some degree of maturation occurs and gradual improvement takes place. In the case of keloids, the overreactive proliferation of fibroblasts continues for weeks or months. By the time it ceases, an actual tumor is present that typically extends well beyond the limits of the original scar, involves the surrounding skin, and may become quite large. Maturation with spontaneous improvement does not usually occur.

Hypertrophic scars and keloids can be differentiated by histopathologic methods. Clinical observation of the course of the scar is also a practical means of differentiation.

Treatment

Since nearly all hypertrophic scars undergo some degree of spontaneous improvement, they do not require treatment in the early phases. If the scar is still hypertrophic after 6 months, surgical excision and primary closure of the wound may be indicated. Improvement may be expected when the hypertrophic scar was originally produced by excessive endothelial and fibroblastic cell proliferation, as is present in open wounds, burns, and infected wounds. However, little or no improvement can be anticipated if the hypertrophic scar followed uncomplicated healing of a simple surgical incision. Improvement of hypertrophic scars across flexion surfaces such as the antecubital fossa or the fingers requires a procedure such as a Z-plasty to change the direction of the scar.

Pressure may help flatten a potentially hypertrophic scar. It is particularly useful for burn scars. A measured elastic garment or face mask (Jobst) is applied to the scarred area and provides continued pressure that causes realignment and remodeling of the collagen bundles. Pressure should be applied early, continuously, and for 6–12 months. Use of intermittent pressure (eg, only at night) or after the hypertrophic scar is established (6–12 months) is of little value.

Additional methods of decreasing the thickness of hypertrophied scars include silicone sheeting applied early and continuously for weeks or months. More recently, early use of the potassium-titanyl-phosphate (KTP) laser has been advocated to decrease scar redness as well as hypertrophy. This instrument appears to work by decreasing capillary supply. There have as yet been no prospective or comparative studies of the procedure.

The treatment of choice for keloids and intractable hypertrophic scars is injection of triamcinolone acetonide, 10 mg/mL (Kenalog-10 Injection), directly into the lesion. This will also help control itching associated with these lesions. In the case of larger lesions, injection is made into more than one site. There is evidence that keloids may respond better to early than to late treatment.

Lesions are injected every 3–4 weeks, and treatment should not be carried out longer than 6 months. The following dosage schedule is used:

Size of Lesion	Dose per Injection
1–2 cm^2	20–40 mg
2–6 cm^2	40–80 mg
6–10 cm^2	80–110 mg

For larger lesions, the maximum dose should be 120 mg. The maximum doses for each treatment for children are as follows:

Age	Maximum Dose
1–2 years	20 mg
3–5 years	40 mg
6–10 years	80 mg

There is a tendency to inject the drug into the scar too often or in too high a dosage—or into the subjacent tissue, which may produce too vigorous a response, resulting in excessive atrophy of the skin and subcutaneous tissues surrounding the lesion and in depigmentation of darker skins. Both of these adverse responses may improve spontaneously in 6–12 months, but not necessarily completely. The response varies greatly; some lesions become flat after two or three injections, and some fail to respond at all. Topical corticosteroid therapy is of no value.

Before the advent of corticosteroid injection therapy, surgical excision and radiation therapy were the only methods of treatment of keloids. Both methods are disappointing; surgical resection usually leads to recurrence of a larger lesion; with very few exceptions, radiation therapy produces an unpredictable result and has obvious potential side effects, including neoplastic degeneration. At present, surgical excision is used only in conjunction with intralesional corticosteroid therapy. Excision is usually confined to the larger lesions in which steroid therapy would exceed safe dosages. (The wound is injected at the time of surgery and then postoperatively according to the schedule recommended above.) Care should be taken so that surgical incisions are not extended into the normal skin around the keloid, since the growth of a new keloid may occur in these scars. It has been reported that intramarginal excisions yield better results than extramarginal excisions.

Niessen FB et al: On the nature of hypertrophic scars and keloids: a review. Plast Reconstr Surg 1999;104:1435.

Niessen FB et al: The use of silicone occlusive sheeting (Sil-K) and silicone occlusive gel (Epiderm) in the prevention of hypertrophic scar formation. Plast Reconstr Surg 1998;102:1962.

CONTRACTURES

Contraction is a normal process of wound healing. Contracture, on the other hand, is a pathologic end stage related to the process of contraction. Generally, contractures develop when wounds heal with too much scarring and contraction of the scar tissue results in distortion of surrounding tissues. Although scar contractures can occur in any flexible tissue, such as the eyelids or lips, contractures usually occur across areas of flexion, such as the neck, axilla, or antecubital fossa. The contracted scar brings together the structures on either side of the joint space and prevents active or even passive extension. Exceptions to this pattern of flexion contractures are extension contractures of the toes and MP (metacarpophalangeal) joints of the digits. Contraction is thought to occur via smooth muscle contractile elements in myofibroblasts, but the mechanism is not well understood. In one vertical abdominal scar there may be an area of normal scar formation and an area of hypertrophic scar formation with visible con-

tracture. Contracture can occur in response to the presence of foreign material such as Silastic or saline breast implants. Overall, there is a 10% incidence of some form of breast capsular contracture. Myofibroblasts are thought to play an important role, but the actual cause is not known. Some patients have a soft, excellent result on one side but significant contracture on the other. Clinical practice with a newer-type of implant by changing the surface from smooth to textured have yielded unclear results as to whether there is a decrease in capsular contracture with the textured surface. Polyurethane-coated silicone implants which did show a decrease in the rate of capsular contracture are no longer available for clinical use.

The best treatment of contractures is prevention. Incisions should not be made at right angles to flexion creases or should be reoriented by Z-plasties. Wounds in areas of flexion can be covered with flaps or grafted early with thick split-thickness or full-thickness grafts to stop the process of contraction. Such wounds should also be splinted in a position of extension during healing and for 2–3 weeks after healing is complete. Vigorous physical therapy may also be helpful.

Once a contracture is established, stretching and massage are rarely beneficial. Narrow bands of contracture may be excised and released with one or more Z-plasties. Larger areas must be incised from the medial to the lateral axis across the flexion surface and completely opened up to full extension. The resulting defect can be extensive and must be resurfaced with a skin flap or skin graft. In recurrent contractures a fasciocutaneous flap is the treatment of choice. If a skin graft is used, the area must be splinted in extension for approximately 2 weeks after the graft has healed. Less aggressive surgery is likely to result in recurrence.

Achauer GM, Spenler CW, Gold ME: Reconstruction of axillary burn contractures with the latissimus dorsi fasciocutaneous flap. J Trauma 1988;28:211.

Collis N et al: Ten-year review of a prospective randomized controlled trial of textured versus smooth subglandular silicone gel breast implants. Plast Reconstr Surg 2000;106:786.

SKIN TUMORS*

Tumors of the skin are by far the most common of all tumors in humans. They arise from each of the histologic structures that make up the skin—epidermis, connective tissue, gland, muscle, and nerve elements—and are correspondingly numerous in variety. Skin tumors are classified as benign, premalignant, and malignant.

---

* Melanoma is discussed in Chapter 47.

BENIGN SKIN TUMORS

The many benign tumors that arise from the skin rarely interfere with function. Since most are removed for aesthetic reasons or to rule out malignancy, they are quite commonly treated by the plastic surgeon. The majority are small and can be simply excised under local anesthesia following the principles of elliptical excision and wound closure discussed above. General anesthesia may be necessary for larger lesions requiring excision and repair by skin grafts or flaps or those occurring in young children.

When the diagnosis is not in doubt, most superficial lesions (seborrheic keratoses, verrucae, squamous cell papillomas) can be treated by simple techniques such as electrodesiccation, curettage and electrodesiccation, cryotherapy, and topical cytotoxic agents.

Seborrheic Keratosis

Seborrheic keratoses are superficial noninvasive tumors that originate in the epidermis. They appear in older people as multiple slightly elevated yellowish, brown, or brownish-black irregularly rounded plaques with waxy or oily surfaces. They are most commonly found on the trunk and shoulders but are frequently seen on the scalp and face.

Since the lesion is raised above the epidermis, treatment usually consists of shave excision. Care should be exercised to avoid shaving a melanoma because if that is done it will interfere with the determination of the depth of invasion by the Breslau or Clark classifications. If there is any question about a pigmented lesion, it is preferable to do an excisional biopsy rather than to shave it.

Verrucae

Verrucae (common warts) are usually seen in children and young adults, commonly on the fingers and hands. They appear as round or oval elevated lesions with rough surfaces composed of multiple rounded or filiform keratinized projections. They may be skin-colored or gray to brown.

Verrucae are caused by a virus and are autoinoculable, which can result in multiple lesions around the original growth or frequent recurrences following treatment if the virus is not completely eradicated. They may disappear spontaneously.

Treatment by electrodesiccation is effective but is frequently followed by slow healing. Repeated applications of bichloroacetic acid, liquid nitrogen, or liquid CO_2 are also effective. Surgical excision is not recommended, since the wound may become inoculated with the virus, leading to recurrences in and around the scar.

Because recurrences are common despite thorough treatment, it is reasonable to delay treatment of asymptomatic lesions for several months to determine if they will disappear spontaneously.

Cysts

A. EPIDERMAL INCLUSION CYST

Although sebaceous cyst is the commonly used term, these lesions more properly should be called epidermal inclusion cysts, since they are composed of thin layers of epidermal cells filled with epithelial debris. True cysts arising from sebaceous epithelial cells are uncommon.

Epidermal inclusion cysts are soft to firm, usually elevated, and are filled with an odorous cheesy material. Their most common sites of occurrence are the scalp, face, ears, neck, and back. They are usually covered by normal skin, which may show dimpling at the site of skin attachment. They frequently present as infected cysts.

Treatment consists of surgical excision.

B. DERMOID CYST

Dermoid cysts are deeper than epidermal cysts. They are not attached to the skin but frequently are attached to or extend through underlying bony structures. They may appear in many sites but are most common around the nose or the orbit, where they may extend to meningeal structures, necessitating CT scans to determine their extent.

Treatment is by surgical excision, which may necessitate sectioning of adjacent bony structures.

Pigmented Nevi

Nevocellular nevi are groups of cells of probable neural crest origin which contain melanocytes that form melanin more rapidly upon stimulation than surrounding tissue. These cells migrate to different parts of the skin to give different types of nevi. They may also be distinguished by their clinical presentation.

A. JUNCTIONAL NEVI

Junctional nevi are well-defined pigmented lesions appearing in infancy. They are usually flat or slightly elevated and light brown to dark brown. They may appear on any part of the body, but most nevi seen on the palms, soles, and genitalia are of the junctional type. Histologically, a proliferation of melanocytes is present in the epidermis at the epidermal-dermal junction. It was formerly thought that these nevi give rise to malignant melanoma and that all junctional nevi should be excised for prophylactic reasons. However, most investigators now feel that the risk is very slight. If there is no change in their appearance, treatment is unnecessary. Any change such as itching, inflammation, darkening in color, halo formation, increase in size, bleeding, or ulceration calls for immediate treatment.

Surgical excision is the only safe method of treatment.

B. INTRADERMAL NEVI

Intradermal nevi are the typical dome-shaped, sometimes pedunculated, fleshy to brownish pigmented moles that are characteristically seen in adults. They frequently contain hairs and may occur anywhere on the body.

Microscopically, melanocytes are present entirely within the dermis and, in contrast to junctional nevi, show little activity. They are rarely malignant and require no treatment except for aesthetic reasons.

Surgical excision is nearly always the treatment of choice. Pigmented nevi should never be treated without obtaining tissue for histologic examination.

C. COMPOUND NEVI

Compound nevi exhibit the histologic features of both junctional and intradermal nevi in that melanocytes lie both at the epidermal-dermal junction and within the dermis. They are usually elevated, dome-shaped, and light- to dark-brown in color.

Because of the presence of nevus cells at the epidermal-dermal junction, the indications for treatment are the same as for junctional nevi. If treatment is indicated, surgical excision is the method of choice.

D. SPINDLE CELL-EPITHELIOMA CELL NEVI

These nevi, formerly called benign juvenile melanomas, appear in children or adults. They vary markedly in vascularity, degree of pigmentation, and accompanying hyperkeratosis. Clinically, they simulate warts or hemangiomas rather than moles. They may increase in size rapidly, but the average lesion reaches only 6–8 mm in diameter, remaining entirely benign without invasion or metastases. Microscopically, the lesion can be confused with malignant melanoma by the inexperienced pathologist. The usual treatment is excisional biopsy.

E. BLUE NEVI

Blue nevi are small, sharply defined, round, dark blue or grayish-blue lesions that may occur anywhere on the body but are most commonly seen on the face, neck, hands, and arms. They usually appear in childhood as slowly growing, well-defined nodules covered by a smooth, intact epidermis. Microscopically, the melanocytes that make up this lesion are limited to (but may be found in all layers of) the dermis. An intimate association with the fibroblasts of the dermis is seen, giving

the lesion a fibrotic appearance not seen in other nevi. This, together with extension of melanocytes deep into the dermis, may account for the blue rather than brown color.

Treatment is not mandatory unless the patient desires removal for aesthetic reasons or fear of cancer. Surgical excision is the treatment of choice.

F. GIANT HAIRY NEVI

Unlike most nevi arising from melanocytes, giant hairy nevi are congenital. They may occur anywhere on the body and may cover large areas. They may be large enough to cover the entire trunk (bathing trunk nevi). They are of special significance for several reasons: (1) Their large size is especially deforming from an aesthetic standpoint; (2) they show a predisposition for developing malignant melanoma; and (3) they may be associated with neurofibromas or melanocytic involvement of the leptomeninges and other neurologic abnormalities.

Microscopically, a varied picture is present. All of the characteristics of intradermal and compound nevi may be seen. Neurofibromas may also be present within the lesion. Malignant melanoma may arise anywhere within the large lesion; the reported rate of occurrence ranges from 1% to as high as 13.7% in one study. Malignant melanoma with metastases rarely arises in childhood or infancy.

The only full treatment is complete excision and skin grafting. Large lesions may require excision and grafting in stages. Some lesions are so large that excision is not possible and the most effective approach is using tissue expansion in combination with flaps. Split-thickness excision or dermabrasion has been successful when done in infancy.

Gur E, Zuker R: Complex facial nevi: a surgical algorithm. Plast Reconstr Surg 2000;106:25.

Hemangioma

It is confusing to attempt to classify hemangiomas on the basis of their histology. For example, the histologic term capillary hemangioma is used for both the common involuting hemangioma of childhood that disappears by age 7 and the port wine stain that persists into adulthood. The term cavernous is used to designate several types of hemangiomas that behave quite differently. Some hemangiomas are true neoplasms arising from endothelial cells and other vascular elements (such as involuting hemangiomas of childhood, endotheliomas, and pericytomas). Others are not true neoplasms but rather malformations of normal vascular structures (eg, port wine stains, cavernous hemangiomas, and arteriovenous fistulas).

A simple classification based upon whether or not the hemangioma undergoes spontaneous involution is proposed in Table 44–3.

A. INVOLUTING HEMANGIOMA

Involuting hemangiomas are the most common tumors that occur in childhood and constitute at least 95% of all the hemangiomas that are seen in infancy and childhood. They are true neoplasms of endothelial cells but are unique among neoplasms in that they undergo complete spontaneous involution.

Typically, they are present shortly after birth or appear during the first 2–3 weeks of life. They grow at a rather rapid rate for 4–6 months; then growth ceases and spontaneous involution begins. Involution progresses slowly but is complete by 5–7 years of age.

Involuting hemangiomas appear on all body surfaces but are seen more often on the head and neck. They are seen twice as often in girls as in boys and show a predisposition for fair-skinned individuals.

Three forms of involuting hemangioma are seen: (1) superficial, (2) combined superficial and deep, and (3) deep. Superficial involuting hemangiomas appear as sharply demarcated, bright-red, slightly raised lesions with an irregular surface that has been described as resembling a strawberry. Combined superficial and deep involuting hemangiomas have the same surface characteristics, but beneath the surface, a firm bluish tumor is present that may extend deeply into the subcutaneous tissues. Deep involuting hemangiomas present as deep blue tumors covered by normal-appearing skin.

The histologic findings in involuting hemangiomas are quite different from those seen in other types of hemangiomas. There is a constant correlation between the histologic picture and the clinical course. During the growth phase, the lesion is composed of solid fields of closely packed round or oval endothelial cells. As would be expected during the growth phase, cellular division with mitotic figures is seen, so that the lesion is sometimes called a hemangioendothelioma by the pathologist. This term must not be used, however, since it is commonly used to denote the highly malignant angiosarcoma that is seen in adults.

As the phase of involution progresses, the histologic picture changes, with the solid fields of endothelial cells breaking up into closely packed, capillary-sized, vessel-like structures composed of several layers of soft endothelial cells supported by a sparse fibrous stroma. These vascular structures gradually become fewer and spaced more widely apart in a loose, edematous fibrous stroma. The endothelial cells continue to disappear, so that by the time involution is complete the histologic picture is entirely normal, with no trace of endothelial cells.

Treatment is not usually indicated, since the appearance following spontaneous regression is nearly always superior to the scars that follow surgical excision. Complete surgical excision of lesions that involve important structures such as the eyelids, nose, or lips results in unnecessary disfigurement that is difficult to repair.

Partial resection of a portion of a hemangioma of the brow or eyelid is indicated when the lesion is large enough to prevent light from entering the eye—a condition that will lead to blindness or amblyopia. The same type of treatment may be necessary for lesions of the mucosal surfaces of the lips when they project into the mouth and are traumatized by the teeth. In these cases, surgery should be very conservative—only enough of the lesion should be resected to alleviate the problem, and the remaining portions should be allowed to involute spontaneously.

In approximately 8% of cases, ulceration will occur. This may be accompanied by infection, which is treated by the use of compresses of warm saline or potassium permanganate and by the application of antibiotic powders and lotions. Bleeding from the ulcer is not common; when it does occur, it is easily controlled by the application of pressure. In rare cases, the platelet trapping of these lesions leads to the clinical picture of disseminated intravascular coagulopathy called **Kasabach-Merritt syndrome.**

Table 44–3. Proposed classification of hemangiomas based on appearance and clinical course of lesion.

Proposed Term	Terms in Common Use[1]
Involuting hemangioma Superficial	Strawberry nevus Nevus vasculosus Capillary hemangioma
Combined superficial and deep	Strawberry nevus Capillary hemangioma Capillary and cavernous hemangioma
Deep	Cavernous hemangioma
Noninvoluting hemangioma Port wine stain	Port wine stain Capillary hemangioma Nevus flammeus
Cavernous hemangioma	Cavernous hemangioma
Venous racemose aneurysm	Cavernous hemangioma
Arteriovenous fistula	Arteriovenous fistula

[1]Confusing because different terms are used to denote the same lesion and because the same term is sometimes used to denote different lesions.

After involution of large lesions, superficial scarring may be present or the involved skin may be thin, wrinkled, or redundant. These conditions may require conservative plastic surgery procedures.

The application of local agents such as dry ice to the surface of these lesions has been popular. This type of treatment has no effect on the deep portions of the hemangioma. It will destroy superficial lesions but results in severe scarring. Injections of sclerosing agents have minimal effect. There is no place for radiation therapy in the treatment of these benign lesions. Corticosteroids given systemically or intralesionally have been used with varying success. Anecdotal evidence exists in favor of compression to speed up the involution process and give a better final result. Innovative treatments have recently been proposed for the most serious hemangiomas. They include the insertion of a laser probe deep into the lesion so that the heat generated by the laser produces contracture of the hemangioma. Systemic interferon treatment of life-threatening hemangiomas of the head and neck area obstructing the airway have produced varying results.

B. Noninvoluting Hemangioma

Most noninvoluting hemangiomas are present at birth. In contrast to involuting hemangiomas, they do not undergo rapid growth during the first 4–6 months of life but grow in proportion to the growth of the child. They persist into adulthood and may cause severe aesthetic and functional problems. Some, such as arteriovenous fistulas, may cause death due to cardiac failure.

Unfortunately, treatment of noninvoluting hemangiomas is difficult and usually far from satisfactory.

Port wine stains are by far the most common of the noninvoluting hemangiomas. They may involve any portion of the body but most commonly appear on the face as flat patchy lesions that are reddish to purple in color. When present on the face, they are located in areas supplied by the sensory branches of the fifth cranial nerve. The light-red lesions may fade to a varying degree but persist into adulthood. Some of the deep red or purplish lesions that have a stippled appearance show a propensity for growth later in life, in which case they become raised and thickened, with nodules appearing on the surface.

Microscopically, port wine stains are made up of thin-walled capillaries that are arranged throughout the dermis. The capillaries are lined with mature flat endothelial cells. In the lesions that produce surface growth, groups of round proliferating endothelial cells and large venous sinuses are seen.

Results following treatment of the port wine stain have up to now been uniformly disappointing. Since most lesions occur on the face or neck, patients seek treatment for aesthetic reasons. The simplest and still most effective method of treatment is camouflaging. Unfortunately, this is difficult because the port wine stain is darker than the surrounding lighter skin.

Tattooing with skin-colored pigments may offer some measure of disguise in the lighter lesions but generally is unsatisfactory because the pigment deposited in the skin looks artificial and tends to be absorbed unevenly, producing a mottled appearance.

Superficial methods of treatment such as dry ice, liquid nitrogen, electrocoagulation, and dermabrasion are ineffective unless they destroy the upper layers of the skin, which produces severe scarring.

Radiation therapy, including the use of x-rays, radium, thorium X, and grenz x-rays, is to be condemned. If it is administered in doses high enough to destroy the vessels involved, it also destroys the surrounding tissues and the overlying skin and the cancer incidence after radiotherapy for skin hemangioma increases. The best treatment for early port-wine stains lighter red in color is with the laser. The pulsed dye and Candela lasers are especially useful. The beam is selectively absorbed by red-pigmented material such as hemoglobin, and the treated area becomes whiter. Multiple treatments are necessary to obtain a satisfactory result. In darker and more advanced nodular lesions, the laser is less effective and probably contraindicated because of the severe scarring and hyperpigmentation that may develop.

If the lesion is small, surgical excision with primary closure is possible. Unfortunately, most lesions are large. Sometimes the best choice is no treatment. Certain fast-growing capillary or primarily arterialized hemangiomas have been managed successfully with superselective embolization, either alone or in conjunction with surgery. This is performed under fluoroscopic control and with an expert team. There have been reports of slough of large portions of the face as a result of misdirected embolizations.

C. Cavernous Hemangioma

Cavernous hemangiomas are bluish or purplish lesions that are usually elevated. They may occur anywhere on the body but, like other hemangiomas, are more common on the head and neck. They are composed of mature, fully formed venous structures that are present in tortuous masses which have been described as feeling like a bag of worms.

Cavernous hemangiomas are usually present at birth but do not usually grow except to keep pace with normal body growth. In many cases, growth occurs later in life and may interfere with normal function.

Microscopically, cavernous hemangiomas are made up of large dilated, closely packed vascular sinuses that are engorged with blood. They are lined by flat endothelial cells and may have muscular walls like normal veins.

Treatment is difficult. In only a few cases is the lesion small enough or superficial enough to permit complete surgical excision. Most lesions involve deeper structures—including muscle and bone—so that complete excision is impossible without radical surgery. Since most lesions are no more than aesthetic problems, radical surgery is rarely indicated. Occasionally, the injection of sclerosing agents directly into the venous channels may lead to some involution or may make surgical excision easier. Great care must be used so that areas of overlying skin do not slough.

Mulliken JB, Fishman SJ, Burrows PE: Vascular anomalies. Curr Probl Surg 2000;37:517.

PREMALIGNANT SKIN LESIONS

Actinic (Solar) Keratoses

Actinic keratoses are the most common of the precancerous skin lesions. They usually appear as small, single or multiple, slightly elevated, scaly or warty lesions ranging in color from red to yellow, brown, or black. Since they are related to sun exposure, they occur most frequently on the face and the backs of the hands in fair-skinned Caucasians whose skin shows evidence of actinic elastosis.

Microscopically, actinic keratoses consist of well-defined areas of abnormal epithelial cells limited to the epidermis. Approximately 15–20% of these lesions become malignant, in which case invasion of the dermis as squamous cell carcinoma occurs.

Since the lesions are limited to the epidermis, superficial treatment in the form of curettement and electrodesiccation or the application of chemical agents such as liquid nitrogen, phenol, bi- or trichloroacetic acid, or fluorouracil is curative. The application of fluorouracil (5-FU) cream is of particular benefit in preventive treatment in that it will destroy lesions of microscopic size—before they can be detected clinically—without causing damage to uninvolved skin.

Chronic Radiation Dermatitis & Ulceration

There are two distinct types of radiation dermatitis. The first and most common follows the acute administration of relatively high dosages of ionizing orthovoltage radiation over relatively short periods—almost always for the treatment of cancer. Dermatitis is characterized by an acute reaction that begins near the third week of therapy, when erythema, blistering, and sloughing of the epidermis start to occur. Burning and hyperesthesia are commonly present. This initial reaction is followed by scarring characterized by atrophy of

the epidermis and dermis along with loss of skin appendages (sweat glands, sebaceous glands, and hair follicles). Marked fibrosis of the dermis occurs, with gradual endarteritis and occlusion of the dermal and subdermal vessels. Telangiectasia of the surface vessels is seen, and areas of both hypo- and hyperpigmentation occur.

The second type of radiation dermatitis follows chronic exposure to low doses of ionizing radiation over prolonged periods. It is usually seen in professional personnel who handle radioactive materials or administer x-rays or in patients who have been treated for dermatologic conditions such as acne or excessive facial hair. Therefore, the face and hands are most commonly involved. The acute reaction described above does not usually occur, but the same process of atrophy, scarring, and loss of dermal elements occurs. Drying of the skin becomes more pronounced, and deepening of the skin furrows is typically present. Fortunately, this second type of radiation dermatitis is rarely seen today.

In both types of radiation dermatitis, late changes such as the following may occur: (1) the appearance of hyperkeratotic growths on the skin surface, (2) chronic ulceration, and (3) the development of either basal cell or squamous cell carcinoma. Ulceration and cancer, however, are seen much less commonly in the first type of radiation dermatitis than in the second. When malignant growths appear, basal cell carcinomas are seen more frequently on the face and neck and squamous cell carcinomas more frequently on the hands and body.

Newer radiotherapeutic methods using megavoltage and electron beam techniques have a sparing effect on the skin. However, marked scarring and avascularity of deeper, more extensive areas may present more difficult problems.

Surgical excision is the treatment of choice. Excision should include all of the irradiated tissue including the area of telangiectasia, whenever possible, and the defect should be covered with an appropriate axial or musculocutaneous flap to provide a new blood supply.

Primary wound closure is feasible for only the smallest lesions, and even so at some risk. Free skin grafting is usually unsuccessful because of the damage to the vascular supply of the subcutaneous structures. Adjacent random flaps are unreliable because they depend upon blood supply from the surrounding irradiated area.

MALIGNANT LESIONS

1. Intraepidermal Carcinoma

Intraepidermal carcinoma includes Bowen's disease and erythroplasia of Queyrat.

Bowen's Disease

Bowen's disease is characterized by single or multiple, brownish or reddish plaques that may appear anywhere on the skin surface but often on covered surfaces. The typical plaque is sharply defined, slightly raised, scaly, and slightly thickened. The surface is often keratotic, and crusting and fissuring may be present. Ulceration is not common but when present suggests malignant degeneration with dermal invasion.

Histologically, hyperplasia of the epidermis is seen, with pleomorphic malpighian cells, giant cells, and atypical epithelial cells that are limited to the epidermis.

Treatment of small or superficial lesions consists of total destruction by curettement and electrodesiccation or by any of the other superficially destructive methods (cryotherapy, cytotoxic agents). Excision and skin grafting are preferred for larger lesions and for those that have undergone early malignant degeneration and invasion of the dermis.

Erythroplasia of Queyrat

Erythroplasia of Queyrat is almost identical to Bowen's disease both clinically and histologically but is confined to the glans penis and the vulva, where the lesions appear as red, velvety, irregular, slightly raised plaques. Treatment is as described for Bowen's disease.

2. Basal Cell Carcinoma

Basal cell carcinoma is the most common skin cancer. The lesions usually appear on the face and are more common in men than women. Since exposure to ultraviolet rays of the sun is a causative factor, basal cell carcinoma is most commonly seen in geographic areas where there is significant sun exposure and in people whose skins are most susceptible to actinic damage from exposure, ie, fair-skinned individuals with blue eyes and blond hair. It may occur at any age but is not common before age 40.

The growth rate of basal cell carcinoma is usually slow but nearly always steady and insidious. Several months or years may pass before the patient becomes concerned. Without treatment, widespread invasion and destruction of adjacent tissues may occur, producing massive ulceration. Penetration of the bones of the facial skeleton and the skull may occur late in the course. Basal cell carcinomas rarely metastasize, but death can occur because of direct intracranial extension or erosion of major blood vessels.

Typical individual lesions appear as small, translucent or shiny ("pearly") elevated nodules with central umbilication and rolled, pearly edges. Telangiectatic vessels are commonly present over the surface, and pigmentation is sometimes present. Superficial ulceration occurs early.

A less common type of basal cell carcinoma is the **sclerosing** or **morphea carcinoma,** consisting of elongated strands of basal cell cancer that infiltrate the dermis, with the intervening corium being unusually compact. These lesions are usually flat and whitish or waxy in appearance and firm to palpation—similar in appearance to localized scleroderma.

The superficial **erythematous basal cell cancer** ("body basal") occurs most frequently on the trunk. It appears as reddish plaques with atrophic centers and smooth, slightly raised borders. These lesions are capable of peripheral growth and wide extension but do not become invasive until late.

Pigmented basal cell carcinomas may be mistaken for melanomas, because of the large number of melanocytes present within the tumor. They may also be confused with seborrheic keratoses.

Treatment

There are several methods of treating basal cell carcinoma. All may be curative in some lesions, but no one method is applicable to all. The special features of each basal cell cancer must be considered individually before proper treatment can be selected.

Since most lesions occur on the face, aesthetic and functional results of treatment are important. However, the most important consideration is whether or not therapy is curative. If the basal cell carcinoma is not eradicated by the initial treatment, continued growth and invasion of adjacent tissues will occur. This will result not only in additional tissue destruction but also in invasion of the tumor into deeper structures, making cure more difficult. Adequate treatment of basal cell carcinoma by different modalities achieves a cure rate of approximately 95%.

The principal methods of treatment are curettage and electrodesiccation, surgical excision, and radiation therapy. Chemosurgery, topical chemotherapy, and cryosurgery are not often used but may have value in selected cases.

A. Curettage and Electrodesiccation

Curettage plus electrodesiccation is the usual method of treatment for small lesions. After infiltration with suitable local anesthetic, the lesion and a 2- to 3-mm margin of normal-appearing skin around it are thoroughly curetted with a small skin curette. The resultant wound is then completely desiccated with an electrosurgical unit to destroy any tumor cells that may not have been removed by the curette. The process is then repeated once or twice if necessary. The wound is left open and allowed to heal secondarily.

When used as treatment for superficial basal cell carcinoma, curettage and electrodesiccation is a simple, quick, and inexpensive procedure that will cure nearly all superficial lesions. However, this method of treatment should not be used in the deeper infiltrative and morphea type lesions. These lesions should be treated by surgical excision, x-ray therapy, or chemosurgery.

B. Surgical Excision

Surgical excision, following the principles outlined earlier in this chapter, offers many advantages in the treatment of basal cell carcinoma: (1) Most lesions can be quickly excised in one procedure. (2) Following excision, the entire lesion can be examined by the pathologist, who can determine if the tumor has been completely removed. (3) Deep infiltrative lesions can be completely excised, and cartilage and bone can be removed if they have been invaded. (4) Lesions that occur in dense scar tissue or in other poorly vascularized tissues cannot be treated by curettage and desiccation, radiation therapy, or chemosurgery, since healing is poor. Excision and flap coverage may be the only method for treatment in these conditions. (5) Recurrent lesions in tissues that have been exposed to maximum safe amounts of radiation can be excised and covered.

Small to moderate-sized lesions can be excised in one stage under local anesthesia. The visible and palpable margins of the tumor are marked on the skin with marking ink. The width of excision is then marked 3–5 mm beyond these margins. If the margins of the basal cell carcinoma are vague, the width of excision will have to be wider to ensure complete removal of the lesion. The lines of incision are drawn around the lesion as a circle. This tissue is excised, taking care to leave a margin of normal-appearing subcutaneous tissue around the deep margins of the tumor. Frozen sections may be obtained at the time of excision to aid in determining whether tumor-free margins have been obtained. This is minimized with experience. It is better to err on the side of removing more normal tissue than necessary rather than to run the risk of including tumor at the margins. Closure of the wound is accomplished in the direction of minimal skin tension, usually along the skin lines. The dog-ears are removed appropriately.

Wounds resulting from the excision of some moderate-sized tumors and nearly all large tumors may necessitate for optimum reconstruction of function and appearance, the use of local, regional and free flaps. This can nearly always be performed in one stage.

The disadvantages of surgical excision are as follows: (1) Specialized training and experience are necessary to master the surgical techniques. (2) Whereas curettage and desiccation may be performed in the office, surgical excision requires specialized facilities. (3) In lesions with vague margins, an excessive amount of normal tissue may have to be excised to ensure complete removal. (4) Structures that are difficult to reconstruct, such as the eyelids, nasal tip, and lips, have to be sacrificed when they are extensively infiltrated and immediate reconstruction to cover vital structures is indicated. To overcome some of these objections, Mohs described in 1941 a new technique that allows for serial excisions and microscopic examination of chemically fixed tissue. Newer developments have obviated the cumbersome fixation techniques, but it may still take several hours to scan an area for suspected malignant cells. The procedure is nevertheless quite useful for recurrent lesions and in areas in which maximal preservation is desirable. Nonetheless, there are no prospective comparative studies to indicate that the so-called microscopically controlled removal of tumor by the Mohs technique, which amounts to excision of the lesion with serial review by fresh frozen section, is superior to surgical excision. An additional problem is that there is no quality control because the excising physician is also the one who evaluates the pathology slides. Some of the lesions treated with the Mohs technique do require secondary reconstruction.

C. X-ray Therapy

X-ray therapy is as effective as any other in the treatment of basal cell carcinoma. Its advantages are as follows: (1) Structures that are difficult to reconstruct, such as the eyelids, tear ducts, and nasal tip, can be preserved when they are invaded by but not destroyed by tumor. (2) A wide margin of tissue can be treated around lesions with poorly defined margins to ensure destruction of nondiscernible extensions of tumor. (3) It may be less traumatic than surgical excision to elderly patients with advanced lesions. (4) Hospitalization is not necessary.

The disadvantages are as follows: (1) Only well-trained, experienced physicians can obtain good results. (2) Expensive facilities are necessary. (3) Improperly administered radiation therapy may produce severe sequelae, including scarring, radiation dermatitis, ulceration, and malignant degeneration. (4) In hair-bearing areas, epilation will result. (5) It may be difficult to treat areas of irregular contour (ie, the ear and the auditory canal). (6) Repeated treatments over a period of 4–6 weeks may be necessary.

X-ray therapy should not be used in patients under age 40 except in unusual circumstances, and it should not be repeated in patients who have failed to respond to radiation therapy in the past.

3. Squamous Cell Carcinoma

Squamous cell carcinoma is the second most common cancer of the skin in light-skinned racial groups and the most common skin cancer in darkly pigmented racial groups. As with basal cell carcinoma, sunlight is the most common causative factor in whites. The most common sites of occurrence are the ears, the cheeks, the lower lip, and the backs of the hands. Other causative factors are chemical and thermal burns, scars, chronic ulcers, chronic granulomas (tuberculosis of the skin, syphilis), draining sinuses, contact with tars and hydrocarbons, and exposure to ionizing radiation. When a squamous cell carcinoma occurs in a burn scar, it is called a **Marjolin ulcer.** This lesion may appear many years after the original burn. It tends to be aggressive, and the prognosis is poor.

Since exposure to the sun is the greatest stimulus for the production of squamous cell carcinoma, most of these lesions are preceded by actinic keratosis on areas of the skin showing chronic solar damage. They may also arise from other premalignant skin lesions and from normal-appearing skin.

The natural history of squamous cell carcinoma may be quite variable. It may present as a slowly growing, locally invasive lesion without metastases or as a rapidly growing, widely invasive tumor with early metastatic spread. In general, squamous cell carcinomas that develop from actinic keratoses are more common and are of the slowly growing type, whereas those that develop from Bowen's disease, erythroplasia of Queyrat, chronic radiation dermatitis, scars, and chronic ulcers tend to be more aggressive. Lesions that arise from normal-appearing skin and from the lips, genitalia, and anal regions also tend to be aggressive.

Early squamous cell carcinoma usually appears as a small, firm erythematous plaque or nodule with indistinct margins. The surface may be flat and smooth or may be verrucous. As the tumor grows, it becomes raised, and, because of progressive invasion, becomes fixed to surrounding tissues. Ulceration may occur early or late but tends to appear earlier in the more rapidly growing lesions.

Histologically, malignant epithelial cells are seen extending down into the dermis as broad, rounded masses or slender strands. In squamous cell carcinomas of low-grade malignancy, the individual cells may be quite well differentiated, resembling uniform mature squamous cells having intercellular bridges. Keratinization may be present, and layers of keratinizing squamous cells may produce typical round "horn pearls." In highly malignant lesions, the epithelial cells may be extremely atypical; abnormal mitotic figures are common; intercellular bridges are not present; and keratinization does not occur.

As with basal cell carcinomas, the method of treatment that will eradicate squamous cell carcinomas and produce the best aesthetic and functional results varies with the characteristics of the individual lesion. Factors that determine the optimal method of treatment include the size, shape, and location of the tumor as well as the histologic pattern that determines its aggressiveness.

Treatment consists of surgery or irradiation. The advantages and disadvantages of each type of therapy are discussed above. Since basal cell carcinomas are relatively nonaggressive lesions that rarely metastasize, failure to eradicate the lesion may result only in local recurrence. Although this may result in extensive local tissue destruction, there is rarely a threat to life. Aggressive squamous cell carcinomas, on the other hand, may metastasize to any part of the body, and failure of treatment may have fatal consequences. For this reason, total eradication of each lesion is the imperative goal of treatment.

Because the overall incidence of lymph node metastasis is relatively low, most authorities agree that node resection is not indicated in the absence of palpable regional lymph nodes except in the case of very aggressive carcinomas of the genitalia and anal regions.

Alam M, Ratner D: Cutaneous squamous-cell carcinoma. N Engl J Med 2001;344:975.

Arbuckle HA, Morelli JG: Pigmentary disorders: update on neurofibromatosis-1 and tuberous sclerosis. Curr Opin Pediatr 2000;12:354.

Kanzler MH, Mraz-Gernhard S: Treatment of primary cutaneous melanoma. JAMA 2001;285:1819.

Lentsch EJ, Myers JN: Melanoma of the head and neck: current concepts in diagnosis and management. Laryngoscope 2001; 111:1209.

Stadelmann WK et al: Cutaneous melanoma of the head and neck: advances in evaluation and treatment. Plast Reconstr Surg 2000;105:2105.

SOFT TISSUE INJURY

The plastic surgeon is often involved in emergency room assessment and treatment of soft tissue injuries. Many aspects of wound management must be considered in even a relatively simple facial laceration.

If possible, the following factors should be determined in patients with soft tissue injuries: (1) the type of wound or wounds (abrasion, contusion, etc); (2) the cause of injury; (3) the age of the injury; (4) the location of injured tissues; (5) the degree of contamination of the injured area before, during, and after trauma; (6) the nature and extent of associated injuries; and (7) the general health of the patient (eg, any chronic or acute illnesses or any allergies; any medications being taken).

The location of the wound must be noted because different healing characteristics are present in various types of skin. The face and scalp are highly vascular and therefore resist infection and heal faster than other areas, but there are many important structures in and around the face, and scars and defects are noticeable. Skin of the trunk, upper arms, and thighs is fairly thick and heals more slowly than facial or scalp skin and is more susceptible to infection. Scarring is less noticeable. The hands are a critical area because there are important structures near the surface, and the destruction caused by infection can be devastating. The lower legs are a particular problem area because the relatively poor blood supply can cause skin loss, and infection is more likely to occur.

Treatment

The type of wound must be determined so that proper treatment can be given. Contusions and swelling require ice packs for 24 hours, rest, and elevation. Abrasions should be cleaned and dressed in a sterile manner as for a skin graft donor site or must be washed daily until a dry scab forms or healing takes place. Ground-in dirt or gravel must be entirely scrubbed out or picked out with a small blade within 24 hours after injury, or foreign material will be sealed in and traumatic tattooing will result. Extensive local anesthesia may be required to accomplish this. Imbedded particulate matter from an explosion must be removed in a similar manner. Hematomas may be treated with ice bags and pressure until stable. Evacuation is then indicated if vital structures such as the ear or nasal septal cartilage are in danger of being injured or destroyed. Lacerations over bony prominences and various types of cuts require special care that will be detailed below. Treatment must be meticulous if optimal results are to be achieved. Puncture wounds and bites are notoriously innocuous in appearance but may result in severe destruction or tetanus or gas gangrene. Antibiotic coverage, irrigation, open treatment, and observation are indicated. Most bites on the face, however, can be cleaned and safely closed. Wounds that create flaps of skin or avulsions are difficult to manage. Careful debridement and judicious use of full- or split-thickness grafts from the avulsed tissue are recommended. Timing is the first factor to consider.

Wound contamination can be caused by bacteria on the surface of the wounding agent, such as rust on a nail or saliva on a tooth, or bacteria that enter the wound when the skin is broken. Bacteria driven into tissue become more established as time passes, and it is therefore important to know the age of the wound at the time of the presentation for treatment. Other injuries associated with cuts almost always take precedence in treatment. In general, wounds other than those on the face or scalp should not be closed primarily if they occurred 8–12 hours or longer before presen-

tation unless they were caused by a very clean agent and have been covered by a sterile bandage in the interim. Delayed primary closure as described previously is an excellent and safe alternative. Nearly any facial wound up to 24 hours old can be safely closed with careful debridement, irrigation, and antibiotic coverage.

The surgeon must decide whether or not antibiotic treatment is indicated. In general, wounds treated appropriately and early do not call for antibiotic therapy. Antibiotics should be given for wounds with delayed presentation or those for which treatment is delayed by choice (eg, wounds with known contamination; wounds in compromised patients, such as very young or old persons, debilitated persons, or persons with general ill health; wounds in areas where infection may have serious consequences, such as the lower legs and the hands; and wounds in persons in whom bacteremia might have serious sequelae, such as those with prosthetic heart valves or orthopedic appliances). Antibiotics should be started before debridement and closure. Only a few days of coverage are necessary—usually until the wound is checked at 2–3 days and found to be free of infection. Penicillin or a substitute is appropriate for wounds involving the mouth, such as through-and-through lip lacerations and bites. Other wounds are usually contaminated by *Staphylococcus aureus,* and an antibiotic effective for penicillin-resistant *S aureus* is therefore appropriate. If gram-negative or anaerobic contamination is suspected, wound closure is risky, and hospitalization of the patient for treatment with parenteral antibiotics should be considered. Tetanus prophylaxis should be routinely given for patients who have not received current immunizations or who have wounds likely to lead to tetanus. Guidelines for this are detailed in Chapter 8.

Anesthesia is an important part of adequate soft tissue wound care and closure. Local anesthesia with either 0.5% or 1% lidocaine with epinephrine 1:200,000 or 1:100,000 is recommended for all wounds. Smaller amounts of lidocaine and epinephrine may be used in areas of appendages, such as earlobes, toes, and the penis. The injection may be given through the wound edge before debridement and irrigation for maximum patient comfort. Complete epinephrine vasoconstrictor effect occurs within 7 minutes. Overdose of epinephrine and lidocaine injection into vessels or use of the drugs in patients sensitive to these agents should be avoided.

The importance of irrigation cannot be overstated. Over 90% of bacteria in a recently sustained and superficially contaminated wound can be eliminated by adequate irrigation. Ideally, a physiologic solution such as lactated Ringer's solution or normal saline should be forcefully ejected from a large syringe with a 19-gauge needle or from other equipment designed for this purpose such as a water-jet apparatus. The wound is irrigated once to remove surface clots, foreign material, and bacteria and is then debrided and irrigated again. Detergents and antiseptic solutions are toxic to exposed tissue and should not be used.

Debridement must include removal of all obviously devitalized tissues. In special areas such as the eyelids, ears, nose, lips, and eyebrows, debridement must be done cautiously, since the tissue lost by debridement may be difficult to replace. Where tissues are more abundant, such as in the cheek, chin, and forehead areas, debridement may be more extensive. Small irregular or ragged wounds in these areas can be excised completely to produce clean, sharply cut wound edges which, when approximated, will produce the finest possible scar. Because the blood supply in the face is plentiful, damaged tissues of questionable viability should be retained rather than debrided away. The chances for survival are good.

Following adequate anesthesia, debridement, and irrigation, the wound is ready for final assessment and closure. Lighting must be adequate, and appropriate instruments should be available. The patient and the surgeon must be positioned comfortably. The skin surrounding the wound is prepared with an antiseptic solution, and the area is draped. A final check of the depth and extent of the wound is made, and vital structures are inspected for injury. Hemostasis must be achieved by use of epinephrine, pressure, cautery, or suture ligature. Important structures in facial wounds include the parotid duct, lacrimal duct, and branches of the facial nerve. These should be repaired in the operating room by microsurgical techniques.

Layers of tissue—usually muscle—in the depth of the wound should be closed first with as few absorbable sutures as possible, since sutures are foreign material within the wound. If possible, dead space should be closed with judicious use of fine absorbable sutures. If dead space cannot be closed, external pressure or small drains are sometimes effective. Skin closure should begin at the most important points of the laceration (eg, the borders of the ears and nose; the vermilion border or margins of the lip; the margins of the eyebrow [which should never be shaved]; and the scalp hairline). Subcuticular sutures are very helpful. Skin edges can be approximated without tension or strangulation with 5-0 or 6-0 monofilament suture material as outlined earlier under wound closure.

Complicated lacerations, such as complex stellate wounds or avulsion flaps, often heal with excessive scarring. Because of the associated subcutaneous tissue injury, U-shaped or trap-door avulsion lacerations almost always become unsightly as a result of wound contracture. Small lacerations of this type are best excised and closed in a straight line initially; larger flaps that must

be replaced usually require secondary revision. Extensive loss of skin is generally best treated by initial split-thickness skin grafting followed later by secondary reconstruction. Primary attempts to reconstruct with local flaps may fail because of unsuspected injury to these adjacent tissues. The decision to convert avulsed tissues to free grafts that may not survive and thus delay healing requires sound surgical judgment.

Small or moderate-sized closures on the face may be dressed with antibiotic ointment alone. The patient may cleanse the suture lines with hydrogen peroxide to clear away crusts and dirt and then reapply the ointment. Elsewhere, closures benefit from the protection of a sterile bandage. Pressure dressings are useful in preventing hematoma formation and severe edema that may result in poor wound healing. Dressings should be changed early and the wound inspected for hematoma or signs of infection. Hematoma evacuation, appropriate drainage, and antibiotic therapy based on culture and sensitivity studies may be required. Removal of sutures in 3–5 days, followed by splinting of the incision with sterile tape, will minimize scarring from the sutures themselves.

The final result of facial wound repair depends on the nature and location of the wounds, individual propensity to scar formation, and the passage of time. A year or more must often pass before resolution of scar contracture and erythema results in maximum improvement. Only after this time can a decision be made regarding the desirability of secondary scar revision.

In wounds involving the major joints the extracapsular soft tissue and the intracapsular structures should be considered individually to assess accurately the magnitude of the injury and to provide a prognosis. Open joint injuries that are single penetrating and without extensive soft tissue damage, permit uncomplicated joint and wound closure. Injuries that are single or multiple penetrations with extensive soft-tissue disruption (flaps, avulsions, degloving) often require secondary operations to attain closure. In injuries which show open periarticular fractures with extension through the adjacent intra-articular surface and with associated nerve or vascular injury requiring repair, the cornerstone for successful management is debridement, antibiotic therapy properly timed and performed, joint closure and aggressive treatment of the bony injury. Newer techniques such as free tissue transfer can expedite wound care, decrease morbidity and spare some limbs from amputation.

FACIAL BONE FRACTURES

Because of the aesthetic and functional importance of the face, fractures of the facial bones—though rarely life-threatening—are best treated by surgeons who have extensive experience with facial injuries and reconstruction. Operation is most successful when performed in the acute setting, usually within the first week, because reconstruction becomes much more difficult if surgery is delayed.

Facial bone fractures are usually caused by trauma from a blunt instrument, such as a fist or club, or by violent contact with the steering wheel, dash-board, or windshield during an automobile accident. Particularly in the latter case, the patient should be assessed for associated injuries. For example, cervical spine injuries are present in up to 12% of automobile accident patients and should be treated or stabilized before facial bone injuries are attended to. Injuries to the brain, eyes, chest, abdomen, and extremities must also be assessed and may require earlier treatment.

The diagnosis of facial fractures is made primarily on clinical examination. Ideally, the examination should be done immediately, so that swelling will not obscure the findings. The mechanism and the line of direction of injury are important. If conscious, the patient should be asked about previous facial injuries, areas of pain and numbness, whether the jaw opens properly and the teeth come together normally, and whether vision in all quadrants is normal.

Most facial fractures can be palpated, or at least the abnormal position of bones can be noted. Beginning along the mandibular rims, feel for irregularities of the facial bones. The dental occlusion is noted. With bimanual palpation, placing the thumbs inside the mouth, one can elicit bony crepitus if there is an associated fracture. The maxilla and mid face can be rocked forward and backward between the thumb and the index finger in the presence of a midfacial fracture. Nasal fractures may be detected by palpation. Irregularities and step-offs along the infraorbital border, lateral orbital rim, or zygomatic arch regions indicate a depressed zygomatic fracture.

Radiologic studies are only an adjunct to the diagnosis of facial fractures. Rarely is a significant fracture seen on x-ray that is not also clinically evident. Helpful views include the Waters and submentovertex projections and oblique views of the mandible. If available, the Panorex view of the mandible is very useful. CT scans of facial bones, with appropriate biplanar and three-dimensional reconstructions so that bones can be viewed through several planes, are helpful in assessing the extent of fractures in posterior areas such as the ethmoid area, posterior and inferior orbit, pterygoid plates, and base of the skull. CT scans have supplanted plain x-rays in the evaluation of facial fractures.

The bones of the nose are the most commonly fractured facial bones. Next in frequency are the mandible, the zygomatic-malar bones, and the maxilla.

NASAL FRACTURES

Fractures may affect the nasal bones, cartilage, and septum. Fractures occur in two patterns, caused by lateral or head-on trauma.

With lateral trauma, the nasal bone on the side of the injury is fractured and displaced toward the septum; the septum is deviated and fractured; and the nasal bone on the side away from the injury is fractured and displaced away from the septum, so that the upper part of the nose, as a whole, is deviated. Depending upon the degree of violence, one or more of these displacements will be present, and the degree of comminution is variable.

Head-on trauma gives rise to telescoping and saddling of the nose and broadening of its upper half as a result of the depression and splaying of the fractured nasal bones. This of course produces severe damage to the septum, which usually buckles or actually suffers a fracture. The diagnosis of a fractured nose is made on clinical grounds alone, and x-rays are unnecessary.

Nasal fractures requiring reduction should be treated with a minimum of delay, for they tend to become fixed in the displaced position in a few days. The surgical approach depends on whether the fracture has resulted in deviation or collapse of the nasal bones. Local anesthesia is preferred; either topical tetracaine or cocaine intranasally or lidocaine for infiltration of the skin can be used. The nasal bones may be disimpacted with intranasal forceps or a periosteal elevator and aligned by external molding or pressure. Collapsed nasal fractures can be repositioned with Walsham's nasal forceps, introduced into each nostril and placed on each side of the septum, which is then elevated to its proper position. A septal hematoma should be recognized and drained to prevent infection and subsequent necrosis of the cartilaginous septum with associated collapse of the entire nose. Compound fractures of the nose require prompt repair of the skin wound and, if possible, early reduction of the displaced nasal bones.

External splinting, which is essentially a protective dressing, and intranasal packing using nonadhering gauze are appropriate after reduction. The intranasal packing provides support for the septum in its reduced position and helps prevent development of a hematoma. It also provides counter pressure for the external splint immobilizing the nasal bones and prevents them from collapsing. The packing is usually removed within 48 hours.

In severe comminuted nasal fractures, the medial canthal ligaments, which are easily felt by applying lateral traction to the upper eyelid, may have dislodged. If they have been avulsed, they should be reattached in position to prevent late deformities. For these severe fractures involving the entire naso-orbital and ethmoid complex, the coronal approach, which offers wide exposure, allows for proper anatomic reduction of all small nasal fragments as well as repositioning of the canthal ligaments and correction and elevation of the telescoped bone fragments at the root of the nose and glabella.

The lacrimal apparatus is commonly disrupted in these injuries and should be repaired and stented appropriately.

MANDIBULAR FRACTURES

Mandibular fractures are most commonly bilateral, generally occurring in the region of the mid body at the mental foramen, the angle of the ramus, or at the neck of the condyle. A frequent combination is a fracture at the mental region of the body with a condylar fracture on the opposite side. Displacement of the fragments results from the force of the external blow as well as the pull of the muscles of the floor of the mouth and the muscles of mastication. The diagnosis is suggested by derangement of dental occlusion associated with local pain, swelling, and often crepitation upon palpation. Appropriate x-rays confirm the diagnosis. Special views of the condyle, including tomograms, may be required. Sublingual hematoma and acute malocclusion are usually diagnostic of a mandibular fracture.

Restoration of functional dental occlusion is the most important consideration in treating mandibular fractures. In patients with an adequate complement of teeth, arch bars or interdental wires can be placed. Local nerve block anesthesia is preferable for this procedure, though certain patients may require general anesthesia. Intermaxillary elastic traction will usually correct minor degrees of displacement and bring the teeth into normal occlusion by overcoming the muscle pull. When the fracture involves the base of a tooth socket with suspected devitalization of the tooth, extraction of the tooth should be considered. Particularly in the incisor region, such devitalized teeth may be a source of infection, leading to the development of osteomyelitis and nonunion of the fracture.

Patients with more severe mandibular injuries require anatomic reduction and fixation of the fracture by the open, direct technique. These include compound, comminuted, and unfavorable fractures. An unfavorable fracture is one that is inherently unstable because muscle pull distracts the fracture segments. In this situation, intermaxillary fixation alone is insufficient. Edentulous patients also benefit from the open technique, although proper dentures or dental splints are useful to maintain normal occlusion.

Metal wire fixation of fractured segments and intermaxillary fixation for 6 weeks is a proved and popular method of fracture treatment. The recent resurgence in popularity of the screw-plate system is due to a number of advantages over wiring. The screw plate usually achieves rigid fixation in three dimensions, providing adequate stability; it eliminates the need for intermaxillary fixation in most cases; it is useful in complex, comminuted fractures; and it is quite easy to use after familiarity with the technique has been acquired.

With bilateral parasymphysial fractures, anterior stabilization of the tongue may be lost, so that it may fall back and obstruct the airway. Anterior stabilization and splinting must be accomplished early in these cases.

Open reduction is rarely advised in condylar fractures; simple intermaxillary fixation for 4–6 weeks is sufficient. Indications for open reduction are severely displaced fractures, which may prevent motion of the mandible because of impingement of the coronoid process on the zygomatic arch. In children, the fracture may destroy the growth center of the condyle, resulting in maldevelopment of the mandible and gross distortion.

ZYGOMATIC & ORBITAL FRACTURE

Fractures of the zygomatic bones may involve just the arch of the zygomatic bone or the entire body of the zygoma (the malar eminence) and the lateral wall and floor of the orbit. The so-called tripod fracture characteristically occurs at the frontozygomatic and zygomaticomaxillary sutures as well as at the arch. Displacement of the body of the zygoma results in flattening of the cheek and depression of the orbital rim and floor.

Important diagnostic signs are subconjunctival hemorrhage, disturbances of extraocular muscle function (which may be accompanied by diplopia), and loss of sensation in the upper lip and alveoli on the involved side as a result of injury to the infraorbital nerve. Reduction of a displaced zygomatic fracture is seldom an emergency procedure and may be delayed until the patient's general condition is satisfactory for anesthesia. Local anesthesia will suffice only for reduction of fractures of the zygomatic arch. More extensively displaced fractures usually require general anesthesia. At least two-point fixation with direct interosseous wiring is necessary for these fractures. Here again, delicate miniplates have been used with success, providing anatomic reduction and rigid fixation.

Depressed fractures of the zygomatic arch can best be elevated using the Gillies technique. Through a temporal incision above the hairline, an instrument is passed beneath the superficial layer of the temporalis fascia and under the arch and the body of the zygoma. The fracture can also be elevated percutaneously with a hook in conjunction with overlying palpation to achieve accurate reduction.

Extensive disruption should be suspected in conjunction with the zygomatic fracture when significant diplopia and enophthalmos and posterior displacement of the globe are present. Orbital fat and extraocular muscles may herniate through the defect and become entrapped, giving rise to the signs and symptoms. A "blowout" fracture is similar disruption of the orbital floor due to blunt trauma to the globe but not associated with a fracture of the zygoma or orbital rim. Treatment in both cases demands exploration, reduction of herniated contents, and repair of the floor. The most direct approach is through a lower lid subciliary incision, which provides excellent visualization. A buccal transantral (Caldwell-Luc) approach can be used, and blind antral packing for support has been described. This is quite hazardous, because bony spicules may be pushed into the ocular globe and perhaps cause injury or blindness. In cases where there is extensive communication or loss of bony fragments of the floor, use of local autogenous bone or cartilage as a scaffold is ideal. A thin sheet of alloplastic material such as Silastic has also been satisfactory.

Even with careful anatomic reduction and repair of the orbital floor, ocular problems—particularly enophthalmos—may persist. This may be due to an undiagnosed fracture, especially a medial ethmoidal blowout fracture. These can be properly evaluated with CT scanning. Treatment requires reduction and repair of the defect. The injury can at times cause ischemia of herniated soft tissue and subsequent atrophy and scarring. This may result in enophthalmos, which is almost impossible to resolve completely.

MAXILLARY FRACTURES

Maxillary fractures range in complexity from partial fractures through the alveolar process to extensive displacement of the midfacial structures in conjunction with fractures of the frontonasal bones and orbital maxillary region and total craniofacial separation. Hemorrhage and airway obstruction require emergency care, and in severe cases, tracheostomy is indicated. Mobility of the maxilla can be elicited by palpation in extensive fractures. "Dish-face" deformity of the retrodisplaced maxilla may be disguised by edema, and careful x-ray studies are necessary to determine the extent and complexity of the midfacial fracture. Treatment may have to be delayed because of other severe injuries. A delay of as long as 10–14 days may be safe before reduction and fixation, but the earliest possible restoration of maxillary position and dental occlusion is desirable to prevent late complications.

In the case of unilateral fractures or bilateral fractures with little or no displacement, splinting by intermaxillary fixation for 4 weeks may suffice. Fractures are usually displaced inferiorly or posteriorly and require direct surgical disimpaction and reduction. Early reduction may help control bleeding, as torn, stretched vessels are allowed to reestablish their normal tension. In certain severe cases, external traction may be necessary. Manipulation is directed toward restoring normal occlusion and maintaining the reduction with intermaxillary fixation to the mandible in association with direct fixation or supporting wires from other intact facial or cranial bones. Complicated fractures may require external fixation utilizing a head cap and intraoral splints in conjunction with multiple surgical incisions for direct wire fixation. Coexisting mandibular fractures usually necessitate open reduction and fixation at the same time.

Antonyshyn O, Gruss JS: Complex orbital trauma: the role of rigid fixation and primary bone grafting. Plast Reconstr Surg 1988;7:61.

Krsarai L et al A biomechanical analysis of the orbital zygomatic complex in human cadavers: examination of load sharing and failure patterns after fixation with titanium and bioresorbable systems. J Craniofac Surg 1999;10:400.

Thaller SR, Kawamoto HK: A histologic evaluation of fracture repair in the midface. Plast Reconstr Surg 1990;85:196.

Thaller SR, Mabourakh S: Pediatric mandibular fractures. Ann Plast Surg 1991;26:511.

Yaremchuk MJ: Vascularized bone grafts for maxillofacial reconstruction. Clin Plast Surg 1989;16:29.

CONGENITAL HEAD & NECK ANOMALIES

CLEFT LIP & CLEFT PALATE

Cleft lip, cleft palate, and combinations of the two are the most common congenital anomalies of the head and neck. The incidence of facial clefts has been reported to be 1 in every 650–750 live births, making this deformity second only to clubfoot in frequency as a reported birth defect.

The cleft may involve the floor of the nostril and lip on one or both sides and may extend through the alveolus, the hard palate, and the entire soft palate. A useful classification based on embryologic and anatomic aspects divides the structures into the primary and the secondary palate. The dividing point between the primary palate anteriorly and the secondary palate posteriorly is the incisive foramen. Clefts can thus be classified as partial or complete clefts of the primary or secondary palate (or both) in various combinations. The most common clefts are left unilateral complete clefts of the primary and secondary palate and partial midline clefts of the secondary palate, involving the soft palate and part of the hard palate.

Most infants with cleft palate present some feeding difficulties, and breast feeding may be impossible. As a rule, enlarging the openings in an artificial nipple or using a syringe with a soft rubber feeding tube will solve difficulties in sucking. Feeding in the upright position helps prevent oronasal reflux or aspiration. Severe feeding and breathing problems and recurrent aspiration are seen in Pierre Robin syndrome, in which the palatal cleft is associated with a receding lower jaw and posterior displacement of the tongue, obstructing the oropharyngeal airway. This is a medical emergency and is a cause of sudden infant death syndrome (SIDS). Nonsurgical treatment includes pulling the tongue forward with an instrument and laying the baby prone with a towel under the chest to let the mandible and tongue drop forward. Insertion of a small (No. 8) nasogastric tube into the pharynx may temporarily prevent respiratory distress and may be used to supplement the baby's feedings. Several surgical procedures that bring the tongue and mandible forward have been described but should be employed only when conservative measures have been tried without success.

Treatment

Surgical repair of cleft lip is not considered an emergency. The optimal time for operation can be described as the widely accepted "rule of ten." This includes body weight of 10 lb (4.5 kg) or more and a hemoglobin of 10 g/dL or more. This is usually at some time after the 10th week of life. In most cases, closure of the lip will mold distortions of the cleft alveolus into a satisfactory contour. In occasional cases where there is marked distortion of the alveolus, such as in severe bilateral clefts with marked protrusion of the premaxilla, preliminary maxillary orthodontic treatment may be indicated. This may involve the use of carefully crafted appliances or simple constant pressure by use of an elastic band.

General endotracheal anesthesia via an orally placed endotracheal tube is the anesthetic technique of choice. A variety of techniques for repair of unilateral clefts have evolved over many years. Earlier procedures ignored anatomic landmarks and resulted in a characteristic "repaired harelip" look. The Millard rotation advancement operation that is now commonly used for repair employs an incision in the medial side of the cleft to allow the cupid's bow of the lip to be rotated down to a normal position. The resulting gap in the medial side of the cleft is filled by advancing a flap from the lateral side. This principle can be varied in placement of the incisions and results in most cases in a symmetric lip with normally placed landmarks. Bilateral clefts, because of greater deficiency of tissue, present more challenging technical problems. Maximum preservation of available tissue is the underlying principle, and most surgeons prefer approximation of the central and lateral lip elements in a straight line closure, rolling up the vermilion border of the lip (Manchester repair).

Secondary revisions are frequently necessary in the older child with a repaired cleft lip. A constant associated deformity in patients with cleft lip is distortion of the soft tissue and cartilage structures of the ala and dome of the nose. These patients often present with deficiency of growth of the structures of the mid face. This has been attributed to intrinsic growth disturbances and to external pressures from the lip and palate repairs. Some correction of these deformities, especially of the nose, can be done at the initial lip operation. More definitive correction is done after the cartilage and bone growth is more complete. These may include scar revisions and rearrangement of the cartilage structure of the nose. Recent approaches involve degloving of the nasal skin envelope with complete exposure of the abnormal cartilage framework. These are then rearranged in proper position with or without additional grafts. Maxillary osteotomies (Le Fort I with advancement) will substantially correct the midfacial depression. A tight upper lip due to severe tissue deficiency can be corrected by a two-stage transfer of a lower lip flap known as an Abbe flap.

Palatal clefts may involve the alveolus, the bony hard palate, or the soft palate, singly or in any combination. Clefts of the hard palate and alveolus may be either unilateral or bilateral, whereas the soft palate cleft is always midline, extending back through the uvula. The width of the cleft varies greatly, making the amount of tissue available for repair also variable. The bony palate, with its mucoperiosteal lining, forms the roof of the anterior mouth and the floor of the nose. The posteriorly attached soft palate is composed of five paired muscles of speech and swallowing.

Surgical closure of the cleft to allow for normal speech is the treatment of choice. The timetable for closure depends on the size of the cleft and any other associated problems. However, the defect should be closed before the child undertakes serious speech, usually before age 2. Closure at 6 months usually is performed without difficulty and also aids in the child's feeding. If the soft palate seems to be long enough, simple approximation of the freshened edges of the cleft after freeing of the tissues through lateral relaxing incisions may suffice. If the soft palate is too short, a pushback type of operation is required. In this procedure, the short soft palate is retrodisplaced closer to the posterior pharyngeal wall utilizing the mucoperiosteal flaps based on the posterior palatine artery.

Satisfactory speech following surgical repair of cleft palate is achieved in 70–90% of cases. Significant speech defects usually require secondary operations when the child is older. The most widely used technique is the pharyngeal flap operation, in which the palatopharyngeal space is reduced by attaching a flap of posterior pharyngeal muscle and mucosa to the soft palate. This permits voluntary closure of the velopharyngeal complex and thus avoids hypernasal speech. Various other kinds of pharyngoplasties have been useful in selected cases.

CRANIOFACIAL ANOMALIES

These are congenital deformities of the hard and soft tissues of the head. Particular problems of the brain, eye, and internal ear are treated by the appropriate specialist. The craniofacial surgeon often needs the collaboration of these specialists when operating on such patients.

Serious craniofacial anomalies are relatively rare, although mild forms often go undiagnosed or accepted as normal variants. A classification is therefore difficult, although many have been proposed. Tessier has offered a numerical classification based on clinical presentation. He considers a cleft to be the basis of the malformation, which involves both hard and soft tissues. Other classifications are based on embryologic and etiologic features. With greater understanding and continued investigation, classification efforts will no doubt be more satisfactory.

There are well-known chromosomal and genetic aberrations as well as environmental causes that can lead to craniofacial deformity. The cause in most cases, however, is unknown. Arrest in the migration and proliferation of neural crest cells and defects in differentiation characterize most of these deformities. We will describe some of the more common ones in brief terms.

Crouzon's syndrome (craniofacial dysostosis) and **Apert's syndrome** (acrocephalosyndactyly) are closely related, differing in the extremity deformities present in the latter. Both are autosomal dominant traits with variable expression. Both present with skull deformities due to premature closure of the cranial sutures. The cranial sutures most affected will determine the type of skull deformity. Exophthalmos, midfacial hypoplasia, and hypertelorism are also features of these two syndromes.

The facial organs and tissues proceed in great measure from the first and second branchial arches and the first branchial cleft. Disorders in their development lead to a spectrum of anomalies of variable severity. **Treacher-Collins syndrome** (mandibulofacial dysostosis) is a severe disorder characterized by hypoplasia of the malar bones and lower eyelids, colobomas, and antimongoloid slant of the palpebrae. The mandible and ears are often quite underdeveloped. The presentation

is bilateral and is an autosomal dominant trait. A unilateral deformity known as **hemifacial microsomia** presents with progressive skeletal and soft tissue underdevelopment. The Goldenhar variant of hemifacial microsomia is a severe form associated with upper bulbar dermoids, notching of the upper eyelids, and vertebral anomalies.

Some of these patients show mental retardation, but in most cases intelligence is not affected. The psychosocial problems are serious and most often related to how the patients look. Within the past 2 decades, craniofacial surgery has progressed so that previously untreatable deformities can now be corrected. With the anatomic work of Le Fort as a basis—and guided by the incomplete attempts of Gillies and others—Paul Tessier, in the late 1960s, proposed a set of surgical techniques to correct major craniofacial deformities. Two basic concepts soon emerged from his work: (1) Large segments of the craniofacial skeleton can be completely denuded of their blood supply, repositioned, and yet survive and heal; and (2) the eyes can be translocated horizontally or vertically over a considerable distance with no adverse effect on vision. The tendency today is to operate at approximately 6–9 months of age (not later than 9 months) for cranial vault remodeling and fronto-orbital advancement.

A bicoronal scalp incision is utilized to expose the skull and facial bones with an intra- or extracranial approach. The cut bones are then reshaped, repositioned, and fixed with a combination of wires or miniplates and screws. The latter have the advantage of rigid fixation and less need to maintain large movements with bone grafts. Autogenous inlay and onlay bone grafts can be used to improve contour. The entire operation is usually completed in one stage, and complications are surprisingly few. Miniplates have been used extensively in the last few years. In infants, fixation with absorbable suture material such as Maxon can replace the usual steel wires and avoid any radiologic tracks.

Craniofacial surgery has improved the treatment not only of major congenital deformities but also of major complex facial fractures, chronic sequelae of trauma, isolated exophthalmos, fibrous dysplasia, and aesthetic facial sculpturing.

MICROTIA

Microtia is absence or hypoplasia of the pinna of the ear, with a blind or absent external auditory meatus.

The incidence of significant auricular deformity is about one in 8000 births and is usually spontaneous. Ten percent of these defects are bilateral, and boys are afflicted twice or three times as commonly as girls. Because the ear arises from the first and second branchial arches, the middle ear is always involved, and many patients have other disorders of the first and second arches. The inner ear structures are usually spared.

Generally, correction of conductive hearing by an otologist has not been long-lasting or helpful, and surgery for this problem is reserved for bilateral cases.

Reconstruction of the external ear usually involves a multistage procedure beginning at preschool age. Autogenous rib cartilage or cartilage from the opposite ear is used to construct a framework to replace the absent ear. The cartilage is imbedded under the skin in the appropriate area, and after adjustments are made in local tissue to reposition or recreate the earlobe and conchal cavity, the framework is elevated posteriorly and the resulting sulcus grafted to obtain projection. In cases where local tissue is poor or unavailable, the neighboring superficial temporalis fascia is dissected and placed over the cartilage framework. This is then skin-grafted with adequate tissue. The opposite (normal) ear is occasionally altered to provide better symmetry. Excellent results have been achieved. Silastic frameworks for ear cartilage have also been used, and although their use eliminates donor site problems, rates of infection and extrusion have been unacceptable.

Lesser deformities, such as overly large, prominent, or bent ears, are corrected by appropriate resection of skin and cartilage, "scoring" of the cartilage to alter its curve, and placement sutures to aid in contouring.

Cohen SR: Craniofacial distraction with a modular internal distraction system: evolution of design and surgical techniques. Plast Reconstr Surg 1999;103:1592.

McCarthy JG: The timing of surgical intervention in craniofacial anomalies. Clin Plast Surg 1990;17:161.

Nocini PF et al: Vertical distraction of a free vascularized fibula flap in a reconstructed hemimandible: case report. J Craniomaxillofac Surg 2000;28:20.

ANOMALIES OF THE HANDS & EXTREMITIES

The most common hand anomaly is syndactyly, or webbing of the digits. This may be simple, involving only soft tissue, or complex, involving fusion of bone and soft tissue. The fusion may be partial or complete. Surgical correction involves separation and repair with local flaps and skin grafts. Correction should be done before growth disturbance of the webbed digits takes place. Other anomalies such as extra digits (polydactyly), absence of digits (adactyly), and cleft hand also exist.

Flexion contractures of the hands or digits may require surgical release and appropriate skin grafting. Congenital ring constriction of the extremities may be associated also with congenital amputation. The ring constrictions are best treated by excision and Z-plasty.

Poland's syndrome consists of a variable degree of unilateral chest deformity—usually absence of the pectoralis major muscle—associated with hand symbrachydactyly. The hand deformity is treated according to the severity. The latissimus dorsi muscles can be transposed to replace the absent pectoralis major, simulating the sites of origin and insertion. In more severe cases and in women requiring breast and chest reconstruction, the transverse rectus abdominis island flap can be used to replace the deficit.

POSTABLATIVE RECONSTRUCTION

HEAD & NECK RECONSTRUCTION

Many of the tumors discussed in Chapter 15 require surgical excision as a primary form of therapy. This often involves removal of large areas of composite tissue, such as the floor of the mouth, the maxilla, part of the mandible, or the lymph-bearing tissue of the neck. Reconstruction after such resections can be very challenging and may require special skill.

A salient advance in the complete treatment of the patient with a head or neck tumor is reconstruction, usually done in the same setting. Free flaps with microvascular techniques are the most appropriate methods even though they require a high level of skill and are time-consuming. The free flaps most commonly used following ablative procedures in the head and neck include the radial forearm flap for resurfacing the floor of the mouth; and the composite fibular flap, which includes fibula as well as skin to reconstruct the mandible and the floor of the mouth. For larger defects, judicious use of the rectus abdominis muscle, latissimus dorsi, or other musculocutaneous flaps have also been helpful. For pharyngoesophageal reconstruction, either the tubed radial forearm flap or the free jejunum is most successful.

Since no two surgical resections for tumor in the head and neck are identical, the key to effective treatment is preoperative planning. Probable extent of resection, areas that will require pre- or postoperative radiation therapy, incision and flaps created by neck dissections, and available donor areas must all be carefully assessed. Tissue attached to an adequate blood supply must be used to ensure early and watertight healing in the mouth and oropharynx, in areas of radiation injury, and over metal or other alloplastic implants.

Useful musculocutaneous flaps in the head and neck are the sternocleidomastoid, platysma, trapezius, pectoralis major, and latissimus dorsi muscles. Useful axial skin flaps can be obtained from the forehead, deltopectoral, and cervicohumeral areas. When these flaps are insufficient or unavailable for the reconstructive needs of the patient, free tissue transfer must be used. Many flaps with acceptable donor sites exist. The deep circumflex iliac vessels provide an osteocutaneous flap quite useful in mandible reconstruction. The forearm and scapular areas are also good sites for composite free flaps. Healing is quick, so that radiation, if necessary, may be started as early as one month after surgery.

Pearl RM et al: An approach to mandibular reconstruction. Ann Plast Surg 1988;21:401.

Santamaria E et al: Sensation recovery on innervated radial forearm flap for hemiglossectomy reconstruction by using different recipient nerves. Plast Reconstr Surg 1999;103:450.

Yamamoto Y et al: Superiority of end-to-side anastomosis with the internal jugular vein: the experience of 80 cases in head and neck microsurgical reconstruction. Br J Plastic Surg 1999; 52:88.

BREAST RECONSTRUCTION

Reconstruction of the female breast after mastectomy is becoming common in the USA as new techniques have become available and more women have become aware of this option. Most insurance carriers now pay for this procedure as part of the treatment for breast cancer. Even women with significant defects in the anterior chest wall as a result of radical mastectomy and radiation therapy can undergo reconstructive surgery if they are otherwise appropriate candidates.

As the modalities for surgical treatment of breast cancer have changed, so has the reconstructive aspect. The modified radical mastectomy, which preserves the pectoralis major and minor muscles appears, to be the standard as far as local recurrence is concerned. Lumpectomy followed by irradiation, initially tried for relatively small tumors, has now expanded to larger tumors and may thus result in considerable distortion and concavity in the treated breast. These defects also, at times, require reconstruction. Most recently, there is an increasing use of the skin-sparing mastectomy.

Through a keyhole access made by removal of the nipple and areola, the oncologic surgeon removes the entire breast tissue with the cancerous mass, in some cases followed by sentinel node biopsy or axillary sampling through a separate axillary incision. By saving most of the breast skin, reconstruction of the breast mound is facilitated and superior aesthetic results are obtained.

The methods of reconstruction include the use of saline implants or expanders and flaps for coverage such as a latissimus dorsi flap or the transverse rectus abdominis musculocutaneous (TRAM) flap for autologous reconstruction.

Following mastectomy, simple placement of an implant is usually unsatisfactory except in a few thin patients with relatively small contralateral breasts. The implant is usually placed in the submuscular position,

utilizing the remaining pectoralis major muscle and occasionally the serratus anterior muscle for adequate muscle coverage. This results in a hard, rounded type of reconstruction and does not simulate the soft "teardrop" appearance of the normal breast. Even when adequate skin has been saved following a skin-sparing mastectomy, placement of an implant is unsatisfactory because of the high rate of complications due to skin necrosis of the saved overlying skin, which results in exposure of the implant. When doing an immediate reconstruction with implant following a skin-sparing mastectomy, it is preferable to transpose the latissimus dorsi muscle to provide another layer of cover for the implant so that if there is necrosis of the skin from the skin-sparing mastectomy, the implant will not be exposed.

The use of skin expanders is also a popular method of breast reconstruction. A partially filled silicone envelope with a separate valve is inserted under the chest skin and muscle, and at intervals over a period of 6 weeks to 3 months the bag is progressively inflated with saline percutaneously. The expander is inflated at least 25% more than the desired volume. A period of time—approximately 3 months—is advisable as a waiting period to prevent the "recall phenomenon," which is the shrinking that may occur following removal of the expander as it is replaced by a permanent implant. The disadvantages of this method include the rare occurrence of the hemispheric expansion of the skin, which may result in a hard, rounded breast mound; the necessity for a second operation; and problems with infection, deflation, exposure of the prosthesis, and occasional skin necrosis when expansion is too rapid.

The latissimus dorsi myocutaneous flap is used most often for reconstruction of the breast with an implant. The myocutaneous unit is outlined with a skin island transversely so that the scar will be transverse and covered by the brassiere. The unit is freed up completely except for its insertion at the humerus, thus preserving the neurovascular pedicle. It is transposed as a pendulum through the anterior chest wall. The superior portion of the latissimus dorsi is sutured to the pectoralis major muscle and the lower edge is secured to the lower skin flap as far down as it will reach. The implant is then inserted, having been covered by the latissimus dorsi inferiorly and by two layers of muscle superiorly—the latissimus dorsi and the pectoralis major. The skin island is utilized in its entirety, if necessary, or is deepithelialized appropriately, maintaining only the skin portion that is needed. This method is most suitable for patients who do not have a large amount of abdominal skin, are relatively thin, and do not object to the use of implants, which sometimes may even be inserted in the opposite breast in an effort to achieve symmetry.

The transverse rectus abdominal flap based on the superior epigastric vessel has been successfully used to provide adequate tissue so that an implant is not required in reconstructing the breast. This is the most versatile method of reconstruction in that one can obtain as much tissue as necessary to match the opposite breast and to contour it and position it to simulate the shape as well as the size of the opposite breast. The incision at the donor site is similar to that of an abdominoplasty operation along the lower abdomen. This method of reconstruction produces the most normal and natural breast in appearance and feel, but it requires a longer operating time as well as a longer period of hospitalization.

In some patients, the opposite (noncancerous breast) may be altered to better match the reconstructed breast. A breast that is hypertrophic may be reduced, and a ptotic breast may be elevated.

The nipple-areola complex can also be reconstructed, and since reconstructions are more natural at this time, the great majority of patients accept this second stage in the reconstructive process. It is advisable that the cancerous breast be reconstructed at the initial operation and that the opposite breast be altered (if necessary) so that the second operation will consist of reconstruction of the nipple-areola complex along with whatever touch-ups are needed to achieve symmetry. In this manner, symmetric positioning of the nipple and areola can be achieved. The current technique for nipple reconstruction utilizes adjacent flaps from the area where the nipple is to be positioned, taking variable amounts of underlying fat if a TRAM flap has been used or hugging skin and lesser amounts of subcutaneous tissue if the latissimus dorsi flap was used. For the areola, it is preferable to tattoo it, thus avoiding the need for skin grafts, which in the past were taken from the groin. Occasionally, both the newly created as well as the contralateral normal areola need to be tattooed to be made similar in appearance.

Prophylactic total mastectomies are performed in some patients. Indications for the procedure include high risks of cancer in the opposite breast, eg, a strong family history of breast cancer—particularly a mother and sister with premenopausal bilateral breast cancer. Screening for the breast cancer gene (BRCA1) is available, but the test is expensive and there are no long-term studies verifying its clinical utility.

It should be stressed that prophylactic mastectomy and reconstruction should not be made available as a cosmetic procedure. Scarring and contour defects in sensitive areas may result, and the implant problems may be significant.

Bostwick J III: Breast reconstruction after mastectomy. Semin Surg Oncol 1988;4:274.

Hartrampf CR Jr: The transverse abdominal island flap for breast reconstruction: a 7-year experience. Clin Plast Surg 1988; 15:703.

Lejour M, Jabri M, Deraemaecker R: Analysis of long-term results of 326 breast reconstructions. Clin Plast Surg 1988;15:689.

Nieminen T et al: Free microvascular tram flaps: report of 185 breast reconstructions. Scand J Plast Reconstr Surg Hand Surg 1999;33:295.

LOWER EXTREMITY RECONSTRUCTION

Probably one of the most difficult areas for which to provide wound coverage and closure is the lower extremity, particularly the distal leg and foot areas. Tenuous and unstable skin grafts or poorly vascularized local or cross-leg skin flaps were once the only tissues available for resurfacing of these parts of the body. When large segments of bone were exposed or missing or when infection had become established, these grafts or flaps often were inadequate and amputation was the only recourse. Use of musculocutaneous flaps and particularly free flaps has greatly improved coverage in the lower extremities.

Generally, wound problems in the lower leg, ankle, and foot involve orthopedic injuries, such as compound ankle or distal tibial fractures. Incisions and metal screws and plates associated with open reduction and fixation of fractures may lead to increased scarring and make coverage more difficult. Other injuries requiring reconstruction are avulsion loss of the skin of the leg, heel, or sole of the foot and ischemic or venous stasis skin loss.

Treatment depends on the extent of tissue loss and the depth of the wound. Fairly extensive wounds around the knee and upper third of the leg can be covered with a (usually medial) gastrocnemius muscle flap and a split-thickness skin graft. The middle third of the leg can be covered in a similar manner by the soleus muscle in many cases. Large middle third and distal third defects are more difficult to reconstruct. Although there are small muscles that end in tendons in the foot, such as the peroneus brevis, flexor hallucis longus, and extensor digitorum muscles, they can provide only limited coverage. If there is a suitable recipient artery remaining in the leg, better coverage is generally provided by a free muscle flap such as the gracilis muscle for small and medium-sized defects or the latissimus dorsi or rectus abdominis muscle for larger defects.

Large areas of the heel or the sole of the foot are difficult to replace because skin in these regions is specially constructed to bear the weight of the body without shearing or breaking down. Free muscle flaps surfaced with skin grafts can be used, but protective sensation is missing. The use of free neurovascular axial skin flaps, such as the inferior gluteal thigh flap and the deltoid flap, may help provide coverage with some sensation. Neurosensory flaps—and specifically the sural flap, distally based on one of the lower septocutaneous perforators from the lateral aspect of the leg and supplied by the sural artery, which accompanies the sural nerve—have been used to resurface defects around the ankle and heel. The procedure provides good skin and fascia for a weight-bearing area such as the heel, but it usually does not provide protective sensibility.

Small segments of missing tibia can be replaced by soft tissue coverage followed by bone grafting. Free microvascular fibula or iliac crest transplants have been used to replace larger segments of missing bone.

Osteomyelitis of the tibia or bones in the foot may be devastating and often uncontrollable. Probably because of poor vascularity in the area, even long-term antibiotic treatment has often failed to control bone infections in the leg. Recently, effective surgical treatment for bone infections has been developed. The bone is surgically debrided and covered with a microvascular free muscle flap such as the gracilis or rectus abdominis muscle. Apparently, the muscle tissue with its excellent blood supply not only covers the exposed bone but assists natural defenses in controlling infection. Antibiotics are also used, but the well-vascularized muscle flap appears to be the deciding factor in control of infection. Bone grafts can be added later if needed. For tibial fractures where there is segmental bone loss injury to the soft tissue, a combination of the bone transport system of Ilizaroff and coverage with a free microvascular muscle flap has been most effective in replacing bone segments up to 6 cm in length. The bone transport method of Ilizaroff consists of performing a cortical osteotomy proximal to the site of injury and then applying a distraction apparatus, which in effect lengthens the bone 1 mm per day by appropriate adjustment screws.

Cronewett JL et al: Limb salvage despite extensive tissue loss: free tissue transfer combined with distal revascularization. Arch Surg 1989;124:609.

Erdmann MW, Court-Brown CM, Quaba AA: A five-year review of islanded distally based fasciocutaneous flaps on the lower limb. Br J Plastic Surg 1997;50:421.

Kuran I et al: Gulgonen A: Comparison between sensitive and non-sensitive free flaps in reconstruction of the heel and plantar area. Plast Reconstr Surg 2000;105:574.

Park S, Han SH, Lee TJ: Algorithm for recipient vessel selection in free tissue transfer to the lower extremity. Plast Reconstr Surg 1999;103:1937.

PRESSURE SORES

Pressure sores—often less precisely called bedsores or decubitus ulcers—are another example of difficult wound problems that can be treated by plastic surgery.

Pressure sores generally occur in patients who are bedridden and unable or unwilling to change position; patients who cannot change position because of a cast or appliance; and patients who have no sensation in an area that is not moved even though they may be ambulatory. The underlying cause of sores in these patients is ischemic necrosis resulting from prolonged pressure against the soft tissue overlying bone. There is also some evidence that local factors in denervated skin predispose to pressure breakdown because there is atrophy of the skin and subcutaneous tissue.

Absence of normal protective reflexes must be compensated for. Prevention is clearly the best treatment for pressure sores. Casts and appliances must be well padded, and points of pressure or pain should be relieved. Bedridden patients must be turned to a new position at least every two hours. Water and air mattresses, sheepskin pads, and foam cushions may help relieve pressure but are not substitutes for frequent turning. The introduction of the flotation bed system, which distributes pressure uniformly over a large surface area, has greatly aided in the management of these patients. The pressure on the skin at any time is less than the capillary filling pressure, avoiding many ischemic problems. Paraplegics should not sit in one position for more than two hours. Careful daily examination should be made for erythema, the earliest sign of ischemic injury. Erythematous areas should be freed from all pressure. The use of electrical stimulations, biomaterials, and growth factors are additional modalities to expedite wound repair, but the results are variable.

Once pressure necrosis is established, it is important to determine whether underlying tissues such as fat and muscle are affected, since they are much more likely than skin to become necrotic. A small skin ulcer may be the manifestation of a much larger area of destruction below. If the area is not too extensive and if infection and abscess due to external or hematogenous bacteria are not present, necrotic tissue may be replaced by scar tissue. Continued pressure will not only prevent scar tissue from forming but will also extend the injury. A surface eschar or skin may cover a significant abscess.

If the pressure sore is small and noninfected, application of drying agents to the wound and removal of all pressure to the area may permit slow healing. Wounds extending down to bone rarely heal without surgery. Infected wounds must be debrided down to clean tissue. The objectives at operation are to debride devitalized tissue, including bone, and to provide healthy, well-vascularized padded tissue as a covering. All of the original tissue that formed the bed of the ulcer must be excised.

When the patient's nutritional status and general condition of health are optimal, definitive coverage can be performed. Coverage is usually accomplished with a muscle, musculocutaneous, or, sometimes, an axial flap. Well-vascularized muscle appears to help control established low-grade bacterial contamination. The muscle flaps used for the more common bedsores are as follows: greater trochanter—tensor fasciae latae; ischium—gracilis, gluteus maximus, or hamstrings; sacrum—gluteus maximus. Occasionally, it is possible to provide sensibility to the area of a pressure sore with an innervated flap from above the level of paraplegia. The most common example is the tensor fasciae latae flap with the contained lateral femoral cutaneous nerve from L4 and L5, which is used to cover an ischial sore. Rarely, an innervated intercostal flap from the abdominal wall may be used to cover an insensible sacrum. Unfortunately attempts to provide protective sensibility with sensory flaps have not had good results. The tissue expansion techniques should not be the primary surgery treatment of decubitus ulcers but can be used in difficult cases where available tissue is insufficient to close the wound.

Postoperatively, the donor and recipient areas must be kept free of pressure for 2–3 weeks to allow for complete healing. This puts significant demands on other areas of the body that may be equally at risk or may already have areas of breakdown. The use of the air-fluidized bed has greatly aided such situations.

In spite of excellent padding provided by musculocutaneous flaps, recurrence of pressure sores is still a major problem, because the situation that caused the original breakdown usually still exists. Prevention of sores is even more important for these patients.

Bruck JC et al: More arguments in favor of myocutaneous flaps for the treatment of pelvic pressure sores. Ann Plast Surg 1991; 25:85.

Goodman CM et al: Evaluation of results and treatment variables for pressure ulcers in 48 veteran spinal cord-injured patients. Ann Plast Surg 1999;42:665.

AESTHETIC SURGERY

Aesthetic surgery is an integral part of plastic surgery. In fact, the two terms have become almost synonymous even though aesthetic surgery is only one band in a broad spectrum. Increased interest and curiosity about the specialty results in part from increased demands for its services by an aging population but also from the development of more predictable, lasting, and safer techniques. A number of specialists other than plastic surgeons have also performed and contributed to cosmetic surgery. A skilled surgeon can perform such cosmetic operations safely and with maximum benefit to the patient.

Patient selection is probably as important as any other factor. Not all patients are good candidates for aesthetic procedures, and such operations are contraindicated in others. Age or poor general health of the patient may be a reason for delay or avoidance of purely elective procedures. Two other major factors must be considered. The first factor is the anatomic feasibility of the procedure. Can the alterations be made successfully and safely? Which technique will best accomplish the goal? The second factor is the psychologic makeup of the patient. Does the patient fully understand the nature of the proposed procedure and its risks and consequences? Are the patient's expectations realistic? Cosmetic changes in appearance will generally not save a failing marriage, help to procure a new job, or substantially improve a person's station in life, and persons with such expectations should not undergo aesthetic surgery. Surgery should be postponed for persons experiencing severe stress, such as is associated with divorce, death of a loved one, or other periods of emotional instability.

The ideal candidate for cosmetic surgery is an adult or mature younger person who has a realistic idea of what is to be accomplished, is not under pressure from others to have the operation done, and does not expect major changes in interpersonal relations or career potential following surgery. Personal satisfaction is a valid reason for seeking aesthetic refinements.

The more common aesthetic procedures are discussed below. Some procedures involve correction of functional problems as well and are therefore not always considered purely cosmetic procedures.

RHINOPLASTY

Surgical alterations of nasal structures are done for relief of airway obstruction (usually secondary to trauma) and to reshape the nose because of undesirable characteristics, such as a prominent dorsal hump, bulbous or drooping tip, or overly large size. There is often a combination of problems.

Procedures are generally performed through intranasal incisions. The nasal skin is usually temporarily freed from its underlying bony and cartilaginous framework, so that the framework can be altered by removal, rearrangement, or augmentation of bone or cartilage. The skin is then redraped over the new foundation. The nasal septum and lower turbinate can also be altered to reestablish an open airway. A better understanding of nasal physiology has enabled surgeons to correct internal valve dysfunction by inserting spreader grafts—often following modification of the bony radix of the nose. Spreader grafts are small pieces of cartilage placed next to the septum and under the upper lateral cartilages. They serve to open up the internal valve in somewhat the same was as the external "breathe easy" appliances utilized by athletes.

Surgery can be done under local or general anesthesia; in either case, topical and injectable vasoconstrictors and anesthetic agents are commonly used. Hospitalization may or may not be indicated. Nasal packing is often used for hemostasis and support of the nasal mucosa during initial healing, as incisions are usually only minimally sutured with absorbable sutures. External nasal splints are placed to control swelling and provide some protection, particularly if osteotomy of the nasal bones is performed.

Convalescence requires 10–14 days before most swelling and periorbital ecchymosis subside; however, several months are often required before completely normal sensation returns, and all swelling resolves.

Nasal procedures are very commonly performed, generally quite safe, and usually effective. Complications include bleeding, internal scarring, recurrence of airways obstruction, and irregularities of contour. Infections are rare except with the use of alloplastic nasal implants.

RHYTIDECTOMY (Facelift)

The combined effects of gravity, sun exposure, and loss of elasticity due to aging result in varying degrees of wrinkles and sagging of skin along the cheeks, jawline, neck, and elsewhere in the facial area. These natural signs of aging can be removed to a great extent by a facelift procedure. Not all wrinkles can be removed, however; those in the forehead, around the eyes, in the nasolabial area, and around the lips are not significantly corrected without additional procedures.

Rhytidectomy is a major procedure requiring extensive incisions hidden in the scalp and in front of and behind the ears and occasionally in the submental region. The first such operations consisted of freeing up the skin and then stretching it and resuturing as it was drawn cephalad and laterally. This gave a mask-like and unnatural appearance. In the last few years, there has been a significant change in the concept of the facelift procedure, so that now it consists of elevation of the soft tissues—particularly the jowls and malar fat pads— to where they were at a younger age, giving more prominence to the cheek bones and better delineating the jawline. Undermining of the skin is done only to approach the soft tissues to be elevated, and the excess skin is now removed and reapproximated without tension. This approach to the mid face has given more natural and lasting results and provides also a three-dimensional type of restoration of the soft tissues, giving a more youthful appearance.

For the double neck, extensive freeing up of the skin over the neck from the jawline down to the hyoid is performed, and the fat overlying the platysmal muscle is removed either by suctioning or directly with scissors. The platysma itself is tightened laterally as well as centrally to provide an effect similar to a hammock that will give a more defined neck and jaw angle.

Drains are used particularly in the neck, as well as a padded circumferential dressing to protect the face and provide light pressure during healing. The introduction of fat aspiration procedures (liposuction) has been adapted to the neck but is not recommended for the face since it may produce abnormal lines ("railroad tracks of demarcation"). In appropriate patients, liposuction in the neck does give fine definition to the chin and jawline and may substantially correct the double chin appearance.

Either local or general anesthesia may be used for this often lengthy (3–4 hours) procedure. Local vasoconstrictors are routinely used.

Complications include hematoma, skin slough, injuries to branches of the facial nerve or greater auricular nerve, scars, and asymmetry. Signs of aging often recur years later.

Endoscopy

Endoscopy has become an integral part of plastic surgery, particularly for procedures involving the face or the breast. Smaller endoscopes are now utilized as well as different methods of achieving a desired optical field other than by distention of natural cavities with fluid or gases. In the face and in the breast, the optical cavity is usually obtained by tractioning the skin with appropriate elevators or sutures.

Endoscopy has been most effective for the forehead, where it has replaced the coronal incision which goes from ear to ear, peeling the scalp down to the supraorbital rims. By means of endoscopy, the forehead lift becomes a more physiologic operation in that one frees up the forehead skin at the subperiosteal level, dividing the periosteum at the supraorbital rim and then removing the depressors of the eyebrows (the procerus and corrugator muscles in the glabella region), thus allowing the frontalis muscle to act unopposed to elevate the eyebrows. The key to the procedure appears to be the division of the periosteum, which by itself frees up the eyebrows and elevates them for at least 5–10 mm. In addition, removal of the glabellar muscles seems to ameliorate in a lasting way the vertical wrinkles in the glabella region. For suspension of the elevated eyebrows, different methods have been advocated that include soft tissue to bony anchoring, the use of temporary screws in the skull as well as miniplates, or, most simply, by providing external traction tied in between staples with nylon sutures. It appears that it is only necessary to maintain that elevation for a short period of time (3–5 days) until the periosteum reattaches at the higher level.

Endoscopy has also been effectively utilized to do a midface lift, and this procedure is applicable to younger patients where there is no excess skin in the face or neck and where scars will be unattractive.

Endoscopy is also utilized for the breasts—particularly for insertion of breast implants in the submammary or subpectoral plane through an axillary incision. An endoscope attached to a right-angle retractor allows perfect visualization of the cavity where the implant is to be inserted, and it allows the development of a pocket inferiorly down to—and if necessary below—the submammary fold and also the division of the lower portion of the origin of the pectoralis major muscle from the sternum to permit insertion of a saline implant and to provide acceptable cleavage. Appropriate instruments for dissection as well as hemostasis have been developed for this procedure, which recently has gained in popularity.

BLEPHAROPLASTY

Blepharoplasty involves removal of redundant skin of the upper and lower eyelids and removal of periorbital fat protruding through sagging orbital septa. It is done alone or as part of a facelift procedure.

Incisions are made in the upper lids surrounding previously marked redundant skin, which is removed. A subciliary incision is generally used in the lower lids. The orbicularis oculi muscle may be altered if necessary. The periorbital fat compartments are opened, and protruding fat is removed. The extent of redundant skin in the lower lid is gauged, and the skin is resected. External sutures are used. Minimal or no dressing is required.

Local anesthesia in the form of lidocaine with epinephrine is usually adequate. Swelling and ecchymosis subside in 7–10 days, and sutures are removed in 3–4 days.

Complications include bleeding, hematoma formation, epidermal inclusion cysts, ectropion, and asymmetry. Patients are usually satisfied with the results. Recurrence is much less of a problem than with facelift procedures.

In recent years there have been changes in the concept of the blepharoplasty procedure. For the upper lids, the change consists of the recognition of senile ptosis due to either disruption or stretching of the levator mechanism. This can be corrected by imbrication of the levator mechanism with sutures.

The second concept is with respect to the orbicularis muscle, which is disrupted when doing the traditional blepharoplasty. In an effort to avoid any injury to the orbicularis muscle, subconjunctival removal of fat has been advocated and is particularly applicable to young patients with congenital fat hernias. The subconjunctival approach is also utilized in conjunction with the laser, which has the effect of tightening the skin of the lower lid and ameliorating the periorbital wrinkles.

However, the most important change in the concept of blepharoplasty is the recognition that due to gravity the skin of the lid, which is distinct from the cheek skin, has dropped down below the infraorbital rim. With the midface procedure, the skin of the lid is restored to its youthful position above infraorbital rim, thus necessitating on occasion the removal of skin only and tightening of the uninjured and undivided orbicularis muscle.

MAMMOPLASTY

Aside from procedures related to breast cancer, surgery of the female breast is generally done for one of the following reasons: to increase the size of the breasts (augmentation mammoplasty), or to lift the breasts (mastopexy). Augmentation, lifting of the breasts, and correction of asymmetry are nearly always done for cosmetic reasons. Reduction of hypertrophied breasts may, however, be done for functional reasons, since such breasts can cause poor posture, back and shoulder pain, and discomfort due to grooves from brassiere straps.

Augmentation Mammoplasty

In procedures for augmentation of the breasts, a silicone bag filled with saline solution, air, or a combination of saline and air is placed beneath the breast tissue in the submammary or subpectoral plane. Incisions are concealed in the periareolar margin, inframammary fold area, or axilla. Dissection is then carried out above or below the pectoralis major muscle, and the implant is placed in the pocket created. Drains are not generally used, and a padded dressing providing light pressure is applied. The subpectoral plane is preferred by most surgeons for augmentation mammoplasty because it does not interfere with mammography, but it does necessitate division of the lower portion of the origin of the pectoralis major muscle up to approximately 3 o'clock in relation to the nipple to provide adequate cleavage.

The procedure can be done on an outpatient basis with local anesthesia, although this may not be satisfactory when subpectoral implants are used. General anesthesia is often used for augmentation procedures.

Although patient satisfaction is excellent in most cases, a significant rate of capsular contracture remains a problem in about 10%. Scar tissue around the implant may contract in variable degrees even in the same patient. Control of this process is difficult even though the best possible environment for healing is provided (ie, appropriate implants are used, infection is controlled, bleeding is not present, debris is removed, and movement is restricted). Implants placed in the subpectoral position appear to be associated with a lesser degree of capsular contracture and less severe deformity if contracture occurs. Deflation of saline implants occurs at a rate of 1% per year.

Other complications include hematoma, infection, exposure of the implant, deflation or rupture of the implant, asymmetry of the breasts, and external scars. Breast function and sensation are usually not altered in any way.

Silicone gel was used as an implant material for 30 years. Although the matter has recently become controversial, there is no definitive scientific evidence that silicone gel is carcinogenic or that it produces collagen type diseases. In fact, there is now sufficient evidence to warrant it as a safe substance, but even so its use is at present limited to investigational status.

Mastopexy

Mastopexy is another common procedure used for correction of sagging or ptotic breasts. Although some breasts develop in a ptotic manner, most cases are caused by normal relaxation of aging tissues, gravity and atrophy after pregnancy and lactation. It is not clear whether use of a brassiere alters this process in any significant manner. The degree of deformity is defined by the relationship of the areola to the inframammary fold and the direction of the nipple. A ptotic breast will have a nipple which is below the inframammary line and pointing down towards the toes.

Correction may be done with simultaneous reduction or augmentation. An incision must be made around the areola, and the breast tissue itself is imbricated or, better still, an inferiorly based flap of breast tissue is designed and placed underneath the remnant superior part of the breast and over the pectoralis major muscle, serving as an autoaugmentation as one brings the lateral breast columns together. This procedure gives a more lasting effect than merely decreasing the skin envelop. Attempts at making more lasting corrections of ptosis of the breasts through the periareolar incision, which decreases the scarring, have included wrapping the breast with prosthetic material such as polyglycolic meshes or, more recently, by wrapping it around with segments of pectoralis major muscle.

Nonetheless, significant scarring may occur, particularly around the periareolar incision.

General anesthesia is usually necessary, and recovery from mastopexy may take 7–10 days. Complications include bleeding, infection, tissue loss, altered sensation or loss of function of the nipple and areolar areas, scars, and asymmetry of the breasts.

Patient satisfaction with the results is often not as great as with other procedures. Satisfaction often depends on how well the patient is prepared to accept the resulting scars.

Reduction Mammoplasty

Reduction mammoplasty is similar to mastopexy, since nearly all hypertrophic breasts are ptotic and must be lifted during correction. Enlargement can occur during puberty or later in life. Massive breasts can become a significant disability to the patient.

Although various techniques have been developed for breast reduction, nearly all require a pedicle to carry the nipple areola to its new position and a circumareolar incision as well as an inverted T incision beneath the areola. In gigantomastia, the nipple-areola is often removed as a free full-thickness graft and positioned appropriately. Most tissue is removed from the center and lower poles of the breast.

Vertical reduction mammoplasty has aroused considerable recent interest because of the decrease in amount of scarring. It can be accomplished through an incision made circumferentially around the areola and then a vertical incision that extends to and sometimes slightly below the inframammary fold. Resection of the breast tissue is done from below as well as from the lateral aspect of the breast. Considerable wrinkling of the skin occurs in an effort to avoid "T-ing off" the incision at the inframammary fold, but pleating of the skin usually resolves over a period of weeks. General anesthesia is nearly always required because dissection is considerable, but blood loss can be minimized by the use of epinephrine as a vasoconstricting agent. Transfusions are rarely indicated, and postoperative drains are often not used. The procedure is done on an outpatient basis.

General anesthesia is nearly always required, as dissection and blood loss can be significant. Transfusions may be indicated as well as operative drains and hospitalization for several days.

Although problems with nipple-areola loss, bleeding, infection, asymmetry of breasts, and scarring may occur; these women are generally among the most satisfied and appreciative of patients.

ABDOMINOPLASTY & OTHER AESTHETIC PROCEDURES

Other procedures usually classified as aesthetic are abdominoplasty and other operations for removal of excess tissue from the lower trunk, thighs, and upper arms. Patients with sagging tissue due to aging, pregnancies, multiple abdominal operations, or significant weight loss are usually good candidates for body contour procedures. Surgery can benefit the occasional patient with an isolated excessive deposit of fat below the lower abdominal skin, in the thighs (trochanteric lipodystrophy), or elsewhere. The typical case of generalized obesity, however, is not amenable to surgical correction of contour deformity.

Abdominoplasty usually involves removal of a large ellipse of skin and fat down to the wall of the lower abdomen. Dissection is carried out in the same plane up to the costal margin. The naval is circumscribed and left in place. After the upper abdominal flap is stretched to the suprapubic incision, excess skin and fat are excised. The fascia of the abdominal wall midline can be plicated and thus tightened. The umbilicus is exteriorized through an incision in the flap at the proper level, and the wound is closed over drains with a long incision generally in an oblique line or W shape just above the os pubis and out to the area below the anterior iliac crests (so-called bikini line).

Spinal anesthesia is used in some cases. Hospitalization may be required for a few days. Blood transfusions are sometimes necessary.

Complications involve blood or serum collections beneath the flap, infection, tissue loss, and wide scars. Results are generally very good, with excellent patient satisfaction in properly selected cases.

Various surgical procedures have been devised to remove excess skin and fat from the upper arms, buttocks, and thighs. Unfortunately, nearly all of these procedures result in significant scarring, and there may be difficulty in achieving a smooth transition between the end point of the contour alteration and normal tissue. The use of a suction apparatus fitted with appropriate cannulas to remove localized excess fat deposits has become widespread. It is clear, however, that patient selection and judicious use of liposuction are necessary to avoid complications, including hypovolemia due to blood loss, hematoma formation, skin sloughs, and waviness and depressions in the operative site. Used with discretion, liposuction can offer definition to areas of the abdomen, flanks, thighs, and buttocks.

SUCTION-ASSISTED LIPECTOMY

Suction-assisted lipectomy, or liposuction, has now become the most common cosmetic procedure performed in the United States. As presently practiced, it consists of infiltration of a solution of Ringer's lactate with the addition of 1 mg of epinephrine per 1000 mL of Ringer's and 250 mg of lidocaine—the former to provide vasoconstriction and the lidocaine to provide a certain amount of anesthesia and thus reduce the depth of general anesthesia. Some surgeons perform the entire operation under local anesthesia, necessitating the use of larger amounts of lidocaine.

Once the solution has been infiltrated sufficiently to produce tumescence, a small cannula is introduced through a small incision and suction is applied either with a syringe or with a suction machine. The fat that has been enlarged by the injection of tumescent solution dislodges easily and disrupts much faster than the blood vessels and the nerves.

Suction-assisted lipectomy is effective in removing abnormal bulges throughout the body, particularly in the trochanters or the abdomen and flanks, but it is not considered a weight reduction technique.

The procedure is safe when done by well-trained surgeons respecting sterility and in adequately equipped operating rooms. Safety in the use of up to 35 mg of lidocaine per kilogram has been established by clinical studies. Although fatalities have been reported with suction-assisted lipectomy—which is almost unacceptable in an entirely elective procedure—they are due to pulmonary embolization, perforation of the intestines, or severe infections of the abdominal wall. Fortunately, fatalities have markedly decreased since the American Society of Plastic and Reconstructive Surgeons established safety guidelines requiring that suctioning not exceed 5000 mL at a setting and that combined procedures should be cautiously undertaken.

Complications of suction-assisted lipectomy include irregularities of contour, dimpling, and, rarely, local infection at the entrance points.

Ultrasonic liposuction, external and internal, has also been advocated. External ultrasonic liposuction has the effect of a massage to disperse the infiltrated tumescent solution. Internal liposuction, on the other hand, dilutes the fat with ultrasonic energy, which produces heat, so that this diluted fat needs to be suctioned with standard suctioning equipment. The problems with ultrasonic liposuction include seroma formation, the need for larger portals of entrance, the possibility of burns of the skin if the cannula accidentally touches the skin, and, more importantly, problems with postoperative pain due perhaps to demyelinization of the sensory nerves as an effect of the ultrasonic energy.

Burk RW 3rd, Guzman-Stein G, Vasconez LO: Lidocaine and epinephrine levels in tumescent technique liposuction. Plast Reconstr Surg 1996 Jun; 97: 1379-84.

Cardoso de Castro C: The changing role of platysma in face lifting. Plast Reconstr Surg 2000;105:764.

Chajchir A: Fat injection: long-term follow-up. Aesthetic Plast Surg 1996;20:291.

Matarasso A, Hutchinson OH: Evaluating rejuvenation of the forehead and brow: an algorithm for selecting the appropriate technique. Plast Reconstr Surg 2000;106:687.

Pitanguy I: Facial cosmetic surgery: a 30-year perspective. Plast Reconstr Surg 2000;105:1517.

TELANGIECTASIAS
(Spider Veins)

When there is no trace of primary or secondary varicosities, most telangiectasias, or spider veins, are viewed as a cosmetic problem. However, one should be aware that in some cases spider veins may be an indication of deep venous valvular insufficiency. Factors that may play a role in the formation of spider veins include venostasis with decreased flow rate due to atony of the venous wall, chronic venous inflammation, hormonal influences, or venous compression at the saphenofemoral valve.

Treatment of spider veins is with sclerosing agents, which may include hypertonic saline, sodium tetradecyl, and hydroxypolyethoxydodecan (Sclerovein). These agents are injected directly into the spider veins with the objective of creating intimal damage that will result in fibrosis and obliteration of the lumen. The technique is simple and effective, but when the sclerosing agent extravasates it might produce superficial skin necroses.

Hand Surgery

David M. Young, MD, Mahesh Mankani, MD, John T. Alexander, MD,
Eugene S. Kilgore, MD, William P. Graham III, MD, & Robert E. Markison, MD

Both in industry and in the home, the hand is the most commonly injured part of the body. A disorder of the hand rarely jeopardizes life but often impairs vocational capacity.

Introduction

The prime functions of the hand are feeling (sensibility) and grasping. Sensibility is important on the radial sides of the index, long, and ring fingers and on the opposing ulnar side of the thumb, where one must feel and be able to pinch, pick up, and hold things. The ulnar side of the small finger and its metacarpal, upon which the hand usually rests, must register the sensations of contact and pain to avoid burns and other trauma.

Mobility is critical for grasping. The upper extremity is a cantilevered system extending from the shoulder to the fingertips. It must be adaptable to varying rates and kinds of movements. Stability of proximal joints is essential for good skeletal control distally.

The specialization of the thumb ray has endowed humans with superior aptitudes for defense, work, and dexterity. The thumb has exquisite sensibility and is a highly mobile structure of appropriate length, with a well-developed adductor and thenar (pronating) musculature. It is the most important digit of the hand, and every effort must be made to preserve its function.

The **position of function** of the upper extremity favors reaching the mouth and perineum as well as comfortable, forceful, and unfatiguing grip and pinch. The elbow is held at or near a right angle, the forearm neutral between pronation and supination, and the wrist extended 30 degrees with the fingers furled to almost meet the opposed (pronated) tip of the thumb (Figure 45–1A). This is the desired stance of the extremity if stiffness is likely to occur, and it should be maintained when joints are immobilized by splinting, arthrodesis, or tenodesis.

Opposite to the position of function is the **position of rest,** in which the flexed wrist extends the digits, making grip and pinch awkward, uncomfortable, weak, and fatiguing (Figure 45–1B). The forearm is usually pronated, and the elbow may be extended. This habitus is assumed, without intention, after injury, paralysis, and the onset of painful state; it is also called the **position of the injury.** Stiffening in this attitude jeopardizes function.

ANATOMY

All references to the forearm and hand should be made to the radial and ulnar sides (not lateral and medial) and to the volar (or palmar) and dorsal surfaces. The digits should be identified as the thumb, index finger, long finger, ring finger, and small finger or referred to as rays I, II, III, IV, and V.

Skin is the elastic outer sleeve and glove of the arm and hand. Sacrifice of its surface area or elasticity by debridement and fibrosis can severely curtail range of motion and constrict circulation. In the adult hand, the dorsal skin stretches about 4 cm in the longitudinal and in the transverse planes when the palm is flattened and spread. The long finger can easily have 48 cm^2 of skin cover, and the whole hand (exclusive of digits) is 210 cm^2.

Fascia anchors palmar skin to bone to make pinch and grip stable; the midlateral fibers of "Cleveland's and Grayson's ligaments" keep the skin sleeve from twisting about the digit (Figure 45–2). In the form of sheaths and pulleys, fascia holds tendons in the concavity of arched joints to convey mechanical efficiency and power. The fascial sleeve of the forearm, hand, and digits must sometimes be slit along with skin to prevent or relieve congestion (eg, compartment syndrome). Any fascial compartment of the hand provides a space for infection or an avenue for its dissemination.

Each finger has four joints (MC, MP, PIP, and DIP), any two of which may be fused and still leave adequate overall function. The thumb has only three joints (MC, MP, and IP), and every effort must be made to preserve at least two. The position of the wrist stretches and governs the efficiency of extrinsic muscle contraction. The wrist is the "key joint" of the hand, governing motion of the digits, and must be included in the immobilization process required for any major digital problem. The stability of the digital joints and their planes of motion are governed by the length of the ligaments and the anatomy of their articulating surfaces. The longitudinal and transverse arches of the hand (Figure 45–3) are architectural prerequisites to

Figure 45–1. Positions of function *(A)* and rest (injury) *(B)*.

Figure 45–3. Longitudinal *(top)* and transverse *(bottom)* arches.

gripping, pinching, and cupping and are maintained by the active contraction and passive tone of intact muscles. The arches create the position of function. When the arches are collapsed, the hand assumes the position of injury. Loss of these arches is most often initiated by edema. They may be preserved by splinting in the position of function, elevation without constriction, and early restoration of active and vigorous joint motion.

Each MP and PIP joint has a distally anchored volar trapdoor called the volar plate (Figure 45–4) in addition to collateral ligaments stabilizing the joint on either side (Figure 45–5).

Figure 45–4. Volar plate.

Figure 45–2. *A:* Cleland's ligament. *B:* Transverse retinacular ligament.

Figure 45–5. Collateral ligaments.

Figure 45–6. Carpal tunnel and no-man's-land.

The extrinsic flexor tendons are contained in fibrous **sheaths** to prevent bowstringing and preserve mechanical efficiency as the digits furl into the palm. Pulleys (hypertrophied sections of the sheath) resist the points of greatest tendency to bowstring. Sheaths are inelastic and relatively avascular. Therefore, they crowd and congest any swollen, inflamed, or injured tendons and curtail glide by friction, constriction, and the generation of inelastic adhesions. **"No-man's-land"** is the zone from the middle of the palm to just beyond the PIP joint, wherein the superficialis and profundus lie ensheathed together and where recovery of glide is so difficult after wounding (Figure 45–6).

Across the wrist, the dense volar carpal ligament closes the bony carpal canal (**carpal tunnel**) through which pass all eight finger flexors as well as the flexor pollicis longus and median nerve (Figure 45–6). The **ulnar bursa** is the continuation of the synovium around the long flexors of the small finger through the carpal tunnel, encompassing the other finger flexors which interrupted their separated bursa at the mid palm level. The **radial bursa** is the synovium around the flexor pollicis longus contained through the carpal tunnel. These two bursas may intercommunicate. **Parona's space** is the tissue plane over the pronator quadratus in the distal forearm deep to the radial and ulnar bursas.

The extensor tendons are ensheathed in six compartments at the wrist beneath the extensor retinaculum

(Figures 45–7 and 45–8), which predisposes to adhesions. Its role as a pulley is not vital and can be dispensed with.

The nerves of greatest importance to hand function are the musculocutaneous, radial, ulnar, and median nerves. The importance of the musculocutaneous and radial nerves combined is forearm supination and of the radial nerve alone is innervation of the extensor muscles. The ulnar nerve innervates 15 of the 20 intrinsic muscles. The median nerve, by its sensory innervation, is "the eye of the hand"; through its motor innervation, it maintains most of the long flexors, the pronators of the forearm, and the thenar muscles. Figure 45–9 shows the sensory distribution of the ulnar, radial, and median nerves.

CLINICAL EVALUATION OF HAND DISORDERS

The presenting complaint must be recorded explicitly and in complete detail with regard to its mechanisms of onset, evolution, aggravating factors, and relieving factors. Age, sex, hand dominance, occupation, preexisting

Figure 45–7. **A:** Extensor retinaculum over six tendon compartments. **B:** Juncturae tendinum (conexus intertendineus).

A: Middle extensor tendon
B: Intrinsics
C: Lateral extensor tendon
D: Terminal extensor tendon

Dorsal   **Lateral**

Figure 45–8. Extensor hood mechanism.

hand problems, and relevant matters pertaining to the patient's general health and emotional and socioeconomic status must be recorded also.

The examination should follow an orderly routine. Observe the neck, shoulders, and both upper extremities and the action and strength of all muscle groups, and be certain that all parts can pass painlessly and coordinately through a normal range of motion, starting with the head and neck and working down to the fingertips. Compare both upper extremities and keep detailed immediate notes, diagrams, and measurements of the case. Having the patient reach for the ceiling and simultaneously open and close both fists and then spread and adduct the fingers and, finally, oppose the thumbs sequentially to each fingertip will immediately demonstrate any abnormalities.

Observe habitus, wasting, hypertrophy, deformities, skin changes, skin temperature, scars, and signs of pain (including when the patient attempts to bear weight on the palms). Feel the wrist pulses and the sweat of the finger pads, and test reflexes and the sensibility of the median, ulnar, and radial nerves.

Serial x-rays and laboratory procedures may clarify a problem with an indolent evolution (eg, Kienböck's aseptic necrosis of the lunate, causing unexplained wrist pain). Contralateral and multiple-view x-rays in different planes (even CT scans) are often helpful. This is especially true in patients who have persistent perplexing bone and joint pain or limited motion or in patients who have not attained adult growth. In the case of wrist problems, arthrograms and arthroscopy may be of diagnostic value. MRI can also be quite helpful in the diagnosis of subtle carpal bone problems.

The diagnosis is often made by noting the response to therapy. This is particularly true in the case of local corticosteroids injected at the site of noninfectious inflammatory conditions (eg, carpal tunnel syndrome, trigger finger).

GENERAL OPERATIVE PRINCIPLES

A bloodless field (eg, by tourniquet ischemia) is essential for accurate evaluation, dissection, and management of tissues of the hand. This is achieved by elevat-

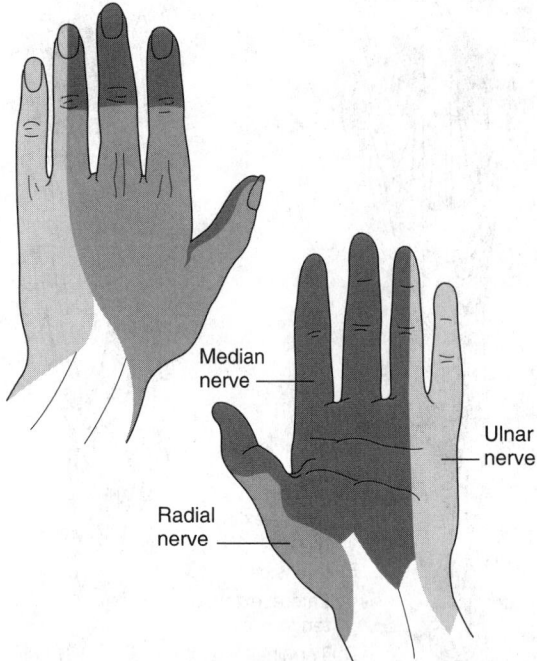

Figure 45–9. Sensory distribution in the hand. Dotted area, ulnar nerve; diagonal area, radial nerve; darker area, median nerve.

ing or exsanguinating the extremity and then inflating a padded blood pressure cuff around the arm to 100 mm Hg above systolic pressure. This is readily tolerated by the unanesthetized arm for 30 minutes and by the anesthetized arm for 2 hours.

Incisions (Figure 45–10) must be either zigzagged across lines of tension (eg, must never cross perpendicularly to a flexion crease) or run longitudinally in "neutral" zones (eg, connecting the lateral limits of the flexion and extension creases of the digits); and, whenever possible, must be designed so that a healthy skin-fat flap is raised over the zone of repair of a tendon, nerve, or artery.

Proper evaluation and treatment of a fresh injury often requires extension of the wound. Normal structures can then be recognized and traced into the zone of injury, where blood and trauma so often make their identification difficult or impossible.

Constriction and tension by dressings must be avoided at all costs. The dressing should be applied evenly to the skin without wrinkles. The wound should be covered with a single layer of fine-mesh gauze followed by a wet spongy medium (fluffs, Rest-On, Kling, or Kerlix). Wetness facilitates the drainage of blood into the dressing, which should be applied with gentle pressure to curtail dead space.

Splinting and immediate elevation are paramount in controlling swelling and pain and favoring healing. In general, plaster (fast-setting) or fiberglass is preferred because of its adaptability to specific requirements. More often than not, the wrist requires immobilization along with any other part of the hand (Figures 45–11 and 45–12).

Figure 45–10. Proper placement of skin incisions.

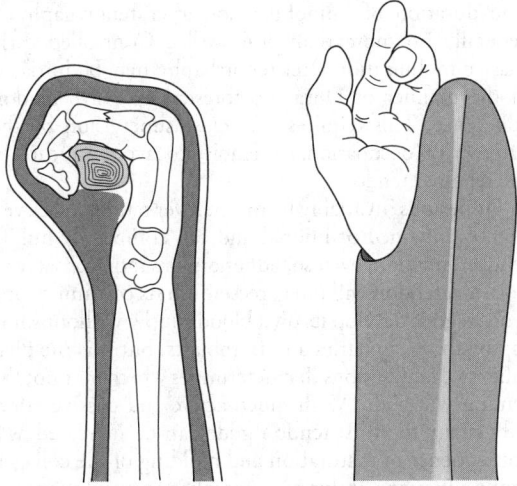

Figure 45–11. Casting.

It must be appreciated that effective immobilization of a finger most often requires concomitant immobilization of one or more adjacent fingers, usually in the position of function. Straight splints such as tongue blades involve a hazard of digital stiffness and distortion and should not be used across the MP joint.

Persistence of pain signifies inadequate immobilization and, if throbbing is present, congestion. Congestion must be promptly relieved by elevation and sectioning of the cast and dressing and, if necessary, the skin and fascia.

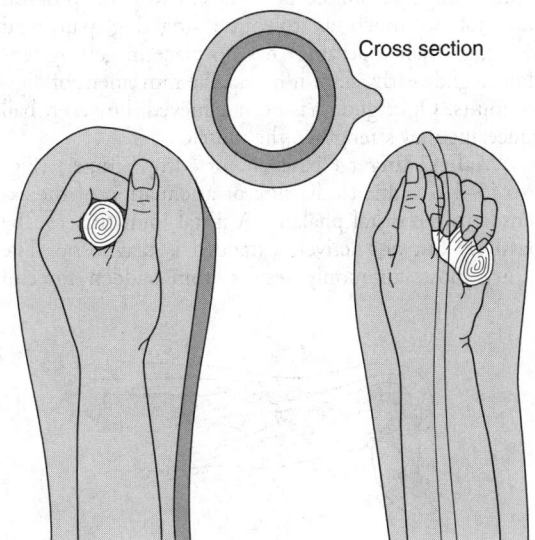

Cross section

Figure 45–12. Casting.

CONGENITAL ANOMALIES OF THE HAND

Major congenital hand anomalies are not rare, with approximately one in 700 live births affected. When minor deformities are included, approximately 3% of all births are affected. Camptodactyly ("bent"), polydactyly ("many"), and syndactyly ("together") are the most common malformations. Newborns with hand anomalies should be carefully examined for other malformations because multisystem syndromes can be present in 5% (eg, VACTERL syndrome with radial head dysphasia).

Anomalies may be inherited, caused by environmental factors affecting the womb (drugs, viral infections, irradiation, alcohol), or may be of unknown cause. Major genetic or major environmental causes are infrequently found, suggesting that the cause of most defects is multifactorial.

In order to simplify an extremely complex clinical problem, the American Society for Surgery of the Hand and all major international hand societies have adopted a single classification system that divides anomalies into six main categories: failures of formation (absent digits, phocomelia [seal limb]), failures of differentiation (syndactyly), duplication (polydactyly), undergrowth (brachydactyly), overgrowth (macrodactyly), and constriction ring syndrome (focal necrosis, intrauterine amputation). There is considerable overlap in the categories, as might be expected.

Ideally, surgery is performed early in the first two years of life, but timing is individually tailored to the problem.

McCarroll HR: Congenital anomalies: a 25-year overview. J Hand Surg [Am] 2000;25:1007.

Watson S: The principles of management of congenital anomalies of the upper limb. Arch Dis Child 2000;83:10.

TENDON DISORDERS OF THE HAND

Movement of the muscles of the hand and arm are transmitted into finger and wrist motion by the tendons. The tendons are strong, compact units that glide within their individual compartments. Disruption of the tendon by trauma or loss of tendon gliding by inflammation hinders tendon excursion and therefore limits active motion of the joints. Passive motion of the joint is still possible with an isolated tendon problem and distinguishes tendon disorders from joint disorders, when both active and passive motion are limited.

Tendon disruption can result from any penetrating injury and can be diagnosed by physical examination. A tendon injury should be suspected when the patient is unable to actively move a joint. Certain tendon lacerations, such as an isolated flexor digitorum superficialis disruption, may be masked because the profunda tendon can still move the entire finger. Blocking of profunda function by blocking flexion in the neighboring fingers (the profunda tendons are joined in the palm) reveals the injury to the superficialis when the injured PIP joint cannot be flexed.

The state of the wound and the complexity of the injury are the principal issues the hand surgeon must weigh in choosing between a primary or secondary tenorrhaphy. Tidy wounds generally favor primary tenorrhaphy. Primary tenorrhaphy is defined as one that is done within 24–72 hours after injury. When wounds are untidy, contaminated, or complicated by fracture or ischemia, formal tenorrhaphy may have to be delayed for weeks or months until the tendon bed is more favorable to healing and glide. However, interim tacking of the tendons—together, to tendon sheaths, or to bone—to maintain the fiber length of a muscle may be done as a preliminary procedure.

Preoperative treatment of fresh lacerations consists of wound closure, immobilization, and prophylactic antibiotics. Such cases can be deferred for definitive primary repair for 24 hours or more. The timing of delayed secondary procedures depends upon the resolution of wound edema and fibrous callus (ie, how soft and pliable it is). After 6–8 weeks, tendons that retract over 2.5 cm may defy full excursion because muscle elasticity has been lost or because the tendon is recoiled and congealed in scar.

Tenorrhaphy must be done without surface trauma along the tendon or its bed. The repair is made end-to-end or by weaving one tendon with the other, using nylon or wire sutures. A flexor tendon graft is anchored distally to bone (Figure 45–13). Tenodesis will occur if the surface of the tendon and the surface where adherence is desired are roughened. The position of immobilization should relieve tension on the tendon juncture.

The duration of immobilization after tenorrhaphy is generally no more than 3–4 weeks. Controlled early passive mobilization after tenorrhaphy may be initiated in the manner of Duran to forestall excessive tendon adherence. This requires very close supervision by the surgeon or occupational therapist to avoid rupture of the repaired tendon.

Adhesions invariably form wherever tendons are even slightly inflamed or injured and can completely nullify tendon function; even so, adhesions are indispensable to repair. A tendon will rarely reestablish its continuity or a tendon graft develop its own blood supply without some ingrowth of capillaries and fibroblasts, but it is the pliability of the adhesions that determines whether or not the tendon will glide. With much active and passive effort over many months, tendon glide can be increased as a consequence of maturation and molding of the collagen in the adhesions. If this does not take place and the adhesions remain thick and short, tendon excursion fails and tenolysis needs to be performed.

The access to tenolysis should be through a wound offering effective exposure and placed where the immediate active and passive joint motion that must follow will not jeopardize healing of the wound by undue stretching or direct pressure. The most common causes of failure are immobilization of the tendon for longer than 24 hours after lysis; failure of the musculotendinous unit; carrying out a concomitant procedure requiring immobilization (eg, neurorrhaphy); and separation of the tendon.

The patient must understand that musculotendinous and joint mobilization after tendon surgery is a time-consuming process, often taking many weeks or months. Exercise—eg, squeezing a sponge after flexor tendon surgery—should be sufficient to make progress but not so much as to cause lingering pain and swelling. "Ball squeezing" has no place in getting tendon to glide early, since it blocks the movement of digital joints. Once glide has been achieved, however, ball squeezing may strengthen the muscles.

"Mallet" finger ("baseball" or "drop" finger) (Figure 45–14) is due to division or attenuation of the extensor to the distal phalanx. A distal joint that can be passively but not actively extended is diagnostic. The injury most commonly results from sudden forceful

Figure 45–13. Flexor tenorrhaphy by advancement or graft. Pulleys are saved.

Figure 45–14. Mallet finger with swan-neck deformity.

flexion of the digit when it is held in rigid extension. Either the extensor is partially or completely ruptured or the dorsal lip of the bone is avulsed. Less frequently, the injury is due to direct trauma such as a laceration or a crush force. An x-ray should be taken to determine the presence and extent of any fracture.

Treatment may not be necessary if the loss of active extension is less than 15 degrees and any existing fracture is only a chip. More severe injury requires 6 weeks of continuous splinting in full distal joint extension (not hyperextension)) with or without 40 degrees of PIP joint flexion. Joint fixation internally with fine Kirschner wire or externally with padded aluminum, plastic, or even plaster splints is equally effective. A lacerated tendon should be delicately reapproximated. When a significantly displaced fracture fragment represents one-third or more of the surface of the joint, it should be reduced if necessary by wiring or pinning. In selected cases, smaller fracture fragments may be removed. If there is sufficient articulator disruption, one may consider joint fusion. Tendon grafting is difficult and easily leads to a poor cosmetic and functional result. It should be done only rarely.

Swan-neck deformity (Figure 45–14) is a frequent complication of mallet finger, but it may also be the result of disparity of pull between the extrinsic flexors and extensor hood with or without attenuation of the DIP joint extensor. It is seen in congenitally hypermobile joints, spastic and rheumatoid states, and following resection of the superficialis tendon. The dorsal hood acts to extend the distal joint but is held back by its insertion at the base of the middle phalanx, which it therefore hyperextends ("PIP joint recurvatum"). This in turn increases the tension on the profundus, which hyperflexes the DIP joint. If the mallet deformity is 25 degrees or less and there is some active distal joint extension, it may be treated by undermining and elevating the extensor hood at the PIP joint and severing its insertion on the base of the middle phalanx. Otherwise, the deformity may be corrected by tethering PIP joint extension with one slip of the flexor digitorum superficialis threaded through the flexor pulley of the proximal phalanx with the PIP joint flexed 20 degrees.

The **"buttonhole,"** or **"boutonnière," deformity** (Figure 45–15) appears as the opposite of the swan neck deformity: hyperextension of the DIP joint and flexion of the PIP joint. There is attenuation or separation of the dorsal hood, so that the middle extensor tendon becomes ineffective and the lateral extensor tendons shift volar to the PIP joint axis and the joint buckles dorsally. The entire extrinsic-intrinsic force on the hood passes onto the lateral extensor tendons, which flex the PIP joint and hyperextend the DIP joint. This deformity may develop suddenly or, more often, insidiously after closed blunt or open trauma over the dorsum of the PIP joint.

Figure 45–15. Buttonhole deformity.

To avoid this complication, sutured extensor tendon lacerations and severe contusions over the PIP joint should always have the PIP joint alone splintered in extension for 3–4 weeks. A small oblique Kirschner wire provides an alternative form of immobilization. Established deformities can be treated by such immobilization but more often require operative correction.

Tendon rupture, subluxation, and drift. The most frequent rupture of a healthy tendon is that of the distal joint extensor of one of the fingers as a result of sudden forceful flexion (see mallet finger, above), or avulsion of the profundus from the distal phalanx in violent flexion. Other tendons rupture where they have been weakened by division and suture, partial transection, crushing, or attritional fraying over roughened bone. The synovial thickening, degenerative tendon nodularity, and roughening of articular bone seen in the rheumatoid hand easily dispose to rupture by mechanical abrasion and circulatory depletion of tendons. Much can be done prophylactically in rheumatoid disease by synovectomy, sectioning of constricting tendon sheaths, and resection of bony spurs and tendon nodules. If correction of any form of tendon rupture is indicated, the methods of doing so include suture, tendon graft, tendon transfer, or tenodesis.

The most common subluxations and drifts of tendons are twofold: (1) volar drift of the intrinsic tendons as they pass the PIP joint of the fingers, causing the "buttonhole" deformity (see above); and (2) ulnar drift of the extrinsic middle extensors (central slips) as they pass the MP joints. The latter may result from trauma that divides or attenuates the lateral expansion (sagittal band) or the extensor hood on the radial side of the central slip. It more commonly results from attenuation of the entire extensor hood over the MP joint as a consequence of marked distension of the joint space and thickening of the synovium in rheumatoid arthritis. Treatment of ulnar drift involves repositioning of the extensor tendon to a point central to the MP joint and holding it by appropriate reefing of the sagittal band fibers of the hood on the radial side.

STENOSING TENOSYNOVITIS

In stenosing tenosynovitis there is a disproportion between the clearance inside a tendon pulley or tunnel and the diameter of the tendon or tendons that must glide through it. Any pulley or tunnel may be implicated. The more common sites are as follows:

(1) The proximal digital pulleys in the distal palm, causing **trigger finger** or thumb (stenosing flexor tenosynovitis). There is local tenderness of the pulley; pain, which may be referred to the PIP joint; and (usually but not always) locking of the digit in flexion with a painful jog as it goes into extension (ie, as the bulge in the tendon or tendons passes through the tight pulley).

(2) The pulley over the radial styloid housing the abductor pollicis longus and extensor pollicis brevis, causing **De Quervain's tenosynovitis.** Local tenderness and pain if these tendons are actively stretched (eg, Finkelstein's test).

Relief of the symptoms can be achieved by local injections of triamcinolone mixed with lidocaine and splinting the extremity. Immediate surgery is justified if the constriction is so tight that no tendon glide is possible. Surgical section of the constricting tendon sheath is also indicated if symptoms persist or recur. When releasing the flexor tendon, care is taken not to resect more than the section of sheath restricting the tendon or else the tendon will pull away from the finger like a bowstring and weaken the grip.

Anderson B, Kaye S: Treatment of flexor tenosynovitis of the hand ("trigger finger") with corticosteroids. Arch Intern Med 1991;151:153.

Coons MS, Green SM: Boutonnière deformity. Hand Clin 1995;11:387.

Crosby CA, Wehbe MA: Early motion after extensor tendon surgery. Hand Clin 1996;12:57.

Ingari JV, Pederson WC: Update on tendon repair. Clin Plast Surg 1997;24:161.

Taras JS, Lamb MJ: Treatment of flexor tendon injuries: surgeons' perspective. J Hand Ther 1999;12:141.

Turowski GA, Zdankiewicz PD, Thomson JG: The results of surgical treatment of trigger finger. J Hand Surg [Am] 1997; 22:145.

Wang AW, Gupta A: Early motion after flexor tendon surgery. Hand Clin 1996;12:43.

■ SKELETAL INJURIES OF THE HAND

Injuries to the bones and joints of the hand are the most common skeletal injuries treated by physicians. Recognition of the injury, appropriate diagnostic tests, and timely treatment are essential for minimizing the complications of these injuries. Some patients may neglect obvious fractures and dislocations in hope of spontaneous recovery. More subtle injuries to the wrist are more often neglected by the patient and sometimes even missed by physicians until further damage is done. The use of the portable minifluoroscope, found in many offices, greatly enhances the surgeon's ability to diagnose fractures. The machine allows real-time assessment of the bones as part of the physical examination. A common late sequela of skeletal injury at the articular surfaces is osteoarthritis, which is difficult to treat. Patients with symptoms related to the hand or wrist but without a discernible cause should be referred early to a hand specialist.

METACARPALS & PHALANGES

Fractures

Fractures of the metacarpal and phalangeal bones such as distal phalanx tuft of the fingers caught in closing doors and metacarpal shaft fractures of the ulnar side of the hand (boxer's fractures) create an obvious deformity and are easy to diagnose. Adequate x-rays of the specific site of the fracture with frontal, lateral, and oblique views are essential for developing a treatment plan. An order to the radiology technician for generic radiographs of the hand is often unhelpful.

Fractures of the shaft can usually be treated with closed reduction and a cast or splint holding the hand in the position of function (Figure 45–1) for 3–4 weeks. Residual angulation of a metacarpal shaft fracture of up to 30 degrees in the fifth finger and 20 degrees in the fourth finger is functionally well tolerated, although a dorsal bump may be aesthetically unpleasant. However, even a small rotational misalignment of the fracture at the metacarpal bone results in crossing of the fingers in flexion and causes severe dysfunction.

When fractures do not remain reduced, fixation with Kirschner pins placed through the skin are required. Placement of more than one pin is usually needed to keep the fracture reduced. The pins are removed after the fracture is healed. Displaced and comminuted fractures may require opening of the fracture site and reduction under direct visualization. Pins and, more recently, very small and thin metal plates and screws are used to maintain reduction. Metal plates provide strong support to the fracture site and allow earlier mobilization of the hand. However, plates are more difficult to place in small bones and occasionally interfere with tendon function.

Fractures through an articular surface need to be carefully evaluated. Nondisplaced fractures can be treated by casting. Displaced fractures require open reduction and accurate pin or lag screw fixation since discrepancies of the articular surface will eventually result in degenerative arthritis.

Fractures of the distal phalanx from crush injuries require attention to the disrupted nail bed. The nail is removed to decompress the painful subungual hematoma, irrigation of the open fracture, and careful reapproximation of the nail matrix. Large disruptions in the nail matrix may result in deformity of the regenerating nail. The nail is replaced under the nail fold as a splint. A protective splint is placed over the finger to hold the distal fragment in extension.

An intra-articular fracture of the base of the thumb metacarpal bone with subluxation (displacement) of the metacarpal leaving a volar pyramidal shaped fragment attached to the trapezium is called a **Bennett fracture.** The anterior oblique ligament, responsible for stability of the thumb base, is left attached to the pyramidal fragment. The remainder of the thumb metacarpal is unstable and limits use of the thumb. The fracture must be reduced and stabilized with Kirschner pins or a lag screw. Accurate reduction of the articular surface is crucial in reducing complications. Even despite adequate treatment, most patients eventually develop arthritis.

Dislocations

Dislocations are most common in the PIP joint. Injuries are classified according to the position of the distal digit as hyperextension, dorsal displacement, or volar displacement. The type of dislocation determines which structures, such as the volar plate, collateral ligaments, and extensor tendon, are likely to be disrupted.

The MP and MC joints are better protected by surrounding soft tissue but can still be dislocated. The MP joint of the thumb is most frequently injured by forced abduction. The ulnar collateral ligament is torn, as occurs with forced use of a ski pole or as historically described in gamekeepers when twisting the neck of birds ("gamekeeper's thumb"). Of the MC joints, the fifth is most commonly injured. A fracture analogous to Bennet's fracture can occur. Examination to determine injury to the deep motor branch of the ulnar nerve in this area should be done.

Radiographs are occasionally useful for diagnosis, but the physical examination is most important. Since pain often limits the extent of the examination, regional anesthesia with a wrist or finger block allows a more detailed examination. Partial tears of ligaments without dislocation or instability are treated by splints. Dislocations can usually be reduced, and the need for surgical therapy is determined by the stability of the joint after reduction. Stable reductions are treated with early mobilization to decrease stiffness.

Fracture dislocations usually require surgical repair. Instability after reduction can be treated by repair of the torn collateral ligament or volar plate. Severe dislocations of the PIP and MP joints can result in interposition of disrupted soft tissue in the joint, making closed reduction impossible. The joint must be opened and the trapped soft tissue removed and repaired to correct the dislocation. A complete disruption of the ulnar collateral ligament in a gamekeeper's thumb injury can result in interposition of the adductor aponeurosis between the torn ends of the ulnar collateral ligament. The ends of the ligament must be reduced and repaired under direct vision.

WRIST & FOREARM INJURIES

Fractures

Fractures in the wrist and forearm usually result from falls on the outstretched hand. The distal radius is most commonly fractured. Many classification systems and eponyms have been used based on the extent and displacement of the fracture and involvement of the articular surface. The hyperextended wrist also exposes the scaphoid bone to injury in a fall. Since the scaphoid is crucial to wrist motion, displacement of the fracture is poorly tolerated. In addition, the blood supply enters the distal part of the bone and makes ischemic necrosis of the proximal fragment a problem.

Diagnosis of radial fractures is not difficult, but scaphoid fractures can easily be missed. Special radiographic views of the wrist or CT scans may be needed in difficult cases. If the clinical picture is suspicious but the radiographs are inconclusive, the wrist should be immobilized. Repeat radiographs in 2 weeks may demonstrate the fracture. Untreated scaphoid fractures lead to debilitating arthritis of the wrist.

Radial fractures are treated by reduction and immobilization. As with other fractures, articular irregularities and unstable fractures need to be treated operatively. Use of bone grafting and external fixation devices to initially treat the fracture has been advocated. Scaphoid fractures require careful and prolonged immobilization. Displaced fractures or nonhealing fractures require operative treatment with screw immobilization, bone grafts, or scaphoid replacement.

Dislocations & Sprains

Dislocations and ligamentous (sprain) injuries of the wrist are the most difficult hand injuries to diagnose and treat. Wrist injuries often present as a painful wrist after minor trauma. Routine radiographs are often normal, and physical findings can be unimpressive. Still, these injuries can lead to chronic problems. Special stress radiographs, fluoroscopy, and physical maneuvers (scaphoid shift test) help delineate the injury.

The scaphoid lunate ligament is most often injured. Instability of the joint is best treated by repair or reconstruction of the ligament. Injury of the ligaments of the radiocarpal-radioulnar joint is likewise difficult to determine. Surgical treatment involves repair of the disrupted ligament.

Cohen MS: Fractures of the carpal bones. Hand Clin 1997;13:587.

Corley FG Jr, Schenck RC Jr: Fractures of the hand. Clin Plast Surg 1996;23:447-62.

Divelbiss BJ, Baratz ME: The role of arthroplasty and arthrodesis following trauma to the upper extremity. Hand Clin 1999; 15:335.

Eustace S, Denison W: Pictorial review: magnetic resonance imaging of acute orthopaedic trauma to the upper extremity. Clin Radiol 1997;52:338.

Katarincic JA: Fractures of the wrist and hand. Occup Med 1998; 13:549.

Kozin SH, Thoder JJ, Lieberman G: Operative treatment of metacarpal and phalangeal shaft fractures. J Am Acad Orthop Surg 2000;8:111.

Metz VM, Wunderbaldinger P, Gilula LA: Update on imaging techniques of the wrist and hand. Clin Plast Surg 1996; 23:369.

Wolf JM, Weiss AP: Portable mini-fluoroscopy improves operative efficiency in hand surgery. J Hand Surg [Am] 1999;24:182.

NERVE DISORDERS

Nerve disorders of the hands are conveniently organized into compression neuropathies, injuries of peripheral nerves, and various problems located more proximal to the upper extremities (spinal cord or central nervous system). For nerve dysfunction due to strokes, cerebral palsy, and spinal cord injury, readers are referred to more specific textbooks on hand surgery.

Compression Neuropathies

Compression of the nerves of the upper extremities due to an increase in surrounding tissue pressure occurs in specific locations and causes predictable signs and symptoms. Tissue edema from a variety of causes such as crushing injuries, vascular disorders, and prolonged repetitive hand motions can compress nerves traveling within tight compartments of the arm and produce nerve ischemia. Prolonged ischemia results in axonal destruction and sensory and motor dysfunction.

The median nerve can be compressed by local structures at the elbow (pronator syndrome), the anterior interosseous branch, and the wrist (carpal tunnel syndrome). Compression of the median nerve at the elbow causes forearm pain and sensory changes in the radial four fingers. The anterior interosseous branch of the median nerve is purely a motor nerve, and lesions produce only weakness of thumb and index finger flexion and no pain. Carpal tunnel syndrome presents with weakness in the hand, sensory abnormalities of the fingers sparing the little finger, and exacerbation of symptoms on forced flexion of the wrist (Phalen's sign) or tapping the nerve at the wrist (Tinel's sign). Shoulder, elbow, and forearm pain is also common. Atrophy of thenar muscles occurs in long-standing cases.

The ulnar nerve can be compressed at the elbow (cubital tunnel syndrome) or the wrist (Guyon's canal). Sensory abnormalities in the little finger and weakness of intrinsic hand muscles occur with compression in either area. Segmental nerve conduction velocity tests help to localize the abnormality to one site or the other. Compression of the radial nerve occurs most frequently from fractures of the humerus. Compression of the nerve along the proximal radius (radial tunnel syndrome) causes diffuse pain around the elbow but occurs rarely.

Abnormal findings on electrodiagnostic studies and clinical manifestations of nerve compression are adequate for diagnosis. Electromyography demonstrating denervation patterns in the corresponding muscles or slowing of nerve conduction velocities indicates injury to the nerve. Although helpful, these tests only compliment the physical examination since electrodiagnostic tests can occasionally be inaccurate.

Early or mild cases of compression are treated by controlling tissue swelling. Resting the extremity with splints, nonsteroidal anti-inflammatory medications, and local injection of steroids often resolve the problem. If repetitive motions, such as typing, are thought to be the cause, changing the motion or hand position should help. If clinical manifestations are severe or if nonsurgical therapy fails, surgical decompression of the nerve is advocated.

Carpal tunnel syndrome is the most common type of compression neuropathy and one of the most common hand disorders. Surgical therapy of median nerve entrapment in the carpal tunnel or any of the compression neuropathies requires detailed knowledge of the anatomy. Division of the constricting structures results in partial or complete reversal of the abnormalities. In the carpal tunnel, the median nerve is surrounded on three sides by carpal bones. Incision of the transverse carpal ligament, which forms the roof of the tunnel, decompresses the nerve. Occasionally, internal fibrosis of the nerve occurs and endoneurolysis is required to allow the nerve to recover. Endoscopic release of the carpal tunnel through a smaller skin incision has been advocated.

Nerve Injuries

Injury to individual peripheral nerves of the arm results in predictable and defined deficits. More proximal injuries to the brachial plexus have more variable manifestations. Nerve conduction can be disrupted in the absence of structural changes due to compression, blunt injury, or ischemia (neurapraxia or axonapraxia). More severe injury results in disruption of the axon with preservation of the epineurial covering of the nerve (axonotmesis). Both types of injury are followed by spontaneous recovery of function of good quality. Complete disruption of the nerve (neurotmesis), as with a laceration, requires surgical repair. Wallerian degeneration of the distal nerve occurs in both neurotmesis and axonotmesis, and recovery depends upon the growth of the cut axon to the end organ. However, with neurotmesis, orientation of the proximal and distal axons are lost and recovery may be incomplete, especially in mixed motor and sensory nerves. Methods to differentiate sensory from motor fascicles have been used during repairs with some benefit.

A patient with loss of the radial nerve is unable to extend the fingers or wrist, and a wrist drop is noticeable. The sensory loss to the dorsum of the hand is well tolerated. Median nerve dysfunction causes problems with opposition of the thumb and grip of the fingers. Sensory loss is to the radial four digits and can significantly impair use of the hand. An ulnar neuropathy causes dysfunction of the intrinsic muscles of the hand, clawing of the ulnar two digits, and weakness in gripping a key. Sensation is lost along the ulnar side of the hand.

Diagnosis of nerve injury is mainly by the physical examination. Understanding the functional anatomy of the peripheral nerves allows adequate evaluation of nerve loss. Electrodiagnostic studies are used to distinguish between partial and complete lesions and to follow functional recovery.

Obvious and complete disruption of the nerve is treated best by early surgical exploration and repair. An incomplete lesion or questionable disruption of nerve integrity is best treated with close observation, splinting to prevent contractures, and surgical exploration if no recovery occurs. Segmental loss of nerves requires nerve grafts, usually taken from a minor sensory nerve, such as the sural nerve, to bridge the gap. Results of primary repair are better than the results of grafts, and repairs done soon after injury are better than delayed repairs. Recovery of protective sensation of the hand is crucial for good functional recovery.

Motor dysfunction due to nerve damage can be treated by arthrodesis (stabilization of flail joints) and tendon transfers. Tendon transfers work best when the transferred muscle is unaffected by the nerve injury, has direction of force and excursion similar to those of the damaged muscle, and produces no further deficits due to loss of the donor muscle. For radial nerve palsy, the pronator teres to extensor carpi radialis transfer provides wrist extension, flexor carpi radialis to extensor digitorum communis transfer gives finger extension, and the palmaris longus or flexor digitorum superficialis of the fourth finger transfer to the extensor pollicis longus extends the thumb. Restoration of thumb opposition is most important with median nerve palsies, and the use of several donor muscles to achieve this result has been described. Tendon transfers to control claw deformity and strengthen key pinch are used for ulnar nerve palsies.

Brandsma JW, Ottenhoff-De Jonge MW: Flexor digitorum superficialis tendon transfer for intrinsic replacement. Long-term results and the effect on donor fingers. J Hand Surg [Br] 1992;17:625.

Deutinger M et al: Clinical application of motorsensory differentiated nerve repair. Microsurgery 1993;14:297.

Nagal D, Harris G, Foley M: Prospective review of 278 endoscopic carpal tunnel releases using the modified Chow technique. Arthroscopy 1994;10:259.

Nagano A: Treatment of brachial plexus injury. J Orthop Sci 1998;3:71.

Novak CB, Kelly L, Mackinnon SE: Sensory recovery after median nerve grafting. J Hand Surg [Am] 1992;17:59.

Sloan EP: Nerve injuries in the hand. Emerg Med Clin North Am 1993;11:651.

Weiss AP, Sachar K, Gendreau M: Conservative management of carpal tunnel syndrome: a reexamination of steroid injection and splinting. J Hand Surg [Am] 1994;19:410.

■ HAND INFECTIONS

Small breaks in the skin or nails of the hand can lead to widespread infection and abscess. Sometimes the original injury cannot be identified. Poor venous and lymphatic drainage of the upper extremity, especially when held in a dependent position, aggravate the situation. Immunocompromised patients (diabetics, AIDS patients) are prone to develop extensive infections very quickly and should be treated more carefully.

The hallmark of infection (pain, swelling, and erythema) may be widespread in the hand and make localizing the infection difficult. Swelling of the dorsum of the hand is common even with palmar infections, and knowledge of the tissue planes of the hand is crucial to understanding how infections spread. Red lymphatic streaks (lymphangitis) extending up the arm indicate rapid extension of the infection and must be treated urgently.

Oral antibiotics effective against staphylococcus and common anaerobic organisms (ie, first-generation cephalosporins and penicillin) are adequate to treat most infections. Infections from animal bites (*Pasteurella multocida*) and human bites (oral flora) also respond to penicillin. The intravenous route is reserved for severe infections or for those not responsive to oral antibiotics. Once the situation improves, oral antibiotics are given for 7–10 days. Equally as important, the infected hand needs to be immobilized and elevated. Pillows and trapezes help to elevate the arm, but slings aggravate the dependent position of the arm and should not be used. The best results are obtained when the patient is convinced that elevation of the extremity is beneficial.

Once treatment of a hand infection is begun, improvement within 24 hours is expected. If prompt improvement does not occur, a hidden abscess may be present. Obvious abscesses should be drained at the point of maximum tenderness or the point of maximum fluctuation, where the overlying tissues are thinnest. The drainage wound should run parallel to and not across the paths of nerves, arteries, and veins. Wounds should be made long enough and should be zigzagged, when necessary, to avoid secondary contractures. Ultrasonography may be useful when a definite abscess cannot be located.

Pyogenic Granuloma

Pyogenic granuloma is a mound of granulation-like tissue 3–20 mm (or more) in diameter. It usually develops under a chronically moist dressing and may form around a suture. A small granuloma (6–7 mm in diameter) exposed to the air will soon dry up and epithelialize, whereas larger ones should be scraped flush with the skin under local anesthesia and covered with a thin split-thickness skin graft. If the granuloma is adjacent to the nail and the nail is acting as a foreign body aggravating the reaction, the nail must be removed.

Nail Infections

The nail fold is often traumatized and becomes secondarily inflamed, leading to a **paronychia** on the radial or ulnar side. The lesion is called an **eponychia** if it involves the base of the nail; a **"runaround"** if the entire fold is involved; and a **"subungual abscess"** if pus develops and extends under the nail plate. Because of the early and unrelenting tissue tension that develops, these entities are quite painful. Early treatment before abscess formation is by means of soaking, elevation, immobilization, and antibiotics. Most abscesses can be drained painlessly with a scalpel without drawing blood; the insensible necrotic skin cap should be cut through where it points (Figure 45–16). Sagittal incisions, which form a "trapdoor" of the eponychium, should be reserved for the long-standing case in which a dense fibrous callus of the nail fold must be excised. Occasionally the nail must be basally excised or totally avulsed, after which the eponychial fold should be separated from the nail matrix by a thin, loose pack. Chronically wet nails of dishwashers may develop tissue changes and nail deformities which are best treated by removing the nail plate. Fungal infections should be diagnosed and treated, and the fingers should be protected from water or excessive sweating.

Deep Space Abscess

An abscess in the pulp of the fingertip, a **felon,** is often deep and very painful. Untreated or inadequately drained abscesses may lead to osteomyelitis of the distal phalanx. Wide incision and drainage with disruption of the many vertical fibrous septa of the pulp space are required to adequately drain the abscess (Figure 45–17). The traditional fishmouth incision is no longer recommended for drainage since it may expose the underlying bone and because it often heals in a tender scar. Instead, lateral through-and-through incisions or direct incisions on the pulp, where the abscess points, have better results (Figure 45–18).

The **web spaces** are the path of least resistance for pus from infected distal palm calluses, puncture wounds, and infections of the lumbrical canals. Infection and abscess formation in the dorsum of the thumb web may be the result of extension from the volar thenar space (collar button). A dorsal incision is usually made between the fingers to drain both spaces. A dorsal incision in the web of the thumb may be zigzagged to prevent contracture (Figure 45–10).

The **midpalmar space** becomes infected by direct puncture or by extension of infections from the flexor sheaths of rays II, III, or IV (Figure 45–6). Only the skin should be incised over the point of fluctuation. The rest of the dissection should be carried out by gentle spreading with a blunt clamp to avoid injury to arteries, nerves, and tendons. Infection spreads easily

Figure 45–16. Incision and drainage of paronychia.

Figure 45–17. Cross section of distal phalanx.

Figure 45–19. Drainage and irrigation for septic tenosynovitis. The antibiotic solution drips in through the distal catheter and drains out through the proximal one.

from this space along the lumbrical canals and to the thenar space.

A hypothenar space abscess is usually a product of a penetrating wound and should be drained where it points. The same is true for a thenar space abscess, which may point in the palm rather than the thumb web.

Infection within the synovium of the flexor tendon is difficult to diagnose. **Pyogenic tenosynovitis** spreads easily down the tendon sheath to affect the other fingers. Untreated, the infection causes adhesions of the tendon to the surrounding soft tissues and permanently limits movement of the fingers.

The signs of flexor tendon infection described by Kanaval include fusiform swelling of the digit, severe pain on passive finger extension, a fixed flexed position of the finger, and, most importantly, tenderness over the extent of the tendon sheath into the palm. Ultrasonography of the distal palm can also be helpful when the diagnosis is unclear. The probe is held across the palm and reveals swelling of the involved tendon and fluid around the tendon at the proximal flexor sheath.

Only unresponsive, tensely swollen, and toxic cases need immediate incision and drainage. With rest, elevation, and antibiotics, it is safe to observe most cases for several hours. The preferred method of incision and drainage (Figure 45–19) is to make a short sagittal

midline distal wound immediately over the tendon and introduce a small plastic catheter into the synovial bursa for irrigating with an antibiotic solution. The catheter should pass through the sheath and exit by a counterincision in the palm to allow for drainage of the fluid. These incisions do not cross flexion creases. The hand should then be elevated and immobilized in the position of function and covered by a dressing. Phlegmonous tenosynovitis usually requires opening of the entire synovial sheath (often through a lateral mid axial digital incision, or longitudinally across the wrist for extensor sheath infections) and, frequently, excision of necrotic tendon and sometimes amputation of a digit.

Other Infections

Necrotizing soft tissue infections of the upper extremity are rare but devastating when they occur. The condition has been called many different names such as necrotizing fasciitis, Meleney's ulcer, and streptococcal gangrene. The organisms responsible include clostridium species, *Streptococcus pyogenes,* and mixed infections. The hallmarks are the rapid spread of infection and the extensive necrosis of soft tissue. Treatment includes wide debridement of the necrotic tissue and intravenous antibiotics.

Human bite wounds of the hand occur most often during altercations when the fist strikes an opponent's tooth. The MP joint can be entered. The injury is often ignored by the patient until infection of the joint has

Figure 45–18. Incision of felon (distal fat pad infection).

begun. The joint must be explored and cleaned and the patient treated with antibiotics to cover oral flora (penicillin). Once the infection reaches the joint, destruction of the cartilage often occurs despite all therapy.

An inordinate amount of pain, with little or no swelling or induration, predating and accompanying the appearance of multiple tiny vesicles suggests **herpes simplex (herpetic whitlow).** The vesicles may appear cyclically. They contain clear fluid and not pus and should be distinguished from paronychias. Antibiotics are not indicated in this self-limited viral infection. Acyclovir 5% ointment applied topically for 7 days decreases the severity and duration of symptoms but is of no value in prophylaxis.

Tuberculous infection of the hand is usually chronic and may be relatively painless. Some cultures take months to become positive. Tuberculosis commonly involves only one hand, which may be the only focus of infection in the body. Bones and joints may be infected, but the process more commonly involves the tendon synovium, which becomes matted to the tendons. Treatment is by synovectomy and antituberculous drug therapy for 6–12 months.

Leprosy causes neuritis of the median and ulnar nerves, resulting in sensory and motor loss to the hand. Crippling claw deformities develop as a result of intrinsic muscle palsy. Open sores appear on the hands as a result of trauma to anesthetic digits. Reconstructive surgery and occupational training are required.

Fungal infections involve primarily the nails. Tinea unguium (onychomycosis) may be caused by many organisms, including *Epidermophyton floccosum,* trichophyton, and *Candida albicans.* Prolonged treatment with antifungal drugs—griseofulvin systemically or nystatin topically—may be necessary, along with daily applications of fungicidal agents such as tolnaftate. Removal of the nail is advocated for chronic intractable cases associated with nail deformity.

Boles SD, Schmidt CC: Pyogenic flexor tenosynovitis. Hand Clin 1998;14:567.

Canales FL, Newmeyer WL, Kilgore ES: The treatment of felons and paronychias. Hand Clin 1989;5:515.

Faciszewski T, Coleman DA: Human bite wounds. Hand Clin 1989;5:561.

Fowler JR: Viral infections. Hand Clin 1989;5:613.

Hitchcock TF, Amadio PC: Fungal infections. Hand Clin 1989; 5:599.

Jebson PJ: Deep subfascial space infections. Hand Clin 1998; 14:557.

Nemoto K, Yanagida M, Nemoto T: Closed continuous irrigation as a treatment for infection in the hand. J Hand Surg [Br] 1993;18:783.

Seltzer DG et al: AIDS in the hand patient: the team approach. Hand Clin 1991;7:433.

■ INFLAMMATORY DISORDERS OF THE HAND

DUPUYTREN'S CONTRACTURE (Palmar Fasciitis)

The cause of Dupuytren's contracture, which is common particularly among white populations of Celtic origin, is not known. It occurs in one of three types (acute, subacute, and chronic), predominately in males over 50 who have been in sedentary occupations, and is bilateral in about half of cases. There is a hereditary influence, and the incidence is higher among idiopathic epileptics, diabetics, alcoholics, and patients with chronic illnesses. The contracture may develop in people who do not work and (in laborers) in the hand that does the least work, so that it is not considered work-related. It is frequently found in the plantar fascia of the instep and occasionally in the penis (Peyronie's disease).

Dupuytren's contracture manifests itself most commonly in the palm by thickening, which may be nodular, and therefore mistaken for a callosity; or cord-like, and therefore mistaken for a tendon abnormality because it passes into the digits and restricts their extension. This process typically involves the longitudinal and vertical components of the fascia but at times seems to exist apart from anatomically distinct fascia. The skin may fuse with it and become raised and rock-hard, or it may be greatly shrunken and sometimes drawn into a deeply puckered crevasse. The disorder invades the palm at the expense of fat but is never adherent to vessels, nerves, or musculotendinous structures (though it may be adherent to flexor tendon sheaths). It has an unpredictable rate of progression, but the earlier it starts in life, the more destructive and recurrent it is apt to be.

Dupuytren's fasciitis may involve any digit or web space, but it affects predominantly the ring and small fingers. In long-standing cases the fingers may be drawn tightly into the palm, resulting in secondary contracture of joint capsule and ligaments, flexor sheaths, and atrophic muscles.

Surgery is indicated when the disorder has progressed sufficiently, especially when it causes more than 30 degrees of flexion at the MP joint or any flexion contracture of the PIP joint. The patient must be warned about the increasing technical difficulty with progressive flexion and adduction contractures and the potential for recurrence after surgery. Fasciectomy is the surgical procedure that gives the best long-term results. In selected cases where only the longitudinal pretendinous fascial band is involved and the skin moves freely over it, subcutaneous fasciotomy done through a small longitudinal incision may release a contracture quite well with only a few days of postoperative disability. In the occasional-case with acute and rapid onset of a tender nodule, local triamcinolone may be used for not only subjective but even objective relief.

Depending upon the amount of cutaneous shrinkage, skin grafts may be required for wound closure after fasciectomy. The overlying dermis has been implicated as an inductive mechanism in this process. Thus, skin grafting may diminish the recurrence rate in severe cases. The hopelessly contracted little finger must sometimes be amputated.

Motion should be started within 3–5 days after surgery. Dynamic splints and postoperative injection of corticosteroids into joints and the zone of surgery may help the well-motivated patient.

The complications of surgery are digital infarction and ischemic skin flaps, hematoma formation, fibrosis and stiffness, anesthesia or neuromatous pain, and recurrence of contractures. Reflex sympathetic dystrophy, a painful debilitating neurologic disorder of the hand, can occur after surgery and must be treated aggressively. In general, the functional reward of the patient is great at any age.

Chick LR, Lister GD: Surgical alternatives to Dupuytren's contracture. Hand Clin 1991;7:715.

Ketchum LD: The use of the full thickness skin graft in Dupuytren's contracture. Hand Clin 1991;7:731.

Rayan GM: Palmar fascial complex anatomy and pathology in Dupuytren's disease. Hand Clin 1999;15:73.

Watson HK, Fong D: Dystrophy, recurrence, and salvage procedures in Dupuytren's contracture. Hand Clin 1991;7:745.

DEGENERATIVE & RHEUMATOID ARTHRITIS

Arthritis of the hand is divided into two categories. **Degenerative changes** are usually due to some trauma resulting in damage to the bone or cartilage or to the supporting ligamentous structures. The increased wear to the joint results in inflammation and damage to the cartilage or underlying bone followed by reactive new bone formation (spurs). The wrists, hips, and knees are most commonly affected. **Rheumatoid arthritis** is a systemic disease characterized by synovial inflammation. The diseased synovium destroys adjacent tendons and joints in a specific way, leading to characteristic deformities in the hand.

Patients with degenerative arthritis complain of pain, aching, and stiffness in the area of the affected joint. Progression of the problem leads to immobility of the joint that affects the entire hand. Radiographic studies demonstrate joint narrowing and periosteal thickening early in the problem, progressing to bone spurs, loss of the articular surface, and bone destruction later. Patients with rheumatoid arthritis often present with very severe deformities without pain. Nodules around the olecranon and dorsum of the hand are often found. Both flexor and extensor tendons at the wrist can be inflamed, limiting tendon movement and resulting in rupture of the tendon. Involvement of the tendons and ligaments at the digits and MP joints results in ulnar deviation of the digits, MP joint destruction and dislocation, and swan neck and boutonnièere deformities. Destruction of the wrist joint is also common.

Arthritis is common among older patients and usually treated by primary care physicians and rheumatologists with anti-inflammatory medications and modification of the patient's activities. In most cases it is only when symptoms greatly hinder the patient's lifestyle that they are referred to a hand surgeon. Physical therapy, splints, and medications are often no longer effective for these patients.

Surgical treatment of painful joints includes replacement with a prosthetic joint and partial or full fusion. Prosthetic joints of metal or Silastic permit near-normal movement but can become unstable and dislocate or degenerate over time. For a durable solution to the problem, fusion of the joint is recommended. Motion is severely limited, but pain relief is complete. There are more therapeutic options for the wrist, such as replacement, local fusion of only the affected carpal bone, or complete excision of the proximal row of carpal bones, leaving motion and stability to the distal carpal bones and ligaments.

Therapy for synovial inflammation in rheumatoid disease includes excision of the synovium to increase tendon excursion and prevent rupture, repair of ruptured tendons, and excision of painful nodules. Tendon balancing procedures can help ulnar deviation of the MP joints and improve joint movement. The most important concept of treating patients with rheumatoid hand disease is that often the patients have adapted well to their functional deficits. Correcting a physical deformity in a well-compensated patient may actually result in more problems for that patient.

Adamson GJ et al: Flexible implant resection arthroplasty of the proximal interphalangeal joint in patients with systemic inflammatory arthritis. J Hand Surg [Am] 1994;19:378.

Bogoch ER: Surgery of rheumatoid arthritis in peripheral joints. Curr Opin Rheumatol 1992;4:191.

Ferlic DC: Rheumatoid flexor tenosynovitis and rupture. Hand Clin 1996;12:561.

Kobus RJ, Turner RH: Wrist arthrodesis for treatment of rheumatoid arthritis. J Hand Surg [Am] 1990;15:541.

Osterman AL, Hood J: Synovectomy, arthroplasty, and arthrodesis in the reconstruction of the rheumatoid wrist and hand. Curr Opin Rheumatol 1991;3:102.

Toledano B, Terrono AL, Millender LH: Reconstruction of the rheumatoid thumb. Hand Clin 1992;8:121.

Wilson RL, DeVito MC: Extensor tendon problems in rheumatoid arthritis. Hand Clin 1996;12:551.

SCLERODERMA & LUPUS ERYTHEMATOSUS

These systemic diseases of unknown cause have distinctive—though not necessarily pathognomonic—manifestations in the hands.

Scleroderma initially produces joint stiffness, hyperhidrosis, and Raynaud's phenomenon. Unchecked, it leads to marked tautness of skin and rigidity of joints with associated osteoporosis (even atrophy and ultimate resorption of the distal phalanges) and soft tissue calcifications.

Lupus erythematosus, which may be initiated or aggravated by certain drugs, foreign proteins, or psychic states, often causes polyarthritis indistinguishable from that of rheumatoid arthritis. It does not usually lead to similar joint destruction. Vasospasm in both lupus and scleroderma can cause severe ischemia of the hand and digits and may require therapy to prevent gangrene.

GOUT

Gout is a metabolic disorder of uric acid metabolism that affects about 1% of the population; approximately 50% of patients with gout have **cheiragra** (gouty hands).

The diagnosis is suggested by a rapid onset of severe pain and inflammatory signs about the joints and musculotendinous structure, simulating a phlegmonous infectious cellulitis with marked induration (most dramatically seen about the elbow). The usual duration of an attack is 5–10 days. The serum uric acid is elevated in 75% of cases. Gout may coexist with rheumatoid disease. The diagnosis is confirmed by identification of uric acid crystals in joint fluid or tissue biopsy.

In time, typical tophi form, consisting of toothpaste-like infiltrates of urate crystals, arising in multilobulated form about soft tissue structures that have been invaded. X-rays show characteristic punched-out lesions at the margins of articular cartilage.

Prophylactic treatment of gouty arthritis consists of diet, colchicine, allopurinol (a urate-blocking agent) or probenecid (a uricosuric agent), and avoidance of stress. Colchicine, 0.6 mg/h with a glass of water for 6–8 doses or to the point of gastrointestinal distress, is the time-honored means of interrupting an attack, but phenylbutazone, topical corticotropin gel, and systemic corticosteroids are also of value.

Surgical measures consist of drainage of abscessed tophi (seldom needed) and tophectomy. The latter procedure is more often of cosmetic rather than functional value. Tophectomy consists of removal of as much tophaceous material as can be fairly easily recovered. The surgeon should be careful not to destroy ligaments, tenoretinacular structures, nerves, and vessels in the process.

Dieppe PA: Investigation and management of gout in the young and the elderly, Ann Rheumat Dis 1991;50:263.

Hauptman HW, Ruddy S, Roberts WN: Reversal of the vasospastic component of lupus vasculopathy by infusion of prostaglandin E$_1$. J Rheumatol 1991;18:1747.

O'Brien BM et al: Radical microarteriolysis in the treatment of vasospastic disorders of the hand, especially scleroderma. J Hand Surg [Br] 1992;17:447.

BURNS & FROSTBITE OF THE HAND

Thermal Burns

The hands are a common site of thermal (including frictional), electrical, chemical, and radiation burns. Function is imperiled in all instances by swelling and scar formation. Prompt measures to preserve existing function are often urgently required. Burns over other areas of the body may be more life threatening and require more urgent attention, but burns of the hand should never be neglected. Delay in therapy leads to irreversible impairment and deformity that are impossible to correct later.

As in other areas of the body, thermal burns are grouped into three degrees. Superficial (first-degree) burns are red and painful; partial-thickness (second-degree) burns develop blisters; and full-thickness (third-degree) burns are insensate and appear like leather or charred tissue. The prognosis and therapy depend upon the location, depth, and extent of the burn.

All burns to the hand cause swelling of the tissues, and the need for elevation of the arm to relieve pain and prevent stiffness cannot be overemphasized. Tetanus immunization should be given. Cold compresses may help alleviate the pain in first-degree burns. Second-degree burns must be watched more carefully. Large blisters restricting motion are broken. Otherwise, since they are sterile, they should be left intact. Treatment with thrice-daily washing and silver sulfadiazine is usually adequate. Patients with third-degree burns or superficial burns that fail to heal and patients unable to care for their burns at home should be admitted to the hospital.

Deeper burns require close observation and more extensive treatment. In the first few hours after injury, circumferential or near-circumferential burns may cause ischemia in the extremity. Since evaluation of sensory function and capillary refill is nearly impossible in these limbs, escharotomies should be performed if compartment syndrome is suspected. If done correctly, escharotomies have few complications since these burns usually require surgical debridement anyway. Incisions are placed to avoid exposure of neurovascular structures.

Partial-thickness burns heal spontaneously. Deeper burns on the dorsum of the hand are best treated with early excision of the eschar and placement of skin grafts to prevent contractures. Palmar burns are best left to heal spontaneously since skin grafts function very poorly in this area. Some hand surgeons believe that excision and grafting of superficial burns should be performed to prevent contractures. This is true in cases where adequate therapy has not been available. In burn units with good rehabilitation services, surgeons are treating superficial second-degree burns without surgery and obtaining results as good as with skin grafting. Pigskin, cadaver homografts, or a number of commercially available biologic dressings can be used to cover the wounds temporarily, decreasing pain and keeping the wound moist until autologous skin grafts are placed.

Neglected burns of the hands result in contracture deformities that often require extensive surgery to restore function. Delayed healing and wound contractures often result in a claw hand with MP hyperextension and fusion of the digits with loss of the web space (syndactyly). Burns on the volar surface leave flexion contractures. Some contractures can be treated with release and skin grafting of the tissue gap. Web space contractures and released contractures with exposed tendons or nerves must be covered with skin or muscle flaps. Web space release is done with skin flaps from the dorsum folded down to create the space. Large flaps can be obtained by attaching the hand to the groin, allowing the tissue to adhere and vascularize before cutting the flap away from the groin. Recently, free tissue transfer from other parts of the body using microsurgical techniques has allowed more extensive reconstruction of severely burned hands.

Electrical Burns

Electrical burns of the upper extremity may not appear extensive on initial inspection. The skin may be burned only in a very small area of the entry point of the current or by ignited clothing. The current tends to spare the skin but damage underlying muscles, vessels, and nerves. Often the extent of dead tissue is not evident for several days.

Initial treatment is the same as for thermal burns. Since muscle damage may be extensive, it is important to prevent renal failure from myoglobinuria by maintaining a high output of alkaline urine. Arteriography, fluorescein injections, and radionuclide studies may help delineate the extent of necrosis. Examination of the patient in the operating room is still the most accurate method of assessing the extent of tissue damage. All obviously dead tissue should be removed during the initial evaluation. Two or three days later, the patient is reexamined in the operating room and any additional debris is removed. The wounds are closed when only clearly viable tissue remains.

Frostbite

Frostbite occurs most often in people under the influence of alcohol or with psychiatric illness. The lower extremity is affected more often than the upper. Freezing tissue causes cellular death and vascular thrombosis. Hypothermia of the entire body must first be treated. The frozen part should be quickly rewarmed by immersion in warm water (40 °C). Elevation of the extremity minimizes edema. Skin wounds are treated like burns with silver sulfadiazine cream. The extent of necrosis may not be obvious for several weeks, and debridement or amputation should be delayed until demarcation of the injury occurs. Sympathectomy may help ameliorate the sequelae of frostbite such as cold sensitivity and pain. Children with frostbite may develop premature closure of phalangeal epiphyses, which creates growth disturbances of the bone.

Achauer B, Appelbaum R, Vander Kam VM: Electrical burn injury to the upper extremity. Br J Plast Surg 1994;47:331.

Robson MC et al: Making the burned hand functional. Clin Past Surg 1992;19:663.

Smith MA, Munster AM, Spence RJ: Burns of the hand and upper limb—a review. Burns 1998;24:493.

Valnicek SM, Chasmar LR, Clapson JB: Frostbite in the prairies: a 12-year review. Plast Reconstr Surg 1993;92:633.

MASSES OF THE HAND

Only 2% of all masses in the hand are malignant lesions; the majority are benign neoplasms, cysts, or a myriad of other masses. Though the clinician must be ever vigilant to identify malignancy, a mass of the hand is highly likely to be benign—excisional biopsies are thus reserved for subcutaneous lesions that are rapidly growing or for skin lesions that may be carcinomas. Otherwise, masses can be observed over a period of time to determine that they are not growing. They may be removed for functional or cosmetic reasons.

Ganglions are formed by herniation of the synovial lining of joints or tendons into the surrounding soft tissue. These cysts are filled with a viscous fluid thought to be modified joint fluid. Trauma to the wrist or hand may cause extrusion of the synovium, but it is more likely that the ganglion was already present and that trauma to that area merely brought the lesion to the surgeon's attention.

Ganglions can arise from any joint of the hand but most commonly appear on the dorsal wrist over the scapholunate ligament and the volar wrist near the radial artery. Tendon ganglions are most common on the flexor sheath at the metacarpal head (A1 pulley). Pain and tenderness are due to compression of adjacent nerves by the mass.

Ganglions have a typical appearance, and diagnosis is simple. If any doubt exists, aspiration with a large-bore needle of the viscous fluid confirms the diagnosis and occasionally cures the lesions. Injection of the empty sac with steroids and lidocaine may help to keep the mass from reappearing, but the majority recur. Ganglions need not be treated unless they cause pain or interfere with hand function. Often, it is enough just to reassure the patient that the mass is benign.

Operative removal of ganglions should be done using loupe magnification and a tourniquet. The entire ganglion should be removed, including all attachments to the joint capsule and the underlying ligament, without injuring the surrounding structures. Prolonged splinting after removal of ganglions does not decrease recurrence rates but does cause hand stiffness. Unfortunately, despite careful surgical removal of the lesion, recurrence of ganglions is relatively common.

Epidermal cysts are rests of epidermis located in the subcutaneous tissue. Many are thought to be due to traumatic disruption of epidermal cells into the soft tissue (inclusion cyst). The cells proliferate just as skin does and form a cyst filled with creamy keratin, the remains of dead epidermal cells that usually desquamate from the skin. Infected cysts become inflamed and form abscesses. Removal of the entire cyst wall is required to prevent abscess formation.

Pyogenic granuloma may form in any chronic wound. Histologically, it consists of vascular tissue identical to granulation tissue. Just as for hypertrophic granulation tissue elsewhere on the body, excision or cautery of the material flush to skin level allows epidermis to migrate over the wound.

Giant cell tumors are benign, multilobulated, solid masses found on the lateral aspects of the finger. They are often attached to the tendon sheath. The mass may be quite complex and extend throughout the adjacent nerves, vessels, tendons, and ligaments. The entire lesion should be removed, but recurrence is relatively common.

The most common bone tumors are **enchondromas.** Multiple enchondromas (Ollier's disease) are associated with other skeletal deformities. The lesion appears on x-ray as thinned cortical bone with speckled calcifications. Fractures through the tumors usually do not heal spontaneously. The tumor should be removed

with a curette. Bone graft taken from the distal radius is used to fill the gap if needed.

A **carpal boss** is due to abnormal bone formation at the base of the second or third metacarpal bones and presents as a hard mass on the dorsum of the hand. The excess growth of bone can be removed if symptomatic.

Glomus tumors are composed of blood vessels and unmyelinated nerves of a heat-regulating arteriovenous malformation. They are usually found in the fingertip or under the fingernail and can be extremely painful. Local excision of the tumor is curative. Occasionally, when the tumor is large and disrupts the nail matrix, a split-thickness nail graft from another digit is needed to reconstruct the defect.

The most common malignant tumor of the hand is **squamous cell carcinoma,** though **basal cell carcinomas** and **melanomas** also occur. Subungual melanomas are often difficult to diagnose because they are difficult to examine. These tumors should be treated just the same as elsewhere on the body. Particular care should be taken to examine for spread of tumor in the lymphatic drainage at the supratrochlear and axillary nodes.

Other tumors include lipomas, fibromas, hemangiomas, arteriovenous malformations, neurofibromas, sarcomas, and various skin lesions. These tumors act no differently in the hand than elsewhere in the body. However, because of the close proximity of the nervous and vascular structures within the small spaces of the hand, these tumors cause compressive signs and symptoms sooner. CT scans or MRI help delineate the extent of soft tissue tumors and may help in preoperative planning.

Babins DM, Lubahn JD: Palmar lipomas associated with compression of the median nerve. J Bone Joint Surg [Am] 1994; 76:1360.

Chakrabarti I, Watson JD, Dorrance H: Skin tumors of the hand. A 10-year review. J Hand Surg [Br] 1993;18:484.

Diao E, Moy OJ: Common tumors. Orthop Clin North Am 1992; 23:187.

Glowacki KA, Weiss AP: Giant cell tumors of tendon sheath. Hand Clin 1995;11:245.

Miller TT, Potter HG, McCormack RR Jr: Benign soft tissue masses of the wrist and hand: MRI appearances. Skeletal Radiol 1994;23:327.

COMPLEX HAND INJURIES

Crush Injuries & Amputations

Recent advances in microvascular surgery have greatly increased our ability to treat complex hand injuries. Mangled and amputated digits, hands, and even entire upper extremities have been replanted or repaired. Complex nerve repairs, microvascular free tissue transfers of muscle flaps, and toe-to-hand reconstructions have made it possible to restore more function to severely injured hands. The end result must be a sensate, painless, and useful extremity. Patients who undergo multiple surgical procedures and prolonged rehabilitation with only marginal results would have benefited from early amputation. A surgeon with extensive experience can best assess the patient's injuries, occupational requirements, and psychosocial needs to determine if salvage is worthwhile.

Complex hand injuries often result from improper use or malfunction of machinery. Heavy machinery in the workplace or motorized cutting tools at home, such as rotary saws, are often cited as the mechanism of injury. Sharply amputated or partially devascularized parts are most likely to be saved. Severe crushing or avulsion of the part produces wider nerve and vessel injury. The extent of this type of damage is difficult to determine and often impossible to repair.

The decision to try to salvage a damaged part must be individualized to each situation, but some general principles apply. The thumb is crucial to hand function, and all efforts are made to save the entire digit or as much length as possible. When multiple digits or half of the hand is damaged or amputated, a greater effort is made to repair the part. Children can recover function in badly damaged extremities far better than adults, and any amputated parts in children should be replanted. Replantation of the entire arm at the elbow and above is controversial. The usefulness of these replanted limbs is limited by the slow nerve regeneration, and some hand surgeons believe that amputations in these cases result in better function.

Patients with complex hand injuries should be immediately referred to a regional center with the staff and facilities to manage the problems. Occasionally, in the rush to transfer patients with these very obvious injuries, intra-abdominal, neurologic, and other less obvious injuries have been overlooked. The entire patient must be evaluated and stabilized prior to transfer. A clean moist dressing should be placed on the wound and the extremity elevated. The amputated part is wrapped in a plastic bag and placed in ice water. The amputated part should never be frozen.

The accepting hand surgeon evaluates the patient's overall condition, potential for rehabilitation, and personal wishes before coming to a decision. To revascularize or replant a part, the patient must be taken urgently to the operating room. Ischemia over 6 hours is often associated with failure of revascularization, but—depending on the metabolic needs of the constituent tissues—extremities that have undergone periods of ischemia longer than this can be successfully replanted.

Bone must first be stabilized with Kirschner wires or metal plates before vascular repairs are performed. Arterial and venous repairs are done with microscopic magnification, and the ischemic tissue is reperfused. Failure of a replanted part is more often due to venous outflow problems than arterial inflow. Systemic and local anticoagulants help to maintain perfusion but are not always needed. Leeches placed on the part release a potent local anticoagulant and can decrease venous congestion. Nerve and tendon repairs must also be performed. When there is inadequate local soft tissue to cover the repaired structures, muscle or skin flaps from a distant site must be transferred using microsurgical methods to the area. Although these operations are not life-threatening, blood loss can be extensive and transfusions are sometimes required.

Secondary procedures to free tendon adhesions, reduce bulky flaps, and transfer tendons in motor nerve injuries may need to be done. Reconstruction of unsuccessful replantations are being done more often. The original method using toes to reconstruct thumbs has also been used to make fingers. These reconstructions give patients the ability to grasp objects. Because these digits are sensate, they can even perform fine movement tasks not possible with prosthetic devices. Patients with loss only of the thumb are better treated with transfer of the index finger to the thumb position (pollicization).

Partial or total loss of a single digit is less critical. Hand function is better without a stiff or painful digit. When a decision is made to amputate a digit, care must be taken to leave a painless stump with good sensate soft tissue coverage. The flexor tendon must not be sutured to the extensor tendon for soft tissue coverage since this will cause the tendons to pull each other rather than move the joint. Local flaps to cover the stump are preferred to skin grafts or cross finger flaps since they usually provide better sensation. A short amputation stump on the long or ring finger is often bothersome since small objects such as coins tend to fall out of the palm, and a ray amputation eliminates the problem. For cosmetic purposes, ray amputations are far less noticeable than partial amputations. The loss of hand breadth with a ray amputation can decrease grip strength, however.

The loss of part of all of the hand can be compensated both functionally and cosmetically by a variety of prostheses. Their use involves careful adaptation to the requirements of the patient, who must receive appropriate training to ensure success.

INJECTION INJURIES OF THE HAND

High-pressure devices used in industry to apply material such as air, grease, paint, and oil cause a unique hand injury. The typical case is injection of the material into the index finger of the nondominant hand of a factory worker. A pinpoint injection site may be the only external evidence of injury, and the hand appears discolored or pale, or swollen due to the injected material.

The examination should include a careful hand evaluation and an x-ray to demonstrate the distribution of material or gas in the hand. All such cases require continued unrelenting scrutiny, even if the part seems completely normal. If there is any evidence of retained foreign material, swelling, or ischemia, early surgical exploration is advocated to release the tourniquet effect of the skin and fascia and to remove as much of the material as possible without injuring healthy tissue. Prophylactic antisludging agents (dextran 40), corticosteroids, and antibiotics may help.

Often the pressure forces the material to spread along the tendon sheaths throughout the hand and even into the forearm. Expansion of the foreign material in a closed space and the chemical irritation cause congestion, inflammation, vascular thrombosis, and gangrene. The injected material is difficult to remove completely, and a foreign body response leads to fibrosis so extensive that it often destroys the function of the hand.

Buncke HJ Jr: Microvascular hand surgery—transplants and replants—over the past 25 years. J Hand Surg [Am] 2000; 25:415.

Das De S, Tai LS, Pho RW: Emergency repair and reconstruction in the severely crushed hand. World J Surg 1991;15:470.

Goldner RD et al: One hundred eleven thumb amputations: replantation vs revision. Microsurgery 1990;11:243.

Lewis HG et al: A 10-year review of high-pressure injection injuries to the hand. J Hand Surg [Br] 1998;23:479.

Partington MT et al: Unrecognized injuries in patients referred for emergency microsurgery. J Trauma 1993;34:238.

Reigstad A et al: Free flaps in the reconstruction of hand and distal forearm injuries. J Hand Surg [Br] 1992;17:185.

■ MINIMALLY INVASIVE HAND SURGERY

The goal of reconstructive hand surgery is return of normal function, including pain-free movement, normal active and passive range of motion, premorbid strength, and intact sensation. Yet the process of incising, dissecting, and sewing is associated with significant scarring and pain. Scarring is especially troublesome in the hand since it leads to stiffness, ligamental tightening, and arthritis. As a result, any procedure in the hand that minimizes postoperative scarring or pain will contribute to an improved result.

Surgical care in the past decade has been revolutionized by the introduction and incorporation of minimally invasive surgical techniques. Laparoscopies and thoracoscopies have permitted the resection of hollow and solid organs through 1 cm incisions, reducing the need for laparotomies and thoracotomies. Likewise, urologists have employed cystoscopy for evaluation and treatment of bladder and kidney disorders, while orthopedic surgeons have used arthroscopy to similar effective ends in the knee, ankle, elbow, and shoulder.

Two areas of hand surgery incorporate minimally invasive techniques: Wrist arthroscopy has expanded the options for evaluating the chronically painful wrist, and endoscopic carpal tunnel release (ECTR) provides a less invasive method than open release for decompressing the median nerve. While ECTR theoretically allows for a faster recovery, it may in fact offer only limited advantages.

WRIST ARTHROSCOPY

Diagnostic wrist arthroscopy was first successfully used in 1970. Over the past 3 decades, it has taken its place among traditional imaging techniques as a low-morbidity method for evaluating chronic wrist pain. As the hardware for examining the wrist has become more sophisticated and as hand surgeons have become more familiar with the arthroscopic view of the wrist, increasingly aggressive attempts have been made to use the arthroscope to treat as well as to diagnose wrist problems.

Indications & Contraindications

Diagnostic wrist arthroscopy is a useful technique to evaluate patients with wrist pain, whether chronic or acute. In patients with chronic pain, this technique can be used to augment information offered by plain radiographs, CT, MRI, or wrist arthrography. It can confirm an uncertain diagnosis or be used to reevaluate a patient who has failed other treatments. In contrast, patients with acute symptoms—such as those suffering from mechanical wrist pain—may complain of pain localized over the joint, catching and popping sensations, and relief with rest. Here, the wrist can be manipulated during arthroscopy to localize the source of the symptoms. In general, the technique is useful for evaluating articular cartilage, ligaments, the triangular fibrocartilage complex (TFCC), and the synovium. Interestingly, diagnostic wrist arthroscopy may provide too comprehensive an examination. Only some of the lesions that are visualized during an examination may be responsible for a patient's symptoms. The hand surgeon must critically correlate arthroscopic findings with the patient's examination to arrive at the appropriate diagnosis.

Therapeutic wrist arthroscopy is useful for the treatment of ligament tears, TFCC lesions, articular cartilage lesions, subtle distal radius and carpus fractures, dorsal wrist ganglions, removal of isolated carpal bones up to and including the proximal carpal row, and disorders of the distal radioulnar joint. It is useful also in the management of lesions arising from rheumatoid arthritis. It has been successfully used in completing synovectomies, proximal row carpectomies in the case of scaphoid nonunion or scapholunate collapse, radial styloidectomy, and isolated symptomatic chondral defects.

Procedure

Equipment for diagnostic wrist arthroscopy includes an apparatus for elevating and distracting the wrist, an arthroscopic telescope, a video camera, a fluid infusion system, and both manual and powered instruments.

Either general or regional anesthesia may be used. A tourniquet is placed at the mid arm to provide a blood-free field during the operation. The distal forearm, wrist, and hand are prepared into the operative field. Traction is applied to the hand, usually via sterile finger traps, and a distraction force is applied across the wrist.

Individual skin incisions are then made at standard portal sites determined by the goal of the operation. Portal sites are described according to their relationship with the radius and ulna, the carpal bones, and the extensor tendons. The relationship to the extensor tendons is indicated by listing the extensor compartments on either side of the incision. Typical portals include the 3–4 radiocarpal, through which the scaphoid and lunate facets can be visualized; the 4–5 radiocarpal, through which the TFCC and the ulnocarpal ligaments can be seen; and the 6R radiocarpal, through which the extensor carpi ulnaris tendon and ulnar wrist are approached. The midcarpal joint is approached through any of three portals, including the midcarpal ulnar, the midcarpal radial, and the scaphotrapezial-trapezoid.

Once abnormalities are identified, therapeutic wrist arthroscopy can be used to effect repairs. Partial ligament tears and tears of the TFCC can be debrided arthroscopically using knife blades and motorized shavers. Carpal bone resections can be completed with miniature osteotomes and powered saw blades.

Outcomes

Operations employing diagnostic and therapeutic wrist arthroscopy typically result in less swelling, less postoperative pain, and less stiffness than comparable open wrist procedures. There is a concomitant earlier return to function and work. Therapeutic wrist arthroscopy even of dorsal wrist ganglia, the most superficial of wrist abnormalities, is followed by fewer—or no more—recurrences than the open technique.

Complications

The rate of complications associated with diagnostic and therapeutic wrist arthroscopy is estimated to be 2% and is due to a variety of causes. The continuous traction nec-

essary to properly distract the wrist can cause problems, including ligamental strain at the MCP joints with concomitant joint edema and stiffness and stretching of peripheral nerves. Establishment of the operative portals can damage articular cartilage, ligaments, tendons, cutaneous nerves, the radial artery, and cutaneous and deep veins. Such injuries include abrasions, contusions, lacerations, and transections. A high proportion of complications of therapeutic wrist arthroscopy are associated with inadequate relief of symptoms or a diminished return of function. A now less common complication of therapeutic wrist arthroscopy results from the fluid infusion. Forearm compartment syndromes have resulted from extravasation of infusion fluid during endoscopic repair of distal radius fractures; this problem is now avoided by circumferential compression of the forearm during the procedure.

ENDOSCOPIC CARPAL TUNNEL RELEASE

Endoscopic release of the transverse carpal ligament is an increasingly popular method of treating carpal tunnel syndrome. Advocates of the procedure claim that it is associated with decreased postoperative morbidity and earlier return to work. Others caution that there is little if any short-term difference between endoscopic and open carpal tunnel release, no long-term difference, and that endoscopic carpal tunnel release is associated with an increased likelihood of significant nerve injury.

Indications & Contraindications

Endoscopic carpal tunnel release is easier to perform in patients with larger wrists. Ease of access to the carpal tunnel correlates with the wrist circumference and the height and age of patients. Surgeons should be aware that the procedure is likely to be more difficult in small patients with small wrists and are advised to maintain a lower threshold for conversion to the open technique to avoid neurologic complications.

Absolute contraindications to endoscopic carpal tunnel release include masses in the carpal canal and other space-occupying lesions, abnormalities in canal anatomy, and wrist stiffness that precludes proper positioning.

Procedure

In the United States, most surgeons use one of two techniques—either Chow or Agee. The two differ primarily in the number of incisions, or portals, needed to gain access. The Chow technique, first described in 1989, employs two portals while the Agee technique requires only one.

Either operation can be performed under local anesthesia with a brachial tourniquet. An initial transverse incision is made proximal to the wrist flexion crease between the palmaris longus and flexor carpi ulnaris tendons. The space between the transverse carpal ligament and the flexor tendons is defined with a dissector. In the Agee procedure, the endoscope is advanced under the transverse carpal ligament, radial to the hook of the hamate along the axis of the ring finger. The ligament is incised along its entire length, with care taken to avoid Guyon's canal and the superficial palmar arch. In the Chow operation, a second transverse incision is made just distal to the transverse carpal ligament along the axis of the ring finger. The wrist is dorsiflexed and a slotted cannula is advanced into the proximal incision, deep to the transverse carpal ligament, and out the distal incision. The endoscope is then used to visualize the ligament while the knife divides it. The wounds are closed, and the patient's wrist placed in dorsiflexion.

Outcomes

Several studies have compared open versus endoscopic carpal tunnel release, focusing upon the incidence of recovery from symptoms, the time span until the patient returns to work, and the incidence of recurrence of symptoms. Overall, both techniques have equivalent outcomes.

Many of the most convincing studies are prospective randomized trials. One such study, comparing open and endoscopic carpal tunnel release among 32 hands in 29 patients, found no difference in postoperative recovery time or surgical result. The only significant difference noted by the authors was transient numbness on the radial side of the ring finger in three endoscopic carpal tunnel release patients.

In another study, the authors compared in a prospective randomized manner the early outcome of carpal tunnel release using either a conventional open carpal tunnel release procedure in 40 patients or a two-portal endoscopic release in 56 patients. They found no statistically significant difference between the groups in postoperative pain, recovery from paresthesias, or time taken to return to work. However, the endoscopic group demonstrated better grip strength recovery at 1 and 3 months. No surgical complications were observed in either group.

Nonrandomized studies have supported this trend. An analysis of 191 consecutive patients undergoing carpal tunnel release with an average 2-year follow-up showed that none of the patients undergoing open release had a recurrence, while 7% of patients undergoing endoscopic release had recurrences. Another study observed a higher incidence of incomplete release of the carpal tunnel with endoscopic techniques than with standard open releases.

The factors identified with poor outcomes in endoscopic carpal tunnel release are similar to those seen in open release. Less satisfactory results were present in workers' compensation cases; patients with normal motor latencies on nerve conduction studies; patients with preoperative hand weakness, widened two-point discrimination, myofascial pain syndrome, or fibromyalgia; and patients involved in litigation, those with multiple compressive neuropathies, and those with abnormal psychologic factors.

Complications

Only a limited number of studies include a sufficient number of patients to compare complication rates and type between endoscopic and open carpal tunnel release. Overall, the types and rates of complications between the two forms of release are similar. Nonetheless, isolated but severe complications from endoscopic release over the past decade tend to dramatize its risk.

The study by Boeckstyns and Sorensen is perhaps the most comprehensive to date. These authors analyzed 54 published series of endoscopic and open releases comprising 9516 and 1203 patients, respectively. Irreversible nerve damage from the procedure occurred in 0.3% of endoscopic and 0.2% of open releases, including such injuries as transection of the median nerve. While reversible nerve injuries were more common with endoscopic release than with open release (4.4% versus 0.9%, respectively, among prospective controlled and randomized studies), tendon lesions, reflex sympathetic dystrophy, hematoma, and wound problems were equally common with either technique.

A less compelling analysis—a retrospective survey of hand surgeons who had performed either open or endoscopic carpal tunnel release over the preceding 5 years—found major complications with either approach, including median nerve lacerations, ulnar nerve lacerations, digital nerve lacerations, vessel lacerations, and tendon lacerations. While the authors could not reach a conclusion about the rate of complications for one procedure versus the other, their results demonstrate the potentially devastating sequelae of carpal tunnel release even in experienced hands.

Carpal tunnel symptoms may persist or recur following either open or endoscopic release. In patients who have persistent symptoms following endoscopic release, many authors recommend open carpal tunnel release as definitive therapy.

Pediatric Surgery

Craig T. Albanese, MD, Roman M. Sydorak, MD, & Michael R. Harrison, MD

The surgical care of children differs markedly from that of the adult in that children have unique physiologic demands that vary according to age and stage of maturation. The neonate's physiologic development is nearer to that of a fetus, while adolescents are more similar to adults in that respect. Infants and children also suffer from congenital abnormalities and diseases not seen in adults, and their management requires intimate understanding of embryology and pathogenesis.

NEWBORN CARE

Neonatal Intensive Care

The newborn infant with a surgically correctable lesion often has other disorders that threaten survival. The care of these babies—particularly the premature and small-for-gestational-age babies, has improved with the emergence of the intensive care nursery. Dramatic advances have been made in the technology of infant monitoring and respiratory support. Tiny babies can now receive ventilatory support from sophisticated infant respirators for prolonged periods in a precisely controlled microenvironment. Temperature is controlled by servoregulation, while pulse and blood pressure are continuously recorded. Ventilation is monitored by transcutaneous O_2 and CO_2 electrodes or by indwelling arterial catheters. The metabolic consequences of prematurity and intrauterine growth retardation are monitored by frequent measurement of glucose, calcium, electrolytes, and bilirubin in microliter quantities of blood. Nutritional requirements for growth and development can be provided by enteral or parenteral routes. This kind of specialized care of critically ill newborns requires trained personnel and specialized equipment. The care of such babies is best accomplished in designated regional centers capable of providing pediatric surgical and neonatal intensive care.

Phibbs CS et al: The effects of patient volume and level of care at the hospital of birth on neonatal mortality. JAMA 1996;276:1054.

Classification

Newborn infants can be classified according to their level of maturation (gestational age) and development (weight). A normal full-term infant has a gestational age of 38–42 weeks and a body weight between the 10th and 90th percentiles for the given gestational age, usually greater than 2500 g. The gestational age of the infant is calculated from the date of the last normal menstrual period. Clinical assessment of gestational age by morphologic and neurologic examination of the small infant is often more accurate than calculation from the menstrual history.

Four signs may be useful in assessing gestational age. Infants of 36 weeks' gestational age or less have (1) fine fuzzy hair with thin, semitransparent skin, (2) ears that lack cartilaginous support, (3) a breast nodule less than 3 mm in diameter, and (4) few transverse creases on the balls of the feet anteriorly. In males, the testicles are in the inguinal canal and the scrotum is small with few rugae. In females, the labia minora are relatively enlarged and the labia majora are small.

Premature infants are those born before 38 weeks of gestation with body weights appropriate for that age. Several physiologic abnormalities exist in preterm infants. Apneic and bradycardic episodes are common and may occur spontaneously or as nonspecific signs of problems such as sepsis or hypothermia. The lungs and retinas of preterm infants are very susceptible to high oxygen levels, and even relatively brief exposures to high oxygen concentrations may result in various degrees of lung damage (hyaline membrane disease) and retinopathy of prematurity. Shunting across a patent ductus arteriosus or foramen ovale is not uncommon. The premature infant may be unable to tolerate oral feeding due to a weak suck reflex, and intragastric tube feeds or total parenteral nutrition may be required. Preterm infants have increased requirements for glucose, calcium, and sodium as well as a propensity for hypothermia, impaired bilirubin metabolism, intraventricular hemorrhage, polycythemia, and metabolic acidosis. These problems are accentuated in low-birth-weight infants (birth weight between 1500 g and 2500 g), very low birthweight infants (birth weight less than 1500 g), and "micropremie" infants (birth weight less than 1000 g).

A small-for-gestational age (SGA) infant is greater than 38 weeks' gestation but less than the tenth percentile in weight for that gestational age. This term differs slightly from the more often used term intrauterine growth retardation (IUGR), which is defined as birth weight below the 25th percentile for a given gestational age. An SGA infant is the product of a pregnancy complicated by any one of several placental, maternal, or fetal abnormalities. Although body weight is low, the body length and head circumference of the SGA infant are age-appropriate. Compared with the premature infant of equivalent weight, the SGA infant is older and developmentally more mature and faces different physiologic problems. Intrauterine malnutrition results in a relative lack of body fat and decreased glycogen stores and, coupled with the relatively large surface area and high metabolic rate, greatly predisposes these newborns to hypothermia and hypoglycemia. SGA infants also have an increased risk of meconium aspiration syndrome. Polycythemia is common and necessitates close monitoring of hematocrits to avoid problems related to hyperviscosity. Because of the adequate length of gestation, retinopathy of prematurity, intraventricular hemorrhage, and hyaline membrane disease are relatively uncommon.

Temperature Regulation

Infants and children are susceptible to heat loss because they have a relatively greater body surface area and a thinner subcutaneous fat layer compared with adults. Heat loss occurring by conduction, convection, evaporation, and radiation is four times that of the adult and may be further increased by prematurity. Heat is generated not by shivering but by metabolizing brown fat reserves (nonshivering thermogenesis). This has practical consequences since brown fat may be rendered inactive by pressors or anesthetic agents and may be depleted by poor nutritional intake. Exposure to cold environments increases metabolic work and caloric consumption. Due to limited energy reserves, prolonged exposure to cold can lead to hypothermia. Resultant catecholamine secretion increases the metabolic rate (particularly in the myocardium) and produces vasoconstriction with impaired tissue perfusion and increased lactic acid production.

It is important to maintain the sick newborn in its optimal thermal environment (thermoneutrality). This is the ambient temperature in which a baby, at a minimal metabolic cost, can maintain a constant and normal body temperature by vasomotor control. To attain such an environment, the gradient between the skin surface and the environmental temperature must be less than 1.5 °C. As the skin surface temperature averages 35.5 °C, the optimal environmental temperature is 34 °C (slightly higher for premature infants). The neonate's environmental temperature is best controlled by placing the infant in an incubator. Either the ambient temperature of the incu-

bator can be monitored and maintained at thermoneutrality, or a servo system can be used. The latter regulates the incubator temperature according to the infant's skin or rectal temperature. Heat loss may be further reduced by wrapping the head, extremities, and as much of the trunk as possible in wadding, plastic wrap, plastic sheets, or aluminum foil.

In the operating room, the temperature of the infant must be continuously recorded by placing a thermistor in the rectum or esophagus. Body heat may be conserved by wrapping the extremities with sheet wadding and by using a circulating heating pad and infrared lamp, but these measures are often not sufficient in small infants. The operating room should be prewarmed and the temperature kept at about 20–27 °C. Wet sponges and drapes exaggerate evaporative heat losses. Plastic drapes against the skin help contain body heat and keep the skin dry. When large volumes of blood are required, the blood should be warmed by circulating it through tubing immersed in warm water or should be prewarmed in the container before being transfused. One of the most effective means of regulating body temperature is to heat and humidify the gases during endotracheal anesthesia.

Albanese CT, Nour BM, Rowe MI: Anesthesia blocks nonshivering thermogenesis in the neonatal rabbit. J Pediatr Surg 1994; 29:983.

Nesher N et al: A novel thermoregulatory system maintains perioperative normothermia in children undergoing elective surgery. Paediatr Anaesth 2000;11:555.

Sauer PJ, Dane HJ, Visser HK: New standards for neutral thermal environment of healthy very low birth weight infants in week one of life. Arch Dis Child 1984;59:18.

Ventilation

Assisted ventilation is often necessary because of underlying disease, medications that affect the central control of respiration (eg, opioids, PGE_2), or due to physiologic changes imposed by a surgical procedure (eg, tight closure of an abdominal wall defect). At birth, the pharynx should be aspirated of mucus, amniotic fluid, or meconium. Respirations should be assisted or controlled with bag and mask. Prolonged respiratory support may require endotracheal intubation. The diameter of the tube should approximate that of the little finger or the nostril, usually between 2.5 and 4 mm. The trachea from the glottis to the carina in the newborn is 7.5 cm long, and placement of the tube into the right or left bronchus must be avoided. An orotracheal tube is preferred to a nasotracheal one to minimize trauma and subsequent infection in the nasal passages. For infants, optimal tube placement can be estimated as follows: 7 cm from the lips in a 1 kg infant; 8 cm in a 2 kg infant; and 9 cm in a 3 kg infant. Once placed, the endotracheal tube is firmly fixed in place and connected to either a modern infant ventilator or a system for continuous positive airway pressure (CPAP) breathing. A small air leak between the endotracheal tube and the airway usually exists and helps minimize laryngeal trauma.

Most infant ventilators are time-cycled flow generators capable of delivering both CPAP and intermittent mandatory ventilation (IMV). IMV is a synthesis of simple mechanical ventilation and CPAP breathing that allows the baby to breathe independently between mandatory breaths provided by the ventilator while a continuous positive pressure is maintained on the airway. CPAP breathing helps keep the terminal airways open and is particularly useful when alveolar collapse develops, such as in hyaline membrane disease or with persistent atelectasis.

The gas mixture flowing into the system should be carefully controlled by an air-oxygen mixing device, and the inspired oxygen concentration should be regulated to maintain the arterial P_{O_2} at 60–80 mm Hg. The gas should be humidified by using a heated nebulizer. Absorption of fluid in the lung may be considerable, and parenteral fluid may have to be restricted. When the arterial P_{O_2} exceeds 80 mm Hg, the inspired oxygen concentration is gradually lowered toward room air, the end-expiratory pressure is lowered to 2 mm Hg, and the rate of IMV is then gradually decreased. In this way, the baby is gradually weaned from oxygen and mechanical ventilation, but CPAP of at least 2 mm Hg should be maintained until the endotracheal tube can finally be removed. Upon removal of the tube, the inspired oxygen concentration should be increased to 10% greater than that during the period of assistance until ventilation becomes normal.

In severe respiratory compromise (eg, congenital diaphragmatic hernia, meconium aspiration), more complex ventilatory strategies are called for. High-frequency ventilation (jet and oscillatory modes) utilizes low tidal volumes at high rates (up to 600 breaths/min) to minimize the deleterious effects of high airway pressure. If this mode of ventilation is ineffective, oxygenation and gas exchange can be accomplished using extracorporeal membrane oxygenation. This temporary bypass unit oxygenates the blood through an external circuit as the lungs are left to mature or recover from the underlying disease process. The use of perfluorocarbons or partial liquid ventilation is being investigated.

Hemmila MR, Hirschl RB: Advances in ventilatory support of the pediatric surgical patient. Curr Opin Pediatr 1999;11:241.

Fluids & Electrolytes

Effective fluid and electrolyte management involves (1) calculating the fluid and electrolyte requirements for maintaining metabolic functions, (2) replacing losses (evaporative, third space, external), and (3) considering preexisting fluid deficits or excesses. Taking these factors into consideration, a tentative program is devised for fluid and electrolyte administration. The patient's response is monitored, and the program is adjusted accordingly.

Monitoring fluid status and acid-base balance can be accomplished by both noninvasive and invasive means. Commonly used noninvasive devices in the operating room and intensive care units include pulse oximetry, transcutaneous CO_2 monitoring, and sphygmomanometry. For critically ill infants, more invasive means are necessary to assess homeostasis. Blood gas analysis via heelstick or arterial catheter is frequently employed. Polyvinyl catheters can be placed through the umbilical artery into the distal aorta with the tip of the catheter positioned at L4 and confirmed radiographically. Indwelling arterial catheters can also be placed in the radial or temporal arteries, either percutaneously or by incision. Blood pressure may be recorded by connecting the catheter to a strain gauge and recorder. Central venous access may assist in cases where monitoring of fluid status, parenteral nutrition, or frequent blood sampling is necessary.

A. Calculating Maintenance Needs

In the newborn infant, the basic maintenance requirement of water is the volume required for growth, renal excretion (renal water), and replacement of losses from the skin, lungs, and stool. Requirements during the first day of life are unique because of the greatly expanded extracellular fluid volume in the newborn baby, which decreases after 24 hours. For example, infants born with intestinal obstruction (eg, intestinal atresia) are not hypovolemic as a result of fluid adjustments across the placenta. In fact, 5–10% of a newborn infant's birth weight is lost in the first 3–7 days; the majority is water loss, with minor contributions from meconium, vernix, and urine. During the first 24 hours of life, basic maintenance fluid should not exceed 90 mL/kg/d in preterm infants weighing less than 1000 g or of less than 32 weeks' gestation, or 65 mL/kg/d in larger infants. This requirement gradually increases to 80 mL/kg/d by 4 days of life in normal infants. For children and adolescents, the most commonly used method of calculating fluid requirements is based on body weight (Table 46–1). However, because of the many factors affecting maintenance requirements, there is no close or constant relationship between body weight and fluid and electrolyte needs.

B. Perioperative Fluid Management

In the surgical patient, fluid, serum electrolyte, and acid-base abnormalities are corrected before operation

Table 46–1. Calculation of maintenance fluid requirements.[1]

Body Weight	Fluid Volume per 24 h
1–10 kg	100 mL/kg
11–20 kg	1000 mL + 50 mL for each kg over 10 kg
> 20 kg	1500 mL + 20 mL for each kg over 20 kg

[1]Reproduced with permission from Albanese CT: Pediatric surgery. In: *Surgery.* Norton JA (editor). Springer, 2000.

except when immediate emergency surgery is necessary. Intraoperative fluid requirements consist of the estimated maintenance requirement plus replacement of preexisting deficits (if uncorrected) plus replacement of estimated intraoperative and electrolyte losses, including blood. The need for intraoperative blood transfusion is determined by the child's clinical condition, pulse, blood pressure, hematocrit, and urine output in relation to measured losses in sponges and suction bottles.

Postoperatively, external losses from intestinal drainage and fistulas are directly measured and replaced volume for volume with an appropriate electrolyte solution (Table 46–2). In neonates, it is wise to measure the electrolytes in the fluid to more accurately guide replacement. Protein-rich losses (eg, from chest tubes) can be replaced with colloid such as an albumin solution or fresh frozen plasma. Internal losses into body cavities or tissues (third space losses) cannot be measured, and adequate replacement of these losses de-

pends on careful monitoring of the patient's vital signs and urine output. Following an operation such as a laparotomy or thoracotomy, the fluid requirement may exceed 150 mL/kg/d for several days postoperatively.

C. ELECTROLYTE CONSIDERATIONS

The basic electrolyte and energy requirements are provided by sodium chloride, 2–3 meq/kg/d (up to 5 meq/kg/d for preterm infants) in 5% or 10% dextrose, with the addition of potassium, 2–3 meq/kg/d, once urine production has been established. Calcium gluconate (200–400 mg/kg/d) may be added, especially in preterm infants. Additional electrolytes such as bicarbonate and magnesium may be added according to the blood chemistry results.

Many stressed newborn infants develop low blood levels of potassium, calcium, magnesium, and glucose. A deficiency of any one of these will produce such signs as vomiting, abdominal distention, poor feeding, apneic spells, cyanosis, limpness, eye rolling, high-pitched cry, tremors, or convulsions. Convulsions and tetany due to hypocalcemia should be treated with intravenous 10% calcium solution given at a rate of 1 mL/min while the ECG is carefully monitored. Although hypocalcemia can be largely eliminated by adding calcium salts to intravenous solutions, caution is required since subcutaneous infiltration may produce severe vasoconstriction and skin necrosis. If there is no response to correction of a documented calcium deficiency, hypomagnesemia should be suspected and a serum magnesium level obtained.

Rapid determination of the blood glucose level can be done in the neonatal unit with blood glucose reagent

Table 46–2. Replacement of abnormal losses of fluids and electrolytes.

Type of Fluid	Electrolyte Content				Replacement
	Na⁺ (meq/L)	K⁺ (meq/L)	Cl⁻ (meq/L)	HCO₃⁻ (meq/L)	

Type of Fluid	Na^+ (meq/L)	K^+ (meq/L)	Cl^- (meq/L)	HCO_3^- (meq/L)	Replacement
Gastric (vomiting)	50(20–90)	10(4–15)	90(50–150)	...	5% Dextrose in half-normal (0.45%) saline plus KCl 20–40 meq/L
Small bowel (ileostomy)	110(70–140)	5(3–10)	100(70–130)	20(10–40)	Lactated Ringer's
Diarrhea	80(10–140)	25(10–60)	90(20–120)	40(30–50)	Lactated Ringer's with or without HCO_3^-
Bile	145(130–160)	5(4–7)	100(80–120)	40(30–50)	Lactated Ringer's with or without HCO_3^-
Pancreatic	140(130–150)	5(4–7)	80(60–100)	80(60–110)	Lactated Ringer's with or without HCO_3^-
Sweat					
Normal	20(10–30)	4(3–10)	20(10–40)	...	...
Cystic fibrosis	90(50–130)	15(5–25)	90(60–120)	...	...

strips. This may be correlated at intervals with serum glucose determinations, the frequency depending on the stability of the infant. Intravenous fluids should contain a minimum of 10% dextrose, and if non-dextrose-containing solutions such as blood or plasma are being administered, close monitoring of the blood glucose level is essential. The treatment of hypoglycemia consists of giving 50% glucose, 1–2 mL/kg intravenously, followed by a continuous infusion of 10–15% glucose solutions at a rate equivalent to that needed for maintenance water requirements.

Coran A, Drongowski R: Body fluid compartment changes following neonatal surgery. J Pediatr Surg 1989;24:829.

Statter MB: Fluids and electrolytes in infants and children. Semin Pediatr Surg 1992;1:208.

Nutrition

Newborns require a relatively large caloric intake because of their high basal metabolic rate, caloric requirements for growth and development, energy needs to maintain body heat, and limited energy reserve. An infant requires calories at a rate of 100–130 kcal/kg/d and protein at a rate of 2–3 g/kg/d to achieve a normal weight gain of 10–15 g/kg/d (Table 46–3). Thirty to 40 percent of the total nonprotein calories should be provided as fat. These requirements decline with age but increase with sepsis, stress, and trauma. Caloric requirements are increased 10–25% by surgery, more than 50% by infection, and 100% by burns.

A. ENTERAL ALIMENTATION

The best means of providing calories and protein is through the gastrointestinal tract. If the gastrointestinal tract is functional, standard infant formulas, blender-

Table 46–3. Caloric requirements of various age groups per 24 hours.[1]

Age	kcal/kg per 24 hours
Newborn term (0–4 days)	110–120
Low birth weight	120–130
3–4 months	100–106
5–12 months	100
1–7 years	75–90
7–12 years	60–75
12–18 years	30–60

[1]Reproduced, with permission, from Albanese CT: Pediatric surgery. In: *Surgery.* Norton JA (editor). Springer, 2000.

ized meals, or prepared elemental diets can be given by mouth, through nasogastric or nasojejunal feeding tubes, or through gastrostomy or jejunostomy tubes placed surgically. Gastric feeding is preferable because it allows for normal digestive processes and hormonal responses, a greater tolerance for larger osmotic loads, and a lower incidence of dumping. The use of nasoduodenal or nasojejunal tubes is reserved for infants who cannot tolerate intragastric feeding (eg, delayed gastric emptying, gastroesophageal reflux, depressed gag reflex).

The availability of nutritionally complete liquid diets of low viscosity allows continuous feeding through small-diameter catheters. Elemental diets made by mixing crystalline amino acids, oligosaccharides, and fats can be completely absorbed in the small intestine with little residue. Their use is limited because they cause diarrhea as a result of the high osmolality of full-strength formulas. This can be avoided by administering dilute solutions by continuous drip. Initially, the volume of dilute solution is gradually increased, and the concentration is then progressively increased in a stepwise fashion—ie, half strength, three-fourths strength, and full strength. Formulas that remain below 500 mosm are best.

Small Silastic or polyethylene catheters such as those used for intravenous infusion can be passed through the nose or mouth into the stomach or jejunum (length: tip of nose to knee) and are well tolerated for long periods. In more complex cases, a surgically placed gastrostomy or jejunostomy may be necessary for postoperative feeding. A variety of techniques and methods are employed in their construction. In the case of a gastrostomy, either a low-profile balloon is used (ie, Foley or Malecott) or a gastrostomy button is placed. Silastic is superior to other plastics because it does not become more rigid when exposed to intestinal contents. Parenteral nutrition combined with enteral feeding is often necessary for infants with short bowel syndrome until intestinal adaptation occurs.

B. PARENTERAL ALIMENTATION

The indications for parenteral alimentation include the following: (1) expected period of prolonged ileus, eg, following repair of gastroschisis or jejunal atresia; (2) intestinal fistulas; (3) supplementation of oral feedings, as in intractable diarrhea, short bowel syndrome, or various malabsorption syndromes; (4) intrauterine growth retardation; (5) catabolic wasting states such as infections or tumors when gastric feedings are inadequate; (6) inflammatory bowel disease; (7) severe acute alimentary disorders (pancreatitis, necrotizing enterocolitis); and (8) chylothorax.

Concentrated solutions (15% glucose or more) thrombose peripheral vessels. Placement of a catheter into the superior vena cava or right atrium allows the large blood flow to dilute the solution immediately. The catheter may be placed percutaneously through the subclavian or internal jugular vein or inserted by cutdown over the external jugular, anterior facial, internal jugular, cephalic, or brachial vein. Tunneling the catheter subcutaneously with a separate exit point on the chest wall may decrease the risk of infection. For long-term use, Broviac or Hickman catheters, with Dacron cuffs positioned near the exit site of the skin, are preferred to minimize infection and to prevent accidental dislodgment.

Intravenous alimentation solutions containing an amino acid source (2–5% crystalline amino acids or protein hydrolysate), glucose (10–40%), electrolytes, vitamins, and trace minerals are used. The electrolyte composition of the protein solution should be known so that the desired composition of the final solution can be adjusted by appropriate additives according to the individual patient's requirements. A standard solution suitable for infants and young children must contain calcium, magnesium, and phosphate to allow for growth. Trace minerals are also added to the basic solution (Table 46–4). These solutions should be infused at a constant rate with an infusion pump to avoid blood

backing up the catheter and clotting and to prevent wide fluctuations of blood glucose and amino acid concentrations. If it is necessary to restrict the volume of infusion, more concentrated glucose solutions can be used to increase the caloric intake.

Complications of prolonged intravenous alimentation are numerous. The most frequent problem is catheter sepsis. Although catheter removal will quickly treat the problem, a trial of antibiotics effective against gram-positive and gram-negative pathogens is indicated. Catheter removal is indicated in the presence of worsening sepsis, three positive blood cultures, or documented yeast infection (with antifungal treatment after catheter removal). Clotting in the catheter may be controlled by adding 1 unit of heparin per milliliter of solution. Emphasis on a constant rate of infusion will minimize hyper- or hypoglycemia. Analysis of serum electrolytes (including calcium and phosphate) may be necessary several times a week initially, but the interval is decreased to once a week when the patient is stable. Patients must be observed for hyperammonemia and for vitamin or trace mineral deficiency. Progressive hepatomegaly and jaundice of uncertain origin can occur after prolonged parenteral alimentation. This syndrome usually subsides when the parenteral solution is discontinued or when it is

Table 46–4. Total parenteral nutrition requirements.[1]

Component	Neonate	6 mo to 10 yr	>10 yr
Calories (kcal/kg/d)	90–120	60–105	40–75
Fluid (mL/kg/d)	120–180	120–150	50–75
Dextrose (mg/kg/min)	4–6	7–8	7–8
Protein (g/kg/d)	2–3	1.5–2.5	0.8–2.0
Fat (g/kg/d)0.5–3.0	1.0–4.0	1.0–4.0	
Sodium (meq/kg/d)	3–4	3–4	3–4
Potassium (meq/kg/d)	2–3	2–3	1–2
Calcium (mg/kg/d)	80–120	40–80	40–60
Phosphate (mg/kg/d)	25–40	25–40	25–40
Magnesium (meq/kg/d)	0.25–1.0	0.5	0.5
Zinc (µg/kg/d)	300	100	3 mg/d
Copper (µg/kg/d)	20	20	1.2 mg/d
Chromium (µg/kg/d)	0.2	0.2	12 mg/d
Manganese (µg/kg/d)	6	6	0.3 mg/d
Selenium (mg/kg/d)	2	2	10–20 mg/d

[1]Reproduced, with permission, from Albanese CT: Pediatric surgery. In: *Surgery*. Norton JA (editor). Springer, 2000.

infused for a period of 12–16 hours and then the infusion is stopped for 8–12 hours (cycling).

Amii LA, Moss RL: Nutritional support of the pediatric surgical patient. Curr Opin Pediatr 1999;11:237.

Holcomb GW 3d, Ziegler MM Jr: Nutrition and cancer in children. Surg Annu 1990;2:129.

Pereira GR: Nutritional care of the extremely premature infant. Clin Perinat 1994;22:61.

Winthrop A et al: Analysis of energy and macronutrient balance in the postoperative infant. J Pediatr Surg 1989;24:686.

Blood Loss

The blood volume of a newborn infant ranges from 50 mL to 100 mL per kilogram body weight (average, 85 mL/kg). This wide variation is due principally to the timing and technique of clamping the umbilical cord. Several hours after birth, plasma shifts out of the circulation and total blood volume and plasma volume decrease. By 1 month of age, premature and full-term infants have a blood volume of approximately 75 mL/kg.

Although not clinically significant, both the prothrombin time and the partial thromboplastin time may be slightly prolonged at birth due to relative deficiencies of clotting factors. Defects in the coagulating mechanism may occur in newborn infants as a result of vitamin K deficiency, thrombocytopenia, inherited disorders, and temporary hepatic insufficiency due to immaturity, asphyxia, or infection.

The blood lost during operation varies greatly according to the extent of the operative procedure, the disease being treated, and the effectiveness of hemostasis. Mild blood loss, amounting to less than 10% of the blood volume, usually does not require transfusion. In a 3.5 kg infant, mild blood loss would be an amount up to 30 mL. Because blood loss greater than 10% should be corrected and because these volumes are quite small, it is imperative to develop methods for closely monitoring the amount of blood lost during operation. Dry sponges should be used and weighed shortly after use to minimize error from evaporation. The suction line, connected to a calibrated trap on the operating table, should be short to diminish the dead space of the tubing and to provide immediate data about accumulated blood loss. Visual observation may be used as a rough guide, but it tends to give a falsely low estimate of the loss. Procedures associated with loss of more than 20% of blood volume should be preceded by placement of a central venous catheter.

Before operation, newborn infants should receive vitamin K, 1–2 mg intravenously or intramuscularly. If an extensive surgical procedure is anticipated, freshly drawn blood should be typed and cross-matched in case transfusion is required. In infants with hematocrits greater than 50%, blood loss may be replaced by infusing lactated Ringer's solution or fresh frozen plasma to compensate for losses of up to 25% of total blood volume. Greater blood losses should be replaced with freshly drawn whole blood or packed red cells. A transfusion of packed red blood cells at a volume of 10 mL/kg usually raises the hematocrit 3–4%. The transfused blood should be prewarmed to body temperature by running it through coiled tubing immersed in water at 37 °C. With excessive blood loss, clotting factors and platelets can be depleted rapidly, and fresh frozen plasma and platelets of identical blood type should be available. A transfusion of 0.1 unit/kg of platelets raises the platelet count by approximately 25,000/μL.

Perioperative Considerations

A. GASTROINTESTINAL DECOMPRESSION

The importance of gastric decompression in the surgical newborn cannot be overemphasized. The distended stomach carries the risk of aspiration and pneumonia and may also impair diaphragmatic excursion, resulting in respiratory distress. For example, oxygenation and ventilation in a neonate with congenital diaphragmatic hernia may become progressively impaired as the herniated intestine becomes distended with air and fluid. With gastroschisis, omphalocele, and diaphragmatic hernia, the ability to reduce the prolapsed intestine into the abdominal cavity is impaired by intestinal distention. A double-lumen sump tube, such as the Replogle tube, is preferred, utilizing low continuous suction. If a single-lumen tube is used, intermittent aspiration by syringe or machine is required. The correct position of the tube in the stomach is confirmed by carefully measuring the tube prior to insertion, by noting the nature of the aspirate, and by radiographs. Careful and adequate taping of the tube is essential to avoid displacement.

B. PREOPERATIVE BLOOD SAMPLING

Blood analyses should be restricted to those studies essential for diagnosis and management. The volume of blood drawn for laboratory tests should be documented as these small volumes cumulatively represent significant blood loss in a small infant. Generally, the only "routine" preoperative blood analyses for a neonate consist of a complete blood count and a blood specimen for type and cross-match (in the case of major newborn surgery). Electrolytes in the first 12 hours of life simply reflect the mother's electrolytes. Coagulation studies (eg, PT, PTT) are virtually never indicated.

C. PREOPERATIVE NPO GUIDELINES

1. Patients younger than 6 months—No food or formula 4 hours prior to the procedure. Children may continue to have breast milk and clear liquids (water, oral electrolyte mixtures, glucose water, or apple juice) until 2 hours prior to the procedure.

2. Patients from 6 months to 18 years—Nothing to eat or drink after midnight except clear liquids (water, apple juice, oral electrolyte mixtures, gelatin dessert, white grape juice), which can be continued until 2 hours prior to the procedure.

3. Patients older than 18 years—Nothing to eat or drink after midnight except clear liquids (water, apple juice, plain gelatin desserts) until 4 hours prior to the procedure.

D. BOWEL PREPARATION INSTRUCTIONS

The bowel is mechanically cleansed for elective bowel resection. Opinion varies about whether a bowel preparation is needed for certain procedures as well as about what to use to accomplish it and whether to do it at home or in the hospital. In-patient regimens generally begin the day prior to surgery and consist of metoclopramide combined with polyethylene glycol-electrolyte solution, 25 mL/kg/h for 4 hours. Outpatient preparations are reserved for patients over 1 year of age. In this setting, bisacodyl suppositories and tap water enemas are given morning and evening on the day before surgery. For children over 5 years of age, magnesium citrate is added (1 oz per year of age up to a maximum of 8 oz) in the morning and evening the day before surgery.

■ LESIONS OF THE HEAD & NECK

DERMOID CYSTS

Dermoid cysts are congenital inclusions of skin and appendages commonly found on the scalp and eyebrows and in the midline of the nose, neck, and upper chest. They present as painless swellings that may be completely mobile or fixed to the skin and deeper structures. Dermoid cysts of the eyebrows and scalp may produce a depression in the underlying bone that appears as a smooth, punched-out defect on radiographs of the outer table of the skull. These cysts contain a cheesy material that is produced by desquamation of the cells of the epithelial lining. Dermoid cysts of the neck may be confused with thyroglossal duct cysts, but they usually do not move with swallowing or protrusion of the tongue as thyroglossal cysts do. Because midline cysts can communicate with the brain, MRI or CT is warranted preoperatively. Dermoid cysts should be excised intact, since incomplete removal will result in recurrence. Those arising on the eyebrows should be

excised through an incision within the hairline. The eyebrows should not be shaved.

McAvoy JM, Zuckerbraun L: Dermoid cysts of the head and neck in children. Arch Otolaryngol 1976;102:529.

BRANCHIOGENIC ANOMALIES

Branchial anomalies are remnants of the branchial apparatus present during the first month of fetal life. Embryologically, the primitive neck develops four external clefts and four pharyngeal pouches that are separated by a membrane. Between the clefts and pouches are branchial arches. The dorsal portion of the first cleft becomes the external auditory canal; the other clefts are obliterated. The pharyngeal pouches persist as adult organs. The first pouch becomes the auditory tube, the middle ear cavity, and the mastoid air cells. The second pouch incompletely regresses and becomes the palatine tonsil and the supratonsillar fossa. The third pouch forms the inferior parathyroid glands and thymus; the fourth forms the superior parathyroid glands.

A tract of branchial origin may form a complete fistula, or one end may be obliterated to form an external or internal sinus, or both ends may resorb, leaving an aggregate of cells forming a cyst (Figure 46–1). Fistulas that arise above the hyoid bone and communicate with the external auditory canal represent persistence of the first branchial cleft. These tracts are always lined by

Figure 46–1. Branchiogenic fistula from second branchial cleft origin. The fistula extends along the anterior border of the sternocleidomastoid muscle and courses between the internal and external carotid arteries and cephalad to the hypoglossal nerve to enter the tonsillar fossa.

squamous epithelium. Cysts and sinuses of second or third branchial origin are lined by squamous, cuboidal, or ciliated columnar epithelium. Fistulas that communicate between the anterior border of the sternocleidomastoid muscle and the tonsillar fossa are of second branchial origin, and those that extend into the piriform sinus are derived from the third branchial pouch. Cysts developing from branchial structures usually appear later in childhood as opposed to sinuses and fistulas. Branchiogenic anomalies occur with equal frequency on each side of the neck, and 15% are bilateral. Second branchial cleft abnormalities are most common, occurring six times more frequently than first cleft anomalies.

Clinical Findings

A sinus or fistulous opening along the anterior border of the sternocleidomastoid muscle is readily seen at birth and usually discharges a mucoid or purulent material. The patient may complain of a foul-tasting discharge in the mouth upon massaging the tract, but the internal orifice is rarely recognized. The cysts are characteristically found anterior and deep to the upper third of the sternocleidomastoid muscle, or they may be located within the parotid gland or pharyngeal wall, over the manubrium, or in the mediastinum. Sinuses and cysts are prone to become repeatedly infected, producing cellulitis and abscess formation.

Differential Diagnosis

Granulomatous lymphadenitis due to mycobacterial infections may produce cystic lymph nodes and draining sinuses, but these are usually distinguishable by the chronic inflammatory reaction that precedes the purulent discharge. Hemangiomas, cystic hygromas, and lymphangiomas are soft, spongy tumor masses that might be confused with branchial cysts, but the latter have a firmer consistency. Cystic hygromas and lymphangiomas transilluminate, and branchial cysts do not. Carotid body tumors are quite firm, are located at the carotid bifurcation, and occur in older patients. Lymphomas produce firm masses in the area where branchial remnants occur, but multiple matted nodes rather than a solitary cystic tumor distinguish these lesions. Mucoid material may be expressed from the openings of branchial sinuses or fistulas, and a firm cordlike tract may be palpable along its course.

Treatment

Almost all branchial abnormalities should be excised early in life since repeated infection is common, making resection more difficult. Infected sinuses and cysts require initial incision and drainage. Excision of these tracts is staged and usually performed approximately 6 weeks later, when the acute inflammatory reaction has subsided. Every effort should be made to excise the entire cyst wall or fistula tract (including the skin punctum, if present) since recurrence and infection are common with incomplete removal. Excision should be undertaken cautiously, as the tracts may lie adjacent to the facial, hypoglossal, and glossopharyngeal nerves as well as the carotid artery and internal jugular vein.

Lin JN, Wang KL: Persistent third branchial apparatus. J Pediatr Surg 1991;26:663.

Roback SA, Talendar RL: Thyroglossal duct cysts and branchial cleft anomalies. Semin Pediatr Surg 1994;3:142.

PREAURICULAR LESIONS

Preauricular sinuses, cysts, and cartilaginous rests probably arise from anomalous development of the auricle and are unrelated to branchial anomalies. They may become infected and may cause a cosmetic deformity. Superficial skin tags and cartilaginous rests can be easily excised under sedation and local anesthesia. Preauricular sinus tracts may be very deceptive in their extent, and the surgeon should be prepared to proceed with extensive dissection under general anesthesia to completely excise these lesions.

LYMPHANGIOMA (Cystic Hygroma)

Lymphangiomas are benign multilobular, multinodular cystic masses lined by endothelial cells. They result from maldevelopment and obstruction of the lymphatic system. Eventually, sequestrations of lymphatic tissue that do not communicate with the normal lymphatic system develop. Fifty to 65 percent appear at birth and 90% by the second year of life. They are located most commonly in the posterior triangle of the neck (75%) (Figure 46–2) and axilla (20%), with the remainder located in the mediastinum, retroperitoneum, pelvis, and groin.

Clinical Findings

Neck hygromas may communicate beneath the clavicle with an axillary hygroma, mediastinal hygroma, or, rarely, both. The majority are asymptomatic, though large lesions invading the floor of the mouth may cause symptoms referable to pharyngeal or upper airway obstruction. The skin is never involved; these lesions grow along fascial planes and around neurovascular structures. Large fetal lesions may be recognized on maternal ultrasound examination, and early delivery may be indicated if fetal airway obstruction and hydrops develop.

Figure 46–2. Typical neonatal lymphangioma arising from the posterior cervical triangle. (Reproduced, with permission, from Filston HC: Hemangiomas, cystic hygromas, and teratomas of the head and neck. Semin Pediatr Surg 1994;3:147.)

Treatment

There are two modes of treatment—sclerotherapy or excision—chosen based on imaging studies (CT, MRI). Intralesional injection of a sclerosing agent is most effective for unilocular cysts. Examples of agents that have been used are OK-432 (a lyophilized mixture of *Streptococcus pyogenes* and penicillin G potassium) and bleomycin. Excision is carried out with bipolar cautery to ensure a hemostatic dissection and decrease the incidence of lymph leak and nerve injury. Nevertheless, postoperative lymph leak is common and is treated by closed suction drainage for days to weeks. Intraoperative cyst rupture increases the difficulty of the dissection since the thin-walled cyst is difficult to identify and the margins are obscured. The recurrence rate is low (10%) if all microscopic disease is resected. When gross disease is left, recurrence occurs very frequently.

Brown RL, Azizkhan RG: Pediatric head and neck lesions. Pediatr Clin North Am 1998;45:899.

Fonkalsrud EW: Congenital malformations of the lymphatic system. Semin Pediatr Surg 1994;3:62.

THYROGLOSSAL DUCT REMNANT

The thyroid gland develops from an evagination in the floor of the primitive pharynx—between the first pair of pharyngeal pouches—during the fourth week of gestation. If the anlage of the thyroid does not descend normally, the thyroid gland may form in the tongue or remain as a mass anywhere in the midline of the neck. If the thyroglossal duct persists, the epithelial tract forms a cyst that usually communicates with the foramen cecum of the tongue. The thyroglossal duct descends through the second branchial arch anlage, which become the hyoid bone, prior to its fusion in the midline. Because of this, the tract of a persistent thyroglossal duct extends through the hyoid bone (Figure 46–3).

Clinical Findings

Lingual thyroid glands may produce dysphagia, dysphonia, dyspnea, hemorrhage, or pain. The most common physical finding is a rounded cystic mass of varying size in the midline of the neck just below the hyoid bone. The acute inflammatory reaction of an infection may herald the presence of a cyst. The fluid in the cyst is usually under pressure and may give the impression of being a solid tumor. Cysts and aberrant midline thyroid glands move up and down with swallowing and with protrusion of the tongue.

Figure 46–3. Thyroglossal cyst and duct course through the hyoid bone to the foramen cecum of the tongue.

Differential Diagnosis

Only lymph nodes, dermoid cysts, and enlarged delphian nodes containing metastases are confused with thyroglossal remnants in the midline of the neck. Dermoid cysts do not move with swallowing. Lingual thyroids may be confused with a hypertrophied lingual tonsil or with a fibroma, angioma, sarcoma, or carcinoma of the tongue. These lesions and thyroglossal cysts may be distinguished from aberrantly located thyroid glands by needle aspiration or by radioiodine scintiscan.

Complications

Thyroglossal cysts are prone to infection, and spontaneous drainage or incision and drainage of an abscess will result in a chronically draining fistula. Excision of an ectopic thyroid may remove all thyroid tissue, producing hypothyroidism. There is some concern over the long-term malignant potential of the dysgenetic thyroid tissue because carcinoma develops more frequently in ectopic thyroid tissue than in normal thyroid glands.

Treatment

Complete excision is indicated because of the risk of acute or chronic infection and the possibility of papillary carcinoma arising from dysgenetic ectopic thyroid tissue later in life. Acute infection in thyroglossal tracts should be treated with local heat and antibiotics. Abscesses should be incised and drained. After complete subsidence of the inflammatory reaction (approximately 6 weeks), a thyroglossal cyst and its epithelial tract should be excised. The mid portion of the hyoid bone should be removed en bloc with the thyroglossal tract to the base of the tongue (Sistrunk procedure). Recurrences occur when the hyoid is not removed or when the cyst was previously infected or drained.

Housawa M et al: Anatomical reconstruction of the thyroglossal duct. J Pediatr Surg 1991;26:766.

Roback SA, Telander RL: Thyroglossal duct cysts and branchial cleft anomalies. Semin Pediatr Surg 1994;3:142.

TORTICOLLIS

Torticollis present with a hard, nontender, fibrosis (mass) within the sternocleidomastoid muscle. It may be present at birth but is usually not noticed until the second to sixth weeks of life. The mass appears with equal frequency in both sexes and on each side of the neck. Rarely, there is more than one mass in the muscle or both sternocleidomastoid muscles are involved. A history of breech delivery is present in 20–30% of these children.

Clinical Findings

Torticollis is manifested when the sternocleidomastoid muscle is shortened, the mastoid process on the involved side is pulled down toward the clavicle and sternum, and the head is tilted and directed toward the opposite shoulder. The shoulder on the affected side is raised, and there may be cervical and thoracic scoliosis. Passive rotation of the head to the side of the involved muscle will be resisted and limited to varying degrees, and the muscle will appear as a protuberant band. Because of persistent pressure when the patient is recumbent, the ipsilateral face and contralateral occiput will be flattened or hypoplastic. Facial hemihypoplasia and plagiocephaly (flattening of the ipsilateral posterior skull) occurs in untreated cases, usually within 6 months.

Treatment

Surgery is rarely necessary for this disorder. Torticollis is treated with active range of motion exercises. The child's shoulders are held flat to a table and the head is tilted and rotated in a full range of motion. This procedure should be performed at least four times a day, usually for 2–3 months. The firm "tumor" often disappears well before the torticollis is cured. If the muscle continues to become progressively shortened, with facial and occipital skull deformity, both heads of the sternocleidomastoid muscle should be divided through a small transverse incision just above the clavicle. This procedure does not reverse the bony changes that have already developed but prevents progression of the process. Recurrence is rare.

Binder H et al: Congenital muscular torticollis: results of conservative management with long-term follow-up in 85 cases. Arch Phys Med Rehabil 1987;68:222.

Bredenkamp JK et al: Congenital muscular torticollis. Arch Otolaryngol Head Neck Surg 1990;116:212.

Celayir AC: Congenital muscular torticollis: early and intensive treatment is critical. A prospective study. Pediatr Int 2000; 42:504.

CERVICAL LYMPHADENOPATHY

PYOGENIC LYMPHADENITIS

Infections in the upper respiratory passages, scalp, ear, or neck produce varying degrees of secondary lymphadenitis. Most of the causative organisms are streptococcal or staphylococcal species. In infants and young children, the clinical course of the suppurative lymphadenitis may greatly overshadow a seemingly insignificant or inapparent primary infection. Scalp or ear infections produce pre- or postauricular and suboccipital lymph node involvement; submental, oral, tonsillar, and pharyngeal infections affect the submandibular and deep jugular nodes.

Clinical Findings

With significant lymphadenitis, the regional lymph nodes become greatly enlarged and produce local pain and tenderness. Enlargement of cervical nodes is most common, followed by occipital and submandibular nodes. Fever is high initially and then becomes intermittent and may persist for days or weeks. The regional nodes may remain enlarged and firm for prolonged periods, or they may suppurate and produce surrounding cellulitis and edema. Subsequently, the nodes may involute or a fluctuant abscess may form, resulting in redness and thinning of the overlying skin.

Differential Diagnosis

A smoldering lymphadenitis that neither resolves nor forms an abscess can be confused with granulomatous lymphadenitis, lymphoma, or metastatic tumor. Excisional biopsy is required to differentiate these lesions. After several weeks, there will usually be a reduction in the size and firmness of pyogenic adenitis, especially after antibiotic treatment has been started.

Treatment

In the acute phase, the patient should be treated with antistaphylococcal antibiotics. In the subacute or chronic phase, the presence of pus in the node may be confirmed by needle aspiration of the mass. When an abscess is present, a general anesthetic should be given and the abscess incised and drained.

GRANULOMATOUS LYMPHADENITIS

Although typical tuberculous cervical adenitis is very rare in the United States, atypical mycobacteria (eg, *Mycobacterium avium-intracellulare*) frequently cause chronic suppuration in the cervical (most common), axillary, and inguinal lymph nodes. Granulomatous lymphadenitis and caseation may occur in the regional nodes draining the inoculation site of BCG). Cat-scratch disease causes a caseating lymphadenitis in regional lymph nodes.

Clinical Findings

Children under age 6 are most frequently affected. The initial manifestation is a painless, progressive enlargement of the lymph nodes in the deep cervical chain and the parotid, suboccipital, submandibular, and supraclavicular nodes. The duration of lymphadenopathy is usually 1–3 months or longer. The nodes may be large and mobile or, with progressive disease, may become matted, fixed, and finally caseate to form an abscess. Incision or spontaneous breakthrough of the skin will result in a chronically draining sinus. In tuberculosis, both sides of the neck or multiple groups of nodes are infected, and the chest radiograph indicates pulmonary involvement. In atypical mycobacterial lymphadenitis, pulmonary disease is rare and the cervical adenitis is unilateral. The tuberculin skin test is weakly positive in over 80% of patients with atypical mycobacterial infection. Skin test antigens from the various strains of atypical mycobacteria are available. A positive skin test helps differentiate granulomatous adenitis from malignant lymphadenopathy. A fluctuant node can be confused with branchial cleft or thyroglossal cysts.

Cat-scratch disease is usually acquired by a bite or scratch from a kitten. It is caused by a pleomorphic gram-negative bacillus (*Bartonella henselae*) that requires a silver stain for detection in tissue. It is an acute illness characterized by fever, malaise, and occasionally a pustular lesion at the site of the scratch. Tender lymph node enlargement usually develops. Two to 4 weeks later, regional lymphadenitis persists, producing painful, fixed suppurative nodes that may develop into a chronically draining sinus.

Treatment

Atypical tuberculous lymphadenitis may be treated with rifampin (10 mg/kg/d), though definitive treatment usually requires nodal excision. Trimethoprim-sulfamethoxazole may shorten the course of cat-scratch disease and prevent suppuration. When antibiotics are ineffective, the procedure of choice is excision of involved nodes before caseation occurs. Once the nodes become fluctuant or a draining sinus forms, a wedge of involved skin should be excised and the underlying necrotic nodes should be curetted out (rather than excised), taking care not to injure neighboring nerves. The wound edges and skin should be closed primarily. The value of continuing chemotherapy is influenced by sensitivity tests on the cultured material. Excision and primary closure usually result in excellent healing with good cosmetic results.

Beiler HA et al: Specific and nonspecific lymphadenitis in childhood: etiology, diagnosis, and therapy. Pediatr Surg Int 1997; 12:108.

Bodenstein L, Altman RP: Cervical lymphadenitis in infants and children. Semin Pediatr Surg 1994;3:134.

Flint D et al: Cervical lymphadenitis due to non-tuberculous mycobacteria: surgical treatment and review. Int J Pediatr Otorhinolaryngol 2000;53:187.

Holley HP: Successful treatment of cat-scratch disease with ciprofloxacin. JAMA 1991;265:1563.

■ CONGENITAL CHEST WALL DEFORMITIES

STERNAL CLEFT

Failure of fusion of the two sternal bars during embryonic development produces congenital sternal cleft, which may involve the upper, lower, or entire sternum. In its severe form, this defect is usually associated with protrusion of the pericardium and heart (ectopia cordis) and congenital heart lesions. Defects may be associated with extracardiac anomalies, including cleft lip, cleft palate, hydrocephalus, and other central nervous system disorders, or may be one component of the pentalogy of Cantrell. Operative correction is performed in the neonatal period since the chest wall is so pliable; it consists of simple suture approximation of the two sternal halves. More complex defects associated with ectopia cordis are often incompatible with life.

PECTUS EXCAVATUM

This depression deformity is the most common congenital chest wall abnormality, occurring in one in 300 live births, with a 3:1 male predominance. It is associated with other musculoskeletal disorders (Marfan's syndrome, Poland's syndrome, scoliosis, clubfoot, syndactyly), and 2% have congenital heart disease. There is a familial form. It results from the unbalanced posterior growth of costal cartilages that are often fused, bizarrely deformed, or rotated. The body of the sternum secondarily exhibits a prominent posterior curvature, usually involving its lower half (Figure 46–4). Commonly, the xiphoid is the deepest portion of the depression. The third, fourth, and fifth costal cartilages are usually affected, though the second to eighth costal cartilages may be involved. The severity of the defect varies greatly from a mild, insignificant depression to an extreme where the xiphoid bone is adjacent to the vertebrae.

Clinical Findings

These patients are typically round-shouldered, with stooped posture, potbelly, and an asthenic appearance. They tend to be withdrawn and refuse to participate in sports activities, particularly if their deformity might be exposed. Few patients complain of easy fatigability or

Figure 46–4. Adolescent with a pectus excavatum deformity. Note that the most pronounced sternal curvature is in the lower half.

inability to compete in exertional activities. Cardiopulmonary function studies rarely demonstrate impairments; this is predominantly a cosmetic deformity with potentially severe psychosocial sequelae.

Treatment & Prognosis

There is no standard age for repair. Traditionally, an open repair is performed in which the abnormal cartilages are resected; the sternum is often fractured and fixed in a corrected position (often with a Kirschner wire or steel strut). Recently, a minimally invasive technique has been used in which a preformed sternal strut (Nuss bar) is passed, either blindly or with thoracoscopic assistance, under the chest wall muscles, into each hemithorax, and across the mediastinum under the sternum via two small incisions in the midaxillary line. The curve bar is passed upside down and "flipped" into position under the sternum, effectively lifting the sternum and chest wall into a corrected position. The bar is left in place for 2 years, and the child can resume activity in 3 months. The recurrence rate for the open procedure is less than 3%; at present there is not enough long-term follow-up to assess the Nuss technique. In general, there is no cardiopulmonary benefit after chest wall repair except in rare instances when the deformity is excessive. Otherwise, the repair is performed solely to improve appearance. However, the psychosocial benefits of repair of this often embarrassing deformity cannot be minimized.

PECTUS CARINATUM

This is a protrusion deformity, also referred to as pigeon breast or chicken chest. It is approximately ten times less frequent than pectus excavatum. It results from the overgrowth of costal cartilages, with forward buckling and secondary deformation of the sternum (Figure 46–5). Atypical and asymmetric forms with ro-

Figure 46–5. Severe pectus carinatum deformity. (Reproduced, with permission, from Albanese CT: Pediatric surgery. In: *Surgery.* Norton JA [editor]. Springer, 2000.)

tation are common. There is a familial form. It is associated with Marfan's disease, neurofibromatosis, Poland's syndrome, and Morquio's disease. Unlike pectus excavatum, the deformity is typically mild or nearly imperceptible in early childhood and becomes increasingly prominent during the rapid growth in early puberty.

Treatment & Prognosis

As with pectus excavatum, there is no cardiorespiratory compromise with this deformity, and repair is performed solely to achieve an improved cosmetic appearance. Mild deformities should be left alone and the patient followed to observe for progression. Moderate to severe defects should be repaired, particularly when the patient or parent indicates a desire for improvement. The deformed cartilages are resected, leaving the costochondral membranes (perichondrium) intact. Sternal fracture is usually not necessary. To ensure that the costal cartilages grow back on a straighter line, reefing sutures are placed in the perichondrium to shorten them. The costal cartilages regenerate within 6 weeks. A thorough procedure will provide an excellent cosmetic result in nearly all cases. Recurrences are rare.

Fonkalsrud EW, Beanes S: Surgical management of pectus carinatum: 30 years' experience. World J Surg 2001;25:898.

Miller KA et al: Minimally invasive repair of pectus excavatum: a single institution's experience. Surgery 2001;130:652.

Morshuis W et al: Pulmonary function before surgery for pectus excavatum and at long-term follow-up. Chest 1994;105:1646.

Nuss D et al: A 10–year review of a minimally invasive technique for the correction of pectus excavatum. J Pediatr Surg 1998; 33:545.

Shamberger RC: Cardiopulmonary effects of anterior chest wall deformities. Chest Surg Clin N Am 2000;10:245.

■ SURGICAL RESPIRATORY EMERGENCIES IN THE NEWBORN

Certain aspects of respiration peculiar to the infant must be appreciated. Except during periods of crying, the newborn baby is an obligate nasal breather. The ability to breathe through the mouth may take weeks or months to acquire. Inspiration is accomplished chiefly by diaphragmatic excursion, and the intercostal and accessory muscles contribute little to ventilation. Impaired inspiration results in retraction of the sternum, costal margin, and neck fossae; the resulting paradoxic motion may contribute to respiratory insufficiency.

The airway is small and flaccid, so that it is readily occluded by mucus or edema, and it collapses readily under slight pressure. Dyspneic infants swallow large volumes of air, and the distended stomach and bowel may further impair diaphragmatic excursion.

Classification

A. UPPER AIRWAY

1. Micrognathia—Pierre Robin syndrome
2. Macroglossia—Muscular hypertrophy, hypothyroidism, lymphangioma
3. Anomalous nasopharyngeal passage—Choanal atresia, Treacher-Collins syndrome, Apert's syndrome, and Crouzon's syndrome
4. Tumors, cysts, or enlarged thyroid remnants in the pharynx or neck
5. Laryngeal or tracheal stenosis, webs, cysts, tumors, or vocal cord paralysis
6. Epiglottitis

B. INTRATHORACIC

1. Atelectasis
2. Pneumothorax and pneumomediastinum
3. Pleural effusion or chylothorax
4. Pulmonary cysts, sequestration, and tumors
5. Tracheal stenosis with complete tracheal rings
6. Tracheomalacia or bronchomalacia
7. Congenital lobar emphysema
8. Diaphragmatic hernia or eventration
9. Esophageal atresia or tracheoesophageal fistula
10. Vascular rings and sling (anomalous origin of left pulmonary artery)
11. Mediastinal tumors and cysts

PIERRE ROBIN SYNDROME

Pierre Robin syndrome is a congenital defect characterized by micrognathia and glossoptosis, often associated with cleft palate. The small lower jaw and strong sucking action of the infant allow the tongue to be sucked back and occlude the laryngeal airway and may be life-threatening.

Infants with mild cases should be kept in the prone position during care and feeding. A nasogastric or gastrostomy tube may be necessary. Nasohypopharyngeal intubation is effective in preventing occlusion of the larynx. If conservative measures fail, prompt attention to maintaining an open airway by tracheostomy is indicated. Feeding by gastrostomy may be necessary. The tongue may be sutured forward (plicated) to the lower jaw, but this frequently breaks down. In time, the lower jaw develops normally. These infants eventually learn how to keep the tongue from occluding the airway.

CHOANAL ATRESIA

Complete obstruction at the posterior nares from choanal atresia may be unilateral and relatively asymptomatic. It may be membranous (10%) or bony (90%). When it is bilateral, severe respiratory distress is manifested by marked chest wall retraction on inspiration and a normal cry.

There is arching of the head and neck in an effort to breathe, and the baby is unable to eat. The diagnosis is confirmed by the inability to pass a tube through the nares to the pharynx. With the baby in a supine position, radiopaque material may be instilled into the nares and lateral x-rays of the head taken to outline the obstruction. A CT scan of the nasopharynx will define bony occlusion.

Emergency treatment consists of maintaining an oral airway by placing a nipple, with the tip cut off, in the mouth. The membranous or bony occlusion may then be perforated by direct transpalatal excision, or it may be punctured and enlarged with a Hegar dilator. The newly created opening must be stented with plastic tubing for 5 weeks to prevent stricture.

CONGENITAL TRACHEAL STENOSIS & MALACIA

There are three main types of congenital tracheal stenosis: generalized hypoplasia; funnel-like narrowing, usually tapering to a tight stenosis just above the carina; and segmental stenosis of various lengths that can occur at any level. Tracheomalacia is a functional obstruction in a "soft" trachea that collapses with inspiration. It is often secondary to external compression by vascular rings, tumors, or from a chronically dilated upper esophageal pouch in those with esophageal atresia.

Diagnosis

The diagnostic approach to an infant with respiratory distress and possible distal tracheal obstruction must be carefully integrated with plans for management of the airway, because the compromised infant airway is easily occluded by edema or secretions. This is especially true in distal tracheal lesions, where an endotracheal or tracheostomy tube may not relieve the distal obstruction. The diagnostic value of every procedure must be weighed against the threat of precipitating airway obstruction. Tracheal lesions can be visualized using esophagography, angiography, or CT scans. Dynamic lesions such as tracheomalacia and vascular compression syndromes are best defined by videotape fluoroscopy or cineradiography with barium in the esophagus. Angiography may be necessary. Flow-volume curves can define the level of obstruction (intrathoracic versus extrathoracic) and the type of obstruction (stenosis versus malacia).

Although bronchoscopy and bronchography often provide the best delineation of tracheobronchial lesions, these more invasive procedures can precipitate acute obstruction from edema or inflammation. A ventilating infant bronchoscope with Hopkins optics should be kept above the critical area to avoid precipitating obstruction. If tracheobronchoscopy is performed, use only a small amount of contrast medium (micropulverized barium mixed in normal saline) or pass a Fogarty catheter, inflating a 1 or 2 mL balloon with 50% diatrizoate meglumine to outline the extent of stenosis and to minimize tracheal irritation.

Treatment

Noncritical stenotic and malacic lesions in infants and children should be managed as conservatively as possible, preferably without intubation. "Temporary" stenting of these lesions is seldom temporary, since the presence of the tube itself ensures continued trauma and irritation such that the tube cannot be removed without airway obstruction. If an infant or child cannot be managed without intubation, surgical correction must be considered. Tracheal reconstruction via resection or a variety of tracheoplasty techniques has proved to be the treatment of choice for tracheal lesions. Severe tracheomalacia is treated by addressing the underlying cause. Aortopexy or an endotracheal stent is often necessary. Tracheostomy is a last resort.

Backer CL et al: Tracheal surgery in children: an 18-year review of four techniques. Eur J Cardiothorac Surg 2001;19:777.

deLorimier AA et al: Tracheobronchial obstructions in infants and children: experience with 45 cases. Ann Surg 1990;212:277.

Rutter MJ, Hartley BE, Cotton RT: Cricotracheal resection in children. Arch Otolaryngol Head Neck Surg 2001;127:289.

CONGENITAL DIAPHRAGMATIC HERNIA

Congenital diaphragmatic hernia is a highly lethal and morbid disease that affects 1 in 2000 live births (Figure 46–6). Anatomically, congenital diaphragmatic hernia results from an embryologic fusion defect, allowing herniation of intra-abdominal contents into the chest. Fusion of the transverse septum and pleuroperitoneal folds normally occurs during the eighth week of embryonic development. If diaphragmatic formation is incomplete, the pleuroperitoneal hiatus (foramen of Bochdalek) persists. There is an almost universal presence of intestinal nonrotation as the bowel herniates

Figure 46–6. Congenital posterolateral (Bochdalek) diaphragmatic hernia. Bowel, spleen, and liver sometimes herniate into the chest and severely compromise lung development in utero and ventilation after birth. (Reproduced, with permission, from Schrock TR: *Handbook of Surgery*, 6th ed. Jones, 1978.)

into the thorax rather than undergoing its normal sequence of rotation and fixation. Severe defects cause pulmonary hypoplasia and pulmonary hypertension. The earlier in gestation the hernia occurs, the more severe the pulmonary hypoplasia.

Clinical Findings

A. SYMPTOMS AND SIGNS

Infants with large diaphragmatic defects are usually symptomatic in the delivery room, with tachypnea, grunting respirations, retractions, and cyanosis, and may require urgent intubation. For smaller defects, symptoms may not appear until the infant is several months old. The abdomen is usually scaphoid. The chest on the side of the hernia may be dull to percussion, but bowel sounds are not usually appreciated. The left side of the diaphragm is affected four or five times as frequently as the right, with a rate of associated anomalies of 20% (chromosomal abnormalities, neural tube defects, and congenital heart disease). When the hernia is on the left, the heart sounds may be heard best on the right side of the chest.

The development of symptoms with CDH correlates with the degree of pulmonary hypoplasia and pulmonary hypertension. Prenatal diagnosis is occurring more and more frequently and allows the mother and the fetus to be referred to an institution where sophisticated perinatal and pediatric surgical units are available.

B. IMAGING STUDIES

A chest radiograph will show a paucity of gas within the abdomen, radiopaque hemithorax if the bowel does not contain a significant amount of gas or if the left lobe of the liver occupies the majority of the hemithorax, loss of normal ipsilateral diaphragmatic contour, bowel in the thorax, contralateral mediastinal shift, and a coiled nasogastric tube in the hemithorax.

Treatment

Repair of the diaphragmatic defect is not a surgical emergency and should be performed once the infant has stabilized and has demonstrated minimal to no pulmonary hypertension (usually over 48 hours postnatally). Early reduction and repair has been shown to transiently worsen pulmonary function by decreasing pulmonary compliance and increasing airway reactivity. A nasogastric tube should be placed in the stomach to aspirate swallowed air and to prevent distention of the herniated bowel, which would further compress the lungs. A transverse abdominal incision should be made and the herniated bowel reduced from the pleural space, though some surgeons prefer a thoracic approach, particularly for right-sided defects. The negative pressure between the bowel and the chest wall may make reduction difficult. This negative pressure may be broken by inserting a tube along the pleura and injecting air through it. Following reduction of the bowel, placement of a chest tube in the pleural space is optional; if used, it is connected to a water seal and not to vacuum. No attempt should be made to expand the collapsed and hypoplastic lung by positive pressure. The diaphragmatic defect should be closed by nonabsorbable sutures. In many instances, a synthetic material is required to close large defects. The abdominal cavity may be too small and underdeveloped to accommodate the intestine and permit closure of the abdominal wall muscle and fascial layers. In such cases, abdominal wall skin flaps should be mobilized and closed over the protruding bowel. The resulting ventral hernia can be repaired later when the infant is thriving.

Continued respiratory support and treatment of hypoxemia, hypercapnia, and acidosis are required postoperatively. Persistent pulmonary hypertension may result in right-to-left shunt and produce severe hypoxemia in the lower aorta. Nitric oxide added to the ventilation gases can induce pulmonary vasodilation, improve pulmonary perfusion, and reverse the right-to-left shunt. The persistent fetal circulation physiology may be treated successfully in many cases by extracorporeal membrane oxygenation and permissive ventilatory strategies (high-frequency ventilation). Hypoxemic myocardiopathy may require infusion of dopamine to enhance cardiac output. For those fetuses with a severe congenital diaphragmatic hernia by ultrasound criteria, intervention before birth is an option and has proved promising.

Prognosis

The death rate for infants with congenital diaphragmatic hernia depends upon the severity of pulmonary hypoplasia, the presence or absence of associated anomalies, and the quality of care provided for these critically ill infants. When diagnosed in utero, prognosis depends on the presence or absence of liver herniation into the hemithorax, the gestational age at diagnosis, and an estimation of lung size (the lung-to-head ratio). Long-term, there are a number of probably clinically insignificant physiologic abnormalities such as a reduction in total lung volume, restrictive or obstructive lung disease, and abnormal lung compliance. A small subset of patients will survive as "pulmonary cripples" and remain oxygen-dependent or ventilator-dependent, often requiring tracheostomies. Since there may be deficient periesophageal muscular tissue or an abnormal orientation of the gastroesophageal junction, gastroesophageal reflux is common. It is most commonly treated nonoperatively, but refractory cases may require an antireflux procedure. Recurrent diaphragmatic hernia occurs in 10–20% of infants and should be considered in any child with a history of congenital diaphragmatic hernia who presents with new gastrointestinal or pulmonary symptoms. Recurrence is most common when a prosthetic patch is used for the repair.

Surgical units that are immediately adjacent to obstetric services report death rates as high as 80%, because infants with severe pulmonary hypoplasia will be recognized and treated immediately. Infants who survive transfer to surgical centers remote from the delivery area usually have less severe disease, and the death rates reported from these facilities are usually under 40%. Prenatally treated infants with severe congenital diaphragmatic hernia can have survival rates approaching 75%.

With improvements in prenatal ultrasonographic imaging, many of these defects can be appreciated early enough so that prenatal intervention or planned delivery is possible.

FORAMEN OF MORGAGNI HERNIA

The foramen of Morgagni is the junction of the septum transversum, the lateral portion of the diaphragm, and the anterior thoracic wall and allows passage of the superior epigastric vessels. This anterior diaphragmatic defect accounts for only 2% of diaphragmatic hernias. It is commonly right parasternal but may be left parasternal, retrosternal, or bilateral. Typically, however, children are asymptomatic and the defect is discovered later in life on a chest radiograph taken for reasons unrelated to the hernia. The lateral chest radiograph demonstrating an air-filled mass extending into the anterior mediastinum is pathognomonic. Repair is indicated in the asymptomatic patient due to the risk of bowel incarceration or strangulation. The viscera are reduced and any associated hernia sac excised. The defect is closed by suturing the posterior rim of diaphragm to the posterior rectus sheath since there is no anterior diaphragm. Rarely, a prosthetic patch closure is required. There is no associated pulmonary hypoplasia or hypertension. This defect, when noted in newborns, can be associated with the pentalogy of Cantrell, a disorder with considerable morbidity and mortality that consists of the diaphragmatic defect, distal sternal cleft, epigastric omphalocele, apical pericardial defect, and congenital heart disease (usually a septal defect). Excluding patients with the pentalogy of Cantrell, survival is nearly 100%.

EVENTRATION OF THE DIAPHRAGM

Diaphragmatic eventration is an abnormally elevated portion of the diaphragm or, most commonly, hemidiaphragm. It may be congenital (usually idiopathic, but can be associated with congenital myopathies or intrauterine infections) or acquired (as a result of phrenic nerve injury during forceps delivery or surgery). There is variable thinning or absence of diaphragmatic muscle, at which point its distinction from congenital diaphragmatic hernia with a persistent hernia sac is obscure. The elevated diaphragm may produce abnormalities of chest wall mechanics with impaired pulmonary function. Respiratory distress and pneumonia are frequent presenting symptoms, although gastrointestinal symptoms such as vomiting or gastric volvulus may occur.

The diagnosis is made by chest radiograph and confirmed by fluoroscopy or ultrasound, which demonstrates paradoxical movement of the diaphragm during spontaneous respiration. Incidentally discovered small, localized eventrations do not need to be repaired. Eventrations that are large or that are associated with respiratory symptoms should be repaired by plicating the diaphragm using interrupted nonabsorbable sutures.

Harrison MR et al: Correction of congenital diaphragmatic hernia in utero IX: fetuses with poor prognosis (liver herniation and low lung-to-head ratio) can be saved by fetoscopic temporary tracheal occlusion. J Pediatr Surg 1998;33:1017.

Puri P: Congenital diaphragmatic hernia. Curr Probl Surg 1994; 31:785.

Tsugawa C et al: Diaphragmatic eventration in infants and children: is conservative treatment justified? J Pediatr Surg 1997; 32:1643.

Wilson JM et al: Congenital diaphragmatic hernia—a tale of two cities: the Boston experience. J Pediatr Surg 1997;32:401.

■ CONGENITAL LOBAR EMPHYSEMA

Lobar emphysema consists of hyperinflation of a single lobe; rarely, more than one lobe is affected. The upper and middle lobes are most frequently involved. There are three kinds of lobar emphysema: (1) hypoplastic emphysema, (2) polyalveolar lobe, and (3) bronchial obstruction.

Hypoplastic emphysema is distinguished by a segment, lobe, or whole lung that has a reduced number of bronchial branches with a diminished number and smaller size of blood vessels. The number of alveoli is abnormally decreased, but the air spaces are too large. The hyperlucent region seen on chest radiograph is normal or small in volume, and since it does not affect the surrounding normal lung, surgical treatment is unnecessary.

Polyalveolar lobe is characterized by a normal size and number of bronchial branches, but there is an abnormal number of alveoli from each respiratory unit. These alveoli are prone to expand excessively, producing emphysema, which encroaches on the surrounding normal lung and therefore requires removal.

Bronchial obstruction may occur either from deficient bronchial cartilage support, redundant mucosa, bronchial stenosis, mucous plug, or bronchial compression by anomalous vessels or other mediastinal lesions. With inspiration, the bronchus opens to allow air into the lung; but on expiration the bronchus collapses, trapping the air, and with each respiratory cycle there is progressive expansion of the lobe.

Clinical Findings

In one-third of patients, respiratory distress is noted at birth; in only 5% of cases do symptoms develop after 6 months. Males are affected twice as frequently as females. The signs include progressive and severe dyspnea, wheezing, grunting, coughing, cyanosis, and difficulty with feedings. Increased dimensions of the chest and retractions may be seen. The chest is hyperresonant, and decreased breath sounds may be noted over the affected lobe. Chest radiographs show radiolucency of the emphysematous lobe, with bronchovascular markings extending to the lung periphery. Compression atelectasis of the adjacent lung, shift of the mediastinum, depression of the diaphragm, and anterior bowing of the sternum can be seen. The emphysematous lobe may continue to expand, compressing adjacent lung and airways and asphyxiating the infant.

Treatment & Prognosis

Occasionally, the emphysema may be due to a mucous plug in the bronchus that may be aspirated by bronchoscopy. Compression of the bronchus by mediastinal masses may be relieved by removal of the tumor or repair of anomalous vessels. Treatment of mildly symptomatic cases may not be necessary.

Many patients with lobar emphysema are severely symptomatic, and pulmonary lobectomy is necessary. Anesthesia should not be started until all personnel are ready for emergency thoracotomy since positive-pressure ventilation may acutely enlarge the emphysematous lobe, thereby compressing the normal lung tissue and heart. The prognosis following surgical relief of the lobar emphysema is excellent. Some patients may show residual disease in the remaining lung. At long-term follow-up, lung volumes are normal, but the air flow rates are diminished.

Martinez-Frontanilla LA et al: Surgery of acquired lobar emphysema in the neonate. J Pediatr Surg 1984;19:375.

Olutoye OO et al: Prenatal diagnosis and management of congenital lobar emphysema. J Pediatr Surg 2000;35:792.

GREAT VESSEL ANOMALIES

Tracheobronchial and esophageal compression by the great vessels may occur as a result of anomalies of the aortic arch or of abnormally located or enlarged pulmonary arteries. While the most common abnormality is an aberrant right subclavian artery, the most important is the double aortic arch, as it often causes serious respiratory distress in young infants (Figure 46–7). Affected infants have a characteristic inspiratory and expiratory wheeze, stridor, or croup. Echocardiography, CT, and MRI can demonstrate the anomalous anatomy. Esophagoscopy and bronchoscopy may be helpful in assessing the degree and level of compression. The surgical approach is through a left thoracotomy. Following removal of the thymus, the aortic arch and its branches are skeletonized and the anatomy identified. For the double aortic arch, the smallest arterial component is divided; an anomalous right subclavian artery is divided at its origin. The accompanying fibrous bands and sheaths constricting the trachea and esophagus must also be divided.

Figure 46–7. Anterior (left) and posterior views of double aortic arch constricting the trachea and esophagus.

Sebening C et al: Vascular tracheobronchial compression syndromes—experience in surgical treatment and literature review. Thorac Cardiovasc Surg 2000;48:164.

Woods RK et al: Vascular anomalies and tracheoesophageal compression: a single institution's 25-year experience. Ann Thorac Surg 2001;72:434.

MEDIASTINAL MASSES

Mediastinal masses are relatively common in infants and children and can be classified according to the compartment of the mediastinum from which they arise. The mediastinum is classically divided into anterior, middle, and posterior compartments. Anatomically, the anterior mediastinum consists of the area between the sternum and the anterior aspect of the trachea and pericardium. The middle compartment contains the trachea, major bronchi, and paratracheal spaces. The posterior segment extends from the posterior aspect of the trachea to the spine.

Anterior mediastinal masses comprise approximately one-third of mediastinal masses. The most common of these masses are teratomas and lymphomas. Teratomas may be cystic or solid and may also be found within the pericardium (middle compartment). Approximately 20% are malignant. The remainder of these tumors include thymic cysts, thymomas, and lymphangiomas. Middle mediastinal masses are rare but when present are most likely to be bronchogenic cysts. Sixty percent of mediastinal masses are located within the posterior compartment. Neurogenic tumors are most common and include neuroblastoma, ganglioneuroblastoma, ganglioneuroma, neurofibroma, and neurofibrosarcoma. Common symptoms include respiratory distress (via tracheal or lung compression), Horner's syndrome, and pain. Enterogenous cysts or duplications are also commonly seen in the posterior compartment. They are termed neurenteric when there is an associated cervical or thoracic vertebral anomaly.

Grosfeld JL et al: Mediastinal tumors in children: experience with 196 cases. Ann Surg Oncol 1994;1:121.

■ CONGENITAL LUNG LESIONS

Congenital lung lesions, which arise from anomalous development of the foregut, are classified as follows: (1) bronchogenic cyst, (2) cystic adenomatoid malformation, (3) pulmonary sequestration, and (4) bronchopulmonary foregut malformation. Embryonic tissues that are destined to form bronchi and lung become anomalous isolated structures within or outside of the lung. These lesions produce symptoms from their size and position, resulting in compression of bronchi or lung parenchyma, or from infection and abscess formation within the cyst and surrounding normal lung.

BRONCHOGENIC CYST

Bronchogenic cysts are lined by cuboidal or ciliated columnar epithelium and are filled with mucoid material. Repeated infection in the cyst may produce squamous epithelial metaplasia. About half arise in the mediastinum and do not communicate with the bronchi. They appear as radiopaque masses on chest radiographs. When located within the lung parenchyma, the cysts usually communicate with the airways and consequently are prone to abscess formation. Bronchogenic cysts arise in the right lung three times more often than in the left. They are more common in the lower lobes but may be found in any lobe. Partial compression of bronchi produces hyperinflation of the involved lung, while complete obstruction produces atelectasis. Rupture of a cyst that communicates with bronchi may present as a tension pneumothorax. Treatment is by excision of the cyst, which may rarely require lobectomy.

CONGENITAL CYSTIC ADENOMATOID MALFORMATION

This lesion is considered a hamartoma in which multiple cysts are lined by a polypoid proliferation of bronchial epithelium surrounded by striated muscle and elastic tissue, but there is an absence of mucous glands and cartilage. They are most often lobar and are classified radiologically based on cyst size: type I are large (> 2 cm) cysts, type II are smaller cysts (< 2 cm), and type III have cysts that are so small as to import a solid appearance. These malformations occur with equal frequency in both lungs, with a slight predominance in the upper lobes. Associated renal and nervous system anomalies may be present.

Clinical Findings

A large lesion can compress the fetal lung, resulting in pulmonary hypoplasia at birth, and may distort or obstruct the esophagus, producing polyhydramnios. In addition, compression of venous return to the heart with exudation of protein into the lung fluid may cause fetal congestive heart failure, hydrops fetalis, and death in utero.

Treatment

If prenatal ultrasound can recognize the presence of this disorder in association with hydrops, resection in utero may be warranted. Children in whom hydrops did not occur before birth may be born asymptomatic (small lesions) or may have variable degrees of respiratory distress due to compression of the ipsilateral normal lung. Asymptomatic children may be observed, but resection (pulmonary lobectomy) is recommended since these lesions often become infected and there are case reports of malignant transformation occurring in untreated, long-standing cysts.

PULMONARY SEQUESTRATION & BRONCHOPULMONARY FOREGUT MALFORMATION

A sequestration consists of normally developed bronchioles and alveoli supplied by systemic rather than pulmonary arteries. Sequestrations occur in the lower chest, most commonly on the left, adjacent to the mediastinum. Rarely, sequestrations may occur in the upper or middle lobes or below the diaphragm. They usually have a systemic arterial blood supply from the aorta, either above or below the diaphragm. On rare occasions, a sequestration will communicate with the esophagus or stomach, a condition termed bronchopulmonary foregut malformation. Sequestrations may be intralobar (in older children) or extralobar. Intralobar lesions drain through the pulmonary veins, are in communication with the tracheobronchial tree, and are prone to infection and to lung abscess formation. Extralobar lesions drain into the azygous venous system, do not communicate with the lung, and are commonly asymptomatic. They are often found in association with congenital diaphragmatic hernia. Histologic evidence suggests that these lesions have embryologic origin similar to that of bronchogenic cysts and congenital cystic adenomatoid malformations. However, unlike the latter, sequestrations rarely grow large enough to produce hydrops and demise in utero. Treatment is by excision of the extralobar sequestration or lobectomy in cases of intralobar sequestration.

Adzick NS et al: Fetal lung lesions: management and outcome. Am J Obstet Gynecol 1998;179:884.

Cass DL et al: Cystic lung lesions with systemic arterial blood supply: a hybrid of congenital cystic adenomatoid malformation and bronchopulmonary sequestration. J Pediatr Surg 1997; 32:986.

Neilson IR et al: Congenital adenomatoid malformation of the lung: current management and prognosis. J Pediatr Surg 1991;26:975.

Nuchtern JG, Harberg FJ: Congenital lung cysts. Semin Pediatr Surg 1994;3:233.

■ CONGENITAL GASTROINTESTINAL LESIONS

ESOPHAGEAL ANOMALIES

The trachea and esophagus are derived from the primitive foregut. Initially, they appear as a common ventral diverticulum at about the nineteenth day of gestation. Beginning several days later, elongation and separation of the diverticulum into the airway and esophagus oc-curs in a caudal to cephalad direction. Errors in this process result in esophageal atresia, tracheoesophageal fistula, and their variants (Figure 46–8).

Classification

A. WITH ESOPHAGEAL ATRESIA

1. There is a blind proximal pouch and a fistula between the distal end of the esophagus and the trachea (type C, 85% of cases).

2. There is a blind proximal esophageal pouch, no tracheoesophageal fistula, and a blind distal esophagus (Type A, 10% of cases). This is referred to as "long gap" atresia.

3. There are fistulas between both proximal and distal esophageal segments and the trachea (Type D, 2% of cases).

4. There is a fistula between the proximal esophagus and the trachea and a blind distal esophagus without fistula (Type B, 1% of cases).

B. WITHOUT ESOPHAGEAL ATRESIA

1. There is an "H" type tracheoesophageal fistula that is usually present in the cervical region (Type E, 4–5% of cases).

2. There is esophageal stenosis consisting of a membranous occlusion (often containing cartilage) between the mid and distal third of the esophagus (rare).

3. There is a laryngotracheoesophageal cleft of varying length, consisting of a linear communication between these structures (very rare).

Figure 46–8. ***A:*** Pure (long gap) esophageal atresia. ***B:*** Esophageal atresia with proximal tracheoesophageal fistula. ***C:*** Esophageal atresia with distal tracheoesophageal fistula. ***D:*** Esophageal atresia with proximal and distal fistulae. ***E:*** Tracheoesophageal fistula without esophageal atresia. (Reproduced, with permission, from Grosfeld JL: Pediatric surgery. In: *Textbook of Surgery.* Sabiston DC [editor]. Saunders, 1991.)

Clinical Findings

Shortly after birth, the infant with esophageal atresia is noted to have excessive salivation and repeated episodes of coughing, choking, and cyanosis. Attempts at feeding result in choking, gagging, and regurgitation. Infants with tracheoesophageal fistula in addition to esophageal atresia will have reflux of gastric secretions into the tracheobronchial tree, with resulting pneumonia. Pneumonic infiltrates are usually noted first in the right upper lobe.

A size 10F catheter should be passed into the esophagus by way of the nose or mouth; if esophageal atresia is present, the tube will not go down the expected distance to the stomach and will coil in the upper esophageal pouch. If a tracheoesophageal fistula connects to the lower esophageal segment, air will be present in the stomach and bowel on plain radiographs. Absence of air below the diaphragm usually means that a distal tracheoesophageal fistula is not present.

Abdominal distention is a prominent finding because the Valsalva effect of coughing and crying forces air through the fistula into the stomach and bowel. The presence and position of the fistula can be determined by bronchoscopy. A general anesthetic is used, and rigid bronchoscopy will demonstrate the majority of fistulas in the lower one-third of the trachea.

Laryngotracheoesophageal cleft produces symptoms similar to those of tracheoesophageal fistula but of much greater severity. Laryngoscopy may show the cleft between the arytenoids extending down the larynx. Bronchoscopy is the best means of outlining the cleft.

There is a 50% incidence of associated anomalies: cardiac (patent ductus arteriosus, septal defects), gastrointestinal (imperforate anus, duodenal atresia), genitourinary, and skeletal. The VACTERL association (vertebral, anorectal, cardiac, tracheoesophageal, renal, and limb anomalies) is present in 25% of cases. Isolated esophageal atresia has been associated with various genetic abnormalities, including trisomy 18 and trisomy 21.

Treatment

A sump suction catheter should be placed in the upper esophageal pouch and the head of the bed elevated. An echocardiogram is required to determine the position of the aortic arch since a right-sided arch makes the standard right thoracotomy repair difficult and is present in 5% of infants. Aspiration pneumonia is treated before surgical treatment is begun. The infant is placed in a humidified incubator, turned from side to side every hour, and stimulated to cry and cough.

The goal of operative therapy is to divide and ligate the fistula and repair the atresia in one stage if possible.

This is usually performed using a right posterolateral thoracotomy with an extrapleural dissection. In infants with H type tracheoesophageal fistulas, the fistula is located above the thoracic inlet in two-thirds of cases. These fistulas may be divided through a left transverse cervical incision. A feeding gastrostomy tube is no longer routinely inserted except when the esophageal repair is under extreme tension, when there is long gap atresia not amenable to single-stage repair, and when there are severe associated anomalies (eg, congenital heart disease). A transanastomotic feeding tube is placed for postoperative feeding pending demonstration of a leak-free anastomosis by esophagogram obtained 7 days after surgery.

Staged operations are reserved for extremely premature babies and those with severe anomalies or long gaps between the esophageal pouches. There are several strategies for repairing these defects. These include cervical esophagostomy, division of the fistula, and insertion of a gastrostomy tube, followed several months later by esophageal replacement (colon or stomach interposition); gastrostomy tube alone with intermittent bougienage and stretching of the upper esophageal pouch, followed by primary esophageal anastomosis; and immediate interposition grafting.

Distal esophageal webs respond readily to esophageal dilation. This is usually accomplished with Hurst or Maloney mercury-weighted bougies. Dilations are repeated until healing occurs without recurrence of the webs. Esophagoscopy and excision of portions of a tough or thick web, using biopsy forceps or the endoscopic laser, may be required in addition to dilation. A lower esophageal stricture containing cartilage will require excision and anastomosis.

Prognosis

The survival rate for a full-term infant without associated anomalies is excellent. However, deaths do occur as a result of pulmonary complications, severe associated anomalies, prematurity, and sepsis due to anastomotic disruption. Anastomotic leaks occur either because of technical problems or because of the extreme weakness of the distal esophageal wall. In performing the anastomosis, the extrapleural approach prevents the development of empyema and confines infection to a small localized area. Swallowing is a reflex response that must be reinforced early in infancy. If establishment of esophageal continuity is delayed for more than 4–6 weeks, it may take many months or years to teach the patient to swallow. Babies with cervical esophagostomies should be encouraged to suck, eat, and swallow during gastrostomy feedings.

Dysphagia may occur for months or years following successful repair of esophageal atresia. Stricture of the anastomosis may require one or more dilations with a filiform and follower or with antegrade or retrograde dilators. Swallowed foreign bodies will lodge at the site of anastomosis and require removal with esophagoscopy. Another cause of dysphagia may be neuromuscular incoordination, usually associated with esophageal anomalies. This frequent problem improves with age.

Most of these infants have an alarming, barking cough and rattling sound on respiration owing to chondromalacia of the tracheal rings at the site of the tracheoesophageal fistula. This frequently improves with age. Reflux esophagitis sometimes follows successful repair and may result in recurrent aspiration pneumonitis and esophagitis. Recurrent anastomotic stricture is usually due to gastroesophageal reflux. A surgical antireflux procedure may be necessary.

Choudhory SR et al: Survival of patients with esophageal atresia: influence of birth weight, cardiac anomaly, and late respiratory complications. J Pediatr Surg 1999;34:70.

McKinnon LJ, Kosloske AM: Prediction and prevention of anastomotic complications of esophageal atresia and tracheoesophageal fistula. J Pediatr Surg 1990;25:778.

INTESTINAL OBSTRUCTION IN THE NEWBORN

Since fetuses continually swallow amniotic fluid into their gastrointestinal tracts and excrete it in the urine, intestinal obstruction may be noted on prenatal ultrasound by the presence of polyhydramnios (increased amniotic fluid level). The presence of polyhydramnios correlates with the level of the obstruction; it is most common with proximal gastrointestinal tract obstruction (eg, esophageal and duodenal atresia), is rarely noted with ileal atresia, and is never noted in association with anorectal obstruction.

After birth, vomiting is the principal symptom, and it is bile-stained if the obstruction is distal to the ampulla of Vater. It is important to note that bilious vomiting in the newborn is pathologic until proved otherwise. On physical examination, the presence and degree of abdominal distention depends on the level of the obstruction and should be noted. For example, there is no significant distention with duodenal obstruction versus massive distention with colonic obstruction (eg, Hirschprung's disease). A careful perineal examination should be performed to determine whether the anus is present, patent, and in the normal location. Meconium, the first newborn stool, passes in the first 24 hours of life in 94% of normal full-term infants and by 48 hours in 98%. Failure to pass meconium may be indicative of lower gastrointestinal tract obstruction. However, 30–50% of newborn infants with intestinal obstruction will pass meconium.

HYPERTROPHIC PYLORIC STENOSIS

Pyloric stenosis is the most common surgical disorder producing emesis in infancy. It results from hypertrophy of the circular and longitudinal muscularis of the pylorus and the distal antrum of the stomach with progressive narrowing of the pyloric canal (Figure 46–9). The cause is not known. The male:female incidence is 4:1. The disorder is more common in first-born infants and occurs four times more often in the offspring of mothers who had the disease as infants than in those whose fathers had the disease. If one monozygotic twin is affected, the other will also have the disorder in two-thirds of cases. A seasonal variation is noted in the occurrence of symptoms, with peaks in spring and fall.

Clinical Findings

A. SYMPTOMS AND SIGNS

Typically, the affected infant is full-term when born and feeds and grows well until 2–4 weeks after birth, at which time occasional regurgitation of some of the feedings occurs. Several days later, however, the vomiting becomes more frequent and forceful. The vomitus contains the previous feeding and no bile. Blood may be seen in the vomitus in 5% of cases, and coffee-grounds or occult blood is frequently present. Shortly after vomiting, the infant acts starved and will feed again. The stools become infrequent and firm in consistency as dehydration occurs. With dehydration, infants often have sunken fontanelles, dry mucous membranes, and poor skin turgor. Weight loss follows progressive starvation. Jaundice with indirect hyperbilirubinemia occurs in fewer than 10% of cases. Gastric peristaltic waves can usually be seen moving from the left costal

Figure 46–9. Hypertrophic pyloric stenosis. Note that the distal end of the hypertrophic muscle protrudes into the duodenum (arrow), accounting for the ease of perforation into the duodenum during pyloromyotomy.

margin to the area of the pylorus. In over 90% of cases, the pyloric "tumor," or "olive" can be palpated when the infant is relaxed. Abdominal relaxation may be accomplished by sedating the infant or by feeding clear fluids and simultaneously aspirating the stomach contents with a nasogastric tube.

B. IMAGING STUDIES

An imaging study is indicated only in the approximately 10% of cases in which a pyloric tumor cannot be palpated. Abdominal ultrasound, the most sensitive test, will identify hypertrophic pyloric stenosis when the muscle thickness is greater than 4 mm and the length of the pylorus is greater than 16 mm. A contrast upper gastrointestinal series can include the following diagnostic signs: (1) outlining of the narrow pyloric channel by a single "string sign" or "double track" owing to folds of mucosa; (2) a pyloric "beak" where the pyloric entrance from the antrum occurs; (3) the "shoulder" sign, in which the pyloric mass bulges into the antrum; and (4) complete obstruction of the pylorus.

Differential Diagnosis

Repeated nonbilious vomiting in early infancy may be due to overfeeding, intracranial lesions, pylorospasm, antral web, gastroesophageal reflux, pyloric duplication, duodenal stenosis, malrotation of the bowel, or adrenal insufficiency.

Complications

Repeated vomiting with inadequate intake of formula results in hypokalemic hypochloremic alkalosis, dehydration, and starvation. Gastritis and reflux esophagitis occur frequently. Aspiration of vomitus may produce pneumonia.

Treatment & Prognosis

The preferred operative treatment is the Fredet-Ramstedt pyloromyotomy, which should be undertaken only after dehydration and the hypokalemic hypochloremic alkalosis have been corrected. There are three approaches to the pyloromyotomy: a right upper quadrant transverse skin incision, a circumumbilical or intraumbilical skin incision, or a laparoscopic approach with the camera in the umbilicus and the two working instruments placed directly through the abdominal wall. If, during the pyloromyotomy, the mucosa is inadvertently entered (usually on the duodenal side), it is closed with fine nonabsorbable sutures and an omental patch. Large perforations are managed by closing the pyloromyotomy, rotating the pylorus 90 degrees, and repeating the myotomy. Successful repair is evident

when the submucosa is seen to herniate out of the myotomy site.

Multiple postoperative feeding schedules have been described, ranging from immediate full feeds to delayed feeds with incremental advances in volume. This has stemmed from the observation that nearly all patients with pyloric stenosis vomit after surgery, presumably due to gastric ileus, gastritis, gastroesophageal reflux, or all of the above. An incomplete pyloromyotomy (usually on the antral side) is suspected when vomiting persists beyond 2 weeks postoperatively.

Pyloric stenosis never recurs, and there is a uniformly excellent outcome.

Forman HP et al: A rational approach to the diagnosis of hypertrophic pyloric stenosis. J Pediatr Surg 1990;25:262.

Leinwald MJ, Shaul DB, Anderson KD: The umbilical fold approach to pyloromyotomy: is it a safe alternative to the right upper-quadrant approach? JACS 1999;189:362.

Rothenberg SS: Laparoscopic pyloromyotomy: The slice and pull technique. Pediatr Endosurg Innov Tech 1997;1:39.

CONGENITAL DUODENAL OBSTRUCTION

The various causes of duodenal obstruction are atresia, mucosal web, annular pancreas, preduodenal portal vein, and peritoneal bands (Ladd's bands) from malrotation. Duodenal atresia is distinguished from more distal gastrointestinal atresias since it is due to failure of recanalization of the duodenum rather than to an embryologic vascular abnormality. Atresia of the duodenum is twice as common as in the jejunum or ileum. In about half of cases, multiple congenital anomalies are present, including Down's syndrome in 30% and congenital heart disease in 20%. Birth weight is less than 2500 g in half of these infants. Mucosal webs or stenoses occur as often as pure atresia. Annular pancreas is almost always associated with hypoplasia of the duodenum at the level of the ampulla. The cause is a developmental defect characterized by circumferential persistence of the gland around the duodenum at the site of the embryonic ventral anlage, leading to duodenal obstruction and an accessory pancreatic duct.

Clinical Findings

In 75% of cases, duodenal obstruction occurs distal to the ampulla of Vater, causing bile to be diverted to the proximal duodenum and stomach. Bilious emesis occurs shortly after birth and during attempted feedings. The upper abdomen may be distended, with visible gastric peristalsis. Meconium is passed in over 50% of cases.

Abdominal radiographs show a distended stomach and duodenum ("double bubble" sign). Gas in the small and large intestine indicates incomplete obstruction. Contrast upper gastrointestinal series identifies the presence or absence of malrotation.

Treatment

The abdomen is either explored through a right upper transverse abdominal incision or laparoscopy is performed. A Kocher maneuver should be performed, with complete mobilization of the third and fourth portions of the duodenum. Obstruction from Ladd's bands requires simple division of the bands and correction of the malrotation (see below). Duodenoduodenostomy is performed for duodenal atresia and annular pancreas. A mucosal web is excised, taking care to avoid injury to the adjacent ampulla. Commonly, the duodenum is hugely dilated above the obstruction, which results in impaired aboral progression of ingested feedings. This problem is resolved by excision of a portion of the antimesenteric wall of the bowel to make the lumen diameter normal (tapered duodenoplasty). Gastrojejunostomy should not be done because the blind duodenal pouch may cause repeated vomiting. In all cases, the distal bowel must be irrigated and assessed for associated intrinsic obstruction and atresia (1–3% incidence). Mortality is related to prematurity and associated anomalies.

Grosfeld JL, Rescorla FJ: Duodenal atresia and stenosis: reassessment of treatment and outcome based on antenatal diagnosis, pathologic variance, and long-term followup. World J Surg 1993;17:301.

Spigland N, Yazbeck S: Complications associated with surgical treatment of congenital intrinsic duodenal obstruction. J Pediatr Surg 1990;25:1127.

ATRESIA & STENOSIS OF THE JEJUNUM, ILEUM, & COLON

Atresia and stenosis of the jejunum, ileum, and colon are caused by a mesenteric vascular accident in utero such as may result from hernia, volvulus, or intussusception, producing aseptic necrosis and resorption of the necrotic bowel. Although atresia may occur in any portion of the intestine, most cases occur in the proximal jejunum or distal ileum. A short area of necrosis may produce only stenosis or a membranous web occluding the lumen (type I) (Figure 46–10). A more extensive infarct may leave a fibrous cord between the two bowel loops (type II), or the proximal and distal bowel may be completely separated with a V-shaped defect in the mesentery (type IIIa). Multiple atresias occur in 10% of cases (type IV). A type III variant (type IIIb) is commonly called apple-peel or Christmas tree atresia, in which there is a blind-ending proximal jejunum, absence of a long length of mid small bowel, and a termi-

Figure 46–10. The anatomic spectrum of intestinal atresia. Type I is a stenosis or mucosal web. Type II, a fibrous cord between two bowel ends. Type IIIa, blind-ending proximal and distal bowel loops with a V-shaped mesenteric defect. Type IIIb (apple peel deformity, Christmas tree deformity) consists of a blind ending proximal jejunum, absence of a large portion of the midgut, and a terminal ileum that is coiled around its ileocolic blood supply. Type IV, multiple atresias of any kind. (Reproduced, with permission, from Grosfeld JL: Pediatric Surgery. In: *Textbook of Surgery.* Sabiston DC [editor]. Saunders, 1991.)

nal ileum coiled around its blood supply from the ileocolic vessels.

Clinical Findings

Vomiting of bile, abdominal distention, and failure to pass meconium indicate intestinal obstruction. The plain abdominal radiograph will give an estimate of how far along the intestine the obstruction exists; small bowel, however, cannot be distinguished from colon in the newborn. No contrast material should be given by mouth to newborn babies with complete intestinal obstruction. A barium enema may be indicated to detect the level of obstruction and the coexistence of anomalous rotation or associated colon atresia. In obstructions that occur in the distal bowel and appear relatively early in gestation, the colon is empty of meconium and appears abnormally narrow. When the obstruction is proximal or when it occurs late in pregnancy, meconium is passed into the colon. Barium enema will then outline a more generous-sized colon with its contents. In older children with evidence of partial intestinal obstruction, a small bowel series may be indicated to identify intestinal stenosis.

Treatment

There are three main goals of operation: (1) to restore the continuity of the bowel; (2) to preserve as much intestinal length as possible; and (3) to retain the ileocecal valve if possible (the minimum length of bowel needed to sustain enteral nutrition doubles in the absence of the ileocecal valve). A transverse upper abdominal incision is preferred. Infants with jejunal atresia usually have greatly dilated bowel from the stomach to the point of obstruction. This overly distended jejunum should be resected—to the ligament of Treitz, if necessary—since it is a source of persistent functional obstruction if it is retained. This same principle applies for membranous atresia, and the temptation to resect the web and perform a Heineke-Mikulicz resection should be resisted. If there is a long segment of abnormally dilated jejunum, the antimesenteric bowel wall should be resected or tapered to a normal diameter toward the intestinal anastomosis. Infants born with extensive small bowel loss may benefit from a Bianchi procedure, where the entire greatly dilated jejunum is divided longitudinally into two lengths of bowel. The end of the jejunum in continuity with the duodenum is anastomosed to the proximal end of the divided bowel.

In patients with ileal atresia, only the most distal blind end is bulbously dilated, and this should be excised. In order to prevent malabsorption, resection of the ileum should not be too extensive. A great discrepancy between the diameter of the segments of intestine proximal and distal to the atresia is the rule. Therefore, the preferred anastomosis will be end-to-oblique or end-to-side. Atresia of the proximal colon should be treated by resection of the dilated bowel and ileocolostomy. Atresia of the distal colon may be treated by proximal end colostomy or by a Mikulicz side-to-side colostomy. Later, the continuity of the distal colon may be established by end-to-end anastomosis.

In contrast to duodenal atresia, associated anomalies are unusual in small bowel and colon atresia. Following repair, return of gastrointestinal function is delayed and may not resume for 7–10 days.

Bianchi A: Autologous gastrointestinal reconstruction. Semin Pediatr Surg 1995;4:54.

Puri P, Fujimoto T: New observations on the pathogenesis of multiple intestinal atresias. J Pediatr Surg 1988;23:221.

Sato S et al: Jejunoileal atresia: a 27 year experience. J Pediatr Surg 1998;33:1633.

Thompson JS et al: Experience with intestinal lengthening for the short-bowel syndrome. J Pediatr Surg 1991;26:721.

DISORDERS OF INTESTINAL ROTATION

The fetal intestine begins as a somewhat straight tube that grows faster than the abdominal cavity and thus herniates out into the body stalk (future umbilicus) at about week 4–6 weeks' gestation. At 10–12 weeks, the bowel returns to the abdominal cavity and undergoes counterclockwise rotation about the superior mesenteric artery axis. The duodenojejunal portion of gut rotates posterior to the superior mesenteric vessels for 270 degrees (T12 level). The duodenojejunal junction becomes fixed at the ligament of Treitz and located to the left of and cephalad to the superior mesenteric artery. The cecocolic portion of the midgut also rotates 270 degrees counterclockwise, anterior to the superior mesenteric artery; and the cecum normally becomes fixed in the right lower abdomen (L5 level).

Classification

Anomalies of rotation and fixation are twice as common in males as in females. They may be classified as (1) nonrotation, (2) incomplete rotation, (3) reversed rotation, and (4) anomalous fixation of the mesentery.

A. NONROTATION

With nonrotation, the midgut is suspended from the superior mesenteric vessels; the small bowel is located on the right side of the abdomen and the large bowel in the left abdomen. No fixation occurs, and adhesive bands are not present. Because its base is so short, the mesentery is narrow, which predisposes to volvulus, with clockwise twisting of the bowel about the superior mesenteric vessels. This anomaly is usually found in patients with omphalocele, gastroschisis, and congenital diaphragmatic hernia.

B. INCOMPLETE ROTATION

Incomplete rotation may affect the duodenojejunal segment, the cecocolic segment, or both. Adhesive bands (Ladd's bands) are usually present. In the most common form, the cecum is located near the origin of the superior mesenteric vessels, and dense peritoneal bands extend from the right flank to the cecum and obstruct the second or third portion of the duodenum or other segments of the small bowel. This predisposes to volvulus (Figure 46–11).

C. REVERSED ROTATION

In reversed rotation, the bowel rotates varying degrees in a clockwise direction about the superior mesenteric axis. The duodenojejunal loop is anterior to the superior mesenteric artery. The cecocolic loop may be

Figure 46–11. Malrotation of the midgut with volvulus. Note cecum at the origin of the superior mesenteric vessels. Fibrous bands cross and obstruct the duodenum as they adhere to the cecum. Volvulus is untwisted in a counterclockwise direction.

prearterial or may be rotated clockwise or counterclockwise in a retroarterial position. In either case, the cecum may be right-sided or left-sided. The most frequent anomaly is retroarterial clockwise rotation, which causes obstruction of the right colon.

D. ANOMALOUS FIXATION OF MESENTERY

Anomalies of mesenteric fixation account for internal mesenteric and paraduodenal hernias, mobile cecum, or obstructing adhesive bands in the absence of anomalous bowel rotation. Excessive rotation of the duodenojejunal junction results in superior mesenteric artery compression of the third portion of the duodenum (superior mesenteric artery syndrome).

Clinical Findings

A. SYMPTOMS AND SIGNS

Anomalies of intestinal rotation may cause symptoms related to intestinal obstruction, peptic ulceration, or malabsorption. Three-fourths of patients develop intestinal obstruction in infancy. Older patients may develop intermittent obstruction. The obstruction is in the duodenum or upper jejunum as a result of adhesive bands or midgut volvulus. Vomiting of bile occurs initially. Older patients may be thin and underweight because of chronic postprandial discomfort or malabsorption. Malabsorption with steamm Hghea may result from partial venous and lymphatic obstruction, which is associated with coarse rugal folds in the small bowel. With duodenal obstruction from bands, abdominal distention is not prominent. Volvulus, however, produces marked abdominal distention. Bloody stools and signs of peritonitis are manifestations of intestinal infarction. Peptic ulcer occurs in 20% of patients, presumably as a result of antral and duodenal stasis.

B. IMAGING STUDIES

With obstructing Ladd's bands, plain abdominal radiographs may show a "double bubble" sign that mimics duodenal stenosis. Distribution of gas throughout the intestines may be normal, although there may be a paucity of it. When volvulus with gangrene occurs, the bowel is distended with gas, and the intestinal walls are thickened. Barium enema demonstrates abnormal position of the cecum. With chronic intermittent symptoms of obstruction and a normal position of the cecum on barium enema, an upper gastrointestinal and small bowel series will show distention of the duodenum, abnormal positioning of the duodenojejunal segment (usually to the right of the midline), and narrowing at the point of obstruction. The small bowel is commonly visualized on the right side of the abdomen and the colon on the left.

Treatment & Prognosis

Through a transverse upper abdominal incision, the entire bowel should be delivered from the abdominal cavity to assess the anomalous arrangement of the intestinal loops. Volvulus should be untwisted in a counterclockwise direction. The Ladd procedure is used for incomplete rotation with obstruction of the duodenum by congenital bands. It consists of division of the bands between the duodenum and proximal colon and the lateral abdominal wall. The mesentery is often folded upon itself due to intermesenteric adhesions, and these are incised. The appendix is removed. The cecum is then placed in the left lower quadrant, and the duodenum is moved to the right lateral abdomen. In essence, one is creating nonrotated intestinal anatomy much like the anatomic situation in early fetal life.

About 30% of infants treated for volvulus die from complications of midgut gangrene. Once the anomaly has been corrected, the long-term results are good.

Some patients tend to form adhesions that cause recurrent intestinal obstruction. Recurrent volvulus is rare after the Ladd procedure.

Bass KD, Rothenberg SS, Chang JH: Laparoscopic Ladd's procedure in infants with malrotation. J Pediatr Surg 1998;33:279.

Prasil P et al: Should malrotation in children be treated differently according to age? J Pediatr Surg 2000;35:756.

Rescorla F et al: Anomalies of intestinal rotation in childhood: analysis of 447 cases. Surgery 1990;108:710.

Torres AM, Ziegler MM: Malrotation of the intestine. World J Surg 1993;17:326.

MECONIUM ILEUS

In 10–20% of infants born with cystic fibrosis, the thick mucous secretions of the small bowel produce obstruction by inspissated meconium. This usually occurs in the mid ileum but may develop in the jejunum or colon. Although there is no clear correlation between pancreatic insufficiency and the development of inspissated meconium, meconium ileus also occurs in patients with pancreatic duct obstruction and pancreatic aplasia. Meconium obstruction with no apparent cause has also been described in newborn infants.

Clinical Findings

A. SYMPTOMS AND SIGNS

The infant typically has a normal birth weight. The abdomen is very distended. No meconium is passed, and bilious emesis occurs early. Loops of thick, distended bowel may be seen and palpated.

B. IMAGING STUDIES

Plain abdominal radiographs show loops of bowel that vary greatly in diameter; the thick meconium gives a ground glass appearance. Air mixed with the meconium produces the "soap bubble" sign, which is usually located in the right lower quadrant. Radiographs taken shortly after the infant has been placed in an upright position may fail to show air-fluid levels because the thick, viscid meconium fails to layer out rapidly. Contrast enema will show microcolon with some meconium flecks. Reflux of contrast medium through the ileocecal valve demonstrates a small terminal ileum containing "pellets" of inspissated mucus; more proximally, the bowel is progressively distended with packed meconium. Antenatal perforation may be detected by the presence of abdominal calcifications.

Complications

Meconium ileus may be complicated by volvulus of the heavy, distended loops of bowel. Depending upon how early in fetal life this occurs, the volvulus may progress to gangrene of the bowel, perforation with meconium peritonitis, or atresia of the ileum—singly or in combination.

Other common complications of meconium ileus are related to the almost universal presence of cystic fibrosis. These infants are susceptible to repeated pulmonary infection with chronic bronchopneumonia, bronchiectasis, atelectasis, and lung abscess. Malabsorption due to pancreatic insufficiency requires pancreatic enzyme replacement. Rectal prolapse and intussusception may be produced by passage of inspissated stools. Nasal polyps and chronic sinusitis are frequent. Biliary cirrhosis and bleeding varices from portal hypertension are late manifestations of bile duct obstruction by mucus.

Treatment & Prognosis

Nonoperative treatment is successful in 60–70% of cases. A nasogastric tube should be inserted and connected to suction. Under fluoroscopic control, enemas containing saline, full-strength diatrizoate meglumine, which is hygroscopic, or acetylcysteine, which is mucolytic, may disperse the meconium in uncomplicated cases. The infant must be well-hydrated, and intravenous infusions must be continued during and after the procedure in order to prevent hypovolemia. If this fails to relieve the obstruction, laparotomy is indicated. The ileum is opened and, if possible, flushed clear. The bowel can be reanastomosed or brought out as a double barrel stoma. Alternatively, a T-tube may be placed in the bowel and brought out the anterior abdominal wall for postoperative irrigations. Compromised intestine is resected, and appendectomy is performed because of the high frequency of appendicitis in patients with cystic fibrosis.

All patients should be evaluated for cystic fibrosis. Pancreatic enzyme replacement may be required. A formula low in long-chain fatty acids and high in medium-chain triglycerides may give better absorption and growth than standard formulas. The patient must be placed in an environment with high humidity to keep tracheobronchial secretions fluid. Ultrasonic mist is preferable. Postural drainage with cupping of the chest should be taught to the parents so that they will continue to maintain tracheobronchial toilet indefinitely. Long-term prophylactic antibiotics are not indicated, since infection with antibiotic-resistant pseudomonas and klebsiella organisms usually develops. Older children and adolescents may develop a meconium ileus-like syndrome termed distal ileal obstruction syndrome. This is ileal obstruction due to inspissated stool (common in those who are not compliant with their medications). Most often, it is successfully treated with hypertonic contrast enema.

Mak GZ et al: T-tube ileostomy for meconium ileus: four decades of experience. J Pediatr Surg 2000;35:349.

Ziegler MM: Meconium ileus. Curr Probl Surg 1994;31:731.

HIRSCHSPRUNG'S DISEASE

Hirschsprung's disease (aganglionic megacolon) is due to failure in the cephalocaudal migration of the parasympathetic myenteric nerve cells into the distal bowel. Therefore, the absence of ganglion cells always begins at the anus and extends a varying distance proximally. The aganglionic bowel produces functional obstruction because the bowel does not have normal propulsive waves and contracts en masse in response to distention. Short-segment aganglionosis involving only the terminal rectum occurs in about 10% of cases; the disease extends to the sigmoid colon in 75%; more proximal colon in 10%; and the entire colon with small bowel involvement in 5%. Extensive involvement of the small bowel is rare.

Males are affected four times more frequently than females when the disease is limited to the rectosigmoid. Females tend to have longer aganglionic segments. A familial association occurs in 5–10% of cases–more frequently when females are affected. The length of involvement tends to be consistent in familial cases. Other anomalies such as Down's syndrome are present in 10–15% of patients.

Clinical Findings

A. SYMPTOMS AND SIGNS

The absence of ganglion cells results in a functional obstruction since the affected area fails to relax due to unopposed sympathetic tone. The symptoms vary widely in severity but almost always occur shortly after birth. The infant passes little or no meconium within 24 hours. Thereafter, chronic or intermittent constipation usually occurs. Progressive abdominal distention, bilious emesis, reluctance to feed, diarrhea, listlessness, irritability, and poor growth and development follow. A rectal examination in the infant may be followed by expulsion of stool and flatus, with remarkable decompression of abdominal distention. In older children, chronic constipation and abdominal distention are characteristic. Passage of flatus and stool requires great effort, and the stools are small in caliber. Children with constipation from Hirschprung's disease do not exhibit soiling of their diapers or undergarments, distinguishing this form of constipation from idiopathic constipation (encopresis). These children are sluggish, with wasted extremities and flared costal margins. Rectal examination in older children usually reveals a normal or contracted anus and a rectum without feces. Impacted stools in the greatly dilated and distended sigmoid colon can be palpated across the lower abdomen.

B. IMAGING STUDIES

Plain abdominal radiographs in infants show dilated loops of bowel, but it is difficult to distinguish small and large bowel in infancy. A contrast enema should be performed. There should be no attempt to clean out the stool before the fluoroscopic examination, for this will obscure the change in caliber between aganglionic and ganglionic bowel. The contrast enema often demonstrates an aganglionic segment that appears relatively narrow compared wih the dilated proximal bowel. The proximal aganglionic intestine can be dilated by impacted stool or enema, giving a false impression of the level of the normal colon. Irregular, bizarre contractions (saw-toothed pattern) that do not encircle the aganglionic portion of the bowel may also be recognized. The dilated proximal bowel may have circumferential, smooth, parallel contractions (similar in appearance to those of the jejunum) that are exaggerated contraction waves. The contrast enema may not show a transition zone in the first 6 weeks after birth, since the liquid stool can pass the aganglionic bowel and the proximal intestine may not be dilated. Lateral radiographs should be taken of the pelvis to demonstrate the rectum, the transition zone, and the irregular contractions that may otherwise be obscured by the redundant sigmoid colon on anteroposterior views. Normally, the neonatal rectum is wider than the rest of the colon (including the cecum), and when the rectum is seen to be narrower than the proximal colon, the diagnosis is Hirschsprung's disease. Radiographs of the abdomen and lateral pelvis should be repeated after evacuation 24–48 hours later. The contrast will be retained for prolonged periods, and saline enemas may be required to evacuate it. The delayed film may show the transition zone and the bizarre irregular contractions more clearly than the initial study.

C. LABORATORY FINDINGS

Definitive diagnosis is made by rectal biopsy. Mucosal and submucosal biopsies may be taken from the posterior rectal wall with a suction biopsy capsule without anesthesia at the bedside. Serial sections may demonstrate the characteristic lack of ganglion cells and proliferation of nerve trunks in Meissner's plexus. If the findings are equivocal, it is necessary to remove a 1 cm or 2 cm full-thickness strip of mucosa and muscularis from the posterior rectum proximal to the dentate line under anesthesia. A sample of this size is sufficient for the pathologist to determine whether ganglion cells are or are not present in Meissner's plexus or in Auerbach's plexus. Manometric studies will show a failure of relaxation of the internal sphincter following rectal distention by a balloon, although this test is rarely performed except in older children.

Differential Diagnosis

Low intestinal obstruction in the newborn infant may be due to rectal or colonic atresia, meconium plug syndrome, or meconium ileus as well as a variety of functional causes such as hypermagnesemia, hypocalcemia, hypokalemia, and hypothyroidism. Hirschsprung's disease in patients who develop enterocolitis and diarrhea may mimic other causes of diarrhea. Chronic constipation due to functional causes may suggest Hirschsprung's disease. Although functional constipation may occur early in infancy, the stools are normal in caliber, soiling is frequent, and enterocolitis is not usually a problem. In functional constipation, stool is palpable in the lower rectum, and a barium enema shows uniformly dilated bowel to the level of the anus. However, short segment Hirschsprung's disease may be difficult to differentiate, and rectal biopsy may be necessary. Segmental dilation of the colon is a rare entity that causes constipation similar to that found in Hirschsprung's disease.

Treatment

Traditionally, the surgical treatment was staged and consisted of a leveling colostomy followed several months later by resection of the aganglionic bowel and performance of a pull-through procedure. The trend recently has been toward performing a single-stage procedure (no colostomy) in the newborn period. This paradigm is as follows: bowel obstruction and enterocolitis (if present) may be relieved by placement of a large (30F) rectal tube and repeated warmed saline irrigations in 10 mL/kg aliquots preoperatively. Infants with moderate to severe enterocolitis should be treated with a diverting colostomy. At the time of surgery, frozen section analysis of the colonic muscle is required in order to establish the correct (ganglionic) level for the stoma. Infants who are not ill may undergo any one of three effective operative procedures: Swenson operation, Duhamel operation, or Soave operation. The main operative principles for these procedures are removal of most or all of the aganglionic bowel—while preserving the surrounding nerves to the pelvic organs—and anastomosing ganglionic bowel (confirmed by frozen section analysis) to the rectum 0.5 cm above the dentate line. In contrast to the Swenson and Soave procedures, the Duhamel operation leaves a cuff of aganglionic rectum along which the ganglionic bowel is stapled, creating a mini-reservoir. Historically, these operations have been performed via a low transverse abdominal incision. However, the laparoscopic approach is the method of choice. A solely transanal mucosectomy has been used for those babies with short-segment disease.

In total aganglionic colon, ileostomy is necessary. Conservative treatment with enemas is ineffective because it does not prevent further obstruction and enterocolitis.

Prognosis

The death rate for untreated aganglionic megacolon in infancy may be as high as 80%. Nonbacterial, nonviral enterocolitis is the principal cause of death. This tends to occur more frequently in infants but may appear at any age. The cause is not known but seems to be related to the high-grade partial obstruction. There is no correlation between the length of aganglionosis and the occurrence of enterocolitis. Perforation of the colon and appendix may result from distal bowel obstruction. Atresia of the distal small bowel or colon also develops secondary to bowel obstruction due to Hirschsprung's disease in utero.

Anastomotic leak with perirectal and pelvic abscess is the most serious problem following definitive surgical treatment. This complication should be treated immediately by proximal colostomy until the anastomosis has healed. Necrosis of the pulled-through colon may occur if the bowel has not been mobilized sufficiently to prevent tension on the mesenteric blood supply.

Patients who are properly treated for Hirschsprung's disease do well. Problems with occasional incontinence and soiling may occur in a few cases. Episodic constipation and abdominal distention are more common, since the aganglionic internal anal sphincter is intact. Patients with these symptoms respond to anal dilation. Occasionally, an internal sphincterotomy may be necessary. Smaller children may still develop enterocolitis after definitive treatment, and they should be vigorously treated with a large rectal tube and enemas.

Albanese CT et al: Perineal one-stage pull-through for Hirschsprung's disease. J Pediatr Surg 1999;34:377.

Coran AG, Teitelbaum DH: Recent advances in the management of Hirschsprung's disease. Am J Surg 2000;180:382.

Georgeson KE et al: Primary laparoscopic-assisted endorectal colon pull-through for Hirschsprung's disease: a new gold standard. Ann Surg 1999;229:678.

Langer JC et al: One-stage versus two-stage Soave pull-through for Hirschsprung's disease in the first year of life. J Pediatr Surg 1996;31:33.

NEONATAL SMALL LEFT COLON SYNDROME (Meconium Plug Syndrome)

This problem of newborn infants consists of low intestinal obstruction associated with a left colon of narrow caliber and a dilated transverse and right colon.

The infants are in most cases otherwise normal, though approximately 30–50% are born to diabetic mothers and are large for gestational age. Most are over 36 weeks' gestational age and have normal birth weights. Two-thirds are male. Hypermagnesemia has been occasionally associated when the mother has been treated for eclampsia by magnesium sulfate injections.

Clinical Findings

Rectal examination may be normal or may reveal a tight anal canal. Little or no meconium is passed, and progressive abdominal distention is followed by vomiting. After thermometer or finger stimulation of the rectum, some meconium and gas may be evacuated. Contrast enema shows a very small left colon, usually to the level of the splenic flexure. Proximal to this point, the colon and commonly the small bowel are greatly distended. In about 30% of cases, a meconium plug is present at the junction of the narrow and dilated portion of the bowel, and the enema (using water-soluble contrast) will dislodge it. There is some risk of bowel perforation with the enema.

Differential Diagnosis

The small left colon syndrome may be confused with Hirschsprung's disease or meconium ileus. These lesions rarely cause obstruction at the level of the splenic flexure, and when the colon readily decompresses without further obstruction, Hirschsprung's disease is unlikely.

Complications

If colonic distention becomes severe, the cecum or appendix may perforate. The difficulty in differentiating small left colon syndrome from meconium ileus and Hirschsprung's disease may lead to inappropriate surgical exploration.

Treatment

A nasogastric tube should be inserted and intravenous fluids started. A contrast enema is required to differentiate the causes of low intestinal obstruction. When the left colon is narrow and contrast material refluxes into the dilated proximal colon, the diagnosis is most likely the small left colon syndrome. The contrast enema is usually followed by evacuation of stool and decompression of the bowel, with resolution of the problem. Persistent symptoms after evacuation of the meconium mandates a suction rectal biopsy to rule out Hirschsprung's disease.

INTUSSUSCEPTION

Telescoping of a segment of bowel (intussusceptum) into the adjacent segment (intussuscipiens) is the most common cause of intestinal obstruction in children under 2 years of age (Figure 46–12). The process of intussusception may result in gangrene of the intussusceptum. The most common form is intussusception of the terminal ileum into the right colon (ileocolic intussusception), but ileoileal, ileocolic, jejunojejunal, and colocolic intussusceptions also occur. In 95% of infants and children, no contributing cause is found. The disease is most common in midsummer and midwinter, and there is a correlation with adenovirus infections. In most cases, hypertrophied Peyer's patches are noted on the leading edge of bowel. Mechanical factors such as Meckel's diverticulum, polyps, hemangioma, enteric duplication, intramural hematoma (Henoch-Schönlein purpura), and intestinal lymphoma are present with increasing frequency in patients over 2 years old. Postoperative intussusception can occur at any age, is usually ileoileal or jejunojejunal, and is due to differential return of bowel motility. The ratio of males to females is 3:2. The peak age is in infants 5–9 months of age; 80% of patients are under the age of 2 years.

Figure 46–12. Intussusception.

Clinical Findings

The typical patient is a healthy child who suddenly begins crying and doubles up because of abdominal pain. The pain occurs in episodes that last for about 1 minute, alternating with intervals of apparent well-being. Reflex vomiting is an early sign, but vomiting due to bowel obstruction occurs late. Blood and mucus produce a "currant jelly" stool. In small infants and in postoperative patients, the colicky pain may not be apparent; these babies become withdrawn, and the most prominent symptom is vomiting. Pallor and sweating are common signs during colic. Repeated vomiting and bowel obstruction will produce progressive dehydration. A mass is usually palpable along the distribution of the colon. A hollow right lower quadrant may be noted. Occasionally, intussusception is palpable on rectal examination. Prolonged intussusception produces edema and hemorrhagic or ischemic infarction of the intussusceptum.

Treatment & Prognosis

The most important test is contrast enema, which is diagnostic and therapeutic in 60–80% of cases (Figure 46–13). Contrast enema (using either barium or air) should not be attempted until the patient has been resuscitated enough to allow an operative procedure to be performed safely. If barium is used, the column of contrast should not stand more than 100 cm above the sedated patient in order to minimize the risk of perforation. Air is pumped into the colon at a pressure of 60–80 mm Hg (certainly not more than 120 mm Hg). A successful study reduces the intussusceptum and demonstrates reflux of barium or air into the terminal ileum. Several attempts should be made before taking the child to surgery. Barium enema will not reduce gangrenous bowel.

Operation is required for unsuccessful enema reduction or signs of bowel perforation and peritonitis. The procedure may be performed either by laparotomy or laparoscopically. When no gangrene is present, reduction is accomplished by gentle retrograde compression of the intussuscipiens, not by traction on the proximal bowel. Resection of the intussusception is indicated if the bowel cannot be reduced or if the intestine is gangrenous. The appendix is usually removed to prevent confusion in later years if abdominal pain occurs and a right lower quadrant scar is present.

Intussusception recurs after 3% of barium enema reductions and 1% of operative reductions. Deaths are rare but do occur if treatment of gangrenous bowel is delayed.

Ong NT, Beasley SW: The leadpoint in intussusception. J Pediatr Surg 1990;25:640.

DiFiore JW: Intussusception. Semin Pediatr Surg 1999;8:214.

Meyer JS et al: Air and liquid contrast agents in the management of intussusception: a controlled, randomized trial. Radiology 1993;188:507.

Figure 46–13. Contrast enema demonstrating obstruction to retrograde flow of barium by a filling defect (intussusceptum) in the mid transverse colon. (Reproduced with permission from Albanese CT: Pediatric surgery. In: *Surgery,* Norton JA [editor]. Springer, 2000.)

ANORECTAL ANOMALIES
(Imperforate Anus)

The normal continence mechanism for bowel control consists of an internal sphincter composed of smooth muscle and the striated muscle complex from the levator ani and external sphincter. The striated muscles assume a funnel shape, originating from the pubis, pelvic rim, and sacrum. These muscles converge at the perineum while interdigitating with the internal and external sphincters. Most of the striated muscle complex consists of horizontal muscles that contract against the wall of the rectum and anus while longitudinal muscle fibers run in a cephalocaudal direction and elevate the anus.

Anomalies of the anus result from abnormal growth and fusion of the embryonic anal hillocks. The rectum is normally developed, and the sphincter mechanism is usually intact. With proper surgical treatment, the sphincter will function normally. Anomalies of the rectum develop as a result of faulty division of the cloaca into the urogenital sinus and rectum by the urorectal septum. In these anomalies, the internal sphincter and striated muscle complex are hypoplastic. Therefore, surgical repair results in varying degrees of continence.

Classification

Physical examination of the perineum and imaging studies determine the extent of malformation of the anus or rectum. When an orifice is evident at the perineum or distal vagina, the anomaly is referred to as a low imperforate anus; the absence of an obvious orifice at the perineal level suggests a high imperforate anus (anorectal atresia; see Figures 46–14 to 46–17.) In most instances, with high imperforate anus, there is a communication (fistula) with the urethra or bladder in the male or with the upper vagina or bladder in the female. Distinguishing between a high and low anomaly may be possible radiologically by determining the position of the rectum in relation to the levator ani or pubococcygeal line.

A. Low Anomalies

In low anomalies, the anus may be ectopically placed anterior to its normal position or it may be in the normal position with a narrow outlet due to stenosis or an anal membrane. There may be no opening in the perineum, but the skin at the anal area is heaped up and may extend as a band in the perineal raphe completely covering the anal opening. A small fistula usually extends from the anus anteriorly to open in the raphe of the perineum, scrotum, or penis in the male or the vulva in the female. These babies often have well-developed perineal and gluteal musculature and rarely have sacral vertebral anomalies.

B. High Anomalies

In high anomalies the rectum may end blindly (10%), but more commonly there is a fistula to the urethra or

Figure 46–15. **A:** High female autonomic anomaly. Low vaginal fistula. **B:** High female anomaly. High vaginal fistula. (Reproduced, with permission, from Pena A: *Surgical Management of Anorectal Malformations.* Springer-Verlag, 1992.)

bladder in the male or the upper vagina in the female. In the female, a very high fistula may extend between the two halves of a bicornuate uterus directly to the bladder. Patients with high imperforate anus often have deficient pelvic and gluteal musculature, a high incidence of sacral anomalies, and a poor prognosis for continence after surgical repair. The most severe of the high deformities is a cloacal anomaly in which there is a common channel between the poorly developed pelvic structures with a single perineal opening.

Clinical Findings

A. Signs

The best means of establishing the type of anorectal anomaly is by physical examination. In low anomalies, an ectopic opening from the rectum can be detected in the perineal raphe in males or in the lower vagina, vestibule, or fourchette in females. A high anomaly exists when no orifice or fistula can be seen upon exami-

Figure 46–14. **A:** Low female anomaly. Perineal fistula. **B:** Low female anomaly. Fourchette/vestibule fistula. (Reproduced, with permission, from Pena A: *Surgical Management of Anorectal Malformations.* Springer-Verlag, 1992.)

Figure 46–16. **A:** Low male anomaly. Perineal fistula. **B:** Low male anomaly. Rectobulbar urethra fistula. (Reproduced with permission from Pena A: *Surgical Management of Anorectal Malformations.* Springer-Verlag, 1992.)

Figure 46–17 *A:* High male anomaly. Rectoprostatic urethra fistula. *B:* High male anomaly. Rectovesical neck fistula. (Reproduced, with permission, from Pena A: *Surgical Management of Anorectal Malformations.* Springer, 1992.)

nation of the perineum or when meconium is found at the urethral meatus, in the urine, or in the upper vagina. Absence of external sphincter contraction with cutaneous stimulation of the anus may also help differentiate between high and low lesions.

B. IMAGING STUDIES

No single test is ideal in the evaluation of imperforate anus, so several studies are used to define the neonatal anatomy. Radiographs are sometimes useful when the clinical impression is unclear. A lateral film of the pelvis with the baby inverted (Wangensteen invertogram), once commonly used, is an inaccurate method of establishing the lower extent of the rectum because swallowed air may not have completely displaced the meconium from the rectum; or the striated muscle complex may be contracted, which obliterates the lumen and makes it look as if the gas in the rectum ends high in the pelvis. With crying or straining, the puborectalis muscle and rectum may actually descend below the ischium, giving a falsely low estimate of rectal height. Gas in the bladder clearly indicates a rectourinary fistula. Lower abdominal and perineal ultrasound, CT, and MRI have been advocated to define the pelvic anatomy and location in relation to the rectal musculature. Anomalies of the vertebrae and the urinary tract occur in two-thirds of patients with high anomalies and in one-third of male patients with low anomalies. Vertebral abnormalities in females invariably indicate a high imperforate anus. Anomalies of the sacrum warrant MRI of the lumbosacral area to identify spinal cord anomalies such as a tethered filum terminale.

Complications

Associated anomalies are frequent, occurring up to 70% of the time in association with high anomalies. The VACTERL and VATER syndromes are important

and require consideration (see Esophageal Anomalies). They include esophageal atresia, anomalies of the gastrointestinal tract, agenesis of one or more sacral vertebrae (agenesis of S1, S2, or S3 is associated with corresponding neurologic deficits, resulting in neuropathic bladder and greatly impaired continence), genitourinary anomalies (most common), and anomalies of the heart and lungs.

Delay in diagnosis of imperforate anus may result in excessively large bowel distention and perforation of the cecum. The presence of a rectourinary fistula allows reflux of urine into the rectum and colon, and absorption of ammonium chloride may cause acidosis. Colon contents will reflux into the urethra, bladder, and upper tracts, producing recurrent pyelonephritis.

Treatment

The three main goals of treatment are (1) to eliminate rectal obstruction, (2) to place the rectal pouch on the perineum in good position, and (3) to close the fistula.

A. LOW ANOMALIES

Low anomalies are usually repaired from the perineal approach in the newborn period using a muscle stimulator to precisely determine the location of the sphincter complex. The anteriorly placed anal opening is mobilized to the level of the levator ani and transferred to the normal position. After healing, the anal opening must be dilated daily for 6–8 months to prevent stricture formation and to allow for growth.

B. HIGH ANOMALIES

Traditionally, a high deformity was treated by a three-stage repair consisting of colostomy and mucous fistula formation, a posterior sagittal anorectoplasty 4–6 weeks later, and closure of the colostomy several months after that. Recently, the staged approach has been challenged and a one-staged repair has been performed by both the posterior sagittal and a laparoscopic approach. Because the anal sphincters are poorly developed—especially the internal sphincter—continence is most dependent upon a functioning striated muscle complex, which requires conscious voluntary contraction. Care must be taken to preserve the afferent and efferent nerves of the defecation reflex arc as well as the existing sphincter muscles. In all cases, the surgically created anus must be dilated for several months to prevent circumferential cicatrix formation.

Prognosis

Surgical complications include damage to the nervi erigentes, resulting in poor bladder and bowel control and failure of erection. Division of a rectourethral fistula some distance from the urethra produces a blind pouch prone to recurrent infection and stone formation, while cutting the fistula too short may result in urethral stricture. Erroneously attempting to repair a high anomaly from the perineal approach may leave a persistent rectourinary fistula. An abdominoperineal pull-through procedure performed for a low anomaly invariably produces an incontinent patient who might otherwise have had an excellent prognosis. Injury to the vas deferens and ureter is possible during repair of high anomalies.

Most patients with imperforate anus also have constipation as an inherent part of the defect. The colon and rectum are usually very dilated and have desultory motility. This is fortunate for individuals who have defective sphincter control, but it requires considerable attention to prevent obturation obstruction and constant soiling. Patients with low anomalies usually have good sphincter function. Children with high anomalies do not have an internal sphincter that provides continuous, unconscious, and unfatiguing control against soiling. However, in the absence of a lower spine anomaly, perception of rectal fullness, ability to distinguish between flatus and stool, and conscious voluntary control of rectal discharge by contraction of the striated muscle complex can be achieved. When the stools become liquid, sphincter control is usually impaired in patients with high anomalies.

Albanese CT et al: One-stage repair of high imperforate anus in the newborn male. J Pediatr Surg 1999;34:834.

Georgeson KE, Inge TH, Albanese CT: Laparoscopically assisted anorectal pull-through for high imperforate anus—a new technique. J Pediatr Surg 2000;35:927.

Hendren WH: Management of cloacal malformations. Semin Pediatr Surg 1997;6:217.

Pena A, Hong A: Advances in the management of anorectal malformations. Am J Surg 2000;180:370.

■ GASTROINTESTINAL TRACT ABNORMALITIES

GASTROESOPHAGEAL REFLUX

Studies of esophageal motility, including manometric measurements of the cardioesophageal junction, show absence of the high-pressure zone (lower esophageal sphincter) in the terminal esophagus in most normal newborns. Evolution to the normal adult pattern of peristalsis and cardioesophageal sphincter function occurs after several months. Until this happens, many infants experience varying degrees of regurgitation after feeding. Rarely, repeated gastric reflux may produce peptic esophagitis and interfere with development of a competent sphincter.

Clinical Findings

A. SYMPTOMS AND SIGNS

Symptoms consist of repeated effortless regurgitation of feedings, particularly when the baby is placed in a recumbent position. The baby will be hungry and will readily feed after regurgitating. Persistent regurgitation may result in poor weight gain, peptic esophagitis with appearance of blood in the vomitus, or occult bleeding, producing anemia. One cause for apnea and sudden infant death syndrome (SIDS) is regurgitation and aspiration. Lesser degrees of aspiration, particularly during sleep, may produce recurrent pneumonia. Stricture formation of the lower esophagus and metaplasia of the mucosa producing, Barrett's esophagus, are possible late effects. Almost half of infants and children with gastroesophageal reflux have neurologic disorders related to perinatal asphyxia or congenital nervous system anomalies. Abnormal motility of the esophagus and gastric dysmotility and impaired gastric emptying are frequently present. Gastroesophageal reflux is associated with esophageal atresia, congenital diaphragmatic hernia, and omphalocele.

B. IMAGING STUDIES

The standard diagnostic test is lower esophageal 24-hour pH monitoring. An upper gastrointestinal series is less sensitive but is useful to rule out other disorders (eg, intestinal malrotation) and to assess for esophageal stricture. Gastric emptying may be assessed by technetium pertechnate scan. There is virtually no role for esophageal manometric studies in children except for those in whom one suspects the relatively rare achalasia or diffuse esophageal spasm.

Treatment

Nonoperative treatment is successful in most cases. Feedings should be thickened with rice cereal, and reflux is lessened if the baby is maintained upright in an infant seat or in a prone position. Persistent symptoms mandate drug therapy with an antacid (eg, H_2 blocker or proton pump inhibitor) with or without a prokinetic agent (eg, metoclopramide). If a prolonged trial of nonoperative therapy fails or if complications of reflux can be documented (ie, esophagitis, stricture, asthma, recurrent aspiration pneumonia, failure to thrive), an antireflux procedure such as the Nissen or Thal fundoplication procedure is indicated. The open operation has been virtually replaced by the more cosmetic and better visualized laparoscopic procedure. Pyloroplasty may be required when there is associated impaired gastric emptying, though there is accumulating evidence suggesting that the "funneling" effect of the fundoplication promotes gastric emptying even in the face of documented delayed emptying.

Georgeson KE: Laparoscopic fundoplication and gastrostomy. Semin Laparosc Surg 1998;5:25.

Johnson DG: The past and present of antireflux surgery in children. Am J Surg 2000;180:377.

Kazerooni NL et al: Fundoplication in 160 children under 2 years of age. J Pediatr Surg 1994;29:677.

ACUTE APPENDICITIS

Acute appendicitis is one of the most common causes of acute abdomen in childhood. This diagnosis must be considered in all age groups, but it is most common between the ages of 4 and 15 years.

Clinical Findings

The diagnosis is most often made by obtaining a careful clinical history and performing a thorough physical examination. In some patients, observation and periodic reexamination by the same physician may be necessary to confirm or exclude the diagnosis. In young children, the diagnosis of appendicitis can be difficult to arrive at as the clinical history may be difficult to elicit. The classic presentation includes the onset of epigastric or periumbilical pain followed by anorexia, nausea, and vomiting. Anorexia is a significant finding, as the child will often refuse favorite foods. A fever will usually develop, and the pain then localizes to the right lower quadrant. Rovsing's sign (right lower quadrant pain during palpation of the left lower quadrant), localized tenderness, and involuntary spasm of the right hemirectus muscle indicate the presence of peritonitis.

A complete blood count with differential and urinalysis should be obtained in all patients. The white blood cell count is greater than $10,000/\mu L$ (often with a left shift) in more than 90% of patients with appendicitis. Radiologic evaluation should include a chest film to exclude pneumonia. Findings on flat and erect abdominal radiographs are often nonspecific, though they may infrequently demonstrate the presence of a fecalith. Ultrasound (particularly in females) and CT scans are being used with increasing frequency, especially for those without the classic history and physical examination results.

Differential Diagnosis

Gastroenteritis is often confused with appendicitis. Vomiting follows periumbilical pain in appendicitis but often precedes abdominal pain in gastroenteritis. In addition, the patient with gastroenteritis commonly has diffuse abdominal pain and frequent copious watery diarrhea. Intussusception, intestinal obstruction and volvulus, mesenteric adenitis, Meckel's diverticulum, ruptured ovarian cyst, and Crohn's disease must also be considered in the differential diagnosis for children. In adolescent girls, information regarding the menstrual cycle, previous episodes of pelvic inflammatory disease, and an accurate sexual history is important to exclude gynecologic causes of acute abdomen.

Treatment

Once the diagnosis is made, fluid resuscitation is performed and antibiotics are administered. Appendectomy is accomplished through a right lower quadrant incision or using the laparoscope. In cases of perforation, the peritoneal cavity is irrigated and aspirated dry but drainage is not performed. The wound is closed in all cases. Antibiotics are continued for 3–7 days or until the white blood cell count and fever normalize. The morbidity and mortality of appendicitis in children have gradually decreased even though the incidence of ruptured appendix at diagnosis remains high. Perforation is present in 25% of children at 24 hours after onset of symptoms, in 50% at 36 hours, and in 80% at 48 hours. Most deaths are noted in the very young when the diagnosis is not considered and long delays in treatment occur and in those with ruptured appendix who are not prepared properly for operation and develop renal failure and sepsis.

Madonna MB, Boswell WC, Arensman RM: Acute abdomen. Outcomes. Semin Pediatr Surg 1997;6:105.

Pearl RH et al: Pediatric appendectomy. J Pediatr Surg 1995; 30:173

DUPLICATIONS OF THE GASTROINTESTINAL TRACT

Duplications may occur at any point along the gastrointestinal tract from the mouth to the anus. Duplications occur (in order of decreasing frequency) in the ileum (50% of cases), mediastinum, colon, rectum, stomach, duodenum, and neck. Intrathoracic and small bowel duplications are usually spherical; colonic duplications are commonly long and tubular (Figure 46–18). Characteristically, the intra-abdominal duplications are within the mesentery and have a common wall with the intestine.

Based on embryology, duplications have been categorized as foregut, midgut, and hindgut. Foregut duplications include the pharynx, respiratory tract, esophagus, stomach, and the first portion and proximal half of the second portion of the duodenum. Midgut duplications include the distal half of the second part of the duodenum, the jejunum, ileum, cecum, appendix, the ascending colon and the proximal two-thirds of the transverse colon. The hindgut is composed of duplications of the

Figure 46–18. Duplications of the gastrointestinal tract. Duplications may be saccular or tubular. They usually arise within the mesentery, having a common wall with the intestine. Thoracoabdominal duplications arise from the duodenum or jejunum and extend through the diaphragm into the mediastinum.

distal third of the transverse colon, the descending and sigmoid colon, the rectum, anus, and components of the urologic system. Combined thoracoabdominal duplications also occur in which the thoracic saccular component extends through the esophageal hiatus or a separate diaphragmatic opening to empty into the duodenum or jejunum. A thoracic duplication, associated with a cervical or thoracic vertebral anomaly, in which the duplication communicates with the subarachnoid space, is called a neurenteric cyst. Associated cardiovascular, neurologic, skeletal, urologic, and gastrointestinal anomalies occur in more than a third of cases. Carcinoma may arise within duplications of the colon.

Clinical Findings

A. Symptoms and Signs

Two-thirds of patients with duplications are symptomatic in the first year of life. Duplications of the neck and mediastinum produce respiratory distress by compression of the airway. Thoracic duplications may also ulcerate into the lung and lead to pneumonia or hemoptysis. Intestinal duplications usually produce abdominal pain owing to spastic contraction of the bowel, excessive distention of the duplication, or peptic ulceration and bleeding resulting from ectopic gastric mucosa in the duplication. Intestinal obstruction due to intussusception, volvulus, or encroachment on the lumen by an intramural cyst also occurs. An isolated asymptomatic mass may be the only finding. Sixty percent of duplications are diagnosed by 6 months of life and 85% by 2 years.

B. Imaging Studies

Studies include radiographs of the chest and thoracolumbar spine, CT scan of the chest and abdomen, contrast enema, esophagography, and gastrointestinal series. If an intraspinal extension of a duplication is suspected, MRI is indicated. Ultrasonography may show a cystic or tubular mass within the mediastinum or abdomen.

Treatment

Duplications not intimately adherent to adjacent organs should be excised. Isolated spherical duplications can be excised with the adjacent segment of bowel and an end-to-end anastomosis of the bowel performed. Long tubular duplications can be decompressed by establishing an anastomosis between the proximal and distal ends of adjacent bowel. Noncommunicating duplications, which would require radical resection of surrounding structures, should be drained by a Roux-en-Y technique. Duplications that cannot be removed completely and which contain gastric mucosa should be opened (without jeopardizing the blood supply of the normal bowel) and the mucosal lining excised. Extension of a mediastinal duplication into the spine or abdomen should be resected. An intra-abdominal extension is closed at the level of the diaphragm, and complete excision by laparotomy is accomplished. Intraoperative radiography, including scintigraphy, ultrasonography, and cholangiography, may be of assistance in identifying anatomic arrangements.

Iyer CP, Mahour GH: Duplications of the alimentary tract in infants and children. J Pediatr Surg 1995;30:1267.

Merry C, Spurbeck W, Lobe TE: Resection of foregut-derived duplications by minimal access surgery. Pediatr Surg Int 1999;15:224.

Stern LE, Warner BW: Gastrointestinal duplications. Semin Pediatr Surg 2000;9:135.

Wilkinson CC et al: Fetal neurenteric cyst causing hydrops: case report and review of the literature. Prenat Diagn 1999;19:118.

OMPHALOMESENTERIC DUCT ANOMALIES

The omphalomesenteric (vitelline) duct is a remnant of the embryonic yolk sac. When the entire duct remains intact postnatally, it is recognized as an omphalomesenteric fistula. When the duct is obliterated at the intestinal end but communicates with the umbilicus at the distal end, it is called an umbilical sinus. When the epithelial tract persists but both ends are occluded, an umbilical cyst or intra-abdominal enterocystoma may develop. The entire tract may be obliterated, but a fibrous band may persist between the ileum and the umbilicus (Figure 46–19).

Figure 46–19. Omphalomesenteric duct anomalies arise from the primitive yolk sac. Remnants include Meckel's diverticulum, enterocystoma, and a fibrous band or fistulous tract between the ileum and the umbilicus.

The most common remnant of the omphalomesenteric duct is Meckel's diverticulum, which is present in 1–3% of the population. Meckel's diverticulum may be lined wholly or in part by small intestinal, colonic, or gastric mucosa, and it may contain aberrant pancreatic tissue. Heterotopic tissue is found in 5% of asymptomatic and 60% of symptomatic cases. In contrast to duplications and pseudodiverticula, Meckel's diverticulum is located on the antimesenteric border of the ileum, 10–90 cm from the ileocecal valve. Meckel's diverticulum occurs with equal frequency in both sexes. It is usually asymptomatic and is seen as an incidental finding during operation for other disease. Of those with Meckel's diverticulum, the lifelong risk of complications is 4%, and 40% of these cases occur in children under 10 years of age.

Clinical Findings

Symptomatic omphalomesenteric remnants (male:female incidence 3:1) produce rectal bleeding in 40%, intussusception in 20%, diverticulitis or peptic perforation in 15%, umbilical fistula in 15%, intestinal obstruction in 7%, and abscess in 3% of cases. Rectal bleeding associated with Meckel's diverticulum is due to peptic ulceration caused by ectopic gastric mucosa. Over 50% of these patients are under 2 years of age. The blood is mixed with stool and is most often dark red or bright red; tarry stools are unusual. A history of a previous episode of bleeding may be elicited in 40% of cases. Occult bleeding from Meckel's diverticulum is very rare. Younger patients tend to bleed quite briskly and may exsanguinate rapidly. Diverticulitis or free perforation will present with abdominal pain and peritonitis similar to acute appendicitis. The pain and tenderness occur in the lower abdomen, most commonly near the umbilicus. Periumbilical cellulitis may be present.

Intestinal obstruction may develop as a result of volvulus of the bowel about a persistent band between the umbilicus and the ileum or as a result of herniation of bowel between the mesentery and a persistent vitelline or mesodiverticular vessel. Obstruction is the most common presentation in adults. An infected umbilical sinus or omphalomesenteric fistula may present with mucoid, purulent, or enteric discharge, recurrent cellulitis, or a deep abdominal wall abscess about the umbilicus. This can be diagnosed by intubation and contrast injection via the umbilical tract.

Upper and lower contrast studies rarely outline the primary defect. Technetium Tc 99m pertechnetate may localize in gastric mucosa lining Meckel's diverticulum and may identify the source of hematochezia or melena. Retention of dye in the mucous and parietal cells is enhanced by giving cimetidine, 30 mg/kg intravenously, 30 minutes before administration of the radionuclide.

Treatment

After depleted blood volume has been restored and fluid and electrolyte disturbances have been corrected, resection can be accomplished by laparotomy or laparoscopy. An omphalomesenteric remnant with a narrow base may be treated by amputation and closure of the bowel defect. In cases where the anomaly has a wide mouth with ectopic tissue or where an inflammatory or ischemic process involves the adjacent ileum, intestinal resection with the diverticulum and anastomosis may be necessary. Involvement of Meckel's diverticulum by tumor would require intestinal resection with the lymphatic pathways of the mesentery.

Fa-Si-Oen PR, Roumen RM, Croiset van Uchelen FA: Complications and management of Meckel's diverticulum and intestinal duplication—a review. Eur J Surg 1999;165:674.

Moore TC: Omphalomesenteric duct malformations. Semin Pediatr Surg 1996;5:116.

NECROTIZING ENTEROCOLITIS

Necrotizing enterocolitis is the most serious and frequent gastrointestinal disorder of predominantly premature infants, with a median onset of 10 days after birth. The incidence is increasing given the recent therapeutic advances in neonatal intensive care that have allowed smaller and smaller babies to survive. It is characterized by necrosis, ulceration, and sloughing of intestinal mucosa, which frequently progresses to full-thickness necrosis and perforation. This process progresses from the submucosa through the muscular layer to the subserosa. Gas-producing bacteria in the intestinal wall may lead to pneumatosis, a finding that may be noted on gross examination as well as on plain abdominal radiographs. The terminal ileum and right colon are usually affected first, followed in descending order of frequency by the transverse and descending colon, appendix, jejunum, stomach, duodenum, and esophagus—in fact, the entire bowel may be necrotic. Eighty percent of cases occur in premature infants weighing less than 2500 g at birth, and 50% are under 1500 g. However, the disorder may also occur in full-term infants. Contrary to earlier impressions, there is no established relationship between necrotizing enterocolitis and stressful perinatal events such as premature rupture of membranes with amnionitis, breech delivery, intrauterine bradycardia, umbilical vessel catheterization with or without exchange transfusion, respiratory distress syndrome, sepsis, omphalitis, and congenital heart disease. An associated patent ductus arteriosus is common. In older infants and children, necrotizing enterocolitis is usually preceded by malnutrition and gastroenteritis. The clustering of cases in nurseries suggests that an infectious agent may be responsible.

Clinical Findings

Clinical findings include increased gastric residual, bilious vomiting, abdominal distention, bloody stools, lethargy, and poor skin perfusion. When intestinal perforation occurs, guarding is evident on abdominal examination, but in weak premature infants this may not be obvious. There are a variety of nonspecific clinical findings that suggest physiologic instability such as apnea, bradycardia, hypoglycemia, and temperature instability. On examination, abdominal distention and fixed loops of intestine may be appreciated. The presence of abdominal wall erythema, edema, and crepitus may be a sign of bowel necrosis. Laboratory evaluation is nonspecific since the white blood cell count may be low or high, but thrombocytopenia and acidosis develop with perforation and sepsis.

Supine and cross-table lateral abdominal radiographs show small bowel distention early, followed by pneumatosis intestinalis and eventually gas within the portal venous system. Serial examinations may show failure of movement of bowel loops. Perforation with peritoneal air develops in 20% of cases. Infants who develop ascites without pneumoperitoneum should have paracentesis and examination of the fluid for bacteria, which would signify perforation. Contrast studies are hazardous and contraindicated as they may easily lead to perforation.

Treatment

Treatment includes cessation of feedings, nasogastric suction, systemic antibiotics, and correction of hypoxemia, hypovolemia, acidosis, and electrolyte abnormalities. The only absolute indication for operation is pneumoperitoneum. Relative indications are portal vein air, clinical deterioration, a fixed intestinal loop on serial radiographs, erythema of the abdominal wall, an abdominal mass, and a paracentesis demonstrating bacteria. At laparotomy, necrotic bowel is resected and the proximal bowel is made into a stoma. Rarely is primary anastomosis safe. Severe disease may not be amenable to operation or require extensive bowel resection, resulting in short bowel syndrome. An alternative treatment option that is gaining acceptance for documented perforation is bedside drainage of the peritoneal cavity in the right lower quadrant using local anesthesia.

In one-third of cases, the disorder resolves without further treatment, and the overall survival rate is more than 50%. Intestinal stricture may occur as a late complication following healing. For this reason, a contrast enema is used to evaluate the defunctionalized distal bowel before closing the stoma.

Andorsky DJ et al: Nutritional and other postoperative management of neonates with short bowel syndrome correlates with clinical outcomes. J Pediatr 2001;139:27.

Ladd AP et al: Long-term follow-up after bowel resection for necrotizing enterocolitis: factors affecting outcome. J Pediatr Surg 1998;33:967.

Noble HG, Driessnack M: Bedside peritoneal drainage in very low birth weight infants. Am J Surg 2001;181:416.

GASTROINTESTINAL BLEEDING

Significant gastrointestinal bleeding in children is rare. When it occurs, it can be alarming and anxiety-provoking for caregivers and parents. The diagnostic approach used in the evaluation of these children is similar to that used in adults, but the causes vary depending on the age of the child. Rarely is the gastrointestinal bleeding massive, and the majority of causes are benign. A diagnosis can be established in over 85% of cases. Usual presenting symptoms include hematemesis, hematochezia, and melena. Depending on the amount of bleeding, the child may have sunken fontanelles, dry mucous membranes, and cool skin. Tachycardia, oliguria, and hypotension may be present. Intravenous access should be obtained, fluid and blood administered as needed, and an evaluation begun. Laboratory tests include serial hematocrits and coagulation studies. Following stabilization and physical examination, evaluation should then proceed to the appropriate diagnostic tests.

Upper Gastrointestinal Bleeding

Upper gastrointestinal bleeding originates above the ligament of Treitz. The presence of melena and the presence of blood on passage of an orogastric tube can help differentiate between upper and lower gastrointestinal bleeding. Upper gastrointestinal bleeding in infants and young children is most often associated with stress ulcers or erosions, but in older children it may also be caused by duodenal ulcer, esophagitis, and esophageal varices in children with underlying liver disease. The majority of these diseases are benign. Evaluation following stabilization of the child begins with flexible esophagoduodenoscopy. Once the diagnosis is made, treatment is usually amenable to antacids (H_2-blockers, proton pump inhibitors) and sucralfate. Variceal hemorrhage may require more aggressive intervention, including the use of octreotide, endoscopic varix sclerosis or band ligation, and, in extreme cases, transjugular intrahepatic portocaval shunt (TIPS), mesocaval shunt, or liver transplantation.

Lower Gastrointestinal Bleeding

Although diverticulitis, cancer, and angiodysplasia are the most common causes of lower gastrointestinal bleeding in adults, those diseases are not present in children. The causes of lower gastrointestinal bleeding in infants and children can be categorized in diagnostic age groups where the age of the patient, the amount of bleeding, and the color of the blood passed provide some guidance to the probable source of bleeding.

Bleeding in the neonate may be caused by swallowing maternal blood at delivery, an anorectal fissure, upper gastrointestinal bleeding secondary to gastritis or ulceration, necrotizing enterocolitis, volvulus, and an incarcerated hernia. The Apt test for maternal blood, physical examination of the rectum and inguinal canal, and evaluation of the upper gastrointestinal tract can quickly rule out most of these causes. Bleeding from necrotizing enterocolitis is rarely life-threatening, and the diagnosis is commonly made based on the premature delivery of the infant and radiologic evaluation. If bleeding from malrotation with midgut volvulus is suspected, prompt laparotomy is indicated.

In infants, anal fissures continue to be the most common cause of rectal bleeding. Other causes include intestinal volvulus, intussusception, intestinal duplication, Meckel's diverticulum, and infectious diarrhea. Contrast studies and appropriate stool cultures guide treatment. Children have a differential diagnosis similar to that of infants with the addition of rectal prolapse and a variety of polyps of the colon (juvenile, Peutz-Jeghers, polypoid lymphoid hyperplasia, and, rarely, adenomatosis). These entities are diagnosed by physical examination and proctosigmoidoscopy. If no source of bleeding is identified, colonoscopy is indicated. Juvenile polyps are the single most common cause of lower gastrointestinal bleeding in children (20–30%). Most juvenile polyps are single (80%) and often pass spontaneously without treatment. However, when bleeding continues to occur, the polyp can be snared and excised endoscopically. Adolescents may manifest signs and symptoms of inflammatory bowel disease (ulcerative colitis, Crohn's disease), familial adenomatous polyposis, and small vascular lesions such as telangiectasias. Diagnosis is made by colonoscopy, and treatment is disease-specific.

Arain Z, Rossi TM: Gastrointestinal bleeding in children: an overview of conditions requiring nonoperative management. Semin Pediatr Surg 1999;8:172.

Oldham KT, Lobe TE: Gastrointestinal hemorrhage in children: a pragmatic update. Pediatr Clin North Am 1985;32:1247.

GASTROINTESTINAL FOREIGN BODIES

Children aged 9 months to 2 years are at particular risk for the ingestion or aspiration of foreign bodies given their newly acquired mobility, curiosity, and the tendency to place objects in their mouths. The type of foreign body and the location in the airway or gastrointestinal tract dictate management.

Esophagal Foreign Bodies

Typical foreign bodies found in the esophagus include coins, food, and small toys. The three most common sites of obstruction are at the level of the cricopharyngeus muscle, at the level of the aortic arch, and at the gastroesophageal junction. Previous areas of repair or injury predispose to obstruction due to scar and narrowing. Common symptoms include drooling, feeding intolerance, dysphagia, and pain. Perforation is rare but is dictated by the ingested object's shape, composition, and time in the esophagus. The diagnosis is easily obtained by anteroposterior chest or lateral neck radiography if the ingested object is radioopaque. Otherwise, esophagoscopy or an upper gastrointestinal series is needed.

Because of the risk of erosion, aspiration, perforation, and late stricture, impacted objects should be removed. Extraction can be performed using balloon catheter retrieval under fluoroscopic control or under direct visualization using esophagoscopy with general anesthesia. The latter technique is generally preferred if the nature of the object is unknown or is sharp or the ingestion was 24–48 hours previously. A Hopkins rod lens endoscopy system allows visualization of the object and retrieval with specially designed forceps for grasping small objects.

Ninety-five percent of foreign bodies that pass beyond the gastroesophageal junction proceed uneventfully through the gastrointestinal tract. Operative retrieval is reserved for batteries, which must be removed, and for cases where ingested objects cause obstruction (bezoars), intestinal injury, or have been in place for more than 1 week.

Tracheal Foreign Bodies

Children, particularly those 1–2 years of age, can occlude the airway by aspiration of a foreign body. The most common objects are peanuts and pieces of popcorn. Obstruction tends to occur at the level of the laryngeal inlet, the subglottis, or the right main stem bronchus. Because this can be a life-threatening problem, witnessed events should be treated with back blows, abdominal thrusts, or the Heimlich maneuver, which may dislodge the object.

Symptoms include coughing, choking, wheezing, dyspnea, and fever. Unilateral wheezing and rhonchi may be present. Air trapping may result when the foreign body forms a ball-valve obstruction leading to hyperinflation of the affected lung and mediastinal shift away from the affected side. On the other hand, complete obstruction may lead to loss of air volume with atelectasis and mediastinal shift to the ipsilateral side. Inspiratory and expiratory radiographs or bilateral decubitus films in infants may demonstrate air trapping; the foreign body is rarely noted on radiographs.

With a worrisome history, a foreign body suggested on a radiograph, or any symptoms, the child should be taken to the operating suite for bronchoscopic evaluation under general anesthesia. Working in tandem with the anesthesiologist to allow ventilation during rigid endoscopy, the foreign body can be readily identified. Lighted grasping forceps made specifically for foreign body extraction are placed through the sheath of the bronchoscope; the foreign body is grasped; and the forceps, foreign body, and sheath are removed as one unit. Rarely, an unrecognized aspirated foreign body presents as chronic lung infection and can require removal of the affected lung.

Baharloo F et al: Tracheobronchial foreign bodies: presentation and management in children and adults. Chest 1999;115:1357.

Kaiser CW et al: Retained foreign bodies. J Trauma 1997;43:107.

■ LIVER & BILIARY TRACT DISORDERS

Jaundice in the first 2 weeks of infancy is usually due to indirect (unconjugated) hyperbilirubinemia. The causes include (1) "physiologic jaundice" due to immaturity of hepatic function; (2) Rh, ABO, and rare blood group incompatibilities, which produce hemolysis; and (3) infections. Jaundice that persists beyond the first 2 weeks in which the indirect and conjugated bilirubin levels are elevated should prompt a more thorough workup aimed at diagnosing potential surgical disorders. The most frequent cause (60%) of prolonged jaundice in infancy is biliary atresia; various forms of hepatitis occur in 35%; and choledochal cyst is found in 5% of cases of obstructive jaundice. Mild indirect hyperbilirubinemia occurs with pyloric stenosis and quickly disappears after pyloromyotomy. Intestinal obstruction can intensify jaundice by increasing the enterohepatic circulation of bilirubin. Finally, jaundice is an early and important sign of septicemia in the newborn.

BILIARY ATRESIA

Biliary atresia is the absence of patent bile ducts draining the liver. Familial cases and frequent association with the polysplenia syndrome indicate a congenital onset. However, biliary atresia probably develops after birth because jaundice is not usually remarkable in the newborn period but becomes evident more than 2 weeks later. Furthermore, conjugated bilirubin is not cleared by the placenta as unconjugated bilirubin is, and jaundice due to conjugated hyperbilirubinemia with biliary obstruction has not been recognized in newborn infants. The atretic ducts consist of solid fibrous cords that may contain occasional islands of biliary epithelium.

The extent of duct involvement varies greatly. There are three anatomic patterns of obstruction: (1) the proximal extrahepatic bile ducts are patent and the ducts distal to the cystic duct are obliterated; (2) the gallbladder, cystic duct, and common bile duct are patent and the proximal hepatic ducts are occluded: and (3) the entire extrahepatic ductal system is obstructed. Liver biopsy demonstrates proliferation of the bile canaliculi containing inspissated bile. Over time, the failure to excrete bile out of the liver results in progressive periportal fibrosis and obstruction of the intrahepatic portal veins, resulting in biliary cirrhosis.

Clinical Findings

A. SYMPTOMS AND SIGNS

The infant with biliary atresia often has an uneventful neonatal course until jaundice is noted at 2–3 weeks of age. Stools may be normal or clay-colored, and the urine may be dark. The stools contain an increased quantity of fat but are of normal consistency and not frothy. The liver may be of normal size early, but it becomes enlarged with time. A hard liver may develop as a consequence of progressive cirrhosis. Splenomegaly usually develops. Ascites and portal hypertension do not become manifest for several months.

B. LABORATORY FINDINGS

The workup of biliary atresia consists of analysis of liver function tests, complete blood count, and metabolic and serologic screening. The bilirubin levels may vary considerably from day to day, but direct bilirubin levels over 3 mg/dL are common. Alkaline phosphatase levels are often elevated to 500–1000 units/L, and γ-glutamyl-transpeptidase levels are greater than 300 units/L.

C. IMAGING STUDIES

Ultrasonography may demonstrate absence or inability to visualize a contracted gallbladder. Serial scintiscans of the right upper abdomen should be obtained after injection of technetium Tc 99m-labeled iminodiacetate compounds (IDA, HIDA, PIPIDA, DISIDA) to observe the intensity of uptake within the liver and evidence of secretion into the bowel. A 2- to 3-day course of phenobarbital should be given prior to the nuclide scan to promote tracer uptake. Needle biopsy of the liver may be safely performed at any age if bleeding and clotting tests are normal. A diagnosis based on needle biopsy is accurate in 60%, equivocal in 16%, and erroneous in 24% of cases. Unless the workup has conclusively diagnosed another entity, all children suspected of having biliary atresia

should undergo operative cholangiography with the intention of proceeding to exploration of the porta hepatis.

Other Causes

Other causes of obstructive jaundice are choledochal cyst, inspissated bile syndrome, and any one of several neonatal hepatitides. A choledochal cyst is identified by the presence of a palpable mass in the right upper quadrant and ultrasonographic confirmation. Inspissated bile syndrome follows a hemolytic process in which a large bilirubin load is excreted into the bile ducts, where it becomes coalesced and impacted, or may occur after a prolonged period of bowel rest with total parenteral nutrition. The syndrome is recognized by abdominal ultrasound. Hepatitis is most commonly of unknown cause. It may be due to a variety of infections, often of maternal origin, such as toxoplasmosis, cytomegalovirus, rubella syndrome, herpes simplex, coxsackievirus, and varicella. Serum should be tested for elevated antibody titers to these agents. Neonatal physiologic jaundice is self-limited and also responds to phototherapy.

Genetic metabolic diseases producing jaundice include alpha-antitrypsin deficiency, galactosemia, and cystic fibrosis. Other rare causes include sepsis, parenteral alimentation cholestasis, Gilbert's disease, and Alagille's syndrome.

Treatment

Surgical exploration for neonatal jaundice is indicated as early in infancy as possible, when biliary atresia is the likely cause. Delayed treatment will result in progressive cirrhosis. Preoperative care includes correction of anemia and administration of intravenous glucose and vitamin K. Fluoroscopy should be available in the operating room. The gallbladder is cannulated through a transverse abdominal incision. Diatrizoate diluted to 25% should be gently instilled into the biliary tree. If the image shows a patent common duct but no reflux into the liver, a rubber-shod bulldog clamp may be placed on the distal common duct and the cholangiogram repeated. During development of the radiograph films, a needle biopsy of each lobe is obtained.

Confirmed biliary atresia requires hepatic portoenterostomy (Kasai procedure). The scarred bile ducts and gallbladder are removed, and a Roux-en-Y limb of jejunum is sutured to an area of the hilum bounded laterally by the hepatic artery branches. A number of variations to this procedure, including use of an intussuscepted antireflux valve using the appendix or jejunal limbs, are used to minimize postoperative cholangitis. The appendix may also be used as a conduit between the porta hepatis and the duodenum.

Prognosis

A good long-term outcome is related to a meticulously performed procedure, age at operation less than 2 months, absence of cirrhosis at the time of operation, the presence of microscopic ductules in the portal plate, and establishment of adequate bile flow. In general, one-third of the infants will have excellent bile flow and do not develop liver failure; one-third never have bile flow and require early liver transplantation; and one-third have initially good bile flow but months to years later develop progressive biliary cirrhosis requiring liver transplantation. The average life span for infants with uncorrectable biliary atresia without transplantation is 19 months. Death is due to progressive liver failure, bleeding from esophageal varices, or sepsis. For those with established bile flow postoperatively, the most common complication is cholangitis, and this may recur. Most often, the cause is unknown and not readily correctable by surgical means.

Delarue A et al: Is the appendix graft suitable for routine biliary surgery in children? J Pediatr Surg 2000;35:1312.

Narkewicz MR: Biliary atresia: an update on our understanding of this disorder. Curr Opin Pediatr 2001;13:435.

Nio M, Ohi R: Biliary atresia. Semin Pediatr Surg 2000;9:177.

Tagge DU et al: A long-term experience with biliary atresia: reassessment of prognostic factors. Ann Surg 1991;214:590.

CHOLEDOCHAL CYST

A choledochal cyst is a dilation or diverticulum of all or a portion of the common bile duct. Estimates of incidence range from 1:2,000,000 to 1:13,000. There is a female predominance (3:1), and the lesions are more common in Asians, with a large majority of the reported cases from Japan. Numerous theories exist as to the cause of this abnormality, including infectious agents, reflux of pancreatic enzymes into the bile duct via a long common channel, genetic factors, and biliary autonomic dysfunction.

Choledochal cysts are classified into one of five subtypes. Type I is a fusiform dilation of the extrahepatic bile duct. Type II is a saccular outpouching of the common bile duct. Type III is referred to as a choledochocele and is a wide mouth dilation of the common duct at its confluence with the duodenum. Type IV is cystic dilation of both the intra- and extrahepatic bile ducts. Type V consists of lakes of multiple intrahepatic cysts with no extrahepatic component and when associated with hepatic fibrosis is termed Caroli's disease. Type I and type IV are the most common lesions, with type I cysts accounting for 85% of these abnormalities. Caroli's disease appears to be a congenital syndrome and often follows an autosomal recessive pattern of inheritance in association with various other anomalies such as polycystic kidney disease and renal tubular ectasia.

If left untreated, a choledochal cyst may cause cholangitis and cholangiocarcinoma. The risk of cholangiocarcinoma in the first decade of life is only 0.7%; however, this increases to 14% at 20 years and is postulated to increase even further throughout life. It has been suggested that type III cysts, or choledochoceles, represent a form of duodenal duplication and therefore do not share the malignant potential of other bile duct cysts.

Clinical Findings

The clinical manifestations of a choledochal cyst are recurrent abdominal pain, episodic jaundice, and a right upper quadrant mass, though in most cases one of these features is missing. As children grow older, the cyst may become painful or infected. On rare occasions, children have been described with bile peritonitis secondary to perforation of a cyst. In adults, an abdominal mass is rarely appreciated, and patients present more commonly with symptoms of cholangitis or pancreatitis. Gallstones and cholangitis may develop due to biliary stasis.

The diagnosis is most often established by the clinical presentation and abnormal ultrasonography. Technetium Tc 99m-labeled IDA scan, MRI, endoscopic retrograde cholangiopancreatography, upper gastrointestinal tract barium studies, and operative cholangiography may be necessary. Ultrasonography is increasingly responsible for detecting choledochal cysts in the fetus.

Treatment

In the past, the cysts were drained into a limb of intestine, but many of these patients developed carcinoma in the cyst years later. Presently, the treatment is complete excision with Roux-en-Y hepaticojejunostomy. The duodenal end of the bile duct should be oversewn without injury to the anomalous entry of the pancreatic duct, limiting the amount of residual biliary tissue at risk for malignancy. Side-to-side choledochoduodenostomy is not recommended because it is followed by a high incidence of stricture of the anastomosis and recurrent cholangitis. Cholecystectomy is always performed. Biliary cirrhosis and portal hypertension, occurring from prolonged ductal obstruction, may be assessed with liver biopsy. The results of choledochal cyst excision with hepaticojejunostomy reconstruction are consistently excellent, but these children do require lifelong follow-up because of the risk of anastomotic stricture and intrahepatic stone formation.

Han S et al: Acquired choledochal cyst from anomalous pancreaticobiliary duct union. J Pediatr Surg 1997;32:1735.

Lipsett PA et al: Choledochal cyst disease: a changing pattern of presentation. Ann Surg 1994;220:644.

Miyano T, Yamataka A: Choledochal cysts. Curr Opin Pediatr 1997;9:283.

O'Neill J: Choledochal cyst. Curr Probl Surg 1992;29:365.

■ INGUINAL & SCROTAL DISORDERS

INGUINAL HERNIA & HYDROCELE

Inguinal hernia is a common condition in infancy and childhood occurring in 1–3% of all children. Unlike hernias in adulthood, these nearly always result from a patent processus vaginalis (indirect hernia) and not from a weakness in the floor of the inguinal canal (direct hernia). The processus vaginalis follows the descent of the testis into the inguinal canal. Failure of obliteration of the processus may lead to a variety of anomalies, including hernia, communicating hydrocele, noncommunicating hydrocele, hydrocele of the spermatic cord, and hydrocele of the tunica vaginalis (Figure 46–20).

The processus vaginalis remains patent in over 80% of newborn infants. With increasing age, the incidence of patent processus vaginalis diminishes. At 2 years, 40–50% are open, and in adults 25% are persistently patent. Actual herniation of bowel into a widely patent processus vaginalis develops in 1–4% of children; 25% occur within the first year of life. Indirect inguinal hernia occurs four to six times more frequently in males. Direct and femoral hernias occur in children but are very rare.

Figure 46–20. Spectrum of inguinoscrotal disorders. ***A:*** Normal anatomy. The processus vaginalis is obliterated and there is a small remnant, the tunica vaginalis, adjacent to the posterior surface of the testis. ***B:*** Scrotal hydrocele. ***C:*** Communicating hydrocele. Note the proximal patency of the processus vaginalis. ***D:*** Hydrocele of the spermatic cord. ***E:*** Inguinal hernia. ***F:*** Inguinoscrotal hernia. (Reproduced, with permission, from Sheldon CA: Inguinal and scrotal disorders. In: *Essentials of Pediatric Surgery.* Rowe MI et al [editiors]. Mosby, 1995.)

Hernias are found on the right side in 60% of cases, on the left side in 30%, and bilaterally in 10%. Conditions associated with an increased risk of inguinal hernia include prematurity, family history, history of an abdominal wall defect (eg, gastroschisis), cryptorchidism, intersex anomalies, connective tissue disorders, and ascites. The processus vaginalis may be obliterated at any location proximal to the testis or labium.

Clinical Findings

The incidence of a clinically detectable inguinal hernia varies with gestational age: 9–11% in preterm infants and 3–5% for full-term infants. The diagnosis of hernia in infants and children can be made only by the demonstration of an inguinal bulge originating from the internal ring. The bulge often cannot be elicited at will, and signs such as a large external ring—the "silk glove" sign (thickening of the spermatic cord)—are not dependable. The hernia is often appreciated when the child strains or cries. Under these circumstances, a reliable history alone may be sufficient. One must always locate the position of the testis during examination for a hernia since an inguinal bulge due to an undescended or retractile testis may be mistaken for a hernia.

Incarcerated inguinal hernia accounts for approximately 10% of childhood hernias, and the incidence is highest in infants. In 45% of girls with incarcerated hernia, the contents of the sac consist of various combinations of adnexal structures. These structures are usually a sliding component of the sac.

Because hydroceles almost always represent peritoneal fluid trapped in a patent processus vaginalis, they are commonly called communicating hydroceles. A hydrocele is characteristically an oblong, nontender soft mass. With a noncommunicating hydrocele, the processus vaginalis has closed proximally and the fluid is most commonly trapped around the testicle or it can extend into the inguinal area. The normal spermatic cord can also be palpated above the level of the hydrocele. Transillumination is not reliable in the newborn since intestine and fluid transilluminate equally well.

Differential Diagnosis

A hydrocele under tension is often confused with an incarcerated inguinal hernia. The sudden appearance of fluid confined to the testicular area may represent a noncommunicating hydrocele secondary to torsion of the testis or testicular appendage or to epididymo-orchitis. Rectal examination and palpation of the peritoneal side of the inguinal ring may distinguish an incarcerated hernia from a hydrocele or other inguinoscrotal mass.

Complications

Failure to treat an inguinal hernia in infancy shortly after the diagnosis has been made may allow the hernia to become incarcerated and subsequently strangulated. About a third of incarcerated inguinal hernias in infancy show evidence of strangulation, and in 5% of cases the bowel is gangrenous. Compression of the spermatic vessels by an incarcerated hernia may produce hemorrhagic infarction of a testicle.

Treatment

In general, hydroceles that do not communicate with the peritoneal cavity are physiologic and the vast majority resolve within 1 year. Those that persist after 1 year or those that demonstrate changes in size (communicating hydroceles) should be repaired.

Inguinal hernia in infancy and childhood should be repaired soon after diagnosis to prevent incarceration, strangulation, or injury to the ipsilateral testis from compression of the spermatic cord by the incarcerated bowel. In premature infants under constant surveillance in the hospital, hernia repair may be deferred until the baby is ready to be discharged. High ligation of the hernia sac by obliteration of the internal ring (leaving enough space for the spermatic cord) is all that is required. Historically, it was recommended that all boys under 2 years of age and all girls under 5 years undergo operative exploration of the contralateral inguinal canal in search of a clinically silent patent processus vaginalis. This approach has been replaced, in large part, by laparoscopic exploration. This is performed either through the ipsilateral hernia sac, through the umbilicus, or in-line with the internal ring (at the lateral border of the rectus muscle) using a needlescope. If a patent processus vaginalis is demonstrated, a second inguinal incision is made and the procedure is repeated as described above. The incidence of complications from uncomplicated inguinal hernia repair (recurrence, wound infection, and damage to the spermatic cord) should be 2% or less.

An incarcerated hernia in an infant can usually be reduced initially before operation. This is accomplished by sedation and by elevation of the foot of the bed to keep intra-abdominal pressure from being exerted against the inguinal area. When the infant is well-sedated, the hernia may be reduced by gentle constant pressure over the internal ring in a manner that milks the bowel into the abdominal cavity. If the bowel is not reduced within an hour, operation is required. If the hernia is reduced, operative repair should be delayed for 48 hours to allow edema in the tissues to subside. An incarcerated ovary may not be able to be reduced but is usually asymptomatic, and repair at the next available operating room time is sufficient since torsion is rare and the blood supply, unlike that of the intestine, is not compromised by being trapped in the canal. Bloody stools and edema and red discoloration of the skin around the groin suggest a strangulated hernia, and reduction of the bowel should not be attempted. Emergency repair of incarcerated inguinal hernia is technically difficult because the edematous tissues are friable and tear readily. When gangrenous intestine is encountered, the bowel should be resected and an end-to-end intestinal anastomosis performed.

Fuenfer MM et al: Laparoscopic exploration of the contralateral groin in children: an improved technique. J Laparoendosc Surg 1996;1:S1.

Kapur P, Caty MG, Glick PL: Pediatric hernias and hydroceles. Pediatr Clin North Am 1998;45:773.

Yerkes EB et al: Laparoscopic evaluation for a contralateral patent processus vaginalis: part III. Urology 1998;51:480.

UNDESCENDED TESTIS (Cryptorchidism)

In the seventh month of gestation, the testicles normally descend into the scrotum. A fibromuscular band—the gubernaculum—extends from the lower pole of the testes to the scrotum, and this band probably acts by guiding the path for descent during differential growth of the fetus rather than by pulling the testes down. Undescended testis (cryptorchidism) is a form of dystopia of the testis that occurs when there is arrested descent and fixation of the position of the testis retroperitoneally, in the inguinal canal, or just beyond the external ring. Continued descent of the testes may progress after birth, but descent comes to a halt before 2 years of age.

Another form of dystopia is ectopic testis, in which the gubernaculum may have guided the testis to the pubis, penis, perineum, or thigh or to a subcutaneous position superficial to the inguinal canal. In these instances, the testis has descended beyond the external ring of the inguinal canal, and the vascular supply is sufficiently developed so as to pose little difficulty in operative repair.

Normal spermatogenesis requires the critical cooler temperature range provided in the scrotum. When the testis remains undescended and subjected to normal body temperature, degenerative changes in the seminiferous tubules occur in which the lining cells become progressively atrophic and hyalinized, with peritubular fibrosis. The degenerative changes begin to occur at 2 years of age. Unless the disorder is corrected, all bilaterally cryptorchid adult males become sterile.

The incidence of undescended or partially descended testis is 1–2% in full-term infants and up to 30% in pre-

mature babies. The cryptorchid testis may be located in the inguinal canal, in the peritoneal cavity, or anywhere in the lower abdomen, thigh, and perineum. The right testis is affected in 45% of cases, the left testis in 30%, and both testes in 25%. A patent processus vaginalis is present in 95% of patients with cryptorchidism, and approximately 25% develop a clinical hernia.

Anomalies associated with cryptorchidism occur in about 15% of cases and include a wide variety of syndromes. Fewer than 50% of the anomalies are associated with Klinefelter's syndrome, hypogonadotropic hypogonadism, or germinal cell aplasia. Other anomalies include the prune belly syndrome, horseshoe kidneys, renal agenesis or hypoplasia, exstrophy of the bladder, ureteral reflux, gastroschisis, and cloacal exstrophy.

Clinical Findings

Physical examination demonstrates an "empty hemiscrotum" with absent rugae. Because of the very active cremaster of children under 3 years of age and the small size of the testis, the gonad can retract into the external inguinal ring or within the inguinal canal. The retractile testis usually can be manipulated into the lower scrotum. This differentiation is important since no therapy is required for a retractile testis; it is a variant of normal.

Treatment

Operation is indicated after 12–18 months since degenerative changes begin to take place in these testes that may impair spermatogenesis and lead to malignant transformation. Additionally, cryptorchid testes are more susceptible to trauma and torsion, often have an associated inguinal hernia, and may cause adverse psychosocial effects. The incidence of testicular cancer in a cryptorchid testis (30 times higher than the normal population) is not lessened by repair, but a scrotal testicle can be more reliably examined for a testicular mass later in life.

Orchidopexy is the surgical method for mobilizing the testis—based on the testicular vessels and the vas deferens—from its ectopic location to the scrotum. When the dystopic testis is not palpable preoperatively, 17% are absent, 33% are intra-abdominal, and 50% are in the inguinal canal or just beyond the inguinal ring. If the testis is not palpable when the child is anesthetized, laparoscopy should be performed before making an inguinal incision. This will allow for identification of an abdominal testis or the diagnosis of an absent testis. Very high testes with a short blood supply can be brought into the scrotum by a two-stage repair (dividing the spermatic artery and vein with clips or lasers followed by positioning in the scrotum 6–8 weeks later) based on collateral blood supply via the vas deferens and the gubernaculum. Testes confined in the inguinal canal (25% of cases) can usually be brought into the scrotum in one stage. Ectopic testicles located outside the inguinal canal, such as in the subcutaneous inguinal pouch, occur in over 50% of cases, and the testicular vessels are so well developed that scrotal placement is rarely a problem. The prognosis for fertility following orchidopexy in unilateral maldescent is 80%, whereas fertility after bilateral orchidopexy is about 50%.

Docimo SG: The results of surgical therapy for cryptorchidism: a literature review and analysis. J Urol 1995;154:1148.

Humke U et al: Pediatric laparoscopy for nonpalpable testes with new miniaturized instruments. J Endourol 1998;12:445.

Mayr JM, Lawrenz K, Berghold A: Undescended testicles: an epidemiologic review. Acta Paediatr 1999;88:1089.

Pillai SB, Besner GE: Pediatric testicular problems. Pediatr Clin North Am 1998;45:813.

TESTICULAR TORSION

Testicular torsion is most frequent in late childhood and early adolescence, though the range can include the fetus and the adult. Anatomically, there are two forms of testicular torsion depending on where the spermatic cord is twisted with respect to the tunica vaginalis: intravaginal torsion (bell-clapper deformity), the most common form, and extravaginal torsion that occurs principally in neonates and in children with an undescended testis. Rarely, the testis may twist on a long epididymal mesentery. In children and adolescents, testicular torsion is either idiopathic or occurs after activity or trauma.

Clinical Findings

Acute scrotal or testicular pain that may radiate to the lower abdomen is usually present. Progressive swelling, edema, and erythema of the hemiscrotum occur. The testis is exquisitely tender to palpation. The testicle may be foreshortened, the epididymis may lie anteriorly, and the cremasteric reflex may be absent—though these signs are difficult to elicit. Fetal or neonatal torsion is probably responsible for the "absent" testis noted during the workup of cryptorchidism.

The diagnosis of testicular torsion is based mainly on clinical examination. Although one may utilize Doppler ultrasonography and radionuclide scanning to aid in the diagnosis, these tests are time-consuming and, in the case of ultrasound, not very specific.

Differential Diagnosis

Torsion of the testicular appendices (vestigial müllerian duct structures) and epididymitis may mimic testicular torsion. With epididymitis, there is often pyuria, voiding symptoms, and fever. Torsion of the testicular appendices often has a gradual onset, and careful palpation may reveal point tenderness rather than diffuse tenderness. There may be a visible necrotic lesion on scrotal transillumination (blue dot sign).

Treatment

If the diagnosis is strongly suspected, the best "test" is operative scrotal exploration. The testicular salvage rate if detorsion is performed within 6 hours after onset of symptoms is up to 97%, versus less than 10% if delayed more than 24 hours. At operation, the torsion is corrected and the gonad, if viable, is fixed to the hemiscrotum in three places. Because the paired testicle is at risk for torsion since the testicular anatomy tends to mirror itself, contralateral orchiopexy should be performed in all cases. Torsion of the testicular appendices tends to be self-limiting since necrosis and autoamputation usually occur. Treatment is with warm baths, limited activity, and an anti-inflammatory agent. If significant pain persists after 2–3 days and the appendix has not autoamputated, excision is indicated. Testicular salvage after neonatal torsion is rare.

Kass EJ, Lundak BL: The acute scrotum. Pediatr Clin North Am 1997;44:1251.

■ ABDOMINAL WALL DEFECTS

UMBILICAL HERNIA

A fascial defect at the umbilicus is frequently present in the newborn, particularly in premature infants. The incidence is highest in blacks. In most children, the umbilical ring progressively diminishes in size and eventually closes. Fascial defects less than 1 cm in diameter close spontaneously by 5 years of age in 95% of cases. When the fascial defect is greater than 1.5 cm in diameter, it seldom closes spontaneously. Unlike inguinal hernias, protrusion of bowel through the umbilical defect rarely results in incarceration in childhood. Surgical repair is indicated if the intestine becomes incarcerated, when the fascial defect is greater than 1.5 cm, and in all children over 4 years of age.

OMPHALOCELE

This is a midline abdominal wall defect noted in 1:5000 live births. The abdominal viscera (commonly liver and bowel) are contained within a sac composed of peritoneum and amnion from which the umbilical cord arises at the apex and center (Figure 46–21).

Figure 46–21. Neonate with omphalocele. The liver and bowel herniated through a midline abdominal wall defect and are surrounded by a sac of amnion and chorion from which the umbilical cord emanates. (Reproduced, with permision, from Albanese CT: Pediatric surgery. In: *Surgery*, Norton JA [editor]. Springer, 2000.)

When the defect is less than 4 cm, it is termed a hernia of the umbilical cord; when greater than 10 cm, it is termed a giant omphalocele. Associated abnormalities occur in 30–70% of infants and include, in descending order of frequency, chromosomal abnormalities (trisomy 13, 18, 21), congenital heart disease (tetralogy of Fallot, atrial septal defect), Beckwith-Wiedemann syndrome (large-for-gestational-age baby; hyperinsulinism; visceromegaly of kidneys, adrenal glands, and pancreas; macroglossia, hepatorenal tumors, cloacal extrophy), pentalogy of Cantrell, and prune belly syndrome (absent abdominal wall muscles, genitourinary abnormalities, cryptorchidism). Small omphaloceles are most often linked to chromosomal defects and Beckwith-Wiedemann syndrome, especially when the liver is not in the hernia sac.

Treatment

The primary goal of surgery is to return the viscera to the abdominal cavity and close the defect. With an intact sac, emergency operation is not necessary, so a thorough physical examination and workup for associated anomalies is performed. A nasogastric tube should be placed on suction to minimize intestinal distention. An umbilical artery catheter can be maintained without interfering with the repair.

The success of primary closure depends on the size of the defect and of the abdominal and thoracic cavities and on the presence of associated problems (eg, lung disease). It is wise to leave the sac in situ since primary closure may not be possible, and in this way one has maintained the best biologic dressing for the viscera.

Plastic wrap or a bowel bag can be used to supplement coverage to prevent heat loss. If the viscera reduce but abdominal wall closure is not possible, there are two options: staged repair and prosthetic patch repair. A staged repair aims to create a protective extra-abdominal extension of the peritoneal cavity (termed a silo), allowing gradual reduction of the viscera and gradual abdominal wall expansion using two parallel sheets of reinforced Silastic sheeting sutured to the fascial edges or a new preformed one-piece silo with a collapsible ring at its base for ease of insertion. A prosthetic patch repair bridges the fascial gap with a nonabsorbable material (eg, polytetrafluoroethylene) and the skin is closed over the patch. The silo is progressively compressed to invert the amniotic sac and its contents into the abdomen and to bring the edges of the linea alba together by stretching the abdominal wall muscles. This usually requires 5–7 days, after which the defect is then primarily closed. The intra-abdominal pressure produced by the silo should not exceed 20 cm H_2O to avoid impairing venous return from the bowel and kidneys. When abdominal relaxation is sufficient to allow the rectus muscles to come together, the silo is removed, the amnion is left inverted into the abdominal cavity, and the defect in the linea alba is closed.

In rare cases, nonoperative management is advised for infants with severe associated anomalies. The amnion is allowed to dry and form an eschar. The membrane becomes vascularized beneath the eschar, and contraction of the wound with skin growth covers the defect. A ventral hernia results which is repaired electively when the patient is stable. The survival rate for infants with small omphaloceles is excellent. Deaths associated with larger omphaloceles are principally from wound dehiscence and ensuing infection and from associated anomalies.

GASTROSCHISIS

Gastroschisis is a defect in the abdominal wall that usually is to the right of a normal insertion of the umbilical cord (Figure 46–22). It is believed to arise at the site of involution of the right umbilical vein, though there is some evidence that it results from rupture of an omphalocele sac in utero. It is twice as common as omphalocele. The remnants of the amnion are usually reabsorbed. The skin may continue to grow over the remnants of the amnion, and there may be a bridge of skin between the defect and the cord. The small and large bowel herniate through the abdominal wall defect, and, as is not the case with omphaloceles, the liver is virtually never present in the hernia. Having been bathed in the amniotic fluid and with compression of the blood supply at the abdominal defect, the bowel wall has a very thick, shaggy membrane ("peel") cover-

Figure 46–22. Neonate with a gastroschisis. The defect is to the right of the umbilical cord, and the bowel has no investing sac. Note edema of the bowel wall and the dilated stomach adjacent to the umbilical cord. (Reproduced, with permission, from Albanese CT: Pediatric surgery. In: *Surgery.* Norton JA [editor]. Springer, 2000.

ing it. The loops of intestine are usually matted together, and the intestine appears to be abnormally short. The membrane thickens during delay in surgical closure and compromises the outcome. When the anomaly is discovered in utero by ultrasound, planned delivery at a tertiary care hospital where immediate operation can be performed is possible.

Complications

Since the bowel has not been contained intra-abdominally, the abdominal cavity fails to enlarge, and it frequently cannot accommodate the protuberant bowel. Over 70% of infants with this disorder are premature, but associated anomalies occur in fewer than 10% of cases. Nonrotation of the midgut is present. Associated intestinal atresia occurs in approximately 7% because segments of intestine that have herniated through the defect become infarcted in utero.

Treatment & Prognosis

Unlike omphalocele, urgent repair is necessary. Small defects may be closed primarily after manually stretching the abdominal cavity. A staged approach is frequently required. Initially, the bowel should be covered by forming a tube from silicone-coated fabric and incorporating the protuberant bowel into the tube (silo). As bowel wall edema subsides, the bowel will readily reduce into the abdominal cavity. Reduction is aided by having the infant paralyzed and receiving endotracheal ventilation to relax the abdominal wall and allow it to stretch and accommodate the bowel. When the bowel

has completely returned to within the abdomen (usually 5–7 days), the silo is removed and the abdominal wall is closed in layers.

The death rate for infants with gastroschisis is less than 5%. Poor gastrointestinal function and episodes of sepsis, presumably from compromised bowel, may occur. Prolonged postoperative ileus (more than 2 weeks) is the rule, and total parenteral nutrition is necessary.

Langer JC: Gastroschisis and omphalocele. Semin Pediatr Surg 1996;5:124.

Lunzer H, Menardi G, Brezinka C: Long-term follow-up of children with prenatally diagnosed omphalocele and gastroschisis. J Matern Fetal Med 2001;10:385.

Molik KA et al: Gastroschisis: a plea for risk categorization. J Pediatr Surg 2001;36:51.

■ CUTANEOUS VASCULAR ANOMALIES

Cutaneous vascular anomalies comprise a group of congenital and acquired vascular malformations of the skin. They are present in 2.6% of all newborns. These anomalies are broadly divided into two categories: hemangiomas and vascular malformations. They are most precisely classified by the biologic activity of the endothelium.

HEMANGIOMAS

Hemangiomas demonstrate endothelial hyperplasia and are seen in children and adults but behave differently at different ages. Hemangiomas are much more common than vascular malformations. In the neonatal period, hemangiomas can be subclassified according to their growth phase. A rapid proliferating phase is usually seen during the first few years of life followed by an involuting phase that may last several years.

Clinical Findings

The clinical appearance depends on the depth of the lesion. Superficial dermal lesions (capillary hemangiomas, strawberry hemangiomas) are raised and profoundly erythematous, with an irregular texture; deep lesions (cavernous hemangiomas) are smooth and slightly raised, with a bluish hue or a faint telangiectatic pattern on the overlying skin. Mixed lesions are often noted (capillary-cavernous hemangiomas). Twenty percent of patients have multiple lesions. Complications from hemangiomas consist of ulceration (during the proliferative phase), bleeding, thrombocytopenia (Kasabach-

Merritt syndrome), consumptive coagulopathy, high-output heart failure, visual field encroachment, airway obstruction, and minor skeletal distortions.

Treatment

Fifty percent of hemangiomas will involute without treatment by age 5 years and 70% by 7 years. The remainder will slowly resolve by age 10–12 years. Steroid therapy hastens the rate of proliferation of hemangiomas by 30–90% and is indicated for complicated lesions (ie, those causing severe physiologic or anatomic abnormalities).

CUTANEOUS VASCULAR MALFORMATIONS

Vascular malformations have normal endothelial cell turnover and tend to grow with the child. These lesions are structural anomalies that are considered errors in vascular morphogenesis. They are usually visible at birth but may take years or even decades to become manifest. They are separated into low-flow and high-flow variants and further classified according to the type of vascular channel abnormality: capillary, venous, arterial, and mixed malformations. Capillary and venous malformations are low-flow variants; arterial and mixed arterial and venous ones are high flow variants.

Capillary Malformations

Capillary malformations are nevus flammeus (port wine stain), nevus flammeus neonatorum (angel's kiss), nevus flammeus nuchae (stork bite, salmon patch), angiokeratomas, and telangiectasias (spider, hereditary hemorrhagic telangiectasia [Rendu-Osler-Weber syndrome]). They are prone to infection and are treated aggressively with intravenous antibiotics. A compression garment should be used if anatomically feasible. Some lesions can be excised or injected with a sclerosing solution.

Venous Malformations

Venous malformations have a wide spectrum of appearances ranging from simple varicosities to complex deep lesions that may be located in deeper tissues (eg, bone, muscle, salivary gland). Pain is often related to thrombosis within the lesion. Radiographic imaging delineates the nature and extent of the lesion (angiogram, CT, MRI). Photocoagulation or Nd:YAG laser may be effective for superficial lesions. Resection is the definitive treatment since it can reduce bulk, improve contour and function, and control pain. It is limited by anatomic boundaries, and multiple-staged procedures may be required.

Arterial Malformations

Arterial and arteriovenous malformations are associated with multiple small fistulas surrounded by abnormal tissues and can cause high-output cardiac failure. They are most common in the head and neck region (especially intracerebral). There is pain and overlying cutaneous necrosis. Adjacent osseous structures are often destroyed. Selective embolization is used either as palliation or presurgically to limit hemorrhage. Excision, when possible, is the treatment of choice.

Combined Malformations

Combined vascular malformations and hypertrophy syndromes consist of Klippel-Trenaunay-Weber syndrome (combined capillary-lymphatic venous malformation associated with lower limb hypertrophy), Parkes-Weber syndrome (upper limb arteriovenous shunting), Maffucci's syndrome (low-flow vascular malformations and multiple extremity enchondromas with hypoplastic long bones), and Sturge-Weber syndrome (upper facial port wine stain and vascular anomalies of the choroid plexus and leptomeninges).

Low DW: Hemangiomas and vascular malformations. Semin Pediatr Surg 1994;3:40.

Mulliken JB, Fishman SJ, Burrows PE: Vascular anomalies. Curr Probl Surg 2000;37:517.

■ TUMORS IN CHILDHOOD

NEUROBLASTOMA

Of all childhood neoplasms, neuroblastoma is exceeded in frequency only by leukemia and brain tumors. Approximately 60% of cases occur within the first 2 years of life and 97% within the first 20 years. This tumor is of neural crest origin and may originate anywhere along the distribution of the sympathetic chain. The most common site for primary disease is in the abdomen (adrenal), followed by the thorax, pelvis, and occasionally the head and neck. Neuroblastomas originate in the retroperitoneal area in 75% of cases; 55% arise from the adrenal gland. They may reach massive size and violate tissue planes such that they envelop major blood vessels, their branches, and other important structures (eg, ureters), making initial primary resection potentially hazardous. The biologic behavior varies with the age of the patient, the site of primary origin, and the extent of the disease.

Clinical Findings

A. SYMPTOMS AND SIGNS

Symptoms are site-specific. The most common symptom is pain (from primary or metastatic disease). Nonspecific symptoms include growth retardation, malaise, fever, weight loss, and anorexia. Children frequently appear ill at the time of diagnosis. Constipation and urinary retention are signs of pelvic disease. Orbital metastases commonly present with periorbital ecchymoses and proptosis ("raccoon eyes"). Spinal canal involvement may present with acute paralysis due to compression. Opsomyoclonus syndrome is an acute cerebellar encephalopathy characterized by ataxia, opsoclonus ("dancing eyes"), myoclonus, and dementia. It occurs in association with approximately 3% of all neuroblastomas and is usually associated with a good prognosis, though the neurologic abnormalities tend to persist after successful treatment of the primary tumor. Infants with stage IV-S disease (see below) may display cutaneous metastases ("blueberry muffin" lesions) or respiratory embarrassment secondary to massive hepatomegaly from tumor infiltration. Palpable lesions are often hard and fixed.

In infants, metastases confined to the liver or subcutaneous fat are frequent and bone metastases unusual. In older children, metastases to lymph nodes and bone are found in over 70% of cases at diagnosis. Pain in areas of bony involvement and in joints with associated myalgia and fever mimics rheumatic fever. Eighty-five to 90 percent secrete high levels of the catecholamine metabolites vanillymandelic acid and homovanillic acid. Hypertension and diarrhea may occur as a result of catecholamine and vasoactive intestinal peptide secretion.

B. IMAGING STUDIES

Imaging is aimed at defining the extent of the tumor and determining the presence of metastases to distant sites (most commonly lymph nodes, bone, lung, and liver). Neuroblastoma is the most common abdominal tumor to demonstrate calcifications (50%) prior to chemotherapy. CT scan of the area of tumor involvement helps to identify the relationship to surrounding structures and determine resectability. CT myelography is useful in assessing tumor within the spinal canal and spinal cord compression. MRI is as sensitive as CT scanning in terms of assessing tumor size and resectability but has the added advantage of being superior to CT in assessing vessel encasement, vessel patency, and spinal cord compression. MRI can also demonstrate bone marrow involvement in selected cases. Metaiodobenzylguanidine (MIBG) or somatostatin receptor scintigraphy is very sensitive in detecting tumors which concentrate catecholamines and has been useful in the diagnosis of primary, residual, and metastatic disease in patients with neuroblastoma. For retroperitoneal tumors, an intravenous urogram may show displacement or compression of the adjacent kidney without distortion of the renal calices. Bone scans may be useful in detecting osseous metastases.

Prognostic Factors

Favorable prognostic factors include diagnosis before age 1, a thoracic primary lesion, and low stage. In addition, several molecular and cellular characteristics of neuroblastic tumors are prognostically important. The most important is the high incidence of amplification of the proto-oncogene N-*myc*, seen in approximately 30% of tumors. Amplification of N-*myc* (more than 10 copies) adversely correlates with prognosis independently of clinical stage. Using the histologic Shimada index, well-differentiated, stroma-rich tumors have a favorable prognosis. An elevated ratio of vanillymandelic acid to homovanillic acid correlates with an improved outcome in patients with advanced disease. Other biochemical indicators of advanced disease include neuron-specific enolase, serum ferritin, and serum lactate dehydrogenase. Staging systems are surgically and anatomically based and have prognostic value. The most recent is the International Neuroblastoma Staging System (Table 46–5).

Treatment

Diagnosis depends upon demonstration of immature neuroblastic tissue obtained by tissue or bone marrow aspirate and biopsy. Tissue is obtained by biopsy (either

Table 46–5. Staging of neuroblastoma.

	Survival
I. Tumor confined to site of origin	100%
IIa. Unilateral tumor completely excised. Nodes negative.	80%
IIb. Unilateral tumor, complete or incomplete excision. Nodes positive.	70%
III. Tumor infiltrating across the midline, or a unilateral tumor with contralateral nodes positive.	40%
IV. Remote disease in bone, soft tissue, distant nodes.	15%
IVs. Infants with stage I or stage II primary and remote spread to liver, skin, or bone marrow.	85%

by laparotomy or laparoscopically), which allows accurate determination of resectability and ensures that adequate tissue (1 g or 1 cm^3) is available for determination of tumor markers, cytologic studies, and the special stains required for accurate diagnosis and staging.

A localized neuroblastoma should be excised, and the local area of the tumor should be irradiated only when gross tumor remains. Unresectable neuroblastomas should be biopsied and treated initially by chemotherapy and radiation therapy and then by surgical resection for residual tumor. Removal of all residual disease is the goal, and a more radical approach is warranted. Most neuroblastomas are radiosensitive and respond to 3000 cGy or less of radiation. Patients with disseminated disease should be treated with a combination of chemotherapeutic agents such as cyclophosphamide, vincristine, dacarbazine, doxorubicin, cisplatin, and teniposide. Patients with stage III or stage IV tumors who are at high risk by virtue of their age or of the stage or biologic characteristics of the tumor benefit from total body irradiation followed by either allogeneic or, more commonly, purged autologous bone marrow transplantation.

Chamberlain RS et al: Complete surgical resection combined with aggressive adjuvant chemotherapy and bone marrow transplantation prolongs survival in children with advanced neuroblastoma. Ann Surg Oncol 1995;2:93.

Grosfeld JL: Risk-based management: current concepts of treating malignant solid tumors of childhood. J Am Coll Surg 1999; 189:407.

Matthay KK: Neuroblastoma: a clinical challenge and biologic puzzle. CA Cancer J Clin 1995;45:179.

Shimada H et al: International neuroblastoma pathology classification for prognostic evaluation of patients with peripheral neuroblastic tumors: a report from the Children's Cancer Group. Cancer 2001;92:2451.

WILMS' TUMOR
(Nephroblastoma)

Renal neoplasms account for about 10% of malignant tumors in children. Nephroblastoma (Wilms' tumor), which accounts for 80% of these, consists of a variety of embryonic tissues such as abortive tubules and glomeruli, smooth and skeletal muscle fibers, spindle cells, cartilage, and bone. Seventy-five percent of children with nephroblastoma are under 5 years of age; the peak incidence is at 2—3 years. With current multimodality treatment, the survival rate exceeds 85%.

The left kidney is affected in 50% of cases of Wilms' tumor and the right kidney in 45%. In 5% of cases, the tumors are bilateral; 60% are synchronous and 40% are metachronous. Associated anomalies and their incidence per 1000 cases are aniridia, 8.5; hypospadias, 18; hemihypertrophy, 25; and cryptorchidism, 28. Beck-

with-Wiedemann syndrome and neurofibromatosis occur together occasionally, and renal tumors may also occur in families. The constellation of Wilms' tumor, aniridia, genitourinary anomalies, and mental retardation (WAGR syndrome) is associated with deletion of 11p13.

Clinical Findings

A. SYMPTOMS AND SIGNS

In contrast to what is seen in euroblastoma, children are usually healthy-appearing. Symptoms consist of abdominal enlargement in 60%; pain in 20%; hematuria in 15%; malaise, weakness, anorexia, and weight loss in 10%; and fever in 3%. An abdominal mass, palpable in almost all cases, is usually very large, firm, and smooth, and it does not ordinarily extend across the midline. Hypertension, noted in over half of patients, may cause congestive heart failure.

B. IMAGING STUDIES

Imaging is required to determine the extent of the mass; to assess for bilateral disease, venous invasion, and metastases; and to confirm contralateral renal function. This is accomplished with abdominal ultrasound and a CT scan of the chest and abdomen.

Differential Diagnosis

Abdominal masses may also be caused by hydronephrotic, multicystic, or duplicated kidneys and by neuroblastoma, teratoma, hepatoma, and rhabdomyosarcoma. Ultrasonography and CT scanning can usually distinguish nephroblastoma from these other tumors. Calcification occurs in 10% of cases of nephroblastoma and tends to be more crescent-shaped, discrete, and peripherally situated than the calcifications of neuroblastoma, which are finely stippled.

Treatment & Prognosis

Surgical excision is often accomplished without any preoperative treatment. The aim of surgery is to completely remove the tumor (nephrectomy) and ureter without spill and to determine the tumor stage by virtue of its extent and the presence lymph node involvement (Table 46–6). Stage I is tumor confined to a kidney that has been completely excised; stage II is tumor extending beyond the kidney (perirenal tissues, renal vein or vena cava, biopsy or local spill in the flank) and completely excised; stage III is residual, nonhematogenous tumor confined to the abdomen (lymph node metastases, preoperative or intraoperative diffuse peritoneal deposits, residual tumor at the surgical margins, or unresectable tumor); stage IV is hematogenous

Table 46–6. Wilms' tumor staging system.

Stage I: Tumor limited to kidney and completely excised. The surface of the renal capsule is intact and the tumor was not ruptured prior to removal. There is no residual tumor.
Stage II: Tumor extends through the perirenal capsule but is completely excised. There may be local spillage of tumor confined to the flank, or the tumor may have been biopsied. Extrarenal vessels may contain tumor thrombus or be infiltrated by tumor.
Stage III: Residual nonhematogenous tumor confined to the abdomen: lymph node involvement, diffuse peritoneal spillage, peritoneal implants, tumor beyond surgical margin either grossly or microscopically, or tumor not completely removed.
Stage IV: Hematogenous metastases to lung, liver, bone, brain, etc.
Stage V: Bilateral renal involvement at diagnosis; each kidney should be staged separately.

metastases (lung, liver, bone, and brain); and stage V is bilateral renal involvement.

Irradiation of the tumor bed is indicated if the tumor has extended beyond the capsule of the kidney to involve adjacent organs or lymph nodes or if intraoperative tumor spillage has occurred. Very large tumors may be treated with radiation therapy and chemotherapy preoperatively to reduce their size. A significant reduction in size usually occurs in 7–10 days, after which nephrectomy can be readily performed. Nephrectomy is accomplished through a long transverse or thoracoabdominal incision.

Palpation of the renal veins and inferior vena cava is performed to detect tumor thrombus. The contralateral kidney must be examined and palpated. The treatment of bilateral disease is individualized with the goal of eradicating tumor while preserving the maximal amount of functional renal mass. Bilateral involvement (6%) is a contraindication to primary nephrectomy. Suspicious lesions in the opposite kidney are biopsied. Bilateral disease mandates "nephron-sparing" surgery. If the tumor is too large for safe resection, it is biopsied along with regional lymph nodes. Chemotherapy with or without radiation therapy will usually result in a significant reduction in tumor size and allow subsequent resection. Metastatic foci in the lung or liver may be resected or treated with radiation therapy. Any residual tumor following radiation therapy, including multiple lesions, should be resected.

Overall survival is 85%, and most patients are cured. Survival correlates with stage and histology. The 4-year survival with respect to age and histology is shown in Table 46–7. Tumor rupture with gross spillage portends a sixfold increase in risk of local recurrence and requires the use of postoperative external beam radiation.

Table 46–7. Four-year survival for Wilms' tumor.

Stage I/FH: 98%
Stage I–III/UH: 68%
Stage II/FH: 90–95%
Stage III/FH: 85–90%
Stage IV/FH: 78–86%
Stage IV/UH: 52–58%

FH: Favorable histology
UH: Unfavorable histology

Capra ML et al: Wilms' tumor: a 25-year review of the role of preoperative chemotherapy. J Pediatr Surg 1999;34:579.

Green DM et al: Wilms tumor. CA Cancer J Clin 1996;46:46.

Haase GM, Ritchey ML: Nephroblastoma. Semin Pediatr Surg 1997;6:11.

RHABDOMYOSCARCOMA

Rhabdomyosarcoma is a childhood malignancy that arises from embryonic mesenchyme with the potential to differentiate into skeletal muscle. It is the most common pediatric soft tissue sarcoma and is the third most common solid malignancy. It accounts for 4–8% of all malignancies and 5–15% of all solid malignancies of childhood.

The age distribution is bimodal—the first peak is between 2 years and 5 years, and the second peak is between 15 years and 19 years. Fifty percent present before 5 years, and 6% present in infancy. There is an increased incidence in patients with neurofibromatosis, Beckwith-Wiedemann syndrome, and Li-Fraumeni cancer-family syndrome.

Most studies divide rhabdomyosarcoma into distinct histologic groups: favorable, intermediate, and unfavorable. Favorable types (5%) include the sarcoma botryoides and spindle cell variants. Botryoid tumors typically present in young children from within visceral cavities (eg, vagina), while spindle cell types have a predilection for paratesticular sites. Intermediate-prognosis tumors (50%) are of the embryonal type. Unfavorable-prognosis tumors (20%) include alveolar and undifferentiated tumors. Alveolar tumors arise from the extremities, trunk, and perineum. Undifferentiated tumors arise from the extremity and head and neck sites. Thirteen percent cannot be adequately characterized and are labeled "small, round cell sarcoma, type indeterminate."

Clinical Findings

The clinical presentation varies with the site of origin of the primary tumor, the patient's age, and the presence or absence of metastatic disease. The majority of symptoms are secondary to the effects of compression by the tumor or by the presence of a mass. The most common site is the head and neck region (35%). These are subdivided into orbital (10%), parameningeal (15%), and nonparameningeal (10%) sites. They are usually embryonal and present as asymptomatic masses or functional deficits. Genitourinary rhabdomyosarcoma (26%) are divided into two groups: bladder and prostate (10%) and non-bladder and prostate, including paratesticular sites, perineum, vulva, vagina, and uterus (16%). The most common histologic type is embryonal, though botryoid tumors and spindle cell tumors are seen more frequently here than in any other site. These tumors may be so massive as to make determination of the primary tumor site impossible. There is a propensity for early lymphatic spread in genitourinary primary tumors. Bladder and prostate tumors frequently present with urinary retention or hematuria, while vaginal and uterine tumors present with vaginal bleeding or discharge or with a mass exiting the vagina. Extremity rhabdomyosarcoma (1%) are more common in the lower than in the upper extremity. These are usually alveolar varieties with a high incidence of regional nodal involvement and distal metastases. "Other" sites account for 20%. The most common are the thorax, diaphragm, abdominal and pelvic walls, and intraabdominal or intrapelvic organs.

Staging is determined by the histologic variant, the primary site, and the extent of disease since each has an important influence on the choice of treatment and on prognosis. CT scanning or MRI is essential to evaluate the primary tumor and its relationship to surrounding structures. A clinical grouping system was designed by the Intergroup Rhabdomyosarcoma Study Group to stratify different extents of disease in order to compare treatment and outcome results (Table 46–8). It is based upon pretreatment and operative outcome and does not account for the biologic differences or the natural history of tumors arising from different primary sites.

Treatment & Prognosis

The surgical management is site-specific and includes complete wide excision of the primary tumor and surrounding uninvolved tissue while preserving cosmetic appearance and function. Incomplete excision (beyond biopsy) or tumor debulking is not beneficial, and severely mutilating or debilitating procedures should not be performed. Tumors not amenable to primary excision should be amply biopsied and then treated with neoadjuvant agents; secondary excision is then per-

Table 46–8. Intergroup Rhabdomyosarcoma Study Clinical Group staging system.[1]

Group I: Localized disease, completely removed
  a. Confined to muscle or organ of origin
  b. Infiltration outside organ or muscle of origin; regional nodes not involved.
Group II: Total gross resection with evidence of regional spread
  a. Grossly resected tumor with microscopic residual
  b. Regional disease with involved nodes, completely resected with no microscopic residual
  c. Regional disease with involved nodes, grossly resected, but with evidence of microscopic residual and/or histologic involvement of the most distal regional node in the dissection
Group III: Incomplete resection, or biopsy with presence of gross disease
Group IV: Distant metastases

[1]Reproduced, with permission, from Neville HL et al: Preoperative staging, prognostic factors, and outcome for extremity rhabdomyosarcoma: a preliminary report from the Intergroup Rhabdomyosarcoma Study IV (1991–1997). J Pediatr Surg 2000;35:317.

formed and is associated with a better outcome than partial or incomplete excisions. Clinically suspicious lymph nodes should be excised or biopsied, while excision of clinically uninvolved nodes is site-specific. Primary reexcision has been shown to improve outcome in patients where microscopic margins are positive, where the initial procedure was not a formal "cancer" resection, or where malignancy was not suspected preoperatively.

The 5-year survival for stage I tumors is 90%; for stage II, clinical group I or II, it is 77%; for stage II, clinical group III, it is 65%; and for stage III lesions (group I, II, or III), it is 55%. Stage IV tumors arising from favorable sites of origin are curable, while those from unfavorable sites have a very poor prognosis. The prognosis for recurrent disease is poor.

Andrassy RJ: Rhabdomyosarcoma. Semin Pediatr Surg 1997;6:17.

Neville HL et al: Preoperative staging, prognostic factors, and outcome for extremity rhabdomyosarcoma: a preliminary report from the Intergroup Rhabdomyosarcoma Study IV (1991–1997). J Pediatr Surg 2000;35:317.

Wiener ES: Rhabdomyosarcoma: new dimensions in management. Semin Pediatr Surg 1993;2:47.

TERATOMA

Teratomas are embryonal neoplasms derived from totipotential cells containing tissue from at least two of three germ layers (ectoderm, endoderm, mesoderm). Approximately 80% are found in females. They are typically midline or para-axial tumors and are distributed in the following regions: sacrococcygeal (57%), gonadal (29%), mediastinal (7%), retroperitoneal (4%), cervical (3%), and intracranial (3%). Other sites are rare. Nongonadal teratomas present in infancy, gonadal ones in adolescence. Twenty-one percent are malignant.

The serum alpha-fetoprotein (AFP) level is elevated in tumors containing malignant endodermal sinus (yolk sac) elements. Serial AFP levels are markers for recurrence. Beta-human chorionic gonadotropin (β-hCG) is produced from those containing malignant choriocarcinoma tissue. Rarely, enough β-hCG is produced to cause precocious puberty. Elevated AFP and β-hCG levels in histologically benign tumors indicate an increased risk of recurrence and malignant transformation, particularly with "immature" benign teratomas.

Sacrococcygeal Teratoma

The majority of sacrococcygeal teratomas present in the newborn period and can be detected by prenatal ultrasound. Females predominate; a history of twins is common. Pregnancy may be complicated by high-output cardiac failure via arteriovenous shunting within the tumor, polyhydramnios, and hydrops fetalis leading to fetal demise. Fetal surgery has been utilized successfully in those with hydrops. The tumors are classified according to location: Type I, predominantly external (46%); Type II, external mass and presacral component (35%); Type III, visible externally, but predominantly presacral (9%); and Type IV, entirely presacral, not visible externally (10%).

Treatment is excision of the tumor and coccyx; Type I and II lesions are resected from the perineal approach, Type III and IV lesions require a combined intra-abdominal and perineal resection. The majority (97%) of newborn sacrococcygeal teratomas are benign and do not require adjuvant therapy. Follow-up requires serial AFP levels and physical examinations which include digital rectal examination. Recurrent tumors are excised. The greatest risk factor for malignancy is age at diagnosis. The malignancy rate is approximately 50–60% after 2 months of age. Malignant tumors are often treated with surgery and chemotherapy. The 5-year survival for malignant germ cell tumors arising from a sacrococcygeal teratoma is approximately 50%.

Mediastinal Teratoma

Mediastinal teratomas account for approximately 20% of all pediatric mediastinal tumors. They usually arise in the anterior mediastinum, though intrapericardial and cardiac lesions have been reported. Symptoms include respiratory distress, chronic cough, chest pain, and wheezing. Males with β-hCG-producing tumors may display precocious puberty. Cardiac failure may develop from compression or pericardial effusion. The chest radiograph demonstrates a calcified anterior mediastinal mass in over one-third of cases. Ultrasonography delineates cystic and solid components. General anesthesia should not be induced until a CT scan evaluation of the airway has been obtained since the supine position coupled with a loss of airway tone from anesthetic agents may allow the anterior mass to obstruct the distal trachea, making rapid establishment of an airway all but impossible. If significant airway compression is present, an awake needle biopsy under local anesthesia followed by radiation therapy or chemotherapy is indicated. Complete resection is definitive treatment.

Cervical Teratoma

Cervical teratomas are rare neonatal neck masses that by virtue of their large size frequently cause respiratory distress. Calcifications may be seen on a plain radiograph and a mixed cystic and solid appearance on ultrasound. These tumors are most commonly benign. The most common malignant type is the yolk sac tumor (endodermal sinus tumor). Serum AFP and β-hCG levels can be monitored to detect the presence of recurrent germ cell tumors. The rapid establishment of an endotracheal airway may be necessary. Tracheostomy is hazardous because of the distortion of landmarks by the large mass. Treatment is complete excision. Some malignant tumors respond to radiation therapy. Regardless of the stage of disease, these tumors behave aggressively and should be treated adjunctively with a combination of cisplatin, vinblastine, and bleomycin or with dactinomycin, cyclophosphamide, and vincristine.

Altman RP, Randolph JG, Lilly JR: Sacrococcygeal teratoma: American Academy of Pediatrics Surgical Section Survey-1973. J Pediatr Surg 1974;9:389.

Kerner B et al: Cervical teratoma: prenatal diagnosis and long-term follow-up. Prenat Diagn 1998;18:51.

Rescorla FJ et al: Long-term outcome for infants and children with sacrococcygeal teratoma: a report from the Children's Cancer Group. J Pediatr Surg 1998;33:171.

Tapper D, Lack EE: Teratomas in infancy and childhood: a 54-year experience at the Children's Hospital Medical Center. Ann Surg 1983;198:398.

LIVER NEOPLASMS

Tumors of the liver are uncommon in childhood (2% of all pediatric malignancies). More than 70% of pediatric liver masses are malignant. The majority of hepatic malignancies are of epithelial origin, while most benign lesions are vascular in nature.

1. Hepatoblastoma

Hepatoblastomas account for nearly 50% of all liver masses in children and approximately two-thirds of malignant tumors. The majority are seen in children under 4 years of age, and two-thirds are noted prior to 2 years of age. Beckwith-Wiedemann syndrome, hemihypertrophy, fetal alcohol syndrome, and parenteral nutrition administration in infancy all increase the risk of hepatoblastoma.

Clinical Findings

A. SYMPTOMS AND SIGNS

The most common finding is an asymptomatic abdominal mass or diffuse abdominal swelling in a healthy-appearing child. There may be obstructive gastrointestinal symptoms secondary to compression of the stomach or duodenum or acute pain secondary to hemorrhage into the tumor. Physical examination reveals a nontender, firm mass in the right upper quadrant or midline that moves with respiration. Advanced tumors present with weight loss, ascites, and failure to thrive. Approximately 10% of males present with isosexual precocity secondary to tumor secretion of β-hCG.

B. LABORATORY FINDINGS

Laboratory studies reveal nonspecifically elevated liver function tests and a mild anemia. Thrombocytosis of unknown cause is occasionally seen. AFP is significantly elevated in 90–95%. This marker is also associated with other malignant lesions such as germ cell tumors, but levels are lower. Serial serum AFP measurements are used to monitor patients for tumor recurrence. Levels fall to normal after curative resection.

C. IMAGING STUDIES

Abdominal ultrasound demonstrates a solid, usually unilobar (right lobe most common) lesion of the liver but lacks sufficient detail to determine resectability. Abdominal CT scan using intravenous contrast is currently the imaging procedure of choice both for diagnosis and for planning therapy. The CT scan demonstrates the tumor's proximity to major vascular and hilar structures. The typical CT appearance is a solid solitary mass with lower attenuation levels than those of the surrounding liver. A novel technique, CT arterioportography, holds promise as a reliable means of assessing vascular invasion along with gross tumor distribution. MRI has proved to be very useful in defining the patency of vascular structures.

Differential Diagnosis

One major management problem is the inability to differentiate adenomas from hepatocellular carcinoma. Because of this, hepatic adenoma, despite being a benign lesion, is often excised. Focal nodular hyperplasia is a well-circumscribed, nonencapsulated nodular liver mass. Ultrasonography and CT scan demonstrate a solid mass, but one cannot differentiate it from adenoma or malignancy without a biopsy. If the diagnosis can be made by biopsy (percutaneous or open), no further treatment is needed. Mesenchymal hamartoma is an uncommon benign lesion presenting in the first year of life as an asymptomatic large solitary mass usually confined to the right lobe of the liver. CT scan demonstrates a well-defined tumor margin and minimal to no contrast enhancement. The treatment is surgical wedge resection; lobectomy is rarely required.

Treatment

The definitive diagnosis of hepatoblastoma requires tissue biopsy. Although this can be performed percutaneously, there are reports of "seeding" of the biopsy tract. It is preferable to perform open biopsy of the lesion with assessment of resectability. If the lesion is not primarily resectable, vascular access is obtained during the same anesthetic interval for subsequent chemotherapy. A surgical staging system for childhood hepatic malignancies is set forth in (Table 46–9).

Complete surgical resection is the major objective of therapy and represents the only chance for cure. Approximately 60% of patients will have primarily resectable lesions. Lobectomy or extended lobectomy (trisegmentectomy) is usual, but segmental (nonanatomic) resection of small isolated tumors may be possible. Careful preoperative evaluation and planning have made liver resection in children a safe procedure with a mortality rate of less than 5%. Adequate exposure can be obtained via an extended subcostal or bilateral subcostal incision, although bulky lesions may require extension into the right hemithorax to gain adequate vascular control during dissection. Ascitic fluid is obtained for cytologic examination. If the lesion is deemed unresectable, the tumor is biopsied. If the lesion is made resectable following chemotherapy, lobectomy or trisegmentectomy is performed. Intraoperative cholangiography is helpful to verify the integrity of the remaining biliary tree.

Table 46–9. Hepatic tumor staging.

Stage I: Tumor localized and completely resected
Stage II: Tumor resected with microscopic residual disease
Stage III: Unresectable tumor or gross residual disease
Stage IV: Metastatic disease

Postoperative complications include bleeding, biliary fistula, subphrenic fluid collections or abscess, and inadvertent injury to the biliary tree. Hepatic regeneration occurs quickly, and hepatic insufficiency is rare if 25% or more of the liver parenchyma remains. Hepatic transplantation is used for unresectable disease when chemotherapy has failed to allow complete resection but no demonstrable metastases exist. Long-term follow-up is required before this becomes an accepted alternative treatment.

The overall survival for all children with hepatoblastoma is approximately 50%. The best survival (90%) is seen in patients with stage I tumors who receive adjunctive chemotherapy after complete excision. Survival decreases as the surgical stage increases, though long-term survival approaches 60–70% in patients with unresectable disease who receive chemotherapy.

Tagge EP et al: Resection, including transplantation, for hepatoblastoma and hepatocellular carcinoma: impact on survival. J Pediatr Surg 1992;27:292.

Wheatley JM, LaQuaglia MP. Management of hepatic epithelial malignancy in childhood and adolescence. Semin Surg Oncol 1993;9:532.

2. Hepatocellular Carcinoma

Hepatocellular carcinoma is less common than hepatoblastoma and typically presents in older children and adolescents (median age 10 years). It is associated with preexisting chronic hepatitis, cirrhosis due to hepatitis B virus, and other causes of childhood cirrhosis (tyrosinemia, biliary cirrhosis, α_1-antitrypsin deficiency, type 1 glycogen storage disease, and long-term parenteral nutrition). Signs and symptoms consist of an abdominal mass or diffuse swelling, abdominal pain, weight loss, anorexia, and jaundice. The serum AFP level is elevated in 50%, though the absolute levels are lower than in patients with hepatoblastoma. Diagnostic studies, staging, and treatment are somewhat the same as for hepatoblastoma. Because of multicentricity, bilobar involvement, portal vein invasion, and lymphatic metastases, only 15–20% of hepatocellular carcinomas are resectable. Fibrolamellar hepatocellular carcinoma in younger patients is associated with a high rate of resectability and a better prognosis. The overall long-term survival is poor (15%) even for resectable disease. The role of liver transplantation remains unclear.

3. Liver Hemangioma

This is the most common benign pediatric hepatic lesion. These tumors are solitary (cavernous hemangioma) or multiple (infantile hemangioendothelioma),

involving the bulk of the liver. Isolated cavernous hemangiomas are not often associated with cutaneous hemangiomas, whereas infantile hemangioendotheliomas are commonly associated with hemangiomas in other parts of the body or integument. Patients with a solitary hemangioma frequently have no symptoms or present with a mass. Infrequently there is intratumor hemorrhage or rupture resulting in abdominal pain. Infants with hemangioendothelioma commonly present with massive hepatomegaly and high-output cardiac failure from arteriovenous shunting. Approximately 40% develop Kasabach-Merritt syndrome (thrombocytopenic coagulopathy due to platelet sequestration within the tumor). The diagnosis is made by red blood cell-labeled radionuclide or dynamic abdominal CT scanning. CT scan demonstrates increased filling and a rapid venous phase from arteriovenous shunting. Angiography is unnecessary, and percutaneous biopsy is contraindicated.

Treatment is not necessary in an asymptomatic child. Patients with congestive heart failure or thrombocytopenia are treated with corticosteroids, digoxin, and diuretics. Refractory patients benefit from hepatic artery embolization. External beam radiation reduces hepatic size and controls symptoms. Their large size and diffuse involvement often preclude resection. Indications for surgery include ruptured lesions with hemorrhage, masses with uncertain diagnoses, symptomatic lesions, or disease limited to one lobe. Hemangioendotheliomas may undergo malignant degeneration into angiosarcoma.

Newman KD: Hepatic tumors in children. Semin Pediatr Surg 1997;6:38.

Reynolds M: Pediatric liver tumors. Semin Surg Oncol 1999; 16:159.

Stringer MD: Liver tumors. Semin Pediatr Surg 2000;9:196.

■ BATTERED CHILD SYNDROME

Child abuse is any nonaccidental injury inflicted by a parent, guardian, or other supervising adult. It may be passive, in the form of emotional or nutritional deprivation, but is most readily recognized in the active form, characterized as "battered, bruised, beaten, broken, and burned." It is estimated that 1 million children per year in the United States suffer injuries that qualifying for reporting to the National Center on Child Abuse and Neglect. About 20–50% of children are rebattered after the first diagnosis, resulting in death in 5% and permanent physical damage in 35% when the syndrome is not recognized.

The child abuser is usually a young, insecure, unstable person who had an unhappy childhood and who has unrealistic expectations of the child. Most of these individuals are of low socioeconomic status. The abuser may be a parent, guardian, babysitter, neighborhood child, or other close associate. Active traumatic abuse is usually perpetrated by the father, but passive neglect with failure to thrive from nutritional or emotional deprivation is usually attributable to the mother.

Clinical Findings

In most cases, the battered child is under 3 years of age and is the product of a difficult or premature pregnancy and labor, usually unwanted or born outside of a stable parental relationship. Many battered children have congenital anomalies or are hyperkinetic and colicky. In most cases there is a discrepancy between the history supplied and the magnitude of the injury—or else a reluctance to give a history. Contradictory histories or delay in bringing the child to medical attention—or taking it to many different emergency room visits in different hospitals for unusual reasons—should be regarded with suspicion. A past injury in the child or sibling and almost any injury in an infant under 1 year of age are likely to be the results of child abuse. The parents may be evasive or hostile. They may have open guilt feelings or may be capable of complete concealment. The innocent spouse is usually more protective of the abuser than of the child.

The child is usually withdrawn, apathetic, whimpering, and fearful and shows signs of neglect or growth retardation. Multiple forms of injury may be noted at varying stages of healing. The child should be completely disrobed to enable the clinician to look for welts, bruises, lacerations, bite or belt wounds, stick or coat hanger marks on the head, trunk, buttocks, or extremities, and similar evidence of mistreatment. Cigarette, hot plate, match, or scalding burns may be evident. Subgaleal hematomas may be caused by pulled hair. Retinal hemorrhage or detachment may follow blows to the head. Abdominal injuries may produce ruptured liver, spleen, or pancreas or bowel perforation. Sexual abuse should be identified by determining whether the vaginal introitus or anus is bruised, lacerated, or enlarged and whether aspirated fluid contains sperm or prostatic acid phosphatase.

Even though no obvious fracture may be present, a skeletal radiographic survey should be performed. The bone most commonly fractured is the femur, followed by the humerus in the region of the diaphysis. Rib fractures and periosteal reactions in various stages of heal-

ing will be seen. Skull fractures are most commonly seen in infants less than 1 year old. Suture separation of the skull may indicate subdural hematoma. Neurologic injury may require a brain scan or MRI.

Treatment

The child should be admitted to hospital to be protected until the home environment can be evaluated. Injuries should be documented radiographically and with photographs. The presence of sperm in the vagina or anal canal should be confirmed. Bleeding disorders should be evaluated by a platelet count, bleeding time, prothrombin time, and plasma thromboplastin test to make certain that multiple bruises are not due to coagulopathy. A serologic test for syphilis may be indicated as well as cultures (including pharyngeal) for gonorrhea.

Injuries should be treated. Consultation with ophthalmologists, neurologists, neurosurgeons, orthopedic surgeons, and plastic surgeons may be required.

It is required by law in every state for both the hospital and the physician to report child abuse (suspected as well as documented) to local authorities. The district attorney's office can inform the physician about details of the local law. The physician is the protector of the child and a consultant to the parents and must not assume the role of prosecutor or judge. The most difficult task is to notify the parents without confrontation, accusation, or anger that battering or neglect is suspected. The physician must tell the parents that the law requires reporting injuries that are unexplained or inadequately explained in view of the nature of the injury. A written referral should then be made to other professionals, such as child welfare personnel, hospital social workers, or psychiatrists. The referral should describe the history of past injuries and the nature of current injuries, results of physical examination and laboratory and x-ray studies, and a statement about why nonaccidental trauma is suspected.

Prognosis

The abuser may require careful evaluation for possible psychosis by a psychiatrist. Child welfare personnel and social workers will have to assess the home environment and work with the parents to prevent future abuse. It may be necessary to place the child in a foster home, but approximately 90% of families can be reunited.

Berkowitz CD: New patterns of injury. Emerg Med Clin North Am 1995;13:321.

Duhaime AC et al: Nonaccidental head injuries in infants—the "shaken-baby syndrome". N Engl J Med 1998;338:1822.

REFERENCES

Andrassy RJ (editor): *Pediatric Surgical Oncology.* Saunders, 1998.

Ashcraft KW et al (editors): *Pediatric Surgery,* 3rd ed. Saunders, 2000.

Burg FD et al (editors): *Gellis & Kagan's Current Pediatric Therapy.* Saunders, 1999.

Gray SW, Skandalakis JE: *Embryology for Surgeons: The Embryological Basis for Treatment of Congenital Defects,* 2nd ed. Williams & Wilkins, 1994.

Harrison MR et al: *The Unborn Patient: The Art and Science of Fetal Therapy,* 3rd ed. Saunders, 2001.

O'Neill JA et al (editors): *Pediatric Surgery,* 5th ed. Mosby, 1998.

Rowe MI et al (editors): *Essentials of Pediatric Surgery,* Mosby, 1995.

Rudolph C, Rudolph AM, Hostetter MK (editors): *Rudolph's Pediatrics,* 21st ed. McGraw-Hill, 2002.

Oncology

47

Steven Hunt, MD, & Gerard M. Doherty, MD

Over 1 million individuals in the United States are diagnosed with malignant neoplasms each year. Cancer ranks second only to heart disease as the leading cause of mortality in this country. In 1998, the American Cancer Society estimates that malignancies caused 564,000 deaths, accounting for 23% of all deaths.

The surgeon is intimately involved in the care of cancer patients, since nearly 90% of patients with malignancies require surgical therapy at some time. Surgical resection is the initial curative treatment for nearly three-quarters of cancer patients. Since surgeons are often the first specialists to see newly diagnosed cancer patients, it is imperative that they have an in-depth knowledge of the different types of cancer and the different modalities available for treatment. For many cancers, the surgeon plays a principal role in the orchestration of the patient's care.

Neoplasms may be defined as benign or malignant based on the clinical behavior of the tumor. Benign tumors have lost normal growth regulation but tend to be surrounded by a capsule and do not invade surrounding tissues or metastasize. Malignant tumors invade surrounding tissues and have a propensity to metastasize to distant sites in the host. The term "cancer' is used to denote malignant neoplasms.

Tumor nomenclature is based on the tissue of origin. Benign tumors are generally designated by adding the suffix *-oma* to the name of the cell of origin. The nomenclature of malignant tumors is essentially the same, with additional information about the cell's embryonal tissue origins. Malignant tumors derived from cells of mesenchymal origin are called "sarcomas." These include cancers that derive from muscle, bone, tendon, fat, cartilage, lymphoid tissues, vessels, and connective tissue. Neoplasms of epithelial origin are called "carcinomas." These may be further categorized according to the histologic appearance of the cells. Tumor cells that have glandular growth patterns are referred to as adenocarcinomas, and those that resemble squamous epithelial cells are called squamous cell carcinomas. Cancers composed of undifferentiated cells that bear no resemblance to any tissues are designated as "poorly differentiated" or "undifferentiated carcinomas."

During the course of cancer treatment, it is important to define the progress and outcomes resulting from therapy. The terms complete and partial response are often used as end points to evaluate the efficacy of a particular therapeutic regimen. A complete response is defined as the absence of demonstrable cancer. A partial response refers to a reduction of tumor mass by greater than 50%. Tumor progression signifies a failure of therapy and is defined as a 50% or greater increase in the tumor mass.

It is important also to understand the terms used to define the therapeutic goal of particular treatments. Local control refers to freedom from tumor recurrence at the original site; regional control refers to freedom from recurrence in the region of lymphatic drainage; and systemic control refers to freedom from distant metastases.

GRADING & STAGING OF TUMORS

Comparison of outcomes for various forms of cancer is important both in evaluating different modalities of therapy and in determining appropriate therapy. For this reason, tumors are classified by grading and staging systems that attempt to predict the behavior and prognosis of particular cancers.

Grading of a tumor is a histologic determination and refers to the degree of cellular differentiation. Separate pathologic grading systems exist for each histologic type of cancer. Depending on the type of tumor, these systems are based on nuclear pleomorphism, cellularity, necrosis, cellular invasion, and the number of mitoses. Increasing grades generally denote increasing degrees of anaplasia. In most types of cancer, the grade of the tumor has less prognostic value than its stage. Some notable exceptions to this rule are that tumor grade has great clinical significance in soft tissue sarcoma, astrocytoma, transitional cell cancers of the genitourinary tract, and Hodgkin's and non-Hodgkin's lymphoma.

Tumor staging establishes the extent of disease and has important prognostic and therapeutic implications in most types of cancer. Clinical staging is based on the results of a noninvasive evaluation, including physical examination and various imaging studies. Pathologic staging is based on findings in surgical tumor specimens and biopsies and allows for the evaluation of microscopic disease undetectable by imaging techniques. Pathologic staging may reveal more extensive tumor spread than the clinical evaluation and is the more reli-

1352

able information. Clinicians must be careful when attempting to compare clinically and pathologically staged patients, as the two groups may have dramatically different outcomes.

As with grading, the staging systems vary with different tumor types. Two major staging systems are currently in use, one developed by the Union Internationale Contre le Cancer (UICC), and the other by the American Joint Committee on Cancer (AJCC). The UICC system is based on the TNM classification. T refers to the primary tumor and is based on the size of the tumor and invasion of surrounding structures. Tumors are characterized as T1 to T4 cancers, with the higher T stages for larger and more invasive tumors. N refers to regional lymph nodes, and classifications of N0 to N3 denote increasing numbers or range of lymph node metastases. Finally, M refers to distant metastatic disease, with M0 signifying no distant metastases and M1 and M2 indicating the presence of blood-borne metastatic disease.

The AJCC system divides cancers into stages 0 to IV, with higher stages representing more widespread disease and a poorer prognosis. Like the TNM system, AJCC staging is based on the size of the primary lesion, the presence of regional nodal metastases, and whether or not metastatic disease has occurred.. Regardless of the staging system or the tumor type, higher stages correlate with decreased survival.

AJCC Cancer Staging Manual, 5th ed. Lippincott Williams & Wilkins, 1997.

Cotran CS, Kumar V, Robbins SL (editors): *Robbins Pathologic Basis of Disease,* 6th ed. Saunders, 1999.

Landis SH et al: Cancer statistics, 1999. CA Cancer J Clin 1999; 49:8.

ROLE OF THE SURGICAL ONCOLOGIST

The surgeon is often the first specialist to see a patient with suspected or newly diagnosed cancer. In many cases the surgeon assumes responsibility for orchestrating the overall management of the cancer patient's care. Operation may be required for biopsy, staging, resection for cure or palliation, prophylaxis, or for management of tumor- and treatment-related complications.

A tissue diagnosis is critical to the care of all cancer patients. Depending on the type of tumor and its location, the method of biopsy will vary. Common diagnostic techniques include needle aspiration biopsy, core needle biopsy, incisional biopsy, and excisional biopsy.

Fine-needle aspiration (FNA) is a rapid and minimally invasive technique for the biopsy of palpable superficial tumors. Deeper, nonpalpable lesions may also be sampled by this technique when FNA is combined with various imaging modalities, such as ultrasonography or CT. FNA involves aspiration of cells and atten-

dant fluid from a suspicious mass, followed by cytologic examination of the stained smear. Clinically, FNA is particularly useful in the diagnosis of enlarged lymph nodes, breast lumps, thyroid masses, and lung nodules. While false-positive results from needle aspiration are rare, sampling errors commonly lead to false-negative results. FNA cytology does not allow the pathologist to accurately grade tumors and does not reveal the extent of invasion of a tumor. For tumors that require accurate diagnosis of tumor grade and invasion, the technique may be inadequate.

Core needle biopsy utilizes a needle that cuts a sliver of tissue for analysis. This technique provides more histologic information than FNA because it allows the pathologist to see the histologic architecture of the sample rather than just the cellular characteristics. As with FNA, sampling errors may occur, and a negative result is not definitive. Core biopsies are frequently used for prostate, breast, and liver masses. Again, ultrasound and radiographic imaging may enable the clinician to sample deep-seated or nonpalpable masses. The technique may also be used during surgery to biopsy suspicious masses encountered at operation.

When a larger tumor sample is necessary for accurate grading or staging, an incisional or excisional biopsy is required. Excisional biopsy is defined as the surgical removal of an entire gross lesion, while incisional biopsy involves sampling a representative portion of a suspicious lesion. In general, excisional biopsy is recommended whenever it is possible to excise the entire lesion without damage to surrounding structures. For large (> 5 cm), deep soft tissue masses, incisional biopsy is the preferred method.

Although biopsy techniques are usually simple, the surgeon must adhere to some specific principles when performing a biopsy for a suspected malignancy. The positioning of the needle tract or scar should be such that if further surgery is required, the biopsy site will be included in the excised specimen. This is especially important in biopsies of the breast and extremity. Meticulous hemostasis is imperative, as the formation of a wound hematoma may lead to tumor seeding within the wound and may make subsequent operation more difficult. The surgeon should also pay careful attention to the orientation of the pathologic specimen, as it may prove important in curative surgical procedures. Finally, if radiation therapy is anticipated following the biopsy or staging of a lesion, the surgeon should place radiopaque clips at the margin of resection to guide the radiation oncologist.

Surgeons are often called upon to perform operations that provide staging information for various types of cancer. Such procedures are necessary when the clinical extent of the disease has a direct bearing on the choice of treatment modalities. Examples include staging laparotomy for Hodgkin's lymphoma and ovarian cancer and mediastinoscopy for lung and esophageal cancer. Staging procedures can often help to avert highly morbid procedures in cases where there is little chance for cure.

Surgical resections with curative intent can be divided into three categories: resection of a primary lesion, resection of isolated metastases, and debulking of tumors to increase the chance for a cure by other treatment modalities. In each of these cases, the clinician must strive to reach a balance between the chance for cure and the morbidity of the procedure. Each situation must be evaluated individually, and the patient's wishes must be paramount.

In the resection of a primary lesion, the tumor type guides the extent of the resection. Various tumors require different disease-free margins in order to achieve optimal chances for a cure. It is important that the surgeon have knowledge of other modalities that may be integrated into the management plan to allow for a less ablative surgical procedure. Radiation and chemotherapy are commonly used in combination with surgery and are referred to as adjuvant therapies if used after complete resection with no demonstrable local or systemic disease. If these modalities are used in the preoperative setting, they are called neoadjuvant therapies.

As a general rule, operation for metastatic disease is warranted if there is a reasonable chance for cure with minimal procedure-related morbidity. This is especially true for cancers known to respond poorly to radiation or chemotherapy. Examples include resection of lung metastases in sarcomas, liver metastases in colon cancer, and solitary brain metastases in various cancers. The resection of metastatic disease may not achieve a definitive cure but may give substantial palliation or increase life expectancy.

Palliative surgery is performed for incurable malignancies in order to improve the patient's quality of life. Situations in which palliative procedures should be considered include impending intestinal obstruction, obstruction of the respiratory tract, severe pain, intractable ascites, pathologic fractures, and recurrent pleural effusions.

Finally, the surgeon may be called upon to manage oncologic emergencies. Most of the procedures performed in such situations are palliative, but they can be lifesaving in the short term. Severe hemorrhage and intestinal obstruction or perforation are some of the situations in which surgeons may be called on to emergently intervene in the care of a cancer patient.

SYSTEMIC ANTICANCER THERAPY

Systemic therapy is the treatment of a tumor via the systemic delivery of agents that have antitumor effects. These agents may act directly on the tumor cells, change the hormonal or cytokine milieu in the body, or influence the body's natural defenses against tumors. Generally, systemic therapy is delivered via the enteral, subcutaneous, or intravenous route. In theory, systemic therapy is directed not only at the primary tumor but also at occult or clinically evident sites of metastatic deposit. Included in the broad category of systemic therapy are chemotherapy, hormonal therapy, and immunotherapy.

1. Cytotoxic Chemotherapy

The goal of chemotherapeutic regimens is to deliver pharmacologic agents systemically to eradicate all tumor cells. The ideal tumor drug would kill cancer cells without harming normal tissues. No such agent exists, and most drugs affect normal cells to some extent. The success of chemotherapy relies on the normal cell's greater capacity for repair and survival relative to tumor cells.

A single cancer cell can potentially reproduce to form a lethal tumor. For this reason, the goal of curative chemotherapy must be the complete eradication of all tumor cells. Tumor burden is important in chemotherapy. A large cancer may harbor more than 10^9 tumor cells. If a tolerable dose of an effective drug killed 99.99% of these cells, the tumor burden would still be 10^5 cells. The remaining cells, while clinically undetectable, are likely to continue to grow and lead to a clinical recurrence of cancer. For this reason, most chemotherapy protocols rely on repeated administrations of drugs in order to achieve maximal cell killing. Tumor cells may avoid the cell killing effects of a particular drug because of their stage in the cell cycle, residence in an area protected from the drug (central nervous system), or an inherent resistance to the drug.

As with antibiotics, tumor cells may be resistant to a chemotherapeutic agent. Drug resistance plays a large role in chemotherapy failures. Several mechanisms of tumor resistance are known. The multidrug resistance gene encodes a protein that actively pumps drugs out of tumor cells. This gene confers resistance on a variety of antitumor drugs, including the antibiotics and plant-derived compounds. Other tumor mechanisms of resistance include the alteration of target enzymes, increased production of a target enzyme to overwhelm the drug, and an increased capability for DNA repair. Tumor resistance to a given chemotherapeutic agent can often be overcome by the administration of multiple drugs.

Induction chemotherapy refers to chemotherapy as the sole mode of treatment for a cancer, whether the goal is cure or palliation. Several types of cancers can be cured by induction chemotherapy, including testicular cancer, choriocarcinoma, Wilms' tumor, and Hodgkin's and some non-Hodgkin's lymphomas.

Adjuvant chemotherapy is chemotherapy used in combination with surgery or radiation therapy which has presumably removed all foci of local disease. The goal of adjuvant chemotherapy is to eliminate any microscopic foci of systemic disease. Neoadjuvant chemotherapy is the use of chemotherapy prior to attempts at locoregional control through surgery or radiotherapy. The theoretical advantage of neoadjuvant therapy is that it may facilitate surgical resection by shrinking the primary tumor, or it may convert an unresectable tumor into a resectable tumor. Neoadjuvant therapy also allows the oncologist to observe the primary tumor to determine if it is sensitive to a particular chemotherapeutic regimen.

Classes of Chemotherapeutic Agents

With all forms of curative chemotherapy, the goal is elimination of all tumor stem cells. Cells that are incapable of further division cannot cause progression of a tumor, and the sterilization of a tumor cell is as good as a kill. Chemotherapeutic drugs are generally classified as cell cycle specific (CCS) drugs, which are toxic to actively proliferating cells; or cell cycle-nonspecific (CCNS) drugs, which are capable of killing cells that are not dividing during drug exposure. These two classifications are not absolute, and many drugs may overlap between the two categories.

In order to achieve maximal cell killing, most therapeutic protocols use combination chemotherapy. Agents with differing mechanisms of action and different toxic side effects are used, allowing for relatively high doses of multiple agents. This method of combining agents helps to combat tumor cell resistance and increase the tumor cell killing while avoiding the compounding of toxic effects.

A. ALKYLATING AGENTS

These agents exert their effects by the transfer of alkyl groups to various cellular components, most importantly by the alkylation of DNA. Alkylators can cause DNA strand breaks, cross-linking of DNA strands, or miscoding of DNA during replication. The alkylating agents are considered cell cycle-nonspecific agents but tend to have their greatest effect on proliferating cells. Normal cells are able to avoid many of the lethal affects of alkylating agents because of their ability to repair DNA. The alkylating agents are effective in treatment of the hematologic malignancies and in a variety of solid tumors such as breast, lung, and endometrial cancers. Included in this class are the nitrosoureas (eg, carmustine, semustine, lomustine), cyclophosphamide, chlorambucil, cisplatin, mechlorethamine, dacarbazine, and procarbazine.

B. ANTIMETABOLITES

Rapidly dividing cells require increased synthesis of nucleic acid precursors. This increased synthesis can be exploited pharmacologically by the antimetabolites. These drugs are analogs of nucleic acids or nucleic acid precursors. The antimetabolites may be incorporated into the nucleic acids of a cell and serve as a false messenger. Antimetabolites can shut down the cellular synthetic machinery by binding to and inhibiting enzymes important in the production of nucleic acids. Since this class of drugs affects all rapidly proliferating cells, they are relatively toxic to normal tissues that have a high rate of cell turnover. Antimetabolites are most effective in the hematologic malignancies but are also used in the treatment of solid tumors such as breast and gastrointestinal cancers. They include methotrexate, mercaptopurine, thioguanine, fluorouracil, and cytarabine.

C. PLANT ALKALOIDS

A variety of antitumor drugs are derived from natural plants. Vincristine, vinblastine, and paclitaxel are plant products that work by binding tubulin and poisoning the assembly of microtubules in the mitotic spindle. This leads to mitotic arrest in metaphase, and these compounds are effective only on rapidly dividing cell populations. The plant alkaloids are most useful for hematologic malignancies and breast, renal, testicular, and head and neck cancers.

Another subgroup of the plant alkaloids are the topoisomerase inhibitors, including etoposide, teniposide, and topotecan. These plant derivatives exert their antitumor effects by binding to and inhibiting various forms of the enzyme topoisomerase. Topoisomerases are responsible for the maintenance of DNA structure and are also important in the cleavage and re-ligation of DNA strands. Inhibition of these enzymes leads to DNA strand breakage and structural damage. The topoisomerase inhibitors are also cell cycle-specific agents and have their greatest activity against rapidly proliferating cells. These drugs are used in the treatment of hematologic malignancies and lung, bladder, prostate, and testicular cancers.

D. ANTIBIOTICS

The majority of the drugs in this class are derived from the soil fungus streptomyces. All the antibiotics exert their antitumor effects by interference with the synthesis of nucleic acids. Most of the drugs in this class intercalate in DNA; blocking DNA synthesis and inducing strand breakages. The antibiotics are considered cell cycle-nonspecific, and they have antitumor activity against a wide variety of solid tumors. Included in this class of drugs are doxorubicin, dactinomycin, plicamycin, mitomycin, and bleomycin.

Side Effects of Chemotherapy

Most side effects from chemotherapeutic regimens are the result of toxicities to rapidly dividing normal cell populations—particularly bone marrow and epithelial cells. Bone marrow suppression is an adverse effect of many of these drugs, resulting in neutropenia, thrombocytopenia, and even anemia. Mucosal ulcerations and alopecia also occur in patients treated with cell cycle-specific agents. Intractable nausea and vomiting is another common side effect that can severely effect quality of life. Testicular or ovarian failure can result from chemotherapy, leading to sterility. Many of these drugs also are powerful teratogens and should be avoided in pregnant patients. Finally, many of the alkylating agents have been implicated in the development of secondary cancers, especially hematologic malignancies.

2. Hormonal Therapy

Both sex hormones and adrenocortical hormones have roles in the systemic therapy for several types of cancer. These steroid hormones are normally involved in the differentiation, stimulation, and control of certain tissues, including lymphoid tissue, the uterus, the prostate, and the mammary glands. It follows that tumors arising from these normal tissues may be stimulated or inhibited by manipulations in hormonal balance.

Adrenocortical Hormones

The corticosteroids, particularly the glucocorticoids, have a powerful suppressive effect on lymphoid cells. This lympholytic effect makes them useful in the treatment of acute leukemias, lymphomas, myeloma, and other myeloproliferative disorders. In these diseases, they can cause dissolution of lymphocytes and regression of lymph nodes.

Sex Hormones

The sex hormones include androgens, estrogens, and progesterones. These hormones often promote the proliferation of tumors derived from tissues normally sensitive to sex hormones, but there are a few situations in which the hormones can slow tumor proliferation. At replacement doses, estrogen has been shown to increase the proliferation of most breast and endometrial cancers. Paradoxically, some metastatic breast cancers actually regress when treated with high-dose estrogen. Generally, however, antiestrogen therapy is the hormonal treatment of choice in most breast cancers. Estrogens suppress androgen production and are a useful adjunct in the treatment of some prostate cancers. Progesterone inhibits the proliferation of endometrial cells and is useful in the treatment of endometrial cancers. Finally,

progesterone can inhibit the growth of some breast cancers that possess the progesterone receptor.

Estrogen & Androgen Inhibitors

The most definitive way to block the production of testosterone and estrogen is by surgical castration. Postmenopausal women have functionally inactive ovaries. Even after ablation, androgens and estrogens are still produced to a lesser extent in extragonadal tissues, and further pharmacologic blockade of the sex hormones is often useful.

Tamoxifen is a competitive inhibitor of estrogen at the estrogen receptor. Clinically, it is useful in treating estrogen and progesterone receptor-positive breast cancers and progesterone-resistant endometrial cancers, as these cancers often grow in the presence of estrogen stimulation. Estrogen has a tenfold higher affinity for the estrogen receptor than tamoxifen; hence, tamoxifen therapy is most beneficial in patients with low levels of endogenous estrogen.

Flutamide is a testosterone antagonist used in the treatment of prostate cancer. It works by blocking translocation of the androgen receptor to the nucleus. Although hormonal therapy for prostate cancer is palliative, it can be quite effective in slowing the progression of disease. Hormonal therapy can add several years to the life expectancy of patients with unresectable or metastatic disease. Flutamide is most effective when used in combination with surgical or pharmacologic castration.

Gonadotropin-Releasing Hormone Analogs

The pharmacologic equivalent of castration can be accomplished with leuprolide, an analog of gonadotropin-releasing hormone (GnRH). Normally, GnRH leads to the production of LH and FSH, the physiologic stimulators of sex hormone production. Constant stimulation with leuprolide actually inhibits LH and FSH release and leads to decreased synthesis of the sex steroids. Leuprolide is commonly used to decrease testosterone levels in the treatment of unresectable prostate cancer. In premenopausal women, estrogen levels fall to postmenopausal values with leuprolide administration. For this reason, the drug can be useful in the treatment of estrogen receptor-positive breast cancers in premenopausal women.

Aromatase Inhibitors

Although the ovaries are no longer able to synthesize estrogens in postmenopausal and oophorectomized women, there is continued low-level estrogen production from modification of adrenal steroids in the fat cells. The enzyme involved in this extragonadal estrogen production is called aromatase. Aromatase inhibitors can eliminate functional estrogen in this population of women and may be effective treatment for metastatic breast cancer in women whose tumors contain large numbers of estrogen or progesterone receptors. Aminoglutethimide is an aromatase inhibitor, but it also blocks the synthesis of adrenal steroids by inhibiting the conversion of cholesterol to a steroid precursor. Aminoglutethimide therapy must be administered with glucocorticoid replacement. For these reasons, aminoglutethimide is normally considered second-line therapy in women who have failed tamoxifen therapy.

Recently, a new selective aromatase inhibitor, anastrozole, was approved for the treatment of advanced estrogen or progesterone receptor-positive breast cancers which are no longer responsive to tamoxifen therapy. Reportedly, this new drug has no effects on the adrenal synthesis of steroids and concomitant glucocorticoid replacement is unnecessary.

3. Immunotherapy

Immunotherapy represents an attempt to mobilize the body's natural defense mechanisms against cancer cells, relying on the immune system's ability to differentiate between tumor cells and normal tissues. The science of immunotherapy, or biologic therapy, is relatively new, and the majority of therapies are still in the investigational stages.

The central cell in the immune system is the lymphocyte, including T cells, B cells, and null cells. The immune system can mount an attack by a variety of mechanisms. Cytokines, produced mainly by lymphocytes and macrophages, are soluble proteins that regulate cells through cytokine receptors. Cytokines can function as cell activators, inhibitors, or chemoattractants. These varied responses are dependent on the responding cell type and the particular cytokine involved.

Humoral immunity is mediated by antibodies, which recognize and bind to unique molecules on the surface of cells. Antibodies tag cells for destruction by phagocytic cells or soluble proteins called complement. B cells are the normal source of antibodies.

Cellular immunity refers to cell killing by cytotoxic cells that recognize target cells. T cells and null cells are the effector cells in this arm of the immune system. T cells bind cells expressing specific surface molecules, while the null cells have the ability to recognize and kill a broader array of foreign cells.

The basic premise behind immunotherapy is that malignant cells express relatively unique cell surface molecules, or antigens. The perfect tumor antigen would be found only on tumor cells and not on normal cells. In reality, there is no ideal tumor antigen, but scientists have identified a variety of antigens which are expressed predominantly on tumor cells or are expressed at a much higher concentration on these cells.

The antigens recognized by humoral and cellular immune mechanisms are different. Humoral immunity is directed at certain cell surface molecules (lipids, proteins, and carbohydrates) on the target cell. Cellular immunity antigens are small processed protein fragments presented on the cell surface in association with proteins called MHC molecules.

There are four basic approaches to the biologic therapy of cancer: nonspecific immunotherapy, antibody therapy, adoptive immunotherapy, and active immunotherapy with tumor vaccines.

Nonspecific Immunotherapy

The goal of nonspecific immunotherapy is to activate the entire immune system. Theoretically, if the immune system is jolted into a high level of activity, its surveillance system will subsequently recognize tumors as foreign cells and eliminate them. Early attempts at nonspecific immunotherapy involved the use of BCG, corynebacterium, and levamisole as immune stimulators. Although the systemic delivery of these substances led to a high level of immune activity, their antitumor effects were minimal. Local delivery of these immune stimulators can have some antitumor effects, eg, with bladder instillation of BCG in patients with superficial bladder cancers.

More recently, with the isolation and availability of several cytokines, nonspecific immunotherapy with these soluble factors has received a great deal of attention. Studies initially revealed great promise for tumor necrosis factor (TNF), interferons (IFNs), and IL-2. The interferons were initially isolated as soluble proteins produced by a variety of cells in response to viral infections. These cytokines—IFN-α, IFN-β, and IFN-γ—are now known to have a much broader role in the body's normal immune surveillance and regulation of cell growth and differentiation. The interferons' antitumor effects are thought to result from both immunomodulation and direct antiproliferative effects on malignant cells. A large number of malignancies, both solid and hematologic, are responsive to interferons. Although promising in theory, the practice has proved less satisfactory because the systemic toxicities of these agents are relatively severe. With systemic delivery, IFN-α is better tolerated, and clinical trials with this cytokine have proved successful in the treatment of several tumors, including melanoma and some forms of lymphoma. IFN-γ is poorly tolerated systemically, but laboratory models using this cytokine have yielded an enormous amount of information about tumor growth and cell signaling.

IL-2 is a cytokine produced by activated T cells. Its main function in the immune system is to stimulate the growth of activated lymphocytes. In animals, this cytokine has been shown to mediate regression of established tumors when delivered systemically. By an unknown mechanism, IL-2 can activate lymphoid cells directed at nonspecific tumor cell killing. In the clinical realm, systemic IL-2 therapy has not proved as effective against human tumors, but the cytokine does have some benefit in the treatment of renal cell carcinoma (for which it is FDA-approved) and metastatic melanoma.

Antibody-Mediated (Passive) Immunotherapy

Polyclonal or monoclonal antibodies directed against a large number of relatively specific tumor antigens have been developed. These antibodies can exert antitumor effects by blocking functions of the target molecule, by tagging these cells for elimination, or by tumor cell-specific localization of chemotherapeutic and radioactive agents conjugated to the antibody. Antibody-mediated therapy has proved promising in the treatment of several tumors, particularly lymphomas (tositumomab) and breast cancer (herceptin).

Adoptive Immunotherapy

In adoptive immunotherapy, the patient serves both as the donor and recipient of lymphocytes. The patient's peripheral lymphocytes are removed, activated against tumor cells, and then transferred back to the tumor-bearing patient. The in vitro incubation of lymphocytes with IL-2 produces lymphokine activated killer (LAK) cells that can lyse tumor cells. The LAK cells are not directed against specific tumor antigens, and it is unclear how these cells recognize and lyse tumor cells while sparing normal cells. Trials of adoptive immunotherapy often are done in conjunction with the systemic administration of IL-2, but this approach has not yet proved effective in the clinical setting.

Another approach in adoptive immunotherapy is the expansion of tumor infiltrating lymphocytes (TILs). These cells are produced by the in vitro incubation of the patient's tumor cells with IL-2. Presumably, the gross tumors contain infiltrative lymphocytes that are previously sensitized to specific tumor antigens. While incubating lymphocytes in IL-2, the cells expand in polyclonal fashion, resulting in an activated lymphocyte population with specific recognition of the target tumor cells. This approach has been limited by the fact that TILs can be produced from only a minority of tumors and have had only sporadic antitumor effects.

Tumor Vaccines

The goal of tumor vaccines is to augment the host's specific immune recognition of tumor cells. The theory behind tumor vaccines is similar to that supporting the use of bacterial and viral vaccines—ie, the presentation of tumor antigens to the immune system will elicit a specific response to the tumor. The antigens can be in the form of inactivated tumor cells taken directly from the host or in the form of purified tumor-specific antigens.

The host can theoretically mount a more dramatic response to the tumor antigens if they are presented in the setting of localized inflammation. For this reason, the vaccines are often given in combination with a substance that will elicit a localized inflammatory response.

Although multiple investigative attempts to develop a clinically useful tumor vaccine have been unsuccessful, the present ability to genetically manipulate tumor cells in vitro to a more immunogenic form holds great promise for future therapy.

Abbas AK, Lichtman AH, Pober JS (editors): *Cellular and Molecular Immunology,* 3rd ed. Saunders, 1997.

Katzung BG (editor): *Basic & Clinical Pharmacology,* 8th ed. McGraw-Hill, 2000.

Hardman JG et al (editors): *Goodman and Gilman's The Pharmacologic Basis of Therapeutics,* 9th ed. McGraw-Hill, 1996.

Old LJ: Immunotherapy for cancer. Sci Am 1996 Sep;275:136.

Rosenberg SA: A new era for cancer immunotherapy based on the genes that encode cancer antigens. Immunity 1999;10:281.

REGIONAL THERAPY

Systemic chemotherapy is limited by toxicity to the host. Regional delivery of chemotherapeutic agents via arterial cannulation allows for high levels of drugs in the region of the primary tumor while decreasing systemic toxicity. Regional perfusion techniques are focused primarily on the treatment of cancers in the extremities and liver.

Isolated limb perfusion is an investigational technique for the delivery of chemotherapeutic agents to an extremity with locally advanced cancer. Current investigations are aimed at the treatment of extremity melanoma and sarcoma. In this approach, a tourniquet is applied to the extremity to occlude venous outflow. The major artery perfusing the limb is then isolated, cannulated, and perfused with hyperthermic chemotherapeutic agents using a pump oxygenator as for cardiopulmonary bypass. The perfusion is done in the operating room and lasts for approximately 1 hour. The cannula is then removed. Most protocols involve only a single treatment. Melphalan, an alkylating agent, and the cytokine tumor necrosis factor (TNF) are used today in the treatment of both sarcomas and melanomas. Although evidence in support of this technique is controversial, many oncologists feel that isolated limb perfusion is of some benefit in the treatment of locally recurrent melanoma and unresectable or multifocal sarcoma. In patients with unresectable extremity sarcomas, preoperative limb perfusion can often shrink the tumor and allow for a limb-sparing resection. While decreasing the rate of regional recurrence, this therapy has yet to show a definitive survival benefit.

Another promising investigational approach is isolated hepatic artery infusion for the treatment of unresectable colorectal cancer metastatic to the liver. Metastatic tumors derive nearly all of their blood supply from the hepatic artery, while the normal liver parenchyma derives more than two-thirds of its blood supply from the portal system. This permits the delivery of higher doses of chemotherapeutic agents to the tumor relative to the normal hepatocytes. The drug most commonly used in this protocol is floxuridine, which is almost completely extracted on its first pass through the liver. This allows for relatively low systemic toxicity. Hepatic artery infusion requires the surgical placement of a catheter into the hepatic artery. This catheter is connected to an implanted or external infusion pump, allowing for continuous treatment. While nearly all studies of this technique have shown improved tumor responses in comparison to systemic therapy, the survival benefits have been less dramatic. Some studies, however, have shown improved survival and have stimulated further investigation.

Cascinu S et al: Locoregional treatments of unresectable liver metastases from colorectal cancer. Cancer Treat Rev 1998; 24:3.

Fraker DL: Hyperthermic regional perfusion for melanoma and sarcoma of the limbs. Curr Probl Surg 1999;36:841.

Kemeny NE, Ron IG: Hepatic arterial chemotherapy in metastatic colorectal patients. Semin Oncol 1999;26:524.

Pelosi E et al: Hepatic arterial infusion chemotherapy for unresectable confined liver metastases: prediction of systemic toxicity with the application of a scintigraphic and pharmacokinetic approach. Cancer Chemother Pharmacol 1999;44:505.

RADIATION THERAPY

Radiation therapy is the treatment of malignant tumors with ionizing radiation. Certain tumor types are particularly sensitive to irradiation, while others may be completely resistant. Radiation therapy may be used alone or in combination with surgery and chemotherapy and may be given with curative or palliative intent. Some tumors, such as head and neck cancers, cervical cancer, prostate cancer, and Hodgkin's disease, can often be cured by irradiation alone, eliminating the need for surgical resection or chemotherapy.

Principles of Radiation Therapy

Ionizing radiation is defined as energy that causes ejection of an atomic orbital electron when absorbed. There are two forms of ionizing radiation: electromagnetic radiation and particulate radiation. Electromagnetic radiation consists of gamma rays and x-rays produced by radioisotopes or electrical machines. The bulk of clinical radiotherapy treatments use electromagnetic radiation. Particulate radiation refers to particles that possess finite mass and includes electrons, protons, neurons, atomic nuclei, and alpha and beta particles. Radioisotopes are a clinically useful source of particulate radiation. The radioisotopes used clinically in the treatment of malignancies exert their effects by the emission of beta particles and gamma rays.

The quantification of a radiation dose is based on the amount of energy delivered to a certain mass of tissue. Currently, therapeutic radiation doses are measured in gray (Gy) units, which are equal to the absorption of 1 joule per kilogram of tissue. One gray is equal to 100 rads.

The biologic effects of ionizing radiation are primarily due to the fact that ionization, particularly of intracellular water, yields highly reactive oxygen free radicals. This effect is enhanced in the presence of molecular oxygen. The radicals readily interact with molecules in the irradiated cells to break chemical bonds or directly change molecular structures. Such alterations in molecular structure may damage the cellular DNA or the protein machinery needed for cellular reproduction and metabolism.

The goal of radiation therapy is to kill or to alter the reproductive ability of malignant cells, but these effects are not specific for tumor cells. Radiosensitivity is the susceptibility of a certain cell to damage by ionizing radiation. Rapidly dividing cells tend to be much more radiosensitive than quiescent ones. Normal tissues have a greater capacity to repair sublethal cellular damage than tumor cells, and it is this difference which can be exploited in the radiotherapy of cancer. The DNA repair differences between normal cells and tumor cells are due to rapid tumor cell division and their loss of the machinery necessary for repair. Certain rapidly dividing normal cells (hematopoietic stem cells and epithelial cells) also have a decreased capacity to repair structural damage and therefore suffer greater consequences from radiation. Other tissues such as bone, cartilage, muscle, and peripheral nerves are quite resistant to the effects of radiation.

The dose of therapeutic radiation is limited by the toxicity to the surrounding tissues. Fractionation is the division of radiation doses into smaller units over time, and it takes advantage of the greater capacity for repair in normal tissues relative to tumors. Ideally, fractionation would result in compounding of the radiation damage to the tumor cells while allowing the normal tissues adjacent to the tumor to fully repair sublethal damage and repopulate before the next dose. Cellular damage—both to the tumor and to the surrounding tissues—is based on the total amount of radiation delivered, the size of the fractions, and the duration of time between fractions.

As molecular oxygen enhances the production of free radicals, oxygen must be available for maximal cell killing. Tumor cellular hypoxia in areas of tumor necrosis and fibrosis can facilitate tumor cell survival during radiation therapy. Because the oxygen tension is generally lower at the center of a large tumor, the probability of controlling a tumor with irradiation is inversely related to the size of the tumor.

Locoregional control of tumors often involves both surgical resection and localized radiation. The theoretical advantage of combining these two therapies is based on the mechanisms by which they fail to achieve their purpose. Surgical failures occur at the margins of tumors, while radiation therapy fails in the center of tumors, where the malignant cells are numerous and hypoxic conditions exist. Radiation failures are rare at the periphery of tumors, where cell numbers are low and oxygenation is high. Depending on tumor histology and location, radiation therapy can be used as a surgical adjunct either preoperatively or postoperatively. Preoperative radiation can shrink tumors and increase the chances for complete surgical resection in cancers such as sarcomas, rectal cancers, and superior sulcus lung cancers.

Modes of Delivery

Ionizing radiation can be delivered to tumor cells by a variety of modalities. The most common mode of delivery is through the use of external beam radiation teletherapy (EBRT). EBRT uses a device located some distance from the patient to focus electromagnetic radiation on the tissues of interest. In determining the target volume of tissue, the radiation oncologist must take into account the primary location of the tumor, the type of tumor, the tumor's natural history, the routes of spread, the results of imaging studies, and the operative or pathologic reports. As in all types of radiation therapy, the goal is to deliver maximal radiation to the tumor while sparing as much normal surrounding tissue as possible. The location of the tumor is the most important determinant of the maximal radiation dose that can be delivered by EBRT. In the irradiation of tumors by teletherapy, the radiation passes through all the tissues between the source and the tumor. Although modern techniques allow for relatively precise focusing of the electromagnetic beam, it is not possible to com-

pletely spare the surrounding tissues. Abdominal viscera are relatively sensitive to radiation, and it is difficult to deliver high doses of therapeutic radiation to an abdominal tumor without causing significant toxicity. On the other hand, the muscles and bone of the extremities are relatively resistant to radiation, allowing for delivery of a higher therapeutic dose to extremity tumors.

Given the limitations of EBRT, it is desirable, when possible, to use other modes of delivery in order to precisely target tumor cells. One commonly used modality is brachytherapy. The principle of brachytherapy is to place—either surgically or via the normal body orifices—a radiation source near the site of the primary tumor. This allows for direct delivery of ionizing radiation to the target tissue, with minimal toxicity to the surrounding tissues. Depending on the tumor location, brachytherapy sources may vary. In prostate cancer, it is possible to implant radioactive seeds directly into the gland via a transrectal approach. Other methods of brachytherapy involve the use of catheters that can be filled with radioisotopes. These catheters may be placed noninvasively, as in the radiotherapy of many gynecologic and oropharyngeal tumors. Other tumors are not as easily accessible, and require the surgical placement of brachytherapy catheters. Surgical placement is usually done in conjunction with resection of the primary malignancy and allows for radiation delivery directly to the tumor bed.

Another target-tissue specific mode of delivery is through the use of intraoperative radiation therapy. This technique is used in the operating room after resection of a tumor. External beam radiation or brachytherapy devices are used to deliver radiation directly to the tumor bed while the surrounding tissues are shielded. The advantages of this mode of delivery are obvious, but its practical application is less straightforward. Intraoperative therapy dramatically lengthens the operative time, exposing patients to prolonged anesthesia. A radiation oncologist must be present in the operative suite during the course of the treatment. This method also requires dedicated radiotherapy machinery in an operating room equipped with appropriate shielding. Finally, the complex nature of operative access does not allow for dose fractionation. Such limitations have restricted the use of intraoperative radiotherapy to only a few large cancer centers worldwide.

In certain cancers, it is possible to deliver ionizing radiation directly to tumors via the systemic route. Systemic targeting of selected tumors may take advantage of unique characteristics of the tumor cells, as in the specific uptake of radioactive ^{131}I by certain types of thyroid cancers. Radioimmunotherapy is an experimental mode of systemic delivery in which radioisotopes are bound to antibodies targeted to tumor-associated or tumor-specific antigens. This technique has shown great promise in the treatment of many cancers, including hepatocellular carcinoma, lymphoma, and ovarian cancer. Aside from the relatively tumor-specific delivery of radiotherapy, the advantage of systemic radiotherapy is that it allows for the treatment of tumors which may have metastasized or spread beyond predictable anatomic boundaries.

Complications of Radiation Therapy

Complications of radiation therapy result from damage to normal tissues. The nature of such complications depends upon the type of normal tissues irradiated, the age of the patient, the presence of comorbid disease, the use of adjuvant chemotherapy, and the total dose, fraction, and time course of the treatment.

Early or acute complications include tissue inflammation, edema, erythema, and desquamation of epithelial cells. These complications appear within hours or days after therapy, and therapeutic regimens are titrated to these acute effects.

Late complications occur within weeks or months of treatment. These delayed injuries are usually due to radiation-induced fibrosis or injury to the vascular endothelium. Late complications include chronic edema, tissue necrosis, sterility, chronic ulcerations of skin or mucosal surfaces, intestinal obstruction, fistula formation, gastroenteritis, pericarditis, radiation pneumonitis, and cataracts.

With large doses of radiation, the risk of somatic mutations is also increased. Increased cancer risk after irradiation has been well described for leukemias and malignancies of the breast, thyroid, genitourinary tract, and gastrointestinal tract.

DeNardo GL et al: Strategies for developing effective radioimmunotherapy for solid tumors. Clin Cancer Res 1999; 5:3219s.

Perez CA, Brady LW (editors): *Principles and Practice of Radiation Oncology*, 3rd ed. Lippincott Williams & Wilkins, 1998.

Tobias JS, Thomas PRM (editors): *Current Radiation Oncology*, vol 3. Oxford Univ Press, 1998.

Zelenetz AD: Radioimmunotherapy for lymphoma. Curr Opin Oncol 1999;11:375.

■ SPECIFIC TYPES OF MALIGNANT NEOPLASMS

SOFT TISSUE SARCOMA

Soft tissue sarcomas account for approximately 1% of all new cancer diagnoses. Slightly more than half of all patients diagnosed with the disease eventually die as a result of the cancer. Classically, soft tissue sarcomas present as asymptomatic large masses in the extremities or retroperitoneum, but they also develop with some frequency in the neck and within the abdominal viscera. Fifty percent of these tumors occur in the lower extremity, most commonly in the thigh. Soft tissue sarcomas originate from a wide variety of mesenchymal cell types and include liposarcoma, fibrosarcoma, rhabdomyosarcoma, leiomyosarcoma, and desmoid tumors. While the histopathology of these tumors is highly variable, with some exceptions they tend to behave in a fashion dictated by tumor grade rather than the cell of origin.

Most soft tissue sarcomas arise de novo, and rarely do they result from malignant degeneration of a benign lesion. There are some familial syndromes in which patients are genetically predisposed to the formation of soft tissue sarcomas. Patients with Gardner's syndrome have a tendency to form desmoid tumors, and those with Recklinghausen's disease are predisposed to the formation of neurofibrosarcomas. Other proved risk factors exist that may increase the chances of sarcoma formation. It is known that tissue irradiation can predispose a patient to a variety of types of sarcomas. Chronic extremity lymphedema also increases the risk for lymphangiosarcoma. A classic example is the development of upper extremity lymphangiosarcomas in patients with a postmastectomy lymphedematous arm. Other less clear associations link chronic tissue trauma and occupational chemical exposures with an increased risk for sarcoma formation.

The major features of the staging system for soft tissue sarcomas (Table 47–1) are the grade of the tumor, its size, and the presence of metastatic disease. Although the site of the tumor is not considered in staging, patients with retroperitoneal tumors tend to have a worse prognosis. Sarcomas generally metastasize by the hematogenous route, and the metastatic sites of sarcomas are related to the location of the primary tumor. The vast majority of metastases from extremity sarcomas are to the lung, while the majority of retroperitoneal tumors metastasize to the liver. Some epithelioid sarcomas (clear cell sarcoma and synovial sarcoma) can also metastasize to lymph nodes.

Any mass suspected of harboring a soft tissue sarcoma should be imaged prior to operation. Both CT and MRI can be used to image these tumors, but MRI is often more accurate in defining the extent of the tumor and invasion of surrounding structures. A chest x-ray or chest CT should be obtained in order to evaluate for pulmonary metastases in patients with high-grade tumors. In imaging a retroperitoneal tumor, the liver should be examined in the same radiographic study.

The most important prognostic variables for patients with soft tissue sarcoma are the size and grade of the primary tumor. Since grading is based on the cellular archi-

Table 47–1. AJCC staging system for soft tissue sarcoma.

Stage	Description
IA	Low-grade sarcoma; tumor < 5 cm; no nodal or systemic metastases (G1T1N0M0)
IB	Low-grade sarcoma; tumor > 5 cm; no nodal or systemic metastases (G1T2N0M0)
IIA	Moderate-grade sarcoma; tumor < 5 cm; no nodal or systemic metastases (G2T1N0M0)
IIB	Moderate-grade sarcoma; tumor > 5 cm; no nodal or systemic metastases (G2T2N0M0)
IIIA	High-grade sarcoma; tumor < 5 cm; no nodal or systemic metastases (G3T1N0M0)
IIIB	High-grade sarcoma; tumor > 5 cm; no nodal or systemic metastases (G3T2N0M0)
IVA	Any grade sarcoma; any tumor size; regional node metastases, no systemic metastases (any G, any T, N1M0)
IVB	Any grade sarcoma; any tumor size; any nodal status, with systemic metastases (any G, any T, any N, M1)

tecture and invasive nature of the tumor, FNA is not a typically useful biopsy technique for the initial diagnosis of a sarcoma. Core needle biopsies may be performed for large, palpable superficial tumors. For large deep tumors or those adjacent to vital structures, incisional biopsy is usually the diagnostic method of choice. If a tumor is small (< 3 cm) and superficial, excisional biopsy should be performed. All extremity biopsy incisions should be oriented longitudinally, as the biopsy incision scar should be excised in a subsequent definitive resection of the tumor. The role of FNA should be confined to the confirmation of recurrent sarcoma.

Treatment

Surgery is the mainstay of therapy for sarcoma, but these tumors are also relatively sensitive to radiation. A pseudocapsule composed of tumor cells surrounds sarcomas, and local invasion along fascial planes and neurovascular structures is common. Local capsular excision is inadequate for cure, as local recurrence rates for such procedures are greater than 90%.

Historically, amputation was the only form of curative surgical therapy for large extremity sarcomas. Now, with a better understanding of tumor response to radiation therapy, wide local excision in combination with radiation can provide adequate local control, with local recurrence rates of approximately 15% and equivalent survival. This combination therapy has allowed for a high rate of limb preservation. Amputation for soft tissue sarcoma is currently reserved for patients whose tumors cannot be resected adequately by wide local excision, have no evidence of metastatic disease, and have a good prognosis for rehabilitation.

Generally, the margin for wide local excision should be at least 2 cm. The dissection should be carried out at least one fascial plane away from the tumor and may necessitate a compartmental resection. The surgeon should take care to avoid direct visualization of the tumor during the procedure in order to prevent tumor from seeding into the wound. Surgical excision of the tumor may involve resection of important neurovascular structures. In such cases, nerve grafts and arterial reconstruction with autologous or prosthetic conduits may be required. Large soft tissue defects often require the construction of myocutaneous flaps to improve function and cosmesis. Soft tissue sarcomas rarely invade bone or skin, and wide resections of these structures are infrequently necessary. Following wide local excision, metal clips should be placed at all margins of the resection in order to guide subsequent radiotherapy.

Radiation therapy is a necessary adjunct in the local control of sarcomas. Based on the location and size of the tumor, several modes of delivery are used, including EBRT, intraoperative radiation, and brachytherapy. In many centers, small (< 2 cm) low-grade extremity tumors are treated with wide local excision alone. Larger tumors should be treated by wide excision and postoperative radiation therapy, either by EBRT or brachytherapy catheters. Preoperative radiotherapy appears to have distinct advantages in patients with tumors larger than 10 cm, improving local control rates and sometimes shrinking tumors sufficiently to allow for limb-sparing procedures.

Retroperitoneal tumors are generally large at presentation and often invade vital structures; however, the majority of these tumors are resectable. Resection should be carried out en bloc with involved organs and include appropriate margins where possible. Because of the low tolerance of the abdominal and retroperitoneal organs to radiation, delivery of adequate radiotherapy is often difficult. There is encouraging evidence for intraoperative radiation therapy to the tumor bed, but this technique is still considered investigational and can only be performed in select centers.

Multiple trials have been conducted using adjuvant chemotherapy in soft tissue sarcomas, but the results are conflicting and no clear survival benefit has been demonstrated. Currently, the role of adjuvant chemotherapy should be limited to clinical trials.

The vast majority of localized recurrences in soft tissue sarcomas occur in the first 2 years after resection, necessitating close follow-up during that period. A local recurrence is not indicative of systemic disease and, in the absence of evidence of metastases, should be treated aggressively in the same manner as a primary tumor.

The resection of pulmonary metastases should be considered in patients who have fewer than four radiographically detectable lesions and who have achieved apparent local control following resection of the primary tumor. In such circumstances, disease-free survival can approach 25–35%.

Bland KI et al: Application of magnetic resonance imaging and computerized tomography as an adjunct to the surgical management of soft tissue sarcomas. Ann Surg 1987;205:473.

Brennan MF et al: The role of multimodality therapy in soft-tissue sarcoma. Ann Surg 1991;214:328.

Fraker DL: Hyperthermic regional perfusion for melanoma and sarcoma of the limbs. Curr Probl Surg 1999;36:841.

Gadd MA et al: Development and treatment of pulmonary metastases in adult patients with extremity soft tissue sarcoma. Ann Surg 1993;218:705.

Pisters PW et al: Long-term results of a prospective randomized trial of adjuvant brachytherapy in soft tissue sarcoma. J Clin Oncol 1996;14:859.

Rydholm A et al: Limb-sparing surgery without radiotherapy based on anatomic location of soft tissue sarcoma. J Clin Oncol 1991;9:1757.

Williard WC et al: Comparison of amputation with limb-sparing operations for adult soft tissue sarcoma of the extremity. Ann Surg 1992;215:269.

MELANOMA

In the United States, there has been a threefold increase in the incidence of melanoma over the last decade. The incidence of melanoma is increasing faster than that of any other tumor type.

Several risk factors have been identified for melanoma. The presence of multiple or dysplastic nevi can increase the risk of developing melanoma between four- and tenfold. Suspicion of dysplastic nevi is aroused by those moles that are larger than 5 mm and possess two of the following characteristics: variable pigmentation, irregular shape, and indistinct or asymmetric borders. There is a causal relationship between melanoma and exposure to sunlight. Individuals whose first sunburn occurred at an early age have an increased incidence of

Table 47–2. Clinical identification (ABCD) of melanoma.

Asymmetry: Asymmetric shape, color, or contour
Borders: Irregular or ill-defined borders
Color: Black, brown, blue, red, gray, or white
Diameter: Larger than 5 mm

Table 47–3. Breslow classification of melanoma.

Less than 0.75 mm thick
0.76–1.5 mm thick
1.5–4 mm thick
Greater than 4 mm thick

melanoma. Other risk factors include freckles, a fair complexion, reddish or blond hair, blue eyes, and a first-degree relative with melanoma.

The prognosis of melanoma is inversely and dramatically related to the depth of invasion at diagnosis, emphasizing the importance of early diagnosis of this disease. Lesions that are suspicious for melanoma can be identified by their clinical characteristics, often referred to as the ABCDs of Asymmetry, Borders, Color, and Diameter (Table 47–2). The most common site for melanoma in men is on the back and trunk, while the most common site in women is on the lower extremities.

The vertical height of melanoma is the single most important prognosticator for primary tumors. Several classification systems for the microscopic staging of melanomas exist, but the Breslow method provides the most accurate and reproducible prognostic information (Table 47–3). The AJCC and UICC have also developed a clinical staging system that includes both the Breslow thickness and the presence of regional or systemic metastases (Table 47–4).

Melanoma generally metastasizes by the lymphatic route in a predictable and orderly fashion. In most cases, the first site of metastatic disease is to the first regional lymph node group. The number of lymph nodes harboring metastatic disease also affects a patient's

Table 47–4. AJCC staging system for melanoma.

Stage	Description
IA	Localized melanoma < 0.75 mm thick; no nodal or systemic metastases (T1N0M0)
IB	Localized melanoma 0.76–1.5 mm thick; no nodal or systemic metastases (T2N0M0)
IIA	Localized melanoma 1.5–4.0 mm thick; no nodal or systemic metastases (T3N0M0)
IIB	Localized melanoma > 4.0 mm thick; no nodal or systemic metastases (T4N0M0)
III	Regional or in-transit metastases; no systemic metastases (any T, N1M0)
IV	Evidence of systemic metastatic disease (any T, any N, M1)

prognosis. Systemic metastases may involve almost any organ system, but they are most common in the liver, lung, brain, bone, adrenals, heart, and bowel. Systemic metastases imply a poor prognosis, with an average survival of 6–9 months after recognition of metastatic spread.

There are four distinct categories of melanoma: superficial spreading, nodular, lentigo maligna, and acral lentiginous melanoma.

Superficial spreading melanoma is the most common presentation, accounting for nearly 70% of all melanomas. These usually occur in sun-exposed areas of the body or in individuals with multiple dysplastic nevi. They generally arise in preexisting nevi and can occur at any age after puberty. The superficial spreading subtype tends to grow in a radial pattern during the earlier stages and converts to a vertical growth pattern during the later stages of development.

Nodular melanomas account for between 15% and 25% of all melanomas. These tend to occur in older individuals and are more common in men. Nodular melanomas generally develop de novo, not in a preexisting nevus. They usually are dome shaped with distinct borders and often resemble a blood blister. Nodular melanomas occur most commonly on the head, neck, and trunk. They lack a significant horizontal growth phase and tend to be deep at the time of diagnosis.

Lentigo maligna melanoma has less propensity to metastasize and thus has a more favorable prognosis relative to the other subtypes. These lesions account for 4–10% of melanomas and occur in an older population. Lentigo maligna almost always develops in sun-exposed areas. They have a long horizontal growth phase and often have very convoluted borders.

Acral lentiginous melanomas account for between 2% and 8% of melanomas in Caucasians but for 30–60% of melanomas in blacks, Asians, and Hispanics. These lesions do not occur in sun-exposed areas; instead, they occur on the sole of the foot, the palm, beneath the nail beds, and in the perineal region. Acral lentiginous melanomas are often large, with an average diameter of 3 cm at the time of diagnosis. They develop relatively rapidly over the course of months to several years and tend to behave very aggressively. The clinical characteristics of these melanomas are often unmistakable, with variegations in color and convoluted borders. Ulceration of these lesions is common.

Treatment

Any suspected melanoma should be removed by excisional biopsy. Given the importance of microscopic staging, shave or curette biopsies are absolutely contraindicated. In occasional cases of large lesions, especially on the face and hands, that cannot be easily excised, a full-thickness incisional biopsy or punch biopsy should be performed.

If the biopsy specimen reveals melanoma, a formal excision with adequate margins is required. Because satellite lesions containing microscopic tumor cells frequently surround primary melanomas, excision with narrow margins often is followed by local recurrence. Traditionally, excision of a melanoma called for 5-cm margins; however, several randomized clinical trials have supported less aggressive excisions. The current standard for lesions less than 1 mm in depth is excision with 1-cm margins. Melanomas between 1mm and 4 mm in thickness should be excised with 2-cm margins. Those deeper than 4 mm should be excised with a 2- to 3-cm margin and may require the resection of underlying fascia.

In the past, there was substantial controversy regarding elective lymph node dissection of the draining nodal basin for melanoma. Melanoma has now been demonstrated to have an orderly progression of nodal metastatic disease. Biopsy of the first draining ("sentinel") lymph node in the regional drainage basin of a lesion allows for accurate staging of the nodal basin. If there is no tumor in the sentinel lymph node, then there is a greater than 95% certainty that there is no metastatic disease in that basin. Sampling only the sentinel lymph node means that patients are spared the morbidity associated with unnecessary extensive lymph node dissections.

The sentinel lymph node biopsy has become the standard of care in the staging and treatment of melanoma. The dominant drainage basins can be identified by lymphoscintigraphy, which involves injection of technetium-99m sulfur colloid in the area around the tumor and a gamma camera to image the sites of lymph node drainage. Immediately following this nuclear imaging, the patient is taken to the operating room, where a handheld gamma counter is used to identify the sentinel lymph node, which is subsequently excised. During surgery, visual guidance and confirmation are facilitated by the injection of vital blue dye around the lesion immediately before the procedure.

Several pathologic techniques of analysis have dramatically increased the sensitivity of the sentinel lymph node biopsy. After removal of the nodes, they are analyzed by serial section, routine H&E staining, immunostaining, and reverse transcription polymerase chain reaction testing. Using these methods of analysis, the pathologist is able to detect even minute numbers of metastatic melanoma cells in the sentinel node. Patients with clinically palpable lymph nodes or a positive sentinel lymph node biopsy should undergo formal lymph node dissection of the entire drainage basin. There is controversy regarding the use of sentinel node biopsies for patients with primary lesions less than 1 mm thick, as these lesions are unlikely to metastasize. The presence of lymph node metastases may signify systemic disease and portends a 5-year survival rate of 40%.

Traditional chemotherapy regimens have proved largely ineffective in the treatment of melanoma; however, the cytokine interferon alfa-2b has been shown to improve disease-free and overall survival in high-risk patients with no evidence of systemic metastases. The duration of therapy is long (12 months) and the toxicities are universal and substantial., but even so, interferon alfa-2b remains the best hope for the chemotherapeutic treatment of melanoma. A large body of research investigating the use of immunotherapy in the treatment of high-risk patients has shown great promise, but such therapies are still in the experimental stage.

There is some evidence that radiation therapy may improve local and regional control of melanoma when combined with surgery.

Local Recurrence & Metastatic Disease

Local recurrence is defined as any melanoma that occurs within 5 cm of the scar of a previously excised lesion. These generally develop within 5 years after removal of the primary. Local recurrence rates are higher with thicker or ulcerated melanomas. Excision with wide (> 2 cm) margins is considered adequate treatment for a single local recurrence. For multiple recurrences, excision followed by hyperthermic isolated limb perfusion with melphalan or cisplatin is recommended. Such combined therapy improves the local recurrence rate but shows no improvement in systemic control of the disease.

Surgery, chemotherapy, and radiation therapy in patients with systemic metastases serve only as palliative treatments, as cure is not a realistic aim. Systemic disease requires systemic therapy, often with cytotoxic chemotherapy or immunotherapy.

Regional and systemic recurrence of melanoma can be latent, and recurrence 10 years after the original diagnosis is not uncommon. This fact necessitates close lifelong follow-up of these patients. Patients with a past history of melanoma have a dramatically increased risk of developing a second primary lesion and require diligent screening for other lesions.

Balch CM et al: Efficacy of 2-cm surgical margins for intermediate-thickness melanomas (1 to 4 mm). Results of a multi-institutional randomized surgical trial. Ann Surg 1993;218:262.

Messina JL et al: Pathologic examination of the sentinel lymph node in malignant melanoma. Am J Surg Pathol 1999; 23:686.

Reintgen D et al: Lymphatic mapping and sentinel node biopsy in patients with malignant melanoma. 1997;84:188.

Reintgen D, Kirkwood J: The adjuvant treatment of malignant melanoma. J Fla Med Assoc 1997; 84:147.

Tucker MA et al: Clinically recognized dysplastic nevi. A central risk factor for cutaneous melanoma. JAMA 1997;277:1439.

LYMPHOMA

Lymphomas are malignant neoplasms that originate from the lymphoid tissues. Two distinct categories of lymphoma exist: Hodgkin's and non-Hodgkin's. The two types not only have different morphologic characteristics but differ also in their clinical behavior and their response to various therapeutic regimens. It is not possible to differentiate Hodgkin's and non-Hodgkin's lymphoma on clinical grounds but only by surgical biopsy. In the diagnosis of a suspected lymphoma, excisional biopsy of the entire lymph node or nodes is imperative, as the architecture has a bearing on the diagnosis and the subsequent treatment of the tumor.

1. Hodgkin's Lymphoma

Hodgkin's lymphoma may occur at any age but is generally a disease of young adults. Modern therapy has allowed for cure of over 70% of patients with this malignancy. Hodgkin's lymphomas are differentiated from non-Hodgkin's lymphomas morphologically by the presence of a distinctive giant neoplastic cell, the Reed-Sternberg cell. This cell is the presumed malignant cell in Hodgkin's disease, but its origin is not well understood. Recent evidence suggests that it originates from B cells. Reed-Sternberg cells are typically surrounded by an inflammatory lymphocytic infiltrate. It is the pattern of the lymphocytic infiltrate that determines the classic subtypes of Hodgkin's disease (see Table 47–5). Although the natural history of the different subtypes is variable, effective modern therapy has reduced the relevance of these histologic classifications.

The cause of Hodgkin's disease is not well understood; however, epidemiologic studies have revealed certain patterns of disease clustering. The incidence appears to be higher with a lower number of siblings, early birth order, siblings with Hodgkin's disease, a decreased number of playmates, certain HLA antigens, single-family dwellings, and patients who have undergone tonsillectomy. The incidence is increased also in persons with immunodeficiencies and autoimmune disorders. This pattern suggests that an oncogenic virus may cause Hodgkin's; however, no candidate viruses have been identified.

Hodgkin's disease normally presents as painless enlargement of lymph nodes. The disease has a characteristic pattern of spread to contiguous lymph node groups. A distinctive array of symptoms, called B symptoms, often accompanies advanced disease. The

Table 47–5. Classic subtypes of Hodgkin's lymphoma.

Subtype	Characteristics
Lymphocyte-predominant	Uncommon (6% of Hodgkin's lymphomas), diffuse lymphocytic infiltrate with few Reed-Sternberg cells, excellent prognosis
Lymphocyte-depleted	Rare (2% of Hodgkin's lymphoma), abundant Reed-Sternberg cells, paucity of lymphocytes, occurs in older males, aggressive clinically
Mixed cellularity	Common (20–25% of Hodgkin's lymphoma), histologically intermediate between above two forms, often presents with disseminated disease
Nodular sclerosis	Most common form (70% of Hodgkin's lymphoma), fibrosis with Reed-Sternberg and lymphoid cells, more common in young women, presents with cervical or mediastinal disease, excellent prognosis

B symptoms consist of weight loss, fever, and drenching night sweats.

Staging

With regard to therapy, the most important prognostic factor in Hodgkin's lymphoma is the disease stage. The currently accepted staging system for Hodgkin's is the Ann Arbor (see Table 47–6). This system is based on the gross anatomic distribution of lymph node involvement with respect to the diaphragm. Although important prognostically, the system makes no allowance for tumor bulk or the invasive nature of the lymphoma.

Table 47–6. Ann Arbor staging system of Hodgkin's lymphoma.

I	Single lymph node region or single extranodal site
II	Two or more nodal groups on same side of diaphragm or two or more contiguous extranodal organs
III	Two or more nodal groups on both sides of diaphragm; may include spleen or sites of localized extranodal involvement
IV	Disseminated involvement of one or more extranodal sites (eg, liver, bone marrow, skin), with or without lymph node involvement

Splenic disease is considered as another site of lymphatic involvement.

As discussed earlier, excisional lymph node biopsy is essential to the diagnosis of Hodgkin's lymphoma. Once the diagnosis is made, disease staging begins with a detailed history and physical examination, with attention to all lymph node beds, B symptoms, and symptoms related to extranodal involvement. A chest radiograph should be obtained to evaluate the mediastinum. If the chest film is abnormal or the patient has any symptoms of mediastinal involvement, CT of the chest is mandatory. An abdominal and pelvic CT scan should also be performed to evaluate the viscera, the retroperitoneal and pelvic lymph nodes, and the spleen. Bone marrow biopsy is also part of the staging evaluation of patients with bony symptoms or cytopenias. Other selectively used imaging techniques include bilateral pedal lymphangiography, gallium scan, and positron emission tomography (PET).

Radiographic evaluation of the spleen is often not adequate to predict histologic involvement. Occasionally, a staging laparotomy is necessary if the anatomic extent of disease in the abdomen is important in guiding therapy. The staging laparotomy includes splenectomy, wedge liver biopsy, and dissection of the para-aortic, iliac, splenic hilar, and hepatic portal lymph nodes. If a female patient is likely to receive pelvic radiotherapy, an oophoropexy is performed. Staging laparotomy is associated with potential morbidity and mortality and delays the initiation of therapy for several weeks. It is purely a staging procedure and provides no direct therapeutic benefit. For these reasons, many oncologists forgo the staging laparotomy unless the procedure is absolutely necessary to guide therapy.

Treatment

The treatment of Hodgkin's lymphoma involves radiation alone or the combination of radiation and chemotherapy, called combined modality therapy. In patients with localized (stage I or stage II) disease, external beam radiotherapy alone is the preferred treatment. Wide field radiation rather than irradiation of involved areas is the current standard. Depending on the extent of disease, mantle, subtotal, or total lymphoid irradiation is performed. Mantle radiation consists of irradiation of the cervical, axillary, mediastinal, and hilar lymph nodes. Subtotal lymphoid irradiation (STLI) is treatment of the mantle plus the upper abdominal, para-aortic, and splenic bed lymph nodes. Total lymphoid irradiation (TLI) refers to irradiation of the pelvic field in addition to STLI.

Most patients with stage I and stage II disease can be successfully managed with radiotherapy alone; however, certain subgroups with a high risk of relapse have been identified. Patients with bulky mediastinal disease or multiple areas of extranodal involvement have a high risk of relapse, and combined-modality therapy is indicated.

Many experimental and standard protocols for adjuvant combination chemotherapy exist; however, two regimens have consistently proved superior in efficacy—MOPP (mechlorethamine, Oncovin [vincristine], procarbazine, and prednisone) and ABVD (doxorubicin [Adriamycin], bleomycin, vinblastine and dacarbazine). The majority of current protocols involve some combination of these two regimens.

In addition to the subgroups discussed above, several other clinical scenarios require combined chemotherapy and radiotherapy. Patients with unfavorable disease stages (stage III and stage IV) or extensive splenic involvement by staging laparotomy should be treated by both modalities. Another group of patients that can benefit from combined therapy are children whose growing bones and muscles cannot tolerate radiation therapy in full doses.

Even though the current therapeutic regimens for Hodgkin's lymphoma are quite efficacious, up to 30% of patients relapse or fail to undergo remission. In these situations, high-dose chemotherapy with stem cell transplant (bone marrow transplant) should be considered, as further radiotherapy is limited by cumulative toxicity and repeated salvage chemotherapy often fails.

Investigational immunotherapeutic regimens also appear to have potential in preventing relapse of higher-stage disease. In contrast to normal cells, Reed-Sternberg cells express large numbers of the surface antigen CD30. Monoclonal antibodies to this antigen have been explored as vehicles for directing cytotoxins to tumor cells; and preliminary results of trials using this immunotoxin appear very promising in decreasing the rate of relapse.

2. Non-Hodgkin's Lymphoma

Non-Hodgkin's lymphoma encompasses a wide spectrum of lymphoid-derived tumors. This heterogeneous group of diseases includes more than ten distinct tumor subtypes with variable biologic behavior and responses to treatment.

Non-Hodgkin's lymphoma can occur in patients of all ages; however, different subtypes tend to have a predilection for certain age groups. Several risk factors have been identified that predispose patients to the development of disease. Patients with congenital disorders such as ataxia-telangiectasia, Wiskott-Aldrich syndrome, and celiac disease have an increased incidence of lymphoma. Certain acquired conditions also predispose patients to lymphoma, including prior chemotherapy or radiotherapy, immunosuppressive therapy, HIV in-

fection, HTLV-1 infection, *Helicobacter pylori* gastritis, Hashimoto's thyroiditis, and Sjögren's syndrome.

Non-Hodgkin's lymphoma may originate from B cells, T cells, or histiocytes. Morphologically, the tumors may appear as nodular clusters or diffuse sheets of lymphoid cells. In contrast to Hodgkin's lymphoma, non-Hodgkin's lymphoma is more likely to spread in a noncontiguous fashion.

Classically, non-Hodgkin's lymphoma presents as nontender enlargement of lymph nodes, but nearly one-third of all cases originate outside the lymph nodes. These extranodal malignancies develop in organs that normally have nests of lymphoid tissue (mucosal surfaces, bone marrow, and skin).

Staging & Classification

Although the Ann Arbor system was developed for Hodgkin's disease, this staging system is also used in non-Hodgkin's lymphoma. The goal of the staging evaluation is to distinguish patients who have localized disease from those with disseminated disease. After pathologic diagnosis, the staging evaluation for non-Hodgkin's lymphoma consists of a detailed history and physical examination, routine laboratory tests, a bone marrow biopsy, and a CT scan of the neck, chest, abdomen, and pelvis. Only in very rare instances are more aggressive staging procedures (laparotomy or liver biopsy) necessary. Although helpful in assessing the anatomic extent of disease, the Ann Arbor system is of minimal clinical value in non-Hodgkin's lymphoma. Instead, prognosis and treatment are more dependent on the grade and type of the malignancy.

Scientists have made countless attempts at developing a universal, clinically relevant classification system for the subtypes of non-Hodgkin's lymphoma, and the merits of the various classifications are an area of hot debate. While still evolving, the most widely accepted classification system is the Revised European-American Lymphoma (REAL) Classification.

In determining the therapeutic approach to patients with non-Hodgkin's lymphoma, a simpler classification system can be utilized. For treatment purposes, these lymphomas can be functionally divided into two groups: indolent (low-grade) and aggressive (high-grade) lymphomas (Table 47–7). The extranodal lymphomas are not amenable to conventional classifications and are generally regarded as a separate entity.

Smaller, differentiated cells characterize the indolent lymphomas, and this class tends to have a follicular architecture. Although the course of these lymphomas is not very aggressive, they are very difficult to cure, and most patients eventually die of their disease. Median survival times with treatment are between 6 years and 12 years. The indolent lymphomas occur in older indi-

Table 47–7. Functional classification
of non-Hodgkin's lymphoma.

Indolent (low-grade) lymphomas
  Follicular small-cleaved
  Follicular mixed small-cleaved and large cell
  Diffuse small lymphocytic
  Diffuse intermediate
  Follicular large cell
  Diffuse small cleaved-cell
Aggressive (high-grade) lymphomas
  Diffuse mixed small-cleaved and large cell
  Diffuse large cell
  Immunoblastic
  Burkitt's
  Lymphoblastic

---

viduals and are extremely rare in young patients. They typically present as localized disease but are often demonstrated to be widely disseminated after staging evaluation—only 10% of the indolent lymphomas are truly localized at presentation. In addition to the nodal sites, disease commonly affects the bone marrow, liver, and spleen. The natural history of indolent lymphomas often involves progression of the tumor cells to a more aggressive subtype. This progression is sometimes heralded by the onset of B symptoms and portends a dismal prognosis.

The aggressive lymphomas behave differently from the indolent ones and demand a different therapeutic approach. Histologically, the aggressive lymphomas spread more diffusely throughout the lymph nodes and consist of larger, less differentiated cell types. This class of lymphomas demonstrates a very rapid growth rate and an increased rate of early mortality. Despite this malignant behavior, this class of non-Hodgkin's lymphoma is often curable. In contrast to the indolent lymphomas, at least one-third of these patients present while the disease is still localized. The aggressive lymphomas can occur in any age group, but almost all childhood non-Hodgkin's lymphomas are of the aggressive type.

The extranodal lymphomas develop outside of the lymph nodes. They can involve any organ but most commonly affect the oropharynx, paranasal sinuses, thyroid, gastrointestinal tract, liver, testicles, skin, and bone marrow. Once considered a rare tumor, central nervous system lymphomas have become more common over the last 20 years, especially in AIDS patients. Of all the extranodal sites, the stomach is most commonly involved, accounting for half of all gastrointestinal lymphomas. Lymphomas of the stomach can result

from primary or secondary involvement. The tumor is considered to be a primary gastric lymphoma if the patient presents with gastric symptoms and the stomach is the predominant site of disease. This tumor is generally a disease of older patients, and its incidence has been strongly linked to *H pylori* gastritis.

Treatment

A. INDOLENT LYMPHOMA

Therapy for non-Hodgkin's lymphoma is generally guided by the functional classification of the disease (Figure 47–1). If the staging evaluation reveals localized disease, radiotherapy may be curative. Relapse rates after radiation therapy for localized disease approach 50%, with most relapses occurring in the first 5 years. For this reason, some institutions combine radiotherapy with adjuvant chemotherapy for localized disease.

The current standard therapies for systemic indolent lymphomas are rarely curative, and the goal of treatment is generally directed at palliation of symptoms. Radiation therapy has no beneficial role in the therapy of systemic indolent lymphomas. At present, a "watch and wait" approach to treatment is recommended. After diagnosis, asymptomatic patients are followed clinically until they have progression to more aggressive disease, B symptoms, or laboratory abnormalities (cytopenia, increased hepatic enzymes, or decreased renal function). Withholding treatment does not reduce survival in patients with non-Hodgkin's lymphoma, and it probably improves quality of life. When treatment is initiated, single-agent chemotherapy with alkylating agents (chlorambucil or cyclophosphamide) has proved as effective as the more toxic combination therapies.

In younger patients with systemic indolent disease, high-dose chemotherapy with autologous bone marrow transplant is currently under clinical investigation.

B. AGGRESSIVE LYMPHOMAS

Despite their aggressive nature, these lymphomas have a better chance for cure than their more indolent counterparts. The consensus therapy for localized disease is radiotherapy with adjuvant chemotherapy.

Systemic disease (stages II–IV) is treated by combination CHOP (cyclophosphamide, doxorubicin, Oncovin [vincristine], and prednisone) chemotherapy. Radiotherapy may be added following chemotherapy for areas of bulky disease. Disease-free survival after aggressive chemotherapy is 30% at 12 years. The therapeutic prognosis is better for younger patients (approaching 50% disease-free survival for patients under 40) and worse for those over age 65. This therapeutic difference

Figure 47–1. Non-Hodgkin's lymphoma treatment algorithm. CHOP, cyclophosphamide, doxorubicin (hydroxydaunomycin), Oncovin (vincristine), and prednisone; XRT, x-ray therapy

is probably related to the older population's poor tolerance of chemotherapy.

Patients who relapse after aggressive treatment have a poor prognosis, with less than 10% long-term survival rates. Currently, high dose cytotoxic therapy and bone marrow transplant should be considered for patients who relapse or fail to enter remission after induction chemotherapy. The treatment-related mortality from bone marrow transplant is approximately 10%—high enough to restrict its use to patients who have failed conventional therapy.

A number of approaches using monoclonal antibodies to different non-Hodgkin's lymphoma tumor-specific antigens have been developed. Of these immunotherapies, anti-CD20 therapy has yielded the most promising clinical results. CD20 is a cell-surface protein involved in the development and differentiation of normal B cells. It is found on the vast majority of B cell lymphomas. Treatment regimens utilizing the anti-CD20 monoclonal antibodies use unmodified antibodies called rituximab or antibodies bound to radionuclides called tositumomab. Rituximab is assumed to work by antibody-mediated cellular cytotoxicity and activation of complement-mediated tumor cell lysis. Tositumomab can activate the cell-killing pathways but also allows for the tumor-specific delivery of cytotoxic [131]I.

Both of these regimens have proved effective in clinical trials, but current protocols use these therapies only in the treatment of relapsed or refractory B cell lymphomas after initial induction chemotherapy has been tried without success.

C. NONLYMPHOID DISEASE

There is no consensus about the proper management of localized nonlymphoid lymphomas since large-scale studies of therapy for this disease have not been conducted. With few exceptions, nonlymphoid disease is managed somewhat in the same way as systemic aggressive lymphomas, using combination CHOP therapy.

The CHOP regimen has the disadvantage of poor penetration of the blood-brain barrier and is thus ineffective in the treatment of primary central nervous system lymphomas. These lymphomas are sensitive to radiation, and current regimens utilize whole brain radiation with some form of adjuvant chemotherapy. Methotrexate is the most common adjuvant treatment in this patient population, and it can be effective when delivered either systemically or intrathecally. Central nervous system lymphomas have a poor prognosis, with approximately 20% 5-year survival rates in treated patients. The combined modalities, while providing modest survival benefits, have significant neurotoxicity, and as many as 50% of patients develop severe dementia. Given this morbidity, clinicians are currently attempting to improve the therapy for this disease, with most efforts directed toward using chemotherapy as the sole modality in the treatment of patients with primary central nervous system lymphomas.

Several extranodal lymphomas, including testicular, paranasal, epidural, and AIDS-related lymphomas, have a predilection for metastasis to the central nervous system. Such tumors require systemic CHOP therapy combined with prophylactic intrathecal methotrexate treatments.

The treatment of gastric lymphomas in particular—and organ-isolated lymphomas in general—is controversial. The data supporting resection of these tumors is debatable; however, many centers continue to perform gastric resections for gastric lymphomas to prevent chemotherapy-related perforation or hemorrhage. Although some studies support gastrectomy as the sole treatment of isolated gastric tumors, many centers treat these patients with adjuvant regimens of radiotherapy or combination chemotherapy (or both). When these tumors are not isolated to the stomach, systemic treatment is required.

Splenectomy in patients with lymphomatous splenic involvement has no demonstrated therapeutic benefit and should be reserved for patients with symptomatic splenomegaly, pain from recurrent splenic infarctions, and hematologic depression from hypersplenism.

Advani RH, Horning SJ: Treatment of early-stage Hodgkin's disease. Semin Hematol 1999;36:270.

DeAngelis LM: Primary CNS lymphoma: treatment with combined chemotherapy and radiotherapy. J Neurooncol 1999; 43:249.

Gopal AK, Press, OW: Clinical applications of anti-CD20 antibodies. J Lab Clin Med 1999;134:445.

Harris NL et al: A revised European-American classification of lymphoid neoplasms: a proposal from the International Lymphoma Study Group. Blood 1994;84:1361.

Jaffe ES et al: World Health Organization Classification of lymphomas: a work in progress. Ann Oncol 1998;(9 Suppl_5:S25.

Jox A et al: Hodgkin's disease—new treatment strategies toward the cure of patients. Cancer Treat Rev 1999;25:169.

Kodera Y et al: The role of radical gastrectomy with systematic lymphadenectomy for the diagnosis and treatment of primary gastric lymphoma. Ann Surg 1998; 227:45.

Mounter PJ, Lennard AL: Management of non-Hodgkin's lymphomas. Postgrad Med J 1999;75:2.

Patte C: Non-Hodgkin's lymphoma. Eur J Cancer 1998;34:359.

Rosen ST: Recent advances and future directions using monoclonal antibodies for B cell malignancies. Semin Oncol 1999;26 (Suppl 14):1.

Vose JM: Antibody-targeted therapy for low-grade lymphoma. Semin Hematol 1999;36:15.

■ PARANEOPLASTIC SYNDROMES

Many tumors develop the ability to elaborate hormones or cytokines that can have deleterious consequences for the host. Host antibodies to tumor antigens are also thought to play a role in the development of paraneoplastic syndromes. These immune effects probably result from cross-reaction with normal tissue antigens and immune complex deposition. Paraneoplastic syndromes can be systemic or can affect only a single organ system. Included in the paraneoplastic syndromes are the common cancer sequelae of hypercoagulopathy, cachexia, fevers, and anemia of chronic disease. More specific effects are summarized in Table 47–8.

Paraneoplastic syndromes occur in approximately 10% of all patients with advanced malignant disease. Rarely, these syndromes represent the earliest manifestations of an occult cancer. The presence of a paraneoplastic syndrome does not necessarily signify incurable disease, and treatment of the primary tumor can eliminate the related symptoms.

Endocrinopathies are familiar paraneoplastic syndromes, and they are readily understood since they result from the elaboration of true hormones or peptides that mimic naturally occurring hormones. The most common endocrinopathy is Cushing's syndrome, which results from tumor production of ACTH or an ACTH-like peptide. The production of these mediators leads to excessive cortisol production and its associated stigmas, including truncal obesity, moon facies, weakness, hypertension, and glucose intolerance. Bronchogenic carcinomas, thymomas, medullary thyroid cancers, and carcinoids are frequent causes of Cushing's syndrome. Direct elaboration of cortisol from adrenal neoplasms may also lead to Cushing's syndrome.

Hypercalcemia is another common paraneoplastic syndrome. Hypercalcemia of malignancy can generally be attributed to one of two causes. Multiple myeloma and cancers that metastasize to bone can raise serum calcium levels through lytic bone metastases. Solid tumors such as breast, lung, and renal cancers can secrete a molecule called parathyroid hormone related peptide (PTHrP) which resembles parathyroid hormone. This molecule can bind parathyroid hormone receptors and mimic the action of parathyroid hormone. PTHrP is not subject to feedback inhibition like parathyroid hormone, and elaboration of large quantities of this molecule can cause severe hypercalcemia.

The neuromyopathic syndromes are presumed to result from cross-reaction of antitumor antibodies with

Table 47–8. Paraneoplastic syndromes.

Endocrinopathies		
Cushing's syndrome	Lung, pancreatic, adrenal, and neural tumors	ACTH or ACTH-like molecules
Syndrome of inappropriate ADH secretion	Lung and intracranial tumors	ADH
Hypercalcemia	Lung, breast, renal, prostate, and ovarian cancers; myeloma	Osteolytic metastases or parathyroid hormone-related peptide
Hypoglycemia	Sarcomas, islet cell tumors, hepatocellular carcinoma	Insulin or insulin-like peptides
Neurologic		
Myasthenia	Thymomas and lung cancer	Autoimmune
Encephalomyelitis	Lung, ovarian, and breast cancer	Autoimmune
Neuropathies	Myeloma; lung, breast, and ovarian cancer	Autoimmune
Cerebellar atrophy	Breast and ovarian cancer	Autoimmune
Dermatologic		
Acanthosis nigricans	Gastric, lung, and uterine cancer	Autoimmune
Dermatomyositis	Lung and breast cancer	Autoimmune
Hematologic		
Venous thrombosis	GI, lung, pancreatic, ovarian, breast, and prostate cancer	Tumor products that activate clotting factors
DIC	Pancreas, lung, stomach, and prostate cancer	Tumor products that activate and consume clotting factors
Osseous		
Hypertrophic osteoarthropathy	Lung cancer	Unknown

neuronal cells. In some cases, neurologic deficits are the first manifestations of an occult cancer. The paraneoplastic syndromes can involve every level of the central and peripheral nervous system from the cerebral cortex to the neuromuscular junction. Individuals may present with symptoms predominantly affecting one particular element of the nervous system, or they may present with diffuse nervous system involvement. Common central nervous system syndromes include cerebellar degeneration, encephalitis, and myelopathies of the spinal cord. Peripheral involvement can be manifested as polyneuropathy, myositis, or myasthenic syndromes similar to myasthenia gravis. The most common cancers causing neuromyopathic syndromes are small cell carcinoma of the lung, breast carcinoma, gynecologic cancers, and thymic tumors.

The etiology of the dermatologic syndromes is unclear, but they are theorized to result from either au-

toimmunity or from tumor elaboration of growth factors. Acanthosis nigricans is characterized by the appearance of gray-black hyperkeratotic patches on the skin. Although these lesions may occur sporadically, they are often associated with neoplasms, including lung cancer, gastric carcinoma, uterine cancer, and melanomas.

Abeloff MD: Paraneoplastic syndromes: a window on the biology of cancer. N Engl J Med 1987; 317:1598.

Cotran CS, Kumar V, Robbins SL (editors): *Robbins Pathologic Basis of Disease*, 6th ed. Saunders, 1999.

Dropcho EJ: The remote effects of cancer on the nervous system. Neurol Clin 1989;7:579.

Posner JB: Paraneoplastic syndromes: a brief review. Ann N Y Acad Sci 1997;835:83.

Salomon JC: Paraneoplastic syndromes. Med Hypotheses 1990; 32:29.

Organ Transplantation

48

John P. Roberts, MD, Nancy L. Ascher, MD, Nicholas J. Feduska, MD, Fraser M. Keith, MD, Juliet Melzer, MD, & Oscar Salvatierra, Jr., MD

The development of human organ transplantation was one of the truly outstanding medical achievements of the twentieth century. Before the availability of renal transplantation and hemodialysis, for example, all patients with end-stage renal failure succumbed to the illness. Working as a team, surgeons, nephrologists, and immunologists can now totally rehabilitate most transplanted patients. Although hemodialysis can prolong survival and provide partial rehabilitation for many patients with end-stage renal disease, only renal transplantation can truly restore them to a normal lifestyle. The success of renal transplantation has been followed by heart and heart-lung transplantation, liver transplantation, and pancreatic transplantation. The indications for and the successes and limitations of these procedures are the subject matter of this chapter.

■ KIDNEY TRANSPLANTATION

The principal biologic impediment to successful transplantation of an organ from one human to another human **(allograft)** is the immunologic rejection reaction that results from the genetic dissimilarity between the two individuals. It is rarely possible to perform a transplant between a genetically identical pair (monozygotic twins) **(isograft).** Transplantation of an organ between species (xenograft) has never been successful.

It was not until the early 1960s that practical immunosuppression became available with the advent of azathioprine and its combined use with prednisone. The success of this regimen ushered in a period of great enthusiasm and utilization of kidney allograft transplants.

Renal diseases responsible for renal failure that can be treated by transplantation are chronic glomerulonephritis, 50%; diabetic nephropathy, 30%; chronic pyelonephritis, 8%; malignant nephrosclerosis, 6%; polycystic kidney disease, 5%; and other renal disease, 6%. In patients age 10 and younger with end-stage renal disease, the incidence of glomerulonephritis is only 30%, and congenital nonobstructive and obstructive uropathies are more common than in adults (30%).

IMMUNOLOGIC RESPONSE

HLA Histocompatibility Antigens

The host response to the donor's histocompatibility antigens is the major biologic obstacle to successful transplantation. A single chromosomal complex of closely linked genes makes up the code for the major histocompatibility antigens. The **major histocompatibility complex (MHC)** in humans is called the **HLA system** (originally for "human leukocyte antigen") and occupies a segment of the short arm of the sixth chromosome. The HLA system is now known to include at least seven histocompatibility loci: HLA-A, HLA-B, HLA-C, HLA-D, HLA-DR, HLA-DQ, and HLA-DP. Each HLA gene locus is highly polymorphic, so that about 8–50 separate antigens are controlled by each locus. The HLA chromosomal complex, including the HLA antigens, is termed a **haplotype,** which is the portion of the phenotype determined by closely linked genes of a single chromosome inherited from one parent.

Histocompatibility antigens are classified in groups according to function and biochemistry as class I antigens (at the A, B, and C loci) and class II antigens (at the D and DR loci). Class I antigens are composed of a 44,000-MW heavy chain carrying the alloantigenic specificity and a 12,000-MW light chain associated with β_2-microglobulin. Class II antigens are composed of a 33,000-MW alpha chain and a 28,000-MW beta chain that carries the HLA specificities. Although both class I and class II antigens can elicit an immunologic response, class I antigens act as targets of cytotoxic T cells, and class II antigens have an important function in antigen presentation in vivo and in stimulation in vitro of the proliferative response of the mixed lymphocyte culture (MLC). Class I and class II antigens are also distributed differently on cells. Class I antigens are present on virtually all nucleated cells in the body, including T and B lymphocytes and platelets; class II antigens are expressed only on B lymphocytes, monocytes, macrophages, some types of endothelial cells, and activated T lymphocytes but are not expressed on platelets or unstimulated T cells. In the kidney, class I antigens are present on glomeruli, the vasculature, and tubules. In contrast, class II antigens appear to be located primarily on interstitial dendritic cells.

Lymphocytes are categorized as T or B cells. The cellular response directed against mismatched HLA antigens is T cell-dependent. Functional T cell subsets are generally divided into (1) helper T lymphocytes, which preferentially recognize class II antigens; (2) cytotoxic T lymphocytes, which preferentially recognize class I antigens; and (3) suppressor cells, which act to enhance graft survival. Allograft rejection is a complex event that results from the cytodestructive effects of activated helper T cells, cytotoxic T cells, B lymphocytes, antibodies, and activated macrophages. Activation of helper T cells by class II antigens stimulates the release of various factors, including interleukin-2 and macrophage-stimulating lymphokine. Cytotoxic T lymphocytes stimulated by class I antigens develop interleukin-2 receptors. Subsequently, stimulated macrophages and other accessory cells release interleukin-1, which in turn also influences the release of interleukin-2. Interleukin-2 then interacts with specific interleukin-2 receptors on activated helper and cytotoxic T cells, initiating DNA synthesis and eventual clonal proliferation of receptor-bearing cells. In addition, the continued viability of activated T cell clones is interleukin-2-dependent. In essence, the activation of helper T cells by alloantigens and interleukin-1 stimulates the release of a variety of lymphokines from helper T cells, and this process in turn activates macrophages, cytotoxic T cells, and antibody-releasing B cells. Although cytotoxic T cells are the dominant cell type infiltrating the allograft during rejection, helper T cells are most important in initiating the process.

The humoral response is also important, especially for class I antigens. Recipients who mount a primary immune response against class I antigens—manifested by the presence of cytotoxic antibodies in the serum—can produce an overwhelming secondary antibody response upon reexposure to the same antigens. The existence of cytotoxic anti-HLA antibody in a recipient at the time of transplantation (with a graft bearing antigen against which the antibodies are directed) results in an immediate destructive hyperacute rejection reaction involving fixation of antibody to the donor vascular endothelium, formation of platelet and fibrin plugs, and ischemic necrosis of the organ. In practice, this is avoided by performing before surgery a complement-mediated cytotoxic crossmatch with pretransplant recipient sera against T lymphocytes from the potential donor.

Histocompatibility Testing, Cross-Matching, & Blood Group Compatibility

When donor and recipient are identical twins, there is no antigenic difference, and grafts are accepted without immunosuppressive therapy, but such transplants are rare. Grafts from HLA-identical siblings give the next best results and constitute the most common privileged immunologic situation in transplantation. Nevertheless, even though there may be perfect matching for the major histocompatibility antigens in an HLA-identical sibling match, immunosuppression is required because of incompatibilities at minor histocompatibility loci. Parents, offspring, and half of siblings will share one HLA haplotype plus many minor antigens, since they have one identical chromosome.

HLA histocompatibility testing is primarily of value in searching for HLA-identical siblings; it has not proved valuable in choosing between parents, offspring, or HLA-non-identical siblings as donors—except to identify the zero-haplotype match sibling. Since cadaver organs are donated by an unrelated person, it is not surprising that many experts question the value of HLA matching for cadaver kidney transplantation. The HLA system is the most polymorphic genetic system known, and it is very unlikely that one will find perfectly matched cadaver kidney donors for prospective recipients. Nevertheless, six-antigen-match (at the A, B, and DR loci) cadaver kidneys do appear to provide better graft survival compared with lesser matched grades.

Regardless of the results of tissue typing and antigen matching, it is essential to determine whether a recipient has preformed antibodies against antigens on the tissues of a potential donor, since their presence would result in an immediate (hyperacute) rejection reaction. These antibodies can be identified by crossmatching the patient's serum against the donor's lymphocytes. Preexisting antibodies have usually developed because of prior exposure to foreign histocompatibility antigens, such as by blood transfusion, pregnancy, or previous transplantation.

Although histocompatibility and crossmatch testing are important, an absolute prerequisite before kidney transplantation is the presence of ABO blood group compatibility.

Klein J, Sato A: The HLA system. (Two parts.) N Engl J Med 2000;343:702, 782.

The Influence of Blood Transfusions on Graft Survival

A. Pretransplant Blood Transfusions

Random third-party blood transfusions given before a first cadaver kidney transplant have a beneficial effect on graft survival in patients treated with immunosuppression using azathioprine and prednisone. The improved graft survival occurs whether or not the patients form cytotoxic antibodies in response to the transfusions. The mechanism of the beneficial effect is still speculative.

Pretransplant transfusions do not benefit recipients of cadaver organs who are treated with cyclosporine preceded by antilymphocyte globulin (sequential therapy) as the primary mode of immunosuppression. A number of multicenter trials report no difference in graft survival rates among patients treated with cyclosporine who did or did not receive pretransplant transfusions, but other reports, including those from our center, showed improved graft survival rates following pretransplant transfusions when sequential therapy was not utilized.

B. Donor-Specific Blood Transfusions (DST)

Living related one-haplotype donor-recipient pairs with a high stimulating MLC have in our experience resulted in a 56% 1-year graft survival rate. In order to select MLC-incompatible related donor-recipient pairs that would experience better graft survival rates, and in an effort to alter the recipient's immune response, patients have received transplants after receiving transfusions from their prospective kidney donors (donor-specific transfusions) before transplantation. Graft survival rates for these patients were 94%, 90%, and 83% at 1, 2, and 5 years, respectively, using azathioprine immunosuppression.

The DST approach has also been applied with promising results with transplants involving poorly matched living nonrelated donors.

Graft enhancement with DST appears to be maximized with an immunosuppressive regimen that allows lower doses of both cyclosporine and prednisone than in non-DST-treated patients. Graft survival in a series of more than 50 patients at this center is essentially 100% at 2 years.

Thus, it appears that MLC-incompatible living related donors—and perhaps living nonrelated donors as well—can now be selected with prospects of excellent graft survival. The posttransplant course of most recipients who receive donor-specific transfusions has been similar to that of two-haplotype matched transplants, and consequently they have required less aggressive corticosteroid therapy. Avoidance of potentially unsuccessful living related transplants is very important. For the potential kidney donor, the process of blood donation has been harmless compared with the risk of donating a kidney that would probably be rejected.

The Influence of Presensitization on Cadaver Graft Survival Rate

The effect of previous blood transfusions and other methods of recipient sensitization on cadaver renal allograft survival has been controversial. Patients with end-stage renal failure often require transfusions and as a result develop antibodies. The more antibodies that form,

the more likely is it that a donor kidney will be incompatible on crossmatch. In our series, graft survival rate seems to be the same as in a nonimmunized recipient as long as extended testing of all reactive sera is carried out. The favorable graft survival rate of the hyperimmunized group is consistent with the theory that if potential recipients have been permitted to form cytotoxic antibodies to histocompatibility antigens, then crossmatch tests will select only those kidneys with antigens to which recipients respond less readily.

The obvious disadvantage of presensitization is that it is more difficult to find a compatible cadaver donor, and the period of waiting for a transplant is therefore prolonged. In general, the duration of the waiting period correlates directly with the level of antibodies. High levels of antibodies do not negate the possibility of a transplant, and in fact a number of successful transplants have been reported in patients with antibody levels as high as 100%.

Immunosuppressive Drug Therapy

The best current immunosuppressive protocol appears to be sequential (quadruple) therapy. This entails initial use of prednisone, azathioprine, and antilymphocyte (or antithymoblast) globulin. The latter drug is used only for induction until approximately 7 days post operation, with introduction of cyclosporine at 5 days post operation (2 days of overlap). If renal function is not good at 5 days (serum creatinine 2.5 mg/dL), cyclosporine introduction and the 2-day overlap of these two medications is delayed. Subsequent tapering of prednisone and cyclosporine dosage levels is then achieved with time. Rejection episodes are initially treated with increased steroid dosages or, in the absence of an immediate response, with monoclonal or polyclonal antibodies as later described.

The primary drugs used for immunosuppression today are azathioprine, corticosteroids (prednisone), cyclosporine, and antilymphocyte or antithymocyte globulins. As a working hypothesis, it is assumed that the closer the histocompatibility match, the less immunosuppression by drugs will be required to achieve graft acceptance. Use of immunosuppressive agents even in lower doses imposes an increased risk of death and complications due to viral, fungal, and bacterial infections.

A. Azathioprine

Azathioprine is one of the mercaptopurine class of drugs and inhibits nucleic acid synthesis. Patients are maintained indefinitely on daily doses of 1 mg/kg or less, with the dosage adjusted in accordance with the white cell count. The drug may cause depression of the bone marrow elements (leukocytes and platelets) and may cause jaundice. In the face of untoward effects or in the presence of infections, the drug is temporarily discontinued or reduced. Azathioprine is never given in increased doses during an acute rejection episode, and the dosage may have to be reduced during rejection when renal function is poor.

B. CORTICOSTEROIDS (PREDNISONE)

Prednisone, which is used in almost all transplant recipients, is usually given in association with azathioprine and cyclosporine. The dosage must be regulated carefully so as to prevent complications such as infection, the development of cushingoid features, hypertension, increased bruisability, and acne. At our center, the initial maintenance prednisone dosage is 0.5 mg/kg/d. This dosage is then further decreased in the outpatient clinic until maintenance levels of about 10 mg/d for adults are reached. In recent years, most transplant centers have used corticosteroids less aggressively than before; this has resulted in fewer problems with infection and in improved patient survival rates.

The exact site of action of corticosteroids on the immune response is not known, but it is believed that they inhibit the inflammatory aspect of rejection.

High daily doses of prednisone in children inhibit growth. This may be circumvented by alternate-day treatment, administering the drug once in the morning every other day. This dosage regimen is usually started after the initial 6-month period of daily corticosteroid administration, before which time there is the greatest risk of graft loss secondary to rejection. The exact dosage has not been precisely defined, but an initial 2 mg/kg in children on alternate days has permitted growth.

Therapy for a rejection episode may consist of increasing the prednisone dosage to 2–3 mg/kg and then tapering the dosage to a maintenance level—or of intravenous administration of larger doses of corticosteroids for a brief period, followed by tapering of dosages to maintenance levels. In general, immunosuppressive therapy should not be increased after the second rejection episode, nor should it be increased after the first rejection episode if renal function does not return to normal or near normal.

C. CYCLOSPORINE

Cyclosporine is a cyclic undecapeptide isolated from a fungus. It is a potent immunosuppressant and the first compound identified that can inhibit immunocompetent lymphocytes specifically and reversibly. Cyclosporine was first of a new generation of important immunosuppressants. Its primary mechanism of action appears to be inhibition of the production and release of interleukin-2 by T helper cells. In addition, it also interferes with the release of interleukin-1 by macrophages as well as with proliferation of B lymphocytes.

Blood levels must be carefully monitored because the drug is nephrotoxic and hepatotoxic and may also increase the incidence of neoplasms, particularly lymphomas.

The graft survival rate at 1 year for recipients of cadaver kidney transplants treated with cyclosporine is greater than 80%—better than the 55–60% rates with conventional immunosuppression (without cyclosporine). Cyclosporine has a major role in kidney transplantation involving related individuals. One-year graft survival rates of more than 90% have been reported for recipients of one-haplotype-matched related transplants in which recipients were treated with cyclosporine and did not receive donor-specific transfusions. The combination of DST with sequential quadruple therapy appears to allow the use of lower cyclosporine and prednisone dosages.

D. ANTITHYMOBLAST OR ANTILYMPHOCYTE GLOBULIN (ALG) AND ANTITHYMOCYTE GLOBULIN (ATG)

Antilymphoblast globulin and antithymocyte globulin are important adjunctive immunosuppressants. They are particularly effective in induction of immunosuppressive therapy and in the treatment of corticosteroid-resistant rejection. Both ALG and ATG can be made by immunizing horses, rabbits, or sheep, but the main source at present is horses. Lymphocytes from human peripheral blood, spleen, lymph nodes, or thymus serve as the immunogen. In the Minnesota antilymphoblast preparation, a human T cell lymphoblastoid cell line is used. After immunization, the serum is recovered and the active globulin fraction is isolated. Some workers have used cultured lymphoblasts for immunization. The IgG fraction is purified and then given intramuscularly or intravenously.

E. MONOCLONAL ANTIBODY THERAPY

The focus of antirejection therapy has been to develop more specific therapy to control the rejection process. An example of such an agent is the monoclonal antibody OKT3 (muromonab-CD3), which is secreted by a hybridoma produced by the technique developed by Kohler and Milstein. This agent may have some advantages over ALG or ATG preparations in management of rejection in that it specifically blocks T cell generation and function. Because it is a monoclonal antibody and reacts with a defined antigen, it can be consistently produced with a defined activity and without unwanted reactivities. Muromonab-CD3 efficacy may be greatest in the treatment of steroid-resistant rejection, where excellent results have been obtained and where further high-dose steroids are obviated.

Carpenter CB: Immunosuppression in organ transplantation. N Engl J Med 1990;322:1224.

Mourad G et al: Induction versus noninduction in renal transplant recipients with tacrolimus-based immunosuppression. Transplantation 2001;72:1050.

Sarwal M et al: Promising early outcomes with a novel, complete steroid avoidance immunosuppression protocol in pediatric renal transplantation. Transplantation 2001;72:13.

SOURCES OF DONOR KIDNEYS

The three sources of kidneys for renal transplantation are living related donors, cadaver donors, and living nonrelated donors. Of all the patients who are acceptable candidates for transplantation, only about 30% have a willing and medically suitable living related donor. The donor must be ABO-compatible with the recipient. Living donors should be in good health both physically and psychologically. Above all, the living donor should be a volunteer and must clearly understand the nature of the procedure so that informed consent to the operation can be given. Donors must be of legal age.

Living Donors

Over the last decade, more than 10,000 people have donated kidneys for transplantation. In young donors, the remaining kidney hypertrophies and in a few months provides 75–80% of the original renal function. Follow-up studies on donors show that they have good renal function and suffer no ill effects from the procedure, either physically or psychologically. Women with one kidney do not have an increased incidence of urinary infections during pregnancy. Some transplant surgeons have advocated removal of the right kidney in women of childbearing age because of the increased chance of the gravid uterus partially obstructing the right ureter during pregnancy.

The main risk to a donor is the anesthesia and the operation itself. The death rate is estimated to be 0.1%—about the same risk as in driving 8–10 thousand miles a year in an automobile.

The most common complication following nephrectomy—except for minor atelectasis—is wound infection, which occurs in less than 1% of cases and is usually superficial.

After the donor has been judged to be a true volunteer and the risks and complications have been explained, special studies are undertaken in the hospital. A detailed history is taken, and a physical examination is performed. The routine workup includes chest x-ray, electrocardiography, urinalysis, complete blood count, fasting blood glucose, serum bilirubin, creatinine clearance, and blood urea nitrogen. If these are normal, an excretory urogram is performed; if that is normal, a renal arteriogram is performed. Kidneys with multiple renal arteries may be transplanted, but care must be

taken in the anastomosis of small accessory vessels. When there are multiple renal veins, the smaller veins may be ligated since there is free communication of the veins within the kidney. If the arteriogram is normal, the patient is an acceptable donor.

Cadaver Donors

Since only 30% of recipients have a suitable living donor, the only way to provide transplantation to most patients is to use cadaver kidneys, which are in short supply, or kidneys from living nonrelated donors. It is essential to the success of the procedure that the transplanted organ be of good quality. This means that the organ must be removed before or immediately after cardiac arrest. Brain death must be established in cadaver donors before organs can be removed. Most states have legislation to the effect that a patient can be declared dead if irreversible cessation of brain function has occurred. The kidneys may be removed for transplantation up to 1 hour after cardiac arrest provided intra-aortic flush with iced solution is used for in situ cooling of the kidneys. It is also important that the donor have relatively normal renal function at the time of death. Phenoxybenzamine or another vasodilator drug is often given to prevent renal vasospasm during the agonal phase.

There are two techniques for short-term preservation of kidneys: simple hypothermia and continuous pulsatile perfusion. With simple hypothermia, the organs are flushed with an appropriate solution, the most common at present being University of Wisconsin (UW) solution and Collins' solution. These solutions contain appropriate amounts of osmotically active but nonpermeable solutes such as glucose, mannitol, or sucrose, and their main beneficial effect is to prevent cellular swelling during hypothermic storage. Kidneys can be successfully preserved by cold storage alone, especially if warm ischemia was minimal during organ removal. However, after 30 hours, there appears to be a progressively increasing incidence of acute tubular necrosis—over 80% in organs preserved for 48 hours. The technique of simple hypothermia is the method of choice for small transplant units that perform fewer than 25 transplants per year.

With continuous hypothermic pulsatile perfusion preservation, kidneys can be stored for up to 3 days—and perhaps longer—with a low incidence of acute tubular necrosis. This method of preservation eases the logistical problems involved in transplantation since patients awaiting kidneys often live a long distance from the transplant center. Another advantage of pulsatile perfusion is that the sudden influx of a large number of cadaver organs can be easily managed.

Patients who are hyperimmunized with high levels of antibodies have a better chance of extended crossmatch testing with perfusion preservation and therefore better graft survival. In addition, the presence of a low ATN rate with perfusion preservation allows maximum efficacy of cyclosporine with little risk of nephrotoxicity or permanent nonfunction of cadaver kidneys.

Enough kidneys and other organs for transplantation will not be available until there is greater public acceptance and support for organ donation. Many United States citizens now carry Uniform Donor Cards that comply with the Uniform Anatomical Gift Act, which has been adopted by all 50 states. In addition in many states, persons may record the desire to donate an organ when they renew their driver's license; this is considered a legal document. The generally accepted age range for cadaver donors is 1-55 years, though donors up to age 70 years have been accepted after close scrutiny of the donor's general medical status. The cadaver donor must have evidence of good kidney function and must be free of systemic infection, cancer (except for primary brain tumors), and other diseases that could be transferred from the donor to the recipient by the transplant. HIV and hepatitis screening are mandatory.

SELECTION OF RECIPIENTS

During the early years of renal transplantation, most of the patients accepted for transplantation were in the age group from 15 to 45 years. In recent years, the age range has been extended in both directions–children below age 1 and adults up to age 70. Children between ages 5 and 15 do as well as adults below age 50. Children below age 5—and especially below age 1—seem to have a higher death rate but do well in centers specializing in infant transplantation. Infants and small children do poorly on dialysis. Although transplantation is not contraindicated in the elderly, the success rate is lower in these patients because associated diseases are more common, resistance to infection is less, and the surgical risks are greater. It appears that success rates for older patients may be improved by the use of sequential immunosuppression, so the number of older patients currently being accepted for transplantation is increasing.

The ideal recipient is one who has no serious infections or lower urinary tract disease, with minimal and reversible systemic disease secondary to renal failure. Recipients with the following primary renal diseases have been successfully transplanted: glomerulonephritis, pyelonephritis, polycystic kidney disease, malignant hypertension, reflux pyelonephritis, Goodpasture's syndrome, congenital renal hypoplasia, renal cortical necrosis, Fabry's syndrome, and Alport's syndrome. Successful transplants have been achieved in patients with certain systemic diseases in which the kidney is one of the end organs (cystinosis, systemic lupus erythematosus, and type 1 diabetes). Renal transplantation is generally contraindicated in oxalosis because the disease recurs in the transplant quickly.

When the bladder is found to be unsuitable for ureteral implantation, a Bricker conduit has been used to obtain satisfactory urinary drainage. However, most long-term defunctionalized bladders can still be utilized for ureteral reimplantation. Patients with a history of peptic ulcer disease may be accepted for transplantation, but those with active or recurring ulcers refractory to medical therapy should first be treated surgically for this problem.

Emotional instability or psychosis has been thought to be a contraindication to transplantation, but successful transplantation may cure these patients if their emotional difficulties were due to uremia or poor response to dialysis. Unfortunately, there is no way to tell if the psychiatric symptoms are a manifestation of the renal disease.

Advanced retinopathy due to uncontrolled hypertension and peripheral neuropathy secondary to uremia often improve after transplantation. Diabetic retinopathy often stabilizes or improves after transplantation, so transplantation is frequently recommended for diabetics with renal disease before they reach end-stage disease.

The decision to accept patients in the poorer risk groups is usually based on the available dialysis facilities and the number of cadaver kidneys offered for transplantation.

Once a patient has been selected as a transplant candidate, either hemodialysis or chronic ambulatory peritoneal dialysis is usually started. If the patient is to receive a transplant from a living related donor, dialysis may not be necessary before the transplant is performed. Recipients awaiting a cadaver kidney will usually require dialysis.

Bilateral nephrectomy prior to transplantation was common in the 1960s but has been performed less frequently in recent years. The indications for preliminary nephrectomy are (1) severe hypertension uncontrolled by dialysis or medication, (2) anatomic abnormalities of the urinary tract with or without infection (eg, hydronephrosis, ureteral reflux), and (3) polycystic kidney disease with documented recurring infections or recurring episodes of gross hematuria requiring transfusions. Only 6% of recipients require preliminary bilateral nephrectomy.

There is no good evidence that splenectomy is of value before transplantation with current immunosuppressive protocols.

OPERATIVE TECHNIQUES

Great care should be taken in removal of the living donor kidney. The major difference between nephrectomy for transplantation and nephrectomy for disease is that the quality of the donor kidney must be preserved. This means that every attempt should be made to minimize renal ischemia and damage to the ureter. Renal ischemia may be minimized by hydrating the donor and administering an osmotic diuretic to promote a urine flow rate of 3–4 mL/min at the time of nephrectomy. Since the blood supply for the ureter arises from the renal artery, the ureter should not be skeletonized and dissected high in the renal pedicle.

Recipient Operation

The surgical technique of renal transplantation involves anastomoses of the renal artery and vein and ureter (Figure 48–1). In adults, the transplant kidney is placed in the iliac fossa through an oblique lower abdominal incision. The iliac and hypogastric arteries and the iliac vein are mobilized as indicated for the proposed specific anastomoses. An end-to-side anastomosis is performed between renal vein and iliac vein; an end-to-end anastomosis can be performed between the renal artery and the hypogastric artery unless the latter is too arteriosclerotic. In that case, the renal artery is anastomosed end-to-side to the common (or external) iliac artery. When multiple arteries are present in cadaver donors, the kidneys are transplanted with anastomoses of a Carrell patch of donor aorta containing the multiple renal arteries to the common (or external) iliac artery.

In small children and infants, a midline abdominal incision is used and the cecum and ascending colon are

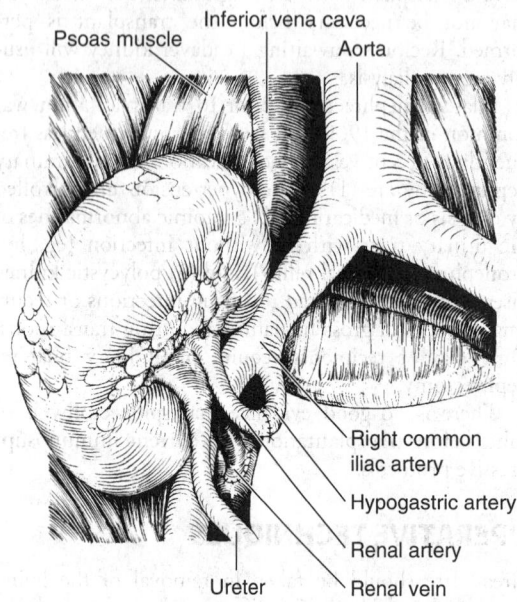

Psoas muscle
Inferior vena cava
Aorta

Right common iliac artery

Hypogastric artery

Renal artery

Ureter
Renal vein

Figure 48–1. Technique of renal transplantation.

mobilized medially, exposing the aorta and vena cava. End-to-side anastomoses of the renal vessels to the vena cava and aorta are then accomplished, and the kidney is secured in its retroperitoneal location by approximating the previously divided posterior parietal peritoneum over the transplanted kidney.

Many centers have been reluctant to use small pediatric cadaver kidneys, and, when used, pediatric kidneys have often been transplanted en bloc with the donor aorta and vena cava anastomosed to the recipient's iliac vessels along with double ureteral anastomoses. We prefer to transplant pediatric cadaver kidneys as single units with the arterial anastomosis consisting of a Carrell patch of donor aorta and a Carrell patch of the vena cava for the venous anastomoses. Direct anastomoses of the small renal vessels to the larger recipient vessels too often result in thromboses. The en bloc transplantation of both kidneys into one recipient provides a larger functioning renal mass that more closely approximates the immediate needs of the recipient, but a single small kidney hypertrophies so fast that its function soon matches the recipient's needs.

Urinary tract continuity can be established by pyeloureterostomy, ureteroureterostomy, or ureteroneocystostomy. We have used ureteroneocystostomy by a modified Politano-Leadbetter submucosal tunnel technique in over 3500 renal transplants with very few complications.

POSTOPERATIVE MANAGEMENT & COMPLICATIONS

Recipients who have received transplants from living donors usually undergo immediate diuresis and natriuresis. The magnitude is related to how hydrated the patient was before transplantation. The diuresis and natriuresis occur because the transplanted kidney is vasodilated, but the glomerular filtration rate as measured by inulin clearance is rarely above that expected for a single kidney. The kidney has been found to have a low PAH (para-aminohippurate) extraction ratio and a low filtration fraction but a normal maximum tubular excretion of PAH. How long vasodilatation persists after transplantation is not known.

Once this phase has passed, the patient maintains a relatively stable weight, though the weight may increase because of increased appetite and food intake. At our center, the urethral catheter is usually left in place from 5 to 7 days to ensure healing of the bladder incision. Most recipients may be started on a solid food diet with no added salt on the first to third postoperative days.

Kidney transplantation can be followed by a variety of postoperative complications that must be recognized and treated early for optimal results. A number of these problems are unique to the operation or to transplantation in general. In 3500 consecutive transplants performed at our center, the incidence of vascular complications was less than 1%. The most common vascular complication is renal artery stenosis, which is usually associated with rejection involving the renal artery. This may result in severe hypertension. It may be treated surgically or in some cases by percutaneous transluminal balloon angioplasty. Urologic complications occur in fewer than 2% of patients, most often urinary extravasation from the cystotomy closure, ureteral necrosis, or ureteral obstruction. These complications can be kept to a minimum by attention to technical details during donor nephrectomy and graft implantation. Early surgical treatment is necessary to avoid infection and loss of the graft. Lymphocele of the transplant bed, formerly a common problem, has now become rare with careful ligation of the adjacent lymphatics during preparation of the recipient blood vessels. Large lymphoceles may obstruct the ureter or the vasculature of the transplanted kidney, and they occasionally become infected. Sterile lymphoceles may be drained into the peritoneal cavity, while infected lymphoceles should be drained externally.

Many complications of transplantation are consequences of immunosuppressive therapy, and they have become less frequent now that immunosuppression is less aggressive. Pulmonary and gastrointestinal complications are most common. Others include cushingoid changes, cataracts, aseptic necrosis of bone, steroid diabetes, and increased frequency of tumors (mainly malignant lymphomas). Pyelonephritis may affect either the transplant or the native kidneys. Preliminary nephrectomy is indicated in patients with an increased risk of pyelonephritis, such as those with vesicoureteral reflux or a history of recurrent infections or calculi.

Cyclosporine may produce nephrotoxicity, hypertension, and hepatotoxicity and, less commonly, hirsutism, tremor, gastrointestinal symptoms, gingival hyperplasia, and neoplasia. Acute nephrotoxicity and hypertension can be obviated by careful monitoring of cyclosporine blood levels, but the long-term effects of cyclosporine therapy are not yet known.

Bacterial pneumonia is now the most common pulmonary complication. Infections with viruses, *Pneumocystis carinii*, and aspergillus are seen much less often than previously. Bacterial pneumonia can usually be treated effectively with antibiotics selected on the basis of drug sensitivity studies.

Gastrointestinal complications may affect all levels of the intestine, and the diagnosis is often difficult because of the masking effect of immunosuppressive drugs. Candidal esophagitis occurs with a higher frequency in diabetic patients and usually responds to oral nystatin.

Peptic ulcer may develop after transplantation despite vigorous prophylactic use of antacids and drugs such as cimetidine or ranitidine. The problem is greatest in the early months following transplantation. Three out of four patients with peptic ulcer disease present with gastrointestinal hemorrhage. Factors related to the occurrence of peptic ulcer are treatment of an acute rejection episode (ie, when corticosteroid dosage is increased) and the presence of sepsis or hepatitis. The incidence of peptic ulcer has decreased dramatically (from 11% to 6%) as the intensity of corticosteroid therapy has been decreased and the use of H_2 blocking agents has been liberalized. Further reductions in corticosteroid dosages are now possible as nonulcerogenic drugs such as cyclosporine have become a mainstay of current immunosuppressive protocols with a marked reduction in the incidence of peptic ulcer disease. The mortality rate of peptic ulcer was once very high (about 50%), whether patients were treated surgically or medically. However, the patients who died often had multisystem disease, with sepsis being the primary cause of death. Medical therapy to prevent peptic ulcers in transplant recipients must therefore be aggressive, and surgical therapy should be performed promptly if medical therapy fails. Prophylactic ulcer operations should be limited to patients with an antecedent history of peptic ulcer refractory to medical therapy.

Hepatitis and **pancreatitis** are other gastrointestinal complications that may occur in transplant patients. Hepatitis may be caused by viral infections (hepatitis B virus, cytomegalovirus) or may be a complication of immunosuppressive drugs (eg, azathioprine). Pancreatitis can also be a direct complication of immunosuppressive drugs (eg, prednisone, azathioprine), but some cases result from gallstone disease. The current incidence of posttransplant pancreatitis is about 1%. The incidence of pancreatitis is no greater in the early months following transplantation than later. More than half of cases of pancreatitis occur in patients with a normally functioning transplant, and only one-fourth occur in association with treatment for rejection. In general, patients with pancreatitis have higher serum cholesterol and triglyceride levels and a higher incidence of nephrosclerosis as the cause of renal disease. Patients with posttransplant pancreatitis have survival rates of 74% and 50% at 1 and 5 years, respectively, compared with 96% and 87% for patients who did not have pancreatitis.

GRAFT REJECTION

The major hazard for the postoperative allograft recipient is rejection. Most rejections occur within the first 3 months. There are four kinds of rejection:

(1) Hyperacute rejection is due to preformed cytotoxic antibodies against donor lymphocytes or renal cells. This reaction begins soon after completion of the anastomosis, and complete graft destruction occurs in 24–48 hours. Initially, the graft is pink and firm, but it then becomes blue and soft, with evidence of diminished blood flow. There is no effective method of treating this reaction, and patients who have preformed antibodies against donor cells should not be transplanted with a kidney from that donor. Pretransplant crossmatch testing can eliminate this type of rejection.

(2) Accelerated rejection usually appears within 5 days after a period of good function. It is believed to be related to subliminal preformed cytotoxic antibodies against donor cells not detected by the usual cytotoxicity techniques. It has also been suggested that sensitized cells could bring about this reaction.

(3) Acute rejection is the most common type of rejection episode during the first 3 months after transplantation. It is primarily an immune cellular reaction against foreign antigens and is characterized by oliguria, weight gain, hypertension, and blood chemical evidence of impaired renal function. Fever and tenderness and enlargement of the graft are less common with cyclosporine immunosuppressive protocols than was the case with prednisone and azathioprine therapy. This type of rejection process may be reversed by increasing the dosage of corticosteroids. If this is unsuccessful, an ALG or ATG preparation or muromonab-CD3 can be used.

(4) Chronic rejection is a late cause of renal deterioration mediated by humoral factors. It is most often diagnosed on the basis of slowly decreasing renal function in association with proteinuria and hypertension. Chronic rejection is resistant to corticosteroid therapy and graft loss will eventually occur, though perhaps not for several years after renal function begins to deteriorate.

Diagnosis

There is no single study that will pinpoint a rejection crisis. However, an elevation of blood urea nitrogen and serum creatinine appears to be the most consistent and reliable means of detecting renal deterioration secondary to rejection. The glomerular filtration rate as measured by creatinine clearance also declines. The urine shows an increase in protein and lymphocytes, and urinary sodium is low. Renal blood flow studies with pertechnetate Tc 99m may be used to confirm rejection and exclude urologic causes of renal function impairment.

Renal ultrasonography is often the first test to help diagnose rejection and to exclude ureteral obstruction as a cause of deterioration of renal function. Prominence of renal pyramids and loss of renal sinus fat are findings consistent with rejection.

Magnetic resonance imaging (MRI) may also be helpful in diagnosing rejection and in distinguishing between rejection and cyclosporine nephrotoxicity. MRI reveals changes in tissue water content and blood flow, variables affected by rejection and cyclosporine nephrotoxicity. With rejection, corticomedullary differentiation is lost, while it is preserved with cyclosporine nephrotoxicity.

The diagnosis is made by analysis of the total clinical and laboratory findings. Although a rejection crisis will be experienced by most patients (HLA-identical siblings tend to have very few), they can usually be successfully treated so the patient will survive with normal renal function. After the first rejection episode, others are less frequent. There is evidence that a blocking antibody is formed which prevents host cells from attacking the graft's vascular endothelium. Whatever the mechanism, most grafts that are lost are rejected within the first 3 months; very few grafts are lost after 2 years.

Since most rejection reactions occur within the first 3 months, the death rate from immunosuppressive drugs is highest during this period.

Differential Diagnosis

There are a number of considerations in the differential diagnosis of rejection, including ureteral obstruction. With the current use of cyclosporine as a major component of immunosuppressive therapy, cyclosporine nephrotoxicity must be excluded as a cause of renal dysfunction. If a high cyclosporine blood level is present, cyclosporine nephrotoxicity is the most likely explanation; this can be confirmed if serum creatinine levels decrease after reducing the cyclosporine dosage. If the diagnosis remains unclear, a renal biopsy is helpful in confirming the presence of rejection.

■ HEART TRANSPLANTATION

The first successful human heart allograft was performed in 1967. At that time, however, immunosuppression with azathioprine and steroids was inadequate to prevent significant numbers of deaths and morbidity from rejection and infection, and the procedure remained confined to an experimental state in selected institutions worldwide. The advent of cyclosporine in 1981 resulted in improved survival, and in 1985 heart transplantation was federally designated as no longer experimental. In 1988, there were 2500 heart transplants performed worldwide—1600 of them in 118 centers in the United States. The 1-year survival rate is 80% and the 5-year survival rate is 74%.

SELECTION OF DONORS

Cardiac donors should be men aged 40 or below or women 45 or below with established brain death. They should be ABO-compatible with the recipient and within 20% of the recipient's body weight. There should be no history of preexistent or intercurrent cardiac disease, which can most often be ruled out by echocardiography. Preferably, there should be no history of cardiac arrest, and the donor should be receiving less than 10 μg/kg/min of dopamine. There should be no evidence of transmissible disease, and donors must have no evidence of bacterial infection and be hepatitis antigen-negative and HIV-negative. Donors should be free of a history of cancer except for primary brain tumor.

At donor cardiectomy, which is performed in conjunction with the harvesting of kidney and usually liver or pancreas, the heart is arrested with cold potassium cardioplegia and stored in a balanced electrolyte solution at 4 °C. Optimal function is obtained when the heart is implanted within less than 4 hours of ischemia. Because of the shortage of donor organs, donor age has been raised and ischemic time extended in some institutions.

SELECTION OF RECIPIENTS

Patients for cardiac transplantation should have end-stage cardiac disease for which there is no other surgical option; should have received maximal medical treatment; and should have a life expectancy of less than 1 year. Most heart transplant candidates have idiopathic dilated cardiomyopathy or ischemic cardiomyopathy. Patients should be less than 55 years of age, have a short duration of illness, have no systemic disease that will be worsened by the immunosuppressive regimen (infection, type 1 diabetes, severe peripheral vascular disease, poorly controlled hypertension), as well as no underlying renal insufficiency that cannot be attributed to low cardiac output. Patients should have pulmonary vascular resistance of less than 5 Wood units, since levels above this or a pulmonary artery systolic pressure of greater than 50 mm Hg or a transpulmonary gradient (mean pulmonary artery pressure – pulmonary capillary wedge pressure) of greater than 15 mm Hg are associated with inadequate donor heart function. A history of compliance with a complex medical regimen and a strong social support system are necessary for long-term success.

The recipient's serum is crossmatched against a random panel of lymphocytes from a number of donors. If the percentage of reactive antibodies is greater than 15%, then a prospective crossmatch between the donor

and the potential recipient is necessary. Although human leukocyte antigen (HLA) typing is performed, there is only time for a retrospective crossmatch. A higher survival rate is reported with one or no HLA-DR antigen mismatches compared with two DR antigen mismatches.

OPERATIVE TECHNIQUE

The operative technique originally developed by Lower and Shumway continues to be used and is shown in Figure 48–2. The recipient heart is removed, and the dilated right and left atria are trimmed. The left atrial anastomosis is performed first and then the right, each with one continuous suture. The aortic and then pulmonary artery anastomoses are then performed. Topical cooling is continued, and the addition of blood cardioplegia after the atrial anastomoses may improve graft function. The implant time is generally 45–60 minutes, and "payback" time of support on total cardiopulmonary bypass after cross-clamp removal is determined by the total ischemic time and visual assessment of cardiac function. The heart rate is supported by atrial pacing or isoproterenol.

IMMUNOSUPPRESSION

Triple immunosuppression with corticosteroids, azathioprine, and cyclosporine is the cornerstone of most immunosuppressive protocols and has allowed lower doses of each drug with fewer drug-related complications. Perioperative induction immunosuppressive therapy may include the three drugs mentioned or may employ T lymphocyte cytolytic therapy with antithymocyte globulin (ATG), antilymphoblast globulin (ALG), or murine antihuman lymphocyte monoclonal antibody (muromonab-CD3; OKT3) in order to avoid the renal toxicity sometimes associated with early high-dose cyclosporine. Rejection is diagnosed on endomyocardial biopsy, which is performed regularly, since rejection may occur in the absence of clinical symptoms. Rejection is treated with pulsed steroids (1 g of methylprednisolone daily for 3 days) and resistant rejection with ATG, ALG, or muromonab-CD3.

FOLLOW-UP CARE

Transplant recipients must be carefully monitored for infection and rejection. Endomyocardial biopsies are performed every other month for the first year, then every 3 months. The incidence of rejection episodes is 0.5–1.5 per patient for the first year. The major infection rate is 1.5 episodes per patient for the first year and then declines. Accelerated coronary atherosclerosis oc-

Levels of transection of
recipient aorta and
pulmonary artery

Posterior view of donor heart
showing incisions connecting
pulmonary vein orifices and
opening of right atrium

Recipient
heart
remnant

Right atrium

Left atrium

L. V. Schaubert

Flaps opened in donor heart

Figure 48–2. ***Top left:*** Recipient heart showing levels of transection across aorta and pulmonary artery. *Lower left:* Implantation site with recipient heart removed. *Top right:* Posterior view of donor heart showing lines of incision connecting pulmonary vein orifices and opening the right atrium in preparation for implantation. *Lower right:* Flaps opened in donor heart in preparation for implantation curs in 30–40% of patients within 5 years after transplantation. The only treatment of severe accelerated coronary atherosclerosis is retransplantation. Progressive renal dysfunction may occur over time and is probably related to the total cyclosporine dose. Patients with decreasing creatinine clearance can be converted to azathioprine and steroids alone with stabilization of renal function but with a higher incidence of rejection.

Goldstein DJ, Oz MC, Rose EA: Implantable left ventricular assist devices. N Engl J Med 1998;339:1522.

Morrow WR: Cardiomyopathy and heart transplantation in children. Curr Opin Cardiol 2000;15:216.

Taylor DO: Immunosuppression therapies after heart transplantation: best, better and beyond. Curr Opin Cardiol 2000; 15:108.

COMBINED HEART-LUNG TRANSPLANTATION

Combined heart-lung transplantation was first performed in 1981. Initially it was felt that rejection of both organs would be evident in the myocardial biopsy. However experience has shown that rejection is dissimilar in the two organs, with heart rejection occurring infrequently and lung rejection, evidenced by obliterative bronchiolitis and arteritis, being a more severe problem. The current indication for heart-lung transplantation is end-stage disease in both organs or end-stage disease in one with poor function in the other prohibiting single organ transplantation. Examples are primary pulmonary hypertension, congenital heart disease with Eisenmenger's physiology, fibrotic lung disease and cor pulmonale, and cystic fibrosis.

The operation consists of en bloc heart-lung transplantation with anastomosis of the trachea, right atrium, and aorta of the donor. Lung perfusion or total body perfusion has allowed long distance procurement, making heart-lung transplantation more practical.

Immunosuppression consists of cyclosporine and azathioprine with no steroids initially in order to promote tracheal wound healing. Heart-lung transplantation currently results in a 70% 1-year survival rate.

LUNG TRANSPLANTATION

Single lung transplantation became clinically successful through a systematic approach by the Toronto Lung Transplant Group to the problem of bronchial disruption, which had made previous attempts unsuccessful.

The addition of an omental wrap to the bronchial anastomosis and the avoidance of steroids during the first 3 weeks allowed bronchial healing and clinical success. Candidates for lung transplantation have end-stage fibrotic lung disease, are oxygendependent, and are likely to die of their disease within 12–18 months. Lung donors are scarce, but the use of one lung for transplantation does not preclude using the heart for another recipient. Long-distance procurement of lungs has been possible since institution of a regimen consisting of pulmonary artery flush with cold Euro-Collins solution following alprostadil (PGE$_1$) via the central venous line to promote pulmonary vasodilatation.

For patients with bilateral pulmonary sepsis, such as cystic fibrosis or bronchiectasis, or patients with emphysema and normal heart function, double lung transplantation has been carried out in a few patients. The advantage is that the patient does not have the potential complications of heart transplant and rejection. Another innovative approach to the lung transplant patient with a normal heart is the operation where a heart-lung block is placed in a patient with end-stage lung disease and a normal heart, and the recipient's heart is extracted and donated to a patient in need of an isolated heart transplantation.

Tralock EP: Lung transplantation for COPD. Chest 1998; 113:269S.

Yankaskas JR, Mallory GB: Lung transplantation and cystic fibrosis: consensus conference statement. Chest 1998;113:217.

LIVER TRANSPLANTATION

After many years of experimental effort, Dr Thomas Starzl performed the first human liver transplantation in 1963. Since then, we have seen markedly improved results (70–90% 1-year patient survival) and markedly increased activity in the field.

Indications

Since the introduction of clinical liver transplantation, the list of indications has rapidly expanded and the list of contraindications has diminished. The diseases for which liver transplant is most often indicated in adults include chronic active hepatitis, primary biliary cirrhosis, sclerosing cholangitis, autoimmune hepatitis, and alcoholic liver disease. Less common indications are Wilson's disease, α_1-antitrypsin deficiency, Budd-Chiari syndrome, and hemochromatosis. Alcoholic cirrhosis, a subject of considerable controversy, is now recognized as an accepted indication for liver transplant if the patient has demonstrated the ability to abstain from alcohol and is clearly committed to continued abstinence. Early reports indicating poor results in alcoholic recipients have been challenged recently by data indicating no difference in their outcomes.

Although chronic active hepatitis B is a frequent indication for liver transplantation (particularly in Europe), there are conflicting reports about the rate and severity of recurrent disease. It appears that nearly every patient with chronic hepatitis B infection and up to 20% of patients with acute hepatitis B infection become reinfected with hepatitis B after transplantation. The severity of the recurrent disease ranges from a new chronic carrier state to fulminant liver failure. A number of approaches have been tried in an attempt to decrease the rate of recurrent hepatitis, including the use of alpha interferon, hyperimmune globulin, and modification of immunosuppression, but none have been successful.

There is controversy also concerning the role of liver transplantation in the treatment of cancer in adults. In primary hepatocellular carcinoma or cholangiocarcinoma confined to the liver and biliary tree without nodal involvement, 5-year survival rates of 30–40% have been achieved; with nodal involvement, the results are poorer. An exception to these relatively poor results is seen with liver transplantation for fibrolamellar carcinoma, where survival exceeds 50%. The high rate of recurrence in cholangiocarcinoma has led the Pittsburgh group to perform cluster transplants in which the liver, pancreas, duodenum, and distal stomach are resected with transplantation of liver, pancreas, and small bowel as one unit. Follow-up of these patients has been short, but the results are promising. The rationale for cluster transplantation is to resect the nodal drainage shared by these organs.

The most common indication for transplantation in children is extrahepatic biliary atresia. Other common diagnoses are chronic active hepatitis, α_1-antitrypsin deficiency, tyrosinemia, and other inborn errors of metabolism.

Portal vein thrombosis, which at one time was a contraindication to transplant, is now managed by using vein grafts to bypass thrombosed vessels. Most transplant surgeons will perform liver transplantation if either the superior mesenteric vein, the portal vein, or the splenic vein is patent. Current absolute contraindications to transplantation are active substance abuse, positive HIV status in the recipient, and evidence of severe irreversible central nervous system disease.

Donor Selection

The donors for liver transplantation are usually young trauma victims who have sustained an irreversible brain injury and have an intact circulation but are being kept alive on a respirator. Contraindications to donation are (1) HIV-positive status, (2) evidence of systemic infection or malignancy, and (3) massive and irreversible hepatic injury. It is not required that the liver size and blood type of the donor and recipient match; blood group incompatibility does not contraindicate donation, and livers can be pared down to accommodate a smaller recipient. Restrictions on donor age have been relaxed because the function of transplanted organs from older donors has been good.

The technique of preserving the liver grafts after removal from the donor is based on decreasing metabolic requirements by keeping the graft cold. Blood is flushed from the organ to prevent vascular occlusion; preservation solution is infused; and the organ is kept on ice at 40 °C. The University of Wisconsin (UW) preservation solution contains high-molecular-weight sugar molecules that do not diffuse into the cell, which keeps the cells from swelling. These sugars and glutamine act as free oxygen radical scavengers, which are thought to prevent injury upon reperfusion of the graft. The UW solution has extended the period of safe in vitro liver preservation from 10 hours to more than 36 hours. The distance a donor liver can be transported is thus expanded, and the extended preservation time has allowed surgeons to pare down livers safely in the cold.

Operative Technique

In general, liver transplantation is an orthotopic procedure: The host liver is removed and the donor organ placed in an orthotopic position. The operation is performed in three phases: the dissection phase, during which the attachments of the diseased liver are dissected and the vascular structures are prepared for resection; the anhepatic phase, which extends from the time the host liver is removed until the time the donor liver is revascularized; and the reperfusion phase, during which blood is circulating through the new organ and the biliary tree is reconstructed.

Vascular instability during the anhepatic phase is avoided using venovenous bypass or preloading to overcome decreased venous return when vena caval flow is interrupted. Recipient portal vein and hepatic artery thrombosis are not contraindications to transplantation; donor iliac vein and artery can be used to bypass thrombosed or stenotic vessels.

The development of the pared-down liver technique to provide tissue for one or two recipients from a single donor organ has expanded the donor pool for small recipients. Although the results are not as good as with unaltered grafts, it seems likely that they will improve with time. The use of a segment (ie, left lateral segment) from a living related liver donor has recently become a reality and undoubtedly will often be resorted to in the future.

The current methods of biliary drainage—choledochocholedochostomy (if the recipient duct is intact) or choledochojejunostomy (if it is not intact)—have decreased the incidence of postoperative biliary leaks and sepsis. The indications for choledochojejunostomy include biliary atresia, sclerosing cholangitis, cholangiocarcinoma, size discrepancy between donor and recipient duct, and excessive bleeding from the recipient duct.

The method of rearterialization of the donor organ depends on the specific arterial supply to the graft. The incidence of aberrant vessels to the right lobe (from the superior mesenteric artery) and to the left lobe (from the left gastric artery) is over 20%. The celiac axis conduit may be used alone if the only variant is a replaced left hepatic artery. If a replaced right hepatic artery exists, the superior mesenteric orifice can be anastomosed to the splenic artery orifice or it can be used as the conduit itself with anastomosis of its most proximal end to the orifice of the celiac axis.

There is renewed interest in heterotopic liver transplantation with the new graft placed beneath the recipient liver. The heterotopic approach is best accomplished with a naturally small or pared-down donor organ because of space limitations when the host liver is not removed. The heterotopic graft requires portal inflow. Whether these grafts will flourish in the absence of vascular compromise to the host liver is unknown. Studies in animals indicate that a heterotopic graft requires both a source of portal inflow and decreased vascular inflow to the native organ in order to avoid atrophy of the allograft.

Immunosuppressive Therapy

The use of cyclosporine as an immunosuppressive agent has greatly improved the results of liver transplantation. Most centers use triple-drug therapy (cyclosporine, prednisone, azathioprine) to take advantage of the synergy between several agents while minimizing toxicity. The dose of each drug is individualized according to the patient's sensitivity and toxicity. There is controversy about whether antilymphocyte preparations (muromonab-CD3 or ALG-antilymphocyte globulin) should be reserved for treatment of rejection or should be used for prophylaxis (to prevent rejection). In one controlled trial using muromonab-CD3 as prophylaxis, a benefit in prevention of rejection was shown without increased mortality or morbidity.

Efforts are under way to develop more powerful immunosuppressive agents with more specific effects. Tacrolimus (FK506) is similar to cyclosporine in that it inhibits interleukin-2 production and release, but it is more potentd and is the basis for new protocols. The agent has been used successfully in first-time transplant recipients and in individuals who are losing their grafts to rejection while receiving conventional immunosuppressive therapy.

Complications

Complications following liver transplantation fall into two groups: technical complications occurring as a result of the transplant procedure and complications resulting from the host immune response or the results of immunosuppressive drugs. Technical complications include bleeding, primary nonfunction of the liver, hepatic artery thrombosis, portal vein thrombosis, biliary stenosis and leaks, and intra-abdominal infection. Immune-related complications include rejection and opportunistic infections of viral, fungal, or bacterial origin, nephrotoxicity, bone marrow suppression, and steroid toxicity.

Primary nonfunction refers to a condition where the new liver does not function and death results unless a second transplant is performed. The incidence varies from 1% up to 20%. This entity occurs as a spectrum ranging from severe dysfunction to conditions where some aspects of liver function remain intact while others do not. The incidence may also reflect the availability of second livers; transplant surgeons with an ample supply of donor organs may be more likely to decide that a poorly functioning graft will not recover. The cause of primary nonfunction is poorly understood: donor injury before retrieval, preservation technique, and recipient immunologic response have all been suggested as contributing factors. Hepatic artery and portal vein thrombosis are fortunately rare early after transplant, as the consequences are often serious without retransplantation. Biliary stenosis or leak are frequent complications (5–20%) but are rarely lethal. The incidence of complications following choledochocholedochostomy is the same as for choledochojejunostomy. These complications can often be successfully treated with transhepatic tube drainage or nasobiliary drainage rather than reoperation.

Rejection—the most frequent complication of liver transplantation—occurs in about 60% of patients. It is characterized by specific histologic findings and usually is associated with abnormalities in liver function tests, though the latter may be nonspecific. The histologic features include a mixed portal infiltrate with injury to bile duct epithelia and inflammation of the central vein endothelia (endothelitis). The hepatic parenchyma is a late target for the rejection response. The pattern of injury mirrors the distribution of major histocompatibility complex (MHC) antigens on the surfaces of the affected cells. Bile duct epithelium and central vein endothelium are rich in class I and class II antigens, whereas there is a relative paucity of class I antigens and no class II antigens on hepatocytes. Rejection can be differentiated histologically from other causes of hepatic dysfunction—such as hepatitis—and graded according to its severity. When diagnosed early and treated aggressively, rejection rarely culminates in a need for retransplantation. Because the principal rejection target is the bile duct epithelium, severe unrelenting rejection is often manifested by destruction and disappearance of bile ducts (vanishing bile duct syndrome). The treatment for rejection depends on its severity. Mild rejection is treated with additional corticosteroids; moderate to severe rejection is treated with an antilymphocyte preparation.

Cytomegalovirus (CMV) infection is an the opportunistic infection seen in about 50% of liver transplant recipients. It is usually mild, consisting of fever, leukopenia, malaise, and viremia, but 15% of patients develop a more serious picture with pneumonitis or hepatitis. Patients most at risk for severe CMV disease are those without previous CMV exposure who receive a liver or blood products from a CMV-positive donor. Treatment for CMV is with ganciclovir. Although relapse is common (20%), repeat treatment is usually successful.

Epstein-Barr virus (EBV) is another common viral pathogen in these patients. Although the systemic illness with EBV infection is usually mild, it may be associated with development of a lymphoproliferative disorder known as "posttransplant lymphoma." Treatment consists of prolonged acyclovir administration and a decrease in immunosuppression.

Since fungal infections may occur, nystatin is used prophylactically to decrease gastrointestinal colonization by *Candida albicans*.

Future Direction of Liver Transplantation

Developments over the past 25 years have made liver transplantation a common treatment for end-stage liver disease. Although liver donation has steadily increased, there is a marked discrepancy between the number of potential donors and the number of recipients, which will stimulate further developments. For example, living related hepatic transplantation using the left lateral segment may become common. Furthermore, hepatocyte transplantation has a potential role in patients with enzyme deficiencies such as α_1-antitrypsin (α_1-antiprotease) deficiency. The optimal technique for cellular transplant and the optimal immunosuppression regimen for this procedure are unknown. Xenotransplantation (the use of organs from other species) would provide additional donor material. The specific mechanisms of xenograft rejection and the appropriate treatment to prevent rejection are still obscure. Previous attempts at xenotransplantation have been uniformly unsuccessful because of uncontrolled rejection.

Disease prevention is another major area that could change liver transplantation. For example, increasing

understanding of hepatitis C may lead to the development of a vaccine that could eliminate the need for transplantation in many patients.

Bussutil RW, Goss JA: Split liver transplantation. Ann Surg 1999; 229:313.

Edwards EB et al: The effect of the volume of procedures at transplantation centers on mortality after liver transplantation. N Engl J Med 1999;341:2049.

Gridelli B, Remuzzl G: Strategy for making more organs available for transplantation. N Engl J Med 2000;343:404.

Neuberger J: Liver transplantation. QJM 1999;92:547.

■ PANCREATIC TRANSPLANTATION

Although pancreatic transplantation involves transplantation of a nonessential organ as compared with the liver, heart, or kidney, it has enormous potential in the management of patients with insulin-dependent diabetes. In this disease, even though insulin and diet are carefully controlled, vascular changes in small arteries continue relentlessly. Many patients develop severe retinopathy at an early age, leading to blindness, renal disease and uremia, and peripheral vascular disease with severe neuropathy or limb loss.

There are approximately 1 million patients with type I (insulin-dependent) diabetes mellitus in the USA, and an additional 10,000 new cases occur each year. Hence, the potential usefulness of pancreatic transplants for treating these patients is obvious. Currently, whole organ pancreas transplantation with implantation of a duodenal cuff containing the pancreatic duct into the bladder appears to be the most promising. With this technique under coverage of cyclosporine therapy, about 65% of transplant patients survive for 1 year.

Much research has dealt with the transplantation of isolated pancreatic islet cells, which could eventually become the procedure of choice. Numerous studies have documented reversal of experimental diabetes by pancreatic islet cell transplantation in a variety of animal models and by several routes of administration. The feasibility of this procedure in humans would be enhanced if the islet cells could be successfully preserved before transplantation and if graft sites more accessible and less hazardous than the portal vein or the peritoneal cavity could be shown to be useful.

Stegall MD et al: Pancreas transplantation for the prevention of diabetic nephropathy. Mayo Clin Proc 2000;75:49.

Sutherland DG et al: Lessons learned from more than 1000 pancreas transplants at a single institution. Ann Surg 2001; 233:463.

Index

Page numbers in boldface indicate a major discussion. Those followed by *t* and *i* indicate tables and illustrations, respectively. Drugs are listed under their generic names; when a trade name is listed, the entry is cross-referred to the generic name.

Abandonment, 74–75
Abbe flap, for lip cancer, 287
Abciximab, for angina pectoris, 413
Abdomen, acute. *See* Acute abdomen
Abdominal abscess, 508*t*
Abdominal aortic aneurysm(s), 829–830
  infrarenal, **830–835**
  ruptured, 208
Abdominal aortic coarctation, **829**
Abdominal apoplexy, 701
Abdominal bleeding, physical findings in, 508*t*
Abdominal crisis, in sickle cell anemia, 53
Abdominal distention
  management of, in acute secondary bacterial
    peritonitis, 520
  in small bowel obstruction, 684
Abdominal injuries, **247–255**
Abdominal mass
  palpation of, 509
  physical findings with, 508*t*
Abdominal pain, 42, **503–507**, 504*t*, 505*f*, 796
  in acute appendicitis, 1328
  in cardiac patients, 514
  character of, 506–507, 506*i*
  chronic, 672
  in Crohn's disease, **690**
  with femoral hernia, 790
  hematologic causes of, 53
  with intestinal duplications, 1329
  with intussusception, 1324
  location of, 503–504
  mode of onset of, 504–506
  progression of, 504–506
  symptoms associated with, 507
Abdominal wall
  anatomy of, 783–784
  congenital defects of, 796, **1339–1341**
  hemorrhage in, 53
  hernias of, 783–791, 1339
    rare types of, 794–795
    traumatic, **795–796**
  injuries to, treatment of, 252
  pain in, **796**
  trauma to, 795–796
  tumors of, 796
Abdominoplasty, **1267–1268**
Ablative surgery, for cancer pain, 950
Abnormal rectal fixation, **764–766**
Abortion
  elective, 1091–1092
  methods of, 1091–1092
  missed, 1113
  therapeutic, 1090–1091
  threatened, 1113

Above-knee amputation, 864, 865
Abscess, 112
  abdominal, 508*t*
  amebic, and chronic mediastinitis, 372
  anorectal, **771–773**
    intersphincteric, 771, 772
    in ulcerative colitis, 743
  appendiceal, 670
  with Bartholin cyst, 1095
  brain, 114, **958–960**
  breast, **343**
  clostridial, 124
  collar-button, 126, 1282
  cutaneous, 125–127
  deep space, of hand, **1282–1283**, 1283*i*
  diagnosis of, 117
  drainage of, 117–118, 384, 525–526, 525*i*,
    639, 664
  epidural, **960**, 1213, 1214*i*
  of gouty tophi, 1286
  hepatic, **593–594**
    causes of, 593
  hypothenar space, 1283
  in infected hand, 1282
  interloop, 524*t*
  intra-abdominal, 24, 36, **521–527**
  intraperitoneal, **521–526**, 522*i*, 523*i*, 524*i*,
    524*t*
  ischiorectal, 772
  liver, 114
    amebic, 593, 594
    cryptogenic, 593, 594
  lung, **383–384**, 384*i*
  midpalmar space, 1282–1283
  of neck, 997
  pancreatic, 632, **638–639**
  paracolostomy, 754
  para-ileostomy, 753*t*
  pelvic, 524*t*
  perianal, in Crohn's disease, 690
  pericholecystic, **608–609**
  perinephric, **1039**
  perirectal, 772
    classification of, 771
    cryptoglandular, **771–773**
  peritonsillar, 988
  pilonidal, 774
  in postoperative parotitis, 30
  psoas, 526
  renal, **1038–1039**
  retrofascial, **526–527**
  retroperitoneal, **526–527**
  in small intestine fistulas, 697
  soft tissue, 1218–1220

  splenic, 664
  spread of, 114
  stitch, 25
  subcutaneous, 125–127
  subdural, **960**
  subpectoral, 352
  subscapular, 352
  subungual, 1282
  treatment of, by incision and drainage,
    117–118
  in vertebral osteomyelitis, 1213, 1214*i*
  wound, 25
Absorption
  in colon, **708–709**, 709*t*
  in small intestine, **677–679**
Acanthosis nigricans, as paraneoplastic syn-
    drome, 1371, 1371*t*
Acceleration-deceleration injury, of brain,
    900–901
Accidental hypothermia, **280–281**
Accidents. *See* Trauma
Accident scene, trauma care at, **232–234**
ACE inhibitors. *See* Angiotensin-converting en-
    zyme inhibitors (ACEI)
Ace of spades deformity, in sigmoid volvulus,
    739, 740*i*
Acetabulum, fractures of, 1127–1128, 1127*i*
Acetaldehyde, in alcoholic pancreatitis, 628
Acetaminophen, for osteoarthritis, 1202
Acetaminophen with codeine, for postoperative
    analgesia, 21
Acetazolamide, in radionuclide imaging, 897
Acetic acid, for otalgia, 979
Acetylcysteine, and cystic fibrosis, 387
Achalasia, 476, **477–479**, 478*i*
Achilles tendon rupture, *versus* deep venous
    thrombosis, 876
Achlorhydria
  gastric ulcer and, 547
  in pancreatic cholera, 650
Acid, gastric. *See* Gastric acid
Acid-base balance, **150–153**, **223–224**
  abnormalities of, 150–153 (*See also specific*
    abnormality)
  mixed disorders of, **153**
  nomogram for, 150, 151*i*
  normal physiology of, 150
  and renal stones, 1042
  respiratory disorders and, 151
Acidosis
  metabolic, **152**
    hyperchloremic, in total parenteral nutri-
      tion, 184*t*
    with respiratory acidosis, 153

Acidosis (*cont.*)
  with respiratory alkalosis, 153
  respiratory, **151**
    with metabolic acidosis, 153
    with metabolic alkalosis, 153
  in total parenteral nutrition, 181
Acids, ocular burns caused by, **1008**
Acinar adenocarcinoma, of lung, 396
Acoustic neuroma, **919–920**
  management of, 976
  resection of, intraoperative neurophysiologic
    monitoring in, 897–898
Acoustic trauma, hearing loss from, 969
Acquired hemolytic anemia, **658**
Acquired immunodeficiency syndrome (AIDS).
    See also Human immunodeficiency
    virus (HIV)
  and fungal infections of lung, 390
  hearing loss in, 974
  immune thrombocytopenic purpura in, 659
  non-Hodgkin's lymphoma in, and small in-
    testine, 702
  nutritional support in, 189–190
  otolaryngology in, 998
  and pneumothorax, 369
Acquired intestinal diverticula, **688,** 688*i*
Acquired short esophagus, 487
Acrocephalosyndactyly, 1259
Acrocyanosis, 843
Acromegaly, pituitary tumor causing, 930,
    931
Acromioclavicular joint, dislocation of, **1129**
Actinic keratitis, **1008**
Actinic (solar) keratoses, **1249**
Actinobacter infection, drug therapy for, 135*t*
Actinomyces israelii, 129
Actinomycosis (*Actinomyces* infection), 112,
    129, 997
  and chronic mediastinitis, 372
  drug therapy for, 136*t*
Activated partial thromboplastin time (aPTT),
    52
  in liver disease, 57
  prolonged, 58
Active core rewarming, for accidental hy-
    pothermia, 281
Activities of daily living, 69*t*
  performance of, by elderly, 69
Acute abdomen, **503–516**
  auscultation of, 509
  causes of, 504*t*
  differential diagnosis of, 513–515
  hematologic disease simulating, 53
  history in, 503–508
  imaging studies in, 511–513
  indications for surgery in, 515, 515*t*
  inspection of, 508–509
  investigative studies for, 510–513, 510*t*
  laboratory studies for, 510–511
  medical causes of, 514–515, 514*t*
  palpation of, 509–510
  percussion of, 509
  physical examination for, 508–510, 508*t*
  preoperative management of, 515–516

Acute necrotizing ulcerative gingivitis,
    984–985
Acute phase response, 103, 105*t*, 108
Acute respiratory distress syndrome, **212**
Acute tubular necrosis, 49, 51
Acyclovir
  for Bell's palsy, 977
  dosage of
    in hepatic failure, 138*t*
    in renal failure, 138*t*
  for herpetic stomatitis, 985
  ototoxicity of, 998
  pharmacology of, 138*t*
Adactyly, 1260
Adamantinomatous craniopharyngioma, 920
Adams forward bending test, 1185
Addisonian crisis, 41, 810
Addison's disease
  hypercalcemia in, 149
  with thyroid disease, 41
Adenitis
  atypical mycobacterial, 997
  mesenteric, 693
  tuberculous, 997
Adenocarcinoma
  of ampulla of Vater, **647–648**
  of appendix, 672–673
  of bile ducts, **617–619**
  chronic pancreatitis and, 641
  definition of, 1352
  duodenal, 562
  of esophagus, 496
  of fallopian tubes, 1110
  follicular, **306,** 307
  of gallbladder, **616–617**
  gastric, 557
  of large intestine, 716–724, 726
  of lung, 396, 396*t*, 399*f*
  mucocele of appendix and, 673
  of pancreas, **644–646**
  papillary, **306,** 307
  renal, **1054–1058,** 1056*i,* 1057*i,* 1058*t*
    versus renal stones, 1043
    versus simple renal cyst, 1076
  of small intestine, 702
  vaginal, 1105, 1106
Adenoidal hypertrophy, 988
Adenoid cystic carcinomas, 397, 404
Adenoidectomy, for otitis media with effusion,
    966
Adenoma(s)
  adrenal
    aldosterone-producing, 798–800
      as adrenal incidentaloma, 811–812,
        812*t*
    in hyperadrenocorticism (Cushing disease,
      Cushing syndrome), 806
    nonfunctioning, as adrenal incidentaloma,
      811–812, 812*t*
  of ampulla of Vater, **647–648**
  of bile ducts, 619
  bronchial, 404
  bronchial gland, 397
  corticotropic, 921

of gallbladder, 619
  gonadotropic, 921
  hepatic, 577, 1348
  of large intestine, 725, 726
  macrocystic, of pancreas, 647
  malignant potential of, 726
  parathyroid, 309
  pituitary, 806, 921, 930–931
    excision of, 809
  pleomorphic, 294
  renal, **1059**
  somatotropic, 921
  thyrotropic, 921
  villous, 563, 727
Adenoma-to-carcinoma sequence, 726
Adenomatous hyperplasia, of gallbladder,
    619
Adenomatous polyposis coli, **727–728.** *See also*
    Familial adenomatous polyposis
    (FAP)
Adenomatous polyps, 560
Adenomyomatosis, of gallbladder, 619
Adenomyosis, **1098–1099**
Adenosine diphosphoribose, 89
Adenosine washout phenomenon, 566–567
Adenosquamous tumors, 397
Adhesiolysis, for small bowel obstruction, 687
Adhesions
  after abdominal surgery, 92–93
  pelvic, pain caused by, 1090
  peritoneal, **529–530**
  and small bowel obstruction, **683,** 683*t*
Adhesive capsulitis, **1198–1199**
Adler's sign, 63
Adnexal mass(es), **1100–1102**
  differential diagnosis of, 1101, 1101*t*
  persistent, 1101–1102
  in pregnant patient, 66–67
Adolescent(s). *See also* Child(ren)
  caloric requirements of, 1297, 1297*t*
  gastrointestinal bleeding in, 1332
Adrenalectomy
  for breast cancer, 334
  in hyperadrenocorticism (Cushing disease,
    Cushing syndrome), 809
  laparoscopic, 797–798, 801, 809
  maintenance therapy after, 809–810
  open, 797–798
  for pituitary tumors, 931
Adrenal glands, **797–812**
  anatomy of, 797, 798*i*
  cancer of, paraneoplastic syndromes with,
    1371*t*
  diseases of, 798–812
  hypersecretory state of, 797 (*See also* Hyper-
    adrenocorticism (Cushing disease,
    Cushing syndrome))
  metastatic disease in, 812
  pathology of, in hyperadrenocorticism
    (Cushing disease, Cushing syn-
    drome), 806
  surgical approaches for, 797–798
  surgical principles for, 797
  tumors of (*See also* Incidentalomas)

feminizing, **811**
virilizing, **810**
Adrenal hyperplasia, 798–799
congenital, 810
macronodular, 806, 809
pigmented micronodular, 806, 809
Adrenal insufficiency
hyperkalemia in, 146
in surgical patient, **41**
Adrenal vein sampling, in hyperaldosteronism,
800
Adrenocortical carcinoma, **811**
as adrenal incidentaloma, 811–812, 812*t*
aldosterone-producing, 799, 800, 811
prognosis for, 810, 811
treatment of, 809, 811
Adrenocortical hormones, anticancer therapy
with, **1356**
Adrenocorticotropic hormone (corticotropin,
ACTH), 103–104, 106
actions of, 167
excess, **805–810**
secretion of, in hyperadrenocorticism (Cushing disease, Cushing syndrome),
806–808, 807*i*
Adriamycin. *See* Doxorubicin
Adriamycin (doxorubicin), bleomycin, vinblastine, and dacarbazine (ABVD) regimen, for Hodgkin's lymphoma,
1367
Adson's test
in subclavian vein thrombosis, 879
for thoracic outlet syndrome, 845
Adult respiratory distress syndrome, in acute
pancreatitis, 633
Advance directives, 81
Adynamic ileus, 677, 683
Aerotitis media, 965
Aesthetic surgery, **1264–1269**
Aflatoxins, and hepatic cancer, 571
African Americans, and sarcoidosis, 395
Aganglionic megacolon, 1321–1322
Age, and organ function, 67–69, 68*t*
Agee technique, for endoscopic carpal tunnel
release, 1291–1292
Age-related cataract, **1004–1005**
Aging. *See* Elderly
Agkistrodon contortrix, 130
Agkistrodon piscivorus, 130
Agnogenic myeloid metaplasia, **663**
Agranulocytic colitis, **750**
AIDS. *See* Acquired immunodeficiency syn-
drome (AIDS)
Air bags, 230–231
Air conduction hearing, 962
Air embolism, **35**
and pulmonary thromboembolism, 880
in total parenteral nutrition, 181
in tracheobronchial injury, 245
Air pollution, and lung cancer, 396
Airway
foreign bodies in, in children, **1333**
Mallampati classification of, 192
management of, 196

in craniocerebral trauma, 903
in depressed consciousness, 889
in primary trauma survey, **236**
at scene of accident, **232–234**, 233*i*
obstruction of
and foreign bodies in larynx and tracheobronchial tree, 990
pediatric, **991–994**
relief of, **232–234**, 233*i*
temporary, establishment of, 233, 233*i*
trauma to, prehospital care for, 232
Alanine, metabolism of, 166, 166*i*
Albendazole, indications for, 129
Albumin
for acute pancreatitis, 633
as blood substitute, 62
intravenous infusion of, in ascites treatment,
590
in pancreatic abscess, 639
in resuscitation, 206
serum levels of, 7, 157*t*, 158, 158*t*
in ascites, 590
Alcohol
and accidental hypothermia, 280
consumption
and chronic pancreatitis, 641
and pancreatitis, 630
and head and neck tumors, 282
for skin antisepsis, 12
Alcoholic liver disease, *versus* choledocholithiasis, 614
Alcoholic pancreatitis, 628
Alcoholism. *See also* Varices
and delirium tremens, 35
esophageal involvement in, 480
and Mallory-Weiss syndrome, 551
portal hypertension in, 578–579
Alcohol withdrawal seizures, in craniocerebral
trauma, 904
Aldehyde oxidase, 164
Aldosterone, 104, 106, 107
actions of, 146, 167–168, 798
adrenal adenomas secreting, 810
excess, 798 (*See also* Hyperaldosteronism)
and hypokalemia, 148
in hypovolemic shock, 203
in shock, 211
Aldosteronoma, 798–800
as adrenal incidentaloma, 811–812, 812*t*
localization of, 800
Alert, definition of, 888
Alkaline gastritis, 544
Alkaline phosphatase, serum levels of
in bile duct malignancies, 617
bone disease and, 602, 602*i*
in choledocholithiasis, 614
in chronic pancreatitis, 641
with hepatic abscess, 593
in hepatobiliary disorders, 602*i*
in jaundice, 602, 602*i*
with liver cancer, 572
with metastatic neoplasms of liver, 574
in pancreatic abscess, 639
in pancreatic adenocarcinoma, 644

Alkalis, ocular burns caused by, **1007–1008**
Alkaloids, plant, anticancer therapy with, 1355
Alkalosis
in hyperaldosteronism, 799
with hypokalemia, 148
metabolic, **152–153**
with respiratory alkalosis, 153
respiratory, **152**
with metabolic alkalosis, 153
Alkylamines, for allergic rhinitis, 978*t*
Alkylating agents, anticancer therapy with,
1355
Allelic losses
and colorectal cancer, 723
in meningiomas, 919
Allen's test, 36, 827
Allergic bronchopulmonary aspergillosis, 393
Alligator hide, 1231
Allograft
definition of, 1372
human, for aortic valve replacement, 428,
429*i*
Allopurinol, for gout, 1286
Alpha-adrenergic blocking agents
for benign prostatic hyperplasia, 1035
for pheochromocytoma, 804
Alpha-fetoprotein, serum levels of
in cancer, 572
in hepatocellular carcinoma, 1349
teratoma and, 1347
in testicular cancer, 1071
Alpha interferon
for bladder tumors, 1065
for hairy cell leukemia, 663
for renal adenocarcinoma, 1057
Alpha toxin, 124
Alprostadil
for aortic coarctation, 446
for patent ductus arteriosus, 458
for pulmonary stenosis, 441
Alteplase. *See* Recombinant tissue plasminogen
activator
Amaurosis fugax, and cerebrovascular disease,
848
Amblyopia, 1007
Ambulance transport, from accident scene, 234
Ambulation
early, for elderly, 68
postoperative, 15
Amebas, 112
Amebiasis
hepatic abscess in, 593, 594
versus ulcerative colitis, 742–743
Amebic abscess, and chronic mediastinitis, 372
American Burn Association, burn severity classification of, 268, 269*t*
American Joint Committee on Cancer (AJCC),
cancer staging system of, 1353
for lung cancer, 398
for melanoma, 1363, 1363*t*
American Society of Anesthesiologists, physical
status classification system of,
191–192, 192*t*

American Spinal Injury Association (ASIA)
  impairment scale used by, 1119
  motor and sensory examination recom-
    mended by, 1118–1119
American trypanosomiasis. *See* Chagas' disease
Amikacin, indications for, 129, 136*t*, 137
Amiloride, indications for, 801
Amino acid(s), 161–162
  absorption of, in small intestine, 678
  aromatic, 161
  branched chain, 161–162, 166
  essential, 161
  metabolism of, 165–166
    in sepsis, 169–170
  neurotransmitter, and hepatic encephalopa-
    thy, 591–592
  nonessential, 161
  sulfur-containing, 161
Aminocaproic acid, for postoperative bleeding,
  436
Aminoglutethimide, 1357
  for breast cancer, 333*t*, 334
  in males, 340
Aminoglycosides. *See also* Amikacin; Gentamicin; Tobramycin
  for acute cholecystitis, 609
  for cholangitis, 612
  dosage of, renal failure and, 137
  for esophageal perforation, 372
  indications for, 135*t*, 136*t*, 137
  nephrotoxicity of, 51
  for preoperative bowel preparation, 755
Aminophylline
  for inhalation injuries, 276
  seizures and, 274
Aminosalicylic acid
  for Crohn's disease, 692, 748
  for tuberculosis, 388*t*
  for ulcerative colitis, 744
Amiodarone
  for atrial dysrhythmias, 437
  toxicity of, 300 (*See also* Hyperthyroidism)
  for ventricular arrhythmias, 437
Ammonia, and hepatic encephalopathy, 592
Amniotic fluid embolism, in pulmonary
  thromboembolism, 880
Amoxicillin
  for acute otitis media, 970
  for acute tonsillitis, 988
  for duodenal ulcer, 541
  for otitis media with effusion, 966
Amoxicillin-clavulanic acid, indications for,
  135*t*
Amphetamine abuse, and vasculitis, 700
Amphotericin B, **140**
  for aspergilloma, 394
  for blastomycosis, 392
  for coccidioidomycosis, 392
  for cryptococcosis, 393
  for invasive aspergillosis, 393–394
  lipid preparations of, **140**
  for lung abscess, 384
  for mucormycosis, 394
  nephrotoxicity of, 51

Ampicillin
  after splenectomy, 666–667
  and antibiotic-associated colitis, 749
  dosage of
    in hepatic failure, 138*t*
    in renal failure, 138*t*
  for gas cysts in small intestine, 701
  for hepatic encephalopathy, 592
  indications for, 135*t*, 136*t*
  pharmacology of, 138*t*
  prophylactic, in valvular heart disease, 45
Ampicillin-sulbactam, for acute secondary bacterial peritonitis, 519
Ampulla of Vater, 625, 626*i*
  adenocarcinoma of, **647–648**
  adenoma of, **647–648**
Ampullary stenosis, **622**
Amputation, **859–870**
  above-knee, 864, 865
  arterial injuries and, 256
  below-knee, 864–865, 865*i*
  for bone tumor, 1222
  Burgess technique for, 864–865
  Chopart's, 863
  congenital, 1260
  in crush injuries of hand, **1288–1289**
  emergency, 861
  forearm, **867**
  forequarter, **867**, 868*i*
  gait analysis after, 870
  goals of, 859
  guillotine, 864
  immediate, in arterial injury, 262
  leg, **864–865**
  level of, 859–860
    determination of, 860–861
  Lisfranc's, 863
  long-term care after, 870
  lower extremity, 859, **861–866**
    rehabilitation after, 869
  medical, 861
  mortality rates and, 868
  for osteogenic sarcoma, 1224
  pain after, **951–952**
  for peripheral arterial insufficiency,
    824
  for peripheral nerve tumors, 929
  phantom limb pain and, **951–952**
  Piroff's, 863
  preparation for, 861
  prostheses and, **869–870**
  ray, **862**, 862*i*
  rehabilitation after, **869**
  toe, 859, **862**, 862*i*
  transhumeral, **867**
  transmetatarsal, **863**, 863*i*
  types of, 861–867
  upper extremity, **866–867**, 867*i*
    rehabilitation after, 869
Amputees, special problems of, **867–869**
Amylase
  in pancreatic pleural effusion, 640
  serum (*See also* Hyperamylasemia)
    in acute cholecystitis, 608

    in acute mesenteric vascular occlusion,
      699
    in acute pancreatitis, 631–632
    in ascites, 590
    in choledocholithiasis, 614
    in chronic pancreatitis, **640**
    in pancreatic abscess, 639
    in pancreatic pseudocyst, 636
  urinary
    in acute pancreatitis, 632
    in chronic pancreatitis, **640**
    in pancreatitis with hyperlipidemia, 628
Amyloidosis, esophageal manifestations in, 480
Anal canal, 756. *See also* Anorectum
  epidermoid (squamous, basaloid, mucoepi-
    dermoid) carcinoma of, **781–782**
  glands of, 771
  tumors of, **781–782**
Anal encirclement procedure, 760, 764
Anal fissure, 767, **768–770**
  in infants, 1332
  in ulcerative colitis, 743
Analgesia. *See also* Pain control
  continuous epidural, **21**
  for diverticulitis, 731
  patient-controlled, **21**, 200
  postoperative, 20–21, 194, **200**
Analgesics
  oral, 20–21
  parenteral
    nonopioid, 20
    opioid, 20
Anal incontinence. *See* Fecal incontinence
Anal margin
  carcinoma of, 779–780
  tumors of, **780–781**
Anal pain, causes of, 763
Anal sphincter mechanism, 756
  artificial, 760
  dysfunction of, 764–766
  external, 756, 757, 757*i*, 759
    normal function of, 758–759
  internal, 756, 757, 757*i*
    normal function of, 758–759
Anal sphincterotomy, lateral internal, 770
Anal stenosis, 762, 764, 769*i*
Anal ulcer, **768–770**
Anal verge, 756, 769*i*
Anaplastic astrocytomas, **918**, 926
Anastomoses
  in coarctation of aorta, 446
  end-to-end, for arterial injuries, 243
  intestinal
    colorectal cancer recurrence in, 718
    for Crohn's disease, 748
    for diverticulitis, 734
    for ulcerative colitis, 745, 745*i*
    for volvulus, 740
  neural
    for facial paralysis, 977
    for peripheral nerve injury, 914
  ureteral, 1050
Anastomotic ulcer, 542–543
Anastrozole, 1357

Ancure, 834, 834*i*
Androgen deprivation therapy, for prostate
     cancer, 1069
Androgen inhibitor(s), anticancer therapy with,
     1356
Androgens, anticancer therapy with, **1356**
  for breast cancer, 334
Anemia, 60–61
  after gastric surgery, 544
  colon cancer and, 719
  in Crohn's disease, **690**
  hemolytic
     acquired, **658**
     autoimmune, **658**
     hereditary nonspherocytic, **657**
     versus hereditary spherocytosis, 656
     immune, secondary, 658, 658*t*
  with hepatic abscess, 593
  megaloblastic, 52
  in myelofibrosis, 663
  pernicious, 52
  in renal adenocarcinoma, 1054–1055
  in renal disease, 49–50
  in surgical patients, **52**
  with uterine leiomyomas, 1100
Anergy, 113–114, 388
  and operative risk, 7–8
Anesthesia, **191–202**
  administration of, preparation for, 194
  for brain tumors, 925
  and cardiac risk, 28
  complications of, **201–202**
  depth of
     monitoring, 197
     signs of, 197*t*
  drugs affecting, 9
  in elderly, 10
  heart disease and, 45
  historical perspective on, 191
  induction of, 194
  in intraoperative cranial nerve monitoring,
     898
  monitoring during, 194
  for outpatient surgery, 200–201, 201*t*
  postoperative care in, 199–200
  preoperative procedures in, 191–194
  selection of, 194
  standby, **199**
  for wound care and closure, in soft tissue in-
     jury, 1253
Anesthesia consultation, preoperative, 10
Anesthetic equipment, improper placement of,
     injuries caused by, 195
Anesthetic risk
  overall, 191
  preoperative evaluation for, 191–193
AneuRx, 834, 835*i*
Aneurysm(s)
  of anterior choroidal artery, 939
  aortic
     abdominal, 829–830
     dissecting, **852**
     infrarenal abdominal, **830–835**
     ruptured, **837**

     suprarenal, **836–837**
     thoracic, **431–432**
  aortic arch, 432
  arterial, **829–843**, 830*i*
  of ascending aorta, 432
  of carotido-ophthalmic artery, 896*i*
  degenerative, 829
     and atherosclerosis, 814
  of descending aorta, 432
  dissecting, 938
  of extracranial carotid artery, **840–841**
  false, 258, 829, **842**
  of femoral artery, **839**
  fusiform, 938
  of great cerebral vein, 934
  of hepatic artery, **841–842**
  iliac, **835–836**, 836*i*
  infected, **838**
  infectious, 938
  inflammatory, **837**
  of internal carotid artery, 939
  intracranial, **937–943**
  left ventricular, 416–417, 418*i*
  neoplastic, 938
  of ophthalmic artery, 939
  of persistent sciatic artery, **839**
  of popliteal artery, **839**
  of posterior communicating artery, 939
  of radial artery, false, **842**
  of renal artery, **842**, 1020, **1076–1077**,
     1077*i*
  saccular, **934**, 938
  of splenic artery, **841**
  of subclavian artery, **842**
  of superior hypophyseal artery, 939
  of superior mesenteric artery, **842**
  and tinnitus, 971
  traumatic, 938
  true, 829
  upper extremity, **842**
  of visceral artery, **841–842**
Aneurysmal bone cyst, **1227–1228**
  of chest wall, 355
Aneurysmectomy
  for infrarenal abdominal aortic aneurysms,
     834
  intraoperative neurophysiologic monitoring
     in, **899–900**
Angina pectoris, 43, **408–415**
  clinical presentation of, 42, 410–412
  as contraindication to surgery, 42
  in elderly, 67–68
  pathology of, 409–410
  prognosis for, 414–415, 415*f*, 415*t*
  risk factors for, 410, 411*t*
  survival rates for, 412, 412*i*, 413*i*
  treatment of, 412–414
Angiodysplasia, **738**
Angiofibroma, juvenile, 989
Angiography, 412. *See also* Arteriography
  in acute abdomen, 512
  in arteriovenous malformations, intraopera-
     tive, 946–947

  carotid artery, percutaneous, 851–852
  complications of, 819
  in craniocerebral trauma, 903
  digital subtraction, **896**
  in insulinoma, 649
  in intracranial aneurysms, 940
  intraoperative, in arteriovenous malforma-
     tions, 946–947
  in kidney injury, 1048
  of liver tumors, 572
  in lower gastrointestinal bleeding, 736, 737*i*
  in neurodiagnosis, 894–895, 895*i*, **896**, 896*i*
  portal, 584
  in pulmonary thromboembolism, 880–881,
     881, 881*i*
  in renal adenocarcinoma, 1055
  screening isotope, in arterial injuries, 260
  in spinal cord tumors, 928
  time-of-flight, 894
Angiokeratoma, 1342
Angiomas
  retinal, 1011
  splenic, 664
Angiomyolipoma, **1059**
Angioplasty
  for acute mesenteric vascular occlusion, 699
  balloon, for intracranial aneurysm, 942–943
Angiosarcoma, 886
  hepatic, 572
Angiotensin, 49
  in hypovolemic shock, 203
Angiotensin-converting enzyme inhibitors
     (ACEI)
  indications for, 801
  and microvascular circulation, 828
  for mitral regurgitation, 423
Angiotensin II, 104, 106
  in shock, 210
Angle-closure glaucoma, **1005**
Anion gap, **152**
Aniridia, Wilms' tumor and, 1344
Anismus, 762
Ankle
  dislocation of, **1171–1172**
  fractures of, 1170–1171
  injuries of, **1170–1172**
     combined patterns of, 1171
  sprain, 1170
"Ankle blowout syndrome," 883
Ankle-brachial index (ABI), 259
  and peripheral arterial insufficiency, 815,
     816*i*, 818
Ankyloglossia, **986**
Annular pancreas, 627
Annuloaortic ectasia, and thoracic aortic
     aneurysms, 431
Annulus, idiopathic calcification of, 422
Anomalous left coronary artery, **468–469**
Anorectal angle, 758, 759
Anorectal manometry, 759–760, 762, 764
Anorectum, **756–782**. *See also* Rectum
  abscess of, **771–773**
     in Crohn's disease, 690
     in ulcerative colitis, 743

Anorectum (*cont.*)
anatomy of, 756–758, 757*i*
anomalies of, **1324–1327,** 1325*i,* 1326*i*
high, 1325–1326, 1325*i,* 1326*i*
low, 1325–1326, 1325*i*
arterial supply of, 757–758
basal cell carcinoma of, **780**
cancer of, 769, **779–780**
staging of, 780, 780*t*
in Crohn's disease, **690**
dysfunction of, 759–771
fistula of, **771–773,** 778
in Crohn's disease, 690
in ulcerative colitis, 743
infections of, **771–778**
lesions of, in Crohn's disease, **690**
lymphatic drainage of, 758
neoplasms of, **779–780**
normal function of, 758–759
squamous cell carcinoma of, 777, **780**
venous drainage of, 758
Anoscopy, 767, 769, 777
in lower gastrointestinal bleeding, 736, 737*i*
Antacids
adverse effects and side effects of, 149
for columnar-lined lower esophagus, 489
for duodenal ulcer, 541
for reflux esophagitis sliding hiatal hernia,
486
Anterior choroidal artery, aneurysms, 939
Anterior cord syndrome, **909**
Anterior cruciate ligament injury, 1163, 1163*i*
Anterior peritoneal reflection, 705
Anthelmintic therapy, for ascariasis, 623
Anthracyclines, for breast cancer, 332
Anthrax, drug therapy for, 136*t*
Anthropometric measurements, 158*t,* 159*t*
in nutritional assessment, 156–158
Antibacterial agents, topical, for burns,
271–272
Antibiogram data, 134, 135*t*–136*t*
Antibiotic-associated colitis, **127, 748–749**
Antibiotics. *See also* Antimicrobial chemotherapy
for acute mastoiditis, 971
for acute mesenteric vascular occlusion, 699
for acute pancreatitis, **633**
for acute secondary bacterial peritonitis, 519
antagonism among, 140
anticancer therapy with, 1355
for appendiceal abscess, 670
for aspiration, 26
for brain abscess, 959
for bronchiectasis, 385
for cellulitis, 123
for cholangitis, 612
for chronic mediastinitis, 373
for chronic osteomyelitis, 1218–1219
for chronic otitis media, 967
for closed disk space infections, 960
for diffuse necrotizing infections, 125
for empyema, 366
for endocarditis, 430
for esophageal perforation, 372

and fungal infections of lung, 390
for hepatic abscess, 594
for hepatic encephalopathy, 592–593
indications for, 118, 126–127
in pulmonary failure, 219
for infected hand, 1281–1282
for infected joint replacement, 1157–1158
for lung abscess, 384
microbial resistance to, 12, 120–121
for nasal trauma, 983
for neck infections, 997
for otitis externa, 969–970
for otitis media with effusion, 966
for pancreatic abscess, 639
for paranasal sinusitis, 979–980
for perforated peptic ulcer, 554–555
for perinephric abscess, **1039**
for pharyngitis, 987–988
in preoperative bowel preparation, 754–755
for primary peritonitis, 527
prophylactic
after splenectomy, 666–667
for appendicitis, 671
indications for, 13, 122
principles of, 120
with prosthetic heart valves, 45
against surgical infections, 120–121
in valvular heart disease, 45
for Wiskott-Aldrich syndrome, 661
for septic arthritis, 1221–1222
for supraglottitis, 993
synergism among, 140
for tonsillitis, 988
for tuberculosis of spine, 961
for ulcerative colitis, 744
for urinary tract infections, 1037
Antibody(ies), against tumor antigens, 1358
Anticancer therapy. *See also* Radiation therapy
regional, **1358–1359**
systemic, **1354–1358** (*See also* Chemotherapy; Immunotherapy)
Anticholinesterase agents, for thymoma, 379
Anticoagulant therapy
and abdominal pain, 507
for acute mesenteric vascular occlusion, 699,
700
after cardiac surgery, 436
for deep venous thrombosis, 876–877
and fresh frozen plasma, 62
for internal carotid dissection, 852
for intra-arterial injections, 858
perioperative management of, 28, 29, **45–46**
for pulmonary thromboembolism, **881**
for superior vena caval syndrome, 374
in surgical patients, **54–55**
Anticonvulsants
for brain tumors, 924
for craniocerebral trauma, 903–904
Anticytokine agents, for rheumatoid arthritis,
1204
Antidiuretic hormone (ADH), 103, 107, 111
actions of, 167–168
inappropriate secretion of, 145
secretion of, 106

Antiemetics, indications for, 194, 199–200
Antiepileptics. *See* Anticonvulsants
Antifibrinolytics, for postoperative bleeding,
436
Antifungal therapy, **140–141**
for onychomycosis, 1284
Antihistamines
for allergic rhinitis, 978*t*
for Meniere's disease, 975
Antihypertensive therapy, perioperative management of, 45
Antilymphoblast globulin, for transplant recipient, 1381
Antilymphocyte globulin, for transplant recipient, 1375, 1385
Antimetabolites, anticancer therapy with, 1355
Antimicrobial chemotherapy, **133–142.** *See
also* Antibiotics
combination regimens, 137–140
dosage of
assessment of, 134–137
oliguria and, 137
renal failure and, 137, 138*t*–139*t*
drug selection for, 133–137, 135*t*–136*t*
for empiric therapy, 134, 135*t*–136*t*
initial, 133–134, 135*t*–136*t*
by laboratory tests, 134, 135*t*–136*t*
duration of, 137
response to, assessment of, 134–137
Antimycobacterial therapy, **141**
Antiperistalsis, 708
Antiphospholipid antibody syndrome, and subclavian vein thrombosis, 878–879
Antiplatelet agents
for angina pectoris, 412
for cerebrovascular disease prevention,
850
Antipsychotic agents, seizures and, 274
Antisepsis, 11–13, 119, 120
Antiseptics, skin, 12
Antisperm antibodies, 1081
Antithrombin III, replacement of, 62
Antithymoblast globulin, for transplant recipi-
ent, **1375**
Antithymocyte globulin, for transplant recipi-
ent, 470, **1375,** 1381
α_1-Antitrypsin deficiency, and bronchiectasis,
384
Antituberculosis drugs, 388*t*
indications for, 136*t*
Antivenin
for snakebite, 131–132
for spider bites, 133
Antiviral agents, **141**
Antral inhibition, of acid secretion, 538
Antrectomy, for duodenal ulcer, 541–542,
542*i*
Anuria
ureteral calculi and, 1046
in ureteral injury, 1049
Anus. *See* Anal; Anorectum
Anusitis, **776–778**
Anxiety
and pain, 19

in surgical patient, 34
and tinnitus, 971
Anxiety attacks, 804
Anxiety neurosis, 301
AO/ASIF classification, of distal radius fractures, 1144, 1144*i*
Aorta, 706*i*
ascending, 432
coarctation of, **445–446,** 829
descending, 432
dissection of, clinical presentation of, 42
overriding of, and tetralogy of Fallot, 460, 460*i*
traumatic rupture of, 257, 257*t*
Aortic allografts, 428, 429*i*
Aortic aneurysms
abdominal, 829–830
infrarenal, **830–835**
dissecting, 852
ruptured, **837**
suprarenal, **836–837**
thoracic, **431–432**
Aortic arch
aneurysms of, 432
anomalies of, **1311,** 1311*i*
double, **1311,** 1311*i*
interrupted, **447**
and aortopulmonary window, 454
Aortic autograft, 428
Aortic insufficiency, **427–428**
Aortic regurgitation, 427–428
Aortic stenosis, 28, 44, **426–427, 441–445,** 441*i,* 442*i*
as contraindication to surgery, 42
Aortic valve, 419–420
replacement of, 428
for aortic insufficiency, 427
for aortic stenosis, 427
Aortoiliofemoral interventions, for peripheral arterial insufficiency, 822–823, 822*i,* 823*i*
Aortoplasty, for aortic coarctation, 446
Aortopulmonary window, 449, **454–455**
APACHE II score, 225
Apathetic hyperthyroidism, 300
APC gene
and colorectal cancer, 717
and familial adenomatous polyposis, 727
Apert's syndrome, 932, 1259
Aphthous stomatitis, **985**
in AIDS, 998
Apical bullectomy, for pneumothorax prevention, 369
Apnea
with gastroesophageal reflux, in children, 1327
obstructive sleep, 988–989
Apoplexy
abdominal, 701
mesenteric, 701
Appeal(s), legal, 73–74
Appendectomy
in acute appendicitis, 668
for appendiceal abscess, 670

for appendiceal tumors, 672–673
for mucocele of appendix, 673
in pregnancy, 64, 669
technique for, 671*i*
and ulcerative colitis, 741
Appendices epiploicae, 705, 707*i*
Appendicitis, 112
in actinomycosis, 129
acute, **668–672**
in children, **1328**
chronic, **672**
versus colorectal cancer, 721
versus Crohn's disease, **691**
differential diagnosis of, 513–514, 515
versus diverticulitis, 733
in elderly, 670
and hepatic abscess, 593
in infants, 670
in pregnancy, 63–64, 514, **669**
Appendix, **668–673**
abscess (mass) of, **670**
anatomy and physiology of, **668**
benign tumors of, 672
carcinoid tumor of, 703
malignant tumors of, **672–673**
mucocele of, 673
tumors of, **672–673**
Appendix epididymis, torsion of, **1080**
Appendix testis, torsion of, **1080**
"Apple core" appearance, of intestinal carcinoma, 720, 720*i*
Apple-peel deformity, 1317, 1317*i*
Aprotinin, for postoperative bleeding, 436
Apudomas
of small intestine, 703
in Zollinger-Ellison syndrome, 544
Arachnoid granulations, 890*i*
Arachnoiditis, hydrocephalus and, 934
Arc burns, 277
Areflexia, and spinal cord injury, 910
Areflexic bladder, **1076**
Argentaffin tumors, of appendix, 672
Arginine
in nutritional support, 162
tumor stimulation with, 162
L-Arginine, for peripheral arterial insufficiency, 821
Arm. *See also* Forearm; Hand(s); Upper extremity
edema of, breast cancer and, 336–337
symptoms in, of subclavian vein thrombosis, 879
Aromatase inhibitors, anticancer therapy with, **1356–1357**
Arrhythmia(s). *See* Dysrhythmia(s)
Arsenic, and lung cancer, 396
Arterial aneurysms, **829–843,** 830*i*
Arterial arcades, of small intestine, 675*i*
Arterial blood gas determination. *See* Blood gases
Arterial emboli, mesenteric, 698
Arterial insufficiency
atherosclerotic, 814
versus chronic venous insufficiency, 884

Arterial occlusion, acute, **825–827**
and emergency amputation, 861
Arterial revascularization, for impotence, 1084
Arterial spasm, 261
Arterial switch procedure, 465
Arteriography. *See also* Angiography
in acute mesenteric vascular occlusion, 699
and amputation level determination, 861
in arterial injuries, 259–260, 259*i*
in arteriovenous malformations, 944–945
complications of, 260
in insulinoma, 649
in ischemic colitis, 750
in large intestine examination, 711
in neck injuries, 242
in pancreatic pseudocyst, 637
in peripheral arterial insufficiency, 819
in renovascular hypertension, 854
Arterioles
constriction of, in shock, 211
systemic, dilation of, in shock, 211
Arteriosclerosis
in elderly, 67–68
and thoracic aortic aneurysms, 431
Arteriovenous fistula, 259, **845–846,** 1246, 1247*t*
congenital, 1020
and varicose veins, 873
Arteriovenous malformation(s), 382, **934–935, 943–947**
in pediatric patients, 1342
and tinnitus, 971
Artery(ies), **813–858.** *See also specific named artery*
dissection of, and arterial occlusion, 825
injuries of, **255–262**
malformations of, 1342
palpation of, in peripheral arterial insufficiency, 817
reconstruction, for peripheral arterial insufficiency, 822
Arthritis. *See also* Osteoarthritis
acute pyogenic, 1220–1222
degenerative, hand involvement in, **1285**
glenohumeral, **1132–1133**
gouty, hand involvement in, 1286
hand involvement in, **1285**
inflammatory, *versus* rheumatoid arthritis, 1203–1204
posttraumatic, of wrist, 1147–1148
septic, **1220–1222**
of hip, **1187–1189,** 1188*i*
osteomyelitis caused by, 1217–1218
Arthrography, of congenital hip dislocation, 1191
Arthroplasty, and deep vein thrombosis, 877
Arthropod bites, **132–133**
Arthroscopy
knee, 1162–1164
wrist, **1290–1291**
for fracture reduction, 1145–1146
Asbestos, and lung cancer, 395
Ascariasis, **623**
Ascending aortic aneurysm, 432

Ascending colon, 706i
Ascending thoracic dissection, 433
Ascites, **528–529**, 579, **590–591**
    chylous, 528–529
    clinical presentation of, 42
    malignant, **529**
    medical treatment of, 590
    pancreatic, **639–640**
    surgical management of, 590–591
    and wound healing, 24
Ascitic leaks, 25
Ascorbic acid. *See* Vitamin C
Asepsis, 11–13
    in venous catheter changes, 36
Aseptic technique, 13
Aspartate aminotransferase (AST, SGOT)
    in choledocholithiasis, 614
    in jaundice, 602
Aspergilloma, 393
Aspergillosis, **393–394**
    invasive, 393
    and thoracic empyema, 361
Aspergillus flavus, 393
Aspergillus fumigatus, 393
Aspergillus glaucus, 393
Aspergillus niger, 393
Aspiration, **26, 213**
    clinical presentation of, 26
    of foreign body, and bronchiectasis, 385
    with gastroesophageal reflux, in children,
        1327
    in near-drowning, 265
    of oropharyngeal contents, and lung abscess,
        383
    prevention of, 26
    risk factors for, 19, 26
    treatment of, 26
    of vomitus, 233
Aspiration pneumonitis, **201**
Aspiration therapy, for brain abscess, 959–960
Aspirin
    for angina pectoris, 412
    for axillary-subclavian venous thrombosis,
        879
    and brain tumors, 924
    for cerebrovascular disease prevention, 850
    and colorectal cancer, 717
    indications for, 34, 44
    for peripheral arterial insufficiency, 821
    and platelet function, 55
Asplenia, 468
Assault, legal definition of, 75
Assisted reproductive techniques, for male in-
        fertility, **1081**
Asthma
    and operative risk, 25
    preoperative management of, 47
Astrocytomas, **917–918**, 926
    anaplastic, **918**, 926
    in children, **935**, 936i
Atelectasis, **25–26**, 213
    clinical manifestations of, 26, 36
    pathogenesis of, 25
    postoperative, 17, 18, 20
    prevention of, 26

risk factors for, 25
treatment of, 26
Atenolol, for angina pectoris, 412
Atherectomy, for peripheral arterial insuffi-
        ciency, 821–822
Atherogenesis, 813
Atheromas, locations of, 813
Atherosclerosis, **813–824**
    and arterial aneurysms, 829
    and cerebral infarction, 847
    collateral development of, 814, 814i
    in heart transplant recipient, 1381–1383
    in hyperaldosteronism, 801
    and renovascular hypertension, 853
    risk factors for, 813–814
    of thoracic aorta, 408
    and thoracic aortic aneurysms, 431
Athletes, arterial injuries in, 262
Atrial dysrhythmias, after cardiac surgery,
        436–437
Atrial isomerism, 468
Atrial myxoma, 42
Atrial septal defect, 449
    and aortopulmonary window, 454
    omphalocele and, 1340
    ostium secundum type, **450**, 450i
Atriopeptin, 103
Atrioventricular (AV) block, 45
Atrioventricular canal, 449
Atrioventricular canal defect, **451–452**, 451i
    complete, 451, 451i, 452
    partial, 451, 452
    and ventricular septal defect, 452
Atrioventricular valves, 419, 419i
Atrophy, in peripheral arterial insufficiency,
        818
Atropine
    for cardiogenic shock, 208
    for Ménétrier's disease, 561
Attractaspidae, 130
Atypical parkinsonism, 948
Audiology, clinical, **962–965**
Audiometry, 963–965, 964i
    brain stem, 965
    impedance, in otitis media with effusion,
        966
Auditory canal, external
    foreign bodies in, 971
    inflammation of, 969–970
    tumors of, 972
Auditory tube (eustachian tube) dysfunction,
        965–966
Augmentation mammoplasty, **1266–1267**
Auricle. *See also* Pinna
    congenital deformities of, 973
    reconstruction of, 973
Auscultation, 4
    in acute abdomen, 509
    in mitral stenosis, 420–421
Autoamputation, 862
Autoclaving, 11, 119
Autodigestion theory, of pancreatitis, 629
Autoimmune disorders, **657–661**
    inner ear disease in, 974
    silicone gel prostheses and, 343

Autoimmune hemolytic anemia, **658**
    versus hereditary spherocytosis, 656
Autonomic blocking agents, shock caused by,
        209
Autotransplantation, splenic, 664
Avascular necrosis, of femoral head, **1201**
Axillary-subclavian venous thrombosis,
        878–880
Axillary vein, 872
Axonapraxia, 1281
Axonotmesis, 913, 1281
Azathioprine
    for Crohn's disease, 692, 748
    in heart transplantation, 470
    for immune thrombocytopenic purpura, 660
    pancreatitis and, 629
    for secondary hemolytic anemia, 658
    for transplant recipient, **1374–1375**, 1381,
        1385
    for ulcerative colitis, 744
Azithromycin
    indications for, 136t
    for perianal chancroid, 778
Azlocillin. *See also* Penicillin, antipseudomonal
    dosage of
        in hepatic failure, 138t
        in renal failure, 138t
    pharmacology of, 138t
Azoles, **141**
    fungistatic, 141
Azoospermia, hormone studies in, 1080
Azotemia, prerenal, 144–145
Aztreonam
    for acute secondary bacterial peritonitis, 519
    dosage of
        in hepatic failure, 138t
        in renal failure, 138t
    indications for, 135t
    pharmacology of, 138t

Bacillary dysentery, *versus* ulcerative colitis,
        742–743
Bacilli
    gram-negative, septic arthritis caused by,
        1220–1222
    infection by, drug therapy for, 136t
Bacitracin, for antibiotic-associated colitis, 749
Back pain, **1210–1215**. *See also* Low back pain
    in lumbar disk syndrome, 956, 957
    mechanical, **1214–1215**
    in pancreatic adenocarcinoma, 644
Backwash ileitis, 741
Baclofen pump, for spastic cerebral palsy, 937
Bacteremia, **115**
    fulminant, after splenectomy, 666
Bacteria
    cholangitis caused by, **612**
    commensal, as source of infection, 119–120
    flesh-eating (*See* Infection(s), diffuse necro-
        tizing)
    gram-negative, pneumonia caused by, 27
    hospital-acquired infection with, 12–13
    host defense against, 113
    prostatitis caused by, **1039–1040**
    septic arthritis caused by, 1220–1222

in small intestine, 679–680
  and gas cysts, 701
Bacterial peritonitis, acute secondary, **517–521**
Bacterial sialadenitis, acute, **986**
Bacteriotherapy, for antibiotic-associated colitis, 749
Bacteriuria, 33
Bacteroides spp.
  gastrointestinal strains, infection by, drug therapy for, 135*t*
  hepatic abscess caused by, 593, 594
  infection by, 112
  oropharyngeal strains, infection by, drug therapy for, 135*t*
  and retroperitoneal abscesses, 526
Bacteroides fragilis
  in cholangitis, 612
  in feces, 710–711
  and peritonitis, 518
Balloon angioplasty
  for supravalvular aortic stenosis, 444
  transluminal, for intracranial aneurysm, 942–943
Balloon dilation
  for large bowel obstruction, 714
  percutaneous, for aortic coarctation, 446
  for valvular aortic stenosis, 443
Balloon tamponade, for variceal bleeding, 581, 582, 582*i*
Balloon test occlusion, for intracranial aneurysm, 941
Balloon valvotomy, percutaneous
  for aortic stenosis, 427
  for mitral stenosis, 421
Balloon valvuloplasty, for congenital mitral valve disease, 448
Banti's syndrome, 579
Barbiturates
  in aneurysm surgery, 899–900
  interactions with anesthetics, 193
  for intracranial hypertension, 905–906
Barium enema, 711, 711*i*, 762, 764, 767
  in acquired intestinal diverticula, 688
  in colorectal cancer, 720, 720*i*
  in Crohn's disease, 690, 691*i*
  in diverticulitis, 732, 733*i*
  in diverticulosis, 730–731
  in ischemic colitis, 750
  in large bowel polyps, **726**
  in lower gastrointestinal bleeding, 736, 737*i*
  in sigmoid volvulus, 739, 740*i*
  in ulcerative colitis, 742, 742*i*, 744*i*
Barium impaction, 31
Barium studies, in acute mesenteric vascular occlusion, 699
Barium swallow, in variceal bleeding, 581
Baroreceptors, 103
Barrett's esophagus, **488–489**
Bartholin cyst, **1095**
Bartholin gland, adenocarcinoma of, 1104
Bartonella henselae, 1304
Barton's fracture, 1144
Basal acid output (BAO), 540, 540*t*
Basal cell carcinoma, **1250–1251**
  anal, **780**

erythematous, 1250
of eyelid, 1011
of hand, 1288
pigmented, 1250
  in skull base, 972
vulvar, 1104
Basal metabolic rate (BMR), 161, 166
Base deficit, 224
Base excess, 224
Basilar artery aneurysms, 939
Basilar impression, **932**
Basilic vein, 872
  transposition of, 872
Bassini repair, for inguinal hernia, 788
Batista procedure, 418
Battered child syndrome, 1177, **1349–1350**
Batteries, ingestion of, **492**
Battery, legal definition of, 75–76
B cells (B lymphocytes), 106–107, 108, 1373
BCG vaccine, for bladder tumors, 1065
Beckwith-Wiedemann syndrome
  omphalocele and, 1340
  Wilms' tumor and, 1344
Bedsores. *See* Pressure sores
Bee stings, 132
Beevor's sign, 1119
Behçet's disease, *versus* Crohn's disease, 748
Bell clapper deformity, in testicular torsion, 1080
Bell's palsy, 977
Below-knee amputation, 864–865, 865*i*
Benign familial hypocalciuric hypercalcemia, 312
Benign lymphogranulomatosis, **394–395**
Benign paroxysmal positional vertigo, **976**
Bennett's fracture, **1149**, 1279
Bentiromide test, 643
Benzalkonium, for skin antisepsis, 12
Benzodiazepines
  for craniocerebral trauma, 903, 904
  indications for, 194
  intravenous, indications for, 133
Benzopyrones, for lymphedema, 886
Beta-blockers (beta-adrenergic blocking agents)
  adverse effects and side effects of, 45
  for angina pectoris, 412
  for atrial dysrhythmias, 437
  for cardiogenic shock, 209
  for coronary artery disease, 44
  for dysrhythmias, with pheochromocytoma, 804, 805
  for hypertrophic obstructive cardiomyopathy, 444
  for ventricular arrhythmias, 437
Beta-lactam-clavulanic acid combination, for primary peritonitis, 527
Bevan repair, for sliding inguinal hernia, 790
Bezoar, **562**
  and small bowel obstruction, 683
Bicarbonate
  absorption of, in small intestine, 678
  for aortic coarctation, 446
  balance, in response to injury, 107
  in pancreatic fluid, 643
  plasma levels of, 150

Bicarbonate ion concentration [HCO$_3^-$], 221*t*, 223–224
Biceps tendinitis, **1198**
Bicuspid aortic valve, and aortic coarctation, 445
Bile
  concentration of, 596, 599*i*
  flow of, **595–596**, 598*i*, 599*i*
    posthepatic obstruction of, 32*t*, 33
  formation of, 598*i*
Bile acids, and colorectal cancer, 717
Bileaflet mechanical heart valve, 428–429, 429*i*
Bile canaliculi, 595, 596*i*
Bile duct(s), 595
  benign tumors of, **619**
  diseases of, **604–624** (*See also specific disease*)
  exploration of
    in choledocholithiasis, 614, 615
    pancreatitis after, 628–629
  hepatic, 566
  injuries to, **619–620**
  malignant tumors of, **617–619**
  obstruction of
    in chronic pancreatitis, **621–622**, 641
    uncommon causes of, **621–624**
  stenosis of, 618
  stones in, **613–615**, 613*i*
  strictures of, **619–620**, 621–622, 623
  tumors of, **617–619**
    versus choledocholithiasis, 614
Bile salts, **596–598**, 599*i*
  for dissolution of gallstones, 606
Biliary atresia, **1333–1335**
Biliary colic, 506, **605–606**
  in choledocholithiasis, 613
Biliary pancreatitis, **627–628**, 634
Biliary surgery, pancreatitis after, 32
Biliary tract, **595–624**. *See also specific structure*
  diagnostic examination of, **599–601**
  diseases/disorders of, in children, 1333–1335
  embryology and anatomy of, **595**, 596*i*, 597*i*
  injuries to, treatment of, 253
  physiology of, **595–598**
Bilirubin, **599**. *See also* Hyperbilirubinemia
  in acute cholecystitis, 608
  after hepatic resection, 568
  in bile duct malignancies, 617, 618
  in choledocholithiasis, 614
  in chronic pancreatitis, 641
  with hepatic abscess, 593
  in hereditary spherocytosis, 656
  in jaundice, 601–602
  in liver cancer, 572
  in metastatic neoplasms of liver, 574
  overload, 32, 32*t*
  in pancreatic adenocarcinoma, 644
  in pancreatitis, 621–622
  in sclerosing cholangitis, 623
Billroth I resection, for duodenal ulcer, 541–542, 542*i*
Billroth II resection
  for duodenal ulcer, 541–542, 542*i*
  pancreatitis after, 629

Biocompatibility, of implantable materials, 95
Biologic heart valves, **428,** 428*i,* 429*i*
Biopsy
  of bone tumor, 1223
  of breast cancer, 319–320, **324–326**
  with bronchoscopy, 349
  core needle, 319, **1353**
  endomyocardial, in heart transplant recipi-
    ent, 1381
  excisional, 319, 1353
  fine-needle aspiration, 283, 319–320, **1353**
  of gastric carcinoma, 558
  of gastric ulcer, 547
  of head and neck tumors, 283
  incisional, 1353
  large-needle (core needle), 319, **1353**
  of liver, in biliary atresia, 1334
  lung, **351**
  mammographic localization, 320
  and mammography, 322–323
  of melanoma, 1364
  needle, **350–351**
  open, 319, **351**
  of pancreatic adenocarcinoma, **645**
  pinch, 283
  pleural, **350–351**
  of prostate cancer, **1068**
  punch, 283
  of renal adenocarcinoma, 1055
  of scalene lymph node, **350**
  of sentinel lymph node, in melanoma,
    1364–1365
  of soft tissue sarcoma, 1362
  testicular, in male infertility, **1080**
  of tumors, **1353**
Biotin, 163
  requirements for, 164*t*
Bird's beak deformity, in sigmoid volvulus,
  739, 740*i*
Bispectral index, 197
Bite(s)
  arthropod, **132–133**
  hand infections from, 1281–1282,
    1283–1284
  human, of hand, 1283–1284
  spider, **132–133**
  venomous, **130–133** (*See also* Snakebite)
  wasp, 132
Biventricular pacing, 418
Black patch syndrome, 34
Black widow spider, 132–133
Bladder
  agenesis of, 1026
  anatomy of, **1015–1017**
    myoneural, **1073**
  anomalies of, **1026–1028**
  areflexic, **1076**
  catheterization of
    prophylactic, 33
    therapeutic, 33
  changes in, in obstructive uropathy, **1030**
  duplication of, 1026
  embryology of, **1013,** 1015*i,* 1016*i*
  endometriosis and, 1096

  exstrophy of, **1027,** 1027*i*
  fistulas of, 1077–1078
  hyperreflexic, 1074*i,* **1075–1076**
  injuries to, 254, **1050–1051,** 1051*i*
  innervation of, **1073–1074**
  myoneurophysiology of, **1074**
  neuropathic (neurogenic), **1073–1076**
    versus benign prostatic hyperplasia, 1034
  obstruction, in elderly men, 69
  overdistention of, 33
  physiology of, **1018**
  stones in, **1046–1047**
  tuberculosis of, 1041
  tumors of, **1062–1066,** 1063*t*
    versus vesical stone, 1047
Bladder outlet, obstruction of, 50
Bladder pressure, during micturition,
  1074–1075
Blalock-Taussig operation, 458, 459*i*
Blalock-Taussig shunt, 465
Blast injury, **264**
Blastomyces dermatidis, 392
Blastomycosis, **392**
  and chronic mediastinitis, 372
  and thoracic empyema, 361
  treatment of, 141
Bleeding
  abnormalities
    screening for, 52
    in surgical patients, **52**
  after cardiac surgery, 436
  with defecation, 769
  in disseminated intravascular coagulation, 58
  gastrointestinal
    in children, **1332**
    with hepatic cirrhosis, 57, 579, 580
  hemorrhoidal, 767
  with hepatic trauma, 569–570
  in leukemia, 53
  in liver disease, 56–57, 579, **580–583**
  with peptic ulcer, 539
  in portal hypertension, 579
  postoperative, 29
  rectal
    history-taking about, 2
    with Meckel's diverticulum, 1330
  in small intestine, 701
  uterine (*See also* Bleeding, vaginal)
    abnormal, **1087–1089**
      with uterine leiomyomas, 1100
    dysfunctional, 1088, 1089
    intermenstrual, 1088, 1107
    postcoital, 1107
  vaginal (*See also* Bleeding, uterine)
    postmenopausal, 1088
      with adenocarcinoma of fallopian tube,
        1110
      in endometrial cancer, 1108
      in pregnancy, with gestational trophoblas-
        tic disease, 1113
  variceal, **580–583**
    clinical findings with, 580–581
    mortality rate for, 580, 581
    in portal hypertension, 579

    with portal venous occlusion, 588
    recurrence of, 583, 584
    signs and symptoms of, 580
    surgery for, 582–583
    treatment of, 581–583
Bleomycin, 47, 1355
  for malignant pleural effusion, 359
Blepharoplasty, **1266**
Blind loop syndrome, **679–680**
Blisters
  with frostbite, 279
  with second-degree burns, 267
Blood
  antibody screen for, 58
  arterial, oxygen saturation of, in mechanical
    ventilation, 216–217
  cross-matching, 58
  preoperative analysis, in newborn surgical
    patient, 1299
  typing, 58
  whole, for transfusion therapy, 60
Blood dyscrasias, and abnormal uterine bleeding, 1087–1089
Blood gases, in pulmonary thromboembolism,
  880
Blood group substances, in gastric juice, 536
Blood loss
  maximum, 107
  in newborn, 1299
Blood oxygen level-dependent contrast imaging, in brain tumors, 923
Blood pressure. *See also* Hypertension; Hypotension
  and amputation level determination, 860
  brachial, in cerebrovascular disease, 849
  in cardiac compressive shock, 206, 207
  control of
    in arteriovenous malformations, 946
    for subarachnoid hemorrhage, 941
  in craniocerebral trauma, 902–903
  elevation of, for subarachnoid hemorrhage,
    942
  in hypovolemia, 203
  in increased intracranial pressure, 890
  in response to injury, 107
Blood substitutes, 62
Blood tests, in acute abdomen, 510–511, 510*t*
Blood transfusion, **58–62.** *See also* Transfusion
  reactions; Transfusion therapy
  allergic reaction to, 60
  amount of blood for
    in adults, 59
    in children, 59
  autologous, prehospital donation for, 61
  bacterial contamination of, 60
  circulatory problems caused by, 60
  complications of, 59–60
  donor-specific, and graft survival in kidney
    transplantation, 1374
  elective, 58
  emergency, 58
  hemolytic reactions in, 59–60
  hepatitis transmission in, 60
  in hypovolemic shock, 205–206

indications for, 49–50, 52
infections transmitted by, 60
intraoperative autotransfusion as, 61
massive, 59
 and fresh frozen plasma, 62
preoperative preparation for, 7
pretransplant, and graft survival in kidney
 transplantation, 1373–1374
rate of, 59
Blood urea nitrogen, 144–145
Blood volume
 expansion of, for subarachnoid hemorrhage,
 942
 intracranial, and intracranial hypertension,
 905–906
Blount's disease, 1184
Blowout fracture, orbital, 1257
Blue dot sign, 1080, 1339
Blue toe syndrome, 50, 827
Blumer's shelf, 718
Blunt trauma
 abdominal, 249–252
 arterial, 257
 to chest, 208
 to neck, 243
 to ocular adnexa, **1009**, 1009*t*
 to orbit, **1009**, 1009*t*
Body cell mass, 159*t*
 assessment of, 156
Body composition
 assessment of, 159*t*
 of elderly, 69–70
 studies of, 156
Body contouring, **1267–1268**
Body mass index (BMI), 159*t*, 190
 assessment of, 156–157
Body temperature. *See also* Fever; Hypothermia; Thermoregulation
 in peripheral arterial insufficiency, 818
 in response to injury, 107, 108
Body weight
 assessment of, 156–158
 ideal, 158*t*
 loss of
 in cancer, 186
 in HIV-infected (AIDS) patients, 189
 in pancreatic cancer, 644
 per unit of time, clinical significance of,
 158*t*
 and surgical risk, 156
 in response to injury, 109, 110
 usual, 158*t*
Boeck's sarcoid, **394–395**
Boerhaave's syndrome, 490
Bogota bag, 520
Boils. *See* Furuncles
BOLD contrast imaging. *See* Blood oxygen
 level-dependent contrast imaging
Bombs, 264
Bone(s)
 cutting cone in, 93
 enchondral formation of, 93
 giant cell tumor of, **1227**, 1227*i*
 growth of, 1176–1177

healing in, 93–94
 manipulation of, 94
 by primary intention, 93–94
 by secondary intention, 93–94
immature, characteristics of, 1177
infection of, 1263 (*See also* Osteomyelitis)
paraneoplastic syndrome involving, 1371*t*
pediatric, systemic disorders affecting,
 1184
in primary hyperparathyroidism, 311, 311*i*
remodeling of, 93
reticulum cell sarcoma of, **1226**
transplantation of, 1237
traumatic bowing of, 1177
tumors of, **1222–1229**
 benign, **1226–1229**
 radiologic characteristics of, 1222
 biopsy of, 1223
 chemotherapy for, 1223
 grading and staging of, 1223
 malignant, **1224–1226**
 radiologic characteristics of, 1222
 metastatic, 1223–1224
 operative technique for, 1222
 radiation therapy for, 1223
 radiologic characteristics of, 1222
Bone conduction hearing, **962–963**
Bone cyst
 aneurysmal, 355, **1227–1228**
 unicameral, **1228–1229**, 1228*i*
Bone grafts, in lower extremity, 1263
Bone marrow
 failure of, in chronic lymphocytic leukemia,
 662
 hyperplasia, in hypersplenism, 654
 in idiopathic myelofibrosis, 663
Bone marrow transplantation (BMT)
 for Hodgkin's lymphoma, 1367
 for non-Hodgkin's lymphoma, 1369
 for Wiskott-Aldrich syndrome, 661
Bone morphogenetic protein, 93
Bone pain, in prostate cancer, 1069
Bony decompression, for increased intracranial
 pressure, **891**
Bony spurs, in cervical disk syndrome, 954
Borborygmus, in colonic obstruction, 713
Borrelia infection, drug therapy for, 136*t*
Botryoid tumors, 1345–1346
Botulinum toxin, indications for, 770
Botulism, 124
Bouttonnière deformity, 1277, 1277*i*
Bowel gas pattern, abnormal, 512
Bowel habits, **709–710**
 change in, history-taking about, 2
 large bowel polyps and, 726
Bowel obstruction. *See* Intestinal obstruction
Bowel preparation, **754–755**
 in pediatric patients, 1300
Bowen's disease, **780–781**, 1249, **1250**
Bowlegs, **1183**
Boyd's perforator, 871, 872*i*
Brachial artery injury, 257
Brachial neuritis, *versus* cervical disk syndrome,
 955

Brachial plexus
 injury to, 1281
 improper positioning and, 195
 pain in, 952
 palsy of, **1184**
Brachial veins, 872
Brachiocephalic vein, 872
Brachydactyly, 1275
Bracing, in osteoarthritis, 1202
Bradycardia
 in craniocerebral trauma, 902–903
 sinus, 45
Brain, 890*i*
 abscess of, 958–960
 blood supply to, 847, 847*i*
 injury of, **900–908**
 surgery, subcortical, for movement disorders,
 947–949
 tumors of, **915–927**, 916*t*, 917*t* (*See also*
 specific tumor)
 in adults, 916*i*
 in children, 915*i*, **935–936**, 936*i*
 investigations for, **923**
 surgery for, intraoperative neurophysiologic monitoring in, 900
 volume of, and intracranial hypertension,
 904–905
Brain stem, tumors in, 915*i*, 916*i*, 923
Brain stem evoked response audiometry, 965
 in skull base surgery, 898
Branchiogenic anomalies, **1300–1301**, 1300*i*
Branham's sign, and arteriovenous fistulas, 846
Brawny edema, 883
BRCA gene mutations
 and adenocarcinoma of fallopian tube, 1110
 and breast cancer, 1111
 and ovarian cancer, 1110–1111
Breach of contract, 75
Breast(s)
 abscess in, **343**
 augmentation, disorders of, **343**
 cancer of (*See* Breast cancer)
 cosmetic surgery of, 1266–1267
 fibroadenoma of, **341–342**
 hypertrophied, reduction of, 1266, 1267
 mass in, evaluation of
 in postmenopausal women, 325, 326*i*
 in premenopausal women, 325–326, 325*i*
 reconstruction of, **337**, **1261–1262**
Breast cancer, **319–337**. *See also* Mastectomy
 and arm edema, 336–337
 bilateral, 329
 biopsy of, 324–326
 breast augmentation and, 343
 diagnosis of
 clinical findings in, 323–326
 tests for, 319–320
 differential diagnosis of, 326
 early detection of, 321–323
 hormone receptor sites for, 329
 imaging of, 324
 incidence of, 320–321
 invasive, 328
 laboratory findings in, 324

Breast cancer (*cont.*)
  during lactation, 328–329
  male, **339–340**
  mymymetastases of, 324
  noninvasive, 328, 329
  paraneoplastic syndromes with, 1371*t*
  pathologic types of, 326–328, 328*t*
  pleural effusion and, 357
  postmenopausal, treatment of, 332, 332*t*,
    334
  pregnancy and, 65–66, 328–329, 337
  premenopausal, treatment of, 331*t*, 332, 334
  prognosis for, 335–336, 335*t*
  recurrence of, 336
  risk factors for, 320–321, 321*t*
  screening programs for, 321–322
  signs of, 319, 323–324
  sites of, 323, 323*i*
  in situ, 328, 329
  special clinical forms of, 328–329
  staging of, 326, 327*i*
  and superior vena caval syndrome, 373
  survival rates of, 335*t*
  symptoms of, 319, 323
  treatment of
    adjuvant, 331–333, 331*t*, 332*t*
    breast-conserving, 330–331
    choice of, 330
    curative, 329–333
    current recommendations for, 331
    follow-up care, 336–337
    palliative, 329–330, 333–335
Breast self-examination, 322
Breathing
  postoperative, 17, 20
  in primary trauma survey, **236–237**
Breath tests
  in blind loop syndrome, 680
  in Crohn's disease, 690
  in gas cysts in small intestine, 701
  in malabsorption, 707
  and orocecal transit time, 677
Breslow classification, of melanoma, 1363,
  1363*t*
Brochardt's triad, 561
Brodie-Trendelenburg test, 873–874
Bronchi
  foreign bodies in, 990
  injuries of, 245
  mucoid impaction of, **387**
  obstruction of
    and bronchiectasis, 385
    in lobar emphysema, 1310
    and lung abscess, 383
    tracheal foreign body and, 990
Bronchial adenomas, 404
Bronchial arteries, 348
  enlargement of, 458
Bronchial gland adenomas, 397
Bronchiectasis, **384–386**
  saccular, 385
  in surgical patient, 47
Bronchitis, 46–47
  chronic, and operative risk, 25
Bronchitis obliterans, 387

Bronchoalveolar carcinoma, 396
Bronchoalveolar lavage, for bronchiectasis, 385
Bronchodilators
  for bronchiectasis, 385
  for inhalation injuries, 276
Bronchogenic cyst, **380**, 1311, **1313**
Broncholithiasis, **386–387**
Bronchopleural fistula, 213
Bronchopneumonia, and bronchiectasis, 385
Bronchopulmonary dysplasia, **380–381**
Bronchopulmonary foregut malformation,
  1313–1314
Bronchoscopy, 26, **349**
  in bronchiectasis, 385
  flexible, 349
  rigid, 349
  in thoracic empyema, 361
  with tracheobronchial foreign body, 990
Brown recluse spider, 133
Brown-Séquard's syndrome, **909**
Brown's sign, 973
Brucella infection, drug therapy for, 135*t*
Bruits
  of cerebrovascular disease, 849
  in peripheral arterial insufficiency, 817
Bryan sign, 64
Budd-Chiari syndrome, 579, **589**
Buerger's disease. *See also* Thromboangiitis
    obliterans
  and small artery occlusive disease, 827
Bulbocavernosus reflex, in spinal cord injury,
  910
Bulking agents
  for diverticulosis, 731
  indications for, 770
Bullectomy, apical, for pneumothorax preven-
  tion, 369
Bundle branch block, left, 45
Bunions. *See* Hallux valgus
Bupivacaine, intercostal block with, 21
Burgess technique, for amputation, 864–865
Burkell's classification, of mediastinum, 347,
  347*i*
Burkholderia mallei infection, drug therapy for,
  135*t*
Burkholderia pseudomallei infection, drug therapy for, 135*t*
Burn(s), **267–270**
  circumferential, 273
  closed therapy for, 272
  depth of, **267–268**, 268*i*
  electrical, **277**
    of hand, **1287**
  first-degree, 267, 268*i*
  flame, 277
  flash, 277, **1008**
  hypermetabolism with, 107
  immunologic factors in, 270
  management of, **270–276**
    acute resuscitation phase, 270–271
    complications of, 273–274
    postresuscitation period, 271
    rehabilitation in, 276
    wound care in, 271–273
  metabolic effects of, 269–270

  nutritional support in, 185–186, 186*t*
  ocular, **1007–1008**
  pathology and pathophysiology of, 268–269
  physiologic response to, 109
  respiratory tract injury and, 274–276
  and response to injury, 103
  second-degree (partial-thickness), 267, 268*i*
  severity of, determination of, 268, 269*i*,
    269*t*
  thermal, of hand, **1286–1287**
  third-degree (full-thickness), 268, 268*i*
  treatment of, 206
Bursitis
  calcific, in shoulder, **1197–1198**
  versus cervical disk syndrome, 955
  of hip, **1200–1201**
  olecranon, **1200**
  subacromial, **1197**
Burst/suppression ratio, in aneurysm surgery,
  899–900
Buschke-Löwenstein tumors, 778
Butchart staging system, for mesothelioma,
  370, 370*t*
Button batteries, ingestion of, **492**
Buttonhole deformity, 1277, 1277*i*
Bypass grafts, for renovascular hypertension,
  855
Bypass surgery
  cardiopulmonary, pancreatitis after,
    628–629
  intestinal, for small bowel obstruction, 687
  for intracranial aneurysm, 941–942
  saphenopopliteal, for chronic venous insuffi-
    ciency, 885

CA 19-9, in pancreatic adenocarcinoma, 644
CA-125
  in endometriosis, 1097
  in ovarian cancer, 1112
  with persistent adnexal masses, 1101–1102
Cachexia
  cancer, 187
    in colorectal cancer, 719
  cardiac, 188
Cadmium, and lung cancer, 396
Café coronary, 990
Caffeine, and mammary dysplasia, 341
Caffeine-halothane contracture test, 202
Calcaneus
  anterior process of, fracture of, **1174**
  body of, fracture of, **1174**
  fracture of, 1118, **1173–1174**, 1173*i*
  tuberosity of, fracture of, **1174**
Calcaneus (term), definition of, 1194
Calcifications
  idiopathic, of mitral valve and annulus,
    422
  in mammography, 322
Calcific tendinitis, in shoulder, **1197–1198**
Calcitonin, 308
  for hypercalcemic crisis, 313
  indications for, 149
Calcitriol
  for hypoparathyroidism, 317
  for hypoparathyroid tetany, 318

Calcium
  absorption of, in small intestine, 678
  for acute pancreatitis, **633**
  balance, **148–149**
  and colorectal cancer, 717
  dietary intake of, 185
  requirements for, 164*t*
  serum levels of, 148 (*See also* Hypercalcemia)
    in acute pancreatitis, 632
Calcium carbonate, indications for, 51
Calcium-channel blockers
  for achalasia, 478
  adverse effects and side effects of, 45
  for angina pectoris, 412
  for atrial dysrhythmias, 437
  for coronary artery disease, 44
  indications for, 801
  for pheochromocytoma, 804
Calcium chloride, and postoperative pancreati-
    tis, 628–629
Calcium gluconate
  for hypoparathyroid tetany, 317
  indications for, 133
  for newborn, 1296
Calcium oxalate calculi
  renal, prevention of, **1044**
  urinary tract, and small bowel syndrome,
    680
Calcium renal stones, prevention of,
    1043–1044
Calculi
  bile duct, **613–615**, 613*i*
  gallbladder, **603–606**, 603*i*
  genitourinary, **1042–1048**
  prostatic, *versus* prostate cancer, 1069
  renal, **1042–1045**
  salivary gland, **987**
  staghorn, 1043*i*
  ureteral, **1045–1046**, 1045*i*
  urinary tract
    ileostomy and, 753*t*
    and small bowel syndrome, 680
  vesical, **1046–1047**
Calf muscle pump, function of, in chronic ve-
    nous insufficiency, 884
Calf vein thrombosis, 875
Callus, 93
Caloric reflex, in craniocerebral trauma, 902
Caloric stimulation test, in assessment of dizzi-
    ness, 975
Calories. *See* Energy
Calretinin stain, 370
Camptodactyly, 1275
Campylobacter infection, drug therapy for, 135*t*
Campylobacter jejuni infection
  enteritis caused by, **694**
  in HIV-associated enteropathy, 693–694
  versus ulcerative colitis, 742–743
Canals of Hering, 595
Cancer. *See also* Metastatic disease
  adjuvant therapy for, 1354
  Barrett's esophagus and, 488
  breast (*See* Breast cancer)
  cervical, **1106–1108**
  colorectal (*See* Colorectal cancer)

and deep vein thrombosis, 875
  definition of, 1352
  differential diagnosis of, 358*t*
  endometrial, 1088, 1089, **1108–1109**
  epidemiology of, 1352
  gastric, **556–559**, 557
    early, 557
    paraneoplastic syndromes with, 1371*t*
    staging of, 558*i*
  gastrointestinal, paraneoplastic syndromes
    with, 1371*t*
  hepatic
    metastatic, **574–576**
    primary, **571–574**
  hypercalcemia in, 149, 311, 1370, 1371*t*
  of lung (*See* Lung cancer)
  metastases of (*See also* Metastatic disease)
    to liver, **574–576**
  nutritional support in, 186–187
  occult, manifestations of, 1370–1371
  ovarian (*See* Ovarian cancer)
  palliative surgery for, 1354
  of prostate (*See* Prostate gland, cancer of)
  serum alpha-fetoprotein levels in, 572
  skin
    basal cell, **1250–1251**
    squamous cell, **1251–1252**
  staging, surgical procedures in, 1353–1354
  surgical resection of, 1354
  testicular, **1070–1072**, 1071*t*
    in cryptorchid testis, 1338
  treatment of (*See also* Radiation therapy)
    biologic (immunotherapy), **1357–1358**
    hormonal, **1356–1357**
    regional, **1358–1359**
    response to, 1352
    role of surgical oncologist in, **1353–1354**
    systemic, **1354–1358** (*See also*
      Chemotherapy)
  uterine (*See also* Cancer, endometrial)
    paraneoplastic syndromes with, 1371*t*
  vaginal, **1105–1106**
  vulvar, 1104–1105
Cancer cachexia, 187
  in colorectal cancer, 719
Cancer family syndrome, 716–717
Cancer pain, **950**
Candida albicans
  and bezoars, 562
  and burn infections, 274*t*
  colitis caused by, 127
  and lung abscess, 383
Candidiasis (*Candida* infection), 112
  drug therapy for, 140
  oral (thrush), **985**
    in AIDS, 998
  treatment of, 141
Canker sores, **985**
  in AIDS, 998
Capillary hemangioma, 1246, 1341
  of eyelid, 1010
Capillary malformations, 1342
Capreomycin, for tuberculosis, 388*t*
Capsulotomy, for cataracts, 1004–1005, 1005*i*
Captain of the ship doctrine, 79

Carbenicillin. *See also* Penicillin,
    antipseudomonal
  dosage of
    in hepatic failure, 138*t*
    in renal failure, 138*t*
  pharmacology of, 138*t*
Carbidopa, for Parkinson's disease, 948
Carbohydrates
  dietary, 184–185
  digestion of, in small intestine, **678**
  and intestinal gas, 707
  metabolism of
    in cancer patient, 186–187
    colonic, 707
Carbon dioxide (CO_2), partial pressure of
  in arterial blood ($PaCO_2$), 214, 221*t*
    elevation of, causes of, 223
  in mixed venous blood ($PmvCO_2$), 221*t*
Carbon monoxide poisoning, 274–275, 274*t*
  treatment of, 275–276
Carbuncles, **125–127**
Carcinoembryonic antigen (CEA), in colorectal
    cancer, 719–720
Carcinogenesis, in large intestine, 717
Carcinoid syndrome, 703–704, 804
Carcinoid tumors, 404, 404*t*
  of appendix, 672, 703
  of bronchial gland, 397
  of large intestine, **729**
  of small intestine, **703–704**
Carcinoma. *See also* Cancer
  adenoid cystic, 397, 404
  adrenocortical, **811**
    as adrenal incidentaloma, 811–812, 812*t*
    aldosterone-producing, 799, 800, 811
    prognosis for, 810, 811
    treatment of, 809, 811
  anal, **781–782**
  bronchoalveolar, 396
  of colon (*See* Colorectal cancer)
  of conjunctiva, **1011**
  Crohn's disease and, 691
  definition of, 1352 (*See also* Cancer)
  of gallbladder, **616–617**
  intraepidermal, **1249–1250**
  poorly differentiated, 1352
  of prostate gland (*See* Prostate gland, cancer
    of)
  of rectum (*See* Colorectal cancer)
  renal cell, **1054–1058**, 1056*i*, 1057*i*, 1058*t*
  undifferentiated, 1352
Carcinoma in situ
  cervical, 1106–1108
  vaginal, 1105
Cardia, of stomach, 533
Cardiac arrest
  posttraumatic, **234**
  treatment of, in field, 232
Cardiac cachexia, 188
Cardiac catheterization, 42, 412
  for aortic insufficiency, 427
  for aortic stenosis, 426–427
  for congenital heart disease, 439
  for mitral regurgitation, 423
  for mitral stenosis, 421

Cardiac catheterization (*cont.*)
  for tricuspid valve disease, 425–426
Cardiac compressive shock, in trauma victim, **240**
Cardiac disease. *See* Heart, diseases/disorders of
Cardiac hemodynamic values, 411, 411*t*
Cardiac index, 220, 221*t*
Cardiac massage, open, 238, 238*i*
Cardiac output
  age-related changes in, 67
  low, after cardiac surgery, 436
  measurement of, 220
  in response to injury, 107
Cardiac stapling, 247, 247*i*
Cardiac surgery
  complications of, management of, 436–437
  future directions in, 471
  postoperative care for, **435–437**
Cardiac tamponade
  after cardiac surgery, 436
  in cardiac trauma, 247
Cardiac tumors, **434–435,** 434*t,* 435*f,* **469–470**
Cardiac (type 2) venous return, 455, 456*i*
Cardiogenic shock, in trauma victim, **240**
Cardiomyopathy
  achalasia and, 479
  hypophosphatemic, in total parenteral nutrition, 181
  surgery for, 417–418, 418*t*
Cardiomyoplasty, 418
Cardiopulmonary arrest, emergency room thoracotomy for, 238–239, 238*i*
Cardiopulmonary bypass, 413
  for atrial septal defect, 450
  for congenital heart disease, 439–440
  pancreatitis after, 32, 628–629
  for thoracic aortic aneurysm, 432
Cardiopulmonary failure, in total parenteral nutrition, 181
Cardiovascular system
  adrenergic discharge, in shock, 210
  age-related changes in, 67–68, 68*t*
  disorders of
    manifestations of, 205*t*
    pleural effusion and, 359–360, 360*i*
    preoperative evaluation for, 42
  in response to injury, 107
  in shock, **203–210**
Carnett's test, 509
Carney's complex, 806
Carnitine, for peripheral arterial insufficiency, 821
Caroli's disease, **621,** 1334
Carotid artery(ies)
  atherosclerosis of, coronary artery atherosclerosis coexistent with, 851
  extracranial, aneurysm of, **840–841**
  injuries to, 257
  internal, 890*i*
    aneurysm of, 939
    dissection of, **852**
    stenosis of, 848*i*
    thrombosis of, 893*i*
  surgery on, and postoperative stroke, 34

Carotid body, tumors of, **840–841,** 841*i*
Carotido-ophthalmic artery aneurysm, 896*i*
Carpal boss, 1288
Carpal tunnel, 1272, 1272*i*
Carpal tunnel syndrome, **1280**
  endoscopic release of, 1280, **1291–1292**
Carpentier annuloplasty ring, 423, 424*i*
Carpometacarpal joint, of small finger, fracture-dislocation of, 1149
Carpus (carpal bone), 1143
  dislocation of, 1147
  dissociation of, 1147
  fracture-dislocation of, 1147–1148
  fractures of, **1146–1148**
  traumatic instability of, 1147–1148
Cartilaginous rests, preauricular, 1301
Castration, for male breast cancer, 340
Catabolic response, 103, 105*t,* 108, 162, 168
  in burn patient, 186
  in cancer patient, 186–187
  in sepsis, 169, 169*i*
Cataract, **1004–1005**
  congenital, **1004**
  extracapsular extraction of, **1004–1005,** 1005*i*
  senile, **1004–1005**
Catecholamines, 106
  assays for, drugs affecting, 803
  excess, with pheochromocytoma, 802
  free, urinary, in diagnosis of pheochromocytoma, 803
  in response to injury, 107
Catheter(s)
  femoral, complications of, 36
  radial, complications of, 36
  Silastic, 36
  suction, for hepatic abscess, 594
  for total parenteral nutrition, 178
    infection of, 181, 182*t*
  venous
    in hypovolemic shock, 205
    and phlebitis, 36
Catheterization. *See also* Central venous catheter/catheterization
  cardiac (*See* Cardiac catheterization)
  urinary
    in benign prostatic hyperplasia, 1035
    in urethral injury, 1052, 1053*i*
    and urinary tract infections, 1036–1037
Cat-scratch fever, 112, 1304
  versus lymphangitis, 887
Cauda equina, motor roots in, intraoperative monitoring of, 899
Cauda equina syndrome, **910,** 953
Cauliflower ear, 970
Causalgia, 914. *See also* Reflex sympathetic dystrophy
Causation
  factual, 78
  proximate (legal), 78
Cavernous hemangioma, 1246, 1247*t,* **1248–1249,** 1341, 1349
  of chest wall, 354, 355
  of eyelid, 1010

Cavernous internal carotid artery, aneurysms of, 939
Cavernous malformations, 934, 945
Cavitating lesions, and lung abscess, 383
C-D-xylose breath test, for blind loop syndrome, 680
Cecal bascule, 738–739
Cecal volvulus, **739,** 740
Cecostomy
  for large bowel obstruction, 715, 715*i*
  for volvulus, 740
Cecum, 706*i*
  perforation of, in large bowel obstruction, 714
Cefazolin
  for acute cholecystitis, 609
  for cholangitis, 612
  dosage of
    in hepatic failure, 139*t*
    in renal failure, 139*t*
  pharmacology of, 139*t*
  renal failure and, 51, 139*t*
Cefixime, indications for, 135*t*
Cefoperazone, indications for, 135*t*
Cefotetan
  dosage of
    in hepatic failure, 139*t*
    in renal failure, 139*t*
  pharmacology of, 139*t*
Cefoxitin
  for cholangitis, 612
  dosage of
    in hepatic failure, 139*t*
    in renal failure, 139*t*
  indications for, 135*t,* 136*t*
  pharmacology of, 139*t*
Ceftazidime
  dosage of
    in hepatic failure, 139*t*
    in renal failure, 139*t*
  indications for, 135*t*
  pharmacology of, 139*t*
Ceftriaxone
  dosage of
    in hepatic failure, 139*t*
    in renal failure, 139*t*
  indications for, 135*t,* 136*t*
  for perianal chancroid, 778
  pharmacology of, 139*t*
Cefuroxime
  dosage of
    in hepatic failure, 139*t*
    in renal failure, 139*t*
  pharmacology of, 139*t*
Celecoxib, 51
  for cervical spondylotic myelopathy, 1209
Celiac plexus block, for chronic pancreatitis, **642**
Cell-mediated immunity. *See* Immunity, cell-mediated
Cell membrane, failure of, in shock, 211
Cell transplantation, for Parkinson's disease, 948
Cellulitis, **123**

versus lymphangitis, 887
orbital, **1003**
Cellulose sodium phosphate, for calcium renal stones, 1044
Centers for Disease Control and Prevention
National Nosocomial Infections Surveillance (NNIS), 121
Rabies Section website, 128
recommendations, for prevention and treatment of tetanus, 127
Central cord syndrome, **909**
Central nervous system (CNS)
age-related changes in, 68*t*, 69
infections of
consciousness in, 888
surgical, 958–961
postoperative complications in, **34**
tumors of, **915–927**, 916*t*, 917*t*
in adults, 916*i*
in children, 915*i*, **935–936**, 935*t*
Central venous catheter/catheterization
cardiopulmonary complications of, 36
in hypovolemic shock, 205
Central venous pressure, postoperative monitoring of, 14
Cephalic phase, of acid secretion, 538
Cephalic vein, 872
Cephalosporin(s)
for acute secondary bacterial peritonitis, 519
and antibiotic-associated colitis, 749
for appendicitis, 671
for cholangitis, 612
indications for, 135*t*
for primary peritonitis, 527
for ulcerative colitis, 744
Cerebellar atrophy, as paraneoplastic syndrome, 1371, 1371*t*
Cerebellar dysarthria, 1209
Cerebellopontine angle, neoplasms of, 915*i*, 916*i*, **923**, 975–976
Cerebellum, 890*i*
tumors in, 915*i*, 916*i*
Cerebral aqueduct, 890*i*
obstruction of, 934
Cerebral arteries, 890*i*
middle, infarction of, 893*i*
Cerebral blood flow, autoregulation of, in elderly, 69
Cerebral edema, in elderly, 69
Cerebral hemispheres, tumors in, 915*i*, 916*i*, **922**
Cerebral hypoxia, 458
Cerebral infarction, 847, 895*i*
Cerebral ischemia, in elderly, 69
Cerebral metabolism, and intracranial hypertension, 905–906
Cerebral palsy, spastic, 937
Cerebral perfusion pressure, 889
Cerebral thrombophlebitis, **960**
Cerebral veins, 890*i*
aneurysms of, 934
Cerebrospinal fluid
absorption of, congenital disorders of, **934**
circulation of, 890*i*
congenital disorders of, **934**

drainage of, for increased intracranial pressure, **891**
examination of
in brain abscess, 959
in brain tumors, 923
in intracranial aneurysms, 940
leakage of
in nasal trauma, 983
in temporal bone fractures, 972
volume of, and intracranial hypertension, **904**
Cerebrovascular accident, postoperative, **34**
Cerebrovascular disease, **846–853**, 848*i*
clinical findings in, 848–849
sites of, 847, 847*i*
surgical results for, 852
treatment of, 849–852
Ceruloplasmin, 158
Cervical collar
for cervical spondylotic myelopathy, 1209
for cervical strain, 1205
for whiplash injury, 1206
Cervical disk syndrome, **953–955**
Cervical dysphagia, 475
Cervical esophageal webs, 481
Cervical fasciitis, necrotizing, 997
Cervical intraepithelial neoplasia, 1106, 1108
Cervical lymphadenopathy, in pediatric patients, **1303–1304**
Cervical mucus penetration test, 1080–1081
Cervical myeloradiculopathy, 1208
Cervical spine
disk degeneration in, **1206–1210**
disk herniation in, **953–955**
differential diagnosis of, 1205
fractures of
odontoid (hangman's), 910
treatment of, 243
imaging of, 1119–1120
injury of, 242
associated injuries, 1118
clinical assessment of, 1117–1118
complications of, 1120
external support for, 1123, 1125*i*
incidence of, 1117
with neurologic injury, 1123
treatment of, 243
pain in, 1204–1205
protection of
in craniocerebral trauma, 903
during intubation, 215
spondylosis, **1206–1210**
differential diagnosis of, 1205
Cervical spondylotic myelopathy, 1207–1208
differential diagnosis of, 1208–1209
prognosis for, 1210
treatment of, 1209–1210, 1210*i*
Cervical spondylotic radiculopathy, 1207
differential diagnosis of, 1208
prognosis for, 1210
treatment of, 1209, 1209*i*
Cervical (muscle) strain, **1204–1205**
Cervicitis, chronic, 1107
Cervix, uterine
carcinoma in situ of, 1106–1108

carcinoma of, **1106–1108**
clinical findings in, 1107
complications of, 1107
differential diagnosis of, 1107
lymph node involvement in, 1106–1107
prevention of, 1107
prognosis for, 1108
staging of, 1106, 1106*t*
treatment of, 1108
cytology of, 1088
Cestodes. *See* Echinococcosis
Chagas' disease, 477
and large intestine volvulus, 738
"Chain of lakes" appearance, of chronic pancreatitis, 641
Chamberlain procedure, **350**
Chancroid, perianal, 778
Charcot deformity, 96
Charcot's triad, 612
Charles procedure, for lymphedema, 887
Chauffeur's fracture, 1144
Chédiak-Higashi syndrome, **661–662**
Cheiragra, **1286**
Chemical burns, of eye, **1007–1008**
Chemoattraction, 113
Chemoembolization, arterial, in primary hepatic cancer, 574
Chemoprevention, for head and neck tumors, 297
Chemoradiotherapy
for cervical cancer, 1108
for epidermoid carcinoma of anal canal, 781
Chemotherapy
adjuvant, 1355
for lung cancer, 403
adverse effects and side effects of, 1356
agents for, classes of, 1355
for bladder tumors, **1064–1065**, **1065**
for bone tumors, 1223
for brain tumors, **926**
for breast cancer, 331, 331*t*, 332*t*, 334–335
male, 340
for colorectal cancer, 723
concomitant, 297
cytotoxic, **1354–1356**
for endometrial cancer, 1109
for esophageal carcinoma, 498
for Ewing's sarcoma, 356
for gastric carcinoma, 559, 560
for gestational trophoblastic disease, 1114–1115
for head and neck tumors, 296–297
for Hodgkin's lymphoma, 1366–1367
induction, 297, 1354
with irradiation, 297
for laryngeal cancer, 291
for lung cancer, 398–401, 402–403
for melanoma, 1365
for metastatic neoplasms of liver, 575
for neuroblastoma, 1344
for non-Hodgkin's lymphoma, 1368–1369
for ovarian cancer, 1112
for pancreatic adenocarcinoma, 646
regional delivery of, **1358–1359**
for renal pelvis and calices tumors, 1061

Chemotherapy (*cont.*)
for sarcomas, 1362
for spinal cord tumors, 928
teratogenicity of, 1356
for testicular cancer, 1072
for thymic carcinoma, 379
for thymoma, 378–379
for thyroid cancer, 307
for tuberculosis, 389
for ureteral tumors, 1062
for Wilms' tumor, 1345
for Zollinger-Ellison syndrome, 546
Chenodeoxycholate, 597
Chest injury. *See also* Thoracic injuries
traumatic, 236–237
Chest pain
in pulmonary thromboembolism, 880
severity of, classification of, 411
with thoracic aortic dissection, 433
Chest wall
anatomy of, **344**, 345*i*, 346*i*
congenital deformities of, **1305–1306**
diseases of, **352**
infections of, **352–353**
physiology of, **344–346**
reconstruction of, **353**
trauma to, **244–245**
tumors of, **353–356**
benign skeletal, 354–355
benign soft tissue, 354
malignant skeletal, 355–356
malignant soft tissue, 354
metastatic, 356, 356*i*
Chest x-ray(s)
in aortic insufficiency, 427
in aortic stenosis, 426
in heart disease, 42
in mitral regurgitation, 423
in pulmonary thromboembolism, 880
in subclavian vein thrombosis, 879
in ventilatory management, 219
Chiari malformations, **932**
Child(ren). *See also* Infant(s); Juvenile; Newborn; Premature infant
abdominal wall defects in, **1339–1341**
abuse of (*See* Battered child syndrome)
acute appendicitis in, **1328**
airway obstruction in, **992–994**
anorectal anomalies in, **1324–1327**
bones of, systemic disorders affecting,
1184
bowel preparation in, 1300
brachial plexus palsy in, 1184
caloric requirements of, 1297, 1297*t*
cervical lymphadenopathy in, **1303–1304**
chest wall deformities in, **1305–1306**
constipation in, 1321–1322
cutaneous vascular anomalies in, **1341–1342**
elbow fractures and dislocations in,
1180–1181
endotracheal intubation in, 1294–1295
enteral alimentation for, 1297
esophageal anomalies in, **1313–1315**, 1313*i*
fluid requirements in
for maintenance, 1295, 1296*t*

perioperative management of,
1295–1296, 1296*t*
foot deformities in, **1194–1196**
forearm fractures in, 1181
gait disorder in, **1183**
gastroesophageal reflux in, **1327–1328**
gastrointestinal bleeding in, **1332**
gastrointestinal foreign bodies in,
1332–1333
gastrointestinal tract in
abnormalities of, **1327–1333**
congenital lesions of, **1313–1327**
duplications of, 1328–1329, 1329*i*
great vessel anomalies in, **1311**, 1311*i*
head and neck lesions in, **1300–1304**
inguinoscrotal disorders in, **1336–1339**,
1336*i*
intussusception in, **1323–1324**, 1323*i*
joints of
inflammation of, 1184
systemic disorders affecting, 1184
juvenile rheumatoid arthritis in, 1184
laryngotracheal stenosis in, 992
limb deformity in, **1183–1184**
liver neoplasms in, **1347–1349**
liver transplantation in, 1384
lobar emphysema in, **1310–1311**
lower extremity of
angular deformity of, 1183–1184
fractures and dislocations in, 1181–1183
lymphadenitis in
granulomatous, **1304**
pyogenic, **1303–1304**
mediastinal masses in, **1311–1312**
necrotizing enterocolitis in, **1331**
neurosurgery in, **931–937**
NPO guidelines for, 1299–1300
orthopedics in, **1176–1197**
parenteral nutrition for, 1297–1299
scoliosis in, **1185–1189**
septic arthritis in, 1220–1222
sinusitis in, 980
spinal deformity in, **1185–1189**
subluxation of radial head in, 1180
temperature regulation in, 1294
total parenteral nutrition for, 1297–1299,
1298*t*
traumatic hip dislocation in, 1181
tumors in, **1342–1349**
upper extremity fractures and dislocations
in, **1179–1181**
ventilation for, 1294–1295
Child-Pugh classification, of functional status
in liver diseases, 582, 583–584,
583*t*
Chlamydial proctitis, 777
Chlamydia pneumoniae infection, drug therapy
for, 136*t*
Chlamydia psittaci infection, drug therapy for,
136*t*
Chlamydia trachomatis infection
versus Crohn's disease, 748
drug therapy for, 136*t*
in epididymitis, 1040
versus ulcerative colitis, 742–743

Chlorambucil, 1355
for thyroid cancer, 307
Chloramphenicol
dosage of
in hepatic failure, 138*t*
in renal failure, 138*t*
indications for, 135*t*, 136*t*
pharmacology of, 138*t*
Chlordiazepoxide, for craniocerebral trauma,
904
Chlorhexidine gluconate, 12
Chloride
absorption of
in colon, 707
in large intestine, 709, 709*t*
in small intestine, 677–678
loss of, in gastrointestinal fluid, 147*t*
Chloride:phosphate ratio, 311
Chlorpropamide, perioperative management
of, 38
Chlorthalidone, indications for, 51
Choanal atresia, **1307**
Cholangiocarcinoma, 571–574
choledochal cyst and, 1334
Cholangiography
in choledocholithiasis, 614, 615
in jaundice, 603
in pancreatitis, 621–622
percutaneous transhepatic
in bile duct malignancies, 617–618
in biliary tree examination, **600**
in jaundice, 602
retrograde, in chronic pancreatitis, 641
Cholangiohepatitis, Oriental (recurrent pyogenic cholangitis), 621, **623**
Cholangiopancreatography, endoscopic retrograde
in acute pancreatitis, 632
in bile duct malignancies, 617–618
for biliary tree examination, **600**
in choledocholithiasis, 614
in gallstone disease, 605–606
in jaundice, 602
in pancreatic adenocarcinoma, **645**
in pancreatic ascites, 639
in pancreatic pseudocyst, 636
in pancreatitis, 621–622
in sclerosing cholangitis, 623
Cholangitis, **612**
bacterial, **612**
choledochal cyst and, 1334
in pancreatic adenocarcinoma, 644
recurrent pyogenic (Oriental cholangiohepatitis), 621, **623**
sclerosing, **623–624**
bile duct malignancies and, 618
suppurative, **612**
Cholate, 597
Cholecystectomy
for acute cholecystitis, 609–610, 610*i*
for acute pancreatitis, 634
bile duct injuries in, **619–620**
complications of, 32
failure of, to relieve symptoms, **615–616**,
622

for gallbladder carcinoma, 616–617
for gallstone ileus, 612
for gallstones, 605, 606
for hereditary spherocytosis, 656
intestinal motility after, 677
laparoscopic, and response to injury, 101
in pregnancy, 64–65
prophylactic, for asymptomatic gallstones,
605
Cholecystenteric fistula, **609**
in gallstone ileus, 611
Cholecystitis
acalculous, 607
acute, **607–610**
chemical, 33
chronic, gallstones and, **605–606**
differential diagnosis of, 515, 540, 554
emphysematous, **611**
ischemic, 33
postoperative, **33**
in pregnancy, 64–65
suppurative, 608
Cholecystitis glandularis proliferans, of gallbladder, 619
Cholecystography
in benign tumors and pseudotumors of gallbladder, 619
for biliary tree examination, **600**
in gallstone disease, 605
Cholecystojejunostomy
for bile duct malignancies, 618
for pancreatic adenocarcinoma, 646
Cholecystokinin
bile flow affected by, 596
pancreatic secretion affected by, 625–626
Cholecystokinin test, **643**
in chronic pancreatitis, 640
Choledochal cyst(s), 1334, **1335**
congenital, **621**
Choledochojejunostomy, for pancreatic adenocarcinoma, 646
Choledocholithiasis (common bile duct
stones), **613–615**, 613i
versus bile duct malignancies, 618
versus biliary stricture, 620
Cholelithiasis (gallstones)
asymptomatic, **604–605**
and chronic cholecystitis, **605–606**
versus colorectal cancer, 721
ileostomy and, 753t
pathogenesis of, **603–604**, 603i
in pregnancy, 64–65
in short bowel syndrome, 682
Cholera
drug therapy for, 135t
pancreatic, **650**
Cholerrheic diarrhea, 679
Cholestasis
benign postoperative intrahepatic, 32
intrahepatic, versus choledocholithiasis, 614
Cholesteatoma, keratinizing aural, in chronic
otitis media, 967
Cholesterol, dietary, 185
Cholesterol gallstones, **603–604**
Cholestyramine, for sclerosing cholangitis, 624

Chondritis, 970
Chondroblastoma, **1229**
Chondroblasts, in fracture healing, 93
Chondroitin sulfate, for osteoarthritis, 1202
Chondroma. See also Enchondroma
of chest wall, 354
Chondrosarcoma
of chest wall, 355
grading of, 1223
primary, **1225**
secondary, 1226
in skull base, 921, 925, **927**
Chopart's amputation, 863
Chordee
in hypospadias, 1028
in Peyronie's disease, 1082
Chordomas, in skull base, 921, 925, **927**
Chorioadenoma destruens, 1112, 1113
Choriocarcinoma, 1072
hydatidiform mole and, 1113–1114
nongestational, mediastinal, 377
ovarian, 1110
Choroid plexus, 890i
carcinoma of, **919**
hemangioma of, 1011
papilloma of, **919**, 924, 926
and cerebrospinal fluid overproduction,
934
Chow technique, for endoscopic carpal tunnel
release, 1291–1292
Christmas tree atresia, 1317, 1317i
Chromium
deficiency of, 164
and lung cancer, 396
requirements for, 164t
Chromosomal abnormalities, omphalocele and,
1340
Chromosome deletions, and lung cancer, 396
Chronic cystic mastitis. See Mammary dysplasia
Chronic lymphocytic leukemia (CLL), 662
Chronic obstructive pulmonary disease
(COPD)
lung transplantation for, 369
operative risk in, 25, 111
postoperative analgesia in, 18
in surgical patient, **47**
Chronic organizing empyemas, 360–361
Chronic venous insufficiency, **883–885**
Chronotropic agents, for cardiogenic shock,
208
Chylopericardium, 247
Chylothorax, 247, 357, **367**
Chylous ascites, 528–529
Chymopapain, for lumbar disk syndrome, 958
Cigarette smoking
and colorectal cancer, 717
and infrarenal abdominal aortic aneurysms,
830
and ulcerative colitis, 741
Ciliary body, blunt trauma to, 1009t
Ciliary muscle, blunt trauma to, 1009t
Cilostazol, for peripheral arterial insufficiency,
821
Cimetidine
for duodenal ulcer, 541

indications for, 26, 194, 201
and postoperative psychosis, 34
for reflux esophagitis sliding hiatal hernia,
486
for Zollinger-Ellison syndrome, 545–546
Cineradiography, 473
Ciprofloxacin
for bronchiectasis, 385
for Campylobacter enteritis, 694
dosage of
in hepatic failure, 138t
in renal failure, 138t
indications for, 135t, 136t
for perianal chancroid, 778
pharmacology of, 138t
Circle of Willis, 896i
Circular muscle, of colon, 707i
Circulation
hyperdynamic, in response to injury, 107
in primary trauma survey, **237–238**
Circulatory hypoperfusion, 814
Circumflex coronary artery, 408, 409i
Cirrhosis, **580**
alcoholic
versus choledocholithiasis, 614
liver transplantation for, 1383–1384
in childhood, 1349
gastrointestinal bleeding with, 57, 579, 580
and hypersplenism, 653–654
and liver cancer, 571–574
mortality rate for, 580
pleural effusion and, 360
and portal hypertension, 578–579
and primary peritonitis, 527
and wound healing, 24
Cisapride, for intestinal pseudo-obstruction,
686
Cisplatin, 1355
Cisterna chyli, 674
Cisternography, 897
Cladribine, for hairy cell leukemia, 663
Clarithromycin
for duodenal ulcer, 541
indications for, 136t
Claudication, intermittent, in peripheral arterial insufficiency, 815–816
Clavicle, fracture of, **1128**, 1129i
Clavulanic acid
amoxicillin and, combined, indications for,
135t
beta-lactam and, combined, for primary
peritonitis, 527
mechanism of action of, 140
ticarcillin and, combined, for acute secondary bacterial peritonitis, 519
Cleft hand, 1260
Cleft lip, **1257–1259**
Cleft palate, **1257–1259**
and auditory tube dysfunction, 965
Pierre Robin syndrome and, 1307
Cleland's ligament, 1270, 1271i
Clindamycin
for acute cholecystitis, 609
for acute secondary bacterial peritonitis,
519

Clindamycin (*cont.*)
  and antibiotic-associated colitis, 749
  for cholangitis, 612
  dosage of
    in hepatic failure, 138*t*
    in renal failure, 138*t*
  indications for, 126–127, 135*t*, 136*t*
  for lung abscess, 384
  pharmacology of, 138*t*
Clipping, of intracranial aneurysm, 941
Cloaca, persistent, 1026–1027
Clofazimine, indications for, 136*t*
Clomiphene, indications for, 1089
Clonidine suppression test, 803
Clonorchis sinensis, and hepatic cancer, 571
Clopidogel, for cerebrovascular disease prevention, 850
Closed-chest catheter, for pneumothorax, 368
Closed disk space infections, **960**
Clostridium spp.
  in emphysematous cholecystitis, 611
  in feces, 710–711
  infection by, 112
    drug therapy for, 136*t*
Clostridium, and peritonitis, 518
Clostridium botulinum, 124
Clostridium difficile
  colitis caused by, **127,** 749
    postoperative, **33**
  diarrhea caused by, in enteral feeding, 174
Clostridium novyi, 124
Clostridium perfringens, 124
  in cholangitis, 612
  colitis caused by, 127
Clostridium ramosum, and lung abscess, 383
Clostridium septicum, 124
Clostridium tetani, 124. *See also* Tetanus
Clotting factor(s)
  concentrates, for transfusion therapy, 61–62
  deficiency of
    in liver disease, 56
    in surgical patients, **56**
    in pulmonary failure, 219
    in stored blood, 59, 60
Clubbing, of fingers and toes, 458
Clubfoot, **1195**
  pectus excavatum with, 1305
"24 cm" perforator, 872*i*
CMV regimen
  for bladder tumors, 1065
  for ureteral tumors, 1062
Coagulation. *See also* Disseminated intravascular coagulation (DIC)
  mediators of, in acute respiratory distress syndrome, 212
  in wound healing, 86–87
Coagulation factor(s). *See* Clotting factor(s)
Coagulation necrosis, 268
Coagulopathy
  in craniocerebral trauma, 903
  postoperative, 29
  and renal disease, 50
  treatment of, 59
Coarctation of the aorta, **445–446**

abdominal, **829**
Cobb method, for measurement of spinal deformity, 1185, 1186*i*
Cobras, 130
Cocaine packets, ingestion of, **492**
Cocci
  in feces, 710–711
  gram-negative, infection by, drug therapy for, 135*t*
  gram-positive, infection by, drug therapy for, 135*t*
Coccidioides immitis, 391
  and thoracic empyema, 361
Coccidioidomycosis (*Coccidioides* infection), 112, **391–392**
  skin tests for, 349
Cochlear implants, for sensorineural hearing loss, 968–969
Cochlear nerve, intraoperative monitoring of, 898
Cockcroft-Gault equation, 49
Cockett perforators, 871, 872*i*
Codman's triangle, 1224, 1225*i*
Coffee bean shape, in volvulus, 739
Cohen procedure, for vesicoureteral reflux, 1026
Coils, for intracranial aneurysm, 942
Coin lesions. *See* Solitary pulmonary nodule
Coins, ingested, **492**
Colchicine, for gout, 1286
Cold, common. *See* Common cold
Colectomy
  for Crohn's disease, 748
  for familial adenomatous polyposis, 728
  ileostomy after, 752*i*
  for lower gastrointestinal bleeding, 737
  for ulcerative colitis, 745, 745*i*, 746
Colic, 506–507
Colic arteries, 705, 706*i*
Colic lymph nodes, 718*i*
Colitis, **740–750.** *See also* Ulcerative colitis (UC)
  agranulocytic, 750
  antibiotic-associated, **127, 748–749**
  Candida albicans, 127
  Clostridium difficile, **33, 127,** 749
  Clostridium perfringens, 127
  collagenous, 743
  Crohn's (granulomatous), **746–748**
  diversion, **743**
  indeterminate, 743
  ischemic, 743, **749–750**
  in large bowel obstruction, 714
  neutropenic, **750**
  pseudomembranous, 749
  Salmonella, 127
  Staphylococcus aureus, 127
  ulcerative, **741–746**
    versus Crohn's disease, **691**
Collagen, in wound healing, 87, 87*i*, 88–89, 90, 90*i*
Collagenase, 90
  for lumbar disk syndrome, 958
Collagen disease, differential diagnosis of, 358*t*

Collagenous colitis, 743
Collar-button abscess, 126, 1282
Colles fracture, 1144
Collis procedure, 487
Colloids, artificial, 62
Colon. *See also* Large intestine; Neonatal small left colon syndrome
  absorption in, **708–709,** 709*t*
  anatomy of, **705,** 706*i*, 707*i*
  atresia and stenosis of, 1317–1318
  cancer of, **716–724,** 716*i* (*See also* Colorectal cancer)
    in colovesical fistula, 735
    Crohn's disease and, 748
    versus diverticulitis, 733
    in ulcerative colitis, 743–744
    versus ulcerative colitis, **743**
  dilation of
    in Crohn's disease, 748
    in ulcerative colitis, **743,** 744*i*
  diseases of, **712–750** (*See also specific disease*)
  diverticular disease of, **730–735,** 730*i*
  duplication of, 1328–1329, 1329*i*
  injuries to, treatment of, 254
  obstruction of, 712–715, 713*i*, 713*t*
  perforation of, in ulcerative colitis, **743**
  physiology of, **707–710**
  polyps of, **725–728,** 725*t*
  preoperative preparation of, **754–755**
  resection of
    for angiodysplasia, 738
    for cancer, 721–722, 722*i*
    for diverticulitis, 734–735, 734*i*
    intestinal motility after, 677
    for lower gastrointestinal bleeding, 736–737
    for volvulus, 740
  strictures of, in ulcerative colitis, **743**
  tumors of, **729**
Colon cutoff sign, in acute pancreatitis, 632
Colonic inertia, 709–710, 762
Colonic lavage, intraoperative, 715
Colonic transit time, 762
Colonoscopy, 762, 764, 767
  for angiodysplasia, 738
  in children, 1332
  for colorectal cancer, 719, **721**
    follow-up, 724
  for colovesical fistula, 735
  for Crohn's disease, 748
  diagnostic, 712
  for diverticulitis, 733
  for diverticulosis, 731
  fiberoptic, **712**
  indications for, 712*t*
  for large bowel polyps, 724, **726,** 727
  for lower gastrointestinal bleeding, 736, 737*i*
  for ulcerative colitis, 742, 744
Color duplex imaging, for peripheral arterial insufficiency, 819
Colorectal cancer, **716–724**
  and colonic obstruction, 713*t*
  direct extension of, 717–718, **723**
  metastases of, 717–718

hematogenous, **718**
intraluminal, **718**
lymph node, **718**, 718*i*
transperitoneal, **718**
screening for, 718–719
staging of, 723, 724*t*
in ulcerative colitis, 746
Colostomy, **752–754**
end (terminal), 752, 754*i*
for large bowel obstruction, 714, 715
loop, 752
sigmoid (iliac), 752
transverse, 715, 753
Colovesical fistula, **735**
Colpectomy, 1093
Colpocleisis, 1093
Colporrhaphy
anterior, 1093
posterior, 1093
Columns of Morgagni, 756
CoLyte. *See* Polyethylene glycol-electrolyte solution
Coma
definition of, 888
differential diagnosis of, 238
in Glasgow Coma Scale, 902
hyperosmolar, postoperative, **40**
myxedema, 40
in trauma victims, **238**
Commissurotomy, for tricuspid stenosis, 426
Common bile duct, 595, 597*i*, 626*i*
exploration of
in choledocholithiasis, 614, 615
complications of, 32
pancreatitis after, 628–629
stones in, **613–615**, 613*i* (*See also* Choledocholithiasis)
Common cold, 46, **978**
Common femoral vein, injuries of, 262
Common hepatic duct, 595
Common peroneal nerve, injury to, improper
positioning and, 195
Common ventricles, and single ventricle, 467
Communicating diverticulitis, 732
Communicating veins, 871
Compartment syndrome, **1143, 1169–1170**
in upper extremity, **1280**
Complete atrioventricular canal defect, 451,
451*i*, 452
Complete vascular rings, 382
Complex regional pain syndrome, 914
Complications
of anesthesia, **201–202**
in elderly, 67
of endotracheal intubation, 196–197
of enteral feeding, 174, 180*t*
of excisional hemorrhoidectomy, 768
of extubation, 197
of hemodynamic monitoring, **35–36**
of hepatic resection, 568
intraoperative, cardiac, 41
of intravenous therapy, **35–36**
of kidney transplantation, 1378–1379
of liver transplantation, 1385–1386

perioperative, pulmonary, 46
postoperative, **23–37**, 199
cardiac, **28–29**, 41
central nervous system, **34**
drain-related, **30**
peritoneal, **29–30**
prevention of, 23
psychiatric, **34–35**
respiratory, **25–27**
urinary, **33–34**
wound, **23–25**
of radiation therapy, 1361
of sliding inguinal hernia repair, 790
of spinal anesthesia, 198
of surgical infections, 114–115
of total parenteral nutrition, 180*t*, 181–184,
182*t*–184*t*
of wrist arthroscopy, 1291
Composite resection, for oral cavity cancer,
287
Compression
pneumatic, for lymphedema, 886
sclerotherapy, for varicose veins, 875
stockings for
for chronic venous insufficiency, 884
for deep vein thrombosis, 877
for lymphedema, 886
for varicose veins, 874, 875
Computed tomography (CT)
abdominal, 37
in trauma, 251
of abscesses, 117
of acute abdomen, 513
of acute mesenteric vascular occlusion, 699
of acute pancreatitis, 632
of adrenal incidentalomas, 811
of adrenal masses, 797
of aldosteronoma, 800
of anorectum, 1326
indications for, 772
of arteriovenous malformations, 944
of bile duct malignancies, 617
of bladder tumors, **1063**
of brain abscess, 959, 960
in cervical disk syndrome, 954
of choledocholithiasis, 614
of chronic otitis media, 967
of colorectal cancer, 720
of colovesical fistula, 735
of congenital hip dislocation, 1191
in craniocerebral trauma, 903
of cystic neoplasms of pancreas, 647
in diverticulitis, 732
of focal nodular hyperplasia of liver, 578
of hand, 1273
helical scan mode for, 892
of hepatic abscess, 593
of hepatic adenomas, 577
of hepatic trauma, 569–570
in Hodgkin's lymphoma, 1366
of hydrocephalus, 934
in hyperadrenocorticism (Cushing disease,
Cushing syndrome), 808
in hyperaldosteronism, 800

of infrarenal abdominal aortic aneurysms,
831
of intracranial aneurysms, 939–940
of intraperitoneal abscesses, 523–524
in ischemic colitis, 750
in jaundice, 602–603
of kidney injury, 1048
of large intestine, 711
of liver cancer, 572
in lumbar disk syndrome, 957
of lung cancer, 398, 405–406
of metastatic neoplasms of liver, 574–575
of neuroblastoma, 1343
in neurodiagnosis, **892–893**, 893*i*
in obstructive uropathy, **1031**
of pancreatic abscess, 639
of pancreatic adenocarcinoma, **645**
of pancreatic ascites, 639–640
of pancreatic pseudocyst, 636, 636*i*
of paranasal sinusitis, 980
pelvic, 37
of pheochromocytoma, 802, 803–804, 805
of prostate cancer, 1067
of pulmonary disorders, 351
of renal adenocarcinoma, **1055**, 1056*i*,
1057*i*
of renal pelvis and calices tumors, 1060
of renal stones, 1042
of small bowel obstruction, 685
of soft tissue sarcoma, 1361
of spinal cord injury, 910
of spinal cord tumors, 928
of spinal injury, 910, 1120
spiral
in acute appendicitis, 669
in pulmonary thromboembolism, 881,
881*i*
of spleen size, 654
of splenic abscesses, 664
xenon, 897
Computed tomography angiography, in intracranial aneurysms, 940
Computed tomography myelography,
895–896
Concussion, 901
Conduction bundle, 466
Conductive hearing loss, **962**, 964*i*, **965–968**
in otosclerosis, 968
Condylomata acuminata, **1082**
anal, **777**
Condylomata lata, 776, 777
Conexus intertendineus, 1273*i*
Confusion
and neurosurgery for movement disorders,
948–949
postoperative, in elderly, 70
Congenital adrenal hyperplasia, 810
Congenital arteriovenous fistulas, 1020
Congenital aural atresia, 973
Congenital cataract, **1004**
Congenital choledochal cysts, **621**
Congenital diaphragmatic hernia, **1308–1309**,
1309*i*
Congenital flaccid larynx, 992

Congenital heart disease, **45, 439–471**
   decreasing pulmonary arterial blood flow,
      458–468
   diagnosis of, 439
   increasing pulmonary arterial blood flow,
      449–458
   management of, 439–440
   postoperative, 440
   omphalocele and, 1340
   transplantation for, 470
Congenital hemolytic jaundice, **655–656**
Congenital malformations
   of abdominal wall, 796, **1339–1341**
   of chest wall, **1305–1306**
   of ear, **973, 1259–1260,** 1301
   of esophagus, **1313–1315,** 1313*i*
   of female reproductive system, **1085–1086**
   of female urinary tract, 1085
   of gastrointestinal tract, **1313–1327**
   of genitourinary tract, **1018–1029**
   of hands, **1260, 1275**
   of head and neck, **1257–1260**
   of nervous system, **931–935**
   of nose, **983–984**
   of oral cavity, **986**
   of rectum, **1324–1327,** 1325*i*, 1326*i*
   of scrotum, 1029
   of vagina, **1085–1086**
Congenital neurovesical dysfunction, **1027**
Congenital subglottic stenosis, 992
Congenital tumors, **920–921**
Congestive heart failure, **44**
   versus chronic venous insufficiency, 884
   differential diagnosis of, 358*t*
   and pleural effusion, 359
   postoperative, 29
Conjoined tendon, 784
Conjunctiva
   foreign bodies in, **1009–1010**
   tumors of, **1011**
Conjunctivitis, 1001*t*, **1002**
Consciousness
   assessment of, **888–891**
   brain abscess and, 959
   depressed states of, **888–891**
   levels of, 888
Consent. *See also* Informed consent
   implied, in emergency, 81
   incompetent patient and, 82
   minors and, 82
   refusal of, 81
   substituted, 82
Constipation, 709–710, 710*t*
   abdominal pain and, 507
   in children, 1321–1322
   in colonic obstruction, 713
Constriction ring syndrome, 1260, 1275
Consultation(s)
   legal definition of, 75
   preoperative, 5, 10
   psychiatric, 3, 34, 35
Continent ileostomy, 751
Continuous epidural analgesia, **21**
Continuous positive airway pressure

for inhalation injuries, 276
   for obstructive sleep apnea syndrome, 989
   for pediatric patients, 1295
Contraception, **1090–1092**
   efficacy of, 1091–1092
   intrauterine (*See* Intrauterine device (IUD))
   oral (*See* Oral contraceptives)
   subdermal implant, 1091
Contracture(s), 90–91, **1244**
   amputation and, 867–868
   flexion, 867–868
Contrast media, in computed tomography, 892
Contrast nephropathy, risk factors for, 50
Contrast x-ray studies, for acute abdomen, 512
Contusion, intraparenchymal, 907
Conus medullaris compression, **910**
Convalescence, 14, 15
Convalescent care, 6
Convulsions, postoperative, **34**
Cooley's anemia, **657**
Cooper's ligament, 784
Cooper's ligament (Lotheissen-McVay) repair
   for femoral hernia, 791
   for inguinal hernia, 788
Copper
   deficiency of, 164
   requirements for, 164*t*
   serum levels of
      high, in total parenteral nutrition, 184*t*
      low, in total parenteral nutrition, 184*t*
Copperhead, 130
Coral snake(s), 130, 132
Cordotomy, for malignant pain, 950
Core needle biopsy, **1353**
Cori cycle, 165–166, 166*i*
Corium, 267
Cornea
   blunt trauma to, 1009*t*
   foreign bodies in, **1009–1010**
   infection of, 1001*t*
   trauma to, 1001*t*
   ulcers of, **1002–1003**
Corneal reflex, in craniocerebral trauma, 902
Corona phlebectatica paraplantaris, 873
Coronary arterial fistula, **455**
Coronary arteriography, 42, 412
Coronary arteriovenous fistulas, 382
Coronary artery(ies)
   atherosclerosis of, 409–410
      carotid artery atherosclerosis with, treat-
         ment of, 851
   distribution of, 465
   origins of, 465
Coronary artery disease, **43–44,** 408
   operative risk in, 43
   reoperation for, 415–416
   risk factors for, 410, 411*t*
Coronary blood flow, 408
Coronary bypass
   for angina pectoris, 413–414, 413*i*
   comparison with other procedures, 415
   graft patency in, 414*t*
   for postinfarction ventricular septal defect,
      416

Coronary revascularization, 412
Coronary stents, 415
Coroner, investigation by, 83–84
Corpus, of stomach, 533
Corpus callosum
   surgery of, for intractable seizures in chil-
      dren, 937
   tumors in, 915*i*, 916*i*
Corrected transposition of the great arteries,
   466–467
Corrosive esophagitis, **493–494,** 494*t*
Corticospinal tract(s), 1117
Corticosteroid(s). *See also* Steroid(s); *specific agent*
   and abdominal pain, 507–508
   adverse effects and side effects of, 41, 1379
   for allergic bronchopulmonary aspergillosis,
      393
   anticancer therapy with, **1356**
   for asthma, 47
   for Bell's palsy, 977
   for brain abscess, 960
   and colonic diverticulitis, 731
   for Crohn's disease, 692
   and fungal infections of lung, 390
   in heart transplantation, 470
   for immune thrombocytopenic purpura, 660
   indications for, 132, 133
   for inhalation injuries, 276
   for intra-arterial injections, 858
   for male breast cancer, 340
   pancreatitis and, 629
   and postoperative psychosis, 34
   for rheumatoid arthritis, 1204
   for sarcoidosis, 395
   for secondary hemolytic anemia, 658
   for thymoma, 379
   for transplant recipient, **1375,** 1381, 1385
   and ulcerative colitis, 743
   for ulcerative colitis, 744
   and wound healing, 16
Corticotropic adenomas, 921
Corticotropin-releasing hormone (CRH),
   103–104
Cortisol, 106
   actions of, 167–168
   adrenal adenomas secreting, 810
   for adrenal insufficiency, 41
   plasma level of, midnight, in hyperadreno-
      corticism (Cushing disease, Cushing
      syndrome), 808
   secretion of, in hyperadrenocorticism (Cush-
      ing disease, Cushing syndrome), 806
   in shock, 210–211
   stress dose of, 41
Cor triatriatum, **448–449**
Corynebacterium diphtheriae infection
   drug therapy for, 136*t*
   pharyngitis caused by, 988
Corynebacterium jeikeium infection, drug therapy for, 136*t*
Corynebacterium parvum, 359
Coryza, **978**
Cosmetic surgery, **1264–1269**
Costal cartilage, infection of, **352–353**

Costochondritis, 353
Costovertebral angle tenderness, 510
Cottonmouth, 130
Coughing, to elicit pain, in abdominal examination, 509
Coumarin
  for acute mesenteric vascular occlusion, 700
  for lymphedema, 886
  in surgical patients, 55
Counseling, preoperative, 34
Courvoisier's sign, 644
Coxa plana. *See* Legg-Perthes disease
Cranial meningiomas, **920**
Cranial nerves. *See also specific nerve*
  assessment of, in craniocerebral trauma, **902**
  dysfunction of, with head and neck tumors, 283
  intraoperative monitoring of, 897–898
Craniocerebral trauma, **900–908**
Craniofacial anomalies, **1259**
Craniofacial dysostosis, 1259
Craniofacial surgery, advances in, 1230, 1259
Craniofacial syndromes, **932**
Craniopharyngioma, 925, **926–927**
  adamantinomatous, 920
  in children, **936**
  papillary, 920
Craniosynostosis, **932**, 932*t*
Craniotomy
  for brain tumors, 925
  for epidural hematoma, 906
  for intracranial aneurysm, 941
  for pituitary tumors, 931
Cranium bifidum, encephalocele with, 933
Creatine kinase, in acute mesenteric vascular occlusion, 699
Creatinine
  in prune belly syndrome, 1027
  serum levels of, 49, 144–145
    in diabetic patient, 38
    in renal failure, 50
    in ureteropelvic junction obstruction, 1032
Creatinine clearance, 49
Creatinine-height index, 158*t*, 159*t*, **160**
Credé's maneuver, for areflexic bladder, 1076
Cremasteric reflex, in spinal cord injury, 910
Cremaster muscle, 783
Crepitus, in necrotizing infections, 124
Cricoid cartilage, fracture of, 991
Cricopharyngeal achalasia, **475**
Cricopharyngeus, foreign bodies in, 492
Cricothyroidostomy, 214, 215
Cricothyroidotomy, in trauma care, 236, 236*i*
Crohn's disease (CD), **689–692, 746–748**
  differential diagnosis of, 769, 772, 778
  and diverticulitis, 733
  fistulas in, 773–774, 1094
  versus ischemic colitis, 750
  "metastatic," 691
  and postoperative convulsions, 34
  rectovaginal fistula in, 773–774
  small bowel involvement in, 689–692
  versus ulcerative colitis, 743, 747*t*
  ulcerative colitis and, 741

Cronkhite-Canada syndrome, **728**
Cross-trigonal repair, for vesicoureteral reflux, 1026
Crotalidae, 130
Crotalus spp., 130
Crouzon's syndrome, 932, 1259
Crush injury(ies), **264**
  of hand, **1288–1289**
Cryohemolysis test, for hereditary spherocytosis, 656
Cryoprecipitate, indications for, 57, 58, 61
"Cryptic" vascular malformations, 945
Cryptococcosis, **392–393**
  drug therapy for, 140
Cryptococcus neoformans, 140, 392
Cryptogenic emboli, and arterial occlusion, 825
Cryptorchidism, **1338–1339**
  and testicular cancer, **1070**
  Wilms' tumor and, 1344
Cryptosporidium, in HIV-associated enteropathy, 693–694
Crypts of Lieberkühn, 674, 677*i*
Crystalloid, 62
  indications for, 205
Cubital tunnel syndrome, 1280
Cubital vein, median, 872
Cuboid bone, fractures of, **1174–1175**
Cullen's sign, in acute pancreatitis, 631
Culling, in spleen, 652
Culture, microbial, in surgical infection, 115–117
Cuneiform bone, fractures of, **1174–1175**
Curettage, plus electrodesiccation, for basal cell carcinoma, 1250–1251
Curling's ulcers, with burns, 273–274
Cushing reflex, 209
Cushing response, 890
  in craniocerebral trauma, 902
Cushing's disease. *See* Hyperadrenocorticism (Cushing disease, Cushing syndrome)
Cushing's syndrome. *See* Hyperadrenocorticism (Cushing disease, Cushing syndrome)
Cushing's ulcer, 556, 890
Customary practice standard, 80
Cutis marmorata, 843
Cutting cone, in bone, 93
Cyanocobalamin. *See* Vitamin B$_{12}$
Cyanosis, right-to-left shunt and, 458
Cyclooxygenase (COX) 2 selective inhibitor(s), 1204
  for cervical spondylotic myelopathy, 1209
Cyclophosphamide, 1355
  for breast cancer, 331–332, 332, 334
  for carcinoid tumor of intestine, 704
  doxorubicin, Oncovin, and prednisone (CHOP) regimen
    for non-Hodgkin's lymphoma, 1368
    for nonlymphoid lymphomas, 1369–1370
  for Ewing's sarcoma, 356
  for gastric carcinoma, 560
  for secondary hemolytic anemia, 658

Cycloserine, for tuberculosis, 388*t*
Cyclosporine
  adverse effects and side effects of, 1379, 1380, 1381, 1383
  for Crohn's disease, 692, 748
  for transplant recipient, **1375**, 1381, 1385
    in heart transplantation, 470
  for ulcerative colitis, 744
Cylindric bronchiectasis, 385
Cylindromas. *See* Adenoid cystic carcinomas
Cyproheptadine, for carcinoid syndrome, 704
Cyst(s), **1245**. *See also* Bone cyst
  Bartholin, **1095**
  branchiogenic, **1301**
  bronchogenic, 380, 1311, **1313**
  of chest wall, 355
  choledochal, 1334, **1335**
    congenital, 621
  corpus luteum, 1101
  dermoid, **1245, 1300**
  echinococcal, and chronic mediastinitis, 372
  epidermal, of hand, 1288
  epidermal inclusion, **1245**
  esophageal, 495
    congenital, 495
  follicular, 1101
  Gartner duct, **1095**
  hepatic, **576–577**
  mediastinal, 376
  mesenteric, **531**
  of omentum, **532**
  ovarian, 1097
    functional, 1101
    rupture of, 1101
  preauricular, 973, 1301
  renal, simple, 1020, **1076**
  retroperitoneal, **531**
  sebaceous, vulvar, **1095**
  splenic, **664**
  thymic, 1311
  thyroglossal, 1302–1303, 1302*i*
  umbilical, 1330
  urachal, 1026
Cystadenocarcinoma
  pancreatic, 637, 647
  papillary, *versus* simple renal cyst, 1076
Cystadenoma, 647
  mucinous, 66
  mucocele of appendix and, 673
  pancreatic, 637
  serous, 66
Cystectomy, for bladder tumors, 1065
Cystic adenomatoid malformation, congenital, **381–382**, 1313
Cystic anomalies, congenital, of lungs, **379–382**
Cystic artery, 597*i*
Cystic duct, 595, 597*i*
Cystic fibrosis, **387**
  and bronchiectasis, 384
  and infection control, 385
  lung transplantation for, 369
  management of, 1320
  meconium ileus in, 1320

Cystic fibrosis (*cont.*)
and small bowel obstruction, **684**
Cystic hygroma, **1301–1302**, 1302*i*
Cystic medial necrosis, and extracranial carotid
artery aneurysm, 840
Cystine renal stones, **1044**
Cystitis, **1039**
interstitial, 1078
postoperative, 33–34
Cystocele, 1093
Cystogastrostomy, for pancreatic pseudocyst,
637
Cystography
in bladder injury, 1051
in urethral injury, 1053*i*
Cystolitholapaxy, for vesical stone, 1047
Cystometrography, 1074*i*
Cystometry, **1074**, 1074*i*
Cystosarcoma phyllodes, 342
Cystoscopy
in bladder tumors, 1064, 1064*i*
in colovesical fistula, 735
in diverticulitis, 733
in interstitial cystitis, 1078
Cystourethrography, in vesicoureteral reflux,
1025, 1025*i*
Cystourethroscopy, for renal pelvis and calices
tumors, 1060
Cytadren. *See* Aminoglutethimide
Cytarabine, 1355
Cytochrome oxidase, 163–164
Cytokines, 115, 116*t*–117*t*, 1357
in burn catabolism, 186
in nonspecific immunotherapy, 1357–1358
in sepsis, 169*i*
in wound healing, 86, 89, 91–92
Cytology
in bladder tumors, 1064
in prostate cancer, 1067–1068
in renal adenocarcinoma, 1055
in renal pelvis and calices tumors, 1060
Cytomegalovirus (CMV) infection
in HIV-associated enteropathy, 693–694
in liver transplant recipient, 1386
Cytopenia, in hypersplenism, 653
Cytoreductive surgery, for brain tumors, 924

Dacarbazine, 1355
for glucagonoma, 651
Dacron graft replacement, for thoracic aortic
aneurysm, 432
Dacryocystitis, **1003**
Dactinomycin, 1355
for Ewing's sarcoma, 356
for gestational trophoblastic disease,
1114–1115
Dalteparin, 54
Damages, in medical negligence actions, 79–80
caps on, 79–80
exemplary (punitive), 80
general, 79
special, 79
Danazol
for endometriosis, 1098

for mammary dysplasia, 341
Dancing eyes, 1343
Dantrolene, for malignant hyperthermia, 202
Dapsone, indications for, 133, 136*t*
Darvocet. *See* Propoxyphene
David procedure, for thoracic aortic aneurysm,
432
DCC gene, and colorectal cancer, 717
D-Dimer plasma levels
in deep venous thrombosis, 876
in pulmonary thromboembolism, 880
Deafened, prelingually or postlingually, 968
Death(s)
attributable to medical error, 84
early, 230, 244
immediate, 230
late, 230
later, 244
leading causes of, 408, 409*i*
pneumonia-related, 26, 27
DeBakey classification scheme, for thoracic
aortic dissection, 432, 433*i*
Debridement
for arterial injuries, 243
for burns, 272–273
in soft tissue injury, 1254
4-Debrisoquine hydroxylase, and lung cancer,
396
Debrisoquine metabolic phenotype, and lung
cancer, 396
Debulking, of brain tumors, 924
Decerebrate posturing, in craniocerebral
trauma, 902
Decompression
bony, for increased intracranial pressure,
891
for cervical disk syndrome, 955
for colonic pseudo-obstruction, 714
for large bowel obstruction, 714
for lumbar disk syndrome, 957
for small bowel obstruction, 687
in spinal cord injury, 912
for spinal cord tumors, 928
for volvulus, 739–740
Decorticate posturing, in craniocerebral
trauma, 902
Decubitus ulcers, **95,** 1118. *See also* Pressure
sores
spinal cord injury and, 912
Deep brain stimulation
for dystonia, 949
for essential tremor, 949
for Parkinson's disease, 948
Deep tendon reflexes
in cervical disk syndrome, 954
in spinal cord injury, 910, 911*i*
Deep venous thrombosis, **875–877**
postoperative, 877
in pulmonary thromboembolism, 880
risk factors for, 9
in spinal cord-injured patient, 1120
Defamation, 76
Defecation
frequency of, 709

obstructed, 709–710, 710*t*, 759, **762–764,**
763*i*, 767
physiology of, 708
Defecography, 760, 762, 764, 767
Defenses, in medical negligence actions, 80
Defibrination syndrome. *See* Disseminated in-
travascular coagulation (DIC)
Degenerative aneurysms, 829
and atherosclerosis, 814
Degenerative diseases, consciousness in, 888
Deglutition, 474, 474*i*
Dehydration
and heat stroke, 278
in small bowel obstruction, 684
Delirium
in elderly, 70
postcardiotomy, **35**
postoperative, 34
Delirium tremens, **35**
Delorme procedure, 764
Deltoid ligament, tear of, 1171–1172
Denis Browne bar splinting, for clubfoot,
1195
Denonvilliers, rectovesical fascia of, 705
Dentate line, 756, 757
Deoxycholate, 597
Depression
and chronic pelvic pain, 1089–1090
postoperative, 34
and tinnitus, 971
De Quervain's tenosynovitis, **1278**
Dermatitis
glucagonoma and, 650–651
radiation, **1249**
Dermatomyositis, as paraneoplastic syndrome,
1371*t*
Dermis, 267
artificial, 1232
Dermoid cyst, **1245, 1300**
Dermoid tumors, **920, 925**
δ-6 Desaturase, 163
Descending aorta aneurysm, 432
Descending colon, 706*i*
Descending perineum syndrome, 759, 762
Descending thoracic dissection, 433–434, 434*i*
Desensitization therapy, for allergic rhinitis,
978
Desert fever, 391
Desert rheumatism, 391
Desflurane, depth of anesthesia with, signs of,
197*t*
Desmoid tumors, 728, 796, 1361
Desmopressin, indications for, 55, 56, 57
Detrusor areflexia, 1075
Detrusor-sphincter dyssynergia, 1075
Developmental anomalies, of genitourinary
tract, **1018–1029**
Developmental anterior-posterior diameter
(DAPD), in subaxial cervical spine,
1207, 1207*i*
Dexamethasone
for acute otitis media, 970
for brain tumors, 924
for laryngotracheobronchitis, 993

Dexamethasone suppression test, 806–808, 807*i*

Dextran(s)
  as blood substitutes, 62
  for intra-arterial injections, 858

Dextrocardia, 468

Dextrose
  5% in saline, 18, 18t
  5% in water, 18t
  for newborn, 1296–1297

Diabetes mellitus
  and adrenal insufficiency, perioperative management of, 41
  and amputations, 859
  anorectal infection in, 772
  carbuncles in, 126
  in chronic pancreatitis, **640–641**
  chronic ulcers in, 96
  esophageal involvement in, 480
  glucagonoma and, 650–651
  immunity in, 114
  intraoperative management of, 38–40
  osteomyelitis in, 1217–1218
  in pancreatic adenocarcinoma, 644
  pancreatic transplantation in, 1386
  postoperative care for, 40
  preoperative management of, 38–40
  and renal disease, 50
  and small artery occlusive disease, 827
  in surgical patient, **38–40**
  type 1 (insulin-dependent), 39–40
  type 2 (non-insulin-dependent), 38–39

Diabetic macular edema, laser treatment for, **1012**

Diabetic nephropathy, kidney transplantation for, 1372

Diabetic retinopathy, proliferative, panretinal photocoagulation for, **1012**

Diabetic vascular disease, **827–828**

Diagnostic workup, 6

Dialysis, indications for, 51, 55, 56

Diapedesis, 113

Diaphanography, 322

Diaphragm, **500–502**
  anatomy of, 500–501, 500*i*
  eventration of, **1310**
  injuries of, **247**
  rupture of, cardiac compressive shock caused by, 206, 207
  tumors of, **502**

Diaphragmatic breathing, 344

Diaphragmatic hernia, congenital, **1308–1309,** 1309*i*

Diarrhea, 709
  abdominal pain and, 507
  in blind loop syndrome, 679
  in carcinoid syndrome, 703
  cholerrheic, 679
  in Crohn's disease, **690**
  in enteral feeding, 174
  in HIV-infected (AIDS) patients, 189
  ileostomy and, 753t
  infectious, in children, 1332
  osmotic, 709

in pancreatic cholera, 650
postoperative, in *Clostridium difficile* colitis, **33**
postvagotomy, 544
in small bowel syndrome, 680, 681
in ulcerative colitis, 741

Diastasis recti, 792

Diastematomyelia, **932**

Diatrizoate sodium, indications for, 31

Diazepam
  for craniocerebral trauma, 903, 904
  indications for, 194
  for Meniere's disease, 975
  for penetrating or perforating ocular injuries, 1008–1009

Diazoxide, for insulinoma, 649

Die punch fracture, 1144

Diet(s), **184–185**
  and colorectal cancer, 717
  for Crohn's disease, 691–692
  diverticulosis and, 731
  elemental, 171
  for excessive intestinal gas, 707
  for ileostomy, 751
  lactose-free, 185
  low-residue, 185
  optimal, 184–185
  postoperative, 15, 19
  progressive, 185
  regular, 185
  in renal stone prevention, 1043, 1044
  for short bowel syndrome, 682
  supplemental, for cancer patients, 187

Diethylenetriamine pentaacetic acid, in radionuclide imaging, 897

Diethylstilbestrol (DES)
  for breast cancer, 333t, 334
  for prostate cancer, 1069

Diffuse esophageal spasm, **475–477,** 476

Diffuse goiter, **304**

Diffuse subaortic stenosis, 443–444

Digestion, 538, **677–679**

Digit(s). *See also* Thumb
  amputation of, in crush injuries of hand, **1288–1289**
  clubbing of, 458
  dislocations of, **1149–1150,** 1150*i*
  ischemic necrosis of, 36
  ligamentous injuries in, **1150**

Digitalis
  for heat stroke, 279
  indications for, 29, 208
  renal failure and, 51

Digital subtraction angiography (DSA)
  for cerebrovascular disease, 849
  in neurodiagnosis, **896**
  for peripheral arterial insufficiency, 819

Digoxin
  adverse effects and side effects of, 45
  for atrial dysrhythmias, 437
  indications for, 29

1,25-Dihydroxyvitamin D (1,25-dihydroxyvitamin D$_3$), 49

Diltiazem, for angina pectoris, 412

Diphenhydramine
  for aphthous stomatitis, 985
  indications for, 132
  seizures and, 274

2,3-Diphosphoglycerate, 221, 221t

Diplopia, 1000
  orbital fracture and, 1256–1257

Direct fluorescent antibody test, in diagnosis of rabies, 128

Disability Rating Scale, 907

Discitis, 1213, 1214*i*

Discography, in lumbar disk syndrome, 957

Disconnective surgery, for intractable seizures in children, 937

Discovery rule, 80

Discrete subaortic stenosis, 443–444

Disease-modifying antirheumatic drugs, for rheumatoid arthritis, 1204

Disinfectants, 119

Diskectomy, lumbar
  closed disk space infection following, 960
  for lumbar disk syndrome, 958, 1214

Disk herniation. *See* Intervertebral disk(s), herniation of

Dislocation(s)
  acromioclavicular, **1129**
  of ankle joint, **1171–1172**
  carpal, **1146–1148**
  in children, **1176–1183**
  of digits, **1149–1150,** 1150*i*
  of distal radioulnar joint, 1146
  elbow, **1133–1135,** 1139–1140, 1139*i*
  with frostbite, 280
  hand, **1148–1150,** 1279
  of hip, **1154–1157,** 1154*i*
    anterior, 1155
    congenital, 1188, **1189–1192,** 1191*i*
    posterior, 1154–1155, 1154*i*
    traumatic, **1154–1157,** 1154*i*
      in children, **1181**
  of knee joint, **1161–1162**
  lunate, 1147–1148
  metacarpal, **1279**
  midtarsal, **1175**
  of patella, **1161**
  pelvic, **1123–1127**
  perilunate, 1147–1148
  of phalanges of toes, **1176**
  of shoulder joint, **1130–1132**
  spinal, **1117–1123**
  sternoclavicular, **1129**
  of subtalar joint, 1172–1173
  of talonavicular joint, 1172–1173
  tarsometatarsal, **1175**
  traumatic, of hip joint, **1154–1157,** 1154*i*
    in children, **1181**
  wrist, **1279–1280**

Dissecting aneurysms, 938
  of aorta, **852**

Dissection
  arterial, and arterial occlusion, 825
  neck (*See* Neck dissection)
  thoracic aortic, **432–434,** 434*i*

Disseminated intravascular coagulation (DIC), 53, 55, **57–58**
in liver disease, 57
as paraneoplastic syndrome, 1371*t*
Distal arterial reconstruction, for peripheral arterial insufficiency, 823–824
Distal ileal obstruction syndrome, 1320
Distraction osteogenesis, 94, 1230
Diuresis, in hemolytic transfusion reaction, 59
Diuretics
for ascites, 590
for cardiogenic shock, 208
indications for, 29, 801
for lymphedema, 886
for mitral regurgitation, 423
osmotic, for increased intracranial pressure, **891**
thiazide
and hypercalcemia, 312
pancreatitis and, 629
for renal stones, 1043
Diversion colitis, 743
Diverticula
colonic, **730–735**
giant, 730
sites of, 730*i*
versus colorectal cancer, 721
duodenal, **562, 622–623**
gastric, **562**
intestinal, acquired, **688,** 688*i*
jejunal, 688, 688*i*
urachal, 1026
urethral, 1028
female, 1079
Diverticulitis, 185
colonic, **731–735**
and colonic obstruction, 713*t*
in colovesical fistula, 735
communicating, 732
and hepatic abscess, 593
noncommunicating, 732
Diverticulosis
colonic, **730–731**
of gallbladder, 619
jejunal, 688
Dizziness. *See also* Vertigo
clinical assessment of, **974–975**
Dobutamine, for cardiogenic shock, 208
Docosahexaenoic acid, 163
Doctor-patient relationship. *See* Physician-patient relationship
Doctrine of proportionality, 81
Dodd's perforator, 871, 872*i*
Dog-ear, correction of, 1241, 1241*i*, 1242*i*
Doll's eye reflex, in craniocerebral trauma, 902
Do-not-resuscitate order, 81–82
Dopamine
for craniocerebral trauma, 903
for heat stroke, 279
indications for, 29, 51
for renal dysfunction after cardiac surgery, 437
Dopamine hydroxylase, 164

Doppler ultrasonic flowmeter, in acute mesenteric vascular occlusion, 699
Doppler ultrasonography
in arterial injuries, 259
in small bowel obstruction, 687
Dorsal root entry zone procedure
for spinal cord injury pain, 952
for spinal nerve root avulsion pain, 952
Dorsal veins, 872
Double bubble sign, 627, 1316, 1319
Double-duct sign, 618
pancreatic adenocarcinoma and, 645
Double-inlet ventricles, and single ventricle, 467
Double-outlet right ventricle, 449, **467**
Double-switch procedure, 467
Double vision, 1000
in brain tumors, 922
Doxorubicin, 1355
for breast cancer, 332, 334
for carcinoid tumor of intestine, 704
for Ewing's sarcoma, 356
for gastric carcinoma, 559
for leiomyosarcoma, 1110
for malignant pleural effusion, 359
for thyroid cancer, 307
Doxycycline
for *Campylobacter* enteritis, 694
indications for, 136*t*
for malignant pleural effusion, 359
for *Yersinia* enteritis, 694
Drain(s)
closed suction, 30
complications of, **30**
latex Penrose, 30
postoperative management of, 15, **16–17**
Silastic, 30
sump, 17
and wound healing, 24
Drainage
of abscess, 117–118, 384, 525–526, 525*i*, 639, 664
for appendicitis, 671
catheter, for retroperitoneal abscesses, 526
of cerebrospinal fluid, for increased intracranial pressure, 891
for chronic pancreatitis, **641–642,** 641*i*
closed, 16–17
for diverticulitis, 734
open, for intraperitoneal abscess, 525, 525*i*
for pancreatic abscess, 639
for pancreatic pleural effusion, 640
for pancreatic pseudocyst, **638**
percutaneous
for intraperitoneal abscess, 525, 525*i*
for lung abscess, 384
for perinephric abscess, **1039**
peritoneal, in acute secondary bacterial peritonitis, 520
postural, for bronchiectasis, 385
of small intestine fistulas, 697
for splenic abscesses, 664
ventricular
for increased intracranial pressure, 891
for subarachnoid hemorrhage, 941

Dressings, 15, 16, 23, 98
for hand, 1274
hygroscopic, 1234
moist, indications for, 96
for skin graft donor site, 1234
for skin graft recipient site, 1233, 1233*i*
in soft tissue injury, 1254
tie-over stent, 1233, 1233*i*
Droperidol, indications for, 200
Drowning, **265**
Drug(s). *See also* Medications
and anesthesia, 9
concurrent therapy with, and anesthetic risk, 192–193, 192*t*
disposition of, in elderly, 69–70
dosage of, in renal failure, 51
in elderly, 10
nephrotoxicity of, 51
and operative risk, 9
perioperative management of, 9, 15
and postoperative psychosis, 34
and renin-angiotensin-aldosterone axis, 799
Drug history, abdominal pain and, 507
Drummond, marginal artery of, 705
Drunk driving, 230
Dry eye, in Bell's palsy, 977
Dry heat
direct inhalation of, 274
for sterilization, 11, 119
D-transposition of the great arteries, **463–466,** 464*i*
Dual-energy x-ray absorptiometry (DEXA), 157
Duct of Santorini, 625, 626*i*
Duct of Wirsung, 625, 626*i*
Ductography, 322
Ductus arteriosus, and aortic coarctation, 445
Duhamel operation, in Hirschsprung's disease, 1322
Dukes classification, of colorectal cancer, 723, 724*t*
Dulcolax, for slow-transit constipation, 710
Dumbbell tumor, 928
Dumping syndrome, 543–544
Duodenal atresia, **1316–1317**
Duodenal diverticula, **562, 622–623**
Duodenal hematoma, 253–254
Duodenal reflux, in pathogenesis of pancreatitis, **630**
Duodenal ulcer(s), **539–544**
bleeding, 550
in children, 1332
recurrent, 542–543
Duodenoscopy, for adenoma and adenocarcinoma of ampulla of Vater, 648
Duodenum, **562–564**
blood supply to, 533, 536*i*
congenital obstruction of, **1316–1317**
mucosal resistance in, 537–538
nerve supply to, 536*i*
regional enteritis of, **564**
superior mesenteric artery obstruction of, **563–564**
tumors of, **562–563**

benign, **563**
   malignant, **562–563**
Duplex ultrasonography
   in chronic venous insufficiency, 883
   in deep venous thrombosis, 876
   in subclavian vein thrombosis, 879
Dupuytren's contracture, **1284–1285**
Durant position, 181, 184*i*
Duty of affirmative disclosure, 74
Du Val procedure, for chronic pancreatitis, 642
Dyclonine, for aphthous stomatitis, 985
Dysentery, bacillary, *versus* ulcerative colitis,
   742–743
Dysequilibrium, geriatric, **976**
Dysfibrinogenemia, acquired, 57
Dysfunctional uterine bleeding, 1088, 1089
Dysgerminoma, 66, 1110
Dysmenorrhea
   differential diagnosis of, 514
   primary, 1089
   secondary, 1089
Dysphagia, 282
   clinical presentation of, 42
Dyspnea
   mitral stenosis and, 420
   pulmonary thromboembolism and, 880
Dysrhythmia(s), **44–45**
   atrial, after cardiac surgery, 436–437
   and cardiogenic shock, 207
   in elderly, 67, 68
   intraoperative, **28**
   with pheochromocytoma, 804, 805
   postoperative, **28**
   supraventricular, 28, 44
   ventricular, 28
      after cardiac surgery, 437
Dystonia, **949**

Ear(s), **962–973**
   abnormalities, in osteogenesis imperfecta,
      974
   atresia of, 973
   congenital anomalies of, **973, 1259–1260,**
      1301
   foreign bodies in, **971**
   injuries to, 264
   pain and (otalgia), **969–970**
   systemic disorders affecting, **974**
Eardrum. *See* Tympanic membrane
Early death, 230, 244
EBRT. *See* External beam radiation teletherapy
   (EBRT)
Ebstein's anomaly, **463**
Echinococcal cysts
   and chronic mediastinitis, 372
   splenic, 664
Echinococcosis, 112, **128–129,** 664
Echinococcus granulosus infection. *See*
   Echinococcosis
Echinococcus multilocularis infection. *See*
   Echinococcosis
Echocardiography
   in aortic insufficiency, 427
   in heart disease, 42
   in mitral stenosis, 421

   preoperative, 42
   in tricuspid valve disease, 425
Echoplanar imaging, 894
Echothiophate, interactions with anesthetics,
   193
Ectasia, submucosal vascular, 738
Ectopia cordis, 1305
Ectopic ACTH syndrome, 806
   prognosis for, 810
Ectopic hyperparathyroidism, 311
Ectopic kidney, 1019
Ectopic spleen, 652
Edema. *See also* Pulmonary edema
   of arm, breast cancer and, 336–337
   brawny, 883
   in chronic venous insufficiency, 883
Edematous pancreatitis, 631–635
Edrophonium (Tensilon), 378
Effort thrombosis, 844, 878, 878*i*, 879–880
Ehlers-Danlos syndrome, diverticulosis and,
   730
Eicosanoids, and immune function, 162–163
Eicosapentaenoic acid, 163
Eisenmenger's syndrome, 449
Ejaculation, retrograde, in male infertility,
   1081
Ejaculatory duct, obstruction of, 1080, 1081
Ejection fraction, in chronic venous insuffi-
   ciency, 884
Elapidae, 130
Elastase, in pancreatitis, 629
Elastic band ligation, for hemorrhoids, 767
Elbow
   acute instability of, **1139–1140,** 1139*i*
   anatomy of, 1133
   biomechanics of, 1133
   dislocation of
      anterior, 1139*i*, 1140
      complications of, 1140
      irreducible, 1140
      lateral, 1139*i*, 1140
      medial, 1139*i*, 1140
      posterior, 1139–1140, 1139*i*
      postreduction care for, 1140
      rehabilitation for, 1140
   fractures and dislocations about, **1133–1135**
      in children, 1180–1181
   nursemaid's, 1180
   pain syndromes of, **1199–1200**
   pulled, 1180
Elderly, **67–71**
   abdominal pain in, 514
   antibiotic therapy for, in pulmonary failure,
      219
   appendicitis in, 670
   avascular necrosis of femoral head in, 1201
   body composition of, 69–70
   cardiac risk in, 29
   cataracts in, **1004–1005**
   delirium in, 70
   drug disposition in, 69–70
   falls in, 70
   fecal incontinence in, idiopathic, 760
   functional status of, 69
   heat stroke in, 278

hernia repair in, 786
infection in, 70
malnutrition in, 70
operative risk in, 17, 25, 111
   factors affecting, 9–10
performance of activities of daily living, 69
postoperative parotitis in, 30
postoperative psychiatric complications in,
   34–35
pressure sores in, 70
special problems in, 69–71, 70*t*
spinal cord injury in, 1117
surgical mortality in, 67
vestibular disorders in, 976
Electrical injury, **277**
Electrocardiography
   in aortic insufficiency, 427
   in aortic stenosis, 426
   in endocarditis, 430
   in mitral regurgitation, 423
   in mitral stenosis, 421
   monitoring by, postoperative, 28
   preoperative, 42
   in pulmonary thromboembolism, 880
   in thoracic aortic dissection, 433
   in tricuspid valve disease, 425
Electrocautery snare, for large bowel polyps,
   727
Electrocoagulation, for colorectal cancer, 722
Electroencephalography, in aneurysm surgery,
   899–900
Electrolytes. *See also* Fluid and electrolyte balance; *specific electrolyte*
   abnormalities of
      in enteral feeding, 174
      in total parenteral nutrition, 181, 183*t*
   absorption of
      in colon, 707, 709*t*
      in small intestine, **677–678**
   administration of
      postoperative, 15, 23
      for small bowel obstruction, **687**
      for small intestine fistulas, **696–697,** 696*t*
   in body fluids, 142, 143*i*
   concentrations of, units for, 142
   depletion of, with volume depletion,
      144–145
   disorders of, 145–150
   in gastric secretion, 536
   loss of
      in gastrointestinal fluid, 146, 147*t*
      in small bowel fistulas, 696
   replacement of, 145
      principles of, 153–154
      rule of thumb for, 154
   requirements for, 164*t*
      in newborn, 1296
      in premature infant, 1296
Electrolyte solutions, as blood substitute, 62
Electromyography
   in fecal incontinence, 760
   in lumbar disk syndrome, 957
   in neuropathic bladder, **1075**
   in skull base surgery, 898
Electron-beam computed tomography, 412

Electroneurography, in facial nerve paralysis, 977

Electronystagmography, in assessment of dizziness, 975

Electrothermal burns, 277

Elliptocytosis, hereditary, **657**

Eloesser procedure, 362

Embolectomy, for pulmonary thromboembolism, 882

Embolism. *See also* Pulmonary embolism
and arterial occlusion, 825, 826
and atherosclerosis, 814
and cerebral infarction, 847
and consciousness, 888
cryptogenic, 825

Embolization
for epistaxis, 981
for hemobilia, 621
for pancreatic pseudocyst, 637
transcatheter, for arterial injury, 260–261

Embryology, of genitourinary tract, **1013–1014**

Embryonal carcinoma
mediastinal, 377
vaginal, 1106

Emergency
implied consent in, 81
scene of, legal definition of, 77
treatment in, legal considerations in, 77

Emergency amputation, 861

Emergency Care for Complication Arising From Prior Care By Another, 77

Emergency physical examination, 4

Emergency room thoracotomy, **238–239**, 238*i*

Emergency surgery, for bleeding peptic ulcers, 551

Emergency tracheotomy, 233, 233*i*

Emesis. *See* Vomiting

Emetogenic esophageal perforation, 490

Emotion, and pain, 19

Emphysema
congenital lobar, **382**
and operative risk, 25
in surgical patient, 47

Emphysematous cholecystitis, **611**

Emphysematous pyelonephritis, **1038**

Empyema, 114, 357, 960
in acute cholecystitis, **608**
thoracic, **360–366**, 360*i*, 361*i*, 362*t*
tuberculous, 390

Encephalitis, as paraneoplastic syndrome, 1371, 1371*t*

Encephalocele
with cranium bifidum, **933**
nasal malformations and, 984

Encephalomyelitis, as paraneoplastic syndrome, 1371*t*

Enchondroma, **1226–1227**
of hand, 1288

Encopresis, 1321

Encrustation hypothesis, of atherosclerosis, 813

Endarterectomy, for cerebrovascular disease prevention, 850–851, 850*i*

End colostomy, 752, 754*i*

End-diastolic volume, 409, 410*i*

Endobronchial neoplasms, and bronchiectasis, 385

Endocardial fibroelastosis, **469**

Endocarditis, 114
bacterial, and hepatic abscess, 593
infective, **430**
prevention of, 120

Endocrine disease
and impotence, **1083**
as paraneoplastic syndrome, 1370, 1371*t*
in surgical patient, **38–41**

Endocrine function, of pancreas, **627**

Endodermal sinus tumor, 1347
ovarian, 1110

Endolymphatic hydrops, **975**

Endometrial ablation, for dysfunctional uterine bleeding, 1089

Endometrial biopsy, 1088

Endometrial cancer, 1088, 1089, **1108–1109**

Endometrioma, 1086
of large intestine, **729**
treatment of, 1097–1098

Endometriosis, 1086, **1095–1098**, 1095*i*
classification of, 1096
clinical findings in, 1096–1097
and ovarian cancer, 1110
pain caused by, 1090
prevalence of, 1096
prevention of, 1097
treatment of, 1097–1098
medical, 1097–1098
surgical, 1098

Endoneurium, 913

Endoprosthesis, hip, 1157
bipolar or universal, 1157

Endorphins, 104, 109

Endosaccular occlusion, for intracranial aneurysm, **942**

Endoscopic retrograde cholangiopancreatography
for acute abdomen, 513
in acute pancreatitis, 632
in bile duct malignancies, 617–618
for biliary tree examination, **600**
in choledocholithiasis, 614
in gallstone disease, 605–606
in jaundice, 602
in pancreatic adenocarcinoma, **645**
in pancreatic ascites, 639
in pancreatic pseudocyst, 636
in pancreatitis, 621–622
in sclerosing cholangitis, 623

Endoscopic retrograde pancreatography
in chronic pancreatitis, 641
in pancreatic ascites, 639

Endoscopy, **349**
for acute abdomen, 510*t*, 513
in benign prostatic hyperplasia, 1034
in bladder tumors, 1064
for bleeding peptic ulcers, 551
for carpal tunnel release, 1280, **1291–1292**
in Crohn's disease, 691

in facelift, **1265–1266**
for neck injuries, 242
in paranasal sinusitis, 980
in renal pelvis and calices tumors, 1060
sphincterotomy and
for acute pancreatitis, **634**
for adenoma and adenocarcinoma of ampulla of Vater, 648
for cholangitis, 612
for choledocholithiasis, **615**
in ulcerative colitis, 742
for upper gastrointestinal hemorrhage, 549
in ureteral tumors, 1062
in variceal bleeding, sclerotherapy or ligation via, 581

Endothelioma, 1246
of chest wall, 355–356

Endothelium, vascular, disruption of
in acute respiratory distress syndrome, 212
in shock, 211–212

Endotracheal intubation, 195, 233–234, 233*i*. *See also* Intubation
for burn patients, 270
cardiovascular response to, 196
complications of, 196–197
for craniocerebral trauma, 903
in depressed consciousness, 889
indications for, 196, 196*t*
for inhalation injuries, 276
in pediatric patients, 1294–1295
for respiratory failure, 18
tubes for, cuff types for, 215

Endourology, for renal stones, 1044

Endovascular coils, for intracranial aneurysm, 942

Endovascular management
of arterial injury, 260–261
of peripheral arterial insufficiency, 821–822

Endovascular stents, for peripheral arterial insufficiency, 821

Energy
requirements for
in burn patient, 186, 186*t*
determination of, **160–161**
in pediatric patients, 1297, 1297*t*
sources of, in nutritional support, 161

Enophthalmos, orbital fracture and, 1257

Enoxaparin, 54

Entacapone, for Parkinson's disease, 948

Entamoeba histolytica
in HIV-associated enteropathy, 693–694
and thoracic empyema, 361

Enteral feeding, **170–174**
benefits of, 170
for burn patient, 186
in cancer patient, 186, 187
complications of, 174, 180*t*
contraindications to, 170
cost of, 170
delivery methods for, 170–171
formulas for, 171, 172*t*–173*t*
immunologic effects of, 170
implementation of, 170–171

indications for, 110, 170
initiation of, 171
monitoring during, 171–174
for pediatric patients, 1297
safety of, 170
Enteric hyperoxaluria, 680
prevention of, 682
Enteric nervous system, 675–676
Enteritis
acute, **693**
Campylobacter, **694**
in intestinal tuberculosis, 694–695
regional, **689–692** (*See also* Crohn's disease (CD))
of stomach and duodenum, **564**
Yersinia, **694**
Enterobacter aerogenes, and thoracic empyema, 361
Enterobacter infection
drug therapy for, 135*t*
and peritonitis, 518
Enterobius vermicularis. See Pinworm
Enterocele, anterior, 1093
Enterochromaffin cells, 674
Enteroclysis, for small bowel obstruction, 685
Enterococcal infection
cholangitis caused by, 612
drug therapy for, 135*t*
hepatic abscess caused by, 593, 594
Enterocolitis, 693
neutropenic, 750
Enterocystoma, 1330*i*
Enterocystoplasty
augmentation, for genitourinary tuberculosis, 1041
for hyperreflexic bladder, 1075
Enterohepatic circulation, of bile salts, **596–598,** 599*i*
Enteroliths, and duodenal diverticula, 562
Enteropathy
HIV-associated, 189, **693–694**
necrotizing, 750
nonsteroidal anti-inflammatory drugs causing, **695**
protein-losing, 188
radiation, **695**
Enterostomal therapist, 751
Enterostomy therapy, 751
Enterotomy
for gallstone ileus, 611–612
for small bowel obstruction, 687
Entrapment, *versus* peripheral nerve tumors, 929
Environmental modifications, in accident prevention, 231
Enzymes
for lumbar disk syndrome, 958
pancreatic, supplements of, for short bowel syndrome, 682
Eosinophilic granuloma, **1229**
of chest wall, 354–355
Ependymomas, 917, **918,** 924, 926
of spinal cord, 928

Epidermal growth factors, and lung cancer, 396
Epidermal inclusion cyst, **1245**
Epidermis, 267
Epidermoid tumors, **920,** 925
Epididymectomy, for genitourinary tuberculosis, 1041
Epididymis
anatomy of, 1017
obstruction of, in male infertility, 1081
Epididymitis, 1339
acute, **1040**
versus spermatic cord torsion, 1079–1080
Epidural abscess, **960**
Epidural anesthesia
advantages and disadvantages of, 110
intraoperative management of, **198–199**
Epidural hematoma, **906,** 906*i*
Epigastric artery, inferior, 784
Epilepsy, 34, 894*i*
surgery for, in children, 937
Epinephrine, 103
actions of, 167–168
for bleeding peptic ulcers, 551
indications for, 132
for laryngotracheobronchitis, 993–994
plasma, in diagnosis of pheochromocytoma, 803
in shock, 210–211
Epineurium, 913
Epiphrenic diverticulum, **482**
Epiphysial fracture(s), 1177–1179
Epiphysial separations, 1177–1179
Epispadias, **1028**
Epistaxis, **981**
Epithelialization, in wound healing, 90
Eponychia, **1282**
Epstein-Barr virus (EBV) infection
in liver transplant recipient, 1386
treatment of, 141
Equinus, definition of, 1194
Equivalent (eq), 142
Erb's palsy, 1184
Erectile dysfunction. *See* Impotence
Erections, impotence and, 1082–1084
Erythromycin
for bronchiectasis, 385
for *Campylobacter* enteritis, 694
for chlamydial proctitis, 777
dosage of
in hepatic failure, 138*t*
in renal failure, 138*t*
indications for, 135*t,* 136*t*
for lung abscess, 384
pharmacology of, 138*t*
for preoperative bowel preparation, 755
Erythromycin base, for perianal chancroid, 778
Erythroplakia, in oral cavity cancer, 286
Erythroplasia of Queyrat, 1249, **1250**
Erythropoietin (EPO), 49
indications for, 56
recombinant, indications for, 61
Escharotomy, for circumferential burns, 273

Escherichia coli
in feces, 710–711
infection by
in cholangitis, 612
in cystitis, 1039
drug therapy for, 135*t*
in emphysematous cholecystitis, 611
hepatic abscess caused by, 593, 594
and infected aneurysms, 838
and lung abscess, 383
and peritonitis, 517–518, 518, 527
and retroperitoneal abscesses, 526
and thoracic empyema, 361
versus ulcerative colitis, 742–743
Esmolol, for thoracic dissection, 433
Esophageal atresia, 1313–1315, 1313*i*
Esophageal bands, **499–500**
Esophageal diverticula, **480–482**
Esophageal motility
disorders of, **475–479**
studies of, 485
Esophageal perforation, 247, **489–491**
and acute mediastinitis, 371–372
dilation and, 479
instrumental, 490, 491*i*
spontaneous, 490
Esophageal rings, **499–500**
Esophageal transection, for variceal bleeding, 583
Esophageal varices, 873
in children, 1332
Esophageal webs, **499–500**
Esophagectomy, for esophageal carcinoma, 498
Esophagitis
in children, 1332
corrosive, **493–494,** 494*t*
endoscopic grading system for, 485, 485*t*
Esophagogastrectomy, for gastric carcinoma, 559
Esophagogastroduodenoscopy, in lower gastrointestinal bleeding, 736
Esophagogastroscopy, of variceal bleeding, 580–581
Esophagogastrostomy, for gastric carcinoma, 559
Esophagus, **472–500**
anatomy of, 472, 473*i*
carcinoma of, **496–499,** 497*i*
annular, 496, 497, 497*i*
fungating, 496, 497, 497*i*
congenital anomalies of, **1313–1315,** 1313*i*
foreign bodies in, in children, **1333**
function of, 473
injuries to, 242, **247**
treatment of, 243
lower, columnar-lined, **488–489**
physiology of, 472–474
tumors of, **494–499**
benign, **494–495,** 495*i*
Essential tremor, **949**
Esthesioneuroblastoma, 292
Estrogen(s)
for abnormal uterine bleeding, 1089
adrenal tumors producing, 811
anticancer therapy with, **1356**

Estrogen(s) (*cont.*)
  for male breast cancer, 340
  for prostate cancer, 1069
  conjugated, indications for, 55, 56
  and endometrial cancer, 1108
  pancreatitis and, 629
Estrogen inhibitor(s), anticancer therapy with, **1356**
Estrogen receptors, breast cancer and, 329
Etanercept, for rheumatoid arthritis, 1204
Ethambutol
  indications for, 136*t*, 141
  for tuberculosis, 388*t*, 389
    of spine, 961
Ethanolamines, for allergic rhinitis, 978*t*
Ethanol injection
  for bleeding peptic ulcers, 551
  in primary hepatic cancer, 573
Ether, and lung cancer, 396
Ethionamide
  indications for, 136*t*
  for tuberculosis, 388*t*
Ethylene oxide, as sterilizing agent, 11, 119
Etidronate, for hypercalcemic crisis, 313
Etoposide, 1355
Eustachian tube (auditory tube) dysfunction, 965–966
Euthyroid sick syndrome, 106
Evisceration
  definition of, 24
  recurrence of, 25
  wound dehiscence with, 24–25
Ewing's sarcoma, 1223, **1225–1226**
  of chest wall, 355–356
Excision(s)
  for colorectal cancer, **722**
  for pancreatic pseudocyst, **637–638**
  and primary closure, in plastic surgery, 1241–1242
Exercise, response to, in peripheral arterial insufficiency, 818
Exercise rehabilitation, for peripheral arterial insufficiency, 820
Exercise testing, 42
Exertional rhabdomyolysis, 277
Exocrine function, of pancreas, **625–626**
  tests of, **643**
    in chronic pancreatitis, **640**
Exophthalmos, 301, 302–303, 1001
Exostoses, bony. See Osteochondroma
Exotoxin(s)
  clostridial, 124
  streptococcal, 124–125
Expectorants, for bronchiectasis, 385
Expiration, 344
Exposure, trauma victim and, **238**
Exposure therapy, for burns, 272
Extensor posturing, in craniocerebral trauma, 902
Extensor retinaculum, 1272, 1273*i*
External beam radiation teletherapy (EBRT), 1360
External iliac artery, 706*i*
External inguinal ring, 785, 785*i*
External oblique muscle, 783

Extracellular fluid (ECF), electrolyte composition of, 142, 143*i*
Extracorporeal membrane oxygenation (ECMO), 1295
Extracorporeal shock wave lithotripsy
  for chronic pancreatitis, 642
  for gallstones, **606**
  for renal stones, **1044**
Extralobar sequestration, 381
Extravaginal torsion, **1029**
Extremity peripheral microemboli, **827**
Extubation, **218–219**
  complications of, 197
Exudates, 357
Exudative empyemas, acute, 360–361
Eye(s), **999–1012**
  anterior segment of
    blunt trauma to, 1009*t*
    inspection of, **999–1000**
  blood supply to, 847, 847*i*
  blunt trauma to, 1009*t*
  burns of, **1007–1008**
  discharge from, **1001**
  diseases/disorders of, **1002–1007**
    laser treatment for, **1012**
    symptoms and signs of, 1000–1001
  displacement of, **1001**
  examination of, **999–1000**
  in Graves' disease, 302–303
  injuries to, 264
  movements of, **1000**
  pain in, **1000–1001**
  redness of, **1001**, 1001*t*
  trauma to, **1008–1010**
  tumors of, **1010–1012**
Eyelid(s). See also Blepharoplasty
  blunt trauma to, 1009*t*
  gold weight implant of, for facial paralysis, 977
  lacerations of, 1009
  swelling of, **1001**
  tumors of, **1010–1011**, 1010*i*
    benign, 1010
    malignant, 1011
Eye-opening, in craniocerebral trauma, **902**

Face
  bones of, fractures of, **1254–1257**
  expression lines and wrinkles of
    facelift for, 1265–1266
  incisions corresponding to, 1241, 1241*i*
  wounds on, repair of, 1253–1254
Facelift, **1265–1266**
Facet(s)
  dislocation of, 1121
  perching of, 1121
Facetectomy, for spinal cord tumors, 928
Facet syndrome, **1214–1215**
Facial bone(s), fractures of, **1254–1257**
Facial nerve
  intraoperative monitoring of, 897–898
  paralysis of, **977**
  and salivary gland cancer, 295
Facial wound repair, 1253–1254
Factor V, in stored blood, 59

Factor V Leiden mutation, and subclavian vein thrombosis, 878–879
Factor VIII
  concentrate
    dosage and administration of, 56
    for transfusion therapy, 61
  deficiency of, 56
  in stored blood, 59
Factor IX
  deficiency of, 56
  replacement of, 62
Factor XI, deficiency of, 56
Factor XII, replacement of, 62
Fallopian tubes
  abnormalities of, 1086–1087
  adenocarcinoma of, **1110**
  adhesive disease of, 1087
  obstruction of, 1086–1087
  reanastomosis of, 1087
  repair of, 1087
  surgical occlusion of, for female sterilization, 1091
  tumors of, 1110
Falls, 900
  in elderly, 70, 976
False aneurysms, 258, 829
  of radial artery, **842**
False imprisonment, 76
Falx inguinalis, 784
Famciclovir, **141**
Familial adenomatous polyposis (FAP), 702, **727–728,** 727*t*
  in adolescent, 1332
  cancer screening in, 719
  large bowel cancer and, 726
Familial hemolytic anemia, **655–656**
Familial Mediterranean fever, differential diagnosis of, 519
Familial pancreatitis, 628
Familial paroxysmal polyserositis. See Familial Mediterranean fever
Familial polyposis coli, 702
Familial visceral myopathy, and intestinal pseudo-obstruction, 686
Familial visceral neuropathy, and intestinal pseudo-obstruction, 686
Family history, 2
  acute abdomen and, 508
Fascia, closure of, 24, 97
Fasciitis
  Dupuytren's, **1284–1285**
  necrotizing, 114, **124–125**
    of upper extremity, 1283
  palmar, **1284–1285**
Fasciotomy, in arterial trauma, 262
Fasting
  metabolic response to, 164–165, 165*i*
  preoperative, 194
Fat
  absorption of, in pancreatic insufficiency, 643
  body, estimation of, 158
  dietary, 162–163, 184–185
    and colorectal cancer, 717
    digestion of, in small intestine, **678–679**

Fat embolism syndrome, **27**, 212, 880
Fat necrosis, of breast, **343**
Fatty acids
    absorption of, in small intestine,
        678–679
    free, 165
        in sepsis, 169
    medium-chain, 163
    in nutritional support, 162–163
    polyunsaturated, 163
    ω-3, 163, 185
    ω-6, 163
Fear, in surgical patient, 34
Fecal continence, 758
Fecal fat balance test, **643**
Fecal flora, **710–711**
Fecal impaction, 763, **779**
    postoperative, **31**
Fecal incontinence, 759–762
    causes of, 759
    clinical findings in, 759–760
    complete, 759
    diagnosis of, 760, 761*i*
    differential diagnosis of, 760
    epidemiology of, 759
    idiopathic, in elderly, 760
    imaging in, 759–760
    laboratory findings in, 759–760
    partial, 759
    prognosis for, 760
    signs and symptoms of, 759
    treatment of, 760, 761*i*
Fecal markers, in Crohn's disease, 690
Fecal mass, preoperative reduction of, 754
Fecal occult blood testing, 718–719
Fecaluria, with colovesical fistula, 735
Feet. *See* Foot
Felon, **1282**, 1283*i*
Felty's syndrome, **660**
Female reproductive system, embryology of,
    1013–1014, 1016*i*
Female urethral caruncle, **1079**
Female urethral diverticulum, **1079**
Female urethritis, **1078–1079**
Feminization, tumors causing, 811
Femoral adenopathy, 790
Femoral artery aneurysm, **839**
Femoral canal, 784
Femoral neck, fracture of, **1150–1151**
    stable, 1150–1151
    unstable, 1150–1151
Femoral nerve, 784
    greater saphenous vein and, 871, 872*i*
Femoral rings, in acute abdomen, 510
Femoral veins, 871, 872*i*
Femoropopliteal reconstruction, for peripheral
        arterial insufficiency, 823, 823*i*
Femur. *See also* Slipped capital femoral epiph-
            yses
    distal
        fractures of, 1159–1160
        growth plate of, fractures of, in children,
            1182
    fractures of
        condylar, 1160

extra-articular, 1159, 1160*i*
        intercondylar, 1160
        intra-articular, 1160
        supracondylar, 1159, 1160*i*
    head and neck resection in, 1156
    head of
        avascular necrosis of, **1201**
        in Legg-Perthes disease, 1193–1194,
            1194*i*
    proximal
        fractures of, in children, **1181–1182**
        osteomyelitis of, 1188
    shaft of, fracture of, 1158–1159, 1158*i*
        in children, **1182**
Fenretinide, chemopreventive, 297
Fentanyl
    advantages and disadvantages of, 110
    indications for, 196
    renal failure and, 51
Fever
    in acute abdomen, 508
    with atelectasis, 26, 36
    with brain abscess, 959
    in pneumonia, 27
    postoperative, **36–37**
    in response to injury, 108
    in transfusion reaction, 60
Fiber
    dietary, 678
        and colorectal cancer, 717
        intake of, 185
    diverticulosis and, 731
Fiberoptic colonoscopy, **712**
Fibrillary astrocytomas, low-grade, 917–918
Fibrin, 114
    in wound healing, 86–87
Fibrin glue, 61–62, 252
    for nasal trauma, 983
    for small intestine fistulas, 697
Fibrinolysis, primary, in liver disease, 57
Fibrinolytic agents, for deep venous thrombo-
        sis, 877
Fibrinopurulent empyemas, 360–361
Fibroadenoma, of breast, **341–342**
Fibroblastoma, perineurial, 929. *See also* Nerve
        sheath tumors (schwannomas)
Fibroblasts
    in fracture healing, 93
    in wound healing, 87, 90–91
Fibrocystic disease. *See* Mammary dysplasia
Fibroelastosis, endocardial, **469**
Fibroepithelial polyps, ureteral, 1061
Fibroma(s)
    cardiac, 435, 469
    of chest wall, 355
    of lung, 404
    renal, 1059
Fibromuscular dysplasia, **852**
    and extracranial carotid artery aneurysm,
        840
    and renovascular hypertension, 853
Fibroplasia, in wound healing, 87
Fibrosarcoma(s), **1226**, 1361
    of chest wall, 354
Fibrosing mediastinitis, 372, 373

Fibrosis
    of penis, 1082
    retroperitoneal, **531–532**
Fibrous bands, between ileum and umbilicus,
        1330–1331, 1330*i*
Fibrous dysplasia, of chest wall, 354
Fibrous skeleton, of heart, 419
Fibula
    distal epiphyses of, fracture of, in children,
        1182–1183
    fracture of, in children, 1182
    shaft of, fracture of, 1167–1169, 1168*i*
Filariasis, in lymphedema, 885
Film screen radiography, in mammography,
        322
Fine-needle aspiration, **1353**
    of breast cancer, 319–320
    of head and neck tumors, 283
Fingernail(s), infections of, **1282**, 1282*i*
    fungal, 1282, 1284
Fingers. *See* Digit(s)
Firearms, 231. *See also* Gunshot wound(s)
Fireman's carry, in spinal cord injury, 910
First-degree burns, 267, 268*i*
Fisher scale, for subarachnoid hemorrhage,
        939*t*
Fissures
    in Crohn's disease, 689–690
    of lungs, 347
Fistula(s), 114–115
    anorectal, **771–773**
        in Crohn's disease, 690
        in ulcerative colitis, 743
    arteriovenous, 259, **845–846**
        congenital, 1020
        and varicose veins, 873
    of bladder, 1077–1078
    branchiogenic, **1300–1301**, 1300*i*
    cholecystenteric, **609**
        in gallstone ileus, 611
    colovesical, 735
    diverticulitis and, 733
    enterocutaneous, nutritional support with,
        189
    gastrocolic, 543
    gastrointestinal, nutritional support with, 189
    gastrojejunocolic, 543
    omphalomesenteric, 1330–1331, 1330*i*
    para-ileostomy, 753*t*
    rectovaginal, **773–774**, **1094**, 1107
    sigmoidovaginal, **1094**
    of small intestine, **696–697**, 696*t*
    ureterovaginal, 1093–1094
        versus ureteral injury, 1050
    urethrovaginal, 1093–1094
    urinary tract, **1093–1094**
    vesical, 1077–1078
    vesicocutaneous, 1077–1078
    vesicointestinal, 1077
    vesicovaginal, 1077, 1093–1094, 1107
        versus ureteral injury, 1050
Fistula-in-ano, 771, 772
Fitz-Hugh-Curtis syndrome, *versus* acute chole-
            cystitis, 608
Five Ps, of arterial occlusion, 825–826

FK506, in heart transplantation, 470
Flaccid larynx, congenital, 992
Flail chest, 212, 237, 237*i*, 244–245
Flame burns, 277
Flaps, **1234–1237**
  axial pattern, 1235
  for breast reconstruction, 1261
  classification of, 1234
  closure technique for, 1239–1241, 1240*i*
  deltoid, for lower extremity, 1262
  elevation of, 1239
  fasciocutaneous, **1237**
  free, 1230, **1237**
    in head and neck, 1260
  indications for, by wound type, 1239*t*
  inferior gluteal thigh, for lower extremity,
    1262
  motor, 1237
  muscle, 1235–1237
    for pressure sores, 1264
  musculocutaneous, 1235–1237, 1235*i*
    in head and neck, 1260
  neurocutaneous, **1237**
  neurosensory, for lower extremity,
    1262–1263
  osteocutaneous, for mandible reconstruc-
    tion, 1261
  perforator, 1230, **1237**
  random pattern, 1234–1235
  selection of, 1238–1239, 1239*t*
  sensory, 1237
  sural, 1230
    for lower extremity, 1262–1263
  techniques for, 1230
  transposition of, 1239
Flash burn, 277, **1008**
Flatfoot, **1196**
  flexible, 1196
  rigid, 1196
Flexion contracture, amputation and, 867–868
Flexor posturing, in craniocerebral trauma,
  902
Flexor tenorrhaphy, in hand, 1276, 1276*i*
Flow cytometry, of bladder tumors, 1064
Fluconazole, **141**
  for coccidioidomycosis, 392
  for cryptococcosis, 393
  dosage of
    in hepatic failure, 138*t*
    in renal failure, 138*t*
  pharmacology of, 138*t*
Flucytosine, **140–141**
  for cryptococcosis, 393
Fludarabine, for hairy cell leukemia, 663
Fluid(s)
  administration of
    for acute pancreatitis, **633**
    for burn patients, 270–271
    for lung injuries, 246
    postoperative, 15, 18–19
    principles of, 153–154
    in resuscitation, 205–206, 207
    for small bowel obstruction, **687**
    for small intestine fistulas, **696–697,** 696*t*

gastrointestinal, loss of, volume and electrolyte content of, 146, 147*t*
intake of, for renal stones, 1043
intravenous, composition of, 18, 18*t*
loss of (*See also* Hypovolemia)
  with ileostomy, 751
  perioperative, in children, 1295–1296,
    1296*t*
  postoperative, 18
  and replacement therapy, 154
  in small intestine fistulas, 696
overload, and cardiac complications, 28, 29
requirements for
  factors affecting, 153
  for maintenance, 153
    in newborn, 1295, 1296*t*
  postoperative, 18–19
shift, in shock, 211
in small bowel obstruction, 684
therapy with, principles of, 153–154
Fluid and electrolyte balance. *See also specific*
    electrolyte
  management of, **142–155**
    in newborn, **1295–1297**
    in volume disorders, 144–145
Fluid-attenuated inversion recovery, 894, 894*i*,
    895*i*
  in epidermoid tumors, 920
Fluid balance
  perioperative, in children, management of,
    1295–1296, 1296*t*
  postoperative
    in children, management of, 1295–1296,
      1296*t*
    factors affecting, 18
    management of, **18–19**, 23
    monitoring of, 14, 19
Fluorescein test
  in acute mesenteric vascular occlusion, 699
  in pancreatic insufficiency, 643
  in small bowel obstruction, 687
Fluoride, requirements for, 164*t*
2-[^{18}F]Fluoro-2-deoxy-D-glucose, in radionu-
    clide imaging, 897
Fluoroscopic imaging, in deep venous throm-
    bosis, 876
Fluorouracil, 1355
  for actinic (solar) keratoses, 1249
  for breast cancer, 331–332, 332, 334
  for carcinoid tumor of intestine, 704
  for colorectal cancer, 723
  for gastric carcinoma, 559
  and intestinal wound healing, 92
  for malignant pleural effusion, 359
  for Zollinger-Ellison syndrome, 546
Flutamide, anticancer therapy with, **1356**
Focused Assessment with Sonography for
    Trauma (FAST), 249–250, 250*i*
Folic acid, 163
  deficiency of, 52
  requirements for, 164*t*
Follicle-stimulating hormone, in male infertil-
    ity, 1080, 1081
Follicular adenocarcinoma, **306,** 307

Fontan procedure, 459
  for hypoplastic left heart syndrome, 448
Foot
  care of, in peripheral arterial insufficiency,
    820–821
  deformities of, in children, **1194–1196**
  injuries of, **1172–1176**
  pain in, **1215–1217**
Foramen of Bochdalek hernia, **501,** 501*i*
Foramen of Luschka, 890*i*
Foramen of Magendie, 890*i*
Foramen of Morgagni hernia, **501,** 501*i*,
    1309–1310
Foraminotomy, for lumbar disk syndrome,
    957–958
Forced expiratory volume at 1 minute (FEV$_1$),
    postoperative, 17
Forearm
  amputation of, **867**
  fractures of, **1140–1141**
    both-bone, 1142–1143
    in children, 1181
  injury to, **1279–1280**
Forefoot
  adduction of, 1194–1195
  eversion of, 1194
  hooking of, 1195–1196
  inversion of, 1194
Foreign bodies
  aspiration of, 385
    by children, **1333**
  conjunctival, **1009–1010**
  corneal, **1009–1010**
  in ear, **971**
  esophageal, in children, **1333**
  ingestion of, **491–493**
    in children, **1332–1333**
  in larynx, **990**
  nasal, **977–978**
  in pharynx, **989–990**
  and small bowel obstruction, **683**
  in tracheobronchial tree, **990**
    in children, **1333**
Forequarter amputation, **867,** 868*i*
Formaldehyde, and lung cancer, 396
Fosphenytoin, for craniocerebral trauma, 903
Fothergill's sign, 796
Fourth ventricle, 890*i*
Fracture(s)
  acetabular, 1127–1128, 1127*i*
  angulation of, 1116
  ankle joint, 1170–1171
  arterial injuries and, 261
  in battered child syndrome, 1350
  Bennett's, **1149,** 1279
  blowout, orbital, **1009,** 1257
  buckle (torus), 1177
  burst, of lumbar spine, 1118
  calcaneal, 1118, **1173–1174,** 1173*i*
  carpal, **1146–1148**
  in children, **1176–1183**
  clavicular, **1128,** 1129*i*
  comminuted, 1116
  cricoid cartilage, 991

cuboid bone, **1174–1175**
cuneiform bone, **1174–1175**
delayed healing of, **1176**
displaced, 1116
distal femoral growth plate, in children,
1182
distal femur, 1159–1160, 1160*i*
distal humerus, 1133–1135
distal radius, 1144–1146, 1144*i*, 1145*i*,
1279
distal tibia, 1171, 1172*i*
elbow, **1133–1135**
epiphysial, 1177–1179
facial bone, **1254–1257**
fatigue, of metatarsal shafts, **1175**
femoral neck, **1150–1151**
femoral shaft, 1158–1159, 1158*i*
in children, **1182**
fibular, in children, 1182–1183
fibular shaft, 1167–1169, 1168*i*
fifth metatarsal tuberosity, **1176**
forearm, **1140–1141, 1279**
both-bone, 1142–1143
with frostbite, 280
Galeazzi's, 1141
greenstick, 937, 1177
growth plate, 1177–1179
hamate, **1147**
hand, **1148–1150**
healing of, 93–94
humeral shaft, **1133**
immobilization of, at accident scene, 234
intertrochanteric, 1152–1153, 1152*i*
lunate, **1147**
mandibular, **1256**
maxillary, **1257**
metacarpal, **1148–1149, 1278–1279**
metatarsal shaft, **1175**
Monteggia's, 1139, **1141–1142,** 1142*i*
nasal, **1255–1256**
nasal bone, 982, 983
navicular, **1174**
nightstick, 1141
nonunion of, **1176**
odontoid (hangman's), 910
open, 1116
orbital, **1256–1257**
patellar, **1160–1162**
pathologic, with bone tumors, 1224
pelvic, **1123–1127**
and bladder injury, 1050
classification of, 1126–1127
nonunion of, 1126
treatment of, 1126–1127
and urethral injury, 1053*i*
phalangeal, **1278–1279**
of toes, **1176**
proximal femur, in children, **1181–1182**
proximal humerus, **1130,** 1130*i,* 1131*i*
in children, **1179**
proximal radius, **1138–1139,** 1138*i*
proximal tibia, **1164–1166**
proximal ulna, **1137–1138,** 1137*i*
radial head, **1138–1139,** 1138*i*

radial shaft, **1141**
reduction of, 1116
scaphoid, **1146–1147,** 1147*i,* **1279**
scapular, **1129–1130**
sesamoid, of great toe, **1176**
skull, 937
open, **907**
spinal, **1117–1123**
classification of, 1118
stability of, 1118
stable, 1120
unstable, 1120–1121, 1123
without neurologic deficit, 1120–1121
subtrochanteric, 1153, 1153*i*
talar, 1173
temporal bone, **972**
thoracolumbar, 1121
tibial, 1118, 1263
in children, 1182–1183
tibial eminence, 1166
tibial plateau, 1164–1166, 1165*i*
tibial shaft, 1167–1169, 1168*i*
tibial tuberosity, 1166
trochanteric, **1151–1153**
ulnar shaft, **1141–1143**
ulnar styloid, 1146
upper extremity, in children, **1179–1181**
vertebral, 1118
wrist, **1279**
zygomatic, **1256–1257**
Fragility test, incubated, for hereditary spherocytosis, 656
Frank-Starling property, 409
Fredet-Ramstedt pyloromyotomy, for pyloric
stenosis, 1316
Free flaps. *See* Flaps, free
Free hepatic venous pressure, 584
Free perforation
in acute cholecystitis, **609**
in diverticulitis, 733
Fresh frozen plasma, for craniocerebral trauma,
903
Frontal lobe, tumors in, 922
Frontal sinusitis, acute, 980
Frostbite, **279–280**
deep, 279
of hand, **1287**
rewarming for, 1287
superficial, 279
Frostnip, 279
Frozen shoulder, **1198–1199**
Fructose, seminal, in male infertility, 1080
Frykman classification, of distal radius frac-
tures, 1144, 1144*i*
Fulguration
for bladder tumors, **1064**
for colorectal cancer, 722
Full-thickness burns. *See* Third-degree burns
Functional congenital disorders, **937**
Functional residual capacity (FRC), postopera-
tive, 17
Fundus, of stomach, 533
Fungi
brain abscesses caused by, 959

and bronchiectasis, 385
host defense against, 113
and infected aneurysms, 838
infection by, 112
of fingernail, 1282, 1284
and lung abscess, 383
in lung infections, **390–394**
and thoracic empyema, 361
Fungus balls. *See* Aspergillosis
Furosemide
for hypercalcemic crisis, 313
indications for, 51, 149
for renal dysfunction after cardiac surgery,
437
Furuncles, 112, **125–127**
Furunculitis, in nasal vestibulitis, 978
Furunculosis, 125, 126
Fusiform aneurysms, 938

Gadolinium, in magnetic resonance imaging,
894
Gag reflex, in craniocerebral trauma, 902
Gait
analysis of, after amputation, 870
disorders of, in children, **1183**
Galeazzi's fracture, **1141**
Gallbladder
benign tumors of, **619**
carcinoma of, **616–617**
diseases of, **604–624** (*See also specific disease*)
embryology and anatomy of, 595, 597*i*
empyema of, and hepatic abscess, 593
injuries to, treatment of, 253
pseudotumors of, **619**
ultrasound of, 64
Gallbladder colic, **605–606**
in choledocholithiasis, 613
Gallstone ileus, **611–612**
and small bowel obstruction, **683**
Gallstones (cholelithiasis)
asymptomatic, **604–605**
and chronic cholecystitis, **605–606**
versus colorectal cancer, 721
dissolution of, 606
ileostomy and, 753*t*
pathogenesis of, **603–604,** 603*i*
Galveston Orientation and Amnesia test, 907
Gamekeeper's thumb, 1279
Gamma-aminobutyric acid (GABA), and hepatic encephalopathy, 591–592
Ganciclovir
dosage of
in hepatic failure, 138*t*
in renal failure, 138*t*
pharmacology of, 138*t*
Ganglion(s), of hand, **1287–1288**
Ganglioneuroblastoma, 1312
Ganglioneuroma, 1312
Gangrene
and autoamputation, 862
midgut, 1319–1320
streptococcal, 124, 1283
treatment of, 125
Gardner's syndrome, 702, 727–728, 1361

Gartner duct cysts, 1095
Gas, intestinal, **707**
Gas cysts
  in large intestine, **701**
  in small intestine, **701**
Gas gangrene, 124
  drug therapy for, 136*t*
Gas sterilization, 11
Gas stoppage sign, 507
Gastrectomy
  for gastric carcinoma, 559
  subtotal, for duodenal ulcer, 542
Gastric acid
  hypersecretion, in short bowel syndrome,
    681
  in pancreatic cholera, 650
  secretion of
    and duodenal ulcer, 539
    inhibition of, 538
    parietal cells and, 536–537, 537*i*
    regulation of, 538
    stimulation of, 538
Gastric analysis, of duodenal ulcer, 540, 540*t*
Gastric cancer, **556–559**
  adenocarcinomas, 557
  early, 557
  paraneoplastic syndromes with, 1371*t*
  staging of, 558*i*
Gastric dilation, postoperative, **31**
Gastric diverticula, **562**
Gastric feeding, 170–171
Gastric juice, **535–536**
Gastric mucosa, prolapse of, **561**
Gastric peristalsis, postoperative, 19, 30
Gastric phase, of acid secretion, 538
Gastric polyps, **559–560**
Gastric suction
  for acute pancreatitis, **633**
  for perforated peptic ulcer, 554–555
Gastric ulcer(s), **546–547**
  increased intracranial pressure and, 890
  type I, 546
  type II, 546–547
  type III, 547
Gastric vein(s), 565, 567*i*
Gastric volvulus, **561**
Gastrin, 535
  inhibition of, 538
  serum levels of
    in duodenal ulcer, 540
    in Zollinger-Ellison syndrome, 545
Gastrinoma. *See* Zollinger-Ellison syndrome
Gastritis
  acute hemorrhagic, **556**
  alkaline, 544
  hypertrophic, 561
Gastrocnemius muscle flap, **1236–1237**
  for lower extremity, 1262
Gastrocolic fistula, 543
Gastrocolic response, 708
Gastroduodenal ulcers. *See also* Duodenal ulcer(s)
  in burn patient, 273–274
Gastroduodenitis, stress, **555**
Gastroduodenoscopy, for acute abdomen, 513

Gastroenteritis, 693
  Yersinia, 694
Gastroenterostomy, for perforated peptic ulcer,
    554
Gastroepiploic artery, 626*i*
Gastroepiploic vein, 626*i*
Gastroesophageal reflux
  caused by hiatal hernia, in pregnancy, 65
  in children, **1327–1328**
  and chronic laryngitis, 995
Gastroesophageal sphincter, 472, 473–474
Gastrointestinal fluid loss, volume and elec-
    trolyte content of, 146, 147*t*
Gastrointestinal hemorrhage, acute lower,
    736–737
Gastrointestinal ischemia syndromes,
    856–857, 856*i,* 857*i*
Gastrointestinal tract
  congenital lesions of, **1313–1327**
  diseases/disorders of
    nutritional support in, 188–189
    in transplant recipient, 1379
  duplications of, 1328–1329, 1329*i,* 1332
  foreign bodies in, in children, **1332–1333**
  injuries to, 249
    treatment of, 253–254
  postoperative care of, **19**
Gastrojejunocolic fistula, 543
Gastrojejunostomy
  for duodenal ulcer, 541
  for pancreatic adenocarcinoma, 645, 646
Gastroparesis, chronic, after gastric surgery,
    544
Gastroschisis, **1340–1341,** 1341*i*
Gastroscopy
  in gastric carcinoma, 558
  in gastric ulcer, 547
Gastrostomy, in acute secondary bacterial peri-
    tonitis, 520
Gastrostomy tube, 19
Gaucher's disease, **661**
Gelatin, as blood substitute, 62
Gemcitabine, for pancreatic adenocarcinoma,
    646
General anesthesia
  induction of, 195–196
    combined intravenous-inhalation, 196
    inhalation, 195–196
    rapid-sequence, 195
  intraoperative management of, 195–198
  maintenance of, 197–198
Generalized juvenile gastrointestinal polyposis,
    728
Genes, in colorectal cancer, 717
Gene therapy, for peripheral arterial insuffi-
    ciency, 821
Genitalia. *See also* Genitourinary tract; Repro-
    ductive system
  external, differentiation of, 1014
  male (*See also specific anatomic entity*)
    injuries to, 254
Genitofemoral nerve, 784
Genitourinary tract
  acquired lesions of, **1029–1036**

anatomy of, 1014–1017
developmental anomalies of, **1018–1029**
diseases/disorders of, **1076–1084**
embryology of, **1013–1014**
injuries to, treatment of, 254–255
physiology of, **1017–1018**
trauma to, **1048–1054**
tuberculosis of, **1040–1042**
tumors of, **1054–1073**
Gentamicin
  indications for, 135*t,* 137
  for infection control, 385
  for ulcerative colitis, 744
Genu varum, 1183
  pathologic, **1183–1184**
Geriatric dysequilibrium, **976**
Germ cell tumor(s)
  central nervous system, **920–921, 927**
  mediastinal, 376–377
  ovarian, 1110, 1112
  testicular, **1070**
Gerota's fascia, renal adenocarcinoma in,
    1057
Gestational age, assessment of, 1293
Gestational trophoblastic disease, **1112–1115.**
    See also Hydatidiform mole
  clinical findings in, 1113
  complications of, 1113–1114
  differential diagnosis of, 1113
  FIGO staging of, 1113, 1113*t*
  persistent
    risk of, WHO scoring system for, 1113,
      1114*t*
    treatment of, 1114
  prognosis for, 1115
  treatment of, 1114–1115
Giant cell arteritis. *See* Takayasu's arteritis
Giant cell tumor
  of bone, **1227,** 1227*i*
  of hand, 1288
Giardia lamblia, in HIV-associated enteropa-
    thy, 693–694
Gigantism, 930, 931
Gillies technique, for depressed zygomatic frac-
    tures, 1256
Gingivitis, **984–985**
  acute necrotizing ulcerative, **984–985**
Girdlestone arthroplasty, in hip, 1156, 1157
Glanders, drug therapy for, 135*t*
Glasgow Coma Score, 225
  in craniocerebral trauma, **902**
  in subarachnoid hemorrhage, 939*t*
Glasgow Outcome Scale, 907–908
  in intracranial aneurysm, 943
Glaucoma, 1001*t*
  acute (angle-closure), **1005**
  chronic simple (open-angle), **1005–1006**
Gleason scale, in prostate cancer, 1068
Glenn operation, 459, 459*i*
Glenohumeral joint
  arthritis of, **1132–1133**
  dislocation of, **1130–1132**
  inflammation in, and painful arc syndrome,
    1197

Glial cell tumors, **926**
Glioblastoma multiforme, **918,** 926
Gliomas, **917–919**
   and cerebrospinal fluid obstruction, 934
Gliosis, and cerebrospinal fluid obstruction, 934
Glipizide, perioperative management of, 38
Glomerular filtration, 1017
Glomerular filtration pressure, 1017
Glomerular filtration rate (GFR), 49
   in elderly, 68–69
Glomerulonephritis
   chronic, kidney transplantation for, 1372
   and pleural effusion, 360
Glomus tumor
   in hand, 1288
   jugulare, 972–973
   tympanicum, 972–973
   vagale, 973
Glossectomy, for oropharyngeal cancer, 288
Glossoptosis, 1307
Glottis
   cancer of, 282
   and swallowing, 474
Glucagon, 106, **627**
   actions of, 165, 165*i*, 167–168
   in response to injury, 107–108
   in shock, 210–211
Glucagonemia, in response to injury, 108
Glucagonoma, **650–651**
Glucocerebrosidase, recombinant, for Gaucher's disease, 661
Glucocorticoid(s), 106
   adverse effects and side effects of, 189
   for hypercalcemic crisis, 313
Gluconeogenesis, hepatic, 165–166, 165*i*, 166*i*
Glucosamine, for osteoarthritis, 1202
Glucose
   blood levels of (*See also* Hyperglycemia; Hypoglycemia)
      after hepatic resection, 568
      in diabetic patient, 38
         and postoperative care, 40
      factors affecting, 38
      intraoperative monitoring of, 39
      monitoring, in diabetic patient, 38–39
      neonatal, 1296–1297
   cerebral utilization of, 166
   depressed consciousness and, 889
   extracellular concentration of, in shock, 210–211
   intolerance
      in response to injury, 108
      in trauma, 168, 168*i*
   metabolism of, 165, 165*i*, 166*i*
      in cancer patient, 186–187
      in sepsis, 169
   uptake, in radionuclide imaging, 897
Glucose 6-phosphate dehydrogenase (G6PD) deficiency, **657**
Glucosuria, 49
Glue ear, 965
Glutamate, in brain injury, 901

Glutamine
   absorption of, in small intestine, 678
   analogs of, as antineoplastic agents, 187
   metabolism of, 166
      in cancer patient, 187
   in nutritional support, 162
   protective effects of, 187
   for radiation enteropathy prevention, 695
   and small bowel syndrome, 681
   supplementation of, for cancer patients, 187
Glutathione peroxidase, 164
Gluteal muscle flap, **1236**
   for anorectal dysfunction, 760
   for pressure sores, 1264
Glyburide, perioperative management of, 38
Glycolysis, anaerobic, 108
Glycoprotein IIB/IIIA inhibitors, for angina pectoris, 413
Glycopyrrolate, indications for, 194
Goblet cells, intestinal, 674, 676*i*
Goblet sign, in ureteral tumors, 1061, 1061*i*
Goiters, 298
   diffuse, **304**
   evaluation of, 303–304
   multinodular, **304**
   simple/nontoxic, **304**
   substernal, and superior vena caval syndrome, 373
Goldenhar variant of hemifacial microsomia, 1259
Goldman Index, 42–43
Gold weight eyelid implant, for Bell's palsy, 977
GoLYTELY. *See* Polyethylene glycol-electrolyte solution
Gonadotropic adenomas, 921
Gonadotropin-releasing hormone (GnRH) analog
   anticancer therapy with, **1356**
   for endometriosis, 1099
Gonads, differentiation of, **1013–1014,** 1016*i*
Gonococcal infection
   drug therapy for, 135*t*
   perihepatic, *versus* acute cholecystitis, 608
   pharyngitis caused by, 988
   proctitis caused by, **776–777**
      versus ulcerative colitis, 742–743
   septic arthritis caused by, 1220–1222
Good Samaritan Acts, 77
Gout, hand involvement in, 1286
G6PD deficiency. *See* Glucose 6-phosphate dehydrogenase (G6PD) deficiency
Gracilis muscle flap, **1236**
   for lower extremity, 1262
   for pressure sores, 1264
Gracilis procedure, for anorectal dysfunction, 760
Grafts
   for aortic coarctation, 446
   for arterial injury, 261
   for burns, 272–273
   dermal, 1232
   epithelial, cultured, 1232
   for head and neck tumors, 295

   skin, **1231–1234**
   for thoracic aortic aneurysm, 432
Gram-negative organisms, and infected aneurysms, 838
Granisetron, indications for, 200
Granulation tissue, 86n
   of bone, 93
   in wound healing, 86, 89, 89*i*
Granulocyte colony-stimulating factor (G-CSF), 116*t*
Granulocyte-macrophage colony-stimulating factor (GM-CSF), 116*t*
Granulocytes, 113
   in fracture healing, 93
   in wound healing, 87, 87*i*
Granulocytosis, after splenectomy, 666
Granuloma(s)
   in Crohn's disease, 689–690
   of esophagus, 494
Granulomatous colitis, **746–748.** *See also* Crohn's disease (CD)
Granulomatous lymphadenitis, in pediatric patients, **1304**
Granulomatous mediastinitis, 372, 373
Granulomatous peritonitis, **528**
Granulosa-theca cell tumors, 1110
Graves' disease, 300. *See also* Hyperthyroidism
   ocular manifestations of, 302–303
Grayson's ligament, 1270
Greater trochanter, fracture of, 1151–1152
Great toe, sesamoids of, fracture of, **1176**
Great vessels
   anomalies of, **1311,** 1311*i*
   injuries of, 242
   malposition of, 464, 468
   transposition of, 449, 452, 458, **463–467,** 464*i*
Greenfield filter, for pulmonary thromboembolism, 881, 882*i*
Greenstick fracture, 1177
Greenstick skull fractures, 937
Grey Turner's sign, in acute pancreatitis, 631
Growth factors, 115, 116*t*–117*t*
   in fracture healing, 93
   in wound healing, 86–89, 90, 91
Growth failure, in Crohn's disease, 690
Growth hormone (GH)
   actions of, 167
   in response to injury, 105
Grynfelt, space of, dorsal hernia into, 794–795, 794*i*
Guarding, in acute abdomen, 509
Gubernaculum, 1338
Guglielmi coils, for intracranial aneurysm, 942
Guillotine amputation, 864
Gunshot wound(s), 231, 247, 257, 900, 901
   history-taking about, 2
Gynecologic history, abdominal pain and, 507
Gynecology, **1085–1115**
Gynecomastia, and breast cancer, 339

Haemophilus infection
   of aneurysms, 838
   drug therapy for, 135*t*

Haemophilus influenzae infection
    after splenectomy, 666, 667
    and bronchiectasis, 385
    in paranasal sinusitis, 979, 980
    septic arthritis caused by, 1220–1222
    type B, in acute otitis media, 970
Hairy cell leukemia, **662–663**
Hairy leukoplakia, in AIDS, 998
Haldol. *See* Haloperidol
Hallpike caloric stimulation test, in assessment
        of dizziness, 975
Hallpike positional testing, in benign paroxys-
        mal positional vertigo, 976
Hallux valgus, **1216–1217**
Haloperidol
    for agitated elderly patient, 70
    for postcardiotomy delirium, 35
Halstead-Reitan Neuropsychological Battery,
        908
Halsted repair, for inguinal hernia, 788
Halter traction, for cervical strain, 1205
Hamartoma(s)
    cardiac, 469
    large bowel polyps and, 728
    of large intestine, 725*t*
    of lung, 404
    mesenchymal, 1348
    of small intestine, 702
    of spleen, 664
Hamate, fracture of, **1147**
Hamman's sign, in esophageal perforation, 371
Hamstring muscle flap, for pressure sores, 1264
Hand(s)
    amputation of, 866, 867*i*
        in crush injuries, **1288–1289**
    anatomy of, 1270–1272, 1271*i*, 1272*i*,
            1273*i*, 1274*i*
    basal cell carcinoma of, 1288
    bone tumors of, 1288
    burns of
        electrical, **1287**
        thermal, **1286–1287**
    carpal boss in, 1288
    casting of, 1274, 1275*i*
    complex injuries of, **1288–1289**
    compression neuropathies of, **1280**
    congenital anomalies of, **1260, 1275**
    crush injuries of, **1288–1289**
    deep space abscess of, **1282–1283**, 1283*i*
    degenerative arthritis of, **1285**
    disorders of, clinical evaluation of,
            1272–1273
    Dupuytren's contracture of, **1284–1285**
    enchondroma in, 1288
    epidermal cysts of, 1288
    extensor tendons of, 1272, 1273*i*
    fractures and dislocations about,
            1148–1150, 1278–1280
    frostbite of, **1287**
    ganglions of, **1287–1288**
    giant cell tumor of, 1288
    glomus tumors in, 1288
    gout in, 1286
    incisions for, 1274, 1274*i*, 1282, 1283

infections of, **1281–1284**
    tuberculous, 1284
inflammatory disorders of, **1284–1290**
injection injuries of, **1289–1290**
innervation of, 1272, 1274*i*
joints of, 1270–1271, 1271*i*, 1272*i*
ligaments of
    collateral, 1271, 1272*i*
    injury to, **1279–1280**
    longitudinal arch of, 1270–1271, 1271*i*
in lupus erythematosus, 1286
masses of, **1287–1288**
melanoma of, 1288
minimally invasive surgery for, **1290–1292**
nerves of, 1272, 1274*i*
    injuries to, 1280–1281
no-man's-land of, 1272, 1272*i*
operative principles for, 1273–1275
phlegmonous tenosynovitis of, 1283
physical examination of, 3–4, 1272–1273
position of function, 1270, 1271*i*
position of injury, 1270
position of rest, 1270, 1271*i*
pyogenic granuloma of, **1282**, 1288
pyogenic tenosynovitis of, 1283, 1283*i*
rheumatoid arthritis of, **1285**
in scleroderma, 1286
skeletal injuries of, **1148–1150, 1278–1281**
squamous cell carcinoma of, 1288
stenosing tenosynovitis in, **1278**
tendons of, 1272, 1273*i*
    disorders of, **1275–1278**
    drift of, 1277
    flexor
        infections of, 1283
        tenorrhaphy for, 1276, 1276*i*
        rupture of, 1277
        sheath of, 1272
        subluxation of, 1277
    transverse arch of, 1270–1271, 1271*i*
web spaces of
    abscess of, 1282
    contracture of, postburn, 1287
Hand-Schüller-Christian disease, 355
Hand scrub routine, 12
Hand washing, 13
    in infection control, 118–119, 120
Hangman's fracture, 910
Haplotype, 1372
Haptoglobin, in hereditary spherocytosis,
        656
Hartmann procedure
    for colorectal cancer, 722–723
    for diverticulitis, **734,** 734*i*
    for large bowel obstruction, 715
Hashimoto's thyroiditis, 305
Haustra, 705, 707*i*
β-hCG. *See* Human chorionic gonadotropin
        (HCG), beta subunit of
Headache
    in arteriovenous malformations, 944
    in brain abscess, 959
    in brain tumors, 915
    in intracranial aneurysm, 938

in paranasal sinusitis, 979
    post-dural puncture, 198
Head and neck
    congenital anomalies of, **1257–1260**
    lesions of, in pediatric patients, **1300–1304**
    reconstructive surgery for, **1260–1261**
    tumors of, **282–297**
        biology of, 282
        biopsy in, 283
        cervical lymph nodes in, 284
        chemoprevention for, 297
        chemotherapy for, 296–297
        diagnosis of, 282–284
        neck mass workup in, 284–285, 284*t*
        physical examination in, 283
        radiation therapy for, 295–296
        reconstruction for, 295
        reconstructive surgery for, 1260–1261
Head and neck surgery, **962–998**
    for ear disorders, **962–973**
    for facial nerve paralysis, 977
    for laryngeal disorders, **990–998**
    for nose and paranasal sinus disorders,
            977–984
    for oral cavity disorders, **984–986**
    for pharyngeal disorders, **987–990**
    for salivary gland disorders, **986–987**
    for vestibular system disorders, 974–976
Head injury
    in children, **936–937**
    mechanical ventilation in, 214
    prehospital care for, 232
    pulmonary edema with, 214
    shock caused by, 209
    survival in, prediction of, 225
Healing. *See also* Wound healing
    intestinal, 92–93
Healing ridge, 24
Health assessment, preoperative, 6–7
Hearing, **962**
    air conduction, **962**
    bone conduction, **962–963**
Hearing aids, for otosclerosis, 968
Hearing loss
    conductive, **962,** 964*i,* **965–968**
        in otosclerosis, 968
    evaluation of, **962–965,** 963*t*
        in infants, 964–965, 965*t*
    with head and neck tumors, 282–283
    high-risk criteria for, 965*t*
    in Meniere's disease, 975
    sensorineural, **962–963,** 964*i,* **968–969**
        in AIDS, 998
        in infants, 969
Heart. *See also* Cardiac
    accidental hypothermia and, 280
    conduction abnormalities, **44–45**
    diseases/disorders of (*See also* Heart failure)
        abdominal pain in, 514
        acquired, **408–437**
        anesthetic selection in, 45
        congenital (*See* Congenital heart disease)
        contraindications to surgery in, 42–43
        ischemic, **408–418**

masquerading as surgical illness, 42
nutritional support in, 188
shock caused by, 207–208
in surgical patient, 41–46
valvular, 28, **44**, 45
fibrous skeleton of, 419
injuries of, **246–247**
postoperative complications in, **28–29**
noncardiac complications and, 28
risk factors for, 28
transplantation of, 417–418, **1380–1383**
donor for, selection of, 1381
follow-up care for, 1381–1383
graft rejection in, 470, 1381
immunosuppression for, 1381
operative technique for, 1381, 1382i
pediatric, **470**
recipient for, selection of, 1381
survival rate with, 1380
tumors of, **434–435**, 434t, 435f, **469–470**
Heart block, 466
bifascicular, 45
complete, postoperative, 28
Heartburn, and reflux esophagitis, 485
Heart failure
arteriovenous malformations and, 944
clinical presentation of, 42
as contraindication to surgery, 42
in elderly, 67–68
postoperative, **29**
in elderly, 68
right, clinical presentation of, 42
Heart-lung transplantation, combined, **1383**
Heart murmur
with aortic insufficiency, 427
with aortic stenosis, 426
with mitral stenosis, 421
with tricuspid valve disease, 425
Heart muscle, metabolic activity of, 408–409
Heart rate
in cardiogenic shock, 207–208
in craniocerebral trauma, 902–903
in hypovolemia, 204
in increased intracranial pressure, 890
Heart valves, 419–420
diseases/disorders of, 28, **44**, 45
prosthetic, **428–430**
antibiotic prophylaxis with, 45
biologic, **428,** 428i, 429i
mechanical, **428–429,** 429i
replacement of
for congenital mitral valve disease, 448
for endocarditis, 430
indications for, 429–430
for valvular aortic stenosis, 443
Heat cramps, 277
Heat exhaustion, 278
Heat loss, in burn patients, 270
Heat stroke, **277–279**
Height, assessment of, 156–158
Heimlich maneuver, 990
Heimlich valve, for pneumothorax, 368
Heineke-Mikulicz procedure, for duodenal
ulcer, 541, 542i

Heister, spiral valve of, 595
Helicobacter pylori
and duodenal ulcer, 539, 541
and gastric carcinoma, 556
and gastric lymphoma, 1368
and gastric ulcer, 547
and peptic ulcer, 539
and Raynaud's syndrome, 843
Heller myotomy, for achalasia, 479
Helmets, as safety precaution, 231
Hemangioblastomas, of spinal cord, 928
Hemangioendothelioma
of chest wall, 355–356
infantile, 1349
Hemangioma, **1246–1249**
capillary, 1246, 1341
cavernous, 1246, 1247t, **1248–1249,** 1341,
1349
of chest wall, 354, 355
of eyelid, 1010
choroidal, 1011
classification of, 1246–1247, 1247t, 1341
of eyelid, 1010
hepatic, **576**
angiography of, 572, 576
in childhood, **1349**
involuting, 1246, **1247–1248,** 1247t,
1341–1342
combined superficial and deep, 1247,
1247t
deep, 1247, 1247t
superficial, 1247–1248, 1247t
noninvoluting, 1247t, **1248**
in pediatric patients, **1341–1342**
renal, 1059
subglottic, 992
Hematemesis, 548
abdominal pain and, 507
in children, 1332
history-taking about, 2
Hematochezia, 548
abdominal pain and, 507
in children, 1332
history-taking about, 2
in rectal cancer, 719
Hematocolpos, 1085
Hematocrit
in acute pancreatitis, 631
in hypovolemia, 204, 205
with metastatic neoplasms of liver, 574
Hematogenous dissemination
of colorectal cancer, **718**
and lung abscess, 383
Hematologic disease
malignant, in surgical patient, **53–54**
simulating acute abdomen, 53
in surgical patient, **52–62**
Hematoma(s)
duodenal, 253–254
epidural, **906,** 906i
in fracture healing, 93
lung, 246
perirenal, 255
postoperative, **23**

of rectus sheath, **796**
septal, 982–983
and small bowel obstruction, **684**
subdural, **906–907,** 907i
venous epidural, 906
wound, and wound healing, 24
Hematometra, 1085
Hematuria
abdominal pain and, 507
in renal adenocarcinoma, 1054, 1056
in renal pelvis and calices tumors, 1059
in ureteral tumors, 1061
Hemiarthroplasty, in hip, 1157
Hemicolectomy
for angiodysplasia, 738
right, for tumors of appendix, 672–673
for volvulus, 740
Hemifacial microsomia, 1259
Hemigastrectomy, for gastric ulcer, 547
Hemihypertrophy, Wilms' tumor and, 1344
Hemipelvectomy, **866,** 866i
Hemivagina, 1085
Hemobilia, 570, **621**
with hepatic abscess, 594
Hemoconcentration, in acute mesenteric vascular occlusion, 699
Hemodilution, 57
for subarachnoid hemorrhage, 942
Hemodynamic instability, in craniocerebral
trauma, management of, **903**
Hemodynamic monitoring, 45
complications of, **35–36**
indications for, 51
Hemoglobin, 220–222
in hereditary spherocytosis, 656
Hemoglobinopathies, *versus* hypersplenism,
654
Hemoglobinuria, in hemolytic transfusion reaction, 59
Hemolysis
in hereditary spherocytosis, 656
increased, 32, 32t
Hemolytic anemia
acquired, 658
autoimmune, **658**
hereditary nonspherocytic, **657**
versus hereditary spherocytosis, 656
immune, secondary, 658, 658t
Hemoperitoneum, 249
postoperative, **29–30**
Hemophilia A, 56, 61
Hemophilia B, 56, 61
Hemophilia C, 56
Hemopneumothorax, 245i, 367
Hemoptysis, in pulmonary thromboembolism,
880
Hemorrhage. *See also* Bleeding; Hematoma
abdominal wall, 53
arterial injury causing, 258, 260
in arteriovenous malformations, 934, 944,
947
postoperative, 946
epidural, 906i
gastrointestinal, lower, **736–737,** 737i

Hemorrhage (*cont.*)
in head and neck tumors, 282
hepatic, 252
in trauma, 569–570
in intracranial aneurysm, 938, 939*t*
normal perfusion pressure, 946
and pancreatic pseudocyst, **637**
with pelvic fracture, 1126
in peptic ulcer, **550–551**
perirenal, in kidney injury, 1049
postpartum, 58
sentinel, 938, 940
subdural, 907*i*
in trauma victim, 237–238, 569–570
in ulcerative colitis, **743**
upper gastrointestinal, **548–550**
Hemorrhagic gastritis, acute, **556**
Hemorrhagic pancreatitis, 631–635
Hemorrhagic shock. *See* Shock, hypovolemic
Hemorrhagic stroke, and neurosurgery for
movement disorders, 948
Hemorrhoid(s), 758, **766–768**, 873
external, 766
thrombosed, 767–768
internal, 766
classification of, 766–767
prolapse of, 764
Hemorrhoidal arteries, 705–706, 706*i*
Hemorrhoidal veins, 706*i*
Hemorrhoidectomy, excisional, 768
Hemostasis, preoperative evaluation of, 52
Hemothorax, 244, 245, 245*i*, 347, 357,
366–367
Hemotoxin, in snake venom, 130–131
Henderson-Hasselbalch equation, 150, 223
Henoch-Schönlein purpura, 53
Heparin
for acute mesenteric vascular occlusion, 699
for angina pectoris, 412
for arterial injury, 261
for burn patients, 271
for deep venous thrombosis, 876, 877
in elderly, 68
for glucagonoma, 651
indications for, 54
for intra-arterial injections, 858
low-molecular-weight, **54**
for deep venous thrombosis, 877
for pulmonary thromboembolism, 881
neutralization of, 54
perioperative management of, 28, 46
for pulmonary thromboembolism, 881
in surgical patients, **54**
unfractionated, 54
Heparin-induced thrombocytopenia with
thrombosis syndrome (HIT/TS),
54–55
Hepatectomy. *See* Liver, resection of
Hepatic artery(ies), 565–566, 595, 597*i*
aneurysms of, **841–842**
angiographic embolization of, for metastatic
neoplasms of liver, 575
infusion chemotherapy, 1359
for metastatic neoplasms of liver, 575

ligation of, for metastatic neoplasms of liver,
575
Hepatic blood flow, 566–567
Hepatic ducts, 595, 597*i*
Hepatic encephalopathy, 188, **591–593**
laboratory findings in, 592
pathogenesis of, 591–592, 591*t*
prevention of, 592
treatment of, 592–593
Hepatic flexure, of colon, 706*i*
Hepaticojejunostomy, for choledochal cyst,
1334
Hepatic portoenterostomy, for biliary atresia,
1334
Hepatic vein(s), 565, 567*i*
injuries of, 252
thrombosis of, 589
Hepatitis
alcoholic, *versus* choledocholithiasis, 614
neonatal, 1334
in renal transplant recipient, 1379
viral
and hepatic cancer, 571
liver transplantation for, 1384
transfusion-related, 60
Hepatoblastoma, 571
in pediatric patients, **1348–1349**
Hepatocellular carcinoma (HCC), 571–574
and Budd-Chiari syndrome, 589
in childhood, **1349**
endocrinopathy with, 573
paraneoplastic syndromes with, 1371*t*
screening for, 572
Hepatocellular insufficiency, 32, 32*t*
Hepatocholangioma, 571–574
Hepatocyte transplantation, 1386
Hepatoduodenal ligament, 565, 597*i*
Hepatoma, **571–574**
diffuse, 571
fibrolamellar, 571
massive, 571
metastases of, 571
nodular, 571
Hepatomegaly
in idiopathic myelofibrosis, 663
in pancreatic adenocarcinoma, 644
Hepatopancreatic ampulla, stenosis of, **622**
Hepatorenal failure, nutritional support in,
188
Herceptin, 1358
Hereditary disorders, splenectomy and,
655–657
Hereditary elliptocytosis, **657**
Hereditary flat adenoma syndrome, 728
Hereditary hemorrhagic telangiectasia, 736
Hereditary nonpolyposis colorectal cancer
(HNPCC), 716–717
Hereditary nonspherocytic hemolytic anemia,
657
Hereditary site-specific colon cancer (HSSCC),
716–717
Hereditary spherocytosis, **655–656**
versus hypersplenism, 654
Hering, canals of, 595

Hernia(s), **783–796**
of abdominal wall, 783–791
rare types of, 794–795
traumatic, **795–796**
bowel strangulation with, 786
complete, 783
diaphragmatic
congenital, **1308–1309**, 1309*i*
traumatic, **501–502**
dorsal, 794–795, 794*i*
epigastric, **791–792**, 792*i*
femoral, 784, **790–791**, 1336
causes of, 784
foramen of Bochdalek, **501**, 501*i*
foramen of Morgagni, **501**, 501*i*, **1309–1310**
of groin, 783–791
causes of, 784
classification of, 784–785
hiatal
paraesophageal, **482–483**, 483*i*
in pregnancy, 65
reflux esophagitis sliding, **484–488**, 484*i*,
487*i*, 488*i*
incisional, **792–793**
large, 793
small, 793
inguinal, 33, **1336–1338**, 1336*i*
Bassini repair for, 788
bilateral repair of, 787
clinical findings with, 785, **1337**
complications of, 1337
Cooper's ligament (Lotheissen-McVay)
repair for, 788
differential diagnosis of, 785–786, **1337**
direct, 784, **785–789**, 1336
causes of, 784
funicular type, 784, 786
treatment of, 787, 787*i*
Halsted repair for, 788
incarcerated, 1337–1338
indirect, 783, **785–789**, 1336 (*See also*
Hernia(s), inguinal, sliding)
causes of, 784
repair of, 786–787, 786*i*
Marcy repair for, 787
nonsurgical management of, 788
open mesh repair for, 788
operative treatment of, **1337–1338**
principles of, 786–787
procedures for, 787–788
in pregnancy, 65
prognosis for, 788–789
recurrent, 787, 788–789
risk factors for, 1337
Shouldice repair for, 788
signs and symptoms of, 785, 785*i*
sliding, **789–790**, 789*i*, 790*i*
strangulation of, 1337
treatment of, 786–788, **1337–1338**
pre- and postoperative course in, 788
preperitoneal approach for, 788
prosthetic materials for, 788
by simple high ligation of sac, 787
truss for, 788

inguinoscrotal, 1336*i*
internal (mesenteric), 31
interparietal, 795
irreducible (incarcerated), 783, 786
Littre's, 794
lumbar, 794–795, 794*i*
   acquired, 795
   congenital, 795
lung, **352**
mediastinal, 347
obstructed, 783
obturator, 795
pantaloon, 784
paracolostomy, 753–754
parasternal, **501**, 501*i*
perineal, 795
pleuroperitoneal, **501**, 501*i*
in pregnancy, 65
reducible, 783
retrosternal, **501**, 501*i*
Richter, 783
sciatic, 795
and small bowel obstruction, **683**, 683*t*
spigelian, 794
strangulated, 783
umbilical, **1339**
   in adults, **791**
   in pregnancy, 65
ventral, **792–793**
   in pregnancy, 65
Herniation
   tonsillar, **891**
   transtentorial, **891**, 891*t*
Herniography, 785–786
Herpes proctitis, **776**
Herpes simplex virus (HSV) infection
   hand involvement in, 1284
   treatment of, 141
   type 2, and cervical cancer, 1106
   versus ulcerative colitis, 742–743
Herpes zoster, 796
   treatment of, 141
Herpes zoster oticus syndrome, in AIDS,
   998
Herpetic stomatitis, **985**
Herpetic whitlow, 1284
Hesselbach's triangle, 784
Hetastarch, as blood substitute, 62
Heterotaxia, **468**
HHH (hypervolemia, hypertension hemodilu-
   tion) therapy, for subarachnoid hem-
   orrhage, 942
Hiatal hernia. *See* Hernia(s), hiatal
Hibiclens. *See* Chlorhexidine gluconate
HIDA scan. *See* Radionuclide scan
Hidradenitis suppurativa, **126–127**, 772
Hidradenoma, **1095**
High-frequency ventilation, for pediatric pa-
   tients, 1295
Hilar lymphadenopathy, and bronchiectasis,
   385
Hip(s). *See also* Legg-Perthes disease; Slipped
   capital femoral epiphyses
   arthrodesis in, 1155

arthroplasty of, and deep vein thrombosis,
   877
bursitis of, **1200–1201**
congenital dysplasia of, **1189–1192**
disarticulation of, **865**
dislocatable
   detection of, 1190, 1190*i*
   treatment of, 1192
dislocated
   detection of, 1190–1191, 1190*i*
   treatment of, 1192
dislocation of, **1150–1155**
   congenital, 1188, **1189–1192**, 1191*i*
   traumatic, **1154–1157**, 1154*i*
      in children, **1181**
endoprosthesis for, 1157
   bipolar or universal, 1157
fractures of, **1150–1155**
   sequelae of, surgical management of,
      1155–1157
Girdlestone arthroplasty in, 1156, 1157
hemiarthroplasty in, 1157
intertrochanteric fractures of, 1152–1153,
   1152*i*
osteotomy in, 1155
pain syndromes of, **1200–1204**
replacement, total, 1156–1157, 1156*i*
septic arthritis of, **1187–1189**, 1188*i*
snapping, **1201**
subtrochanteric fractures of, 1153, 1153*i*
tendinitis of, **1200–1201**
transient synovitis of, **1189**
traumatic dislocation of, **1154–1157**, 1154*i*
   in children, **1181**
trauma to, **1154–1157**, 1154*i*
   and avascular necrosis of femoral head,
      1201
   in children, **1181**
trochanteric fractures of, 1151–1153
Hippel-Lindau syndrome, 1054
Hirschsprung's disease, **1321–1322**
Histamine (H₂) antagonists
   for columnar-lined lower esophagus, 489
   for duodenal ulcer, 541
   indications for, 194, 201
   for Ménétrier's disease, 561
   for pancreatic insufficiency, 643
   prophylactic, indications for, 568
   for reflux esophagitis sliding hiatal hernia,
      486
   for short bowel syndrome, 682
   for small intestine fistulas, 697
   for stress ulcers, 556
   for upper gastrointestinal hemorrhage, 549
   for Zollinger-Ellison syndrome, 545–546
Histocompatibility antigens, 1372–1373
   class I, 1372
   class II, 1372
Histoplasma capsulatum, 390, 392
   and thoracic empyema, 361
Histoplasmosis (*Histoplasma* infection), 112,
   390–391
   and broncholithiasis, 386
   and chronic mediastinitis, 372

skin tests for, 349
treatment of, 141
History, **1–3**
   in anesthetic risk evaluation, 192
   family, 2
   in female infertility, 1086
   in heart disease, 42
   in nutritional assessment, 156, 157*t*
   past, 2–3
   in pulmonary dysfunction, 8
HIV. *See* Human immunodeficiency virus
   (HIV)
HLA-DR, 107
HLA system, 1372–1373
HNPCC (hereditary nonpolyposis colorectal
   cancer), 716–717
Hoarseness, 282, 990
Hodgkin's lymphoma, **1365–1367**
   B symptoms of, 1365–1366
   mediastinal, 377
   staging of, 1366, 1366*t*
   subtypes of, 1365, 1366*t*
   and superior vena caval syndrome, 373
   treatment of, 1366–1367
Hollenhorst plaques, and cerebrovascular disease, 848
Homan's sign, in deep venous thrombosis,
   876
Homografts (human skin), 272
Hordeolum, acute, **1002**
Hormone(s)
   anticancer therapy with, **1356–1357**
   counterregulatory (catabolic), 106
   in male infertility, **1080**
   metabolically active, in shock, 210–211
   therapy with, for breast cancer
      in females, 331, 331*t*, 332*t*, 333–334,
         333*t*
      in males, 340
   vasoactive, in shock, 210
   volume-conserving, in shock, 211
Hormone receptor sites, breast cancer and,
   329
Hormone replacement therapy (HRT)
   after hysterectomy, 1098
   uterine bleeding with, 1089
Horner's syndrome, with head and neck tumors, 283
Horseshoe kidneys, 1019, 1019*i*
Hospital environment, control of, in infection
   control, 12–13
Houston, rectal valves of, 705
Howship-Romberg sign, 795
HSSCC (hereditary site-specific colon cancer),
   716–717
Human chorionic gonadotropin (HCG)
   beta subunit of, in testicular cancer, 1071
   in ectopic pregnancy, 1102–1103
   in gestational trophoblastic disease, 1113
   serum levels of, teratoma and, 1347
   tumors secreting, 300 (*See also* Hyperthy-
      roidism)
Human fetal substantia nigra allografts, for
   Parkinson's disease, 948

Human immunodeficiency virus (HIV). *See also* Acquired immunodeficiency syndrome (AIDS)
  and anal cancer, 779
  and fungal infections of lung, 390
  infection
    enteropathy with, **693–694**
    hearing loss in, 974
    thrombocytopenia and, 659
  and pneumocystosis, 394
  transmission of, transfusion-related, 60
  and tuberculosis, 387
Human leukocyte antigen(s) (HLA). *See* HLA system
Human papillomavirus (HPV), 777–778. *See also* Condylomata acuminata
  and anal cancer, 779
  and cervical cancer, 1106
  in recurrent respiratory papillomatosis, 994
  venereal, 1082
  and vulvar cancer, 1104
Human T-cell lymphotropic virus (HTLV), transmission of, transfusion-related, 60
Humerus
  capitellum, fractures of, 1136, 1136*i*
  distal, fractures of, 1133–1135
  epicondylitis of, **1199–1200**
  fractures of
    condylar, 1135, 1135*i*
    epicondylar, 1135
    intercondylar, 1136–1137, 1136*i*
    intra-articular, 1135–1137
    supracondylar
      in adults, 1135
      in children, 1134–1135, 1134*i*, **1179–1180**
  proximal, fractures of, **1130,** 1130*i*, 1131*i*
    in children, **1179**
  shaft of, fractures of, **1133**
Humidification, for bronchiectasis, 385
Humoral immunity. *See* Immunity, humoral
Hunter's perforator, 871, 872*i*
Hunt-Hess Scale, for subarachnoid hemorrhage, 939*t,* 943
Hydatid disease. *See* Echinococcosis
Hydatidiform mole, 1112. *See also* Gestational trophoblastic disease
  complete, 1113
  frequency of, 1113
  invasive, 1112
  partial, 1113
Hydration. *See also* Fluid(s)
  perioperative, 50
  preoperative, 49–50
Hydrocele, 786, **1336–1338,** 1336*i*
  communicating, 1336, 1336*i*, 1337
  noncommunicating, 1336, 1337
  scrotal, 1336*i*
  of spermatic cord, 1336, 1336*i*
Hydrocephalus, 934
  progressive, 891
  in subarachnoid hemorrhage, 940

Hydrochloric acid
  in gastric secretion, 536
  secretion of, 152
Hydrochlorothiazide, for renal stones, 1043
Hydrocodone with acetaminophen, for postoperative analgesia, 21
Hydrocortisone
  for aspiration, 26
  indications for, 809–810
  for ulcerative colitis, 744
Hydrocortisone suppression test, 311
Hydrogen
  and gas cysts in small intestine, 701
  in intestinal gas, 707
Hydrogen ion concentration [H⁺], 150, 221*t*, 223
  conversion of pH to, 224, 224*t*
Hydromorphone, 20
Hydronephrosis
  in kidney injury, 1049
  and pleural effusion, 360
  ureteral calculi and, 1045*i*
Hydrops, endolymphatic, **975**
Hydrosalpinx, 1087
Hydrotherapy, for burns, 272
Hydrothorax, **357–360**
  in cirrhotic patient with ascites, 591
  with malignancy, 357–359, 359*i*
5-Hydroxyindoleacetic acid, in carcinoid syndrome, 703–704
21-Hydroxylase deficiency, 810
Hydroxyurea, indications for, 53
Hydroxyzine, 20
Hymen, imperforate, **1085**
Hymenotomy, 1085
Hypaque. *See* Diatrizoate sodium
Hyperadrenocorticism (Cushing disease, Cushing syndrome), **805–810,** 930–931
  complications of, 808–809
  imaging in, 808
  laboratory diagnosis of, 806–808, 807*i*
  manifestations of, 798*t*, 806
  medical therapy for, 809
  as paraneoplastic syndrome, 1370, 1371*t*
  pathology of, 806
  preclinical, as adrenal incidentaloma, 811–812, 812*t*
  prognosis for, 810
  treatment of, 809–810
Hyperaldosteronism
  familial, 799
    type 1, 800
  glucocorticoid-remediable, 800
  idiopathic
    with adrenal hyperplasia, 798
    differential diagnosis of, 799–800
  primary, **798–801**
    confirmatory test for, 799
    differential diagnosis of, 799–800
    laboratory diagnosis of, 799
    medical therapy for, 801
    screening test for, 799
    signs and symptoms of, 799
    treatment of, 800–801

secondary, 798
Hyperalimentation
  for pancreatic ascites, 639
  preoperative, 7
Hyperamylasemia
  chronic, 632
  postoperative, 32
Hyperbaric oxygen therapy
  for arterial/ischemic ulcers, 96
  for diffuse necrotizing infections, 125
Hyperbilirubinemia
  neonatal, 1333–1334
  postoperative, 32
Hypercalcemia, **148–149**
  benign familial hypocalciuric, 312
  causes of, 310–311, 310*t*
  and hyperparathyroidism, 309
  laboratory evaluation of, 310*t*
  malignancy-associated, 149, 311, 1370, 1371*t*
  marked, 313
  in pancreatic cholera, 650
  and pancreatitis, **628**
  as paraneoplastic syndrome, 1370, 1371*t*
  in total parenteral nutrition, 183*t*
Hypercalcemic crisis, 313
Hypercalciuria, in renal stones, 1042, 1044
Hypercapnia, 223
  and cardiac complications, 28
Hypercholesterolemia, and atherosclerosis, 813
Hypercoagulability
  and axillary-subclavian venous thrombosis, 878, 879
  and deep vein thrombosis, 875
Hyperemia, reactive, in peripheral arterial insufficiency, 817
Hyperextension injury, cervical disk syndrome and, 955
Hyperglycemia
  in enteral feeding, 174
  hyponatremia in, 146
  in response to injury, 108
  in total parenteral nutrition, 181, 182*t*–183*t*
Hyperhomocysteinemia, 50
Hyperkalemia, **147**
  emergency treatment of, 147
  in renal failure, 146
  in response to injury, 107
  in total parenteral nutrition, 183*t*
Hyperlipidemia
  hyponatremia with, 145–146
  and pancreatitis, **628**
  and peripheral arterial insufficiency, 820
Hypermagnesemia, **149**
  in total parenteral nutrition, 183*t*
Hypermenorrhea, 1088, 1089
Hypermetabolism, in response to injury, 107
  in burn patient, 185–186
Hypernatremia, 144, 145
  and intracranial hypertension, 905
  in total parenteral nutrition, 183*t*
Hyperosmolar coma, postoperative, **40**
Hyperostosis, in meningiomas, 919
Hyperoxaluria, enteric, 680
  prevention of, 682

Hyperparathyroidism
    ectopic, 311
    normocalcemic patient with, 312
    primary, **308–315**
    recurrence rate of, 315
    secondary, **316**
    tertiary, **316**
Hyperphosphatemia, **150**
    in total parenteral nutrition, 183*t*
Hyperprolactinemia
    in impotence, 1083
    in male infertility, 1081
    in pituitary tumors, 921, 930, 931
Hyperproteinemia, hyponatremia with,
        145–146
Hyperreflexic bladder, **1075–1076**
Hypersensitivity reactions, and granulomatous
        peritonitis, 528
Hypersplenism, **653–655**
    primary, 653
    secondary, 653, 654*t*
    versus splenomegaly, 653
Hypertension, **45**. *See also* Portal hypertension
    causes of, differential diagnosis of, 804
    as contraindication to surgery, 42
    corticosteroid therapy and, 41
    in craniocerebral trauma, 902–903
    in elderly, 68
    in endotracheal intubation, 196
    in hyperaldosteronism, 799, 800, 801
    and infrarenal abdominal aortic aneurysms,
        830
    intracranial (*See* Intracranial pressure, ele-
        vated)
    in kidney injury, 1049
    and mitral regurgitation, 422
    and mitral stenosis, 420
    and peripheral arterial insufficiency, 820
    with pheochromocytoma, 802, 804
    renovascular, **853–856**, 853*i*
    shock caused by, 207–208
Hypertensive lower esophageal sphincter, 476
Hyperthyroidism, **300–303**, 300*t*
    apathetic, 300
    differential diagnosis of, 312
    iodine-induced, 301
    in surgical patient, **40–41**
Hypertrophic gastritis, 561
Hypertrophic obstructive cardiomyopathy,
        444–445
Hypertrophic osteoarthropathy, as paraneoplas-
        tic syndrome, 1371*t*
Hyperuricosuria, and renal stones, 1043–1044
Hyperventilation
    and delirium tremens, 35
    for intracranial hypertension, 905
    with respiratory alkalosis, 152
    for subarachnoid hemorrhage, 941
Hypoaldosteronism, hyporeninemic, 38
Hypocalcemia, **148**
    in acute pancreatitis, 633
    in blind loop syndrome, 679
    neonatal, 1296
    in total parenteral nutrition, 183*t*

Hypogastric artery, 706*i*
    injury to, in urethral injury, 1051–1052
Hypoglycemia
    with insulinoma, 649
    neonatal, 1297
    as paraneoplastic syndrome, 1371*t*
    postoperative, in diabetic patient, 40
    signs and symptoms of, 40
    in total parenteral nutrition, 181, 183*t*
Hypogonadotropic hypogonadism, in male in-
        fertility, 1081
Hypokalemia, 146, **147–148**, 153
    and cardiac complications, 28
    corticosteroid therapy and, 41
    in hyperaldosteronism, 798–799, 800
    and hyperglycemia, 38
    in pancreatic cholera, 650
    in total parenteral nutrition, 183*t*
Hypomagnesemia, **149**
    in acute pancreatitis, 633
    neonatal, 1296
    in total parenteral nutrition, 183*t*
Hyponatremia, 145–146, 153
    in hyperglycemia, 146
    with hyperlipidemia, 145–146
    with hyperproteinemia, 145–146
    in response to injury, 107
    in total parenteral nutrition, 183*t*
Hypoparathyroidism, **317–318**
    chronic, 318
    and hypocalcemia, 148
Hypopharynx, cancer of, 282, **289–290**
Hypophosphatemia, **149–150**
    in total parenteral nutrition, 181, 183*t*
Hypophysectomy, for breast cancer, 334
Hypoplastic left heart syndrome, **447–448**
    and single ventricle, 467
Hypospadias, **1028**, 1028*i*
    Wilms' tumor and, 1344
Hypotension
    and cardiac complications, 29
    in cardiac compressive shock, 206
    in craniocerebral trauma, 902
    in hypovolemia, 204
    postural
        in cardiac compressive shock, 206
        in elderly, 68
        in hypovolemia, 203, 204
        supine, in hypovolemia, 204
Hypothalamic-pituitary-adrenocortical axis, in
        response to injury, 103, 105*i*
Hypothenar space, abscess of, 1283
Hypothermia. *See also* Frostbite
    accidental, **280–281**
    in cardiopulmonary bypass, 439–440
    in near-drowning, 265
Hypothyroidism
    iodide-induced, 301
    in surgical patient, **40–41**
Hypovolemia. *See also* Shock, hypovolemic
    with aspiration, 26
    clinical classification of, 203–204, 204*t*
    clinical manifestations of, 29
    inebriation and, 204, 205*t*

with pheochromocytoma, 804
    postoperative, 18
    in small bowel obstruction, 684
Hypovolemic shock. *See* Shock, hypovolemic
Hypoxemia
    in acute pancreatitis, 633
    in acute respiratory distress syndrome, 212
    and cardiac complications, 28, 29
Hypoxia, tissue, and wound healing, 89, 91, **91**
Hysterectomy
    for adenomyosis, 1099
    for chronic pelvic pain, 1090
    for dysfunctional uterine bleeding, 1089
    for endometrial cancer, 1109
    for endometriosis, 1098
    for leiomyomas, 1100
    in ovarian cancer, 1112
    vesicovaginal fistula after, 1094
Hysterosalpingography, 1086
    of tubal abnormalities, 1087
Hysteroscopy, 1088

Iatrogenic arterial trauma, **858**
Iatrogenic pancreatitis, **628–629**
Icterus. *See also* Jaundice
    in bile duct malignancies, 617
ICU syndrome, **35**
Ideal body weight, 158*t*
Idiopathic hypertrophic subaortic stenosis,
        441*i*
Idiopathic mucosal ulcerative colitis. *See* Ulcer-
        ative colitis (UC)
Idiopathic myelofibrosis, **663**
Idiopathic pancreatitis, **629**
Idiopathic thrombocytopenic purpura (ITP),
        659–660
"Ileal brake" reflex, 679
Ileal pouch-anal anastomosis
    for familial adenomatous polyposis, 728
    for ulcerative colitis, 745, 746
Ileitis
    backwash, 741
    ileostomy and, 753*t*
Ileoanal anastomosis
    for familial adenomatous polyposis, 728
    for ulcerative colitis, 745, 745*i*
Ileocecal syndrome, 750
Ileocecal valve, and intestinal obstruction, 713,
        713*i*
Ileocolic artery, 706*i*
Ileocolic lymph nodes, 718*i*
Ileorectal anastomosis, for Crohn's disease, 748
Ileostomy, 709*t*, **751–752**, 752*i*
    complications of, 753*t*
    for Crohn's disease, 748
    for ulcerative colitis, 745
Ileum, 674
    atresia and stenosis of, 1317–1318
    duplication of, 1328–1329, 1329*i*
    resection of, consequences of, 680–682, 681*i*
    tumors of, 701–704
Ileus
    gallstone, **611–612**
    and small bowel obstruction, **683**

Ileus (*cont.*)
paralytic (adynamic), 31, 677, 683
versus large bowel obstruction, **714**
versus small bowel obstruction, 686
postoperative, 24, 30
Iliac artery, 872*i*
aneurysms of, **835–836**, 836*i*
external, 706*i*, 784
internal, 705–706
stenosis of, treatment of, 822, 822*i*
Iliac colostomy, 752
Iliac veins, 871, 872*i*
Iliofemoral thrombectomy, 877
Iliofemoral venous thrombosis, 876
Ilioinguinal nerve, 784
Iliopsoas sign, 509
Iliopsoas tendon, snapping of, 1201
Iliotibial band, snapping hip caused by, 1201
Ilizarov technique
for bone transport, 1263
of linear distraction osteogenesis, 94
Imaging. *See also* Chest x-ray(s); Computed tomography (CT); Magnetic resonance angiography (MRA); Magnetic resonance imaging (MRI); Ultrasonography
in acute abdomen, 511–513
of anorectal anomalies, 1326
of blast injuries, 264
in cervical muscle strain, 1205
in chronic osteomyelitis, 1218
of congenital diaphragmatic hernia, 1309
of congenital hip dislocation, 1191, 1191*i*
in degenerative cervical disk disease, 1208, 1208*i*
of facial fractures, 1255
of focal nodular hyperplasia of liver, 578
of gastroesophageal reflux, in children, 1327
of hand, 1273
of hepatic abscess, 593
of hepatic adenomas, 577
of hepatic hemangioma, 572, 576
of hepatic trauma, 569–570
of hepatoblastoma, 1348
in Hirschsprung's disease, 1321
in Hodgkin's lymphoma, 1366
in hyperadrenocorticism (Cushing disease, Cushing syndrome), 808
in infection, 117
of intestinal duplications, 1329
of intestinal malrotation, 1319
of liver cancer, 572
in low back pain, 1211
in lumbar disk syndrome, 1213
of meconium ileus, 1320
of metastatic neoplasms of liver, 574–575
of neuroblastoma, 1343
in osteoarthritis, 1202
postoperative, 15
of pyloric stenosis, 1316
in rheumatoid arthritis, 1203
in septic arthritis, 1221
of spinal deformity, 1185
of spinal injury, 1119–1120

in surgical patient, 5
in trauma management, 240
of uterine leiomyomas, 1100
in whiplash injury, 1206
of Wilms' tumor, 1344
Imipenem
for acute cholecystitis, 609
for acute pancreatitis, 633
dosage of
in hepatic failure, 138*t*
in renal failure, 138*t*
indications for, 129, 135*t*
pharmacology of, 138*t*
renal failure and, 51
Imipenem-cilastatin, for acute secondary bacterial peritonitis, 519
Immediate death, 230
Immersion foot, 279
Immigration, and tuberculosis, 387
Immobilization
at accident scene, **234**
of hand, 1274–1275
for spinal fracture, 1120–1121, 1123
Immune competence, preoperative assessment of, 7–8
Immune deficiency. *See also* Acquired immunodeficiency syndrome (AIDS); Immunocompromised patient
and operative risk, 7–8
risk factors for, 7–8
Immune function
dietary fats and, 162–163
in malnutrition, 157*t*, 158*t*, 159*t*, 160
of spleen, 652–653
Immune hemolytic anemias, secondary, 658, 658*t*
Immune-mediated inner ear disease, 974
Immune thrombocytopenic purpura, **659–660**
Immunity
cell-mediated, 106, 1357, 1372–1373
in burn patients, 270
in diabetes mellitus, 114
humoral, 1357, 1373
impaired, and operative risk, 7–8
innate (*See* Immunity, nonspecific)
nonspecific, 107, **113**
and organ transplantation, 1372–1375
specific, 106, 108, **112–113**
Immunization, in asplenic patients, 666–667
Immunocompromised patient
anorectal infection in, 772
Bowen's disease in, 780
lung abscess and, 383
Immunoglobulin(s)
deficiency of, and bronchiectasis, 384
IgG
autoantibodies, in autoimmune disorders, 657
in Felty's syndrome, 660
IgM, autoantibodies, in autoimmune disorders, 657
Immunoproliferative small intestinal disease, 702

Immunosuppression, 112
after injury, 108
carbuncles in, 126
for Crohn's disease, 748
and fungal infections of lung, 390
for heart transplantation, 470, 1381
for immune thrombocytopenic purpura, 660
for kidney transplantation
complications of, 1379
drugs for, **1374–1375**
for liver transplantation, 1385
for organ transplantation, 470, 1372, 1374–1375, 1379, 1381, 1385
for retroperitoneal fibrosis, 531–532
and superinfection, 115
for ulcerative colitis, 744
Immunotherapy
for allergic rhinitis, 978
anticancer, **1357–1358**
active, with tumor vaccines, **1358**
adoptive, **1358**
antibody-mediated (passive), **1358**
nonspecific, **1357–1358**
for bladder tumors, 1065
for Hodgkin's lymphoma, 1367
for lung cancer, 403
for non-Hodgkin's lymphoma, 1369
for renal adenocarcinoma, 1057
Imodium, for short bowel syndrome, 682
Impact injury, of head, **901**
Impedance audiometry, in otitis media with effusion, 966
Imperforate anus, **1324–1327**, 1325*i*
Implantable materials
for augmentation mammoplasty, 1266–1267
biocompatibility of, 95
for breast reconstruction, 1261
infection with, 95
Impotence, **1082–1084**
and peripheral arterial insufficiency, 817
postoperative, 35
in urethral injury, 1051
Incentive spirometry, 26
Incidentalomas, **811–812**
Incision(s), in hand, 1274, 1274*i*
Incomplete vascular rings, 382
Incontinence
fecal (*See* Fecal incontinence)
urinary (*See* Urinary incontinence)
Incubated fragility test, for hereditary spherocytosis, 656
Indigestion, differential diagnosis of, 540
Indigo carmine, in ureteral injury, 1049
Indirect calorimetry, 160–161
Indole, 710
Indomethacin, for patent ductus arteriosus, 453
Induction chemotherapy, 297
for lung cancer, 403
Induction therapy, in heart transplantation, 470
Infant(s). *See also* Child(ren); Newborn; Premature infant
airway obstruction in, **992–994**

appendicitis in, 670
dacryocystitis in, **1003**
pain in, 19
risk of hearing impairment in, 965, 965*t*
sensorineural hearing loss in, 969
Infarction
cerebral, 847, 895*i*
of middle cerebral arteries, 893*i*
myocardial (*See* Myocardial infarction)
omental, **532**
pulmonary, with pulmonary thromboembolism, 880
renal, **1077**
versus renal stones, 1043
Infection(s). *See also* Sepsis; Wound infection
after appendectomy, 671–672
after injury, 109, 111
and aneurysms, **838**
anorectal, **771–778**
bacterial
acute secondary peritonitis caused by,
517–521
cholangitis caused by, **612**
and hepatic abscess, 593
hospital-acquired, 12–13
host defense against, 113
prostatitis caused by, **1039–1040**
septic arthritis caused by, 1220–1222
sialadenitis caused by, **986**
biliary, and hepatic abscess, 593
in burn patient, 186
of burn wounds, 273, 274*t*
catheter site, in total parenteral nutrition,
181, 182*t*
of central nervous system, consciousness in,
888
of chest wall, **352–353**
and chronic ulcers, 96
determinants of, 119
diffuse necrotizing, **123–125**
classification of, 123, 124*t*
clostridial, **123–124**
nonclostridial, **124–125**
in elderly, 70
fingernail, **1282,** 1282*i*
fungal, 1282, 1284
fungal
of fingernails, 1282, 1284
and hepatic abscess, 593
of lung, **390–394**
peritonitis caused by, 141
treatment of, **140–141,** 1284
of hand, **1281–1284**
hospital-acquired, 12–13
epidemiology of, 13
with implantable materials, 95
inflammatory response in, 107
of joint replacement, **1157–1158**
lower respiratory tract, acute, 46–47
and male infertility, 1081
mediators of, 103, 103*t*
necrotizing, 114
and neurosurgery for movement disorders,
949

nosocomial, **118–121**
occult
in diabetic patient, 40
diagnosis of, 117
orthopedic, **1217–1222** (*See also* Osteomyelitis)
and pancreatic pseudocyst, **637**
postoperative, fever in, 36
primary line (catheter), in total parenteral
nutrition, 181, 182*t*
prognosis for, 118
pyogenic, **960**
recovery from, nucleotides and, 162
risk factors for, 7–8
soft tissue, *versus* lymphangitis, 887
source of
determination of, 117
operating room as, 119
patient as, 119–120
personnel as, 118–119
of spleen, **664**
spread of
via bloodstream, 114
via lymphatics, 114
of stitch, 25
superficial, 114
surgical, **112–118**
antibiotic prophylaxis against, 120–121
closed space and, 114
complications of, 114–115
diagnosis of, 115–117
host factors in, 112–114
infectious agent in, 112
pathogenesis of, 112–114
spread of, 114
surgical site, **121–123** (*See also* Wound infection)
risk factors for, 121, 122*t*
types of, 121, 121*t*
transfusion-related, 60
treatment of
antibiotics for, 118
circulatory enhancement in, 118
by excision, 118
by incision and drainage, 117–118
nutritional support in, 118
upper respiratory tract, acute, 46
of urinary tract (*See* Urinary tract, infections
of)
vertebral, 1213, 1214*i*
Infection control, **118–121**
in hospital, 121
Infectious aneurysms, 938
Infectious hypothesis, of atherosclerosis, 813
Infective endocarditis, 42, 422, **430**
Inferior mesenteric artery, 705, 706*i*
Inferior mesenteric vein, 706*i*
Inferior pancreatic vein, 626*i*
Inferior vena cava, 565, 567*i,* 871
compression of, cardiac compressive shock
caused by, 206, 207
interruption of, for pulmonary thromboembolism, **881,** 882*i*
membranous obstruction of, 589

Infertility
definition of, 1086
endometriosis and, 1097
female, tubal abnormalities and, **1086–1087**
male, **1080–1081,** 1086
varicocele and, 1079
uterine leiomyomas and, 1100
Inflammation, 100, **112–121**
hand involvement in, 1284–1290
and impaired wound healing, 91–92
in wound healing, 86–87
Inflammatory aneurysms, **837**
Inflammatory bowel disease (IBD)
in adolescent, 1332
and Crohn's disease, 689
fistulas in, 1094
nutritional support in, 188
and small bowel obstruction, **684**
Inflammatory carcinoma, of breast, **328**
Inflammatory mediators, 103, 103*t,* 104*t,*
105*t,* 111, 115, 116*t*–117*t*
in acute respiratory distress syndrome, 212
Inflammatory polyps
of esophagus, 494
of large intestine, 725
in ulcerative colitis, 741
Inflammatory proctitis, **778**
Inflammatory thyroid disease, **304–305**
Inflatable penile prosthesis, 1084
Infliximab
for Crohn's disease, 692
for rheumatoid arthritis, 1204
Influenza, and bronchiectasis, 385
Informed consent, 11, 76, 78, **80–82**
in acute abdomen, 515–516
for anesthesia, 193–194, 193*t*
Infracardiac (type 3) venous return, 455–456,
456*i*
Infracolic compartment, abscess in, 522, 523*i*
Inframalleolar perforator, 871
Infrarenal abdominal aortic aneurysms,
830–835
clinical findings in, 831
endovascular repair of, 834–835, 834*i,* 835*i*
natural history of, 831–832
treatment of, 832–834, 832*i,* 833*i*
Infravesical obstruction, in obstructive uropa-
thy, **1031**
Infundibular atresia, and tetralogy of Fallot,
460, 460*i*
Infundibular muscle, spasm of, 458
Infundibular pulmonary stenosis, 441, 441*i*
Infundibular stenosis, and tetralogy of Fallot,
460, 460*i*
Inguinal canal, 783
Inguinal hernia, **1336–1338,** 1336*i*
Inguinal (Poupart) ligament, 784
Inguinal rings, in acute abdomen, 510
Inhalation injury, **274–276**
Injection injuries, of hand, **1289–1290**
Injection sclerotherapy, for hemorrhoids, 768
Injury. *See also* Trauma
anabolic phase (phase 3) of, 101*t,* 110
definition of, 100

Injury (*cont.*)
  endocrine withdrawal phase of, 109
  hormonal mediator changes with, 103, 104*t*, 105*t*
  injury phase (phase 1) of, 101–109, 101*t*, 108–109
  late anabolism (phase 4) in, 101*t*, 110
  metabolic response to, **100–111**, 101*t*
  neuroendocrine response to, **100–111**, 102*i*
  response to, 167–169, 168*i*
    afferent pathways of, 102*i*, 103
    decreasing, methods for, 110–111
    efferent pathways of, 103–104, 105*i*, 105*t*
    phases of, 100–111, 101*t*
    variations in, 111
  stimuli caused by, 101, 101*t*, 102*i*
  systemic effects of, 103, 105*t*
  thermal (*See* Burn(s))
  turning point (phase 2) of, 101*t*, 109
In-line traction, for craniocerebral trauma, 903
Inokuchi shunt, 587
Inotropic agents
  for cardiogenic shock, 208
  for heat stroke, 279
Inspection, 4
  of acute abdomen, 508–509
Inspired oxygen concentration (FiO₂), in mechanical ventilation, 216
Inspissated bile syndrome, 1334
Insufflation, for malignant pleural effusion, 359
Insular string sign, 893*i*
Insulin, **627**
  actions of, 164–165, 165*i*, 167
  administration of, intraoperative, conventional procedure for, 39
  in glucose solution, intravenous administration of, intraoperative, 39
  in insulinoma, 649
  intraoperative therapy with, 39
  piggy-backed into glucose solution, intraoperative administration of, 39–40
  in response to injury, 106, 114
Insulin-like growth factor, and lung cancer, 396
Insulinoma, **648–650**
Insulin resistance, in response to injury, 107–108
Insulin shock, 204–205, 205*t*
Insurance
  claims made policy for, 82
  liability, 82
  long tail coverage in, 82
  malpractice, 82
  occurrence policy for, 82
Integumentary changes, in peripheral arterial insufficiency, 818
Intensive care, 6
Intercostal block, for postoperative analgesia, **21**
Interferon(s) (IFN), 116*t*. *See also* Alpha interferon
  for bladder tumors, 1065
  for carcinoid syndrome, 704

  for hairy cell leukemia, 663
  for melanoma, 1365
  in nonspecific immunotherapy, 1357–1358
  for renal adenocarcinoma, 1057
Interleukin(s) (IL)
  IL-1, 116*t*
    in response to injury, 108
  IL-2, 116*t*
    arginine and, 162
    in nonspecific immunotherapy, 1357–1358
    in production of lymphokine-activated killer cells, 1358
    in production of tumor-infiltrating lymphocytes, 1358
    for renal adenocarcinoma, 1057
  IL-4, 116*t*
  IL-6, 116*t*
  IL-8, 116*t*
  IL-1ra, 116*t*
Interloop abscess, causes of, 524*t*
Intermediate care, 6
Intermittent claudication, in peripheral arterial insufficiency, 815–816
Intermittent mandatory ventilation (IMV), 217
  for pediatric patients, 1295
Intermittent positive-pressure breathing (IPPB), 17, 26
Intermuscular space, 771*i*
Internal carotid artery, 890*i*
  bifurcation aneurysms, 939
  thrombosis of, 893*i*
Internal iliac artery, 705–706
Internal inguinal ring, 783
Internal jugular vein, 890*i*
Internal oblique muscle, 783
Internal pudendal artery, 705–706
International Federation of Gynecology and Oncology (FIGO) staging
  of endometrial cancer, 1108, 1109*t*
  of gestational trophoblastic tumors, 1113, 1113*t*
  of ovarian cancer, 1111, 1112*t*
  of vaginal cancer, 1105, 1105*t*
  of vulvar cancer, 1104, 1104*t*
"Intern vein," 872
Interrupted aortic arch, **447**
  and aortopulmonary window, 454
Interstitial cystitis, 1078
Interstitial fluid, electrolyte composition of, 142, 143*i*
Intervertebral disk(s)
  anatomy of, **952**
  disease of, **952–958**
  herniation of, 1121
    cervical, **953–955**, 1205
    lumbar, **956–958** (*See also* Lumbar disk syndrome)
    thoracic, **955–956**
Intestinal adaptation, 681
Intestinal bypass, complications of, 32
Intestinal diverticula, acquired, **688**, 688*i*
Intestinal gas, **707**

Intestinal inhibition, of acid secretion, 538
Intestinal ischemia
  chronic, radiation enteropathy and, 695
  nonocclusive, **700**
Intestinal obstruction
  closed loop, 683
  in colorectal cancer, 723
  differential diagnosis of, 514
  diverticulitis and, 733
  endometriosis and, 1096–1097
  ileostomy and, 753*t*
  of large intestine, **712–715**
    versus small bowel obstruction, 686
    in volvulus, 738
  mechanical, 683
  in newborn, **1315**
  with omphalomesenteric duct anomalies, 1330
  physical findings in, 508*t*
  postoperative, **31**
    and wound healing, 24
  in pregnancy, 65
  simple, 683, **684–685**, 685*i*, 686*i*
  of small intestine, **683–687**, 683*t*, 685*i*, 686*i*
    versus large bowel obstruction, **714**
  strangulation, 683, **685–686**
    versus acute mesenteric vascular occlusion, 699
    and closed loop obstruction, 684
  in volvulus, 738
Intestinal phase, of acid secretion, 538
Intestinal pseudo-obstruction
  of colon, **714**
  of small intestine, **686**
Intestinal rotation
  disorders of, **1318–1320**
  incomplete, **1318**, 1319*i*
  nonrotation, 1318
  reversed, **1318–1319**, 1319*i*
Intestinal stomas, **751–754**
Intestinal transit, in short bowel syndrome, 682
Intestine(s)
  atresia and stenosis of, **1317–1318**, 1317*i*
  healing of, 92–93
Intimal cell mass hypothesis, of atherosclerosis, 813
Intoe gait, in children, **1183**
Intra-abdominal abscess, **521–527**
Intra-abdominal pressure, and wound healing, 24
Intra-arterial injections, **858**
Intracellular fluid (ICF), electrolyte composition of, 142, 143*i*
Intracranial aneurysms, **937–943**
Intracranial compartments, 890*i*
Intracranial mass, in elevated intracranial pressure, 889
Intracranial pressure, elevated, **889–891**, 890*i*, 891*i*
  in brain tumors, 922, 924
  in craniocerebral trauma, **904–906**
  pulmonary edema with, 214
Intracranial pressure monitors, 904

Intracranial tumors, **915–927**
  in adults, 916*i*
  in children, 915*i*
  and consciousness, 888
  paraneoplastic syndromes with, 1371*t*
Intraepidermal carcinoma, **1249–1250**
Intrahepatic vena caval injuries, 252
Intralobar sequestration, 381
Intraocular pressure, 1006
Intraocular tumors, **1011**
Intraoperative monitoring, neurophysiologic, **897–900**
Intraparenchymal contusion, **907**
Intraperitoneal abscess, **521–526**
  causes of, 524*t*
  clinical findings in, 522–525
  pathophysiology of, 521, 522*i*
  prognosis for, 525–526
  sites of, 521–522, 523*i*, 524*i*, 524*t*
  treatment of, 525
Intrauterine device (IUD)
  adverse effects and side effects of, 1091
  efficacy of, 1091
  levonorgestrel-containing, 1089, 1091
  safety of, 1091
Intrauterine growth retardation (IUGR), 1294
Intravaginal torsion, **1079–1080**
Intravenous (IV) therapy
  at accident scene, **234**
  for acute secondary bacterial peritonitis, 519
  for burn patients, 270–271
  complications of, **35–36**
  for short bowel syndrome, 681–682
Intrinsic factor, **535–536**
Intubation. *See also* Endotracheal intubation; Extubation
  indications for, 214
  nasogastric, 19
    in acute abdomen, 515
    for gastric decompression, 31
  nasotracheal, 214–215, 233*i*
  orotracheal, 214–215
    in trauma care, 233*i*, 236
  translaryngeal
    advantages and disadvantages of, 215
    conversion to tracheostomy, 215
  of trauma patient, 1118
  types of, 214–215
Intussusception, 1332
  internal, 762, 763–764, **764–766**
  in pediatric patients, **1323–1324**, 1323*i*
  small bowel, **31**
  and small bowel obstruction, **683**
Inverse ratio ventilation (IRV), pressure control mode with, 217–218
In vitro fertilization (IVF), 1087
  and ectopic pregnancy, 1102
Iodine
  deficiency of, 164
  requirements for, 164*t*
  for skin antisepsis, 12
Iodophor, for skin antisepsis, 12
Ipratropium bromide, for vasomotor rhinitis, 979

Iridocyclitis, in juvenile rheumatoid arthritis, 1184
Iris, blunt trauma to, 1009*t*
Iritis, 1001*t*
Iron
  absorption of, in small intestine, 678
  and colorectal cancer, 717
  deficiency of, 52, 163
  requirements for, 164*t*
Irrigation
  of colostomy, 753
  of wound, in soft tissue injury, 1253–1254
Irritable bowel syndrome
  versus colorectal cancer, 721
  and diverticular disease, 730
Ischemia
  arterial injury causing, 258
  and atherosclerosis, 814
  cerebral, in elderly, 69
  gastrointestinal, **856–857**, 856*i*, 857*i*
  intestinal
    chronic, radiation enteropathy and, 695
    nonocclusive, **700**
    physical findings in, 508*t*
  of lower extremity, nonatherosclerotic disorders causing, **828–829**
  myocardial (*See* Myocardial ischemia)
  and peripheral nerves, 258
  in residual limb, 869
Ischemic colitis, 743, **749–750**
  versus ulcerative colitis, 743
Ischemic heart disease, **408–418**
Ischemic injury, in acute mesenteric vascular occlusion, 698
Ischemic mitral regurgitation, 422
Ischemic rest pain, and peripheral arterial insufficiency, 816–817
Ischiorectal space, 771*i*
Islet cells, transplantation of, 1386
Islet cell tumors, **648–651**. *See also specific tumor*
  in α₂ cells, 650–651
  non-beta, of pancreas, 650
  nonfunctioning, **648**
  paraneoplastic syndromes with, 1371*t*
Isoflurane, depth of anesthesia with, signs of, 197*t*
Isograft, definition of, 1372
Isolated limb perfusion, 1358–1359
Isolation, 13
  procedures for, 120
Isoniazid
  indications for, 136*t*, 141
  for tuberculosis, 388*t*, 389
    in spine, 961
Isoproterenol
  for cardiogenic shock, 208
  for heat stroke, 279
Isosthenuria, 49
Isotope studies. *See* Radionuclide scan
Isotretinoin
  chemopreventive, 297
  indications for, 127
Itching, perianal, 775–776

Itraconazole, **141**
  for blastomycosis, 392
  for coccidioidomycosis, 392
  for cryptococcosis, 393
  for histoplasmosis, 390

Jaundice, **601–603**
  abdominal pain and, 507
  causes of, 1334
  cholestatic, 32
  congenital hemolytic, **655–656**
  fluctuating, in choledocholithiasis, 614
  neonatal, 1333–1335
  in pancreatic adenocarcinoma, 644
  in pancreatitis, 621–622
  postoperative, causes of, 32–33, 32*t*
  prehepatic, 32, 32*t*
Jaw, reconstruction of, with head and neck tumors, 295
Jejunal diverticula, 688, 688*i*
Jejunal diverticulosis, 688
Jejunoileal bypass, 190
Jejunostomy tube, 19
Jejunum, 674
  atresia and stenosis of, 1317–1318
  resection of, consequences of, 680–682, 681*i*
  tumors of, 701–704
Jergesen tube system, 1219*i*
Jodbasedow, 300, 301. *See also* Hyperthyroidism
Joint(s)
  debridement, for osteoarthritis, 1202
  digital, 1270
    collateral ligaments of, 1271, 1272*i*
  fusion of
    for osteoarthritis, 1203
    for rheumatoid arthritis, 1204
  inflammation of, in children, 1184
  pain in (*See* Osteoarthritis; Rheumatoid arthritis)
  pediatric, systemic disorders affecting, 1184
  prosthetic, in osteoarthritis, 1203
  reconstruction of, in osteoarthritis, 1203
  reduction of, 1116
  transplantation of, 1237
Joint fluid, examination of, in septic arthritis, 1221
Joint replacement
  with avascular necrosis of femoral head, 1201
  hip, total, 1156–1157, 1156*i*
  infections associated with, **1157–1158**
  knee, total, **1166**, 1167*i*
  in osteoarthritis, 1203
  for rheumatoid arthritis, 1204
Juncturae tendinum, 1273*i*
Juvenile angiofibroma, 989
Juvenile laryngeal papillomatosis. *See* Respiratory papillomatosis, recurrent
Juvenile polyposis coli, 728
Juvenile polyps, 702
Juvenile rheumatoid arthritis (JRA), **1184**

Kanamycin, for tuberculosis, 388*t*

Kaposi's sarcoma, in HIV-infected (AIDS) patients
of ear, 998
oral, 998
Kartagener's syndrome, and bronchiectasis, 384
Kasabach-Merritt syndrome, 1247, 1341–1342
Kasai procedure, for biliary atresia, 1334
Kawasaki's disease, and abdominal aortic coarctation, 829
Keloids, 91, **1243–1244**
Kenalog-10 Injection. *See* Triamcinolone acetonide
Keratitis, actinic, **1008**
Ketoconazole, **141**
for coccidioidomycosis, 392
for histoplasmosis, 390
Ketones, 165*i*, 166, 167*i*
Ketorolac tromethamine, 20
indications for, 200
Kidney(s). *See also* Renal
abscess of, **1038–1039**
agenesis of, 1019
age-related changes in, 68–69, 68*t*, 70
anatomy of, **1014**
anomalies of, **1019–1021**
cadaver
graft survival rate, presensitization and, 1374
preservation of, **1376**
transplantation of, **1376–1377**
calculi in, **1042–1045**
developmental anomalies of, **1019–1021**
disease of
assessment of, 49–50
versus chronic venous insufficiency, 884
operative risk in, 111
pleural effusion and, 360
in surgical patient, **48–52**
hazards of, 50
dysfunction of (*See also* Renal failure)
after cardiac surgery, 437
ectopic, 1019
embryology of, **1013**, 1014*i*
functions of, 142–143
horseshoe, 1019, 1019*i*
infarction of, **1077**
versus renal stones, 1043
injury to, 254–255, **1048–1049**
versus bladder injury, 1051
in neuropathic bladder, 1076
medullary sponge, **1020**
multicystic dysplastic, **1020**
physiology of, **1017–1018**
polycystic, **1019–1020,** 1020*i*
size of, 50
transplantation of, **1372–1380** (*See also* Organ transplantation)
cadaver graft for, **1376–1377**
presensitization and, 1374
complications of, 1378–1379
contraindications to, 1377
graft rejection in, **1379–1380**
diagnosis of, 1380

differential diagnosis of, 1380
graft survival in, blood transfusions and, 1373–1374
immunosuppressive drug therapy for, **1374–1375**
indications for, 1377
living-donor, **1376, 1377–1378**
operative techniques for, 1377–1378
pancreatitis after, 32, **1379**
recipient
operative technique for, 1378, 1378*i*
postoperative management of, 1378–1379
selection of, 1377
sources of donor kidneys for, **1376–1377**
survival rate with, 1374, 1379
and transfusion therapy, 50, 1373–1374
tuberculosis of, 1041
versus renal stones, 1043
tubular reabsorption in, 1017
tubular secretion in, **1017–1018**
tumors of, **1054–1061**
benign, **1059**
malignant
primary, **1054–1058**
secondary, **1058–1059**
versus ureteral calculi, 1046
vascular abnormalities of, **1020**
Wilms' tumor of, 1344–1345
Kienböck's disease, 1147
Klatskin tumors, 617–618
Klebsiella infection, 112
in cholangitis, 612
drug therapy for, 135*t*
and primary peritonitis, 527
and retroperitoneal abscesses, 526
Klebsiella pneumoniae
and bronchiectasis, 385
hepatic abscess caused by, 593, 594
and lung abscess, 383
and thoracic empyema, 361
Klippel-Trenaunay syndrome, *versus* varicose veins, 874
Klippel-Trenaunay-Weber syndrome, 1342
Klumpke's paralysis, 1184
Knee (joint)
angular deformity of, in children, 1183–1184
arthroplasty of, and deep vein thrombosis, 877
cartilage of, injuries to, 1164, 1164*i*
dislocation of, **1161–1162**
injuries of, **1159–1162**
ligamentous reconstruction of, 1164
ligaments of, injuries to, 1163–1164, 1163*i*
locking of, 1162–1163
menisci of, injuries to, 1162–1163
replacement of, total, **1166,** 1167*i*
Knock-knees, **1183**
Kock pouch, 751
Konno procedure, 444
Kraits, 130
Krukenberg tumor, 1110

Kussmaul sign, 207

Laboratory examination(s)
in anesthetic risk evaluation, 193
postoperative, 15
in surgical patient, 5
in trauma management, 240
Labyrinthectomy, for Meniere's disease, 975
Labyrinthitis, **976**
Lacerations
of ocular adnexa, **1009**
peripheral nerve, 913
scalp, **907**
Lacrilube, for Bell's palsy, 977
Lacrimal sac, infection of, 1003
Lactate
metabolism of, 165, 166*i*
in wound healing, 86–87, 88*i*, 89, 91–92
Lactate dehydrogenase (LDH)
in ascites, 590
in testicular cancer, 1071
Lactated Ringer's solution, 18, 18*t*
Lactation, breast cancer and, **328–329**
Lactic acid, in hypovolemic shock, 205
Lactic acidosis
in cancer patient, 187
in short bowel syndrome, 680
and wound healing, 91
Lactitol, 592
Lactobacillus bifidus, in feces, 710–711
Lactose intolerance, 185
in short bowel syndrome, 682
Lactrodectism, 132–133
Lactulose
for hepatic encephalopathy, 592–593
for slow-transit constipation, 710
Lactulose breath hydrogen test, 677
Lacunar (Gimbernat) ligament, 784
Ladd procedure, 1319–1320
Ladd's bands, 1316–1317, 1319
Laminectomy
for lumbar disk syndrome, 1214
for malignant pain, 950
for spinal cord tumors, 928
Laminotomy, for lumbar disk syndrome, 957–958
Langer's lines, 1241
Lansoprazole, for duodenal ulcer, 541
Laparoscopic surgery (Laparoscopy)
for abdominal trauma, 251–252
for acute abdomen, 513
for adnexal mass, 67
for adrenal disorders, 797–798, 801, 809
advantages and disadvantages of, 46, 110
for appendectomy, in pregnancy, 64
for cholecystectomy, in pregnancy, 64–65
for chronic pelvic pain, 1090
for colorectal cancer, 721–722, 723
common bile duct exploration by, in choledocholithiasis, 615
in endometriosis, 1097
for female sterilization, 1091
for hepatic cysts, 577
for incisional hernia repair, 793

for large bowel polyps, 727
for pancreatic adenocarcinoma, 646
for perforated peptic ulcer, 554
in pregnancy, 63–65
for rectal prolapse, 764
for renal adenocarcinoma, 1057
and response to injury, 101
for sliding inguinal hernia, 790
for small bowel obstruction, 687
for splenectomy, 666
of tubal abnormalities, 1087
of uterine anomalies, 1086
Laparotomy
for abdominal trauma, 252
for acute pancreatitis, 634
for bile duct malignancies, 618
for cholangitis, 612
for diverticulitis, 734
for gallstone ileus, 611–612
and peritoneal adhesions, 529
for stress ulcers, 556
for volvulus, 740
Laplace's law, 713
diverticulosis and, 730
and infrarenal abdominal aortic aneurysms, 831
Large cell carcinoma, of lung, 396
Large intestine, **705–755**. *See also* Colon; Rectum
absorption in, **708–709**, 709*t*
anatomy of, **705–706**, 706*i*, 707*i*
blood supply to, **705–706**, 706*i*
cancer of, **716–724**, 716*i* (*See also* Colorectal cancer)
diseases of, **712–750** (*See also specific type*)
gas cysts in, **701**
lymphatic drainage of, **705–706**
microbiology of, **710–711**
motility of, **708**
nerve supply to, **706**
obstruction of, **712–715**
in colorectal cancer, **723**
versus small bowel obstruction, 686
in volvulus, 738
perforation of, in colorectal cancer, **723**
physiology of, **707–710**
polyps of, **725–728**, 725*t*
sacculations of, 705
tumors of, **729**
x-rays of, **711**
Large-needle (core needle) biopsy, for breast cancer, 319
LaRoque repair, for sliding inguinal hernia, 790
Laryngeal mask airway, 196
Laryngectomy, for laryngeal cancer, 291
Laryngitis
acute, **995**
chronic, **995**
Laryngomalacia, 992
Laryngoscope, fiberoptic, 196
Laryngoscopy, **349**
Laryngotracheal stenosis, pediatric, 992

Laryngotracheobronchitis, 992*t*, 994*i*
acute, 993
Larynx, **990–998**
cancer of, 282, **290–292**, 296
congenital flaccid, 992
foreign bodies in, **990**
functions of, 990
injuries to, 241
treatment of, 243
trauma to, **991**
Lasègue's test, 1213
Laser Doppler studies, and amputation level determination, 860
Laser photocoagulation
for large bowel obstruction, 714
panretinal, 1012
Laser therapy
for adenoma and adenocarcinoma of ampulla of Vater, 648
for bladder tumors, **1064**
for correction of refractive error, **1012**
for large bowel obstruction, 714
for ocular disease, **1012**
for port wine stain, 1248
for retinal detachment, 1006
for scarring, 1243
for villous adenomas of large intestine, 727
Late death, 230
Lateral collateral ligament, injury to, 1163
Lateral femoral cutaneous nerve, 784
Lateral ventricles, 890*i*
Later death, 244
Latissimus dorsi flap, **1235–1236**
for breast reconstruction, 337, **1261**
for lower extremity, 1262
Law
adversary system and, 73
civil, **72–73**, 74
common, 74
criminal, **72–73**, 74
tort, 75–76
Laxatives, and bowel habits, 709–710
L cells, 674–675
Lead pipe appearance, in ulcerative colitis, 742*i*
Lead poisoning, 53
Lean body mass, 159*t*
Leapfrog Group, 84
Left atrial pressure, 220
Left coronary artery, 408, 409*i*
Left lower quadrant, abscess of, causes of, 524*t*
Left subhepatic space, abscess in, 521, 523*i*
Left-to-right shunt, 449, **455**
Left ventricular aneurysm, 416–417, 418*i*
Left ventricular failure, postoperative, 29
Left ventricular-right atrial shunt, **455**
Leg. *See also* Lower extremity
amputation of, **864–865**
chronic ulcers of, hereditary spherocytosis and, 656
Legal principles, of medical practice, **72–85**
Legg-Calve-Perthes disease. *See* Legg-Perthes disease
Legg-Perthes disease, **1193–1194**, 1194*i*
Legionella infection

and bronchiectasis, 385
versus ulcerative colitis, 742–743
Legionella micdadei, and lung abscess, 383
Legionella pneumophila infection
drug therapy for, 135*t*
and lung abscess, 383
Leiomyoma(s)
of esophagus, 495, 495*i*
gastric, **561**
of large intestine, **729**
of lung, 404
renal, 1059
uterine, **1099–1100**
bleeding caused by, 1088–1089
differential diagnosis of, 1099, **1100**
Leiomyosarcoma, **561**, 1109–1110, 1361
duodenal, 562
in small intestine, 703
Lens
blunt trauma to, 1009*t*
intracapsular extraction of, for senile cataract, **1004–1005**
Lepirudin, 55
Leprosy, hand involvement in, 1284
Leptospira infection, drug therapy for, 136*t*
Leriche's syndrome, 816
Lesioning surgery
for dystonia, 949
for essential tremor, 949
for Parkinson's disease, 948
Lesser trochanter, fracture of, 1151
Letter bombs, 264
Letterer-Siwe disease, 355
Leucovorin, for breast cancer, 332
Leukemia
chronic lymphocytic, **662**
hairy cell, **662–663**
versus hypersplenism, 654
myeloblastic, and neutropenic colitis, 750
in surgical patient, 53–54
Leukocoria, **1002**
Leukocyte count
in acute appendicitis, 669
in ascites, 590
with hepatic abscess, 593
Leukocytes, in wound healing, 86
Leukocytosis
in acute cholecystitis, 608
in acute mesenteric vascular occlusion, 699
in acute pancreatitis, 631
in choledocholithiasis, 614
in pancreatic pseudocyst, 636
in sickle cell anemia, 53
Leukoplakia
hairy, in AIDS, 998
in oral cavity cancer, 286
Leuprolide, anticancer therapy with, **1356**
Levamisole, for colorectal cancer, 723
Levator ani muscle, 756–757, 757*i*, 758
LeVeen shunt, in ascites, 590–591
Levels of consciousness, 888–891. *See also* Consciousness, levels of
Levocardia, 468
Levodopa, for Parkinson's disease, 948

Levothyroxine, 40–41
LHRH agonists. *See* Luteinizing hormone-releasing hormone agonists
Liability, vicarious, 79
Liability insurance, 82
Lichen planus, **984**
Lidocaine
    and arterial spasm, 261
    for dysrhythmias, 28
    indications for, 196
Lieberkühn, crypts of, 674, 677*i*
Life support, cessation of, 81
Ligaments, of spleen, 652
Ligation, for venous injuries, 243
Lincomycin, and antibiotic-associated colitis, 749
Linea alba, 783
Linitis plastica, 557
Linoleic acid, 163
α-Linolenic acid, 163
Lipase, serum, in acute pancreatitis, 631
Lipectomy
    suction-assisted, **1268** (*See also* Liposuction)
    ultrasonic, **1268**
Lipid insudation hypothesis, 813
Lipids, serum. *See* Hyperlipidemia
Lipiodol, 572, 574
Lipodystrophy, mesenteric, **531**
Lipoma
    of chest wall, 354, 355
    of large intestine, **729**
    renal, 1059
Lipomeningocele, of spinal cord, 928
Liposarcoma, 1361
    of chest wall, 354
Liposuction, **1268**
    applications of, 1268
    in neck, 1265
Lips, cancer of, 286–287
Lisfranc's amputation, 863
Listeria infection, drug therapy for, 136*t*
Listeria monocytogenes, and primary peritonitis, 527
Lithocholate, 597
Lithoptysis, 386
Lithotripsy
    for chronic pancreatitis, 642
    for gallstones, **606**
    for renal stones, **1044**
    for vesical stone, 1047
Litigation, 73–74
Littre's hernia, 794
Livedo reticularis, 843
Liver. *See also* Hepatic
    abscess of, **593–594**
    adenomas of, 577
    age-related changes in, 70
    angiosarcoma of, 572
    arterial blood supply of, 565–566
    benign tumors of, **576–578**
    biliary drainage of, 566
    biopsy of
        with liver tumor, 572
        with metastatic neoplasms of liver, 574
        in sclerosing cholangitis, 623

cancer of
    and hepatic abscess, 593, 594
    liver transplantation for, 1384
    metastatic, **574–576**
    primary, **571–574**
        differential diagnosis of, 573
        laboratory diagnosis of, 572
        liver scan in, 572
        prognosis for, 574
        signs and symptoms of, 572
        treatment of, 573–574
        tumor markers in, 572
    cirrhosis of, **580**
        gastrointestinal bleeding with, 57, 579, 580
        and liver cancer, 571–574
        and portal hypertension, 578–579
        and wound healing, 24
    cysts of, **576–577**
    diseases/disorders of, **569–594**
        alcoholic, 578–579
        in children, 1333–1335
        versus chronic venous insufficiency, 884
        functional status in, Child-Pugh classification of, 582, 583–584, 583*t*
        operative risk in, 111
        in surgical patients, **56–57**
    failure
        antibiotic dosage in, 138*t*–139*t*
        nutritional support in, 188
        peripheral parenteral nutrition solution in, 178
        total parenteral nutrition in, 181
    focal nodular hyperplasia of, 577–578, 1348
    hemangioma of, **576**
        angiography of, 572, 576
    injuries to, treatment of, 252–253
    and intestinal carcinoid tumor, 704
    lobectomy in, 568, 568*i*
    lobes of, 565, 566*i*
    lobules of, vascular anatomy of, 566–567, 567*i*
    lymphatics of, 566
    malignancy of, in childhood, staging of, 1348, 1348*t*
    neoplasms of, in childhood, **1347–1349**
    physiology of, 566–567
    postoperative dysfunction of, **32–33**
    regeneration of, 567
    resection of, **567–569**
        for bile duct malignancies, 618
        for carcinoma of gallbladder, 616–617
        complications of, 568
        extent of, 568, 568*i*
        indications for, 567
        with metastatic neoplasms, 575
        postoperative course in, 568
        preoperative evaluation for, 567–568
        in primary hepatic cancer, 573
    segments of, 565, 566*i*
    spontaneous rupture of, 571
    surgical anatomy of, 565–566, 566*i*, 567*i*
    transplantation of, **1383–1386**
        advances in (future directions for), 1386
        complications of, 1385–1386

contraindications to, 1384
donor selection for, 1384
graft rejection in, 1385–1386
immunosuppressive therapy for, 1385
indications for, 589, 1383–1384
living-related donor for, 1386
for nonbleeding varices, 585
operative technique for, 1384–1385
in primary hepatic cancer, 573
primary nonfunction after, 1385–1386
for sclerosing cholangitis, 624
survival rate with, 1383
transfusion therapy in, 57
    trauma to, **569–571**
        clinical findings in, 569–570
        mechanism of injury in, 569
        postoperative complications in, 570
        prognosis for, 570
        staging of, 569, 569*t*
        treatment of, 570
    venous blood supply of, 565, 567*i*
Liver fluke, and hepatic cancer, 571
Liver Injury Scale, 569, 569*t*
Lobar emphysema
    congenital, **1310–1311**
    hypoplastic, 1310
Lobectomy
    cerebral, for intracranial hypertension, 904–905
    pulmonary, for lung cancer, 402
Lobes, of lungs, 347, 348*i*
Locality rule, 77
Longitudinal muscle, of colon, 705, 707*i*
Loop colostomy, 752
Lop-ear, 973
Loperamide, for short bowel syndrome, 682
Lorazepam, for craniocerebral trauma, 903
Lotheissen-McVay repair
    for femoral hernia, 791
    for inguinal hernia, 788
Low back pain, **1210–1211**
Lower esophageal sphincter, and reflux esophagitis, 484
Lower extremity
    amputation of, 859, **861–866**
        rehabilitation after, 869
    angular deformity of, in children, **1183–1184**
    atherosclerosis in, 815
    ischemia of, nonatherosclerotic disorders causing, **828–829**
    pain in (*See* Lumbar disk syndrome)
    reconstruction of, **1262–1263**
Lower motor neuron disorders, 1186
Lower motor neuron lesion, in neuropathic bladder, 1075
Loxoscelism, 133
L-transposition of the great arteries, **466–467**
Lumbago, in lumbar disk syndrome, 956
Lumbar diskectomy
    closed disk space infection following, 960
    for lumbar disk syndrome, 958
Lumbar disk syndrome, **956–958, 1211–1214**
Lumbar puncture
    in arteriovenous malformations, 944

in brain abscess, 959
in intracranial aneurysms, 940
Lumbar spine
  disk herniation in (*See* Intervertebral disk(s),
    herniation of)
  injury to, associated injuries, 1118
Lumbar strain, **1210–1211**
Lumbar sympathectomy, for peripheral arterial
  insufficiency, 824
Lumpectomy, 330
Lunate, 1143
  dislocation of, 1147–1148
  fracture of, **1147**
Lung(s). *See also* Pulmonary
  abscess of, **383–384**, 384*i*
  anatomy of, **347–349**, 348*i*
  biopsy of, 351
  closing volume of, 25
  congenital cystic anomalies of, **379–382**
  congenital lesions of, 1312–1313
    vascular, **382–383**
  diseases/disorders of, **379–395**
    and operative risk, 17
    preoperative treatment of, 47
    restrictive, preoperative management of,
      47
    and surgical site, interaction between, 47
  function
    age-related changes in, 67, 68*t*
    impaired, and gas cysts in small intestine,
      701
    and operative risk, 8
    postoperative, 17
    preoperative evaluation of, 47–48
  fungal infections of, **390–394**
  hematoma of, 246
  hypoplasia of, 380–381 (*See also* Lobar em-
    physema, hypoplastic)
    with congenital diaphragmatic hernia,
      1308–1309
  increased intracranial pressure and, 890
  injuries of, **246**, 264
  lacerations of, 246
  metastases to, 356
  neoplasms of, unusual, 404, 404*t*
  reexpansion of, for pneumothorax, 368
  resection of
    contraindications to, 401*t*
    empyemas following, 362, 364*i*
    for lung cancer, 401–402
  suppurative diseases of, **383–390**
  transplantation of, 369, **1383**
    for cystic fibrosis, 387
Lung cancer, **395–407**
  paraneoplastic syndromes with, 1371*t*
  pleural effusion and, 357, 359*i*
  primary, **395–403**
    chemotherapy for, 402–403
    clinical presentation of, 397
    diagnosis and workup of, 398, 399*i*
    immunotherapy for, 403
    locations of, 396*t*
    paraneoplastic syndromes associated with,
      397, 397*t*
    pathology of, 396–397

prognosis for, 403, 403*t*
  radiation therapy for, 402
  staging of, 398, 400*t*
  surgical treatment of, 401–402
  targeted therapy for, 403
  treatment of, 398–403
secondary, **406–407**
sputum analysis in, 351
and superior vena caval syndrome, 373
unusual neoplasms in, 404, 404*t*
Lung hernia, **352**
Lung stone, 386
Luria-Nebraska Neuropsychological Battery,
  908
Luschka, foramen of, 890*i*
Luteinizing hormone, in male infertility,
  1081
Luteinizing hormone-releasing hormone agonists, for prostate cancer, 1069
Luteotropic hormone, in testicular cancer,
  1071
Lyme disease
  drug therapy for, 136*t*
  facial nerve paralysis in, 977
Lymphadenectomy
  for penile cancer, **1072**
  regional, for carcinoma of gallbladder,
    616–617
  for testicular cancer, 1071–1072
Lymphadenitis
  acute suppurative, 997
  caseating, 1304
  granulomatous, in pediatric patients, **1304**
  mesenteric, **693**
  pyogenic, in pediatric patients, **1303–1304**
  tuberculous, in pediatric patients, 1304
Lymphangiography, in lymphedema, 886
Lymphangioma, **1301–1302**, 1302*i*, 1311
  of chest wall, 354
Lymphangiosarcoma, 886, 1361
Lymphangitis, 114, 123, **887**
  in infected hand, 1281
Lymphatic drainage, 349
  of colon, 718*i*
Lymphatic system, 349, **885–887**
  fluid dynamics of, 885
Lymphedema, **885–887**, 886*i*
  versus chronic venous insufficiency, 884
Lymphedema praecox, 885
Lymphedema tarda, 885
Lymph nodes
  cervical
    examination of, 284
    and hypopharyngeal cancer, 289, 290
    and laryngeal cancer, 290
    and nasal cavity cancer, 292
    and oral cavity cancer, 289
    and oropharyngeal cancer, 289
    radiation therapy for, 296
  in head and neck tumors, 283, 283*i*
  metastases to, in colorectal cancer, **718**, 718*i*
Lymphocele, of transplant bed, in kidney transplant recipient, 1379
Lymphocyte(s). *See also* B cells (B lymphocytes); T cells (T lymphocytes)

in renal adenocarcinoma, 1057
tumor-infiltrating, 1358
Lymphocytic leukemia, chronic, **662**
Lymphocytosis, after splenectomy, 666
Lymphoepithelioma, 292
Lymphogranulomatosis, benign, **394–395**
Lymphogranuloma venereum (LGV), 777
Lymphokine-activated killer (LAK) cells,
  1358
Lymphoma, **1365–1370**. *See also* Hodgkin's
  lymphoma; Non-Hodgkin's lym-
  phoma (NHL)
  of bone, **1226**
    primary, 1223
  central nervous system, 1369–1370
  of chest wall, 356
  versus Crohn's disease, **691**
  duodenal, 562
  gastric, **560**, 1368
    treatment of, 1370
  versus hypersplenism, 654
  of large intestine, **729**
  mediastinal, 376, 377, 1311
  nonlymphoid, 1369–1370
  pleural effusion and, 357
  posttransplant, 1386
  of small intestine, 702
  splenic involvement in, 1366, 1370
  in surgical patient, 53–54
  of thyroid gland, 307
Lymphosarcoma
  mediastinal, 377
  and superior vena caval syndrome, 373
Lymphoscintigraphy, in lymphedema, 886
Lynch syndrome, 716–717
  cancer screening in, 719
Lysine analogs, for postoperative bleeding, 436
Lysolecithin, in pancreatitis, 629
Lysosomes, 113
Lysyl hydroxylase, 89
Lysyl oxidase, 164
  and arterial aneurysms, 830

Macroamylasemia, 632
Macrocystic adenomas, of pancreas, 647
Macrocytic anemia, in blind loop syndrome,
  679
Macrodactyly, 1275
Macroglobulinemia, 54
Macroglossia, **986**
Macrolides, indications for, 135*t*, 136*t*
Macrophage colony-stimulating factor
  (M-CSF), 116*t*
Macrophages
  in fracture healing, 93
  in wound healing, 86–87, 87*i*
Macula
  degeneration of, photodynamic therapy for,
    1012
  detachment of, 1006
  diabetic edema of, laser treatment for, **1012**
Madura foot, 129
Mafenide, for burns, 272
Maffucci's syndrome, 1342
Magendie, foramen of, 890*i*

Magnesium
  absorption of, in small intestine, 678
  for acute pancreatitis, **633**
  balance, **149**
  for hypoparathyroid tetany, 318
  replacement therapy, 149
  requirements for, 164*t*
  serum levels of, 149 (*See also* Hypermagne-
    semia; Hypomagnesemia)
Magnesium-ammonium-phosphate renal
  stones, prevention of, **1044**
Magnetic resonance angiography (MRA)
  of craniocerebral trauma, 903
  of intracranial aneurysms, 940
  in neurodiagnosis, 894–895, 895*i*, 896*i*
  of peripheral arterial insufficiency, 819
  of pulmonary thromboembolism, 881
  of renal adenocarcinoma, **1055**
Magnetic resonance imaging (MRI)
  of adnexal masses, 1101
  of adrenal incidentalomas, 811–812
  of adrenal masses, 797
  of aldosteronoma, 800
  of anorectal anomalies, 1326
  of anorectum, indications for, 772
  of arteriovenous malformations, 944
  of bladder tumors, 1063
  of brain abscess, 959, 960
  of brain tumors, 923
    in children, 936*i*
  of cervical disk syndrome, 954
  of closed disk space infections, 960
  of colorectal cancer, 720
  of craniocerebral trauma, 903
  of epidermoid tumors, 920
  of facial nerve paralysis, 977
  of hand, 1273
  in hyperadrenocorticism (Cushing disease,
    Cushing syndrome), 808
  of intraperitoneal abscess, 524–525
  of knee, 1162–1164, 1163*i*
  of large intestine, 711
  of liver cancer, 572
  of lumbar disk syndrome, 957
  of metastatic neoplasms of liver, 574–575
  of neuroblastoma, 1343
  in neurodiagnosis, **893–895**
  of osteomyelitis, 1217
  of pheochromocytoma, 802, 803–804,
    805
  of pituitary tumors, 931
  of prostate cancer, 1068, 1068*i*
  of pulmonary disorders, 351–352
  of renal adenocarcinoma, **1055**, 1056*i*
  of renal transplant, 1380
  of soft tissue sarcoma, 1361
  of spinal cord injury, 910
  of spinal cord tumors, 928
    in children, 936
  of spinal deformity, 1185
  of spinal injury, 1120
  of spinal tumor, 1213
  of uterine leiomyomas, 1100
  of vertebral osteomyelitis, 1213, 1214*i*

Magnetic resonance venography
  of deep venous thrombosis, 876
  in neurodiagnosis, 896
Magnetoencephalography, in neurodiagnosis,
  897
Major histocompatibility complex (MHC),
  1372
Malabsorption, **643**
  in blind loop syndrome, 679–680
  in short bowel syndrome, 189
  in small bowel syndrome, 680, 681*i*
Malacoplakia
  versus Crohn's disease, 748
  versus ulcerative colitis, 743
Male infertility, **1080–1081**, 1086
  varicocele and, 1079
Male reproductive system, embryology of,
  1013–1014, 1016*i*
Malignant ascites, **529**
Malignant hyperthermia, **201–202**
Malignant melanoma. *See* Melanoma
Malignant pain, **950**
Malignant pleural effusion, 335, 357–359,
  359*i*
Mallampati classification, of airway, 192
Malleolus
  lateral, fracture of, 1171
  medial, fracture of, 1170–1171
Mallet finger, 1276–1277, 1276*i*
Mallory-Weiss syndrome, **551–552**
Malnutrition
  and achalasia, 478
  in blind loop syndrome, 679
  in cancer patient, 186
  clinical staging of, 158, 158*t*
  in Crohn's disease, **690**
  in elderly, 70
  in HIV-infected (AIDS) patients, 189–190
  incidence of, 156, 157*t*
  myocardial dysfunction in, 188
  and operative risk, 7
  pathophysiology of, **164–170**
  in small intestine fistulas, 696
  total parenteral nutrition in
    rate of, 181
    and refeeding syndrome, 181
  and wound healing, 92
Malposition of the great arteries, 464, 468
Malpractice, **84**
Malpractice insurance, 82
Mamba, 130
Mammary dysplasia, 319, **340–342**
Mammographic localization biopsy, for breast
  cancer, 320
Mammography, 321–322, **322–323**
Mammoplasty, **1266–1267**
  augmentation, **1266–1267**
  reduction, **1267**
Mandible, fractures of, **1256**
Mandibulofacial dysostosis, 1259
Manganese
  deficiency of, 164
  requirements for, 164*t*
Manganese superoxide dismutase, 164

Mannitol
  colonoscopy and, 707
  for heat stroke, 279
  for hemolytic transfusion reaction, 59–60
  for intracranial hypertension, 905
  for renal dysfunction after cardiac surgery,
    437
Manometry, 472–473
  for achalasia, 478
  for diffuse esophageal spasm, 476
Mantle radiation, for Hodgkin's lymphoma,
  1366
Marcy repair, for inguinal hernia, 787
Marfan's syndrome
  and diverticulosis, 730
  and extracranial carotid artery aneurysm, 840
  pectus carinatum in, 1306
  pectus excavatum with, 1305
  and thoracic aortic aneurysms, 431
  and thoracic aortic dissection, 432
Marginal artery of Drummond, 705
Marginal (mucocutaneous) space, 771*i*
Marginal ulcer, 542–543
Marjolin ulcer, 1252
Marlex mesh, in chest wall reconstruction, 353
Marshall's test, 1078
Mass movement, in colon, 708
Mast cell disease, systemic, **663**
Mast cells, 674–675
Mastectomy, 330
  breast reconstruction after, **1261–1262**
  prophylactic, 1262
Mastocytosis, 663
Mastoidectomy, 971
  for chronic otitis media, 968
Mastoiditis, acute, **971**
Mastopexy, **1267**
Maxilla, fractures of, **1257**
Maxillary ligation, internal, for epistaxis, 981
Maxillectomy, 293
Maximal acid output (MAO), 540, 540*t*
Maximum intensity projection, 894
May-Husni procedure, for chronic venous in-
  sufficiency, 885
May-Thurner syndrome, 871
M cells, 674–675
McGoon ratio, 461
MCT (medium-chain triglycerides), for pan-
  creatic insufficiency, 643
Mean arterial pressure (MAP), 69
Measles, and bronchiectasis, 385
Meat impaction, **492**
Mechanical heart valves, **428–429**, 429*i*
Mechanical obstruction, intestinal, 683
Mechanical ventilation, **214–219**. *See also* Ven-
  tilator(s)
  assist (control) mode, 217
  indications for, 214
  for inhalation injuries, 276
  and lobar emphysema, 382
  for lung injuries, 246
  for pediatric patients, 1294–1295
  pressure control, with inverse ratio ventila-
    tion (IRV), 217–218

pressure support, 217–218
pulmonary failure caused by, 212–213
weaning from, **218**
Mechlorethamine, 1355
for malignant pleural effusion, 359
vincristine, procarbazine, and prednisone
(MOPP) regimen, for Hodgkin's
lymphoma, 1367
Meckel's diverticulum, 1330–1331, 1330*i*,
1332
and Littre's hernia, 794
Meconium ileus, **1320**
Meconium plug syndrome, **1322–1323**
Medial collateral ligament, injury to, 1163
Medial perforators, of foot, 872*i*
Median arcuate ligament syndrome, 856
Median nerve, 1272, 1274*i*
compression of, 1280
injury to, 1281
in endoscopic carpal tunnel release,
1292
Mediastinal arteries, enlargement of, 458
Mediastinal cystic lesions, 376
Mediastinal herniation, 347
Mediastinal masses, **375–377,** 375*t*
in pediatric patients, **1311–1312**
Mediastinal tumors, and superior vena caval
syndrome, 373
Mediastinitis, **371–373**
acute, **371–372**
chronic, **372–373**
and esophageal trauma, 242
fibrosing, 372, 373
granulomatous, 372, 373
Mediastinoscopy, **349–350**
anterior, 350
cervical, 349
extended cervical, 349–350
Mediastinum
anatomy of, **346–347,** 347*i*
anterior, 347, 347*i*
compartments of, **1311**
diseases of, **371–379**
displacement of, 347
middle, 347, 347*i*
posterior, 347, 347*i*
Medical amputation, 861
Medical consultation, preoperative, 5, 10
Medical examiner. *See* Coroner
Medical record, legal aspects of, 80
Medications. *See also* Drug(s)
for acute pancreatitis, **634**
for brain tumors, **924**
colitis caused by, **748–749**
impotence caused by, **1083**
for islet cell tumors, **649**
management of, in pregnancy, 63
ototoxic, in AIDS treatment, 998
pancreatitis caused by, 629
for Parkinson's disease, 948
perioperative management of, 45
preoperative (*See* Premedication)
in secondary hemolytic anemia, 658
Mediterranean anemia, **657**

Medium-chain triglycerides (MCT), for pancreatic insufficiency, 643
Medroxyprogesterone, for renal adenocarci-
noma, 1057
Medroxyprogesterone acetate
for endometriosis, 1098–1099
indications for, 1089
Medtronic-Hall heart valve, 428–429, 429*i*
Medullary carcinoma, **306,** 307
Medullary compression, 891
Medullary sponge kidney, **1020**
Medulloblastoma, 917, **918–919,** 926
in children, **935–936**
Megace. *See* Megestrol acetate
Megacolon
in sigmoid volvulus, 739
toxic
in Crohn's disease, 748
in ulcerative colitis, 743, 744*i*, 745
Megaureter, primary obstructive, 1021,
1021*i*
Megestrol acetate, for breast cancer, 333*t*,
334
Melanocytes
in basal cell carcinoma, 1250
in nevi, 1245–1246
Melanocytic nevi
of eyelid, 1010
intraocular, 1011
Melanoma, **1363–1365**
acral lentiginous, 1364
biopsy of, 1364
Breslow classification of, 1363, 1363*t*
clinical identification (ABCD) of, 1363,
1363*t*
of eyelid, 1011
giant hairy nevi and, 1246
of hand, 1288
intraocular, 1011
lentigo maligna, 1364
local recurrence of, 1365
metastases of, 1363–1365
nodular, 1364
of pinna, 972
recurrence of, 1365
risk factors for, 1363
sentinel lymph node biopsy in, 1364–1365
small bowel metastases of, 703
staging of, 1363, 1363*t*
superficial spreading, 1364
and superior vena caval syndrome, 373
treatment of, 1364–1365
vaginal, 1106
vulvar, 1104
Melena, 548
in children, 1332
Meleney's ulcer, 1283
Melioidosis, drug therapy for, 135*t*
Melphalan, 1358
Ménétrier's disease, **561**
Meniere's disease, **975**
Meningioma, **919,** 919*t*, **926**
cranial, **920,** 924
of spinal cord, 927–928

Meningitis
in acute otitis media, 970
in chronic otitis media, 967
Meningocele, **933**
nasal malformations and, 984
Meningococci. *See also Neisseria meningitides*
infection by, drug therapy for, 135*t*
Menorrhagia, 1088
Menstrual disorder(s), 1087–1089
Menstrual history, abdominal pain and, 507
Menstruation, retrograde, 1096
Mental distress, infliction of, 76
Mental status, in cardiac compressive shock,
206
Meperidine, 20
nephrotoxicity of, 51
for penetrating or perforating ocular injuries,
1008
and postoperative psychosis, 34
Mercaptopurine, 1355
for Crohn's disease, 692, 748
for ulcerative colitis, 744
Mesalamine
for Crohn's disease, 692, 748
for inflammatory proctitis, 778
for ulcerative colitis, 744
Mesenteric adenitis, 693
Mesenteric apoplexy, **701**
Mesenteric arteries
emboli of, 698
inferior, 705, 706*i*
superior, 705, 706*i*
pancreas supplied by, 625, 626*i*
small intestine supplied by, 674
thrombosis of, 698
Mesenteric fixation, anomalies of, **1319**
Mesenteric lipodystrophy, **531**
Mesenteric lymphadenitis, **693**
Mesenteric lymph nodes, 718*i*
Mesenteric panniculitis, **531**
Mesenteric vascular occlusion, acute,
698–700
Mesenteric vein(s)
inferior, 565, 567*i*, 706*i*
superior, 565, 567*i*, 626*i*, 706*i*
thrombosis of, 698
Mesentery, 674
cysts of, **531**
vascular lesions of, **698–701**
Mesh repair(s)
for incisional hernia, 793
for inguinal hernia, 788
Mesoatrial shunt, 589
Mesoblastic nephroma, **1059**
Mesocaval shunt, 586, 586*i*
in Budd-Chiari syndrome, 589
Mesocolon, 707*i*
Mesothelioma
diffuse malignant pleural, **369–371**
peritoneal, **530**
MESS (Mangled Extremity Severity Score),
861
Metabolic acidemia, in hypovolemic shock,
205

Metabolic acidosis, **152**
  hyperchloremic, in total parenteral nutrition, 184*t*
  with respiratory acidosis, 153
  with respiratory alkalosis, 153
Metabolic alkalosis, **152–153**
  and delirium tremens, 35
  with respiratory alkalosis, 153
Metabolic disorders, **661–662**
  and depressed consciousness, 888
Metabolic renal stones, prevention of, **1044**
Metabolism. *See also* Hypermetabolism
  alteration of, in response to injury, 107–108
  in burn patient, 185–186, 269–270
  cerebral, and intracranial hypertension, 905–906
  in renal failure, 187
  in response to trauma and surgery, **100–111**
  surgical, **156–190**
Metacarpal fractures, **1148–1149, 1278–1279**
Metachronous cancer, of large intestine, 716, 728
[123I]Metaiodobenzylguanidine scan, of pheochromocytoma, 376
[131I]Metaiodobenzylguanidine scan, of pheochromocytoma, 804, 805
Metanephrines
  assays, factors affecting, 803
  plasma, in diagnosis of pheochromocytoma, 802–803
  urinary, in diagnosis of pheochromocytoma, 802–803
Metaphysial-diaphysial angle, in children, 1183–1184
Metastatic disease
  in abdominal wall, 796
  in adrenals, 812
  of bone, 1223–1224
  versus cervical disk syndrome, 955
  in colorectal cancer, **718**
  in epidermoid carcinoma of anal canal, 781–782
  intracranial, **921, 927**
  in liver, **574–576**
  ovarian, 1110
  spinal involvement in, 1213
  surgical management of, 1354
  vaginal, 1106
  vulvar, 1104
Metatarsal(s)
  fifth, tuberosity of, fracture of, **1176**
  fractures and dislocations of, **1175–1176**
  shafts of
    fatigue fracture of, 1175
    fracture of, **1175**
Metatarsalgia, **1216**
Metatarsus adductus, **1195–1196**
Metatarsus varus, 1216. *See also* Metatarsus adductus
Methadone, 20
Methane, in intestinal gas, 707
Methanobrevibacter smithii, in feces, 710–711
Methimazole, for hyperthyroidism, 301
Methotrexate, 1355

for breast cancer, 331–332, 334
for ectopic pregnancy, 1103
for gestational trophoblastic disease, 1114–1115
for nonlymphoid lymphomas, 1369–1370
for rheumatoid arthritis, 1204
Methoxyflurane, nephrotoxicity of, 51
3-Methylhistidine, urinary excretion of, 160
Methyl methacrylate, in chest wall reconstruction, 353
Methylprednisolone
  injection, and painful arc syndrome, 1197
  for spinal cord injury, 909, **912,** 1118
Methysergide, and retroperitoneal fibrosis, **1033**
Metoclopramide, indications for, 201
Metolazone, indications for, 51
Metronidazole
  for acute secondary bacterial peritonitis, 519
  in antibiotic-associated colitis, 749
  for brain abscess, 959
  for cholangitis, 612
  for Crohn's disease, 692, 748
  dosage of
    in hepatic failure, 138*t*
    in renal failure, 138*t*
  for gas cysts in small intestine, 701
  for hepatic encephalopathy, 593
  indications for, 127, 135*t*, 136*t*
  pharmacology of, 138*t*
  for preoperative bowel preparation, 755
  for ulcerative colitis, 744
Metroplasty, 1086
Metrorrhagia, 1088
Metyrosine, for pheochromocytoma, 804
Mezlocillin. *See also* Penicillin, antipseudomonal
  dosage of
    in hepatic failure, 138*t*
    in renal failure, 138*t*
  pharmacology of, 138*t*
Micelles, **597–598,** 678–679
Microemboli
  in extremity, **827**
  recurrent, and small artery occlusive disease, 827
Micrognathia, 1307
Microplatelets, in Wiskott-Aldrich syndrome, 661
Microtia, 973, **1259–1260**
Microvilli, intestinal, 676*i*
Micruroides euryxanthus, 130
Micrurus fulvius, 130
Micturition, bladder pressure during, 1074–1075
Mid-arm muscle circumference (MAMC), 157, 158*t*, 159*t*
Midazolam, indications for, 194
MID-CAB (minimally invasive direct coronary artery bypass), 414
Middle ear
  effusions of, 965
  tumors of, 973
Middle lobe syndrome, **386**

Midgut, malrotation of, **1318–1320,** 1319*i*
Midpalmar space, infections of, 1282–1283
Migrating myoelectric complex (MMC), interdigestive, 676
Migratory thrombophlebitis, in pancreatic adenocarcinoma, 644
Miliary coccidioidomycosis, 391
Milk-alkali syndrome, 311–312
Milrinone, for cardiogenic shock, 208
Milroy's disease, 885
Minerals, abnormalities of, in total parenteral nutrition, 181, 183*t*–184*t*
Minimal bactericidal concentration (MBC), 134
Minimal inhibitory concentration (MIC), 134
Minimally invasive surgery, for hand, **1290–1292**
Minocycline, indications for, 135*t*, 136*t*
Mist, for inhalation injuries, 276
Mitchell's causalgia. *See* Reflex sympathetic dystrophy
Mitomycin, 1355
Mitoxantrone, for malignant pleural effusion, 359
Mitral regurgitation, **422–424,** 423*i*
  survival rates with, 424, 425*i*
Mitral ring annuloplasty, 424, 424*i*
Mitral stenosis, 44, **420–422**
  as contraindication to surgery, 42
  rheumatic fever and, 420
Mitral valve, 419
  allograft, 429*i*
  annuloplasty, 418
  congenital disease of, **448**
  idiopathic calcification of, 422
  prolapse of, 44, 422
  repair of, for mitral regurgitation, 423–424, 424*i*, 425*i*
  replacement of, for mitral regurgitation, 423–424, 424*i*, 425*i*
Mittelschmerz, 1089–1090
Mixed bronchiectasis, 385
Mixed tumors of the salivary gland type, 397
Mobilization
  early, 23
  postoperative, 15, 17
Mohs technique, for basal cell carcinoma removal, 1251
Molar (M), 142
Molybdenum
  deficiency of, 164
  requirements for, 164*t*
Mondor's syndrome, **353**
Monitored anesthetic care, **199**
Monitoring
  during anesthesia, 194
  cardiovascular, in elderly, 68
  in enteral feeding, 171–174
  hemodynamic, 45
    complications of, **35–36**
  intraoperative, neurophysiologic, **897–900**
  postoperative, 14
Monoclonal antibody(ies) (MAb)
  in heart transplantation, 470

for transplant recipient, 470, **1375**, 1381
in treatment of non-Hodgkin's lymphoma, 1369
against tumor antigens, 1358
Monoclonal hypothesis, of atherosclerosis, 813
Monocyte chemotactic and activating factor (MCAF), 116t
Monocyte chemotactic peptide-1 (MCP-1), 116t
Monocytes, in fracture healing, 93
Monocytosis, after splenectomy, 666
Monopolar electrocautery, for bleeding peptic ulcers, 551
Monosaccharides, absorption of, in small intestine, 678
Monro-Kellie doctrine, 889
Monteggia's fracture, 1139, **1141–1142,** 1142i
Moraxella catarrhalis infection, drug therapy for, 135t
Morphea carcinoma, 1250
Morphine
    advantages and disadvantages of, 110
    adverse effects and side effects of, 20
    for cardiogenic shock, 208–209
    epidural, 21
    parenteral, 20
    for penetrating or perforating ocular injuries, 1008
    renal failure and, 51
    spinal, for malignant pain, 950
Morquio's disease, pectus carinatum in, 1306
Morton's neuroma, **1215**
Motility (gastrointestinal)
    disorders of
        in intestinal pseudo-obstruction, 686
        in jejunal diverticulosis, 688
        postoperative complications caused by, **30–31**
    of large intestine, **708**
    of small intestine, **675–677**
Motility studies, for sphincter of Oddi dysfunction, 622
Motorcycle accidents, 231
    pain in, 952
Motor evoked potential
    neurogenic, in spinal cord surgery, 898
    transcranial, in spinal cord surgery, 898–899
Motor function, assessment of, in craniocerebral trauma, **902**
Motor pathways, mapping of, **900**
Motor response, in craniocerebral trauma, **902**
Motor vehicle accidents, 230–231, 900
Mounier-Kuhn syndrome, and bronchiectasis, 384
Mouth. *See* Oral cavity
Movement disorders, **947–949**
Mucinous cystadenomas, of pancreas, 647
Mucocele
    of appendix, **673**
    frontal sinus, 980
Mucoepidermoid carcinoma, 294, 397, 404
Mucoid impaction of bronchi, **387**
Mucolytics, for bronchiectasis, 385
Mucormycosis, **394**

Mucosa
    of colon, 707i
    of small intestine, **674–675,** 676i, 677i
Mucosa-associated lymphoid tissue (MALT), 560
Mucosal resistance, in stomach and duodenum, 537–538
Mucosectomy, rectal, for ulcerative colitis, 745
Mucous cell, intestinal, 676i
    of small intestine, 674–675
Mucous gland adenoma, 397
Mucus, **535**
"Mulberry" appearance, of cavernous malformations, 945
Multicystic dysplastic kidney, **1020**
Multinodular goiter, **304**
Multi-organ system failure, in acute mesenteric vascular occlusion, 698
Multiple endocrine neoplasia (MEN)
    and pheochromocytoma, 802, 805
    type I, 309
        insulinoma and, 650
        intestinal carcinoids and, 703
    type II, 309
        intestinal carcinoids and, 703
    and Zollinger-Ellison syndrome, 544–545
Multiple myeloma (MM), 54, **1224**
    spinal involvement in, 1213
Multiple organ dysfunction syndrome (MODS), 111, 115, 124
Multiple organ failure, 109, 111, 118
Multiple sclerosis
    differential diagnosis of, 1208–1209
    esophageal manifestations in, 480
Multiple telangiectases, 469
Muromonab-CD3, for transplant recipient, **1375,** 1381, 1385
Murphy's sign, 509, 608
Muscle, breakdown of, in response to injury, 108
Muscle relaxants, in ventilatory management, 219
Muscularis, intestinal, 675
Muscularis mucosae, 756
Muscularis propria, 705
Muscular sinusoids, 871
Musculoaponeurotic fibromatoses, 796
Musculocutaneous flaps, in chest wall reconstruction, 353
Musculocutaneous nerve, 1272
Mustard operation, 465
M-VAC regimen, for bladder tumors, 1065
Myasthenia, as paraneoplastic syndrome, 1371, 1371t
Myasthenia gravis, **377–379**
Mycetoma, 129. *See also* Aspergillosis
Mycobacteria
    and bronchiectasis, 385
    infection by, drug therapy for, **141**
Mycobacterium avium, 387
Mycobacterium avium-intracellulare
    granulomatous lymphadenitis caused by, 1304

in HIV-associated enteropathy, 693–694
    infection by, drug therapy for, 136t
Mycobacterium bovis, 387
Mycobacterium fortuitum-chelonei infection, drug therapy for, 136t
Mycobacterium kansasii infection, drug therapy for, 136t
Mycobacterium leprae infection, drug therapy for, 136t
Mycobacterium tuberculosis infection, 387
    drug therapy for, 136t, 141
    genitourinary, 1041
    intestinal, 694–695
    and retroperitoneal abscesses, 526
Mycoplasma infection, drug therapy for, 136t
Mycoplasma pneumoniae, in pharyngitis, 987
Myeloblastic leukemia, and neutropenic colitis, 750
Myelofibrosis, idiopathic, **663**
Myelography
    in cervical disk syndrome, 954
    in lumbar disk syndrome, 957
    in neurodiagnosis, **895–896**
    in spinal cord tumors, 928
Myeloid metaplasia, agnogenic, **663**
Myeloma
    of chest wall, 355
    paraneoplastic syndromes with, 1371t
    and spinal cord, 928
    in surgical patient, 53–54
Myelomeningocele (spina bifida aperta), **933,** 933i
Myeloproliferative disorders, 53
Myenteric plexus, 675
Myoblastoma, of lung, 404
Myocardial contusion, management of, 247
Myocardial infarction, 43–44
    after cardiac surgery, 437
    clinical presentation of, 42
    as contraindication to surgery, 42
    postoperative, **28–29**
        risk factors for, 29
Myocardial ischemia
    in cardiac compressive shock, 206
    in elderly, 67–68
    shock caused by, 207–208
    in surgical patient, 41
    symptoms of, 410–411
Myocardiopathy, and cardiogenic shock, 207
Myocarditis, and cardiogenic shock, 207
Myocardium, contusion of, 208
Myochosis coli, 730
Myoma. *See* Leiomyoma(s)
Myomectomy, 1100
Myopathy
    familial visceral, and intestinal pseudo-obstruction, 686
    and spinal deformity, 1186–1187
Myositis
    clostridial, treatment of, 118
    as paraneoplastic syndrome, 1371
Myotomy, for cricopharyngeal achalasia, 475
Myotoxin, in snake venom, 131

Myringotomy
for acute otitis media, 970–971
for otitis media with effusion, 966, 966*i*
Myxedema, esophageal manifestations in, 480
Myxedema coma, 40
Myxochondromas, of chest wall, 354
Myxoma
atrial, and superior vena caval syndrome, 373
cardiac, 434–435, 435*i*, 469

Nafcillin
dosage of
in hepatic failure, 139*t*
in renal failure, 139*t*
pharmacology of, 139*t*
Nakata index, 461
Narcotics, with nitrous oxide, 197
Nasal bones, fractures of, 982, 983
Nasal cavity, cancer of, 282, **292–293**
Nasal packing, for epistaxis, 981, 982*i*
Nasal polyps, in allergic rhinitis, 978, 979
Nasal vestibulitis, **978**
Nasogastric feeding. *See also* Enteral feeding
protocol for, 174
Nasogastric intubation, 19
for acute abdomen, 515
for gastric decompression, 31
Nasogastric suction
for small bowel obstruction, **687**
for ulcerative colitis, 744
Nasolacrimal duct, obstruction of, 1003
Nasopharynx, cancer of, 282, **292–293**, 296
Nasotracheal intubation, 214–215, 233*i*
National Acute Spinal Cord Injury Studies, 909
National Health Interview Survey, 900
National Nosocomial Infections Surveillance
(NNIS), 121
National Practitioner Data Bank, 84–85
National Surgical Adjuvant Breast Project
(NSABP), 330
Nausea, postoperative, **199–200**
Navicular, fracture of, **1174**
N cells, 674
Near-drowning, **265**
Neck
abscesses of, 997
immobilization of, at accident scene, 234
inflammatory masses of, 997
injuries of, **241–243**
pain syndromes of, **1204–1210**
surgery of, **962–998** (*See also* Head and neck surgery)
veins of
in cardiac compressive shock, 206
in hypovolemia, 204
whiplash injury of, **1205–1206**
zones of, 241, 241*i*
Neck dissection
for head and neck tumors, 284–285
for laryngeal cancer, 291
for oral cavity cancer, 287, 287*t*
for oropharyngeal cancer, 289
for thyroid cancer, 307
Neck mass, workup of, 284–285, 284*t*

Necrosectomy, for acute pancreatitis, 634
Necrosis
pancreatic, 632
in peripheral arterial insufficiency, 818
Necrotizing cervical fasciitis, 997
Necrotizing enterocolitis, **1331**, 1332
Necrotizing enteropathy, 750
Necrotizing fasciitis, 114, **124–125**
of upper extremity, 1283
Necrotizing pancreatitis, 634–635
Necrotizing ulcerative gingivitis, acute,
984–985
Needle biopsy, **350–351**
of lung, **351**
Negligence, 72, 76–78
comparative, 80
contributory, 80
imputed, 79
liability aspect of, 78
reporting of, 83
res ipsa loquitur doctrine and, 78–79
Neisseria meningitides infection, after splenectomy, 666
Nelson's syndrome, 809, 930
Neodymium:YAG laser surgery
for adenoma and adenocarcinoma of ampulla of Vater, 648
for bladder tumors, 1064
for bleeding peptic ulcers, 551
for lung cancer, 402
for mucormycosis, 394
for villous adenomas of large intestine, 727
Neomycin
for hepatic encephalopathy, 592–593
for preoperative bowel preparation, 755
Neonatal intensive care, 1293
Neonatal small left colon syndrome,
1322–1323
Neonate. *See* Newborn
Neoplasm(s). *See also* Tumor(s)
anal, **779–780**
perianal, **779–780**
Neoplastic aneurysms, 938
Neoplastic diseases, **662–664**
Neostigmine, for colonic pseudo-obstruction, 714
Neostigmine bromide, for thymoma, 379
Neoureterocystostomy, 1050
Nephrectomy
for genitourinary tuberculosis, 1041
in recipient, before kidney transplantation, 1377
for renal adenocarcinoma, 1057
for xanthogranulomatous pyelonephritis, 1038
Nephric system, embryology of, 1014*i*
Nephroblastoma. *See* Wilms' tumor
Nephrocalcinosis, 1047–1048
Nephrolithotomy, for renal stones, 1044, 1045
Nephroma, mesoblastic, **1059**
Nephrosclerosis, malignant, kidney transplantation for, 1372
Nephroscopy, for renal stones, 1044
Nephrostomy, for renal stones, 1044

Nephrotic syndrome, and pleural effusion, 360
Nephroureterectomy, for renal pelvis and calices
tumors, 1060
Nerve(s)
anastomosis of
for facial paralysis, 977
for peripheral nerve injury, 914
healing of, 92
injuries to
improper positioning and, 195
treatment of, 243
Nerve block(s), **199**
Nerve crossover procedures, for facial paralysis,
977
Nerve entrapment syndromes, *versus* cervical
disk syndrome, 955
Nerve grafts, for peripheral nerve injury, 914
Nerve palsy, in brain tumors, 922
Nerve roots
anatomy of, and intervertebral disk disease,
952–953
injury of, **909**
Nerve sheath tumors (schwannomas), **919–920**,
925, 926
of facial nerve, 973
of peripheral nerves, 929
of spinal cord, **927**, 928
vestibular, 919–920, **975–976**
Nerve stimulation, for chronic benign pain, 951
Nervous system
congenital malformations of, **931–935**
paraneoplastic syndromes involving,
1370–1371, 1371*t*
Nesbit procedure, for Peyronie's disease, 1082
Netilmicin. *See* Aminoglycosides
Neuralgia, traumatic. *See* Reflex sympathetic
dystrophy
Neural monitoring, intraoperative, **897–900**
Neural placode, 933*i*
Neural tube, incomplete formation of, **932–934**
Neurapraxia, 913, 1281
Neurectomy, vestibular, for Meniere's disease,
975
Neurilemmomas, 929. *See also* Nerve sheath tumors (schwannomas)
Neuritis
brachial, *versus* cervical disk syndrome, 955
versus peripheral nerve tumors, 929
Neuroblastoma, 1312, **1342–1344**
metastases of, 1343
prognosis for, 1343
signs and symptoms of, 1343
of spinal cord, 928
staging of, 1343, 1343*t*
treatment of, 1343–1344
Neurodiagnostic procedures, **892–897**. *See also*
specific procedure
Neuroendocrine response to injury, **100–111**,
167–169, 168*i*
afferent pathways of, 102*i*, 103
in burn patient, 185–186
in cancer, 186
clinical correlates of, 108–109
magnitude of, 107
physiologic correlates of, 107–108

Neurofibroma, 1312
  of lung, 404
  of peripheral nerves, 929
  of spinal cord, 927, 928
Neurofibromatosis, 929–930
  pectus carinatum in, 1306
Neurofibrosarcoma, 1312
  of chest wall, 354
Neurogenic motor evoked potential, in spinal
    cord surgery, 898
Neurogenic shock, 1118
  in trauma victim, **239–240**
Neurogenic tumors
  chest wall, 354
  mediastinal, 375, 376
Neuroglial cells, tumors of, **917–919**, 924
Neurologic deficits
  after near-drowning, 265
  in arteriovenous malformations, 944
  in brain abscess, 959
  in cerebrovascular disease, 847, 848
  in impotence, **1082–1083**
  in trauma victims, **238**
Neurologic effects, of increased intracranial
    pressure, 890
Neurologic episodes, transient, in cerebrovascu-
    lar disease, 848
Neurologic examination
  of consciousness, **888**
  of head and neck tumors, 283
Neurologic instability, in craniocerebral
    trauma, management of, **903–906**
Neurolysis, for peripheral nerve injury, 914
Neuroma, 913
  acoustic, **919–920**
    management of, 976
    resection of, intraoperative neurophysio-
      logic monitoring in, 897–898
  interdigital nerve (Morton's), **1215**
  of wound, 25
Neuromodulation, for chronic benign pain,
    951
Neuromuscular blocking drugs, **197–198**
  drug interactions with, 192–193, 192*t*
Neuromuscular transfer, for facial paralysis,
    977
Neuromyopathy, as paraneoplastic syndrome,
    1370–1371
Neuropathic bladder, **1073–1076**
  versus benign prostatic hyperplasia, 1034
Neuropathic pain, 914, 950
Neuropathy
  familial visceral, and intestinal pseudo-ob-
    struction, 686
  as paraneoplastic syndrome, 1371*t*
  peripheral, *versus* peripheral nerve tumors,
    929
  traumatic, **913–914**
Neurophysiologic monitoring, intraoperative,
    897–900
Neurorrhaphy, for nerve injuries, 243
Neurospinal compression, differential diagnosis
    of, 816
Neurosurgery, **888–961**
  for arteriovenous malformation, 943–947

for brain abscess, 958–960
for brain tumors, **915–927**
for craniocerebral trauma, **900–908**
for intervertebral disk disease, 952–958
for intracranial aneurysms, 937–943
intraoperative neurophysiologic monitoring
    in, **897–900**
for movement disorders, 947–949
for pain, **950–952**
for Parkinson's disease, 947–949
pediatric, **931–937**
for peripheral nerve tumors, 929–930
for pituitary tumors, 930–931
for spinal cord injury, 908–913
for spinal cord tumors, **927–928**
for traumatic peripheral nerve lesions,
    913–914
Neurotmesis, 913, 1281
Neurotoxin(s)
  in snake venom, 130–131
  synergistic, and hepatic encephalopathy,
    592
Neurotransmitters
  amino acid, and hepatic encephalopathy,
    591–592
  false, and hepatic encephalopathy, 592
  in response to injury, 105
Neurovesical dysfunction, congenital, **1027**
Neutropenia, in Felty's syndrome, 660
Neutropenic colitis, **750**
Neutropenic enterocolitis, 750
Neutropenic typhlitis, 750
Nevi
  bathing trunk, 1246
  blue, 1246
  compound, 1246
  congenital, 1246
  dysplastic, 1363
  giant hairy, 1246
  intradermal, 1246
  junctional, 1245–1246
  and melanoma, 1363
  nevocellular, 1245
  pigmented, **1245–1246**
  spindle cell-epithelioma cell, 1246
Nevus flammeus. *See* Port wine stain
Nevus flammeus neonatorum, 1342
Nevus flammeus nuchae, 1342
Newborn. *See also* Infant(s); Premature infant
  airway obstruction in, 992
  antibiotic dosage in, 137
  blood loss in, 1299
  care of, **1293–1300**
  classification of
    by gestational age, 1293–1294
    by weight, 1293–1294
  electrolyte requirements in, 1296
  female, reproductive tract of, examination
    of, 1085
  gastrointestinal bleeding in, 1332
  gastrointestinal decompression in, **1299**
  gestational age of, assessment of, 1293
  hepatic rupture in, 571
  intestinal obstruction in, **1315**
  jaundice in, 1333–1335

meconium plug (small left colon) syndrome
    in, 1322–1323
NPO guidelines for, 1299–1300
nutrition for, **1297–1299**
pain in, 19
preoperative blood analysis in, 1299
respiratory emergencies in, **1306–1310**
  classification of, 1307
small-for-gestational-age (SGA), 1293–1294
temperature regulation in, 1294
transfusion therapy in, 1299
uterine bleeding in, 1087
ventilation for, 1294–1295
New York Heart Association (NYHA), 411
Niacin, 163
  requirements for, 164*t*
Nicotine, for ulcerative colitis, 744–745
Nifedipine, for angina pectoris, 412
Nightstick fractures, 1141
Nimodipine, for subarachnoid hemorrhage,
    942
Nipple-areola complex, reconstruction of, 1262
Nipple discharge, **342**
  in breast cancer, 319, 339–340
  cytologic examination of, 326
Nipple erosion, with breast cancer, 319
Nissen fundoplication, 487, 487*i*
Nitrates, for coronary artery disease, 44
Nitrogen
  balance
    arginine and, 162
    determination of, 158–160, 159*t*, 160*i*
    in renal failure, 187, 187*t*
    in response to injury, 109, 110
  excretion of, 166
    in burn patient, 185
  in intestinal gas, 707
  loss, in response to injury, 108
  retention of, in cancer patient, 186
  in small bowel obstruction, 684
  total body, 159*t*
Nitroglycerin
  for anal fissure, 770
  for angina pectoris, 412
  and arterial spasm, 261
  for cardiogenic shock, 208–209
  for intra-arterial injections, 858
Nitroprusside
  for cardiogenic shock, 208–209
  for dysrhythmias, with pheochromocytoma,
    805
  indications for, 29
Nitrosoureas, 1355
Nitrosurea-based compounds, for brain tu-
    mors, 926
Nitrous oxide, 197
  indications for, 195
  plus ketamine, depth of anesthesia with,
    signs of, 197*t*
  plus narcotic, 197
    depth of anesthesia with, signs of, 197*t*
Nobel plication procedures, 687
Nocardiosis (*Nocardia* infection), 112, **129**
  and chronic mediastinitis, 372
  drug therapy for, 136*t*

Nociceptors, 103
No code order, 81–82
Noise, hearing loss from, 969
Nolvadex. *See* Tamoxifen
No-man's-land, of hand, 1272, 1272*i*
Nonatherosclerotic disorders, causing lower
        limb ischemia, **828–829**
Noncommunicating diverticulitis, 732
Non-glial cell tumors, **919–921**, 924, **926–927**
Non-Hodgkin's lymphoma (NHL), 560,
        1367–1370
  aggressive (high-grade), 1368*t*
    characteristics of, 1368
    treatment of, 1368–1369
  AIDS-associated, and small intestine, 702
  classification of, 1367–1368, 1368*t*
  indolent (low-grade), 1368*t*
    characteristics of, 1367–1368
    treatment of, 1368
  risk factors for, 1367
  staging of, 1367
  treatment of, 1368–1369, 1369*i*
Noninvasive tests
  for cerebrovascular disease, 849
  for peripheral arterial insufficiency, 818–819
Nonocclusive intestinal ischemia, **700**
Nonprotein respiratory quotient (RQ), 159*t*,
    161
  in sepsis, 169
Nonrelaxing puborectalis syndrome, 762,
    763–764
Nonseminomatous cell tumors, **1072**
Nonspecific esophageal motor disorder, 476
Nonspherocytic hemolytic anemia, hereditary,
    657
Nonsteroidal anti-inflammatory drugs
    (NSAIDs)
  adverse effects and side effects of, 20, 51
  for chronic pelvic pain, 1090
  and colonic diverticulitis, 731
  and colorectal cancer, 717
  contraindications to, 50
  enteropathy caused by, **695**
  nephrotoxicity of, 51
  for osteoarthritis, 1202
  for painful arc syndrome, 1197
  parenteral, for postoperative analgesia, 20
  and platelet function, 55
  for rheumatoid arthritis, 1204
  and ulcerative colitis, 743
Nontoxic goiter, **304**
Noonan's syndrome, 988
Norepinephrine
  actions of, 167
  for craniocerebral trauma, 903
  for neurogenic shock, 209
  plasma, in diagnosis of pheochromocytoma,
    803
Norethindrone acetate, for endometriosis,
    1098–1099
Norethynodrel, for endometriosis, 1098–1099
Normal perfusion pressure hemorrhage, and ar-
    teriovenous malformations, 946
Normothermia, in surgery, 110

Nose, **977–984**. *See also* Nasal; Rhinoplasty
  bleeding of (epistaxis), **981**
  congenital malformations of, **983–984**
  foreign bodies of, **977–978**
  fractures of, **1255–1256**
  trauma to, **982–983**
Noxious chemicals, in smoke inhalation, 275,
    275*t*
NPO guidelines, for pediatric patients,
    1299–1300
Nucleotides, in nutritional support, 162
Numbness, with spinal cord tumors, 927
Nuss bar, 1305–1306
Nutcracker esophagus, 476
Nutrition
  disorders of, pathophysiology of, **164–170**
  for newborn, **1297–1299**
  and wound healing, 16
Nutritional assessment, **156–161**
  preoperative, 7
Nutritional support, **170–181**. *See also* Enteral
    feeding; Parenteral nutrition
  for acute pancreatitis, **634**
  after injury, 108, 110
  after small bowel resection, 680
  in AIDS, 189–190
  arginine in, 162
  in burn patient, 185–186, 186*t*, 271
  in cancer patient, 186–187
  in cardiac disease, 188
  for Crohn's disease, 691–692
  energy requirements in
    determination of, 160–161
    sources for, 161
  fatty acids in, 162–163
  in gastrointestinal disease, 188–189
  glutamine in, 162
  in hepatic failure, 188
  in hepatorenal failure, 188
  in infections, 118
  nucleotides in, 162
  nutrient requirements in, 161–164
  in obesity, 190
  in pancreatic disease, 189
  protein requirements in, sources for,
    161–162
  in renal failure, 187–188
  in short bowel syndrome, 189
  for small bowel syndrome, 681–682
  for small intestine fistulas, 696*t*, **697**
  vitamins in, 163, 164*t*
Nutritional therapy, evaluation for, 3
Nystagmus, in dizziness, 975
Nystatin, for bezoars, 562

Oat cell carcinoma. *See* Small cell carcinoma
Obesity
  complications of, 190
  and incisional hernia, 793
  morbid, 190
  nutritional support in, 190
  and operative risk, 10, 17, 23
  pulmonary involvement in, preoperative
    management of, 47

  and wound healing, 24
Obstipation
  abdominal pain and, 507
  in colonic obstruction, 713
Obstructed defecation, 709–710, 710*t*
Obstruction, intestinal. *See* Intestinal
    obstruction
Obstructive congenital heart lesions, **440–449**
Obstructive pancreatitis, 629
Obstructive sleep apnea syndrome, 988–989
Obstructive uropathy, **1029–1032**
Obturator canal, herniation through, 795
Obturator sign, in acute abdomen, 509
Occipital lobe, tumors in, **923**
Occult blood, tests for, 548
Occupational exposure, and lung cancer, 396
Octreotide
  for blind loop syndrome, 680
  for carcinoid syndrome, 704
  indications for, 189
  for variceal bleeding, 582
Ocular adnexa, **999–1012**. *See also* Eye(s)
  blunt trauma to, **1009**, 1009*t*
  diseases of, **1002–1007**
  inspection of, **999–1000**
  lacerations of, **1009**
Ocular burns, **1007–1008**
Ocular diseases/disorders, **1002–1007**
  laser treatment for, **1012**
  symptoms and signs of, 1000–1001
Ocular lubricants, for Bell's palsy, 977
Ocular pain, **1000–1001**
Ocular trauma, **1008–1010**
Ocular tumors, **1010–1012**
Oculocephalic reflex, in craniocerebral trauma,
    902
Oculomotor nerve, in intracranial aneurysm,
    939
Oculopharyngeal muscular dystrophy, 475
Oculovestibular reflex, in craniocerebral
    trauma, 902
Oddi, sphincter of, dysfunction of, 622
Odontoid fracture, 910
Odynophagia, 282
Ofloxacin, indications for, 136*t*
Ogilvie's syndrome, **714**
OKT3 therapy, for transplant recipient, **1375**,
    1381
Older patient. *See* Elderly
Olecranon bursitis, **1200**
Oligodendrogliomas, **918–919**, 926
Oligospermia, hormone studies in, 1080
Oliguria
  in cardiac compressive shock, 206
  definition of, 204
  in hemolytic transfusion reaction, 59
  in hypovolemia, 204
  in response to injury, 108, 111
  in ureteral injury, 1050
Ollier's disease, 1288
Omentum, 517
  cysts of, **532**
  disorders of, **532**
  infarction of, **532**

infection of, **532**
torsion of, **532**
tumors of, **532**
Omeprazole
  for duodenal ulcer, 541
  for Ménétrier's disease, 561
  for reflux esophagitis sliding hiatal hernia, 486
  for short bowel syndrome, 682
  for upper gastrointestinal hemorrhage, 549
  for Zollinger-Ellison syndrome, 546
Omphalocele, **1339–1340**, 1340*i*
Omphalomesenteric duct anomalies, **1330–1331**, 1330*i*
Oncocytoma(s), 294
  renal, **1059**
Oncology, **1352–1371**
Ondansetron
  indications for, 200
  for penetrating or perforating ocular injuries, 1009
Onychomycosis, 1284
Oophorectomy
  bilateral, for breast cancer, 334
  for persistent adnexal masses, 1101–1102
OPCAB (off-pump coronary artery bypass), 414
Open-angle glaucoma, **1005–1006**
Open biopsy
  for breast cancer, 319
  of lung, **351**
Open cardiac massage, 238, 238*i*
Open heart surgery, postoperative management, 440
Open pneumothorax, 237, 347, 367
Operation history, acute abdomen and, 508
Operative permit, 11
Ophthalmic artery, aneurysms, 939
Ophthalmoplegia, 301
Ophthalmoscopy, **1000**
Opioids
  for cardiogenic shock, 208
  for chronic benign pain, 951
  endogenous, 104
  epidural, 21
  gastrointestinal effects of, 19
  indications for, 194
  intestinal motility and, 677
  intramuscular, 20, 21
  intravenous, 20, 21
    indications for, 133
  for malignant pain, 950
  mechanism of action of, 20
  with nitrous oxide, 197
  parenteral, 20
Opportunistic infection, and lung abscess, 383
Optic chiasm, tumors in, 915*i*, 916*i*
Optic nerve
  intraoperative monitoring of, 898
  tumors in, 915*i*, 916*i*, 923
Oral candidiasis, **985**
Oral cavity, **984–986**
  cancer of, 282, **286–287**, 296
  congenital malformations of, 986

herpetic lesions of, **985**
white lesions of, **984**
Oral cholecystography, for biliary tree examination, 600
Oral contraceptives
  and abdominal pain, 507
  for chronic pelvic pain, 1090
  for control of abnormal uterine bleeding, 1089
  for endometriosis, 1099
  and nipple discharge, 342
  and prevention of ovarian cancer, 1111
Oral feedings, in short bowel syndrome, 682
Orbit
  blunt trauma to, **1009**, 1009*t*
  floor of, blowout fracture of, **1009**
  fractures of, **1256–1257**
  tumors of, **1011–1012**
Orbital cellulitis, **1003**
Orbital pain, **1000–1001**
Orchidopexy, in cryptorchidism, 1338–1339
Orchiectomy
  for prostate cancer, 1069
  for testicular cancer, 1071
Orchiopexy, for testicular torsion, 1339
Orchitis, *versus* spermatic cord torsion, 1079–1080
Organ dysfunction, 115
Organ function, age-related changes in, 67–69, 68*t*
Organ transplantation. *See also* Heart, transplantation of; Kidney(s), transplantation of; Liver, transplantation of; Lung(s), transplantation of; Pancreas, transplantation of
  blood group compatibility and, 1373
  cross-matching for, 1373
  donors for, 1376–1377
  graft rejection in, 470, 1373, **1379–1380,** 1385–1386
    accelerated, 1380
    acute, 1380
    chronic, 1380
    hyperacute, 1379–1380
  histocompatibility testing for, 1373
  immunosuppression for, 470, 1372, 1374–1375, 1379, 1381, 1385
Oriental cholangiohepatitis (recurrent pyogenic cholangitis), 621, **623**
Orocecal transit time, 677
Oropharynx, cancer of, 282, **288–289**, 296
Orotracheal intubation, 214–215
  in trauma care, 233*i*, 236
Orthopedics, **1116–1229**
  bone tumors and, 1222–1229
  congenital dysplasia and dislocation of hip and, 1189–1192
  foot deformities in children and, 1194–1196
  fractures and, 1117–1176
  gait disorders and, 1183
  infections in, 1217–1222
  joint dislocations and, 1117–1176
  Legg-Perthes disease and, 1193–1194
  limb deformity and, 1183–1184

osteomyelitis and, 1217–1220
pain syndromes and, 1197–1217
pediatric, 1176–1197
scoliosis and, 1185–1187
septic arthritis and, 1220–1222
septic arthritis of hip and, 1187–1189
slipped capital femoral epiphysis and, 1192–1193
spinal deformity and, 1185–1187
terminology for, 1116
Orthophosphates, for renal stones, 1043
Orthotics
  for hallux valgus, 1217
  for metatarsalgia, 1216
Ortolani's test, for congenital hip dislocation, 1190–1191, 1190*i*
Osler-Weber-Rendu disease, and arteriovenous fistulas, 845
Osmolality, 142–143
Osmoreceptors, 106
Osmotic diarrhea, 709
Osmotic diuretics, for increased intracranial pressure, 891
Osmotic fragility, in hereditary spherocytosis, 656
Osteoarthritis, **1201–1203**
  differential diagnosis of, 816
  primary, 1202
  versus rheumatoid arthritis, 1203–1204
  secondary, 1202
Osteoblasts, in fracture healing, 93
Osteochondroma, **1226**
  of chest wall, 354
Osteogenesis imperfecta, ear abnormalities in, 974
Osteogenic sarcoma, of chest wall, 355
Osteomalacia, in short bowel syndrome, 682
Osteomas, of chest wall, 355
Osteomyelitis, 93, 1263
  adjacent soft tissue infection and, **1217–1218**
  chronic, **1218–1220**
    malignant degeneration in, 1218
  diagnosis of, 117
  hematogenous, 1221
  of proximal femur, 1188
  of ribs, **352**
  sternal, **352**
  vertebral, 1213, 1214*i*
Osteophyte, in cervical disk syndrome, 954
Osteoporosis, and hyperparathyroidism, 309
Osteotomy, for osteoarthritis, 1202
Ostomy. *See* Stoma
Otalgia, 282, **969–970**
Otitis externa, **969–970**
Otitis media
  acute, **970–971**
  chronic, **967–968**
    intracranial complications in, 967
  with effusion, **965–966**
  nonsuppurative, 965
Otolaryngology, **962–998**. *See also* Head and neck surgery
  in HIV-infected (AIDS) patients, 998

Otoplasty, for congenital deformities of ear, 973
Otorrhea, in chronic otitis media, 967
Otosclerosis, **968**
Otosyphilis, in AIDS, 998
Ototoxic drugs, in AIDS treatment, 998
Outcome scales, for craniocerebral trauma, 907–908
Outpatient surgery, anesthesia for, 200–201, 201t
Ovalocytosis, **657**
Ovarian cancer, **1110–1112**
  clear cell, 1110
  clinical findings in, 1111
  differential diagnosis of, 1111
  endometrioid, 1110
  epithelial, 1110
  FIGO staging of, 1111, 1112t
  germ cell, 1110
  hormonally active, 1110
  mucinous, 1110
  paraneoplastic syndromes with, 1371t
  in pregnant patient, 66
  prevention of, 1111
  prognosis for, 1112
  serous, 1110
  stromal, 1110
  transitional cell, 1110
  treatment of, 1111–1112
  types of, 1110
  undifferentiated adenocarcinoma, 1110
Ovarian cyst, 63
  endometrial, 66
Ovarian remnant syndrome, 1090
Ovary(ies)
  dystrophy of, 1090
  embryology of, 1013–1014, 1016i
  lesions of, differential diagnosis of, 514
  torsion of, 1101
    in pregnant patient, 66–67
  tumors of, 1110 (*See also* Ovarian cancer)
    differential diagnosis of, 1111
    in pregnant patient, 66–67
Ovulation
  pain at, 1089–1090
  suppression of
    for abnormal uterine bleeding, 1088–1089
    for chronic pelvic pain, 1090
Oxalate renal stones, prevention of, **1044**
Oxidative killing, 113
Oxycodone
  with acetaminophen, for postoperative analgesia, 21
  with aspirin, for postoperative analgesia, 21
Oxygen
  consumption
    determination of, 220, 221t
    normal value for, 221t
    in response to injury, 107
  content
    in arterial blood (CaO_2), 220–223, 221t
    in mixed venous blood ($CmvO_2$), 221t
  partial pressure of

    in arterial blood (PaO_2), 214, 220–223, 221t
      low, causes of, 223
      and SaO_2, correlation of, 222, 222i
    in mixed venous blood ($PmvO_2$), 221t
  return, 221t
  saturation
    in arterial blood (SaO_2), 221t
      and PaO_2, correlation of, 222, 222i
    in mixed venous blood ($SmvO_2$), 221t
  transport, 221t
Oxygen tension
  and amputation level determination, 860
  and antibacterial capacity of granulocytes, 113
  tissue
    and infection, 121–122
    and wound healing, 86–87, 88i, 90
Oxygen therapy
  for acute pancreatitis, **633**
  for gas cysts in small intestine, 701
Oxyhemoglobin dissociation, **220–223**, 222i
Oxytinic gland area, of stomach, 533, 535i

PABA excretion test, **643**
Paced Auditory Serial Addition Test, 907
Pacesetter potentials, of small intestine, 675
Packed red blood cells, for craniocerebral trauma, 903
Paclitaxel, 1355
Paget's carcinoma, **328**
Paget-Schroetter syndrome, 844, 878, 878i, 879–880
Paget's disease, **781**
Pain, **950–952**. *See also* Pain syndromes
  abdominal, 42, **503–507**, 504t, 505f, 796
    in acute appendicitis, 1328
    in cardiac patients, 514
    character of, 506–507, 506i
    chronic, 672
    in Crohn's disease, **690**
    with femoral hernia, 790
    hematologic causes of, 53
    with intestinal duplications, 1329
    with intussusception, 1324
    location of, 503–504
    mode of onset of, 504–506
    progression of, 504–506
    symptoms associated with, 507
  in abdominal wall, **796**
  in acute mesenteric vascular occlusion, 698–699
  amputation and, 867–868, **951–952**
  of anal fissure, 769
  anorectal, 763
  of anorectal abscess, 771
  in back, **1210–1215**
    in lumbar disk syndrome, 956, 957
    mechanical, **1214–1215**
    in pancreatic adenocarcinoma, 644
  bone, in prostate cancer, 1069
  in brachial plexus injury, 952
  in breast cancer, 319
  cancer, **950**

  and cardiac complications, 28
  in cervical disk syndrome, 954
  of cervical strain, **1204–1205**
  chest
    in pulmonary thromboembolism, 880
    severity of, classification of, 411
    with thoracic aortic dissection, 433
  chronic benign, **951**
  in chronic pancreatitis, 640
  in colonic obstruction, 713
  in Crohn's disease, **690**
  with defecation, 769, 776
  of duodenal ulcer, 540
  elbow, **1199–1200**
  epigastric, 796
    with epigastric hernia, 792
  evaluation of, 1
  in eye, **1000–1001**
  in foot, **1215–1217**
  of gastric ulcer, 547
  in gastrointestinal ischemia syndromes, 857
  groin, differential diagnosis of, 785–786
  in hand, in arthritis, 1285
  of head and neck tumors, 282
  hemorrhoidal, 767
  hip, **1200–1204**
    in young children, 1189
  history-taking about, 1
  incisional, 796
  with inguinal hernia, 785
  leg, 956, 957
  low back (*See* Low back pain)
  in lumbar disk syndrome, 956, 957
  malignant, **950**
  in mammary dysplasia, 341
  management of, in elderly, 68
  of nail infections, 1282
  neck, **1204–1210**
  neuropathic, 914, 950
  neurosurgical procedures for, **950–952**
  orbital, **1000–1001**
  in osteoarthritis, 1202
  ovulatory, 1089–1090
  in pancreatic adenocarcinoma, 644
  in pancreatic pseudocyst, 636
  parietal, 503
  pelvic, 1089–1090
  of peptic ulcer, 539
  of peripheral arterial insufficiency, 816–817
  pleural, 356
  postoperative, **19–21, 950–951**
    factors affecting, 19
    management of, 20–21, **200**
    physician-patient communication and, 20
    physiology of, 19
    and postoperative complications, 20
  rectal, 777
  referred, 503, 505i
  in renal adenocarcinoma, 1056–1057
  and respiratory function, 17, 18
  shifting, 504, 505i
  shoulder, **1197–1199**
  of spigelian hernia, 794
  in spinal cord injury, **952**

of spinal cord tumors, 927, 928
spreading, 504, 505*i*
sympathetically maintained, 914
with umbilical hernia, 791
of ureteral calculi, 1045
visceral, 503, 504*t*, 505*f*
wound, 25
Pain control (pain relief). *See also* Analgesia
for chronic pancreatitis, 641–642
neurosurgery for, **950–952**
for penetrating or perforating ocular injuries, 1008–1009
Pain syndromes, 951–952. *See also* Pain
Palliative therapy
for colorectal cancer, **722–723**
for prostate cancer, **1069**
Pallidotomy, for Parkinson's disease, 947–948
Pallor
in acute arterial occlusion, 825
in peripheral arterial insufficiency, 817
Palma procedure, for chronic venous insufficiency, 885
Palmar fasciitis, **1284–1285**
Palmaz type stents, for peripheral arterial insufficiency, 821
Palpation, 4
of abdominal mass, 509
of acute abdomen, 509–510
in breast cancer diagnosis, 323, 323*i*, 324*i*
of cerebrovascular disease, 849
of head and neck tumors, 283
Pancoast's tumor, 399*i*
Pancolitis, 741
Pancreas, **625–651**, 706*i*
abscess of, 632, **638–639**
anatomy of, **625**, 626*i*
annular, **627**, 1316
cancer of, **644–646**
paraneoplastic syndromes with, 1371*t*
cystic neoplasms of, 637, **647**
disease of, nutritional support in, 189
divisum, 629
embryology of, **625**
endocrine function of, 627
exocrine function of, 625–626
tests of, **643**
in chronic pancreatitis, 640
injuries to, treatment of, 253
physiology of, **625–627**
resection of, for pancreatic adenocarcinoma, 645
rupture, pancreatic pseudocyst and, **637**
transplantation of, **1386**
Pancrease, for pancreatic insufficiency, 643
Pancreatectomy
for chronic pancreatitis, **642**
distal subtotal, 642
partial, for insulinoma, 650
total, 642
for pancreatic adenocarcinoma, 646
Pancreatic ascites, **639–640**
Pancreatic cholera, **650**
Pancreatic ducts, 595, 625, 626*i*
back diffusion across, and pancreatitis, 630

obstruction of, and pancreatitis, 629
Pancreatic enzymes, 626
supplements of, for short bowel syndrome, 682
Pancreatic insufficiency, **643**
Pancreatic islet cell tumors, **648–651**
Pancreatic juice, 625–626
Pancreatic necrosis, 632
Pancreaticoduodenal arteries, 625, 626*i*
Pancreaticoduodenal veins, 626*i*
Pancreaticoduodenectomy
for adenoma and adenocarcinoma of ampulla of Vater, 648
for bile duct malignancies, 618
for chronic pancreatitis, 642
for pancreatic adenocarcinoma, 645–646, 646*i*
Pancreaticojejunostomy
distal, for chronic pancreatitis, 642
longitudinal, for chronic pancreatitis, 641–642, 641*i*
Pancreatic phlegmon, 632
Pancreatic pleural effusion, **639–640**
Pancreatic pseudocyst, **635–638**
Pancreatic vein, inferior, 626*i*
Pancreatitis, **621–622, 627–642**
acute, 627, **631–635**
versus acute cholecystitis, 608
nutritional support in, 189
relapsing, 627
versus acute mesenteric vascular occlusion, 699
alcoholic, **628**
autodigestion theory of, 629
back diffusion across pancreatic duct in, **630**
biliary, **627–628**
chronic, 627, **640–642**
relapsing, 627
common channel theory of, **630**
differential diagnosis of, 540, 554
drug-induced, **629**
duodenal reflux in, **630**
edematous, 631–635
etiology of, 627–629
familial, **628**
gallstone-induced, 64
hemorrhagic, 631–635
hypercalcemia and, **628**
hyperlipidemia and, **628**
idiopathic, **629**
necrotizing, 634–635
obstruction-secretion theory of, **629–630**
obstructive, **629**
pathogenesis of, **629–631**
pleural effusion and, 360
postoperative, **31–32**
postoperative (iatrogenic), **628–629**
protein deficiency and, **628**
in renal transplant recipient, 32, 1379
subacute, 627
systemic manifestations of, **630–631**
Pancreatography
endoscopic retrograde
in chronic pancreatitis, 641

in pancreatic ascites, 639
in pancreatic adenocarcinoma, 645
Pancrelipase replacement, for pancreatic insufficiency, 643
Pancreolauryl test, **643**
Pancytopenia, in hypersplenism, 654
Paneth cells, 674
Panhypopituitarism, in surgical patient, 41
Panniculitis, mesenteric, **531**
Panretinal photocoagulation, **1012**
Pantothenic acid, 163
requirements for, 164*t*
Papaverine
for acute mesenteric vascular occlusion, 699
and arterial spasm, 261
for intra-arterial injections, 858
for intracranial aneurysm, 943
for nonocclusive intestinal ischemia, 700
Papillary adenocarcinoma, 305, **306**, 307
of lung, 396
Papillary craniopharyngioma, 920
Papillary cystadenocarcinoma, *versus* simple renal cyst, 1076
Papillary-cystic neoplasm, of pancreas, 647
Papillary muscle rupture, 422
Papillary necrosis, **1038**
versus renal stones, 1043
Papillary sloughs, *versus* ureteral calculi, 1046
Papilledema, in brain tumors, 915, 922
Papilloma
of bile ducts, 619
of esophagus, 494
of larynx, **994**
Papillomatosis, respiratory recurrent, **994**
Pap smear, in Bowen's disease, 780
Paracentesis
for acute abdomen, 513
of ascitic fluid, 590
Paracolic lymph node, 718*i*
Paracolostomy hernia, 753–754
Paradoxical pelvic floor contraction, 762
Paradoxic pulse, 207
Paraesophageal hiatal hernia, **482–483**, 483*i*
Paralysis
of facial nerve, **977**
of vocal cords, **995–996**
Paralytic ileus, 677, 683
versus large bowel obstruction, **714**
physical findings in, 508*t*
versus small bowel obstruction, 686
Paramedics, in trauma care, 232
Paranasal sinus(es), **977–984**
cancer of, **292–293**
Paranasal sinusitis, **979–980**
Paraneoplastic syndromes, **1370–1371**, 1371*t*
Paraphimosis, **1082**
Parasellar region, tumors in, 915*i*, 916*i*, **923**
Parasites
and chronic mediastinitis, 372
and thoracic empyema, 361
Parasitic cysts, of spleen, 664
Parasternal hernia, **501**, 501*i*
Parathyroid gland(s), **307–308**
adenoma of, 309

Parathyroid gland(s) (*cont.*)
  anatomy of, 307–308
  carcinoma of, 309
  diseases of, **308–318**
  embryology of, 307–308
  physiology of, 308
  surgery on, pancreatitis after, 32
  tumors of, localization of, 313, 314*i*
Parathyroid hormone (PTH), 308, 310
Parathyroid hormone-related peptide (PTHrP),
    1370
Parathyromatosis, 309
Paratibial perforators, 872*i*
Parenteral nutrition, **175–181**
  in gastrointestinal disease, 189
  for pediatric patients, 1297–1299
  peripheral, **175–178**
    administration of, 177
    characteristics of, 176*t*
    complications of, 181
    contraindications to, 176*t*, 178
    in hepatic failure, 178
    indications for, 175, 176*t*
    in nonoliguric renal failure, 178
    orders for, 177, 177*i*
    solution formulation of, 175, 177*t*
    special solutions for, 177–178
  total, 175, **178–181**
    for acute pancreatitis, 634
    administration of, 178
      in pediatric patients, 1297–1298
    in cancer patient, 186, 187
    catheter for, 178
      for pediatric patients, 1297–1298
    characteristics of, 176*t*
    complications of, 180*t*, 181–184,
        182*t*–184*t*
      in pediatric patients, 1298–1299
    contraindications to, 176*t*
    daily nutrient requirements in, 178
      for pediatric patients, 1298, 1298*t*
    in gastrointestinal disease, 189
    for glucagonoma, 651
    in hepatic failure, 188
    indications for, 176*t*, 178
      for pediatric patients, 1297
    in liver failure, 181
    orders for, 178, 179*i*
    in pancreatic disease, 189
    in renal failure, 179–181
    for small intestine fistulas, 697
    solution formulation for, 178, 179*t*
      for pediatric patients, 1298
    special solutions for, 179–181
    tapering schedule for, 184
Parietal cells, and acid secretion, 536–537,
    537*i*
Parietal cell vagotomy, for duodenal ulcer, 541,
    542*i*
Parietal lobe, tumors in, **922**
Parietal pain, 503
Parietal peritoneum, 517
Parietal pleurectomy, for pneumothorax pre-
    vention, 369

Parinaud's syndrome, 920–921
Parkes-Weber syndrome, 1342
Parkinsonism, atypical, 948
Parkinson's disease, **947–949**
Parona's space, 1272
Paronychia, **1282,** 1282*i*
Parotitis, postoperative, **30**
Partial-thickness burns. *See* Second-degree
    burns
Pasteurella infection, drug therapy for, 135*t*
Past history, 2–3
Patella
  dislocation of, **1161**
  fracture of, **1160–1162**
    comminuted, 1161
    transverse, 1160–1161
Patellar ligament, tear of, **1161**
Patellar tendon-bearing prosthesis, 869
Patent ductus arteriosus, 449, **453–454,** 458
Patent foramen ovale, and aortic coarctation,
    445
Patient
  approach to, **1–5**
  emotional background of, 3
  history-taking from, 1–3
  imaging studies in, 5
  information for, 10–11
  laboratory examination in, 5
  physical examination of, 3–4
  special examinations for, 5
Patient-controlled analgesia (PCA, PCEA), **21,**
    200
Patient Self-Determination Act, 81
"Pearly tumors," **920**
Pectoralis major flap, **1236**
Pectus carinatum, **1306,** 1306*i*
Pectus excavatum, **1305,** 1305*i*
Pediatric surgery, **1293–1356**. *See also*
    Child(ren)
Pelvic abscess, causes of, 524*t*
Pelvic examination
  in acute abdomen, 510
  for chronic pelvic pain, 1090
  for endometriosis, 1097
  indications for, 1086, 1088
Pelvic floor, 756
  anatomy of, 1092, 1124–1125
  dysfunction of, 762
  normal function of, 758
  obstetric injuries to, 1092
Pelvic floor muscle (Kegel) exercises, 1093
Pelvic inflammatory disease (PID)
  and appendicitis, 670
  and ectopic pregnancy, 1102
Pelvic organ prolapse
  measurement of, 1092–1093
  treatment of
    nonoperative, 1093
    surgical, 1093
  and urinary incontinence, 1092–1093
Pelvic pain, chronic, **1089–1090**
Pelvirectal (supralevator) space, 757*i*, 771*i*
Pelvis
  anatomy of, 1124–1125

  in bladder exstrophy, 1027, 1027*i*
  fractures and dislocations of, **1123–1127**
    and bladder injury, 1050
    and urethral injury, 1053*i*
  stability of, 1125
Penetrating trauma
  abdominal, 249
  arterial, 256–257
  cardiac, 247
  of head, **901**
  ocular, **1008–1009**
Penicillamine, for renal stones, 1044
Penicillin
  for acute cholecystitis, 609
  after splenectomy, 666–667
  for anorectal syphilis, 776
  and antibiotic-associated colitis, 749
  antipseudomonal, indications for, 135*t*
  for burn patients, 271
  indications for, 135*t*, 136*t*
  for lung abscess, 384
  penicillinase-resistant, indications for,
      135*t*
  seizures and, 274
Penicillin G
  dosage of
    in hepatic failure, 139*t*
    in renal failure, 139*t*
  pharmacology of, 139*t*
Penile-brachial index, in impotence, 1083
Penile prosthesis, for impotence, 1084
Penis
  anomalies of, **1028–1029**
  injuries to, **1052–1053**
  plastic induration of, 1082
  tumors of, **1072**
Pentagastrin, in carcinoid syndrome, 704
Pentalogy of Cantrell, 1305
  omphalocele and, 1340
Pentamidine, for lung abscess, 384
Pentostatin, for hairy cell leukemia, 663
Pentoxifylline, for peripheral arterial insuffi-
    ciency, 821
Pepsinogen, **535**
Peptic ulcer, **539**
  versus acute cholecystitis, 608
  versus colorectal cancer, 721
  hemorrhage from, **550–551**
  perforated, 539, **553–555**
    differential diagnosis of, 515
  pyloric obstruction in, **552–553**
  in transplant recipient, 1379
Peptide histidine isoleucine, in pancreatic
    cholera, 650
Peptococci, and lung abscess, 383
Peptostreptococci, and lung abscess, 383
Percocet. *See* Oxycodone, with acetaminophen
Percodan. *See* Oxycodone, with aspirin
Percussion, of acute abdomen, 509
Percutaneous balloon dilation, for aortic coarc-
    tation, 446
Percutaneous balloon valvotomy
  for aortic stenosis, 427
  for mitral stenosis, 421

Percutaneous carotid artery angiography, 851–852

Percutaneous nephrolithotomy, for renal stones, 1044

Percutaneous nephroscopy, for renal stones, 1044

Percutaneous nephrostomy, for renal stones, 1044

Percutaneous transhepatic cholangiography
in bile duct malignancies, 617–618
for biliary tree examination, **600**
in jaundice, 602

Percutaneous transluminal angioplasty (PTA)
for peripheral arterial insufficiency, 821
for renovascular hypertension, 855

Percutaneous transluminal coronary angioplasty (PTCA), comparison with other procedures, 415

Perforated viscus, physical findings in, 508t

Perforating injuries, ocular, **1008–1009**. See also Penetrating trauma

Perforating veins, 871, 872i
ligation of, for chronic venous insufficiency, 884

Perforation
in acute cholecystitis, **608–609**
appendicitis and, **670**
in diverticulitis, 733
of large intestine, in colorectal cancer, **723**

Pergolide, for Parkinson's disease, 948

Perianal (subcutaneous) space, 771i

Pericardial tamponade, cardiac compressive shock caused by, 206–207

Pericardiocentesis, 247

Pericardium
injuries of, **246–247**
lacerations of, 247

Pericholecystic abscess, **608–609**

Perichondritis, 970

Pericytoma, 1246

Peridiverticulitis, colonic, 731–732

Perihepatitis, gonococcal, *versus* acute cholecystitis, 608

Perimetry, 999

Perinephric abscess, **1039**

Perineum, in urethral injury, 1052

Perineurial fibroblastoma, 929. See also Nerve sheath tumors (schwannomas)

Perineurium, 913

Periodic peritonitis. See Familial Mediterranean fever

Periodontitis, acute, **985**

Periorbital skin, lacerations of, 1009

Peripheral arterial insufficiency, **815–825**, 815i
clinical findings in, 815–817
noninvasive vascular tests for, 818–819
prognosis for, 819–824, 820i
risk factors for, 815, 816i
reduction of, 820
treatment of, 819–824

Peripheral nerves
injury to, **913–914**
versus spinal cord injury, 910–912
ischemia and, 258

traumatic lesions of, **913–914**
tumors of, **929–930**

Peristalsis, 30, 474
gastrointestinal, postoperative, 19, 30
postoperative return of, and diet, 185
retrograde, 708
in small bowel obstruction, 684
of small intestine, 675, 676
in stomach, 534–535

Peristaltic waves, 474, 474i

Peritoneal adhesions, **529–530**

Peritoneal bands. See Ladd's bands

Peritoneal cavity, **517–532**

Peritoneal lavage
in acute pancreatitis, **633–634**
in acute secondary bacterial peritonitis, 520
diagnostic, in abdominal trauma, 250–251, 251i, 251t

Peritoneal mesothelioma, **530**

Peritoneal reflection, anterior, 705

Peritoneovenous shunting, for malignant ascites, 529

Peritoneum, 674
adhesions in, 92–93
disease and disorders of, **517–532**
drainage of, in acute secondary bacterial peritonitis, 520
functions of, **517**
tumors of, **530–531**

Peritonitis
and abdominal trauma, 252
in acute mesenteric vascular occlusion, 698–699
acute secondary bacterial, **517–521**
causative organisms, 518
clinical findings in, 518–519
complications of, 520–521
differential diagnosis of, 519
laboratory findings in, 518–519
prognosis for, 518t, 521
symptoms and signs of, 518
treatment of, 519–520
appendicitis and, **670**
in diverticulitis, 732
fungal, treatment of, 141
granulomatous, **528**
physical findings in, 508t
in pregnancy, 64
primary, **527**
secondary, 517
tuberculous, **527–528**
versus ureteral injury, 1050

Peritonsillar abscess, 988

Periurethral glands, in benign prostatic hyperplasia, 1033, 1034i

Periurethritis, **1078–1079**

Permit, operative, 11

Persistent left superior vena cava, **469**

Persistent sciatic artery aneurysm, **839**

Petit's triangle, hernia into, 794–795, 794i

Peutz-Jeghers syndrome, 702, **728**

Peyer's patches, 674

Peyronie's disease, **1082**, 1284

Pfeffer loop, 629, 630

P53 gene, and colorectal cancer, 717

pH
of arterial blood, 221t
conversion to hydrogen ion concentration, 224, 224t
esophageal, 473, 485–486, 486t
and hydrogen ion concentration [H$^+$], 150
and renal stones, 1042
of urine, 49

Phacoemulsification, for cataracts, 1005

Phagocytosis, 113

Phalanx
distal, cross-section of, 1283i
fractures of, **1149**, 1149i, **1278–1279**

Phalen's sign, 1280

Phantom limb pain, 867–868, 951–952

Pharyngitis, 46, **987–989**

Pharyngoesophageal (Zenker's) diverticulum, **480–481**, 481i

Pharyngoesophageal sphincter, 472, 473

Pharynx, **987–990**
benign neoplasms of, **989**
foreign bodies in, 492, **989–990**
and swallowing, 474

Phenothiazines
for heat stroke, 279
seizures and, 274

Phenoxybenzamine, for pheochromocytoma, 804

Phenylephrine
for craniocerebral trauma, 903
for eye examination, 999
for neurogenic shock, 209

Phenytoin
for craniocerebral trauma, 903
renal failure and, 51

Pheochromocytoma, **802–805**
as adrenal incidentaloma, 811–812, 812t
complications of, 804
differential diagnosis of, 804
hypertensive crisis with, 804
laboratory diagnosis of, 803, 803i
localization of, 803–804, 805
malignant, 802, 805
mediastinal, 376
medical therapy for, 804
pathology of, 802
in pregnancy, 804
prognosis for, 805
signs and symptoms of, 802–803
surgery for, 805
treatment of, 804–805

Phimosis, **1082**

Phlebitis, **36**
suppurative, **36,** 126

Phlebography
in chronic venous insufficiency, 884
in deep venous thrombosis, 876

Phleboliths, *versus* prostate cancer, 1069

Phlegmasia alba dolens, 876

Phlegmasia cerulea dolens, 876

Phlegmon, 114
pancreatic, 632

Phlegmonous tenosynovitis, of hand, 1283
Phocomelia, 1275
Phosphate. *See also* Hyperphosphatemia; Hy-
    pophosphatemia
    absorption of, in small intestine, 678
    in acute mesenteric vascular occlusion, 699
Phospholipase A, 626
    in pancreatitis, 629
Phosphorus
    balance, **149–150**
    requirements for, 164*t*
Photocoagulation
    for large bowel obstruction, 714
    panretinal, **1012**
Photodynamic therapy
    for colorectal cancer, 722
    for lung cancer, 402
    for macular degeneration, **1012**
Physial injuries, **1177–1179**
    Salter-Harris classification of, 1177–1178,
        1178*i*
Physical examination
    in acute abdomen, 508–510, 508*t*
    of anal fissure, 769
    in anesthetic risk evaluation, 192
    of arterial injuries, 259
    of body orifices, 4
    of diabetic patient, 38
    elective, 3–4
    emergency, 4
    in heart disease, 42
    in nutritional assessment, 156, 157*t*
    of pelvic injury, 1126
    preoperative, 7
    of rectal prolapse, 764
    of spinal deformity, 1185
    in surgical infection, 115
    of surgical patient, 3–4
Physical therapy, for peripheral nerve injury,
    914
Physician-patient relationship
    contract basis of, 74–75
    intentional formation of, 77
    termination of, 74–75
Phytobezoars, 562
Pickwickian syndrome, 988–989
Pierre Robin syndrome, 1258, **1307**
Pigeon toe, **1183**
Pigment gallstones, **604**
    hereditary spherocytosis and, 656
Pilocytic astrocytomas, 917
Pilonidal disease, 772, **774–775**
Pinch biopsy, in head and neck tumors, 283
Pineal region, tumors in, 915*i*, 916*i*, **923**, 925
Pinna. *See also* Auricle
    tumors of, 972
Pinworm, 775–776
Piperacillin. *See also* Penicillin, an-
    tipseudomonal
    dosage of
        in hepatic failure, 138*t*
        in renal failure, 138*t*
    pharmacology of, 138*t*
Piriform sinus, cancer of, 289

Piroff's amputation, 863
Pitting, in spleen, 652
Pituitary gland
    adenomas of, 921
    region of, tumors in, 915*i*, 916*i*
    surgery of, **888–961**
    tumors of, **921, 930–931**
Pituitary hormones, in response to injury, 105
Pituitary insufficiency, in surgical patient, 41
Pit vipers, 130, 132
Plague, drug therapy for, 135*t*
Plain films
    abdominal
        in acute abdomen, 510*t*, 511–512
        in acute appendicitis, 669
        in acute cholecystitis, 608
        in acute mesenteric vascular occlusion,
            699
        in acute pancreatitis, 632
        for biliary tree examination, **599–600**
        in cecal volvulus, 739
        in choledocholithiasis, 614
        in diverticulitis, 732
        in emphysematous cholecystitis, 611
        in gallstone ileus, 611
        in large intestine examination, 711
        in sigmoid volvulus, 739
        for small bowel obstruction, 684–685,
            686*i*
        for splenic abscesses, 664
        in ulcerative colitis, 742
    for arterial injuries, 259
    chest, in acute abdomen, 511
    for infrarenal abdominal aortic aneurysms,
        831
    in neurodiagnosis, **892**
    skull, 892
    spinal, 892
        in cervical disk syndrome, 954
        in closed disk space infections, 960
        in lumbar disk syndrome, 956–957
        in spinal cord tumors, 928
Plaintiff, definition of, 72
Plant alkaloids, anticancer therapy with, 1355
Plantar keratoses (callosities), **1216**
Plasma
    electrolyte composition of, 142, 143*i*
    fresh frozen, indications for, 57, 59, 62
    sodium concentration (P_{Na}) in, 143
    for transfusion therapy, 62
Plasmacytoma, solitary, of chest wall, 355
Plasmapheresis
    for secondary hemolytic anemia, 658
    for thrombotic thrombocytopenic purpura,
        661
Plasma proteins, for burn patients, 271
Plasminogen factor, and adhesions, 93
Plastic and reconstructive surgery, **1230–1269**
    advances in, 1230
    aesthetic, **1264–1269**
    for basal cell carcinoma removal, 1251
    for burn patients, 276
    for contractures, 1244
    for craniofacial anomalies, **1259**

    for facial bone fractures, **1254–1257**
    fetal, 1230
    flaps for, 1234–1237
    grafts for, 1231–1234
    of head and neck, for congenital anomalies,
        1257–1260
    for hypertrophic scars, 1243–1244
    for keloids, 1243–1244
    for mandibular fractures, **1256**
    for maxillary fractures, **1257**
    for nasal fractures, **1255–1256**
    for orbital fractures, **1256–1257**
    for pressure sores, 1263–1264
    principles of, 1230
    for scarring, 1243–1269
    for skin tumors, 1244–1252
    for soft tissue injury, **1252–1254**
    tissue coverage in, selection of, 1238–1239,
        1239*t*
    wound care in, principles of, 1237–1243
    for zygomatic fractures, **1256–1257**
Platelet count, 52, 53, 61
    in idiopathic myelofibrosis, 663
    in immune thrombocytopenic purpura,
        659
    in Wiskott-Aldrich syndrome, 661
Platelets
    after splenectomy, 666
    defects of, 53
        qualitative, in surgical patients, 55–56
    disorders of, in surgical patients, **55–56**
    substitutes for, 62
    transfusion of, 61
        indications for, 56, 58, 59
Pleomorphic adenoma, 294
Plethysmography, 818
    in chronic venous insufficiency, 883–884
    in deep venous thrombosis, 876
Pleura
    anatomy of, **344**, 345*i*
    biopsy of, **350–351**
    diseases of, **356–371**
    physiology of, **344–346**
Pleural effusion, **357–367**, 358*t*
    and cardiovascular disease, 359–360, 360*i*
    and cirrhosis, 360
    differential diagnosis of, 358*t*
    and malignancy, 335, 357–359, 359*i*
    pancreatic, **639–640**
    and pancreatitis, 360
    postoperative, **27**
    and renal disease, 360
    and thromboembolism, 360
Pleural irrigation, for accidental hypothermia,
    281
Pleural pain, 356
Pleural space, 344
    fluid formation and reabsorption in,
        344–346, 346*i*
    injuries of, **245–246**
    physiology of, **344–346**
    pressure in, 344
Pleural tumors
    diffuse malignant, **369–371**

localized fibrous, **369**
primary, **369–371**
Pleurectomy
for malignant pleural effusion, 359
parietal, for pneumothorax prevention, 369
Pleurodesis, for pneumothorax, 368–369
Pleuroperitoneal hernia, **501,** 501*i*
Plicae circulares, 674, 675*i*
Plicamycin, 1355
for hypercalcemic crisis, 313
indications for, 149
Plombage therapy, for tuberculosis, 389
Plummer's disease, 300. *See also* Hyperthy-
roidism
PMN chemotactic activity, in burn patients,
270
Pneumatic antishock garment, 206
Pneumatosis, fulminant, 701
Pneumatosis coli, **701**
Pneumatosis cystoides intestinalis, **701**
Pneumaturia, in colovesical fistula, 735
Pneumocystis carinii, 394
and lung abscess, 383
Pneumocystosis, **394**
Pneumonectomy
empyemas following, 362–366, 365*i*, 366*i*
for lung cancer, 402
Pneumonia, 46–47, **213**
aspiration, 26
bacterial, in renal transplant recipient, 1379
and bronchiectasis, 385
chronic, and lung abscess, 383
and coccidioidomycosis, 391
differential diagnosis of, 358*t*
host defenses against, 27
inhalation injury and, 275
and middle lobe syndrome, 386
necrotizing, and lung abscess, 383
postoperative, 26, **26–27**
clinical manifestations of, 27
mortality rate for, 26, 27
prevention of, 27
risk factors for, 26
treatment of, 27
Pneumonitis, and hepatic abscess, 593
Pneumoperitoneum, for laparoscopic surgery,
46
Pneumoretinopexy, for retinal detachment, 1006
Pneumothorax, 245–246, **367–369,** 367*i*
open, 237, 347, 367
postoperative, **27**
spontaneous, 367–368, 367*i*
tension, 236–237, 237*i*, 244, 246, 367
Pointed objects, ingestion of, **492**
Poland's syndrome, 1260
pectus carinatum in, 1306
pectus excavatum with, 1305
Polidocanol, for bleeding peptic ulcers, 551
Poliomyelitis, 1186
Politano-Leadbetter procedure, for vesi-
coureteral reflux, 1026
Polyalveolar lobe, in lobar emphysema, 1310
Polyarteritis nodosa, and vasculitis, 700
Polyarthralgia, 1221

Polycystic kidney disease, **1019–1020,** 1020*i*
kidney transplantation for, 1372
Polycythemia vera, 53–54
Polydactyly, 1260, 1275
Polyethylene glycol
in preoperative bowel preparation, 754
for small bowel obstruction, 687
Polyethylene glycol-electrolyte solution, indications for, 31
Polymenorrhea, 1088
Polymorphonuclear leukocytes, 107
Polyneuropathy, as paraneoplastic syndrome,
1371
Polyp(s)
adenomatous, 560
cervical, 1107
colonic, **725–728,** 725*t*
in children, 1332
juvenile, 1332
endometrial, 1088, 1089
esophageal, 494
of gallbladder, 619
gastric, **559–560**
hyperplastic, 559
of large intestine, 725
inflammatory
of esophagus, 494
of large intestine, 725
in ulcerative colitis, 741
juvenile (retention), 702
nasal, in allergic rhinitis, 978, 979
rectal, **725–728,** 725*t*
of small intestine, 702
in ulcerative colitis, 741
ureteral, 1061
Polypectomy, 726
for large bowel polyps, 727
Polypoid adenoma, of large intestine, 725
Polypoid carcinoma, 557
Polyposis (polyposis coli)
familial adenomatous, 702, **727–728,** 727*t*
cancer screening in, 719
large bowel cancer and, 726
generalized juvenile gastrointestinal, 728
juvenile, 728
Polysomnography, for obstructive sleep apnea,
989
Polysplenia, 468
Polytetrafluoroethylene (PTFE), 823
Popliteal artery
aneurysm of, 830*i*, **839**
cystic degeneration of, **829**
injuries to, 257
Popliteal artery entrapment syndrome, 262,
828–829
Popliteal vein, injuries of, 262
Porcine heart valves, 428, 428*i*
Porcine xenografts, 272
Porphyria
abdominal findings in, 53
acute intermittent, 53
variegate, 53
Portacaval shunt
in ascites, 590

emergency, for variceal bleeding, 582–583
end-to-side, 586, 586*i*
for nonbleeding varices, 585–587
selection of, 587
side-to-side, 586, 586*i*
in Budd-Chiari syndrome, 589
types of, 586–587, 586*i*
Porta hepatis, 565
Portal circulation, 565, 567*i*
collaterals in, in portal hypertension, 579
Portal decompression, for hypersplenism, 654
Portal hypertension, **578–580,** 587, 588, 589
collateral channels in, 579
etiology of, 578, 578*t*
pathophysiology of, 578–579
portal flow and pressure measurements in,
578–579, 584
Portal pressure, measurement of, 578–579,
584
Portal vein, 597*i*, 626*i*
anatomy of, 565, 567*i*
angiography of, 584
extrahepatic occlusion of, **588**
flow in, assessment of, 578–579, 584
preduodenal, 1316
thrombosis
after splenectomy, 666
idiopathic, **588**
and liver transplantation, 1384
Portal venous sampling, transhepatic, for insulinoma, 649
Portal venous system, suppurative thrombophlebitis of, appendicitis and,
670–671
Portasystemic shunts
central splenorenal, 586, 586*i*
distal splenorenal (Warren), 586–587, 586*i*,
588, 592
end-to-side, 586, 586*i*
Inokuchi, 587
mesocaval, 586, 586*i*, 589
for nonbleeding varices, 585–587
results with, 587
selection of, 587
selective, 586–587, 586*i*
side-to-side, 586, 586*i*
total, 586, 586*i*
types of, 586–587, 586*i*
Portography, CT or MRI, with metastatic neoplasms of liver, 574–575
Port wine stain, 1246, 1247*t,* **1248,** 1342
Positional testing, in benign paroxysmal positional vertigo, 976
Positioning of patient
improper, nerve injuries caused by, 195
intraoperative, **195**
postoperative, 15
Positive end-expiratory pressure
in mechanical ventilation, 216
physiologic, 216
Positive-pressure ventilation, adverse cardiac effects of, 206–207
Positron emission tomography (PET)
for lung cancer, 398

Positron emission tomography (PET) (cont.)
in neurodiagnosis, 897
in pulmonary disorders, 352
Postanesthesia care, 14
Postanesthesia care unit (PACU), **199**
Postanesthetic observation, 6
Postcholecystectomy syndrome, **615–616,** 622
Posterior arch vein, 872i
Posterior communicating artery, aneurysm of,
939
Posterior cruciate ligament, injury to, 1164
Posterior fossa, tumors in, **923,** 924
Postmenopausal women
breast cancer in, treatment of, 332, 332t,
334
breast mass evaluation in, 325, 326i
Postoperative care, 6, **14–22**
anesthesia-related, 199–200
for diabetic patient, 40
and wound healing, 97–98
Postoperative orders, 14
Postoperative pain, **19–21, 950–951**
factors affecting, 19
management of, 20–21, **200**
physician-patient communication and, 20
physiology of, 19
and postoperative complications, 20
Postoperative pancreatitis, **628–629**
Posttraumatic sympathetic dystrophy. See Reflex sympathetic dystrophy
Postural drainage, for bronchiectasis, 385
Postural hypotension. See Hypotension
Postural stimulation test, in hyperaldosteronism, 800
Postural therapy, for superior mesenteric artery
obstruction of duodenum, 564
Potassium
absorption of
in large intestine, 709, 709t
in small intestine, 678
administration of
for newborn, 1296
postoperative, 18
balance, 144t, **146–148,** 152–153
in response to injury, 107
deficiency of, 146–147
dosage and administration of, 148
excretion of, 148
loss of
in gastrointestinal fluid, 147t
with ileostomy, 751
metabolism of, factors affecting, 146
serum levels of, 146 (See also Hyperkalemia;
Hypokalemia)
and fluid therapy, 153
and total body potassium stores, 146,
146i, 153–154
for small bowel obstruction, 687
total body, 159t
Potassium chloride, indications for, 153
Pott's anastomosis, 458, 459i
Pott's disease, **960–961**
Pouchitis, 751
Pramipexole, for Parkinson's disease, 948

Prazosin, for pheochromocytoma, 804
Prealbumin, serum levels of, 157t, 158, 159t
Preauricular cysts, 973
Preauricular lesions, 1301
Preauricular sinus tracts, 973
Prednisolone, for ulcerative colitis, 744
Prednisone
for aphthous stomatitis, 985
for breast cancer, 332
for Crohn's disease, 692
for immune thrombocytopenic purpura, 660
for retroperitoneal fibrosis, 531–532
for sensorineural hearing loss, 969
for transplant recipient, **1375,** 1385
Pregnancy
appendicitis in, 63–64, 514, 669
breast cancer and, 65–66, **328–329,** 337
cholecystectomy in, 64–65
cholecystitis in, 64–65
cholelithiasis in, 64–65
ectopic, 63, **1102–1103**
signs and symptoms of, 1102
treatment of, 1103
hepatic rupture in, 571
hernia in, 65
heterotopic, 1102
intestinal obstruction in, 65
laparoscopic surgery in, 63–65
loss, recurrent, uterine anomalies and, 1086
medication management in, 63
molar, 1112–1115
outcome of, uterine anomalies and, 1086
ovarian torsion in, 66–67
ovarian tumors in, 66–67
peritonitis in, 64
pheochromocytoma in, 804
radiological examination in, 63
in surgical patient, **62–67**
tubal, 1087, 1102
ultrasonography in, 64
vaginal bleeding in, with gestational
trophoblastic disease, 1113
volvulus in, 738
Prehn's sign, 1040
Prehospital trauma care, 232
Premature infant
antibiotic dosage in, 137
electrolyte requirements in, 1296
intensive care for, 1293
necrotizing enterocolitis in, **1331**
problems of, 1293
temperature regulation in, 1294
Premedication, **194,** 201
Premenopausal women
breast cancer in, treatment of, 331t, 332,
334
breast mass evaluation in, 325–326, 325i
nipple discharge in, 342
Preoperative care, **6–13.** See also Preoperative
evaluation; Preoperative preparation
for anesthesia, 194–195
for diabetic patient, 38
Preoperative evaluation, **6–13.** See also Preoperative preparation

for anesthetic risk, 191–193
for cardiovascular disease, 42
definition of, 6
of elderly, 9–10
of hemostasis, 52
for hepatic resection, 567–568
of pulmonary function, 47–48
Preoperative note, 10
Preoperative preparation, **10–13.** See also Pre-
operative evaluation
definition of, 6
Prepyloric ulcer, 546–547
Prerenal azotemia, 49, 51
Presacral neurectomy, 1090
Presbycusis, 968
Pressure, for scar treatment, 1243
Pressure sores. See also Decubitus ulcers
in elderly, 70
plastic surgery for, 1263–1264
prevention of, 1263
Pressure-volume relationships, ventricular, 409,
410i
Priapism, **1082**
Prima facie case, 72
Primitive neuroectodermal tumors, 935–936
Primordial tests, and atherosclerosis, 813
Pringle's maneuver, 570
for hepatic hemorrhage, 252
Privacy, invasion of, 76
Probenecid
for gonococcal proctitis, 776
for gout, 1286
Procainamide
for atrial dysrhythmias, 437
for ventricular arrhythmias, 437
Procaine penicillin G, for gonococcal proctitis,
776
Procarbazine, 1355
Processus vaginalis, 1336, 1336i
Proctalgia fugax, 763
Proctitis, **776–778**
chlamydial, 777
gonococcal, **776–777**
herpes, **776**
inflammatory, **778**
radiation, **778**
Proctocolectomy
for Crohn's disease, 748
sexual consequences of, 752
for ulcerative colitis, 745, 746
Proctosigmoidoscopy, 711, 769, 777
for acute abdomen, 513
in colorectal cancer, **720**
in Crohn's disease, 746
Progesterone
anticancer therapy with, **1356**
serum levels, in ectopic pregnancy, 1103
Progesterone receptors, breast cancer and, 329
Progestins
for endometrial cancer, 1109
in endometrial cancer prevention, 1109
for endometrial sarcoma, 1110
for endometriosis, 1098–1099
indications for, 1089

in subdermal implant contraception, 1091
Prognostic nutrition indicator (PNI), 160
Proinsulin, in insulinoma, 649
Prolactin. *See also* Hyperprolactinemia
    pituitary adenoma secreting, 930, 931
Prolactinomas, 921
Proliferative diabetic retinopathy, panretinal
    photocoagulation for, **1012**
Prolyl hydroxylase, 89
Pronator syndrome, 1280
Proparacaine, for eye examination, 999
Propofol, for intracranial hypertension,
    905–906
Propoxyphene, for postoperative analgesia,
    21
Propranolol
    for angina pectoris, 412
    for hypertrophic obstructive cardiomyopa-
        thy, 444
    for nonbleeding varices, 584–585
Proptosis, 1001
Propylthiouracil, 40
    for hyperthyroidism, 301
Prostaglandin(s) (PG)
    for peripheral arterial insufficiency, 821
    PGE₁
        for aortic coarctation, 446
        for pulmonary stenosis, 441
    PGE₂, 106–107, 108
Prostaglandin inhibitors, for patent ductus ar-
    teriosus, 453
Prostatectomy
    for benign prostatic hyperplasia, 1035
    for prostate cancer, 1069
Prostate gland
    anatomy of, **1017**
    benign hyperplasia of, **1033**, 1034*i*
        and prostate cancer, 1066, 1069
    calculi of, *versus* prostate cancer, 1069
    cancer of, **1066–1069**, 1067*i*, 1067*t*
        versus benign prostatic hyperplasia, 1034
        paraneoplastic syndromes with, 1371*t*
    embryology of, **1013**
    fibrosis of, *versus* prostate cancer, 1069
    sarcoma of, **1070**
Prostate-specific antigen
    in benign prostatic hyperplasia, 1034
    in prostate cancer, **1066–1067**
Prostatic hyperplasia, 786
Prostatic hypertrophy, 33
Prostatic urethra, 1017
Prostatitis, **1039–1040**
    acute
        bacterial, **1039–1040**
        versus benign prostatic hyperplasia, 1034
    chronic, **1040**
Prostheses, **869–870**
    penile, 1084
    upper extremity, 866
Prosthetic heart valves, **428–430**
    antibiotic prophylaxis with, 45
    biologic, **428**, 428*i*, 429*i*
    mechanical, **428–429**, 429*i*
Protamine sulfate, 54

Protease inhibitors, for postoperative bleeding,
    436
Protein
    deficiency of, and pancreatitis, **628**
    dietary, restriction of, in hepatic en-
        cephalopathy, 592
    digestion of, in small intestine, **678**
    quality of, 161
    requirements for, in burn patient, 186, 186*t*
    serum, in jaundice, 602
    sources of, in nutritional support, 161–162
Protein reserve(s)
    somatic (skeletal), 157
    visceral, 158
Proteinuria, 49
    nephrotic range, 50
Proteoglycans, in wound healing, 87*i*, 88–89
Proteus infection
    and cholangitis, 612
    and peritonitis, 518
    and retroperitoneal abscesses, 526
    and thoracic empyema, 361
Proteus mirabilis infection, drug therapy for,
    135*t*
Proteus vulgaris infection, drug therapy for,
    135*t*
Prothrombin time (PT), 52
    abnormal, fresh frozen plasma for, 62
    in liver disease, 57
    prolonged, 58
Proton pump blockers, for duodenal ulcer, 541
Proto-oncogenes, and lung cancer, 396
Providencia infection, drug therapy for, 135*t*
Prune belly syndrome, **1027**
    omphalocele and, 1340
Pruritus
    in choledocholithiasis, 614
    in jaundice, 601
Pruritus ani, **775–776**
Pseudoaneurysm, 829
Pseudobronchiectasis, 385
Pseudocyst, pancreatic, 632, **635–638**
Pseudohypoparathyroidism, **318**
Pseudolymphoma, gastric, **560**
Pseudomembranous colitis, 749
Pseudomonas aeruginosa infection
    and burn infections, 274*t*
    and corneal ulcers, 1003
    drug therapy for, 135*t*
Pseudomonas infection, 112
    and bronchiectasis, 385
    in cholangitis, 612
    and lung abscess, 383
    and thoracic empyema, 361
Pseudomyxoma peritonei, **530**
Pseudo-obstruction
    of colon, *versus* large bowel obstruction, **714**
    of small intestine, **686**
Pseudopolyps, in ulcerative colitis, 741
Pseudopseudohypoparathyroidism, **318**
Pseudotumor
    of gallbladder, **619**
    in ischemic colitis, 750
    of spleen, 664

Pseudotumor cerebri, 891
Psittacosis, 112
Psoas abscess, 526
Psychiatric consultation, 3
Psychogenic impotence, **1083**, 1084
Psychoneuroimmunologic system, 106–107
Psychosis, postoperative, **34–35**
Pterygium, **1004**
Pterygoid muscles, cancer of, 282
Puborectalis muscle, 756–757, 759, 762
Pudendal artery, 872*i*
    injury to, in urethral injury, 1051–1052
    internal, 705–706
Pudendal nerve
    injury to, 760
        and fecal incontinence, 759
    latency studies, 764
        in fecal incontinence, 760
Pudendal vein, 872*i*
Puestow procedure, for chronic pancreatitis,
    641–642, 641*i*
Pulmonary agenesis, 380
Pulmonary aplasia, 380
Pulmonary arterial banding, 449
Pulmonary arterial blood flow
    congenital heart lesions decreasing, **458–468**
    congenital heart lesions increasing, **449–458**
Pulmonary arterial pressure
    diastolic, 220
    mean, 220, 221*t*
    systolic, 220
Pulmonary arterial wedge pressure, 220
    mean, 221*t*
Pulmonary arteriovenous fistula, **469**
Pulmonary artery(ies), 348
    anomalies of, **1311**
Pulmonary artery band, 465
Pulmonary artery catheter, **220**
Pulmonary aspiration. *See* Aspiration
Pulmonary atresia
    with intact ventricular septum, **462**
    and tetralogy of Fallot, 460–461, 460*i*
Pulmonary care, postoperative, 17, 18
Pulmonary complications, postoperative, pre-
    vention of, 23
Pulmonary contusion, **213**, 246
Pulmonary edema
    in acute respiratory distress syndrome, 212
    with burns, 275
    cardiogenic, **213–214**
    in elderly, 69
    hemorrhagic, in increased intracranial pres-
        sure, 890
    neurogenic, **214**
    postoperative, 17, 29
Pulmonary embolism, **213**, **880–882**
    with burns, 275
    differential diagnosis of, 358*t*
    risk factors for, 9
    in spinal cord-injured patient, 1120
Pulmonary failure
    acute, **212–214**
    adjuvant treatment of, **219**
    case examples of, 225–228

Pulmonary failure (*cont.*)
    evaluation of, **220–225**
    mechanical, **212–213**
    in surgical patients, causes of, 212–214
Pulmonary fibrosis
    and operative risk, 25
    preoperative management of, 47
Pulmonary function testing, 47–48
    preoperative, 8
Pulmonary infarction, 42
    with pulmonary thromboembolism, 880
Pulmonary sequestration, **381, 1313–1314**
Pulmonary stenosis, **440–442,** 441*i*
    and tetralogy of Fallot, 460, 460*i*
Pulmonary thromboembolism, **880–882**
    postoperative, 877
Pulmonary trauma, prehospital care for, 232
Pulsatile tinnitus, 971
Pulsion diverticula, 562
Pulsus paradoxus, 207
Punch biopsy, in head and neck tumors, 283
Punch tenderness, abdominal, 509–510
Pupillary reflex
    assessment of, **1000**
    in craniocerebral trauma, 902
Purified protein derivative (PPD) test, 349, 388
Purine nucleoside analogs, for hairy cell
        leukemia, 663
Purpura
    Henoch-Schönlein, 53
    idiopathic thrombocytopenic, **659–660**
    immune thrombocytopenic, **659–660**
    nonthrombocytopenic, 53
    thrombotic thrombocytopenic, 55, 62
Pyelography, in renal pelvis and calices tumors,
        1060, 1060*i*
Pyelolithotomy, for renal stones, 1045
Pyelonephritis
    acute, **1037–1038**
    chronic, **1038**
        kidney transplantation for, 1372
    emphysematous, **1038**
    postoperative, 33–34
    versus renal stones, 1043
    in renal transplant recipient, 1379
    versus ureteral calculi, 1046
    vesicoureteral reflux and, 1024, 1025
    xanthogranulomatous, **1038**
Pyelophlebitis, appendicitis and, **670–671**
Pyloric gland, 533
Pyloric obstruction, with peptic ulcer,
        552–553
Pyloric stenosis, hypertrophic, **1315–1316,**
        1315*i*
Pyloromyotomy, for pyloric stenosis, 1316
Pyloroplasty
    for duodenal ulcer, 541, 542*i*
    for gastric ulcer, 547
    for perforated peptic ulcer, 554
    for stress ulcers, 556
Pylorus, 533
Pyoderma gangrenosum, 96
Pyogenic cholangitis, recurrent (Oriental
        cholangiohepatitis), **623**

Pyogenic granuloma, of hand, **1282,** 1288
Pyogenic infections, 960
Pyogenic lymphadenitis, in pediatric patients,
        1303–1304
Pyogenic tenosynovitis, of hand, 1283, 1283*i*
Pyopneumothorax, 367
Pyospermia, in male infertility, 1081
Pyothorax, 357, **360–366,** 360*i,* 361*i,* 362*t*
Pyrazinamide
    indications for, 136*t,* 141
    for tuberculosis, 388*t*
        of spine, 961
Pyridoxine. *See* Vitamin B$_6$
Pyruvate, metabolism of, 166, 166*i*
Pyruvate carboxylase, 164
Pyruvate kinase deficiency, **657**
Pyuria
    in epididymitis, 1040
    in genitourinary tuberculosis, 1040, 1041

Quadriceps tendon, tear of, **1161**
Quinacrine, for malignant pleural effusion, 359
Quinsy, 988

Rabies, **128**
Raccoon eyes, 1343
Radial artery false aneurysms, **842**
Radial bursa, 1272
Radial nerve, 1272, 1274*i*
    compression of, 1280
    injury to, 1281
        improper positioning and, 195
Radial tunnel syndrome, 1280
Radiation dermatitis, **1249**
    chronic, 1249
Radiation enteropathy, **695**
Radiation proctitis, **778**
Radiation therapy, **1359–1361**
    adjuvant, 296
    adverse effects of, 296
    for basal cell carcinoma, 1251
    for bladder tumors, **1065**
    for bone tumors, 1223
    for brain tumors, **925–926**
    for breast cancer, 333
    for cervical cancer, 1107, 1108
    chemotherapy with, 297
    in children, 935
    for colorectal cancer, **723**
    complications of, 1361
    definitive, 1360
    delivery of, 1360–1361
    dose fractionation in, 1359–1360
    for endometrial cancer, 1109
    for esophageal carcinoma, 498, 499
    external beam, for epidermoid carcinoma of
        anal canal, 781
    for head and neck tumors, **295–296**
    for Hodgkin's lymphoma, 1366–1367
    for hypopharyngeal cancer, 290
    intraoperative, 1360
    for laryngeal cancer, 291
    localized, 1360
    for lung cancer, 398–401, 402

    for melanoma, 1365
    for nasal cavity cancer, 293
    for non-Hodgkin's lymphoma, 1368
    for oral cavity cancer, 287
    for oropharyngeal cancer, 289
    palliative, 296
    principles of, 1359–1360
    for prostate cancer, 1069
    for renal adenocarcinoma, 1057
    for salivary gland cancer, 295
    for sarcomas, 1362
    for spinal cord tumors, 928
    for superior vena caval syndrome, 374
    systemic, 1360–1361
    for testicular cancer, 1072
    urinary tract fistulas caused by, 1093–1094
    and wound healing, 9
Radioactive colloidal gold and chromium phos-
        phate, for malignant pleural effusion,
        359
Radioactive iodine (RAI), in thyroid evalua-
        tion, 298–300
Radioactive seed placement, for prostate can-
        cer, 1069
Radiofrequency ablation
    of metastatic neoplasms of liver, 575
    in primary hepatic cancer, 574
Radiography. *See* Plain films; X-rays
Radioimmunoscintigraphy, in colorectal can-
        cer, 720
Radioimmunotherapy, 1360–1361
Radioiodine (^{131}I), for hyperthyroidism,
        301–302
Radionuclide scan. *See also* Scintigraphy
    for acute abdomen, 513
    in acute cholecystitis, 608
    for biliary tree examination, **600–601**
    in infection, 117
    for intraperitoneal abscess, 524
    in lower gastrointestinal bleeding, 736, 737*i*
    in neurodiagnosis, **897**
    in obstructive uropathy, **1031**
    in renal adenocarcinoma, **1055**
    for spermatic cord torsion, 1079
    in ulcerative colitis, 742
    voiding studies, in vesicoureteral reflux,
        1025
Radiosurgery
    for arteriovenous malformations, 946–947
    for brain tumors, 925–926
    for trigeminal neuralgia, 951
Radioulnar joint, distal, 1143
    dislocation of, 1146
Radius
    distal, 1143
        fractures of, 1144–1146, 1144*i,* 1145*i,*
        1279
    fractures of, **1279**
    head of, subluxation of, in children, 1180
    proximal, fractures of, **1138–1139,** 1138*i*
    shaft of, 1143
        fractures of, **1141**
Radon, and lung cancer, 395
Ramsay Hunt's syndrome, in AIDS, 998

Rancho Los Amigos Cognitive Functioning Scale, 907
Ranitidine
  for duodenal ulcer, 541
  for reflux esophagitis sliding hiatal hernia, 486
  for Zollinger-Ellison syndrome, 545–546
Ranson's criteria, in acute pancreatitis, 633*i*
Ranula, **986**
Rash, in breast cancer, 319
Rastelli procedure, 465–466
Ray, amputation of, **862,** 862*i*
Raynaud's disease, esophageal manifestations in, 480
Raynaud's syndrome, 843
Reactive hyperemia, in peripheral arterial insufficiency, 817
Rebleeding
  of peptic ulcers, 551
  in upper gastrointestinal hemorrhage, 550
Receptive relaxation, 534–535
Recklinghausen's disease, 1361
  and pheochromocytoma, 802
  and spinal cord tumors, 927
Recombinant glucocerebrosidase enzyme, for Gaucher's disease, 661
Recombinant tissue plasminogen activator
  for axillary-subclavian venous thrombosis, 878*i*, 879
  for deep venous thrombosis, 877
  for pulmonary thromboembolism, 881
Reconstructive surgery, **1230–1269.** *See also* Plastic and reconstructive surgery
  of breast, **1261–1262**
  for head and neck, 1260–1261
  for head and neck tumors, **295–296**
  lower extremity, **1262–1263**
  postablative, **1260–1262**
  venous, for chronic venous insufficiency, 884
Recovery
  convalescent phase of, 14, 15
  immediate postoperative period of, 14–15
  intermediate postoperative period of, 15
Rectal bleeding, **736–737,** 737*i*
  cancer and, 719
  in large bowel polyps, 726
  in ulcerative colitis, 741
Rectal examination, in acute abdomen, 510
Rectal mucosectomy, for ulcerative colitis, 745
Rectal pain, 777
Rectal procidentia, 762
Rectal prolapse, **764–766,** 767
  incontinence associated with, 760
Rectal ulcer, 767
  solitary, 762
Rectal valves of Houston, 705
Rectoanal inhibitory reflex, 758
Rectocele, 1093
Rectopexy, 764
Rectosigmoid, 706*i*
Rectosigmoid junction, 756, 757*i*
Rectovaginal fistula, **773–774, 1094**
Rectovesical fascia of Denonvilliers, 705

Rectum. *See also* Abnormal rectal fixation; Anorectum
  anatomy of, 705, 706*i*
  bleeding from, history-taking about, 2
  cancer of, 716–724, 716*i,* **719, 721–723**
    in ulcerative colitis, 743–744
  congenital anomalies of, **1324–1327,** 1325*i,* 1326*i*
  digital examination of, 762, 764
  diseases of, **712–750**
  duplication of, 1328–1329, 1329*i*
  hemorrhage from (*See* Rectal bleeding)
  innervation of, 757
  polyps of, **725–728,** 725*t*
  resection of, for cancer, 721–722
  tumors of, **729**
Rectus abdominis muscle, 783
Rectus abdominis muscle flap, **1236**
  for lower extremity, 1262
Rectus femoris flap, **1236**
Rectus sheath, hematoma of, **796**
Recurrent pyogenic cholangitis (Oriental cholangiohepatitis), 621, **623**
Red-backed spider, 133
Red blood cells
  packed, for transfusion therapy, 60–61
  substitutes for, 62
Red cell count
  after splenectomy, 666
  in hereditary spherocytosis, 656
Redness, of eyes, **1001,** 1001*t*
Red pulp, of spleen, 652
5α-Reductase inhibitors, for benign prostatic hyperplasia, 1035
Reduction mammoplasty, **1267**
Reduction of joint or fracture, 1116
  closed (nonsurgical), 1116
  open (surgical), 1116
Reduplications, of esophagus, 495
Reed-Sternberg cell, 1365, 1367
Refeeding syndrome, 181
Referral, legal definition of, 75
Referred pain, 503, 505*i*
Reflexes, assessments of, in craniocerebral trauma, **902**
Reflex sympathetic dystrophy, **844**
Reflux
  duodenal, in pathogenesis of pancreatitis, 630
  gastroesophageal, in chronic laryngitis, 995
  venous, in chronic venous insufficiency, 883, 884
  vesicoureteral, **1023–1026,** 1023*i,* 1024*i,* 1025*i*
Reflux esophagitis sliding hiatal hernia, **484–488,** 484*i,* 487*i,* 488*i*
Refractive error, correction of, LASIK surgery for, **1012**
Regeneration, after peripheral nerve injury, 914
Regional anesthesia
  intraoperative management of, **198–199**
  shock caused by, 209
Regional enteritis, **689–692.** *See also* Crohn's disease (CD)

Rehabilitation
  after amputation, **869**
  for burn patients, 276
Reid sleeves, for lymphedema, 886
Rejection
  of heart transplant, 470, 1381
  of kidney transplant, **1379–1380**
  of liver transplant, 1385–1386
Relapsing fever, drug therapy for, 136*t*
Renal abscess, **1038–1039**
Renal adenocarcinoma, **1054–1058,** 1056*i,* 1057*i,* 1058*t*
  versus renal stones, 1043
Renal adenoma, **1059**
Renal agenesis, 1019
Renal anomalies, **1019–1021**
Renal artery
  aneurysm of, **842,** 1020, **1076–1077,** 1077*i*
  occlusion of, **1077**
  stenosis of, in transplant recipient, 1379
Renal calices
  anatomy of, **1015**
  changes in, in obstructive uropathy, **1030**
  tumors of, **1059–1061**
    versus renal stones, 1043
Renal cell carcinoma, **1054–1058,** 1056*i,* 1057*i,* 1058*t*
Renal cysts, simple, **1020, 1076**
Renal failure
  acute, 50
    causes of, 50
    definition of, 50
    diagnosis of, 50–51
    oliguric *versus* nonoliguric, 50, 51
    treatment of, 50–51
  antibiotic dosage in, 137, 138*t*–139*t*
  chronic, 50
  in diffuse necrotizing infection, 125
  and drug therapy, 51
  in hemolytic transfusion reaction, 59–60
  in hyperaldosteronism, 800
  hyperkalemia in, 146
  and hypermagnesemia, 149
  kidney transplantation for, 1372
  nitrogen balance in, 187, 187*t*
  nonoliguric, peripheral parenteral nutrition solution in, 178
  nutritional support in, 187–188
  platelet dysfunction in, 55, 56
  postoperative, in elderly, 69
  in prune belly syndrome, 1027
  spinal cord injury and, 912
  total parenteral nutrition in, 179–181
Renal function, normal, 49–50
Renal infarction, **1077**
  versus renal stones, 1043
Renal oncocytoma, **1059**
Renal parenchyma
  anatomy of, **1014–1015**
  changes in, in obstructive uropathy, **1030,** 1031
Renal pelvis
  anatomy of, **1015**
  anomalies of, **1020–1021**

Renal pelvis (*cont.*)
changes in, in obstructive uropathy, **1030**
tumors of, **1059–1061**
versus renal stones, 1043
versus ureteral calculi, 1046
Renal sarcoma, **1058**
Renal stones, **1042–1045**
prevention of, **1043–1044**
Renal tuberculosis, *versus* renal stones, 1043
Renal vascular abnormalities, 1020
Renal vein renin ratio (RVRR), 854
Renal veins, 871
thrombosis of, **1077**, 1078*i*
Rendu-Osler-Weber syndrome, 469, 736, 1342
Renin, 49
plasma, in hyperaldosteronism, 798–799
Renin-angiotensin-aldosterone axis, drugs affecting, 799
Renovascular hypertension, **853–856**, 853*i*
clinical findings in, 854
prognosis for, 855
treatment of, 855
Repair (wound). *See* Wound healing
Reperfusion injury, in acute mesenteric vascular occlusion, 698, 699
Reperfusion syndrome, 258
Replantation, 866
Reporting
National Practitioner Data Bank, 84–85
statutes governing, 76
Reproduction, assisted techniques of, for male infertility, **1081**
Reproductive system
embryology of, 1013–1014, 1016*i*
female, congenital anomalies of, **1085–1086**
Reservoir ileostomy, 751
Residual limb, trauma to, 869
Residual volume function, in chronic venous insufficiency, 884
Res ipsa loquitur, 78–79
Respiration
control of, for increased intracranial pressure, **891**
in increased intracranial pressure, 890
mechanics of, 344
neonatal, 1306–1307
Respiratory acidosis, **151**
with metabolic acidosis, 153
with metabolic alkalosis, 153
Respiratory alkalosis, with metabolic alkalosis, 153
Respiratory care
postoperative, 15, 23, 26, 27
preoperative, 47
Respiratory disease
risk factors for, 46
in surgical patient, **46–48**
Respiratory failure
postoperative, **17–18**
diagnosis of, 17–18
early, 17
late, 17
prevention of, 18

respiratory acidosis in, 151
in tonsillar herniation, 891
Respiratory function, postoperative, 17, 20
intercostal block and, 21
Respiratory papillomatosis, recurrent, **994**
Respiratory support. *See also* Mechanical ventilation
for pediatric patients, 1294–1295
Respiratory tract
development of, 379–380
injury to, burns and, **274–276**
postoperative complications in, **25–27**
Respondeat superior, 79
Response to injury hypothesis, of atherosclerosis, 813
Resting energy expenditure
in burn patient, 185
in cancer patient, 186
in response to injury, 107, 161
in sepsis, 169
Rest pain, ischemic, and peripheral arterial insufficiency, 816–817
Resuscitation, in hypovolemic shock, 205–206
Resuscitation phase, of trauma management, **239–240**
Retention polyps, 702
Reticular veins, 873
Reticulum cell carcinoma, mediastinal, 377
Reticulum cell sarcoma of bone, **1226**
Retina
angioma of, 1011
blunt trauma to, 1009*t*
congenital hypertrophy of, familial adenomatous polyposis and, 728
detachment of, **1006**
Retinoblastoma, intraocular, 1011
13-*cis*-Retinoic acid, chemopreventive, 297
Retinol. *See* Vitamin A
Retinol-binding protein, serum levels of, 157*t*, 158, 159*t*
Retinopathy, proliferative diabetic, panretinal photocoagulation for, **1012**
Retractile mesenteritis, 531
Retrofascial abscess, **526–527**
Retrograde cholangiography, in chronic pancreatitis, 641
Retrograde ejaculation, 1081
Retrograde peristalsis, 708
Retroperitoneal abscess, **526–527**
Retroperitoneal cysts, **531**
Retroperitoneal fibrosis, **531–532, 1033**
Retroperitoneal space
anterior portion of, 526
posterior portion of, 526
Retroperitoneum, tumors of, **530–531**
Retropubic urethropexy, 1093
Retrosternal hernia, **501**, 501*i*
Reversed-3 sign, 645
Reverse transcription-polymerase chain reaction (RT-PCR), in diagnosis of rabies, 128
Rewarming
for accidental hypothermia, 281

for frostbite, 1287
for near-drowning, 265
Rhabdomyolysis, exertional, 277
Rhabdomyoma, cardiac, 469
Rhabdomyosarcoma, **1345–1346**, 1361
embryonal, 1346
of extremity, 1346
genitourinary, 1346
of head and neck, 1346
staging of, 1346, 1346*t*
Rheumatic heart disease, 420, 422
Rheumatoid arthritis, **1203–1204**
differential diagnosis of, 358*t*
esophageal manifestations in, 480
in Felty's syndrome, 660
hand involvement in, **1285**
versus osteoarthritis, 1203–1204
Rheumatoid factor (RF), in rheumatoid arthritis, 1203
Rhinitis
acute, **978**
allergic, **978–979**, 978*t*
medicamentosa, **979**
vasomotor, **979**
Rhinoliths, 977–978
Rhinoplasty, **1264–1265**
Rhinorrhea, cerebrospinal fluid
in nasal trauma, 983
in temporal bone fractures, 972
Rhizopus arrhizus, **394**
Rhizotomy
for hyperreflexic bladder, 1075–1076
for spastic cerebral palsy, 937
for trigeminal neuralgia, 951
Rhytidectomy, **1265–1266**
Riboflavin. *See* Vitamin B₂
Ribonucleases, 626
Ribs
fracture of, 244
osteomyelitis of, **352**
resection of, for axillary-subclavian venous thrombosis, 879
Rickettsial infection, drug therapy for, 136*t*
Riedel's thyroiditis, 305
Rifampin
indications for, 135*t*, 136*t*, 141
for tuberculosis, 388*t*, 389
of spine, 961
Right atrial pressure, 220
mean, 221*t*
Right coronary artery, 408, 409*i*
Right lower quadrant, abscess of, causes of, 524*t*
Right subhepatic division, abscess in, 521, 523*i*
Right to die, 81
Right-to-left shunt, 458
Right to refuse treatment, 81
Right ventricular hypertrophy, and tetralogy of Fallot, 460, 460*i*
Ringer's solution, lactated, for craniocerebral trauma, 903
Rinne test, 963
Risk, operative, factors affecting, 7–10

Risk assessment, in critically ill surgical patient, 224–225
Rituximab, 1369
RNA, dietary, 162
Rods
  acid-fast, infection by, drug therapy for, 136t
  gram-negative, infection by, drug therapy for, 135t
  gram-positive, infection by, drug therapy for, 136t
Rofecoxib, for cervical spondylotic myelopathy, 1209
Ross-Konn procedure, 444
Ross procedure, 428
Rotator cuff tear(s), **1132,** 1132i
Rotator cuff tendinitis, **1197**
Roux-en-Y choledochojejunostomy
  for bile duct malignancies, 618
  for recurrent pyogenic cholangitis, 623
Roux-en-Y cystojejunostomy, for pancreatic pseudocyst, 638
Roux-en-Y hepaticojejunostomy
  for bile duct injuries, 620
  for bile duct malignancies, 618
  for sclerosing cholangitis, 624
Rovsing's sign, 1328
Rubor, in peripheral arterial insufficiency, 817–818
Rule of nines, 269i
Runaround, 1282
Ryanodine receptor gene, 202

Saccharomyces boulardii, for antibiotic-associated colitis, 749
Sacrocolpopexy, 1093
Saddle nose deformity, 983
Sagittal sinus, 896i
  thrombosis of, 896i
St. Jude bileaflet mechanical heart valve, 428–429, 429i
St. Jude Medical stentless porcine aortic valve, 428, 428i
Saline
  indications for, 153
  isotonic, indications for, 149
Saline load test, 552, 553
Salivary glands, **986–987**
  diseases of, 293t
  stones in, **987**
  trauma of, **987**
  tumors of, **293–295**
Salmonella infection
  colitis caused by, 127
  drug therapy for, 135t
  and thoracic empyema, 361
  versus ulcerative colitis, 742–743
Salmonella typhi, **695**
Salmonella typhimurium, in HIV-associated enteropathy, 693–694
Salmon-Goodsall rule, 772–773, 772i
Salpingitis
  differential diagnosis of, 514
  and ectopic pregnancy, 1102

  pain caused by, 1089–1090
Salpingo-oophorectomy
  in ovarian cancer, 1112
  in ovarian cancer prevention, 1111
Salpingostomy, for ectopic pregnancy, 1103
Salter-Harris classification, of physial injuries, 1177–1178, 1178i
Salt retention
  dietary, 185
  in response to injury, 107
Sampling reflex, 758
Santorini, duct of, 625, 626i
Saphenofemoral junction, 871
Saphenopopliteal bypass, for chronic venous insufficiency, 885
Saphenous nerve, 872i
Saphenous veins, 871, 872i
  grafts of, for intracranial aneurysm, 941–842
  stripping of, 874, 874i
Sarafotoxin, 130
Sarcoidosis, **394–395,** 395t, **662**
  hypercalcemia in, 149
Sarcoma. *See also* Ewing's sarcoma
  cardiac, 435, 469
  cervical, 1106
  definition of, 1352
  Ewing's (*See* Ewing's sarcoma)
  osteogenic, 1223, **1224,** 1225i
    of chest wall, 355
  paraneoplastic syndromes with, 1371t
  of prostate, **1070**
  renal, **1058**
  soft tissue, **1361–1363**
    biopsy of, 1362
    grading of, 1223, 1361–1362
    pulmonary metastases of, 1363
    recurrence of, 1362–1363
    staging of, 1361, 1362t
    treatment of, 1362–1363
  of thyroid gland, 307
  treatment of, 1362–1363
  uterine, **1109–1110**
  vaginal, 1106
  vulvar, 1104
Scalenectomy, for axillary-subclavian venous thrombosis, 879
Scalene lymph node biopsy, **350**
Scalp lacerations, **907**
Scanning speech, 1209
Scaphoid, 1143
  fractures of, **1146–1147,** 1147i, **1279**
Scaphoid lunate ligament, injury to, 1280
Scaphoid shift test, 1280
Scapholunate dissociation, 1147
Scapula, fractures of, **1129–1130**
Scar(s)
  abdominal, 796
  with burns, 273, 276
  hypertrophic, 91
    plastic surgery for, **1243–1244**
  prevention of, in plastic surgery, 1241, 1241i, 1242i
Scarpa's fascia, 783
Schatzki's ring, 500

Schilling test, in blind loop syndrome, 679–680
Schistosomiasis, 579
Schmidt's syndrome, 41
Schwannomas (nerve sheath tumors), **919–920,** 925, 926
  of facial nerve, 973
  of peripheral nerves, 929
  of spinal cord, **927,** 928
  vestibular, 919–920, **975–976**
Sciatica, in lumbar disk syndrome, 956
Sciatic nerve, injury to, improper positioning and, 195
Scintigraphy. *See also* Radionuclide scan
  in acquired intestinal diverticula, 690–691
  adrenal, of adrenal masses, 797
  of biliary atresia, 1334
  for estimating small bowel transit time, 677
  in gastroesophageal reflux, 486
  of neuroblastoma, 1343
  test, in hepatopancreatic ampulla stenosis and dysfunction, 622
Scleroderma, **843**
  and blind loop syndrome, 680
  esophageal manifestations in, **479–480**
  hand involvement in, 1286
  and lung cancer, 396
Sclerosing agents, for spider veins, 1269
Sclerosing carcinoma, 1250
Sclerosing cholangitis, **623–624**
  bile duct malignancies and, 618
Sclerotherapy
  for lymphangioma, 1302
  for nonbleeding varices, 584
  for variceal bleeding, 581
  for varicose veins, 875
Scoliosis, **1185–1189**
  congenital, 1185, **1187**
  correction of, intraoperative neurophysiologic monitoring in, 898, 899
  idiopathic, 1185–1186
  neuromuscular, 1186–1187
  pectus excavatum with, 1305
Screening program
  for colorectal cancer, 718–719
  for infants at risk of hearing impairment, 965, 965t
  for prostate tumors, 1066
Scrotal thermography, in male infertility, 1081
Scrotum
  anomalies of, **1029**
  congenital lesions of, 1029
  disorders of, in pediatric patients, **1336–1339,** 1336i
  injuries to, **1053**
  lesions of, 1029
Sea snake, 130
Seat belts, 230
Seborrheic keratosis, 1245
Second-degree burns, 267, 268i
Second opinion, 10
Secretin
  and acid inhibition, 538
  and pancreatic secretion, 625–626

Secretin test, **643**
  in chronic pancreatitis, 640
Secretion, in small intestine, **677–679**
Secretory otitis media, 965
Sedation, preoperative, 194
"Seeding" of colorectal cancer, 718
Segmental limb pressure measurements, and
        peripheral arterial insufficiency,
        818–819
Segmentation, in colon, 708
Seizures. *See also* Epilepsy
  arteriovenous malformations and, 944
  brain abscess and, 959
  brain tumors and, 918, 922, 923–924
  burns and, 274
  craniocerebral trauma and, **903–904**
  delirium tremens and, 35
  surgery for, in children, **937**
Seldinger technique, for peripheral arterial in-
        sufficiency, 819
Selenium
  deficiency of, 164
  requirements for, 164*t*
Sellar region, tumors in, 915*i*, 916*i*, **923**
Semen analysis, in male infertility, **1080**
Semilunar line, 783
Seminal emission, lack of, in male infertility,
        1081
Seminoma, 1072
  mediastinal, 377
Semirigid penile prosthesis, 1084
Sengstaken-Blakemore tube, 582, 582*i*
Senile cataract, **1004–1005**
Senning operation, 465
Senokot, for slow-transit constipation, 710
Sensorineural hearing loss, **962–963**, 964*i*,
        968–969
  in AIDS, 998
  in infants, 969
Sensory loss
  of head and neck tumors, 283
  peripheral arterial insufficiency and, 817
Sentinel Event Policy, of JCAHO, 83
Sentinel hemorrhage, 938
  in intracranial aneurysms, 940
Sentinel loop, in acute pancreatitis, 632
Sentinel pile, 769, 769*i*
Sepsis, 152. *See also* Infection(s); Shock, septic
  in acute mesenteric vascular occlusion, 698
  after splenectomy, **666–667**
  with anorectal abscess, 771
  with burns, 273, 273*t*, 274*t*
  control of, in acute secondary bacterial peri-
        tonitis, 519
  definition of, 111, 115
  intra-abdominal, case example of, 226–227
  manifestations of, 210
  metabolic response to, 169–170, 169*i*
  mortality rate for, 118
  postoperative jaundice in, 33
  postoperative pulmonary edema in, 17
  prognosis for, 118
  in small intestine fistulas, 696
    control of, **697**

Sepsis syndrome, 111
Septal dermoplasty, for epistaxis, 981
Septal deviation, 983
Septal hematoma, 982–983
Septal perforations, 983
Septicemia, in acute secondary bacterial peri-
        tonitis, care for, 519
Septic thrombophlebitis, 883
Septum primum atrial septal defect, 451
Sequestration, pulmonary, **381**
Serine protease inhibitors, for postoperative
        bleeding, 436
Seroma, **23**
  and wound healing, 24
Serosa, intestinal, 674, 675
Serotonin, in carcinoid syndrome, 703
Serous effusions, 357
Serous otitis media, 965
Serratia infection, 112
  drug therapy for, 135*t*
Sertoli-Leydig cell tumors, 1110
Sevoflurane, depth of anesthesia with, signs of,
        197*i*
Sex hormones, anticancer therapy with, **1356**
Sexual dysfunction, postoperative, **35**
Sexual impairment
  after ileostomy, 752
  after proctocolectomy, 752
Shaken baby syndrome, 936–937
Sharp objects, ingestion of, **492**
Shaving, preoperative, 12
Sheath(s), tendon, in hand, 1272
Shifting pain, 504, 505*i*
Shigella infection (shigellosis)
  drug therapy for, 135*t*
  in HIV-associated enteropathy, 693–694
  versus ulcerative colitis, 742–743
Shingles. *See* Herpes zoster
Shock, 108, **203–212**
  in acute mesenteric vascular occlusion,
        698–699
  with bee or wasp sting, 132
  cardiac compressive, **206–207**, 240
  cardiogenic, 206, **207–209**, 240
    case example of, 227
  cardiovascular involvement in, **203–210**
  case examples of, 225–228
  cellular response to, 210–212
  control of, in depressed consciousness, 889
  evaluation of, **220–225**
  hemorrhagic (*See* Shock, hypovolemic)
  hypovolemic, **203–206, 239**, 252
    case example of, 227
    causes of, 203
    diagnosis of, 203–205
    mild, 203, 204*t*
    moderate, 204, 204*t*
    nonhemorrhagic, treatment of, 206
    pathophysiology of, 203
    severe, 204, 204*t*
    in trauma victim, 205–206, **239**
    treatment of, 205–206
  neurogenic, **209, 239–240**
  neurohumoral response to, 210–212

  and peritonitis, 518
  septic, 118, 124, 125
    high-output, **209–210**
    low-output, **210**
    in small bowel obstruction, 684
  snakebite and, 131
  spinal, 1119
    spinal cord injury and, 910
    in trauma victim, **239–240**
Shock phase, of spinal cord injury, 209, 1075
Shone's syndrome, and aortic coarctation, 445
Short bowel syndrome, **680–682**, 681*i*
  nutritional support in, 189
Shoulder
  calcific tendinitis in, **1197–1198**
  dislocation of, **1130–1132**
  frozen, **1198–1199**
  injury to, **1128–1133**
  multidirectional instability of, 1131
  pain syndromes of, **1197–1199**
  voluntary dislocation of, 1131
Shoulder-hand syndrome. *See* Reflex sympa-
        thetic dystrophy
Shouldice repair, for inguinal hernia, 788
Shunt(s)
  for hydrocephalus, 934
  for increased intracranial pressure, 891
  peritoneovenous, for malignant ascites, 529
  for spinal cord tumors, 928
Sialadenitis
  acute bacterial, **986**
  chronic, **986–987**
  viral, **986**
Sialolithiasis, **987**
Sickle cell anemia, 52, **53**
Sigmoidal vessels, 706*i*
Sigmoid colon, 706*i*, 757*i*
  resection of, 764
Sigmoid colostomy, 752
Sigmoidoscopy, **712,** 769
  in antibiotic-associated colitis, 749
  and colorectal cancer, 718–719
  in colovesical fistula, 735
  in diverticulitis, 732–733
  for familial adenomatous polyposis, 728
  in lower gastrointestinal bleeding, 737*i*
  rectal valve and, 705
  in ulcerative colitis, 741–742
Sigmoidovaginal fistula, **1094**
Sigmoid volvulus, 738, **739,** 739*i*, 740*i*
Silicone gel prostheses, and autoimmune disor-
        ders, 343
Silver sulfadiazine, for burns, 272
Simple goiter, **304**
Simple obstruction, intestinal, 683, **684–685,**
        685*i*, 686*i*
Sinemet, for Parkinson's disease, 948
Single ventricle, **467–468**
Sinuses, paranasal, **977–984**
  cancer of, **292–293**
Sinusitis
  acute frontal, 980
  paranasal, **979–980**
  pediatric, 980

Sinus of Valsalva, 420
  ruptured, 449, **455**
Sinus tracts, 114–115
  branchial, 1300–1301
  preauricular, 973, 1301
Sinus venosus defects, 450, 450*i*
Sipple's syndrome, and hyperparathyroidism, 309
Sistrunk procedure, for lymphedema, 887
Sistrurus spp., 130
Situs, abnormalities of, **468**
Situs inversus totalis, 468
Sitz bath, indications for, 770
Sjögren's syndrome, esophageal manifestations in, 480
Skatole, 710
Skin
  anatomy and physiology of, **267**
  antiseptics for, 12
  arterial malformations in, 1342
  capillary malformations in, 1342
  in cardiac compressive shock, 206
  care of, for lymphedema, 886
  in hypovolemia, 204
  irritation of, ileostomy and, 753*t*
  mixed vascular malformations in, 1342
  operative field on, preparation of, 12
  paraneoplastic syndromes involving, 1371, 1371*t*
  premalignant lesions of, **1249**
  preparation of, in operating room, 12
  tumors of, **1244–1252**
    benign, **1245–1249**
    malignant, **1249–1252**
  vascular anomalies of (*See also* Hemangioma)
    in pediatric patients, **1341–1342**
  venous malformations in, 1342
Skin cancer
  basal cell, **1250–1251**
  squamous cell, **1251–1252**
Skin expanders, for breast reconstruction, 1261
Skin expansion techniques, for burn patients, 276
Skin fluorescence, and amputation level determination, 860
Skin grafts, **1231–1234**
  color match for, 1234
  composite, 1232
  donor area for, 1231, **1233–1234**
  donor site
    healing, thickness of graft and, 1234
    management of, 1234
  full-thickness, 1231–1232, 1231*i*, 1232*t*
  for giant hairy nevi, 1246
  indications for, by wound type, 1239*t*
  for lower extremity, 1262–1263
  meshed, 1231
  obtaining, 1232
  recipient area for, 1231, **1232–1233**
  for scrotal injury, 1053
  split-thickness, 1231, 1231*i*, 1232*t*
  thickness of, and donor site healing, 1234
  types of, 1231–1232

Skin perfusion
  and amputation level determination, 860, 861
  in hypovolemic shock, 239
Skin substitutes
  permanent, for burns, 272–273
  temporary, for burns, 272
Skin temperature, and amputation level determination, 861
Skin tests
  in malnutrition, 158*t*, 159*t*
  in pulmonary disorders, 349
Skull
  fracture of, 901
    open, **907**
  malformations of, **932**
Skull base
  surgery of, intraoperative neurophysiologic monitoring in, **897–898**
  tumors in, **921**, 927
    neoplastic, **972–973**
Sleep apnea, obstructive, 988–989
Sling procedures, for stress incontinence, 1093
Slipped capital femoral epiphyses, **1192–1193**, 1192*i*
Slow-transit constipation, 709–710
Sludge, in gallbladder, 600
Small artery occlusive disease, **827**
Small cell carcinoma, of lung, 396, 396*t*, 399*f*
  prognosis for, 403, 403*t*
  treatment of, 402, 403
Small-for-gestational-age (SGA) infant, 1293–1294
Small intestine, **674–704**
  absorption in, **677–679**
  anatomy of, **674–675**, 675*i*
    gross, 674
    microscopic, **674–675**
  carcinoid tumors of, **703–704**
  digestion in, **677–679**
  fistulas of, **696–697**, 696*t*
  gas cysts in, **701**
  inflammatory diseases of, **693–695** (*See also* Enteritis)
  injuries to, treatment of, 254
  intussusception, **31**
  metastatic disease of, 703
  motility of, **675–677**
  obstruction of, **683–687**, 683*t*, 685*i*, 686*i*
    versus large bowel obstruction, **714**
  peristalsis in, postoperative, 19, 30
  physiology of, **675–679**
  pores in, 677
  secretion in, **677–679**
  stricture of, and obstruction, **684**
  tumors of, **701–704**
    benign, **702**
    malignant, **702–703**
    obstruction caused by, **683**, 683*t*
  ulcerative diseases of, **693–695**
  vascular lesions of, **698–701**
Smith's fracture, 1144
Smoke inhalation, 274–275, 275*t*
Smoking
  and cervical cancer, 1107

  cessation
    benefits of, 47
    preoperative, 8, 23
  and coronary heart disease, 410
  and operative risk, 17
Snake(s)
  identification of, 130
  venom of, 130–131
Snakebite, **130–132**
Snapping hip, **1201**
Snellen chart, 999
Snow blindness, **1008**
Soave operation, in Hirschsprung's disease, 1322
Sodium
  absorption of
    in colon, 707
    in large intestine, 708–709, 709*t*
    in small intestine, 677–678
  balance, 144*t*, **145–146**
    in response to injury, 107
  excess, estimation of, 144
  fractional excretion of, 50–51
  loss of
    in gastrointestinal fluid, 147*t*
    with ileostomy, 751
  renal handling of, 142–143
  serum levels of (*See also* Hypernatremia; Hyponatremia)
    and fluid therapy, 153
    and intracranial hypertension, 905
  urinary levels of, and ascites treatment, 590
Sodium bicarbonate, indications for, 51, 152
Sodium carboxymethylcellulose, for aphthous stomatitis, 985
Sodium chloride
  for craniocerebral trauma, 903
  0.9% intravenous solution, 18t
  0.45% intravenous solution, 18t
  3% intravenous solution, 18t
  for newborn, 1296
Sodium citrate, indications for, 201
Sodium nitroprusside. *See* Nitroprusside
Sodium phosphate, in preoperative bowel preparation, 754
Sodium-potassium citrate solution, for renal stones, 1044
Sodium sulfate
  indications for, 149
  in preoperative bowel preparation, 754
Sodium tetradecyl sulfate, for varicose veins, 875
Soft tissue infections, *versus* lymphangitis, 887
Soft tissue injury, plastic surgery for, **1252–1254**
Soft tissue sarcoma, **1361–1363**
Soleal venous sinusoids, 873
Soleus muscle flap, for lower extremity, 1262
Solid-and-papillary neoplasm, of pancreas, 647
Solid ankle cushion heel (SACH) prosthesis, 869
Solitary pulmonary nodule, **405–406**, 405*i*
Solitary rectal ulcer, 762
Solute balance(s), normal, 143, 144*t*

Somatomedins, actions of, 167
Somatosensory evoked potentials
  in aneurysm surgery, 899–900
  in skull base surgery, 898
  in spinal cord surgery, 898–899
Somatostatin
  for blind loop syndrome, 680
  for glucagonoma, 651
  for pancreatic ascites, 639
  for pancreatic cholera, 650
  for pituitary tumors, 931
  for small bowel obstruction, 684
  for small intestine fistulas, 697
Somatostatinoma, **651**
Somatotropic adenomas, 921
Sonohysterogram, 1088
Sound, physics of, **962**
Spastic cerebral palsy, **937**
Spectinomycin
  for gonococcal proctitis, 776
  indications for, 135*t*
Speech discrimination score, 964, 964*i*
Speech perception, evaluation of, 963–964,
    963*t*, 964*i*
Speed limits, 231
Spermatic cord
  lipoma of, 786
  torsion of, **1079–1080**
Spermatic vein, in varicocele, 1079
Spermatocele, **1079**
Sperm penetration assay, 1080
Sperm washing, for male infertility, 1081
Spetzler-Martin system, for arteriovenous mal-
    formations, 945–946, 946*t*
Spherocytosis, hereditary, **655–656**
  versus hypersplenism, 654
Spherules, 391
Sphincter of Oddi, dysfunction of, 622
Sphincteroplasty
  for chronic pancreatitis, 642
  for obstructive pancreatitis, 629
Sphincterotomy
  endoscopic
    for acute pancreatitis, **634**
    for adenoma and adenocarcinoma of am-
      pulla of Vater, 648
    for ascariasis, 623
    for cholangitis, 612
    for choledocholithiasis, **615**
    for chronic pancreatitis, 642
    for hepatopancreatic ampulla stenosis and
      dysfunction, 622
  pancreatitis after, 628–629
  for sphincter of Oddi dysfunction, 622
Spider bites, **132–133**
Spider veins, 873, 875, **1269**
Spigelian hernia, 794
Spina bifida aperta (myelomeningocele), **933,**
    933*i*
Spina bifida occulta, **932–933**
Spinal anesthesia
  advantages and disadvantages of, 110
  intraoperative management of,
    198–199

Spinal cord
  anatomy of, 1117
    and intervertebral disk disease, **952–953**
  central canal of, 890*i*
  cervical, neoplasm of, 1209
  in cervical stenosis, 1207–1208
  motor and sensory levels of, 911*i*
  surgery of, intraoperative neurophysiologic
    monitoring in, **898**
  tumors of, **927–928**
    in children, **936**
Spinal cord injury, 242, **908–913**
  in children, **937**
  with complete neurologic deficit,
    1122–1123
  complications of, 1120
  epidemiology of, 1117
  incidence of, 1117
  with incomplete neurologic deficit,
    1121–1122, 1122*i*
  methylprednisolone for, 1118
  motor levels with, determination of, 1119
  neurologic injury with, classification of,
    1118–1119
  and neuropathic bladder, 1075
  pain in, **952**
  sensory levels with, determination of, 1119
  shock caused by, 209, 1075
  stability in, 912
  treatment of, 243
Spinal-epidural anesthesia, combined, 199
Spinal nerve roots
  anatomy of, 1117
  avulsion, pain of, **952**
Spinal reflex center, injury to, in neuropathic
    bladder, 1075
Spinal shock, 1119
  spinal cord injury and, 910
Spinal taps, for increased intracranial pressure,
    891
Spine
  anatomy of, 1117
  bony injury in, classification of, 1118
  deformity of, in children, **1185–1189**
  fixation of, 1121
  flexion-distraction injury of, 1121
  fractures and dislocations of, **1117–1123**
    imaging of, 1119–1120
    with neurologic deficit, 1121–1123
    without neurologic deficit, 1120–1121
  fusion procedures for, 1121–1123
  immobilization of, at accident scene, 234
  metastases to, 1213
  tuberculosis of, **960–961**
  tumors of
    extradural, 1213
    intradural, 1213
Spinothalamic tract(s), 1117
Spiral computed tomography, in pulmonary
    thromboembolism, 881, 881*i*
Spiral valve of Heister, 595
Spirochete infection, drug therapy for, 136*t*
Spirometer, incentive, 17
Spirometry, 48

Spironolactone
  adverse effects and side effects of, 801
  for ascites, 590
  indications for, 800–801
Splanchnicectomy, thoracoscopic, for chronic
    pancreatitis, 642
Splanchnic nerve
  pancreas innervated by, 625
  small intestine innervated by, 674
Splanchnic vasoconstriction, in nonocclusive
    intestinal ischemia, 700
Spleen, **652–667**
  abscesses of, **664**
  accessory, 652
  anatomy of, **652,** 653*i*
  cysts of, **664**
  ectopic (wandering), 652
  function of, evaluation of, 654
  infections of, 664
  injury of, treatment of, 253
  physiology of, **652–653**
  size of, evaluation of, **654**
  tumors of, **664**
Splenectomy, **665–667,** 665*i*
  for autoimmune disorders, 657–661
  and autoimmune hemolytic anemias, 658
  for chronic lymphocytic leukemia, 662
  for cysts and tumors of spleen, 664
  disorders potentially amenable to, **655–664**
  for gastric carcinoma, 559
  for Gaucher's disease, 661
  hematologic effects of, **666**
  for hereditary disorders, **655–657**
  for hereditary spherocytosis, 656
  for hypersplenism, 655
  for idiopathic myelofibrosis, 663
  for immune thrombocytopenic purpura, 660
    in AIDS patients, 659, 660
  indications for, 655*t*
  laparoscopic, 666
  for massive splenomegaly, 665–666
  for metabolic disorders, 661–662
  for neoplastic diseases, 662–664
  for portal pressure reduction, 587
  postoperative problems of, **666–667**
  for pyruvate kinase deficiency, 657
  for secondary hemolytic anemia, 658
  sepsis after, **666–667**
  for splenic abscesses, 664
  in splenic vein thrombosis, 588–589
  for systemic mast cell disease, 663
  for thalassemia major, 657
  for Wiskott-Aldrich syndrome, 661
Splenic artery, 625, 626*i*, 652
  aneurysms of, **841**
  ligation of, 587
Splenic autotransplantation, **664**
Splenic flexure, of colon, 706*i*
Spleniculi, 652
Splenic vein, 565, 567*i*, 626*i*
  in portal hypertension, 579
  thrombosis of, 579, **588–589,** 641
Splenomegaly
  evaluation of, 654

in Felty's syndrome, 660
hypersplenism *versus*, 653
in idiopathic myelofibrosis, 663
massive, defined, 665–666
pancreatic adenocarcinoma and, 645
physiology of spleen in, 652, 653
in systemic mast cell disease, 663
Splenorrhaphy, 665
Splenosis, **664**
Splinting
    for rheumatoid arthritis, 1204
    in trauma management, 234
Spondylolytic anterior-posterior diameter
        (SAPD), in subaxial cervical spine,
        1207, 1207*i*
Spondylosis, 954
Spontaneous peritonitis. *See* Peritonitis, pri-
        mary
Spontaneous pneumothorax, 367–368, 367*i*
Sports-related injuries, 900
Sprain(s)
    ankle, 1170
    wrist, 1143–1144, **1279–1280**
Spreading pain, 504, 505*i*
Sputum analysis, **351**
Squamous cell carcinoma, **1251–1252**
    and achalasia, 478
    anal, 777, **780**
    cervical, 1106–1108
    definition of, 1352
    of esophagus, 496
    of eyelid, 1011
    of hand, 1288
    of head and neck, 282, 284
        chemotherapy for, 296–297
        development of, 282
        and hypopharyngeal cancer, 289
        and laryngeal cancer, 290
        and nasal cavity cancer, 292
        oral cavity, 286
        oropharynx, 288
        staging of, 285, 286*i*
    of lung, 396, 396*t*
    penile, **1072**
    in renal pelvis and calices, 1059
    in skull base, 972
    vaginal, 1105–1106
    vulvar, 1104–1105
Stab-avulsion technique, for varicose veins, 874
Stab wound(s), 247, 249
    history-taking about, 2
Staff privileges, 82–83
Staged reconstruction, for hypoplastic left heart
        syndrome, 448
Staging. *See also* TNM staging system
    of anorectal cancer, 780, 780*t*
    of bladder tumors, 1063*t*, 1064
    of breast cancer, 326, 327*i*
    of cervical cancer, 1106, 1106*t*
    of colorectal cancer, 723, 724*t*
    of endometrial cancer, 1108, 1109*t*
    of gastric cancer, 558*i*
    of gestational trophoblastic tumors, 1113,
        1113*t*

of lung cancer, 398, 400*t*
of melanoma, 1363, 1363*t*
of neuroblastoma, 1343, 1343*t*
of non-Hodgkin's lymphoma, 1367
of ovarian cancer, 1111, 1112*t*
of prostate cancer, **1066–1067**, 1067*t*, 1068
of renal adenocarcinoma, 1058*t*
of rhabdomyosarcoma, 1346, 1346*t*
of soft tissue sarcoma, 1361, 1362*t*
of squamous cell carcinoma of head and
        neck, 285, 286*i*
of testicular cancer, 1071*t*
of tumors, **1352–1353**
of vaginal cancer, 1105, 1105*t*
of vulvar cancer, 1104, 1104*t*
of Wilms' tumor, 1344, 1345*t*
Standard of care, 77
    locality rule for, 77
    minimum, 78
Standby anesthesia, **199**
Stanford classification scheme, for thoracic aor-
        tic dissection, 432–433, 433*i*
Stapedectomy, for otosclerosis, 968
Stapedotomy, for otosclerosis, 968
Staphylococcal infection
    carriers, and infection control, 13
    furunculitis caused by, in nasal vestibulitis,
        978
    hepatic abscess caused by, 593
    hospital-acquired, 12
    and infected aneurysms, 838
    and lymphangitis, 887
    methicillin-resistant, drug therapy for, 135*t*
    in nasal trauma, 983
    non-penicillinase-producing, drug therapy
        for, 135*t*
    penicillinase-producing, drug therapy for,
        135*t*
    pneumonia caused by, complications of,
        362*t*
    in splenic abscesses, 664
    and thoracic empyema, 361, 362*t*
Staphylococcus aureus infection, 112
    and acute hordeolum (sty), 1002
    and breast abscess, **343**
    and bronchiectasis, 385
    and burn infections, 274*t*
    in closed disk space infections, 960
    colitis caused by, 127
    and endocarditis, 430
    and lung abscess, 383
    in paranasal sinusitis, 979–980
    and retroperitoneal abscesses, 526
    septic arthritis caused by, 1220–1222
Starch, digestion of, in small intestine, 678
Stare decisis, 74
Starling equation, 344
Starvation, 111
    adjustment to, 108
    cardiac effects of, 188
    pathophysiology of, **164–167**, 167*i*
Status epilepticus, in craniocerebral trauma,
        903–904
Statute of limitations, 80

Stauffer's syndrome, 1054
Steal syndrome, 895*i*
Steatorrhea, **643**
    in blind loop syndrome, 679
    in cholecystenteric fistula, 609
    in small bowel syndrome, 680
Stenosing tenosynovitis, in hand, **1278**
Stenosis
    aortic, **426–427, 441–445,** 442*i*
    iliac artery, 822, 822*i*
    infundibular, 441, 441*i*, 460, 460*i*
    mitral, **420–422,** 448
    pulmonary, **440–442,** 441*i*, 460, 460*i*
    subaortic, 441*i*, **443–444**
    supravalvular, 441*i*, **444**
    tricuspid, 425
    valvular aortic, 441*i*, **443**
    valvular pulmonary, 441, 441*i*
Stenotrophomonas maltophilia infection, drug
        therapy for, 135*t*
Stent(s)
    for bile duct malignancies, 618
    carotid artery, 851–852
    for chronic pancreatitis, 642
    coronary, comparison with other procedures,
        415
    endovascular, 821
    for gallbladder cancer, 616–617
    for large bowel obstruction, 714
    laryngeal, 243
    Palmaz type, 821
    for pancreatic adenocarcinoma, 646
    for peripheral arterial insufficiency, 821
    for small bowel obstruction, 687
    for thyroid cartilage injuries, 243
    Wallstent, 821
Stented pericardial valve, 428, 428*i*
Stented porcine bioprosthesis, 428
Stentless porcine valve, 428, 428*i*
Stereotactic neurosurgery, for Parkinson's dis-
        ease, 948
Sterilization
    for contraception, 1090–1091
    in infection control, 119
        of instruments and supplies, methods for,
            11
Sternal cleft, **1305**
Sternal osteomyelitis, **352**
Sternal wound infection, after cardiac surgery,
        437
Sternoclavicular joint, dislocation of, **1129**
Sternocleidomastoid muscle, in torticollis,
        1303
Steroid(s). *See also* Corticosteroid(s); Glucocor-
        ticoid(s)
    for allergic rhinitis, 978
    for Crohn's disease, 748
    for lymphedema, 886
    for ulcerative colitis, 744
    withdrawal, in heart transplant recipient,
        470
Steroid retention enema, for inflammatory
        proctitis, 778
Stewart-Treves syndrome, 886

Still's disease, 1184
Stimulated-gracilis procedure, for anorectal
    dysfunction, 760
Stings, arthropod, **132–133**
Stoma, intestinal, **751–754**
Stomach, **533–562**. *See also* Gastric
    anatomy of, 533–534, 534*i*, 535*i*, 536*i*
    blood supply to, 533, 536*i*
    decompression of, 553
    duplication of, 1328–1329, 1329*i*
    leiomyoma of, **561**
    lymphoma of, **560**
    motility of, 534–536
    mucosal resistance in, 537–538
    nerve supply to, 533–534, 536*i*
    physiologic function of, integration of, 538
    physiology of, 534–538
    pseudolymphoma of, **560**
    regional enteritis of, **564**
Stomal ulcer, 542–543
Stomatitis
    aphthous, **985**
    herpetic, **985**
Stool
    examination of, for fat, 643
    volume of, in pancreatic cholera, 650
Stool softeners, indications for, 770
Stool tests, in acute abdomen, 510*t*, 511
Strabismus, **1001–1002, 1007,** 1007*i*
Straddle injury, 1052
Straight leg raising test, 1212–1213
Strangulation obstruction, intestinal, 683,
    685–686
    versus acute mesenteric vascular occlusion,
        699
    and closed loop obstruction, 684
    physical findings in, 508*t*
Streptococci (*Streptococcus* spp.)
    anaerobic
        in emphysematous cholecystitis, 611
        hepatic abscess caused by, 593, 594
    empyema caused by, 361, 361*i*
    group A, 124
        beta-hemolytic, in pharyngitis, 987
        infection by, drug therapy for, 135*t*
    group B, infection by, drug therapy for, 135*t*
    group C, infection by, drug therapy for,
        135*t*
    group G, infection by, drug therapy for,
        135*t*
    hemolytic, infection by, drug therapy for,
        135*t*
    and infected aneurysms, 838
    infection by, 112
        diffuse necrotizing, 124–125
    in lymphangitis, 887
    and peritonitis, 518
    and primary peritonitis, 527
    in splenic abscesses, 664
Streptococcus faecalis, in feces, 710–711
Streptococcus pneumoniae
    in acute otitis media, 970
    after splenectomy, 666
    and infected aneurysms, 838

infection by, drug therapy for, 135*t*
    in paranasal sinusitis, 979, 980
    resistant, in acute tonsillitis, 988
Streptococcus pyogenes, and lung abscess, 383
Streptococcus viridans, infection by, drug ther-
    apy for, 135*t*
Streptomycin
    indications for, 135*t*
    for tuberculosis, 388*t*, 389
Streptozocin
    for carcinoid tumor of intestine, 704
    for glucagonoma, 651
    for insulinoma, 649
    for pancreatic cholera, 650
    for Zollinger-Ellison syndrome, 546
Stress
    injury-related, 100
    in surgical patient, 34
Stress gastroduodenitis, **555**
Stress incontinence, urinary, **1078,** 1092, 1093
Stress testing, 42
Stress ulcer(s), **555–556,** 555*i*
    after hepatic trauma, 570
    in children, 1332
    with partial hepatectomy, 568
    postoperative prevention of, 15
Strictureplasty, for Crohn's disease, 692
Strictures, in ulcerative colitis, **743**
Stridor, in pediatric airway obstruction,
    991–992
String sign, in Crohn's disease, 690, 691*i*
Stroke, 895*i*
    completed, 848
    postoperative, **34**
    prevention of, 849–852
Stuporous, definition of, 888
Sturge-Weber syndrome, 1342
Sty, 1002
Subacromial bursitis, **1197**
Subaortic stenosis, 441*i*, **443–444**
    diffuse, 443–444
    discrete, 443–444
Subarachnoid hemorrhage, 894*i*
    in intracranial aneurysms, **938–943,** 939*t*
Subarachnoid space, 890*i*
Subclavian artery
    aneurysm of, **842**
    injury to, treatment of, 243
    occlusion of, 895*i*
Subclavian steal syndrome, 851, 851*i*
Subclavian vein, 872
    thrombosis of, **878–880**
Subdiaphragmatic abscess, 521, 523*i*
Subdural abscess, **960**
Subdural hematoma, **906–907,** 907*i*
Subglottic hemangioma, 992
Subglottic stenosis, congenital, 992
Subjective global assessment (SGA), 160
Subluxation provocation test, for congenital
    hip dislocation, 1190, 1190*i*
Submucosa
    of colon, 707*i*
    intestinal, 675
Submucosal plexus, of small intestine, 675

Submucous space, 771*i*
Subpectoral abscess, 352
Subphrenic abscess, causes of, 524*t*
Subpyloric vein, 626*i*
Subscapular abscess, 352
Subtalar joint, dislocation of, 1172–1173
Subtotal lymphoid irradiation (STLI), for
    Hodgkin's lymphoma, 1366
Subungual abscess, 1282
Succinylcholine, indications for, 195
Sucking chest wound, 246. *See also* Open
    pneumothorax
Sucralfate, for stress ulcers, 556
Suction
    in airway management, 233
    endotracheal, 26
    nasogastric, for small bowel obstruction, 687
Suction curettage, in ectopic pregnancy, 1103
Suction-irrigation, in chronic osteomyelitis,
    1219–1220, 1219*i*
Sudden infant death syndrome (SIDS), with
    gastroesophageal reflux, 1327
Sudeck's atrophy. *See* Reflex sympathetic dys-
    trophy
Sulfasalazine
    adverse effects and side effects of, 189
    for Crohn's disease, 692, 748
    for ulcerative colitis, 744
Sulfonamides
    indications for, 129, 135*t*, 136*t*
    mechanism of action of, 140
Sulfonylureas, perioperative management of,
    38
Sulfur, requirements for, 164*t*
Sulfur granules, 129
Sulindac, for familial adenomatous polyposis,
    728
Superficial femoral vein, injuries of, 262
Superficial spreading carcinoma, 557
Superficial thrombophlebitis, **882–883**
    versus lymphangitis, 887
Superinfection, 134
    immunosuppression and, 115
Superior hypophyseal artery, aneurysms, 939
Superior mesenteric artery, 705, 706*i*
    aneurysm of, **842**
    and duodenal obstruction, **563–564**
    injuries to, 257
    small intestine supplied by, 674
        pancreas supplied by, 625, 626*i*
Superior mesenteric artery syndrome, 1319
Superior mesenteric vein, 626*i*, 706*i*
Superior sagittal sinus, 890*i*
Superior vena caval syndrome, **373–374**
Superoxide anion injuries, 258
Suppurative cholangitis, **612**
Suppurative cholecystitis, 608
Supracardiac (type 1) venous return, 455, 456*i*
Supraglottitis, 992–993, 992*t*, 993*i*
Suprahiatal repair, for vesicoureteral reflux,
    1026
Suprahyoid neck dissection, for oral cavity can-
    cer, 287, 287*t*
Suprarenal aortic aneurysms, **836–837**

Supravalvular aortic stenosis, 441*i*
Supravalvular stenosis, **444**
Supravesical obstruction, in obstructive uropathy, **1031**
Surgery
  elective, metabolic response to, 167–169, 168*i*
  metabolic response to, **100–111**, 167–169, 168*i*
  for nonbleeding varices, 585–587, 585*t*
  outpatient, anesthesia for, 200–201, 201*t*
  for variceal bleeding, 582–583
Surgical care, continuum of, 6
Surgical oncologist, role of, **1353–1354**
Survival, of critically ill surgical patient, prediction of, 224–225
Sutures, 24–25, **94**, 97, 97*i*, 122
  buried half-mattress (flap), 1239, 1240*i*
  for cardiac lacerations, 247
  catgut, 94
  for diaphragmatic injuries, 247
  placement of, 24
  postoperative care for, 15–16
  for primary closure, in plastic surgery, 1242
  silk, 94
  stainless steel wire, 94
  staples as, 94
  synthetic absorbable, 94
  synthetic nonabsorbable, 94
  tapes as, 94
Swallowing, 474
Swan-Ganz catheter, **220**
  complications of, 36
  indications for, 207, 208
Swan-neck deformity, 1276*i*, 1277
Sweat glands, 267
Swenson operation, in Hirschsprung's disease, 1322
Switch procedure
  arterial, 465
  double, 467
Syme's amputation, **863–864**, 863*i*
Sympathectomy
  for intra-arterial injections, 858
  lumbar, for peripheral arterial insufficiency, 824
Synchronized intermittent mandatory ventilation (SIMV), 217
Syndactyly, 1260
  congenital, 1275
  pectus excavatum with, 1305
  postburn, 1287
Syndrome of inappropriate antidiuretic hormone secretion (SIADH)
  with brain tumors, 924
  as paraneoplastic syndrome, 1371*t*
Synovectomy, for rheumatoid arthritis, 1204
Synovitis, transient, of hip, 1189
Syphilis
  anorectal, **776**
  and chronic mediastinitis, 372
  drug therapy for, 136*t*
Syringomyelia, in spinal cord tumors, 928

Systemic diseases, esophageal manifestations in, **479–480**
Systemic inflammatory response syndrome (SIRS), 92, 111, 115
Systemic lupus erythematosus
  esophageal manifestations in, 480
  hand involvement in, 1286
  and vasculitis, 700
Systemic mast cell disease, **663**
Systemic vascular resistance, 221*t*

T$_3$. *See* Triiodothyronine (T$_3$)
T$_4$. *See* Thyroxine (T$_4$)
Tachycardia
  with atelectasis, 26
  in craniocerebral trauma, 902–903
  in endotracheal intubation, 196
Tachypnea
  with atelectasis, 26
  in pneumonia, 27
Tacrolimus, for transplant recipient, 470, 1385
Taeniae coli, 705, 707*i*
Takayasu's arteritis, **852**
Takayasu's disease, and abdominal aortic coarctation, 829
Talc
  for malignant pleural effusion, 359
  for pneumothorax, 368–369
Talofibular ligament, tear of, 1172
Talonavicular joint, dislocation of, 1172–1173
Talus
  body and head of, fractures of, 1173
  fracture of, 1173
  injuries of, **1172–1173**
  lateral process of, fracture of, 1173
  neck of, fracture of, 1173
Tamoxifen
  anticancer therapy with, **1356**
  for breast cancer, 321, 329, 332, 333*t*, 334
    in males, 340
  for retroperitoneal fibrosis, 532
Tapeworm. *See* Echinococcosis
Targeted therapy, for lung cancer, 398–401, 403
Tarsometatarsal dislocation(s), **1175**
Taxanes, for breast cancer, 332–333
T cells (T lymphocytes), 106–107, 108, 1373
  arginine and, 162
  cytotoxic, 1373
  helper, 1373
Telangiectasia, 873, 875, **1269**, 1342
  in adolescent, 1332
  hereditary hemorrhagic, 736, 1342
Temozolomide, for brain tumors, 926
Temperature. *See* Body temperature
Temporal bone, fractures of, **972**
Temporalis muscle flap, **1236**
Temporal lobe, tumors in, **922–923**
Temporary airway, establishment of, 233, 233*i*
Tendinitis
  biceps, **1198**
  calcific, in shoulder, **1197–1198**
  of hip, **1200–1201**
  rotator cuff, **1197**

Tendon transfer, for upper extremity nerve injury, 1281
Teniposide, 1355
Tennis elbow, **1199–1200**
Tenolysis, in hand, 1276
Tenorrhaphy, in hand, 1276, 1276*i*
Tenosynovitis
  phlegmonous, of hand, 1283
  pyogenic, of hand, 1283, 1283*i*
  stenosing, in hand, **1278**
Tension pneumothorax, 236–237, 237*i*, 244, 246, 367
  cardiac compressive shock caused by, 206, 207
Tensor fasciae latae flap, **1236**
  for pressure sores, 1264
Teratodermoids, mediastinal, 376
Teratoma, **1346–1347**
  benign cystic, 66, 1110
  cardiac, 469
  cervical, **1347**
  immature, ovarian, 1110
  mediastinal, 377, 1311, **1347**
  sacrococcygeal, **1347**
Terlipressin, for variceal bleeding, 581–582
Terminal colostomy, 752, 754*i*
Testicular appendices, torsion of, **1080**, 1339
Testicular cancer, **1070–1072**, 1071*t*
  in cryptorchid testis, 1338
Testicular torsion, **1339**
  of appendages, **1080**, 1339
  versus epididymitis, 1040
  intravaginal, **1079–1080**
  neonatal (extravaginal), **1029**
Testicular vein, and varicocele, 1079
Testimony, expert. *See* Witness(es), expert
Testis
  anatomy of, **1017**
  anomalies of, **1029**
  ectopic, 1338, 1339
  embryology of, 1013–1014, 1016*i*
  injuries to, **1053**
  masses of, 1071
  tumors of, **1070–1072**, 1071*t*
    versus epididymitis, 1040
  undescended, 786, **1338–1339**
Testosterone
  for impotence, 1083
  in male infertility, 1081
Tetanus, 124, **127–128**
  drug therapy for, 136*t*
  immunization/prophylaxis against, 134, 134*t*
Tetany, with hypoparathyroidism, 317–318
Tetracaine, for eye examination, 999
Tetracycline
  for aphthous stomatitis, 985
  for chlamydial proctitis, 777
  for chronic prostatitis, **1040**
  dosage of, renal failure and, 137
  indications for, 127, 135*t*, 136*t*
  for malignant pleural effusion, 359
  pancreatitis and, 629

Tetracycline (*cont.*)
  pleurodesis using, for pneumothorax, 368–369
  as sclerosant, 23
Tetralogy of Fallot, 458, **460–462**, 460*i*
  omphalocele and, 1340
  and ventricular septal defect, 452
Thalamotomy, for Parkinson's disease, 947–948
Thalassemia
  major, **657**
  minor, 657
Thallium scintigraphy, 42
  reversible defect on, significance of, 44*t*
Thermal injuries. *See also* Burn(s)
  of eye, **1008**
  pathology and pathophysiology of, 268–269
Thermogenesis, in pediatric patients, 1294
Thermography, 322
  scrotal, in male infertility, 1081
Thermoregulation
  for increased intracranial pressure, **891**
  in pediatric patients, 1294
  in response to injury, 107
Thiamin. *See* Vitamin B$_1$
Thiazide diuretics
  and hypercalcemia, 312
  pancreatitis and, 629
  for renal stones, 1043
Thioguanine, 1355
Thiopental
  in aneurysm surgery, 899–900
  indications for, 195
Thiotepa
  for bladder tumors, 1064–1065
  for malignant pleural effusion, 359
Third-degree burns, 268, 268*i*
Third spacing, 107, 109
Third ventricle, 890*i*
Thompson procedure, for lymphedema, 887
Thoracentesis, for thoracic empyema, 361
Thoracic aorta
  aneurysms of, **431–432**
  atherosclerotic disease of, 408
  disease of, **431–434**
  dissection of, **432–434**
  injuries to, 257, 257*t*
Thoracic duct, injuries of, **247**
Thoracic empyema, **360–366**, 360*i*, 361*i*, 362*t*
  bacteriology of, 361, 361*i*
  treatment of, 362–366, 363*i*, 364*i*, 365*i*
Thoracic injuries, **244–248**
Thoracic outlet syndrome, **844–845**
  in subclavian vein thrombosis, 879
Thoracic spine
  disk disease of, **955–956**
  disk herniation in, **955–956**
Thoracoepigastric vein, thrombophlebitis of, **353**
Thoracolumbar spine
  fractures of, 1121
  imaging of, 1120
  injury to
    associated injuries, 1118

complications of, 1120
    external support for, 1123
    with neurologic injury, 1123, 1124*i*
Thoracoscopy
  for hemothorax, 245
  and response to injury, 101
  for splanchnicectomy, for chronic pancreatitis, 642
Thoracotomy
  emergency room, **238–239**, 238*i*
  for esophageal perforation, 372
  for lung abscess, 384
  for spinal cord tumors, 928
Thorax, anatomy of, 345*i*
Three-stage procedure, for diverticulitis, **734**
Thrombectomy
  for acute mesenteric vascular occlusion, 699
  iliofemoral, 877
Thromboangiitis obliterans, **828**
  and small artery occlusive disease, 827
Thrombocytopenia. *See also* Heparin-induced thrombocytopenia with thrombosis syndrome (HIT/TS)
  in HIV-positive patients, 659
  in liver disease, 57
  with or without platelet dysfunction, 56
  in surgical patients, 54–55, **55**
  in uremia, 56
  in Wiskott-Aldrich syndrome, 661
Thrombocytopenic purpura
  idiopathic, **659–660**
  immune, **659–660**
  thrombotic, **660–661**
Thrombocytosis
  after splenectomy, 666
  essential, 53
Thromboembolism. *See also* Embolism
  after splenectomy, 666
  amputation and, 867
  in elderly, 67–68
  pleural effusion and, 360
  prevention of, 28
  pulmonary, **880–882**
    postoperative, 877
  risk factors for, 9
  in spinal cord-injured patient, 1120
  venous, prevention of, 23
Thrombolysis, in subclavian vein thrombosis, 879
Thrombophlebitis
  cerebral, 960
  migratory, in pancreatic adenocarcinoma, 644
  septic, 883
  superficial, **882–883**
    versus lymphangitis, 887
  suppurative, appendicitis and, 670–671
  of thoracoepigastric vein, **353**
  Trousseau's, 882
Thrombosis. *See also* Embolism; Heparin-induced thrombocytopenia with thrombosis syndrome (HIT/TS)
  and arterial occlusion, 825, 826
  and atherosclerosis, 814

calf vein, 875
  consciousness in, 888
  in disseminated intravascular coagulation, 58
  effort, 878, 878*i*
  of internal carotid artery, 893*i*
  mesenteric, 698
  of renal vein, **1078**, 1078*i*
  of sagittal sinus, 896*i*
  and superior vena caval syndrome, 374
  venous
    axillary-subclavian, **878–880**
    calf, 875
    deep, **875–877**
      postoperative, 877
    in pulmonary thromboembolism, 880
Thrombotic thrombocytopenic purpura (TTP), **660–661**
Thrush, **985**
Thumb
  functions of, 1270
  gamekeeper's, 1279
Thurston-Holland sign, 1178
Thymectomy, 378–379
Thymoma, **377–379**, 1311
  mediastinal, 376
  paraneoplastic syndromes with, 1371*t*
  and superior vena caval syndrome, 373
Thymus
  carcinoma of, **379**
  cyst of, 1311
  tumors of, **377–379**
Thyroglossal duct remnant, **1302–1303**, 1302*i*
Thyroid cartilage, injuries to, 243
Thyroidectomy, 307
  for hypoparathyroidism, 317
  subtotal, for hyperthyroidism, 302
  survival rates after, 306, 306*i*
Thyroid gland
  anatomy of, **298**, 299*i*
  benign tumors of, **305**
  cancer of, 304
    and superior vena caval syndrome, 373
    types of, **306–307**
  diseases of, **300–307**
    in surgical patient, **40–41**
  ectopic, 1302–1303
  embryology of, **298**
  evaluation of, 298–300
  inflammatory disease of, **304–305**
  lingual, 1302
  malignant tumors of, **305–307**
  physiology of, **298**
Thyroid hormone(s), actions of, 167–168
Thyroiditis
  acute suppurative, 304–305
  Hashimoto's, 305
  Riedel's, 305
  subacute, 305
Thyroid nodules, evaluation of, 303–304, 303*i*
Thyroid-stimulating hormone (thyrotropin, TSH), 106
  actions of, 167
  assays, 298

pituitary tumors secreting, 300 (*See also* Hyperthyroidism)
Thyroid storm, 40, 302
Thyrotoxicosis, 40. *See also* Hyperthyroidism
Thyrotropic adenomas, 921
Thyrotropin (TSH), 298
Thyrotropin-releasing factor (TRF), 298
Thyrotropin-releasing hormone (TRH) test, 301
Thyroxine (T_4), 106, 298
Thyroxine (T_4) pseudothyrotoxicosis, 300
Tibia
  distal, fractures of, 1171, 1172*i*
  distal epiphyses of, fracture of, in children, 1182–1183
  fracture of, 1263
    in children, 1182
  proximal, fractures of, **1164–1166**
  shaft of, fracture of, 1167–1169, 1168*i*
Ticarcillin. *See also* Penicillin, antipseudomonal
  dosage of
    in hepatic failure, 139*t*
    in renal failure, 139*t*
  pharmacology of, 139*t*
Ticarcillin-clavulanic acid, for acute secondary bacterial peritonitis, 519
Ticlodipine hydrochloride, for cerebrovascular disease prevention, 850
Tidal volume, in mechanical ventilation, 216
Tietze's syndrome, **353**
Tilting disk mechanical heart valve, 428–429, 429*i*
Time-of-flight angiography, 894, 896*i*
Timolol, for angina pectoris, 412
Tinea unguium, 1284
Tinel's sign, 1280
Tinel's test, for thoracic outlet syndrome, 845
Tinnitus, **971–972**
  in Meniere's disease, 975
Tinzaparin, 54
Tissue engineering, 1230
Tissue transfer, for head and neck tumors, 295
Titrofiban, for angina pectoris, 413
TNM staging system, 285, 286*i*, 1353
  of bladder tumors, 1063*t*
  for breast cancer, 326, 327*i*
  of colorectal cancer, 723, 724*t*
  for lung cancer, 398, 400*t*
  for mesothelioma, 370, 370*t*
  of prostate cancer, 1067*t*
  of renal adenocarcinoma, 1058*t*
  for testicular cancer, 1071*t*
Tobacco
  and head and neck tumors, 282
  and lung cancer, 395
Tobramycin. *See also* Aminoglycosides
  indications for, 137
  for infection control, 385
Toe(s)
  amputation of, 859, **862**, 862*i*
  clubbing of, 458
  great, sesamoids of, fracture of, **1176**
  phalanges of, fractures and dislocations of, **1176**

TOF angiography. *See* Time-of-flight angiography
Tolazoline
  and arterial spasm, 261
  for intra-arterial injections, 858
Tongue, cancer of, 282
Tongue-tie, **986**
Tonometry, **999**
Tonsillar herniation, **891**
Tonsillectomy, for chronic tonsillitis, 988
Tonsillitis, 46
  acute, 988
  chronic, 988
Tonsilloadenoidal hyperplasia, 988
Tonsils, cancer of, 282, 296
Tophectomy, in hand, 1286
Topoisomerase inhibitors, 1355
Topotecan, 1355
Torsion
  of spermatic cord, **1079–1080**
  testicular
    versus epididymitis, 1040
    intravaginal, **1079–1080**
    neonatal (extravaginal), **1029**
  of testicular appendages, **1080**
Torticollis, **1303**
Tort law, 75–76
Torts
  intentional, 75–76
  negligent, 76–78
Torus mandibularis, **986**
Torus palatinus, **986**
Tositumomab, 1358, 1369
Total anomalous pulmonary venous connection (TAPVC), **455–457**, 456*i*
Total-contact suction socket prosthesis, 870
Total energy expenditure (TEE), 160, 161, 161*t*
Total extraperitoneal mesh placement (TEP), for inguinal hernia repair, 788
Total lymphocyte count, 157*t*, 158*t*, 160
Total lymphoid irradiation (TLI), for Hodgkin's lymphoma, 1366
Total parenteral nutrition. *See* Parenteral nutrition, total
Tourniquet
  and amputation, 864
  for hemorrhage control, 237–238
Tourniquet tests, 874
Toxic chemicals, in smoke inhalation, 275, 275*t*
Toxic megacolon
  in Crohn's disease, 748
  in ulcerative colitis, 743, 744*i*, 745
Toxic shock syndrome, streptococcal, 124
Toxin(s). *See also* Exotoxin(s); Hemotoxin; Myotoxin; Neurotoxin(s)
  botulinum, indications for, 770
  clostridial, 124
Toxoplasma brain abscesses, 959
Trabeculectomy, for chronic glaucoma, 1006
Trabeculoplasty, for chronic glaucoma, 1006
Trace elements, in nutritional support, 163–164, 164*t*

Trachea
  congenital stenosis of, **1307–1308**
  foreign bodies in, **990**
    in children, **1333**
  injuries to, 241, 245
    treatment of, 243
  trauma to, 991
Tracheal diverticula, 380
Tracheitis, 46–47
Tracheobronchial atresia, **380**
Tracheoesophageal fistula
  with esophageal atresia, 1313–1315, 1313*i*
  without esophageal atresia, 1313–1315, 1313*i*
Tracheomalacia, **1307–1308**
Tracheostomy, 214, 215
  in depressed consciousness, 889
  for inhalation injuries, 276
Tracheotomy
  emergency, 233, 233*i*
  for spinal cord injuries, 243
Traction, for spinal fracture, 1120–1121, 1123
Trail Making Test B, 907
TRAM flap. *See* Transverse rectus abdominis musculocutaneous (TRAM) flap
Transabdominal intraperitoneal onlay of mesh (IPOM), for inguinal hernia repair, 788
Transabdominal preperitoneal mesh technique (TAPP), for inguinal hernia repair, 788
Transaortic balloon pump, for cardiogenic shock, 209
Transcranial motor evoked potential, in spinal cord surgery, 898–899
Transcutaneous electrical nerve stimulation, for chronic benign pain, 951
Transcutaneous tracheal airway, for craniocerebral trauma, 903
Transesophageal echocardiography
  intraoperative, 45
  for mitral regurgitation, 423, 423*i*
Transfer, of patient with spinal cord injury, 910
Transferrin
  serum levels of, 7, 157*t*, 158, 158*t*, 159*t*
  in small intestine fistulas, 697
Transferrin-like growth factor, and lung cancer, 396
Transfusion reactions
  allergic, 60
  hemolytic, 59–60
Transfusion therapy, **58–62**. *See also* Blood transfusion
  coumarin anticoagulants and, 55
  in newborn, 1299
  in pulmonary failure, 219
  serologic considerations in, 58
  for upper gastrointestinal hemorrhage, 549–550
Transhepatic portal venous sampling, for insulinoma, 649
Transhumeral amputation, **867**

Transient ischemic attack (TIA), 847–848
  prevention of, 849–852
Transitional atrioventricular canal defect, 451
Transitional cell tumors
  of bladder, 1062, 1064
  renal, *versus* renal stones, 1043
  of renal pelvis and calices, 1059, 1060, 1060*i*
  of ureter, 1061
Transit time
  colonic, slow, 709–710
  intestinal, in short bowel syndrome, 682
  orocecal, 677
Transjugular intrahepatic portosystemic shunt (TIPS), for variceal bleeding, 582
Transluminal balloon angioplasty, for intracranial aneurysm, 942–943
Transluminal percutaneous devices, for atrial septal defect, 450
Transmetatarsal amputation, **863**, 863*i*
Transmyocardial laser revascularization, 414
Transperitoneal metastasis, of colorectal cancer, **718**
Transplant coronary artery disease, 470
Transportation, from accident scene, **234**
Transposition of the great arteries, 449, 458
  corrected, **466–467**
  letter designations of, 464
  normal ventricular arrangement, **463–466,** 464*i*
  and ventricular septal defect, 452
Transrectal ultrasonography
  in male infertility, 1081
  for prostate cancer
    monitoring, 1067, 1068*i*
    screening, 1066
Transtentorial herniation, **891,** 891*t*
Transthoracic echocardiography, for aortic stenosis, 426
Transudates, 357
Transureteroureterostomy, 1050
Transurethral incision of prostate, for benign prostatic hyperplasia, 1035
Transversalis fascia, 783
Transverse colon, 706*i*
Transverse colostomy, 753
  for large bowel obstruction, 715
Transverse rectus abdominis musculocutaneous (TRAM) flap, for breast reconstruction, 337, 1261–1262
Transverse sinus, 890*i*
Transversus abdominis muscle, 783
Trapezius muscle flap, **1236**
Trapped lung, 368
Trash foot, 827
Trauma, **230–266**
  abdominal wall hernia caused by, **795–796**
  acoustic, 969
  acute, case example of, 225–226
  arterial, iatrogenic, **858**
  and aspiration, 26
  bile duct, **619–620**
  blunt
    abdominal, 249–252

arterial, 257
chest, 208
to neck, 243
to ocular adnexa, **1009,** 1009*t*
to orbit, **1009,** 1009*t*
brain injury in, **900–908**
  outcome with, 908
cardiac arrest following, 234
cardiac compressive shock in, **240**
cardiogenic shock in, **240**
in children, **936–937**
consciousness in, 888
corneal, 1001*t*
craniocerebral, **900–908**
and emergency amputation, 861
epidemiology of, 230
evaluation in, **234–241**
genitourinary tract, **1048–1054**
hepatic, **569–571**
history-taking in, 2
hypovolemic shock in, 205–206, **239**
initial management of, 1117–1118
intestinal changes following, 678
laryngeal, **991**
management of
  at accident scene, 232–234
  airway and, 232–234, 233*i,* 236, 236*i*
  breathing and, 236–237, 237*i*
  circulation in, 237–238
  emergency room thoracotomy in, 238–239, 238*i*
  exposure and, 238
  imaging studies in, 240
  immobilization in, 234
  intravenous therapy in, 234
  laboratory studies in, 240
  prehospital care in, 232
  prehospital transport in, 234
  primary survey in, 236–240
  priorities in, 240–241
  resuscitation phase of, 239–240
  secondary survey in, 240–241
  triage and, 232, **234,** 235*i*
  vascular access in, 238
metabolic response to, **100–111,** 167–169, 168*i*
multiple injuries in, 240–241
nasal, **982–983**
neurogenic shock in, **239–240**
neurologic disability and, 238
nonaccidental, 936–937
penetrating (*See* Penetrating trauma)
to peripheral nerves, **913–914**
physical examination of patient in, 4
prevention of, 230–231
pulmonary failure in, 212
to residual limb, 869
rewarming after, 110
salivary gland, **987**
and sepsis, case example of, 227–228
shock and, 239–240
spinal injury in, clinical assessment of, 1117–1118

survival in, prediction of, 225
tracheal, 991
Trauma centers, 231–232
Trauma systems, **231–232**
Traumatic aneurysms, 938
Traumatic arterial occlusion, 825, 826–827
Traumatic diaphragmatic hernia, **501–502**
Traumatic neuralgia. *See* Reflex sympathetic dystrophy
Traumatic taps, *versus* subarachnoid hemorrhage, 940
Travel history, acute abdomen and, 508
Treacher-Collins syndrome, 1259
Treadmill testing, for peripheral arterial insufficiency, 819
Tremor, essential, **949**
Trench foot, 279
Trendelenburg's position, 206, 209
Treponema infection, drug therapy for, 136*t*
TRH test. *See* Thyrotropin-releasing hormone (TRH) test
Triage, **232, 234,** 235*i*
Triamcinolone acetonide
  for aphthous stomatitis, 985
    in AIDS, 998
  for keloids and hypertrophic scars, 1243–1244
Triceps skinfold thickness, 158, 158*t,* 159*t*
Trichobezoars, 562
Tricuspid atresia, **463**
  and single ventricle, 467
Tricuspid endocarditis, 426
Tricuspid insufficiency, 466–467
Tricuspid regurgitation, 424–425
Tricuspid stenosis, 425
Tricuspid valve, 419
  disease of, **424–426**
  replacement of, for tricuspid stenosis, 426
Trigeminal neuralgia, **951**
Trigeminal schwannoma, **926**
Trigger finger, **1278**
Triglycerides
  digestion of, in small intestine, 678–679
  medium-chain, for pancreatic insufficiency, 643
Triiodothyronine (T₃), 298
  reverse, 106
Triiodothyronine (T₃) suppression test, 301
Triiodothyronine (T₃) toxicosis, 300
Trimethoprim-sulfamethoxazole
  for bronchiectasis, 385
  dosage of
    in hepatic failure, 139*t*
    in renal failure, 139*t*
  indications for, 129, 135*t,* 136*t*
  for lung abscess, 384
  mechanism of action of, 140
  ototoxicity of, 998
  pharmacology of, 139*t*
  for pneumocystosis, 394
  for *Yersinia* enteritis, 694
Triquetrum, fracture of, 1147
Trismus, 282
Tropicamide, for eye examination, 999

Tropisetron, indications for, 200
Trousseau's thrombophlebitis, 882
True aneurysm, 829
Truncus arteriosus, 449, **457–458**, 457*i*
  and ventricular septal defect, 452
Trypsin, in pancreatitis, 629
T tube, in choledocholithiasis, 615
Tubectomy, sterilization by, 1091
Tube feeding. *See* Enteral feeding
Tubercle bacilli, and lung abscess, 383
Tuberculosis, **387–390**, 389*i*
  anal, 769, 772
  and bronchiectasis, 385
  and bronchiolithiasis, 386
  and chronic mediastinitis, 372
  versus Crohn's disease, **691**
  differential diagnosis of, 358*t*
  drug therapy for, 141
  genitourinary, **1040–1042**
  hand involvement in, 1284
  intestinal, **694–695**
  renal, 1041
    versus renal stones, 1043
  skin tests for, 349
  spinal, **960–961**
Tuberculous adenitis, 997
Tuberculous empyema, 388
Tuberculous peritonitis, **527–528**
Tuboplasty, 1087
Tularemia, 112
  drug therapy for, 135*t*
Tumor(s)
  of abdominal wall, 796
  adrenal, as incidentalomas, **811–812**
  anal, **781–782**
  benign, 1352
  biopsy of, **1353**
  bone, **1222–1229**
    of hand, 1288
  botryoid, 1345–1346
  cardiac, **434–435**, 434*t*, 435*f*, **469–470**
  childhood, **1342–1349**
  congenital, **920–921**
  desmoid, 728, 796, 1361
  endodermal sinus, 1347
    ovarian, 1110
  Ewing's (*See* Ewing's sarcoma)
  glomus
    in hand, 1288
    jugulare, 972–973
    tympanicum, 972–973
    vagale, 973
  grading of, **1352**
  of hand, 1287–1288
  of head and neck, reconstructive surgery for,
    1260–1261
  intracranial, **915–927**
    in adults, 916*i*
    in children, 915*i*
    and consciousness, 888
    paraneoplastic syndromes with, 1371*t*
  islet cell, paraneoplastic syndromes with,
    1371*t*
  of liver, in childhood, **1347–1349**

malignant, 1352 (*See also* Cancer)
mixed mesodermal, of uterus, 1109–1110
neural, paraneoplastic syndromes with,
  1371*t*
neurogenic
  chest wall, 354
  mediastinal, 375, 376
nomenclature for, 1352
progression of, 1352
skin, **1244–1252**
  benign, **1245–1249**
  malignant, **1249–1252**
  premalignant, **1249**
spinal, 1213
staging of, **1352–1353**
virilizing, 810
yolk sac, 1347
Tumor antigen(s), 1357
Tumor infiltrating lymphocytes (TIL), 1358
Tumor markers
  in liver cancer, 572
  in pancreatic adenocarcinoma, 644
Tumor necrosis factor (TNF), 117*t*
  anticancer therapy with, 1358–1359
  in nonspecific immunotherapy, 1357–1358
  in response to injury, 108
Tumor suppressor gene mutations, and lung
  cancer, 396
Tumor vaccine(s), **1358**
Tunica albuginea, rupture of, 1053
Tuning fork tests, of hearing loss, 963
Turcot's syndrome, 727–728
Turner's syndrome, and aortic coarctation, 445
Two-stage procedure
  for diverticulitis, **734**, 734*i*
  for large bowel obstruction, 715
Tylenol No. 3. *See* Acetaminophen with
  codeine
Tylox. *See* Oxycodone, with acetaminophen
Tympanic membrane, perforation of,
  967–968, 967*f*, 967*i*
Tympanometry, in otitis media with effusion,
  966
Typhoid, intestinal manifestations of, **695**

Ulcer(s)
  in achalasia, 478
  anal, **768–770**
  anastomotic, 542–543
  arterial, 96
  in burn patient, 273–274
  chronic, 95–96
    in diabetes, 96
  chronic radiation dermatitis and, 1249
  corneal, **1002–1003**
  in Crohn's disease, 689–690
  Curling's, in burn patient, 273–274
  Cushing's, 556, 890
  decubitus, **95**, 1118 (*See also* Pressure sores)
    spinal cord injury and, 912
  in diabetic patient, 96
  duodenal, **539–544**
    bleeding, 550
    in children, 1332

    recurrent, 542–543
  gastric, **546–547**
    increased intracranial pressure and, 890
    type I, 546
    type II, 546–547
    type III, 547
  gastroduodenal, in burn patient, 273–274
  ischemic, 96
  leg, chronic, hereditary spherocytosis and,
    656
  marginal, 542–543
  Marjolin, 1252
  Meleney's, 1283
  nonhealing, and peripheral arterial insuffi-
    ciency, 817
  peptic (*See* Peptic ulcer)
  in peripheral arterial insufficiency, 818
  prepyloric, 546–547
  rectal, 767
    solitary, 762
  stomal, 542–543
  stress, **555–556**, 555*i*
    after hepatic trauma, 570
    in children, 1332
    with partial hepatectomy, 568
    postoperative prevention of, 15
  trophic, osteomyelitis caused by, 1217
  venous, 95–96
Ulcerating carcinoma, 557
Ulcerative colitis (UC), **741–746**
  cancer screening in, 719
  versus Crohn's disease, 691, 747*t*
  extracolonic manifestations of, 743
  idiopathic mocosal, **741–746**
  and postoperative convulsions, 34
Ulcerative proctitis, 741
Ulna
  coronoid process, fractures of, 1137–1138,
    1137*i*
  distal, 1143
  olecranon, fractures of, 1137
  proximal, fractures of, **1137–1138**, 1137*i*
  shaft of, 1143
    fractures of, **1141–1143**
  styloid, fractures of, 1146
Ulnar bursa, 1272
Ulnar nerve, 1272, 1274*i*
  compression of, 1280
  injury to, 1281
    improper positioning and, 195
Ultrasonic lipectomy, **1268**
Ultrasonography
  in acute abdomen, 510*t*, 512–513
  in acute appendicitis, 669
  in acute cholecystitis, 608
  in acute pancreatitis, 632
  of adrenal incidentalomas, 811
  of anorectal anomalies, 1326
  of arterial injuries, 259
  of bile duct malignancies, 617
  of biliary atresia, 1334
  of biliary tree, **600**
  of bladder tumors, **1063**
  in breast cancer, 66, 320, 322

Ultrasonography (*cont.*)
of choledochal cyst, 1334
in colorectal cancer, 720
Doppler, in small bowel obstruction, 687
duplex
in chronic venous insufficiency, 883
in deep venous thrombosis, 876
in portal flow and pressure measurement, 578–579, 584
in subclavian vein thrombosis, 879
endorectal, 781
of gallbladder, in pregnancy, 64
in gallstone disease, 605
of hepatic abscess, 593
of hepatic adenomas, 577
of infrarenal abdominal aortic aneurysms, 831
of insulinoma, intraoperative, 649
of intraperitoneal abscesses, 523
in jaundice, 602–603
of liver cancer, 572
in male infertility, 1081
of neck injuries, 242
in neurodiagnosis, **892**
in obstructive uropathy, **1031**
in occult infection, 117
of pancreatic pseudocyst, 636
in pregnancy, 64
in prostate cancer
monitoring, 1067, 1068*i*
screening, 1066
renal, 50
in renal adenocarcinoma, **1055,** 1056*i*
of renal transplant, 1380
in strangulation obstruction of small bowel, 686
in testicular cancer, 1071
transrectal, 760, 771–772
transvaginal
in ectopic pregnancy, 1102–1103
of endometrium, 1088
of uterine adnexa, 1101
in ureteral injury, 1049
of uterine anomalies, 1086
of uterine leiomyomas, 1100
Ultraviolet radiation, ocular burns caused by, **1008**
Umbilical cyst, 1330
Umbilical hernia, **1339**
Umbilical sinus, 1330
Undescended testis, **1338–1339**
Undifferentiated carcinoma, of thyroid gland, 305, **306–307,** 307
Unicameral bone cyst, **1228–1229,** 1228*i*
Unified Parkinson's Disease Rating Scale, 948
Unifocalization, 461
Union Internationale Contre le Cancer (UICC)
cancer staging system of, 1353
lung cancer staging system of, 398
Universal precautions, 12, 120
Upper esophageal sphincter dysfunction, **475**
Upper extremity. *See also* Hand(s)
amputation of, **866–867,** 867*i*

rehabilitation after, 869
aneurysms in, **842**
atherosclerosis in, 815
compression neuropathies of, **1280**
fractures and dislocations of, in children, **1179–1181**
necrotizing soft tissue infections of, 1283
nerve injuries in, 1280–1281
position of function, 1270, 1271*i*
position of injury, 1270
position of rest, 1270, 1271*i*
prosthesis for, 866
Upper gastrointestinal hemorrhage, **548–550**
causes of, 549, 549*t*
Mallory-Weiss syndrome and, 551
Upper gastrointestinal series
for pancreatic abscess, 639
for pancreatic adenocarcinoma, **645**
for pancreatic pseudocyst, 636
Upper motor neuron disorders, 1186–1187
in neuropathic bladder, 1075
Urachal anomalies, 1026
Urachal cyst, 1026
Urachal diverticulum, 1026
Uracil, dietary, 162
Urea, 166
Urea nitrogen appearance (UNA), in renal failure, 187–188, 187*t*
Uremia, platelet dysfunction in, 56
Ureolysis, in colon, 707
Ureter
anatomy of, **1015, 1017**
anomalies of, **1021–1023**
changes in, in obstructive uropathy, **1030**
congenital obstruction of, **1021,** 1021*i*
division of, anastomosis of, 1050
duplication of, **1021,** 1022*i*
injuries to, 255, **1049–1050**
obstruction of, 50
resection of, 1050
stenosis of, **1032–1033**
stones in, **1045–1046,** 1045*i*
tuberculosis of, 1041
tumors of, **1061**
versus ureteral calculi, 1046
Ureteral bud, development of, 1015*i*
Ureteral orifice, ectopic, **1021–1022,** 1022*i*
Ureterocele, **1022–1023,** 1023*i*
Ureterolysis, for retroperitoneal fibrosis, 532
Ureteropelvicaliceal system
changes in, in obstructive uropathy, **1030**
physiology of, **1018**
Ureteropelvic junction, obstruction of, 1020–1021, **1032,** 1032*i*
Ureteroplasty, extravesical, for vesicoureteral reflux, 1026
Ureteropyelography, in ureteropelvic junction obstruction, 1032, 1032*i*
Ureterotrigonal complex, 1024*i*
Ureterovaginal fistula, *versus* ureteral injury, 1050
Ureterovesical junction
physiology of, **1018**

reflux in, 1023–1026
Urethra
anatomy of, **1017**
anomalies of, **1028–1029**
changes in, in obstructiveuropathy, **1030**
diverticulum of, **1028**
embryology of, **1013,** 1015*i,* 1016*i*
injuries to, 254, **1051–1052,** 1051*i,* 1053*i*
prostatic, 1017
stricture of, **1028, 1035**
versus benign prostatic hyperplasia, 1034
in urethral injury, 1051
tuberculosis of, 1041
tumors of, **1070**
Urethral caruncle, female, 1079
Urethral diverticulum, 1079, 1093
Urethral meatus
in epispadias, 1028
in hypospadias, 1028, 1028*i*
Urethral sphincter, intrinsic deficiency of, 1092, 1093
Urethral valves, posterior, **1029**
Urethritis, female, **1078–1079**
Urethrography, in bladder injury, 1051
Urethroplasty, for obstructive uropathy, **1031**
Urethrotomy
for obstructive uropathy, **1031**
for urethral stricture, 1035
Urethrovesical angle, in urinary stress incontinence, 1078
Urge incontinence, 1075, 1092, 1093
Uric acid renal stones, 1044
Urinalysis, 49, 142, 143
in acute abdomen, 510*t,* 511
in bladder tumors, 1063, 1064
in hypovolemia, 204
in renal adenocarcinoma, 1054
in renal pelvis and calices tumors, 1060
Urinary bladder. *See* Bladder
Urinary catheter, in acute abdomen, 515
Urinary diversions
for bladder tumors, 1065
for neuropathic bladder, 1076
suprapubic, 1076
supravesical, 1076
Urinary incontinence
mixed, 1092
overflow, 1092
pelvic organ prolapse and, 1092–1093
stress, **1078,** 1092, 1093
treatment of, 1093
urge, 1075, 1092, 1093
Urinary retention, postoperative, **33**
Urinary tract. *See also* Genitourinary tract; *specific organ or structure*
calculi in
ileostomy and, 753*t*
and short bowel syndrome, 680
female, congenital anomalies of, 1085
fistulas of, **1093–1094**
infections of, **1036–1042**
catheterization and, 1036–1037
classification of, 1036

postoperative, **33–34**
spinal cord injury and, 912
urologic instrumentation or surgery and, 1036–1037
in vesicoureteral reflux, 1024, 1025
lesions of, differential diagnosis of, 514
postoperative complications in, **33–34**
surgery of, and urinary tract infections, 1036–1037
Urine
in acute appendicitis, 669
cell casts in, 49
composition of, 142, 143, 144*t*
electrolytes in, 153
extravasation of
in bladder injury, 1051
in ureteral injury, 1049
in urethral injury, 1053*i*
osmolality of, 49
pH of, 49, 153
red blood cells in, 49
residual volume of, in hyperreflexic bladder, 1075
specific gravity of, 49
volume of, 142, 143
white blood cells in, 49
Urine output, in hypovolemic shock, 239
Urobilinogen, 599
in hereditary spherocytosis, 656
Urodynamics, **1074–1075**
studies of, in benign prostatic hyperplasia, 1034
Uroflowmetry, **1074**
Urography
in bladder injury, 1051
in bladder tumors, 1063, 1063*i*
in kidney injury, 1048
in obstructive uropathy, **1031**
in prostate cancer, 1067
in renal adenocarcinoma, 1055, 1055*i*
with renal stones, 1042, 1043*i*
in retroperitoneal fibrosis, **1033**
in testicular cancer, 1071
with ureteral calculi, 1045, 1045*i*
in ureteral injury, 1049
with ureteral tumors, 1061, 1061*i*
in ureteropelvic junction obstruction, 1032
Urology, 1013–1084
Uropathy, obstructive, **1029–1032**
Ursodiol
for dissolution of gallstones, 606
for sclerosing cholangitis, 624
Uterine artery embolization, for leiomyomas, 1100
Uterine bleeding. *See also* Vaginal bleeding
abnormal, **1087–1089**
with uterine leiomyomas, 1100
dysfunctional, 1088, 1089
intermenstrual, 1088, 1107
postcoital, 1107
Uterine nerve ablation, 1090
Uterus
absence of, 1085
bicornuate, 1086

duplication defects of, 1086
injuries of, 254
sarcomas of, **1109–1110**
septate, 1086
Uterus didelphys, 1086

Vaccine(s)
for bronchiectasis, 385
tumor, 1358
VACTERL syndrome, 1275, 1314, 1326
Vagina
absence of, **1085–1086**
adenocarcinoma of, 1105
artificial, 1086
carcinoma in situ of, 1105
carcinoma of, **1105–1106**
congenital anomalies of, **1085–1086**
duplication of, **1085**
prolapse of, 1093
septum of
longitudinal, 1085
transverse, **1085**
tumors of, benign, 1095
urinary leakage from, 1094
Vaginal bleeding. *See also* Uterine bleeding
postmenopausal, 1088
with adenocarcinoma of fallopian tube, 1110
in endometrial cancer, 1108
in pregnancy, with gestational trophoblastic disease, 1113
Vagotomy
diarrhea after, 544
for duodenal ulcer, 541, 542*i*
for gastric ulcer, 547
for perforated peptic ulcer, 554
proximal gastric, for duodenal ulcer, 541
selective, for duodenal ulcer, 542*i*
for stress ulcers, 556
truncal, for duodenal ulcer, 542, 542*i*
Vagus nerve
pancreatic innervation by, 625
small bowel innervation by, 674
stimulator, for intractable seizures in children, 937
Valacyclovir, **141**
for Bell's palsy, 977
Valgus
definition of, 1116, 1194
of knee, 1183
Valves, venous, 871, 873
Valves of Houston, 756, 757*i*
Valvotomy, for valvular aortic stenosis, 443
Valvulae conniventes, 674, 675*i*
Valvular heart disease, 408, **419–428**
Valvuloplasty, for chronic venous insufficiency, 884
Vancomycin
for antibiotic-associated colitis, 749
for brain abscess, 959
dosage of
in hepatic failure, 139*t*
in renal failure, 137, 139*t*
indications for, 127, 135*t*, 136*t*

pharmacology of, 139*t*
prophylactic, in valvular heart disease, 45
resistance to, 120
prevention of, 137
spread of, control of, 137
Varicella-zoster virus (VZV), infection by, treatment of, 141
Varices
bleeding from
in children, 1332
clinical findings with, 580–581
in liver disease, 579, **580–583**
mortality rate for, 580, 581
with portal venous occlusion, 588
recurrence of, 583, 584
signs and symptoms of, 580
surgery for, 582–583
treatment of, 581–583, 581*t*
esophageal
bleeding from, in portal hypertension, 579
surgery for, 585–587, 585*t*
gastric, bleeding from, in portal hypertension, 579
ileostomy and, 753*t*
nonbleeding, **583–587**
devascularization of, 587
evaluation of, 583–584
operative risk with, severity of hepatic disease and, 583–584
in patients who have previously bled, management of, 584–585
prophylactic therapy for, 584
surgery for, 585–587, 585*t*
treatment of, 584–587
saphenous, 790
Varicocele, 873, **1079**
and male infertility, 1081
Varicose bronchiectasis, 385
Varicose veins, **873–875**
stripping of, 874*i*
Varus
definition of, 1116, 1194
of knee, 1183–1184
Vasa recta, 705
Vascular abnormalities, renal, 1020
Vascular access, in trauma victim, **238**
Vascular disorders
in impotence, **1083**
of small intestine and mesentery, **698–701**
Vascular endothelial growth factor (VEGF), for peripheral arterial insufficiency, 821
Vascular flow map, 894
Vascular impotence, 1083
Vascular injury, in urethral injury, 1051–1052
Vascular malformations, **934–935**
"cryptic," 945
Vascular occlusions, consciousness in, 888
Vascular reconstruction, for acute mesenteric vascular occlusion, 699
Vascular rings, 382
Vascular trauma, epidemiology of, 256
Vascular volume, replenishment of, in shock, 211

Vasculitis, **700**
and small artery occlusive disease, 827
Vas deferens
anatomy of, **1017**
obstruction of, in male infertility, 1081
Vasectomy, 1091
for genitourinary tuberculosis, 1041
Vasoactive intestinal polypeptide (VIP),
675–676
in pancreatic cholera, 650
Vasoconstriction
cerebral, for intracranial hypertension, 905
intranasal, abuse of, 979
in pulmonary thromboembolism, 880
splanchnic, in nonocclusive intestinal ischemia, 700
Vasoconstrictive disorders, **843–844**
Vasoconstrictors
for cardiogenic shock, 209
for neurogenic shock, 209
for stress ulcers, 556
Vasodilators
for aortic insufficiency, 427
for cardiogenic shock, 208–209
for intra-arterial injections, 858
for nonocclusive intestinal ischemia, 700
Vasoepididymostomy, for male infertility, 1081
Vasography, in male infertility, 1080
Vasomotor rhinitis, **979**
Vasopressin, 103
in hypovolemic shock, 203
for lower gastrointestinal bleeding, 736
in shock, 210, 211
for stress ulcers, 556
for variceal bleeding, 581–582
Vasospasm, in subarachnoid hemorrhage,
942–943
Vasovasostomy, for male infertility, 1081
Vater
ampulla of (*See* Ampulla of Vater)
papilla of, 625
VATER syndrome, 1326
Veins, **871–885**. *See also Venous; specific named
vein*
anatomy of, **871–872**, 872i
diseases of, **873–885**
endothelial injury of, 875
function of, in chronic venous insufficiency,
884
injuries to, **262**
treatment of, 243
malformations of, 1342
perforating, 871, 872i
physiology of, **872–873**, 872i
varicose, **873–875**
Vena cava, inferior, 871
Venography
in chronic venous insufficiency, 884
in deep venous thrombosis, 876
in male infertility, 1081
in neurodiagnosis, 896
in subclavian vein thrombosis, 879
Venolysis, for axillary-subclavian venous
thrombosis, 879

Venom
arthropod, 132
snake, 130–131
spider, 132
Venomous bite injury, **130–133**
Venous claudication, in chronic venous insufficiency, 883
Venous epidural hematoma, 906
Venous filling index, in chronic venous insufficiency, 884
Venous insufficiency
chronic, **883–885**
versus varicose veins, 874
Venous pressure, 872–873, 872i
measurements of, in deep venous thrombosis, 876
Venous racemose aneurysm, 1247t
Venous reflux, in chronic venous insufficiency,
883, 884
Venous segment transfer, for chronic venous
insufficiency, 884
Venous sinusoids, soleal, 873
Venous stasis, 875
in chronic venous insufficiency, 883
prevention of, 15
versus varicose veins, 874
Venous thrombosis
axillary-subclavian, **878–880**
calf, 875
deep, **875–877**
postoperative, 877
iliofemoral, 876
as paraneoplastic syndrome, 1371t
Venous ulcer(s), 95–96
Venous valves, 871, 873
Ventilating tubes, for otitis media with effusion, 966
Ventilation/perfusion mismatch, 26
Ventilation-perfusion scan, in pulmonary
thromboembolism, 880–881
Ventilator(s). *See also* Mechanical ventilation
pressure, 215, **217–218**
modes for, 217–218
volume, **215–217**
modes for, 217
parameters for, 216–217
Ventilatory support. *See also* Mechanical ventilation
after cardiac surgery, 436
for aortic coarctation, 446
for pediatric patients, 1294–1295
for respiratory failure, 18
Ventricles
fourth, 890i
lateral, 890i
third, 890i
tumors in, 915i, 916i
Ventricular arrhythmias, after cardiac surgery,
437
Ventricular catheter, 904
Ventricular drainage
for increased intracranial pressure, 891
for subarachnoid hemorrhage, 941
Ventricular ectopy, 44

Ventricular premature beats, 28
Ventricular reduction surgery, 418
Ventricular septal defect, **452–453**, 453i
and aortic coarctation, 445
and aortopulmonary window, 454
closure of, 461, 466
and double-outlet right ventricle, 467
postinfarction, 416, 416i, 417i
and tetralogy of Fallot, 460, 460i
and truncus arteriosus, 457
Ventricular septum, 449
intact, pulmonary atresia and, **462**
Ventricular tachycardia, 44
Ventriculocisternostomy, third, for hydrocephalus, 934
Ventriculostomy
for intracranial hypertension, 904
for subarachnoid hemorrhage, 940, 941
Venturi effect, 873
Verapamil
for angina pectoris, 412
for atrial dysrhythmias, 437
Verbal response, in craniocerebral trauma, **902**
Verrucae, 1245
Vertebral artery, injuries to, 257, 1118
treatment of, 243
Vertebral column. *See also* Spine
anatomy of, 1117
malformations of, **932**
stabilization, for spinal cord tumors, 928
Vertebrectomy, for spinal cord tumors, 928
Vertebrobasilar disease, 848–849
Vertigo. *See also* Dizziness
benign paroxysmal positional, **976**
in labyrinthitis, 976
Vesical fistulas, 1077–1078
Vesical stones, **1046–1047**
Vesicocutaneous fistula, 1077–1078
Vesicointestinal fistula, 1077
Vesicolithotomy, for vesical stone, 1047
Vesicoureteral reflux, **1023–1026**, 1023i,
1024i, 1025i
Vesicovaginal fistula, 1077
versus ureteral injury, 1050
Vestibular schwannoma, 919–920, **926,
975–976**
Vestibular system, **974–976**
Vestibulitis, nasal, **978**
Vibrio infection, drug therapy for, 135t
Vicarious liability, 79
Vicodin. *See* Hydrocodone with aceta-
minophen
Video-assisted thoracoscopic surgery (VATS),
350
Vigorous achalasia, 477
Villi, intestinal, 674, 676i, 677i
Villous adenomas
duodenal, 563
of large bowel, 727
Vinblastine, 1355
for renal adenocarcinoma, 1057
Vincent's gingivitis, **984–985**
Vincristine, 1355
for Ewing's sarcoma, 356

for immune thrombocytopenic purpura, 660
for thyroid cancer, 307
Viomycin, for tuberculosis, 388*t*
Viral sialadenitis, **986**
Virchow's triad, 875
Virilization, tumors causing, 810
Virtual colonoscopy, in large intestine examination, 711
Visceral artery aneurysms, **841–842**
Visceral myopathy, familial, and intestinal pseudo-obstruction, 686
Visceral neuropathy, familial, and intestinal pseudo-obstruction, 686
Visceral pain, 503, 504*t*, 505*f*
Visceral peritoneum, 517
Vision
  disturbances in, **1000**
  double, **1000**
  in pituitary tumors, 930
Visual acuity
  decrease in, **1000**
  in increased intracranial pressure, 890
  testing of, **999**
Visual episodes, transient, in cerebrovascular disease, 848
Visual evoked potentials, in skull base surgery, 898
Visual field, testing of, **999**
Vital capacity, postoperative, 17
Vital signs
  in craniocerebral trauma, **902–903**
  postoperative monitoring of, 14
Vitamin(s). *See also specific vitamin*
  digestion of, in small intestine, 679
  fat-soluble, 163
    in hepatic failure, 188
  in nutritional support, 163, 164*t*
  water-soluble, 163
    in hepatic failure, 188
Vitamin A, 163
  for burn patients, 271
  deficiency, and lung cancer, 396
  requirements for, 164*t*
  and wound healing, 91
Vitamin B$_1$, 163
  requirements for, 164*t*
Vitamin B$_2$, 163
  requirements for, 164*t*
Vitamin B$_6$, 163
  for genitourinary tuberculosis, 1041
  for renal stones, 1044
  requirements for, 164*t*
Vitamin B$_{12}$ (cyanocobalamin), 163
  absorption of
    in pancreatic insufficiency, 643
    in small intestine, 679
  deficiency of, 52
  requirements for, 164*t*
  for short bowel syndrome, 682
Vitamin C, 163
  for burn patients, 271
  requirements for, 164*t*

Vitamin D, 163, 308
  intoxication, hypercalcemia in, 149
  requirements for, 164*t*
Vitamin E, 163
  for burn patients, 271
  for mammary dysplasia, 341
  requirements for, 164*t*
Vitamin K, 163
  indications for, 58
    in newborn, 1299
  requirements for, 164*t*
Vitamin K$_1$, 55
Vitreous, blunt trauma to, 1009*t*
Vocal cords, paralysis of, **995–996**
Vocal nodules, **995**
Voiding studies, in vesicoureteral reflux, 1025
Volar plate, 1271, 1271*i*
Volatile anesthetics, 197
  indications for, 195
Volume depletion, 153–154
  diagnosis of, 144
  with electrolyte depletion, 144–145
  and metabolic alkalosis, 152
  treatment of, 144
Volume overload, 145
Volume replacement, 144, 145
Volume resuscitation, for craniocerebral trauma, 903
Volume status, determination of, 50–51
Volvulus, 1332
  and colonic obstruction, 713*t*
  gastric, **561**
  with intestinal malrotation, 1318–1320, 1319*i*
  of large intestine, **738–740**, 739*i*, 740*i*
  with meconium ileus, 1320
  with omphalomesenteric duct anomalies, 1330
  and small bowel obstruction, **683**
Vomiting
  abdominal pain and, 507
  in brain tumors, 915
  in colonic obstruction, 713
  gastroesophageal sphincter and, 474
  history-taking about, 1–2
  Mallory-Weiss syndrome and, 551
  postoperative, **199–200**
Vomitus, aspiration of, 233
von Hippel-Lindau disease, and pheochromocytoma, 802
von Willebrand's disease, 55–56, 61
  and angiodysplasia, 738
Vulva
  carcinoma of, **1104–1105**
    staging of, 1104, 1104*t*
  Paget's disease of, 1104
  tumors of, benign, 1095
Vulvar intraepithelial neoplasia (VIN), 1104–1105

WAGR syndrome, 1344
Waldeyer's sheath, 1023, 1023*i*, 1024*i*
Wallstent stents, for peripheral arterial insufficiency, 821

Wandering spleen, 652
Wangansteen invertogram, 1326
Warfarin
  for axillary-subclavian venous thrombosis, 879
  for deep venous thrombosis, 876–877
  reversal of, 55, 62
Wart(s)
  common, 1245
  venereal, **1082**
Warthin's tumor, 294
Wasp envenomation, 132
Water
  absorption of
    in colon, 707, 708–709, 709*t*
    in small intestine, **677–678**
  body
    distribution of, 142–144
    as percentage of body weight, 142, 143*t*
  deficit
    pure, 144
    treatment of, 144
  excretion of, renal regulation of, 142–143
  extracellular, 159*t*
  intake of, 144*t*
    ileostomy and, 751
  limiting of, in brain tumors, 924
  loss of
    extrarenal (insensible), 143
    and fluid therapy, 154
    in gastrointestinal fluid, 146, 147*t*
  retention of, in response to injury, 107
  total body, 159*t*
Water intoxication, 107
Water moccasin, 130
Waterston anastomosis, 458, 459*i*
WDHA syndrome (watery diarrhea, hypokalemia, and achlorhydria), **650**
Weakness, spinal cord tumors and, 927, 928
Weber test, 963
Wedged hepatic venous pressure, 578–579, 584
Weight. *See* Body weight
Weir formula, 159*t*, 161
Welder's arc burn, **1008**
Werner's syndrome, and hyperparathyroidism, 309
WFNS Scale. *See* World Federation of Neurological Surgeons Scale
Wheat bran, for diverticulosis, 731
Whiplash injury, **1205–1206**
Whipple procedure
  for bile duct malignancies, 618
  for chronic pancreatitis, 642
  for pancreatic adenocarcinoma, 645–646, 646*i*
Whipple's triad, 649
Whitaker test
  in obstructive uropathy, 1031
  in ureteropelvic junction obstruction, 1032
White blood cell count
  in idiopathic myelofibrosis, 663
  in lymphangitis, 887
White pulp, of spleen, 652, 653

Whole-gut lavage, 754
Wide field laryngectomy, for laryngeal cancer, 291
Williams-Beuren syndrome, 444
Williams-Campbell syndrome, and bronchiectasis, 384
Willis, circle of, 896*i*
Wilms' tumor, **1344–1345**
  versus mesoblastic nephroma, 1059
  staging of, 1344, 1345*t*
  survival rate for, 1345, 1345*t*
Winter procedure, for priapism, 1082
Wirsung, duct of, 625, 626*i*
Wiskott-Aldrich syndrome, **661**
Witness(es)
  expert, 73, 77–78, 79
    compensation for, 83
  to fact (percipient), 73, 83
World Federation of Neurological Surgeons Scale, for subarachnoid hemorrhage, 939*t*
Wound(s). *See also* Wound care; Wound healing; Wound infection
  abdominal, dehiscence of, 24
  chronic, 95–96
  clean, 121
  clean-contaminated, 121
  closure of, **96–97,** 97*i*
    adequacy of, 24
    delayed primary, 122
  complications of, **23–25**
  contamination of, 1253
  contraction of, 90–91, 1244
    with burns, 273
  contracture (stricture) of, 90–91, **1244**
  dehiscence of, **24–25,** 96
    diagnosis of, 24–25
    with evisceration, 24–25
    management of, 24–25
    partial, 25
    risk factors for, 24
    technical causes of, 96
    without evisceration, 25
  healing of (*See* Wound healing)
  heavily contaminated, 121
  hormonal mediators of, 103, 104*t*, 105*t*
  infection of (*See* Wound infection)
  laparotomy, dehiscence of, 24
  nonhealing, and peripheral arterial insufficiency, 817
  as organ, 103
  pain in, 25
  sternal, dehiscence of, 24
  stretching of, 90–91
  surgical
    aseptic technique for, 13
    tensile strength of, 16
  tensile strength of, 92, 92*i*
  thoracic, 24

  tissue coverage for, selection of, 1238–1239, 1239*t*
Wound care
  for burns, **271–273**
  in plastic and reconstructive surgery, principles of, 1237–1243
  postoperative, 15–16
  in soft tissue injury, 1253–1254
Wound closure
  dog-ear in, correction of, 1241, 1241*i*, 1242*i*
  for flaps, 1239–1241, 1240*i*
  for head and neck tumors, 295
  with impaired healing, 97
  layered cutaneous, 1239, 1240*i*
  primary
    delayed, 16, 86, 97
    in plastic surgery, 1241–1242
    suture technique for, 1242
  by second intention (secondary), 16, 86
  in soft tissue injury, 1253–1254
  Z-plasty for, 1241–1242, 1242*i*
Wound healing, 15–16, **86–98, 108**
  anemia and, 60
  angiogenesis in, 89–90, 89*i*
  arginine and, 162
  coagulation in, 86–87
  completion of, 91
  components of, 86, 87*i*
  delayed, risk factors for, 8–9
  epithelialization in, 90
  factors affecting, 8–9, 97, 98*t*
  fibroplasia in, 87
  by first intention (primary), 86
  forms of, 86
  in hematologic disorders, 54, 60
  impairment of
    closures with, 97
    in disorders of inflammation, 91–92
  inflammation in, 86–87
  malnutrition and, 92
  matrix deposition in, 88–89
  mediators of, 103, 103*t*
  primary, delayed, 16, 86, 97
  by second intention (secondary), 16, 86
  at skin graft donor site, 1234
  in soft tissue injury, 1252–1253
  suppression of, by infection, 115
  surgical technique and, 96–97
Wound infection, 25, 121, 273, 274*t. See also* Infection(s), surgical site
  after cardiac surgery, 437
  clinical findings in, 122
  delayed, 97–98
  differential diagnosis of, 122
  prevention of, 11–13, 98, 122
  prognosis for, 123
  risk factors for, 23, 121, 122*t*
  treatment of, 122–123
Wrist
  anatomy of, 1143

  arthroscopy of, **1290–1291**
  disarticulation of, **867**
  dislocations, **1279–1280**
  extensor retinaculum at, 1272, 1273*i*
  function of, 1270
  injury to, **1143–1146, 1279–1280**
  ligaments of, 1143
    injury to, 1147–1148, 1279–1280
  posttraumatic arthritis of, 1147–1148
  sprain injuries of, 1143–1144, **1279–1280**

Xanthine oxidase, 164
Xanthogranulomatous pyelonephritis, **1038**
Xenograft(s), 1372, 1386
  porcine, 272
Xenon computed tomography, 897
Xenon-133 studies, and amputation level determination, 860
Xeroradiography, in mammography, 322
Xiphoid, infection of, **352–353**
X-rays. *See also* Plain films
  of congenital hip dislocation, 1191, 1191*i*
  for evaluation of spleen size, 654
  of hepatic abscess, 593
  of intraperitoneal abscesses, 523
  of kidney injury, 1048
  of large intestine, **711**
  of mitral stenosis, 421
  of neck injuries, 242
  in neurodiagnosis, **892**
  of obstructive uropathy, 1031
  of prostate cancer, 1067
  of spinal cord injury, 910
  in surgical patient, 5
  upper gastrointestinal series, in diagnosis of variceal bleeding, 581

Yaws, drug therapy for, 136*t*
Yersinia enterocolitica, enteritis caused by, **694**
Yersinia infection, drug therapy for, 135*t*
Yolk sac tumor, 1347
  mediastinal, 377

Zenker's diverticulum. *See* Pharyngoesophageal diverticulum
Zidovudine, ototoxicity of, 998
Zinc
  for burn patients, 271
  deficiency of, 163
    in Crohn's disease, 690
  requirements for, 164*t*
  serum levels of
    high, in total parenteral nutrition, 183*t*
    low, in total parenteral nutrition, 183*t*
Zollinger-Ellison syndrome, **544–546**
Z-plasty, 1241–1242, 1242*i*
Zygomatic fractures, **1256–1257**
Zymogen, 535

For Reference

Not to be taken from this room